COMPREHENSIVE LEARNING AND TEACHING RESOURCES

The supplements that accompany *Contemporary Psychiatric–Mental Health Nursing* enhance learning and teaching.

PEARSON HEALTH MEDIALINK CD-ROM

The CD-ROM accompanying this textbook provides an interactive study program that allows students to practice answering NCLEX-RN®-style questions with rationales for right and wrong answers. It also contains an Audio Glossary, animations and video clips, and a link to the Companion Website.

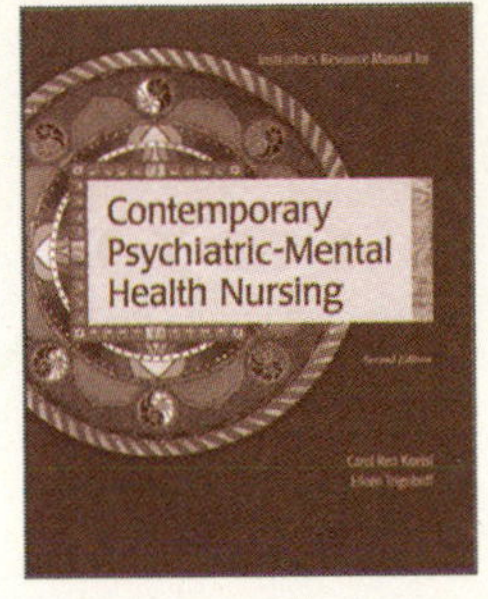

INSTRUCTOR'S RESOURCE MANUAL

This manual contains a wealth of material to help faculty plan and manage the mental health nursing course. For each learning outcome in a chapter, it includes Concepts for Lecture ideas, PowerPoint lecture slides, and Classroom and Clinical Activities. The IRM also includes a complete test bank and answers to the textbook critical thinking exercises.

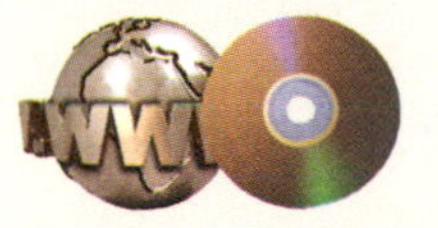

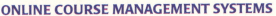

COMPANION WEBSITE

www.prenhall.com/kneisl

This on-line study guide is designed to help students apply the concepts presented in the book. Each chapter-specific module features objectives, Audio Glossary, chapter outline, NCLEX-RN®-style questions, case studies, care plan activities, class discussion questions, MediaLinks, and Nursing Tools, such as Standards of Psychiatric–Mental Health Nursing Practice, and more.

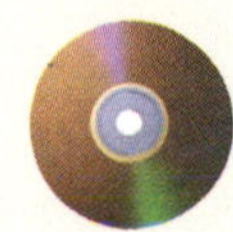

INSTRUCTOR'S RESOURCE DVD-ROM

This useful resource provides illustrations and lecture slides in PowerPoint for use in classroom lectures. It also contains an electronic test bank, answers to the textbook critical thinking challenges, and animations and videos from the CD-ROM that accompanies the textbook. This supplement is available to faculty free upon adoption of the textbook.

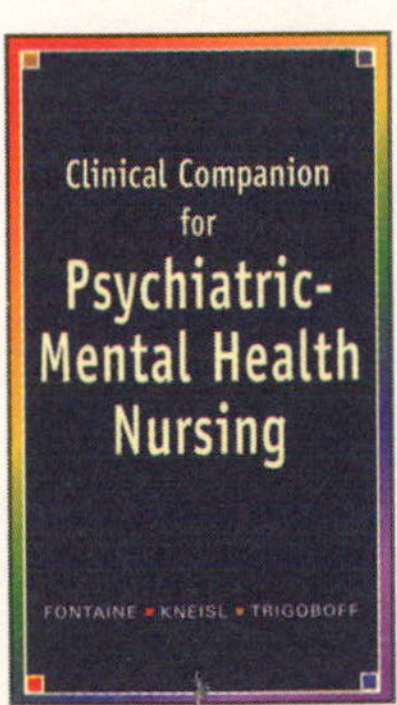

CLINICAL COMPANION FOR PSYCHIATRIC-MENTAL HEALTH NURSING

This clinical companion serves as a portable quick-reference to psychiatric–mental health nursing. Topics include DSM-IV-TR classifications, common diagnostic studies, more than 20 clinical applications for mental health disorders, medications, and much more. This handbook will allow students to bring the information they learn from class into any clinical setting.

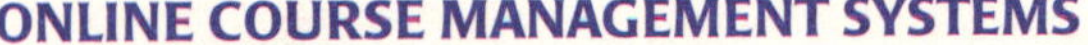

ONLINE COURSE MANAGEMENT SYSTEMS

Also available are all major online course management systems, including Blackboard, WebCT, Moodle, Angel, and eCollege.

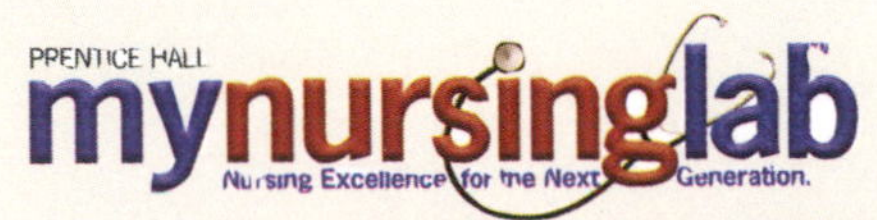

MyNursingLab is a user-friendly site that gives students the opportunity to test themselves on key concepts and skills in psychiatric–mental health nursing. By using MyNursingLab, students can track their own progress through the course and use the personalized, media-rich, study plan activities to help them achieve success in the classroom, in clinical, and ultimately on the NCLEX-RN®. MyNursingLab can also help instructors monitor class progress as students move through the curriculum. To take a tour and see the power of MyNursingLab, go to **www.mynursinglab.com**.

Ask your Pearson Education sales representative for more information and packaging option for including MyNursingLab and online course management systems in your curriculum.

CONTENTS IN BRIEF

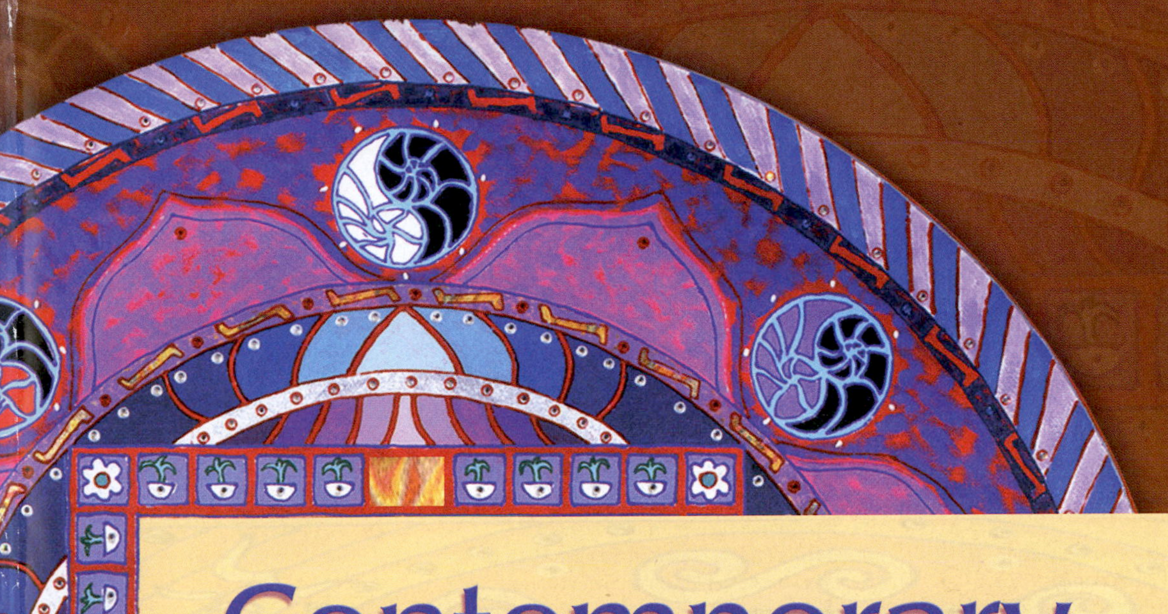

Contemporary Psychiatric–Mental Health Nursing

Second Edition

Carol Ren Kneisl
Eileen Trigoboff

PEARSON
Prentice Hall
Upper Saddle River, New Jersey 07458

Library of Congress Cataloging-in-Publication Data

Kneisl, Carol Ren.
Contemporary psychiatric-mental health nursing / Carol Ren Kneisl, Eileen Trigoboff.--
2nd ed.
p. ; cm.
Includes bibliographical references and index.
ISBN-13: 978-0-13-243489-8
ISBN-10: 0-13-243489-X
1. Psychiatric nursing.
[DNLM: 1. Mental Disorders--nursing. 2. Psychiatric Nursing--methods. WY 160 K68c
2009] I. Trigoboff, Eileen. II. Title.
RC440.K646 2009
616.89 ' 0231--dc22
2008015620

Publisher: Julie Levin Alexander
Assistant to Publisher: Regina Bruno
Editor-in-Chief: Maura Connor
Assistant to the Editor-in-Chief: Marion Gottlieb
Executive Acquisitions Editor: Pamela Lappies
Assistant to the Executive Acquisitions Editor: Sarah Wrocklage
Development Editor: Elizabeth Tinsley
Editorial Art Manager: Patrick Watson
Media Product Manager: John J. Jordan
Director of Marketing: Karen Allman
Senior Marketing Manager: Francisco del Castillo
Marketing Specialist: Michael Sirinides

Managing Editor, Production: Patrick Walsh
Production Editor: Lynn Steines, S4Carlisle Publishing Services
Production Liaison: Anne Garcia
Media Project Manager: Stephen Hartner
Manufacturing Manager: Ilene Sanford
Senior Design Coordinator: Maria Guglielmo
Interior Design: Christine Cantera
Cover Design: Christine Cantera
Cover Illustration: Conscious Living by Paul Heussenstamm
Composition: S4Carlisle Publishing Services
Printer/Binder: Quebecor World Color
Cover Printer: Phoenix Color

Credits: page 2: Aurora Photos, Inc., David McLain; page 64: Photolibrary.com, Wiley/Wales, Amy & Chuck; page 192: Photo Researchers, Inc., William W. Bacon III; page 294: Creative Eye/MIRA.com, David Sanger; page 614: Peter Arnold, Inc., Sebastian Bolesch/DAS FOTOARCHIV; page 772: Creative Eye/MIRA.com, Bill Parsons; ICONS: Getty Images/Stock Illustration Source, Todd Davidson.

Notice: Care has been taken to confirm the accuracy of information presented in this book. The authors, editors, and the publisher, however, cannot accept any responsibility for errors or omissions or for consequences from application of the information in this book and make no warranty, express or implied, with respect to its contents.

The authors and publisher have exerted every effort to ensure that drug selections and dosages set forth in this text are in accord with current recommendations and practice at time of publication. However, in view of ongoing research, changes in government regulations, and the constant flow of information relating to drug therapy and reactions, the reader is urged to check the package inserts of all drugs for any change in indications or dosage and for added warning and precautions. This is particularly important when the recommended agent is a new and/or infrequently employed drug.

Pearson Education Ltd., London
Pearson Education Singapore, Pte. Ltd
Pearson Education Canada, Inc., Toronto
Pearson Education—Japan
Pearson Education Australia PTY, Limited
Pearson Education North Asia, Ltd., Hong Kong
Pearson Educación de Mexico, S.A. de C.V.
Pearson Education Malaysia, Pte. Ltd.
Pearson Education Upper Saddle River, New Jersey

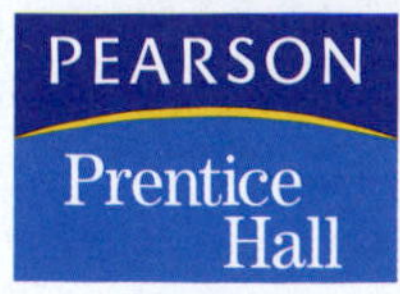

10 9 8 7 6 5 4 3 2 1
ISBN-13: 978-0-13-243489-8
ISBN-10: 0-13-243489-X

This book is dedicated to Isaac James Kneisl,
born on October 13, 2007.

With you I will rediscover the excitement, mystery, and joy
of the world in which we live.

ABOUT THE AUTHORS

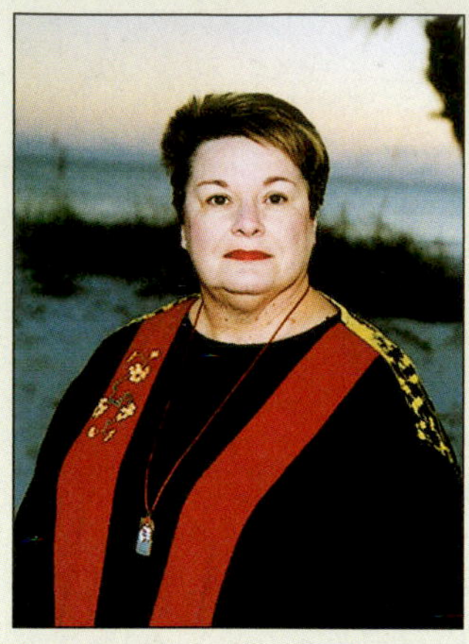

CAROL REN KNEISL, RN, MS, DABFN, has had a variety of psychiatric–mental health nursing experiences. She has taught psychiatric–mental health nursing in a diploma school, a baccalaureate program, and a master's program that prepared clinical specialists in psychiatric–mental health nursing. She has been a staff nurse, a nurse manager, a nursing supervisor, and has supervised the group therapy of clinical nurse specialists and psychiatry medical residents.

Carol is also a nurse entrepreneur. She was the President and Education Director of Nursing Transitions, a corporation that provided continuing education for psychiatric–mental health and corrections/forensic nurses. Her company sponsored the first national nursing conference focused on AIDS. She is a national and international speaker and consults with nurses and mental health and forensic agencies on topics such as group therapy, stress management, self-awareness issues and strategies, implementation of client rights, competency to stand trial, and negligence and malpractice in psychiatric–mental health nursing.

Carol has authored or contributed to 22 nursing textbooks and several nursing journals. She has been an associate editor of a psychiatric nursing review journal and has served on several editorial boards. She is a Diplomate in the American College of Forensic Examiners Board of Forensic Nurse Examiners.

Carol was among the first nurses in the country to develop clinical specialist certification in conjunction with nurses from New York and New Jersey. Their work formed the basis for the national certification granted through the American Nurses Credentialing Center of the American Nurses Association.

She is a graduate of one of the oldest diploma schools in the country, the Millard Fillmore Hospital School of Nursing in Buffalo, New York, from which she received the Alumna of the Century award on the occasion of the school's 100-year anniversary. Carol has a BS in nursing from the University of Buffalo, an MS in nursing from the University of California at San Francisco, and holds a certificate in community mental health administration from the State University of New York at Buffalo.

Carol is the mother of two adult children—a daughter who is a right-brained special effects artist and a son who is a left-brained mathematician and the father of her first grandchild. She writes and consults from her home on the beach in Orange Beach, Alabama.

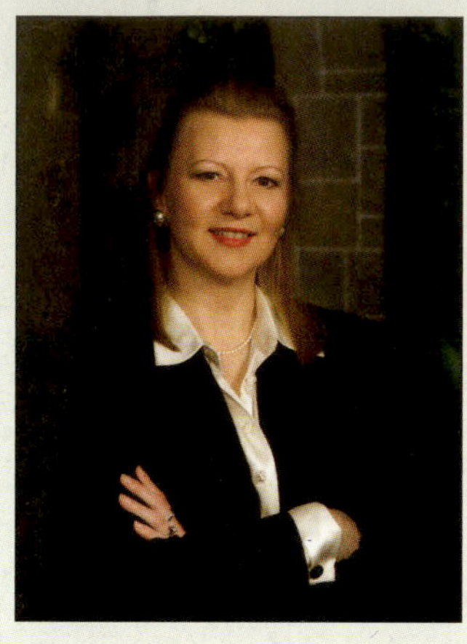

EILEEN TRIGOBOFF, RN, APRN/PMH-BC, DNS, DABFN, CIP, is a Clinical Nurse Specialist with a specialty in Adult Psychiatry–Mental Health in a private psychotherapy practice in western New York. An important part of her practice is the national and international interdisciplinary supervision of, and consultation with, other mental health and health care professionals. Dr. Trigoboff is the research coordinator at the Buffalo Psychiatric Center in Buffalo, New York, and is the Liaison for the Office of Mental Health's Institutional Review Board. She has taught associate degree, bachelor's degree, and graduate-level nursing students on all aspects of the nursing process, research methodologies, statistics, and pharmacology.

Dr. Trigoboff earned her BSN, her MS as a Clinical Nurse Specialist in psychiatric nursing, and her Doctorate in Nursing Science (DNS) in psychiatric nursing from the State University of New York at Buffalo. She received a National Institutes of Mental Health Individual National Research Service Award Pre-Doctoral Research Fellowship for her dissertation research on medication teaching and psychopharmacology. Eileen's research interests include cognitive behavioral nursing interventions with seriously and persistently mentally ill clients and the safety and efficacy of neuroleptics. She is a Diplomate and Fellow in the American College of Forensic Examiners, on the American Board of Forensic Nursing, and is board certified as an Institutional Review Board Professional (CIP) and in hospital and program accreditation.

Eileen is author, coauthor, and contributor to 13 books and numerous journal articles. She has presented internationally on a wide variety of clinical, research, and professional topics to health care, governmental, and corporate organizations. She continues to be an international speaker and consultant on topics including professional issues, assessment, psychopathologies, and interventions. She also serves on the editorial boards of several professional journals and on the editorial panel for a magazine on anxiety and depression. She is active in community service venues, including clinical settings and family support groups. She also serves as a computer systems and statistical consultant and belongs to numerous professional nursing organizations.

Eileen enjoys her clinical psychologist husband, her Congo African Grey parrot, a large and loving family, good friends, international travel, reading, and gardening.

CONTRIBUTORS

Carol Bradley-Corpuel, APRN, BC
Adjunct Clinical Faculty, Orvis School of Nursing
University of Nevada, Reno
Psychiatric Clinical Nurse Specialist
Saint Mary's Regional Medical Center
Reno, Nevada
Chapter 27: Adolescents

Kay K. Chitty, EdD, RN
Adjunct Professor
Medical University of South Carolina
Charleston, South Carolina
Chapter 17: Mood Disorders
Chapter 21: Eating Disorders

Sue DeLaune, MN, RN
Assistant Professor
William Carey University
New Orleans, Louisiana
Chapter 18: Anxiety and Dissociative Disorders
Chapter 19: Somatoform and Sleep Disorders
Chapter 22: Personality Disorders
Chapter 35: Intervening in Violence in the Psychiatric Setting

Karen Lee Fontaine, RN, MSN, AASECT
Professor
Purdue University Calumet
Hammond, Indiana
Chapter 20: Gender Identity and Sexual Disorders
Chapter 21: Eating Disorders
Chapter 24: Persons at Risk for Abuse or Violence

Pamela Marcus, RN, APRN/PMH-BC
Associate Professor of Nursing
Prince George Community College
Largo, Maryland
Nurse Psychotherapist; Clinical Specialist Private Practice
Upper Marlboro, Maryland
Chapter 6: Psychobiology, Behavior, and Mental Disorders

Beth Moscato, RN, PhD, CNS
Research Assistant Professor
University at Buffalo
Department of Social & Preventive Medicine
School of Public Health and Health Professions
Buffalo, New York
Chapter 9: Mental Health, Mental Disorder, and Cultural Competence
Chapter 29: Counseling the Individual

Sandra Niemann, BSN, MA, MDiv, PhD (cand)
Doctoral Candidate
University of California, San Francisco
San Francisco, California
Chapter 26: Children

Sandra J. Weiss, PhD, DNSc, FAAN
Professor, Department of Community Health Systems
Eschbach Endowed Chair in Mental Health Nursing
Director, Graduate Program in Child and Family Psychiatric-Mental Health Nursing
University of California, San Francisco
San Francisco, California
Chapter 26: Children

STUDENT AND INSTRUCTOR RESOURCE WRITERS

Melissa Black
Greenville Technical College
Greenville, South Carolina

Jane Bostick
University of Missouri
Columbia, Missouri

Jennifer Brown
Virginia Commonwealth University
Richmond, Virginia

Denice Davis
National Park Community College
Hot Springs, Arkansas

Mary Louise Fleming
University of California, San Francisco
San Francisco, California

Patricia Freed
Saint Louis University
St. Louis, Missouri

Diane Gardner
University of West Florida
Pensacola, Florida

Elizabeth Harris
New York-Presbyterian Hospital
White Plains, New York

Dana Hillyer
Clinical Nurse Specialist
Helena, Montana

Rose Kutlenios
Wheeling Jesuit University
Wheeling, West Virginia

Dimitra Loukissa
North Park University
Chicago, Illinois

Marina Martinez-Kratz
Jackson Community College
Jackson, Mississippi

Barbara Maxwell
SUNY Ulster
Stone Ridge, New York

Victoria Menzies
Virginia Commonwealth University
Richmond, Virginia

Marci Miller
San Diego State University
San Diego, California

Virginia Osting
Radford University
Radford, Virginia

Marita T. Peppard
Austin Community College
Austin, Texas

Patricia Posey-Goodwin
University of West Florida
Pensacola, Florida

Cathy Weitzel
Wichita State University
Wichita, Kansas

Deborah Wilson
Howard University
Washington, DC

THANK YOU!

The authors and publisher are grateful for the expertise provided by nursing faculty and clinicians who gave of their time to review chapters for this book and the material that accompanies it. Thank you for your generosity in sharing your insightful comments with us.

Elizabeth M. Andal
California State University, Bakersfield, California

Robert L. Anders
University of Texas at El Paso, El Paso, Texas

Mary J. Baukus
Western Michigan University, Kalamazoo, Michigan

Judy A. Bourrand
Samford University, Birmingham, Alabama

Noreen R. Brady
Case Western Reserve University, Cleveland, Ohio

Sandra L. Brisendine
Seward County Community College, Liberal, Kansas

Diane M. Burgermeister
Madonna University, Livonia, Michigan

Virginia L. Byer
Community College of Baltimore County, Catonsville, Maryland

Harlene Caroline
Curry College, Milton, Massachusetts

Beth Clark
Husson College, Bangor, Maine

Tara L. Clark
Morehead State University, Morehead, Kentucky

Barbara Cornett
Otterbein College, Westerville, Ohio

Connie K. Cupples
Union University, Germantown, Germantown, Tennessee

Janet Dahm
Saint Xavier University, Chicago, Illinois

Jan Dalsheimer
Texas Woman's University, Dallas, Texas

Shirlee P. Davidson
Santa Fe Community College, Santa Fe, New Mexico

Denice A. Davis
National Park Community College, Hot Springs, Arkansas

Teri Davis
Western Michigan University, Kalamazoo, Michigan

Susan Decker
University of Portland, Portland, Oregon

Leona F. Dempsey
University of Wisconsin Oshkosh, Oshkosh, Wisconsin

Katherine Detherage
Nazareth College, Rochester, New York

D. Michele Ellis
Southeastern Louisiana University, Baton Rouge, Louisiana

Amanda S. Eymard
Nicholls State University, Thibodaux, Louisiana

Theresa M. Fay-Hillier
Drexel University, Philadelphia, Pennsylvania

Jim W. Flahive
The University of Texas at El Paso, El Paso, Texas

Meredith Flood
University of North Carolina at Charlotte, Charlotte, North Carolina

Denise Fuhrmann
University of Southern Maine, Portland, Maine

Laurie Galatas
Texas Woman's University, Dallas, Texas

Mary Ann Glendon
Southern Connecticut State University, New Haven, Connecticut

Diane Graff
Drexel University, Philadelphia, Pennsylvania

Sheila Green
Tennessee Technological University, Cookeville, Tennessee

Kimberly M. Gregg
University of North Dakota, Grand Forks, North Dakota

Diane E. Greslick
Saint Joseph's College of Maine, Standish, Maine

Betsy D. Gulledge
Jacksonville State University, Jacksonville, Alabama

Krystyna Z. Hopkinson
Abington Memorial Hospital Dixon School of Nursing, Willow Grove, Pennsylvania

Phyllis M. Jacobs
Wichita State University, Wichita, Kansas

Marilyn Jaffe-Ruiz
Pace University, New York, New York

Mada Hodgson Janosik
Youngstown State University, Youngstown, Ohio

Shelley Johnson
LaSalle University, Philadelphia, Pennsylvania

Mary Justice
University of Cincinnati, Cincinnati, Ohio

A. Leah Kelly
Ocean County College, Toms River, New Jersey

Nancy Kupper
Tarrant County College, Fort Worth, Texas

Rose M. Kutlenios
Wheeling Jesuit University, Wheeling, West Virginia

Melissa Lickteig
Georgia Southern University, Statesboro, Georgia

Elizabeth Taber Loran
Spartanburg Community College, Spartanburg, South Carolina

Susan C. Maloney
Edinboro University of Pennsylvania, Edinboro, Pennsylvania

Marina Martinez-Kratz
Jackson Community College, Jackson, Mississippi

Barbara Maxwell
SUNY Ulster, Stone Ridge, New York

Nancy Miller
Minneapolis Community and Technical College, Minneapolis, Minnesota

Ronda D. Mintz-Binder
Los Angeles City College, Los Angeles, California

Virginia Osting
Radford University, Radford, Virginia

Cindy Parsons
University of Tampa, Tampa, Florida

Patricia Patterson
University of Western Ontario, London, Ontario, Canada

Marita T. Peppard
Austin Community College, Austin, Texas

Leslie K. Robbins
New Mexico State University, Las Cruces, New Mexico

Terri L. Schwenk
Ivy Tech Community College, Terre Haute, Indiana

Marcia Rucker Shannon
Saginaw Valley State University, University Center, Michigan

Janet A. Sobczak
Binghamton University, Binghamton, New York

Louise Suit
Regis University, Denver, Colorado

Jane Trainis
Community College of Baltimore County, Catonsville, Maryland

Diane Vines
University of Portland, Portland, Oregon

Mendy Gearhart Wright
Jacksonville State University, Jacksonville, Alabama

Richard Yakimo
Southern Illinois University Edwardsville, Edwardsville, Illinois

Jean Yockey
University of South Dakota, Vermillion, South Dakota

PREFACE

Millions of people worldwide face the challenges that mental health disorders bring. In fact, new studies by World Health Organization international researchers document that four of the ten leading causes of disability in the world today are psychiatric in nature. Worldwide, depression is the number-one health problem, followed by alcohol and drug abuse disorders and dementia of the Alzheimer's type. Fully 15% of patients with a medical illness have a co-occurring psychiatric illness, and almost half of all health-related disability can be directly attributed to psychiatric disorders.

Psychiatric–mental health nursing is a specialized area that employs a wide range of explanatory theories and research on human behavior as its science and the purposeful use of self as its art. Understanding people who are searching for meaning through interaction in complex times demands the most authoritative and contemporary knowledge and clinical competence. It is through the power of knowledge and clinical competence that psychiatric–mental health nurses can help clients from diverse cultures to live with uncertainty, unfamiliarity, and unpredictability and to pursue creative healing on psychobiologic and spiritual levels.

Our goal for this textbook, ***Contemporary Psychiatric–Mental Health Nursing,*** and its companion supplements is to provide students and practicing psychiatric–mental health nurses with the most up-to-date, evidence-based, culturally competent, authoritative, and comprehensive resource available and to present it in an accessible, clinically relevant, and professional format.

UNDERLYING THEMES

Throughout this edition, we as authors remain true to the values of clinical competence, cultural competence in an increasingly diverse society, client-centered care, the relevance of meaning to shaping behavior and treatment choices, and the need to improve quality and access to mental health care so that all people can pursue creative healing on psychobiologic and spiritual levels. We emphasize the importance of empathy and empowerment in the nurse–client relationship. We believe that psychiatric–mental health nursing is concerned with the quality of human life and its relationship to optimal psychobiologic health, feelings of self-worth, personal integrity, self-fulfillment, spirituality, and creative expression.

The psychiatric–mental health nurse's scope of practice is broad enough to include issues such as alienation, identity crises, sudden life changes, and troubled family relationships. It may involve issues of poverty and affluence, cross-cultural disparities in access to health care, and the human experiences of birth, death, and loss. Psychiatric–mental health nursing is concerned with sustaining and enhancing the mental health of both the individual and the group, while its practice locale is often found in the community.

In exploring the theme of global mental health, each unit of this book opens with compelling photographs and stories of individuals from around the world who face a variety of mental health issues. By presenting the readers with this global perspective, we hope to promote awareness of the relevance of those same global issues in our own culturally diverse society.

Along these lines, we selected a mandala to represent the essence of this book. "Mandala" is the Sanskrit word for circle and symbolizes wholeness or organization around a unifying center. The goal of this book is to explore science, art, and spirituality as a path toward our shared vision of global mental health. It is a synthesis of elements important to a holistic view. However, without the involvement of readers, students, and teachers, the mandala is incomplete. The mandala used throughout this book and on its cover was created by Paul Heussenstamm and is titled "Conscious Living." The title is reflective of the degree of awareness the nurse must maintain to act compassionately and appropriately with clients, and to provide nursing care based on sound evidence.

CONTEMPORARY TRENDS

The themes, ideas, knowledge, tools, and organization of this textbook were expressly designed for psychiatric–mental health nursing students and clinicians who are committed to developing the habits of mind, responsibility, and practice that will make a difference in view of contemporary trends. Specifically, this text prepares students to tailor and humanize interventions for traditional as well as "new" psychiatric–mental health clients often encountered in forensic settings, homeless shelters, and in other community-based and rehabilitation-oriented settings. Furthermore, because advances in neuroscience and the study of the human genome are redefining our conception of the basis for mental disorders, a solid grounding in psychobiology is threaded throughout the book. Brain imaging assessment and concise yet comprehensive information on the expanding array of psychopharmacologic treatment is yet another strong emphasis.

We recognize that psychiatric–mental health clients are racially and culturally diverse and include growing numbers of mentally ill elders, children, adolescents, and people with coexisting substance use disorders or comorbidities with other chronic illnesses such as HIV/AIDS. Therefore, we devote separate chapters to each of the above topics. We feel confident in titling this book ***Contemporary Psychiatric–Mental Health Nursing*** because of its explicit links to contemporary trends in our field.

ORGANIZATION

The book is divided into six units. Unit 1 introduces you to the clients you will most likely encounter and to those who become psychiatric–mental health nurses, the professional and personal attributes that enable artful therapeutic practice, as well as the importance of basing nursing action on evidence. Unit 2 clusters five chapters that provide comprehensive coverage of the theoretic basis for psychiatric–mental health nursing. In Unit 3, we address topics traditionally associated with psychiatric–mental health nursing, such as therapeutic communication, assessment, creating a therapeutic environment, advocacy, clients' rights, and legal and forensic issues. Unit 4 focuses on caring for clients with specific DSM-IV-TR mental disorders. In it, we first outline the defining characteristics of each disorder, then cover the biopsychosocial theories necessary to understand them, and finally apply the nursing process to caring for clients with these disorders. Unit 5 shifts the focus to vulnerable populations that require comfort and care from psychiatric–mental health nurses. These populations include people at risk for self-destructive behavior, abuse, or violence, psychiatric–mental health clients with HIV/AIDS, and specific age groups. Unit 6 of the book provides authoritative coverage of nursing intervention strategies and desired outcomes—including a wide range of modalities from individual, group, and family interventions—to psychopharmacology, crisis intervention, alternative and complementary healing practices, and violence in psychiatric settings. Throughout the book, experts contributed their knowledge and skills on all the topics covered.

NEW TO THIS EDITION

For the second edition we have written two new chapters. In Chapter 1: Psychiatric–Mental Health Clients: Who Are They? we examine the diversity of people served by the psychiatric–mental health nurse, and in doing so explode some of the myths that persist about those who have mental illness. In Chapter 7: The Science of Psychopharmacology we provide a current and in-depth examination of this important element of nursing care.

In this edition we introduce several new features. "Why I Became a Psychiatric–Mental Health Nurse" boxes present the personal stories of why the authors and chapter contributors chose this nursing specialty over all others. The new feature "What Every Specialty Nurse Should Know" demonstrates that psychiatric–mental health nursing skills are essential for all nurses—in child health, emergency departments, hospices, general hospitals, post-surgical recovery, public health, primary care, and women's health, for example—by applying psychiatric–mental health nursing knowledge and skills to other areas of nursing practice. Also new to this edition are concept maps that relate to and follow every nursing care plan and aid visual learners in understanding the nursing process. We have prepared NCLEX-RN® review questions to conclude each chapter, and the answers with rationales are included in Appendix C so that students may test their learning as they progress through the textbook.

We strongly believe that it is our responsibility as authors to present all material in clear and understandable language and formats that appeal to a range of learning styles, and many of the changes in this edition promote that purpose.

THE TEXTBOOK AS A MAP, A COMPASS, AND AN INSPIRATION

Psychiatric–mental health nursing is poised at a crossroads. We are challenged to bring complex thinking to a complex world if we are to actualize our contribution to global mental health—the vision to which this text is dedicated. This book has been crafted to provide you with the best possible evidence generated in research to help you achieve your goal of excellence in practice. It offers a fully integrated biopsychosocial perspective rather than relying on any single theory or ideology. It encourages you to become personally, professionally, and spiritually willing to muster the courage and hope necessary to forge proactive steps in our future and to make a commitment to work globally in a contemporary landscape and mindscape.

We have the opportunity to forge a new synthesis of professional wisdom in the face of tough mind-body-spirit problems and needs. We need to face critical transitions with intelligence, stamina, wit, creativity, skill, and moral courage. Global mental health can become a shared emergent vision constructed in a way that is respectful of the rich diversity of the citizens of our contemporary world. We created this book to provide you with a map, a compass, and the inspiration to succeed in your current work. We hope that it encourages you to become a participant and leader in facing the broader challenges ahead of us.

Carol Ren Kneisl
Eileen Trigoboff

ACKNOWLEDGMENTS

Producing a book isn't anything like singing a solo—it rather resembles singing in a choir. We wish to thank the many people in our choir who helped us create this textbook.

First, heartfelt thanks to Elizabeth Tinsley, our truly extraordinary and very talented Developmental Editor. Elizabeth nurtured this book, and its authors, with skill, sensitivity, and a warm heart.

The talented professionals at Prentice Hall, Pearson Health Sciences, are friends of nursing as well as an incredibly savvy team. We appreciate Julie Alexander, Publisher, and Maura Connor, Editor-in-Chief, who continue to support us and our work. We are grateful to have had the opportunity to work with Pamela Lappies, Executive Editor. She has been gracious and encouraging. Her editorial assistant, Sarah Wrocklage, has ably managed myriad small, but vital, details. Our Production Editor, Anne Garcia, has shepherded this book through the complexities of the production process as smoothly as possible given the last-minute changes and additions she had to deal with. The beautiful and reader-friendly design of the book, which adds to the book's appeal, results from the energy provided by Maria Guglielmo, Senior Designer. John Jordan, Media Production Manager, and Stephen Hartner, Media Project Director, coordinated the excellent media supplements. Travis Moses-Westphal headed the team responsible for MyNursingLab, and Barbara Gallagher was the Developmental Editor for that outstanding student resource.

Our professional colleagues and friends, Carol Bradley-Corpuel, Kay Chitty, Sue DeLaune, Karen Fontaine, Pam Marcus, Beth Moscato, Sandra Niemann, and Sandra Weiss, generously shared the power of their collective wisdom and clinical expertise in many chapters.

We also wish to acknowledge the efforts of the writers listed on page vi who developed content for the CD-ROM, Companion Website, NCLEX-RN® review questions, and instructor and student resources, including MyNursingLab.

Our thanks go to the many reviewers of the manuscript and the supplements for helping us to prepare a book that is useful for students and faculty alike, accurate in content, and relevant to every specialty area. We always welcome the thoughtful comments of nursing faculty, nursing students, and practicing psychiatric–mental health nurses. We have tried to make this book a reflection of what they want in a psychiatric–mental health nursing text.

A GUIDE TO CONTEMPORARY PSYCHIATRIC–MENTAL HEALTH NURSING

KEY TERMS

Key Terms alert you to the vocabulary used in the chapter. The page numbers indicate where the term is defined. You can also find them in the Audio Glossary found on the Student CD-ROM or the Companion Website.

LEARNING OUTCOMES

Learning Outcomes indicate what important information or skills you will have after studying the chapter.

CRITICAL THINKING CHALLENGE

The Critical Thinking Challenge at the beginning of each chapter presents a brief, care-based scenario that asks you to analyze an issue or an assertion related to the chapter topic. Questions that follow stimulate critical thinking. Analysis and discussion points for the Critical Thinking Challenge appear in the Instructor's Resource Manual accompanying this text.

MEDIALINK

The MediaLink is a reminder of the related media content on the accompanying CD-ROM and Companion Website. Specific information appears at the end of the chapter.

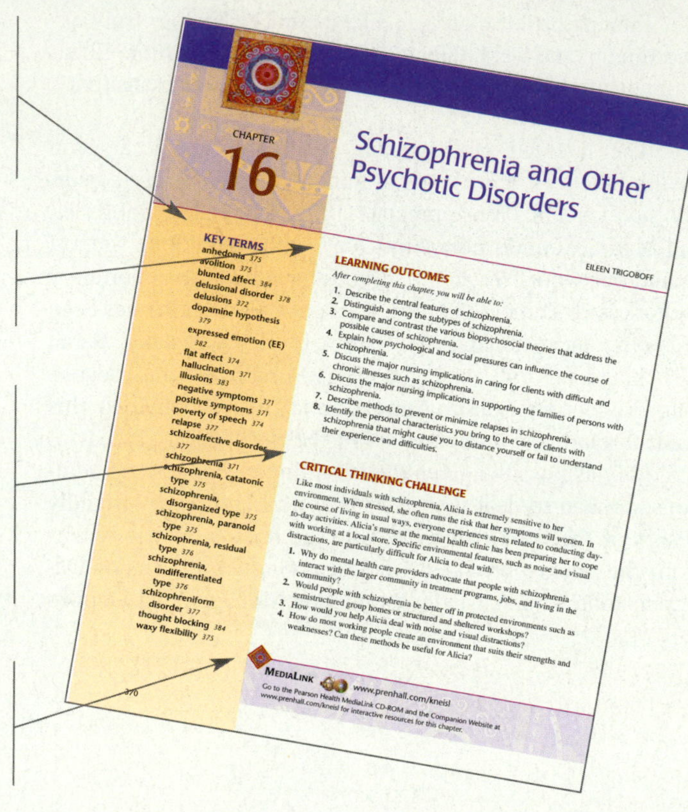

CHAPTER 16

Schizophrenia and Other Psychotic Disorders

EILEEN TRIGOBOFF

KEY TERMS

anhedonia 375
avolition 375
blunted affect 384
delusional disorder 378
delusions 372
dopamine hypothesis 379
expressed emotion (EE) 382
flat affect 374
hallucination 371
illusions 383
negative symptoms 371
positive symptoms 371
poverty of speech 374
relapse 377
schizoaffective disorder 377
schizophrenia 371
schizophrenia, catatonic type 375
schizophrenia, disorganized type 375
schizophrenia, paranoid type 375
schizophrenia, residual type 376
schizophrenia, undifferentiated type 376
schizophreniform disorder 377
thought blocking 384
waxy flexibility 375

LEARNING OUTCOMES

After completing this chapter, you will be able to:

1. Describe the central features of schizophrenia.
2. Distinguish among the subtypes of schizophrenia.
3. Compare and contrast the various biopsychosocial theories that address the possible causes of schizophrenia.
4. Explain how psychological and social pressures can influence the course of schizophrenia.
5. Discuss the major nursing implications in caring for clients with difficult and chronic illnesses such as schizophrenia.
6. Discuss the major nursing implications in supporting the families of persons with schizophrenia.
7. Describe methods to prevent or minimize relapses in schizophrenia.
8. Identify the personal characteristics you bring to the care of clients with schizophrenia that might cause you to distance yourself or fail to understand their experience and difficulties.

CRITICAL THINKING CHALLENGE

Like most individuals with schizophrenia, Alicia is extremely sensitive to her environment. When stressed, she often runs the risk that her symptoms will worsen. In the course of living in usual ways, everyone experiences stress related to conducting day-to-day activities. Alicia's nurse at the mental health clinic has been preparing her to cope with working at a local store. Specific environmental features, such as noise and visual distractions, are particularly difficult for Alicia to deal with.

1. Why do mental health care providers advocate that people with schizophrenia interact with the larger community in treatment programs, jobs, and living in the community?
2. Would people with schizophrenia be better off in protected environments such as semistructured group homes or structured and sheltered workshops?
3. How would you help Alicia deal with noise and visual distractions?
4. How do most working people create an environment that suits their strengths and weaknesses? Can these methods be useful for Alicia?

MEDIALINK www.prenhall.com/kneisl

Go to the Pearson Health MediaLink CD-ROM and the Companion Website at www.prenhall.com/kneisl for interactive resources for this chapter.

370

EVIDENCE-BASED PRACTICE

In addition to a full chapter devoted to evidence-based psychiatric–mental health nursing practice (Chapter 4), each chapter includes a clinical vignette illustrating how research evidence shapes the plan of care for a particular client. Critical thinking questions follow each vignette.

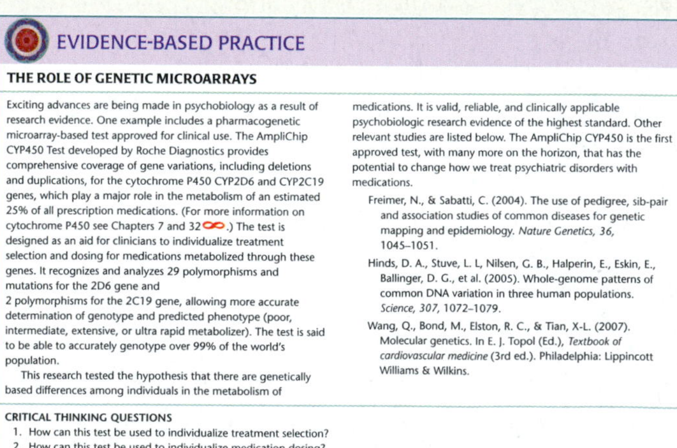

EVIDENCE-BASED PRACTICE

THE ROLE OF GENETIC MICROARRAYS

Exciting advances are being made in psychobiology as a result of research evidence. One example includes a pharmacogenetic microarray-based test approved for clinical use. The AmpliChip CYP450 Test developed by Roche Diagnostics provides comprehensive coverage of gene variations, including deletions and duplications, for the cytochrome P450 CYP2D6 and CYP2C19 genes, which play a major role in the metabolism of an estimated 25% of all prescription medications. (For more information on cytochrome P450 see Chapters 7 and 32.) The test is designed as an aid for clinicians to individualize treatment selection and dosing for medications metabolized through these genes. It recognizes and analyzes 29 polymorphisms and mutations for the 2D6 gene and 2 polymorphisms for the 2C19 gene, allowing more accurate determination of genotype and predicted phenotype (poor, intermediate, extensive, or ultra rapid metabolizer). The test is said to be able to accurately genotype over 99% of the world's population.

This research tested the hypothesis that there are genetically based differences among individuals in the metabolism of medications. It is valid, reliable, and clinically applicable psychobiologic research evidence of the highest standard. Other relevant studies are listed below. The AmpliChip CYP450 is the first approved test, with many more on the horizon, that has the potential to change how we treat psychiatric disorders with medications.

Freimer, N., & Sabatti, C. (2004). The use of pedigree, sib-pair and association studies of common diseases for genetic mapping and epidemiology. *Nature Genetics, 36*, 1045–1051.

Hinds, D. A., Stuve, L. L, Nilsen, G. B., Halperin, E., Eskin, E., Ballinger, D. G., et al. (2005). Whole-genome patterns of common DNA variation in three human populations. *Science, 307*, 1072–1079.

Wang, Q., Bond, M., Elston, R. C., & Tian, X.-L. (2007). Molecular genetics. In E. J. Topol (Ed.), *Textbook of cardiovascular medicine* (3rd ed.). Philadelphia: Lippincott Williams & Wilkins.

CRITICAL THINKING QUESTIONS

1. How can this test be used to individualize treatment selection?
2. How can this test be used to individualize medication dosing?
3. How do clients benefit when nurses are knowledgeable about genetic testing?

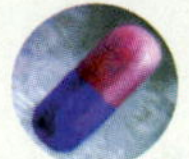

Medication icons throughout identify sections of the text that discuss psychopharmacology.

Culture Awareness icons call your attention to the significant impact of cultural heritage on the manifestation of mental disorders and responses to treatment, issues of mental health disparity, and the importance of developing cultural competence in psychiatric-mental health care.

WHAT EVERY SKILLED NURSING FACILITY NURSE SHOULD KNOW

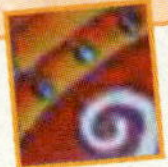

Primary Symptoms of Schizophrenia

A skilled nursing facility (SNF) nurse needs to be familiar with the primary symptoms of schizophrenia—delusions, hallucinations, agitation, and general decompensation. There are two reasons SNF nurses should be familiar with these symptoms:

1. These symptoms are part of a disease process that require treatment.
2. The presence of these symptoms can distort or mask the presentation of symptoms of physical illnesses, and severe psychiatric distress can impair healing from medical and surgical procedures and injuries.

When an SNF resident represents symptoms that appear to include behavioral and psychiatric features, the SNF nurse should be prepared and able to document, classify, and report these symptoms correctly, and to help ensure the resident receives necessary treatment. Knowing the interventions, pharmacol and nonpharmacological, can speed stabilization and in the quality of life the residents experience.

WHAT EVERY SPECIALTY NURSE SHOULD KNOW

These boxes provide examples to illustrate that regardless of the specialty, psychiatric–mental health practices are a part of it. They emphasize the importance of recognizing mental health problems and applying these practices in all nursing situations.

PARTNERING WITH CLIENTS AND FAMILIES

TEACHING ABOUT THE GENETIC BASIS OF SUBSTANCE-RELATED DISORDERS

When someone is diagnosed with a substance-related disorder such as alcoholism, your involvement with that client and the family revolves around teaching. The genetic basis for alcohol dependence includes heritability and a predisposition for offspring to be alcohol dependent as well. While the immediate concern is for the client, a future concern will be the life-impacting ramifications that a substance-related disorder will have for the client's children.

Whether the client's children are biologically related or adopted, there are also complex contributions from environmental conditions. Once a blood relative has been identified as alcohol dependent, there is a presumed genetic predisposition to alcoholism. You may introduce the topic and explain how genetics can serve as advance notice for people to take action. A proactive environment helps the at-risk individual maximize coping skills without turning to substances and begins the process of prevention for future generations.

Your role can include mapping out how an at-risk person reacts when exposed to a stressor. Is the reaction adaptive? These are all healthy responses:

- Learning
- Exploring options
- Thinking about consequences
- Reviewing how well one's coping skills worked in a situation
- Making changes when things don't turn out well
- Adjusting and fine-tuning the changes made

If you detect less-than-ample adaptive coping skills in an at-risk individual, you would proceed with shoring up the weaker areas to prevent (or at least minimize the possibility of) maladaptive coping such as substance abuse. These are some client-centered strategies to promote better coping:

- Become actively involved in shaping a personal support system.
- Identify stressors:
  - Timing—time of year, holidays, anniversaries, schedule disruptions, varying work shifts
  - Interpersonal issues—arguments, intimacy, loneliness, crowding, demands from others, financial problems
  - Intrapersonal issues—feelings of anger, incompetence, fatigue, frustration, fear
- Rehearse and practice healthy responses to difficult situations.
- Develop an array of activities or behaviors that minimize or reduce stressful times and situations.

PARTNERING WITH CLIENTS AND FAMILIES

These boxes emphasize the value of including the family in psychiatric–mental health care. Families play an important role in the treatment of a family member. Understanding the characteristics of the disorder and how it may arise during family interactions improves the client's ability to function and make family life more comfortable. This feature provides key topics to discuss with families.

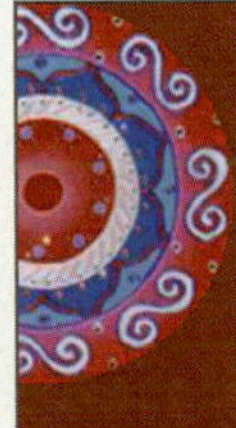

CARING FOR THE SPIRIT

Can Culturally Adapted Interventions Make a Difference in Outcome?

Schizophrenia is a difficult illness with many presentations. The distress people experience during symptom exacerbation motivates the search for treatments that are effective and useful in fulfilling the needs of the client. The search for answers has taken a variety of pathways, including the realm of spirituality and cultural sensitivity.

The quality of mental health services available to people who have schizophrenia are greatly enhanced when the relevant content of both psychoeducational and mental health interventions are culturally linked. Think about the last time you spoke with somebody about a problem you were having. If that person had an understanding of both your culture and your value system, such as spirituality, you probably had an easier time explaining your problem. Now think about a time when you spoke with somebody about a problem you were having and that person had no idea what you were talking about. How would you describe that experience? As you can imagine, this happens quite often with people who have schizophrenia when their symptoms are unusual or they are not able to articulate them clearly.

Culture, spirituality, and a value system are intricately interwoven. They form the fabric for a system of meaning. Symptom expression, stressors, coping mechanisms, and interactions with others arise from this system. Keeping the cultural and spiritual context of a client's experience in mind while interacting around psychiatric symptoms and treatment reduces the client's frustrations and increases the effectiveness of your communication.

CARING FOR THE SPIRIT

These boxes reinforce the belief in the interconnection of mind, body, and spirit. They appear throughout the book and are designed to promote the understanding of the client's essence, meaning, and purpose in life, as well as the nurse's role in supporting spirituality.

WHY I BECAME A PSYCHIATRIC–MENTAL HEALTH NURSE

In this feature the authors and contributing authors for this text share the reasons and events that led them to enter the field of psychiatric–mental health nursing.

WHY I BECAME A PSYCHIATRIC–MENTAL HEALTH NURSE

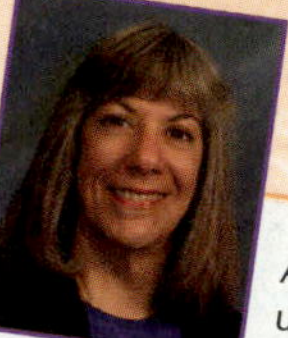

Pamela Marcus
Contributor, Chapter 6

As a very young nurse, I worked in a burn unit. One of my clients was only 7 years old—a young boy who had attempted suicide by grabbing a live electrical wire. When I took care of him, he had full-thickness electrical burns over 90% of his body. His physical care was full of pain for him and I was consumed with worry that his comfort needs would not be met.

Al... after h... My int... atric nu... on suic...

M... risk of ... care, w... outpati... in peo... their di...

YOUR SELF-AWARENESS

These boxes engage the reader in a process of introspection and self-questioning that is essential to the therapeutic use of self.

YOUR SELF-AWARENESS Countertransference

Look for the following cues in your own behavior that signal the presence of countertransference:

- Irrational friendliness toward the client
- Irrational concern about the client
- Reacting with annoyance or irrational hostility toward the client
- Feeling uneasy during or after meeting with the client
- Dreaming about or fantasizing about the client
- Being preoccupied with thoughts of the client during leisure time
- Any actions that are out of line with standard expectations for therapist behaviors

DSM-IV-TR DIAGNOSTIC CRITERIA

The most current diagnostic criteria from the APA 2000 *Diagnostic and Statistical Manual of Mental Disorders* (DSM-IV-TR) are provided in each of the disorders chapters in Unit 4.

DSM-IV-TR Diagnostic Criteria for Schizophrenia Subtypes

PARANOID TYPE

A type of Schizophrenia in which the following criteria are met:

A. Preoccupation with one or more delusions or frequent auditory hallucinations.

B. None of the following is prominent: disorganized speech, disorganized or catatonic behavior, or flat or inappropriate affect.

DISORGANIZED TYPE

A type of Schizophrenia in which the following criteria are met:

A. All of the following are prominent:
1. disorganized speech
2. disorganized behavior
3. flat or inappropriate affect

B. The criteria are not met for Catatonic Type.

CATATONIC TYPE

A type of Schizophrenia in which the clinical picture is dominated by at least two of the following:

1. motoric immobility as evidenced by catalepsy (including waxy flexibility) or stupor
2. excessive motor activity (that is apparently purposeless and not influenced by external stimuli)
3. extreme negativism (an apparently motiveless resistance to all instructions or maintenance of a rigid posture against attempts to be moved) or mutism
4. peculiarities of voluntary movement as evidenced by posturing (voluntary assumption of inappropriate or bizarre postures), stereotyped movements, prominent mannerisms, or prominent grimacing
5. echolalia or echopraxia

UNDIFFERENTIATED TYPE

A type of Schizophrenia in which symptoms that meet Criterion A are present, but the criteria are not met for the Paranoid, Disorganized, or Catatonic Type.

RESIDUAL TYPE

A type of Schizophrenia in which the following criteria are met:

A. Absence of prominent delusions, hallucinations, disorganized speech, and grossly disorganized or catatonic behavior.

B. There is continuing evidence of the disturbance, as indicated by the presence of negative symptoms or two or more symptoms listed in Criterion A for Schizophrenia, present in an attenuated form (e.g., odd beliefs, unusual perceptual experiences).

Source: Reprinted with permission from the *Diagnostic and Statistical Manual of Mental Disorders,* Fourth Edition, Text Revision. (Copyright 2000). American Psychiatric Association.

USING DSM-IV-TR

Health care providers often use language unfamiliar to clients and their families. Reword this DSM statement to make it easier for clients and family members to understand: "Preoccupation with one or more delusions or frequent auditory hallucinations."

RX COMMUNICATION

These boxes offer sample dialogues between nurses and clients. In addition, we provide the rationale for at least two different but helpful alternatives. This feature is designed to provide students with a beginning repertoire of communication interventions useful when interacting with psychiatric–mental health clients.

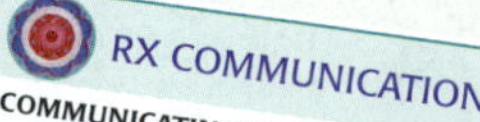

RX COMMUNICATION

COMMUNICATING WITH THE ANGRY, NONVERBAL CLIENT

CLIENT: Flares his nostrils and glares at the nurse.

NURSE RESPONSE 1: "Steven, you look angry today."

RATIONALE: Stating an observation, such as how the client appears, as well as using a feeling word, encourages communication. Talking about feeling angry may decrease the need to act out anger.

NURSE RESPONSE 2: "Steven, I can tell that you are upset. What's going on with you?"

RATIONALE: When you know a client is upset, this direct approach creates an opportunity for the client to discuss the feelings and thoughts with you.

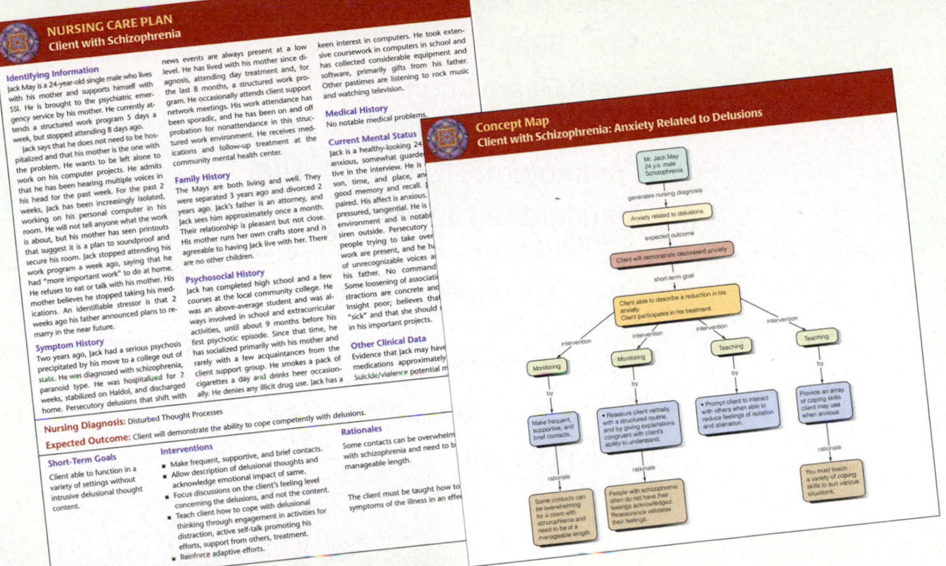

NURSING CARE PLANS and related **CONCEPT MAPS** are included in the chapters dealing with specific disorders. They represent two ways to view care for clients diagnosed with specific mental disorders according to the DSM-IV-TR, fostering critical thinking and analysis for students with different learning styles.

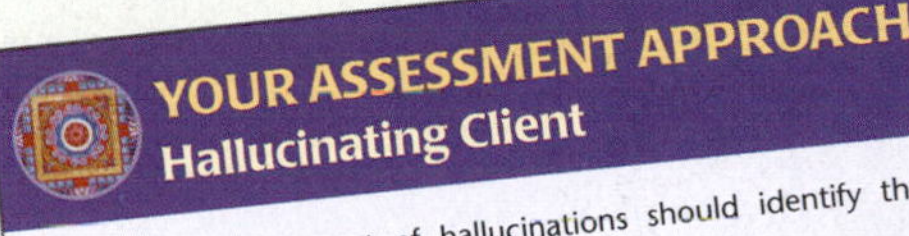
YOUR ASSESSMENT APPROACH
Hallucinating Client

A complete assessment of hallucinations should identify the following:

- Whether the hallucinations are solely auditory or incl
  other senses
- How long the client has experienced the hallucinatio
  the initial hallucinations were like, and whether they
  changed
- Which situations are most likely to trigger hallucinatio
  which times of day they occur most frequently
- What the hallucinations are about (Are they just soun
  voices? If the client hears voices, what do they say?)
- How strongly the client believes in the reality of the
  hallucinations
- Whether the hallucinations command the client to do
  something, and if so, how potentially destructive the
  commands are
- Whether the client hears other voices contradicting
  commands received in hallucinations
- How the client feels about the hallucinations
- Which strategies the client has used to cope with the
  hallucinations and how effective the strategies were

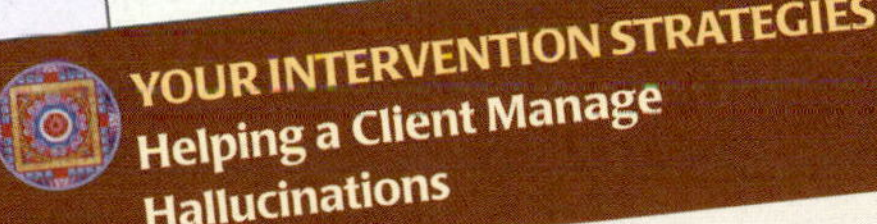
YOUR INTERVENTION STRATEGIES
Helping a Client Manage Hallucinations

- Determine the kind of hallucinations (auditory, visual, etc.).
- Can the symptom be managed with current coping?
- Access resources (advocacy groups, peers, staff, literature) for fresh ideas, better management techniques.
- Discuss options and success rate with professionals.
- Select options for coping with the stimuli:
  Distraction
  Resisting
  Calming
  Treatment (such as medication)
- Practice using an option to cope.
- Use a technique based on the success you have with it.
- Be ready to replace coping styles when they don't work anymore.

YOUR ASSESSMENT APPROACH and **YOUR INTERVENTION STRATEGIES** present clinically relevant strategies in a succinct, user-friendly format. Your Assessment Strategies contain lists of assessment points. Your Intervention Strategies list specific nursing intervention strategies along with their rationales.

OTHER FEATURES

CLINICAL EXAMPLES provide real-life scenarios that students may encounter and point out the challenges involved.

CROSS REFERENCES pinpoint specific content linked to supporting chapters when more depth is required. The icon ∞ refers the reader to content in other sections of the book.

END OF CHAPTER FEATURES

EXPLORE MEDIALINK. At the end of each chapter, this feature encourages students to use the CD-ROM and Companion Website (www.prenhall.com/kneisl) to apply their learning in case studies and care plans, to practice NCLEX-RN® questions, and to use additional resources. Special MediaLink tabs in the margins throughout the chapters refer students to the topics and activities on the media supplements.

NCLEX-RN® REVIEW QUESTIONS. Each chapter concludes with 10 NCLEX-RN®-style questions. Answers and rationales are in Appendix C.

REFERENCES. Each chapter includes a bibliography of the most up-to-date resources on the topic.

MediaLink RESOURCES

SPECIAL FEATURES

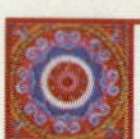

Your Self-Awareness

Evidence-Based Practice

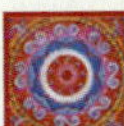

Caring for the Spirit

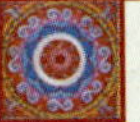

Partnering with Clients and Families

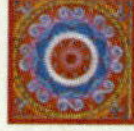

What Every Specialty Nurse Should Know

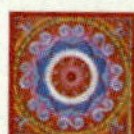

DSM-IV-TR Diagnostic Criteria

Rx Communication

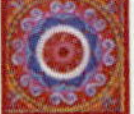

Why I Became a Psychiatric–Mental Health Nurse

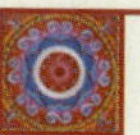

Your Assessment Approach

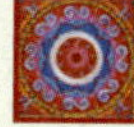

Your Intervention Strategies

DETAILED CONTENTS

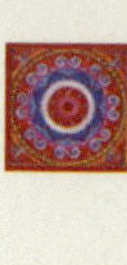

UNIT 1 • The Strength and Structure of Psychiatric–Mental Health Nursing 3

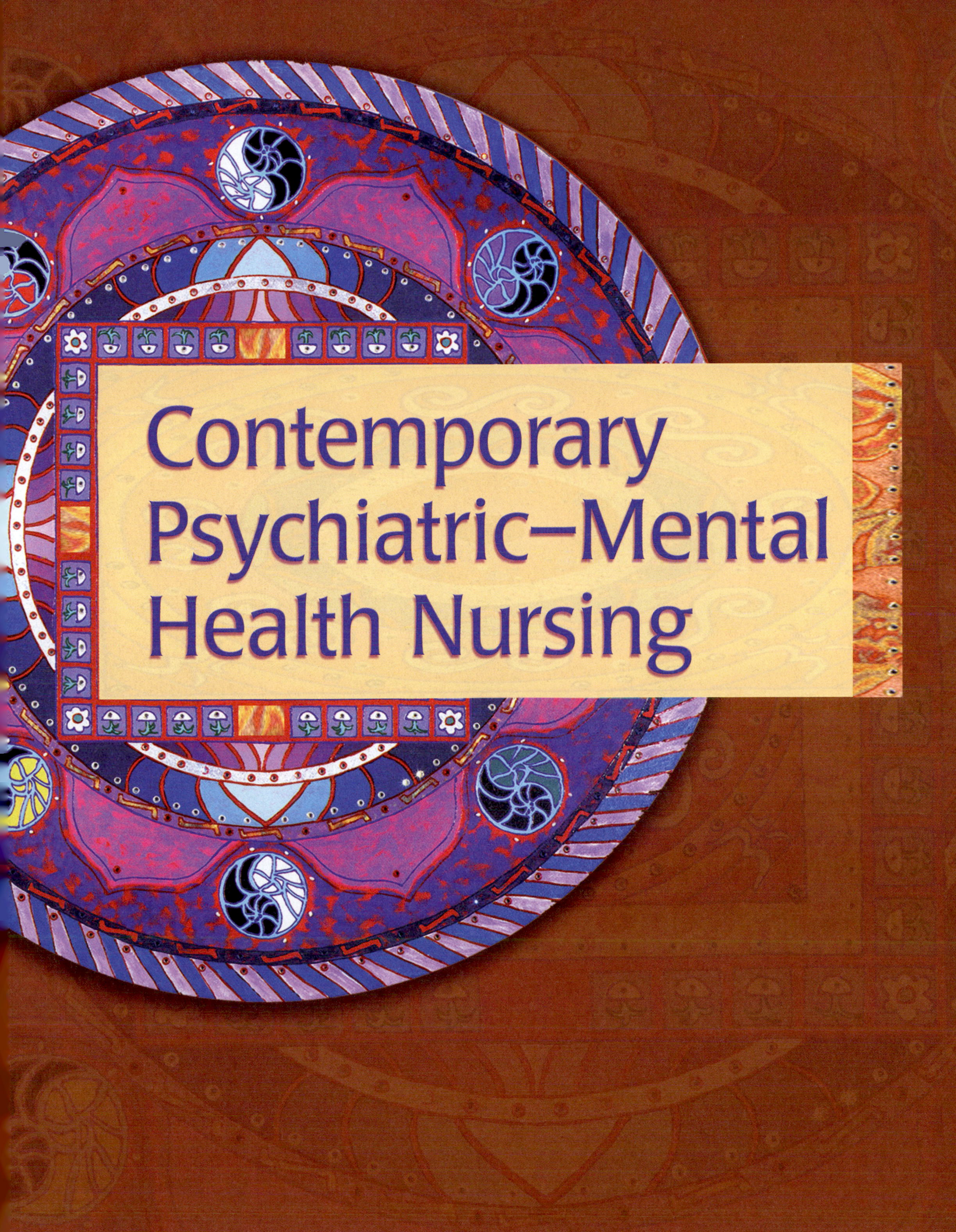
Contemporary
Psychiatric–Mental
Health Nursing

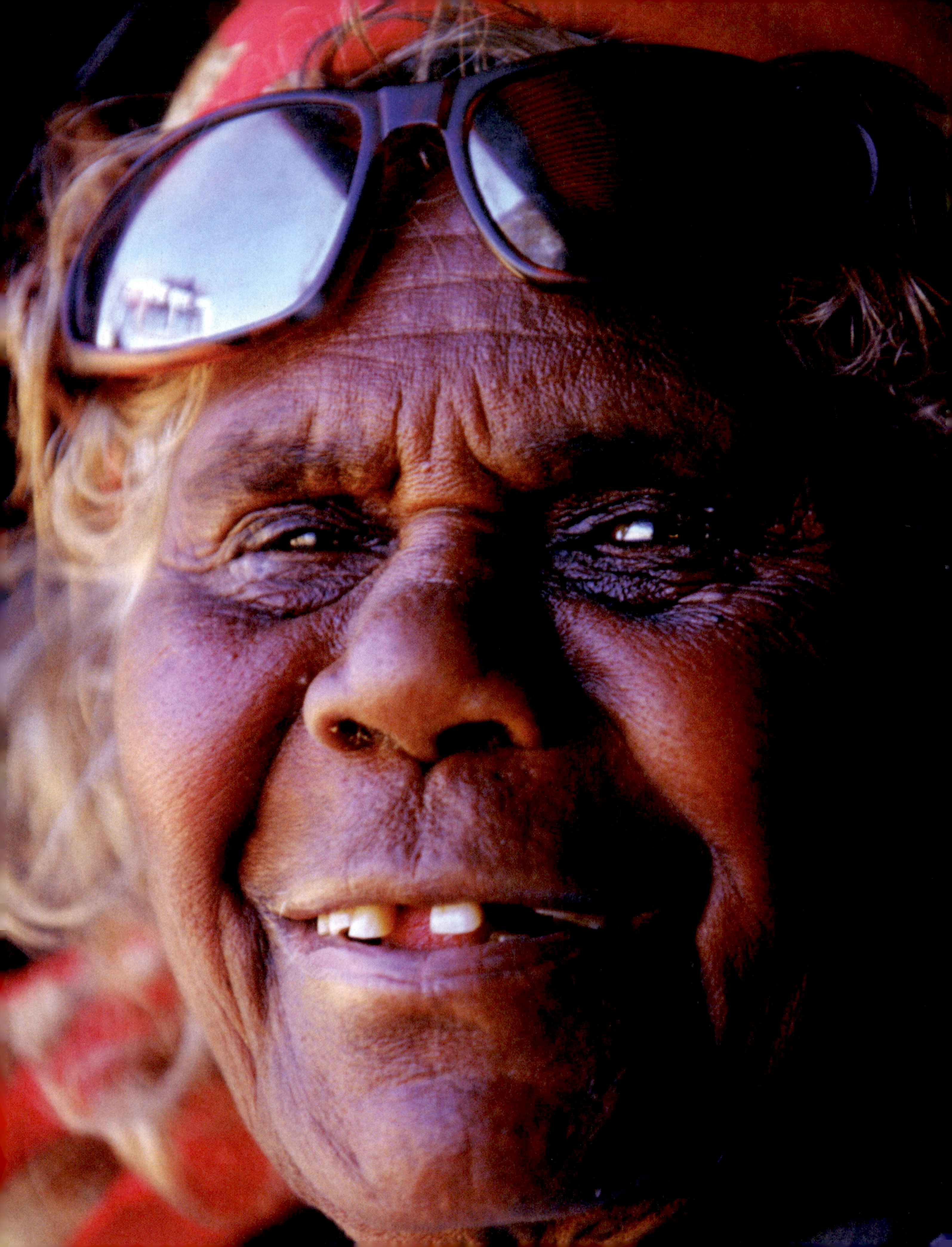

Unit 1

THE STRENGTH AND STRUCTURE OF PSYCHIATRIC–MENTAL HEALTH NURSING

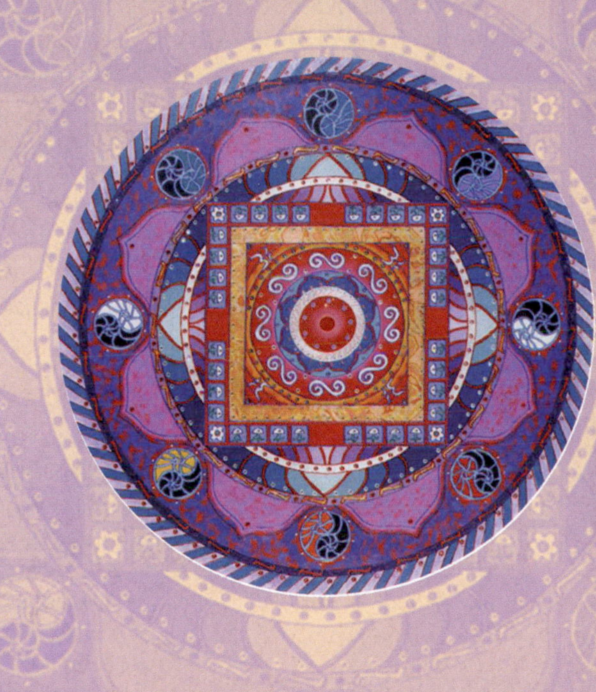

DOLLY, a member of the Anangu Aboriginal people originally from Australia's central desert region, lives with ten other people in a flat in Brisbane. Dolly finds joy and comfort in teaching her grandchildren how to play the didgeridoo, the world's oldest wind instrument and the national instrument of Australia's Aboriginal people. She holds out hope that her 16-year-old grandson, a musician who plays Aboriginal rock, will be able to climb out of poverty.

The Aboriginal people are facing a crisis of social and cultural disintegration. They are twice as likely to report poor or only fair health and twice as likely to have a disability or long-term health condition. Dementia is 26 times more likely in Aboriginal communities, and alcoholism, drug abuse, schizophrenia, and suicide are on the increase. For urbanized indigenous Australians like Dolly, social pressures prevent access to mental health services. In their daily lives they battle violent crime, domestic and sexual abuse, unemployment, and homelessness. A goal in our search for improved global mental health is to correct cultural inequities and promote quality of life for people like Dolly.

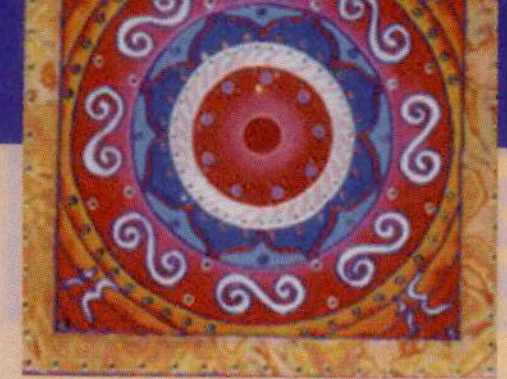

CHAPTER

1

Psychiatric–Mental Health Clients: Who Are They?

CAROL REN KNEISL

KEY TERMS

crazy *5*
deviance *5*
mental disorder *6*
nervous breakdown *5*
psychopathology *6*

LEARNING OUTCOMES

After completing this chapter, you will be able to:

1. Define and explain *mental disorder*.
2. Analyze why the term *deviant behavior* lacks a definition that covers all situations.
3. Discuss how definitions of *mental disorder* have shifted throughout history.
4. Name the mental disorders that rank among the top ten causes of disability worldwide.
5. Identify the major mental health problems in the United States according to the *Healthy People 2010* report.

CRITICAL THINKING CHALLENGE

Your Aunt Lisa and Uncle Bob are worried about your upcoming mental health clinical experiences. Frightened by the many television programs and movies that portray violent acts committed by supposedly mentally deranged people, they point to dramas whose protagonists are forensic scientists or criminal profilers who solve gory cases based on bizarre circumstances. They worry that the mental health settings for your clinical experiences are full of the sorts of characters they have seen on television and in the movies.

1. How will you deal with Aunt Lisa's and Uncle Bob's concerns?
2. What information would be helpful to them?
3. If you have similar concerns, what can you do to attain a sense of comfort in this clinical experience?

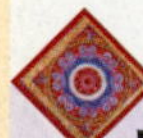

MEDIALINK 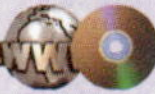 www.prenhall.com/kneisl

Go to the Pearson Health MediaLink CD-ROM and the Companion Website at www.prenhall.com/kneisl for interactive resources for this chapter.

You are about to enter upon a journey unlike any other you have had to date in your nursing program. Facing the unknown in a psychiatric–mental health setting invites a variety of feelings and may prompt you to ask yourself several questions:

- What kinds of people will I encounter in the mental health settings I will visit?
- Will they be hard to talk to?
- What do I have in common with them?
- What if they can't, or won't, control themselves?
- How do I know that what I say won't harm them?
- What are they all about and how can I ever figure them out?

You will undoubtedly hear about, and see, deviant behavior. We use the sociological definition of **deviance**—behavior outside the social norm of a specific group—in this text. Think back to your introductory sociology courses and recall that in its social context, *deviant* does not mean "bad." Behavior that is considered bizarre or unreasonable in one cultural context may be considered desirable in another. Further, your expectations for your clinical experiences are likely to be influenced by your upbringing, what you have seen in your own communities and neighborhoods, have read about in newspapers or magazines, or have seen and read about on the Internet.

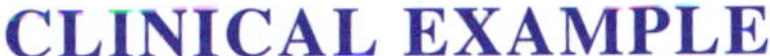

CLINICAL EXAMPLE

A psychiatric–mental health nurse, recalling her childhood experiences with community deviants, commented on the intense and sometimes morbid excitement that she and her friends found in taunting "Crazy Helen" to run out on her porch and shout incoherently at them, or in telling stories about "Lester the Molester" who hung around the school, the playground, and the community pool and occasionally exposed himself to the children.

The interest these characters held for the children, along with "Vince the Window Peeper," "Eddie the Drunk," and other community deviants, was reawakened in her as she approached her first psychiatric–mental health nursing experience. It was all very frightening, yet intriguing at the same time.

What do you have in common with psychiatric–mental health clients? How can you ever hope to understand them? There are many approaches to understanding people—history, sociology, anthropology, philosophy, anatomy, physiology, and psychology, among others. Each is like a searchlight, illuminating some facts while leaving others in shadow. One of the challenges you will face in your clinical experiences, in your classroom lectures and discussions, and in the reading of this textbook is answering these questions by judiciously and appropriately blending knowledge from these diverse areas. Our goal is to help you achieve a sense of comfort in your clinical work with psychiatric–mental health clients. The strategies we present in this book are designed to help you become a comfortable, successful, and safe psychiatric–mental health nurse.

You will also find that, unlike the bizarre characters described in the clinical example, most psychiatric–mental health clients are everyday, ordinary people. They are your neighbors, your friends, your family members; your teacher, pharmacist, or physician; or even yourself. It is highly likely that you know someone who has been diagnosed with a mental disorder or has sought mental health counseling to deal with problems in living.

MediaLink Critical Thinking Exercise: First Clinical Day

Given the right circumstances, anyone can have a mental health problem or disorder, ranging from a mild, temporary increase in anxiety to the most severe of psychoses. Fame, status, and money do not ensure mental health or happiness, at least not according to the celebrities we hear about—actors, sports stars, authors, musicians, singers, movie directors, and scientists. Many celebrities are speaking out about their experiences with mental illness. People who openly discuss their mental health problems or write books about their experiences increase public awareness. They make it easier for others to reveal their own struggles and seek help.

This chapter discusses the concept of mental disorder; reviews the attitudes and philosophic viewpoints that have influenced our understanding and approach to "madness" throughout history; and identifies the global burden of mental disorder in our country, around the world, in our neighbors and friends, and in the celebrities we hear about every day. Our goals are to encourage you to think seriously about what constitutes mental health and mental illness, to appreciate the humanity of people who experience mental illness, and to approach your psychiatric–mental health experience with confidence.

In addition to any anxiety, trepidation, or self-doubt you have, we encourage you to approach this experience as we do, with energetic enthusiasm and an eagerness to relate to people whose behavior may be unusual, offensive, socially inappropriate, or even frightening. By doing so, you will find the humanity, creativity, caring, and joy inherent in your clients.

THE CONCEPT OF MENTAL DISORDER

We believe that concepts such as "mental disorder" and "mental health" are interactional and derive their meaning not only from changes in brain structure and biochemistry but also from how we define certain behavior by certain people. Therefore, we also advocate taking a critical look at the social conditions under which someone is called "mentally ill."

MediaLink Care Plan: Managing Personal Anxiety

Many terms have been used to describe aberrant behavior or mental disorder. In the earlier clinical example, the neighbor lady was called "Crazy Helen." **Crazy** is an informal, denigrating, and stigmatizing term for "mentally ill" that carries with it unfounded and negative implications. People probably described "Crazy Helen" as having had a **nervous breakdown**—a general, nonspecific term for an incapacitating but otherwise unspecified type of mental disorder. Most of the terms that society uses to describe aberrant behavior have a convoluted history and have traveled over time and between languages. The terms, their origins, and their meanings have been studied by Dalby (1993) and are discussed in Table 1-1 ■ on page 6.

You may have used some or all of these terms yourself, and you may hear them used in mental health settings and the

TABLE 1-1 ■ **Terms of Madness and Their Historical Origins**

Term	Origin	Meaning
Berserk	From the Old Norse *bersekr*	Used originally to describe warriors who developed battle madness and killed without mercy, reason, or fear; now means frenzied behavior
Crazy	Originally of Scandinavian origin; its English use occurred in the 16th century	Used originally to describe unsound pitchers or ships liable to fall to pieces; its colloquial use broadened to encompass notions such as unrestrained, confused, and even enthusiastic
Delirium	Originally of Latin origin; its English use occurred in the late 16th century	Its root, *lira*, in Old English originally denoted a furrow or tract. Delirium literally meant going out of the furrow or track and became associated with temporary or transient losses of reason
Delusion	Of Latin origin; appeared in English in the early 16th century	Referred to deceiving, fooling, or cheating with a lie or a false belief
Dementia	Of Greek origin	Originally synonymous with insanity; the term blended madness and loss of intellect
Fury	Derived from Greek and Roman mythology	Originally used to describe female creatures who pursued persons guilty of terrible, unavenged crimes until they went mad. The original connotation changed over time as *fury* was equated with insanity; it now means intense or violent anger
Hallucination	Derived from Latin and Greek roots	Often interchanged with "confusion" until the late 18th century, when it came to mean false impression or perception
Insane	From the Latin *insanus*; appeared initially in the early 16th century	Originally was the equivalent of mad or could mean senseless, idiotic, or irrational; now it has a formal legal, rather than clinical, use
Lunacy	Derived from *Luna,* the Roman moon goddess	Synonymous with madness or cyclical insanity caused by exposure to the moon
Madness	Derived from the Goths and Old German and Old English roots	Denoted foolishness, the pathological loss of reason, or bizarre behavior
Melancholy	From the Greek	Originally meant sullenness, sadness, or general insanity
Nervous	Of Indo-European origin	Originally denoted "twist" or "wind"; later used to describe muscle or sinew; then the system of nerves, which was seen as similar to sinews
Obsession	From Latin	In the early 16th century it meant sitting on or against, describing a siege; in the 17th century it meant being beset by an evil spirit; later meant a "fixed idea"
Paranoia	Of Greek origin	Originally used to denote a lack of mental soundness; it underwent many variations and later connoted fear and delusions of persecution
Psychosis	Of Greek origin	Originally referred to the principle of life or animation and later meant a condition or disease of the mind or the soul

community at large. It is important that you become familiar with the words and their meanings so that you can advocate for others to treat clients respectfully and ethically. We discuss the ethics of stigmatizing labels in Chapter 13∞.

Mental illness and mental health, we believe, are outgrowths of intrapersonal (within the mind or self) and interpersonal (between self and others) processes. Determining that someone is mentally ill is often a matter of judgment, even when brain chemicals are altered. The appropriateness of behavior depends on whether it is judged plausible or not according to a set of social, ethical, and legal rules that define the limits of appropriate behavior and reality. For example, if a man on a street corner says he is Napoleon, people will not believe him and will consider his statement symptomatic or disturbed. If a man at a masquerade party says he is Napoleon, people reach a different conclusion.

With the preceding as philosophic background, we support the concept of **mental disorder** as a psychological group of symptoms, such as a pattern or a syndrome, in which the individual experiences distress (a painful symptom), disability (impairment in one or more important areas of functioning), or a significantly increased risk of suffering, pain, loss of freedom, or death. These signs and symptoms of mental disorder are known as **psychopathology** (literally, pathology of the mind). Mental health professionals refer to mental disorders as psychopathological conditions. According to the American Psychiatric Association (APA), a mental disorder is other than an expected and culturally accepted response to a particular event such as the death of a loved one (APA, 2000). Mental disorders are identified, standardized, and categorized in the *Diagnostic and Statistical Manual of Mental Disorders* published by the APA (2000). Later, in

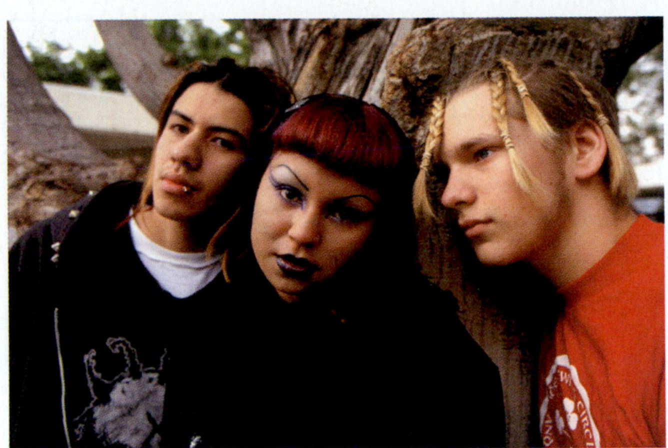

FIGURE 1-1 ■ Nonconforming behavior or appearance that flouts social norms is an example of social deviance—not evidence of psychopathology or abnormal behavior.

Source: PhotoEdit Inc., Michael Newman.

TABLE 1-2 ■ **Prevalence Rates for Various Mental Disorders**

	Women		Men	
	1-year	**Lifetime**	**1-year**	**Lifetime**
Phobic disorder	12.9	17.8	6.3	10.4
Alcohol abuse/ dependence	2.2	4.6	11.9	23.8
Major depression	4.0	7.0	1.4	2.6
Antisocial personality	0.4	0.8	2.1	4.5
Obsessive-compulsive disorder	1.9	3.2	1.4	2.0
Panic disorder	1.2	2.1	0.6	1.0
Schizophrenia	1.1	1.7	0.9	1.2
Bipolar mood disorder	0.8	0.9	0.6	0.7

Chapter 13, in the Your Self-Awareness Feature on page 265, we ask you to consider whether standardized terminology use in psychiatric settings conflicts with individualized client care.

We would not label deviant political, religious, or sexual behavior, or conflicts primarily between an individual and society (see FIGURE 1-1 ■) as mental disorders unless the deviance or conflict is a symptom of dysfunction in the individual. Like many concepts in the human sciences, the concept of mental disorder lacks a definition that covers all situations. In addition, definitions of mental disorder have shifted throughout history. The final section of this chapter reviews the historical shift in attitude and philosophic viewpoints from preliterate cultures to the present day. The history of psychiatric–mental health nursing is reviewed in Chapter 2 and the history of psychiatric treatment in Chapter 5.

THE INCIDENCE OF MENTAL DISORDER WORLDWIDE

How common are mental disorders? Researchers have found surprisingly high incidences of mental disorder in patients seen for physical illnesses in primary health care settings in the United States. Estimates have ranged from 25% to 64% of patients seen in doctors' offices and clinics. Recent research indicates that 29% of patients seen in primary care had a mental disorder (Jackson, Passamonti, & Kroenke, 2007). Another study found that 19% had at least one anxiety disorder (Kroenke, Spitzer, Williams, Monahan, & Lowe, 2007). Of this number, 41% were not receiving treatment. Two other scientifically rigorous studies give us more information about the incidence of mental disorders.

In the 1980s, a large-scale epidemiologic study (the study of the frequency and distribution of disorders within a population) known as the Epidemiologic Catchment Area (ECA) study interviewed approximately 20,000 people in five major metropolitan areas in the United States. The ECA study determined that mental disorders are experienced by many people at some point in their lives. The data in TABLE 1-2 ■ refer to the *prevalence* of active cases of specific mental disorders in a population during a specific period of time (one year). *Lifetime prevalence* is the total proportion of the population that has been affected by mental disorder at some point in their lives. FIGURES 1-2 ■ below and 1-3 ■ on page 8 also illustrate these data in yet another way. Figure 1-2 identifies the lifetime prevalence rates for the major categories of non-substance

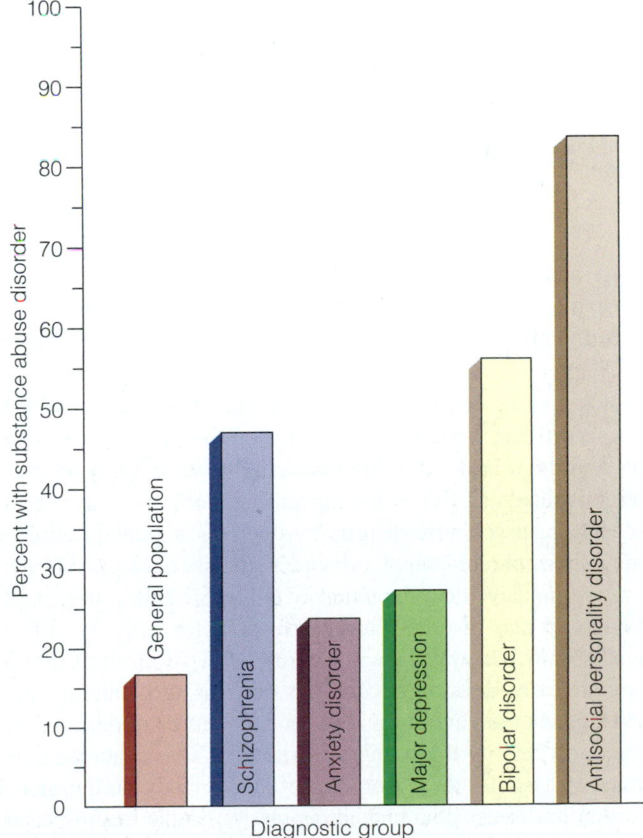

FIGURE 1-2 ■ Lifetime prevalence rates for non-substance abuse disorders.

Source: Based on data from *Epidemiologic Catchment Area Study*, Regler et al., 1990.

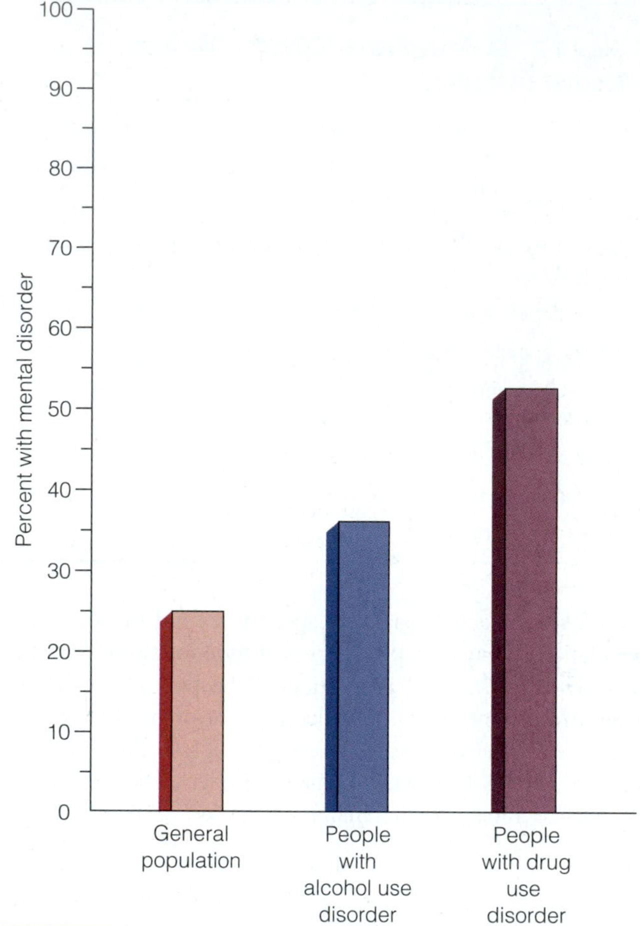

Figure 1-3 ■ Lifetime prevalence rates for substance abuse disorders.

Source: Based on data from *Epidemiologic Catchment Area Study,* Regler et al., 1990.

abuse mental disorders, while Figure 1-3 identifies the rates for substance abuse disorders. What we have learned about mental disorders through epidemiology is discussed more specifically in Chapter 9∞.

A major study by the World Health Organization (WHO) has shown that we have underestimated the incidence of mental disorder worldwide. The *Global Burden of Disease* study demonstrated that five of the top ten causes of disability worldwide were psychiatric disorders—depression (ranked number one), schizophrenia, bipolar disorder, alcohol abuse, and obsessive–compulsive disorder (Murray & Lopez, 1996). In fact, although mental disorders are responsible for only 1% of all deaths, they account for a staggering 47% of all disability in economically developed countries such as the United States and Canada (and are the second leading source of disease burden), and 28% of all disability worldwide. These data are illustrated in Table 1-3 ■. A more recent WHO study on the global burden of disease also ranked depression as the leading cause of disability in people ages 15 and older (Moussavi et al., 2007). These researchers also determined that depression is the factor that produced the greatest decrement in health when compared with the chronic physical diseases of angina, arthritis, asthma, and diabetes. The burden of mental disorders is likely to have been underestimated because of inadequate appreciation of the connection between mental illness and other health conditions (Prince et al., 2007). As these researchers say, there is no health without mental health.

Table 1-3 ■ **Leading Causes of Mental Disability in the World**

Mental Disorder	Percent of Total Disability
1. Unipolar major depression	10.7
4. Alcohol use	3.3
6. Bipolar disorder	3.0
9. Schizophrenia	2.6
10. Obsessive-compulsive disorders	2.2

The prediction of the WHO investigators is that the burden of mental disorders will increase even more by the year 2020. According to WHO, global mental health resources remain low, and improvements in 2001–2004 (the most recent years for which figures are available) were minimal at best (Saxena, Sharan, Garrido, & Saraceno, 2006). Clearly, mental disorders are one of global health's greatest challenges.

Healthy People 2010, a report by the United States Department of Health and Human Services (USDHHS) (2002), identified the 10 major public health/mental health problems in the United States and determined specific mental health objectives to be achieved by the end of this decade. These mental health problems are identified and ranked in Box 1-1. The Healthy People 2010 Mental Health Objectives are listed in Box 1-2.

A second important report was the U.S. Surgeon General's report on mental health and mental illness (USDHHS, 1999). This report underscored the importance of understanding that mental disorders are "real" illnesses, that people should be educated to seek help for symptoms of mental disorder, and that we have an obligation to provide safe and effective treatment for all citizens by improving the delivery of mental health care services. All three reports and studies emphasize the importance of promoting and maintaining mental health and improving mental health delivery systems around the world.

Throughout this text, we will continue to remind you of these serious concerns. We will remind you of the humanity of those diagnosed with a mental disorder—of the family, friends, neighbors, and celebrities we know. We will also continue to remind you that the experience of mental disorder not only has devastating effects on the lives of those affected, but also can encourage extraordinary clarity, insight, and creative potential.

HISTORICAL PERSPECTIVES

People who have been called "mentally ill" have been with us throughout history—to be feared, marveled at, ignored, banished, laughed at, pitied, or tortured. A historical review of the place of the "mentally ill," however they have been de-

Box 1-1 Healthy People 2010 Mental Health Problems

- High suicide rate, especially among adolescents
- Homeless adults with serious mental illness (SMI)
- High relapse rates for persons with eating disorders including anorexia nervosa and bulimia nervosa
- Persons seen in primary health care who do not receive mental health screening and assessment
- Children with mental health problems who do not receive treatment
- Lack of screening for mental health problems of new admissions in juvenile justice facilities
- Adults with mental disorders who do not receive treatment
- Persons with co-occurring substance abuse and mental disorders who do not receive treatment for both disorders
- Inadequate number of community-based jail diversion programs for adults with SMI
- Failure of states and territories to operationalize mental health plans that address cultural competence
- Inadequate number of states and territories with an operational mental health plan that addresses mental health crisis interventions, ongoing screening, and treatment services for elderly persons
- Worksites that fail to provide programs to prevent or reduce employee stress

Source: U.S. Department of Health and Human Services. (2002). *Healthy people 2010*. Retrieved August 20, 2002, from http://www.healthypeople.gov. These data can be found on the USDHHS website (www.dhhs.gov; www.healthypeople.gov), or through a direct resource link on the Companion Website for this book.

Box 1-2 Healthy People 2010 Mental Health Objectives

- Reduce the suicide rate.
- Reduce the rate of suicide attempts by adolescents.
- Reduce the proportion of homeless adults who have serious mental illness (SMI).
- Increase the proportion of persons with SMI who are employed.
- Reduce the relapse rates for persons with eating disorders including anorexia nervosa and bulimia nervosa.
- Increase the number of persons seen in primary health care who receive mental health screening and assessment.
- Increase the proportion of children with mental health problems who receive treatment.
- Increase the proportion of juvenile justice facilities that screen new admissions for mental health problems.
- Increase the proportion of adults with mental disorders who receive treatment.
- Increase the proportion of persons with co-occurring substance abuse and mental disorders who receive treatment for both disorders.
- Increase the proportion of local governments with community-based jail diversion programs for adults with SMI.
- Increase the number of states and the District of Columbia that track consumers' satisfaction with the mental health services they receive.
- Increase the number of states, territories, and the District of Columbia with an operational mental health plan that addresses cultural competence.
- Increase the number of states, territories, and the District of Columbia with an operational mental health plan that addresses mental health crisis interventions, ongoing screening, and treatment services for elderly persons.
- Increase the proportion of worksites employing 50 or more persons that provide programs to prevent or reduce employee stress.

Source: Department of Health and Human Services. (2002). *Healthy people 2010*. Retrieved August 20, 2002, from http://www.healthypeople.gov.

MediaLink Healthy People 2010

fined in societies during different periods, brings up these central points:

- Dominant social attitudes and philosphic viewpoints have influenced the understanding and approach to "madness" throughout recorded history, and probably before.
- Ideas that may be considered contemporary at one time often have roots in earlier centuries.
- The modern medical concept of "madness" as an illness is open to the same scrutiny as interpretations of the past, such as beliefs about witchcraft or mysticism.

Era of Magico–Religious Explanations

In preliterate cultures, mental and physical suffering were not differentiated. Both were attributed to forces acting outside the body. Consequently, no distinctions were made between medicine, magic, and religion. All were variously directed against some mortal or superhuman force that had cruelly inflicted suffering on another. Primitive healers quite logically dealt with the spirits of torment with appeal, reverence, prayer, bribery, intimidation, appeasement, confession, punishment, exorcism, magical ritual, and incantation.

Behavior considered "mental illness" by modern Western cultures was attributed in preliterate cultures to the violation of taboos, the neglect of ritual obligations, the loss of a vital substance from the body (such as the soul), the introduction of a foreign and harmful substance into the body (such as evil spirits), or witchcraft.

Era of Organic Explanations

In the 4th century BCE, Hippocrates proposed a medical concept to explain mental suffering. He rejected demonology and proposed that psychiatric illnesses were caused mainly by imbalances in body humors: blood, black bile, yellow bile, and phlegm. For example, an excess of black bile was thought to cause melancholy.

One important consequence of these beliefs was that psychiatric suffering came within the realm of medical practice to include words (interpretation of dreams and talking) and medicines (purging, bloodletting, and ritual purification).

Era of Alienation

At the height of their civilization, the citizens of ancient Greece found their inner security in knowledge and reason. The Romans adopted the intellectual heritage of Greece but placed greater reliance on their social institutions and the rational organization of society supported by law and military might. When these institutions disintegrated and the Roman Empire went into a decline, fear tore apart the fabric of society.

The collapse of Rome signaled a general return to the magic, mysticism, and demonology from which people had retreated during the age of Greek rationality. During the Middle Ages, the period between approximately 400 CE and the Renaissance (1300–1600 CE), madness was seen as a dramatic encounter with secret powers. Troubled minds were thought to be influenced by the moon (*lunacy* literally means a disorder caused by the moon). (See FIGURE 1-4 ■.)

In the Arab world, the insane were believed to be divinely inspired and not victims of demons. An asylum for the mentally ill was built in Fez, Morocco, early in the 8th century. Other asylums were soon established in Baghdad, Cairo, and Damascus. The care in these asylums was usually benevolent and kindly.

The first European hospital devoted entirely to mental patients was built in 1409 in Valencia, Spain. The problems of the mind, however, remained the domain of clerical scholars. A book called *Malleus Maleficarum* (*The Witches' Hammer,* 1487) became the basis for witch hunts. The *Malleus* details the destruction of dissenters, heretics, and the "mentally ill," most of whom were women and all of whom were labeled *witches*. Theologic rationalizations and magical explanations were used to justify burning witches at the stake.

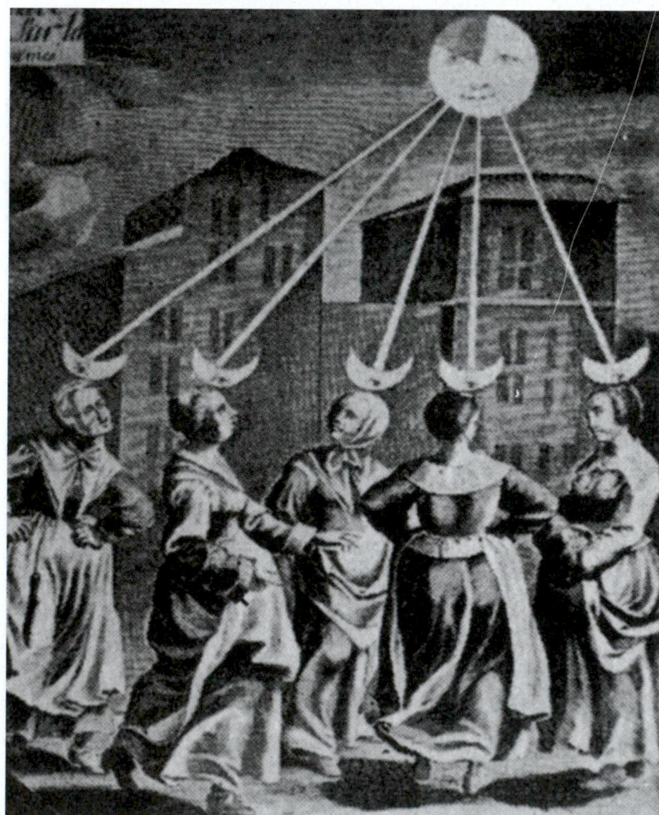

FIGURE 1-4 ■ Moonstruck women dancing in a 17th-century square. This activity is the source for the word *lunatic*.

Source: Philosophical Library.

The violent insane were shackled in prisons. Others were sent on voyages of symbolic importance. The "ships of fools" were boatloads of mad people sent out to sea to search for their reason. In this phase of ritualized social exclusion, social abandonment was thought to provide the opportunity for spiritual reintegration.

Era of Confinement

Unlike the Middle Ages, when the insane were generally driven out of or excluded from community life, during the Renaissance they were confined. Tamed, retained, and maintained, madness was reduced to silence through a system of mutual obligation between the afflicted and society. Mad persons had the right to be fed but were morally constrained and physically confined.

Seventeenth-century society created enormous houses of confinement. In these asylums were gathered the mad, the poor, and various deviants. A landmark date is 1656, when by decree the Hôpital Général in Paris was founded. It was not a medical establishment, but rather a threatening institution complete with stakes, irons, and dungeons. The "insane" were completely under the jurisdiction of the institution and had no recourse to appeal their incarceration. The Hôpital Général and other, similar institutions were established to maintain social order. In London, the hospital of St. Mary of Bethlehem became famous as *Bedlam* (see FIGURE 1-5 ■), where, for the entertainment of onlookers on a Sunday afternoon outing, mad persons were publicly beaten and tortured.

Those chained to cell walls were no longer considered people who had lost their reason or sick persons, but rather beasts seized by a frenzy. Madness was less than ever linked to medicine during this period and could be overcome only by discipline and brutality.

Era of Moral Treatment

The 18th and early 19th centuries were an era characterized by internal contradictions. Although the insane were un-

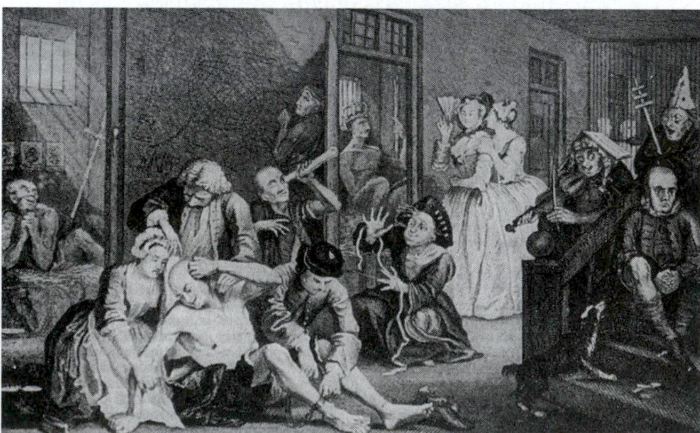

FIGURE 1-5 ■ A ward in Bethlehem Hospital about 1745. A patient is being chained in the foreground, and in the background are two Sunday visitors on an entertainment outing.

Source: Philosophical Library.

chained, the medical treatment they received consisted of torture with special paraphernalia. To grasp the incredible inhumanity with which the mentally disordered were treated in what became known as "the era of enlightenment," consider the following:

- The nature of mental disorders could not be explained by any of the prevailing concepts—black humors could not be seen, demons or animal spirits could not be observed, and knowledge of anatomy could not be applied to the workings of the mind.
- Because mental disorders could not be satisfactorily explained, the deeply felt dread of the insane could not be dispelled.
- Mental disorders were believed to be incurable, and mad persons were thought to be dangerous.

During this period, the emphasis was on the classification of symptoms of mental disorder. Even the most sensitive physicians did not try to understand the sources of mental suffering. Because they had no way to explain or understand mental disorders, they focused on elaborate and detailed systems of classification.

At the same time, a general spirit of reform and humanitarianism swept western Europe and the United States. Physicians developed a zeal for social reform and moral enrichment and began to release inmates from their chains, abolish systematized brutality with chains and whips, feed them nourishing foods, and treat them with kindness. This movement was first led by Philippe Pinel (1745–1826) (see FIGURE 1-6 ■) in France and the Quakers in England under William Tuke (1732–1822). Moral treatment in the United States—led by Benjamin Franklin, Benjamin Rush (called "the father of American psychiatry," 1745–1813), and others—was an alternative to mere confinement. Despite his association with humanitarianism and moral treatment, Rush was a major follower of the ideas of Scotland's William Cullen (1710–1790). Cullen believed that mental disorder was due to decay, either of the intellect or of the involuntary nervous system, that is, a matter of disordered physiology. Rush advocated bloodletting, the restraining chair (see FIGURE 1-7 ■), the gyrating chair, and other devices that we now consider inhumane.

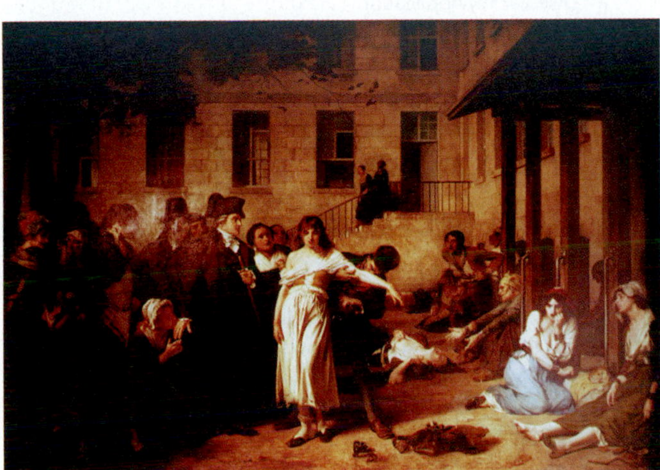

FIGURE 1-6 ■ A landmark event—Philippe Pinel unchaining the insane in the Bicêtre Hospital in Paris.
Source: Photo Researchers, Inc., Charles Ciccione.

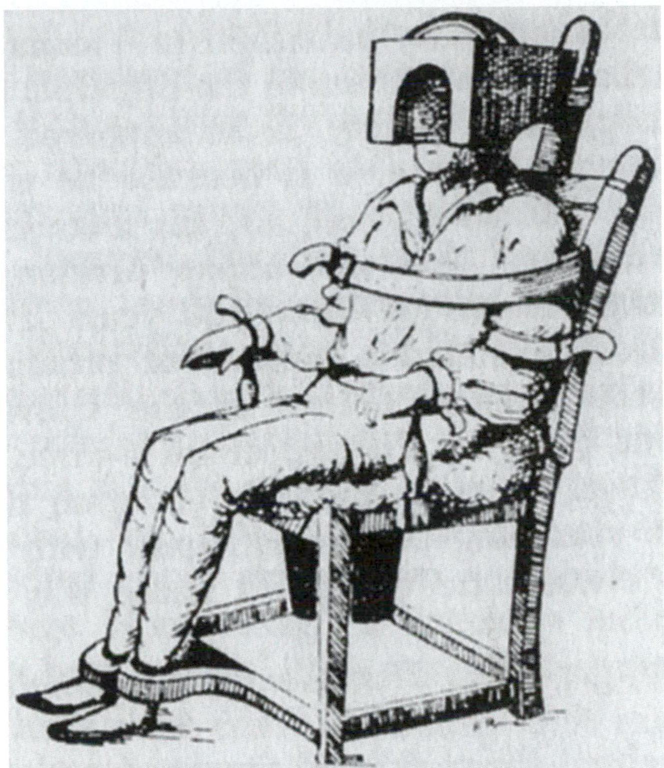

FIGURE 1-7 ■ Benjamin Rush, the "father of American psychiatry" and an idealist and humanitarian, nevertheless favored physical theories such as "excitement of the brain" to explain mental illness. He was preoccupied with somatic treatments such as bleeding and purging and developed the tranquilizing chair to quiet the insane.
Source: Philosophical Library.

Era of Psychoanalysis

During the late 19th and early 20th centuries, the number of mental hospitals, both private and government-run, grew. Beliefs about mental disorder began to change again. Insanity was linked to faulty life habits and treated with new forms of physical or somatic therapies. Other clinicians were inclined toward an organic, neurophysiologic explanation of mental disorders. The emphasis on the classification of distinct disease entities continued.

These developments formed the background for the work of one of the most influential figures in the history of psychiatry, Sigmund Freud (1856–1939). He succeeded in explaining human behavior in psychologic terms. Freud's contributions to psychiatry are discussed in greater detail in Chapter 5 ∞.

Contemporary Developments

By the mid-20th century, psychiatric thinking was expanding and moving toward an emphasis on the importance of the social dimension. Dissatisfaction with psychoanalytic explanations for mental disorder became more common, and drug treatment for mental illness was being developed. Research into chemotherapy and the etiology of mental illness increased.

The primary innovation of the 1990s was the so-called biologic revolution: the collaboration of science and technology to expand concepts of mental disorder proposed by psychologic and behavioral theories. During this period, a quantum leap was made in understanding the brain. For example, research on brain dysfunction in mental disorders has resulted in a major reconceptualization of the diagnosis and treatment of several mental disorders. Researchers have discovered a variety of brain dysfunctions, including ventricular enlargement, cerebral atrophy, and disturbances in neurotransmitters (discussed more thoroughly in Chapter 6 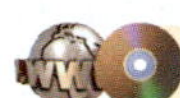).

This up-to-date, research-based knowledge is reflected in contemporary psychiatric and psychiatric–mental health nursing literature, including this text. Research in the 21st century will focus on such areas as:

- The bases of mental disorders
- The continuing development of newer generations of medications with fewer side effects to treat mental disorders
- The effects of various medications on neurotransmitters in the brains of clients with psychiatric disorders
- The role of nutrients in modifying brain function
- The influence on mood and behavior of disruptions of biologic rhythms
- The role of viruses in mental disorders
- The influence of the endocrine system on the brain and behavior
- The role of the brain in producing physical illnesses
- The identification of biologic markers that might alert clients and clinicians to the onset of a mental disorder
- The prevention of major mental illnesses
- The interrelationship between genetics and mental disorder

We can expect that, as the result of contemporary research, our conceptualizations of mental disorder will continue to shift.

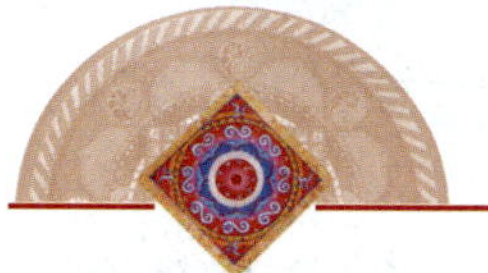

EXPLORE MEDIALINK www.prenhall.com/kneisl

For NCLEX-RN® review questions, case studies, and other resources for this chapter see the Pearson Health MediaLink CD-ROM that accompanies this book and the Companion Website at www.prenhall.com/kneisl.

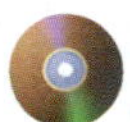

CD-ROM
Audio Glossary
NCLEX-RN® Review Questions

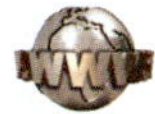

Companion Website
Audio Glossary
NCLEX-RN® Review Questions
Critical Thinking Exercise
- *First Clinical Day*

Case Study
- *Mentally Ill or Different?*

Care Plan
- *Managing Personal Anxiety*

MediaLinks
MediaLink Application
- *Overcoming the Stigma*

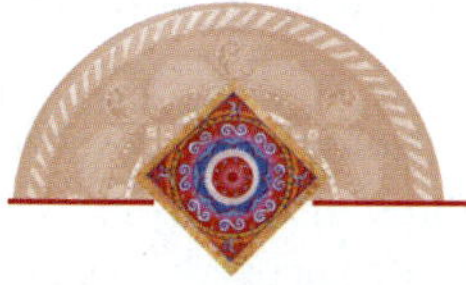

NCLEX-RN® REVIEW QUESTIONS

1. Which of the following is a defining characteristic of a mental disorder?
1. A psychological group of symptoms associated with disability
2. A psychological group of symptoms associated with distress
3. A response that is other than that expected and culturally accepted to an event
4. A psychological group of symptoms associated with suffering, pain, loss of freedom, or death

2. "Deviant behavior" itself does not define mental disorders, unless the deviance or conflict is symptomatic of the individual's dysfunction. "Deviant" behavior is defined by which of the following? (Select all that apply.)
1. Historical and social norms
2. Situational context
3. Peer relationships
4. Understanding of human behavior
5. Political norms

3. One of the obstacles in describing mental disorders is that the phrase "deviant behavior":
   1. Has a pejorative connotation.
   2. Derives its meaning from the culture.
   3. Is used colloquially.
   4. Is value-free.

4. In the early 19th century, individuals with mental disorders were believed to be:
   1. Controlled by evil spirits.
   2. Influenced by the moon.
   3. Incurable and dangerous.
   4. Divinely inspired.

5. Mental disorders were conceptualized as disordered neurology under the purview of medicine by:
   1. Freud.
   2. Pinel.
   3. Hippocrates.
   4. Rush.

6. The nurse is assessing the client for a possible mental disorder using contemporary beliefs about mental illness as a theoretical base for practice. Given this approach, the nurse would definitely ask about:
   1. Current medications and recent stressors.
   2. Early childhood experiences and dreams.
   3. Religious practices.
   4. Recent blood transfusions.

7. Which mental disorders rank among the top ten causes of disability worldwide? (Select all that apply.)
   1. PTSD
   2. Antisocial personality disorder
   3. Bipolar affective disorder
   4. Anxiety disorders
   5. Schizophrenia

8. Which mental disorder ranks first among the top ten causes of disability worldwide?
   1. Depression
   2. Insomnia
   3. Schizoaffective disorder
   4. Chemical dependency

9. According to the *Healthy People 2010* report, major mental health problems do not include clients with which of the following? (Select all that apply.)
   1. A primary diagnosis of chemical dependency
   2. PTSD
   3. Eating disorders
   4. Major mental illness with incarceration
   5. Co-occurring mental disorders and traumatic brain injury

10. The *Healthy People 2010* report suggests that the mental health problems listed are associated with which of the following? (Select all that apply.)
    1. Ignorance associated with the etiology of mental disorders
    2. Availability of secondary care
    3. Stigma associated with mental disorders
    4. Availability of primary care (illness prevention and identification of at-risk populations)
    5. Paucity of psychoactive medications with FDA-approved indications for childhood and adolescent disorders

See Appendix C for answers.

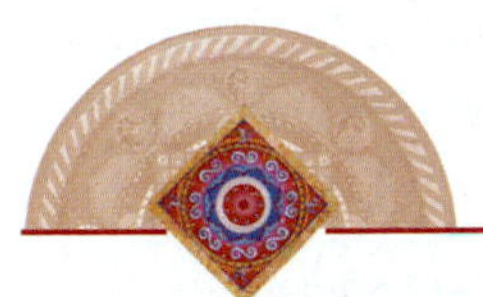

REFERENCES

American Psychiatric Association. (2000). *Diagnostic and statistical manual of mental disorders* (4th ed., Text Revision) (DSM-IV-TR). Washington, DC: Author.

Dalby, J. T. (1993). Terms of madness: Historical linguistics. *Comprehensive Psychiatry, 34*, 392–395.

Jackson, J. L., Passamonti, M., & Kroenke, K. (2007). Outcome and impact of mental disorders in primary care at 5 years. *Psychosomatic Medicine, 69*(2), 217–229.

Kroenke, K., Spitzer, R. L., Williams, J. B., Monahan, P. O., & Lowe, B. (2007). Anxiety disorders in primary care: Prevalence, impairment, comorbidity, and detection. *Annals of Internal Medicine, 146*(5), 317.

Moussavi, S., Chatterji, S., Verdes, E., Tandon, A., Patel, V., & Ustun, B. (2007). Depression, chronic diseases, and decrements in health: Results from the World Health Surveys. *Lancet, 370*(9590), 851–858.

Murray, C. J., & Lopez, A. D. (1996). Evidence-based health policy: Lessons from the global burden of disease study. *Science, 274*, 740–761.

Prince, M., Patel, V., Saxena, S., Maj, M., Maselko, J., Phillips, M. R., et al. (2007). No health without mental health. *Lancet, 370*(9590), 859–877.

Regler, D. A., Farmer, M. E., Rae, D. S., Locke, B. Z., Keith, S. J., Judd, L. L., et al. (1990). Comorbidity of mental disorders with alcohol and other drug abuse: Results from the Epidemiologic Catchment Area (ECA) Study. *Journal of the American Medical Association, 264*(19), 2511–2518.

Saxena, S., Sharan, P., Garrido, M., & Saraceno, B. (2006). WHO's Mental Health Atlas 2005: Implications for policy development. *World Psychiatry, 5*(3), 179–184.

U.S. Department of Health and Human Services. (1999). *Mental health: A report of the surgeon general.* Rockville, MD: National Institute of Mental Health.

U.S. Department of Health and Human Services. (2002). *Healthy people 2010.* Retrieved August 20, 2002, from http://www.healthypeople.gov.

ADDITIONAL REFERENCES

Horwitz, A. V. (2003). *Creating mental illness.* Chicago: University of Chicago Press.

McHugh, P. R., & Slavney, P. R. (1998). *The perspectives of psychiatry* (2nd ed.). Baltimore: Johns Hopkins University Press.

Porter, R. (2003). Madness: *A brief history.* London: Oxford University Press.

Shorter, E. (1998). *History of psychiatry: From the era of the asylum to the age of Prozac.* New York: John Wiley & Sons.

Torrey, E. F., & Miller, J. (2001). *Invisible plague.* Rutgers, NJ: Rutgers University Press.

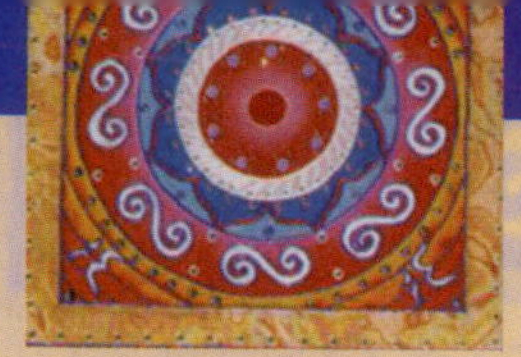

CHAPTER

2

Psychiatric–Mental Health Nurses: Who Are They?

CAROL REN KNEISL

KEY TERMS

advance practice registered nurse (APRN) *21*
certification *21*
psychiatric–mental health nursing *15*

LEARNING OUTCOMES

After completing this chapter, you will be able to:

1. Apply knowledge of current practice and professional performance standards to the delivery of contemporary psychiatric–mental health nursing.
2. Compare and contrast the differences and similarities among the roles of the psychiatric–mental health nurse and other members of the mental health team.
3. Analyze the factors that influence the success with which the mental health team achieves collaboration among its members and with clients and their significant others.
4. Describe how the role of the psychiatric–mental health nurse changed over the years from that of custodian to a multifaceted role.
5. Discuss the nursing theory concepts and principles that have shaped psychiatric–mental health nursing most directly.
6. Explain why you should be capable of functioning in all theories of care.

CRITICAL THINKING CHALLENGE

You find your psychiatric–mental health nursing clinical experience professionally challenging, intellectually stimulating, and personally rewarding. You are considering becoming a psychiatric nurse upon graduation and have discussed your feelings with a classmate, a neighbor, and your primary care physician.

Your classmate says you won't be a real nurse and that you'll forget all the skills you learned in school. Your neighbor, a critical care nurse, thinks you'll be bored as a psychiatric–mental health nurse. The critical care unit, with its high drama, split-second decisions, and high-tech atmosphere, she says, is the setting where a good student like you would be happiest and make the greatest contribution. Your physician suggests that you be cautious. With the explosion in psychobiologic research and the discovery of more effective psychopharmacologic agents, she thinks that in a few years there may be no need for psychiatric–mental health nurses and you'll be out of a job.

1. What do you think about what they have said? Are they right?
2. What elements of psychiatric–mental health nursing provide excitement, challenge, art, and science?
3. In what ways are psychiatric–mental health nurses valuable to their clients?

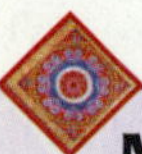

MEDIALINK 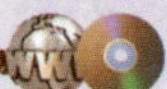 www.prenhall.com/kneisl

Go to the Pearson Health MediaLink CD-ROM and the Companion Website at www.prenhall.com/kneisl for interactive resources for this chapter.

What does it mean to be a psychiatric–mental health nurse? According to a coalition of professional groups (American Nurses Association [ANA], American Psychiatric Nurses Association [APNA], & International Society of Psychiatric–Mental Health Nurses [ISPN], 2007), **psychiatric–mental health nursing** is committed to promoting mental health through the assessment, diagnosis, and treatment of human responses to mental health problems and psychiatric disorders. It is a specialized area of nursing practice and a core mental health discipline that employs explanatory theories of, and research on, human behavior as its science and the purposeful use of self as its art. Essential components of the specialty practice of psychiatric–mental health nursing include:

- Health and wellness promotion though identification of mental health issues
- Prevention of mental health problems
- Care of mental health problems
- Treatment of persons with psychiatric disorders (ANA, APNA, & IPSN, 2007, p. 14)

On a more personal level, this specialty is the only one in which your voice, face, body language, and what cannot be seen—the mind, neurotransmitters, self-esteem, and the like—shape your work. The authors and contributors to this textbook share their personal reasons for choosing psychiatric–mental health nursing in the Why I Became a Psychiatric–Mental Health Nurse features sprinkled throughout this book. We hope that you will join us in rehumanizing mental health care in a technologic society. It requires of you a judicious blending of "high-touch" with "high-tech"—a person-to-person human experience.

EMERGENCE OF THE DISCIPLINE

The role of the psychiatric–mental health nurse has changed over the years from that of custodian to a multifaceted role, and the settings in which psychiatric–mental health nurses practice have expanded from inside the hospital to all of the communities in which people live. This section discusses the history of psychiatric–mental health nursing, which is summarized in the timeline in FIGURE 2-1 ■ on pages 16 and 17.

Although nursing functions have existed since ancient times, the profession of nursing, particularly psychiatric–mental health nursing, is a product of the late 19th and 20th centuries. Theodor and Friedericke Fliedner founded the first systematic school of nursing in Germany in 1836. It was this school at Kaiserwerth that Florence Nightingale visited in 1851 before organizing a school to educate nurses in England after the Crimean War. Her school, Saint Thomas Hospital in London, stressed the importance of providing an optimum environment for clients. Although it is true that in the context of her time she emphasized the physical environment, Nightingale was among the first to note that the influence of nurses on their clients goes beyond physical care and has psychologic and social components.

Early Psychiatric Nursing Education

In the early 1870s, the first three American nursing schools, organized in the pattern of Saint Thomas Hospital, were opened in New York, Boston, and New Haven. Linda Richards—sometimes called "the first American psychiatric nurse"—spent a significant part of her career developing better nursing care in psychiatric hospitals. She opened the first American school for psychiatric nurses at the McLean Psychiatric Asylum in Waverly, Massachusetts, in 1880. By 1890, there were 35 such schools in asylums. Unlike graduates of general hospital schools of nursing, these nurses could find employment only in asylums.

By the end of the 19th century, psychiatric nurses attended mainly to the physical needs of clients and did not pursue systematic interpersonal work with them. Psychiatric theory in this period emphasized providing a physical environment that would promote recovery. Thus, nurses administered medications such as chloral hydrate and paraldehyde, supervised the use of hydrotherapy, and oversaw the nutrition and physical care of clients. Much of psychiatric nursing practice was custodial, mechanistic, and directed by psychiatrists. A ratio of 1 trained nurse to 140 clients was not unusual, and some large mental hospitals hired no registered nurses at all.

The notion that nurses caring for clients with physical disorders should be trained in general hospitals and those caring for clients with mental disorders should be trained in psychiatric hospitals dominated nursing education for over half a century. In 1913, the school of nursing at Johns Hopkins Hospital in Baltimore included a psychiatric nursing component in its curriculum, heralding the beginning of a slow, but important, change in the structure of nursing programs. The first psychiatric nursing text, *Nursing Mental Diseases,* was written in 1920 by Harriet Bailey, the Assistant Superintendent of Nurses at the psychiatric service at Johns Hopkins Hospital. It was, for 20 years, the standard textbook in psychiatric nursing. Prior to this time, psychiatric textbooks were written by psychiatrists who devoted only a few pages to the instruction of nurses in procedures such as tube feeding and preparing treatment trays.

In the years between the two world wars, mental hospitals were seriously understaffed. In an effort to cope with understaffing, mental hospitals opened schools of nursing at an incredible rate—67 in 1936 alone.

Moving into the Mainstream

In 1937, the National League for Nursing Education (now the National League for Nursing [NLN]) recommended, but did not require, that psychiatric nursing content and clinical experience be a part of the curriculum in all basic nursing programs. The NLN also took over from psychiatrists the tasks of standardizing and accrediting psychiatric nursing education in single-focus schools for psychiatric nurses. The American Psychiatric Association, rather than a nursing organization, had been involved since 1906 in monitoring this aspect of nursing.

Psychiatric nursing moved into the mainstream of nursing in the 1940s, and nurses began to assume increasing responsibility for educating their own. However, the focus of

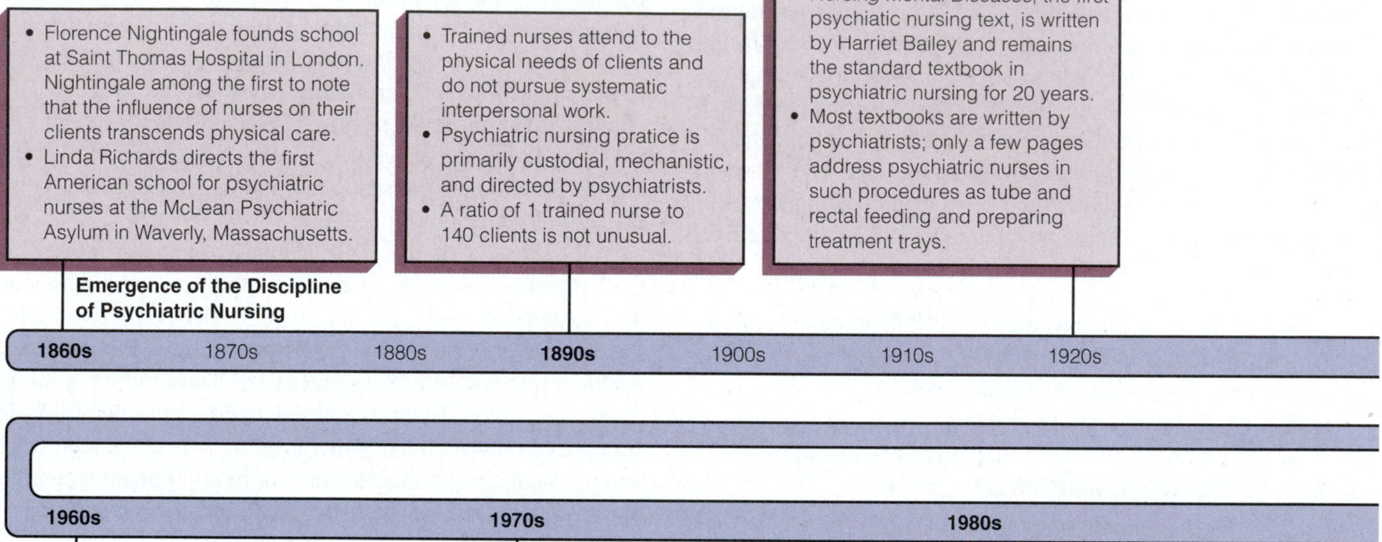

1960s

Confirmation of Specialist Roles

- The Community Mental Health Centers Act pushes trend in psychiatric nursing toward expanded and specialized roles.
- First textbook to address group therapy techniques in nursing practice written by Shirley Armstrong and Sheila Rouslin.
- Shirley Burd and Margaret Marshall write and edit the first compilation of psychiatric nursing papers suitable for graduate students in psychiatric nursing.
- First psychiatric nursing journals—*Perspectives in Psychiatric Care* and *Journal of Psychiatric Nursing and Mental Health Services* published.

1970s

- The first certification programs for advanced psychiatric nursing practice are developed by the New Jersey and New York State Nurses Associations.
- The psychiatric nurses who developed and implemented the early certification programs (Marian Pettingill, Sheila Rouslin Welt, and Carol Ren Kneisl) recognized the need to acknowledge expertise, distinguish generalist from specialist roles, and safeguard the public.
- Certification in psychiatric nursing becomes the responsibility of the ANA.
- *Standards of Psychiatric-Mental Health Nursing* published by ANA.
- *Issues in Mental Health Nursing* published.

1980s

Period of Decline and Retrenchment

- ANA Council of Specialists in Psychiatric and Mental Health Nursing develops a classification system for Psychiatric Nursing Diagnosis.
- *Standards of Child and Adolescent Psychiatric and Mental Health Nursing* and *Standards of Addictions Nursing Practice* published by ANA.
- American Psychiatric Nurses Association formed.
- *Archives of Psychiatric Nursing* and *Journal of Child and Adolescent Psychiatric and Mental Health Nursing* published.
- Psychiatric nursing leaders recommend incorporating new psychobiologic knowledge into clinical practice.

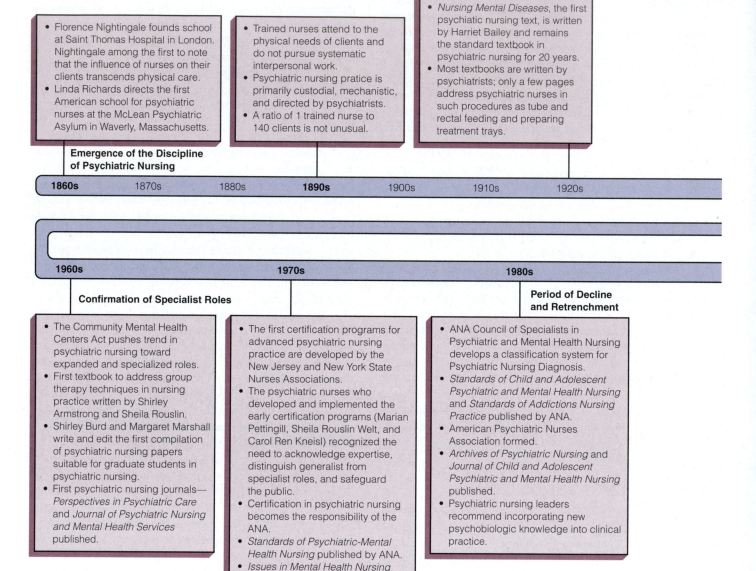

FIGURE 2-1 The history of psychiatric nursing.

psychiatric nursing activities continued to be providing kind, but custodial, nursing care. Nurses supervised or were responsible for providing housekeeping tasks such as scrubbing floors and counting mops and sheets; feeding, clothing, and bathing clients; assisting physicians with treatments; and keeping the keys to locked wards, locked cabinets, even locked toilet tissue containers.

The specialty grew slowly during the 1940s. In the meantime, psychiatric theory expanded to encompass the interpersonal and emotional dimensions of mental illness. During these years, Sigmund Freud published his works on psychoanalysis, Adolph Meyer's *commonsense psychiatry* had great impact in the United States and Great Britain, and Harry Stack Sullivan introduced the concept of *milieu therapy* as a new approach to treating hospitalized psychiatric patients. These ideologic changes in psychiatry, discussed further in Chapter 5, did not have a noticeable influence on psychiatric nursing care until the early 1950s.

1930s — **Movement of Psychiatric Nursing into the Mainstream of Nursing**

- National League for Nursing Education recommends that psychiatric nursing content and clinical experience be part of the curriculum in all basic nursing programs.
- Psychiatric nursing activities continue to be custodial nursing care, including housekeeping tasks and keeping the keys to locked wards, cabinets, and even toilet tissue containers.

1940s

- New medical surgical procedures (deep sleep therapy, insulin shock therapy, psychosurgery, and electroshock therapy) promote the role of psychiatric nurses as participants in psychiatric treatment.
- Nursing leaders recommend elimination of single-focus schools marking the beginning of the mainstreaming of psychiatric nursing.
- National Institute of Mental Health (NIMH) established; National Mental Health Act helps develop psychotherapeutic roles for nurses.

1950s — **Confirmation of Psychiatric Nursing as a Specialty**

- Hildegard Peplau emphasizes psychodynamic concepts and counseling techniques; Gwen Tudor Will demonstrates nursing interventions with a sociopsychiatric base.
- Frances Sleeper advocates psychiatric nurses as psychotherapists.
- First doctoral program in nursing is based on June Mellow's system of psychiatric nursing therapy.
- National League for Nursing introduces the concept of psychiatric nurse specialist; first NIMH grants to integrate mental health concepts into nursing curriculum.

1990s — **Decade of the Brain**

- Several psychiatric nurses appointed to President Clinton's task force on health care reform.
- *Standards of Psychiatric Consultation Liaison Nursing* published by ANA.
- Revised *Standards of Psychiatric–Mental Health Clinical Nursing Practice* published by ANA.
- *Psychopharmacology Guidelines for Psychiatric–Mental Health Nurses*, intended to increase knowledge of psychopharmacology and improve patient care, published by ANA.
- *Journal of the American Psychiatric Nurses Association* published.
- Psychiatric nursing leaders urge nurses to use the challenging circumstances posed by burgeoning information, reduced funding, and health care reform to clarify nursing's unique contribution to mental health care.

2000s — **Beginning of a New Millennium**

- American Nurses Association, in collaboration with the American Psychiatric Nurses Association and the International Society of Psychiatric–Mental Health Nurses, publishes (2000) and revises (2007) the *Scope and Standards of Psychiatric–Mental Health Nursing Practice*.
- An increase in the numbers and types of alternative and nontraditional treatment settings provide new opportunities for psychiatric–mental health nurses to provide mental health care in primary care environments as well as in psychiatric settings.
- As knowledge continues to explode in psychobiology, genetics, and human behavior, psychiatric nursing leaders focus on the need to integrate the biological, psychological, social, spiritual, and environmental realms of the human experience into mental health services while remaining centered in the nursing domain with its focus on caring.
- Primary care becomes a significant point of entry for psychiatric care.
- Nurse practitioner and clinical nurse specialist titles for APRNs.

Although the somatic treatments in use at the time controlled dramatically bizarre client behavior and made clients more available for interpersonal interactions, it was not until 1946, with passage of the National Mental Health Act (the government's response to growing recognition of mental illness as a national health problem), that any systematic development of psychotherapeutic roles for nurses began. Most psychiatric clients were being cared for in large state mental hospitals where small numbers of staff were expected to manage large numbers of clients living in crowded conditions. Somatic treatments, rather than psychotherapy, were more practical in these settings. Psychotherapy was often reserved for the private clients of psychiatrists in private psychiatric hospitals or in private practice settings.

Psychiatric Nursing as a Specialty

During World War II, 43% of all people discharged from the army were classified as having a psychiatric disability, creating a sharp increase in the demand for psychiatric services. The National Mental Health Act, enacted in 1946 to cope with the surge in the need for psychiatric services, provided for the following:

- Establishment of the National Institute for Mental Health (NIMH) to be added to the National Institutes of Health in Bethesda, Maryland
- Development of programs to train professional psychiatric personnel, including psychiatric nurses
- Support for psychiatric research
- Assistance in developing mental health programs

With the establishment of the NIMH, psychiatric nursing was added to psychiatry, psychology, and social work as a field in which the highest priority became the preparation of clinically capable persons for positions of leadership. Before this time, fewer than a dozen psychiatric nurses held master's degrees in the United States. The psychiatric nursing education given most students consisted of a few weeks of observation on a psychiatric ward.

Because of new funding, nine universities received grants to expand and improve graduate programs in 1948. The number increased gradually and steadily. These programs prepared many of the nursing leaders who later developed theoretical frameworks for one–to–one relationship work. Because of its wide-ranging effects, the National Mental Health Act of 1946 is probably the most significant piece of legislation affecting the development of psychiatric–mental health nursing.

Nursing leaders began to question the wisdom of single-focus schools of psychiatric nursing. In 1948, a report entitled *Nursing for the Future* (Brown, 1948) recommended their elimination. The needs of nursing could best be served, the report indicated, if the psychiatric hospitals conducting schools of nursing made their facilities widely available instead to students in basic schools of nursing. Shortly thereafter, in 1955, the NLN made the provision of a clinical experience in psychiatric nursing a requirement for the accreditation of nursing schools. Requiring both coursework and hands-on clinical experience further cemented the mainstreaming of psychiatric nursing.

Until the early 1950s, psychiatric nurses formulated only vague concepts about how nurses might participate in one–to–one relationships with clients. Some pressed for trained postgraduate nurses to provide psychotherapy and become functioning members of an interdisciplinary treatment team that would include psychologists and social workers. Ambiguity about professional psychiatric nursing roles characterized this period.

Role Clarification

The 1950s and early 1960s were a period of role clarification. Three important milestones in psychiatric nursing occurred in 1952.

First, Hildegard Peplau published *Interpersonal Relations in Nursing,* the first systematic theoretic framework in psychiatric nursing, a milestone in the development of psychiatric nursing theory and practice (1952). She delineated several skills, activities, and roles for psychiatric nurses and emphasized the interpersonal nature of nursing and the need for nurses to understand and use psychodynamic concepts and counseling techniques in their practice. Under Peplau's leadership, the first graduate degree in psychiatric–mental health nursing was awarded in 1954 by Rutgers University. Peplau has had greater impact on psychiatric nursing than any other nursing theoretician to date. Peplau's theoretical contributions are discussed in greater detail later in this chapter.

Second, Gwen Tudor (Will) published an article in the journal *Psychiatry* (a major feat in itself since the journal for psychiatrists had never published an article by a nurse and no psychiatric nursing journals existed at the time) demonstrating that nurses can promote emotional growth in clients. She used sociopsychiatric theory to explain a mutual pattern of avoidance that emerged among the nursing staff, physicians, and one particular female client (Tudor, 1952). Tudor designed a nursing intervention to disrupt the pattern of avoidance by closing the gap between herself and the client and then engaging her in activities. To test the reliability of her intervention, Tudor taught it to a nursing student and supervised her in reversing a pattern of mutual withdrawal with another client. Tudor's unique contribution demonstrated that:

- Psychiatric nurses can have a profoundly positive or a profoundly negative effect on the client.
- The social milieu of the psychiatric ward can maintain deviant patterns of behavior.

WHY I BECAME A PSYCHIATRIC–MENTAL HEALTH NURSE

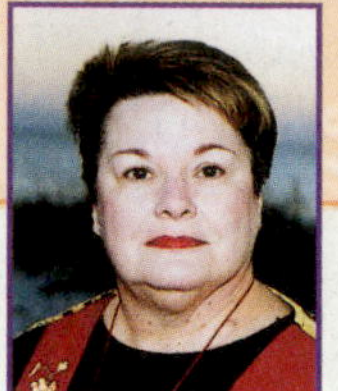

Carol Ren Kneisl
Textbook Author

I love challenges. As a beginning nursing student, I thought the excitement and high-tech atmosphere of a large general hospital was the best and most challenging of all worlds. It was in this setting that I discovered that although I could perform the technical skills without a problem, physical care was not enough for many of the clients I saw.

In this medical-surgical setting, I learned that an effective personal coping style, emotional stability, family support, and resilience and hardiness on the client's part; and the comfort, concern, and commitment provided by caring nurses helped people get well or overcome their circumstances. This is most likely when I realized that through artful therapeutic practice, I could create a common ground with my clients and provide a nurturing, healing milieu. What could be more challenging?

The practice of psychiatric–mental health nursing has brought me the excitement and the challenge I crave. I know, as an optimistic person, that all people, no matter their circumstances, have the capacity for personal responsibility, growth, and change. It is personally satisfying to know that as a psychiatric–mental health nurse, I know how to help them in their search for happier and mentally healthier lives.

- The psychotherapeutic nursing role can be taught to others.
- Nurses can carry out scholarly research.

Hers is the classic scholarly psychiatric nursing research study, significant for its dramatic impact on nursing and its contribution to an understanding of the effects of the milieu.

Third, Frances Sleeper, in an address to the American Psychiatric Association, advocated the use of psychiatric nurses as psychotherapists. Her advocacy ushered in a heated, 10-year controversy over caretaker versus psychotherapist roles for psychiatric nurses.

Clinical Nurse Specialist Role

The Community Mental Health Centers Act in 1963, which encouraged the closing of large mental hospitals in favor of treatment in the community, further encouraged the trend in psychiatric nursing toward expanded and specialized roles. Clinical nurse specialists (CNSs), prepared at the graduate level in psychiatric–mental health nursing, began providing individual, group, and family psychotherapy in a wide variety of settings and obtaining third-party reimbursement in some states. Psychiatric nurses broadened their practice to include schools, outreach clinics, transitional services, jails, alternative treatment settings, and private practice as well as the traditional mental hospital.

The launching in 1963 of *Perspectives in Psychiatric Care*—the first psychiatric nursing journal that was edited and published by Alice Clarke, a psychiatric nurse—provided a forum for airing issues and sharing psychiatric nursing knowledge. A second journal, the *Journal of Psychiatric Nursing and Mental Health Services,* began later that same year and changed its name in 1981 to the *Journal of Psychosocial Nursing and Mental Health Services.* Clinical and research papers by psychiatric nursing leaders in these journals and in the *American Journal of Nursing* further established the counseling role as the basis of psychiatric nursing, whether it was defined as psychotherapy or not.

Shortly thereafter, the first textbook to address group therapy techniques in nursing practice was written by Shirley Armstrong and Sheila Rouslin (1963). Shirley Byrd and Margaret Marshall (1963) wrote and edited the first compilation of psychiatric nursing papers suitable for graduate students in psychiatric nursing.

A 1967 ANA position paper on psychiatric nursing endorsed the assumption by clinical specialists of the role of therapist in individual, group, family, and milieu work (ANA, 1967). By 1969, a psychiatric nurse had, as Peplau predicted a few years before, moved into private practice.

The first master's level certification program for advanced psychiatric nursing practice was developed by the New Jersey Nurses' Association in 1971, followed in two years by the New York State Nurses Association. The psychiatric nurses who developed and implemented these early certification programs—Sheila Rouslin Welt, Carol Ren Kneisl, Marian Pettingill, Marian Krizinofski, and others—recognized the need to acknowledge expertise, distinguish generalist from specialist roles, and safeguard the public. By the mid-1970s, certification at both the generalist and the specialist levels in psychiatric nursing became the responsibility of the ANA.

In 1973, the ANA published the first standards of psychiatric–mental health nursing practice, which were statements to serve as guidelines for providing the desired quality of care. These standards of practice, revised several times since then, delineate psychiatric–mental health nursing roles and functions and are the focus of the next section of this chapter. The clinical specialist role was further legitimized in 1973 when the ANA formed a specialty subgroup, the Council of Specialists in Psychiatric and Mental Health Nursing.

President Jimmy Carter's 1977 Commission on Mental Health, unlike earlier commissions on mental health and mental illness that were dominated by physicians, included a nurse (Martha Mitchell, the chairperson of the ANA Division on Psychiatric and Mental Health Nursing Practice), and three other professional nurses who served on adjunct committees. The Commission's report had special significance for psychiatric nurses. It was hailed as the first official high-level document to give visibility to the professional competence of nurses in mental health care (Hadley, 1978).

According to Osborne (1984), the publication in 1979 of *Psychiatric Nursing* by Holly Skodol Wilson and Carol Ren Kneisl signaled a significant change in psychiatric nursing textbooks and psychiatric nursing thinking. This was the first in a new era of psychiatric nursing textbooks to provide and consistently use a major conceptual theme based on humanistic interactionism advocating negotiated goals between nurse and client, client advocacy, and political sensitivity, as well as caring and compassion. Since that time, other psychiatric nursing textbooks have followed in the tradition of Wilson and Kneisl. Another psychiatric nursing journal, *Issues in Mental Health Nursing,* also began in 1979.

Fiscal Decline and Retrenchment

After two decades of apparently unlimited support from the NIMH in the form of money for educational programs and traineeships for psychiatric nurses at the graduate level, funding for psychiatric nursing education was cut. A major concern for psychiatric nurses in the 1980s was the decrease in the number of nurses selecting psychiatric nursing as a specialty and a shortage of clinical training funding. Psychiatric nursing found itself on the verge of a period of retrenchment that remains to this day.

In 1984, recognizing the need for a set of psychiatric nursing diagnoses to supplement those identified by the North American Nursing Diagnoses Association (NANDA), the ANA Council of Specialists in Psychiatric and Mental Health Nursing appointed a panel of six nursing leaders—Marie Scott Brown, Anita Werner O'Toole, Maxine Loomis, Holly Skodol Wilson, Patricia Pothier, and Patricia West—to develop a classification system for psychiatric nursing. The panel identified relevant and useful categories for psychiatric nursing diagnosis and synthesized its findings with those of NANDA. Psychiatric nursing diagnoses are now an integral part of the NANDA classification system.

In early 1987, another new psychiatric nursing journal, *Archives of Psychiatric Nursing,* made its debut. The purpose of the journal was to provide a forum in which psychiatric nursing clinician-scholars can suggest theoretic linkages between diverse areas of practice and shape public policy for the delivery of psychiatric and mental health nursing services.

Decade of the Brain

The 1990s were designated the "Decade of the Brain" by Congress and the NIMH. During this period, psychiatry underwent a paradigm shift to include the neurobiologic domains. Research studies that focused on psychobiology provided new biologic strategies for assessments and interventions.

Nursing was also challenged to shift and integrate psychobiologic concepts with traditional practice to provide holistic care for both clients and their families in the 1994 revised ANA standards for psychiatric–mental health nursing practice. Psychiatric nursing leaders urged the inclusion of biologic therapies along with the use of more traditional psychotherapy, psychosocial therapies, and combination therapies. McBride cautioned psychiatric–mental health nurses to stop devaluing biologic knowledge and to become fundamentally reassociated with care and caring (1990). Peplau (1989) made additional recommendations: to promote political savvy in advocating psychiatric–mental health care resources; to continue developing out-of-hospital services, including those offered on a private practice basis; to pursue evaluation and outcome clinical studies; to inform the public and others of the work we do; and to keep emphasizing the human aspects of mental health work even as psychiatry moves in the direction of psychobiologic practice. These and other nursing leaders believed that the specialty needed to create a new image for psychiatric–mental health nurses, foster cultural diversity among psychiatric–mental health nurses, and integrate philosophic and theoretic perspectives in both practice and research.

Health care reform was a political concern during the 1990s, and nursing organizations figured prominently in advocating for reform. A coalition of psychiatric nursing organizations proposed a plan to provide essential mental health services through health care reform (Krauss, 1993). The goals of the plan were to demonstrate the willingness and ability of psychiatric–mental health nurses to staff mental health care delivery systems in indirect as well as direct roles; to conduct mental health promotion and mental illness prevention programs; to provide case management for clients with serious mental disorders; and to bring the neurobiological, behavioral, and psychosocial aspects of care together with a holistic perspective that addresses the challenges of daily living in the community. The report advocated for equitable access to basic mental health care equal to general health care, a goal that has not yet been met.

During this period, there was tremendous growth in the development of new psychopharmacologic treatments for mental disorder. The ANA named a task force, the Psychiatric–Mental Health Nursing Psychopharmacology Project, to study the issues and strategies associated with the administration of psychopharmacologic agents. The task force published a set of psychopharmacology guidelines for psychiatric–mental health nurses in 1994 (ANA, 1994). The guidelines recommended integrating current data from the neurosciences, demonstrating knowledge of psychopharmacologic principles, and providing safe and effective clinical management of clients taking these medications.

A specialty organization for psychiatric–mental health nurses, the American Psychiatric Nurses Association (APNA), was established in the 1990s and began publication of a new psychiatric nursing journal, the *Journal of the American Psychiatric Nurses Association.*

The New Millennium

In 2000, the beginning of the new millennium, the ANA collaborated with the APNA and the International Society of Psychiatric–Mental Health Nurses to revise the standards for the practice of psychiatric–mental health nursing. In 2007, these guidelines were revised into the most forward-looking set of standards developed to date (American Nurses Association, American Psychiatric Nurses Association, & International Society of Psychiatric–Mental Health Nurses, 2007).

The knowledge explosion in psychobiology continues, characterized by a broader understanding of the biology of the mind and the biologic foundations of behavior and temperament. Significant knowledge about the genetic basis of inherited mental disorders has resulted from the genetic research undertaken at the NIMH. A growing arsenal of psychopharmacologic agents with fewer side effects helps clients enjoy a higher quality of life. The greatest challenge that psychiatric–mental health nursing faces is integrating psychobiologic knowledge into clinical practice while maintaining a focus on the caring dimension.

Other trends, early in this new millenium, have sparked several significant changes in the delivery of mental health services and provide new challenges for the practice of psychiatric–mental health nursing. For one, a cadre of psychiatric–mental health nurses has been concerned with the physical health problems of psychiatric clients, a sometimes overlooked dimension of care. In particular, Chafetz and her associates (Chafetz, White, Collins-Bride, & Nickens, 2005) have been concerned about the physical health of severely and persistently mentally ill clients who live in community settings and have developed wellness clinics especially for them.

Another important trend is the shift to primary care as a point of entry for psychiatric care (Jackson, Passamonti, & Kroenke, 2007; Kroenke, Spitzer, Williams, Monahan, & Lowe, 2007). This trend was discussed earlier in Chapter 1 ∞.

In response to these challenges, graduate programs in psychiatric–mental health nursing have undergone a curriculum shift. The shift encompasses an increased emphasis on comprehensive health assessment, management of common physical health problems, and a focus on meeting the requirements for prescriptive authority for advanced practice nurses. Accordingly, we are seeing a shift at the advanced

MEDIALINK Case Study: The Multifaceted Role

level of practice toward the use of psychiatric–mental health nurse practitioner as a title. The role competencies for psychiatric–mental health nurse practitioners have been clearly delineated (National Panel for Psychiatric–Mental Health NP Competencies, 2003). Advanced-practice psychiatric–mental health nurses now practice under the clinical nurse specialist or nurse practitioner titles, but share the same core competencies.

The settings for psychiatric–mental health nursing practice continue to expand from hospitals and traditional psychiatric settings to alternative and nontraditional settings. At the same time, in most schools, nursing students receive only brief and limited exposure to mental health clients and mental health settings. It is difficult to appreciate a specialty when you do not experience its many facets. This textbook will, we hope, enhance those limited clinical experiences. We hope not only to challenge you but also to awaken in you a sense of excitement about the possibilities for professional fulfillment that psychiatric–mental health nursing holds.

PROFESSIONAL ROLE

Two sets of standards guide professional psychiatric–mental health nursing practice. The Standards of Practice are reproduced in Box 2-1. The Standards of Professional Performance are reproduced in Box 2-2 on page 22. The chapters in this textbook are firmly guided by the Standards of Practice and the Standards of Professional Performance and demonstrate client-centered care in this specialty area. The chapters go beyond what you have learned in your nursing program to date; they identify how you would assess, diagnose, identify outcomes, plan, implement, and evaluate the care of clients with mental health disorders in nonpsychiatric as well psychiatric settings. Standard 5 specifically discusses the unique role functions of the psychiatric–mental health nurse.

Basic Level of Practice

The *basic level psychiatric–mental health nurse* (PMH) may have received basic nursing preparation in a diploma, associate degree, or baccalaureate program. Essentially a generalist who works in a specialized setting, this nurse provides the bulk of the nursing care to clients. Registered nurses offer direct and indirect care through the nurse–client relationship. They have major responsibility for the milieu and have contact with clients at all stages of daily life. Nurses at this level may seek **certification** as generalists through the ANA's American Nurses Credentialing Center (ANCC). Certification by a professional nursing organization recognizes competence and also protects the consumer of mental health services. Credentialing information can be found on ANCC's website (www.ana.org/ancc) and accessed through the Companion Website for this book.

Advanced Level of Practice

According to the ANA, APNA, and ISPN (2007), the **advanced practice registered nurse** in psychiatric–mental health (APRN-PMH) is a licensed registered nurse who is

Box 2-1 Psychiatric–Mental Health Nursing Standards of Practice

The six standards of practice describe a competent level of nursing care organized around the nursing process. Note that Standards 5E, 5F, and 5G apply to advanced practice psychiatric mental health nurses only.

Standard 1. Assessment The Psychiatric–Mental Health Registered Nurse collects comprehensive health data that is pertinent to the patient's health or situation.

Standard 2. Diagnosis The Psychiatric–Mental Health Registered Nurse analyzes the assessment data to determine diagnoses or problems, including level of risk.

Standard 3. Outcomes Identification The Psychiatric–Mental Health Registered Nurse identifies expected outcomes for a plan individualized to the patient or to the situation.

Standard 4. Planning The Psychiatric–Mental Health Registered Nurse develops a plan that prescribes strategies and alternatives to attain expected outcomes.

Standard 5. Implementation The Psychiatric–Mental Health Registered Nurse implements the identified plan.

Standard 5 A. Coordination of Care The Psychiatric–Mental Health Registered Nurse coordinates care delivery.

Standard 5 B. Health Teaching and Health Promotion The Psychiatric–Mental Health Registered Nurse employs strategies to promote health and a safe environment.

Standard 5 C. Milieu Therapy The Psychiatric–Mental Health Registered Nurse provides, structures, and maintains a safe and therapeutic environment in collaboration with patients, families, and other health care clinicians.

Standard 5 D. Pharmacological, Biological, and Integrative Therapies The Psychiatric–Mental Health Registered Nurse incorporates knowledge of pharmacological, biological, and complementary interventions with applied clinical skills to restore the patient's health and prevent further disability.

Standard 5 E. Prescriptive Authority and Treatment (APRN only) The Psychiatric–Mental Health Advanced Practice Registered Nurse uses prescriptive authority, procedures, referrals, treatments, and therapies in accordance with state and federal laws and regulations.

Standard 5 F. Psychotherapy (APRN only) The Psychiatric–Mental Health Advanced Practice Registered Nurse conducts individual, couples, group, and family psychotherapy using evidence-based psychotherapeautic frameworks and nurse-patient therapeutic relationships.

Standard 5 G. Consultation (APRN only) The Psychiatric–Mental Health Advanced Practice Registered Nurse provides consultation to influence the identified plan, enhance the abilities of other clinicians to provide services for patients, and effect change.

Standard 6. Evaluation The Psychiatric–Mental Health Registered Nurse evaluates progress toward attainment of expected outcomes.

Source: Reprinted with permission from American Nurses Association, American Psychiatric–Mental Health Nurses Association, & International Society of Psychiatric–Mental Health Nurses. *Psychiatric–mental health nursing: Scope and standards of practice,* © 2007. Silver Spring, MD: Nursesbooks.org.

MediaLink American Nurses Credentialing Center

Box 2-2 Psychiatric–Mental Health Nursing Standards of Professional Performance

The nine standards of professional performance describe a competent level of behavior in professional role activities.

Standard 7. Quality of Practice The Psychiatric–Mental Health Registered Nurse systematically enhances the quality and effectiveness of nursing practice.

Standard 8. Education The Psychiatric–Mental Health Registered Nurse attains knowledge and competency that reflect current nursing practice.

Standard 9. Professional Practice Evaluation The Psychiatric–Mental Health Registered Nurse evaluates one's own practice in relation to the professional practice standards and guidelines, relevant statutes, rules, and regulations.

Standard 10. Collegiality The Psychiatric–Mental Health Registered Nurse interacts with and contributes to the professional development of peers and colleagues.

Standard 11. Collaboration The Psychiatric–Mental Health Registered Nurse collaborates with patients, family, and others in the conduct of nursing practice.

Standard 12. Ethics The Psychiatric–Mental Health Registered Nurse integrates ethical provisions in all areas of practice.

Standard 13. Research The Psychiatric–Mental Health Registered Nurse integrates research findings into practice.

Standard 14. Resource Utilization The Psychiatric–Mental Health Registered Nurse considers factors related to safety, effectiveness, cost, and impact on practice in the planning and delivery of nursing services.

Standard 15. Leadership The Psychiatric–Mental Health Registered Nurse provides leadership in the professional practice setting and the profession.

Source: Reprinted with permission from American Nurses Association, American Psychiatric–Mental Health Nurses Association, and International Society of Psychiatric–Mental Health Nurses. *Psychiatric–mental health nursing: Scope and standards of practice*, © 2007. Silver Spring, MD: Nursesbooks.org.

educationally prepared as a clinical nurse specialist or a nurse practitioner at the master's or doctorate degree level in the specialty of psychiatric–mental health nursing. Advanced practice psychiatric–mental health nurses may also seek certification at the advanced level through ANCC. They may use the initials CS (certified specialist). The advanced-level certification is a means of protecting consumers. In addition to the basic-level role functions, several advanced-level role functions are listed in Box 2-1.

THE MENTAL HEALTH TEAM

The psychiatric–mental health nurse is an integral and important part of the mental health team. Of all the disciplines involved in mental health care, nursing is the one most likely to have an overall view of the client's situation.

Mental health services are provided by a variety of professionals—psychiatric–mental health nurses, psychiatrists, clinical psychologists, psychiatric social workers, marriage and family therapists, occupational therapists, recreational therapists, creative arts therapists—who have received many forms of specialized training. These professions require formal academic instruction, often at the graduate level, and extensive clinical experience. Psychosocial rehabilitation workers also provide mental health services and may have formal or on-the-job training. Table 2-1 ■ identifies the estimated number of mental health professionals in the United States. In general, the number of professionals who supply mental health services has expanded dramatically since the 1990s, while the number of psychiatric–mental health nurses has declined (U.S. Department of Labor, 2002). Most of the growth has occurred among nonphysicians (Scheffler, Ivey, & Garrett, 1998).

Role definitions that were traditionally assigned to specific disciplines have become increasingly blurred. Psychiatric–mental health nurses, social workers, and psychologists, among others, have more direct influence than ever before. Roles are less specifically defined, and in many community settings, mental health professionals take on whichever functions they do best.

The descriptions in Table 2-2 ■ of the education and functions of mental health team members reflect more traditional distinctions. Keep in mind that many of the functions are now shared across disciplines when the team member has been appropriately educated for the task and when laws and regulations permit the sharing of functions.

Partnership and Collaboration on the Mental Health Team

Psychiatric–mental health nurses, wherever they practice, must plan and share with others to deliver maximum mental health services to clients and their families. The purpose of partnering and collaborating with others is to make the best use of the different abilities of mental health team members so that the client and the family receive the most effective service available.

Cooperation versus Competition

Relationship problems among mental health team members must be resolved to avoid distorting the team's efforts. The key to working together on a problem with a common pur-

Table 2-1 ■ Estimated Number of Mental Health Workers in the United States

Profession	Number
Psychiatric–mental health nurses	11,300
Psychiatrists	21,280
Clinical psychologists	56,200
Psychiatric social workers	79,740
Marriage and family therapists	19,420
Psychosocial rehabilitation workers	84,100

TABLE 2-2 ■ **The Mental Health Team**

Team Member	Education/Preparation	Role
Psychiatric–mental health nurse	A registered nurse with specialized preparation in psychiatric–mental health nursing; level of expertise depends on education, which may include up to the doctoral level	Responsible for the nursing care of mental health clients; has major responsibility for the milieu
Psychiatrist	A medical physician whose specialty is mental disorders; has completed an approved psychiatric residency	Responsible for diagnosis and treatment of persons with mental disorders
Clinical psychologist	A psychologist specially educated and trained in mental health; certification requires completion of an approved doctoral program and a clinical internship	Performs psychotherapy; plans and implements programs of behavior modification; selects, administers, and interprets psychological tests
Psychiatric social worker	A graduate of a master's program in social work with an emphasis in mental health; may have a doctoral degree	Helps clients and their families cope more effectively; identifies appropriate community resources; may perform counseling and psychotherapy
Marriage and family therapist	May be a member of any mental health discipline, usually prepared at the master's or doctoral level	Provides psychotherapy usually focusing on couples or families
Occupational therapist	Prepared in occupational therapy at the baccalaureate or master's level with a specialty in mental health care	Uses manual and creative techniques to elicit desired interpersonal and intrapsychic responses; teaches self-help activities, helps clients prepare to seek employment
Recreational therapist	May be prepared at informal or formal levels in university physical education and health education programs	Plans and guides recreational activities to provide socialization, healthful recreation, and desirable interpersonal and intrapsychic experiences
Creative arts therapist	May be prepared at informal or formal levels in colleges and universities	Uses art, music, dance, and literature to facilitate interpersonal experiences and increase social responses and self-esteem
Psychosocial rehabilitation worker	Most have either a high school education or a bachelor's degree	Teaches clients practical, day-to-day skills for living in the community and provides case management services

pose is cooperation rather than competition. Working together in cooperation ensures movement toward the common goal, whereas inappropriate competition hinders goal achievement and may be destructive to the competing individuals.

Most of our present understanding of cooperative and competitive behavior has come from the efforts of game theorists, who have researched player behavior. According to game theorists, players can be identified and placed in categories as follows:

- Maximizers—those interested only in their own gain
- Rivalists—those interested only in defeating their partners
- Cooperators—those interested in helping both themselves and their partners

Mental health providers who are maximizers jeopardize the client's welfare because they put themselves first and the client last. Rivalists direct their energies toward being "one up" through put-downs of others. They also are concerned not with the client but with the process of winning. Cooperators are interested in helping both themselves and their colleagues to aid the client. Participants who actively recognize the importance of each individual member of the mental health team can influence maximizers and rivalists to become cooperators.

Effective collaboration is based on respect for the position from which another participant acts. Our values and our culture direct our beliefs and the climate in which we operate. Knowing this, we can become aware of the values and culture of others, and, in turn, respect them. For a full discussion of culture and what it means to be culturally competent, refer to Chapter 9.

Unfortunately, the process of socialization into a profession may make it difficult for a person to respect, accept, and trust the position of another. As students become committed to a profession through the process of socialization, they tend to view members of other disciplines with suspicion. Review the lessons on collaboration in Box 2-3 on page 24. They will help you to collaborate effectively with others.

Administrative and peer support creates an atmosphere in which nurses are free to share their knowledge, skills, and evolving ideas. Such support increases creativity, depth, and perspective in nursing. Self-exploration and self-assessment, through reading and dialogue with other nurses and mental health team members, can help nurses embrace a spirit of cooperation.

MEDIALINK Care Plan: Enhancing Skill with Collaboration

MEDIALINK Critical Thinking Exercise: Unity vs. Autonomy

Box 2-3 Lessons on Collaboration

1. First, as we often remind you in this text, know your own reality. Determine your values, biases, and goals.
2. Value diversity and turn differences into assets.
3. Acknowledge that conflict is natural and develop constructive conflict resolution skills.
4. Recognize your own power base and share it with others (colleagues and clients and their families).
5. Master interpersonal communication skills and processing skills.
6. Approach collaboration as lifelong learning. The more you collaborate with others, the better you get at it.
7. Place yourself in interdisciplinary situations whenever possible—be present, both physically and mentally, at team forums.
8. Appreciate that collaboration is often spontaneous and you must be ready to seize the moment.
9. Balance unity with autonomy. That is, work neither exclusively as a member of a team (collaboration is not required for all decisions) nor in isolation.

Partnership and Collaboration with Clients and Family

Family and friends are a central influence in each person's life. Partnership includes clients and their significant others in the collaborative process of the mental health team whenever possible. Clients' participation in their own health care assures nurses that their clients are informed consumers of mental health services. To help you develop partnerships with your clients and their families we have provided a special feature entitled "Partnering with Clients and Families," which you will find throughout this textbook.

Clients and family members can also be invited to participate in case conferences. These conferences often have an important place in the functioning of mental health agencies and may have a number of purposes. Encourage clients to participate in case conferences involving collaboration among several agencies or several mental health care workers moving toward similar goals.

Consult the client about the information to be shared with family members and other members of the mental health team. It is not always easy for the nurse to determine exactly how much to share and with whom. When the boundaries of confidentiality are not clear, confer with your nursing instructor or a supervisor to determine what should be shared. Decisions should take into consideration what agreement exists between nurse and client about sharing information and how the person or agency receiving information will use that information in the client's best interest. Refer to Chapter 13 for a thorough discussion of client rights as they relate to confidentiality.

NURSING'S THEORETIC HERITAGE

The concept of nursing as primarily technologic has been replaced by the idea that nursing is theory-based. We use theories to organize assessment data, identify problems, plan interventions, generate goals and nursing actions, and determine and evaluate outcomes.

A few of the best-known nursing theorists and the concepts and principles of their theories or models most relevant to psychiatric–mental health nursing are examined in this section. Each of the early nursing theorists has revisited her original formulation to move closer to psychiatric–mental health nursing values of humanism, interactionism, cultural competence, the relevance of meaning, and the importance of empathy and empowerment in the nurse–client relationship. Hildegard Peplau, Joyce Travelbee, Josephine Paterson, Loretta Zderad, and Jean Watson are theorists whose existential and interactional origins and subsequent conceptualizations are particularly congruent with the philosophy of psychiatric–mental health nursing advocated in this text. The notion of choosing a theory upon which to base your practice is discussed in the Your Self-Awareness feature.

Peplau

Hildegard Peplau (see FIGURE 2-2 ■) published her nursing theory in the classic book *Interpersonal Relations in Nursing* (1952). She defined nursing as a significant therapeutic interpersonal process. Peplau was strongly influenced by the psychiatrist Harry Stack Sullivan and the learning theorist Carl Rogers (see Chapter 5).

Peplau conceptualized the one–to–one nurse–client relationship as the situation in which clients can accomplish developmental tasks such as learning to trust or learning to collaborate and practice healthy communication and behaviors. The core concepts of Peplau's theory of interpersonal relations (1997) were the four phases of what she identified as the nurse–client relationship:

1. Orientation
2. Identification

YOUR SELF-AWARENESS
Choosing a Theory

Psychiatric–mental health nurses use one or a combination of the theories presented in this chapter to interpret the meaning of client behavior and to apply the nursing process to their practice. In clinical work the selection of theories for practice may be influenced by a variety of factors. Ask yourself these questions:

- What theory do you rely on to interpret the meaning of client behaviors?
- What theory most accurately conceptualizes the client outcomes and interventions you use?
- How has your education influenced your choice of theories?
- How does the service setting (including the recording and payment systems) influence your choice of theories?
- How does the need to be efficient and practical influence your choice of theories?
- How do attributes such as the race, ethnicity, age, gender, and social class of clients influence your choice of theories?

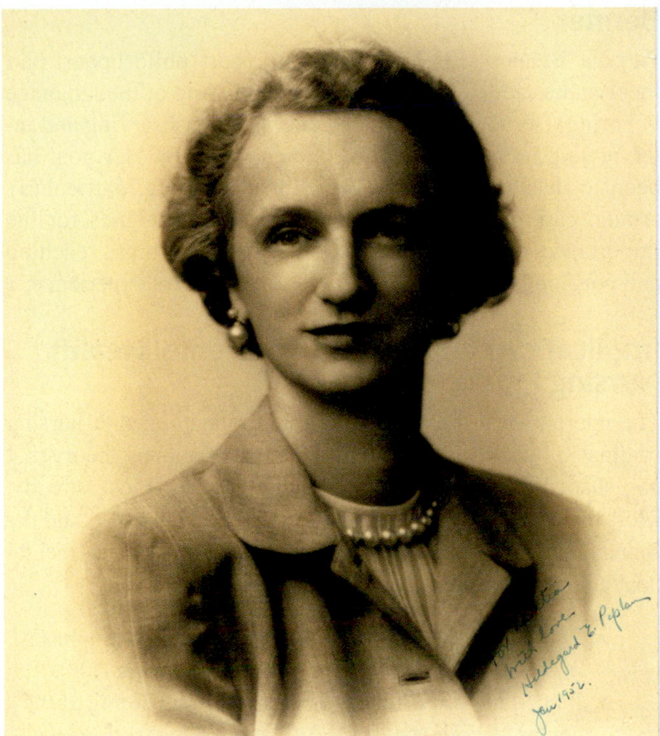

FIGURE 2-2 ■ Hildegard Peplau. Peplau's teaching continues to guide the heart of psychiatric–mental health nursing practice.
Source: Letitia Anne Peplau.

3. Exploitation (or working)
4. Resolution

Some say that these phases are ancestors of the phases of the nursing process.

One of Peplau's major contributions was the development of a step-by-step nursing intervention into anxiety. To this day this classic nursing intervention remains an important strategy in the psychiatric–mental health nurse's armamentarium. Peplau's step-by-step nursing intervention into anxiety is discussed in detail in Chapter 18.

Memorial tributes to Peplau upon her death in 1999 by nurses around the world recognized her as the "mother of psychiatric nursing" (Barker, 1999; Haber, 1999). Psychiatric–mental health nurses continue to use Peplau's teachings to understand and guide decisions in the one–to–one therapeutic relationship. Refer to Chapter 29 for details on individual counseling.

Orem

Dorothea Orem's (1971) theory of self-care was originally introduced around 1959 and identified ten universal self-care requisites, divided into six categories that encompass both physical and psychosocial human needs. Orem also introduced a second order of concepts, originally called *health deviation self-care demands,* to refer to care required in the event of illness, injury, or disease. Nursing, a second key component of her scheme, was divided into compensatory, partially compensatory, and supportive–educational systems of care that could be matched to the client's assessed level of self-care functioning in each area.

This theory firmly established the notion of a goal of self-care as integral to the discipline of nursing's perspective on the meaning of health (Orem, 1995). Orem's theory is particularly well adapted to meeting the nursing care needs of the severely and chronically mentally ill because of its focus on the client's abilities to perform self-care to maintain life, health, and well-being.

Rogers

Martha Rogers (1970) drew on knowledge from anthropology, sociology, religion, philosophy, mythology, and general systems theory to define nursing as a holistic science of unitary human beings. Rogers' key nursing principles, called the principles of homeodynamics, view human beings holistically. Changes in life processes are irreversible, nonrepeatable, and rhythmic and indicate patterns of increasing complexity and organization.

Most of her concepts have counterparts in general systems theory, but she has added the notions of life processes, change, and human–environmental interaction to the concepts central to nursing. Rogers' work gives psychiatric–mental health nurses a mandate to use holistic principles as a guide to practice and to consider human being and environment interactions and change.

Roy

Sister Callista Roy's (1976) adaptation theory views people as psychosocial beings who are constantly faced with the need to adapt to internal and external demands. She identifies four modes of human adapting: *physiologic needs, self-concept, role function,* and *interdependence.* Obviously, these adaptive modes include physiologic, psychologic, and social aspects of people. The notion of coping or adapting to stimuli relates to people in interaction with their environment. Recent versions of Roy's adaptation theory have incorporated humanistic assumptions about the dignity of human beings and the role of nurses in promoting integrity (Roy & Andrews, 1999).

Orlando

Ida Jean Orlando's theory (1961) grew out of dissatisfaction with the possibility that nursing care was governed by organizational rules rather than attention to client needs. She emphasized the importance of deliberative nursing action based on the meanings that are validated between the nurse and client.

Wiedenbach

Ernestine Wiedenbach (1964) was influenced by the work of Orlando. Her theory was also developed around the client's need for help and the validation of such need through client perceptions. She was particularly interested in problems of discomfort and the nurse's role in observing, assessing, exploring, and validating feelings, thoughts, and fears.

Travelbee

Joyce Travelbee is another nurse theorist who, along with Orlando and Weidenbach, focuses on the meaning in nurse–client interactions. Travelbee (1966) explains in detail the concepts of sympathy, rapport, and suffering and emphasizes the importance of communication and stages of nurse–client relationships. Her view of humanity, uniqueness, existential encounters, and nursing is highly congruent with values in psychiatric–mental health nursing.

Paterson and Zderad

Paterson and Zderad's 1976 book, republished in 1988, reflected the contemporary nature of their original ideas. They were a decade ahead of their time in rejecting a mechanistic cause-and-effect view of nursing science and urged instead that observations of the experience of nurses in practice should be the basis of any useful nursing theory.

Their theory portrays nursing as a lived dialogue that incorporates an intersubjective transaction in which both nurse and client are present in the experience in an existential way that includes mutuality and intimacy. Their theory relies heavily on existential philosophers and emphasizes the freedom of human choice and responsibility for one's actions. It is a highly abstract theory with a major focus on the process of interaction (or dialogue) between nurse and client.

Watson

Jean Watson's theory of human caring was influenced by Jungian psychology, feminist theory, and Maslow's psychologic concept of self-actualization (Watson, 1988). This classic work is in the process of being updated (Watson, 2007). Caring–healing within Watson's framework is based on values such as kindness, concern, love of self and others, and the ecology of the earth and involves what she terms *carative* factors: a humanistic–altruistic value system, faith–hope, and sensitivity of self and others (Watson, 1999).

Her theory emphasizes sensitivity to self and values clarification regarding personal and cultural beliefs that might pose barriers to transpersonal caring. Establishing a helping–trusting human care relationship is pivotal to Watson's theory. She credits much of her thinking on therapeutic relationships and communication to the work of Carl Rogers, identifying congruency, empathy, and warmth as foundational to a caring relationship that conveys authenticity and genuineness and facilitates the client's expression of emotions.

In her recent work, Watson (2005) also develops the notion of spiritual environment and the interconnectedness of all things, including the connection between natural healing approaches, self-knowledge, self-control, self-caring, self-healing potential, and caring, healing relationships with self and others. Watson's theory is philosophically congruent with contemporary global approaches to health and health promotion (Falk-Rafael, 2000; Pilkington, 2007).

Benner

Patricia Benner (1983, 1996, 1999), part philosopher, part theorist, has added to nursing's understanding of the language of caring. Her ideas have been generated by observing and interviewing nurses engaged in clinical practice. Her goal has been to disclose the nature of clinical wisdom, particularly around caring and comforting practices. She argues for the importance of forming nurse–client relationships, teaching and coaching, and bearing witness to the illness experience.

Implications for Psychiatric–Mental Health Nursing Practice

The interpersonal theory of psychiatric–mental health nursing originated by Hildegard Peplau remains the nursing theory that has shaped psychiatric–mental health nursing most directly. More contemporary nurse theorists, however, have also laid the foundation for concepts that are central to psychiatric–mental health nursing practice. Nursing theorists have:

- Differentiated nursing from medicine with emphases on caring and comforting rather than curing
- Placed the importance of interpreting meaning at the center of their theories
- Focused on interaction between the nurse and the client
- Advocated humanistic and existential values of client dignity and nurse authenticity as crucial to quality of care

A review of nursing theories indicates some clear differences in emphasis and perspective and some intriguing similarities. From these theories the parameters of our discipline emerge. Such parameters provide the beginnings for directing practice, focusing nursing research, and providing a framework of concepts integral to the preparation of professional students.

Approaches associated with two or more different theories are often used in combination. For example, bizarre, self-destructive behavior may be controlled with medications so that the client is more available for a caring, healing relationship with a psychiatric–mental health nurse. Such a combined or eclectic approach demands that you be capable of functioning according to all theories of care, depending on which is best for the client and best fits the resources and limitations of the situation. If you give adequate consideration to the theoretic framework of your psychiatric–mental health nursing, you will foster practice-oriented research and clinical judgments that can be articulated and taught to others. Research is a tool for developing psychiatric–mental health nursing theory that synthesizes the most useful elements of these theories.

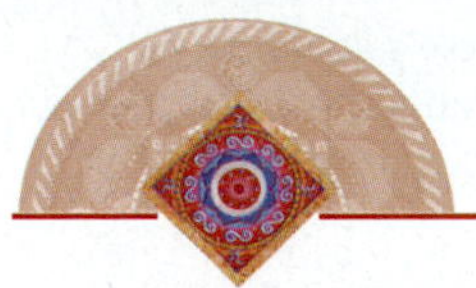

EXPLORE MEDIALINK

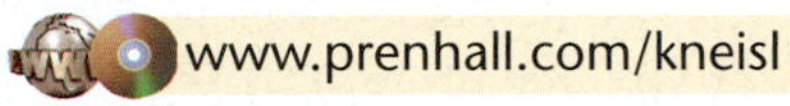

www.prenhall.com/kneisl

For NCLEX-RN® review questions, case studies, and other resources for this chapter see the Pearson Health MediaLink CD-ROM that accompanies this book and the Companion Website at www.prenhall.com/kneisl.

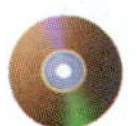

CD-ROM
Audio Glossary
NCLEX-RN® Review Questions

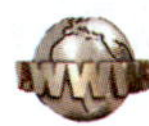

Companion Website
Audio Glossary
NCLEX-RN® Review Questions
Critical Thinking Exercise
- *Unity vs. Autonomy*

Case Study
- *The Multifaceted Role*

Care Plan
- *Enhancing Skill with Collaboration*

MediaLinks
MediaLink Application
- *Applying Theory*

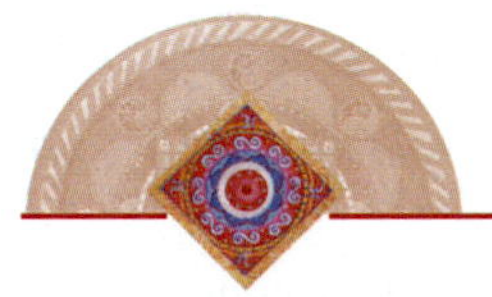

NCLEX-RN® REVIEW QUESTIONS

1. Consequences of the modification of the ANA *Psychiatric–Mental Health Nursing Scope and Standards of Practice* include which of the following?
1. Continued development of the multifaceted role of the nurse
2. Increased blurring with roles of other mental health professionals
3. Recommendations for augmentation of the nurse's role in inpatient settings
4. Recommendations for increases in nurses' entry-level salaries

2. Consequences of the blurring of roles include which of the following? (Select all that apply.)
1. Flexibility and variety within settings based on education and experience (as laws and regulations permit)
2. Increased group cohesiveness
3. Rivalist behavior
4. Increased cohesiveness of the health care team
5. Frustration and burnout

3. Each health care team member's role includes:
1. Postdischarge follow-up care.
2. Milieu management.
3. Psychobiological interventions.
4. Teaching and counseling.

4. Within the health care team, the nurse's holistic, client-centered approach to assessment and care positions the nurse to function as which of the following? (Select all that apply.)
1. A cooperative, integral member
2. A team member who can influence others to cooperate
3. A rivalist and "underdog champion"
4. A leader
5. A maximizer and "captain of the ship"

5. Which factors served to broaden the scope of psychiatric nursing practice? (Select all that apply.)
1. Influx of World War II veterans with psychiatric disabilities
2. The development of milieu therapy as a treatment modality
3. Separation of psychiatric–mental health nursing from the nursing school curriculum
4. Psychiatric nursing textbooks and journals
5. Discovery of new psychopharmacological agents

6. Which of the following is *not* a consequence of the National Mental Health Act?
1. Development of programs to train mental health professionals
2. Prescriptive privileges for nursing
3. Support for psychiatric research
4. Graduate programs in psychiatric nursing

7. Peplau's intervention for anxiety and Tudor's intervention for avoidance:
1. Were presented as alternatives to psychopharmacological intervention.
2. Opposed the medical model of mental illness.
3. Demonstrated that psychiatric–mental health nursing strategies could be articulated and taught to other practitioners.
4. Resulted in direct conflict with other practitioners.

8. Roy modified her adaptation theory to incorporate the "intrinsic human dignity" and the role of the nurse in promoting integrity. This modification is an example of:
1. Peplau's humanistic approach and existential values influencing general nursing theory.
2. The influence of Orem's self-care theory.
3. The incorporation of systems theory.
4. Maslow's contributions to nursing theory.

9. Central to psychiatric–mental health nursing theories are the concepts of:
1. Value of psychobiological interventions.
2. Attention to the nurse–client interaction.
3. Attention to intrapersonal phenomena.
4. Value of an eclectic approach.

10. In the inpatient hospital setting, a master's-prepared psychiatric nurse formulates nursing interventions utilizing Orlando's theory. With her long-term individual therapy clients, this nurse formulates interventions based on Rogers' theory of unitary human beings. The nurse's assumptions about the nature of the nurse–patient relationship are based on Peplau's theory. This nurse's approach demonstrates flexibility based on:
1. Likelihood of the client's recovery.
2. The worldviews of the other professionals in the setting.
3. Day-to-day fluctuations in unit milieu.
4. Resources, limitations, and client needs.

See Appendix C for answers.

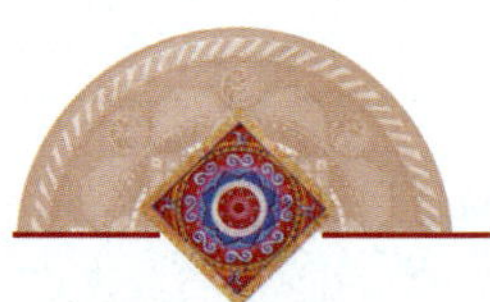

REFERENCES

American Nurses Association. (1967). *Statement on psychiatric nursing practice.* Washington, DC: Author.

American Nurses Association, American Psychiatric Nurses Association, and International Society of Psychiatric-Mental Health Nurses. (2007). *Psychiatric–mental health nursing: Scope and standards of practice.* Silver Spring, MD: Nursesbooks.org.

American Nurses Association Task Force on Psychopharmacology. (1994). *Psychiatric–mental health nursing psychopharmacology project.* Washington DC: Author.

Armstrong, S. W., & Rouslin, S. (1963). *Group psychotherapy in nursing practice.* New York: Macmillan.

Barker, P. (1999). Hildegard E. Peplau: The mother of psychiatric nursing. *Journal of Psychiatric and Mental Health Nursing, 6*(3), 175–176.

Benner, P. (1983). Uncovering the knowledge embedded in clinical practice. *Image: Journal of Nursing Scholarship, 15*(2), 36–41.

Benner, P. (1996). *Expertise in nursing practice: Caring, clinical judgment and ethics.* New York: Springer.

Benner, P. (1999). *Clinical wisdom and interventions in critical care: A thinking-in-action approach.* Philadelphia: Saunders.

Brown, E. L. (1948). *Nursing for the future.* New York: Russell Sage Foundation.

Byrd, S., & Marshall, M. (1963). *Clinical approaches to psychiatric nursing.* New York: Macmillan.

Chafetz, L., White, M., Collins-Bride, G., & Nickens, J. (2005). The poor general health of the severely mentally ill: Impact of schizophrenic diagnosis. *Community Mental Health Journal, 41*(2), 169–184.

Falk-Rafael, A. R. (2000). Watson's philosophy, science, and theory of human caring as a conceptual framework for guiding community health nursing practice. *Advances in Nursing Science, 23*(2), 34–49.

Haber, J. (1999). Hildegard Peplau. The mother of psychiatric nursing. *Nursing and Health Care Perspectives, 20*(4), 228.

Hadley, R. (1978). President's commission sets national mental health goals. *American Nurse, 10,* 1.

Jackson, J. L., Passamonti, M., & Kroenke, K. (2007). Outcome and impact of mental disorders in primary care at 5 years. *Psychosomatic Medicine, 69*(2), 217–229.

Krauss, J. B. (1993). *Health care reform: Essential mental health services.* Washington, DC: American Nurses Publishing.

Kroenke, K., Spitzer, R. L., Williams, J. B., Monahan, P. O., & Lowe, B. (2007). Anxiety disorders in primary care: Prevalence, impairment, comorbidity, and detection. *Annals of Internal Medicine, 146*(5), 317.

McBride, A. B. (1990). Psychiatric nursing in the 1990s. *Archives of Psychiatric Nursing, 4*(1), 21–27.

National Panel for Psychiatric-Mental Health NP Competencies. (2003). *Psychiatric–mental health nurse practitioner competencies.* Washington, DC: National Organization of Nurse Practitioner Faculties. Retrieved September 24, 2007, from http://www.nonpf.com/finalcomps03.pdf

Orem, D. E. (1971). *Nursing: Concepts of practice.* New York: McGraw-Hill.

Orem, D. E. (1995). *Nursing: Concepts of practice* (5th ed.). New York: McGraw-Hill.

Orlando, I. (1961). *The dynamic nurse–patient relationship.* New York: G. P. Putnam's Sons.

Osborne, O. H. (1984). Intellectual traditions in psychiatric–mental health nursing: A review of selected textbooks. *Journal of Psychosocial Nursing and Mental Health Nursing, 22*(11), 27–32.

Paterson, J. G., & Zderad, L. T. (1988). *Humanistic nursing* (Publication No. 41–2218). New York: National League for Nursing.

Peplau, H. E. (1952). *Interpersonal relations in nursing.* New York: Putnam.

Peplau, H. E. (1989). Future directions in psychiatric nursing from the perspective of history. *Journal of Psychosocial Nursing, 27*(2), 18–27.

Peplau, H. E. (1997). Peplau's theory of interpersonal relations. *Nursing Science Quarterly, 10*(4), 162–167.

Pilkington, F. B. (2007). Envisioning nursing in 2050 through the eyes of nurse theorists: Leininger and Watson. *Nursing Science Quarterly, 20*(1), 8.

Rogers, M. E. (1970). *The theoretical basis in nursing.* New York: F. A. Davis.

Roy, C. (1976). *Introduction to nursing: An adaptation model.* New York: Prentice Hall.

Roy, C., & Andrews, H. A. (1999). *The Roy adaptation model: The definitive statement.* Norwalk, CT: Appleton & Lange.

Scheffler, R. M., Ivey, S. L., & Garrett, A. B. (1998). Changing supply and earning patterns of the mental health workforce. *Administration and Policy in Mental Health, 26,* 85–99.

Travelbee, J. (1966). *Interpersonal aspects of nursing.* Philadelphia: Davis.

Tudor, G. (1952). A sociopsychiatric nursing approach to intervention in a problem of mutual withdrawal on a mental hospital ward. *Psychiatry, 15,* 174+.

U.S. Department of Labor. (Bureau of Labor Statistics. (2002). *Mental health occupations statistics.* Retrieved March 4, 2007, from http://www.USDL/mentalhealthoccu.gov

Watson, J. (1988). New dimensions in human caring theory. *Nursing Science Quarterly, 1*(4), 175–181.

Watson, J. (1999). *Postmodern nursing and beyond.* New York: Churchill Livingstone.

Watson, J. (2005). *Caring science as sacred science.* Phildelphia: F. A. Davis.

Watson, J. (2007). *Nursing: The philosophy and science of caring.* Boulder: University Press of Colorado.

Wiedenbach, E. (1964). *Clinical nursing: A helping art.* New York: Springer.

Wilson, H. S., & Kneisl, C. R. (1979). *Psychiatric nursing.* Menlo Park, CA: Addison-Wesley.

ADDITIONAL REFERENCES

McBride, A. B. (1996). Psychiatric–mental health nursing in the 21st century. In A. McBride & J. Austin (Eds.), *Psychiatric–mental health nursing: Integrating the behavioral and biological sciences.* Philadelphia: Saunders.

Peplau, H. E. (1980). The psychiatric nurse—accountable? To whom? For what? *Perspectives in Psychiatric Care, 18*(3), 128–134.

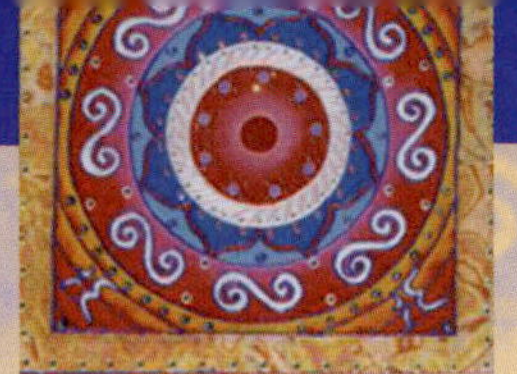

Artful Therapeutic Practice

CHAPTER
3

CAROL REN KNEISL

LEARNING OUTCOMES

After completing this chapter, you will be able to:

1. Explain how self-knowledge and self-reflection are important to psychiatric–mental health nurses.
2. Discuss the concept of personal integration and how it relates to psychiatric–mental health nursing practice.
3. Describe the qualities that enable psychiatric–mental health nurses to practice the use of self artfully in therapeutic relationships.
4. Provide examples of how the concepts of blame and control affect artful therapeutic practice.
5. Foster culturally competent care for clients with psychiatric–mental health disorders by understanding the influence of your own sociocultural background on your nursing practice.
6. Demonstrate empathy in psychiatric–mental health clinical practice.
7. Maintain a respectful attitude toward clients, their families, and colleagues.
8. Demonstrate a commitment to practicing self-care and connecting with self and others.

KEY TERMS

aggressive behavior *37*
assertive behavior *37*
burnout *35*
critical thinking *41*
empathy *41*
nonassertive behavior *37*
self-awareness *31*
spirituality *39*
therapeutic alliance *36*

CRITICAL THINKING CHALLENGE

Ruby Ann is a 19-year-old African-American mother of three small children. She lives with her boyfriend in a one-bedroom mobile home in a rough area of a major Southern city. Ruby Ann has been treated several times in the city hospital's emergency department for bruises, lacerations, and broken bones. She has called 911 four times in the past year because her boyfriend was threatening to kill her and her children. Your assessment interview upon her arrival at the battered women's shelter reveals that Ruby Ann is anxious and depressed and has experienced frequent, severe verbal and physical abuse. She reports that she is unable to sleep, has no appetite, and has lost 20 pounds over the past 9 months. Ruby Ann also confides that her spiritual beliefs have sustained her in her suffering and distress. She says, "If God wasn't with me, I wouldn't have got outta there, but I'm startin' to doubt Him 'cause how could He let all this happen to my babies?"

1. Based on this data, what specific type of spiritual assistance would you offer Ruby Ann? Does it matter if you and Ruby Ann are of different faiths?
2. What feelings do you think Ruby Ann might be experiencing? How would spiritual support help to reduce untoward feelings?

MEDIALINK 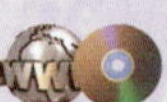 www.prenhall.com/kneisl

Go to the Pearson Health MediaLink CD-ROM and the Companion Website at www.prenhall.com/kneisl for interactive resources for this chapter.

The value of self-knowledge is a recurring theme in both popular and professional literature. Libraries are stocked with volumes dealing with the undiscovered self, the expansion of human awareness, spirituality and the care of the soul, strategies for self-realization, and the like. A common thread in all these is the idea that the quality and nature of a person's relationships with others are strongly influenced by the person's self-view. Consider the comments made by students in their psychiatric nursing clinical experience in the following clinical example.

CLINICAL EXAMPLE

Laurie: "I just can't take it. I feel myself getting confused about who is the crazy one. There's such a fine line. Sometimes I think I'll be a patient here."

Eric: "I hated psych—it just didn't seem like nursing to me. I really like to keep busy. When you change someone's dressing, you really feel like you've helped them. Here it's all so uncertain."

Makayla: "All I kept thinking about was that a lot of the patients had done really weird things. This one guy had lived in an apartment with his dead mother's body for 3 months before they brought him in. Another had tried to shoot the governor. I never felt safe turning my back on them."

Throughout this text, you will be encouraged to attend to the mind–body–spirit of your clients. This chapter explores some dimensions of self-knowledge through the examination of personal integration, recurring problems that pertain to the nurse's identity, the personal qualities on which the artful use of self in therapeutic relationships is based, and strategies for taking care of your mind–body–spirit.

PERSONAL INTEGRATION

Many students and practitioners faced with relating to people whose behavior they view as offensive, frightening, curious, or socially inappropriate find that their personal attitudes, expectations, myths, and values make it difficult for them to fulfill their professional roles. This was the case in the following clinical example.

CLINICAL EXAMPLE

Penny, a baccalaureate nursing student, had selected a clinical placement at a substance abuse clinic in the community. Despite her initial interest, she developed a pattern of absences from the clinic. When her faculty adviser discussed this observation with her, Penny blurted out that, much to her surprise, she was unable to assist with the group meetings for pregnant heroin addicts. The thought of addicting babies before they were born—babies who would ultimately suffer because of their mothers' self-indulgence—horrified Penny. She found herself judging their choices constantly and avoiding interaction with them. "I feel like they should be shot instead of given all this free support and sympathy."

For many nurses, confrontation with deviance (defined in Chapter 1 ∞ as behavior outside the social norm of a specific group; should not be construed to mean negative behavior) reinforces a personal sense of stability. Others are threatened by such confrontation.

Recall the clinical example of "Crazy Helen," "Vince the Window Peeper," "Eddie the Drunk," and "Lester the Molester" on page 5 in Chapter 1 ∞. Dealing with people whose personal integration is fragmented, dissolving, divided, or alienated puts the nurse's own identity on the line as well. To respond with both compassion and the critical distance necessary to be effective, psychiatric professionals must confront their own identity; separate it from another's identity, which may indeed be dissolving; and finally integrate different values and behaviors comfortably in the therapeutic relationships they develop with clients.

This personal quality is called *detached concern*—the ability to distance oneself in order to help others. It is an essential quality not only in avoiding *burnout*, a problem discussed later in this chapter, but also in using appropriate *assertiveness* when collaborating with colleagues, and in maintaining *empathic abilities* in highly stressful situations.

In the conventional focus on the client, the nurse is regarded as the caregiver, the provider of services, the counselor or therapist. Little attention is paid to the stresses psychiatric nurses experience in attempting to relate fully to clients while maintaining their own personal integration.

Creating a Common Ground

Nurses often find that encounters with psychiatric clients are a distancing experience. We become acutely aware of our difference and separateness from clients. We reaffirm our own subjective view of reality and rationalize our actions to keep these actions consistent with our sense of self as healthy, normal people.

Because people are constantly building and protecting their own self-images, they try to get others to see their image of themselves. However, it is impossible to see another's self-image or worldview exactly as that person experiences it. Despite this fact, psychiatry has traditionally attempted to get certain people, labeled *crazy*, to assume the perspective of certain other people, called *therapists*.

A more acceptable alternative seems to lie in the creation of some common ground, a mutually understood, negotiated reality. Even to this common ground the nurse and the client bring their own conceptions, feelings, and attitudes toward and images of each other and themselves. In many instances, our image of the client—how we expect the client to act or feel—is not the same as the client's self-image. This is confusing to both client and nurse and hinders our attempts to establish therapeutic relationships and communicate effectively.

Searching for Meaning

Psychiatric–mental health nurses work with clients in a search for meaning in clients' lives. It is essential that we establish our own personal meaning and integration of self, for these are key resources in treatment. In order to be effective, we must already possess the personal skills to deal with the client's symptoms. And, we must have personally worked through any problems that resemble those of the client. For example, nurses who cannot cope with their own feelings of depression cannot be effective with severely depressed clients.

Feelings: The Affective Self

The ultimate effectiveness of efforts to relate to and communicate with others depends on how well people know themselves **(self-awareness)** and develop the ability to be sensitive to and care about others. In the following clinical example, Josh's limited self-awareness hampers him in his clinical work.

CLINICAL EXAMPLE

Josh is a middle-aged man who sought out nursing as a career. Although he is highly proficient in technical skills and charming and engaging in relationships with most clients, he has discovered a surprising intolerance for some of the tears, complaints, and self-preoccupation of depressed clients. He finds himself responding with admonitions to stop it, to bite the bullet, to grow up. He personally has seldom allowed himself to experience his own sadnesses and jokingly characterizes himself as a firm believer in repression and denial. The need to empathize with people unable to control their feelings evokes discomfort, and he is unable to work with such clients.

Self-awareness and caring seem to go hand in hand. At the root of social interaction is people's ability to understand and care about each other's attitudes and feelings. Because each human being is unique, this ability, called *empathizing,* is a difficult and challenging task. (Empathy is discussed in greater detail later in this chapter, and empathy as a communication skill is discussed in Chapter 10.) One way to develop this ability is to practice it. Learning to be aware of your responses to the expression of feelings from another person is a starting point.

Self-Awareness of Feelings

Feelings are like icebergs: Only the tips stick up into consciousness, and the deeper parts are submerged (FIGURE 3-1 ■). One such feeling is fear. The conscious part may be experienced as dislike, avoidance, or reluctance. At a deeper level, the feeling is reported as anxiety. Even deeper, the person may acknowledge, "I feel scared." Deeper yet, the person may experience genuine panic. Such an iceberg may well explain Josh's attitude toward tearful, depressed clients. His annoyance, irritation, sarcasm, and disdain may represent the tip of the iceberg of Josh's fear of depression.

The iceberg comparison also applies to other feelings, such as love, hurt, and guilt. A person feeling love may be aware only of a liking or attraction for another. Beneath the tip of that iceberg are feelings of warmth and affection. Deeper are feelings of love, and at the deepest level may be feelings of fusion or ecstasy.

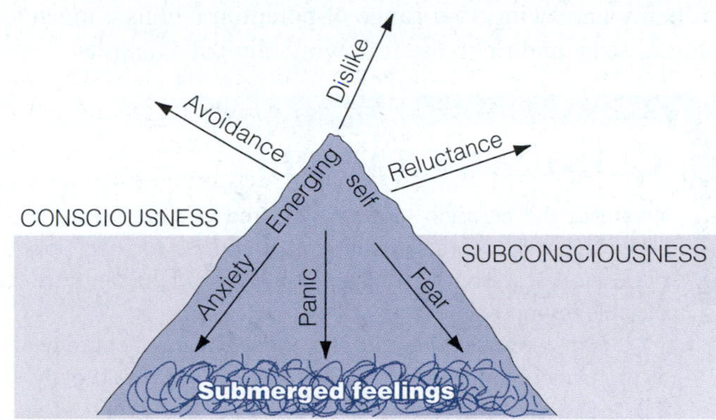

FIGURE 3-1 ■ Self-awareness of feelings. Superficial feelings are visible; deeper feelings are submerged.

Problems with Submerged Feelings

One characteristic of icebergs of feeling is that at the tip the feelings lose their experiential quality and are translated into impulses to act. For example, a person with submerged guilt may express it by frequent worrying and may be completely unaware of the underlying feelings. The behavior is the only outward manifestation.

People lose touch with their feelings over time as they shape their sense of self. They hear such messages as "boys don't cry" or "girls are too sensitive" and incorporate these injunctions into their emerging self-system, especially into the "me" or "self for others." Not being sufficiently aware of one's feelings has several disadvantages:

- What people don't know *can* hurt them. Repressed feelings may reappear in behaviors that are difficult to alter. For example, hidden anger may emerge in migraine headaches or the use of sarcasm. (See the Caring for the Spirit feature in Chapter 8, which discusses repressed memories.)
- People who are not aware of their feelings find it difficult to make decisions. It is hard to tell a "should" from a wish. Without some awareness of their real wants, they may have trouble saying no or requesting something they need. They are more likely to rely on others—experts, authorities, rules and regulations, and so forth—for guidance.
- People who, like Josh, are "out of touch with" or unaware of their feelings may find it difficult to be really close to and empathic toward others. Intimacy and empathy demand the expression of here-and-now feelings, whether positive or negative.

Most people realize the value of thinking clearly. They understand that it is a learned ability and takes practice. Feeling clearly (authentically) can also be practiced and learned.

Dominant Emotional Themes

In order to be effective, we need to explore the dominant emotional themes in our personalities. If you find that you respond to many situations with the same feelings, you are probably narrowing your range of potential feelings, much as Marge, Joan, and Ed in the following clinical example.

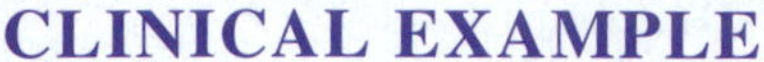

CLINICAL EXAMPLE

Whatever the occasion, Marge was tired or bored. Fatigue and chronically depressed states were routine for her. Holidays, vacations, dinner engagements all evoked the same predictable response.

Joan was afraid of everything. When she met her brother at the plane, her first question was, "Aren't you afraid of flying?" She was afraid driving home from the airport. The prospect of starting back to school also frightened her.

Regardless of the circumstances, Ed always questioned the intentions of his wife, his children, his coworkers, and his friends. According to Ed, the motives for their behavior were always up for debate.

People who feel the same way in a variety of situations may be missing a lot of what is happening in those situations. They perceive only what will fit a narrowed range of feelings. Becoming aware of limited emotional themes is a way to begin to widen one's range of feelings.

Acceptance of Disapproved Feelings

Most people have been taught to block off awareness and expression of certain feelings. Children are taught that being rude or ungrateful or cranky is rarely acceptable. To retain love and approval, they usually comply, not by stopping the feelings but by acting as if they didn't have them. Nursing students often get similar messages from their teachers. That is, it is not acceptable to find a client repulsive, to dislike someone who is sick and dependent, or to express anger at or criticism of the teacher. Positive feelings of attraction and love may also seem unacceptable. Failure to recognize these feelings can interfere with interactions.

Recognizing and accepting our own feelings make us less vulnerable to other people's ideas about how we should feel. Nurses often feel guilty when they don't feel what others imply they should feel. Nurses who can allow themselves the right to their own feelings can also allow clients the right to have and express theirs.

Beliefs and Values

Our personal values are the "ought to's" and "shoulds" that direct our behavior. Beliefs and values take three major forms:

1. Rational beliefs are beliefs that are supported by available evidence.
2. Blind belief is belief in the absence of evidence.
3. Irrational belief is belief held despite available evidence to the contrary.

Dogmatic Belief

Dogmatic belief (opinions or beliefs held as if they were based on the highest authority) includes both blind and irrational belief. Dogmatically held beliefs are not based on personal experience. Operating on the basis of dogmatically held beliefs often causes us to distort our personal experiences of the world to fit our preconceptions. The following are examples of some strongly held beliefs about behaviors that are labeled "mental illness":

- Most clients in mental hospitals are dangerous.
- People who seek counseling are mentally disordered.
- If parents loved their children more, there would be fewer mental disorders.
- When a person has a worry, it is best not to think about it.
- Many people become mentally disordered just to avoid the problems of life.
- People would not become mentally disordered if they avoided bad thoughts.
- Anyone who is in a hospital for a mental disorder should not be allowed to vote.
- To become a psychiatric client is to become a failure in life.
- One of the main causes of mental disorders is a lack of moral strength.

There are two issues at work here. They are discussed in the following section.

Issues of Blame and Control

Inherent in the strongly held beliefs listed earlier are the issues of *blame* and *control*. Believing that people cause their own problems involves the issue of blame. Believing that people are responsible for solutions to their problems involves the issue of control. Your assumptions about personal responsibility affect the way in which you go about your clinical work. FIGURE 3-2 ■ illustrates four models of helping based on the issues of blame and control.

For artful therapeutic practice, you need to be aware of the models from which you operate as well as your client's orientation. The help you offer may not be effective if the person desiring help and the person offering help have different views on personal responsibility. If you believe that people do not create their problems or are responsible for solving them, according to Brickman et al. (1982), you operate from the Medical model. If you believe that people should not be blamed for their problems but should take steps to solve them, you operate from the Compensatory model. If you believe that people are responsible for creating their own problems but need to rely on others to solve them, you operate from the Enlightenment model. If you believe that because people cause their own problems they should also be responsible for developing solutions to them, you operate from the Moral model.

Most research on strongly held beliefs indicates that people usually know more about the things they believe than about those they don't believe. By staying ignorant about anything they don't already agree with, they can avoid changing. This posture cuts off personal growth and learning that could be derived from the unknown. Obviously, clients are better served by nurses who are aware of their own dogmatically held beliefs and then challenge those beliefs.

Attitudes and Opinions

A feeling is a transitory experience. A feeling held over a period of time is called an *attitude*. An attitude linked to an idea or belief becomes an *opinion*. An opinion, then, involves both thinking and feeling. Research in this area has shown that people are more comfortable when their beliefs are consistent with their attitudes. People do several things to keep their attitudes and beliefs consistent:

- They repress any belief or attitude that seems inconsistent.
- They distract their awareness from conflict either physically (such as by leaving the room) or psychologically (such as by daydreaming).
- They distort their perceptions to fit an existing attitude or belief.

These maneuvers take place in an attempt to keep actions consistent with attitudes or beliefs.

Arriving at Values

Every day, each person meets life situations that call for thought, opinion forming, decision making, and action. At every turn in our personal and professional lives, we are faced with choices. Our choices are based on the values we hold, but often those values are not really clear. People actively value something to the degree that they are willing to put energy into doing something about it. Their values are demonstrated in their interests, preferences, decisions, and actions, as in the following clinical example.

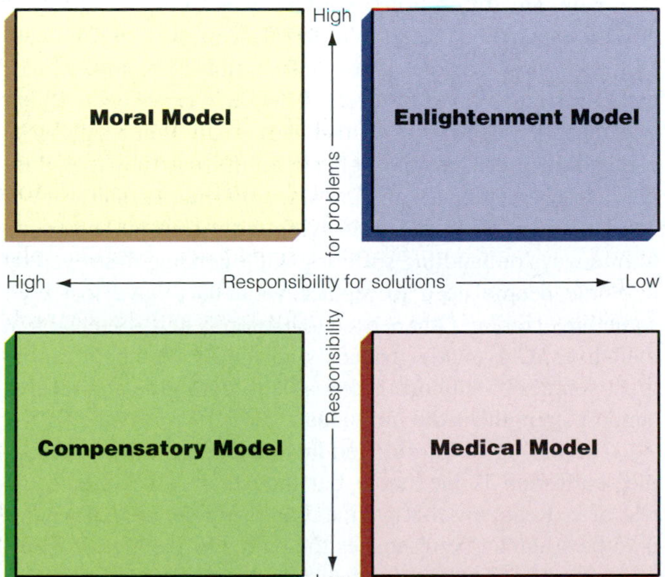

FIGURE 3-2 ■ Four models of helping based on the issues of blame and control.

CLINICAL EXAMPLE

In talking with colleagues, Susan, a psychiatric–mental health nurse, claims to value interacting with clients more than doing paperwork. Yet a quick assessment of how she spends her time—all excuses taken into account—reveals that she acts on other values.

Mel, a nurse working in a state hospital unit for profoundly developmentally disabled children, says that he believes these clients are human beings, despite their uncommunicative, immobile forms. He demonstrates this value in the hours he spends trying to communicate his presence and concern for them, using acupressure and touch performed slowly and with genuine feeling.

The distinction in the above examples is between *cognitive* and *active values*. Susan verbally subscribes to values but fails to act on them. These are cognitive values. Mel's actions demonstrate that he gives more than lip service to the idea of the dignity of all living beings. He follows active values.

Culture and Social Class

Cultural and social class differences between you and the client may impede your best intentions. Gaining awareness of sociocultural differences requires that you first come to understand your own background and the influence of that background on your practice. Nurses are better able to meet the sociocultural needs of a client when they acknowledge that a culture and a society influence their beliefs, values, attitudes, and behavior. Quality nursing care is culturally sensitive; that is, aware of cultural issues that are important to the client and may affect the client's response to treatment.

In planning nursing interventions, do not follow a predetermined plan, but plan care that is culturally competent for each person. For example, if a Hispanic teenage girl is obese and wants to lose weight, you would not hand her a printed 1000-calorie diet plan but would work with her and a nutritionist to plan a diet based on the foods she prefers. If an Asian client who is a Buddhist wants time each day to meditate, you would allow for that time in the care plan rather than filling every hour with "constructive," "growth-producing" activity. Taking a client's culture into consideration when planning care is not an easy task. It is time-consuming and requires patience, insight, and creativity.

Sociocultural Heritage

The questions in the Your Self-Awareness feature on page 34 are designed to facilitate acknowledgment of your own sociocultural heritage. Answering these questions honestly and completely will help you to understand which sociocultural factors impact upon your ability to communicate in a culturally sensitive way.

Avoiding Misdiagnosis

Clients from different cultures may be misdiagnosed by Western health care providers. Culturally competent nurses can

YOUR SELF-AWARENESS
Influence of Sociocultural Heritage

- What ethnic group, socioeconomic class, religion, age group, and community do you belong to?
- What experiences have you had with people from ethnic groups, socioeconomic classes, religions, age groups, or communities different from your own?
- What were those experiences like? How did you feel about them?
- When you were growing up, what did your parents and significant others say about people who were different from your family?
- What about your ethnic group, socioeconomic class, religion, age, or community do you find embarrassing or wish you could change? Why?
- What sociocultural factors in your background might contribute to your being rejected by members of other cultures?
- What personal qualities do you have that will help you establish interpersonal relationships with persons from other cultural groups?
- What personal qualities may be detrimental?
- What assumptions do you hold about the people who populate our world?

play a role in assessing clients' social, psychologic, and behavioral symptoms in light of clients' own cultural norms. For example, a psychiatrist may diagnose a man who talks to the dead as schizophrenic, but for a Puerto Rican who believes in *espiritismo*, talking to the dead is a common practice. A client who is a charismatic Christian may lapse into an altered state of consciousness and speak in tongues. To interpret these behaviors as evidence of schizophrenia is inappropriate. Obtaining a cultural profile helps to prevent misdiagnosis. Culturally competent psychiatric–mental health nursing practice is more thoroughly discussed in Chapter 9∞.

TAKING CARE OF THE SELF

Knowing who you are is just a beginning. Taking care of others requires that nurses respect and care for themselves. Assertiveness, the need for solitude, maintaining physical health, attending to cues of personal stress, and avoiding burnout are all actions crucial to preserving personal integration.

Solitude

Most people need time alone to assimilate what has happened in time spent with other people. They also need it for relief from responding to the demands of others. Aloneness need not mean physical distance. People can be alone in a crowded library. The crucial factors are that they are making no demands on others and that no one is making demands on them. After a sanctioned time away, most people return refreshed to their relationships, work, and usual circumstances. Planning for time alone is highly preferable to reaching a breaking point and then aggressively and irresponsibly running away from others.

Physical Health

An important way of taking care of oneself is to provide for the physical health of the body. A proper diet, adequate rest, and exercise rejuvenate and restore the body. All these activities potentially make nurses more alive and better able to share themselves with their clients.

Attending to Internal Stress Signals

Nursing students who read about mental disorders in their textbooks or encounter emotionally disturbed clients commonly begin seeing in themselves all the "symptoms" about which they are learning. This perception is probably due more to the heightened awareness of and attention to the emotional aspects of their lives than to anything else. However, it is important for us to learn to recognize and respond to our own genuine stress signals. All people have times in their lives when they feel a little "crazy." They may become very upset at small disturbances or see things out of proportion to their ultimate importance. These feelings are significant warning signals that one is not coping adequately with stress.

"Crazy" times can be important turning points in people's lives. They are strong messages that change is needed. It is foolish to ignore these messages. In their daily lives, nurses are often tempted to handle their own symptoms of stress by suppressing them with tranquilizers or other drugs. They could serve themselves better by really experiencing their feelings and attending to what the signals are saying. Help in managing stress creatively is the subject of Chapters 8 and 33∞. Using the strategies and therapies recommended in these chapters will help nurses to gain control of their lives and ease tension before it becomes unmanageable.

Pain and suffering are sources of some of the most intensely experienced stresses in life. Events such as the death of loved ones, divorce, illness, separation from loved ones, and failure are all part of the cycle of life's experience. Being told that they deserve it, or that they really don't have it so bad and therefore have no right to feel the way they feel, does not help people cope with pain and suffering. People want to continue what *was* instead of living with what *is*. They need to find ways of handling suffering without being destroyed by it. Some people need to replace what they have lost with something similar. Others need to explore a new dimension in their lives. Classmates, friends, and family members can be great sources of support. Being able to both give and receive support strengthens the individual.

According to an old Buddhist teaching, a third of people's suffering is inevitable but they themselves create the rest of it. Realizing that pain and hardship are part of what it is to be a human being makes the pain a bit gentler. It is important to attend to genuine feelings about loss or prospective loss. The alternative to experiencing pain is to live on the surface, out of touch with the joyful experiences in life as well as the painful ones. A more life-enhancing approach is to experience all aspects of life.

Burnout

The nurse in the following clinical example verbalizes one of the possible consequences of working intensely with troubled people.

CLINICAL EXAMPLE

"After hours, days, and months of listening to other people's problems, something inside you can go dead and you don't care anymore. That's when you'd rather sit at the desk and do the paperwork than be out talking to clients on the floor."

Burnout is the name given to this phenomenon, a condition in which health care professionals lose their concern and feeling for their clients and come to treat them in detached or even dehumanized ways. Burnout happens to poverty lawyers, social workers, clinical psychologists, childcare workers, prison personnel, and others who struggle to retain both their objectivity and their concern for the people with whom they work. It is an attempt to cope, by distancing oneself, with the stresses of intense interpersonal work. It hurts not only clients but also mental health professionals, in that they become ineffective and dissatisfied.

In many cases, burning out involves not only thinking in derogatory terms about clients but also believing that somehow clients deserve any problem they have. Benner and Wrubel (1989), who have studied both caring and burnout, caution us not to make the mistake of thinking that caring is the cause of burnout and thus try to prevent the "disease" of burnout by protecting ourselves from caring. According to them, the sickness is the loss of caring, and the return of caring is the recovery.

There is little doubt that burnout plays a major role in the poor delivery of psychiatric care. It is also a key factor in low staff morale, absenteeism, and high job turnover.

Cues to Burnout

Cues to burnout can be found in the language used to describe clients. Burnout victims may refer to their clients as "crocks," "vegetables," "wackos," and so forth, or they may become highly analytic and abstract: "That's just a manifestation of his primary process thinking." Another cue is lack of involvement with clients. Some nurses "hide" in the nurses' station or staff conference room to avoid interacting. Some openly reject bids for human contact. "Going by the book" rather than considering the unique factors in a situation is a way of minimizing personal involvement with the client. By rigidly applying the rules, one can avoid thinking about the client's specific problems. Burnout can transform an original and creative nurse into a mechanical bureaucrat.

Another cue to burnout is joking put-downs, such as those in the following clinical example, which make mental health work seem less frightening and overwhelming.

CLINICAL EXAMPLE

When the nurse is asked where Mr. Grant is, she laughingly reports that he's taking a shower in preparation for his MMPI test. Everyone in the nurses' station breaks up in gales of laughter.

In a discharge conference, the psychiatrist says he'd like to discharge Earl, a young male client with a history of violent outbursts. The nurse replies, "With or without a baseball bat?" and everyone chuckles.

Reducing Burnout

Most research, such as that referred to in the Evidence-Based Practice feature on page 36, indicates that the causes of professional burnout are rooted not in the permanent psychologic characteristics of individuals but rather in the social context of their work. Most nurses usually expect the presence of negative conditions: large client loads, time pressures, and daily confrontation with suffering, pain, and death. It is the absence of positive factors—a sense of significance, rewarding interpersonal relationships, the appreciation of others, challenge, and variety—that is most distressing. The strategies listed in the Your Intervention Strategies feature can be used to reduce and modify the occurrence of burnout.

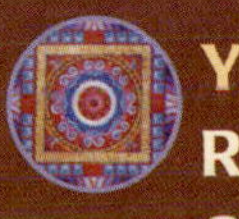

YOUR INTERVENTION STRATEGIES
Reduce and Modify the Occurrence of Burnout

- Request a lower staff–client ratio. You can then give more attention to each client and have time to focus on the positive, nonproblematic aspects of the client's life.
- Recognize that no one is perfect. Your clients deserve the best care you can provide; it may not always be perfect care, and it isn't 24-hours-a-day, 7-days-a-week care.
- Take all sanctioned breaks rather than guilt-provoking escapes from the work situation.
- Talk over your problems to get advice and support when you need it.
- Express, analyze, and share your feelings about burning out. This lets you get things off your chest and gives you the chance to get constructive feedback from others and perhaps a new perspective as well.
- Understand your own motivations in pursuing a psychiatric–mental health nursing career and recognize your expectations for work with clients. Deal with your clients' problems, not your own.
- Attend to your own internal stress signals.
- Pursue happiness and satisfaction in your personal life through family, friends, social or spiritual organizations, and hobbies and recreational interests.

MEDIALINK Care Plan: Managing Burnout on the Unit

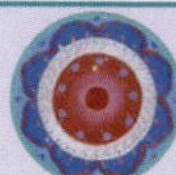

EVIDENCE-BASED PRACTICE

IMPROVING PRACTICE AND AVOIDING BURNOUT

You and a colleague work in the medication clinic of a community mental health center. Both of you have talked about your increasing dissatisfaction with your job. You feel burdened. There are too many clients and too little time. You feel that you don't get enough feedback on your performance from the more experienced nurses. The improvements you would like to make—medication education groups for family members, for example—are impossible to implement given the workload. Neither you nor your colleague feels that you are doing the best you can for your clients and their families. You decide to approach the administration to ask for the following:

1. Hiring another nurse to decrease the workload
2. Regularly scheduled time for clinical supervision by the more experienced nurses
3. Adding a weekly medication education group for family members

Your requests are based on the following nursing research:

Begat, I., Ellefsen, B. & Severinsson, E. (2005). Nurses' satisfaction with their work environment and the outcomes of clinical nursing supervision on nurses' experiences of well-being—a Norwegian study. *Journal of Nursing Management, 13*(3), 221–230.

Edwards, D., Burnard, P., Hannigan, B., Cooper, L., Adams, J., Juggessur, T., et al. (2006). Clinical supervision and burnout: The influence of clinical supervision for community mental health nurses. *Journal of Clinical Nursing, 15*(8), 1007–1015.

CRITICAL THINKING QUESTIONS

1. What relationship do you see between your experience at the medication clinic and the issue of burnout?
2. How do you deal with feeling that you are not doing the best you can for your clients and their families?
3. What are the essential elements to keep in mind when approaching the administration to make your requests?

QUALITIES FOR INTERPERSONAL COMPETENCE

Self-awareness, empathy, and moral integrity all enable psychiatric nurses to practice the use of self artfully in therapeutic relationships. Some characteristics of artful therapeutic practice are respect for the client, availability, spontaneity, hope, acceptance, sensitivity, vision, accountability, advocacy, spirituality, empathy, critical thinking, and self-disclosure. These personal characteristics make a therapeutic alliance with the client possible. A **therapeutic alliance** is a conscious, growth-facilitating relationship between a helping person (the psychiatric–mental health nurse) and the client. The use of the therapeutic alliance in one-to-one work with individual clients is the subject of Chapter 29.

MEDIALINK Case Study: Therapeutic Alliance

Respect for the Client

Respect emerges from the value that human beings have inherent worth and dignity. The behavior of many mental health clients demonstrates their loss of self-respect. Some may appear dirty and disheveled. Others may plead, beg, or cry. Still others may try to do physical harm to themselves or others. A relationship in which they experience a sense of dignity and receive messages of respect from you is of inestimable value. You can convey respect in relationships with clients by:

- Holding personal judgments in check
- Taking the time and energy to listen
- Taking care not to invalidate clients' experience of their world with comments such as "It's not so bad," "Don't be that way," "Time heals all wounds," or "Keep a stiff upper lip."
- Giving clients as much privacy as possible during examinations and treatments or when they are upset
- Minimizing experiences that humiliate clients and strip them of identity, thus allowing them to make as many of their own choices and be in control of as much of their own lives as possible
- Being honest with clients about medicines, treatments, privileges, length of stay, and so on, even when the truth may be difficult to handle
- Holding an inherent but realistic belief in the client's capabilities

Creating an atmosphere that conveys permission for the client to express pain and pleasure also provides an opportunity to demonstrate respect for the client. Expressions of joy and assessments of client abilities, talents, and capabilities are often neglected, but are an essential and respectful element of artful therapeutic practice.

Availability

Of all the members of the mental health team, the nurse has the richest opportunity to be available to clients when needed. Because we are with clients on a relatively constant basis, nurses have the responsibility for:

- Creating a nurturing, healing milieu
- Assisting suffering clients to meet their basic human needs
- Collecting and conveying crucial data about clients that will influence decisions around them

Spontaneity

Many nurses have come to believe that therapeutic relationships with psychiatric clients require them to be stiff, stilted robots uttering clichés from a list of unnatural-sounding communication "techniques." Nurses who are comfortable with themselves, aware of therapeutic goals, and flexible about using a repertoire of possible interventions for any particular clinical problem find that being natural and spontaneous, while keeping therapeutic goals uppermost in their minds, is their most effective "technique." Clients experience such nurses as authentic, that is, showing their real selves, rather than hiding behind the role of nurse. You are unique and necessarily bring your own personal style to practice. We have different ways of putting the words together to convey to clients that we accept and care about them. Sometimes we say it with nonverbal behavior: keeping promises, being on time, touching, and staying with a client who needs someone. We need to trust our own natural styles, combined with sound communication principles such as those discussed in Chapter 10∞, in working toward therapeutic goals.

Hope

Effective mental health–psychiatric nursing practice is characterized by hope and optimism that all clients, no matter how debilitated, have the capacity for growth and change. Even clients whose most marked attributes are chronicity and deterioration can be helped to some optimal level of well-being by a nurse who believes in their possibilities and is willing to search for some strengths on which to build. In a day treatment center, a client joined in a partnership with a creative nurse to assist less able clients toward self-care. This strategy—increasing the connectedness between client and nurse and between client and other clients—decreases the feeling of aloneness while emphasizing the client's ability to manage his illness. It is not unusual in such a situation for the healing to become a source of help to the healer–client.

The primary obstacle to instilling hope is stigma. Remember that many people lead fulfilling lives despite fairly disabling mental illness. You can have a negative impact on clients if you fail to believe in the client's eventual recovery; if you fail to see the client as a person; if you fail to lobby to reduce stigma in both the public and the health care communities; or if you fail to persevere with clients in their journey of recovery.

Acceptance

There is a distinction between acceptance and approval. Acceptance means refraining from judging and rejecting a client who may behave in a way that makes you uncomfortable or that you personally dislike. Clients may feel offended if they perceive the nurse as rejecting them (Hem & Heggen, 2004). Therapeutic work requires that clients be able to examine, explore, and understand their coping mechanisms without feeling the need to cover up or disguise them to avoid negative judgments or punishments. Nurses who tell clients what they should say or do or feel deny these clients the acceptance they need to explore their problems.

Sensitivity

Genuine interest and concern provide the basis for a therapeutic alliance. Clients recognize the falseness of memorized phrases and assumed postures. You convey general interest and concern by trying to understand the client's perspective, working with the client on mutually formulated goals, and persisting even when breakthroughs and improvements are subtle and slow instead of dramatic and quick. A study by Shattell, McAllister, Hogan, and Thomas (2006) determined that understanding the client's perceptions and concerns helps us to connect with our clients, acknowledges their importance, and facilitates the relationship between nurse and client.

Assertiveness

Assertiveness is the ability to express one's feelings, thoughts, and beliefs openly even if doing so is emotionally difficult or personal risk is involved. Assertiveness is a style of interacting with others that protects your rights without depriving others of theirs. It involves standing up for yourself in a nondestructive manner even if your stance is unpopular.

Being assertive in a therapeutic context with clients means that you are able to take advantage of opportunities to make interpersonal contact with clients. Confident nurses are assertive nurses. They recognize that assertiveness and caring are compatible (McCartan & Hargie, 2007).

Often people are either so timid that they do not get what they want or so aggressive and belligerent that they offend and alienate others. Being assertive in one's professional life builds upon being assertive in one's personal life. **Assertive behavior** is asking for what one wants or acting to get it in a way that respects other people. It is midway between **nonassertive behavior** (timid holding back) and **aggressive behavior** (inconsiderate, offensive aggression).

Compare the nonassertive, aggressive, and assertive behaviors listed in the Your Self-Awareness feature on page 38 to see which descriptions best characterize your behavior with others. Fortunately, old behaviors can be unlearned, and new behaviors can be learned.

Passive Behavior

Fear tends to be the major feeling in passive responses—fear of being embarrassed, of disappointing someone, or making someone angry. Because of fear, passive people frequently say "yes" at the expense of their own happiness or well-being, even when they want to say "no." To these individuals, everyone else's feelings and needs are more important than their own. Imagine what could happen if four passive individuals arrive at a four-way stop at approximately the same time. Believing that the others have more important things to do and places to be, none takes the initiative. All are fearful of angering or insulting the others. They sit there, waving one another on. People who consistently give up control are often left with resentment in their interpersonal relationships.

MediaLink Application: Consumers and Psychiatric Nurses in Dialogue

YOUR SELF-AWARENESS
Comparing Your Own Nonassertive, Aggressive, and Assertive Behaviors

Determine which of the following descriptions most closely match your behavior. Once you have finished, develop a personal plan for adopting a wider range of assertive behaviors in both your personal and professional life.

Nonassertive	Aggressive	Assertive
"I'm not angry (but I am scared)!"	"I'm not scared (but I am angry)!"	"I'm both angry and scared!"
"I always do everything wrong."	"They always do everything wrong."	"Neither one of us is perfect, and there's nothing wrong with that."
"I'll try to make it (but I don't intend to because I'm resentful of your demands)."	"You must be crazy if you think I'll be there. Who do you think you are?"	"We should spend some time together and talk about our relationship."
"I never achieve my goals."	"The only way I can achieve my goals is by forcing others to agree with my way of thinking."	"I almost always achieve the goals I set for myself."
"I wish someone else would speak up."	"Be quiet and let me speak. You always monopolize the conversation."	"We can both have a chance to speak."

Aggressive Behavior

Aggressive responses are at the other end of the continuum of interaction. The three hallmarks of aggressive behavior are:

1. The major feeling is anger.
2. The person says "no" even when "yes" could, or should, be said.
3. The aggressive person believes that his or her feelings are more important than the feelings of others.

Generally speaking, people who feel in the least control can be the most aggressive (Dupre & Barling, 2007). Some examples are: a bully, a subordinate at work with little control over others, or someone who shouts angrily, talks over others, and insists there is only one way to do something. Imagine what could happen if four aggressive individuals arrive at a four-way stop at the same time. Each believes that he or she has the most important thing to do or place to be. Each is angry with the others and attempts to be the first to cross the intersection. Perhaps all four crash in the middle of the intersection.

Assertive Behavior

People who focus on neither anger nor fear, respect their own and others' feelings, and say "yes" and "no" appropriately, behave assertively. Imagine what could happen if four assertive individuals arrive at a four-way stop at the same time. Recognizing traffic rules and the rights of others, each allows the person on the right to proceed first.

Everyone has assertiveness potential, but not everyone has learned how to be assertive. You can teach clients and families how to behave assertively by incorporating the guidelines in the Partnering with Clients and Families feature.

Vision

Because psychiatric–mental health nurses focus their work on enhancing the quality of life for all human beings, they must come to terms with a personal and professional vision of what quality means. Some conditions of life associated with high quality are influence or power, freedom, accountability, self-determinism, openness to gratifying experience, action, mastery, a sense of purpose or meaning, privacy, hope, stability, nonviolence, and intimacy.

Accountability

According to Peplau (1980), the need for personal accountability—professional integrity—is greater in psychiatric practice than in any other type of health care. Clients in mental health settings are usually more vulnerable and defenseless than are clients in other health care settings, particularly because their conditions hinder their thinking processes and their relationships with others. Psychiatric–mental health nurses are accountable for the nature of the effort they make on behalf of clients and answerable to clients for the quality of their efforts. As Peplau put it, "Personal accountability is an attitude—a quality of the heart and mind of those professionals who are competent and determined that every psychiatric patient will have the best problem-resolving assistance possible" (1980, p. 133).

Psychiatric–mental health nurses are accountable to themselves, their peers, their profession, and the public in the following ways:

- Accountability to self involves bringing personal behavior under conscious control so that the nurse becomes the person-as-nurse she or he wants to be.
- Accountability to peers involves engaging in peer review with nurse colleagues to give and receive feedback intended to improve the quality of care.
- Accountability to the profession involves clarifying the role of the mental health–psychiatric nurse, keeping current with changes in the field, and

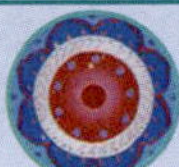

PARTNERING WITH CLIENTS AND FAMILIES

TEACHING ABOUT ASSERTIVENESS

Discuss the following elements of assertive behavior with clients and their families in order to encourage self-confidence and self-control.

1. Identify your usual patterns of behavior. Are you passive, aggressive, or assertive in dealing with others?
2. Deliberately work on changing your pattern of thinking. Assertive people do not respond automatically; they take time to look at a situation and plan their response. Avoid being pressured into a quick decision. Instead, say "I need some time to think about that."
3. Choose not to be responsible for the feelings of others when you know your actions were reasonable. In other words, avoid feeling guilty about being assertive.
4. Stand firm without precipitating an argument. Use the broken-record technique—calmly repeat an assertive statement over and over ("I really don't like violent movies") until the other person hears you.
5. Recognize that it is unrealistic to expect others to read your mind. Instead, use assertive statements of feeling such as: "Something is bothering me. I feel as if my movie preferences don't matter to you."
6. Choose to remain in control of yourself. Focus on remaining relaxed and calm. Breathe deeply, consciously relax your muscles, make eye contact, and speak in an even tone of voice.
7. Use "I" statements, such as: "I am feeling on the spot. I want to have a nice evening with you, but I also want to see a movie I can enjoy." By making it clear that you are expressing your own feelings and opinions you help the other person to be nondefensive and able to listen to what you are saying.
8. Be patient, give yourself a chance, and don't expect too much too soon. Change comes about slowly with repeated practice.
9. Begin with small steps. A few successes will give you confidence. Go slowly and build a solid foundation.
10. Remember to give yourself due credit for successfully asserting yourself. Ask for qualified help—a teacher, a counselor, an assertive person—when you need it.

encouraging self-regulation to protect the public and enhance the quality of care.

- Accountability to the public requires keeping abreast of knowledge in the field, becoming credentialed according to level of competence, applying the ANA standards of psychiatric–mental health nursing practice (discussed in Chapter 2∞), and protecting the rights of clients and their families (discussed in Chapter 13∞).

The personally accountable psychiatric–mental health nurse will insist on clinical supervision. Supervision provides novice as well as experienced nurses with the opportunity to learn therapeutic techniques and attitudes. It enables them to receive validation, insight, and support during the difficult times that may accompany therapeutic relationships (Laskowski, 2001) and enables them to analyze how they affect the outcome of the relationship.

Advocacy

Throughout history, psychiatric–mental health nurses have been ardent supporters of a neglected, ignored, and forgotten population—the mentally ill. In the 21st century, there is a need for new energy and political activism. In this era of health care reform, there is an especially important concern—ensuring that the needs and the rights of mentally disordered people are not overlooked or ignored while the explosion of knowledge in science and technology revolutionizes how nurses practice mental health care.

Nurses are more politically aware than ever before. A newly energized political activism calls for nurses to speak out publicly for the health, welfare, and safety of their clients; to take steps to protect client rights; to write articles for the popular press; to lobby their congressional representatives on behalf of better mental health for all people; and to run for political office. The power that such a large group of citizen nurses could wield on behalf of their clients would be awesome.

Successful advocacy is a positive experience for nurses as well as for clients. Clients derive a benefit, and we feel good about our ability to be agents of change. Be aware, however, that not all advocating will be successful. Sometimes, despite our most earnest and well-intentioned efforts, we fail in our attempt to advocate for positive change for our clients. Be prepared—according to Austin, Bergum, and Goldberg (2003), unsuccessful advocating may lead to frustration, anger, burnout, and moral distress for you.

Spirituality

Spirituality, the search for meaning and purpose in life through a connection with others, nature, and/or a belief in a higher power (Buck, 2006), is at the core of each person's existence. Spirituality varies in strength from person to person. Some people already have a meaningful philosophy of life. Others, on a spiritual journey, search for life's meaning and purpose. Still others experience hopelessness, despair, and spiritual distress. Helping clients find meaning and purpose in their lives empowers them.

For some clients, their spirituality becomes a central focus in their treatment. They may attempt to resolve internal conflicts or conflicts with others through religious rituals or practices. Other clients will have maladaptive behavior that involves religiosity. (To differentiate between religiosity

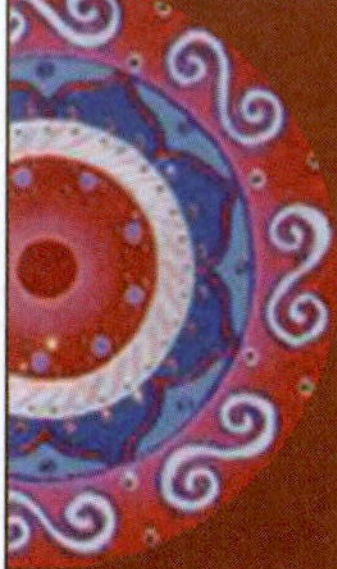

CARING FOR THE SPIRIT

Spirituality: The Connection Between Mental Health and Mental Illness

Spirituality is the third part of the triad known as mind–body–spirit in the holistic practice of nursing. In ancient times, spirit meant breath—as essential to life as air. Spirituality is that part of every person that yearns to share the beauty, love, and joyfulness of the universe.

We take our spirituality from many sources: Nature, God, Buddha, Higher Power, Goddess, Krishna, B'ahaullah, Mohammed, Yahweh, and others. Although many of these sources are incorporated into organized religions, spirituality is not religion, nor is religion spirituality. Religion is the organization of a set of beliefs, practices, and rituals, whereas spirituality is a reflection of one's "spirit" and its relationship to the rest of the universe.

Some people develop their spirituality throughout life with prayer, meditation, and reflection. Others may leave the spiritual path because of conflicts with religious beliefs, values, and practices, because of toxic family relationships, or because they are too busy trying to survive physically and mentally.

Even though spirituality is one of the three central aspects of the holistic practice of nursing, the physical, emotional, mental, and social aspects get most, if not all, of the mental health specialist's attention.

Spirituality may be an important connection between mental health and mental illness. In mental illness, most clients describe feeling "disconnected" from their families, their friends, the universe itself, and from their "faith." For example, clients describe depression as similar to being in a gray or black tunnel with a profound sense of disconnectedness.

Imagine what it would be like to go for 24 hours or longer without sleep. How would you look? Would you feel disconnected or disoriented? Ask someone with mania what that's like. Have you ever awakened suddenly and not known where you are? How would it be to feel like that for an hour, a whole day, or a month? Ask someone with schizophrenia what that's like. Perhaps you've driven down the road and realized that you're confused about where you are and how you got there. And what if you had voices inside your head at the same time? Would this be frightening? Would you feel disconnected?

It may be that a psychiatric crisis has also brought forth a spiritual crisis. The client may, for the first time, be faced with looking at the three spiritual questions of life.

1. "What have I placed on life's altar? Of what value is my life? Why was I born, anyway? I have nothing to give." These are the words of someone who is depressed or actively suicidal.
2. "What do I hold to be sacred?" What things are important to the client, what things have meaning?
3. "How do I know what's true?" The client with anxiety or psychosis has great difficulty sorting out what's real and what's not real, determining what's true and what's not true. Life as we know it has many dichotomies. The unanswerable becomes even more of a challenge when a psychiatric crisis emerges.

Recall what happened to your relationships with friends and family when you were in a personal crisis. Did the relationships change? Our cognitive sphere, our affective sphere, and our relational sphere are all affected. We lose our centering of purpose, of sacredness, of reality. We lose our spirit and become disconnected. Do you think your clients' relationships change when they are in a crisis?

Helping clients rediscover their spiritual path is a fulfilling role for psychiatric–mental health nurses. You can help clients find out who they really are, beyond, for example, simply husband, father, lover, police officer. Help them identify the source of their inner energy and how to get in touch with their "center" or their "soul." Keep in mind that spirituality is a deeply personal inner experience as opposed to a set of behaviors tied to an externally imposed doctrine or ritual. By offering a simple spirituality inventory, such as that in the Caring for the Spirit: Spiritual Health Assessment box in Chapter 11 ∞, you will encourage clients to look at the strength of their faith, which will help them with their recovery. Faith is a way of being—being open to possibilities, and to healing.

and spirituality, see the Caring for the Spirit feature.) Recent research indicates that the connection between mind, body, and spirit is complex and that spirituality is influenced by culture (Baldacchino, 2006).

You need to be aware of the client's concept of God, the client's source of hope and strength, the significance or insignificance of religious practice and rituals in the client's life, the client's thinking about the relationship between spiritual beliefs and mental health, and the client's fear of alienation, loneliness, or solitude (Wilkinson, 2007).

Helping clients in their search for meaning and purpose is possible when nurses have beliefs that sustain them rather than beliefs that are sources of conflict (Taylor, 2002). You must meet your own spiritual needs satisfactorily before you can have a meaningful relationship with your clients. Take the time to carefully consider the questions in Caring for the Spirit: Your Personal Journey of Spiritual Growth to determine whether you meet your own spiritual needs satisfactorily.

Empathy

Comprehension of and ability to use the process of empathy is one strategy for responding to the feelings of aloneness often experienced by people who are psychiatric clients. Perhaps the most important function of empathic understanding is to give the client the very precious feeling of being understood and cared about.

Empathy is a pervasive phenomenon in the life experience of all people. **Empathy** can be defined as the ability to feel what others feel and respond to and understand the experience of others on their terms. A nurse who empathizes with a client momentarily abandons the personal self and relives the emotions and responses of someone else. People in everyday life tend to empathize most with those to whom they feel closest. In mental health work, we must seek to empathize with those from whom we feel most separate or whose closeness threatens our own sense of integration.

The capacity for empathy relies on personal integration. A firm sense of self is necessary for a person to be a good empathizer. As we continue to interact with others, we learn to be sensitive to others without losing our own integration. Empathy is also discussed in Chapter 10∞.

Critical Thinking

The ability to think critically is crucial for psychiatric–mental health nurses. Critical thinking is the means by which we transfer nursing knowledge into clinical practice (Wilkinson, 2007). It is a purposeful mental activity in which ideas are produced and evaluated and judgments are made. A critical thinker analyzes information before drawing conclusions about it. **Critical thinking** can be defined as purposeful, reasonable, reflective thinking that drives problem solving and decision making and aims to make judgments based on evidence (Alfaro-LeFevre, 2001). To encourage you to think critically, we have provided critical thinking challenges at the beginning of every chapter and critical thinking questions at the end of every Evidence-Based Practice feature. To develop effective, critical thinking habits, implement the strategies that are suggested in the Your Intervention Strategies feature on page 42.

MEDIALINK Critical Thinking Exercise: Empathy and Respect

Self-Disclosure

Self-disclosure means being open to personal feelings and experiences, being "real" as opposed to hiding behind a professional facade.

How much should a nurse share with a client? Under what circumstances is it appropriate? The wisdom of disclosing personal information to clients has been the subject of much debate. Some argue that self-disclosure impedes therapeutic work; others argue just the opposite—that self-disclosure facilitates therapeutic work. A study by Barrett and Berman (2001) of clients at a university counseling center revealed that clients not only liked self-disclosing therapists more but also reported lower levels of symptom distress. A study that examined how community mental health nurses promoted wellness with young adult clients who were experiencing an early episode of psychotic illness found that revealing oneself put both clients and nurses at ease and helped to dispel clients' perception that they take part in a one-sided relationship (McCann & Baker, 2001). How much to share, and under what circumstances, remains an area for further research.

It may be helpful to view self-disclosure on a continuum. One end represents underdisclosure; the other overdisclosure. When evaluating any self-disclosure at a given time, ask yourself the questions in the Your Self-Awareness feature on page 42.

Facilitative self-disclosure must be judiciously used within the context of the therapeutic relationship, where attention is given to its timing, appropriateness, and degree. For example, use self-disclosure cautiously with a severely dysfunctional client with poor ego boundaries. This client may not be able to separate thoughts and feelings that belong to the client from those that belong to the nurse. The client might misinterpret the nurse's self-disclosure or might not be able to make sense of the disclosure. The client may also fear engulfment; that is, the nurse's feelings might be perceived as so threatening that they overwhelm the client. Self-disclosure

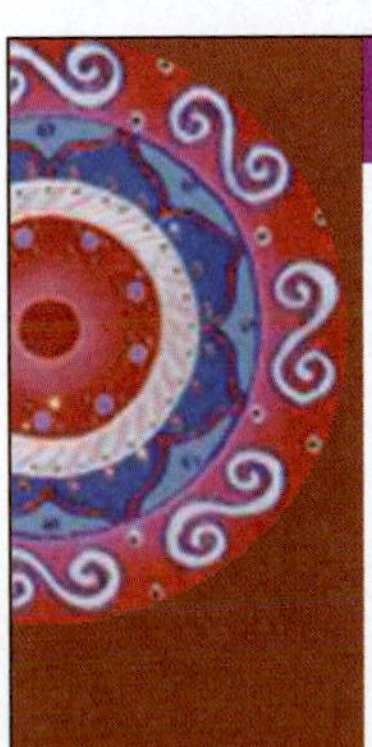

CARING FOR THE SPIRIT

Your Personal Journey of Spiritual Growth

To help you on your personal journey of spiritual growth, contemplate these questions:

1. What gives the greatest meaning or purpose to your life?
2. How do you express your spirituality or your philosophy of life?
3. How does God/Higher Power/Ultimate Other/The Transcendent function in your personal life?
4. What kinds of confusion or doubt do you have about your religious beliefs?
5. What do you do to show love for yourself?
6. What brings you joy and peace in your life?
7. How do you heal your spirit?
8. What art, music, or literature nurtures your spirit?
9. How does your spirituality affect your experience as a nurse?

Answering these questions, eventually fully, and asking yourself how you can change your situation will make you a spiritual activist for yourself and for your clients.

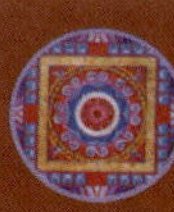

YOUR INTERVENTION STRATEGIES
Promote Critical Thinking

Strategy	Rationale
Anticipate questions others might ask, such as "What will my supervisor or instructor want to know?"	This helps identify a wider scope of questions that must be answered to gain relevant information.
Ask "What if" questions like "What if something goes wrong?" or "What if we try?"	This helps you be proactive and creative.
Look for flaws in your thinking. Ask questions like, "What's missing?" "Have I recognized my biases?" "How could this be made better?"	Such questions help you evaluate your thinking and make improvements.
Ask someone else to look for flaws in your thinking.	You're usually too close to your own work to be objective; others bring a fresh eye and possibly new ideas and perspectives.
Develop "good habits of inquiry" (habits that aid in the search for the truth, such as always keeping an open mind, verifying information, and taking enough time).	These habits can make critical thinking more automatic.
Develop interpersonal skills, such as conflict resolution and getting along with those who have different communication styles.	If you don't have good interpersonal skills, you're unlikely to get the help or information you need to think critically.
Replace "I don't know" and "I'm not sure" with "I'll try."	This demonstrates you have the ability to find answers and mobilizes you to locate resources.
Turn errors into learning opportunities.	We all make mistakes; they're stepping stones to maturity and new ideas. If you aren't making mistakes, maybe you're not trying hard enough.

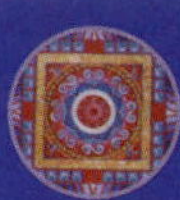

YOUR SELF-AWARENESS
Self-Disclosure

Determining whether or not to self-disclose will be made clearer by answering these questions:

- What is the purpose of the revelation; who is this self-disclosure for?
- Does this self-disclosure meet the client's therapeutic goals, or does it meet my needs?
- Will this self-disclosure take the focus away from the client?
- Does this self-disclosure foster the development of a more productive therapeutic relationship?
  1. Will it encourage the client to disclose what the client has withheld or suppressed?
  2. Will it encourage the client's cooperation?
  3. Will it help the client to consider another point of view?
  4. Will it support the client's positive movement in addressing life problems?
  5. Will it encourage empathic understanding?

should foster the development of the therapeutic relationship rather than threaten its continuance. Beginning nurses should always discuss self-disclosure with an instructor/supervisor first.

When the nurse discloses personal information, evaluation must follow. The client's reaction and subsequent exploration together can be a gauge for measuring how this client perceives and responds to self-disclosures by the nurse. As the nurse expresses feelings about the evolving relationship, the client may feel free to reciprocate. At times, the nurse may choose to role-model emotive expression.

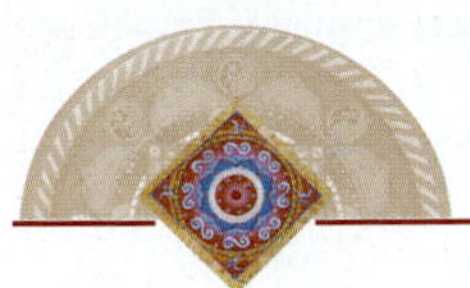

EXPLORE MediaLink 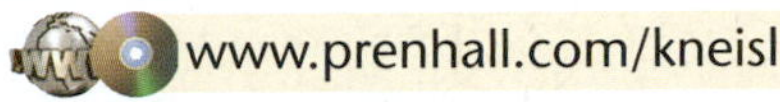

For NCLEX-RN® review questions, case studies, and other resources for this chapter see the Pearson Health MediaLink CD-ROM that accompanies this book and the Companion Website at www.prenhall.com/kneisl.

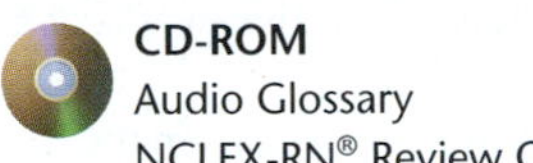

CD-ROM
Audio Glossary
NCLEX-RN® Review Questions

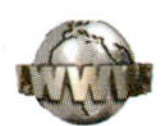

Companion Website
Audio Glossary
NCLEX-RN® Review Questions
Critical Thinking Exercise
- *Empathy and Respect*

Case Study
- *Forming a Therapeutic Alliance with Clients*

Care Plan
- *Managing Burnout on the Unit*

MediaLinks
MediaLink Application
- *Consumers and Psychiatric–Mental Health Nurses in Dialogue*

NCLEX-RN® REVIEW QUESTIONS

1. The concept of blaming as the cause of mental illness is based on the belief that:
1. A higher authority is responsible for the onset of symptoms.
2. Mental illness is hereditary.
3. People cause their own problems.
4. Individuals are responsible to solve their own problems.

2. Detached concern means that the nurse:
1. Willingly agrees to do something even though he or she does not want to.
2. Emotionally distances himself or herself in order to help others.
3. Believes people do not create their own problems.
4. Represses beliefs or attitudes that are inconsistent with the client's.

3. The Enlightenment Model of Thinking reflects the belief that:
1. People create their own problems but need to rely on others to solve them.
2. People do not create their own problems and are not responsible for solving them.
3. People cause their own problems and should be responsible for finding solutions to them.
4. People should not be blamed for their problems, but should be involved in the problem-solving process.

4. To address the cultural needs of a client, the nurse will:
1. Provide the same care that has been provided to other clients.
2. Ask other nurses what the client's needs are.
3. Ask clients what cultural issues are important to them.
4. Read current literature on a specific culture.

5. The nurse can reduce the risk of burnout by:
1. Teaching clients to accept responsibility for their illness.
2. Acknowledging that the nurse's own feelings are more important than the feelings of others.
3. Recognizing and responding to his or her own internal stress signals.
4. Planning time alone with limited social contacts and interactions.

6. The nurse is teaching a group of clients how to use assertive behavior to increase their self-confidence. The nurse explains that assertive behavior includes:
1. The belief that other people's needs are more important than your own.
2. A timid, reserved demeanor.
3. Demanding that you be heard before others have a chance to speak.
4. The ability to ask for what you want while respecting other people.

7. ________ in psychiatric–mental health involves maintaining current knowledge and self-regulation to protect the quality of client care.
   1. Advocacy
   2. Self-awareness
   3. Accountability
   4. Critical thinking

8. The nurse conveys a caring, respectful attitude toward a client when the nurse says:
   1. "Why did you do that?"
   2. "I want to make sure I understood what you said."
   3. "The doctor knows what is best for you."
   4. "Don't worry about those symptoms; they are normal for your illness."

9. Which of the following statements reflects empathy for a client?
   1. "I know exactly how you feel. The same thing happened to me."
   2. "Don't worry. I know things will get better soon."
   3. "I don't know how you feel, but I hear what you are saying."
   4. "It may feel overwhelming now, but things could be worse."

10. To effectively address a client's spiritual needs the nurse should be knowledgeable about:
   1. The significance of religious practices and rituals in the client's life.
   2. The client's prognosis for recovery.
   3. The client's specific religious affiliation.
   4. The nurse's own individual spirituality.

See Appendix C for answers.

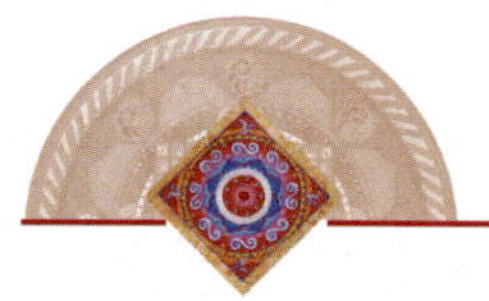

REFERENCES

Alfaro-LeFevre, R. (2001, March). Improving your ability to think critically. *Nursing Spectrum*, 25–30.

Austin, W., Bergum, V., & Goldberg, L. (2003). Unable to answer the call of our patients: Mental health nurses' experience of moral distress. *Nursing Inquiry, 10*(3), 177–183.

Baldacchino, D. R. (2006). Nursing competencies for spiritual care. *Journal of Clinical Nursing, 15*(7), 885–896.

Barrett, M. S., & Berman, J. S. (2001). Is psychotherapy more effective when therapists disclose information about themselves? *Journal of Consulting Clinical Psychology, 69*(4), 597–603.

Begat, I., Ellefsen, B., & Severinsson, E. (2005). Nurses' satisfaction with their work environment and the outcomes of clinical nursing supervision of nurses' experiences of well-being—a Norwegian study. *Journal of Nursing Management, 13*(3), 221–230.

Benner, P., & Wrubel, J. (Eds.) (1989). Coping with caregiving. In *The primacy of caring: Stress and coping in health and illness* (pp. 365–406). Menlo Park, CA: Addison-Wesley.

Brickman, P., Rabinowitz, V. C., Karuza, J., Coates, D., Cohn, E., & Kidder, L. (1982). Models of helping and coping. *American Psychologist, 37*(4), 368–384.

Buck, H. G. (2006). Spirituality: Concept analysis and model development. *Holistic Nursing Practice, 20*(6), 288–292.

Dupre, K. E., & Barling, J. (2007). Predicting and preventing supervisory workplace aggression. *Journal of Occupational Health, 11*(1), 13–26.

Edwards, D., Burnard, P., Hannigan, B., Cooper, L., Adams, J., Juggessur, T., et al. (2006). Clinical supervision and burnout: The influence of clinical supervision for community mental health nurses. *Journal of Clinical Nursing, 15*(8), 1007–1015.

Hem, M. H., & Heggen, K. (2004). Rejection—a neglected phenomenon in psychiatric nursing. *Journal of Psychiatric and Mental Health Nursing, 11*(1), 55–63.

Laskowski, C. (2001). The mental health clinical nurse specialist and the "difficult" patient. *Issues in Mental Health Nursing, 22*(1), 5–22.

McCann, T. B., & Baker, H. (2001). Mutual relating: Developing interpersonal relationships in the community. *Journal of Advanced Nursing, 34*(4), 530–537.

McCartan, P. J., & Hargie, O. D. W. (2007). Assertiveness and caring: Are they compatible. *Journal of Advanced Nursing, 13*, 707–713.

Peplau, H. E. (1980). The psychiatric nurse—accountable? To whom? For what? *Perspectives in Psychiatric Care, 18*(3), 128–134.

Shattell, M. M., McAllister, S., Hogan, B., & Thomas, S. P. (2006). "She took the time to make sure she understood": Mental health patients' experiences of being understood. *Archives of Psychiatric Nursing, 20*(5), 234–241.

Taylor, E. J. (2002). *Spiritual care*. Upper Saddle River, NJ: Prentice Hall.

Wilkinson, J. M. (2007). *Nursing process and critical thinking*. Upper Saddle River, NJ: Prentice Hall.

ADDITIONAL REFERENCES

Graber, D. R., & Mitcham, M. D. (2004). Compassionate clinicians: Taking patient care beyond the ordinary. *Holistic Nursing Practice, 18*(2), 87–94.

Gustafson, C., & Fagerberg, I. (2004). Reflection, the way to professional development? *Journal of Clinical Nursing, 13*, 271–280.

Hart, S. E. (2005). Hospital ethical climates and registered nurses' turnover intentions. *Journal of Nursing Scholarship, 37*(2), 173–177.

Hem, M. H., & Heggen, K. (2003). Being professional and being human: One nurse's relationship with a psychiatric patient. *Journal of Advanced Nursing, 43*(1), 101–108.

Spector, R. E. (2006). *Cultural diversity in health and illness* (6th ed.). Upper Saddle River, NJ: Prentice Hall.

Engaging in Evidence-Based Practice

CHAPTER

4

EILEEN TRIGOBOFF

LEARNING OUTCOMES

After completing this chapter, you will be able to:

1. Explain how evidence-based practice translates into how we function as nurses.
2. Describe an evidence-based practice in contemporary psychiatric–mental health nursing.
3. Explain why critical thinking skills are essential to evidence-based practice.
4. Identify the steps in developing evidence-based psychiatric nursing care.
5. Determine how to find the best evidence on which to base your practice.
6. Discuss how to evaluate evidence.

KEY TERMS

best practices *48*
clinical algorithms *49*
critical pathways *49*
ethnography *58*
evidence-based practice *47*
meta-analyses *49*
practice guidelines *50*
randomized clinical trials *58*

CRITICAL THINKING CHALLENGE

The world of research has a variety of designs for exploration and explanation. One of these designs is the placebo-controlled, double-blind study, in which one or more groups of participants receive a placebo instead of an active medication and neither the participants nor the researchers know which participants are receiving a placebo. The results of a placebo-controlled double-blind study are far less likely to be influenced by opinion, bias, or preconceived notions. You work in an inpatient behavioral health unit in a medical center. Five clients on your unit are participating in a placebo-controlled, double-blind study evaluating the clinical effectiveness of a new medication for schizophrenia.

1. What are your thoughts on giving a placebo to participants who have been diagnosed with a mental disorder?
2. Do the benefits of the information gained by this design balance out the risks of not giving an active medication that would treat the disorder?
3. Following the study's completion, do you think participants and clinicians should have access to information about whether an active medication or a placebo was used during the study?
4. Another issue within evidence-based practice is the value of the evidence. If a study is conducted with mildly to moderately ill outpatients, will it have relevance for your practice in an inpatient behavioral health unit in a medical center? How would you determine what was useful?

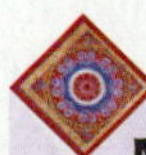

MEDIALINK 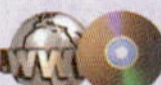 www.prenhall.com/kneisl

Go to the Pearson Health MediaLink CD-ROM and the Companion Website at www.prenhall.com/kneisl for interactive resources for this chapter.

There are many ways to enhance your nursing skills and make your practice effective and meaningful. Learning about mental disorders throughout your career contributes to your skill level, helps you assess the impact of your interventions, and stimulates you to think about what recipients of care might need. One of your main learning resources will be nursing research. Examples of what you can learn include teaching the chronically mentally ill to wash their own clothes and shop for their own food, inviting dancers and musicians into geropsychiatric settings to provide stimulation and enhance quality of life, consulting about what psychotropic medications are safe to give to a dehydrated homeless person in the emergency room, leading groups in which grieving parents feel free to express their feelings, and establishing therapeutic relationships with individuals who struggle through personal crises.

Nurses accept the challenge of questioning, documenting, measuring, and determining—with evidence—the outcomes of their interventions and the degree to which they succeed and fail. Conditions in the contemporary mental health care environment demand that our caring be linked with accountability for client outcomes as well as cost containment. We must, to the extent possible, base psychiatric–mental health nursing on sound, convincing evidence.

In this textbook you will find one perspective of what evidence-based practice means and how to engage in it. Each chapter presents: (a) a clinical case example in which existing research can help guide decisions for care (e.g., Evidence-Based Practice feature); (b) a critical thinking challenge that prompts you to improve your critical thinking skills; (c) a bibliography of current and selected classic references that offers you the most contemporary resources about what is known; and (d) information, examples, strategies, interventions, and summaries of the best evidence currently available presented in a variety of styles (text, boxes, figures, tables, and a website that links to other online resources) to fit the way you learn.

Psychiatric–mental health nursing does not yet have sufficient evidence from traditional science to guide all our practices. The research evidence available may answer your questions to some extent, and may give you enough information to ask better questions. However, our needs exceed what is available, and many areas need to be explored through research to provide the evidence that guides practice. When that evidence becomes available, evaluating the usefulness of a particular piece of research evidence requires some skepticism. FIGURE 4-1 ■ illustrates the steps of traditional science in which hypotheses are tested by conducting controlled experiments and a conclusion is reached about a scientific question. This chapter will guide you through the process of finding, evaluating, and using evidence on which to base your best practices.

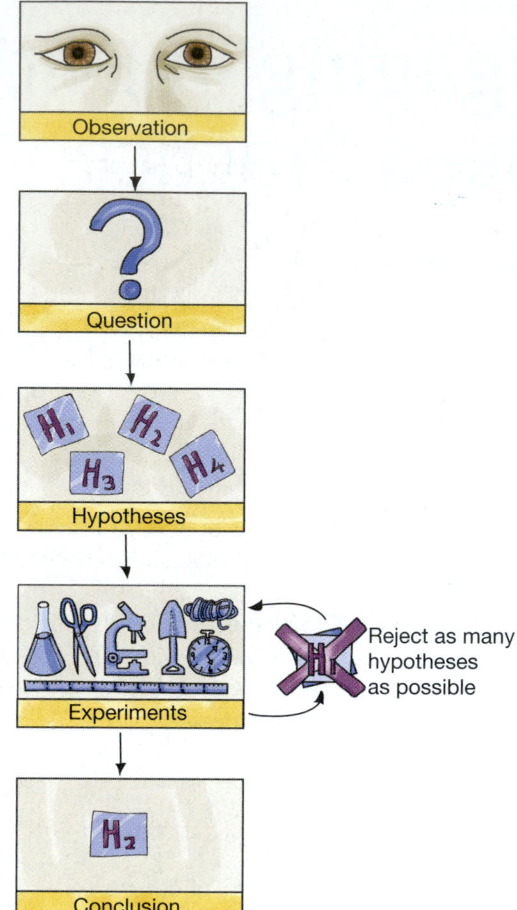

FIGURE 4-1 ■ The traditional scientific method for testing hypotheses to answer questions.

CONTEMPORARY CONDITIONS MANDATING EVIDENCE-BASED PRACTICE

Health care reform in the 21st century has had a profound effect on the way psychiatric care is delivered throughout the world. The length of hospital stays has decreased while client acuity has increased. A knowledge explosion in the neurosciences has contributed to our conception of the basis of each mental disorder. Innovations in technology have broadened diagnostic practices, including sophisticated brain imaging. The array of psychopharmacologic treatments available is continually expanding. The study of stem cells and genome research encourages us to look forward to a time when medications specifically target an individual's disease, yet inspire continuing ethical debate. Spirituality has become an active treatment area for clients in psychiatric–mental health settings as well as other specialty areas in nursing. A global economy continues to transform the way mental health care is provided to diverse populations and particularly the way information, including research evidence, is communicated and disseminated. All of these conditions continue to shape the specialty area of psychiatric–mental health nursing.

Populations of psychiatric clients have changed recently. They have become more racially and culturally diverse and include growing numbers of young people with serious mental illnesses, mentally ill elders, people with coexisting substance use disorders, and comorbidities with other mental illnesses and chronic illnesses such as HIV/AIDS. The streamlining of psychiatric services and sites where psychiatric–mental health nurses practice has expanded to include, besides rehabilitation-oriented inpatient units and psychiatric hospitals, services that are community-based, including those in homeless shelters, nursing homes, on the streets, and in the forensic settings of jails and prisons. As members of interdisciplinary teams, psychiatric–mental health nurses are challenged to tailor and humanize technologies for clients within these conditions.

It is intriguing and satisfying to move through the process of research. Each step, from the opening idea to the end result, where conclusions are discussed and considered, offers an opportunity to clarify your questions and shape your nursing care. In this way, research paves the way for better practice. Evidence-based practice that arises from a team of nurses and other professionals conducting inpatient and outpatient research and developing effective programs promotes high-quality client care (Bauer-Wu, Epshtein, & Reid Ponte, 2006), which is the goal of every professional.

WHAT IS EVIDENCE-BASED PRACTICE?

Evidence-based practice is the integration of individual clinical expertise with the best available external clinical evidence from systematic research. Research produces outcomes and evidence that must be evaluated for usefulness and application to your situation. The Joanna Briggs Institute (JBI), the international research and development unit of Royal Adelaide Hospital in Australia, identifies evidence as coming from a diverse range of sources including experience, expertise, and all forms of rigorous research. The translation, transfer, and use of the best available evidence into health care practice is best accomplished with a logical system that grades evidence based on its usefulness. The categories developed by JBI in 2006 identify the level of evidence and describe a way to grade any recommendations the research outcome suggests. For example, if a study is scientifically sound and chances of error have been reduced to a minimum, it would receive a better grade than a study that examined too few people or had multiple explanations for the outcomes. Research results are given letter grades ranging from the highest, A (effectiveness established to a degree that merits application), through the lowest, E (effectiveness not established). The letter grades are explained in TABLE 4-1 ■. This

TABLE 4-1 ■ Levels of Evidence and Grades of Recommendation

Levels of Evidence	Grades of Recommendation
Studies are categorized based on the strength of the evidence. The source of the evidence (type of study) gives it a certain value, graduated from Level I down through Level IV.	These are based on the JBI grades of effectiveness.
Level I	**Grade A**
Evidence obtained from a systematic review of all relevant randomized, controlled trials	Effectiveness established to a degree that merits application
Level II	**Grade B**
Evidence obtained from at least one properly designed randomized, controlled trial	Effectiveness established to a degree that suggests application
Level III a	**Grade C**
Evidence obtained from well-designed pseudorandomized, controlled trials (alternate allocation or some other method of assignment)	Effectiveness established to a degree that warrants consideration of applying the findings
Level III b	**Grade D**
Evidence obtained from comparative studies with concurrent controls and allocation not randomized (cohort studies), case control studies, or interrupted time series with a control group	Effectiveness established to a limited degree
Level III c	**Grade E**
Evidence obtained from comparative studies with historical control, two or more simple arm studies, or interrupted time series with a parallel control group.	Effectiveness not established
Level IV	
Evidence obtained from case series, either posttest or pretest and posttest.	

Adapted from *Evidence-Based Practice Information Sheets for Health Professionals, Best Practice,* Joanna Briggs Institute, Australia.

grade provides a guide for whether or not to recommend the research-generated assessment, diagnosis, intervention, or evaluation based on the established effectiveness. The combined results from clinically relevant research, clinical expertise, and client preferences plus the grade given the research produce the best evidence for ensuring effective, yet individualized, client care.

The outcome of an evidence-based practice system is often found in the form of practice guidelines (practice guidelines for psychiatric–mental health nursing are discussed in Chapter 2∞), critical pathways (also called clinical pathways), and clinical algorithms, discussed later in this chapter. These forms are designed to specify the best procedures or practices for clinical problems and psychiatric diagnoses, in addition to tracking both the process and the outcomes of care.

WHY IS EVIDENCE-BASED PRACTICE IMPORTANT?

Evidence-based practice is important when you are involved in a situation that raises questions: "Is this a routinely recognized symptom?" "Why is this happening?" "What is the best way to address this issue?" or "How could we intervene differently?" Experienced psychiatric–mental health nurses may be able to provide half the answer to many of these questions from their knowledge base. Access to symptom presentation and treatment modes, however, would be limited by geography, local cultures, and professional systems. The answers to these questions are accummulated from both experience and research. Neither experience nor research alone would be sufficient in making yours the best possible nursing practice. Remember that both are necessary.

Nursing science evolves from the unique combination of nursing research and nursing practice. You are in a position to contribute to nursing's knowledge base with every piece of research you conduct. Ideas are generated from almost every clinical contact, activity, and therapeutic intervention you engage in during your workday. Regardless of your specialty area, people being treated for a clinical problem need information about their problem and its clinical solution. Treatment ideas occur to you, but you want to maximize the effects and streamline your efforts. Available evidence does not answer all your questions. For example, how do you deduce that a particular intervention is likely to be helpful? Your answer might come from considering any one, or several, of the general and specific questions listed below:

1. What type of nursing research will provide solid data that can be used in evidence-based interventions?
2. How do people with certain types of symptoms learn?
3. In what order would you make clinical decisions when you assess whether a client needs a PRN medication for agitation, is having side effects from a medication, is anxious, or is trying to communicate?
4. How do you anticipate a client's needs when he or she is having severe symptoms and is unable to communicate due to apathy and difficulty with associative thought mechanisms?
5. Which client populations can benefit from humor?
6. Which stress management interventions are most effective for someone with panic disorder versus someone in crisis?
7. What early interventions in circadian disruption can promote healing for abused individuals?
8. Does caffeine trigger physiologic arousal in people with post-traumatic stress disorder as it does in people with panic disorder?

To assess how ready you are to engage in evidence-based practice, see the Your Self-Awareness feature. As you accumulate experience, you will be able to determine when you do not have enough information, what you need to do to obtain that information, and how the information will affect your nursing practice.

Best Practices Based on Evidence

Interest in the concept of best practices can be traced to concerns about avoiding nursing and medical mistakes and enhancing safety for clients. **Best practices** are broad consensus statements about values, attitudes, skills, knowledge, and approaches. To avoid mistakes, clinicians need to know the correct course of action. Prior to evidence-based practice, professional knowledge was based on:

- Traditions and customs established in specific settings as part of the collective culture or the ideas of those in charge
- Trial and error if professionals did not necessarily know all the possible approaches and were uncertain what the safest, most effective course of action would be
- Clinical judgment, the accumulated knowledge that inquiring professionals actively, systematically, and intentionally extract from their practice experience
- Authority governed by regulations that accrediting agencies or third-party payers required

YOUR SELF-AWARENESS
How Ready Am I to Engage in Evidence-Based Practice?

If you see the need for more information about intervening therapeutically with clients, ask yourself the following questions to determine your readiness to engage in evidence-based practice:

1. Do I know how to locate sources of best practices based on evidence?
2. Have I had the supports and resources necessary to access evidence-based information?
3. Do I feel confident about my ability to evaluate the usefulness of best practices in my clinical setting?
4. Has my clinical area been open to accepting valuable change?

MEDIALINK Application: When Do Research Results Apply Clinically?

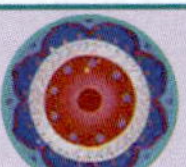

EVIDENCE-BASED PRACTICE

SMOKING CESSATION FOR PSYCHIATRIC INPATIENTS

Matthew is a 26-year-old male who has been diagnosed with schizophrenia. His symptoms include difficulty organizing his thoughts, indistinct auditory hallucinations every couple of days, and lack of motivation to do even those things he used to enjoy. He has been a two-pack-per-day cigarette smoker for the past 6 years, but as an inpatient he smokes as few as six cigarettes a day because of the national hospital ban on smoking. He tells you that during and after smoking he feels he "can think without all that jangling getting in the way" and feels relief from his symptoms for a few minutes. When he is not smoking at his usual level, such as when he is in the hospital as he is now, he is more irritable and is easily agitated.

Nicotine addiction is a reality for Matthew, as are the withdrawal symptoms he routinely experiences when he has a little of the substance (nicotine) he depends on, then has none for long periods. Matthew needs you to try to understand. His experiences with psychiatrists and psychiatric–mental health nurses included very little information or support for his predicament. He was told repeatedly that occasional or low-level smoking while an inpatient should not be a problem for him. He has also been told by staff that smoking was a self-harming activity and he needed to stop.

Your nursing care plan must include all the structural supports that will ensure Matthew has the information he needs about his tobacco dependence and how to safely address the issue. Beyond that immediate goal you must attempt to understand Matthew's own reality, situation, and need for strategies to deal with both the dependence and the impact nicotine has on his symptoms. The study cited below emphasizes that lack of understanding about nicotine use by people with schizophrenia and attitudes about smoking combine to make smoking cessation less likely and less successful for these clients. Although action should be based on more than one study, this research suggests that without psychiatric nursing interventions, psychiatric care is compromised and smoking cessation is unsupported.

Prochaska, J. J., Gill, P., & Hall, S. M. (2004). Treatment of tobacco use in an inpatient psychiatric setting. *Psychiatric Services, 55*(11), 1265–1270.

CRITICAL THINKING QUESTIONS

1. Is it ethical to infringe on a client's right to smoke?
2. Matthew is less irritable and less easily agitated when he smokes at his usual level. Why does he need to stop?

The movement toward evidence-based best practices places nursing care on a more solid scientific foundation by integrating these features with research evidence. Consequently, nurse researchers are conducting clinical trials and outcome studies designed to generate evidence on which to base practice decisions. Others are summarizing this accumulating body of evidence in textbooks such as this, in **meta-analyses** (analyzing the analysis of studies) that are found in "State of the Science" features in nursing journals, and in books in which identified experts collect original research evidence and summarize and evaluate it using identified criteria. The National Institute of Nursing Research (NINR) funds studies designed to summarize research evidence organized around specific topics.

Critical Thinking and Evidence-Based Practice

Closing the gap between evidence and practice requires not only nursing research and critical syntheses of the research, but also competencies among clinical nurses that have at their core the ability to think critically about the evidence. These competencies include the ability to:

- Find meaningful research evidence.
- Conduct an intelligent critique of studies once they are located.
- Summarize studies to accumulate a body of evidence focused on a topic or clinical problem.
- Implement a system for change to evidence-based practice in an organizational setting that includes involving all members of the team to ensure full participation in the design and implementation of new practice guidelines or protocols.
- Follow up and document the impact of changes and adopt, adapt, or discard changes based on additional evidence.

Engaging others in an ongoing discussion about practice and the implications of our science for everyday care ensures the health and vitality of nursing. Using the grading system described earlier contributes to critically thinking about the evidence. The Evidence-Based Practice feature in this section illustrates how research evidence can influence psychiatric–mental health nursing care.

Clinical Algorithms, Critical Pathways, and Practice Guidelines

As evidence accumulates, psychiatric–mental health nurses have the opportunity to develop strategies for care called clinical algorithms, critical pathways, and practice guidelines. **Clinical algorithms** show a logical progression of decisions and activities that are designed to standardize quality care for a particular clinical intervention (see Chapter 30∞, Figure 30-6 as an example).

Critical pathways provide a means of accurate documentation and shift the emphasis from depicting nursing as a series of tasks (e.g., monitoring medication side effects, taking vital signs, etc.) to interventions connected to a purpose or client outcome. They offer us an opportunity to best represent our role in treatment. We must be clear and specific about the manner in which psychiatric–mental health nurses contribute to client outcomes such as:

- Stabilization of acute psychotic symptoms
- Restoration of cognitive function
- Establishment of social support for caregivers
- Management for symptoms of depression
- Safety from harm
- Sense of spiritual solace

FIGURE 4-2 ■ offers an example of a critical pathway for a client experiencing panic disorder.

Practice guidelines are professional mandates for clinical practice. You can find examples of practice guidelines for

Critical Pathway for a Client with Panic Disorder: Outpatient Treatment

Expected length of treatment: 8 weeks

	Date ____________ Weeks 1–2	**Date ____________ Weeks 3–6**	**Date ____________ Weeks 7–8**
Weekly outcomes	Client will: • Identify initial goals for therapy. • Contract for ongoing treatment. • Participate in treatment plan. • Begin to identify sources of anxiety/panic.	Client will: • Identify ongoing goals for therapy. • Maintain contract for ongoing therapy. • Participate in treatment plan. • Identify strategies to manage anxiety and panic.	Client will describe ongoing strategies to manage panic disorder. Client will demonstrate ability to cope with ongoing feelings of panic. Client will describe strategies to cope with an inability to cope with stressors.
Assessments, tests, and treatments	Psychosocial assessment to include mental status, mood, affect, behavior, and communication. Assist client to explore factors that precipitate panic attacks.	Psychosocial assessment. Assess recent history of anxiety and panic attacks. Explore contributing factors. Discuss effectiveness of cognitive restructuring strategies.	Psychosocial assessment. Assess recent history of anxiety and panic attacks. Explore contributing factors. Discuss effectiveness of cognitive restructuring strategies.
Knowledge deficit	Orient client to therapy program. Assess learning needs of client. Review initial plan of care. Assess understanding of teaching. Discuss the etiology and management of anxiety and panic disorders. Discuss the physical symptoms of panic and the importance of understanding the meaning of anxiety and panic disorders. Instruct client to maintain journal of anxiety and panic attacks.	Review therapy program and treatment objectives. Review journal of recent panic attacks. Assist client to identify the early signs of anxiety and panic attacks. Discuss strategies to cope with early signs and symptoms of panic attacks, including talking or activity. Discuss additional strategies to cope with panic attacks including expressing anger, positive self-talk, or guided imagery. Teach principles of cognitive restructuring and practice during session. Teach relaxation techniques and practice during session. Discuss use of exercise to alleviate anxiety/panic. Assist client to explore problem-solving strategies. Assess understanding of teaching.	Review plan of care. Review principles of cognitive restructuring. Assess understanding of teaching.
Diet	Nutritional assessment. Encourage well-balanced diet from all food groups. Contract with client to avoid stimulants.	Encourage a well-balanced diet from all food groups. Encourage the avoidance of stimulants.	Encourage a well-balanced diet from all food groups. Encourage the avoidance of stimulants.
Activity	Discuss the importance of regular aerobic exercise. Contract for regular exercise program. Sleep pattern assessment. Discuss strategies to provide sleep-enhancing atmosphere for 45 minutes prior to sleep.	Review ability to begin and continue exercise program. Maintain contract for regular exercise programs. Encourage client to practice relaxation response. Discuss effectiveness of sleep-enhancing strategies.	Review ability to continue exercise program. Maintain contract for regular exercise programs. Discuss effectiveness of sleep-enhancing strategies.

FIGURE 4-2 ■ Critical pathway for panic disorder.

(continued on page 51)

Critical Pathway for a Client with Panic Disorder: Outpatient Treatment (continued)			
Expected length of treatment: 8 weeks			
	Date ____________ Weeks 1–2	**Date ____________ Weeks 3–6**	**Date ____________ Weeks 7–8**
Psychosocial	Approach with nonjudgmental and accepting manner. Observe and monitor behavior. Assist client to understand relationship of unexpressed feelings to anxiety and panic experience. Encourage client to express feelings, thoughts, ideas, and beliefs.	Approach with nonjudgmental and accepting manner. Observe and monitor behavior. Encourage client to express feelings, thoughts, ideas, and beliefs. Provide positive feedback for efforts to incorporate coping strategies into daily life. Assist client to understand relationship of feelings to panic. Assist client to realistically identify strengths and limitations. Explore ways of reframing limitations in a positive manner. Assist client to practice and implement effective coping strategies. Assist client to identify potentially stressful situations and role-play coping strategies.	Approach with nonjudgmental and accepting manner. Encourage client to review strategies to manage anxiety and panic.
Medications	Identify target symptoms.	Assess target symptoms. Assess need for medications and refer as indicated. Routine medications as ordered.	Assess target symptoms. Routine medications as ordered.
Consults and discharge plan	Family assessment. Establish objectives of therapy with client.	Review with client progress toward therapy objectives.	Review with client progress toward therapy objectives. Make appropriate referrals to support groups.

FIGURE 4-2 ■ Critical pathway for panic disorder. *(continued)*

psychiatric–mental health nursing in Chapter 2 and practice guidelines for ethical practice in Chapter 13.

It is not possible to remember all the clinical algorithms, critical pathways, or practice guidelines, therefore psychiatric–mental health nurses need to learn to use systems that consistently provide what they want. An example of technologic support for such systems is the personal digital assistant (PDA). A growing number of nurses use these devices (also called Palm Pilots) to ensure quick, easy access to assessment data, evidence-based clinical guidelines, medication information, and other applications. Drug reference software such as Epocrates® allows clinicians to access information on medications such as when a drug has been recalled or has new indications. Docking a PDA to a personal computer with an Internet connection, a technique known as hotsyncing, allows you to download the latest information about medications in a handy and convenient way.

Clinical Culture Affects Research Utilization

Throughout this chapter you will read about how to grow in the science of nursing by using research to generate evidence-based practice. To do this, you must consider the culture of the clinical environment. Pepler et al. (2006) note that characteristics of the culture in which care is given contribute to research-based practice and include a supportive environment, adequate facilitation of involvement in research, expert nurse clinicians to establish the link between relevant research and practice, and encouragement to attend conferences. If a clinical practice area is to benefit from research, then the area must be able to respond to change. Research use in the clinical setting results in continually changing practice in light of new information. Assessing the culture of a clinical enviroment will tell us the ease with which change can be made.

A review of the contemporary literature identified a number of requirements for evidence-based practice to flourish. These practice conditions are:

1. Attitudes of open-mindedness to, and knowledge of, research on the part of psychiatric–mental health nurses
2. Access to contemporary and regularly updated research reports or state of the science resources
3. Administrative support from nurse managers and higher-level executives
4. Assistance through expert consultants to become critical consumers of research and to use findings in practice

OBTAINING THE EVIDENCE

How do you obtain the evidence that evidence-based practice is built on? Evidence is the outcome of a research project, and there are progressive steps culminating in achieving research outcomes. Research must be designed and described so that an Ethics Committee (EC) or an Institutional Review Board (IRB) can review the proposed research and determine whether it can be conducted. The composition of these oversight committees is federally regulated. A minimum of five people with various perspectives—including scientific, nonscientific, community representative, and expert in the study area—ensure that research subjects are protected and the study is worth doing. Guidance and regulations for this function come from two main sources:

- The Office for Human Research Protections (OHRP, http://www.hhs.gov/ohrp/)—includes the Department of Health and Human Services regulations 45 CFR 46 (Code of Federal Regulations section 46) and what is known as the Common Rule
- Food and Drug Administration (FDA, http://www.fda.gov/)—Department of Health and Human Services regulations 21 CFR 56 (Code of Federal Regulations section 56); the FDA establishes parameters for research on medications, substances, and medical devices.

MEDIALINK Federal Regulations

Institutional Review Boards are responsible for protecting the rights and welfare of human research subjects. They have the authority to approve, require modifications in, or disapprove all research activities within their jurisdiction.

The Belmont Report

An excellent resource for research basics is the Belmont Report, generated by the National Commission for the Protection of Human Subjects of Biomedical and Behavioral Research in 1979. It is a short (approximately eight pages), easily readable statement on the three main principles on which research is focused:

- Respect for persons
- Beneficence
- Justice

MEDIALINK Office of Civil Rights—HIPAA

Respect for Persons

Respect for persons includes the ethical consideration of autonomy: the research subject is valued; the researcher acknowledges boundaries; and there is respect for the subject's body, family, culture, and community as well as freedom from coercion. The practical demonstration of this principle is seen in the Informed Consent document for studies that involve intervening, or having a certain level of contact, with research participants. The respect-for-persons concept is necessary for ethical research, but it is not sufficient by itself. You must include the other ethical considerations.

Beneficence

Beneficence, the second principle, means doing good. Researchers must inflict no harm (nonmaleficence), prevent or remove harm, and promote good for research subjects. Our profession explicitly states our beneficence role as nurses (described further in Chapter 13∞) in our ethics code. As researching nurses we have to keep the risk/benefit analysis in mind; in other words, are the risks of the study balanced by the benefits to be gained? Further aspects of beneficence include minimizing exploitation. We must make sure we are not taking advantage of people willing to be research participants. Criteria for beneficence are given in the websites and federal regulations mentioned earlier.

Justice

The final principle of the Belmont Report is justice. This principle focuses on how a person should be treated during research, making sure we have provisions for what is fair, given what is due or what is owed. It also provides specific guidelines for the selection of subjects and protects vulnerable subjects (such as children, people who have mental disorders, prisoners). Researchers must seek out subjects who are prepared to bear the burden of research and have not been overutilized. It is best to use a broadly inclusive approach in selecting research subjects. Justice as an ethical mandate is also discussed in Chapter 13∞.

Advantages of Doing Research

What are the advantages of doing research in psychiatric–mental health nursing when all these factors must be kept in mind? Research can help remove some of the stigma of mental illness by studying it as other illnesses are studied. Research asserts that people who have a mental illness are also competent people free to choose to participate in studies to help others. Exploring new perspectives and approaches engenders hope for treating mental illness and leads to new treatments.

Security Protection for Data

An important consideration for all of health care, but particularly relevant for research, is the Health Insurance Portability and Accountability Act (HIPAA) of 1996. This act created uniform standards for electronic health care transactions (EDI) and provides for security protections for data that are electronically stored and transmitted. As so much of health care and research involves electronic information, it is vital that information be responsibly safeguarded. Information on how to protect the privacy rights of individuals regarding their personally identifiable health information is available at http://www.hhs.gov/ocr/hipaa. Researchers include sections within Informed Consent documents and in applications to conduct research that specifically state how HIPAA issues will be addressed.

Research Template

The following is a general template you can use to conduct your research.

1. Establish your research question. What do you want to discover? (For example, can the Nurses

Observation Scale for Inpatient Evaluation [NOSIE] predict whether a newly admitted client will be violent? Will teaching clients how to address side effects increase adherence to prescription medications?)
2. Determine the best approach for obtaining the answer to your question. Would qualitative or quantitative data be most helpful?
3. Write your proposal and apply to the IRB or EC. Each IRB/EC has its own application procedure. Contact the administrator or chairperson; some programs/schools/clinical areas have websites with specific directions for how to proceed.
4. Communicate with the IRB/EC throughout your study, as you may have questions, regular reporting responsibilities, or updating to complete.
5. Conduct your study.

When the Institutional Review Board has approved the study, data collection begins. Statistical analyses are done on numerical data such as test scores or ratings of improvement or worsening of symptoms. This is called *quantitative research.* In *qualitative research,* data are interpreted in a way that examines the qualities of the experience for the participants. Following the analysis, the outcomes of the study are written up and submitted for publication, conference presentation, or other venues for sharing outcomes with other nursing professionals, who can then make a decision about altering practice based on the evidence presented.

RESEARCH INSTITUTES AND MODELS FOR BEST PRACTICES BASED ON EVIDENCE

Evidence-based practice is essential for clinical excellence and measurable nursing interventions. A number of institutes, organizations, and conceptual models are resources for best practices based on evidence. These resources combine evidence-based practice with an interest in quality care and reduced costs, and the need to remain competitive in the current health care environment. See Box 4-1 for international journals and resources generated by these institutes and models.

Box 4-1 International Nursing Research Resources

The following are examples of useful resources for evidence-based practice in nursing. (*Note*: This is *not* an all-inclusive list.)

Websites

Evidence-Based Nursing Online www.evidencebasednursing.com	An international online journal of nursing research; 24 different summaries in each issue, with expert commentators for each. Sponsored by the Royal College of Nursing in the United Kingdom.
The Joanna Briggs Institute www.joannabriggs.edu.au	An international research collaboration for evidence-based nursing; publishes best-practice information summary sheets on individual and group therapy, long-term confusion, effectiveness of suicide prevention programs, music as an intervention, and other topics. Based at the Royal Adelaide Hospital and Adelaide University in Australia with collaborating centers in Australia, New Zealand, and Hong Kong.
McMaster University, Toronto, Canada http://hiru.mcmaster.ca/epc	Extensive resources for teaching, with implications for evidence-based practice in nursing and other disciplines.
National Institute of Nursing Research at the U.S. National Institutes of Health www.ninr.nih.gov	See in-text discussion.

Research Listings

ClinicalTrials.gov www.clinicaltrials.gov/	This site helps you search for clinical trials by disease, location, treatment, sponsor, and other specific search fields. It provides definitions, explanations, and descriptions of clinical trials; lists studies in the news; contains consumer health information, including genetics; and lists research supported by the National Institutes of Health.
CenterWatch Clinical Trials Listing Service www.centerwatch.com/	This site contains information about clinical research, including listings of more than 41,000 active industry and government-sponsored clinical trials, as well as new drug therapies in research and those recently approved by the FDA. Information is available for research professionals and for people interested in participating as research subjects.

Journals

International Journal of Mental Health Nursing	Fully refereed journal that examines current trends and development in mental health practice and research. Official journal of the Australian and New Zealand College of Mental Health Nurses, Inc.
International Journal of Evidence-Based Healthcare	Fully refereed journal that publishes scholarly work from the Joanna Briggs Institute Collaboration.
Journal of Nursing Scholarship	Fully refereed journal that publishes international nursing research.

MediaLink Nursing Research Resources

MEDIALINK Critical Thinking Exercise: Treating Families of the Mentally Ill

Change to Evidence-Based Practice

Now that we have defined evidence-based practice, identified the contemporary conditions in the mental health/psychiatric care environment that have required it, and examined the competencies to establish it, the section that follows provides a model to guide you in its direction. Evidence-based practice is not a new concept to most nurses; it has been referred to as *using research in nursing*. However, the growth in nursing science and research literature, and our enhanced access to it, have intensified the mandate that we use it to discover the most effective approaches to achieve identified client outcomes.

High-quality health care requires delivery based on sound scientific evidence and continuous innovation of new health care practices and approaches. The 2004 Surgeon General's Report focused on the health consequences of smoking. Smoking is considered a mental health issue as nicotine is a highly addictive substance that individuals use to self-medicate for several different psychiatric symptoms. The report provides a synthesis of the state of the art of research in the field. It does not make evidence-based recommendations for practice, but it does serve to put psychiatric–mental health nurses on alert that we have much to contribute to the growing body of knowledge in mental health care and mental health care policy. Smoking cessation with people who have a major mental illness is especially difficult, and our work in this direction can contribute to better health outcomes. It is expected that nurses in the future will substantiate their practice with research-based evidence. We must learn to assess client outcomes and clearly link them to nursing interventions.

New findings from clinical research have brought a variety of choices in nursing interventions to psychiatric–mental health nurses. The list of available options expands with each new piece of nursing research. Standardized language according to the North American Nursing Diagnosis Association International (NANDA-I), the Nursing Outcome Classification (NOC), and Nursing Intervention Classification (NIC) groups have made such options readily available. Detailed discussion of these standardized nursing languages appears in Chapter 13. When you intervene with a client, you have made a choice from all the options available. Doubtless your choice is based on the value of the research evidence, your expertise in the area, and the details of the clinical situation. By making such a choice you signal your ability to make a change in practice. Box 4-2 illustrates one way nurses can recognize that change is needed and make the mental moves necessary to accomplish evidence-based changes in practice. The mental flexibility to make changes is important throughout all aspects of your professional and personal life.

Challenging the Status Quo

The very nature of research challenges standing policies and client care interventions. Nurses involved in using research evidence can offer the best possible care to their clients. Be aware that there is a notable gap between research results and their use in practice. The validated scale, the Barriers to Research Utilization Scale (BARRIERS Scale) developed by Funk et al. in 1991, assesses the barriers to research use. This scale has contributed enormously to our understanding of the obstacles to bridging the gap between research and practice. Hutchinson and Johnston (2006) examined the body of research that used the BARRIERS Scale to determine the barriers to using research in practice. Attributes of a clinical environment that would overcome these barriers include offering ready access to technology to enable access to research evidence, encouraging critical thinking, ensuring that nurses have the authority to change their practice, and providing interdisciplinary support for suggested changes.

The Your Self-Awareness feature in this section challenges you to locate yourself on the ladder of research-use expectations for nurses, which was developed by Aurora Health Care, Milwaukee, Wisconsin.

Box 4-2 How to Change

Making a change involves specific steps. Picture this scenario: A nurse is walking down a particular street and falls into a huge hole. This happens over and over again; the nurse walks down the same street and falls into the same hole. Imagine the hole is a therapeutic intervention with a client that doesn't work well.

Making something different happen with your nursing interventions will not be an automatic or instantaneous event. Change is a process and requires progressive steps of mental action.

Think of these five steps to making a change.

1. At some point you realize you are unsatisfied with a particular behavior and you want it to change. "I keep doing this and I don't want to. I need to make a change." *The idea that change is needed is an important first step.*
2. Now you walk down the street with the huge hole in it and try to see the hole before you fall in it. *You may very well continue to perform the original, unsuccessful nursing intervention, but this step encourages you to recognize that you use it even though it doesn't work.*
3. Try to see the hole as soon as you walk down the street, then continue walking and fall in the hole. *The goal is to progress to anticipating earlier and earlier in the process your use of the unsuccessful nursing intervention.*
4. Walk down the street, see the hole as soon as you begin walking, and walk around the hole when you get to it. *This is an exciting step. You start the interaction with the client, recognize your tendency to use the original nursing intervention, and use the evidence-based intervention instead.*
5. Walk down a street that does not have a huge hole in it. *From now on you will use the evidence-based intervention in your practice. You have successfully made a change in your practice.*

PROCHASKA TRANSTHEORETICAL MODEL FOR CHANGE

Nurses continue to synthesize their experiences and the results from nursing research into a psychiatric–mental health nursing practice that is evidence-based. Initially, this practice area

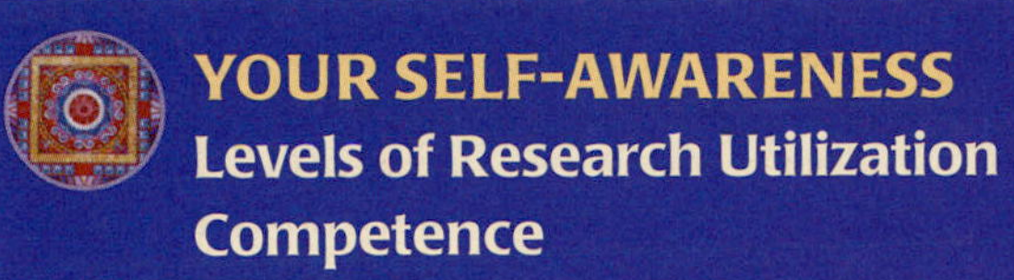

YOUR SELF-AWARENESS
Levels of Research Utilization Competence

Level 1 Am I aware of the research basis for policies, procedures, and assessment tools that I use in my practice?

Level 2 Do I follow organizational policies and procedures and use valid assessment tools and research-based recommendations to effect positive client and family outcomes?

Level 3 Am I able to apply research-based findings to develop individualized plans of care?

Level 4 Am I able to integrate and translate research-based knowledge into well-designed practice guidelines that help achieve positive client and family outcomes?

Level 5 Do I collaborate with other caregivers to challenge current practices and to synthesize research findings to develop systems for achieving desired client and family outcomes?

Level 6 (Advanced-practice nurse) Do I participate in expanding the scientific basis of nursing practice by conducting, using, and disseminating research?

Level 7 (Manager or director) Do I create an environment for practice that assures research-based nursing (e.g., through budgeting, releasing staff time, and integrating research into organizational goals)?

Source: Adapted from Van Mullem, C., Burke, L. J., Dohmeyer, K., Farrell, M., Harvey, S., John, L., et al. (2001). Integrating research into practice. *American Journal of Nursing, 101*(4), 24E.

was anecdotally driven. As an example, a new psychiatric–mental health nurse sees an expert nurse refocusing a client who provides too much information or too many topics. The expert nurse's success in that situation forms the basis for the new nurse's decision to refocus when facing a similar situation. Over time, the nurse observes and conducts further refocusing, but also attends conferences, reads articles, and incorporates research evidence on refocusing. The nurse's practice is evidence-based as a result. Adjustments to practice are continuous as expertise is accrued, more research is conducted, and the outcomes are incorporated into a change process. This section presents one model that can be used to guide nurses through this change process.

The Transtheoretical Model (TTM) of change formulated by Prochaska and DiClemente (1986) suggests five stages of change through which people progress when behavior modifications are desired. These stages are: precontemplation, contemplation, preparation, action, and maintenance. As the words imply, successful change involves thought and action before, during, and after change. The theoretical concept was examined within an addictions framework; however, more general applications are useful.

The five stages of TTM change are summarized in Figure 4-3 ■ on page 56. Movement through the stages of change waxes and wanes throughout the spiral that represents the progression of human behavior. While people tend to progress toward change, slipping back into familiar patterns of previous behaviors—and to a previous stage of change—is expected, especially during times of stress. When health-related behaviors are involved, this slipping back is referred to as *relapse*. If we applied the concept of relapse to the use of evidence-based practices, you may see nurses who become frustrated, annoyed, and even demoralized at the amount of effort required for change, reverting to old, maladaptive behavior or thinking at various points in the change process.

TTM can be applied to professional and clinical situations. Murphy (2005) used TTM in research with individuals who had addictions and comorbid psychiatric disorders. Those who have psychiatric illnesses in combination with substance abuse pose a particularly difficult clinical problem. Conceptualizing treatment programs and therapeutic approaches for this group is best performed along the lines of an organized change model such as TTM. Ample opportunities exist in this field for research. Stage-based treatment highlights the role and impact of choice on treatment outcomes.

Another study (Evers et al., 2006) used TTM in a stress management intervention. Both the treatment group and a control group were assessed for the effectiveness of their stress management skills. Using this model, stress management interventions had a significant impact on stress, depression, and specific behaviors.

Realistic and Attainable Change

Nurses need support to make changes. What kind of support would you need to begin the process of changing to evidence-based practice? Your expectations must be realistic and attainable, keeping in mind they are no different from what you expect from your clients. Change is not immediate, instantaneous, or initially permanent. Use the TTM stages to think about evidence-based practice and surround yourself with the resources necessary to achieve it.

ROSSWURM AND LARRABEE MODEL FOR CHANGE TO EVIDENCE-BASED PRACTICE

Rosswurm and Larrabee (1999) used theoretical and research literature related to evidence-based practice, research utilization, standardized language, and change theory to generate a model that guides clinicians through the process of developing and integrating a change to evidence-based practice. They developed and tested the usefulness of their model at a regional medical center that provides acute care, but its use can be generalized to other settings. Their model endorses quantitative research data, clinical expertise, and contextual evidence as well as qualitative research methodolodgies. It consists of the steps summarized in Figure 4-4 ■ on page 57.

Steps for Change

The six steps of this model are:

- Assessing the need for change
- Linking the problem with interventions and outcomes
- Synthesizing the best evidence

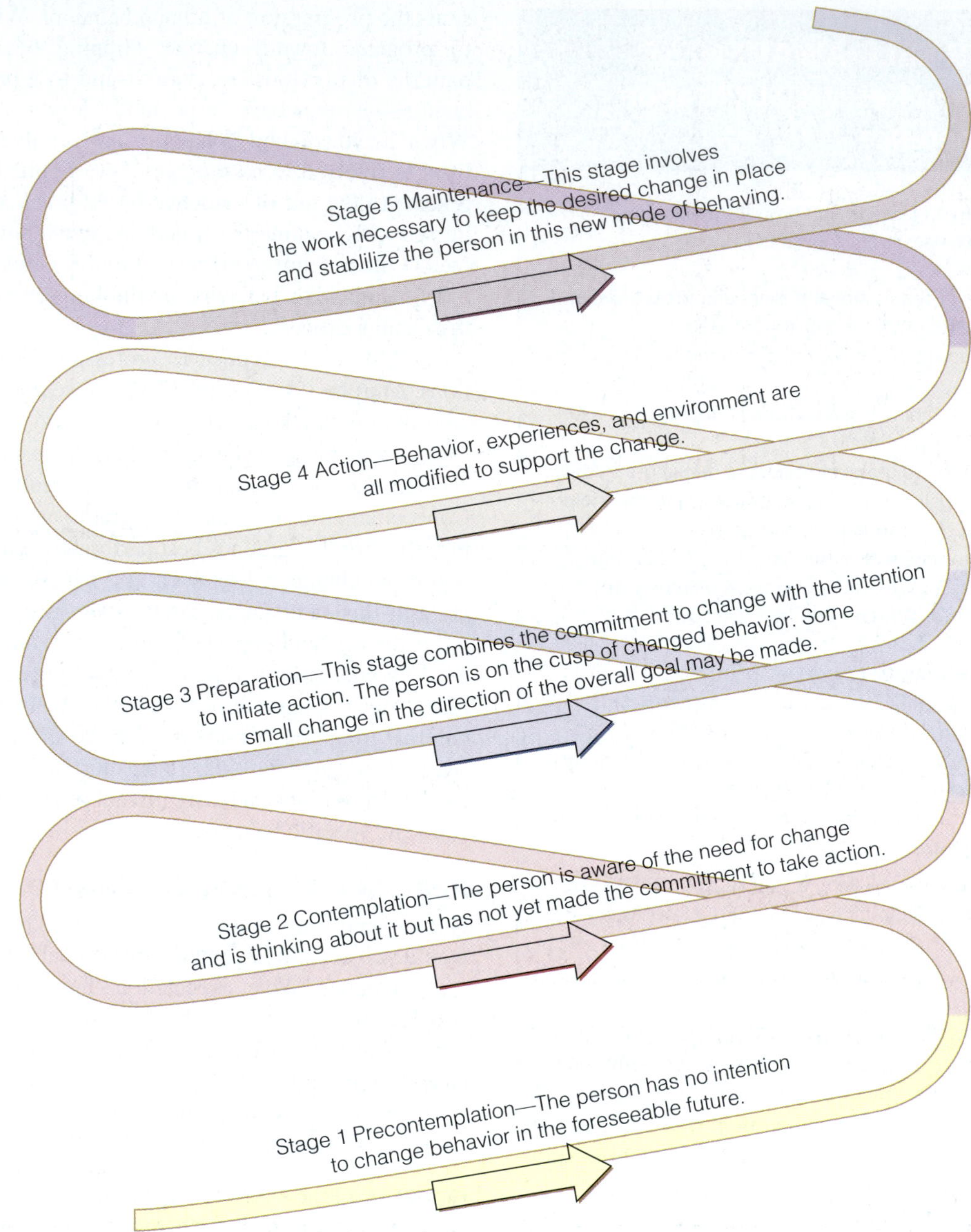

FIGURE 4-3 ■ Prochaska's stages of change.

- Designing the change in practice
- Implementing and evaluating the change in practice
- Integrating and maintaining the change in practice

You can see the similarities in the models for change. TABLE 4-2 ■ illustrates how Rosswurm and Larrabee applied the six-step model to create an evidence-based protocol for clients with acute confusion.

Protocols such as this one must be concisely written and widely shared in order to become integral to any practice environment. This is accomplished in a number of ways, including computer file sharing and electronic charting. Changing to an evidence-based practice system offers a superb opportunity for clinical psychiatric–mental health nurses and nurse researchers to collaborate on their shared concern for clients' well-being.

BUILDING A KNOWLEDGE BASE FOR EVIDENCE-BASED PSYCHIATRIC NURSING PRACTICE

Developing a knowledge base for evidence-based psychiatric nursing practice requires new research ideas, clinical trials, synthesis of research results, and a summary of findings based on the research.

Discovering the Evidence

Research continues to confirm that new nursing knowledge improves practice. The National Institute of Nursing Research (NINR) supports research studies that are creating a cumulative knowledge base that can improve the quality of client care. Examples of NINR-funded studies relevant to psychiatric–mental

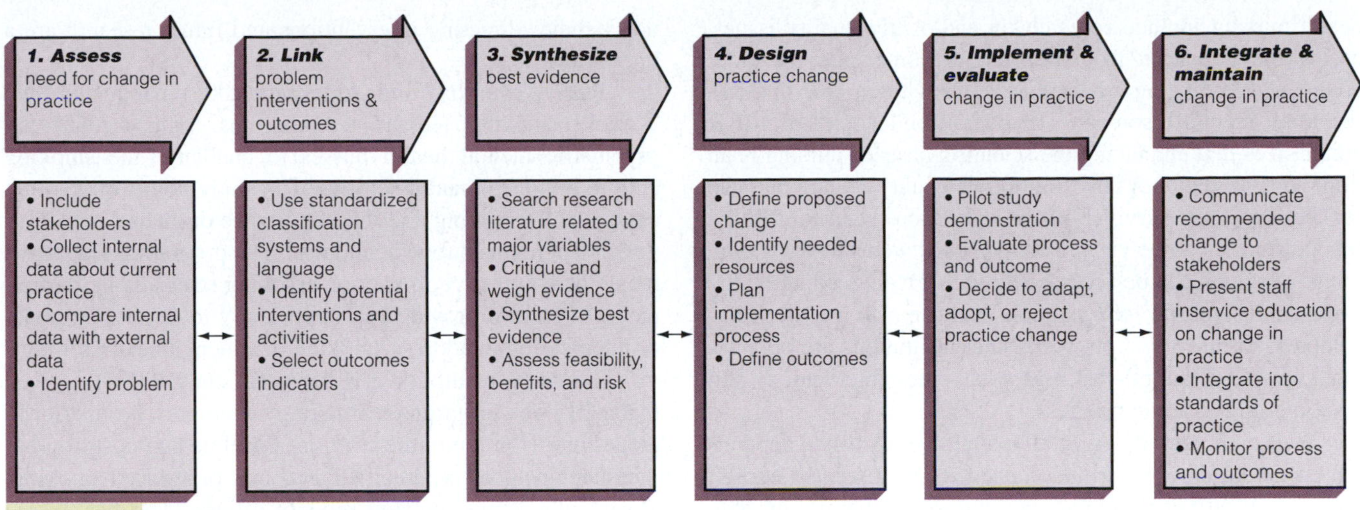

FIGURE 4-4 ■ Model for evidence-based practice.

Source: Rosswurm, M. A., & Larrabee, J. H. (1999). A model for change to evidence-based practice. *Image: Journal of Nursing Scholarship, 31*(4), 318. Reprinted with permission from Sigma Theta Tau International.

TABLE 4-2 ■ **Application of the Model: Evidence-Based Protocol for Clients with Acute Confusion**

Step 1. Assess need for a change

- Discussed clinical problem of acute confusion with nurse managers and nurses
- Reviewed PI/QM data on associated adverse events, i.e., falls, restraints
- Derived from data that patients > 65 years comprised more than 50% of hospital population and were at highest risk for confusion and adverse events
- Assessed nursing knowledge about delirium in elderly patients
- Compared internal data with external data from similar medical centers
- Identified from findings the need to improve nursing staff's knowledge and care of elderly patients at risk for developing confusion during hospitalization

Step 2. Link problem with interventions and outcomes

- Linked acute confusion with the NIC intervention of delirium management
- Included delirium management activities in an acute-confusion protocol
- Identified outcomes of cognitive orientation and safety as measured by a confusion scale, fall rates, and restraints

Step 3. Synthesize best evidence

- Reviewed literature focused on delirium management and safety
- Included nurses in critiquing research literature using worksheets
- Synthesized quantitative research evidence
- Combined quantitative research evidence with qualitative data, clinical judgment, and contextual data
- Assessed system feasibility, patients' benefits, and risks of protocol

Step 4. Design a change in practice

- Included nurses from pilot study units in drafting the evidence-based protocol
- Prepared forms for pilot study and its evaluation with input from unit nurses
- Identified tools for measuring outcomes of cognitive orientation, fall rates, and use of restraints
- Educated all nurses on the pilot study units in use of the evidence-based protocol

Step 5: Implement and evaluate the practice change

- Implemented the pilot study on the two selected hospital units
- Monitored use of the protocol throughout the pilot period
- Collected data and analyzed findings
- Recommended adoption of protocol with minor revisions

Step 6. Integrate and maintain the practice change

- Met with staff nurses on pilot study unit to review revisions
- Presented evidence-based protocol to standards and practice council
- Communicated information to administration and collaborating practitioners
- Conducted inservice education for all nursing staff about the protocol
- Planned ongoing monitoring of outcomes on all units

Source: Rosswurm, M. A., & Larrabee, J. H. (1999). A model for change to evidence-based practice. *Image: Journal of Nursing Scholarship, 31*(4), 319. Reprinted with permission from Sigma Theta Tau International.

MEDIALINK Case Study: Are Control Groups Ethical?

MEDIALINK National Institute of Nursing Research

MEDIALINK Centers for Disease Control and Prevention

health nursing include research on end-of-life quality issues, easing the transition from hospital to home care for older adults, and family caregiving for clients with chronic diseases including mental disorders. The overall philosophy of NINR emphasizes that enhancing the scientific basis of nursing is an important strategy not only to improve quality of care but also for the long-term survival of our profession. Data for NINR-funded studies can be viewed on the NINR website (www.ninr.nih.gov), which can be accessed through a resource link on the Companion Website for this book. You can also use the Companion Website to find out what other institutions are organizing knowledge summaries and what other intervention and outcome studies are in progress.

Research can be designed in a number of ways, depending on the kinds of information needed. As described earlier, quantitative studies involve the numerical nature of data (such as rating scales measuring increases or decreases in symptom level, measurements of weight and height, scored answers to questionnaires) and the statistical quantities determined from the data collected during each study. Qualitative studies use interviews, field notes, and observations to generate, rather than test, hypotheses and/or to interpret meaning under natural conditions. Studies in this category of descriptive **ethnography** (the study of human beings and their culture) attest to the recognized contribution of studies that are not designed as **randomized clinical trials** (studies designed to test hypotheses using the traditional experimental approach of randomly assigning subjects to treatment and control groups and then comparing them on identified and measureable outcomes in quantifiable terms). Psychiatric–mental health nursing benefits from methodological diversity as we continue to build our knowledge base.

Synthesizing Research Data to Understand Smoking

Tobacco use is considered one of the most preventable causes of premature morbidity and mortality. The Centers for Disease Control and Prevention (CDC) have noted repeatedly in research that no amount of tobacco use is safe (see the CDC's website at http://www.cdc.gov/).

Nurses in the psychiatric–mental health field are acutely aware of this as the percentage of smokers with a mental disorder is double to quadruple the rates seen in the general population (Prochaska, Gill, & Hall, 2004). The combination of tobacco use and mental illness produces a mentally ill chemical abuser (MICA). The addiction to nicotine, while difficult for anyone to overcome, has a special hold on people with a major mental illness. Nicotine has been shown to promote the release of a variety of neurotransmitters, including glutamate (Levin, Tizabi, et al., 2005; Levin, Petro, & Caldwell, 2005), thus producing a calming effect. Nicotine is thought to mimic the neurological impact of optimal functioning for a brief period of time.

Smoking cessation is difficult to accomplish for individuals with mental illness because the cognitive benefits of nicotine are real. As a significant percentage of the recipients of psychiatric–mental health nursing services use tobacco products, studies directing interventions and future research are a high priority.

Reilly, Murphy, and Alderton (2006) conducted two 9-week smoking cessation programs with groups of psychiatric–mental health nurses to challenge the smoking culture in mental health settings. The study points out the necessity of intervening and the importance of nurses' active involvement in this public health role. The programs' supportive theme had a positive impact on smoking rates among participants. They also provided an opportunity to develop a model of intervention to address smoking in a mental health setting.

Similarly, results of a Horn et al. study (2004) showed that a 10-week program on smoking cessation was superior to a one-time 15-minute intervention. Baseline and postprogram measures included whether subjects quit or reduced smoking, along with depression and anxiety ratings. The health and longevity of recipients of psychiatric–mental health services can be promoted through smoking cessation programs involving nicotine replacement. Recommendations for further studies of cessation programming would benefit from the inclusion of coping and stress management skills and mental health referral protocols as significant program components.

Nursing research in the area of smoking cessation in psychiatry is relatively limited. Wewers, Sarna, and Rice (2006) assert that intervention by nurses can be extremely effective in smoking cessation programs. It would be an excellent application of evidence-based practice to conduct smoking cessation studies in psychiatric–mental health nursing settings and incorporate the results into your practice. Support and encouragement for such studies are available. As a result of the Master Settlement Agreement with the tobacco industry in the United States, there will be a reliable and decades-long funding mechanism for tobacco-related research, especially research dealing with smoking cessation. Conducting research in this and other areas would contribute to building a body of research evidence relevant to psychiatric–mental health nursing practice.

Designing a Clinical Trial

Research can be conducted in a variety of designs. Each design for collecting data and interpreting the results is related to how the study's value is evaluated. There are different styles of design for different kinds of data.

It is beyond the scope of this chapter to discuss study methodology in detail; however, it should be mentioned that there is a range of types of studies within quantitative research design. At one end of this range is a description of the numbers, called *descriptive statistics*. At the other end are *inferential statistics,* in which inferences are drawn about larger groups from a smaller group under study (Kranzler, 2007). There are options for studying the smaller group. You can compare a group in a wellness program who receive a special session to a group who do not. If you decide who gets the special session and who does not by randomly assigning group members, you are testing your hypothesis about comparative outcomes between the study groups in a randomized clinical trial—considered by many the *gold standard* or highest level of scientific evidence.

Your wellness program study could also look at the qualities of wellness or each subject's experience of belonging to a wellness program—qualitative research. The data collected for this type of study design could be interviews, open-ended questions on a survey, videotaped recordings, fieldwork observations, or discussion groups. Ethnographic studies such as the one Cleary conducted with psychiatric–mental health nurses (2004) promote an understanding of how nurses view their current role. These research findings are relevant within the context of current debates about nurses' roles and can be used to enhance the understanding of contemporary acute mental health nursing practice.

Summarizing the Evidence

As this chapter emphasized from the outset, psychiatric–mental health nursing research focused on client outcomes must be conducted, located, read, and understood before it can be applied systematically in clinical practice. Familiarity with research outcomes and publications is one of your responsibilities as a health care provider. Research evidence must be summarized, critiqued, and synthesized if it is to affect policy development, contribute meaningfully to interdisciplinary knowledge development, and shape standardized practice guidelines.

The purpose of research publications is to make it easier for clinical nurses to locate sources of evidence. The number of journals in which psychiatric–mental health nursing research appears is proliferating. In addition to the specialty psychiatric–mental health nursing journals—*Journal of the American Psychiatric Nurses Association, Journal of Child and Adolescent Psychiatric Nursing, Archives of Psychiatric Nursing,* and *Perspectives in Psychiatric Care*—additional publications that are valuable resources include *Evidence-Based Nursing* and *Evidence-Based Mental Health* (both published in the United Kingdom), *Worldviews in Evidence-Based Nursing,* and the Cochrane Collaboration, an electronic library available on the Internet. You can also access professional organizations such as the American Psychiatric Nurses Association, Association of Child and Adolescent Psychiatric Nurses, International Society of Psychiatric–Mental Health Nurses, and Sigma Theta Tau International for relevant research. The websites for these organizations can be accessed via the Companion Website for this book.

Evaluating the Evidence

It is essential for all psychiatric–mental health nurses who engage in evidence-based practice to become intelligent consumers and evaluators of the growing body of science in our field. It is critical that you learn how to access this information as it evolves and refine your own critical thinking skills so that you can evaluate it with confidence. The extent of what you comprehend in a report of research findings often depends on the amount of active thinking you put into reading research. Box 4-3 offers you some helpful tips for the active reading of research.

Box 4-3 Techniques for Active Reading

Active reading is the process of actively questioning the material you read. Before you can address the questions "Is it any good?" and "What does it mean?" you must understand what you are reading. Here are some helpful tips:

1. Quickly read the title page, preface, or abstract to get an idea of the topic of the article or book and categorize it in your mind. Is it really a report of research findings, or is it an anecdotal account of somebody's isolated experience? Case studies and case histories count as qualitative research.
2. Study the table of contents or the headings in the article to get a sense of its structure. This alerts you in advance about what to expect.
3. Read any boldface excerpts or boxed summaries (like this one) to ascertain the main points or ideas.
4. Leaf through the whole article, dipping in here and there to follow the logic.
5. Find important and unfamiliar words and use a glossary or dictionary to determine their meaning.
6. Highlight key points or conclusions by underlining, tagging the area with a removable tab, or writing notes in the margins.
7. Think of alternative explanations for the conclusions drawn by the author(s).
8. Be able to say with certainty that you understand what you have read before you criticize it.
9. Compare what you have read in one study with what you have read cumulatively on the topic.

MediaLink Professional Organizations

General criteria useful in evaluating evidence that appear consistently across all research sources include:

1. Is the purpose of the study clear and relevant to a significant nursing problem?
2. Is the study problem stated in such a way as to be researchable (can the investigator collect data about it)?
3. Is the literature adequate and current, and does it reflect a mastery of current knowledge of the topic of inquiry?
4. Is there a match among the study purpose, the study design, and the methods? Are all well detailed and justified?
5. Are the sampling procedures and sample well described and appropriate for the study question and study design?
6. Has the investigator used the correct analytic procedures, whether qualitative or quantitative?
7. Are the findings clear and supported by the research data?

The nursing literature abounds with research textbooks that offer guidelines for becoming an intelligent consumer of nursing research evidence. A quick search of the *Cumulative Index to Nursing and Allied Health Literature (CINAHL)*, the

International Nursing Index, and the *Cumulative Medical Index*, as well as a MEDLINE literature search online, will reveal many other books with helpful formats for discovering and digesting research.

Using the Evidence in Practice

To date, most psychiatric–mental health nursing practice continues to be based on what has been termed *received wisdom* found in tradition, unsystematic trial and error, and authority rather than on evidence. Received wisdom is passive, taken-for-granted knowledge. Studies of research utilization and attitudes toward research reveal that even when psychiatric–mental health nurses report positive attitudes toward research, they rarely state that they use research in daily practice. At present, the goal of evidence-based practice is not fully realized in psychiatric–mental health nursing. In this chapter, you have read that evidence-based practice depends on a number of factors, including nurses' attitudes toward and knowledge of research, the availability of and access to relevant research, and an environmental context that provides sufficient resources and managers' support.

LOOKING TO THE FUTURE

Psychiatric–mental health nurses have joined the movement of evidence-based practice, and your reading has introduced you to this culture. You know that research evidence is not only established in experiments and randomized clinical trials but is generated from a variety of sources. Psychiatric–mental health nurses deal with less readily apparent client problems and interventions that are more difficult to quantify and measure. Our history values the intuitive aspects of the interpersonal relationship and caring, and also incorporates that which will provide best practices and positive outcomes. The authors of this textbook believe that a broad definition of what constitutes legitimate evidence, including clinical wisdom, client preference, and solid qualitative (nonnumeric) research findings, melds with the values we attribute to evidence-based practice.

Future psychiatric–mental health nursing research will likely follow the target topics for federal funding. Many of the clients with whom we work are among the chronically ill. As our population ages, so do those older adults who have been mentally disordered since youth, and so does the number of older clients who are cognitively impaired due to diseases of the brain. The growing chasm between the rich and the poor in the United States, along with growing populations of ethnically diverse clients, put vulnerable populations, including adolescents and children, at risk for violence and drug abuse. The movement of psychiatric clients away from inpatient care has created a new population in need of our attention—those in jails, in shelters, in group homes, in emergency rooms, in hospice care, and on the streets.

Refer to the Companion Website for resources and activities designed to keep you informed about contemporary advances in evidence-based psychiatric–mental health nursing practice. The future of research for psychiatric–mental health nursing is to take this movement not only to our traditional psychiatric clients but also to the jails, shelters, hospice care centers, outreach clinics, drug treatment centers, and the streets. Studies conducted under these natural conditions will help us to learn how what we do makes a difference for client outcomes, to build our body of evidence, and to demonstrate it to others in our clinical practice.

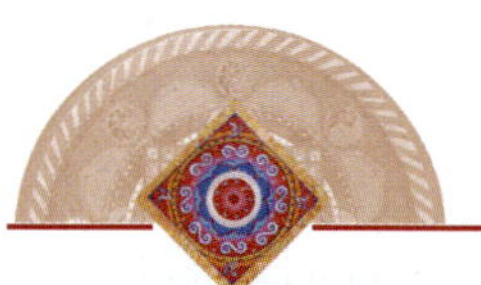

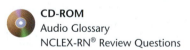

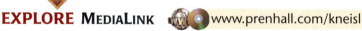

EXPLORE MediaLink 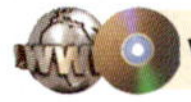 www.prenhall.com/kneisl

For NCLEX-RN® review questions, case studies, and other resources for this chapter see the Pearson Health MediaLink CD-ROM that accompanies this book and the Companion Website at www.prenhall.com/kneisl.

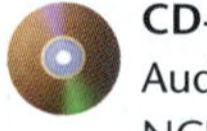

CD-ROM
Audio Glossary
NCLEX-RN® Review Questions

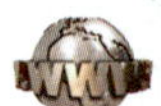

Companion Website
Audio Glossary
NCLEX-RN® Review Questions
Critical Thinking Exercise
- *Treating Families of the Mentally Ill*

Case Study
- *Are Control Groups Ethical?*

Care Plan
- *Antidepressants and Increased Risk of Suicide*

MediaLinks
MediaLink Application
- *When Do Research Results Apply Clinically?*

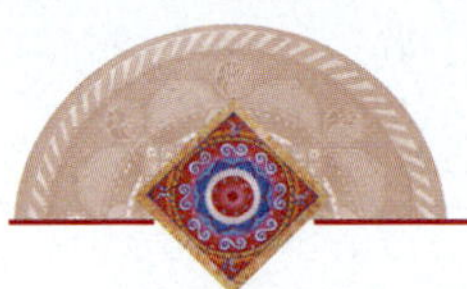

NCLEX-RN® REVIEW QUESTIONS

1. The basis for evidence-based practice is:
1. The nursing process.
2. Clinical research and practice.
3. Critical thinking.
4. Clinical algorithms.

2. An outcome of evidence-based practice includes:
1. Practice guidelines.
2. Standardized care.
3. Reduced hospital length of stay.
4. Reduced workload for nurses.

3. Which of the following critical thinking competencies is *not* applicable to evidence-based practice?
1. Identifying meaningful research evidence
2. Critically and objectively critiquing research findings
3. Integrating personal experiences and beliefs into the process
4. Developing a plan of care based on research findings

4. A benefit of critical pathways is that they:
1. Clearly define skills required to care for clients.
2. Reflect client outcomes based on nursing interventions.
3. Are professional mandates to clinical practice.
4. Are based on trial-and-error nursing.

5. Which step in the nursing process is necessary to initiate a change to evidence-based practice?
1. Assessment
2. Planning
3. Implementation
4. Evaluation

6. The nurse knows that to maintain an evidence-based practice model of care, the nurse will:
1. Follow traditions and customs that have been practiced for years.
2. Rely on trial–and-error to determine the safest method of care.
3. Follow the agency's policies and procedures of care.
4. Review current nursing research.

7. A nurse's first scientific responsibility in conducting research is to:
1. Identify what research questions to pursue.
2. Apply to the Institutional Review Board (IRB) for permission to conduct research.
3. Identify the participants in the study after the study has been approved.
4. Select members of the oversight committee.

8. In determining a nurse's readiness to engage in evidence-based practice, the nurse will:
1. Ask other staff members what their beliefs are related to evidence-based practice.
2. Identify resources needed to access evidence-based information.
3. Recognize the value of maintaining the status quo.
4. Let other staff initiate the change process.

9. To objectively evaluate the findings of a research study, the nurse will:
1. Compare the findings to a similar study.
2. Rely on clinical experience and knowledge.
3. Replicate the study to determine if similar results are obtained.
4. Establish criteria to be used in the evaluation process.

10. The best evidence on which to base your clinical practice is based on:
1. Standards of nursing care.
2. Outcomes of a research project.
3. Practice guidelines.
4. Critical pathways.

See Appendix C for answers.

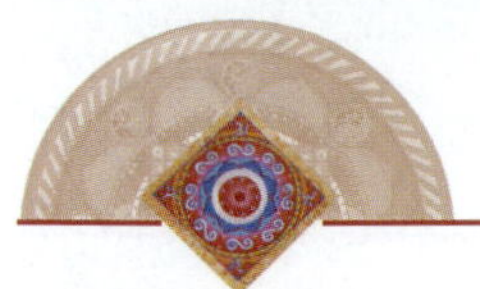

REFERENCES

Bauer-Wu, S., Epshtein, A., & Reid Ponte, P. (2006). Research reflections. Promoting excellence in nursing research and scholarship in the clinical setting. *Journal of Nursing Administration, 36*(5), 224–227.

Cleary, M. (2004). The realities of mental health nursing in acute inpatient environments. *International Journal of Mental Health Nursing, 13,* 53–59.

Evers, K. E., Prochaska, J. O., Johnson, J. L., Mauriello, L. M., Padula, J. A., & Prochaska, J. M. (2006). A randomized clinical trial of a population- and transtheoretical model-based stress-management intervention. *Health Psychology, 25*(4), 521–529.

Funk, S. G., Champagne, M. T., Wiese, R. A., & Tornquist, E. M. (1991). BARRIERS: The barriers to research utilization scale. *Applied Nursing Research, 4*(1), 39–45.

Horn, K., Dino, G., Kalsekar, I., Massey, C., Manzo-Tennant, K., & McGloin, T. (2004). Exploring the relationship between mental health and smoking cessation: A study of rural teens. *Behavioral Science, 5*(2), 113–126.

Hutchinson, A. M., & Johnston, L. (2006). Beyond the BARRIERS scale: Commonly reported barriers to research use. *Journal of Nursing Administration, 36*(4), 189–199.

Kranzler, J. H. (2007). *Statistics for the terrified* (4th ed.) Upper Saddle River, NJ: Pearson Prentice Hall.

Levin, E. D., Petro, A., & Caldwell, D. P. (2005). Nicotine and clozapine actions on pre-impulse inhibition deficits caused by N-methyl-D-aspartate (NMDA) glutamatergic receptor blockade. *Progressive Neuropsychopharmacological Biological Psychiatry, 29*(4), 581–586.

Levin, E. D., Tizabi, Y., Rezvani, A. H., Caldwell, D. P., Petro, A., & Getachew, B. (2005). Chronic nicotine and dizocilpine effects on regionally specific nicotinic and NMDA glutamate receptor binding. *Brain Research, 1041*(2), 132–142.

Murphy, S. A. (2005). Innovative roles. Integration of multiple nursing roles using the stages of change conceptual framework: An interview with Deborah Finnell, DNS, RN, NPP, CARN-AP, APRN-BC. *Journal of Addictions Nursing, 16*(1–2), 69–71.

Pepler, C. J., Edgar, L., Frisch, S., Rennick, J., Swidzinski, M., White, C., et al. (2006). Strategies to increase research-based practice: Interplay with unit culture. *Clinical Nurse Specialist, 20*(1), 23–33.

Prochaska, J. J., Gill, P., & Hall, S. M. (2004). Treatment of tobacco use in an inpatient psychiatric setting. *Psychiatric Services, 55*(11), 1265–1270.

Prochaska, J. O., & DiClemente, C. C. (1986). Toward a comprehensive model of change. In W. Miller & N. Heather (Eds.), *Treating addictive behaviors* (pp. 3–27). New York: Plenum Press.

Reilly, P., Murphy, L., & Alderton, D. (2006). Challenging the smoking culture within a mental health service supportively. *International Journal of Mental Health Nursing, 15,* 272–277.

Rosswurm, M. A., & Larrabee, J. H. (1999). A model for change to evidence-based practice. *Image: Journal of Nursing Scholarship, 31*(4), 317–322.

Van Mullem, C., Burke, L. J., Dohmeyer, K., Farrell, M., Harvey, S., John, L., et al. (2001). Integrating research into practice. *American Journal of Nursing, 101*(4), 24E.

Wewers, M. E., Sarna, L., & Rice, V. H. (2006). Nursing research and treatment of tobacco dependence: State of the science. *Nursing Research, 55*(Suppl. 4S), 11–15.

ADDITIONAL REFERENCES

Cleary, M., & Walter, G. (2006). Educating mental health nurses in clinical settings: Tackling the challenge. *Contemporary Nurse, 21*(1), 153–157.

Engelke, M. K., & Marshburn, D. M. (2006). Collaborative strategies to enhance research and evidence-based practice. *Journal of Nursing Administration, 36*(3), 131–135.

Fanning, M. F., & Oakes, D. W. (2006). A tool for quantifying organizational support for evidence-based practice change. *Journal of Nursing Care Quality, 21*(2), 110–113.

Fitzpatrick, J. J. (2006). Challenges: The continued gap between research and professional practice. *Applied Nursing Research, 19*(1), 1.

LoBiondo-Wood, G., & Haber, J. (2006). *Nursing research: Method and critical appraisal for evidence-based practice* (6th ed.). St. Louis, MO: Mosby.

Marchiondo, K. (2006). Teaching tools. Planning and implementing an evidence-based project. *Nurse Educator, 31*(1), 4–6.

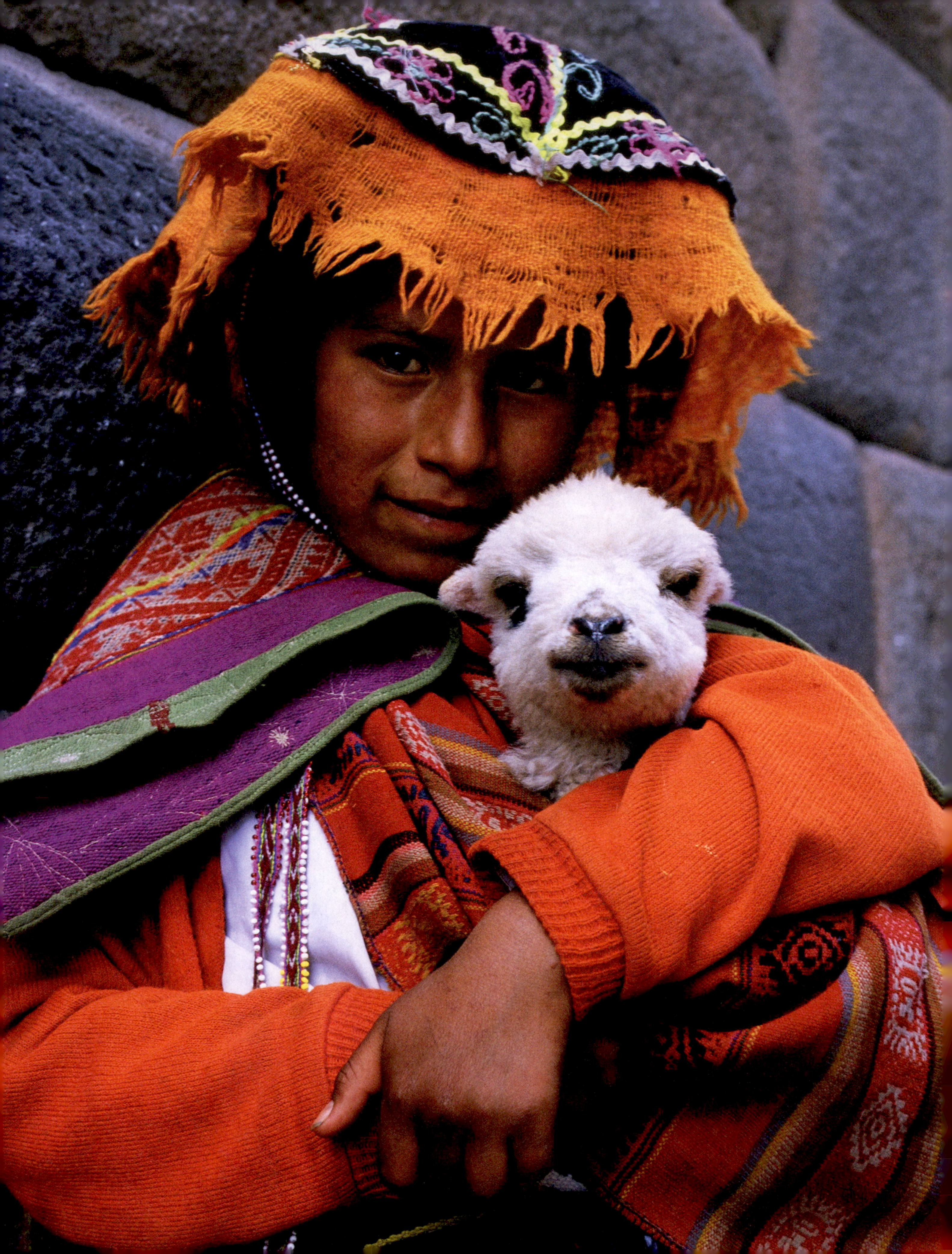

Unit 2

THEORETICAL BASIS FOR PSYCHIATRIC–MENTAL HEALTH NURSING

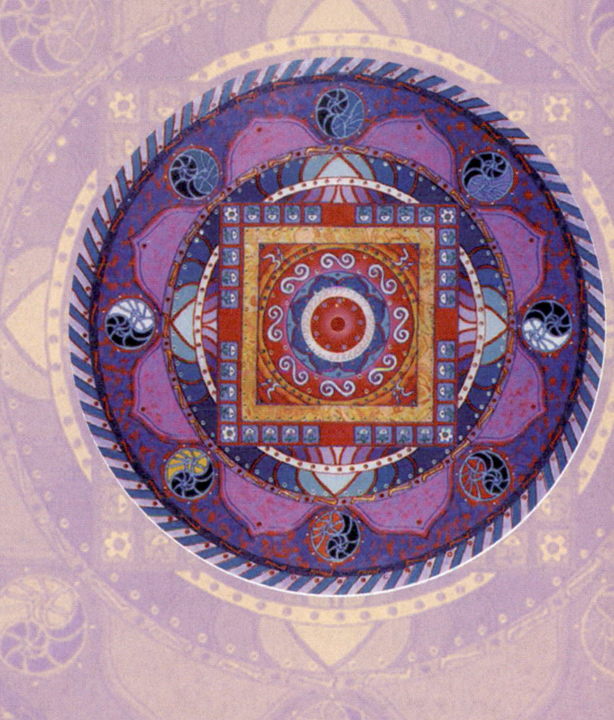

GUADALUPE is a descendant of the Incas and of the Spaniards who once colonized Peru. She lives in the coastal town of Piscas, south of Lima, the capital. In August 2007, a nearby 8.0 magnitude earthquake in the foothills of the Andes caused casualties and extensive damage, leveling her home, her church, and much of the town. The Andes are beautiful but are also one of the world's most unstable mountain regions where earthquakes, landslides, and flash floods are common. Over half the population, including Guadalupe's family, lives below the poverty level. Pedro, her father, injured both legs in the earthquake and is unable to return to work as a fisherman. He is considering work in the cocaine trade as a seagoing ship captain. Peru is the second largest producer of coca leaf, much of which is shipped to Colombia for processing into cocaine. Guadalupe has nightmares and fears she will lose more family and friends if another earthquake strikes or if violence erupts in the coca trade. Chaos, crisis, and emotional distress occur in every corner of the world and remind us of our responsibility to make a difference in world mental health issues.

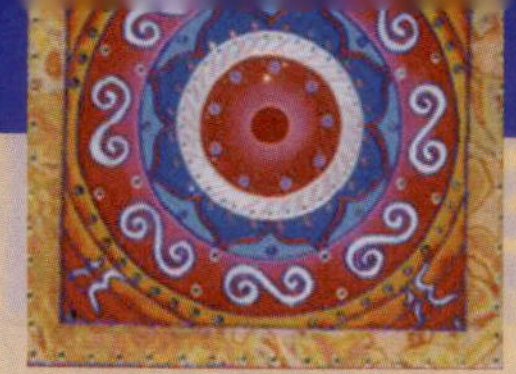

CHAPTER

5

Philosophy and Theories for Interdisciplinary Psychiatric Care

CAROL REN KNEISL

KEY TERMS

cognitive behavior theory *74*
conditioned response *74*
conditioning *75*
conscious *71*
ego *71*
general systems theory *77*
holistic *69*
humanism *69*
id *71*
interpersonal theory *76*
negative reinforcement *75*
operant conditioning *75*
positive reinforcement *75*
psychoanalysis *71*
psychoanalytic theory *71*
psychobiology *69*
reflected appraisals *76*
reinforcement *74*
self-system *76*
shaping *75*
superego *71*
symbolic interactionism *67*
token economy *76*
unconscious *71*

LEARNING OUTCOMES

After completing this chapter, you will be able to:

1. Discuss the major ideas of interactionism.
2. Discuss the major principles of humanism.
3. Describe the influence of the knowledge explosion in psychobiology.
4. Explain how the premises of human interactionism and psychobiology relate to psychiatric–mental health nursing.
5. Compare the assumptions and key ideas of medical–psychobiologic, psychoanalytic, cognitive behavioral, and social–interpersonal theories.
6. Discuss the implications of each theory for the practice of psychiatric–mental health nursing.

CRITICAL THINKING CHALLENGE

Sonia Jones, a 38-year-old musician, comes to the psychiatric clinic complaining of depression, anxiety, and fear about her increasing use of methamphetamines (speed) and alcohol. Sonia's reason for seeking help to is get clean and sober. Some members of the treatment team, however, cite a randomized clinical trial and a psychobiologic theory that support treating the depression prior to addressing Sonia's coexisting addictive disease. Your own clinical wisdom and past experience convince you that both conditions must be addressed simultaneously.

1. When you don't have established theory or clear research findings to guide your clinical decisions, how important are clinical preferences and clinical wisdom?
2. Do you think they constitute evidence on which to base practice?

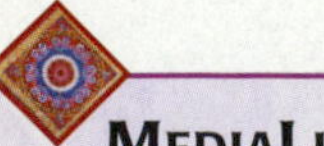

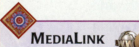

MEDIALINK 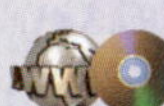 www.prenhall.com/kneisl

Go to the Pearson Health MediaLink CD-ROM and the Companion Website at www.prenhall.com/kneisl for interactive resources for this chapter.

To practice psychiatric–mental health nursing humanistically, you must devote yourself to understanding what makes people human, how they express their joy of living, their sadness, their desire to love, their hopes for growth. Understanding these phenomena becomes even more crucial when psychiatric nurses must explain how the joy of living suddenly turns to the desire to die, how love of self and others turns to violence and hate, how the hope for growth turns to withdrawal and despair, and how alterations in the brain relate to these human experiences.

This chapter introduces you to a holistic philosophy that includes humanism, interactionism, and the knowledge explosion in psychobiology. In this chapter, we also compare the basic assumptions and implications for practice in the dominant theories for interdisciplinary psychiatric care. These are:

- Medical–psychobiologic theory
- Psychoanalytic theory
- Cognitive behavioral theory
- Social–interpersonal theories

Clinicians often say they are *eclectic*, that is, they choose one or a combination of these theories in determining what information to assess about clients, what intervention outcomes and approaches to recommend, and what ultimate evaluation criteria to set. We believe that clinicians *should* be eclectic, choosing strategies based on scientific evidence about their effectiveness for any given client. The best strategies based on the best available evidence are reviewed in every chapter of this book.

Your approach to understanding psychiatric–mental health clients is influenced by your philosophy. We believe, further, that humanistic interactionism is the philosophy that fits best with psychiatric–mental health nursing goals. Theories such as those discussed in this chapter provide the conceptual tools to formulate that understanding and to interpret clinical data. Blend an understanding of these theories with the nursing theories discussed in Chapter 2∞, especially the psychiatric–mental health nursing theory of Hildegard Peplau.

SCOPE OF PSYCHIATRIC–MENTAL HEALTH NURSING PRACTICE

All nurses are concerned with the quality of human life and its relationship to health. The psychiatric–mental health nurse is especially concerned with the relationship between the individual's optimal psychobiologic health and feelings of self-worth, personal integrity, self-fulfillment, and creative expression. Just as important are the satisfying of basic living needs, comfortable relationships with others, and the recognition of human rights. These elements collectively define mental health.

The psychiatric nurse's scope of practice is broad enough to include issues such as alienation, identity crises, sudden life changes, and troubled family interactions. It may deal with poverty and affluence, the experiences of birth and death, the loss of significant others, or the loss of body parts. It is concerned with sustaining and enhancing the individual and the group. Yet it also must address basic life issues of eating, sleeping, grooming, and hygiene shared by psychiatric clients. This broad-ranging, humanistic, interactional, and psychobiologic view of the scope of psychiatric–mental health nursing is dramatically different from the exclusively medical or behavioral science orientation of the last 50 years.

Psychiatric–mental health nurses are concerned with the care of clients who have identified mental disorders. However, our concerns extend to the wide range of human responses to mental distress, disability, and disorder. For example, an addicted parent may not only suffer from shame, unemployment, and abusive outbursts of anger but may also lose a sense of purpose and meaning and experience a disturbed self-concept and spiritual distress. These responses have detrimental effects on the health of children, partners, and other significant people in the person's life.

Like many concepts in the human sciences, the concept of mental disorder lacks a definition that covers all situations. Faced with such a diverse array of human problems, the psychiatric–mental health nurse is challenged to synthesize a holistic philosophy for practice that can be the basis for care.

HUMANISTIC INTERACTIONISM AND PSYCHOBIOLOGY: THE MIND–BODY–SPIRIT CONNECTION

The classic psychiatric and psychologic approaches have described and classified signs and symptoms of *illness*, then accounted for it by individual psychologic dynamics such as character disorder, weak ego, or failed defense mechanisms. The basis for this text is a synthesis of psychosocial and psychobiologic knowledge required for practice in the 21st century.

Basic Premises of Interactionism

One central idea in the approach we advocate has come to be known as **symbolic interactionism**, a term introduced by Herbert Blumer (1969) to describe an approach to the study of human conduct. It is based on the three philosophic premises identified in Box 5-1.

Box 5-1 Symbolic Interactionism: Philosophic Premises

1. Human beings act toward things (other people, events) on the basis of the meaning that the things have for them. Life experiences may have different meanings for different people.
2. The meaning of things in a person's life is derived from the social interactions that person has with others. We learn meanings during our experiences with others.
3. People handle and modify the meanings of the things they encounter through an interpretive process. They come to their own conclusions.

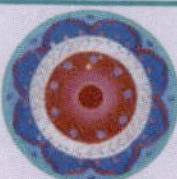

EVIDENCE-BASED PRACTICE

STRATEGY OF PROTECTIVE EMPOWERING

Lorelei is the nurse manager on an alcohol detoxification unit. James, a 55-year-old man with a 30-year history of alcohol abuse and cigarette smoking, is admitted for alcohol detoxification. Because he had pulled out his IV fluids on the preceding shift, managed to get hold of a cigarette lighter in order to smoke, and fallen out of bed, the night shift put him in soft restraints. Every time one of the night shift nurses came into his room, James cursed at them.

Lorelei assigned Kevin, who was newly hired and still in the process of orientation, to James's care. Lorelei and Kevin's joint assessment of James's current mental status, background history, and mental status examination results convinced them that he is at risk for harming himself. Although hospital policy justifies the use of soft restraints, Lorelei cautioned Kevin not to take James's cursing personally. Lorelei felt strongly that James could be kept safe with one-to-one supervision rather than with soft restraints and that the presence of a staff member would be more comforting and less anxiety-provoking for him. Among the goals that Lorelei and Kevin formulated cooperatively were relating to John in a respectful way, keeping him safe, and encouraging him to regain greater self-control. Although action should be based on more than one study, their strategy of protective empowering was based on the following grounded theory research:

Chiovitti, R. F. (2006). Nurses' meaning of caring with patients in acute psychiatric hospital settings: A grounded theory study. *International Journal of Nursing Studies, 43*(7), 831–841.

CRITICAL THINKING QUESTIONS

1. How is protective empowerment in sync with the basic premises of humanistic interactionism?
2. How is protective empowerment in sync with the basic premises of psychobiologic theory?
3. How is protective empowerment in sync with the basic premises of cognitive behavioral theory?

Implications for Psychiatric–Mental Health Nursing Practice

Interactionism offers psychiatric–mental health nursing a perspective of human beings as having purpose and control over their lives, even if they have altered brain structure and chemistry and stressful environments. Interactionism as interpreted here provides the premise for a philosophy of caring with a strong humanistic cast, such as that described in the Evidence-Based Practice feature. Interactionism acknowledges the interaction of psychology, psychobiology, and sociocultural contexts.

The First Premise: Different Meanings for Different People We believe that all behavior has meaning. The psychiatric–mental health nurse must be wary of interventions that ignore, discount, or discredit the meaning an experience has for the client in favor of the nurse's own definition of the situation. Thus, you must develop skill in observing, interpreting, and responding to the client's lived experiences in the hope of arriving at a common ground of negotiated meanings and authentic communication.

The Second Premise: Meanings Arise in One's Social World We believe meanings arise in the *process* of interaction with others. It is essential, therefore, that psychiatric–mental health nurses take into account the social and cultural environment of each client. A holistic assessment of a client accounts for the interaction patterns in that person's social world.

A shaved head, tattoos, baggy denim pants worn low on the hips, and a woolen cap, which appear deviant in a milieu of business suit–wearing bankers and executives, may represent a close adherence to the dress and demeanor codes of some street gang subcultures.

Similarly, it is within interpersonal interaction that clients can learn new definitions for life situations and new repertoires for action. This is the heart of the psychiatric–mental health nurse's therapeutic and caring role. The sensitive, intelligent, and humanistic use of self within interpersonal relationships is a key part of the psychiatric–mental health nurse's skill. You have the potential for helping clients redefine their experiences in more satisfying ways, learn new patterns of coping with stress, and generally enhance the quality of their lives and social worlds. Such is the essence of psychiatric–mental health nursing.

The Third Premise: Meaning Is a Basis for Behavior We believe that people handle situations in terms of what they consider vitally important about the situation. To understand clients' actions, the psychiatric–mental health nurse must identify the meanings those actions have for them.

You need to keep this premise in mind when responding to an expression of human distress. A nurse may say, "I wouldn't worry about it," or "Don't feel that way," "You are reacting inappropriately," or "It's not so bad." Such clichés are not usually helpful, not because they are inherently "untherapeutic" but because in voicing them the nurse invalidates the basic premise that people interpret the world in their own way to act in a specific situation.

Basic Premises of Humanism

One of the purposes of this chapter is to specify a philosophic basis for subsequent chapters. The three premises of interactionism provide us with a partial orientation. A theory of life centered on human beings, termed **humanism**, adds to the philosophic perspective. The humanistic perspective has eight central propositions (Lamont, 1967) identified in Box 5-2.

The central concept of humanism is that the chief end of human life is to work for well-being within the limitations of life in today's world. Humanism is a philosophy of service to benefit humanity through reason, science, and democracy.

Implications for Psychiatric–Mental Health Nursing Practice

As a philosophy underlying psychiatric–mental health nursing practice, humanism means devotion to the interests of human beings wherever they live and whatever their status or culture. It reaffirms the spirit of compassion and caring toward others. It is a constructive philosophy that wholeheartedly affirms the joys, beauty, and values of human living.

The subsequent chapters in this text attempt to show how these basic premises can be put to use in psychiatric–mental health nursing practice. Some fundamental concepts are described briefly in the following sections.

A Holistic View of the Mind–Body Relationship Our humanistic interactional view is that physical and mental factors are interrelated and that a change in one may result in a change in another. For example, anger may result in increased blood pressure. An invading organism, a decrease in a neurotransmitter, or a structural change in the body can alter thought processes. Low self-esteem can result in hunched shoulders and severe skeletal muscle contractures.

The implications for psychiatric–mental health nursing are clear. Healing and caring must be approached in a **holistic** manner. The psychiatric–mental health nurse deals with the biologic aspects of a primarily psychologic or emotional pattern and the psychologic or emotional aspects of biologic experiences, as in the following clinical example.

Box 5-2 Humanism: Philosophic Premises

1. The human being's mind is indivisibly connected with the body.
2. Human beings have the power or potential to solve their own problems.
3. Human beings, while influenced by the past, possess freedom of creative choice and action and are, within certain limits, masters of their own destinies.
4. Human values are grounded in life experiences and relationships, and our highest goal must be the happiness, freedom, and growth of all people.
5. Individuals attain well-being and a high quality of life by harmoniously combining personal satisfactions with activities that contribute to the welfare of the community.
6. We should develop art and awareness of beauty so that the aesthetic experience becomes a pervasive reality in people's lives.
7. We should apply reason, science, and democratic procedures in all areas of life.
8. We must continually examine our basic convictions, including those of humanism.

CLINICAL EXAMPLE

Kate S., a prominent television personality who wants to remain anonymous, is hospitalized for a severe eating disorder on an integrated behaviorial unit, and you are assigned to provide her care. She weighs under 90 pounds for her 5′7″ frame and is dehydrated, malnourished, and obsessed with getting back to work and looking good in an industry that expects bone-thin women anchors for the news.

As a nurse educated to recognize both her physical and psychosocial needs, you are challenged to formulate a holistic, integrated care plan.

Psychiatric–mental health nursing care is given not only in mental health care settings but also in general health care settings and may be directed toward clients whose immediate problems are primarily physical.

An Expanded Role for Nurses The humanistic interactional perspective on mental disorders implies an expanded role for psychiatric–mental health nurses. We believe that psychiatric nurses should be prepared to work for change within social and political systems. Psychiatric–mental health nursing can no longer be limited to client-oriented activities designed exclusively to control symptoms and increase the capability of individuals to adjust satisfactorily to the existing social condition. Instead, psychiatric–mental health nursing must be involved in social goals that advance health holistically. Because psychiatric–mental health nursing has political consequences, it is essential that you begin to develop a philosophic and ethical framework to guide and evaluate the political outcome of therapeutic intervention.

Negotiation and Advocacy In this book, the model for intervention and change is one of negotiation and advocacy. The responsibility for change remains with the person who seeks psychiatric help or consultation. Clients are held accountable for their own behavior. They are not the passive recipients of care given by psychiatric professionals. Instead, they are empowered in the process of developing new perspectives and encouraged to weigh alternatives and make self-directed choices. They and their families are educated about their disorder and its treatment.

Basic Premises of Psychobiology

The last decades have seen major breakthroughs in knowledge about the brain, the mind, the spirit, and behavior. This knowledge explosion has been termed **psychobiology**. Research has generated new understanding of how genetics, immunology, biorhythms, brain structure, and brain biochemistry influence mental disorders.

MEDIALINK Care Plan: Humanism: A Basis for Care

MediaLink Critical Thinking Exercise: Nursing: Art or Science?

New imaging techniques make it possible to view what has never been seen before. Neuroscientists have found that our thoughts, sensations, joys, and aches consist of physiological activity in the 100 billion neurons in the tissues of the brain. They can almost read people's thoughts from the blood flow in their brains. They can tell whether a person is thinking about a face or a place, or whether the person is looking at a bottle or a shoe.

New medications to correct biochemical imbalances in the brain are being prescribed. Psychobiologic interventions such as exposure to bright light and white noise, and the restriction of nutrients and nonnutrients believed to affect behavior, have become commonplace.

Implications for Psychiatric–Mental Health Nursing Practice

Some authorities argue that psychiatric–mental health nurses should continue to focus on the human aspects of care as psychiatry moves toward "remedicalization." They fear that by embracing the biologic sciences we will diminish the art of psychiatric–mental health nursing. Others, ourselves included, contend that, to bring a contemporary holistic perspective to psychiatric–mental health nursing care, we must integrate the rapidly accumulating knowledge in psychobiology. We do not give up our humanistic, psychosocial, and interactional premises simply because we recognize the value of the breakthroughs being made in psychobiology. Instead, as we redefine the traditional art of psychiatric–mental health nursing care and caring in the new millennium, our practice and research must integrate "high tech" and "high touch," nature and nurture, the biologic sciences and the behavioral sciences.

THEORIES FOR INTERDISCIPLINARY PSYCHIATRIC CARE

Dominant social attitudes and philosophic viewpoints have influenced the understanding of and approaches to mental disorder throughout history, and concepts that may be considered modern may have roots in earlier eras. See Figure 5-1 ■, a timeline for the shifting approaches to mental disorder throughout history. A timeline for the development of psychiatric–mental health nursing is illustrated in Figure 2-1 on pages 16–17.

Medical–Psychobiologic Theory

The medical–psychobiologic model in psychiatry originated in the era of classification. The classification of mental disturbances brought the emotional and behavioral aspects of people into the domain of the medical doctor. During this period, the systematic observation, naming, and classification of symptoms were emphasized. Emil Kraepelin's monumental descriptive diagnostic classification system is acknowledged as the first comprehensive medical model (Shorter, 1996). It included the notions that the cause of mental illness was organic, that it was located in the central nervous system, that the disease followed a predictable course, and that treatment should be based on accurate diagnosis. Contemporary research findings in the field of psychobiology lend support to some of these early ideas but advance them and make them specific in important ways.

Assumptions and Key Ideas

Medical–psychobiologic theories view emotional and behavioral disturbances like any physical disease. Thus, abnormal behavior is directly attributable to a disease process, a lesion, a neuropathologic condition, a toxin introduced from outside the body, or (most recently) a biochemical abnormality of neurotransmitters and enzymes or a genetic predisposition. The medical–psychobiologic position can be summarized as follows:

- The individual suffering from emotional disturbances is sick and has an illness or defect.
- The illness can, at least presumably, be located in some part of the body (usually the brain's limbic system and the central nervous system's synapse receptor sites). Factors related to mental disorders include excesses or deficiencies of certain brain neurotransmitters; alterations in the body's biologic rhythms, including the sleep-wake cycle; and genetic predispositions.
- The illness has characteristic structural, biochemical, and mental symptoms that can be diagnosed, classified, and labeled.
- Mental diseases run a characteristic course and have a particular prognosis for recovery.
- Mental disorders respond to physical or somatic treatments, including drugs, chemicals, hormones, diet, or surgery.
- Psychobiologic explanations of mental disorders can reduce the stigma often associated with them, and can discourage claims that mental disorders result from a lack of willpower or moral character.

Implications for Psychiatric–Mental Health Nursing Practice

Nurses who were first involved in the care of psychiatric clients were primarily responsible for the client's physical well-being. Their responsibilities included administering medications prescribed by the physician and caring for clients undergoing treatments such as insulin shock, electroshock therapy, or hydrotherapy.

Psychobiologic theories are the conceptual basis for the continued use of biologic therapies in the care of mental health clients, the hospital as the setting for care, research into the genetic transmission of mental illness, research on biochemical and metabolic variables among diagnosed psychiatric clients, and dominance of the medical doctor—the psychiatrist—in the mental health team. As long as psychiatric clients are admitted to and reimbursed for care according to medical diagnoses, knowledge of this framework is crucial. Furthermore, as long as psychobiologic knowledge expands, psychiatric–mental health nurses are responsible for translating that knowledge into care practices that recognize the biologic factors related to mental disorders. Chapter 6 ∞ of this text provides an authoritative source of such contemporary psychobiologic knowledge. Advances in psychobiologic theory and research are also integrated throughout specific disorders and interventions chapters.

Psychoanalytic Theory

Psychoanalytic theory is usually credited to the Viennese physician Sigmund Freud (1962b). Freud believed that all psychologic and emotional events, however obscure, were understandable. For the meanings behind behavior, he looked to childhood experiences that he believed caused adult neuroses. Psychoanalytic therapy consists of clarifying the meaning of events, feelings, and behavior and thereby gaining insight about them. Freud's work shifted the focus of psychiatry from classification to a dynamic view of mental phenomena.

Assumptions and Key Ideas

The basic principles of psychoanalytic theory are discussed in the following section.

Psychic Determinism Psychic determinism states that no human behavior is accidental. Each psychic event is determined by the ones that preceded it. Events in people's mental lives that seem random or unrelated to what went before are only apparently so. Thus, psychoanalysts never dismiss any mental phenomenon as meaningless or accidental. They always search for what caused it, why it happened. For example, people commonly forget or misplace things. They usually view this as just an accident. Psychoanalysts seek to demonstrate that the accident was caused by a wish or intent of the person involved. Psychoanalysts also view dreams as subject to the principle of psychic determinism, each dream and each image in each dream bearing some relationship to the rest of the dreamer's life.

Role of the Unconscious The distinction between conscious and unconscious thought was made famous by Freud. Some kinds of information in the brain—your plans for the day, the faces of the people near you, your pleasures and your pains—are **conscious**. You think about them, discuss them, and let them guide your behavior. Others—the control of your heart rate and the sequence of muscle contractions that allow you to turn the pages of this book—are **unconscious**. They are in your brain someplace, but are sealed off from your planning and reasoning circuits. Any mental event that occurs outside of conscious awareness represents the unconscious region.

Significant unconscious mental processes occur frequently in normal as well as abnormal mental functioning. Much of what goes on in people's minds is unknown to them, and this accounts for the apparent discontinuities in their mental life. If the unconscious motivation of some behavioral symptoms is discovered, the apparent discontinuities disappear, and the cause becomes clear.

Psychoanalysis The most powerful method for studying the unconscious is the technique that Freud evolved over several years called **psychoanalysis**. The basic logic behind psychoanalysis is as follows:

1. The client underwent a *traumatic experience* that stirred up intense and painful emotion.
2. The traumatic experience represented to the client some ideas that were incompatible with the dominant ideas constituting the ego. Thus, the client experienced a *neurotic conflict*.
3. The incompatible idea and the neurotic conflict associated with it force the ego to bring into action *defense mechanisms*. Chapter 8 ∞ describes in detail common defense mechanisms.
4. Therapy is directed toward resolving the conflict by uncovering its roots in the unconscious. If the client is able to release the repressed feelings associated with the conflict, the symptoms disappear.

Strategies used in psychoanalysis are hypnosis, the interpretation of dreams, and *free association*, in which the client is encouraged to express every idea that comes to mind—no matter how insignificant, irrelevant, shameful, or embarrassing—ignoring all self-censorship and suspending all judgment.

Structure of the Mind With the publication of *The Ego and the Id* in 1923, Freud introduced the *structural model* of the mind (1962a). The structural model of the mind contends that there are three distinct entities: the id, the ego, and the superego. The **id** is a completely unorganized reservoir of energy derived from drives and instincts. The **ego** controls action and perception, controls contact with reality, and, through defense mechanisms, inhibits primary instinctual drives. One of its fundamental functions is also the capacity for developing mutually satisfying relationships with others. The **superego** is concerned with moral behavior. Frequently, the superego allies itself with the ego against the id, imposing demands in the form of conscience or guilt feelings.

The id in a child operates according to what Freud called the *pleasure principle:* the tendency to seek pleasure and avoid pain. This is not always possible, so the demands of the pleasure principle have to be modified by the *reality principle.* The reality principle is a learned ego function by which people develop the capacity to delay the immediate release of tension or achievement of pleasure. The relationship between Freud's levels of awareness and his concepts of id, superego, and ego is often depicted as an iceberg (see FIGURE 5-2 ■). In this image, the id is completely below the water's surface and the superego partially below and partially above the surface. In comparison to the superego, the ego is more fully above the surface in the realm of conscious awareness.

Drives Freud believed that psychic energy was derived from drives. He used the word *cathexis* to refer to the attachment of psychic energy to a person or a thing. The greater the cathexis, the greater the psychologic importance of the person or object.

Freud accounted for the instinctual aspects of a person's mental life by assuming the existence of two drives, the *sexual drive* and the *aggressive drive*. The former gives rise to the erotic component of mental activity, and the latter gives

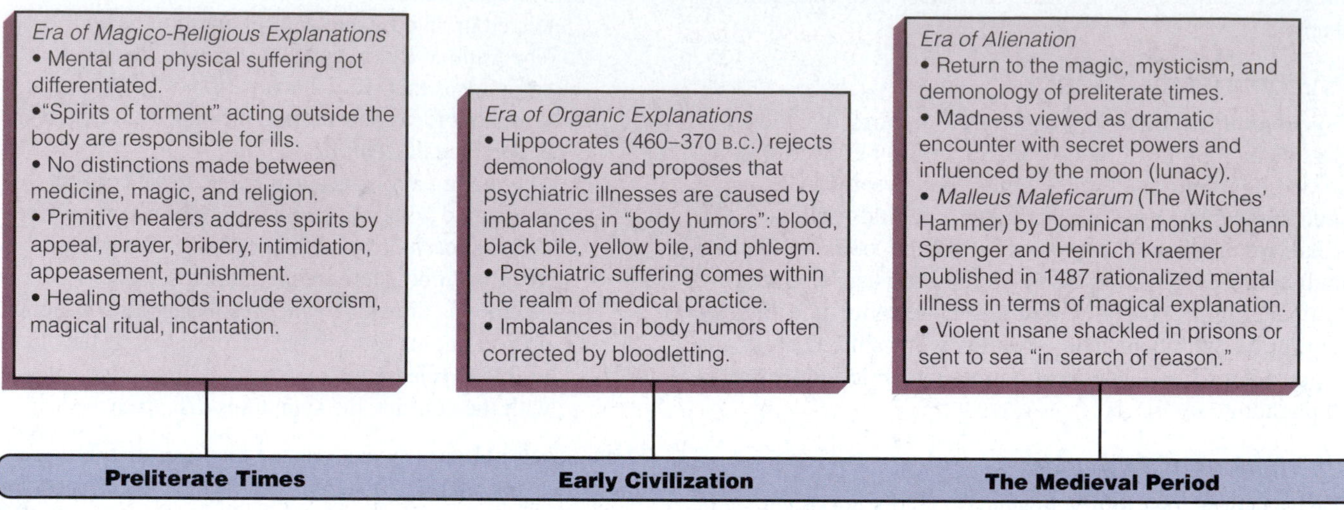
Era of Magico-Religious Explanations
• Mental and physical suffering not differentiated.
•"Spirits of torment" acting outside the body are responsible for ills.
• No distinctions made between medicine, magic, and religion.
• Primitive healers address spirits by appeal, prayer, bribery, intimidation, appeasement, punishment.
• Healing methods include exorcism, magical ritual, incantation.
Era of Organic Explanations
• Hippocrates (460–370 B.C.) rejects demonology and proposes that psychiatric illnesses are caused by imbalances in "body humors": blood, black bile, yellow bile, and phlegm.
• Psychiatric suffering comes within the realm of medical practice.
• Imbalances in body humors often corrected by bloodletting.
Era of Alienation
• Return to the magic, mysticism, and demonology of preliterate times.
• Madness viewed as dramatic encounter with secret powers and influenced by the moon (lunacy).
• *Malleus Maleficarum* (The Witches' Hammer) by Dominican monks Johann Sprenger and Heinrich Kraemer published in 1487 rationalized mental illness in terms of magical explanation.
• Violent insane shackled in prisons or sent to sea "in search of reason."
Preliterate Times
Early Civilization
The Medieval Period

Early 20th Century | **Mid-20th Century** | **Late 20th Century**

Era of Psychoanalysis
- Emil Kraepelin (1856–1926) creates system of distinct disease entities and differentiates bipolar disorder from schizophrenia.
- Sigmund Freud (1856–1939) explains human behavior in psychological terms and demonstrates that behavior can be changed through psychoanalysis.

Era of Ideologic Expansion
- From the mid-1940s to the mid-1950s, a strong rift between biologic orientation and dynamic orientation develops.
- By the early 1950s several drugs for the treatment of mental disorder were in common use.
- In 1946 the National Institute of Mental Health (NIMH) opened for research, training, and provision of preventive, therapeutic, and rehabilitative psychiatric services.
- Harry Stack Sullivan (1892–1949) developed the interpersonal theory of psychiatry.
- By 1960 family therapy had become both a diagnostic tool and a mode of treatment.
- Erik Erikson formulated his psychosocial theory of development.
- Psychotropic drugs help staff members manage large numbers of clients in crowded conditions.
- Group therapy and short-term therapy recognized as options to costly long-term therapy or hospitalization.
- Milieu therapy developed by Maxwell Jones in England.

Deinstitutionalization and the Community Mental Health Movement
- In 1961 the Joint Communication on Mental Illness and Health presented Action for Mental Health to Congress calling for a shift from institutional to community-based care; more equitable distribution of mental health services; preventive services; consumer participation in planning and delivery of mental health workers; education of more mental health professionals; public support for research; shared federal, state, local funding for construction; and operation of community mental health centers.
- Congress passed the Mental Retardation Facilities and Community Mental Health Centers Construction Act.
- Between 1955 and 1975 the number of resident clients in state mental hospitals decreased nearly 66 percent.
- The Community Mental Health Systems Act of 1980 authorized funding of community mental health centers, services to high-risk populations, ambulatory mental health care centers, rape research and services, but was repealed in 1981 and replaced by the Omnibus Budget Reconciliation Act, placing mental health programs into an alcohol, drug abuse, and mental health services block grant.

FIGURE 5-1 ■ A schematic of the history of psychiatry.

The Renaissance

Era of Confinement
- In 1656 Hôpital Générale in Paris founded to confine the mad, poor, and various deviants.
- The "insane" have no recourse to appeal.
- Madness not linked to medicine; could only be mastered by discipline and brutality.
- Radical physicians like Johann Weyer (1515–1588) believed that "those illnesses whose origins are attributed to witches come from natural causes."

Late 18th and Early 19th Centuries

Era of Moral Treatment
- Physicians classify symptoms of mental disorders without understanding the sources of mental suffering.
- In 1794 Philippe Pinel (1745–1826) treated inmates in the French institutions Bicetre and Salpetriere with humanity and was thus considered mad.
- In England, William Tuke (1732–1822) focused on "moral treatment" in a humane milieu called the York Retreat.
- In America, Benjamin Rush (1746–1813) focused on humanitarianism and moral treatment at the Pennsylvania Hospital.

Late 19th and Early 20th Centuries

Era of Public Mental Hospitals
- Dorothea L. Dix (1802–1887) founds or enlarges over 30 mental hospitals.
- Moral treatment replaced by custodial care.
- Clifford Beers (1876–1943) published his book describing his own intense suffering and mental anguish, leading to the development of preventative psychiatry and the formation of child guidance clinics.

The 1990s

The Decade of the Brain
- The primary innovation of the 1990s is the "biologic revolution": collaboration of science and technology to expand concepts of mental disorder proposed by psychological, behavioral, and psychoanalytic theories.
- A report by the National Advisory Health Council calls the gains made in research-based knowledge about the epidemiology, diagnosis, treatment, and prevention of major mental illnesses a "quantum leap in understanding the brain."
- Client advocacy groups welcome psychiatry's shift toward psychosocial rehabilitation for client self-care.
- The National Alliance for the Mentally Ill (NAMI), establishes a separate research foundation to study the biologic basis of major mental illness.

The New Millennium

Era of Health Care Reform
- Reform of psychiatric care has decreased length of hospital stays and increased client acuity.
- The advancing explosion in neuroscience has reshaped our conception of the bases of mental disorders.
- Innovations in technology have informed diagnostic practices such as brain imaging.
- The array of psychopharmacologic treatments available continues to expand.
- Populations of psychiatric clients include growing numbers of mentally ill elders, more people with coexisting substance use disorders, more comorbidities with chronic illnesses including HIV/AIDS, and expanding racial and cultural diversity.
- A yearning for spirituality has been reawakened in clients as well as health care providers.
- The study of genomes and the biology of the brain touch ethical, moral, and political nerves.

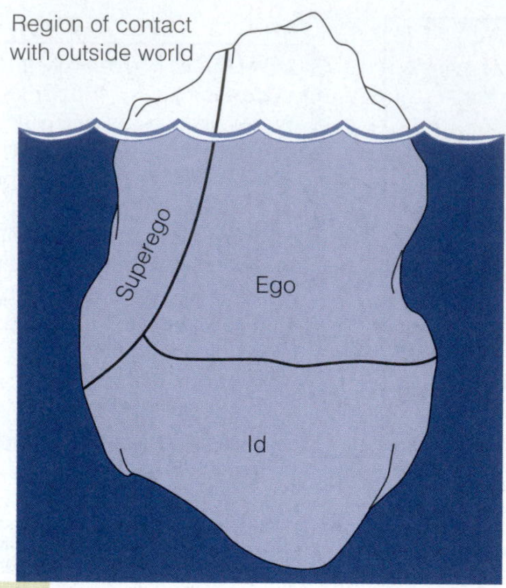

FIGURE 5-2 ■ Levels of awareness in relation to id, ego, and superego.

rise to the destructive component. The sexual drive came to be known as the *libido*. TABLE 5-1 ■ presents the stages of psychosexual development according to Freud.

Decline of Freudian Psychoanalysis

The past 40 years has seen a steady decline in the reliance on psychoanalytic theory and psychoanalysis as a treatment measure. Several critics such as Crews (1998) and Webster (1995) note that psychoanalytic theory is based on inferences (not proof) from clinical experiences, no single verifiable cure exists, and psychoanalysis is the costliest and most time-consuming treatment. In addition, because it requires a person to be relatively well functioning, introspective, and financially secure, psychoanalysis is not accessible to many mental health clients. People with psychotic disorders or personality disorders are especially unlikely to benefit. However, as you will see later in this chapter, variations on Freudian theory led to the development of various insight-oriented therapies such as those described in the section on social–interpersonal theories.

Implications for Psychiatric–Mental Health Nursing Practice

Psychoanalytic theory has historically provided an extremely limited treatment role for the nurse. Psychoanalytic clients are usually seen in the analyst's office as private clients. With the emergence of psychoanalytically oriented private hospital treatment settings such as Chestnut Lodge in Rockville, Maryland, nurses became somewhat more involved, sharing at least in the psychoanalytic language, concepts, and speculations about client dynamics and personality development, but usually not in a psychotherapeutic treatment role.

Cognitive Behavior Theory

Cognitive behavior theory focuses on the present rather than the past. Behaviorist theory in psychiatry has its roots in psychology and neurophysiology. The term *behavior therapy* has largely been replaced by the term *cognitive–behavior therapy,* although they may be used interchangeably throughout this text.

To the behaviorist, symptoms associated with neuroses and psychoses are clusters of learned behaviors that persist because they are somehow rewarding to the individual. One of the most important contributions to this framework was made by Pavlov (1849–1936), who in 1902 discovered a phenomenon he called the **conditioned response** in a famous experiment with a dog and a bell. The basic principle of the conditioned response is this:

1. A response is a reaction to a stimulus.
2. If a new and different stimulus is presented with or just before the original stimulating event, the same response reaction can be obtained.
3. Eventually the new stimulus can replace the original one, so that the response occurs in reaction to the new stimulus alone.

The conditioned or learned response is viewed as the basic unit of all learning, the unit on which more complex behavioral patterns are constructed. Such construction occurs through a process called **reinforcement**, in which behaviors are rewarded and persist. Pavlov's theories have influenced contemporary cognitive behavioral therapists and are valued

TABLE 5-1 ■ **Freud's Psychosexual Stages**

Stage	Age Span	Task	Key Concept
Oral	0–18 months	Satisfaction and anxiety management from oral activity	Oral activity gives pleasure and is a source for learning
Anal	18 months–3 years	Learning muscle control for toilet training	Delayed gratification and rule internalization
Phallic	3–6 years	Gender identification and genital awareness	Repression of attraction to the opposite-sex parent, leading to same-sex identification
Latency	6–12 years	Repression of sexuality	Oedipal conflict resolved with a shift to other interests and friends
Genital	12 years–young adult	Channeling sexuality into relationships with members of the opposite sex	Reemerging sexuality to motivate behavior

for their simplicity, concreteness, and objectivity. Some behaviorists see them as the key to understanding and controlling the whole range of undesirable human behavior.

Assumptions and Key Ideas

The fundamental premises of cognitive–behaviorial theory are as follows:

- The self in humans is the sum or repository of past conditionings or simply the behavioral repertoire. Therapists can know clients only by the clients' behavior.
- Behavior is the way in which a person acts. It can be observed, described, and recorded.
- There is no autonomous person. People are what they do and what they are reinforced for doing by conditions in their environment.
- The self is a structure of stimulus–response chains or hierarchies of habit. It is possible to know and predict conditions under which behavior will occur.
- The symptoms of a mental disorder are, in fact, the substance of that person's troubles. There is no hidden motive, no underlying cause, no internal pathogenic process. There is only the symptom or the behavior, and the aim of cognitive–behaviorial therapy is to change the behavior.
- The therapist determines what behavior should be changed and what plan should be followed. Change comes about by identifying events in the client's life that have been critical stimuli for the behavior and then arranging interventions for *extinguishing* those behaviors. A changed way of acting precedes a changed way of thinking, according to behaviorist theory.

Both Joseph Wolpe (1956) and B. F. Skinner (1971) are associated with psychiatric treatment approaches that represent one form of **conditioning** and reflect the above assumptions. Wolpe defined *neurotic behavior* as unadaptive behavior acquired in anxiety-generating situations. He based his therapeutic method on the introduction of a response that inhibits anxiety when situations occur that ordinarily evoke anxiety. Relaxation, for example, was considered incompatible with anxiety and, therefore, effective in inhibiting it. Thus, Wolpe would direct his intervention to a counterconditioning technique, usually putting the client under hypnosis and using various techniques for gradual *desensitization.* For example, a man afraid of dying might gradually attempt to overcome his anxiety at seeing a coffin, attending a funeral, and so on, by trying to relax in these situations.

Skinner's approach, called **operant conditioning**, emphasizes discovering why the behavioral response was elicited in the first place and what actively reinforces it. The key concept in operant conditioning is reinforcement. Skinner originally used the term **positive reinforcement** to describe an event that increases the probability that the response will recur—a reward for behavior. A **negative reinforcement** was defined as an event likely to decrease the possibility of recurrence because it penalizes the behavior.

Other contemporary cognitive–behaviorists have redefined Skinner's original terms and introduced some new ones. Positive reinforcement is still an environmental event that rewards and thus increases the probability of a behavioral response. Negative reinforcement can mean removal of an adverse stimulus (such as an electric shock to animals or the restriction of people's privileges) to increase the likelihood of a behavior's recurrence. *Positive punishment,* in contrast, is the introduction of aversive stimuli to decrease the likelihood of the recurrence of a behavior. *Negative punishment* removes something that has been a prior reinforcer, thus again decreasing the likelihood of such behaviors as smoking, drug abuse, truancy, temper outbursts, and abuse. TABLE 5-2 ■ lists examples of each of these behaviorist concepts.

The term for an intervention designed to change a person's behavior is **shaping**. It is a procedure of manipulating reinforcement to bring the person closer to the desired behavior. According to Skinner, there are times in a client's life when responses are accidentally reinforced by a coincidental pairing of response and reinforcement. This accidental pairing may play a role in the development of phobias (irrational fears) and other distressing and/or dysfunctional behaviors.

In addition to these classics, contemporary cognitive behavioral therapists use a vast array of techniques based on basic psychological science and developed out of psychological research and validated in thousands of treatment outcome studies. Cognitive behavioral therapy is more fully discussed in Chapter 31 ∞.

TABLE 5-2 ■ Examples of Some Cognitive Behaviorist Concepts

Concept	Purpose	Example
Positive reinforcement	Increase recurrence of the behavior through reward	Leave of absence from the hospital, per contract with the client
Negative reinforcement	Increase recurrence of the behavior by removing aversive consequences	Removal of restrictions on phone calls or visitors, per contract with client
Positive punishment	Decrease the behavior by adding aversive consequences	Quiet time
Negative punishment	Decrease the behavior by withdrawing a reinforcer or reward	Withdrawal of privileges, such as recreational outings in a residential milieu

Implications for Psychiatric–Mental Health Nursing Practice

Most psychiatric–mental health nurses acknowledge that the application of principles of behavior modification is quite complex. The use of this approach raises issues of control, responsibility for behavior, and the morality of using negative or punitive stimuli in a therapeutic context, to name only a few. Therapists who successfully resolve such basic philosophic issues have designed and implemented successful behavior modification plans with disturbed, overtly aggressive children, developmentally disabled clients, and violently self-destructive people.

In many institutional environments, clients follow prescribed schedules for daily living that include a **token economy**. Clients are rewarded for desired behavior by token reinforcers, such as food, candy, and verbal approval. The movement toward community-based psychiatric treatment has made plain some of the shortcomings and economic realities of therapies aimed toward resolving everyone's intrapsychic conflicts. The movement has instead attempted to replace maladaptive behavior with behavior that allows people to function effectively within their natural environment. When parents or others in the client's environment are taught to implement the behavior change procedures, therapy moves away from the artificial situation of the therapist's office into the client's total environment. It no longer requires the presence of highly trained, often expensive experts and thus makes treatment more affordable.

Psychiatric–mental health nurses have had a special role in teaching behaviorist principles to people with little training so that they can act as change agents. Nonprofessional staff can be taught the effective use of behaviorist principles to eliminate chronic, maladaptive behavior. Hyperactive children or children with borderline intelligence can be treated in the home by their parents when nurses teach the parents to use approaches such as frequency counts on specific behaviors to be modified, time-outs (short periods of isolation) for undesired behavior, and the bestowal of attention, praise, and affectionate physical contact as rewards.

Cognitive behavioral interventions focus on the individual—what that person feels, thinks, and assigns meanings to—and empowers clients to learn new skills. How psychiatric–mental health nurses can use cognitive behavioral strategies, such as behavioral contracting, in their clinical practice is the subject of Chapter 31.

MEDIALINK Case Study: Through the Developmental Looking Glass

Social–Interpersonal Theories

Social–interpersonal theories of psychiatry grew out of a general dissatisfaction with approaches that account for mental illness in terms of either intrapersonal mechanisms (the symptoms of a disease) or individual personality dynamics such as anxiety, ego strength, and libido. Advocates of this perspective assert that other theories neglect the crucial social processes and cultural variation involved in the development, identification, and resolution of disturbed human responses.

Assumptions and Key Ideas

Two separate but philosophically congruent schools of thought contribute to social–interpersonal theories. These are the interpersonal–psychiatric and the general systems approaches. The assumptions and key ideas of each are discussed in the following section.

Interpersonal–Psychiatric Theory Psychiatrists Adolf Meyer (1948–1952) and Harry Stack Sullivan (1953) made significant contributions to social–interpersonal theory in the first half of the 20th century. Sullivan trained with William Alanson White and Adolf Meyer rather than with Freud. He is viewed as the least reductionist of psychiatric theorists and emphasizes **interpersonal theory** (the client's past and present relationships with others and modes of interaction) as the real focus of psychiatric inquiry. Sullivan became the theoretic and ideologic leader of the interpersonal school of psychiatry often associated with the William Alanson White Foundation.

One concept that plays a crucial role in the organization of behavior, according to Sullivan, is the **self-system** or *self-dynamism.* The self-system provides tools that enable people to deal with the tasks of avoiding anxiety and establishing security. The self is a construct built from the child's experience. It is made up of **reflected appraisals** the person learns in contact with significant others. The self develops in the process of seeking physical satisfaction of bodily needs and security. To feel secure, the self essentially requires feelings of approval and prestige as protection against anxiety.

Rewarding appraisals from others yield what Sullivan calls the *good-me* aspect of the self. Anxiety-producing appraisals result in the *bad-me*. The *not-me* exists normally in dreams and in aspects of experience that are poorly understood and later experienced as dread, horror, and loathing among mentally disordered people. In summary, Sullivan emphasizes the pervasive interaction between the organism and the environment as well as the developmental tasks of the personality (TABLE 5-3 ■). Nonetheless, Sullivan has little to say about the impact on behavior of specific variations in the social or cultural scene.

Like Sullivan, other advocates of the interpersonal school of psychiatry, such as Karen Horney (1950) and Erich Fromm (1941), stress the general climate in the immediate family. Alfred Adler (1971), however, attempts to understand more of the social and cultural conditions influencing behavior. The interpersonal school of psychiatry in general takes a developmental–interpersonal view of the self.

The *self-actualization* and hierarchy-of-needs theories of Abraham Maslow (1962) belong squarely in this school (FIGURE 5-3 ■). Maslow proposed an order, or hierarchy, of basic human needs. According to Maslow, physiological needs must be met before higher-level needs such as self-esteem and self-actualization.

Erik Erikson also formulated a developmental theory of personality that attempted to take into account not just biologic instincts (in this sense, he can be called a neo-Freudian)

TABLE 5-3 ■ Sullivan's Stages of Interpersonal Development

Age	Stage	Task/Key Concept
Birth–18 months (to appearance of speech)	Infancy	Experiences anxiety in interaction with mother figure; learns to use maternal tenderness to gain security and avoid anxiety
18 months–6 years (from first speech to need for playmates)	Childhood	Learns to delay gratification in response to interpersonal demands; uses language and action to avoid anxiety
6–9 years	Juvenile	Develops peer relationships and uses environment outside the family to shape self
9–12 years	Preadolescence	Develops a caring relationship with same-sex peer, chum relationship
12–14 years	Early adolescence	Develops interest in opposite-sex relationships
14–21 years	Late adolescence	Has satisfying relationships; directs sexual impulses
21 years +	Adulthood	Establishes a love relationship

but also cultural and interpersonal tasks that have to be accomplished in order to move forward developmentally. Erikson's developmental theory is considered more optimistic than Freud's because he believed that clients in therapy could return to a developmental task that had not been accomplished and relearn it (Erikson, 1963). Erikson's eight developmental stages are discussed in TABLE 5-4 ■ on page 78.

General Systems Theory **General systems theory**, when applied to living systems (people), provides a conceptual framework for integrating the biologic and social sciences with the physical sciences. In psychiatry, it offers a resolution of the mind–body dichotomy, an integration of biologic and social approaches to the nature of human beings, and an approach to psychopathology, diagnosis, and therapy. Karl Menninger (1963) views normal personality functioning and psychopathology in terms of general systems theory. His work addresses four major issues:

1. Adjustment or individual–environment interaction
2. The organization of living systems
3. Psychologic regulation and control, known as *ego theory* in psychoanalysis
4. Motivation, which is often called *instinct* or *drive* in the psychoanalytic framework

A salient point of Menninger's theory is the idea of *homeostasis* (equilibrium). He asserts that the greater the threat or stress on a system, the greater the number of system components involved in coping with or adapting to it. Therefore, pathology can exist at various levels:

- The cell and organ level: an example might be the behavioral changes that follow cellular

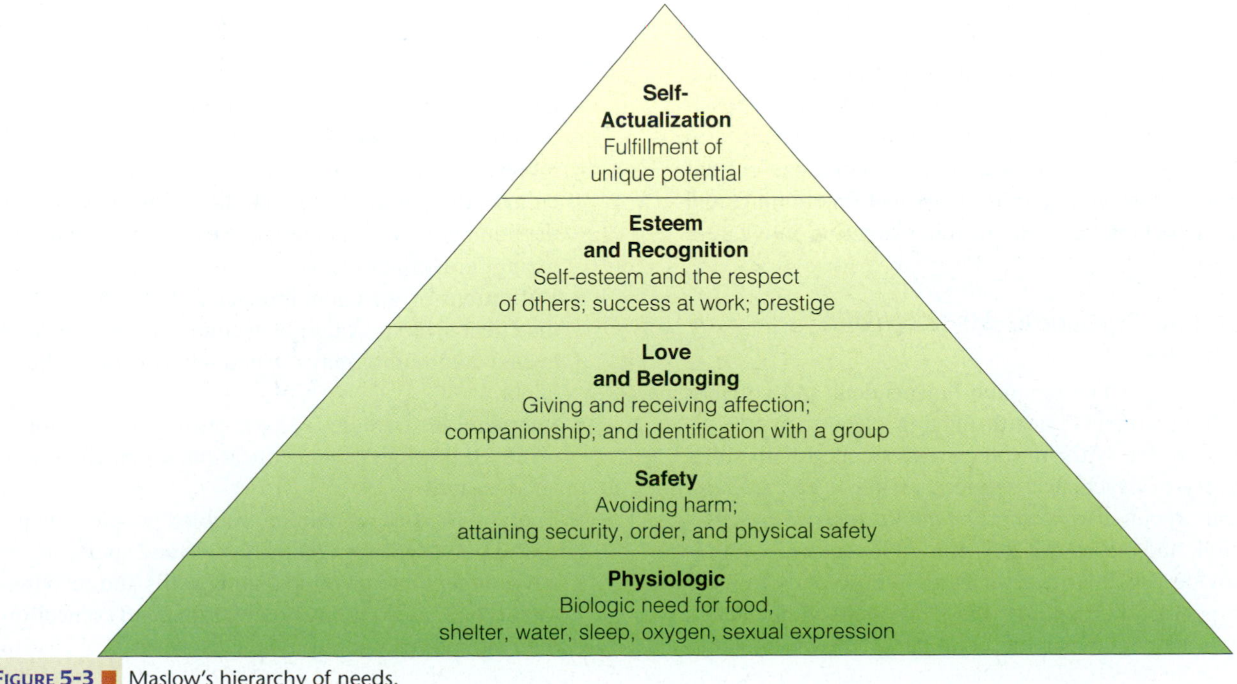

FIGURE 5-3 ■ Maslow's hierarchy of needs.

Table 5-4 ■ Erikson's Eight Developmental Stages

Age	Stage of Development	Task/Area of Resolution	Concepts/Basic Attitudes
Birth–18 months	Infancy	Trust versus mistrust	Ability to trust others and a sense of one's own trustworthiness; a sense of hope; withdrawal and estrangement
18 months–3 years	Early childhood	Autonomy versus shame and doubt	Self-control without loss of self-esteem; ability to cooperate and to express oneself; compulsive self-restraint or compliance; defiance, willfulness
3–5 years	Late childhood	Initiative versus guilt	Realistic sense of purpose; some ability to evaluate one's own behavior; self-denial and self-restriction
6–12 years	School age	Industry versus inferiority	Realization of competence, perseverance; feeling that one will never be "any good," withdrawal from school and peers
12–20 years	Adolescence	Identity versus role diffusion	Coherent sense of self; plans to actualize one's abilities; feelings of confusion, indecisiveness, possibly antisocial behavior
18–25 years	Young adulthood	Intimacy versus isolation	Capacity for love as mutual devotion; commitment to work and relationships; impersonal relationships, prejudice
25–65 years	Adulthood	Generativity versus stagnation	Creativity, productivity, concern for others; self-indulgence, impoverishment of self
65 years to death	Old age	Integrity versus despair	Acceptance of the worth and uniqueness of one's life; sense of loss, contempt for others

alterations due to addictive drugs, to a blood clot, or to a tumor

- The group level: an example is family violence
- The community level: examples are overpopulation, pollution, homelessness, and poverty

In general systems theory, all represent abnormalities or stresses on matter–energy processes and would be included within the domain of psychiatric professionals.

In Menninger's view, a system's well-being depends on the amount of stress on it and the effectiveness of its coping mechanisms. He asserts that mental illness is an impairment of self-regulation in which comfort, growth, and production are surrendered for the sake of survival at the best level possible but at the sacrifice of emergency coping devices. Therapists using the general systems approach emphasize current conflicts, restoration of impaired systems of functioning, and subsequent reintegration of the restored function into future coping strategies.

Implications for Psychiatric–Mental Health Nursing Practice

Social–interpersonal theories give independent and collaborative psychiatric–mental health nursing clear theoretic direction and support. Nursing roles are associated with shifts in the delivery of psychiatric services variously termed *case management, social psychiatry, community psychiatry, psychoeducation*, and *milieu therapy*. All are associated with efforts to provide psychiatric services more efficiently to large groups of people, particularly those previously neglected, and attempts to counteract the debilitating effects of long-term institutionalization. All are also associated with a movement to address the client's social context in providing psychiatric care.

According to these orientations, all social, psychologic, and biologic activity, including research developments in psychobiology, affecting the mental health of the population is important to professionals in community psychiatry. Therapeutic interventions may include programs for social change, political involvement, community organization, social planning, family support groups, and education about medications, symptom management, genetic risk, and family environment. Many implications for practice can be derived from this theoretic model:

- Clients are approached in a holistic way, reflecting the interrelationship and interaction between the biophysical, psychologic, and socioeconomic–cultural dimensions of human life. This increases the number of factors the nurse must assess when caring for a client.
- Definitions of the client must include the concept of the client system. A family, a couple, an aggregate, or even a community may collectively constitute the client.
- Intervention strategies include primary prevention achieved through psychoeducation, social change, and research.
- Therapy focuses on helping troubled people gain a useful perspective on their lifestyle and social environment and develop coping skills and resources, rather than on exclusively repressing and controlling their symptoms.

- The psychiatric–mental health nurse must be prepared to function as an autonomous member of the mental health team and to assume more responsibilities in the shift away from the dominance of the physician in decision making and toward diffusion of roles. Practitioners' roles are based less on background discipline than on availability and interest in helping the client. For example, a cadre of mental health professionals who could become chronic care experts is sorely needed, particularly those who can synthesize psychobiologic knowledge with psychosocial rehabilitation skills and psychoeducation.

Once clients are viewed as becoming dysfunctional in the context of unhealthy or problem-filled interpersonal relationships, establishing healthy, constructive interpersonal relationships becomes important in their care. Psychiatric–mental health nurses can apply concepts of milieu therapy, primary prevention, social psychiatry, community psychiatry, and psychobiologic interventions to implement this fundamental idea. The following clinical example is an illustration.

CLINICAL EXAMPLE

Mrs. Seminara is a 67-year-old, upper-middle-class woman in good physical health. She has become increasingly untidy, forgetful, reclusive, sad, and suspicious since the death of her aggressive, bank-president husband from a heart attack 6 months ago. She recently sold the large house where she had lived for the past 45 years and moved into a two-bedroom apartment in a nearby town. Because of apartment rules, she was unable to take her 12-year-old cat. She sold the house because her husband had told his lawyers that she should do so. (He had made all the family decisions while he lived.) Mrs. Seminara has taken to skipping meals except for candy bars because she must rely on a friend to drive her to the grocery store. (Her husband believed she did not need to learn to drive.) Her younger sister (age 59), seeking advice about Mrs. Seminara's behavior, phoned the community mental health center at the suggestion of the family physician.

The social–interpersonal psychiatric–mental health nurse assessing this situation would tend not to view Mrs. Seminara's symptoms as psychologic conflicts reflecting her ambivalence toward her dead husband or as manifestations of a mental disorder, such as major, single-episode depression. Instead, the nurse would focus on the way Mrs. Seminara is functioning in her current interpersonal situation and her holistic human responses to it. In this analysis, the nurse does not view Mrs. Seminara as "diseased" and therefore in exclusive need of a somatic treatment such as medication.

Instead, treatment consists of helping Mrs. Seminara develop strategies for coping with her new situation and satisfying her needs. The nurse would seek out the younger sister and other family members in an attempt to enhance Mrs. Seminara's social support network. Efforts may be directed toward mobilizing other environmental forces (including the nurse) to provide company, stimulation, and proper nutrition for Mrs. Seminara, since the absence of all three contributes to her symptoms and discomfort.

The clinical situation would undoubtedly reinforce the psychiatric nurse's political efforts to point out the potential consequences of lifelong passive dependence of some adult women. The nurse may also become involved in community organizations working for better services for older clients.

Table 5-5 ■ presents a comparison of the traditional psychiatric theories discussed in this chapter upon which psychiatric–mental health nurses base their plans of care. While the approaches suggested by these theories appear to be very different, it is up to the individual psychiatric–mental health nurse to use the best aspects of each approach in clinical practice. For example, a biologically oriented clinician can see the value of psychotherapy or cognitive behavior therapy, as well as medication, for a man who has a fear of flying, and a cognitive behavioral therapist can appreciate the anxiety-reducing effects of medication for the client.

Table 5-5 ■ Comparison of Major Features of Traditional Psychiatric Theories

Theory	Assessment Base	Problem Statement	Goal	Dominant Interventions
Medical–psychobiologic	Individual client symptoms	Disease	Symptom management; cure	Psychopharmacology and other biologic therapies
Psychoanalytic	Intrapsychic; unconscious	Conflict	Insight	Psychoanalysis
Cognitive behavioral	Behavior	Learning deficit	Behavior change	Behavior modification or conditioning
Social–interpersonal	Interactions between individual and social contexts	Interpersonal dysfunction	Enhanced awareness and quality of interpersonal interactions	Group, family, and milieu therapies

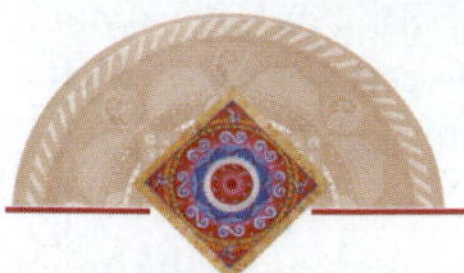

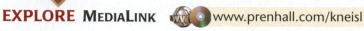

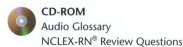

EXPLORE MEDIALINK 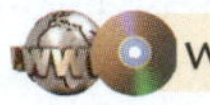 www.prenhall.com/kneisl

For NCLEX-RN® review questions, case studies, and other resources for this chapter see the Pearson Health MediaLink CD-ROM that accompanies this book and the Companion Website at www.prenhall.com/kneisl.

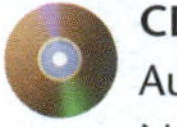

CD-ROM
Audio Glossary
NCLEX-RN® Review Questions

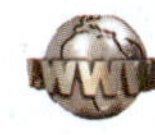

Companion Website
Audio Glossary
NCLEX-RN® Review Questions
Critical Thinking Exercise
- *Nursing: Art or Science?*

Case Study
- *Through the Developmental Looking Glass*

Care Plan
- *Humanism: A Basis for Care*

MediaLinks
MediaLink Application
- *Communicating Competence*

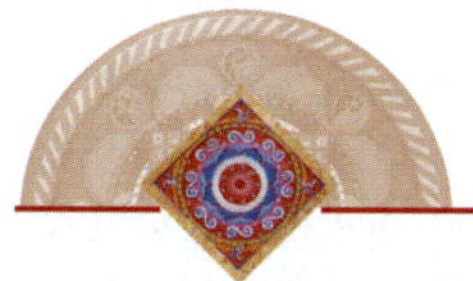

NCLEX-RN® REVIEW QUESTIONS

1. The nurse and physician are discussing a therapeutic approach for a client experiencing depression. The nurse states that clients have control over their own lives. What therapeutic approach does this opinion represent?
1. Humanism
2. Psychoanalysis
3. Interactionism
4. Conditioning

2. A philosophy of service to benefit humanity through science, reason, and democracy is:
1. Symbolic interactionism.
2. Psychobiology.
3. Humanism.
4. Psychic determinism.

3. Which of the following are characteristics of a holistic approach to psychiatric–mental health nursing care? (Select all that apply.)
1. The biological aspect of illness is considered.
2. Physical symptoms are interrelated with mental factors.
3. Mental illness does not impact physiologic homeostasis.
4. The client's socioeconomic status is considered in planning care.
5. The client's spiritual needs are not considered when planning nursing care.

4. The psychiatric–mental health nurse is utilizing interactionism as a therapeutic modality for clients. In using this model, the nurse understands that:
1. The underlying cause of mental illness is organic and located in the central nervous system.
2. Each psychic event is determined by the ones that preceded it.
3. All behavior has meaning.
4. The focus of treatment is on the present rather than the past.

5. According to psychoanalytic theory, the superego is concerned with:
1. The desire to seek pleasure while avoiding pain.
2. The ability to delay an immediate release of tension or achievement of pleasure.
3. Moral behavior.
4. Mutually satisfying relationships with others.

6. The role of the nurse in a humanistic interactional therapeutic model includes:
1. Participating in political systems to promote a holistic approach to mental health care.
2. Advanced knowledge of client dynamics and personality development.
3. Implementing a token economy to reward desirable client behavior.
4. Outreach and case management to a large group of clients with chronic mental illness.

7. The nurse asks the client to describe what the client was feeling prior to an outburst of aggressive behavior during group therapy. The nurse is utilizing what theoretical framework?
1. Medical–psychobiologic
2. Psychoanalytic
3. Cognitive behavioral
4. Social–interpersonal

8. The nurse explains to a group of clients that they will receive an additional 30 minutes of recreation time if they actively participate in group therapy. What is this an example of?
1. Conditioned response
2. Reinforcement
3. Operant conditioning
4. Positive punishment

9. The belief that emotional and behavioral disturbances are the result of a disease process reflects which theory?
1. Psychic determinism
2. Shaping
3. Symbolic interactionism
4. Psychobiology

10. In the general systems theory framework, nursing care is based on the belief that:
1. Mental illness is caused by an organic disease process.
2. Clients need to understand the meaning of their behavior before they can overcome it.
3. Individuals have the capacity to avoid anxiety and establish security.
4. A holistic approach to care includes the client system.

See Appendix C for answers.

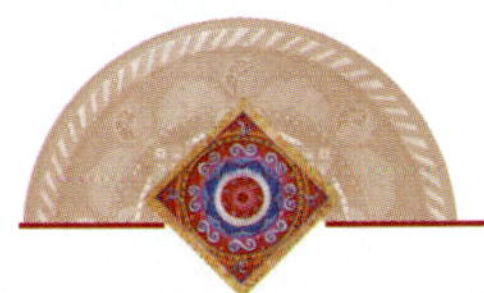

REFERENCES

Adler, A. (1971). *The practice and theory of individual psychology.* New York: Humanities Press. Trans.

Blumer, H. (1969). *Symbolic interaction: Perspective and method.* New York: Prentice Hall.

Chiovitti, R. F. (2006). Nurses' meaning of caring with patients in acute psychiatric hospital settings: A grounded theory study. *International Journal of Nursing Studies, 43*(7), 831–841.

Crews, F. C. (1998). *Unauthorized Freud: Doubters confront a legend.* New York: Viking Press.

Erikson, E. (1963). *Childhood and society* (2nd ed.). New York: Norton.

Freud, S. (1962a). *The ego and the id.* New York: Norton.

Freud, S. (1962b). *The standard edition of the complete psychological works of Sigmund Freud* (24 vols). New York: Hogarth Press.

Fromm, E. (1941). *Escape from freedom.* New York: Irvington.

Horney, K. (1950). *Neurosis and human growth.* New York: Norton.

Lamont, C. (1967). *The philosophy of humanism.* New York: Frederick Ungar.

Maslow, A. (1970). *Motivation and personality* (2nd ed.). New York: Harper & Row.

Maslow, A. (1962). *Toward a psychology of being.* New York: Van Nostrand.

Menninger, K. (1963). *The vital balance.* New York: Viking Press.

Meyer, A. (1948–52). *Collected papers of Adolf Meyer, 1–4.* Baltimore: Johns Hopkins University Press.

Shorter, E. (1996). *A history of psychiatry: From the era of the asylum to the age of Prozac.* New York: John Wiley.

Skinner, B. F. (1971). *Beyond freedom and dignity.* New York: Prentice Hall.

Sullivan, H. S. (1953). *The interpersonal theory of psychiatry.* New York: W. W. Norton.

Webster, R. (1995). *Why Freud was wrong: Sin, science, and psychoanalysis.* New York: Basic Books.

Wolpe, J. (1956). Learning versus lesions as the basis of neurotic behavior. *American Journal of Psychiatry, 112,* 923–931.

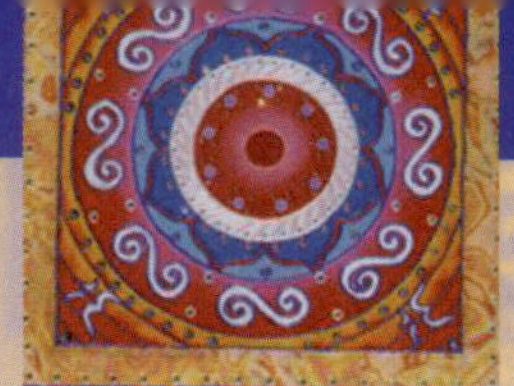

CHAPTER

6

Psychobiology, Behavior, and Mental Disorders

EILEEN TRIGOBOFF
CAROL REN KNEISL
PAMELA MARCUS

KEY TERMS

amygdala *85*
brain stem *89*
cerebellum *88*
cerebrum *83*
dexamethasone suppression test (DST) *97*
DNA *90*
dopamine *95*
genotype *90*
hippocampus *86*
hypothalamus *88*
limbic system *85*
neurons *93*
norepinephrine *96*
neurotransmitters (NTs) *93*
phenotype *90*
serotonin *96*

LEARNING OUTCOMES

After completing this chapter, you will be able to:

1. Describe how neuroanatomic structures affect thought, behavior, memory, understanding of consequences, and emotions.
2. Systematically compare and contrast alterations of the neuromessengers that occur in major psychiatric disorders, such as schizophrenia, bipolar disorder, and major depression.
3. Provide examples of genetic contributions to mental disorder.
4. Identify the ways in which the communication between the endocrine and immune systems affects a person's mood and behavior.
5. Explain how understanding the biologic contribution to emotional problems contributes to your nursing practice.
6. Partner with clients and families to teach the biologic implications of psychiatric illnesses.
7. Develop an awareness of how your own personal feelings, opinions, or beliefs about psychobiology can enhance or diminish your ability to be a support person and advocate for clients and their families.

CRITICAL THINKING CHALLENGE

Imagine you are the nurse at a family care clinic, and Kay, a 30-year-old woman with mood swings, is being assessed. During your clinical interview you discover she is currently a caretaker for several family members: her father, who has dementia of the Alzheimer's type; her mother, who is depressed and unable to function; and her 38-year-old brother, who has severe symptoms of paranoid schizophrenia. Major psychiatric illnesses are now understood as brain diseases that affect behavior, cognition, learning, and emotion. This knowledge has ramifications as it relates to your role, since the interventions that are aimed at improving overall functioning must consider Kay's unique biologic, environmental, and psychosocial strengths and weaknesses.

1. How can you integrate the understanding of the biologic components of Kay's functioning when providing comprehensive care?
2. Do you have a responsibility to integrate the biologic information with the behavioral and affective components of Kay's life?

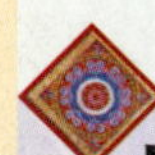

MEDIALINK 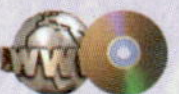 www.prenhall.com/kneisl

Go to the Pearson Health MediaLink CD-ROM and the Companion Website at www.prenhall.com/kneisl for interactive resources for this chapter.

Psychobiology is neither a new concept nor a recent discovery. It has existed since the birth of humankind and has been a subject of discussion for at least the last 2,000 years. What *is* new in psychobiology is a broader understanding of the biologic basis of the mind and behavior. This understanding lowers the likelihood that people with psychiatric disorders will experience stigma. Current knowledge about the biologic components of behavior is revolutionizing not only psychiatry but also our view of behavior, temperament, and psychiatric disorders and their treatment.

Psychobiology encompasses an enormous amount of information that is growing at a tremendous pace, based on current research. The study of the brain structures, biochemical foundations, molecular and genetic influences on cognition, mood, emotion, affect, and behavior and the interactions among them make up the realm of psychobiology. This comprehensive view takes into consideration both internal and external influences across a person's life span, including genetics, the effects of other body systems such as the endocrine and immune systems, temperament, resiliency to stress, and the environment.

A major barrier that inhibits clients and families from seeking care is stigma. Stigma results from lack of knowledge, misunderstanding how a severe mental disorder comes about, and not a small contribution from media sources that sensationalize events and demonize those who are ill. Parenting styles and lack of character can no longer be blamed for contributing to mental disorders. Understanding the working hypotheses of psychobiology is important for removing the guilt and stigma associated with psychiatric disorders. Teaching clients and families about the biologic aspects of the disorder increases their understanding of the illness and its treatment, and can increase the client's motivation to continue to seek appropriate treatment.

The standards of practice for psychiatric–mental health nursing (American Nurses Association, American Psychiatric Nurses Association, & International Society of Psychiatric–Mental Health Nurses, 2007) urge the inclusion of biologic therapies along with the use of the more traditional psychotherapy, psychosocial therapies, and combination therapies in the ongoing shift to a community-based care system. Excellence-based psychiatric–mental health nursing integrates psychobiologic concepts with our traditional practice to provide holistic caring for both clients and their families. Our understanding of the role biologic factors play in the client's illness and recovery can assist the client in adhering to medication regimens and other therapeutic interventions through psychoeducation and partnerships.

In this chapter we highlight the psychobiologic principles that can be used in the nursing care of a client. It is not possible in one chapter to even touch upon all of the facets of psychobiology in any detail. The goal of this chapter is to help you apply basic psychobiologic principles in your professional work. To help integrate these psychobiologic principles into your clinical practice, this chapter will focus on structure and function and how they both play key roles in behavior and emotional communication.

BRAIN, MIND, AND BEHAVIOR

Communication is a vital aspect of psychiatric–mental health nursing. Through neurobiologic discoveries we now know that communication, behaviors, and thought patterns have a molecular, anatomic, and chemical basis. Who we are originates from order or disorder at any of these levels.

The brain encodes or decodes information through complex interactions of neuromessengers, chemical processes, and anatomic systems. When clients say that health care providers told them their symptoms were "a nervous breakdown" or "all in your head," you can reframe those messages using current neurobiologic knowledge. For example, panic attacks are real; they result from the triggering of an overreactive alarm center in the brain, which sends a message of fear via the release of a neurotransmitter, causing a racing heart and shortness of breath.

Certain portions of the brain function in concert with other parts to create a system with a given function; the limbic system is a good example. Other systems that are of special interest to psychiatric–mental health nurses include the reticular activating system and the extrapyramidal system, discussed later in this chapter.

Neuroanatomy

Volumes have been written about the anatomy of the brain and the other components of the nervous system. The definition that best suits the perspective of this chapter is that the brain is a part of the central nervous system (CNS; that also includes the spinal cord) encapsulated by the skull. The brain is the core of our humanity. Intercommunication among different parts of the brain yields the experiences of love, hate, joy, fear, silliness, and sadness. The brain provides the underlying biology for will, determination, hopes, and dreams as well as the ability to problem-solve, to establish memory, and to learn and use acquired knowledge productively. The major features of the brain discussed here are the cerebrum, diencephalon, mesencephalon, pons, medulla oblongata, and cerebellum.

Cerebrum

The cerebrum includes the following structures and functions:

- Cerebral hemispheres
- Conscious thought processes, intellectual functions
- Memory storage and processing
- Conscious and subconscious regulation of skeletal muscle contractions

If you were to dissect the brain, you would see only indistinguishable gray matter, layer after layer. It is remarkable that such homogenous-looking tissue can be fundamentally varied. An atlas of the brain may be viewed on the website of Harvard Medical School (www.med.harvard.edu/AANLIB), which can be accessed on the Companion Website for this book.

MediaLink Whole Brain Atlas

The **cerebrum** comprises the largest part of the human brain. It is divided into two components, the *cerebral hemispheres.* The deep furrow that divides the hemispheres is known as the *longitudinal sulcus.* A small but important piece of tissue, the *corpus callosum,* connects the two hemispheres

Box 6-1 **Tools of Psychobiology**

Brain Imaging

- ***Computed tomography (CT).*** An x-ray beam (radiation exposure) is passed through serial sections of the brain to look at structural images.
- ***Magnetic resonance imaging (MRI).*** Reconstructs detailed images of cerebral anatomy from multiple perspectives, including subcortical structures, using radiofrequency signals emitted by relaxing hydrogen atoms. It delineates gray and white matter. New instruments image elements other than hydrogen, allowing MRI to be used for structural, functional, and metabolic imaging. Contraindicated for clients with any metal objects in their bodies such as pacemakers, due to the presence of a magnetic field.
- ***Positron emission tomography (PET).*** Imaging of active neurochemical substrates and physiologic processes; regional localization of metabolic functions through the measurement of radioactive labels or tags attached to molecules as glucose; density of neuroreceptors; regional cerebral blood flow (rCBF) of the brain. Operates on the principle that blood rushes to the busiest area of the brain to deliver oxygen and nutrients to the active neurons.
- ***Single photon-emission computed tomography (SPECT).*** Measures rCBF; visualizes and measures the density of neuroreceptors, using tracer isotopes such as xenon, a gas; iodine 123; or technetium.

Neurophysiologic Techniques

- ***Electroencephalogram (EEG).*** Measures electrical activity patterns of the brain from leads connected to surface electrodes placed on the scalp and nasopharyngeal area.
- ***Polysomnography (sleep EEG).*** Measures electrical brain activity data during all-night sleep.
- ***Brain electroactivity mapping (BEAM).*** Extends the EEG by generating computerized maps of brain electrical activity to produce images; permits visualization of the brain performing tasks or specific functions. Useful with children.
- ***Event-related potential (ERP).*** Repeated auditory or visual stimuli associated with tiny electrical events in the cerebral cortex or subcortical structures, measured by surface electrodes.

Pharmacologic Challenge

The use of a medication to provoke (challenge) a neuronal system for better understanding of its physiologic effects and changes. Examples are the dexamethasone suppression test (DST), thyrotropin-releasing hormone (TRH) challenge, or giving a medication known to have specific receptor affinity such as clonidine to examine the alpha-2-adrenergic system in panic disorder.

Molecular Genetics

- ***Linkage map.*** A genetic map that represents the relationship between two genes, often revealed by the inheritance of traits in families, to determine the relative position of genes on a given chromosome.
- ***Restriction fragment length polymorphisms (RFLPs).*** Method of molecular genetics using restriction enzymes, which cuts a DNA strand at sites where the enzyme recognizes a sequence between coding information. Differences in the lengths of these restriction fragments are believed to be inherited. The transmission can be mapped within families and a genetic pattern of transmission identified.
- ***Candidate genes.*** Identification of a specific gene thought to have pathophysiologic relevance to the illness being studied.

medially and allows communication between them through networks of neurologic fibers. In the past, scientists believed that each hemisphere had separate functions, such as logic or creativity and spatial accommodation. With technologies such as positron-emission tomography (PET) it is now possible to assess metabolic activity in the brain as it occurs (see Box 6-1). Scientists are able to observe brain activity and have concluded that creative as well as logical activities require input from both cerebral hemispheres.

The cerebral hemispheres are divided into four lobes, named after the parts of the skull under which they lie: frontal, parietal, temporal, and occipital (see Box 6-2 and FIGURE 6-1 ■). The lobes have pairs on each side of the corpus callosum, which splits the brain in half. These lobes make up the *neocortex*. The neocortex is involved in the subjective experience of emotion, motivation, learning, memory, and gross motor skills. Each lobe has unique functions that contribute to a person's ability to move, process information, and have thoughts and feelings.

The frontal lobe has functional responsibilities for muscular movement and *vegetative effects* (slowing effects) on respiration and circulation. The frontal lobe also receives in-

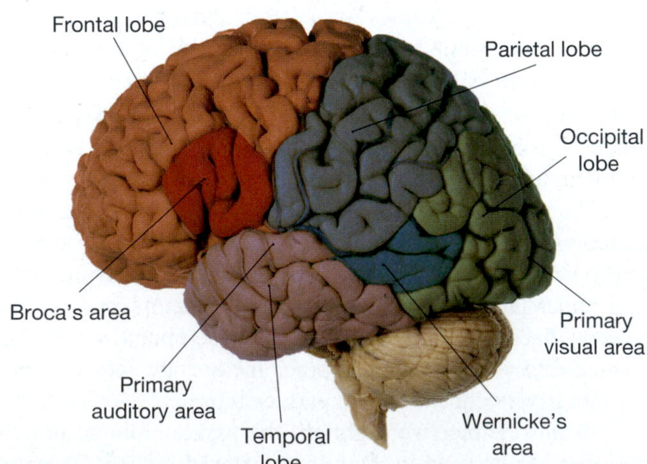

FIGURE 6-1 ■ The brain comprises four major lobes: frontal, parietal, occipital, and temporal. Broca's area (found on the left frontal lobe) is the area responsible for the ability to speak but not the comprehension of speech. Wernicke's area in the left temporal lobe relays speech comprehension information to the frontal lobe.

Source: Smock, T. K. (1999). *Physiological psychology: A neuroscience approach.* Upper Saddle River, NJ: Prentice Hall.

Box 6-2 Functions of the Cerebral Lobes

Frontal Lobes

- Responsible for movement; the right frontal lobe controls the left side of the body's movements, and vice versa
- Contain the premotor cortex, which organizes complicated movement
- Contain prefrontal fibers with capacities for planning and problem solving; also responsible for social judgment, volition, attention, learning, spontaneity, thinking, and affect
- Responsible for executive functioning, which determines how information is interpreted, starting and stopping certain functions (such as verbal exchanges), and filtering and screening out extraneous information

Parietal Lobes

- Contain the sensory cortex, which interprets contact sensations such as touch and pressure
- Facilitate spatial orientation

Temporal Lobes

- Involved in hearing, memory, language comprehension, and emotions
- Connect with the limbic system (the "emotional brain") to allow for the expression of such emotions as rage, fear, sexual and aggressive behavior, and possibly love. Damage to temporal lobes is sometimes seen as extreme and inappropriate expressions of these feelings

Occipital Lobes

- Facilitate the interpretation of visual images and visual memory
- Involved in language formation
- Collaborate with many other brain structures in the formation of memory

formation from the limbic system that results in an effect on thinking, motivation, and understanding consequences to behavior. You may have already seen in your clinical rotations how lesions in the frontal lobe lead to a host of problems. See Box 6-3 on page 86 for information on the practical impacts of frontal lobe damage or a lesion.

The temporal lobe is the emotional center and is involved with memory and cognition. This lobe is also important to understanding the acoustic aspects of language. It is the primary auditory cortex. The limbic system, which is involved in emotions, memory, and thought patterns, will be covered in depth later in this chapter.

The parietal lobe facilitates complex motor and cognitive skills, such as a mastery of visual and spatial balance, mathematical ability, and spelling. The parietal lobe is also the primary somatosensory area receiving input from the thalamus—you know what your body is trying to tell you because the parietal lobe is working. The occipital lobe is involved in visual perception and recognition (D'Amico & Barbarito, 2007). All the lobes contain many gyri (ridges), fissures, and sulci (grooves) that maximize the surface area of the brain.

The brain in general, and the cerebral hemispheres in particular, are well protected not only by the skull but also by a protective fluid, called cerebrospinal fluid (CSF), that circulates around and within the brain. Deep within the brain are three spaces, or ventricles, that aid in the circulation of CSF. Normal CSF volume is about 125 mL in an average adult and is replaced approximately four times in 24 hours. The CSF reflects neurochemical activity of the brain and is one method for studying in vivo (within the living organism) communication. The purposes of spinal taps are to measure the volume and pressure of the CSF; to look for trauma, blood, or infection; and to measure metabolites, which are the products or substances produced from the breakdown of metabolic processes of the brain's neuromessengers.

The cerebral hemispheres consist of both white and gray matter. Gray matter consists of fibers that are referred to as nerves; bundles of nerves are called tracts. The cerebral cortex consists solely of gray matter with underlying white matter. The white matter is an indication of myelination. The white matter increases with age, while gray matter decreases with age. The corpus callosum, a white matter structure, grows in size about 1.8% each year between the ages of 3 and 18 years. This structure integrates the activity between the left and right cerebral hemispheres. The increase in corpus callosum may be a sign of an increased ability for problem-solving (Thomann, Wustenberg, Pantel, Essig, & Schroder, 2006). The cerebral cortex produces results much like those produced by the central processing unit of a computer. The cortex is the part of the brain that makes sense out of the volumes of input. It processes and synthesizes information, thought, reasoning, will, and choice. Dreams come from the cortex.

Limbic System

The **limbic system**, often referred to as the "emotional brain," is believed to be responsible for the experience and expression of emotion, as well as memory and some aspects of attention. The limbic system is not a cohesive structure located in one place in the brain; it is a functional grouping rather than an anatomic one. The limbic system consists of structures from the cerebral hemispheres and the *diencephalon,* a part of the brain located between the cerebrum and midbrain (see Box 6-4 on page 86).

Two limbic structures play an especially important role in how emotions and memories are generated:

1. Amygdala
2. Hippocampus

Learning and memory are two aspects of the interaction between the amygdala and the hippocampus.

The limbic structures also include the olfactory area. If the olfactory sensors determine a scent, the memory of the event will include this cue. For example, does the smell of baking cookies trigger a pleasant memory of being in a kitchen when cookies are being baked? This is the combined effect of amygdalar and hippocampal functions using the cue of the smell of cookies as the stimulus for the memory.

Amygdala The **amygdala** gauges certain emotional reactions and plays a role in social behavior. It serves as the behavioral

Box 6-3 **Practical Impacts of Frontal Lobe Damage or Lesion**

The frontal lobe organizes various aspects of everyday interactions and functioning. Examples of the effects of damage to this lobe are given below.

Abnormalities of Speech

- In a slow-moving supermarket line, someone with frontal-lobe damage might curse and shout at others in line in a way not typical of that person prior to the injury
- The capacity to restrain or inhibit expressions of strong emotion may be impaired, regardless of the circumstances. The person will make inappropriate sexual comments, ask rude questions, or say things that others may think but do not say, such as "You're not too bright, are you?" or "Your breath really stinks."
- The person may have difficulty comprehending a moderately abstract idea, such as an assignment to oversee an area or a process.

Motor and Voluntary Movement Abnormalities

- The person with frontal-lobe damage may have trouble with sucking (using a straw), groping for objects, and gripping them (objects are often dropped).

Loss of Drive and Motivation

- The person loses energy to participate in activities.
- Hygiene activities are neglected or not completed.

Difficulty in Thinking

- The person reacts to a situation without trying to think it through because it is too demanding.

Difficulty in Planning

- The person has difficulty in developing and keeping to a schedule.
- Arranging transportation (with bus schedules, calling for a ride) is challenging.

Disruptions to Concentration

- The person is forgetful.
- The person is unable to track events that occur in his or her environment.

Disruptions to Ability to Sort Out What Is Happening in the Environment

- Stimuli are disorganized.
- The person is easily overwhelmed.

Trouble Shifting from One Mental Activity to Another

- The person finds it difficult to make the shift in activity from watching TV to conversing with another person.

Behavioral Changes

- The person easily loses self-control and has temper tantrums.
- Mood changes are common.
- Apathy (not caring about events or ideas) is another common characteristic.

Box 6-4 **The Limbic System**

Functions

The limbic system is sometimes referred to as the emotional brain, the primitive brain, or the reptilian brain. It is responsible for some of our most basic skills, such as the processing of memories and the creation of emotional states, drives, and behaviors associated with feelings and motivations.

Cerebral Components of the Limbic System

Cortical areas: Limbic lobe (cingulate gyrus, dentate gyrus, and parahippocampal gyrus)

Nuclei: Hippocampus, amygdaloid body

Tracts: Fornix

Diencephalic Components of the Limbic System

Thalamus: Forward (anterior) nuclear group

Hypothalamus: Center for emotions, appetites (thirst, hunger), and related behaviors

Other Components of the Limbic System

Reticular formation: Network of nuclei throughout the brain stem

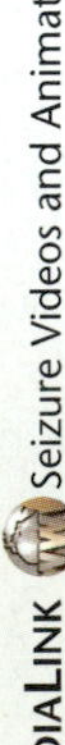
MEDIALINK Seizure Videos and Animation

awareness center and helps pattern appropriate emotional and behavioral responses such as fear, sexual desire, rage, and appetite. It is hypothesized that the amygdala is also important in seeking love and sustaining long-term emotional memories. See FIGURE 6-2 ■ for a cross-sectional view of the structures of the brain.

Hippocampus The **hippocampus** is also involved in emotional reactions and in learning by helping to process, store, and retrieve information in memory. It provides new information for permanent storage. Hallucinations may, in part, originate from hyperexcitability of psychomotor effects of olfactory, visual, auditory, and tactile stimulation in this region (Kring, Davison, Neale, & Johnson, 2007). Weak stimuli in the hippocampus can cause epileptic seizures.

The limbic system has numerous functions beyond those addressed here, and the neuronal connections are so widespread and intricate within the brain that their complex interactions involve many different areas. Other neuronal groups that participate with the limbic system are the thalamus, hypothalamus, and pituitary gland.

Reticular Activating System The reticular activating system (RAS) consists of nerve pathways that originate in the spinal cord and connect in the reticular formation, a system of neu-

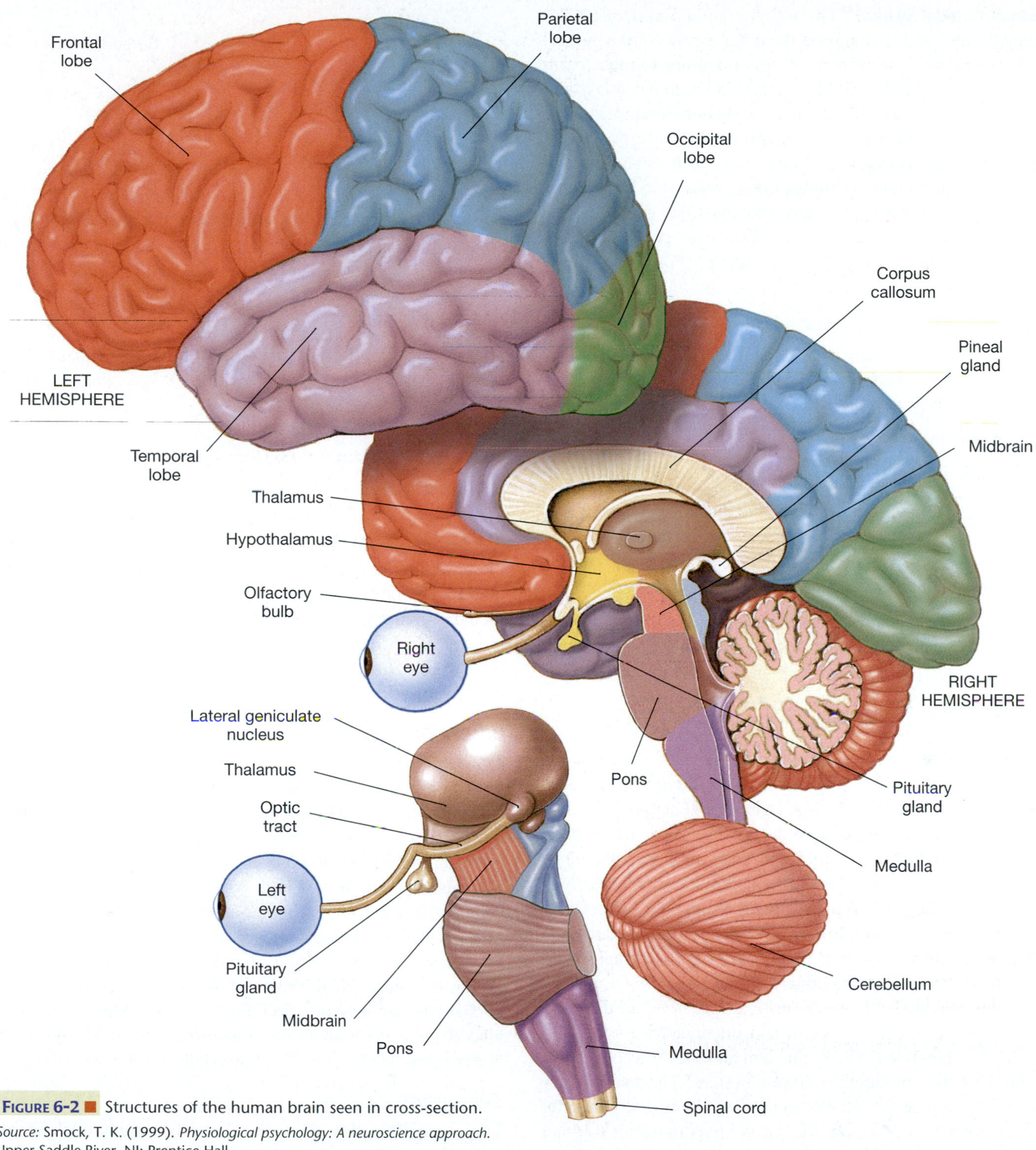

FIGURE 6-2 ■ Structures of the human brain seen in cross-section.

Source: Smock, T. K. (1999). *Physiological psychology: A neuroscience approach.* Upper Saddle River, NJ: Prentice Hall.

rons that modulates awareness and states of consciousness. By screening stimulation from the environment and helping us filter out what we don't need at the moment, the RAS enables us to concentrate. The RAS also permits us to not pay attention for a period of time, allowing us to sleep. During sleep, excitatory neurons of the RAS gradually become more and more excitable because of prolonged rest, while inhibitory neurons of sleep centers become less excitable because of overactivity, leading to a new cycle of wakefulness. This helps explain the rapid transitions between sleep and wakefulness. Arousal, as experienced by people with psychiatric conditions, can be the insomnia that occurs when a person's mind becomes preoccupied with a thought. In states of mental disorder, there is obviously some biologic disequilibrium of the RAS because it involves motivation and levels of arousal. However, the details of this imbalance are complex and not yet well understood.

Extrapyramidal System The extrapyramidal system (so labeled because it lies alongside the outer aspects of the pyramidal system) consists of tracts of motor neurons from the brain to parts of the spinal cord. This system has complex relays and connections to areas of the cortex, cerebellum, brain stem, and thalamus. The tracts play an important role in gross movements and responses of emotional tone, such as smiling and frowning. Antipsychotic medications create side effects that affect the extrapyramidal system and are called *extrapyramidal side effects (EPSE).* The four general classes of EPSE are:

1. Parkinsonism
2. Dyskinesias and dystonias
3. Akathisia
4. Tardive dyskinesia

A complete discussion of extrapyramidal side effects is in Chapters 7 and 32.

Diencephalon

The diencephalon is composed of the thalamus and the hypothalamus. The thalamus functions as a relay and processing center for sensory information. The hypothalamus controls emotions, autonomic functions, and hormone production.

Thalamus The thalamus functions as a relay station, receiving impulses from the spinal cord, brain stem, and cerebellum. With the aid of numerous connections in the cerebral hemispheres and cortex, the thalamus regulates activity and movement, sensory experience (except smell), and emotional expression.

Hypothalamus The **hypothalamus** is a "hub" between the mind and body, giving physical form to thoughts and emotions. It weighs approximately 4 grams and accounts for less than 1% of the total volume of the brain. Its size, however, is not a good indication of its importance. The hypothalamus regulates many of the body's critical activities, including hormone levels, appetite (hunger), body temperature (thermoreceptors), sex drive (libido), water balance (thirst), circadian rhythms, pleasure, and pain. See FIGURE 6-3 ■ for a graphic representation of the hypothalamus as a hub.

The hypothalamus is the critical link between the cerebral cortex, the limbic system, and the endocrine system. It serves as a pipeline to the brain stem and acts as a conduit for control of the autonomic nervous system. The mammillary bodies, located at the back of the hypothalamus, help transfer information about the activities of the hypothalamus to other parts of the brain. The amygdala controls hypothalamic impulses due to the direct neurologic connection. This control is important in the regulation of hunger, thirst, sexual behavior, rage, and/or pleasure.

The infundibulum, a narrow stalk, connects the hypothalamus to the pituitary gland, a part of the endocrine system. The hypothalamus is involved in hormonal balance along with the pituitary gland, which is crucial when the individual experiences a stress response (Smock, 1999). The thalamus and hypothalamus, as well as the pituitary gland, are illustrated in Figure 6-3.

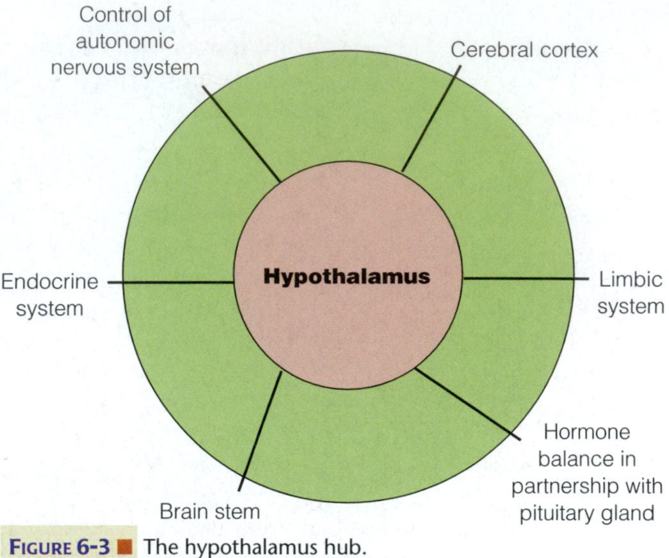

FIGURE 6-3 ■ The hypothalamus hub.

Pituitary Gland

The pituitary gland, under the direction of the hypothalamus, secretes hormones. These hormones are carried through the bloodstream and trigger the activities of other endocrine glands. The pituitary also receives input from the fornix and includes connections to the thalamus, which in turn communicates to and from the frontal cortex (see Figure 6-3). The pituitary gland is the primary link between the nervous and endocrine systems.

Basal Ganglia

The basal ganglia are collectively a complex of structures that include the caudate nucleus, putamen, globus pallidus, and substantia nigra. Their functions include starting and stopping movements, planning motor activities, mediating hallucinations and delusions, and processing emotions and memories. The basal ganglia have a high concentration of dopamine receptors, acetylcholine, gamma-aminobutyric acid, and peptides. A deficit of dopamine in this area is associated with Parkinson's disease. Parkinson's disease is characterized by rhythmic tremors of the extremities, slurred speech, and an unchanging facial expression. Former boxer Muhammad Ali, who demonstrates all these symptoms, sustained numerous blows to his head that resulted in damage to the basal ganglia.

Cerebellum

The **cerebellum** lies below the posterior section of the cerebrum. It is the second largest structure within the brain. Like the cerebral hemispheres, the cerebellum has an outer layer of gray matter and is mainly composed of underlying white matter. The main function of this highly specialized part of the brain is movement, posture, balance, and sensory–motor coordination. The hand–eye coordination of a diamond cutter, the fluid movements of a ballerina, and the success of a quarterback's moves all depend on cerebellar functions. The cerebellum also coordinates complex somatic motor patterns and adjusts the output of other somatic motor centers in the brain and spinal cord.

Brain Stem

Beneath the limbic system is the **brain stem**. The brain stem consists of three smaller structures: the medulla oblongata, the pons, and the midbrain (see Figure 6-3).

Medulla Oblongata The medulla oblongata (Latin for "oblong marrow," or the inner, oblong portion of the organ) relays sensory information to the thalamus and other portions of the brain stem. As the connecting piece of tissue between the brain stem and the spinal cord, it functions as the autonomic center for the regulation of visceral function (cardiovascular, respiratory, and digestive system activities). It is less than 5 cm long but is responsible for controlling many vital functions, including respiration, regulation of blood pressure, and partial regulation of heart rate. It also controls vomiting, swallowing, some aspects of talking, and the perception of pain. Incoming fibers from the spinal cord cross over in the medulla; thus, the left cerebral hemisphere controls the right side of the body, and vice versa.

Pons The pons (Latin for "bridge") contains conduction paths between the spinal cord and the brain, relaying sensory information to the cerebellum and thalamus and serving as a visceral and motor center. Thus, bridging is its function. It also contains reflex centers that mediate sensations of the face, chewing, abduction of the eyes, facial expressions, balance, and the regulation of respiration. Located within the pons is the locus ceruleus, a tiny oval structure that contains 70% of the neurons (nerve cells) that release norepinephrine, a neurotransmitter affecting the entire brain. One projection of the pons is to the amygdala, resulting in emotional and cardiovascular control. Activation of the locus ceruleus is associated with fear, pain, and alarm.

Midbrain The midbrain, also called the mesencephalon, is located above the pons and below the cerebral hemispheres. The midbrain processes visual and auditory data and is a reflex center for the regulation of eye movement, visual accommodation, and regulation of pupil size. The midbrain is also essential for relaying impulses to the cerebral cortex, generating reflexive somatic motor responses (sending behavior-producing messages back to the rest of the body), and maintaining consciousness.

Autonomic Nervous System Within the brain stem is an area of the autonomic nervous system (ANS) known as the parasympathetic division. In stressful emotional circumstances, the sympathetic division of the ANS (also called the sympathetic nervous system), located in the spinal cord, prepares for fight or flight; the parasympathetic initiates the relaxation response with the aid of the endocrine system. Prolonged stress can weaken the immune system and may trigger mood disorders (Akiskal, 2006). Chapter 8∞ includes a complete review of stress reactions. The goal of meditation and other forms of stress management is to inhibit the sympathetic response and strengthen the parasympathetic response.

Genetics

Clients may tell you that others in their family experience "moodiness," "crazy thoughts," or that they "worry constantly for no reason." These disclosures are important clues about how major psychiatric disorders tend to run in families. A new area of research, genomics, explores genetic material for clues to a possible heritable basis of behavior in order to answer the question: What are the molecular consequences of abnormal genes? Applying genetic strategies to clinical practice will bring many new challenges and ethical dilemmas (some of these ethical dilemmas are discussed in Chapter 13∞). Alterations in genetic coding, or designer genes, are currently being used with diseases such as cancer and cystic fibrosis to supply healthy genes or block a defective gene. In the future, perhaps the following questions will be answered for psychiatric–mental health practitioners:

- How can understanding the biological markers determine what medications may help an individual?
- What specific steps can a family take to decrease the incidence of a severe mental disorder if there is a high genetic loading based on history?
- How can nurses help clients understand the role genetics may play in emotional illness?
- Do the same genes, but a different environment, result in depression or an anxiety disorder?
- Does a stressful life event trigger genetically vulnerable neurons to promote rapid-cycling mood disorder or panic disorder?

To begin to answer these questions, a review of the chemical composition of genes and certain aspects of cell structure and function is necessary.

WHY I BECAME A PSYCHIATRIC–MENTAL HEALTH NURSE

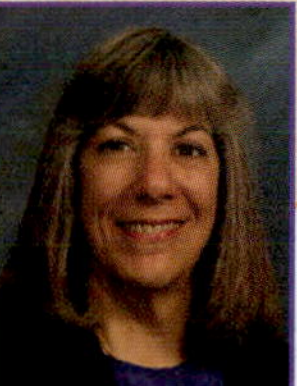

Pamela Marcus
Contributor, Chapter 6

As a very young nurse, I worked in a burn unit. One of my clients was only 7 years old—a young boy who had attempted suicide by grabbing a live electrical wire. When I took care of him, he had full-thickness electrical burns over 90% of his body. His physical care was full of pain for him and I was consumed with worry that his comfort needs would not be met.

Although he later died, this young boy's struggle to live after his suicide attempt made an indelible impression on me. My interest in suicide prevention grew, and I became a psychiatric nurse. In that role I developed nursing care plans for clients on suicide prevention protocols.

Most recently, I developed a staging protocol to predict the risk of suicide potential and determine the appropriate level of care, whether inpatient hospitalization, partial hospitalization, or outpatient treatment. I believe that hope plays an important role in people's lives, and try to instill hope in suicidal persons so that their dilemma is not so overwhelming.

Gene Structure

In 1990, the Human Genome Project was established to discover gene structure, provide a map of how genes work, and locate the chemical base pairs that make up DNA and the spaces between the chemical pairs, to determine abnormal or disease-linked genes.

The gene is the functional unit of information within the chromosome. The human genome consists of 23 pairs of chromosomes, one from each parent; 22 pairs are the somatic chromosomes, and one pair is the sex chromosome (XX female, XY male). Genes are segments of **DNA** (deoxyribonucleic acid), the complex molecule that makes up chromosomes, and are found in all of the body's cell nuclei. Each cell uses the complement of genes selectively. The genes make proteins that are necessary for the cell to do its assigned task. For example, a bone cell gene differs from a brain cell gene in structure and function. Our **genotype**, or our genetic makeup, differs from our **phenotype**, how our genes are actually expressed.

RNA (ribonucleic acid) is another complex molecule that plays a role in translating DNA's coding instructions for making protein. Each strand of the complex molecule of DNA is compactly formed into a double helix. The strand of DNA is composed of chemical nucleotides consisting of one sugar molecule (DNA or RNA), one phosphate group, and one of four nitrogen bases. The nucleotides are:

- Adenine (A)
- Thymine (T)
- Guanine (G)
- Cytosine (C)

The nucleotides line up next to each other like two sides of a zipper, with the phosphate and sugar forming the outer strand; the bases (A, T, G, and C) act like interlocking teeth (see Figure 6-4 ■). The sequence of amino acids, which are proteins, is coded by genes. The sequence or code is like a language and is not arbitrary. The nucleotides, or two sides of the zipper, can fit together in only one way: A pairs with T, and G pairs with C. This base pairing allows for the known sequence of one strand to predict the partner strand. Each strand of the double helix thus specifies its complement and allows for the duplication of genetic information in dividing cells.

Gene Function

Variations in the chemical composition of the genes can produce abnormal structural proteins or enzymes, altering the sending or receiving of signals and resulting in dysfunction or disease. The main component of all living matter is protein, which consists of large molecules or long chains of amino acids linked together. The sequence of amino acids along the chain determines each protein's physical and biologic properties, acting as information molecules.

The transfer of DNA from the nucleus requires messenger RNA (mRNA), which serves as the instructor for the making of proteins outside the nucleus. Ribosomes, which float in the cytoplasm or sit on the rough endoplasmic reticulum, translate the mRNA into proteins. Also in the cytoplasm are the mitochondria, which generate energy, via ions and adenosine triphosphate (ATP), from the oxidation of fats and sugars, and also contain RNA and DNA. The process of protein synthesis is illustrated in Figure 6-5 ■.

Instructions for the synthesizing and metabolizing of the molecular messengers of the brain are coded in the DNA. A typical protein has a useful life of about 2 days; thus, new protein molecules are constantly being synthesized. Genes can be mutated by a single mismatch of the wrong base in the DNA, or a piece of the DNA can be mistakenly repeated, deleted, or altered. This error could cause the cell to function in a changed manner. This may help explain how a client's symptoms or behavioral expression can change over time. New messages among the complex combinations of proteins change the code

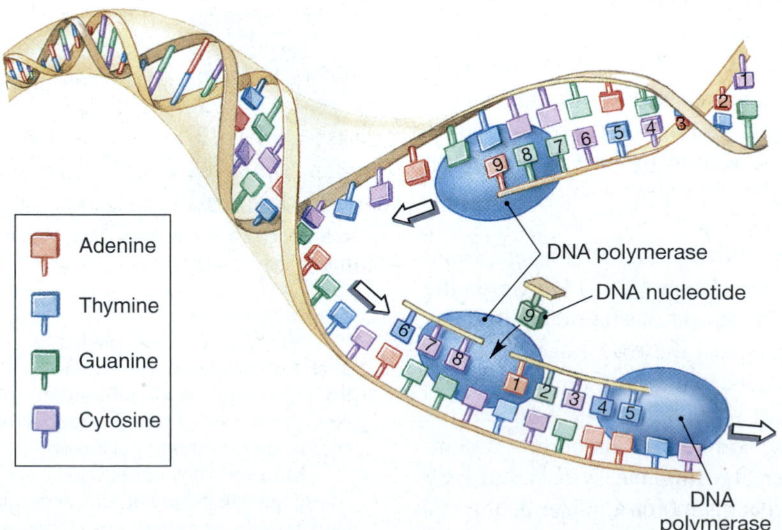

Figure 6-4 ■ The structure of DNA shows how each strand of the complex molecule is compactly formed into a double helix and the strand of DNA is composed of the chemical nucleotides adenine (A), thymine (T), guanine (G), and cytosine (C), which fit together like the teeth of a zipper.

Source: Martini, F. H. (2001). *Fundamentals of anatomy and physiology.* Upper Saddle River, NJ: Prentice Hall.

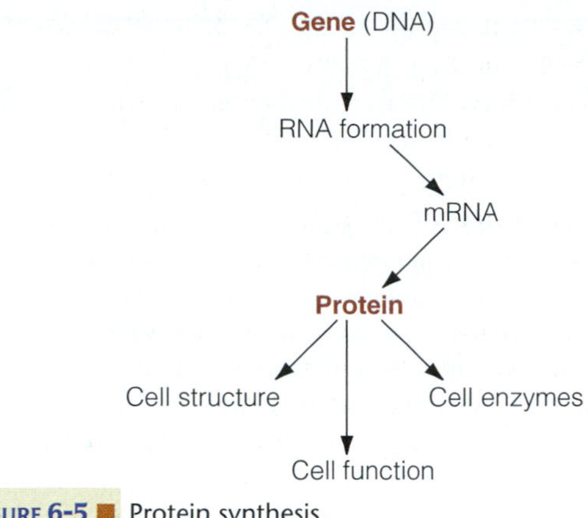

FIGURE 6-5 ■ Protein synthesis.

in the physical environment, resulting in different expressions of temperament, behavior, and individuality.

New technologies enable researchers to modify DNA and RNA so that both the messages and the expression of the messages can be manipulated experimentally. DNA markers, from fragments of DNA (restriction fragment length polymorphisms, or RFLPs), are making it possible to identify and localize the genes involved in a disease process. RFLPs represent a direct reflection of the DNA sequence and can be used to determine accuracy on kinship and group relationships. RFLP separation has led to a large library of DNA sequence markers and a human mutation database. This information has assisted researchers in determining the probability that a mutation can take place at any specific area of the genome (Baker, 2006; Bjorklund, 2006). The data gathered in the mutation database help us to understand the pathophysiology of a disease and its treatment and possibly, in the future, its prevention.

The polymerase chain reaction (PCR) is another technology used with DNA. Even a single cell would be enough to start the process of analyzing a DNA fragment with PCR, as the amounts needed for analysis can be generated from that cell. This process reproduces individual fragments of DNA and is used in genetic engineering efforts and research investigations (Du, Bakish, Ravindran, & Hrdina, 2004). PCR was used to develop a number of diagnostic tests to detect disease-causing agents, and it is used in determining paternity. Also, in forensic medicine, PCR has proved indispensable for criminal investigations.

Genetic Research

Psychiatric-focused genetic studies are conducted by examining the blood of family members who have mental disorders. Linkage studies are a type of genetic blood study used to locate genes that are thought to be involved in susceptibility to emotional illness. These studies examine the inheritance patterns of known DNA markers. This research assists in understanding the possible location of a suspect gene for an identified disorder, although the results thus far have not shown one particular gene as the culprit for any major mental disorder.

In linkage-disequilibrium studies, isolated populations are used to examine suspected genes for an identified disorder that is thought to have come from a few members of the study population (Fehr et al., 2006). The population investigated in a linkage-disequilibrium study may be a geographic or cultural group with possibly fewer variations of the disease gene. Association studies are used to test the hypothesis that a specific gene or group of genes influences a particular disorder.

The National Human Genome Research Institute (NHGRI), part of the National Institutes of Health (NIH), is encouraging research that would lower the cost of sequencing a mammalian-sized genome. Lower costs would enable researchers to sequence the genomes of hundreds or even thousands of people to identify genes that contribute to common, complex diseases. If the cost of whole-genome sequencing is cut to a manageable level, sequencing individual genomes may become part of routine medical care and would allow us to tailor diagnosis, treatment, and prevention to each person's unique genetic profile.

Ethics in Genetic Research

When a genetic loading component has the potential to create a mental disorder, the ethical implications can be controversial:

- How should a mental health professional proceed in discussions about heritability of the illness?
- What treatments are offered if, in the future, a gene is identified as causing a mental disorder and a child with no symptoms has that gene?

The ethical dilemmas include waiting until the child experiences symptoms and treating at that point, or treating before any symptoms appear. These are not clear choices. But overall, action taken by nurses includes the need to be familiar with the biologic mechanism of the illness to help clients make decisions about their care, their choices about childbearing, and to avoid the potential stigma associated with the genetics of mental disorders. See the Evidence-Based Practice feature on page 92 for a perspective on this issue.

The ethics of genetic research is another area under examination. Consent for study participation includes being given information about the study and understanding the risks and benefits of the research, what is involved in study participation, and what will be done with the genetic information obtained during the course of the study. Researchers must define how the information that is gathered during the study is secured, how the client's identity will be protected, and what will be reported. Confidentiality in keeping the genetics of the study sample anonymous is an essential consideration for the participants. Study participants have the right in every study to ask questions of the principal investigator (Williams, Skirton, & Masny, 2006). Questions might include, among others:

1. What do the individual results mean?
2. What implications may the genetic results have for children?
3. What implications may the genetic results have for developing physical illnesses?

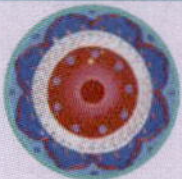

EVIDENCE-BASED PRACTICE

GENETIC TESTING

Your work in a maternal–child health clinic has given you the idea of incorporating genetic testing into the clinic's program. Women who had children with physical and emotional illnesses have been seen in this clinic for a number of years. Questions asked of you typically focus on whether the family can have another child when one child already has a problem, or whether adoption of a child from a parent with a known disease increases the risk of the child becoming ill.

Genetic testing is a fairly new concept in mental health care, although it has been used for some time in the medical nursing specialties. How open your clients are to genetic testing, how well informed they may be, and how interested they would be in the results will determine whether a genetic testing program would be feasible. One study design is to ask your clients about these issues to shape your next steps. Being informed of the current risk estimates may be sufficient for your clients. On the other hand, conducting research to delve into their specific needs for information could offer your clients a service with lifelong impacts. Action should be based on more than one study, but the following nursing study on genetic testing would serve as a useful basis for designing a survey for your clinic.

Barnoy, S., Appel, D., Peretz, C., Meiraz, H., & Ehrenfeld, M. (2006). Genetic testing, genetic information, and the role of the maternal child health nurses in Israel. *Journal of Nursing Scholarship, 38*(3), 219–224.

CRITICAL THINKING QUESTIONS

1. What ethical questions does genetic testing raise?
2. What legal questions does genetic testing raise?
3. Why should the ethical and legal issues raised by genetic testing be of concern to psychiatric–mental health nurses?

4. How do these results compare to those of other participants in the research?
5. How do these results compare to those of people in the general population?

More on this topic is included in Chapter 13.

The Genetic Basis of Psychiatric Illness

The field of genetics has expanded in all areas of human physiology; thus mapping the genetics of psychiatry is more complete with each year. Research on the genetic basis of inherited psychiatric illnesses has been a focus of the Office of Human Genetics and Genomic Resources in the National Institute of Mental Health (NIMH). This group supports research on the identification, localization, function, and expression patterns of genes that produce susceptibility to mental disorders. Research projects supported by the group use DNA and cDNA arrays, gene chips, protein chips, gene expression neuroinformatics, functional genomics, mutation detection, cloning, single nucleotide polymorphisms (SNPs), imprinting, unstable expanding repeats, gene therapy, linkage analysis, candidate gene approaches, and haplotype analysis.

Research findings will set the stage for future understanding of the complexity of the genetic and environmental influences of mental disorder. In all the genetic models, the roles of environmental influences, perinatal events, trauma, infections, and stress have to be considered. When evaluating clients and families for possible genetic links to an emotional disorder, it is important to consider the interaction between the genetic factors and the environment (Mansour et al., 2006).

Scientists have discovered that:

1. There is no single gene responsible for a mental disorder.
2. There may be several susceptibility genes that interact with one another.
3. Environmental influences interact with genes to increase the risk of developing a mental disorder.

Genetic research is often done with twin studies to predict the impact of heredity. The rate of occurrence of the emotional disorder is compared between monozygotic (MZ—identical) twins and dizygotic (DZ—fraternal) twins. If the illness occurs more in MZ twins than in DZ twins, then heredity is an important factor to consider in the development of the mental disorder. See TABLE 6-1 ■ for the most current genetic risks estimated for mental illnesses.

Current research is developing in two directions. The Human Genome Project and genetic mapping have enabled researchers to look for chromosomes that may be implicated in a disease. For example, one group of researchers has identified eight circadian genes associated with bipolar I disorder, schizoaffective disorder, and schizophrenia (Mansour et al., 2006). The second area of current study involves altering the genetic material of mouse brains to understand the structure and behavior patterns demonstrated in these altered animals. This body of research is useful in testing hypotheses about the nature of mental disorders as well as in testing new medications.

Neurons, Synapses, and Neurotransmission

The brain's structural complexity increases as one considers the biochemical processes that occur with every thought, emo-

TABLE 6-1 ■ **Empiric Genetic Risk Estimates for Mental Illnesses (in percentages)**

Disorder	Population Risk	MZ Twin Studies	DZ Twin Studies	Risk to Offspring–Both Parents Have Disorder	1st-Degree Relatives	2nd-Degree Relatives	Heritability
Anxiety Disorders	15–25	22–73	0–17		8–31		40
OCD	3	53–87	22–47		Onset <18 y.o. 10–35 Onset > 18 y.o. no increased risk 3–15		
Major Depressive–Unipolar Depression	Women 10–25; Men 5–12	40	11		5–30		20–80; meta-analysis 31–42
Bipolar Disorder	0.8–1.6	40–70	5–10	50–65; 50–75 for any major affective disorder	5–20; 20–30 for any major affective disorder	5	60
Schizophrenia	1	40–60	10–16	46	5–16	2–6	80
Schizoaffective Disorder	0.5–1				1–6; 1–27 for any major affective disorder		
Attention Deficit Disorder	5–10				15–60	3–9	70–80
Autism Spectrum	1	36–60	0–30		6–30		>90

(Blank areas = no information available at time of printing)

Adapted from Empiric Risks by the National Society of Genetic Counselors. Retrieved March 2, 2007, from http://www.nchpeg.org/cdrom/empiric.html

tion, memory, dream, or hope. Thoughts and feelings are made possible by the complex interplay and communication between cells in the central nervous system (CNS) in response to stimuli in the environment.

The specialized cells of the nervous system are called **neurons**. Like other cells in the body, each neuron has a cell body that contains cytoplasm and a nucleus. Unlike other cells, a neuron has at least two other extensions: an axon and one or more dendrites. An axon is the portion of a neuron that conveys electric impulses from the cell body to other neurons. Axons are covered with a white myelin sheath and are the white matter in the brain and spinal cord. Dendrites are unmyelinated and conduct electrical messages to the cell body. There are approximately 100 billion neurons in the brain and nearly an equal number of supporting (glia) cells.

Neurons are classified according to the direction in which they conduct impulses. Sensory neurons, also known as afferent neurons, send messages from the peripheral body parts to the brain. For example, if you place your foot into a tub of scalding water, the message that the water is too hot is sent to your brain via sensory neuron pathways. Motor neurons, or efferent neurons, carry messages that originate in the brain and yield a behavioral change in the peripheral body parts. When your foot is in the hot water, the message from your brain is to remove the foot (quickly!); this message travels via motor neuron pathways, causing your foot to jerk out of the water.

Communication among and between neurons is complex and specific and is believed to be the basis of behavior. Each neuron forms anywhere from 1,000 to 10,000 synaptic connections. The synapse is a gap in the synaptic cleft between neurons. See FIGURE 6-6 ■ on page 94 for a structural view of how a neuron conveys its messages. These reciprocal synapses form positive and negative feedback loops. Neurons are arranged in networks or pathways whereby neuronal communication is facilitated by repetition. Interneuron communication is electrical and chemical and occurs at synapses, or points of contact between neurons, as well as along the neuron itself.

MEDIALINK Neurological Synapse Animation

Synaptic Transmission

Neuromessenger is a collective, generic term for neurotransmitters, neuromodulators, and neurohormones. **Neurotransmitters (NTs)** are neuromessengers that are rapidly released at the presynaptic neuron on stimulation, diffuse across the synapse between two neurons, and have either an excitatory or inhibitory effect on the postsynaptic neuron (see FIGURE 6-7 ■ on page 94). The membrane of the axon terminal of a neuron contains many saclike projections called synaptic vesicles, which contain the NT molecules that transmit messages across the synapse.

Neurons are encased in cell membranes that function as a complex regulation site. The membranes contain proteins, some of which are phospholipids, enzymes, and ion channels.

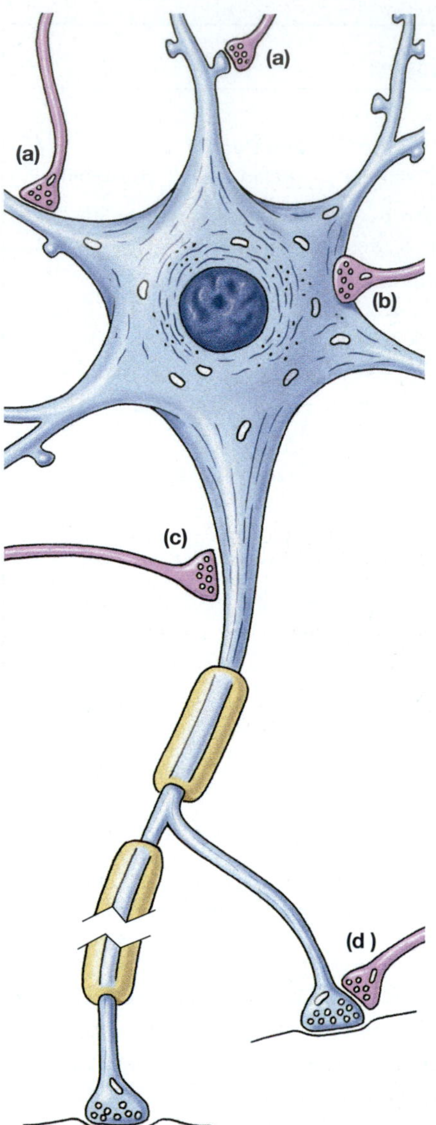

FIGURE 6-6 ■ A neuron is capable of making many different types of synaptic contacts. Shown here are: (a) a synapse onto a dendrite, called axodendritic contact; (b) a contact on the soma, called axosomatic contact; (c) a synapse onto another axon, called axoaxonic contact; and (d) an area where signals are sent and received, called axosynaptic contacts.

Source: Smock, T. K. (1999). *Physiological psychology: A neuroscience approach*, p. 23. Upper Saddle River, NJ: Prentice Hall.

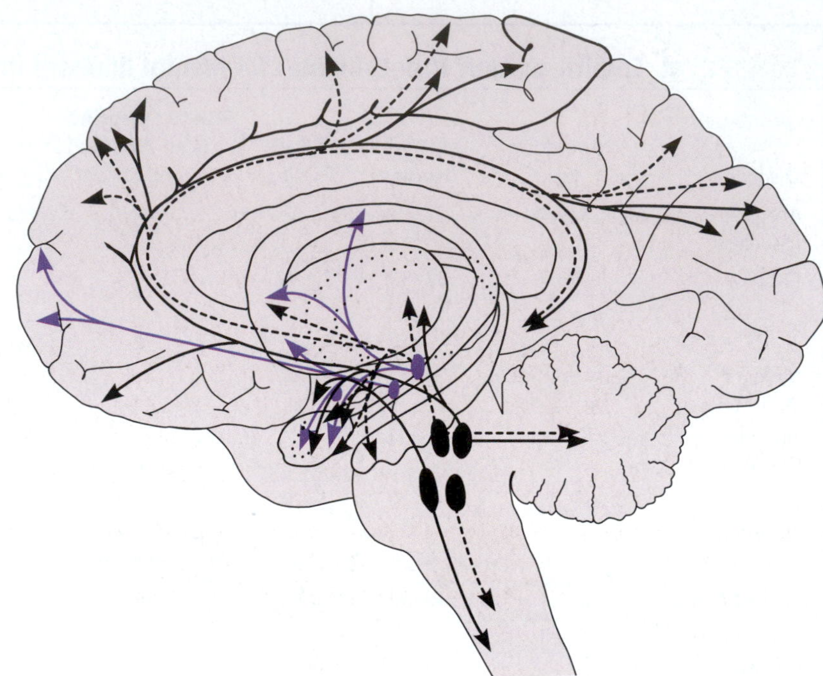

FIGURE 6-7 ■ Common neurotransmitter pathways. Purple = DA, black = NE, dashed line = 5-HT. Dotted line indicates pons.

Ion channels are water-filled molecular tunnels that pass through the cell membrane and allow electrically charged atoms (ions) or small molecules to enter or leave the cell. The neuron exists in a state of tension because of the various ions in its membrane. Changes in ion concentrations cause the nerve impulse, or *action potential,* which transmits information between the neurons. The four major ions are sodium, potassium, calcium, and chloride. Each ion passes in or out of the neuron via its own channel. Nerve impulses involve the opening or closing of the ion channels by gates.

Once the action potential reaches the end of the axon, the electrical transfer of the information ends, and messages are then conveyed by chemicals, the NT molecules. The signal is mediated by binding to specific receptors on the cell surface (Stewart et al., 2007). Depending on the type of channel, the action potential can be:

- Excitatory, influencing the neuron to fire; or
- Inhibitory, preventing it from firing.

Presynaptic axon terminals contain large numbers of calcium channels, which determine the quantity of NT that is released into the synaptic cleft.

At the synapse, the membrane of the postsynaptic neuron contains receptor proteins. Receptors are highly specialized proteins embedded in the membrane of the neuron that are in part exposed to the extracellular fluid and recognize the neuromessenger. Receptors are located on the axon (presynaptic) or on the dendrite (postsynaptic). Neurotransmitters and receptors vary in their affinity for each other, depending on the NT involved. They may bind like a lock and key, or the outcome may depend on what is available. Every neuron is more or less sensitive to a constant amount of neuromessenger, and this is an important principle in pharmacology. The NT that remains in the synapse after the postsynaptic response is either dissolved by synaptic enzymes or reabsorbed for recycling by the presynaptic neuron, a process known as reuptake.

Neurotransmitters

Neurotransmitters include three classes—biogenic amines (monoamines), amino acids, and peptides—as well as dissolved gases and a number of other compounds. Neurotransmitters are discussed in TABLE 6-2 ■.

Table 6-2 ■ The Major Known Neurotransmitters

Neurotransmitter	Function
Biogenic Amines (Monoamines)	
Acetylcholine (Ach) Precursor: choline	Attention; memory; promotes preparation for action; conserves energy; thirst; defense and/or aggression; sexual behavior; mood regulation; REM sleep; voluntary movement of the muscles; stimulates parasympathetic division of the ANS; controls muscle tone in balance with DA in the basal ganglia
Dopamine (DA) Precursor: tyrosine	Integrates thoughts and emotions; regulates pleasure and reward-seeking stimuli; control of complex movements; motivation; cognition; stimulates hypothalamus to release hormones affecting adrenal, thyroid, and sex hormones
Histamine (H) Precursor: histidine	Mediates allergic and inflammatory responses; smooth muscle constriction; stimulates gastric acid secretion; role in biorhythms and thermoregulation; role in second messenger transmission
Norepinephrine (NE) or noradrenalin Precursor: tyrosine	Stimulates sympathetic division of the ANS; role in stress response; fluctuates with sleep and wakefulness; role in attention and vigilance, arousal, ability to focus or learn, feeling of reward, regulation of mood and anxiety
Serotonin (5-HT) Precursor: tryptophan	Inhibits activity and behavior; role in level of arousal; increases sleep time; reduces aggression, play, sexual, and eating activity; temperature regulation; pain control; mood states; role in circadian rhythms; sensory regulation; helps focus the brain; regulates pituitary
Amino Acids	
Aspartate	Excitatory
Gamma-aminobutyric acid (GABA), also written as γ-aminobutyric acid Precursor: glutamic acid	Reduces aroused aggression, anxiety, and excitation; sedation; motor behavior; anticonvulsant and muscle-relaxant properties
Glutamate	Excitatory; role in learning and memory; neural degeneration
Glycine Precursor: serine	Inhibitory; spinal reflexes; motor behavior
Peptides (Neuromodulators)	
Cholecystokinin (CCK)	Role in schizophrenia; eating and movement disorders; panic disorder
Corticotropin-releasing hormone (CRH)	Stress, mood, memory, and anxiety
Neurotensin	Role in schizophrenia
Opioids: endorphins and enkephalins	Alter emotional behavior; pain control; hallucinations; pleasure; motor coordination; water balance
Somatostatin	Mood disorders; Alzheimer's disease; negative feedback control of thyrotropin secretion; role in positive symptoms of schizophrenia; excites limbic neurons
Substance P	Excitatory; role in pain syndromes, mood, and movement disorders
Vasopressin	Role in mood disorders

The biogenic amines include:

- Dopamine (DA)
- Norepinephrine (NE)
- Epinephrine
- Serotonin (5-hydroxytryptamine, or 5-HT)
- Acetylcholine (ACh)
- Histamine (H)

Biogenic amines are synthesized in the axon terminals and released into the synapse. The era of neuropsychopharmacology began with the identification of these neurotransmitters.

Functional imaging techniques now enable researchers and clinicians to visualize the pathways of neuron clusters at work and better understand their functional association with behavior. The original belief that a neuron contained only one NT is no longer valid. Figure 6-7 illustrates the basic pathways of three of the major biogenic amines.

Dopamine **Dopamine** (DA) is released in many areas in the brain, where it influences how we interact in the world. One example of the excitatory effects of DA is when cocaine inhibits the removal of DA from the neuronal synapse. This

MediaLink Application: Schizophrenia and Imbalance in Dopamine Pathways

Table 6-3 ■ Dopamine Location and Function

Area/Location	Dopamine Is Associated with	
Basal ganglia area	The control of complex movement	
Limbic system	Memory	Pleasure
	Mood	Motivation
	Reward	
Hypothalamic tract	Endocrine functions	Food and water intake
	Circadian rhythms	Temperature
Frontal cortex pathway	Insight	Inhibition
	Judgment	Social awareness
	Problem solving	

causes a rise in the concentration of DA at those synapses, the excitatory impact takes effect, and the "high" associated with cocaine use is created.

Because of the presence of DA pathways in all of these areas of the brain, DA disturbance is involved in psychosis. See Table 6-3 ■ for specific DA areas and functions. The efficacy of neuroleptic or antipsychotic medications used to treat psychoses is correlated with the medication's ability to block DA receptors, although the newer antipsychotics have shown us that DA receptor blockade is not the only effective treatment for psychosis.

MediaLink Serotonin Reuptake Inhibition Animation

Norepinephrine **Norepinephrine** (NE) is also called noradrenalin, and synapses that release NE are adrenergic synapses. Receptors for the neurotransmitter norepinephrine are widespread in the brain. Locations of the receptors for NE are listed in Table 6-4 ■. NE plays a major role in mediating mood and anxiety. Normally NE is considered to have an excitatory impact. Regulation of norepinephrine has been examined closely in the treatment of mood and anxiety disorders and contributes to current psychopharmacologic interventions.

Serotonin The **serotonin** (referred to as 5-HT) neurons arise in the raphe nuclei and project to the same areas as the NE pathways. A raphe, anatomically, refers to a seam in the tissue. A raphe nucleus is a moderate-sized cluster of nuclei found in the brain stem. This cluster releases serotonin to the rest of the brain. Selective serotonin reuptake inhibitor (SSRI) antidepressants are believed to act on these nuclei. Serotonin appears to be a modulator. Its effects influence the temperature, sensory, sleep, and assertiveness areas of the brain. Serotonin serves as a chemical mediator in pain perception, normal and abnormal behaviors, moods, drives, the regulation of food intake, and neuroendocrine functions. Receptor subtypes decrease cerebral blood flow during a migraine episode and increase the response to pain.

Table 6-4 ■ Norepinephrine Location and Function

Area/Location	Norepinephrine Is Associated with	
Pons, specifically locus ceruleus	Stress response Arousal	Alertness
Cerebral cortex	Cognitive functioning	
Limbic system	Emotional responses	Regulation of mood
	Ability to focus or learn	Pleasure
	Reward	
Hypothalamus	Endocrine functions	Appetite
	Temperature	Biological rhythms

Acetylcholine The first chemical to be identified as a true neurotransmitter, acetylcholine (ACh) is the "grandparent" of neurotransmitters. Dopamine and ACh share a concentration of activity within the basal ganglia, and medications used to block EPSE are cholinergic stimulants, suggesting a reciprocal relationship between these two neurotransmitters in the modulation of movement and possibly the development of psychosis. ACh plays a major role in the encoding of memory and in cognition. It also plays a mediation role in mood disorders, stress, and sleep regulation. It is considered to be highly significant in neuromuscular transmission.

Histamine The role of histamine (H) in psychiatric illness is less understood. It is a chemical messenger that mediates a wide range of cellular responses, including allergic and inflammatory reactions, gastric acid secretions, and neurotransmission. Some psychiatric medicines block H receptors, resulting in the side effects of sedation, weight gain, and drowsiness (Barinaga, 2000).

Amino Acids These neurotransmitters are natural substances found throughout the brain and body and in the proteins of the food we eat. The amino acid gamma-aminobutyric acid (GABA) is the most prevalent inhibitory NT. GABA neurons are widely distributed in the CNS. Glycine, also an inhibitory NT, exists primarily in the brain stem, spinal cord, and cerebellum. GABA has a prominent role in arousal; when the neuron is stimulated, GABA acts as a brake, decreasing neuronal excitability. Benzodiazepines act by binding with GABA and benzodiazepine receptors to produce antianxiety, sedative, anticonvulsant, and muscle-relaxant properties.

Glutamate and aspartate are the two primary excitatory amino acid neurotransmitters. Glutamate is primarily located in the cerebral cortex and hippocampus and has a role in long-term memory and learning. Too much glutamate can be a neurotoxin, as seen in Huntington's chorea and phencyclidine (PCP) psychosis.

Psychopharmacologic strategies are becoming more specific with increased understanding of signal transduction. When the NT receptor complex creates a direct change in the membrane potential, it is called first messenger transmission. A rapid, direct membrane change can also initiate a series of intracellular reactions, triggering a second messenger transmission. Guanine proteins are large families of receptors that are the links in second messenger cascades. Second messengers are membrane proteins that relay nerve signals from the NT complex through a chain of chemical reactions to the nucleus. Medications acting at this level allow for greater selectivity in targeting specific enzymes associated with behavior. This cascade of signals is a major mechanism for switching proteins on or off.

Psychoendocrinology and Psychoneuroimmunology

This section examines the interaction of the brain with two body subsystems: the endocrine system and immune system. The interaction of the brain with the endocrine system is known as *psychoendocrinology*. The interaction of the brain with the immune system is known as *psychoneuroimmunology*.

Endocrine System

The endocrine system functions through neurochemical messengers in the bloodstream called hormones. The endocrine system is a communication system. Hormones secreted from the hypothalamus instruct the pituitary to stimulate the target tissues, endocrine glands. The major endocrine glands are the adrenals, the gonads, and the thyroid; their primary function is releasing hormones. Hormones act as triggers. Each component of the neuroendocrine axis can feed back into any other component of the system, including the cortex and limbic system. The amount of hormone produced is partly regulated by a negative feedback mechanism. Feedback regulation exists at all levels of the axis. Thus, the rise or fall in the blood level of one hormone can cause an increase or decrease in the level of another hormone. The immune and endocrine systems are integrated through a shared set of hormone receptors. Hormones have a broader range of responses than nerve impulses and require seconds to days to cause a response that may last from weeks to months.

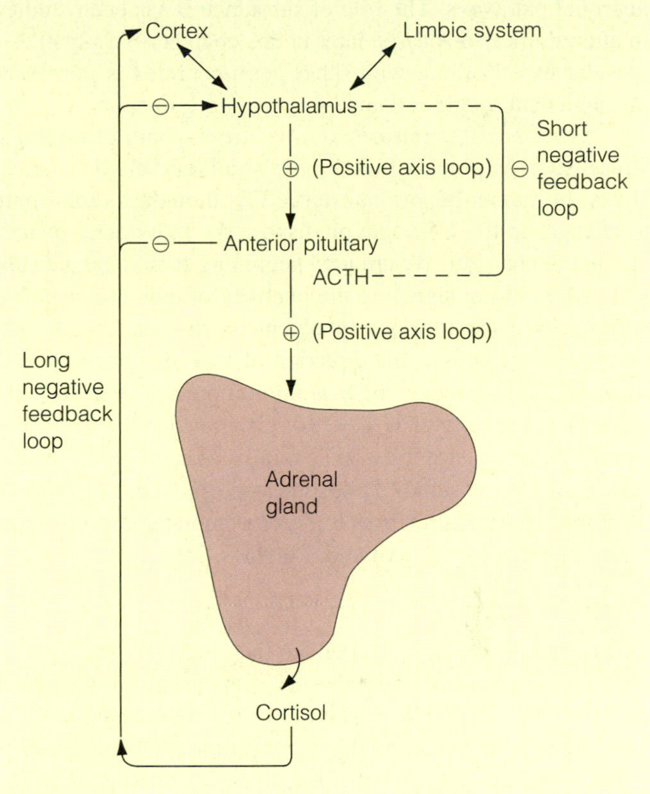

FIGURE 6-8 ■ Example of neuroendocrine feedback. The positive loop in the axis is depicted by the hypothalamus. Upon stimulation from the cortex or limbic system, the release of trophic peptide CRH (corticotropin-releasing hormone) tells the pituitary gland to signal the adrenal cortex, via ACTH (adrenocorticotropic hormone), to release the glucocorticoid cortisol. Cortisol released into the bloodstream provides negative feedback to the hypothalamus or anterior pituitary. Additionally, ACTH can provide negative feedback to the hypothalamus.

Irregularities of Neuroendocrine Function Irregularities of neuroendocrine function have been linked to depression, postpartum psychosis, schizophrenia, polydipsia in clients with psychosis, panic disorder, obsessive–compulsive disorder, anorexia nervosa, dementia of the Alzheimer's type (DAT), and circadian rhythms.

Psychopharmacologic challenge tests, described in Box 6-1 earlier in this chapter, enhance our understanding of the pathophysiology of these conditions. One such test is the **dexamethasone suppression test (DST),** which attempts to assess the hypothalamic–pituitary–adrenal (HPA) axis (FIGURE 6-8 ■). Dexamethasone, a synthetic glucocorticoid, is given by mouth at 11:00 P.M. to "challenge" the axis. By measuring blood samples of the hormone cortisol drawn at 4:00 P.M. the day before the pill is taken, and at 8:00 A.M. (highest level of normal rhythm), 4:00 P.M. (lowest level of rhythm), and 11:00 P.M. the day after the pill is taken, one can assess the relationship between the pituitary and the hypothalamus.

Dexamethasone "turns off" adrenocorticotropic hormone (ACTH) secretion at the pituitary, which in turn suppresses cortisol secretion from the adrenals. In a normally functioning axis, cortisol is reduced for the next 24 hours. However, in many psychiatric conditions, nonsuppression, or "escape," is observed by a rise in the 4:00 P.M. level, when it should be low. There are no side effects or long-lasting changes as a result of taking dexamethasone. The results are not diagnostic of the illness, but suggest some pathology in the HPA axis function.

Neuropeptides Hormones secreted by the hypothalamus and pituitary are neuropeptides, which are large, complex chains of amino acids linked together and synthesized by ribosomes in the neuronal cell body through the transcription of DNA. Their physiology is complex; they bind to specific receptors, modulating the response of the postsynaptic cell to the NT. These effects are slow, involving such prolonged actions as changes in the number of receptors, synapses, and closures of ion channels. They also have an important role in the memory process (Kring et al., 2007). The most commonly understood neuropeptides are summarized in Table 6-2 on page 95.

Researchers have been studying the effect substance P has on human beings. Substance P is a prototype neuropeptide that is thought to co-transmit with serotonin in the

MEDIALINK Occupation of Receptor Sites by Agonists/Antagonists Animation

neuronal pathways. The role of substance P has been studied in altered mice (discussed later in this chapter). The synthesis of substance P along with other neuropeptides is necessary during a neurogenic inflammatory response in mice.

Substance P is released during stress—both physiologic stress, such as pinching the mouse's tail, and environmental stress. In human beings, substance P is thought to contribute to changes in the CNS that predispose the individual to anxiety and depression. We are now beginning to understand substance P's role in signaling the intensity of pain and aversive stimuli and substance P's involvement with depression and psychological stress. The direction of this research will lead to the development of medication compounds that are substance P antagonists that may treat diseases that have an emotional response to aversive stimuli. Antagonists of the neuropeptide substance P, vasopressin, and neuropeptide Y represent a departure from traditional monoamine receptor-based mechanisms (Norman & Burrows, 2007).

Immune System

Psychoneuroimmunology (PNI) is the study of the links between thoughts, emotions, the nervous system, and the immune system. The relationships between these systems have been known to clinicians for a long time. New research is being dedicated to further the *why* of the interactions. The National Institutes of Health (NIH) National Center for Complementary and Alternative Medicine (NCCAM) investigates methods and techniques of complementary and alternative treatments. The goal for most practitioners is to combine effective treatments from complementary and alternative options with commonly understood mainstream medicine to provide the best care. This combination is referred to as an integrative approach. An enormous reservoir of choice for promoting health for an individual can be opened up by determining how these, and other, complementary and alternative techniques discussed in Chapter 33 can influence the healing process:

- Ethnic healing practices
- Therapeutic touch
- Massage
- Guided imagery
- Relaxation
- Magnetic stimulation of the brain

This field holds great potential for nurses and clinicians in all specialties including psychiatry as we strive to understand the influence stress has on mental disorders (Abercrombie, Zamora, & Korn, 2007). The most common psychological problems reported by clients seeking medical consultation are depression and anxiety. These two psychological clusters of symptoms increase the usage of medical diagnostic services. Stress-related symptoms account for 60% of all primary care visits.

Our understanding of chemical communication between the brain and immune system comes from the study of receptors. Cells in the limbic system have many receptors for neuropeptides such as endorphins, and immune system cells contain receptors for endorphins and other peptides such as corticotropin-releasing hormone (CRH).

The brain can directly influence the immune system by sending messages along nerve cells. The series of communication affects the cell nucleus, producing changes in the DNA and RNA that alter the shape of the neuron or even cause cell death. In the fight-or-flight response, immune system function is slowed, and energy is directed toward helping the body meet the immediate challenge.

Kindling and Behavioral Sensitization

Kindling is the repeated administration of a subconvulsant stimulus, such as repeated stress, to the neuron. The stimulus can come from a variety of sources and may be a chemical cascade from stress. When stress occurs over and over, it can sensitize the neuron rather than creating a tolerance to the stimulus. The theory about kindling includes the idea that stress induces symptomatic episodes and, as the illness progresses, the individual becomes more and more vulnerable to stress and further episodes. Soon only a slight stressor tips the person into a symptomatic episode (Altman et al., 2006).

Behavioral sensitization is a chemical phenomenon in which changes occur in the person's behavior. Short-term and long-term memory are affected. Following a series of these "behavioral seizures," the neuron requires less stimulus to produce the seizure-like response. Kindling appears to be a kind of learning, independent of cognition, and it can set off an autonomous process.

Although kindling has not been demonstrated definitively in humans, there is indirect support for these biologic interactions. Alcohol withdrawal, post-traumatic stress disorder (PTSD), panic disorder, and rapid-cycling mood disorders are all similar in that stress or a chemical substrate produces kindled seizures in the amygdala region of the brain, which, over time, produces behavior changes (Bockting et al., 2006; McIntyre & Gilby, 2006; Tass & Majtanik, 2006).

Carbamazepine, an anticonvulsant, and the benzodiazepines act on kindled episodes. Future clinical implications of this research require more formal conceptualization. However, it applies as a working hypothesis because bipolar disorder correlates with a stressful life event around the first episode more than 60% of the time. Thus, repetitions of illness (episode sensitization) may trigger further psychopathology and also provide some explanation for why people with rapid-cycling mood disorders become refractory to medications over time. The neuron actually goes through changes, so different medications or combinations of medications are required to stabilize the progressive course (Altman et al., 2006).

Circadian Rhythms

Biologic rhythms, or biorhythms, program our 24-hour day–night cycles. Chronobiology is the relationship between time and biologic rhythms and their effect on living systems. There are rhythms in endocrine secretion, NT synthesis, receptor number, enzyme levels and affinities, brain electrical activity, duration of cell cycle times, and the transcription regulation of DNA. Rhythms can have different cycle lengths:

- Ultradian: less than 24 hours
- Circadian: 24 hours
- Infradian: more than 24 hours

Plasma cortisol, core body temperature, and growth hormones are all paced in a particular manner. There may be familial influences, suggesting heritability (Mansour et al., 2006). *Zeitgebers* are time cues or synchronizers, environmental cues about timing, and they set the biological rhythms. See Box 6-5 for examples of zeitgebers.

One of the major functions of circadian timing is organizing and prioritizing metabolic and physiologic events. The suprachiasmatic nucleus (SCN), a cluster of neurons in the hypothalamus, is the body's own internal synchronizer for temperature and sleep. External influences work as cues to your body and include the light–dark cycle, mealtime patterns, and work schedules.

One theory of depression is that it represents a phase advance disorder (as evidenced by early morning awakening), decreased onset of rapid eye movement (REM) sleep, and neuroendocrine changes. Mechanisms of sleep, both normal and pathologic, are covered in Chapter 19∞. Research into the question of whether estrogen shortens the circadian period, lengthening the sleep phase, advancing sleep onset, and consolidating sleep, would help our understanding of the phenomenology of depression and menopause related to changes in the sleep–activity cycle for women. Symptoms of people with seasonal affective disorder (SAD) vary, but common symptoms are increased sleep and appetite, decreased energy, weight gain, low self-esteem, and negativism. A common treatment for this desynchronization is exposure to broad-spectrum light. Melatonin, synthesized from tryptophan in the pineal gland, allows the individual to become drowsy and promotes sleep. Light suppresses melatonin production. Therefore, broad-spectrum light can decrease the physiologic source of increased sleep.

Box 6-5 Zeitgebers

Zeitgebers are the external environmental synchronizers that help us adjust to a 24-hour day and include:

- Light
- Eating schedules
- Work
- Sounds (birds chirping, clocks chiming)
- Dark
- Social activities
- Smells (coffee brewing)
- Other time-enforced activities

The solar light–dark cycle is considered the most important environmental cue.

Nurses can teach clients who have a recurrent pattern of winter depression (seasonal affective disorder; see Chapter 17∞) to begin preparing for their symptoms by seeking light treatment in the early fall. Usually, exposure to a light of 10,000 lux for 30 minutes in the morning (Lam et al., 2006) is sufficient to promote a change. Additional strategies include:

- Cautioning individuals with bipolar disorder not to stay up all night studying or partying, as that disrupts the sleep–wake cycle
- Helping postpartum mothers with a history of mood disorders prepare for night feedings to avoid becoming sleep deprived
- Advocating that people with mood disorders not work irregular shift patterns

The Americans with Disabilities Act (ADA) supports the idea that people with psychiatric disabilities should have a "reasonable" work schedule. This could include stable shift assignments.

As our understanding of biorhythms grows, we can expect that certain clinical decisions, such as the optimal time to administer medications or perform surgery, will change. Knowing a client's circadian patterns will help you administer appropriate medication dosages, resulting in greater efficacy and minimal side effects.

PSYCHOBIOLOGY AND MENTAL DISORDERS

This section examines current hypotheses about the psychobiologic basis of schizophrenia, mood disorders (major depression and bipolar disorder), anxiety disorders (panic disorder and OCD), dementia of the Alzheimer's type (DAT) personality disorders, and substance-related disorders. Research is continuing to examine most major psychiatric problems for issues related to biologic changes. The disorders described in this section are examples of how biologic research helps us to understand and treat these disorders.

Schizophrenia

The evolution of the diagnosis of schizophrenia has been dramatic, shifting from a narrowly focused definition of the illness to one with specific criteria that acknowledges the many ways this illness is manifested. No single neurobiologic hypothesis as the source of schizophrenia exists. The variability of the psychopathology requires the implementation of multifaceted, or multifocal, treatments.

Neuron Loss

Researchers are trying to determine why there is a loss of neurons in the brain tissue of people with schizophrenia (Kring et al., 2007). While there are fewer nerve cells overall, there are more pyramidal cells (containing DA, ACh, and glutamate) that are excitatory in nature, bringing sensory inputs (sights, sounds, thoughts) to the cerebral cortex. This suggests that the illness may result from an increased flow of

MediaLink Case Study: Alterations in Psychobiology

activity up to the cortex and may explain why people with schizophrenia become overwhelmed by stimuli such as hallucinations and misperceptions.

Cognitive Abnormalities

Changes in electroencephalograms (EEGs) may indicate a deficit in the processing of data in individuals with schizophrenia. Abnormalities in the GABAminergic system can result in cognitive abnormalities such as hallucinations, and association problems in the thought pattern. Studies of DA receptors, especially DA type II (D_2) receptors, provide clues to the neuropathology of schizophrenia. Most D_2 receptors are in the basal ganglia, as observed with neuroimaging studies. The presence of D_2 receptors in structures with receptors having connections to the limbic and cortical pathways helps link the functions or behaviors of the cognitive and emotional aspects of schizophrenia. Postmortem studies using PET scans are trying to unravel the issue of whether the postmortem findings are a result of antipsychotic medication treatment or primary to the pathophysiology of the disease syndrome (Minzenberg et al., 2006).

Molecular Genetics

The conventional and less frequently used antipsychotic medications, haloperidol and fluphenazine, bind to block D_2 receptors in the basal ganglia and target the symptoms of hallucinations, delusions, and loose associations (also referred to as positive symptoms). From the application of molecular genetics techniques, the cloning of other DA receptors (D_3, D_4, and D_5) has led to the development of more specific psychotropic medications. The newer antipsychotics (sometimes referred to as atypical antipsychotics)—clozapine, risperidone, olanzapine, quetiapine, ziprasidone, aripiprazole, and paliperidone—target such behaviors as restricted emotional expression, attention deficit, poor grooming, lack of motivation, social withdrawal, and poverty of speech (collectively called negative symptoms). These medications are referred to as atypical because they select receptor subtypes other than D_2 as the conventional, more typical antipsychotics do and are less likely to cause EPSE.

MEDIALINK Care Plan: Genetic Implications

Structural Brain Abnormalities

A second major hypothesis about schizophrenia is that structural brain abnormalities are associated with the syndrome. Brain computed tomography (CT) scans show enlarged ventricles and widened sulci and fissures that appear to have been present from the onset of symptoms and are thus not a result of treatment. When a twin has schizophrenia, the nonaffected twin's ventricles appear normal in size; the ventricles of the twin with schizophrenia are larger. A prenatal injury, postnatal maturational change in brain cells, or delayed myelination of nerve cells may explain the delay of the syndrome until adolescence. Myelin forms the insulating lining of axons and is associated with the maturation of behavior during normal development. Myelination is thought to assist with the emotional component of cognition and behavior. The ability to think abstractly is related to myelination in the limbic system and is thought to be established by midadolescence, with full maturity taking place during adulthood. A decrease in myelination would cause an increase in anxiety, difficulty socializing, abrupt or muted styles of interacting, and difficulty in modulating affect.

Genetic Alterations

Genetic polymorphisms—many genetic alterations as opposed to a single gene mutation—are now generally thought to be responsible for the development of schizophrenia. Recent research has concentrated on determining the specific chromosomal locations of those genes. For example, genes 1q22–q24 and 1q42 demonstrate that genetic changes in the brain increase the likelihood of developing schizophrenia or bipolar disorder. Research on genetic location may assist in determining genetic counseling and treatment, and true genotype variants for schizophrenia could be discovered in the near future. Such a discovery would allow us to predict who will get the illness and who will respond to which specific medications. The variable expression of the illness likely occurs through epigenetic modification of gene activation (DeLisi & Fleischhaker, 2007; Keltner, 2005). As mentioned previously, there is evidence of this variability in monozygotic twins when only one twin has schizophrenia even though they have the same genes; in the difference in the risk for schizophrenia between dizygotic twins and siblings, when both share about the same percentage of parental genes; in the considerable drop in elevated risk for schizophrenia from first-degree to second-degree relatives; as well as in multiple documented environmental factors of modest but elevated risk. See the Partnering with Clients and Families feature.

Stress–Diathesis Model

Contemporary treatment of schizophrenia is influenced by a stress–diathesis model (a biologic predisposition to a disease that is activated by stress). We know that merely having a predisposition for the illness does not necessarily mean the individual will develop the illness. Resiliency in response to stress can make the difference between developing the illness or not. These interactions between psychobiologic vulnerability and environmental events can stress the person's adaptive abilities and precipitate the onset of the syndrome or the recurrence of symptoms. Nurses can target interventions that alter the neurochemical systems with pharmacotherapy and psychosocial treatments (such as social skills, case management, client and family education). Chapter 16 includes a thorough discussion of nursing interventions for clients with schizophrenia.

Mood Disorders

Because of the variability in both the genetics and the symptoms of major depression and bipolar disorder, the psychobiologic basis of mood disorders is difficult to determine. Research has focused on 5-HT and NE receptors. Brain stem nuclei that project to the amygdala, hippocampus, mammillary bodies, and cerebral cortex help account for the symp-

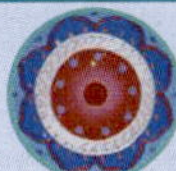

PARTNERING WITH CLIENTS AND FAMILIES

TEACHING ABOUT GENETIC TESTING FOR SCHIZOPHRENIA

At present there is no definitive test for schizophrenia, so genetic testing with schizophrenia as the primary interest would likely take place in a research setting. A reliable test using blood and other body cells is sure to be developed in the not-too-distant future. Your discussions with clients and families should include the science of genetics to familiarize them with this leading edge of genetic diagnosis, treatment, and risk reduction.

If your clients and their family members have the opportunity to be involved in genetic research, Informed Consent documents for participation in such studies explain in detail what is being tested, how the sample will be used, and how long the sample will be kept following the research. Clients and their family members should know that research does not necessarily help study subjects who have the illness. After hundreds of genetic samples have been examined, however, we have the potential for a clear picture of the genetics of schizophrenia. Helping clients and families understand the benefits of genetic research now will shape what happens for future generations of people with schizophrenia.

toms of appetite change, insomnia, depressed affect, loss of interest and pleasure (anhedonia), decreased problem-solving skills, and suicide attempts. Postmortem findings show reduced 5-HT reuptake sites in the hypothalamus and hippocampus. The association of decreased 5-HT with aggression may account for the suicide potential of this population.

Neuroendocrine challenge tests report increased cortisol, blunted ACTH response, hypothalamic–pituitary–thyroid axis alterations, and a higher-than-expected rate of autoimmune thyroiditis. When clients ask you, as their nurse, what these results indicate, you can emphasize they are state-dependent findings, that is, markers that occur while the person is in a depressed mood (state), and not diagnostic or a genetic characteristic of the illness.

Recent NT studies suggest that complex interactions among NE, 5-HT, DA, ACh, GABA, peptides, and second messengers contribute to bipolar disorder. There may be as many as six different types of bipolar disorders; further research to distinguish among them will refine our assessments and clinical treatments. Bipolar disorder tends to accelerate over time if left untreated. Early episodes tend to be precipitated by stress, but once recurrent episodes have occurred, the illness accelerates independently of external causes. Even with a genetic predisposition, there can also be changes in gene expression based on life experiences.

Because of the various clinical symptoms associated with mood disorders, the nurse has an excellent opportunity to assess clients for their unique psychobiologic profile. The outcome of this specific assessment with each client over time will promote improved efficacy of treatment for the target symptoms and potentially prevent disruptive episodes. Promoting client self-care, which involves the client's becoming aware of his or her symptoms in order to report clinical changes early in a recurrence of the depression, will assist in limiting the severity of the mood disorder (see Chapter 17∞).

Electroconvulsive Therapy (ECT)

Somatic therapies other than medications are used in the treatment of mood disorders. Electroconvulsive therapy (ECT) is used for psychotic depression and mania. Exactly how ECT works is not well understood. Evidence suggests that it may resynchronize circadian rhythms, like a "brain defibrillator"; it may act as an anticonvulsant like carbamazepine; it may restore the equilibrium between cerebral hemispheres; or it may help prioritize function over depressive thoughts. Historically, ECT caused some controversy, probably due to its crude beginnings. Current use, known as modified ECT, is not the intense physiologic event it used to be because of the use of muscle relaxants and short-acting anesthetic agents. Contrary to popular belief, ECT causes no tissue damage or neuronal cell loss (structural brain damage). Most ECT clients report positive associations with the treatment and general improvement in cognition, in addition to relief from depression for several weeks following ECT.

Repetitive Transcranial Magnetic Stimulation (rTMS)

Repetitive transcranial magnetic stimulation (rTMS) involves the use of short pulses of magnetic energy to stimulate nerve cells in the brain. rTMS uses magnetic fields to stimulate the brain with an indirect electric current (ECT uses a direct electric current). This stimulation disrupts neuronal firing and is being examined as an alternative to ECT. rTMS is an emerging therapy, still experimental in the United States at this printing but demonstrated to be useful in treating a number of conditions. It is not a precise tool for targeting areas of the brain but may create enough of a disruption to change patterns of thinking. There is no seizure and no need for anesthesia. Preliminary results from active research indicate that there may even be less memory loss with this treatment than with ECT.

The range of applications for rTMS encompasses severe depression, mania, hallucinations, several anxiety disorders, migraine headaches, tinnitus, disturbances in neural circuitry, select neurological conditions, and neuropathic pain. The recent version of rTMS is built on magnetic stimulation of amphibian sciatic nerves (Kolin, Brill, & Broberg, 1959), human muscle impacts from pulsed magnetic stimulation (Bickford et al., 1987), and finally central nervous system (CNS) stimulation by magnetic fields (Kouijzer et al., 1985).

There are two types of rTMS:

- High-frequency stimulation using more than 5 hertz (Hz), also referred to as fast rTMS. High-frequency stimulation induces cortical excitability.

- Low-frequency stimulation using less than 5 Hz, also referred to as slow rTMS. Low-frequency stimulation induces neural inhibition (Rossini & Rossi, 2007).

Treatment with rTMS is a noninvasive strategy. Clients are awake, alert, and require no sedation during treatment sessions. Treatment can be offered in office settings and, as there is no anesthesia or sedation, it can be conducted at any time and does not require the client to fast. Clients complete treatments and continue with daily activities without requiring recovery periods.

The side effects of rTMS are categorized into immediate and short-term. These include seizures, cognitive impairment, cardiovascular side effects, auditory function changes, and headache. Long-term risks have not been identified. No neuronal damage has been observed in any of the animal long-term studies, and the seizures and cognitive deficits noted in shorter time frames have had no long-term sequelae.

Anxiety Disorders

Anxiety disorders have many subtypes, discussed in detail in Chapter 18∞, therefore, a complete review will not be undertaken in this chapter. As you know from an earlier discussion in this chapter, the question of whether anxiety disorders are a separate type of disorder or a variant of a depressive spectrum is still unanswered. MRI and PET scans reveal right hippocampal changes, high brain metabolism, and an abnormal sensitivity to hyperventilation in people with panic disorder.

How is your approach with mildly anxious clients different from your approach with clients who have moderate, high, or crisis levels of anxiety? Provided that nurses assess the client's anxiety accurately, how prescriptive are their interventions, and what objective evaluative measures of anxiety control do they use? See the What Every Crisis Response Team Nurse Should Know feature for an example.

Anxiety is a psychobiologic condition that responds to both behavioral and pharmacologic interventions and is recognized as amenable to nursing care. Through the use of nursing science, a nurse conducts a thorough assessment of a client's symptoms of anxiety, using various assessment tools. Cognitive behavioral and supportive approaches have been effective interventions for anxious clients. Clients with any of the anxiety disorders benefit from being taught about the use of medications to decrease anxiety symptoms. Refer to Chapters 8 and 18∞ for further information about caring for an individual with an anxiety disorder.

Panic Disorder

Neurochemical changes are associated with NE, 5-HT, GABA, and peptides in panic disorder. The discharge of NE in the brain stem, chemoreceptors in the medulla, and 5-HT sets off a series of communications that extend through the limbic system, rich in benzodiazepine receptors, to the prefrontal cortex. This pathway may explain why the cortex interprets the rapid pulse from the NE discharge as a life-threatening heart attack. These neural connections allow for a hypervigilant cognitive appraisal or an inability to integrate the sensory information with any biologic sensation. The inappropriate behavioral outcome is anticipatory anxiety and avoidance of stimuli that might be the associated precipitant of the arousal.

WHAT EVERY CRISIS RESPONSE TEAM NURSE SHOULD KNOW

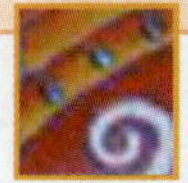

A Client with Psychiatric Symptoms

Imagine that you are the psychiatric nurse on a Crisis Response Team. The team receives a call about a very agitated man who has a history of paranoid delusions and hallucinations. You and the other team members approach the man, who is on his porch mumbling agitatedly to himself.

Your knowledge of the psychobiology of schizophrenia supports the strategy of having only one person speak clearly and simply to this man so as not to overwhelm him. His executive functioning, and therefore his ability to process incoming information, is challenged when symptoms are acute. You interact with him in a calm, straightforward manner, asking what the problem could be. When he answers you in a loud, menacing tone that he must "strike before the irons have cooled beyond their coloration," you ask him to tell you what he wants you to do. In the conversation that follows you discover that he has not been eating or sleeping, that he becomes very upset when people interrupt him (to ask him to eat or try to get some sleep), and that he is exhausted from days of trying to accomplish a delusional task.

When it is apparent that an individual such as this man is experiencing severe symptoms, stabilization is needed to protect him and others. Stabilization can be achieved through a combination of a safe environment, psychopharmacology to balance neurotransmitter functions, and compassionate care to help him through this trauma.

Obsessive Compulsive Disorder (OCD)

PET scans show higher metabolic rates in the left prefrontal cortex and caudate nuclei in people with OCD. The caudate or "gating station" dysfunction may lead to overactive circuits that fail to properly integrate cognitive, emotional, and motor responses to sensory inputs. The prefrontal hyperactivity may be related to the tendency to ruminate and plan excessively, as well as to think in an abstract way. Increased frontal lobe activity manifests as a heightened sense of judgment (guilt and worry), intense affect (depression), and hyperjudgmental rigidity.

Abnormal regulation of the 5-HT subsystem has a role in the pathophysiology of OCD. This possibility is supported by improvement in response to treatment with selective serotonin reuptake inhibitors (SSRIs). In addition, increased levels of arginine, vasopressin, somatostatin, and CRH are found in the CSF of people with OCD. These neuropeptides promote grooming activity and perseverative (repetitive) motor behaviors and increase arousal (anxiety), which are part of the OCD symptomatology.

Eapen, Pauls, and Robertson (2006) describe the genetics of OCD. The complexity of the illness is shown in its various presentations. In a family with a high rate of OCD, the illness will look different clinically as well as genetically among affected family members. A further complication arises with nonfamilial cases of OCD. A reasonable question would be, "Where does OCD come from?" It appears to arise from genetic, neurochemical, neuroanatomical, and environmental influences that are being thoroughly explored. Studies of the genetics of OCD (Kim & Kim, 2006; Perez, Brown, Vrshek-Schallhorn, Johnson, & Joiner, 2006) have found that people who have OCD show differences in their serotonin transporter gene as well as abnormalities in the brain's white matter.

Dementia of the Alzheimer's Type (DAT)

Working with clients suffering from DAT and their family caregivers calls for creativity based on knowledge of the structure and function of the brain. In assessing and intervening with the DAT client, be aware that disorientation results in fear and agitation. Thus any change, such as bed reassignment or facility transfer, is a significant stressor. For those with parietal involvement, walking down a hall with a patterned carpet, stepping up on a weight scale, or managing steps is difficult because they cannot orient themselves in relation to the space around them. Chapter 14 includes a thorough discussion of the nursing care of individuals with DAT.

Neurobiology

People with DAT have decreased cerebral blood flow or metabolic function in the posterior temporoparietal regions. DAT is the only major mental disorder to show this characteristic pattern of hypometabolic function. Thus, PET and SPECT studies may be useful in differentiating DAT from other disorders that include confusion and intellectual deterioration as symptoms. Structural neuronal degeneration occurs, producing neurofibrillary tangles and amyloid deposits, or plaques. Nerve receptor density and distribution studies promise improved diagnostic accuracy.

Decreases in cholinergic neurons in a region of the basal ganglia that connect to the amygdala, hippocampus, and cortex are seen in DAT. Functionally, these decreases result in the short-term memory loss characteristic of the disease. While the deficits are considered central, other NT systems are involved in the pathology, including NE, 5-HT, DA, peptides, and nerve growth factor. If receptors in the limbic structures are affected, depression or labile mood results; a decrease in social skills, inhibition, and impaired judgment can also be a part of the behavioral pattern.

Genetics

DAT research investigates chromosomal abnormalities. Understanding the causal factors in early onset DAT has led to assessing for mutation in presenilin-1. This research used altered mice that lacked the gene for presenilin-1. The mice demonstrated that the presenilin-1 did not cleave in the usual way and the beta-amyloid plaques did not occur. The research concluded that when the gene for presenilin-1 is present and overactive, there is excessive cleaving of the amyloid precursor protein that forms the plaques (Krishnan, 2007; Priller et al., 2007). Further genetic research in DAT is focusing on the effect amyloid-beta-derived diffusible ligands (ADDLs) have on the nerve cells. ADDLs disrupt the neurons responsible for learning and memory, then cause neuronal death. Understanding the changes in the genetic composition of the nerve cells can lead to new medications that block ADDLs or decrease the excessive cleaving of the amyloid precursor protein. Research will contribute to the information needed to develop effective treatments for this complex disease.

Where does AD come from? Inheritance is well documented and accounts for approximately one-third of all cases of AD. Evidence of mutations in at least four genes that can cause AD has now been documented: mutations in the amyloid precursor gene; mutation in a chromosome 14 gene encoding presenilin-1; mutation in a gene on chromosome 1 that encodes presenilin-2; and association with the APOE-4 allele on chromosome 19. Each mutation depicts different aspects of the disease (e.g., early onset, cardiovascular disease). APOE 4-allele confers a risk for both sporadic and familial AD and may be better labeled a risk gene, although there are no widely accepted definitions of risk versus cause. Keep in mind that just the presence of the APOE-4 allele is not necessary or sufficient for the expression of DAT; other yet-to-be-identified environmental or genetic factors may contribute to the development of DAT.

Personality Disorders

Personality disorders, by definition, cause distress and impairment severe enough to lead clients to seek help. You are sure to come in contact with someone with a personality disorder at some point in your practice.

Neurobiology

Recent neurobiologic evidence indicates that the origin of personality disorders rests in biology as well as psychology. There is still a great deal to learn about one of the largest groups of personality disorders, borderline personality disorder (BPD). None of the books and articles published thus far have provided a clear answer to the question of why women are more likely than men to be diagnosed with this disorder. Legitimate gender bias in diagnosis has been found in other mental health disorders (i.e., depression) as well and you will likely become aware of other possible sociocultural factors that influence the development and course of a disorder. Bjorklund (2006) reminds us of the need to understand that mental disorders are complex, interactive, and have multiple determinants. Chapter 22 explores the underlying features of personality disorders in greater detail.

Neurochemistry

The neurochemistry of personality disorders, especially catecholamine activity, differs, depending on the mental health diagnosis. An individual with more than one Axis II personality disorder—also referred to as heterogeneity of diagnosis—will demonstrate a wide variety of clinical symptoms. For example, catecholamine regulates and modulates visual, visiospatial, and verbal working memory tasks. The result of catecholamine activity would likely be different with each individual; the cognitive performance will be improved for some, while others show cognitive impairment (Minzenberg et al., 2006).

Genetics

Both quantitative and molecular approaches are important in understanding the genetics of personality disorders. A comingling of mental disorders, or heterogeneous diagnoses, blurs the picture (Baker, 2006). High comorbidity rates in this group make genetic testing for personality disorders difficult. Hypotheses are being tested for commonalities between mood, behavioral, and personality disorders on a neurobiological substrate. The frequent combination of fear and anger traits among persons with personality disorders suggests a direction for research (Lara & Akiskal, 2006).

Understanding the underlying features of personality disorders contributes to effective goal setting and treatment.

Substance-Related Disorders

The psychobiology of substance abuse is a rich field of study. So many substances are destructive not only to the users' health but also to the integrity of families and communities. Exploring this area to its greatest extent is necessary to promote public health. Research is moving us toward that goal.

Because 4% to 5% of people in Western societies have difficulty with alcohol dependence and the relapse rate is 50% to 80% in a year, understanding its origins and having a reliable genetic analysis are vital. We know from decades of studies that there is heritability and predisposition to alcohol dependence as well as complex environmental influences. The latest research indicates an association of alcohol dependence with a GABA receptor gene, especially in those with a presumed genetic predisposition (Fehr et al., 2006). Identifying the genetic components of the disease helps identify high-risk individuals. Once someone is identified as being at high risk, nurses can intervene on an interpersonal basis. Interventions would include defining weaknesses in stress responses, improving resilience to adversity, and teaching enhancement of support systems. Genetic research has helped to develop meaningful and effective pharmacological treatments. See the Partnering with Clients and Families feature for an example of counseling clients and families about the genetic basis of substance-related disorders.

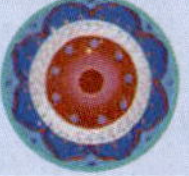

PARTNERING WITH CLIENTS AND FAMILIES

TEACHING ABOUT THE GENETIC BASIS OF SUBSTANCE-RELATED DISORDERS

When someone is diagnosed with a substance-related disorder such as alcoholism, your involvement with that client and the family revolves around teaching. The genetic basis for alcohol dependence includes heritability and a predisposition for offspring to be alcohol dependent as well. While the immediate concern is for the client, a future concern will be the life-impacting ramifications that a substance-related disorder will have for the client's children.

Whether the client's children are biologically related or adopted, there are also complex contributions from environmental conditions. Once a blood relative has been identified as alcohol dependent, there is a presumed genetic predisposition to alcoholism. You may introduce the topic and explain how genetics can serve as advance notice for people to take action. A proactive environment helps the at-risk individual maximize coping skills without turning to substances and begins the process of prevention for future generations.

Your role can include mapping out how an at-risk person reacts when exposed to a stressor. Is the reaction adaptive? These are all healthy responses:

- Learning
- Exploring options
- Thinking about consequences
- Reviewing how well one's coping skills worked in a situation
- Making changes when things don't turn out well
- Adjusting and fine-tuning the changes made

If you detect less-than-ample adaptive coping skills in an at-risk individual, you would proceed with shoring up the weaker areas to prevent (or at least minimize the possibility of) maladaptive coping such as substance abuse. These are some client-centered strategies to promote better coping:

- Become actively involved in shaping a personal support system.
- Identify stressors:
  - Timing—time of year, holidays, anniversaries, schedule disruptions, varying work shifts
  - Interpersonal issues—arguments, intimacy, loneliness, crowding, demands from others, financial problems
  - Intrapersonal issues—feelings of anger, incompetence, fatigue, frustration, fear
- Rehearse and practice healthy responses to difficult situations.
- Develop an array of activities or behaviors that minimize or reduce stressful times and situations.

The combination of substance abuse or dependence and another identified psychiatric problem is common and complicates the picture. The characteristics of one illness meld with the features of another, resulting in a deepening and difficult situation from which few effectively extricate themselves. As you can imagine, people who are alcohol-dependent and have personality disorder characteristics are at increased risk for suicidal behavior (Preuss, Koller, Barnow, Eikmeier, & Soyka, 2006). The impulsivity present in most personality disorders and the disinhibition and judgment problems resulting from alcohol use are a dangerous combination. Psychiatric care settings that address this problem are better equipped to improve outcomes for these clients. See Chapter 15 for detailed discussions of substance-related disorders and their genetics and heritability.

PSYCHOBIOLOGY AND NURSING

We remind you frequently in this text that linking body, mind, brain, and behavior is the essence of a holistic psychiatric–mental health nursing practice. Integrating psychobiologic principles enhances that goal. To function as a professional nurse, it is important to be aware of any personal feelings, opinions, or beliefs that you have, such as those discussed in the Your Self-Awareness feature, that may diminish your ability to be an advocate for and support person to clients and their families.

Your attitude about the underlying neurobiology of behavior can influence therapeutic outcomes. It is important to consider how treatment outcomes are potently influenced by both the style and the knowledge incorporated into nursing interventions. If the comprehensive nursing assessment, interpretation of the assessment, client teaching, and evaluation of the intervention are based on knowledge of the biologic, cognitive, and behavioral factors that affect the client, the client has a greater opportunity for successful reduction of symptoms. If, however, you are ambivalent about the value of biologic or somatic therapies, you will inevitably communicate this attitude to the client and the family, and your interventions may not be as effective as they could be. Remember, you integrate your own viewpoint into client teaching, and its expression can hinder or help your clients and their families.

When performing a comprehensive assessment, it is important to determine the appropriate questions to ask the client in order to obtain information that can lead to an understanding of the client's thoughts and emotional and behavioral patterns. Assess the client with an open mind and interpret and communicate the information to the rest of the multidisciplinary team in a comprehensive manner.

Integrating psychobiology into nursing care involves more than simply administering medications. It enables the nurse to fine-tune assessments, diagnoses, interventions, and evaluations of clients' response patterns. The synthesis of this critical thinking provides clients and families with quality, cost-effective care. The Evidence-Based Practice feature on page 106 is an example of how relevant psychobiologic research can contribute to holistic nursing practice.

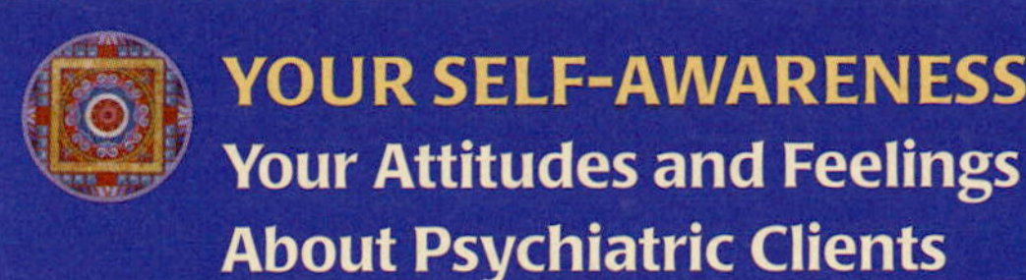

YOUR SELF-AWARENESS
Your Attitudes and Feelings About Psychiatric Clients

To assist you in examining your views about and feelings toward psychiatric clients, answer the following:

- How do you describe an individual with a mental disorder? Do you refer to the person's illness in layman's terms or proper diagnostic nomenclature?
- How would you describe to another team member an individual who walks down the street nude, is hostile, or believes that other people are trying to "clone" him?
- How would you react if a transitional living facility for people with psychiatric problems moved into a house in your neighborhood?
- How do you respond when you think an individual is manipulating you? What do you think causes manipulative behavior?
- Are people with psychiatric problems more violent than the general population?
- Do you become angry with clients who become symptomatic because they have not taken their medication?
- Do you believe that individuals with major mental disorders can be contributing members of their families and society?
- Do you feel hopeless when working with individuals with severe chronic emotional illness?
- Can diet, exercise, and a regular daily pattern of living enhance mental health?
- Do you think that depressed individuals do not try hard enough to "pull themselves up by their bootstraps"?
- Do you think that when people say they are suicidal they are really attempting to receive attention?
- Do you want to work with people who have psychiatric problems?

Being a nurse is an opportunity for you to be flexible, creative, and visionary. Keep a diary of how you made a difference for a client. Was a biologic variable involved? Articulate how you made that difference, and link it with cost-effective care. The care of people who have psychiatric disorders uses technology to find the neuropathology. Technology assists you in determining diagnostic impacts and targeting symptoms in order to effectively intervene as a psychiatric nurse. However, the nurse–client relationship remains the core of your nursing practice.

The exact biologic determinants for psychiatric disorders and behaviors are yet to be discovered. To date, there is no definitive biologic test to identify a psychiatric disorder. We still rely on expert nursing observations and assessment. However, multifocal and multidisciplinary care that incorporates psychobiologic dimensions advances our ability to offer new, more effective assessments and interventions for our clients.

MediaLink Critical Thinking Exercise: Medication Teaching

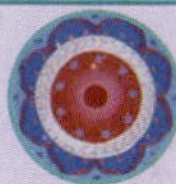

EVIDENCE-BASED PRACTICE

THE ROLE OF GENETIC MICROARRAYS

Exciting advances are being made in psychobiology as a result of research evidence. One example includes a pharmacogenetic microarray-based test approved for clinical use. The AmpliChip CYP450 Test developed by Roche Diagnostics provides comprehensive coverage of gene variations, including deletions and duplications, for the cytochrome P450 CYP2D6 and CYP2C19 genes, which play a major role in the metabolism of an estimated 25% of all prescription medications. (For more information on cytochrome P450 see Chapters 7 and 32.) The test is designed as an aid for clinicians to individualize treatment selection and dosing for medications metabolized through these genes. It recognizes and analyzes 29 polymorphisms and mutations for the 2D6 gene and 2 polymorphisms for the 2C19 gene, allowing more accurate determination of genotype and predicted phenotype (poor, intermediate, extensive, or ultra rapid metabolizer). The test is said to be able to accurately genotype over 99% of the world's population.

This research tested the hypothesis that there are genetically based differences among individuals in the metabolism of medications. It is valid, reliable, and clinically applicable psychobiologic research evidence of the highest standard. Other relevant studies are listed below. The AmpliChip CYP450 is the first approved test, with many more on the horizon, that has the potential to change how we treat psychiatric disorders with medications.

Freimer, N., & Sabatti, C. (2004). The use of pedigree, sib-pair and association studies of common diseases for genetic mapping and epidemiology. *Nature Genetics, 36,* 1045–1051.

Hinds, D. A., Stuve, L. L, Nilsen, G. B., Halperin, E., Eskin, E., Ballinger, D. G., et al. (2005). Whole-genome patterns of common DNA variation in three human populations. *Science, 307,* 1072–1079.

Wang, Q., Bond, M., Elston, R. C., & Tian, X-L. (2007). Molecular genetics. In E. J. Topol (Ed.), *Textbook of cardiovascular medicine* (3rd ed.). Philadelphia: Lippincott Williams & Wilkins.

CRITICAL THINKING QUESTIONS

1. How can this test be used to individualize treatment selection?
2. How can this test be used to individualize medication dosing?
3. How do clients benefit when nurses are knowledgeable about genetic testing?

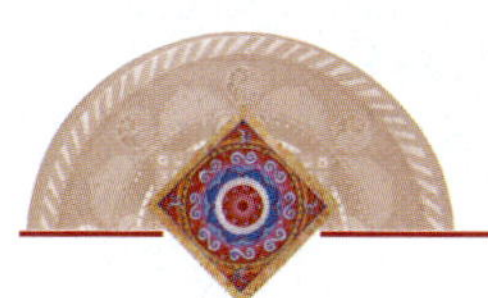

EXPLORE MEDIALINK 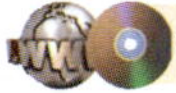 www.prenhall.com/kneisl

For NCLEX-RN® review questions, case studies, and other resources for this chapter see the Pearson Health MediaLink CD-ROM that accompanies this book and the Companion Website at www.prenhall.com/kneisl.

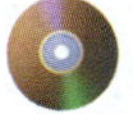

CD-ROM
Audio Glossary
NCLEX-RN® Review Questions
Videos and Animations
- *Seizure*
- *Complex Seizure*
- *Grand Mal Seizure*
- *Neurological Synapse*
- *Serotonin Reuptake Inhibition*
- *Occupation of Receptor Sites by Agonists/Antagonists*

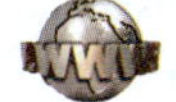

Companion Website
Audio Glossary
NCLEX-RN® Review Questions
Critical Thinking Exercise
- *Medication Teaching*

Case Study
- *Alterations in Psychobiology*

Care Plan
- *Genetic Implications*

MediaLinks
MediaLink Application
- *Schizophrenia-Related Gene Linked to Imbalance in Dopamine Pathways*

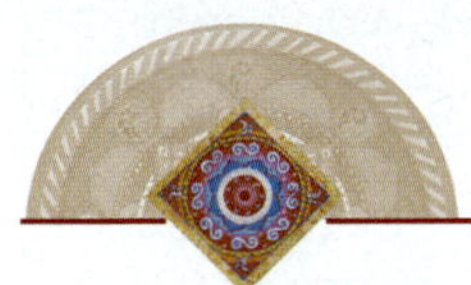

NCLEX-RN® REVIEW QUESTIONS

1. During an assessment, the client is able to perform "serial sevens" and readily adds and subtracts four-digit numbers. To which of the following neuroanatomical areas is this assessment finding related?
1. Temporal lobe
2. Occipital lobe
3. Frontal lobe
4. Parietal lobe

2. A client's wife tells the nurse, "My spouse has developed a shuffling gait and lack of expression that the physician called 'parkinsonism.'" Match this statement with the neuroanatomical area of concern.
1. Reticular activating system
2. Corpus callosum
3. Locus ceruleus
4. Extrapyramidal system

3. One client with depression experiences psychomotor retardation, cognitive dulling, and hypersomnia. Another client experiences depression with hypervigilance, exaggerated startle reflex, and insomnia. Based on your knowledge of the various neuromessengers involved in depression, you hypothesize that the differences in the clients' presentations most likely correlate with differences in availability of which neurotransmitter?
1. Norepinephrine
2. Histamine
3. Acetylcholine
4. Glutamate

4. You are teaching a family support group about the function of dopamine in psychosis. Family members list the client behaviors. Which behaviors are related to increased availability of dopamine? (Select all that apply.)
1. Decreased emotional expression
2. Excessive fluid intake associated with water intoxication
3. Bizarre behavior
4. Avolition
5. Hallucinations

5. A client with schizophrenia asks you, "Is my illness a nature problem or a nurture problem?" In accordance with current practice, your best response is:
1. "No one is born with schizophrenia. It develops as a response to internal and environmental stressors."
2. "We used to think bad parenting could make people schizophrenic, but medications show there's a chemical imbalance."
3. "Individuals with schizophrenia are born with schizophrenia genes that are activated by life stress."
4. "Your medications are going to help, no matter whether it is a nature or nurture problem."

6. A client newly diagnosed with a mood disorder asks you, "I don't want to take medicine if my problem is psychosocial. Is my illness biochemical or psychosocial?" In accordance with current research, your best response includes which of the following? (Select all that apply.)
1. "Your illness is associated with a biochemical imbalance."
2. "Your illness has a lot to do with your upbringing, but you cannot change that."
3. "Stress management early in the course of the illness can lead to fewer illness episodes."
4. "Subsequent illness episodes are preventable if you manage your stress."
5. "Medications help to correct the chemical imbalance."

7. Your client is augmenting his usual pharmacotherapeutic regimen with an experimental substance P antagonist. If the treatment is effective, which of the following is a realistic outcome?
1. Prescriptions for MAOIs will increase.
2. Treatment with substance P will replace pharmacotherapy with SSRIs.
3. In the future, clients will experience decreased side effects from SSRIs with the use of substance P antagonists.
4. The client's level of functioning increases further, as substance P has a different action on the neuronal pathway than traditional monoamine receptor–based pharmacotherapy.

8. A coworker questions the value of the dexamethasone suppression test (DST), since "it is not diagnostic." You explain that the purpose of this test is:
1. To assess the hypothalamic–pituitary–adrenal (HPA) axis.
2. To support the tenet that major depression is a medical disability.
3. To determine if the client has exogenous depression unreceptive to pharmacotherapy.
4. To determine if the client will respond to electroconvulsive therapy (ECT).

9. Your client with bipolar affective disorder had her first episode at age 20 when she lost both parents in a motor vehicle accident. Now 35, the client is unable to identify precipitating factors for her last three episodes. She reports meticulous adherence; however, her longstanding treatment regimen is no longer effective. Her teaching plan should include the concept of:
   1. Tolerance to medication.
   2. Kindling.
   3. Hepatic efficiency changes associated with age.
   4. Honesty in the nurse–client relationship.

10. During a family support group, the nurse compares major mental illness to having hypertension or diabetes. For clients and families, what are the implications for appreciating the biological bases of major mental illnesses? (Select all that apply.)
   1. Increased parental guilt and blame
   2. Decrease in shame and stigma
   3. Acceptance of client responsibility for treatment
   4. Informed family planning
   5. Instillation of hope

See Appendix C for answers.

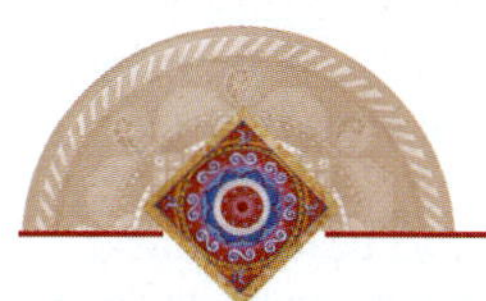

REFERENCES

Abercrombie, P. D., Zamora, A., & Korn, A. P. (2007). Lessons learned: Providing a mindfulness-based stress reduction program for low-income multiethnic women with abnormal Pap smears. *Holistic Nursing Practice, 21*(1), 26–34.

Akiskal, H. S. (2006). Toward an integrative model of the spectrum of mood, behavioral and personality disorders based on fear and anger traits: II. Implications for neurobiology, genetics and psychopharmacological treatment. *Journal of Affective Disorders, 94*(1–3), 89–103.

Altman, S., Haeri, S., Cohen, L. J., Ten, A., Barron, E., Galynker, I. I., et al. (2006). Predictors of relapse in bipolar disorder: A review. *Journal of Psychiatric Practice, 12*(5), 269–282.

American Nurses Association, American Psychiatric Nurses Association, & International Society of Psychiatric–Mental Health Nurses. (2007). *Psychiatric–mental health nursing: Scope and standards of practice.* Silver Spring, MD: nursesbooks.org.

Baker, L. A. (2006). Methods for understanding genetic and environmental influences in normal and abnormal personality. In S. Strack (Ed.), *Differentiating normal and abnormal personality* (2nd ed.) (pp. 257–281). New York: Springer Publishing.

Barinaga, M. (2000). Synapses call the shots. *Science, 290,* 736–738.

Barnoy, S., Appel, D., Peretz, C., Meiraz, H., & Ehrenfeld, M. (2006). Genetic testing, genetic information, and the role of the maternal child health nurses in Israel. *Journal of Nursing Scholarship, 38*(3), 219–224.

Bickford, R. G., Guidi, M., Fortesque, P., & Swenson, M. (1987). Magnetic stimulation of human peripheral nerve and brain: Response enhancement by combined magnetoelectrical technique. *Neurosurgery, 20*(1), 110–116.

Bjorklund, P. (2006). No man's land: Gender bias and social constructivism in the diagnosis of borderline personality disorder. *Issues in Mental Health Nursing, 27*(1), 3–23.

Bockting, C. L. H, Spinhoven, P., Koeter, M. W. J., Wouters, L. F., Visser, I., & Schene, A. H. (2006). Differential predictors of response to preventive cognitive therapy in recurrent depression: A 2-year prospective study. [References]. *Psychotherapy and Psychosomatics, 75*(4), 229–236.

D'Amico, D., & Barbarito, C. (2007). *Health and physical assessment in nursing.* Upper Saddle River, NJ: Prentice Hall.

DeLisi, L. E., & Fleischhaker, W. (2007). Schizophrenia research in the era of the genome, 2007. *Current Opinion in Psychiatry, 20*(2), 109–110.

Du, L., Bakish, D., Ravindran, A., & Hrdina, P. D. (2004). MAO-A gene polymorphisms are associated with major depression and sleep disturbance in males. *Neuroreport, 15*(13), 2097–2101.

Eapen, V., Pauls, D. L., & Robertson, M. M. (2006). The role of clinical phenotypes in understanding the genetics of obsessive-compulsive disorder. *Journal of Psychosomatic Research, 61*(3), 359–364.

Fehr, C., Sander, T., Tadic, A., Lenzen, K. P., Anghelescu, I., Klawe, C., et al. (2006). Confirmation of association of the GABRA2 gene with alcohol dependence by subtype-specific analysis. *Psychiatric Genetics, 16*(1), 9–17.

Freimer, N., & Sabatti, C. (2004). The use of pedigree, sib-pair and association studies of common diseases for genetic mapping and epidemiology. *Nature Genetics, 36,* 1045–1051.

Hinds, D. A., Stuve, L. L., Nilsen, G. B., Halperin, E., Eskin, E., Ballinger, D. G., et al. (2005). Whole-genome patterns of common DNA variation in three human populations. *Science, 307,* 1027–1079.

Keltner, N. L. (2005). Genomic influences on schizophrenia-related neurotransmitter systems. *Journal of Nursing Scholarship, 37*(4), 322–328.

Kim, S. J., & Kim, C. H. (2006). The genetic studies of obsessive-compulsive disorder and its future directions. *Yonsei Medical Journal, 47*(4), 443–454.

Kolin, A., Brill, N., & Broberg, P. (1959). Stimulation of irritable tissues by means of an alternating magnetic field. *Proceedings of the Society for Experimental Biology & Medicine, 102,* 251–253.

Kouijzer, W. J., Stok, C. J., Reits, D., Dunajski, Z., Lopes da Silva, F. H., & Peters, M. J. (1985). Neuromagnetic fields evoked by a patterned on-offset stimulus. *IEEE Transactions on Biomedical Engineering, 32*(6), 455–458.

Kring, A. M., Davison, G. C., Neale, J. M., & Johnson, S. L. (2007). *Abnormal psychology* (10th ed.). Hoboken, NJ: John Wiley & Sons.

Krishnan, K. R. R. (2007). Concept of disease in geriatric psychiatry. *American Journal of Geriatric Psychiatry, 15*(1), 1–11.

Lam, R. W., Levitt, A. J., Levitan, R. D., Enns, M. W., Morehouse, R., Michalak, E. E., et al. (2006). The Can-SAD study: A randomized controlled trial of the effectiveness of light therapy and fluoxetine in patients with winter seasonal affective disorder. *American Journal of Psychiatry, 163*(5), 805–812.

Lara, D. R., & Akiskal, H. S. (2006). Toward an integrative model of the spectrum of mood, behavioral and personality disorders based on fear and anger traits: II. Implications for neurobiology, genetics and psychopharmacological treatment. *Journal of Affective Disorders, 94*(1–3), 89–103.

Mansour, H. A., Wood, J., Logue, T., Chowdari, K. V., Dayal, M., Kupfer, D. J., et al. (2006). Association study of eight circadian genes with bipolar I disorder, schizoaffective disorder and schizophrenia. *Genes, Brain, & Behavior, 5*(2), 150–157.

McIntyre, D. C., & Gilby, K. L. (2006). Parahippocampal networks, intractability, and the chronic epilepsy of kindling. *Advances in Neurology, 97,* 77–83.

Minzenberg, M. J., Xu, K., Mitropoulou, V., Harvey, P. D., Finch, T., Flory, J. D., et al. (2006). Catechol-O-methyltransferase Val158Met genotype variation is associated with prefrontal-dependent task performance in schizotypal personality disorder patients and comparison groups. *Psychiatric Genetics, 16*(3), 117–124.

Norman, T. R., & Burrows, G. D. (2007). Emerging treatments for major depression. *Expert Review of Neurotherapeutics, 7*(2), 203–213.

Perez, M., Brown, J. S., Vrshek-Schallhorn, S., Johnson, F., & Joiner, T. E. (2006). Differentiation of obsessive-compulsive-, panic-, obsessive-compulsive personality-, and non-disordered individuals by variation in the promoter region of the serotonin transporter gene. *Journal of Anxiety Disorders, 20*(6), 794–806.

Preuss, U. W., Koller, G., Barnow, S., Eikmeier, M., & Soyka, M. (2006). Suicidal behavior in alcohol-dependent subjects: The role of personality disorders. *Alcoholism: Clinical & Experimental Research, 30*(5), 866–877.

Priller, C., Dewachter, I., Vassallo, N., Paluch, S., Pace, C., Kretzschmar, H. A., et al. (2007). Mutant presenilin 1 alters synaptic transmission in cultured hippocampal neurons. *Journal of Biological Chemistry, 282*(2), 1119–1127.

Rossini, P. M., & Rossi, S. (2007). Transcranial magnetic stimulation: Diagnostic, therapeutic, and research potential. *Neurology, 68*(7), 484–488.

Smock, T. K. (1999). *Physiological psychology: A neuroscience approach.* Upper Saddle River, NJ: Prentice Hall.

Stewart, S. E., Platko, J., Fagerness, J., Birns, J., Jenike, E., Smoller, J. W., et al. (2007). A genetic family-based association study of OLIG2 in obsessive-compulsive disorder. *Archives of General Psychiatry, 64*(2), 209–214.

Tass, P. A., & Majtanik, M. (2006). Long-term anti-kindling effects of desynchronizing brain stimulation: A theoretical study. *Biological Cybernetics, 94*(1), 58–66.

Thomann, P. A., Wustenberg, T., Pantel, J., Essig, M., & Schroder, J. (2006). Structural changes of the corpus callosum in mild cognitive impairment and Alzheimer's disease. *Dementia and Geriatric Cognitive Disorders, 21*(4), 215–220.

Wang, Q., Bond, M., Elston, R. C., & Tian, X-L. (2007). Molecular genetics. In E. J. Topol (Ed.), *Textbook of cardiovascular medicine* (3rd ed.). Philadelpha: Lippincott Williams & Wilkins.

Williams, J. K., Skirton, H., & Masny, A. (2006). Ethics, policy, and educational issues in genetic testing. *Journal of Nursing Scholarship, 38*(2), 119–125.

ADDITIONAL REFERENCES

Borderline personality disorder: Origins and symptoms. (2006, June). *Harvard Mental Health Letter, 22*(12), 1–3.

Diamond, A., Briand, L., Fossella, J., & Gehlbach, L. (2004). Genetic and neurochemical modulation of prefrontal cognitive functions in children. *American Journal of Psychiatry, 161*(1), 125–132.

Widiger, T., Simonsen, E., Krueger, R., Livesley, W., & Verheul R. (2005). Personality disorder research agenda for the DSM-V. *Journal of Personality Disorders, 19*(3), 315–338.

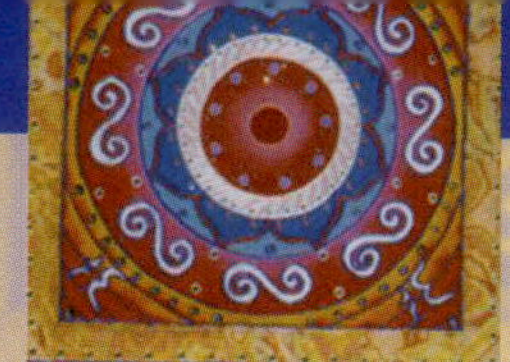

CHAPTER

7

The Science of Psychopharmacology

EILEEN TRIGOBOFF

KEY TERMS

LEARNING OUTCOMES

After completing this chapter, you will be able to:

1. Define psychopharmacology.
2. Describe the chronological development of psychiatric medications.
3. Discuss the biologic impact of medications on ethnically distinct groups.
4. Differentiate psychiatric symptomatology from medication side effects.
5. Document the positive and negative impacts of psychiatric medications on behavior.
6. Compare and contrast the general classifications of medications used for particular psychiatric symptoms.
7. Explain the psychobiologic mechanisms that are important in psychopharmacology.
8. Educate clients and their families about the effects and uses of psychotropic medications.

CRITICAL THINKING CHALLENGE

Medications in psychiatric treatment present an opportunity for the nurse to consider the design of a competent and ethical treatment package. Consider the following situation with a client with schizophrenia. Roberta has symptoms that cause severe difficulties in her thinking, information processing, communication, and relationships. The discomfort she experiences is exceeded only by a sense of demoralization at the realization that she has a chronic and debilitating disease for which there is no cure. Rehabilitating Roberta to a lifestyle with psychotic symptoms, or with fewer or no psychotic symptoms, requires a realistic view of her needs and abilities and specific training to cope with the mental illness and its impact on her life.

1. How would you design a complete treatment protocol for Roberta?
2. Are there times when medications for psychiatric treatment could be used unethically?
3. What steps could you take to reduce the sense of demoralization Roberta feels?

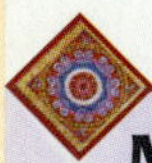

MEDIALINK 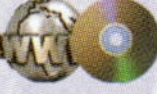 www.prenhall.com/kneisl

Go to the Pearson Health MediaLink CD-ROM and the Companion Website at www.prenhall.com/kneisl for interactive resources for this chapter.

This chapter explores the science of the psychopharmacological agents used to treat symptoms of mental disorders and disabilities. The categories and main effects of these medications are detailed here, as well as some rationales for certain medication choices. Ways to help clients manage their medications and the side effects they may experience are discussed in Chapter 32∞. The science and management of psychopharmacology are intertwined; however, this chapter's discussion of the basics of major medication groups used in psychiatric–mental health nursing can help you create a useful platform on which to build your therapeutic interactions.

Psychopharmacologic nursing interventions deal with the side effects, drug interactions, psychosocial implications, and education activities among you, your clients, and their families. Psychiatric–mental health nursing demands both areas of expertise, but it may be easier to understand psychopharmacology—one of the major tools of your work—in the way we have structured it in this book in two separate chapters.

Psychiatric medications form the primary treatment for many psychiatric diagnoses. As can be seen in the psychopharmacologic timeline in Box 7-1 on page 112, in the years prior to the 1950s (when psychopharmacology became available and widely used), the focus was on behavioral interventions and sedative substances. The past six decades have shown us the beginning use, then enormous leaps of generations of compounds with major impacts, and even success, in treating many of the serious symptoms of mental illness. FIGURE 7-1 ■ illustrates the drop in numbers of inpatients as a result of biologic and pharmacologic interventions. The impacts that psychopharmacology has had on serious mental illness indicate that the physiologic and behavioral outcomes are in response to the physiologic impairment of the mental illness. Just as the symptoms of an endocrine disorder such as diabetes respond to treatment with insulin, mental illness is an imbalance of brain chemicals that can be addressed or corrected with medications.

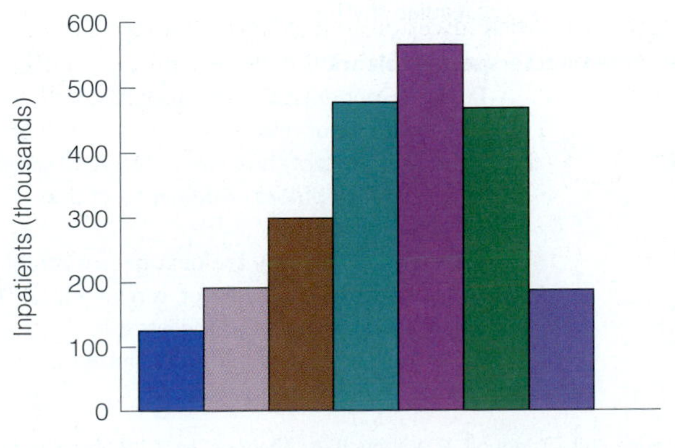

FIGURE 7-1 ■ The great success of biological psychiatry. This graph illustrates the dramatic decrease in psychiatric inpatient numbers since the inception of psychopharmacology.

Psychopharmacology is a primary treatment mode of psychiatric–mental health nursing care and requires nurses to monitor client response as well as identify problems or side effects. Ours is a holistic function, incorporating the client's life, likes and dislikes, and activities along with symptomatology into a comprehensive view of treatment. One of the aims of psychopharmacologic nursing interventions is to teach clients about their medications, including over-the-counter medications and supplements, and what the likely impact will be.

PSYCHOPHARMACOLOGY AND NURSING

The knowledge base of psychopharmacology continues to grow as a result of research and clinical expertise. Psychiatric–mental health nursing has similarly grown, and our responsibilities to recipients of mental health care services involve, to a large degree, psychopharmacologic expertise. Our national professional organization, the American Nurses Association (ANA), examined this issue, and the ANA's Task Force on Psychopharmacology set forth guidelines for this aspect of our nursing practice (ANA, 1994). The guidelines, identified in Box 7-2 on page 113, remain current and delineate three areas that unite the practice of psychiatric–mental health nursing with expertise in psychopharmacology. It is crucial that we:

1. Integrate current data from the neurosciences.
2. Demonstrate knowledge of psychopharmacologic principles.
3. Provide safe and effective clinical management of clients taking these medications through assessment, diagnosis, and treatment.

Psychiatric–mental health nurses must understand current advances in psychobiology to maintain an updated knowledge base for clinical work. The goal of psychopharmacologic interventions is to promote clients' physiologic stability so they can achieve psychologic, social, and spiritual growth.

The word *drugs* conjures up a variety of powerful positive and negative images. Media messages depict the devastating negative effects of IV drug use, alcoholism, and methamphetamine. They also give a picture of people leading productive lives, professionals demonstrating relief of symptoms, and schoolchildren being inoculated against diphtheria, polio, and pertussis. All these images are powerful, and each is backed by truth. But every media representation, positive or negative, must be viewed critically, as misunderstanding and outright ignorance about psychiatric disabilities can lead to inaccurate portrayals of symptoms and treatments. Powerful media messages can influence and interfere with proper care.

Examine your attitudes about medications, in particular psychiatric medications, by looking at the Your Self-Awareness box on page 113. Exploring your personal feelings will be a healthy challenge throughout your psychiatric–mental health nursing practice, and psychopharmacology could evoke very strong feelings in either direction for you. Make sure you are aware of your biases and that your opinions are well-informed so that you give your clients the best possible care.

Box 7-1 Psychopharmacologic Timeline

164 BCE (Before the Common Era) to 1951 CE (Common Era)	Documentation of medicating "insane," "deranged," and mentally ill individuals describes administration of olive oil infused with narcotics, opium, morphine, other sedatives
1948	Discovery of the hallucinogenic effects of lysergic acid diethylamide (LSD)

Antipsychotics

1957	McGill University administers chlorpromazine (Thorazine) to treat psychosis.
1957	Trifluoperazine (Stelazine) is developed and released.
1957	Perphenazine (Trilafon) is developed and released.
1957	Thioridazine (Mellaril) is developed and released.
1959	Fluphenazine (Prolixin) is developed and released.
1967	Thiothixene (Navane) is developed and released.
1967	Haloperidol (Haldol) is developed and released.
1970	Mesoridazine (Serentil) is developed and released.
1973	Loxapine (Loxitane) is developed and released.
1990	Clozapine (Clozaril) is re-released after extensive research to establish safety and use in North America.
1994	Risperidone (Risperdal), an atypical antipsychotic, is developed and released.
1996	Olanzapine (Zyprexa), an atypical antipsychotic, is developed and released.
1997	Quetiapine (Seroquel), an atypical antipsychotic, is developed and released.
2001	Ziprasidone (Geodon), an atypical antipsychotic, is developed and released.
2002	Aripiprazole (Abilify), an atypical antipsychotic, is released in North America.
2003	Risperidone Consta (long-acting injectable Risperdal) is released.
	Geodon Intramuscular (ziprasidone short-acting injection) is released.
2004	Zyprexa Intramuscular (olanzapine as a short-acting injection) is released.
2006	Abilify Intramuscular (aripiprazole as a short-acting injection) is released.

Antidepressants

1952	Tuberculosis treatment with iproniazid caused energetic, even hypomanic and manic, responses. First monoamine oxidase inhibitor.
1987	Fluoxetine (Prozac), first selective serotonin reuptake inhibitor (SSRI), is developed and released.
2000	Fluoxetine (Prozac), indicated for premenstrual dysphoric disorder (PMDD), is released as Sarafem.
2002	Escitalopram (Lexapro) is a single-isomer SSRI. Uses the "S" side (as opposed to the "R" side) of the citalopram molecule.
2004	Duloxetine (Cymbalta) is a serotonin and norepinephrine reuptake inhibitor (SNRI) treating depression and pain.
2006	Selegiline (Emsam) patch is a monoamine oxidase inhibitor (MAOI) that does not require dietary vigilance at lower doses.

Mood Stabilizers

2004	Symbyax is a combination medication, olanzapine (Zyprexa) in combination with Fluoxetine for the treatment of acute mania in bipolar disorder and as maintenance treatment in bipolar disorder and psychotic depression.

Anxiolytics

1960s	Meprobamate (Miltown, Equanil) is the first antianxiety agent to be commonly used.
1993	Zolpidem (Ambien), the first nonbenzodiazepine, is released.
1999	Zaleplon (Sonata), a nonbenzodiazepine, is released.
2004	Eszopiclone (Lunesta) is the first sedative–hypnotic approved by the FDA for long-term treatment of insomnia.
2005	Ramelteon (Rozerem) is a nonbenzodiazepine melatonin receptor agonist for treatment of insomnia; enhances effective functioning of circadian rhythm.

Acetylcholinesterase Inhibitors

1993	Tacrine (Cognex) is the first acetylcholinesterase inhibitor released.
1997	Donepezil (Aricept) is released. Now indicated for use with all phases of dementia of the Alzheimer's type.
1999	Rivastigmine (Exelon), the next generation of acetylcholinesterase inhibitor, is released.
2001	Galantamine (Reminyl) is the latest in acetylcholinesterase inhibitors reported to cause fewer GI disturbances.

Sources: Rosner, F. (1978). *Julius Preuss' biblical and Talmudic medicine.* New York: Sanhedrin Press; Trigoboff, E., Wilson, B. A., Shannon, M. T., & Stang, C. L. (2005). *Psychiatric drug handbook* (1st ed.). Upper Saddle River, NJ: Prentice Hall; Mosnaim, A. D., Ranade, V. V., Wolf, M. E., Puente, J., & Antonieta Valenzuela, M. (2006). Phenothiazine molecule provides the basic chemical structure for various classes of pharmacotherapeutic agents. *American Journal of Therapeutics, 13*(3), 261–273.

Box 7-2 ANA Guidelines on Psychopharmacology

The psychiatric–mental health nurse can perform the following functions relating to psychopharmacology:

1. Describe psychopharmacologic agents.
2. Discuss the actions of psychopharmacologic agents, on a global scale down through cellular responses.
3. Differentiate psychiatric symptomatology from medication side effects.
4. Apply the basic principles of pharmacokinetics and pharmacodynamics.
5. Identify the appropriate use of psychopharmacologic agents in special populations.
6. Involve clients and their significant others.
7. Identify barriers to significant others' involvement.
8. Describe nonpsychopharmacologic interventions.
9. Demonstrate value of standardized rating scales.
10. Synthesize necessary information to develop psychopharmacologic education and treatment plans.

Source: Adapted with permission from American Nurses Association, *Psychiatric–mental health nursing psychopharmacology project,* © 1994. American Nurses Publishing, American Nurses Association, Washington, DC.

YOUR SELF-AWARENESS Your Views on Psychopharmacology

Your cultural inclinations have an influence on your attitudes toward medications. These attitudes have an impact on the major intervention in psychiatry—psychopharmacology. Which of these views do you hold about medications? How will they affect the care you give clients?

- They'll make me healthier.
- This stuff will kill me.
- It's only for a short time.
- They're addictive.
- I'll take meds only if my life depends on it.
- Isn't modern pharmacology a wonderful thing?
- I take the right medication for the problem.
- Taking the meds will mean I'm a bad/weak person because I couldn't battle my disorder on my own.
- Medicine is made from herbs—it's the same thing, so I'd rather take the herbs.
- Medications are too strong for me, so they're too strong for everybody.
- I can't contaminate myself with these chemicals.
- If I take psychiatric medications, people will think I'm crazy.
- What if the people at work find out I'm taking these pills? They'll think I can't do my job.
- It's a flaw in my makeup that I need medication.
- People are more sophisticated these days. They would understand that I'm taking the exact same medications as a well-known public figure.

Biologic Impact on Ethnically Distinct Groups

You may notice in your psychiatric–mental health practice that the effects of medications may differ in ethnically distinct groups. Factors such as medication toxicity levels and autonomic nervous system (ANS) responses are not the same for all groups of individuals (Muñoz & Hilgenberg, 2006; Choi et al., 2006). In a multicultural environment such as mental health care, these are important considerations in assessing responses to psychopharmacologic treatments.

One important factor is the variation in metabolic rates among ethnic groups (an important point in evaluating the effectiveness of a medication). A high metabolic rate may produce effects below the optimal level, resulting in ineffective treatment. A low metabolic rate increases side effects. Because people of Asian extraction have low metabolic rates, almost all Asians (95%) experience extrapyramidal side effects (EPSE) (Ueda et al., 2006), as compared to European- and African-Americans, two-thirds of whom experience EPSE (defined and discussed in Chapter 32). Also because of metabolic differences, the therapeutic range for lithium differs among Asian, African-American, and Caucasian groups. The determination of effective lithium levels must take ethnicity into account.

The relationships between a client with a mental illness and the family have been examined for their psychobiologic impact. Expressed emotion (EE) (discussed in Chapter 16) and its impact on psychiatric–mental health recipients of care is a fertile area of research. A client's perception of the expressed emotionality of his or her family can predict the amount of stress and the outcome of treatment. More than 40 years of research on high expressed emotionality shows a poorer prognosis with more relapses. One study demonstrated that Caucasian and Latino families with high EE, including criticism, were perceived by clients as critical, while African-American high-EE and critical families were not perceived by clients as critical (Weisman, Rosales, Kymalainen, & Armesto, 2006). These results indicate that cultural and ethnic values may influence how high EE (including criticism) is experienced by the people with whom we work.

Recognizing how ethnicity and phenotype determine response to medications promotes the provision of culturally competent care. How ethnicity affects the expression of abnormal biologic processes is a growing field of study. Exploring the related literature will help you to incorporate this expanding knowledge base into your psychiatric–mental health nursing practice and promote your cultural competence.

Neuroleptics and Psychotropics

There has been significant change in recent years in the use of classes of medications for psychiatric symptomatology. Previously, there were clear delineations between what was an antipsychotic and what was not. Empirical data and clinical expertise have led us to a less rigid and much broader application of chemical compounds, with positive results. The complexities of psychiatric disorders and the desire to address the difficulties facing people who have these symptoms have resulted in a number of innovative medication regimens.

MEDIALINK Application: Attitudes Toward Antipsychotic Medications

Research has further expanded our knowledge, and a clearer vision of the capabilities of these compounds is emerging. Now many medications have multiple indications beyond their original ones, which have necessitated more global terms to describe the medication. We still use classification names such as "antipsychotic" and "antidepressant"; however, this is changing and some medications are labeled "neuroleptic" or "psychotropic" with the understanding that they can be used across some diagnostic groups. See TABLE 7-1 ■ for some examples of the changing psychopharmacologic landscape.

One example of this phenomenon is fluoxetine (Prozac), used originally as an antidepressant, indicated as an antiobsessional medication and more recently for the treatment of premenstrual dysphoric disorder (PMDD; a proposed category under study but not yet included in the DSM [Diagnostic and Statistical Manual of Mental Disorders]). A second example is risperidone (Risperdal), an atypical or newer antipsychotic, indicated for use in stabilizing the manic phase of bipolar disorder but also used in dementia. There are clinical applications of psychiatric medications to a different diagnostic

TABLE 7-1 ■ Medications and Their Cross-Diagnostic Uses

	Psychosis	Dementia	Depression	Obsessions/ Compulsions	Mood Instability	PTSD	PMDD	Panic Disorder	Social Phobia	Autism	Convulsions	Cigarette Smoking	Migraine	Pain
Aripiprazole (Abilify)	✓		✓		✓									
Bupropion (Wellbutrin, Zyban)			✓									✓		
Carbamazepine (Tegretol)					✓						✓			
Divalproex (Depakote)		✓			✓						✓		✓	
Duloxetine (Cymbalta)			✓											✓
Fluvoxamine (Luvox)			✓	✓				✓						
Fluoxetine (Prozac, Sarafem)			✓	✓			✓	✓						
Olanzapine (Zyprexa)	✓				✓									
Paroxetine (Paxil)			✓					✓	✓					
Quetiapine (Seroquel)	✓	✓			✓									
Risperidone (Risperdal)	✓	✓			✓					✓				
Sertraline (Zoloft)			✓	✓		✓		✓						
SSRIs			✓					✓						
Tricyclic antidepressants			✓					✓						✓
Ziprasidone (Geodon)	✓		✓		✓									

group, or for a different set of psychiatric symptoms, than originally intended. There may not be a Food and Drug Administration (FDA) indication for the medication in those circumstances; however, clinical appropriateness has established the use pattern. This holds true for risperidone as a treatment for dementia with agitation.

Clinical application of nonpsychiatric medications to treat a psychiatric diagnostic group or a set of psychiatric symptoms also occurs. The complexity of the brain's involvements in physical and emotional problems indicates the need for overlapping and interwoven treatments. One of the most apparent examples is the anticonvulsant class. Valproic acid (Depakote), carbamazepine (Tegretol), and lamotrigine (Lamictal) are all used as mood stabilizers as well as for their original indications.

ANTIPSYCHOTIC MEDICATIONS

The discovery of the first antipsychotic medication, chlorpromazine (Thorazine), is a prime example of the role chance has played in the history of psychopharmacology. Chlorpromazine was initially synthesized as an antihistamine to facilitate operative procedures and was not tried as a tranquilizer for clients with schizophrenia until 1952. Its effects on the behavior, thinking, affect, and perception of clients with schizophrenia were so profound that information about its properties was rapidly disseminated, and it became widely used within 3 to 4 years.

Chlorpromazine's effects on the hospital practice of psychiatry were staggering. Its use contributed to reversing a steady rise in the population in U.S. mental institutions, and that population has progressively decreased ever since (Mosnaim, Ranade, Wolf, Puente, & Antonieta Valenzuela, 2006). One might say that chlorpromazine gave birth to the modern notions of psychiatric treatment—unlocked wards, milieu treatment, occupational and recreational therapy, psychiatric rehabilitation, and supervised living environments. The entire field of community mental health is ultimately linked to its discovery because it enabled clients to return to their lives outside an inpatient facility.

In the decades since that discovery we have learned a great deal about which medications generally work under which circumstances. Studies demonstrated that taking antipsychotic medication is far more effective than taking no medicine, and that taking it regularly is essential to the long-term treatment of schizophrenia. We know that medications alone are not sufficient to cure the disease, but they are necessary to manage it. Every profession needs to take a step back and examine the sum of experiences and knowledge to make sure important features of treatment are not missing. Nurses' goals in the specialty area of psychiatric nursing focus on recovery from mental disabilities, and in order to accomplish this they must have the best possible information.

The National Institute of Mental Health funded a landmark study, the Clinical Antipsychotic Trials of Intervention Effectiveness (CATIE) study (Stroup et al., 2006), that looked at treatment outcomes. This major study was designed to learn whether there were differences among the newer medications and whether they had significant advantages over older medications. The results of the CATIE study are summarized in Box 7-3.

Box 7-3 CATIE Study Summary

The 18-month Clinical Antipsychotic Trials of Intervention Effectiveness (CATIE) study, whose results were published in 2006, involved more than 1,400 participants at 57 sites around the United States. Its findings, based on a wide range of clients in a variety of treatment settings, are considered reliable and relevant to the 3.2 million Americans with schizophrenia. CATIE directly compared an older medication (perphenazine), available since the 1950s, to four atypical antipsychotics (olanzapine, quetiapine, risperidone, and ziprasidone) introduced in the 1990s. The goal of the study was to learn whether there are differences among the newer medications and whether the newer medications hold significant advantages over the older medications. The study was conceptualized before the newest antipsychotic, aripiprazole (Abilify), was available in the United States.

These were the results:

- Several factors, such as adequacy of symptom relief, tolerability of side effects, and treatment cost, influence a person's willingness and ability to adhere to a medication regimen.
- Three fourths of the participants discontinued their antipsychotic medication and changed to another because of intolerable side effects or inadequately controlled symptoms.
- Olanzapine performed slightly better than the other medications but also was associated with significant weight gain and metabolic changes.
- Clients taking olanzapine were less likely to be hospitalized for a psychotic relapse and tended to stay on the medication longer than those taking other medications.
- Quetiapine, risperidone, ziprasidone, and olanzapine had a modest advantage over the older generic medication perphenazine.
- The study's highest olanzapine dose exceeded current label recommendations. Prescribers use higher doses of the other antipsychotics clinically than the study did.
- People taking ziprasidone, on average, experienced no weight gain and fewer of the neurological tremors that can be a serious problem for people with schizophrenia.
- An important issue still to be considered is individual differences in response to these medications.
- Each medication has tradeoffs that must be considered for each client.

Psychobiologic Considerations

Understanding the psychobiology of **antipsychotic medications** (medications used to treat hallucinations, delusions, disorganized thinking, and other psychiatric and nonpsychiatric conditions and symptoms) requires a basic knowledge of the functions of the central nervous system. Chapter 6 provides an inside look at the psychobiologic mechanisms that are important in psychopharmacology. Illustrations and animations are also available on the CD-ROM accompanying this text. Here is an overview of the basic mechanisms of action.

Generally, neuroleptics (medications that work on the central nervous system) work by blocking a variety of central nervous system (CNS) receptors. Medications such as antipsychotics do not work only on one neurotransmitter system. Therefore, it is likely that several types of neurotransmitters and neuromodulators are affected by the administration of a single medication. While most neuroleptics have an affinity for several types of neurotransmitters, others are more specific and work more selectively. These differences account for the effects of the various neuroleptic medications. Blockade of postsynaptic dopaminergic receptors (in other words, receptors that are designed specifically for dopamine are prevented from receiving dopamine) is one way these medications can have their main effect. Other pathways and mechanisms may also contribute. The side effects that result from this mechanism are consistently dry mouth, blurred vision, constipation, urinary retention, and parkinsonian side effects.

Major Effects

The beneficial effects of antipsychotic medications in all psychotic states have been demonstrated beyond question. Multiple and varied criteria have been used to measure improvement. These medications have been used successfully in clients with delusional thinking, hallucinations, confusion, motor agitation, and motor retardation. Antipsychotic medication treatment also decreases formal thought disorder, blunted affect, bizarre behavior, social withdrawal, belligerence, and uncooperativeness.

The most common disintegrative condition treated with antipsychotic medication is the group of symptoms traditionally labeled *schizophrenia*. (See Chapter 16.) The problem of assessment is complicated by the fact that many diseases can cause syndromes with features like those of schizophrenia. For example, delusions may indicate a variety of *DSM-IV-TR* conditions, including schizophrenia, bipolar mania, and dementia of the Alzheimer's type. The finer points of differentiation among these conditions include cognitive functioning and the client's presenting history. (Chapter 14 provides a detailed discussion of delirium, dementia, and related disorders; Chapter 17 describes mood disorders.) All clients manifesting psychotic symptoms should have a thorough review of their medical history and a physical examination to rule out treatable medical illnesses, many of which are accompanied by behaviors considered psychotic or psychobiologic.

MediaLink Food and Drug Administration

The Choice of a Specific Medication

There are currently many older antipsychotic medications and seven newer antipsychotic medications on the market in the United States. One of the newer antipsychotics comes in a long-acting injectable form. Medications have varying success rates as individual responses frequently dictate use. The choice of a particular medication, then, depends on its pharmacologic properties and likely side effects, the client's or a family member's history of response to that medication, and the prescriber's experience with various compounds. Important client variables are past successes with specific medications, a history of allergies, and a history of serious or intolerable side effects. Some medications may have side effects with certain clients (sedation), which, while not necessarily desired by the prescriber, may nevertheless prove helpful in treatment. Expect a certain amount of trial and error with each clinical application.

Table 7-2 ■ lists the major antipsychotic medications. The list is extensive and growing, and it makes sense for each member of the treatment team to become familiar with just a few representative medications, their predictable effects, and their common side effects. Some characteristics of these medications are discussed in the sections that follow.

More than seven distinct chemical classes of antipsychotic medications are now commonly used in the United States. (One class, the phenothiazines, is subdivided into three different types of medications.) As a result, there are choices in terms of side effects and potential client responsiveness. A client who is unresponsive to one class may respond to another that circumvents a problem in absorption, accumulation at neurotransmitter receptor sites, or metabolism. However, there are many people for whom the available medications are not especially helpful, or, if major symptoms are addressed, the side effects reduce the overall benefit of the medication. You will see in the course of your psychiatric–mental health nursing practice that more choices are still needed.

Table 7-2 also shows the wide range among antipsychotic medications in milligram-per-milligram potency. This fact is most relevant when treating clients who require large doses. In such cases, a potent medication is best. Consumer issues and clinician concerns are addressed at www.FDA.gov, the website for the U.S. Food and Drug Administration. You can access the FDA through the Companion Website for this book.

Newer Antipsychotics

The newer antipsychotics (also called atypical antipsychotics) have a drastically different physiologic action than do the traditional or conventional antipsychotics. Conventional antipsychotics primarily affect the positive symptoms of psychotic disorders, with little or no effect on the negative or cognitive symptoms. Their mechanism of action is thought to occur through nonselectively blocking the neurotransmitter dopamine D_2 receptors in the brain. To be clinically effective, these medications occupy between 70% and 90% of the D_2 receptors, while the advent of EPSEs occurs at above 80% occupancy. The newer antipsychotics have a much reduced affinity, or attraction, for D_2 receptors, and they all have an affinity for the serotonin receptors, a profile that appears to mitigate against EPSEs and has an impact on the negative symptoms of psychotic disorders (Haynes et al., 2006; Luby, 2006).

The newer antipsychotics offer a wider range of options for the care and treatment of clients experiencing psychotic conditions. The search continues for more psychopharmacologic treatments for psychoses. Medications are being researched and tested every day, and if they provide relief from symptoms without undue side effects, they will expand our psychopharmacologic set.

There are a variety of atypical antipsychotics (seven in the United States). An overall look at two examples follows.

TABLE 7-2 ■ **Antipsychotic Medications***

Class	Generic Name	Trade Name	Usual Dosage Range (mg/day)
Benzisothiazolyl piperazine derivative	Ziprazidone	Geodon	40–200
Benzisoxazole derivative	Risperidone	Risperdal	4–6
Butyrophenones	Haloperidol	Haldol	2–40
Dibenzodiazepines	Clozapine	Clozaril	12.5–900
Dibenzothiazepine derivative	Quetiapine	Seroquel	300–400
Dibenzoxazepines	Loxapine	Loxitane	10–100
Dichlorophenyl piperazinyl butoxydihydro-quinolin	Aripiprazole	Abilify	10–30
Dihydroindolones	Molindone	Moban	15–225
Phenothiazines			
Aliphatic	Chlorpromazine	Thorazine	150–1500
Piperazine	Trifluoperazine	Stelazine	10–60
	Fluphenazine	Prolixin	3–45
	Perphenazine	Trilafon	12–60
Piperidine	Thioridazine	Mellaril	150–800
Thieno-benzodiazepine	Olanzapine	Zyprexa	10–20
Thioxanthenes	Thiothixene	Navane	10–60
	Chlorprothixene	Taractan	40–600

*Atypical antipsychotics currently not available in the United States: sulpiride, amisulpiride, melperone, sertindole

Clozapine (Clozaril)

The first atypical antipsychotic on the market in the United States was clozapine (Clozaril). Clozapine is an antipsychotic medication with an unusual pharmacologic and clinical profile. It was used in Europe for several years and is now generally used in the United States with clients who cannot tolerate the EPSEs of other antipsychotics, or who have a treatment-resistant or treatment-refractory psychosis, as is the case with certain clients with schizophrenia. Reviews of studies regarding the effectiveness of clozapine have demonstrated its decided impact on both negative and positive symptoms, with improvement evident on follow-up as well.

Serious Side Effects Despite its capacity to ameliorate symptoms of some very recalcitrant clients, clozapine has some serious side effects. The most serious is agranulocytosis (a marked decrease in granulated white blood cells), which occurs in less than 1% of clients taking this medication. It is essential to monitor white blood cell (WBC) counts of clients taking clozapine. Immediately discontinuing the medication when agranulocytosis is detected and before signs of an infection develop will usually resolve the episode. There are specific guidelines for treating a client who experiences agranulocytosis as a result of using clozapine. Clozapine can be reinstituted (called re-challenging) under certain circumstances but not others. This information is clearly explained on the Companion Website.

There is a risk for agranulocytosis with a variety of other psychotropic medications (conventional antipsychotics, benzodiazepines, anticonvulsants); however, there is a higher risk with clozapine. This compound requires blood draws to assess the white blood cell count at varying intervals (currently weekly, biweekly, and monthly). There have been rates of agranulocytosis at significantly lower levels than the currently estimated 1% (i.e., 0.3%, according to Kelly et al., 2006). One of the important questions for clozapine treatment remains, "Is there a specific risk period for agranulocytosis, and if there is, when does it occur?" The risk period establishes the frequency of blood monitoring, which can be an impediment to clients' initial and continued use of the antipsychotic.

Currently, it is estimated that agranulocytosis may occur up to a year following initial treatment with clozapine, although the vast majority of cases appear within 6 months. As a result of these data, blood monitoring for agranulocytosis is completed weekly for the first 6 months of therapy. If WBC levels remain normal and regular use is not interrupted throughout those 6 months, then blood monitoring can be reduced to biweekly frequencies. After another 6 months of regular use and normal blood results, monitoring can be done monthly. Remember that blood monitoring must continue for 4 weeks following the discontinuation of clozapine.

Another serious side effect is the potential for seizure, which seems to be dose-related at over 600 mg/d. Less acute but nonetheless important side effects include sedation,

MEDIALINK Teva Clozapine Patient Registry

tachycardia, sialorrhea (drooling), weight gain, and hypotension. Balancing positive symptom control and negative symptom relief with these side effects—a consideration with all antipsychotic medications—is explored in Chapter 32.

Risperidone (Risperdal)

Risperidone was introduced in the United States in 1994. It was the first of a new class of antipsychotics, benzisoxazole derivatives, that does not clinically relate to any existing antipsychotic medication. Its unique feature is the relative absence of EPSE at the therapeutic dosing level. It addresses the positive, negative, and affective symptoms of schizophrenia and may also alleviate depression and anxiety. Side effects similar to those experienced with haloperidol (Haldol) are seen in doses above 10 mg per day.

Dosage for risperidone has been described as "the 1-2-3" regimen, in which the client receives 1 mg bid, the next increase (slowly titrated according to the client's tolerability and response) is to 2 mg bid, and the next increase after that is to 3 mg bid. This places the client at 6 mg/day, which is in the currently recommended therapeutic window of 4 to 8 mg/day. Doses less than 5 mg/day have been linked with a better outcome than higher doses (Trigoboff, Wilson, Shannon, & Stang, 2005). Risperidone can be administered up to 16 mg/day, but the absence of EPSEs fades over 10 mg/day. Response within 1 to 10 weeks gives the medication a fair trial. Dosage for older clients is lower; the initial dosage is generally cut in half (0.5 mg bid, 1 mg bid, and 1.5 mg bid) and there is at least one full week between dosage changes.

Risperidone has been very useful in the treatment of psychotic symptoms, and the clinical knowledge gained from using it regularly has been valuable. Risperidone is now available in depot injection form. (**Depot injection** is a term used to describe the slow release of a long-term medication given by intramuscular or subcutaneous injection using the body as a temporary storage device for the entire dose.) This compound, called Consta, is injected every 2 weeks. This additional administration mode for risperidone offers another choice in the array of treatments for psychotic symptoms. (See Unique Routes of Administration on page 119.)

Other uses for risperidone include its 2003 indication for treating extreme mood swings in bipolar disorder in addition to its antipsychotic features. In 2006, the orally disintegrating tablets of risperidone, M-tab, received an indication to treat symptoms of irritability in autistic children and adolescents. Aggressiveness, deliberate self-injury, and the temper tantrums associated with autism are also addressed by this medication.

Dosage

Dosage ranges for antipsychotic medications vary widely among clients. Medications must be titrated against the psychotic target symptoms and the appearance of side effects. Most clients are initially given a relatively low dose of an antipsychotic to test for adverse effects for 1 to 2 hours. Consider chlorpromazine, with an initial dose of 20 to 50 mg orally (PO) or 25 mg intramuscularly (IM). Later the medication is typically given in doses of 300 to 400 mg (or IM equivalent) per day, and gradually increased by 25% to 50% each day until maximum improvement is noted or intolerable side effects are encountered. This type of progression is common with the various antipsychotic medications.

Treatment settings frequently influence the medication regimen. In a crowded hospital emergency room, for example, hourly doses of medication may be given until a client is sedated. In more completely staffed, private inpatient units, a client may be observed for several days before medication is given. Symptoms and behavioral problems are addressed by the antipsychotic, but cognitive functioning studies have been inconclusive. When looking at long-term outcome and length of time until eventual remission, neither approach has been found to be superior to the other (McKim, 2007).

Clients who are extremely agitated, violent, severely withdrawn, or catatonic require significant doses during the first few days of treatment, delivered by injection to ensure rapid relief. Chlorpromazine, 50 to 100 mg IM, may be used, particularly if sedation is required. Be aware that this is an irritating medication; injections must be deeply intramuscular in either the buttocks or upper arms, and sites must be rotated. Substantial IM doses of the more potent antipsychotics, such as haloperidol 10 mg or trifluoperazine 10 mg, may be given to agitated clients.

There are options for short-term injections, such as ziprasidone (Geodon), aripiprazole (Abilify), and olanzapine (Zyprexa), that replace the use of older, conventional antipsychotics. Use of an atypical antipsychotic reduces side effects and therefore has a positive impact on a client's perceptions of psychiatric medications. This approach frequently avoids some of the more troublesome side effects while ameliorating behavioral and cognitive symptoms. The role atypical antipsychotics play in helping clients remain on their medications and experience fewer troublesome side effects is discussed more fully in Chapter 32.

After maximum clinical improvement has been obtained, antipsychotic medications are generally reduced in a gradual manner. Continuing to give a client modest doses of an antipsychotic following a psychotic episode lowers the chances of relapse and rehospitalization. Psychotherapy with clients who have schizophrenia may not be particularly effective without maintenance medications in conventional treatment settings, but it does improve psychosocial functioning in clients who are also taking maintenance medications. It is generally believed that clients should be kept on doses of antipsychotics sufficient to suppress symptoms for 3 months to 1 year following an acute episode. After such an interval, the client's course and life situation must be considered and treatment individualized. Some clients recover from a psychotic episode completely within 6 months. Clients with schizophreniform disorder should not receive long-term maintenance medication treatment. For individuals who have already experienced recurrent episodes of psychosis and demonstrate a deteriorating course, it is clearly advantageous to prevent relapses with medications if possible.

MediaLink Care Plan: The Client on Antipsychotic Medication

The Decision to Use a Medication

Today, the following general principles govern antipsychotic medication use:

- Medications are given to treat target symptoms of schizophrenia or other psychotic disorders.
- Initial treatment may require parenteral doses or rapidly dissolving forms. These are changed to oral forms such as pills or liquid concentrate as the behavior disturbance subsides.
- Total dosages are tailored to individual needs; wide variations exist among clients.
- For medications with sedating side effects, divided doses are changed as soon as is practical to a single dose, given at bedtime to maximize the medication's sedative properties.
- Most clients with a chronic course require maintenance doses for sustained improvement and to minimize the number of relapses.

Other considerations for using a particular medication include the use of adjunctive therapies (Haynes et al., 2006). Do the medications needed to treat one problem blend well with any or all of the other medications the client may need? Clients often have more than a single, Axis I diagnosis. Multiple diagnoses require a more complex palette of biologic therapies. See Your Assessment Approach below for antipsychotic medication interactions with other medications and substances to which your client may be exposed.

Special Considerations

The following special considerations apply to the use of antipsychotic medication.

Unique Routes of Administration

The phenothiazines, fluphenazine (Prolixin) and haloperidol (Haldol), are available in long-acting intramuscular injectable forms that behave like timed-release capsules. These medications are gradually released over a long period of time, 2 to 4 weeks. Long-acting fluphenazine and haloperidol are available in decanoate, long-acting depot injection preparations that are oil-based. Risperidone Consta is also a depot medication available for injection every two weeks but instead of being oil-based, the microspheres containing the medication are suspended in water. This injection is easier to tolerate and, because it is an atypical antipsychotic, has fewer side effects and can address the negative symptoms of schizophrenia.

As with any depot medication, the oral form of the same medication must be administered before the depot is used to ensure the client tolerates the medication. The main advantages of depot forms are that they reduce clients' ambivalence about taking medication, eliminate the need for constant pill taking, and can help clients who have illness-related cognitive impairments. Memory and concentration difficulties are typical among those with executive functioning deficits, one of the major impairments that must be overcome by people who have schizophrenia. (Chapter 6∞ discusses executive functioning.) Making sure clients have a steady level of medication in their system minimizes the fluctuations in blood level seen in nonparenteral forms of medication administration. A fluctuating blood level leads to more difficulty managing symptoms, especially if the client is sensitive to minor fluctuations. A depot antipsychotic with considerably fewer side effects than haloperidol and fluphenazine, such as Consta, has the potential to prolong antipsychotic medication use and minimize dissatisfaction with, and discontinuation of, treatment.

The psychiatric–mental health nurse in a community setting may frequently have occasion to administer long-acting fluphenazine, haloperidol, or Consta. With a client whose treatment will include a long-acting medication, a dose of the oral form is taken first to rule out the possibility of allergic reactions. Such reactions can be devastating if discovered after a 2- or 3-week supply of medicine has been given as a depot treatment. If no adverse reactions are noted, the long-acting

YOUR ASSESSMENT APPROACH
Antipsychotic Medication Interactions

Combining One of These	With One of These Antipsychotics	Can Lead to These Problems
Antacids	Phenothiazine antipsychotic	Decreased phenothiazine effect
Anticholinergics	Clozapine	Potentiated anticholinergic effect of clozapine
	Antipsychotic	Increased level of neuroleptic in the system, with extrapyramidal side effects
Benzodiazepines	Clozapine	Respiratory arrest, circulatory difficulties
Carbamazepine	Haloperidol	Decreased effect of either medication
	Clozapine	Additive bone marrow suppression
CNS depressants such as: narcotics, anxiolytics, alcohol, barbiturates, or antihistamines	Antipsychotic	Additive CNS depression
Coffee, tea, milk, or fruit juices	Phenothiazine antipsychotic	Decreased phenothiazine effect

form is injected, usually in the upper outer quadrant of the buttock or the vastus lateralis site.

Better routes for medication administration have been explored by various pharmaceutical companies for years. As a result, there is yet another way to give a number of antipsychotic preparations. Clozapine (Clozaril), risperidone (Risperdal), olanzapine (Zyprexa), and aripiprazole (Abilify) are all available in orally disintegrating tablet formulations. The clozapine version is called FazaClo, risperidone's oral formulation is called M-tab, the olanzapine version is called Zyprexa Zydis, and aripiprazole has a Discmelt product. (You may see the Zydis form of medication used with a variety of compounds in medical–surgical settings.) These tablets begin disintegrating in the mouth within seconds, so they can be swallowed with or without liquid, thus reducing problems with swallowing and cheeking (hiding) behaviors and offering a more discreet option for taking medication during activities. This vehicle for administering full doses of medication promotes adherence.

In the future we will see a variety of innovative and effective technologies for enhancing the administration and absorption of psychiatric medications. Currently research is investigating:

- Multiphase, multicompartment capsules using gelatin, natural hydroxypropyl methylcellulose, and alternative capsule materials
- Quick-dissolving strips and films
- Inhalers
- Implanted pumps

A patch for transdermal delivery of an antidepressant (in selegiline) is currently available, the first in psychiatry, and more are being developed. These opportunities for medication delivery platforms, coupled with research for new compounds to treat disorders, help normalize psychiatric disorders—that is, they are treated just as all other physical disorders are treated—and provide more options. Over the course of your career in psychiatric–mental health nursing, you will see innovative and effective absorption-enhancing delivery systems and routes for administration of medications to treat and improve the quality of life for our clients.

Medication Requirements of Certain Age Groups

In older adult clients, the agitation often associated with delirium, dementia, and related disorders is markedly responsive to antipsychotics. Other sedatives, such as barbiturates and benzodiazepines, may further compromise cerebral functioning, further depressing the level of awareness and concentration, worsening the disorder. Doses of medications are generally reduced for older adults. Risperidone 1 mg/day, trifluoperazine (Stelazine) 5 to 20 mg/day, or haloperidol 1 to 6 mg/day might constitute adequate treatment.

Antipsychotic medications are effective in treating childhood psychoses and in managing the behavior problems associated with mental retardation. The general principle of reduced dosage is again applicable. The upper limit of the usual daily dosage for children under 12 might be 200 mg/day of chlorpromazine or 20 mg/day of trifluoperazine. Amounts of individual IM injections of chlorpromazine must also be kept at 0.25 mg per pound of body weight every 6 to 8 hr, or not over 40 mg/day for up to 50 lb and not over 75 mg/day for children weighing 50 to 100 lb.

Potential Side Effects of Antipsychotic Medications

Continuous contact with clients gives nurses an advantage over other professionals who may see a client only every other day or, at best, once a day. Both the dangerous and the more uncomfortable side effects frequently have a rapid onset and need prompt attention.

The side effects of antipsychotic medications that nurses must recognize can be divided into these classes:

- Autonomic nervous system
- Extrapyramidal
- Other central nervous system
- Allergic
- Blood
- Skin
- Eye
- Endocrine
- Weight gain

See Chapter 32 for details about these side effects and how to help clients manage the side effects they experience.

Metabolizing Psychiatric Medications

A liver enzyme called cytochrome P_{450} and abbreviated as CYP is responsible for metabolizing psychiatric medication out of the client's system. The two main directions that can influence how your clients metabolize psychiatric medications are called inhibition and activation or induction. Inhibition of the enzyme allows the medication and its metabolites to remain in the system longer than usual, accumulating and causing higher blood levels, enhanced effects of the medication, and greater side effects. Imagine a jammed parking lot or gridlock on a city street (see FIGURE 7-2 ■) as the medication is unable to flow out of the system easily.

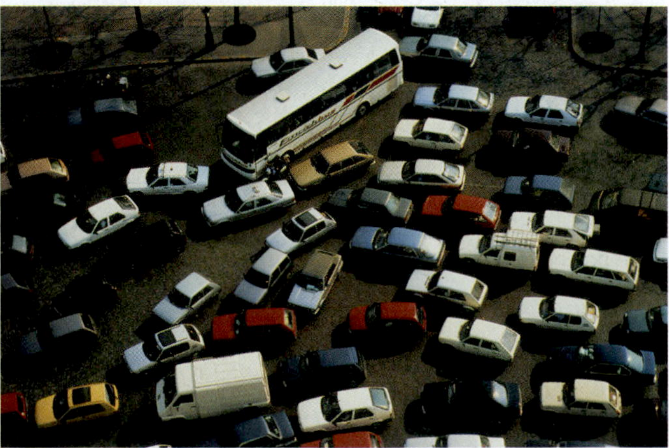

FIGURE 7-2 ■ Inhibited CYP action. The traffic gridlock in this photo represents the difficulty of metabolizing a medication out of the body when the liver enzyme CYP is inhibited.

Source: Getty Images Inc.—Stone Allstock, Will & Deni McIntyre.

MEDIALINK Liver Enzyme Cytochrome P_{450} Animation

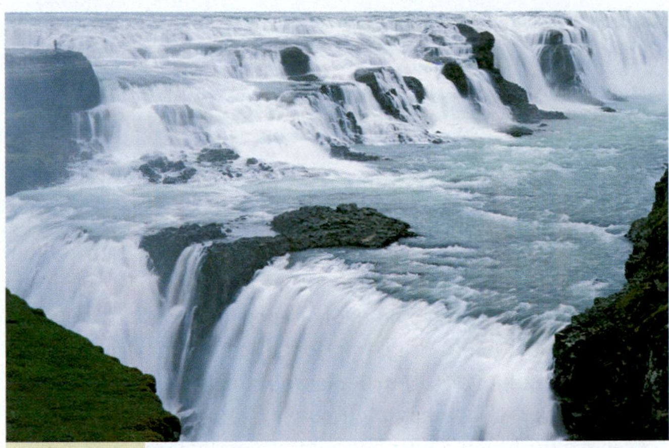

FIGURE 7-3 ■ Induced CYP action. The waterfall in this photo represents how vigorously a medication would be washed out or metabolized out of the system when the liver enzyme CYP is induced or activated.

Source: Dorling Kindersley Media Library, Rowan Greenwood.

Induction or activation of the enzyme speeds the medication and its metabolites out of the system faster than usual. When a medication does not have enough time to take full effect, it may appear that symptoms are not being competently addressed. The medication is considerably less effective in this case than if it had the time to be fully utilized by the body. Picture the medication being washed out of the system faster than intended (see FIGURE 7-3 ■).

Other coadministered medications, your client's genetics, foods eaten, and cigarettes smoked are some of the factors that can induce or inhibit cytochrome P_{450}. The entire field of study on CYPs is an extensive one, covering the intricacies of medication interactions, metabolism, and coadministration cautions.

ANTIDEPRESSANT MEDICATIONS

Classes of **antidepressant medications** (pharmaceutical compounds used to treat the symptoms of depression) that currently exist include: tricyclic antidepressants (TCAs), monoamine oxidase inhibitors (MAOIs), selective serotonin reuptake inhibitors (SSRIs), phenethylamine antidepressants, also known as serotonin and norepinephrine reuptake inhibitors (SNRIs), and atypical antidepressants (so called because of their variety of formulation and actions).

Like antipsychotic medications, the original antidepressant medications were discovered accidentally. In the case of imipramine (Tofranil), the first of the tricyclic antidepressants, investigators were actually searching for effective antipsychotics similar to chlorpromazine. Iproniazid, a MAOI, was discovered when tuberculosis clients regularly treated with a similar medication, isoniazid, became less depressed. Antidepressants have shed considerable light on the biochemical mechanisms of the brain in both normal and abnormal emotional expression. See the Evidence-Based Practice feature regarding psychopharmacology in the treatment of depression.

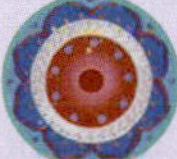

EVIDENCE-BASED PRACTICE

DEPRESSION AND ANTIDEPRESSANT MEDICATIONS

You are working in an acute psychiatric setting with an individual who is severely depressed and is receiving a tricyclic antidepressant. This African-American client, Ryan, told you he feels so much better after only a few doses of medication, although his mouth is uncomfortably dry. You ask a number of questions about his latest symptoms, and he reports significantly less depression. You have a few theories about why this is happening. One is the "flight into health" people sometimes demonstrate, especially those with depressive symptoms. The diagnosis of depression and the need for therapeutic interventions may frighten or disrupt them to the point where they downplay symptoms and declare themselves much better.

Another theory is that the energizing impact of the antidepressant is taking place before a significant difference has been made in depressive thinking, including lethality. This energy can be mobilized into suicide attempts. The third theory for Ryan's improvement is the faster therapeutic response and higher serum concentrations of tricyclics in African-Americans. His dry mouth is evidence that the higher serum concentration is causing more adverse effects than are experienced by other groups.

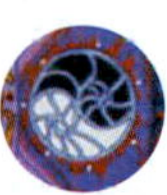

Your discussion with Ryan focuses on his treatment, side effects, and a lethality assessment. You have seen journal articles regarding these issues and are able to assess a depressed individual at this stage of treatment, keeping the possible explanations in mind. Findings from ethnopharmacology research, such as the following reference citation, support anecdotal evidence that the tricyclic can have this particular impact on the client. (Remember that action should be based on more than one study.)

Muñoz, C., & Hilgenberg, C. (2006). Ethnopharmacology: Understanding how ethnicity can affect drug response is essential to providing culturally competent care. *Holistic Nursing Practice, 20*(5), 227–234.

CRITICAL THINKING QUESTIONS

1. How would you go about determining whether Ryan is downplaying his symptoms?
2. How would knowing the racial and cultural differences in main effects and side effects of medications help you assess a depressed client?
3. Why would Ryan's energy level be a helpful indicator of medication effectiveness?
4. How would you go about determining Ryan's suicide risk?
5. Of what value are Ryan's responses to your therapeutic interventions in interpreting whether or not his depressive thoughts have been disrupted?

Psychobiologic Considerations

Knowledge about the pharmacology of antidepressant medications has led to a theory of the biochemistry of depression. Basically, all the true antidepressants make the neurotransmitters norepinephrine (NE) and serotonin (5-HT) more available to the synaptic receptors in the central nervous system. Tricyclics block the reuptake of these substances into the neuron after their release, thereby postponing their degradation. MAOIs interfere with the enzymes responsible for the actual breakdown of the neurotransmitter molecules. Since both are antidepressants, these observations have led to the theory that NE and 5-HT shortages in the brain cause depression, at least the type of depression that responds to medication therapy. The details of the dexamethasone suppression test (DST), an examination of psychoendocrine function in light of depressive behavior, can be found in Chapter 6, which provides an overview of the current psychobiologic theories of depression.

MEDIALINK Methylphenidate Drug Mechanism in Action Animation

The initial distinction to be understood in the psychopharmacology of depression is between true antidepressants and stimulants or euphoriants. TCAs and MAOIs are not stimulants and do not induce euphoria in healthy people. In a single dose, they have a sedative effect. Amphetamines and methylphenidate (Ritalin), on the other hand, are stimulants but not antidepressants in the pharmacologic sense. They can induce an increased sense of well-being in certain individuals, but do nothing to combat depression on a lasting basis.

Tricyclic antidepressants are the "first generation" of antidepressant medications, that is, they were among the first medications identified as effective in the treatment of depression. New developments and ideas in chemical motivations to help treat symptoms of depression are labeled *subsequent generations*.

Since the introduction of the first antidepressants, a number of medications have been developed to treat the symptoms of major depression and the depressive features of schizoaffective disorder. Among these medications are the MAOIs, the SSRIs, and a number of atypical antidepressants with a variety of neurotransmitter actions.

Bupropion (Wellbutrin) is an oral antidepressant medication that is not a TCA and is unrelated to other known antidepressants. Bupropion has been well tolerated in people experiencing orthostatic hypotension when taking TCAs. This medication has a dose-related potential for causing seizures to a greater extent than other antidepressants. It has few anticholinergic side effects and essentially no important cardiovascular effects. Bupropion is also indicated for use as an aid to smoking cessation. Sustained-release formulations of this medication are available under two trade names, Wellbutrin SR and Zyban. For smoking cessation, the medication is used for up to 14 weeks.

Of note is the cross-diagnostic use of medications initially indicated for other conditions (discussed earlier in this chapter and referred to in Table 7-1). Fluoxetine (Prozac) is an antidepressant and was the first SSRI developed. This compound has an indication for another treatment regimen. Under the trade name Sarafem, fluoxetine is used to treat the mood and physical symptoms of PMDD, which is differentiated from depression and other mental disorders. The dosing is flexible, with 10- or 20-mg pulvules available; 20 mg/day is the recommended dose.

As each new group of medications became available, practitioners initially used the new medications to the partial exclusion of the old. When a client is not responding to a medication, it is helpful to have an array of choices from which to select further treatment. The side effect profiles of antidepressants remain one of the linchpins of successful care. If sedation is a side effect and the client is sleeping at a higher-than-preferred level, then a class of medications with less sedating side effects may be a better choice. Experience reinforces the truth that a number of treatment and medication options are necessary to effectively treat psychiatric disorders; therefore, all categories of antidepressants remain useful.

Tricyclic Antidepressants (TCAs)

One of the commonly used classes of antidepressant medications is tricyclic antidepressants (TCAs), named for their consistent triple-ringed chemical structure. These compounds are close in chemical structure to phenothiazines and have many similar side effects, but they have profoundly different effects on mood, behavior, and cognition. TCAs are not antipsychotic agents when given to clients with schizophrenia and may in fact aggravate a disintegrative pattern or precipitate overt symptoms in a client with latent disintegrative behavior. Imipramine (Tofranil) and amitriptyline (Elavil) are the two prime representative TCAs. Desipramine (Norpramin, Pertofrane), nortriptyline (Pamelor), and protriptyline (Vivactil) are compounds prepared in simpler forms (similar to the conversions made in normal metabolism) that are reported to reduce the incidence of side effects.

Monoamine Oxidase Inhibitors (MAOIs)

Clients who do not respond to tricyclic antidepressants may respond to another major class, MAOIs. These medications generally are not as effective as tricyclics and are somewhat slower to act, sometimes requiring a month of treatment before improvement shows. Isocarboxazid (Marplan) is considered the most effective, with phenelzine (Nardil) and tranylcypromine (Parnate) slightly behind. Complicating the decision to use MAOIs is their association with several very severe side effects. Hepatic necrosis, commonly fatal, and **hypertensive crisis** (severe elevation in diastolic blood pressure above 120–130 mm Hg) leading to intracranial bleeding are among the most threatening. The latter reaction, heralded by severe headache, stiff neck, nausea, vomiting, and sharply increased blood pressure, follows the ingestion of foods that contain the amino acid tyramine and the ingestion of sympathomimetic medications.

Introduction of a patch system for treatment with a MAOI, selegiline (Emsam), does not require the dietary restrictions at the lower dose. This transdermal method of delivering an antidepressant dose is also less stigmatizing. See the feature Partnering with Clients and Families: Teaching About a Low-Tyramine Diet in Chapter 32.

Selective Serotonin Reuptake Inhibitors (SSRIs)

Further development of antidepressants has been the result of a scientific search for medications with fewer toxic side effects and greater biologic predictability in the treatment of depression. Newer antidepressants are believed to be more neurotransmitter-specific and better able to treat conditions related to dopamine, serotonin, or norepinephrine dysfunctions. For a look at the variety of antidepressant medications currently available from different classes with differing actions, see TABLE 7-3 ■.

The earlier antidepressants have certain disadvantages. Uncomfortable and sometimes intolerable side effects and a number of use restrictions with certain populations, combined with the dietary restrictions of the MAOIs, make these medications inappropriate for many people.

The next class of antidepressant medications developed was the SSRIs. A profound difference with this group of medications is their side effects. While chemically different, SSRIs inhibit the reuptake (and thus the deactivation) of the neurotransmitter serotonin, allowing for the increased availability of serotonin at synapses. The first SSRI developed was fluoxetine. There are now a number of potent and highly specific medications with this action.

The SSRIs shed light on the workings of synapses. For the first time, psychiatric–mental health nurses were able to see the direct impact of changing neurotransmitter concentrations. FIGURE 7-4 ■ on page 124 shows the structure of the synapse. To see an animation of the synaptic action of these medications, see the DVD accompanying this text.

An important consideration for clients taking SSRIs is the proximity of the administration of MAOIs. Fluoxetine and a MAOI together may cause serious and fatal interactions. The half-life of fluoxetine is such that there must be a 5-week gap between taking fluoxetine and taking a MAOI, and vice versa. Sertraline (Zoloft), paroxetine (Paxil), citalopram (Celexa), and escitalopram (Lexapro) have shorter half-lives, and there must be a 1- or 2-week gap (both directions) between taking these medications and taking MAOIs. Keep in mind that St. John's wort is a naturally occurring MAOI and, although a botanical is much less potent than a pharmaceutical-grade compound, can also interact with an SSRI and cause a negative episode for your client.

FIGURE 7-5 ■ on page 124 illustrates the process of serotonin neurotransmission, so important to the effectiveness of SSRIs. Imagine the movement of neurotransmitters back and forth across the synapse—this is the movement that SSRIs affect.

Serotonin and Norepinephrine Reuptake Inhibitors (SNRIs)

Venlafaxine (Effexor) is the first in a class of new-generation antidepressants called phenethylamine antidepressants, also referred to as SNRIs (serotonin and norepinephrine reuptake inhibitors). They have two mechanisms of action: inhibiting the reuptake of both serotonin and norepinephrine. Anticholinergic-like side effects may occur with venlafaxine. There are also reports of sustained increases in blood pressure with some clients. This last side effect seems to be dose-related, so nursing management of clients taking venlafaxine should include regular blood pressure monitoring. A time buffer is also necessary when the medication is used in conjunction with MAOIs: a 14-day gap after discontinuing a MAOI before starting venlafaxine, and at least a 7-day gap after discontinuing venlafaxine before starting a MAOI.

The recommended starting dosage for venlafaxine is 75 mg/day, administered in two or three divided doses and taken with food. The dose may be increased to 225 mg/day according to clinical needs, and even further increased to 375 mg/day. It is recommended that clients who have been taking venlafaxine for more than 1 week taper the dose when discontinuing the medication. Clients taking it for 6 weeks or more should time this taper over a 2-week period to minimize the risk of symptoms caused by discontinuing the medication. Venlafaxine's new indication for treating adults with panic disorder involves the same dosing amounts and discontinuation regimen.

Another SNRI is duloxetine (Cymbalta). The starting dose is 30 mg/day, usually given for 1 week, with the target therapeutic dose of 60 mg/d. Higher doses have occasionally been used for treatment-resistant neuropathic pain and treatment-resistant depression. Like venlafaxine, duloxetine

MEDIALINK Neurological Synapse Animation

MEDIALINK Fluoxetine Drug Mechanism in Action Animation

TABLE 7-3 ■ **Antidepressant Medications**

TCA	Other Antidepressants	SSRI	MAOI
Amitriptyline (Elavil)	Amoxapine (Asendin)	Sertraline (Zoloft)	Phenelzine sulfate (Nardil)
Desipramine (Norpramin)	Trazodone (Desyrel)	Paroxetine (Paxil)	Tranylcypromine sulfate (Parnate)
Imipramine (Tofranil)	Maprotiline (Ludiomil)	Fluoxetine (Prozac)	Isocarboxazid (Marplan)
Nortriptyline (Aventyl)	Bupropion (Wellbutrin)	Citalopram (Celexa)	Selegiline (Emsam)
Protriptyline (Vivactil)	Venlafaxine (Effexor)	Escitalopram (Lexapro)	
	Mirtazapine (Remeron)		
	Duloxetine (Cymbalta)		

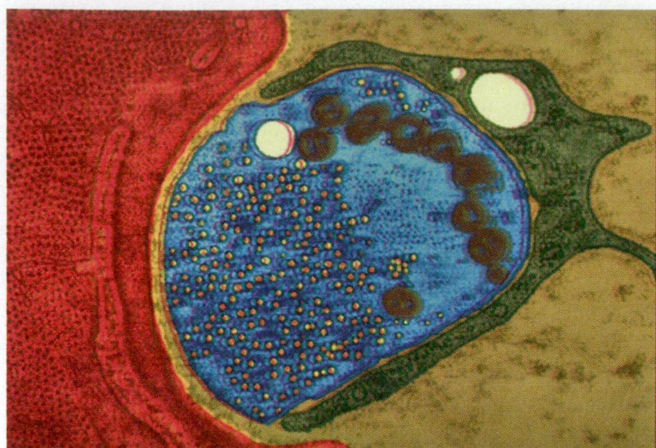

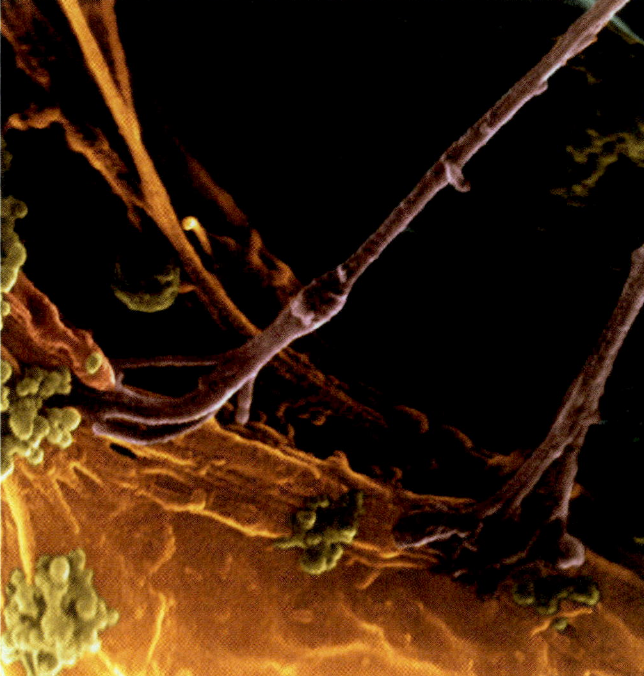

FIGURE 7-4 ■ Structure of the synapse. The synapse at the top has many specialized characteristics. The electron micrograph shows the vesicles containing the synaptic transmitter, the abundance of mitochondria necessary for energy production, and the abundance of protein in the presynaptic and postsynaptic densities. Above are incoming axons (purple) contacting dendrites (yellow) with non-neural cells nearby (green).

Source: Smock, T. K. (1999). *Physiological psychology: A neuroscience approach.* Upper Saddle River, NJ: Prentice Hall.

Source: (top) Photo Researchers, Inc., Don W. Fawcett/Science Source. (bottom) Photo Researchers, Inc., Oliver Meckes & Nicole Ottawa.

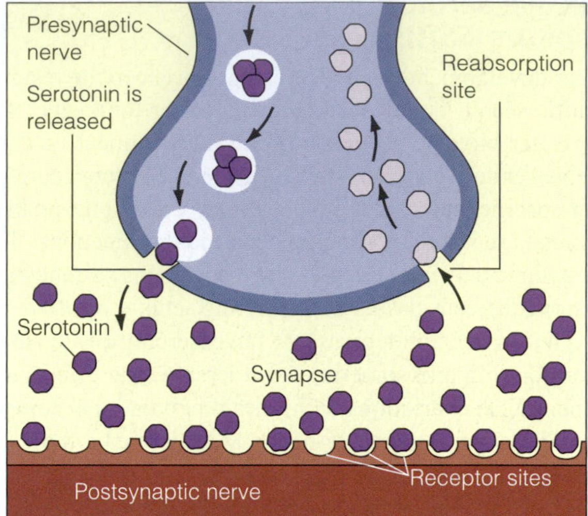

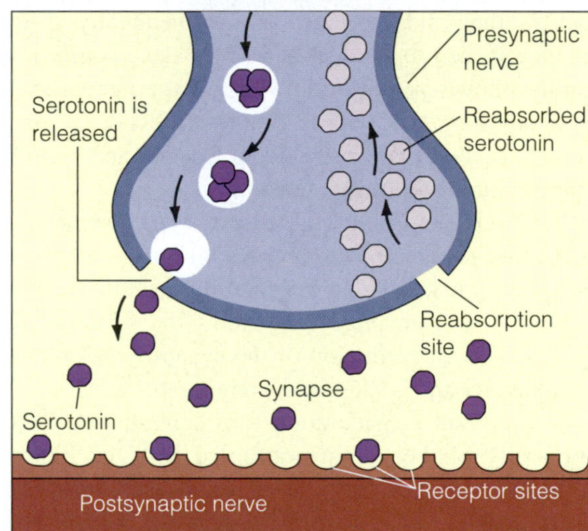

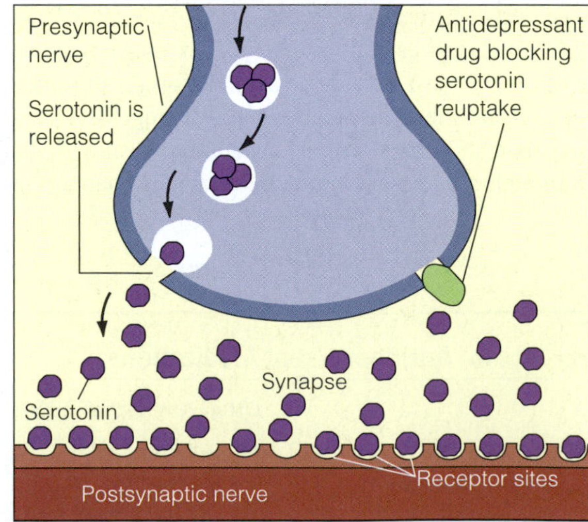

FIGURE 7-5 ■ Serotonin neurotransmission. (A) A highly schematic model of normal serotonin (5-HT) neurotransmission. (B) In depression, there may be a shortage of 5-HT in the synapse. (C) The action of an antidepressant medication blocking 5-HT reabsorption (reuptake)

can occasionally disturb sodium metabolism and disrupt lab values (Glueck, Khalil, Winiarska, & Wang, 2006).

Other Medications Used for Depression

Stimulants, such as amphetamines and methylphenidate (Ritalin), and the phenothiazines are less commonly used antidepressants. Stimulants are not a proven treatment. Phenothiazines may be particularly useful in the presence of agitation. Some clinicians and researchers believe that major depressive episodes with psychotic features (delusional depressions) respond better to a combination of an antidepressant and an antipsychotic agent or to electroconvulsive therapy (ECT) than to antidepressants alone. Others simply recommend higher-than-usual doses of antidepressants.

Age-Related Considerations

Antidepressants have recently been the focus of a number of debates involving client safety. Specifically, the concern has been that the effects of antidepressants on children, adolescents, and adults contribute to an increased risk of suicidal behavior. Following an FDA Public Health Advisory in 2005, all antidepressants now have labeling that indicates that children, adolescents, and adults treated with antidepressants can experience greater suicidal ideation and behavior during the first few months of treatment. While studies are still being conducted at this writing, clients who are new to therapy with these compounds should be assessed for clinical worsening, changes in behavior, or suicidality. See Chapters 23 and 32 ∞ for more information on this topic.

MOOD STABILIZERS

The earliest discovery of a mood-stabilizing medication was made in 1948 by Australian physician John Cade. Cade found that lithium worked to subdue wild behavior in animals. To the astonishment of his colleagues, he went one step further and gave lithium to humans. Lithium was the medication of choice for the treatment of bipolar mood disorder for many years.

The psychopharmacologic treatment of conditions collectively labeled *mania* used to be virtually synonymous with lithium carbonate therapy in the United States. Many well-controlled clinical studies indicated unequivocally that lithium was initially the most effective agent for treating the vast majority of acute manic and hypomanic episodes. In addition, because of the absence of sedative side effects, clients felt much more connected to their environment and able to function normally while under the influence of lithium. See TABLE 7-4 ■ on page 126 for information about which liquids and other medications are, and are not, compatible with lithium.

In the last few years, several medications have been added to the list of pharmacologic treatments for bipolar disorder. The first was carbamazepine, used to control bipolar symptoms in people who either could not take lithium or did not respond therapeutically to it. Recognizing the potential effectiveness of carbamazepine in certain mood disorders, another seizure medication, divalproex (Depakote), was prescribed for clients with diagnoses of bipolar mood disorder or schizoaffective disorder.

Pharmacologic treatments for bipolar disorder have expanded and are a substantial improvement over the clinically efficacious choices available even a decade ago. New guidelines for bipolar treatment have been created and have thus expanded our abilities to care for clients with bipolar disorders. (See Chapter 17 ∞ for more information on treating mood disorders.) Current treatment guidelines for bipolar disorders emphasize these key recommendations:

1. A mood stabilizer is used in all phases of treatment.
2. Atypical, or newer, antipsychotics are preferable to conventionals (first-line use only when mania is accompanied by psychosis).
3. Mild depression is treated initially with a mood stabilizer. Severe depression is treated from the beginning with an antidepressant plus a mood stabilizer.
4. Rapid cycling (mania or depression) is treated from the beginning with a mood stabilizer alone, preferably divalproex.

Divalproex or lithium is the foundation of acute-phase and preventive treatment for mania. An additional treatment feature is the use of atypical antipsychotic medications in the acute manic phase of the disorder. The clinical example on page 128 provides a description of a manic episode with psychotic features. The medications that are effective during the acute manic phase are also used for long-term prevention of mania. Bipolar depression usually necessitates lithium to stabilize clients in monotherapy for depression. If, for some reason, lithium is not used, divalproex or even lamotrigine (Lamictal) can be used.

The various treatments for bipolar disorder necessitate an in-depth view of medication interactions. See the Your Assessment Approach features on page 127 for examples of potential problems.

Dosage

The management of an acute manic episode involves rapid initiation of the selected mood stabilizer, increased to substantial doses during the first week of treatment. Lithium is available only in oral form in capsules and time-release tablets or as a liquid known as lithium citrate. Because lithium is an ion, its concentration can be measured in the blood. In the acute phase the blood level must usually attain a concentration of 1.0 to 1.5 mEq/L. After 1 week to 10 days, as the bipolar symptoms subside, the dosage of lithium can be decreased to 900 to 1,200 mg/day, with the blood level maintained in the range of 0.6 to 1.2 mEq/L for continuing control of symptoms.

The basic principles for lithium medication therapy are as follows:

- Blood levels must be monitored after each dosage increase.
- Blood levels are checked every 2 to 3 months, or sooner if there is evidence of mood instability.

MEDIALINK Case Study: Medication Teaching, Bipolar Disorder

MEDIALINK Critical Thinking Exercise: The Older Client on Divalproex

TABLE 7-4 ■ Lithium and Antipsychotic Medication Compatibility with Liquids and Other Medications

Liquid	Chlor-promazine	Flu-phenazine	Haloperidol	Lox-apine	Mesori-dazine	Thiori-dazine	Thio-thixene	Trifluo-perazine	Lithium citrate
7-Up/Sprite	C	C		C		C		C	C
Apple juice/cider	X	X	C			X	X	X	X
Apricot juice	C	C				U	C	C	C
Coffee	U	X	X	C		X	X	U	C
Cola	U	X	C	C		X	X	C	C
Cranberry juice	X			C	C	C	C		C
Ginger ale		C				C			
Grapefruit juice	C	C	X	C	C	C	C	C	C
Grape juice	X		X		C	X		X	C
Lemonade						C			C
Mellow-Yellow		X				C		C	C
Milk	C	C	X			X	C	C	C
Orange juice	C	C	C	C	C	C	C	C	C
Orange soda	C	C				X		C	C
Pineapple juice		C		C		X	C	C	C
Prune juice	U	C				X	C	C	C
Saline	C	C	X			C		C	C
Soups/pudding	C	C	C				C	C	C
Tang	X			C					C
Tea	U	X	X			X	X	C	C
Tomato juice	C	C	C			X	C	C	C
V-8	C	C				X	X	C	C
Water	C	C	C		C	C	C	C	C
Medication									
Chlorpromazine						X			X
Haloperidol									X
Lithium citrate	X	C	U	C	C	X	C	X	
Thioridazine	X	X	X	X	X		X		X
Trifluoperazine									X

C = compatible; X = incompatible; U = unconfirmed, conflicting data; blank = no data available.

Source: Department of Pharmacy, Buffalo Psychiatric Center, Buffalo, NY, 2000.

For symptoms of breakthrough depression seen with bipolar depression, the dosing of divalproex or lithium must be maximized before other stabilizing or antidepressant agents are added to the regimen. After that episode resolves, the doses of the antidepressant medication are tapered slowly over the following 2 to 6 months. Special assessment skills are called into service during the tapering process to detect any resurgence of depressive symptomatology.

Length of treatment with medication for bipolar disorder is a debated issue. Clinical practice suggests prophylactic use of a mood stabilizer, preferably the compound effective during the acute phase of treatment, for at least 2 years. If the client has no intention of taking the medication for that long a period of time, there may be a premature recurrence of the mania. The following clinical example illustrates the appropriate use of medication in the case of a client with bipolar disorder.

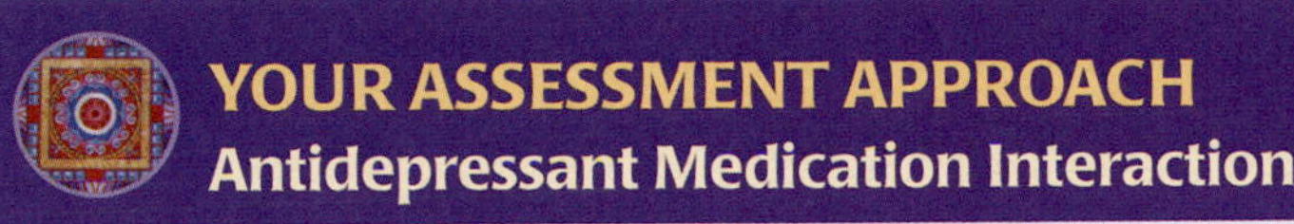

YOUR ASSESSMENT APPROACH
Antidepressant Medication Interactions

Combining One of These	With One of These Antidepressants	Can Lead to These Problems
Antiarrhythmic	TCA	Additive antiarrhythmic effect, myocardial depression
Anticholinergic	TCA	Additive anticholinergic effect
Anticonvulsant	TCA	Decreased TCA effect, lower seizure threshold
Antihypertensive	TCA	Hypertensive crisis
Antipsychotic	TCA	Increased TCA effect, confusion, delirium, ileus
CNS depressants such as: Alcohol Antihistamines Anxiolytics Barbiturates Narcotics	TCA	Decreased TCA effect, additive CNS depression
Foods or medications containing tyramine	MAOI	Hypertensive crisis
Levodopa	MAOI	Hypertensive crisis
MAOI	SSRI	Serotonin syndrome, serious adverse reactions
MAOI	TCA	Hyperpyrexia, severe excitation
Nicotine	TCA	Decreased TCA serum level
St. John's wort (herb)	SSRI	Sedative–hypnotic intoxication
SSRI	TCA	Increased TCA serum levels, elevated nortriptyline serum levels with adverse effects

YOUR ASSESSMENT APPROACH
Mood Stabilizer Medication Interactions

Combining One of These	With One of These Mood Stabilizers	Can Lead to These Problems
Aminophylline	Lithium	Increased lithium secretion
Benzodiazepines	Valproic acid	Excessive CNS depression
Carbamazepine	Lithium	Increased effect of lithium, lithium toxicity
Carbamazepine	Topiramate	Decreased topiramate level
Chlorpromazine	Valproic acid	Valproic acid toxicity
Clozapine	Carbamazepine	Additive bone marrow suppression
CNS depressants	Topiramate	Possible topiramate-induced CNS depression as well as other adverse cognitive and neuropsychiatric effects
Diuretics	Lithium	Increased lithium levels and potential lithium toxicity (monitor electrolytes, especially sodium)
Haloperidol	Carbamazepine	Decreased effectiveness of either compound
Lamotrigine	Valproic acid	Increased lamotrigine levels, decreased valproic levels
MAOI	Lithium	Increased depressant and anticholinergic effects
Marijuana	Lithium	Increased lithium levels and potential lithium toxicity
Neuroleptics	Lithium	Encephalopathy
NSAIDs	Lithium	Increased effect of lithium, lithium toxicity
SSRI	Lithium	Increased effect of lithium, lithium toxicity
Tetracyclines	Lithium	Lithium toxicity
Thyroid hormones	Lithium	May induce hypothyroidism

CLINICAL EXAMPLE

Chris, a 32-year-old legal aide, was brought to the clinic by her sister after she was fired from her position at a law firm. She had been arguing constantly with the lawyers and legal secretaries and stood on the conference room table, loudly telling people how to do their jobs. She had not slept in 3 days and was so irritable that she shoved a court clerk when approached about seeking care. Her sister stated that Chris was grandiose; spoke very quickly, moved from topic to topic in a rapid-fire style; and belittled everyone around her. The family was very concerned. She had not taken any prescription or recreational compounds as far as the family knew. In the past 5 years she had been prescribed lithium, which seemed to help; however, Chris refuses to take it now because it leaves a metallic taste in her mouth.

On interview, Chris spoke about having special powers such as bringing people back from the dead because she was a "sanctioned deity." Her episodes in the past did not include delusional thinking, and this was the first time her family could not contain her. Chris had some awareness that her behavior had frightened her family. She was told she had bipolar disorder with delusions. She was given divalproex sodium (Depakote) 250 mg tid and risperidone (Risperdal) 1 mg bid initially to control the mania and the psychosis. Chris was not hospitalized because her family agreed to supervise her care. After 1 week, the divalproex dosage was increased to 250 mg qid and Chris's behavior was under considerably better control.

The use of anticonvulsants as mood stabilizers has its own unique set of effects and termination-of-treatment issues. Divalproex, carbamazepine, gabapentin, and lamotrigine all have sedation, gastrointestinal (GI) disturbances, and dizziness as side effects, along with others more specific to each compound. The body needs time to adapt to the medication; therefore, some side effects are temporary. However, dosage adjustments can minimize the impact of these side effects so that the quality of life is not shifted downward. An important client teaching point when using anticonvulsants as mood stabilizers is the inability of the body to handle the abrupt discontinuation of these medications. Frank discussions must highlight the increased chance of having a seizure, even if the client has never had one, if the dose is not tapered slowly to discontinuation.

Psychobiology of Lithium

The psychobiology of bipolar disorder has not yet been mapped, but much can be said about the psychobiology of lithium. Lithium, not unlike the antidepressants, affects neurotransmitters, especially norepinephrine and serotonin. In short, lithium aids in the reduction of neurotransmitter release into the synapse and enhances its return, yielding a lower overall amount of the neurotransmitter in the synapse. Behaviorally, these biologic changes can be observed as an absence of mania or depression. What is unclear is why lithium takes up to a few weeks to be fully effective, when its effects can be observed on synaptic activity almost immediately. Also, why do some people with bipolar disorder *not* respond at all to lithium therapy? Many psychobiologists believe that lithium's effects are likely to be based on neurocellular changes that occur over weeks or months after a client begins lithium therapy. A similar explanation may hold true concerning the effectiveness of other mood stabilizers.

ANXIOLYTIC MEDICATIONS

Medications in this class are used to treat a variety of problems from high levels of anxiety and panic to insomnia.

Effects

Anxiolytic medications, or antianxiety agents—sedatives and hypnotics—have very similar pharmacologic attributes. All can be used in small or moderate doses to relieve anxiety and in larger doses to induce sleep. Although they share the major clinical effect of tranquilization or **disinhibition** (loss or reduction of an inhibition) of fear-induced behavior, their side effects, including their addictive potential and overdose sequelae, make certain medications in this category more suitable for routine use and others better reserved for limited, special circumstances.

Antianxiety medications are sometimes called *minor tranquilizers,* but this is a misleading term. Their effects on anxiety have qualities that are different from those of the "major tranquilizers" or antipsychotic medications, but the quantity of the impact is the same.

Medication Classification

The major categories of medication classification separate medications into groups according to their chemical composition and properties.

Meprobamate

Meprobamate (Miltown, Equanil) was the first antianxiety agent to gain popularity in the 1960s. The results of controlled studies of the effects of meprobamate compared to placebos are generally favorable but not overwhelmingly convincing. This, and the addictive and fatal overdose potentials of the medication, prompted investigators to develop more effective and safer medications that have made meprobamate all but obsolete. You will not see the use of this medication very often in clinical settings.

Benzodiazepines and Nonbenzodiazepines

The major class of medications used today in the management of anxiety is benzodiazepines and nonbenzodiazepines. This group, represented by alprazolam (Xanax), lorazepam (Ativan), and others, accounts for a very high percentage of all the psychoactive medications prescribed in the United States. This fact usually evokes a mixed response in professional circles. The easy distribution of medications for such a ubiquitous human phenomenon as anxiety fosters the development of a pill-oriented and pill-dependent society, say critics. Sympathizers focus on the proven effectiveness of the medications, which help people achieve higher levels of functioning, more pleasurable experiences, and even more productive psychotherapies in some instances.

The dosing and timing of an antianxiety medication determine whether the treatment of anxiety is effective or interferes with a client's ability to learn and cope. These are two entirely different pathways in the treatment of anxiety. Anxiety is a normal human response to threats of varying intensities and is not necessarily an experience to be avoided at all costs. At low to moderate levels, anxiety can be motivating and instructive and helps one to be more aware of one's environment. But when anxiety passes these stages and becomes excessive, panic can occur. Extreme feelings of anxiety such as panic are not motivating—in fact, they are immobilizing and make learning impossible (see Chapter 8).

The clinical application and purpose of antianxiety medications is primarily to support clients through episodes of stress and anxiety at moderate to high levels. Medicating so that higher levels of anxiety are prevented allows the individual to have a lower level of anxiety that can be managed with the coping skills taught by nurses, and to gauge the effectiveness of his or her coping skills. If antianxiety medications are given without regard for the actual anxiety level and the individual's need to learn coping skills, it is possible to obliterate the need to learn to cope. Instead, the client learns to rely on the medication to become less anxious. The lesson the client will have learned is: take pills. For a list of currently available benzodiazepines and nonbenzodiazepines, see Table 7-5.

Table 7-5 Generic and Trade Names of Benzodiazepines and Nonbenzodiazepines

Generic Name	Trade Names
Benzodiazepines	
Adinazolam	Deracyn
Alprazolam	Xanax
Bromazepam	Lexotan, Lexotanil, Lexomil
Brotizolam	Lendormin
Camazepam	Albego
Chlordiazepoxide	Librium, Libritabs, Elenium
Clobazam	Frisium
Clonazepam	Klonopin
Clorazepate	Tranxene
Clotiazepam	Clozan, Trecalmo
Cloxazolam	Enadel
Diazepam	Valium
Estazolam	ProSom, Nuctalm
Ethyl loflazepate	Meilax, Victan
Etizolam	Depas
Flunitrazepam	Rohypnol
Flurazepam	Dalmane, Dalmadorm
Halazepam	Paxipam
Ketazolam	Anxon, Unakalm
Loprazolam	Dormonoct
Lorazepam	Ativan
Lormetazepam	Loramet
Medazepam	Nobrium
Midazolam	Versed, Dormicum
Nitrazepam	Mogadon
Oxazepam	Serax
Oxazolam	Tranquit
Pinazepam	Domar
Prazepam	Centrax
Quazepam	Doral, Oniria, Dormalin, Quazium
Temazepam	Restoril
Tetrazepam	Musaril, Myolastan
Tofizopam (tofisopam)	Grandaxin, Seriel, Tavor
Triazolam	Halcion
Nonbenzodiazepines	
Buspirone	BuSpar
Eszopiclone	Lunesta
Meprobamate	Miltown, Equanil
Zaleplon	Sonata
Zolpidem	Ambien

New Medications

In the last decade, anxiety-related research has expanded tremendously, and several new anxiolytic medications have been introduced. The newer benzodiazepines give prescribers a wider range of therapies to target the often idiosyncratic manifestations of anxiety. Some of the new medications have more rapid onsets and shorter half-lives (triazolam, quazepam [Doral]), while others have the usual benzodiazepine onset time and an extended half-life (clonazepam [Klonopin]).

With the recent explosion in psychobiologic knowledge, a great variety of benzodiazepine medications have been used in the treatment of a number of disorders. Benzodiazepines are used for many reasons:

- Anxiety disorders
- Sleep disorders
- Mood disorders
- Anxiety associated with medical illness
- Psychotic symptoms and disorders
- Convulsive disorders
- Involuntary movement disorders
- Spastic disorders and acute muscle spasms
- Intoxication and withdrawal from alcohol and other substances
- Preanesthesia
- Nausea and vomiting associated with chemotherapy
- Anxiolytic, sedative, and amnestic effects in a wide range of stressful diagnostic procedures

Uses for Anxiolytics

There is no question that benzodiazepines offer a rapid, effective, and safe treatment for the emotional state commonly known as anxiety. Caffeine interferes with the effectiveness of these medications, both pharmacologically and as an irritant to the client's mood and systems.

These medications are absorbed much more rapidly and completely from the gastrointestinal tract than from intramuscular injection and are almost always administered orally.

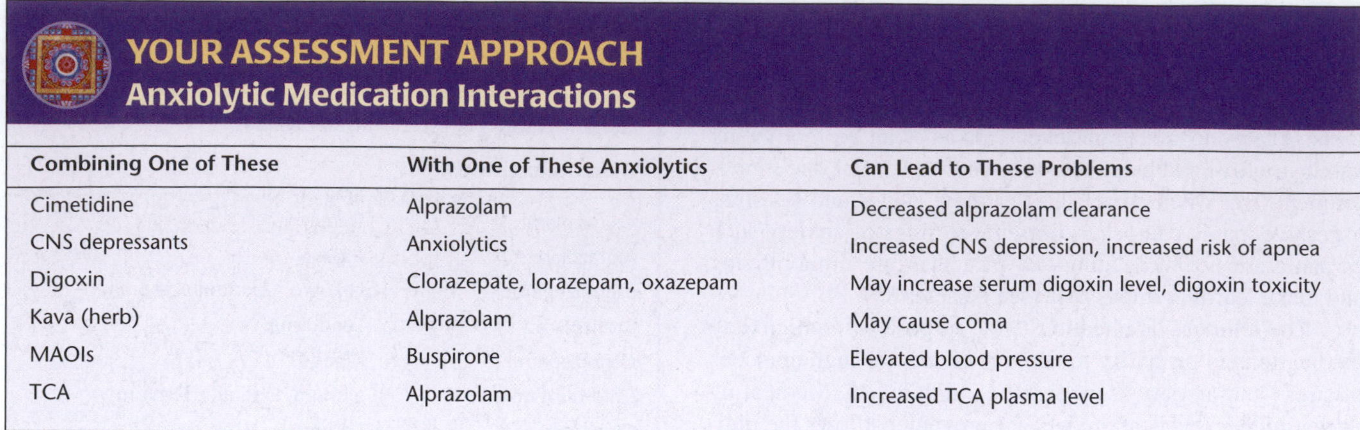

YOUR ASSESSMENT APPROACH
Anxiolytic Medication Interactions

Combining One of These	With One of These Anxiolytics	Can Lead to These Problems
Cimetidine	Alprazolam	Decreased alprazolam clearance
CNS depressants	Anxiolytics	Increased CNS depression, increased risk of apnea
Digoxin	Clorazepate, lorazepam, oxazepam	May increase serum digoxin level, digoxin toxicity
Kava (herb)	Alprazolam	May cause coma
MAOIs	Buspirone	Elevated blood pressure
TCA	Alprazolam	Increased TCA plasma level

MEDIALINK Diazepam Drug Mechanism in Action Animation

Exceptions are the intramuscular injections of lorazepam (Ativan) for extreme agitation and the use of intravenous diazepam (Valium) to induce sleep before anesthesia or to manage status epilepticus. Peak levels of chlordiazepoxide (Librium) are reached in the bloodstream 2 to 4 hours after oral ingestion, and peak levels of diazepam are reached in 1 to 2 hours.

The major side effects of benzodiazepines are related to their sedative qualities. Clients may complain of excessive drowsiness and must be cautioned against driving a car or operating other machinery.

Other medications used to treat anxiety, generally less effectively, include the antihistamines diphenhydramine (Benadryl) and hydroxyzine (Vistaril, Atarax), the beta-blocker propranolol (Inderal), and methaqualone (Quaalude), which is a synthetic nonbarbiturate sedative. Methaqualone has been a much-abused medication, probably because of the intense euphoria associated with peak blood levels.

Another common use of benzodiazepines, especially diazepam and chlordiazepoxide, is in the detoxification of individuals addicted to alcohol. Given adequate doses of benzodiazepines to induce sedation (usually starting at 30 to 40 mg/day of diazepam or 150 to 350 mg/day of chlordiazepoxide), alcoholic clients can be smoothly withdrawn by stepwise reductions in chlordiazepoxide dose over a 1- to 2-week period, without encountering alcohol withdrawal delirium or grand mal seizures.

Psychobiology of Anxiolytic Medications

Antianxiety medications probably work through a process of synaptic activity involving the neurotransmitter gamma-aminobutyric acid (GABA) in the brain and spinal cord. Benzodiazepines most likely potentiate GABA, producing muscle relaxation. This mechanism involves a complex process of presynaptic and postsynaptic receptor activity. The antianxiety effectiveness seen with these medications is related to their impacts on GABA receptors. Recent research has yielded information about the presence of a postsynaptic receptor called the *benzodiazepine receptor*. As the term implies, benzodiazepines bind perfectly and with great specificity to these receptors, allowing for the sensation of relaxation. Two types of benzodiazepine receptors have been identified in the CNS. Type 1 receptors are located in parts of the brain responsible for sedation, and nonbenzodiazepines bind exclusively to the Type 1 receptors. This makes nonbenzodiazepines an excellent choice for the treatment of sleep disturbances. Type 2 receptors are positioned in parts of the brain responsible for cognition, memory, and psychomotor functioning. Benzodiazepines bind with either Type 1 or Type 2 receptors. The Your Assessment Approach feature above points out potential medication interactions between anxiolytics and other medications and substances.

TREATMENT FOR INSOMNIA

The pharmacologic management of insomnia presents an interesting and challenging clinical problem. Many of the truly hypnotic medications tend to have undesirable effects, including physiologic addiction, fatal overdose potential, and dangerous interactions with other medications because of liver enzyme induction. The first principle of treatment is to assess whether the insomnia is related to one of the major mental disorders, such as schizophrenia or major depression. If so, the insomnia can and should be treated as part of the larger problem, and sedative antipsychotics or antidepressants may be given at bedtime for this purpose.

In the management of simple insomnia without an associated major mental disorder, sedative–hypnotics are indicated for short-term treatment. Overall, the available sedative–hypnotics include certain antidepressants, benzodiazepines, nonbenzodiazepines, over-the-counter (OTC) medications, barbiturates, and some miscellaneous substances such as chloral hydrate and alcohol (McKim, 2007). Prescription medications are more effective than OTCs, while barbiturates are rarely, if ever, prescribed due to safety and addiction problems. The benzodiazepine compound flurazepam (Dalmane), 15 to 30 mg at bedtime, is an example of a commonly used historical insomnia treatment. This medication can be used on consecutive nights for about 1 month. Other benzodiazepine compounds that are used for their hypnotic qualities include triazolam and lorazepam.

The rapid absorption of nonbenzodiazepines, within 30 minutes, along with efficient elimination and the minimal hangover effects of sedation the following day, make them the treatment of choice for insomnia. Zolpidem (Ambien), zaleplon (Sonata), and eszopiclone (Lunesta) are newer nonbenzodiazepines that are structurally very different from each other but equally effective in the treatment of insomnia. Fast-acting, competent sleep-inducing, and quickly eliminated medications such as these can be used without the difficulties associated with other commonly used compounds. Eszopiclone is the first sedative–hypnotic medication approved by the FDA for long-term treatment of insomnia. Clients using zolpidem may find it a little more difficult to fall asleep the first night without the medication, but zaleplon is not associated with any withdrawal or rebound effects. Insomnia is discussed in detail in Chapter 19∞.

ACETYLCHOLINESTERASE INHIBITORS

The class of medications with specific abilities for dementia treatment is **acetylcholinesterase inhibitors**, also called cholinesterase inhibitors. The title of this class describes how these compounds affect the CNS. The enzyme responsible for the breakdown of a particular neurotransmitter is inhibited from acting by the medication. The enzyme is acetylcholinesterase, and the neurotransmitter it specifically works on is acetylcholine. The cholinergic system is involved in memory, the ability to logically progress from one step to the next in problem solving, and the identification of objects and people in the environment, among other skills. Clients with dementia of the Alzheimer's type (DAT) have acetylcholine neurotransmitter deficits at the root of some of their problems. When the breakdown of acetylcholine is slowed, it allows more of the neurotransmitter to remain in the synapse, thus promoting acetylcholine's function—transmitting information from one cell to another. In mild to moderately affected individuals, when there is more acetylcholine in the CNS, cognitive functioning and memory improve. This is essentially the path by which these medications slow the progression of dementia in clients with early stage DAT.

Acetylcholinesterase inhibitors are best utilized early in the dementing process when deficits are still mild to moderate in scope. But the best timing and the most effective use of the compounds are frequently thwarted by the realities of human nature. Instituting treatment at early stages may be difficult because many people are not aware they are in the early stages of dementia. Frequently they are unable to grasp their own level of symptomatology and lack information on the early signs, symptoms, or issues of dementia. Confabulation or denial prevents a client or loved ones from noting deficits or recognizing the implications of low-level difficulties. For example, a woman who is unable to tie her shoes may ask her husband to do that for her; both of them attribute her difficulty to arthritis, musculoskeletal problems, or side effects of medications. Another example is the man who stops balancing his checkbook, ostensibly because the bank has always been correct when in reality he has lost the basic math skills required.

Think of this medication class as a treatment for specific symptoms, not a cure. Acetylcholinesterase inhibitors do not alter the course of the underlying disease process or have an impact on the progressive nature of the disease. They are a way to temporarily improve neurotransmission and thus ameliorate memory deficits. The first of the acetylcholinesterase inhibitors was tacrine (Cognex). Although it did not help all clients with DAT, it was the first step in the direction of active treatment for a major portion of people with dementing processes. Problems with this medication included liver toxicity, which could be controlled, and several common side effects including GI disturbances and headache. From this beginning, other compounds were developed. Donepezil (Aricept) and rivastigmine (Exelon) are newer acetylcholinesterase inhibitors with improved impacts and fewer difficulties from side effects. Donepezil (Aricept) is approved for the treatment of all degrees of severity of DAT. GI disturbances occur at a much lower level than with the original compound, and headaches are reported at only a slightly higher level than with clients taking a placebo. There is even hope that these medications can play a role in preventing individuals with cognitive deficits from converting to DAT. See Chapter 14∞ for a discussion of Alzheimer's and its progression.

Another group of medications used to treat dementias, including DAT, are atypical antipsychotics. They are common choices for treating the delusions, hallucinations, aggression, and agitation seen with demented clients. There is ongoing debate about whether the adverse effects of atypical antipsychotics offset the advantages. As these concerns are explored, atypical antipsychotics offer good symptom control with far fewer side effects than haloperidol, the antipsychotic previously used to treat the symptoms of dementia.

Continuing research is focusing on the nutrient CoQ10, or coenzyme Q10, and its effects on dementing processes. At this writing only animal studies have been conducted, but CoQ10 may play a protective role in the development of diseases such as Alzheimer's dementia. CoQ10 had a positive impact on cognitive impairment brought about by damage from free radicals (called oxidative stress or oxidation) (Sahelian, 2005). It remains to be seen if improvements in rat cognitive functioning can be translated to human functioning.

MEDICATION COUNTERFEITING

A fairly new problem has arisen in the world of prescription medications: medication counterfeiting. Counterfeit medications are illegal and inherently unsafe, and are a growing public health problem. A counterfeit medication is a fake medication. It may be contaminated or contain the wrong—or no—active ingredient, be made with the wrong amount of ingredients, or be packaged in phony packaging. Typically a person who cannot afford a particular medication may purchase it over the Internet and unknowingly receive a counterfeit medication instead, with unintended and possibly serious consequences.

The volume of counterfeit medication sales is expected to exceed $75 billion by 2012, an indication that economics plays a large role in this issue (Martello, 2006). To ensure that your clients are receiving safe medications, advocate that they obtain medications only from a licensed pharmacy. Legitimate Internet pharmacies carry accreditation (the Verified Internet

MEDIALINK FDA: Counterfeit Drugs

Pharmacy Practice Sites Accreditation Program, or VIPPS) to show they are a reputable source. The FDA is preparing requirements to track the pedigree of prescription medications from the manufacturer, through the medication distribution chain, to the end retailer. For up-to-date information on this subject, visit the FDA website at www.fda.gov/counterfeit.

HERBAL MEDICINES

Herbal medicines are widely used as an alternative or complementary therapy. (See Chapter 33 for another discussion of these interventions.) One quarter of prescription medications and hundreds of OTC medications are derived from plants. Herbs and plants generally take longer to act than pharmaceuticals, and few have the potency of a prescription. However, many herbal agents have powerful medicine-like actions and side effects.

One of the critical features of safe and effective nursing care is communication about complementary and alternative treatments. Keep in mind the variety of terms used to describe these treatments: complementary, alternative, botanical, nutriceutical, herbal medicine; home remedy, natural remedy, homeopathic remedy; health food, vitamin therapy, dietary supplement, phytomedicine, herbal tea, and others.

The concomitant use of herbal medicines with psychiatric pharmaceuticals can be accomplished safely only when health providers know that their clients use them and the safety and effectiveness for the client's specific condition have been thoroughly appraised. Be sure to assess your clients for the use of herbal medicines.

There are many benefits to using alternative substances. For example:

- Self-treatment can be empowering.
- The very low concentrations of these substances could be helpful and might not be harmful for those who are sensitive to even low doses of pharmaceutical compounds.
- Some people feel safer using "natural" products and distrust chemical formulations.
- Standard labeling and dosing are possible.

However, there are potential problems with the use of alternative substances in psychiatry even though these substances have lower potencies. Psychiatric indications for alternative substances currently exist only for St. John's wort for depression and ginkgo biloba for dementia, although alternative substances are frequently used for several other psychiatric symptoms and disorders. You may encounter clients using ma huang (ephedra) for general malaise, kava for anxiety and stress (see the FDA caution in Table 33-3 on page 887), and ginseng and SAMe for depression. Competent assessment and evaluation requires our awareness of the potential for difficulties with alternative substances. Problems with using herbs may include:

- Contamination of the product
- Dosing inconsistencies
- Delayed absorption of other coadministered medications
- Worsening of high blood pressure, potassium imbalance, and coagulation problems
- Side effects such as nerve damage, kidney damage, and liver damage
- Advertising of unproven claims
- Aggravation of allergic reactions
- Interference with breastfeeding
- Believing that one is treating the problem, when in reality the symptoms could continue to worsen, making effective treatment much more difficult

Assessing Herb Consumption

Many clients do not tell health care providers about their herbal use for fear of being ridiculed or criticized. How do you find out what alternative therapies your clients are taking? Good interviewing skills—tolerance, a nonjudgmental stance, and some expressive questions—will bring much of your client's life into the light. Questions such as "Do you do anything to improve your health?" or "What do you buy at the grocery store or health food store besides food?" can open the subject. See the Rx Communication feature for examples of a conversation about this topic.

Be aware of the client's need to talk to a knowledgeable professional. The client may tell you about someone else who is taking alternatives while watching for your reaction. A nonjudgmental response would include questions about what the client thinks about it, whether it has helped the individual, or whether the client would consider using this particular treat-

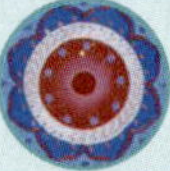

RX COMMUNICATION

COMMUNICATING WITH YOUR CLIENT ABOUT HERBAL MEDICINES

CLIENT: I don't like taking all these chemicals. It's not natural.

NURSE RESPONSE 1: Are you more comfortable taking medicine to help you when you know it's natural?

RATIONALE: This question gathers more data about what the client needs in order to feel better and raises the possibility of alternative substance use.

NURSE RESPONSE 2: Have you had bad experiences with anything in particular?

RATIONALE: This response makes the connection for the client between the idea and a possible result. It may also encourage discussion of recreational substance use.

ment. Not knowing about your client's use of botanicals risks dangerous medication interactions or costly and painful tests or treatments when an herb causes an unrecognized side effect.

Psychopharmacology is an important aspect of the treatment of people who have mental health issues. When you understand the science of pharmacology, you can more easily perform some of the main tasks of psychiatric–mental health nursing—educating clients about medications as a vital part of psychiatric treatment, promoting self-care, and advocating for the best possible outcomes.

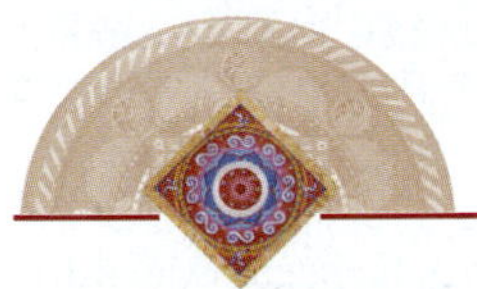

EXPLORE MEDIALINK

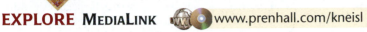

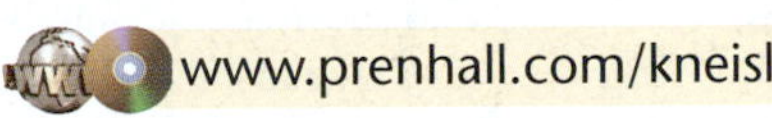

For NCLEX-RN® review questions, case studies, and other resources for this chapter see the Pearson Health MediaLink CD-ROM that accompanies this book and the Companion Website at www.prenhall.com/kneisl.

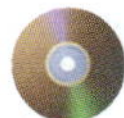

CD-ROM
Audio Glossary
NCLEX-RN® Review Questions
Animations
- *Neurological Synapse*
- *Liver Enzyme (Cytochrome P450) Inhibition and Activation*
- *Fluoxetine (Prozac) Drug Mechanism in Action*
- *Methylphenidate (Ritalin) Drug Mechanism in Action*
- *Diazepam (Valium) Drug Mechanism in Action*

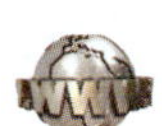

Companion Website
Audio Glossary
NCLEX-RN® Review Questions
Critical Thinking Exercise
- *Family Medication Teaching: The Older Client on Divalproex (Depakote)*

Case Study
- *Family Medication Teaching: The Client with Bipolar Disorder*

Care Plan
- *The Client on Antipsychotic Medication*

MediaLinks
MediaLink Application
- *Attitudes Toward Antipsychotic Medications*

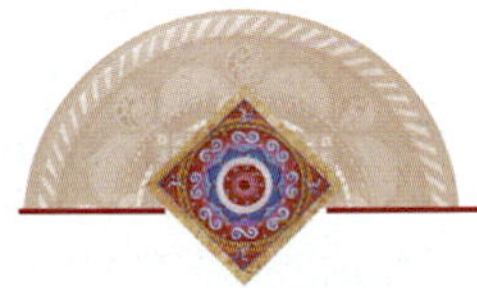

NCLEX-RN® REVIEW QUESTIONS

1. Which of the following treatment team statements are congruent with the text's definition and description of psychopharmacology? (Select all that apply.)
1. "We aim for behavior control through the sedating effects of the medications."
2. "Pharmacologic intervention makes other therapies possible."
3. "The psychiatric–mental health nurse's responsibilities include pharmacologic expertise."
4. "Our goal with pharmacologic interventions is elimination of the illness, whereas other interventions merely 'treat.'"
5. "We consider the client holistically when prescribing a pharmaceutical regimen."

2. Which of the following descriptors accurately describes trends in psychopharmacology?
1. Very specific to less-specific blockage of neurotransmitters
2. Less-comprehensive to more-comprehensive symptom relief
3. Severe side effects to inconsequential side effects
4. Increased use of specific medications for discrete conditions

3. Two clients are participants in a pharmacologic study. They are the same gender and age, and similar in clinical presentation. However, Client 1 requires twice the dosage of the experimental medication to achieve symptom control, while Client 2 experiences debilitating side effects at a much lower dosage. The nurse reviews their histories. Which finding is most helpful in explaining the clients' clinical responses?
1. Client 1 has always required more medication than Client 2 to achieve the same therapeutic effect, and the clients belong to different ethnic groups.
2. Client 2 has always reported more side effects than anyone else in the study.
3. Three years ago, Client 1 had a severe dystonic reaction after a single dose of haloperidol.
4. The psychiatrist reports that Client 2's family is "high-EE."

4. Which of the following family member's statements reflects a therapeutic response to psychoactive medications? (Select all that apply.)
1. "He started the antidepressant less than 1 week ago and already he's more hopeful and future-oriented."

2. "Since the mood stabilizer was started, he complains of sedation and stomach upset."
3. "The lithium has removed the big highs and lows, so that he is on a more 'even keel.'"
4. "Since he started the medication 2 weeks ago, his depression has not changed, but his sleep has increased from 8 to 16 hours per day, and he has gained 20 pounds."
5. "The medication has helped his hallucinations and unrealistic thoughts, but now he just stays in bed all day and doesn't want to do anything."

5. In evaluating the response to psychoactive medication, which of the following client statements indicate a potential for negative impact on behavior? (Select all that apply.)
1. "I feel just like I did before I was hospitalized. I'm getting back to my life as if this was all a bad dream."
2. "My medication regimen enables me to return to work. I just need to watch my stress level more closely."
3. "I feel like myself again. Maybe I don't really need to take this medication anymore."
4. "My therapist wants me to take coping skills and stress management classes, but the medication is enough. I don't need classes."
5. "I still think about death, but at least I don't lie in bed all day."

6. An outpatient client reports that she does not want to pay for her atypical antipsychotic medication because she is experiencing the same side effects as she did on her conventional antipsychotic medication. After reviewing the CATIE Study Summary (Box 7-3), which of the following is essential to consider in the health care team's approach to this client?
1. The health care team must address your individual client's concerns.
2. The majority of the participants changed antipsychotic medications because of intolerable side effects or poor symptom control.
3. The atypical antipsychotic medications demonstrated better symptom control than the conventional antipsychotic medication in the study.
4. Your client may need a higher dose of her atypical antipsychotic medication.

7. Benzodiazepines are used in the treatment of:
1. Alcohol withdrawal and anxiety disorders.
2. Hallucinations and delusions.
3. Bipolar disorder.
4. Depressive disorders.

8. You are preparing for a medication education class for clients with a variety of major mental illnesses. One of your goals is to identify commonalities among clients, their stressors, and their treatments. Which of the following statements is true regarding the mechanism of action of antipsychotic medications, antidepressants, and mood stabilizers?
1. They act like neurotransmitters in the synaptic cleft.
2. They increase production of transmitters, thereby increasing the amount of neurotransmitters in the synaptic cleft.
3. They alter the availability of specific neurotransmitters in the synaptic cleft.
4. They decrease the number of postsynaptic neurons in order to slow transmission and eliminate the target symptoms.

9. Your client with long-term insomnia has been tapered from a benzodiazepine and started on a nonbenzodiazepine sedative–hypnotic. Based on your understanding of psychobiology, what response do you anticipate from this client?
1. "This new medication gave me more of a hangover than I ever had with a benzodiazepine."
2. "This new medication is just as effective."
3. "This new medication works better; it takes longer to work, though."
4. "This new medication doesn't slow down my thinking or relax me as much as the benzodiazepine did."

10. A client with chronic schizophrenia is being discharged on an atypical antipsychotic medication. A family member asks you, "How will I be able to tell if there's a benefit over the conventional antipsychotic medication? It's been prescribed for years." Based on your knowledge of psychopharmacology, which response is most accurate?
1. "There's less potential for tolerance and dependence."
2. "He should experience fewer of the deficit symptoms of the disease."
3. "He's more likely to keep taking these meds."
4. "You won't be able to see a difference, but he will be less likely to develop tardive dyskinesia."

See Appendix C for answers.

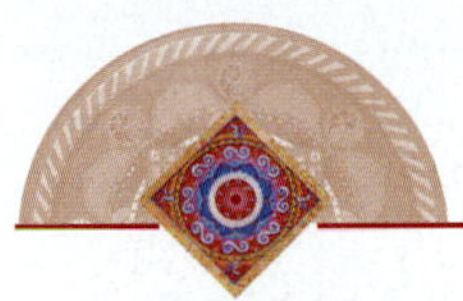

REFERENCES

American Nurses Association Task Force on Psychopharmacology. (1994). *Psychiatric–mental health nursing psychopharmacology project.* Washington, DC: American Nurses Association.

Choi, J. B., Hong, S., Nelesen, R., Bardwell, W. A., Natarajan, L., Schubert, C., et al. (2006). Age and ethnicity differences in short-term heart-rate variability. *Psychosomatic Medicine, 68*(3), 421–426.

Glueck, C. J., Khalil, Q., Winiarska, M., & Wang, P. (2006). Interaction of duloxetine and warfarin causing severe elevation of international normalized ratio. *Journal of the American Medical Association, 295*(13), 1517–1518.

Haynes, R. B., Yao, X., Degani, A., Kripalani, S., Garg, A., & McDonald, H. P. (2006). Interventions for enhancing medication adherence. *The Cochrane Library,* 4–163.

Kelly, D. L., Dixon, L. B., Kreyenbuhl, J. A., Medoff, D., Lehman, A. F., Love, R. C., et al. (2006). Clozapine utilization and outcomes by race in a public mental health system: 1994–2000. *Journal of Clinical Psychiatry, 67*(9), 1404–1411.

Luby, J. L. (2006). Psychopharmacology. In J. L. Luby (Ed.), *Handbook of preschool mental health: Development, disorders, and treatment* (pp. 311–330). New York: Guilford Press.

Martello, K. (2006). Preparing for drug pedigrees. *Drug Delivery Technology, 6*(2), 18–20.

McKim, W. A. (2007). *Drugs and behavior: An introduction to behavioral pharmacology* (6th ed.). Upper Saddle River, NJ: Pearson Education.

Mosnaim, A. D., Ranade, V. V., Wolf, M. E., Puente, J., & Antonieta Valenzuela, M. (2006). Phenothiazine molecule provides the basic chemical structure for various classes of pharmacotherapeutic agents. *American Journal of Therapeutics, 13*(3), 261–273.

Muñoz, C., & Hilgenberg, C. (2006). Ethnopharmacology: Understanding how ethnicity can affect drug response is essential to providing culturally competent care. *Holistic Nursing Practice, 20*(5), 227–234.

Sahelian, R. (2005). Efficacy of coenzyme Q10 in migraine prophylaxis: A randomized controlled trial. *Neurology, 64*(4), 713–715.

Smock, T. K. (1999). *Physiological psychology: A neuroscience approach.* Upper Saddle River, NJ: Prentice Hall.

Stroup, T. S., Lieberman, J. A., McEvoy, J. P., Swartz, M. S., Davis, S. M., Rosenheck, R. A., et al. (2006). Effectiveness of olanzapine, quetiapine, risperidone, and ziprasidone in patients with chronic schizophrenia following discontinuation of a previous atypical antipsychotic. *American Journal of Psychiatry, 163*(4), 611–622.

Trigoboff, E., Wilson, B. A., Shannon, M. T., & Stang, C. L. (2005). *Psychiatric drug handbook* (1st ed.). Upper Saddle River, NJ: Prentice Hall.

Ueda, M., Hirokane, G., Morita, S., Okawa, M., Watanabe, T., Akiyama, K., et al. (2006). The impact of CYP2D6 genotypes on the plasma concentration of paroxetine in Japanese psychiatric patients. *Progress in Neuro-Psychopharmacology & Biological Psychiatry, 30*(3), 486–491.

Weisman, A. G., Rosales, G. A., Kymalainen, J. A., & Armesto, J. C. (2006). Ethnicity, expressed emotion, and schizophrenia patients' perceptions of their family members' criticism. *Journal of Nervous & Mental Disease, 194*(9), 644–649.

ADDITIONAL REFERENCES

Kelly, D. L., & Conley, R. R. (2006). A randomized double-blind 12-week study of quetiapine, risperidone or fluphenazine on sexual functioning in people with schizophrenia. *Psychoneuroendocrinology, 31*(3), 340–346.

Willgerodt, M. A., & Thompson, E. A. (2006). Ethnic and generational influences on emotional distress and risk behaviors among Chinese and Filipino American adolescents. *Research in Nursing & Health, 29*(4), 311–324.

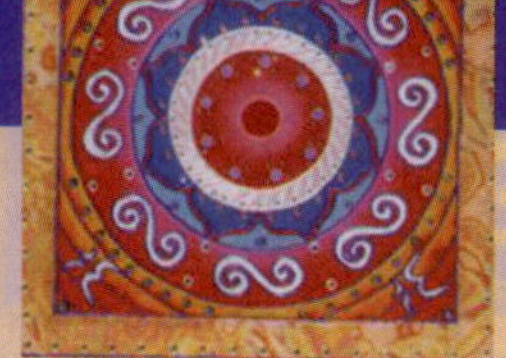

CHAPTER

8

Stress, Anxiety, and Coping

CAROL REN KNEISL

KEY TERMS

anxiety *142*
cardiac neurosis *160*
conflict *137*
coping strategies *146*
defense mechanisms *149*
denial *153*
displacement *155*
dissociation *152*
false memories *151*
fantasy *154*
fight-or-flight *138*
general adaptation syndrome (GAS) *139*
identification *152*
intellectualization *155*
introjection *153*
mental disorder due to a general medical condition *156*
projection *153*
psychological factors affecting medical condition (PFAMC) *156*
psychoneuroimmunology (PNI) *142*
rationalization *154*
reaction formation *155*
recovered memory *151*
repression *150*
selective inattention *144*
stress *137*
stressor *137*
suppression *150*
type A personality *159*

LEARNING OUTCOMES

After completing this chapter, you will be able to:

1. Explain how stress affects an individual.
2. Identify the sources of anxiety.
3. Describe the everyday methods people use to cope with stress and anxiety.
4. Compare and contrast the common defense-oriented behaviors (defense mechanisms) people use to cope with stress and anxiety.
5. Implement nursing intervention strategies specific to each defense-oriented behavior listed.
6. Discuss common medical conditions with an onset or a course influenced by psychological and behavioral factors.

CRITICAL THINKING CHALLENGE

At the scene of an auto accident in which a couple in their eighties lost control of the RV trailer they were towing, the husband remained immobile in the driver's seat, hands firmly fixed to the steering wheel, eyes focused on some distant spot despite the threat of explosion from the smoking car. The wife ran around in circles. She had lost her shoes in the accident, but despite numerous bleeding cuts, she was unaware she was running barefoot through broken glass from the windshield.

The nurses who happened on the scene had differing opinions about which was the healthier response. One said the gentleman's "control" was positive, but the wife's "hysteria" was negative.

1. What is your opinion?
2. Does everyone react in the same way to stress? Anxiety?
3. Are some strategies for handling stress and anxiety better than others? In what ways?

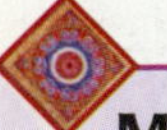

MediaLink 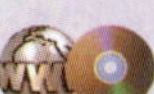 www.prenhall.com/kneisl

Go to the Pearson Health MediaLink CD-ROM and the Companion Website at www.prenhall.com/kneisl for interactive resources for this chapter.

How do we handle the ups and downs of life? Our brains have built-in chemical circuit breakers that shut off stress hormones and networks of nerves whose job is to calm us down. The circuit breakers and the nerves require us to take regular breaks from our everyday routines—that is, we have a biological need to periodically disengage. But what about time-saving devices—cell phones and mobile e-mail devices? The answer is that they make it harder, not easier, to get away, to decompress, or to disengage.

We cannot avoid stress, and there is growing evidence that stress eventually catches up with us. Insurance claims for stress, job burnout, and depression are among the fastest-growing disability categories in the United States.The cost of stress and anxiety can be quite high: They can cost a woman her job; a man, the love and respect of his family. When sufficiently prolonged, stress can kill.

STRESS

Stress is part of being alive. Standing erect stresses the muscles and bones that must work together to keep the body erect; eating stresses the digestive system, which must produce enzymes and absorb nutrients; and breathing stresses the respiratory system, which must exchange carbon dioxide and oxygen. Facing a demanding situation is stressful. More broadly and holistically, **stress** designates a broad class of experiences in which a demanding situation taxes a person's resources or coping capabilities, causing a negative effect.

This broader definition fits more closely with the humanistic perspective of this textbook. In this view, stress is a person–environment interaction. The source of the stress, the demanding situation, is known as a **stressor**. The internal state the stress produces is one of tension, anxiety, or strain. See FIGURE 8-1 ■ for an example of stress as a person–environment situation.

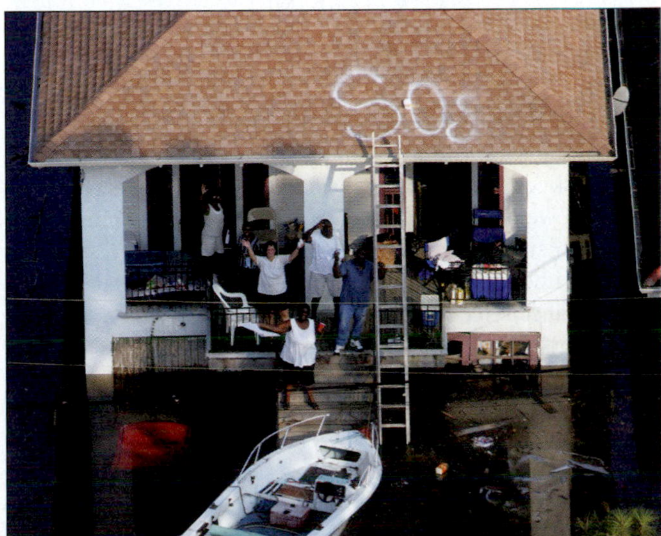

FIGURE 8-1 ■ Although people are no longer being airlifted from roofs, and bodies are no longer being removed from New Orleans houses and buildings toppled by Hurricane Katrina, there are high rates of mental health problems among stressed survivors.

Source: AP Wide World Photos, DAVID J. PHILLIP.

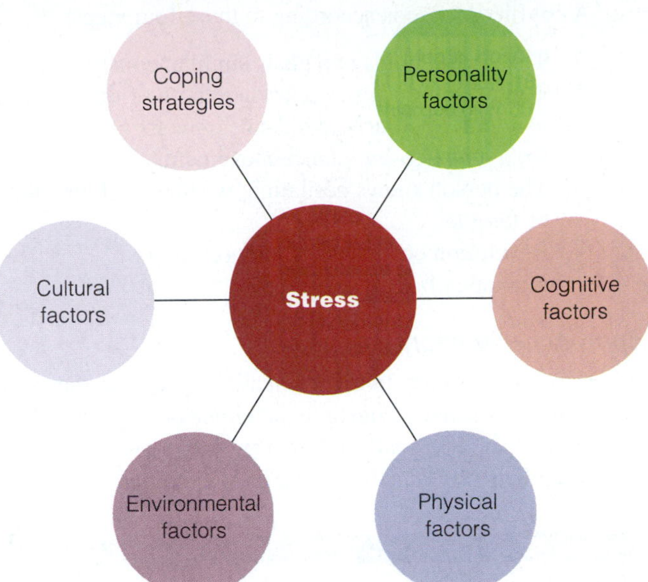

FIGURE 8-2 ■ Factors involved in stress. Several important factors are involved in understanding stress. They include personality factors (such as how we handle anger), cognitive factors (such as whether we perceive an event as a challenge or threat), physical factors (such as how the body responds to stress), environmental factors (such as fog, fire, or snow), cultural factors (such as our learned beliefs about religion, health, and family), and coping strategies (such as what we do to manage stress).

There is no universally accepted definition of stress among stress theorists and researchers. An interactional view of stress, such as the one given above, is consistent with how nurses view human experiences. The theories of stress that follow in this chapter are those in common use. Although they do tell us a great deal about responses to stressful situations, these explanations are not necessarily consistent with nursing's orientation. The causes, the situational context in which the stressful event occurs, and the psychologic interpretation of the demanding situation must be considered in a holistic, humanistic approach to the client. These and other important factors related to stress are illustrated in FIGURE 8-2 ■. Axis IV of the DSM-IV-TR offers some general parameters for assessing the severity of stress (American Psychiatric Association [APA], 2000).

MEDIALINK Stress Webs

Conflict as a Stressor

The concept of conflict is useful in identifying the stresses that help cause disturbed coping patterns. Conflict often explains such behaviors as hesitation, vacillation, blocking, and fatigue. **Conflict**—having opposing desires, feelings, or goals—is frequently seen in the behavior of psychotic clients, who may have difficulty making even the simplest decisions.

These conflicts are the most likely to cause stress:

- Conflicts that involve social relations with significant people
- Conflicts that involve ethical standards
- Conflicts that involve meeting unconscious needs
- Conflicts that involve the problems of everyday family living

A conflict proceeds according to these four steps:

1. The person holds two goals simultaneously.
2. The person moves in relation to both of the goals, using (a) approach–avoidance movements or (b) avoidance–avoidance movements.
3. The person shows hesitation, vacillation, blocking, or fatigue.
4. Resolution occurs either temporarily or permanently.

Approach–Avoidance Conflict

When a person holds two incompatible goals at the same time, the goals usually constitute an either-or situation. If the person chooses one goal, the other goal is rejected or abolished automatically. The following is an example.

CLINICAL EXAMPLE

Mrs. Reynolds holds two goals. She wants to talk with the nurse about her fears of going back to work. At the same time, she wants not to be perceived as weak or "a bother." Mrs. Reynolds makes a movement in relation to her first goal—talking to the nurse—by walking up to her. When the nurse stops and turns toward her, Mrs. Reynolds asks some superficial question about the time of the next group meeting. In this way she avoids discussing her real concerns. When the nurse offers an opening to talk further, Mrs. Reynolds avoids the conversation she needs by saying she wants to rest. An hour later, she approaches the nurse with an apologetic but vague question about her medication.

Vacillation describes Mrs. Reynolds' behavior.

Principles That Explain Vacillation

To understand how vacillation (moving first one way and then another) comes about and what is going on during a conflict situation like the one described above, we need to understand the following four key principles:

1. As you near a desirable goal, the approach tendency is strengthened.
2. As you near an undesirable goal, the avoidance tendency is strengthened.
3. The strength of the avoidance tendency always increases more rapidly with nearness to the goal than does the strength of the approach tendency.
4. An increased need can strengthen both tendencies and intensify the conflict, whereas a decreased need can weaken both tendencies and lessen the conflict.

Avoidance–Avoidance Conflict

In avoidance–avoidance conflict, a person is faced with two undesirable goals at the same time. The person attempts to avoid the nearer of these two goals, but with the retreat from the nearer goal, the tendency to avoid the second goal increases. Unless the tendency to avoid one of the goals overpowers the tendency to avoid the other goal, or unless there is a third way out of the conflict, the person feels trapped by the conflict.

CLINICAL EXAMPLE

Robert Price, the 35-year-old son of well-to-do parents, was strongly attracted to "the good life." He wanted to live in a creative, esthetic environment, read good books, attend the opera, drink quality wine. Simultaneously, he wanted both to avoid working to earn the money for the lifestyle he desired and to not depend on his parents for support. His lifestyle became one of waiting to find a resolution to his conflict. He neither worked nor accepted "handouts" from his family, but his preferred lifestyle became one that he talked about rather than lived.

Using avoidance-oriented strategies can also pose both psychological and physical risks. A study of HIV-positive men and women on HAART (highly active antiretroviral therapy; see Chapter 25∞) demonstrated that those persons with greater negative mood and lower social support were more likely to use avoidance-oriented coping strategies (Weaver et al., 2005). Those who used avoidance-oriented coping strategies were also more likely to have poorer medication adherence and higher viral load.

BIOPSYCHOSOCIAL THEORIES OF STRESS

Each of the theories discussed in this section contributes to our understanding of stress and coping. However, none is complete in and of itself. Psychoneuroimmunology, the final theory discussed in this section, offers a comprehensive framework for understanding stress–disease relationships by taking the best of what the other theories offer and integrating them with the increasing body of evidence on how stress can alter immunologic functioning and, consequently, disease susceptibility and pathology.

The Fight-or-Flight Response to Stress

Beyond the routine and essential stress of everyday life, humans risk encountering undesirable or excess stress that threatens well-being and may even be life-threatening. They cope with such threats through either a fight (aggression) or flight (withdrawal) response. The **fight-or-flight** response was first discussed by the physician Walter Cannon in 1932, when he identified stress as an actual cause of disease.

Consider the following situation of extreme stress: A woman is walking down a dark, deserted street when a man with a knife emerges from the shadows just in front of her. Does she try to defend herself? Does she run away? Whichever action she takes is a result of a variety of physiologic responses to extreme danger. The following signs of adrenaline rush are likely to happen when a person faces such a situation:

- The heart beats strong and fast to circulate the blood more quickly.

- Airways in the lungs dilate so that the extra blood becomes oxygenated.
- Glucose is released into the blood by the liver.
- The blood vessels dilate to permit the oxygen-rich blood to get to where it is needed most.
- The pupils of the eyes dilate to let more light through, making vision more acute.
- Peristalsis in the gastrointestinal system is inhibited so that the energy peristalsis would consume becomes available for other purposes.
- Norepinephrine-containing cells in the central nervous system are active.
- The palms become sweaty; the mouth becomes dry.

Although these physiologic responses seem appropriate, imagine the wear and tear on the body if humans responded to all stress in all of these ways.

Many specialists in the field of behavioral medicine believe the fight-or-flight response to be maladaptive. For example, some forms of hypertension are caused or made worse by chronic activation of the heart due to either an excessive amount of stress or an excessive response to stress. See the section on Psychological Factors Affecting Medical Conditions later in this chapter for a discussion of the relationship between stress and hypertension, heart disease, and a variety of other medical conditions.

Selye's Stress–Adaptation Theory

Hans Selye, a Canadian endocrinologist and the most well-known and widely recognized stress researcher, developed a response-oriented framework for understanding how people respond to stress. According to Selye, each person has a limited amount of energy to use in dealing with stress. How quickly it is used and, therefore, how quickly one adapts to stress depend on several factors such as heredity, mental attitude, and lifestyle, among others.

Selye defined stress as the rate of wear and tear on the body (1956). He disputed the idea that only serious disease or injury causes stress. Selye believed that any emotion or activity requires a response or change in the individual. Stressors can be physical, chemical, physiologic, developmental, or emotional. Playing a game of tennis, going out in the rain without an umbrella, having an argument, and getting a promotion are all examples of stressful events. Life itself is basically stressful because it involves a process of adaptation to continual change.

Though the experience of adaptation is stressful, it is not necessarily harmful. Indeed, it can be exciting and rewarding under certain circumstances; and although we cannot avoid the stress of living, we can learn to minimize its damaging effects.

Selye observed that, regardless of the diagnosis, most physically ill people had certain symptoms in common; they lost their appetite, they lost weight, they felt and looked ill, they were anxious and fatigued, and they had aches and pains in their joints and muscles. A long series of experiments (1956) led to more objective evidence of actual body damage: enlargement of the adrenal glands; shrinkage of the thymus, spleen, and lymph nodes; and the appearance of bleeding gastric ulcers.

Feelings of anxiety, fatigue, or illness are subjective aspects of stress. Though stress itself cannot be perceived, Selye found that it can be objectively measured by the structural and chemical changes that it produces in the body. These changes are called the **general adaptation syndrome (GAS)** because when stress affects the whole person, the whole person must adjust to the changes. The GAS occurs in three stages: alarm, resistance, and exhaustion. The three stages of the GAS are illustrated and summarized in FIGURE 8-3 ■ on page 140.

Exhaustion may be reversible if the total body is not affected and if the person can eventually eliminate the source of stress. However, if stress is unrelieved, or if the body's defenses are totally involved, the person may not regain psychologic stability and may become physically ill.

Selye's theory has stimulated extensive research on the neuroendocrine mechanisms underlying stress. The consequent research into psychoendocrinology has brought Selye's model into question. Now classical research has demonstrated that neuroendocrine response differs for different stressors, and that there is individual variance in the sensitivity to psychosocial stimuli (Lazarus & Folkman, 1984; Smith, 1993). The response-based model of stress is not consistent with nursing's view that each individual is unique and people respond differently to similar situations (Fitzpatrick & Wilke, 2001).

Life Changes as Stressful Events

Most people are accustomed to thinking of untoward events as stressful, but they do not realize that desirable events such as job promotions, vacations, or outstanding personal achievements may also prove stressful. Holmes and Rahe (1967) studied life changes as stressful events to learn the amount of social readjustment required to cope with them. These authors believe that life events that require coping behavior tend to decrease a person's ability to handle illness or subsequent stress. Since Holmes and Rahe began their research, other investigators have raised cautions about applying this stimulus-based explanation indiscriminately. These cautions are discussed later in this section.

Their research assigned ratings to 43 different life changes, called *life change units (LCUs)*. They asked subjects to indicate what life changes had occurred in the past year and then to add up the points assigned to each one. According to these researchers, a low score indicated that the subject was not likely to have an adverse reaction. A "mild" score meant that there was a 30% chance that the person would manifest the impact of stress through physical symptoms. People in the "moderate" category had a 50% chance of a change in health status, and a "high" score meant an 80% chance of major illness in the next two years. High LCU scores also correlated with an increased probability of accidental injury. The following clinical example demonstrates the LCU model.

MEDIALINK Case Study: Midlife Crisis

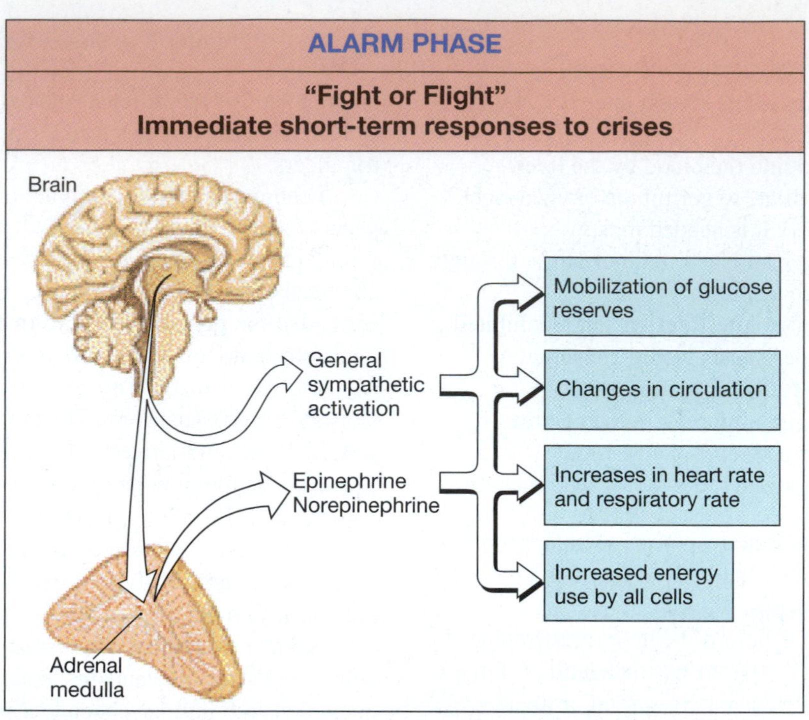

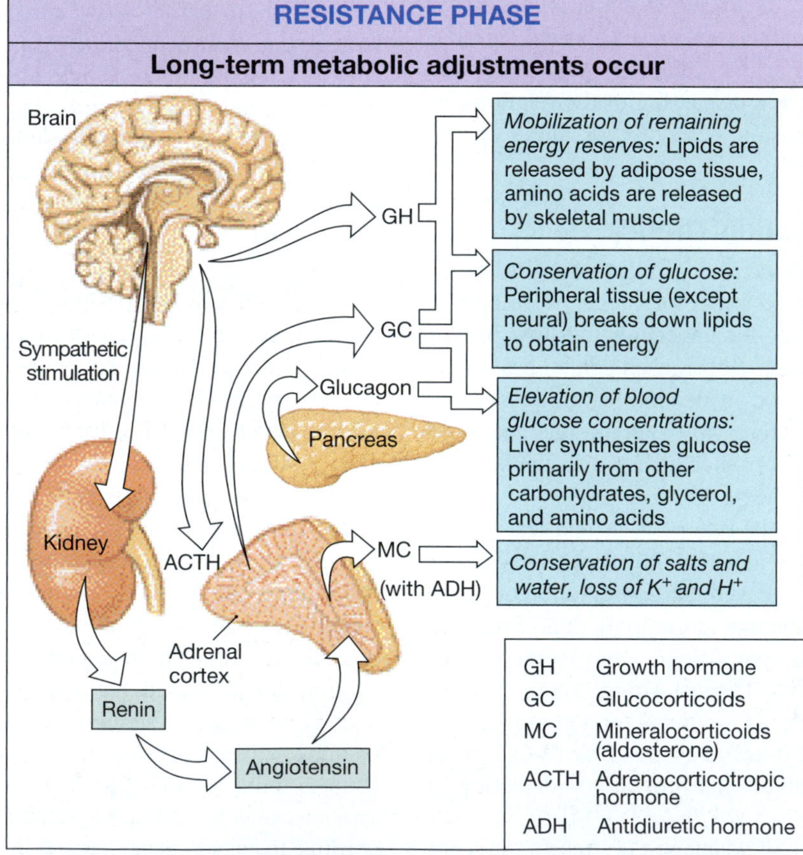

EXHAUSTION PHASE

Collapse of vital systems

Causes may include:
— Exhaustion of lipid reserves
— Inability to produce glucocorticoids
— Failure of electrolyte balance
— Cumulative structural or functional damage to vital organs

FIGURE 8-3 ■ Selye's general adaptation syndrome.

Source: Martini, F. H. (2000). *Fundamentals of anatomy and physiology* (5th ed.) (p. 613). Upper Saddle River, NJ: Prentice Hall.

CLINICAL EXAMPLE

Marcia Montes, a 22-year-old woman in group therapy, had recently been divorced from her husband (LCU 73) after attempting to achieve a marital reconciliation (LCU 45). Marcia's pregnancy (LCU 40) earlier in the year was uneventful, and the couple's healthy son was born on June 2 (LCU 39). At 6 weeks of age, the child suddenly and unexpectedly died in his crib (LCU 63). The couple began to argue frequently (LCU 35) before they made the decision to divorce. After the divorce, Marcia found herself short of funds (LCU 38) and went to work as a waitress in a pizza restaurant (LCU 36). She found it necessary to move to a less expensive apartment (LCU 20). In the period of one year, Marcia accumulated an LCU score of 390 and was in the high-risk group.

In the early 1970s, other researchers correlated life stress events and mental health. In a study of 720 households in a metropolitan area, Meyers (1972) found a relationship between a high number of life changes and changes in the mental status of individuals. For example, an increase in the number of life changes preceded worsening of psychiatric symptoms, whereas a decrease in life changes brought improvement. The more stressful the life changes, the greater the likelihood of mental illness. Meyers also found that entrance-related life events (those involving the addition of a new person into one's social sphere, perhaps through marriage or the birth of a child) produced less symptomatology than did exit-related events (those associated with the loss of a valued individual or status).

A review of the findings of recent research (Tosevski & Milovancevic, 2006) supports classic observations and case reports of a close link between stressful life events and physical health. They also stress the need for early recognition and timely management of stress-induced illnesses.

Application to Clinical Practice

Nurses applying the Holmes and Rahe model should be aware of the following cautions. This model is based on several assumptions that depict a person as a passive recipient of stress.

- It assumes that events affect all people in the same way, regardless of how the individuals perceive the event and regardless of what point they are at in their lives. For example, being pregnant has a much different meaning for an unmarried teenager than it does for a couple eager to conceive a child.
- It assumes that there is a common threshold beyond which disruption occurs.
- It assumes that the same event causes the same amount of stress for everyone.
- It assumes that the same amount of adaptation is required for each event among all people.
- It equates "change" with "stress."
- Some of the life events may be irrelevent to some people. For example, getting divorced or obtaining a mortgage may be irrelevent to most college students.

To understand the effects of life changes on health, you need to identify what each individual perceives as stressful. Only then can you help people become aware of the stress they face in their lives and plan for the future. In the clinical example that follows, we return to the example of Marcia Montes, who had accumulated an LCU score of 390.

CLINICAL EXAMPLE

During the course of group therapy, Marcia shared her desire to return to college and complete the junior and senior years of a medical technology program in which she had been enrolled before her marriage. To do so, she would have to make a number of changes: move to an apartment close to the college because she could not afford to own a car, change her working hours or job so that she could attend day classes, change her sleeping habits, change her recreational and social activities, and reduce her other expenses to pay school costs. The changes required would add almost 200 LCUs to her score.

In group therapy, Marcia was able to consider this information and reevaluate her goals. She decided to delay her return to school until she could get on her feet financially. She chose not to make any other changes in her life for the present time.

Clients can identify the life change events in their lives, much as Marcia did, to help decide when it might be advantageous or disadvantageous to engage in a life change. This knowledge helps them make responsible decisions about the directions their lives will take. The Partnering with Clients and Family feature on page 142 includes some strategies based on the interrelationship between life changes and stressful events.

Stress as a Transaction

Richard Lazarus, a pioneering theorist and researcher in stress, coping, and health, is known for his transaction-based approach to understanding stress. His view is reflected in the definition of stress given at the beginning of this chapter and his transactional model—stress is a process of complex interplay among the perceived demands of the environment and the perceived resources one has for meeting these demands—is consistent with nursing's holistic approach (Lazarus & Folkman, 1984). In the Lazarus model, perceived threat—what the person appraises as taxing or exceeding his or her resources and endangering his or her well-being—is the central characteristic of stressful situations because it threatens a person's most important goals and values (Monat & Lazarus, 1991). Once a person has perceived a threat, the person evaluates it by thinking about it. This process is termed *cognitive appraisal.* According to Lazarus, the process works like this:

1. The person assesses the potential for benefit, harm, loss, threat, or challenge in a situation. This is termed *primary appraisal.*
2. The person then evaluates his or her coping resources and options in the situation. This is termed *secondary appraisal.*

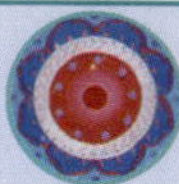

PARTNERING WITH CLIENTS AND FAMILY

TEACHING ABOUT LIFE CHANGES

You can assist clients by incorporating the guidelines below:

- Help clients recognize when a life change occurs.
- Encourage clients to think about the meaning of the change and identify some of the feelings associated with the change.
- Discuss with clients the different ways they might best adjust to the event.
- Encourage clients to take time in arriving at decisions.
- If possible, encourage clients to anticipate life changes and plan for them well in advance.
- Encourage clients to pace themselves. It can be done, even if they are in a hurry.
- Encourage clients to consider the accomplishment of a task as a part of daily living and to avoid looking at such an achievement as a stopping point or a time for letting down.

3. The person applies the coping resources and options at his or her disposal. This is termed *coping*.
4. The person engages in ongoing reinterpretation of the situation based on new information. This is termed *reappraisal*.

Cognitive appraisal and coping style are influenced by the person's culture. Providing culturally competent care requires understanding the client's perspective and recognizing that a client's cognitive appraisal of a situation may, and probably will, differ from your own.

Lazarus believes that stress depends not only on external conditions but also on the person's physical vulnerability and the adequacy of that person's coping styles.

Psychoneuroimmunology Framework

The most comprehensive framework for understanding the relationship between stress and disease and the biopsychosocial nature and complexity of the stress process is the **psychoneuroimmunology (PNI)** framework. As discussed in Chapter 6, PNI is concerned with interaction among the neurologic, endocrine, and immune systems and takes into account the nature of the influence of psychosocial factors on immune function and health outcomes. In other words, the PNI framework integrates the person–environment transactions of the stress process with the psychological and pathophysiological processess involved in stress.

What is emerging is a complex picture of the body's response to stress that involves several related pathways. Over the past few decades, corticotropin-releasing factor (CRF) signaling pathways have been shown to be the main coordinators of the endocrine, behavioral, and immune responses to stress (Taché & Bonaz, 2007). Cortisol, as well as adrenaline (recall the signs of adrenaline rush described earlier on page 138 that helps us to either take flight or to fight in the presence of immediate danger), is a stress hormone. Cortisol, however, is produced more slowly, and lingers longer in the bloodstream. Because it is primarily immunosuppressive, cortisol contributes to reductions in lymphocyte numbers and function and NK-cell activity (natural killer lymphocytes that attack infected cells and tumor cells in the body). In fact, chronic family stress has been shown to be related to increased illnesses in children (Wyman et al., 2007). Neuropeptides, the chemical messengers that are links between the mind and the body, are produced in the brain and in the endocrine and immune systems. The Caring for the Spirit special feature on page 676 in Chapter 25 is an example of the multifaceted nature of the psychoneuroimmunology framework.

Self-Healing Personalities

Neuropeptide manufacture is activated by positive mental states and suppressed by negative mental states. Several stress and coping-related studies have suggested that some people have *self-healing personalities,* while others have *disease-prone personalities*. Self-healers are emotionally stable people who bounce back from stressful situations (Friedman & VandenBos, 1992). These are people whom others describe as enthusiastic, joyful, secure, energetic, alert, and content. They are likable and have close, warm relationships with others. The nurse-theorist Jean Watson, whose nursing theory identifies the centrality of caring and is discussed in Chapter 2, also stresses people's self-healing potential (Pilkington, 2007).

Hardiness and Health

A now-classic study on hardiness and health found that individuals who have strong feelings of confidence in their ability to control circumstances, a willingness to see life events as challenges rather than as obstacles, and a strong commitment to the experiences and demands of daily living have fewer illnesses than those who lack these qualities (Kobasa, 1979). A recent study found that optimism has a stress-buffering effect in women with breast cancer (Ah, Kang, & Carpenter, 2007).

Disease-Prone Personalities

Disease-prone personalities, on the other hand, tend to display negative emotions. They are suspicious of others and tend to be chronically anxious, angry, or depressed. These chronic negative emotional patterns are linked with various physiologic changes such as activation of the sympathetic nervous system, increase in the level of cortisol, and suppression of the immune system, leading to increased vulnerability to illness.

ANXIETY

Anxiety is a state of varying degrees of uneasiness or discomfort. It is frequently coupled with guilt, doubts, fears, and obsessions. Beyond the mild level, anxiety is often described as a feeling of terror or dread; anxiety is believed to be the most uncomfortable feeling a person can experience. In fact, anxiety is so uncomfortable that most people try to get rid of it as soon as possible.

Anxiety is a potent force because the energy it provides can be converted into destructive or constructive action. When used constructively, anxiety can stimulate the action necessary to alter a stressful situation, fill a painful need, or arrange a compromise. A client who understands the source of anxiety is best able to use it constructively.

Neurobiologic Basis of Anxiety

Contemporary thinking about anxiety includes a neurobiologic component. Anxiety is now thought to result, at least in part, from dysregulation of one or more neurotransmitters and their receptors. Most research has focused on the BZ–GABA–chloride complex, although several other neurotransmitters and their receptors such as serotonin, norepinephrine, and the neuropeptide cholecystokinin may play a role in the development of anxiety. Other research using MRIs and PET scans focuses on brain structure itself. The neurobiologic component of anxiety is more fully discussed in Chapters 6 and 18∞.

Sources of Anxiety

Anxiety is an inevitable result of the attempt to maintain equilibrium in a changing world. People experience anxiety in many different situations and interpersonal relationships. However, the general causes of anxiety have been classified into two major kinds of threats, discussed in Box 8-1. It is crucial to understand that *either* actual *or* impending interference may cause anxiety; actual interference with a biologic or psychosocial need is not a necessary condition. All that is necessary is the *anticipation* of one of these major threats.

Threats to biologic integrity or to the fulfillment of such basic human needs as food, drink, warmth, and shelter are a general cause of anxiety. Threats to the security of self are not as easily categorized. In some instances, they are obvious; in others, they are more obscure because each person's sense of self is unique. To one person, power and prestige may be essential; to another, independence; to a third, being of service to others.

Consider the last category—being of service to others.

CLINICAL EXAMPLE

Mrs. C, a nurse, is convinced that a client would feel much better if he expressed his fears to her. But no matter how often she provides the opportunity, he insists, "This is not the time to talk about it," and thwarts her attempt. She is not able to help him in a way that is important to her sense of self. In addition, she believes that the unit's nurse manager (whose skills she admires) expects her to have been successful in this endeavor.

Box 8-1 General Causes of Anxiety

1. Threats to biologic integrity: actual or impending interference with basic human needs such as the needs for food, drink, or warmth
2. Threats to the security of the self:
   a. Unmet expectations important to self-integrity
   b. Unmet needs for status and prestige
   c. Anticipated disapproval by significant others
   d. Inability to gain or reinforce self-respect or gain recognition from others
   e. Guilt, or discrepancies between self-view and actual behavior

Mrs. C is worried and anxious. When unmet needs or expectations related to essential values (such as being of service to the client) are coupled with the actual or anticipated disapproval of others who are important (the nurse manager), anxiety is generated.

Anxiety as a Continuum

Many theorists conceptualize anxiety as a continuum (Figure 8-4 ■). Mild to moderate anxiety can be functionally effective in that it helps us focus our attention and generates energy and motivation. Thus, anxiety is an aspect of problem solving in that it alerts us to the need to concentrate our resources. However, severe anxiety and panic narrow our attention to a crippling degree. Under these conditions alertness is greatly reduced, and learning does not usually take place.

Mild Anxiety

Mild anxiety helps one deal constructively with stress. A mildly anxious person has a broad perceptual field because mild anxiety heightens the ability to take in sensory stimuli. Such a person is more alert to what is going on and can make better sense of what is happening with others and the environment. The senses take in more; the person hears

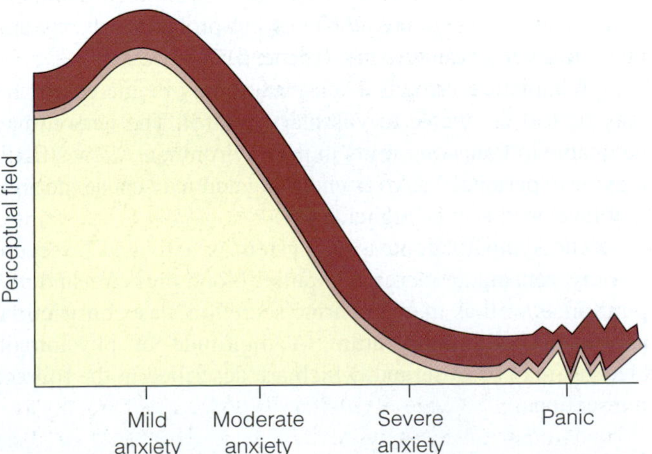

Figure 8-4 ■ The effect of anxiety on the perceptual field. Notice that the perceptual field is increased in mild anxiety, becomes increasingly constricted as anxiety increases, and is completely disrupted at the panic level.

better, sees better, and makes logical connections between events. The person feels relatively safe and comfortable. Because learning is easier when one is mildly anxious, mild anxiety helps clients learn, for instance, how best to administer their own insulin. Mild anxiety can also help a nursing student review psychiatric–mental health nursing before a final examination.

Moderate Anxiety

In moderate anxiety, a person remains alert, but the perceptual field narrows. The moderately anxious person shuts out the events on the periphery while focusing on central concerns.

CLINICAL EXAMPLE

A nursing student who is moderately anxious about the final examination may be able to focus so intently on studying that she or he is not distracted by an argument between roommates, loud music on the stereo, and a rousing chase scene on television. The student shuts out the chaos in the environment and focuses on what is of central personal importance—preparing for the exam.

This process of taking in some sensory stimuli while excluding others is called **selective inattention**.

People also use selective inattention to cope with anxiety-provoking stimuli. This phenomenon may account for the anxious preoperative client who fails to remember what the nurse said about postoperative pain or about the need to cough and deep-breathe after surgery.

Although the perceptual field is narrowed and the person sees, hears, and grasps less, there is an element of voluntary control. Moderately anxious individuals can, with direction, focus on what they have previously shut out.

Severe Anxiety

In severe anxiety, sensory reception is greatly reduced. Severely anxious people focus on small or scattered details of an experience. They have difficulty in problem solving, and their ability to organize is also reduced. They seldom have the complete picture. Selective inattention may be increased and may be less amenable to voluntary control. The person may be unable to focus on events in the environment. New stimuli may be experienced as overwhelming and may cause the anxiety level to rise even higher.

The sympathetic nervous system is activated in severe anxiety, causing an increase in pulse, blood pressure, and respiration as well as in epinephrine secretion, vasoconstriction, and even body temperature. A multitude of physiologic changes may be observed, which are described in the following sections.

Panic

The panic level of anxiety is characterized by a completely disrupted perceptual field. Panic has been described as a disintegration of the personality experienced as intense terror. Details may be enlarged, scattered, or distorted. Logical thinking and effective decision making may be impossible. The person in panic is unable to initiate or maintain goal-directed action. Behavior may appear purposeless, and communication may be unintelligible.

Assessing Anxiety

Anxiety can be assessed in the physiologic, cognitive, and emotional/behavioral dimensions. This observation illustrates the relationship between the mind and the body. Anxiety is a multidimensional phenomenon in that the total person is involved in every aspect of it. Objective data, particularly nursing observations, may be critical because of the nature of anxiety. Selective inattention interferes with the client's awareness of anxiety and ability to give accurate reports. Families and friends also can contribute data useful to the assessment of anxiety.

Physiologic Dimension

Observations of the client's physiologic state are likely to indicate autonomic nervous system responses, particularly sympathetic effects. Sympathetic nervous system dominance is associated with arousal as occurs during anxiety or as the body's response to a physical emergency. The parasympathetic nervous system maintains normal, smooth functioning. Various organs may be affected, such as the adrenal medulla, heart, blood vessels, lungs, stomach, colon, rectum, salivary glands, liver, pupils of the eyes, and sweat glands. FIGURE 8-5 ■ illustrates the sympathetic and parasympathetic nervous systems in detail. Anxious clients may have an increased heart rate, increased blood pressure, difficulty breathing, sweaty palms, trembling, dry mouth, "butterflies in the stomach" or a "lump in the throat," as well as other symptoms.

Laboratory tests are not routinely done to evaluate anxiety because observation is faster and more accurate. However, anxiety affects the results of laboratory tests done for other purposes. Blood studies may show increased adrenal function, elevated levels of glucose and lactic acid, and decreased parathyroid function and oxygen and calcium levels. Urinary studies may indicate increased levels of epinephrine and norepinephrine.

Cognitive Dimension

Assessment of cognitive function may indicate difficulty in logical thinking, narrowed or distorted perceptual field, selective inattention or dissociation, lack of attention to details, difficulty concentrating, or difficulty focusing. The level of anxiety determines the extent to which cognitive function is affected. Mild, moderate, severe, or panic level of anxiety is assessed according to the descriptions earlier in this chapter.

Emotional/Behavioral Dimension

In the emotional/behavioral dimension, clients may be irritable, angry, withdrawn, and restless, or they may cry. The affective response can often be assessed through the client's subjective description. Clients may describe themselves as "on edge," "uptight," "jittery," "nervous," "worried," or "tense."

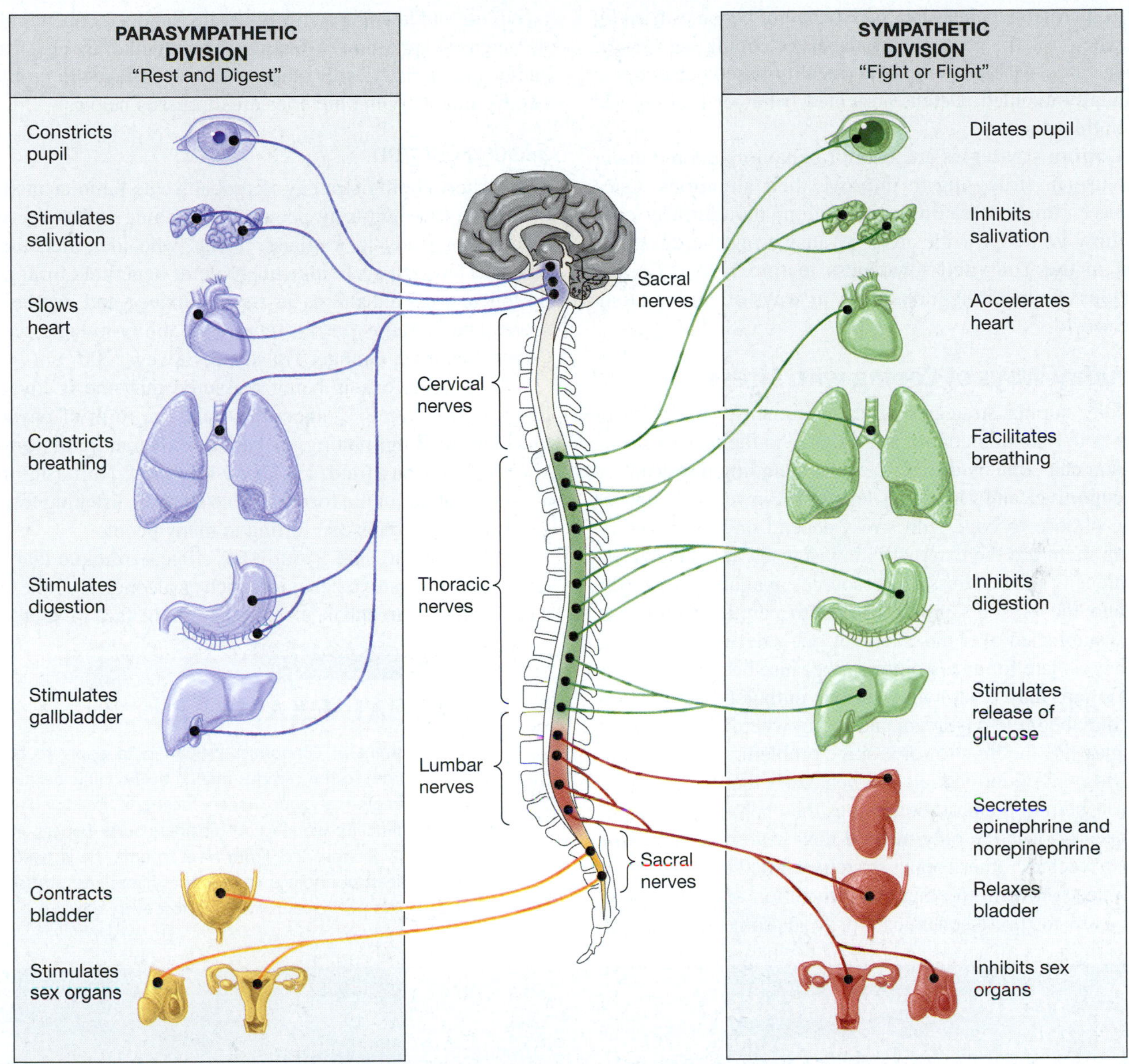

FIGURE 8-5 ■ Involuntary control of bodily functions. The autonomic nervous system has two divisions, the sympathetic and the parasympathetic, which exercise automatic control over the body's organs, generally in opposing ways. The parasympathetic generally has inhibitory or relaxing effects, while the sympathetic has stimulatory effects. Axons of the parasympathetic division emerge not only from the spinal cord, but from the brain as well.

Source: Krogh, D. (2000). *Biology: A guide to the natural world* (p. 515). Upper Saddle River, NJ: Prentice Hall.

They may feel dizzy or faint and may experience a feeling of impending doom as if something terrible were about to happen.

COPING WITH STRESS AND ANXIETY

Nurses can be helpful if they understand the changes their clients are undergoing. Reactions to threatening situations, such as illness and hospitalization, can be divided into two general categories: task-oriented responses and defense-oriented responses.

When we feel competent to deal with stress and the situation is not too threatening to our sense of self, our behavior tends to be *task-oriented*. Task-oriented behavior is geared toward problem solving. Consider the situation of a student who is majoring in mathematics and fails his courses. If he is not too frightened by the possibility that he may not be suited for a career in this field, he can assess the situation and change his major. This is a task-oriented reaction. It is based on a realistic appraisal of the situation and involves a series of carefully thought-out judgments about what course of behavior would be most effective.

When we feel inadequate to cope with stress and the situation is extremely threatening to our sense of self, we tend to engage in *defense-oriented* behavior. The diagnosis of a terminal illness, for instance, may be so overwhelming that a person must temporarily defend against acknowledging this reality. Everyone uses defense-oriented behavior from time to time as a protective measure. Such behavior becomes harmful only when it is the predominant means of coping with stress. In such cases, problem-solving and reality-based behavior are continually avoided. Defense-oriented behavior is discussed later in this chapter.

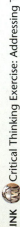

Coping strategies are a set of behaviors people under stress use in struggling to improve their situations. Once you have finished reading this section, thoughtfully consider how you cope with stress by answering the questions posed in the Your Self-Awareness feature below. Coping strategies can be thought of simply as ways of getting along in the world.

Everyday Ways of Coping with Stress

Everyday coping strategies offer an immense repertoire of defenses to maintain control and balance in the face of stress. A person can cope on different levels, including physical, social, cognitive, and emotional levels. However, the devices people choose to cope with stress depend on many factors. Among them are the external circumstances, the suddenness and intensity of the stress, the resources available to the person, and the person's predisposition to certain coping patterns, established over the course of one's development. One man who is late for an appointment because he gets caught in a traffic jam may react with a furious outburst of anger. Another may begin to daydream and forget where he is going. A third may use the time to solve some problem.

Most often, individuals use behaviors that have worked well for them in the past. Sometimes they behave in a certain way because it is the only method they have of coping with stress or because other coping strategies failed to work. Some people learn to turn to others for protection and nurturance; some learn to turn to chemicals or food; some rely on self-discipline and keeping a stiff upper lip; others feel better after the intense expression of feelings; some withdraw physically and/or emotionally; still others exercise or talk the problem out. Common coping methods are discussed below.

Seeking Comfort

The earliest coping strategy is probably the familiar method of turning to a nurturing person for soothing and protecting. In a recent study in England, clients who identified themselves as having psychological problems benefitted from gentle touch, with reductions in stress, anxiety, and depression scores and increases in relaxation and ability-to-cope scores (Weze, Leathard, Grange, Tiplady, & Stevens, 2007).

Receiving love is being reassured that one is lovable. Love from supportive others may take the form of physical touching, rocking, patting, or verbal reassurances of various kinds ("Don't be afraid, I'll stay with you"). Nurturing may also come about in the form of Bible study or listening to religious tapes, which is comforting to many people.

Some people, like Scott in the clinical example that follows, use less positive behaviors such as alcohol, nicotine, and other chemicals to enhance well-being in the face of stress.

CLINICAL EXAMPLE

Scott is a student of economics preparing to apply to law school. He comes to the campus mental health clinic because of difficulty sleeping; a vague, uneasy feeling of dread and apprehension; difficulty working on his final course papers; irritability; and hypervigilance. From time to time, he is sweaty and feels his heart pounding. He describes himself as "stressed out" and smokes pot to calm down almost every day.

MEDIALINK Critical Thinking Exercise: Addressing Teen Anxiety

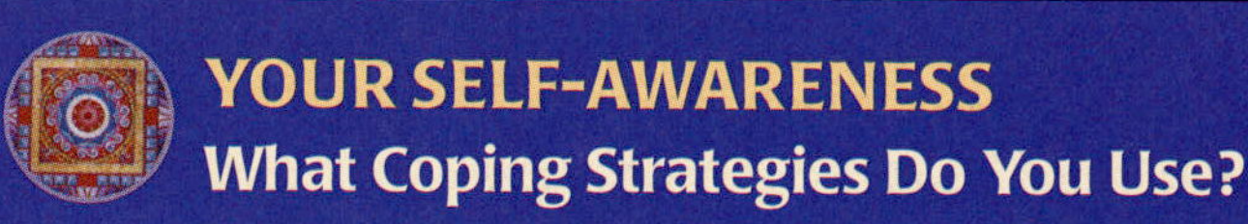

YOUR SELF-AWARENESS
What Coping Strategies Do You Use?

When you are feeling competent to deal with stress and the situation is not too threatening to your sense of self, which task-oriented coping strategies do you use? Review the everyday ways of coping with stress discussed on pages 146–148 and answer the following questions:

- Which everyday ways of coping with stress do you use most often? Be specific.
- Can you identify a pattern or common thread among them?
- What effects do they have on your sense of comfort or well-being?
- What effects do they have on your interpersonal relationships (include professional relationships)?

When you are feeling inadequate to cope with stress and the situation is extremely threatening to your sense of self, which defense-oriented behaviors do you use? Review the defense-oriented ways of coping (defense mechanisms) discussed on pages 149–156 and answer the following questions:

- Which defense-oriented ways of coping do you use most often? Be specific.
- Can you identify a pattern or common thread among them?
- What effects do they have on your sense of comfort or well-being?
- What effects do they have on your interpersonal relationships (include professional relationships)?

Staying healthy and coping adequately with stress are influenced by several factors, called generalized resistance resources (GRRs), that help in managing tension. Review the GRRs discussed on pages 148–149, and answer the following questions:

- Which GRRs most commonly influence the way in which you manage tension? Be specific.
- In which ways have these GRRs influenced your life course?
- How can you mobilize these personal resources to strengthen control over your life and your sense of personal coherence?
- What effects do they have on your interpersonal relationships (including your professional relationships)?

This category also includes eating in times of stress and for general support. While comfort foods can soothe in the short term, they can sabotage the long-term stress response by increasing the number of inflammatory proteins in the body. In addition to comfort foods, alcohol, nicotine, and other chemicals are often used to enhance well-being in the face of stress. Many theorists view these alternatives as substitutes for the dependent comfort of being a baby in the care of a nurturing parent.

Relying on Self-Discipline

Whereas some people under stress tend to turn to the comfort of friendly company, food, or alcohol, all of which are reminiscent of childhood dependence, others rely on self-discipline. Self-control ranks high in the value system of many cultures and subcultures. This coping style involves pride in the ability to laugh off problems, endure frustrations, and discount anxiety. Keep a stiff upper lip, bite the bullet, and get over it are all admonitions that people address to themselves when self-discipline is their patterned response to stress. These people are unlikely to want the company of supportive others and may even push them away. They are often unresponsive when others seek comfort from them, for they see such dependent behavior as weak.

Intense Expression of Feeling

Crying, swearing, and laughing all tend to relieve tension. Swearing loses its usefulness as an escape valve if it becomes a habit. This is less true of both crying and laughing. Crying and laughing tend to release energy and exert a soothing effect on a person who is experiencing tension.

Avoidance and Withdrawal

While some people find it hard to sleep when they are under tension, others react to worries, bad news, or an argument with somnolence. Still others respond with a form of waking sleep like apathy or emotional withdrawal, which accomplishes the same thing.

Talking It Out

Many people relieve tension by talking it out. Talking implies establishing and maintaining a contact of sorts with another human being. In addition, it enables new ideas to emerge and new perspectives to be entertained. Obviously, this device is the medium of most therapeutic intervention. This has profound implications for nursing because nurses are the health care providers who spend the most time with clients. It also has profound implications for clients whose communication is dysfunctional or whose ability to communicate freely is restricted. Psychiatric clients generally fall into these categories.

Privately Thinking It Through

Some people believe that the unexamined life is not worth living. When faced with a problem that causes them anxiety, these individuals become introspective about it. The rationalizations that emerge serve as effective tension relievers.

Working It Off

Physical activity to relieve tension may range from simple gestures such as finger tapping, floor pacing, and door slamming to activities purposely designed to alter the tension-producing circumstances, such as aerobic exercise. In addition, some tense individuals feel a lot of aggressive energy. Physical exertion in the form of demanding sports, like jogging or racquetball, or manual labor, like scrubbing the floor, is a way to use this energy constructively. Even low-impact physical activity resulted in significant improvements in stress, mood, and several quality-of-life indices in a study of older adults (Starkweather, 2007).

Engaging in Self-Healing Mind/Body Practices

Increasing numbers of people are integrating self-healing practices such as yoga, meditation, massage, visualization, and relaxation exercises into their everyday lives. While Western medicine continues its explosive growth in psychobiologic knowledge and technology, more of us are finding that these ancient principles and practices have significant therapeutic value. Meditation has been found to improve the quality and duration of sleep and to improve organ transplant recipients' overall health and well-being (Kreitzer, Gross, Ye, Russas, & Treesak, 2005). It has also been associated with enhanced quality of life and decreased stress symptoms in breast and prostate cancer clients (Carlson, Specca, Patel, & Goodey, 2004), and the relief of depressive symptoms in women with fibromyalgia (Sephton et al., 2007). A thorough discussion of healing practices is in Chapter 32.

MediaLink Care Plan: New Nurse's Worry

Spirituality and Prayerfulness

We define spirituality as the search for self-transcendence—the search for meaning and purpose through connection with others, nature, and/or a Supreme Being. Spirituality may, but does not always, involve religious structure or traditions. Moore (1994) suggests that we "live artfully" in order to find spirituality, that is, to attend to the small things in life that invite contemplation. A failure to let the world in, to perceive it and to engage it fully, leads to the emptiness that some people feel in their lives.

Many people's spirituality includes prayerfulness. Prayer can be individual or communal, private or public. People pray for different reasons—to ask for something for oneself, to ask for something for others, to repent of wrongdoing and ask for forgiveness, to give honor and praise to a Higher Power, to offer thanksgiving. Recent research shows that praying can positively affect high blood pressure, the course and extent of heart attacks, migraine headaches, and anxiety. Further, nursing activities that support prayer as a coping measure may support mental health (Meisenhelder & Chandler, 2000).

Using Symbolic Substitutes

Stress may be relieved by ascribing symbolic values to acts or objects. These acts or objects may or may not have other meanings. There are symbolic devices for the management of tension in religious practices such as confession, prayer, or sacrifice. For some people, the automobile has a symbolic significance; others ascribe symbolic significance to their annual income or their physical appearance.

The list is almost endless, but the principle is always the same. Some people attach a meaning beyond the obvious one to objects, experiences, and people, through which they find a means to reduce their tensions.

Somatizing

Many organs of the body have an expression and communication function. This is sometimes known as *somatizing* or *organ language*. Some organs communicate their messages only to their owner. For example, the heart may communicate by means of palpitation. Other demonstrations are public, such as blushing or stuttering. Urination and defecation, increased sweating, and altered sexual activity are other familiar examples of organ language.

Coping Resources

Early research on coping was concerned with how people respond to specific stresses in a laboratory setting. More recent studies that consider the whole being in interaction with the environment have led to viewing coping as a dynamic process that involves the demands and restrictions on a person as well as the resources available.

Sense of Coherence

According to Antonovsky (1991), the resources that people use to successfully cope with the stresses in life combine and converge to form what Antonovsky terms a sense of coherence. It is this sense of coherence that strengthens resilience and seems to be a health-promoting resource (Eriksson & Lindstrom, 2006). Antonovsky's theory revolves around how people manage to stay healthy, rather than why people get sick.

A sense of coherence comes about when a person has three attributes (Antonovsky, 1996):

1. *Comprehensibility:* the ability to understand the things that happen in life (the cognitive or thinking aspect of coherence)
2. *Manageability:* having trust that things will work out well because one has the resources to meet demands (the behavioral or action aspect of coherence)
3. *Meaningfulness:* the motivation to invest time and energy in life's challenges (the feeling aspect of coherence)

In other words, accenting the positive reduces the negative effects of stressful situations.

Antonovsky's theory fits well with psychiatric–mental health nursing's holistic perspective. The theory is not age-dependent. Both young adults (Hart, Wilson, & Hittner, 2006) and older adults (Schneider, Driesch, Kruse, Nehen, & Heuft, 2006) with a sense of coherence reported a feeling of well-being.

Encouraging a sense of coherence promotes the positive aspects of coping. What are the resources that can be encouraged or enhanced through helpful interventions? People stay healthy or cope adequately with stress because they possess what Antonovsky calls *generalized resistance resources (GRRs),* factors in the person, group, or organization that help in managing tension. The Evidence-Based Practice feature illustrates how nurses can apply Antonovsky's theory in helping clients influence the course of their lives.

Physical and Biochemical GRRs

Physical and biochemical GRRs are physiologic characteristics, such as genetic features and levels of immunity. These GRRs also include interaction of the nervous and endocrine systems that help in adaptation: for example, interactions involving ACTH, thyroid-stimulating hormone (TSH), vasopressin, norepinephrine, and insulin and their influence on human behavior. Not only are individuals different in their genetic and biochemical makeup, but the physiologic effects of illness and stress may also alter a person's ability to use physical and biochemical GRRs positively.

Artifactual and Material GRRs

Material goods and relative wealth constitute the *artifactual and material GRRs;* having these attributes makes it easier to cope with illness. Money helps to ensure the best health care available. Effective coping is often interrelated with one's socioeconomic status simply because the higher the status, the greater the resources to help the person cope. For example, household help not only relieves an ill person's worries but also reduces the practical burden.

Cognitive GRRs

Cognitive GRRs have to do with intelligence and knowledge. When people know about stressors, they can avoid them. They can also predict when periods of stress are imminent and thus reduce their impact. Knowing what community services are available is also a cognitive GRR.

Emotional GRRs

People who are self-aware—who know their own capacities and potentials and have a well-developed sense of themselves—possess *emotional GRRs*. Emotional GRRs determine the extent of psychological hardiness. In general, they have to do with how competent and self-assured one feels.

Valuative and Attitudinal GRRs

Valuative and attitudinal GRRs are the products of a person's culture and environment. People are apt to respond in learned ways. The attitudinal aspect also is related to how flexible, rational, and farsighted the person is. The more rational or accurate one's appraisal of a threatening situation and the more flexible one is in approaching the situation and envisioning the consequences, the greater one's resources for coping.

Interpersonal–Relational GRRs

Interpersonal–relational GRRs are available social support systems. The greater a person's social contacts, the greater the social resources available to augment the ability to deal with stress. Love, affection, and nurturance are hallmarks of interpersonal–relational GRRs.

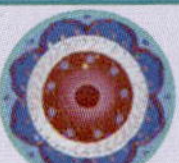

EVIDENCE-BASED PRACTICE

PSYCHOEDUCATION FOR MANAGING STRESS

As the nurse in a day treatment unit located in a suburb of a large city in the southeastern United States, you are especially aware of the difficulty your older clients have in handling stress. Most of your clients are diagnosed with a psychotic disorder and have difficulty maintaining relationships with friends and family and finding or keeping a job. Thus, most have become marginalized, and the day treatment unit has become the core of their daily activities.

You understand that it is important to strengthen life control among those who have become marginalized. People who are in charge of their lives have a sense of coherence. They are more likely to be able to cope with stressful situations in ways that decrease, or even eliminate, their distress. To help your clients develop a sense of coherence and strengthen their resilience to stress, you develop a psychoeducation program for them, focusing on the following:

1. Achieving understanding of the internal environment (what thoughts, feelings, and wishes drive the individual)
2. Achieving understanding of the external environment (what forces affect what an individual is able to accomplish)
3. Exploring human relationships to include client–family, client–friend, client–client, client–employer, client–staff, client–landlord, and whatever other dyads are active relationships or potential relationships in the clients' lives
4. Exploring the meaning of present events, that is, focusing on the here-and-now, rather than the there-and-then, to gain an understanding of what the stressors are in the lives of the clients
5. Partaking in a program of regular physical activity that includes flexibility training and walking in place

The psychoeducation program you developed is based on the following research citations:

Schneider, G., Driesch, G., Kruse, A., Nehen, H. G., & Heuft, G. (2006). Old and ill and still feeling well? Determinants of subjective well-being in > or = 60 year olds: The role of the sense of coherence. *American Journal of Geriatric Psychiatry, 14*(10), 850–859.

Starkweather, A. R. (2007). The effects of exercise on perceived stress and IL.-6 levels among older adults. *Biological Research for Nursing, 8*(3), 186–194.

CRITICAL THINKING QUESTIONS

1. What actual activities would help clients to understand their internal environment and explore human relationships?
2. What does it mean to explore the meaning of present events by focusing on the here-and-now?

Macrosociocultural GRRs

Institutional structures that facilitate coping are called *macrosociocultural GRRs*. These resources include government programs such as Aid to Dependent Children as well as cultural institutions such as death and funeral rites, religious rituals, and ceremonies.

Defense-Oriented Ways of Coping: Defense Mechanisms

The coping strategies described earlier are considered normal. They are simply ways of getting along. In some people, however, what passes for a normal adjustment is actually a very tenuous one with few outlets for controlled aggression, few love objects, few opportunities for satisfaction and growth. These people find it more and more difficult to cope with additional stress. Ultimately, the external stress the person is trying unsuccessfully to ward off is matched by a mounting internal stress. The person suffers both from increased anxiety and from the strain on overworked stabilizers. And what happens to the person who has no one to talk with, who can't jog five miles, or who can't laugh off the problem?

When a person is unable to ward off stress or reduce tension in the usual way, anxiety mounts as the person feels increasingly inadequate to cope with the situation. Under these circumstances, the person is more likely to engage in *defense-oriented behavior*. Defense-oriented behavior is not a specific attempt to solve a problem; it consists of using mental mechanisms to lessen uncomfortable feelings of anxiety and to prevent pain regardless of cost. These characteristic mental mechanisms are commonly called **defense mechanisms**. Defense mechanisms are automatic psychological processes that protect the self by allowing the person to deny or distort a stressful event or to restrict awareness and reduce the sense of emotional involvement. But they can also interfere with rational decision making. People who use defense mechanisms are excluding some information about the situation they are in. They are also denying their own feelings about it.

Defense mechanisms are mostly unconscious and often inflexible coping patterns that protect a person through intrapsychic (coming from within) distortions that are really self-deceptions. The person usually has little awareness of what is happening or even less control over events. Although these reactions may help keep the lid on anxiety, they also limit the ability to grow from and savor the experience, they interfere with rational decision making and the ability to work productively, and they impair and erode interpersonal relationships. Even adaptive devices can go wrong.

Because human behavior is so complex and varied, defense mechanisms can be classified in many ways. Often, they are classified according to whether they are simple or complex, whether they are most likely to arise in a specific phase of development, or whether they are commonly associated with a particular form of psychopathology. Definitions of various defense mechanisms overlap, and the same observed

TABLE 8-1 ■ Defense Mechanisms

Name	Definition	Example
Denial	Blocking out painful or anxiety-inducing events or feelings	A manager tells an employee he may have to fire him. On the way home, the employee shops for a new car.
Displacement	Discharging pent-up feelings on people less dangerous than those who initially aroused the emotion	A student who has received a low grade on a term paper blows up at his girlfriend when she asks about his grade.
Dissociation	Handling emotional conflicts, or internal or external stressors, by a temporary alteration of consciousness or identity	A woman has amnesia for the events surrounding a fatal automobile accident in which she was the speeding driver.
Fantasy	Symbolic satisfaction of wishes through nonrational thought	A student struggling through graduate school thinks about a prestigious, high-paying job she wants.
Identification	Unconscious assumption of similarity between oneself and another	After hospitalization for minor surgery, a girl decides to be a nurse.
Intellectualization	Separating an emotion from an idea or thought because the emotional reaction is too painful to be acknowledged	A man learns from his doctor that he has cancer. He studies the physiology and treatment of cancer without experiencing any emotion.
Introjection	Acceptance of another's values and opinions as one's own	A woman who prefers a simple lifestyle assumes the materialistic, prestige-oriented values of her husband.
Projection	Attributing one's own unacceptable feelings and thoughts to others	A man who is quite critical of others thinks that people are joking about his appearance.
Rationalization	Falsification of experience through the construction of logical or socially approved explanations of behavior	A man cheats on his income tax return and tells himself it's all right because everyone does it.
Reaction formation	Unacceptable feelings disguised by repression of the real feeling and by reinforcement of the opposite feeling	A woman who dislikes her mother-in-law is always very nice to her.
Repression	Unconsciously keeping unacceptable feelings out of awareness	A man is jealous of a good friend's success but is unaware of his feelings.
Suppression	Consciously keeping unacceptable feelings and thoughts out of awareness	A student taking an examination is upset about an argument with her boyfriend but puts it out of her mind so she can finish the test.

behavior may often be explained by more than one type of defense. And people do not use one method of defense at a time; they usually rely on a combination of defenses. For study purposes, the common defense mechanisms discussed here are repression, suppression, dissociation, identification, introjection, projection, denial, fantasy, rationalization, reaction formation, displacement, and intellectualization. They are summarized in TABLE 8-1 ■.

Repression

Repression, the basis of all defense mechanisms, is the dynamic behind much of "forgetting." When people repress, they unconsciously exclude distressing emotions, thoughts, or experiences from awareness. Repression bars access to conscious awareness of feelings and thoughts that would cause anxiety and disrupt the self-concept. It also affords protection from a sudden trauma until the person can deal with the shock. From the individual's point of view, a repressed memory is "forgotten" and cannot be deliberately brought to awareness (see the Caring for the Spirit feature). Although the repressed feelings remain unconscious, they continue to exert pressure for expression. The self tries to maintain the repression, but in people experiencing extreme stress or anxiety, or in febrile (feverish) or toxic states, repression may begin to fail. Clients who are intoxicated by alcohol or drugs or who are emerging from anesthesia may verbalize feelings that they usually repress.

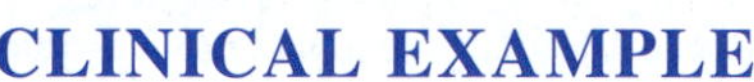

CLINICAL EXAMPLE

Susan was raped. She was brought to an outpatient clinic by her roommate. Susan said she felt very anxious and could not recall the circumstances surrounding her rape or what the rapist looked like. Her use of repression protected her from facing her fears and humiliation.

Nursing Intervention Strategies Nursing intervention in such cases should be supportive and protective of the client's defenses. After the initial shock has lessened and the client's anxiety level has been reduced, you can help the client examine the traumatic event.

Suppression

Suppression is an intentional act that helps keep thoughts, feelings, wishes, or actions that cause anxiety out of conscious awareness. Suppression is the conscious form of repression.

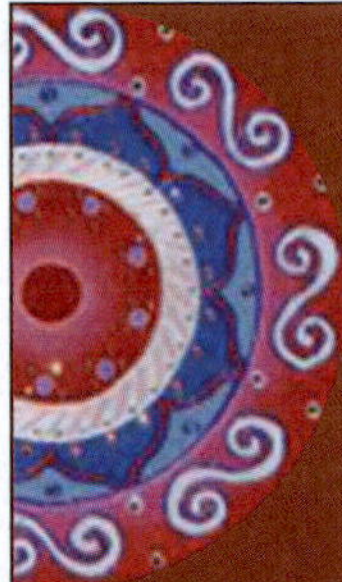

CARING FOR THE SPIRIT

Repressed Memories or False Memories?

Over 100 years ago, Sigmund Freud proposed that we actively and deliberately bury painful or dangerous memories beyond the reach of consciousness. He called this process repression.

According to Freud, repressed memories influence behavior, thinking, and emotions, and produce mental symptoms. Early in his career Freud wrote that sexual abuse in childhood was common and was the cause of repression. This abuse, and the resulting repression, caused the "hysteria" he diagnosed in his patients. After 1897, Freud abruptly abandoned his theory on repression. Instead, he said, children have fantasies of being seduced. These imagined seductions, according to Freud, cause internal conflict, and repression is a way of coping with this internal conflict.

It is unclear why Freud abandoned his theory. Some of his critics believe that Freud bowed to social pressure and the threat of professional ostracism because the notion of rampant childhood sexual abuse was outrageous. Others of his critics believed that Freud himself distorted his patients' stories because of his own psychological problems.

To understand the concept of repression, we need to understand how memory works. Memories are stored in a portion of each of the millions of neurons in the brain. Each neuron represents a little bit of memory. Because the brain is such a complex organ, it parcels out bits and pieces of an experience to different parts of the brain. For example, memories of sound are parceled out to the auditory cortex, memories of appearance to the visual cortex, memories of sensation to the sensory cortex, memories of smell to the olfactory cortex, and source memory to the frontal cortex. All scattered memory fragments remain physically linked. It is the limbic system that takes on the job of assembling these bits and pieces. The limbic system actually acts as a neural file clerk by pulling memory fragments from various file drawers. Intensely traumatic events produce unusually strong nerve connections.

Memory can go awry if the terror of an experience is so great that the biologic processes underlying information storage are disrupted. However, the right biologic stimulus can set the nerve circuits firing and trigger fear. The source of the fear is *not* remembered. Memory blocks come at great cost. They leave a person without an explanation for bewildering emotional distress that causes turmoil.

Memory can also be confounded; that is, snippets of memory from a real event can be interwoven with snippets of an imagined event. Recent research has demonstrated that the mere suggestion that you could have once been lost in a shopping mall can leave a memory trace in the brain. This memory trace can then become linked to the memory of a friend's or sibling's story of being lost or a fairy tale such as Hansel and Gretel, as well as actual memories of shopping malls. Under stress and over time, the knowledge that being lost in a mall was only a suggestion deteriorates. If you're asked at a later time if you were ever lost in a mall, your brain will activate these assorted images, and eventually you "remember" being lost in a mall as a child.

These findings—that memories are open to faulty recollection or that they can be created through a suggestion from another—have caused great distress for survivors of childhood sexual abuse who experience the phenomenon called **recovered memory**. Recovered memories of childhood sexual abuse are those that emerge into consciousness after being repressed for a period of time, sometimes for years. Imagine what it must be like having recalled long-forgotten memories of painful and humiliating sexual abuse by a trusted or loved adult. Imagine further what it must be like to have your unsettling memories viewed with suspicion. You might feel helpless, hopeless, and lost. Your sense of self would be fragmented, and your self-esteem diminished; your spiritual distress would be heightened.

The recent rise in reported cases of recovered memory has led to a large number of lawsuits against perpetrators accused of having committed acts of abuse years ago. Essentially, people who have recovered repressed memories are pitted against alleged perpetrators who claim these memories are actually manufactured **false memories**. Therapists who work to help people recover repressed memories are pitted against memory researchers who claim that false recovered memories are fabricated in the highly charged atmosphere of mental health therapy.

Psychiatric–mental health nurses need to be aware of both sides of the issue. Remember that many persons who have experienced sexual abuse have a history of not being believed by parents or others they love or trust. Expressing disbelief will only cause the client further pain. Being compassionate will help clients in the struggle to examine their own lives.

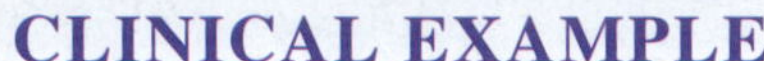

CLINICAL EXAMPLE

A woman who is an only child learns that her elderly widowed mother has been diagnosed with cancer. The woman recognizes that she will be the sole support of her mother during this trying time. She also has some professional responsibilities that cannot be put off. The woman decides to put off worrying about what the future may bring or anticipating her mother's death until her mother's diagnostic studies are completed, an accurate staging of the cancer can be performed, the first chemotherapy sequence has been completed, and a realistic prognosis is made of her mother's chances for a remission. As she puts it: "I've got too much to do and can't afford to fall apart right now."

Clients may refuse to consider their difficulties by saying that they "don't want to talk about it" or that they will "think about it some other time." This, too, is suppression.

Nursing Intervention Strategies Suppression can be dealt with in the same way as repression. Suppression is generally easier to deal with because the material remains conscious. You can be somewhat more directive in assessing why the client avoids talking about a situation. Suggest that the client try to look at the situation because it affects future plans. Offering information about the situation may help clients look at their situations objectively. As they learn more, they may feel less threatened.

Dissociation

In **dissociation**, the individual handles emotional conflicts, or internal or external stressors, by a temporary alteration of consciousness or identity (see Chapter 18 for specific mental dysfunctions in which dissociation is the major mental mechanism). Dissociation resembles repression, but it has a different origin. The self is formed through the process of disapproval and approval from significant other people. Therefore, the self *dissociates,* or refuses awareness of, the expression of personal qualities and experiences of which significant others disapprove. These feelings come to exist separately from the person's self-concept. A little girl with artistic abilities that are not validated by her parents will not think of herself as artistic. She may deny her abilities even when other people point them out.

People who dissociate do not "notice" what they are doing. This limitation of awareness is maintained because they experience anxiety whenever permissible levels for the self are trespassed.

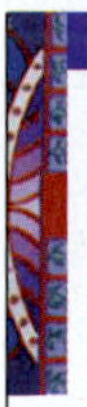

CLINICAL EXAMPLE

Jennifer consciously believes that sexual overtures are wrong, yet she behaves seductively toward men. She cannot understand why men see her behavior as a sexual invitation. The use of dissociation complicates Jennifer's problems. She needs to ignore or deny aspects of her situation to feel comfortable in it. Other people notice and point out Jennifer's seductive behavior, but she cannot recognize it because it is not a part of her self-concept. If Jennifer admitted her sexual feelings, she would experience severe anxiety and personality disorganization.

Nursing Intervention Strategies For a discussion of nursing intervention strategies for dissociation, see Chapter 18.

Identification

Identification is the wish to be like another person and to assume the characteristics of that person's personality. It represents a turning away from our own personality. Identification is unconscious. In this it differs from *imitation,* which is the conscious copying of another person's qualities. Identification with people we admire can serve an important function in maturation by evoking latent qualities. For instance, a little girl who identifies with her mother and sisters learns the behavioral characteristics of womanhood.

The most primitive type of identification is seen in the infant's relationship with the mother. Infants seem to perceive no difference between their mothers and themselves and only gradually become aware that their mothers exist apart from them. Small children deal with people in terms of how these people meet their needs. They do not see them as separate individuals with needs of their own. Such identifications may persist into adult life in people who have not differentiated themselves psychologically from seemingly powerful parents.

One specific manifestation of identification is passiveness in relationships. People who feel they have no resources of their own will overvalue the resources of others and expect to be taken care of. People who are most identified with their parents tend to be people who were not allowed to develop their own individuality. Part of the process of self-realization occurs in adolescence, when we discard, with much anxiety and insecurity, our identification with the parents on whom we have been so dependent. Some clients may not have achieved a degree of self-identity sufficient to do this. Identification can inhibit our usefulness, because it prevents us from focusing on our own capacities.

Identification can be seen in clients who rely heavily on the nurse's advice and support. They expect that all their needs will be met and that nothing will be expected of them.

CLINICAL EXAMPLE

Louie has bipolar disorder and is taking lithium. He is not interested in learning about the medication he must take, dietary recommendations, or blood tests he needs. He expects the nurse to take responsibility for seeing that he gets the right medicine and that everything else is in order. Identification prevents him from being self-reliant.

Nursing Intervention Strategies Nurses who work with clients like Louie should clarify what the client's expectations of the nurse are and then correct any misperceptions about the nurse's role. It is important to help the client increase his own skills and take responsibility for his own care. Initially, you can offer the client collaboration and interdependence. The long-term goal in dealing with identification is for the client to formulate a self-care plan independently.

Introjection

Introjection is closely related to identification. It is the process of accepting another's values and opinions as one's own if they contradict the values one previously held.

CLINICAL EXAMPLE

Joe Kaufmann, a cabinet maker, has worked for a furniture manufacturing company for 10 years. Joe's employer has asked him to cut some corners to help stem the company's financial losses. Afraid of losing his job, Joe compromises his values by providing shoddy workmanship as his employer requests.

Introjection also occurs in severe depression following the death of a loved one. The depressed person may assume many of the deceased person's characteristics, and in so doing lose some self-awareness.

Nursing Intervention Strategies Treat introjection as you would identification, remembering that introjection is more primitive and more intractable. It originates in our experience of being fed as infants. We incorporate people and objects into ourselves in the same way that we swallowed food. We felt a sense of oneness with everything in the external world and could not differentiate ourselves from others. Because thinking processes are not involved in the first experience of introjection, this defense mechanism tends to be difficult to explore on the verbal level.

Projection

Projection is an unconscious means of dealing with personal difficulties or unacceptable wishes by attributing them to others. We blame other people for our shortcomings or see them as harboring our own unacceptable feelings or thoughts. In the course of development, the child, needing parental approval, will identify with the parents and will also deny what they seem to condemn or fail to acknowledge. For instance, if her parents do not openly express and recognize angry feelings, a little girl will tend to regard anger as dangerous. She will then deny awareness of her own anger. Anger in others will disturb her, and she will tend to condemn in others the anger she cannot accept in herself. It is common knowledge that people often tend to criticize others for their own unacknowledged inferiorities. The person who fears being taken advantage of is often an opportunist.

In adult life, projection can be destructive if it interferes with our ability to acknowledge our own feelings. The tendency to attribute our own undesired feelings to others also blurs the boundaries between ourselves and others. This, in turn, makes it difficult to understand other people's feelings. People who make excessive use of projection tend to attribute to others hostile or seductive motives that do not actually exist. This prevents them from forming trusting and reciprocal relationships.

CLINICAL EXAMPLE

Linda is wary and suspicious of every man she meets. Regardless of how they behave toward her, Linda says: "They only want one thing." She interprets their behavior as sexually suggestive but has no awareness of her own sexual interest in them.

A tendency to projection may also interfere with problem solving. A young woman who believes she is failing a course because of her teacher will not focus her energies on her studies.

Nursing Intervention Strategies Clients who must deal with the stress of serious illness may shift the blame for their condition onto you, the nurse. They may complain of poor nursing care to a nurse who is actually very skillful. They may believe that they are being "paid back" for wrongdoing in the past. If such a client is accusing you falsely, do not show anger or retaliate but show, through consistency and attention, that you respect the client and are concerned about his or her welfare.

As clients feel more secure in the nurse–client relationship, encourage them to explore the realistic aspects of their situation. For example, you can help a man who blames his family for his alcoholism objectively explore what is known about the etiology of alcoholism. This may help him come to terms with his feelings of guilt and anger. This type of intervention helps the client separate his own feelings from the objective facts of the situation.

Denial

Denial of reality is one of the simplest of the defense mechanisms. In denial, painful or anxiety-producing aspects of awareness are blocked out of consciousness. The reality of a situation is either completely disregarded or transformed so that it is no longer threatening. Denial is one of the most common defenses against the stress of diagnosis and illness and is typically present in the first few minutes of adjustment to the death of a loved one. It may be helpful as a temporary protection against the full impact of a traumatic event.

CLINICAL EXAMPLE

A father reacts with denial when he shouts, "No, it can't be true; there must be a mistake," when told his 8-year-old son has just died in the trauma unit of injuries incurred when his bicycle collided with an automobile.

A young woman admitted to a psychiatric hospital because of acute anxiety and frightening hallucinations says she just "needs a rest."

Nursing Intervention Strategies Sometimes denial is the best solution for the client. In such situations, support the denial. A terminally ill client who believes she will soon recover and who cannot think about her illness should be allowed the protection of denial. Not all clients need to face up to reality. You should recognize that the use of denial may be preventing serious personality disorganization.

Sometimes, however, denial is directly harmful to the client, as when a man refuses to take medication that is crucial to his survival or to his mental health. In such cases, the motivation for the client's behavior should be assessed. After discovering the protective function the denial is serving, focus on helping the client meet these needs in a way that is not self-destructive. You can also help by not reinforcing patterns of denial but rather focusing on instances when the client seems to be dealing with reality.

Fantasy

Fantasy is a form of nonrational mental activity that enables the individual to temporarily escape the demands of the everyday world. Fantasies are not confined by the reality considerations of cause and effect and time and space. Fantasy normally characterizes the thinking of children before they are able to engage in consensually validated communication. Adults revert to fantasy during times of stress to obtain a symbolic satisfaction of wishes.

CLINICAL EXAMPLE

A businesswoman facing financial difficulties temporarily escapes by daydreaming that she is enjoying a luxurious vacation on a Caribbean island.

Another woman with advanced multiple sclerosis imagines herself a famous ballerina with complete control of her body.

A man whose wife has told him she wants a divorce imagines how much his wife will appreciate him now that he has been diagnosed with cancer.

Fantasy may offer temporary relief from pressures, but people who spend too much time in fantasy may be unable to meet the requirements of reality.

Clients who are very ill may fantasize that when they recover, many good things will happen to them. They may imagine that they will receive special recognition in their work or that they will get along better with their families. These fantasies may help such clients deal with the deprivations caused by illness. However, they may also create unrealistic expectations. The fantasies may make one feel good temporarily but interfere with problem solving.

Nursing Intervention Strategies Clients who engage in fantasy related to their illness need gradual help in assessing the responses others are likely to make and the achievements they themselves may realistically expect. Clients who fail to adjust to reality will be disappointed when their expectations are not met.

A helpful approach that will not devastate clients who need to hold on to some fantasy is to ask them to discuss their specific future plans. Examining the details of work and interpersonal adjustment may help a person relinquish unrealistic expectations and make more realistic plans. For example, the man who believes that a diagnosis of cancer will improve his marriage because his wife will appreciate him more fully must recognize that this is improbable. He needs to examine the real effects his illness will have on her. He must plan how to make specific improvements in their communication by anticipating problem areas.

Imagination does have a creative aspect, however. Fantasies have a richness and variety that is lacking in the everyday world. Certain artists, such as Dalí and Picasso, enriched their works of art through fantasy. Evidence also exists that insights leading to scientific discovery do not come about as the result of step-by-step logical thinking. Rather, they are created through fantasy.

Rationalization

Rationalization is the attribution of "good" or plausible reasons for questionable behavior to justify it or to deal with disappointment. Rationalizing helps us avoid social disapproval and bolster flagging self-esteem.

CLINICAL EXAMPLE

A nurse fails to return to the bedside of a nursing-home client despite a promise to do so before leaving work. She believes her behavior is justified because the client has problems with recent memory and probably wouldn't remember anyway.

Many people use rationalization because they wish to prove to themselves or others that their actions are governed by reason and common sense, even though they may not fully understand the reasons for their own behavior. Such explanations may be essential to maintaining personal integrity. They are not destructive as long as they do not prevent one from solving everyday problems.

Rationalization becomes more of a hindrance when it prevents us from making necessary changes in our behavior by interfering with our ability to examine that behavior. One sign of rationalization is an active search for reasons to justify our behavior or beliefs. Another is an inability to recognize inconsistencies in our beliefs. A third is being upset when our reasons are questioned, since each questioning threatens our defenses.

Clients may use rationalization to soften the blow of losses caused by illness. For instance, a man who is ill may give up work prematurely after rationalizing that he wouldn't have been successful in that field anyway. Such unnecessary restrictions deprive us of possible achievements.

Nursing Intervention Strategies Nurses must respect their clients' need to rationalize fears and insecurities they cannot face. However, hold out to clients the possibility for change.

You can help clients face the reality of their situation by encouraging them to explore ways they can deal with it more effectively. One way is to help them explore past instances in which they did change in order to cope with a stressful situation. Believing and recognizing that we have real strengths helps us face our areas of insecurity.

Reaction Formation

Reaction formation is a defense through which we keep an undesirable impulse out of awareness by emphasizing its opposite. To protect ourselves from recognizing dangerous feelings, we develop conscious attitudes and behavior patterns that are just the opposite of those feelings. For example, the desire to be sexually promiscuous may be concealed behind a moralistic demeanor. Some people who crusade passionately against alcohol or pornography may have an underlying wish to enjoy these things. Hostility may be concealed behind a facade of love and kindness.

CLINICAL EXAMPLE

Sue has been married to Colin for 25 years. Sue's friends and family view Colin as a typical chauvinist. Both of them are professional people—Colin is a banker and Sue is a freelance writer. Colin seldom lifts a hand around the house or drives the children to any of their lessons or sporting events. He drops his clothing all over the bedroom floor and expects Sue to clean up after him. One day, while Sue and her colleague were polishing an article for a travel magazine, Colin arrived home after lunch in a restaurant and rushed upstairs to the bathroom. In a few minutes, he rushed out the door, saying, "Sorry, Susie, but there's a bit of a mess in the upstairs bathroom." Colin had been nauseated and vomited and did not clean the toilet or the towels he used. Although Sue's colleague's astonishment at Colin's behavior turned to anger, Sue remained unnaturally sweet and loving and unable to consider the possibility of being angry with him. Sue is probably using this excess sweetness and loving kindness to counteract an unacceptable (to her) degree of anger.

People who use this defense are not conscious of their true feelings. Clues that reaction formation is occurring are an inappropriate intensity of feeling and the inability to consider alternative points of view.

Nursing Intervention Strategies A client manifesting reaction formation requires essentially the same approach as one manifesting repression. Respect and support the client's defenses while providing a secure relationship in which to explore feelings and new behavioral alternatives. Also be aware that it is easy to be annoyed at clients who cannot face their true feelings. The rigid and excessive display of what seems to be an insincere emotion can be frustrating. Remember that these clients are not "lying" or pretending. They are unconsciously protecting themselves against recognizing threatening feelings.

Displacement

Displacement is the discharging of pent-up feelings, generally hostility, on an object less dangerous than the object that aroused the feelings. This defense is used when emotions are aroused in a situation in which it would be dangerous to express them.

CLINICAL EXAMPLE

John has just failed an important examination. He believes his failure was the instructor's fault. He cannot express the full extent of his anger, because that would get him into worse trouble with the instructor. John goes quietly back to the dormitory. But when his roommate turns the stereo on too loud, John explodes. He doesn't fear retaliation from his roommate—they are peers and friends.

In some cases, we turn our anger toward another person inward upon the self. When this happens, we experience exaggerated self-accusations and guilt.

Nursing Intervention Strategies Clients may express inappropriate anger to the nurse when they are actually angry at someone or something else. The client may feel more secure with the nurse, who offers a safe target for displaced feelings. Displacement differs from projection in that people who use displacement are not distorting their feelings and attributing them to someone else. The feelings are clear, and the person acknowledges them. They are simply being directed at the wrong person. Therefore, it may be easier to help these clients acknowledge the real situation by remaining calm and accepting during an angry outburst. For example, after the outburst is over, say, "You seem so angry; I wonder if you really are angry because your breakfast is cold or if there might be some other reason." Opening up the possibility for a discussion of anger may help these clients to sort out just why and at whom they are angry.

Intellectualization

Intellectualization is the process of separating the emotion aroused by an event from ideas or opinions about the event because the emotion itself is too painful to acknowledge. The painful emotion is avoided by means of a rational explanation that divests the event of any personal significance. Failures are less significant if one believes that the situation could have been worse.

CLINICAL EXAMPLE

A woman whose husband recently died deals with her grief by telling her friends in a rational manner that it was better that he died suddenly by heart attack rather than to have died at the end of a long, chronic illness.

A boy who breaks his pelvis while skiing consoles himself after the accident by saying, "I would rather have a broken hip than a broken neck."

Clients may use intellectualization to blunt the emotional impact of their problems. This may be difficult for the nurse to perceive, because such clients often seem to know a great deal about their condition. They may be able to discuss in great detail the metabolic processes in diabetes or the psychodynamics of anxiety. At the same time, they cannot apply these concepts to their own situation in an emotional sense.

Nursing Intervention Strategies Intellectualization resembles rationalization in that it provides a verbal means of dealing with anxiety. Its use closes off the possibility of accepting and working out problems. Clients often use intellectualization at the onset of a crisis, and the need for this defense may decrease in a supportive nurse–client relationship. You can help the client relate emotionally to a problem by not forcing the expression of feeling. This will only frighten the client further. Asking these clients to explain how their knowledge relates to them personally may encourage them to accept and explore their emotional reactions.

PSYCHOLOGICAL FACTORS AFFECTING MEDICAL CONDITIONS

Physical illnesses with a major emotional component are often referred to as psychophysiologic or psychosomatic disorders. Because these terms are vague and have limited value for diagnosis, treatment, and research, the term **psychological factors affecting medical conditions (PFAMC)** is used in the DSM-IV-TR (APA, 2000) (see the Diagnostic Criteria feature below). The essential feature of this category is the presence of one or more specific psychologic or behavioral factors that adversely affect a medical condition. These factors may influence the course of a medical condition, interfere with the condition's treatment, or constitute an additional health risk. They may be any one or a combination of the following:

- A mental disorder affecting the course or treatment of a general medical condition, such as bipolar I disorder (manic episode) complicating hemodialysis.
- A psychological symptom affecting the course or treatment of a general medical condition, such as anxiety complicating the ability to carry out self-care for diabetes mellitus.
- A personality trait or coping style affecting the course or treatment of a general medical condition, such as denial interfering with the timely treatment of cancer.
- A maladaptive health behavior affecting the course or treatment of a general medical condition, such as a sedentary lifestyle and overeating affecting treatment for coronary artery disease.
- A stress-related physiologic response affecting the course or treatment of a general medical condition, such as stress-related dysrhythmias in a person recovering from myocardial infarction.

According to the DSM-IV-TR (APA, 2000, p. 732), the PFAMC category should be reserved for situations in which:

1. The psychological factors significantly affect the course or outcome of the medical condition, or
2. The psychological factors place the individual at significantly higher risk for an untoward outcome.

In addition, there should be evidence of a relationship between the psychological factors and the medical condition even though it may not be possible to specifically pinpoint the psychological factors as a direct cause or to identify exactly how they operate.

The DSM-IV-TR distinguishes PFAMC from several related disorders. A **mental disorder due to a general medical condition** can be defined as the presence of mental symptoms that are judged to be the direct physiological consequence of a general medical condition. In mental disorder due to a general medical condition, the presumed causality is in the opposite direction. For example, an individual may have catatonic disorder due to a neurologic condition such as a neoplasm, encephalitis, or cerebrovascular disease. Personality change may be due to HIV dis-

DSM-IV-TR Diagnostic Criteria for Psychological Factors Affecting Medical Condition

A. A general medical condition (coded on Axis III) is present.

B. Psychological factors adversely affect the general medical condition in one of the following ways:

1. the factors have influenced the course of the general medical condition as shown by a close temporal association between the psychological factors and the development or exacerbation of, or delayed recovery from, the general medical condition
2. the factors interfere with the treatment of the general medical condition
3. the factors constitute additional health risks for the individual
4. stress-related physiologic responses precipitate or exacerbate symptoms of the general medical condition

Source: Reprinted with permission from the *Diagnostic and Statistical Manual of Mental Disorders*, Fourth Edition, Text Revision. (Copyright 2000). American Psychiatric Association.

USING DSM-IV-TR

Health care providers often use language unfamiliar to clients and their families. Reword this DSM statement to make it easier for clients and family members to understand: "Stress-related physiologic responses precipitate or exacerbate symptoms of the general medical condition."

ease, head trauma, or lupus erythematosus. For situations in which delirium, dementia, amnestic disorder, mood disorder, psychotic disorder, anxiety disorder, sleep disorder, or sexual dysfunction are factors, see the appropriate chapters related to these diagnoses in this text. While somatoform disorders (discussed in Chapter 19∞) are characterized by both psychological and physical symptoms, no medical condition completely accounts for the physical symptoms seen in people with this disorder. Other psychiatric disorders excluded from PFAMC include conversion disorder, hypochondriasis, physical complaints associated with a mental disorder, and substance-related physical complaints.

Holistic Theory of Illness

Because all illnesses may ultimately stem from multiple factors, a holistic theory of illness serves as a basis for understanding all human disorders. As you appreciate the complex, interwoven pattern of emotional and physical elements, you will more fully comprehend the essential unity of the body and the mind. For a partial list of physical conditions having psychological components, see TABLE 8-2 ■.

Clients who come to the attention of health care professionals because of physical complaints frequently have their psychological needs neglected. Those unmet needs may be contributing to the complaint, may be the primary cause of symptom development, or may be the reason for the client's decision to seek help. Even if the most technologically advanced diagnostic and treatment approaches are applied, ignoring the psychological components of illness can be as disastrous as ignoring the biological components. Such psychological components can undermine medically appropriate treatment.

FIGURE 8-6 ■ on page 158 and the following clinical example illustrate these ideas.

CLINICAL EXAMPLE

Peter G., 5 years old, was admitted for the fourth time in 6 months because of an acute asthma attack. While Peter was being treated medically, his parents waited in the family room. Mrs. G. sat crying and wringing her hands while Mr. G. paced the floor with a strained expression on his face. A staff nurse was able to talk to them and trace the sequence of events leading up to Peter's admission to the hospital.

It was a Saturday afternoon, and Mr. and Mrs. G. had been arguing about whether to send Peter to kindergarten in the fall. Two points of view had emerged. Mr. G. was all for it. He wanted Peter to grow up quickly and leave his "babyish ways" behind. Mrs. G. was against it. Peter was the baby of the family, and Mrs. G. felt that her husband was always pushing him to do things too advanced for a 5-year-old. Peter had awakened from his nap to hear his parents shouting at each other. The quarrel ended abruptly when Peter started to wheeze, and both parents rushed to his bedside, united in their concern for him.

What factors brought on Peter's asthma attack at that particular time?

1. The biologic factors include Peter's physiologic makeup. His mother had been asthmatic as a child. She and Peter are both allergic to chocolate, eggs, feathers, and dust. Peter inherited certain genetic features that make him susceptible to certain environmental stressors—in this case, the specific allergens.
2. Sociologic components of Peter's illness revolve around his family's functioning. Mr. and Mrs. G. have different viewpoints on what Peter's role in the

TABLE 8-2 ■ **Examples of Physical Conditions Having Psychological Components**

System	Condition
Cardiovascular	Essential hypertension, angina pectoris, tachycardia, arrhythmia, cardiospasm, coronary artery disease, mitral valve prolapse, myocardial infarction, migraine headache
Gastrointestinal	Irritable bowel syndrome, gastric ulcer, duodenal ulcer, pylorospasm, regional enteritis (Crohn's disease), ulcerative colitis, nausea and vomiting, gastritis, chronic diarrhea
Hormonal	Hypoglycemia, diabetes mellitus, hyperthyroidism, hypothyroidism, hyperparathyroidism, hypoparathyroidism, premenstrual syndrome, obesity
Immune	Allergic disorders, cancer, autoimmune disorders (systemic lupus erythematosus, rheumatoid arthritis, Hashimoto's thyroiditis, myasthenia gravis, psoriasis), AIDS
Integumentary	Neurodermatitis (atopic dermatitis), pruritus, psoriasis, hyperhidrosis, urticaria, alopecia, acne, herpes, genital warts
Neuromuscular/skeletal	Chronic pain, headache, sacroiliac pain, temporomandibular joint (TMJ) pain, rheumatoid arthritis, Raynaud's disease
Respiratory	Asthma, hyperventilation syndrome, tuberculosis

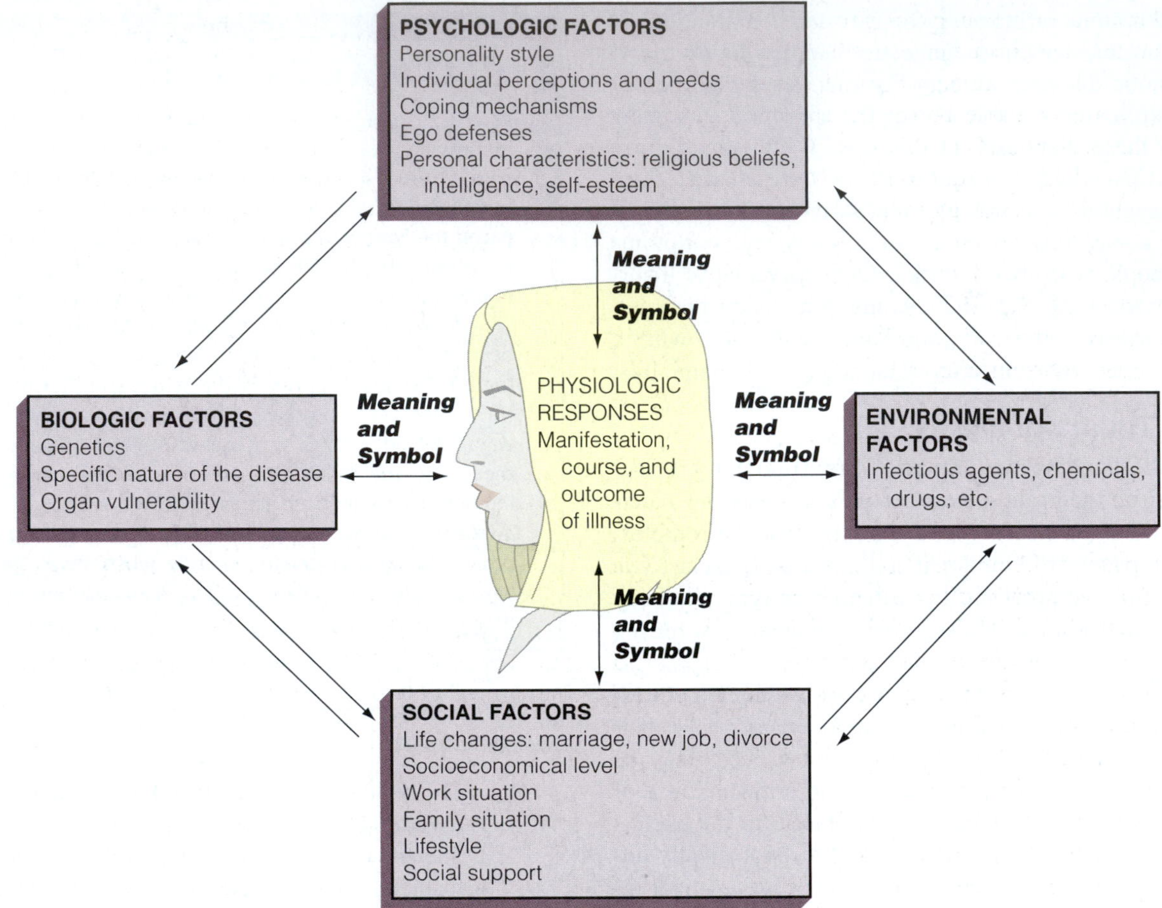

FIGURE 8-6 ■ The multicausational concept of the illness process. The phrase "Meaning and Symbol" refers to the fact that clients interpret all experiences in a highly individual manner according to their specific meaning and the broader meaning in the client's culture.

family should be. Their conflicts create a second source of stress for Peter.

3. A third component is Peter's psychological state. A 5-year-old boy views the integrity of his family as extremely important, and parental conflicts may threaten his sense of security. Peter had discovered that his parents rallied together when he was ill.

In view of these contributing factors, the treatment plan for Peter should not end when Peter stops wheezing. To reduce the number of such emergencies, caregivers need to devise a long-range treatment plan. This plan should encompass the physiologic, psychological, and sociologic components of Peter's asthma attacks. Peter's condition further illustrates the importance of examining cultural, environmental, developmental, genetic, constitutional, and historical factors in all disease processes.

Therefore, in all illness, a holistic approach is necessary if each facet of the client's overall problem is to be addressed. For each of the disorders, we suggest nonmedical interventions that reduce stress while increasing the client's understanding and control over troublesome symptoms. Promoting a healthy lifestyle and advocating lifestyle modifications are important nursing responsibilities regardless of the clinical area in which you practice.

Selected Conditions Affected by Psychological Factors

The following sections review the characteristics of several conditions often considered to be affected by psychological factors. For most of these conditions, an exact etiology is unknown. Current research focuses on the complicated interrelationships among such factors as stress, genetic susceptibility (McCaffery, Snieder, Dong, & de Geus, 2007), personality, environment, and hormones. Treatment is eclectic and holistic, focusing on mind, body, and spirit. Chapter 33 ∞ discusses the complementary and alternative therapies that may be used to help clients with these conditions.

Gastrointestinal Disorders

Gastrointestinal (GI) functional disorders are chronic or recurrent GI symptoms with no identifiable physiological basis. GI symptoms are widespread throughout the population and vary according to such factors as gender and socioeconomic status. Women, for example, tend to more frequently report irritable bowel syndrome or functional constipation, while men more frequently report bloating symptoms. Social, economic, and lifestyle factors all appear to affect susceptibility to GI disorders to varying degrees, although whether such increased susceptibility results from differences in social stress, dietary factors, or other socioeconomic factors is unclear. The medical literature is replete with studies demonstrating a relationship between psychological factors and the GI system, particularly such conditions as irritable bowel syndrome, inflammatory bowel disease (Kunzendorf et al., 2007), dyspepsia, and peptic ulcer, all multifactorial disorders for which stress has been implicated in the pathophysiology (Taché & Bonaz, 2007).

Peptic Ulcer Peptic ulcer disease (PUD) has been one of the most thoroughly studied illnesses thought to be influenced by psychological factors. Most peptic ulcer disease has been attributed to the bacterium *Heliobacter pylori,* which can be treated with antimicrobial medication. However, PUD is prevalent among people with stressful lifestyles and is associated with "getting ahead" in Western cultures. PUD appears to run in families and may be brought on or exacerbated by diet, stress, and certain infections. Duodenal ulcers, seen more frequently in men, are associated with hypersecretion of hydrochloric acid, probably stimulated by stress and anxiety.

Emotions such as anxiety and anger are also associated with the secretion of acid and pepsin, predisposing susceptible individuals to duodenal ulcer formation. Personality features of hostility, irritability, hypersensitivity, and impaired coping ability may also contribute to ulcer formation.

While studies of the relationship between psychological factors and ulcer formation and chronicity are somewhat controversial, psychological intervention is often recommended for PUD clients, especially in the absence of *Heliobacter pylori.* Such intervention is often directed toward resolving dependence conflicts and may include biofeedback and relaxation therapy (see Chapter 33), individual and group educational approaches, and pharmacologic and dietary management.

Inflammatory Bowel Disorders The role of psychological factors in inflammatory bowel disorders is unclear. Autoimmune factors and infections, coupled with psychological factors, may contribute to these disorders (Ringel & Drossman, 2001). Clients with ulcerative colitis tend to have a compulsive personality style with the following features: neatness, orderliness, punctuality, indecisiveness, emotional guardedness, humorlessness, conscientiousness, obstinacy, conformity, moral rigidity, and worry. Recent research, however, raises many questions about the validity of these personality features. Contemporary researchers say that the psychological traits these clients display are similar to those of clients with other chronic illnesses, with dependence being the most common trait. In many cases, onset and flare-ups seem linked to stressful life events, such as separations, failures, and disappointments.

Regardless of the source of the client's illness, treatment should focus on present troublesome areas, particularly concerns about the uncertain nature of the disease. Because of inherent differences between Crohn's disease and ulcerative colitis, the clinician must consider different approaches in planning treatment. The plan may include individual psychotherapy, family therapy, and environmental manipulation along with the medical regimen. These clients do best when they are involved in solid and long-term supportive relationships with nurses and physicians who help them develop coping and self-care skills.

Cardiovascular Disorders

The cardiovascular system is a sensitive indicator of emotional arousal, whether it be fear, anger, or pleasurable excitement. High levels of stress are suspected to have harmful effects on the heart and vascular system, especially if stress is chronic or repeated. Experience, learning, and symbolic meaning, along with their emotional content, can influence heart rate, heart rhythm, and blood pressure. These cardiovascular changes can in turn create emotions, mostly unpleasant, that affect perception and ideation. A number of indicators have been identified as high-risk factors for heart disease. They include genetic, physiologic, social, and psychological influences.

Stress researchers have found that persons who perceive a lack of control over their work situation, and experience high demands at the same time, may be prone to cardiovascular diseases. According to Lützén, Cronqvist, Magnusson, and Andersson (2003), situations such as these, common in nursing, may place nurses at risk for health problems. Another study found that lack of both job resilience and personal resilience, along with age, sex, and family history, correlated with cardiovascular risk (Ferris, Sinclair, and Kline, 2005).

A variety of psychosocial factors are believed to contribute to coronary artery disease (CAD). Many of these have been studied extensively, including affective states, personality or coping style, psychological reaction to environmental stimuli, sociocultural factors, and interpersonal factors. Psychological factors that have been linked to CAD, sudden death, and ventricular arrhythmias include anxiety and depression, a behavior pattern involving feelings of hostility and anger, work overload, life stress, and a lack of social support.

The highly competitive, urgent, impatient, hostile, and driving **type A personality** displays the classic constellation of personality characteristics associated with CAD, angina pectoris, and myocardial infarction. Of all these behaviors, hostility, in particular, is the best predictor of future heart disease (Miller, Smith, Turner, Guijarro, & Hallet, 1996). Adverse conditions in the client's environment, either social or economic, can also create the stress that leads to cardiac dysfunction.

Essential hypertension, cardiac dysrhythmias, and so-called cardiac neurosis are three syndromes of cardiovascular functioning with major psychological inputs. The classical hypothesis in hypertension has been that people have conflict between their dependent and aggressive inclinations. This causes chronic repression of all displays of anger or resentment. The repressed emotions are eventually transformed into disorders of blood pressure regulation. Although this specific hypothesis has been difficult to prove, experiments have shown that fear, anger, frustration, and guilt (along with several medical conditions) all cause rises in diastolic blood pressure in vulnerable individuals. Likewise, anxiety, hostility, depression, interpersonal conflict, and disruptive life events have all been shown to potentially precipitate dysrhythmias, such as sinus tachycardia, paroxysmal atrial tachycardia, and both atrial and ventricular ectopic beats.

Cardiac neurosis is a syndrome consisting of cardiac distress, exercise intolerance, easy fatigability, respiratory discomfort, and dizziness. These features are similar to those found in panic disorder (see Chapter 18) and mitral valve prolapse.

The treatment of cardiac disease must be multifaceted. In addition to medical or surgical treatment, other approaches involve stress management, relaxation training, biofeedback, weight control through diet and exercise, and behavioral interventions to help people give up smoking. More efforts are being geared toward prevention, including programs by industry and corporations to promote healthy lifestyles among employees.

Asthma

Asthma is among the most widely studied illnesses of the respiratory system. Because breathing is essential to life, there has been much speculation about the emotional and symbolic significance that can become attached to the processes of air exchange.

There are allergic, immunologic, and emotional inputs to asthmatic attacks. The emotional components may lead directly to alterations in bronchus size. Contemporary researchers examine the interplay of both psychological and physiologic aspects of asthma such as the relationship between asthma, anger, and quality of life (Nickel et al., 2006) as well as the neurologic and humoral bases of asthma pathogenesis. However, certain personality types are linked by some researchers and clinicians to asthma susceptibility: those with extreme inhibition, covert aggression, marked dependence needs, a high need for affection, and those prone to depression, anxiety, and disturbances of self-esteem.

Asthmatic people may be extremely frightened by asthmatic attacks, particularly in childhood. This fear may make them feel helpless and vulnerable. In response, they often adopt a clinging style of relating. The emotional and physical aspects of the illness seem to interrelate in a complex system of feedback loops. See the clinical profile of Peter G. (page 157) for an example.

Each person with asthma must be assessed individually to determine what factors are contributing to the disease process. A treatment plan may include, along with medication, family therapy, relaxation training, behavior modification, and hypnosis.

Arthritis

Rheumatoid arthritis (RA) has long been identified as an illness that is strongly influenced by emotional life. Its etiology remains uncertain. Psychological stresses are thought to precipitate attacks and flare-ups. The mechanism of transformation from idea or affect into tissue alteration appears to be via hormonal and autonomic nervous system pathways. Specifically, levels of growth hormone, sex hormones, thyroid hormone, and adrenal corticosteroids all change in stages of emotional arousal, and all are involved in the production of connective tissue, especially collagen. The hypothalamus and the limbic system also mediate.

Early psychological studies of individuals with RA attempted to define the "rheumatic personality." These people were described as self-sacrificing, masochistic, inhibited, perfectionistic, and retiring. While a high percentage of people with RA are depressed, they do not differ from others with chronic illness in this respect; that is, chronic illness increases the risk of depression. Thus, in RA, depression may stem from actual and perceived functional and other losses (such as mobility). The diagnosis cannot be based on personality type, however, because there are many exceptions to the rule. Physical findings, deformities, subcutaneous nodules, and blood studies remain the criteria for identification.

A treatment plan for clients with arthritis may include pain control, surgery, drugs, vocational counseling, occupational therapy, and interventions to alleviate or prevent depression and to deal with depression and anger more directly.

Headache

The experience of headache resulting from emotional tension is common. Headaches account for many physician visits and for job absenteeism. Headaches are also highly associated with depressive and anxiety disorders. Headaches may be divided into the five following types:

1. Vascular headache of migraine type
2. Muscle contraction headache (tension headache)
3. Combined vascular–muscle contraction headache
4. Delusional, depressive, conversion, or hypochondriacal headache
5. Structural or disease-related headache

The mechanism of vascular headache seems to involve the release of various vasoactive substances in the brain, such as serotonin, catecholamines, histamine, bradykinin, and prostaglandins. This release frequently occurs with stress. In genetically susceptible individuals, the substances cause vasodilation and inflammation of the arterial walls. There are generally early warning symptoms of migraine attacks. These range from mood changes and GI upset to gross neurologic findings in the visual and contralateral sensorimotor systems. A number of upsets in physiologic functioning can actually be migraine equivalents. These include nausea and vomiting, diarrhea, tachycardia, cyclical edema, vertigo, periodic fever, pain, depression, confusion, and insomnia.

A tension headache results from muscular contraction in the neck, shoulders, face, or scalp. These are steady, persistent headaches with no warning signs that commonly feel like a "band wrapped around the head." Some theorists support the notion that headache sufferers are likely to maintain rigid control over emotions, feel hostility toward others, use introjection as a defense, and be perfectionists.

Structural or disease-related headache arises from systemic infections, primary or metastatic tumors, hematomas, abscesses, cranial infections, cranial nerve inflammations, and eye, ear, nose, sinus, and tooth diseases.

Interventions are based on the diagnosis and the contributing factors that have been identified. Possible treatments and approaches include measures that increase circulation, such as massage or heat application; use of medications; alterations in diet, rest, and exercise patterns; psychotherapy; and biofeedback, meditation, hypnosis, relaxation, and other stress-management approaches.

Endocrine Disorders

A large number of disorders of endocrine functioning are associated with psychologic factors. The endocrine system has particular significance for psychiatry, because there is a close relationship between the emotions and a variety of active chemical substances released in tissues by nerve impulses (Hellhammer & Wade, 1993). In physical medicine, the feedback loop has long been accepted as the model for the functioning of the endocrine organs.

Extensive research on the endocrine feedback system has led to a sophisticated model that includes several kinds of feedback loops. The levels of circulating hormones released by endocrine glands, such as the thyroid and gonads (the sex glands), are controlled by long feedback loops that send information to the cerebral cortex and limbic system. Short feedback loops of pituitary hormones affect the hypothalamus. Very short loops of releasing hormones from the hypothalamus determine their own production and control. Studies on the relationship between emotions and endocrine function have shown that:

- Various neurotransmitters affect hormone-releasing factors.
- Psychoactive medications whose action is mediated by neurotransmitters also affect the release of releasing factors.
- Stress stimulates the autonomic nervous system, which can stimulate the adrenal medulla to produce epinephrine or the pancreas to secrete insulin.
- Corticosteroid production of the adrenal cortex increases greatly during some psychotic episodes in clients with schizophrenia.
- Steroid levels also increase in agitated or anxious depressive people.

It seems fair to conclude that the emotional centers of the brain—the cerebral cortex and limbic system—are intimately tied to the endocrine organs, through the axis of the hypothalamus and the anterior pituitary. Their secretions act as communication messengers. It is not surprising, then, to find expressions of emotional arousal through endocrine changes and major effects on emotional states from endocrine diseases. These are both, in fact, common. Endocrine disorders and their physical and mental symptoms are listed in the Your Assessment Approach feature on page 162.

Adrenal dysfunction characteristically produces prominent mental as well as distinctive physical symptoms. Thyroid disorders are commonly accompanied by cognitive or emotional changes. Stress has been implicated, though inconclusively, in the precipitation of thyrotoxic crises. Stress may influence the course of diabetes, either directly by promoting a flare-up or indirectly by causing the client to neglect a usually rigid medical regimen. So many mental symptoms are associated with hypoglycemia that many clients are classified and treated as "classic neurotics."

It is evident that numerous problems can be caused by endocrine dysfunction. The treatment approach must be individualized to meet the client's physical and psychological needs. An important role for the nurse is primary prevention. Adequately preparing a person for developmental changes by offering accurate information about likely physical and emotional alterations can help prevent severe psychiatric disturbances during these periods. Reliable support and open channels of communication are necessary. New coping strategies can be successful if their design, timing, and presentation are appropriate.

Skin Disorders

Allergic illnesses, particularly those involving the skin, have been shown to have psychological elements in etiology or course (Picardi et al., 2006). The skin, with its critical sensory functions, mediates between the outside world and internal states. Itching (pruritus), excessive sweating (hidrosis), urticaria, and atopic dermatitis are all commonly classified as psychophysiologic conditions. Because of the skin–nervous system interactions, there is a significant psychophysiological or behavioral component to many dermatological conditions (Shenefelt, 2005).

A variety of stressful or emotional states are associated with flare-ups of allergic skin disorders. Attempts have been made to correlate the following specific emotional states or stresses with individual disorders:

- Generalized pruritus: aggression
- Genital and anal pruritus: sexuality (heterosexual and homosexual)
- Hyperhidrosis: anxiety
- Urticaria: anger
- Atopic dermatitis: longing for love

In truth, these feelings and conflicts are seen in normal, disordered, and other psychophysiologic states. Therefore, you should be cautious about accepting these psychopathogenic mechanisms as the only valid explanations.

The location of the lesions has, historically, had symbolic significance. Thus, conflict over an extramarital affair has been associated with dermatitis in the wedding ring area. Head and face locations have been classically associated with conflict over affective display. Affliction of the hands is associated with practical or professional conflicts. A genital distribution of lesions may be associated with sexual concerns.

Resistance to Psychosocial Intervention

Behavioral therapy, cognitive therapy, biofeedback, hypnotherapy, and psychotherapy have all been used successfully with appropriate clients. However, despite the wealth of psychosocial interventions available to people with psychophysiologic

YOUR ASSESSMENT APPROACH
Common Features of Endocrine Disorders

Disease	Physical Symptoms	Mental Symptoms
Addison's disease (adrenal insufficiency)	Weakness, fatigue, anorexia, weight loss, nausea and vomiting, pigmentation of skin, hypotension	Depression, irritability, psychomotor retardation, apathy, memory defect, hallucinations
Cushing's syndrome (adrenal cortex hyperfunction)	Truncal obesity, moon facies, abdominal striae, hirsutism, amenorrhea, hypertension, osteoporosis, weakness	Impotence, decreased libido, anxiety, increased emotional lability, apathy, insomnia, memory deficits, confusion, disorientation
Diabetes mellitus	Polydipsia, polyuria, polyphagia, weight loss, blurred vision, fatigue, impotence, fainting, paresthesia	Stupor, coma, fatigue, impotence
Hyperthyroidism	Exophthalmos, goiter, moist warm skin, weight loss, increased appetite, weakness, tremor, tachycardia, heat intolerance	Anxiety, tension, irritability, hyperexcitability, emotional lability, depression, psychosis, or delirium
Hypoglycemia	Tremor, light-headedness, sweating, hunger, nausea, pallor, tachycardia, hypertension	Anxiety, fugue, unusual behavior, confusion, apathy, psychomotor agitation or retardation, depression, delusions, hallucinations, convulsions, coma
Hypothyroidism	Dull expression, puffy eyelids, swollen tongue, hoarse voice, rough dry skin, cold intolerance	Psychomotor retardation, decreased initiative, slow comprehension, drowsiness, decreased recent memory, delirium, stupor, depression or psychosis
Premenstrual syndrome	Headache, breast engorgement, lower abdominal bloating, GI complaints, increased sweating, craving for sweets, other appetite changes	Irritability, depression, anxiety, emotional lability, fatigue, crying spells

disorders, many are resistant to approaches that are not strictly medical. Reasons for this include:

- These clients are believed to lack insight because they express conflict through somatic complaints rather than verbalization.
- Conflicts over unresolved dependence and aggressive wishes may make it difficult to relate to these clients interpersonally.
- These clients focus steadfastly on their somatic complaints, apparently indicating that alternative defense mechanisms are unavailable or inadequate.
- They are rarely highly motivated to heighten their self-awareness, which is the goal of many forms of psychotherapy.
- Even when they are somewhat motivated, they may be unable or unwilling to delay gratification and thus are impatient with the slow process of growth usually required in psychotherapeutic work.

For these reasons, traditional psychotherapy is not the most useful intervention. Approaches that enhance medical and surgical intervention and allow the client's primary bond to remain with nonpsychiatric health care providers are more successful. Programs geared toward stress management (such as those discussed in Chapter 33) are very useful because they present stress as part of the human condition and the participants do not feel labeled as having psychiatric problems. Cognitive and behavioral approaches have also gained increasing favor in the last decade because they alleviate symptoms over a short period of time and thus prove effective in terms of outcome and cost. Cognitive and behavioral approaches are thoroughly discussed in Chapter 31.

EXPLORE MEDIALINK

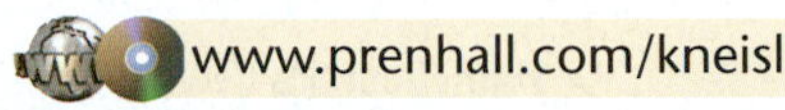

www.prenhall.com/kneisl

For NCLEX-RN® review questions, case studies, and other resources for this chapter see the Pearson Health MediaLink CD-ROM that accompanies this book and the Companion Website at www.prenhall.com/kneisl.

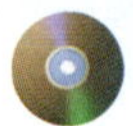

CD-ROM
Audio Glossary
NCLEX-RN® Review Questions

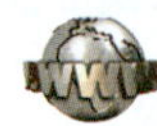

Companion Website
Audio Glossary
NCLEX-RN® Review Questions
Critical Thinking Exercise
- *Addressing Teen Anxiety*

Case Study
- *Midlife Crisis*

Care Plan
- *Revisiting Stress: New Nurse's Worry*

MediaLinks
MediaLink Application
- *Stress Webs*

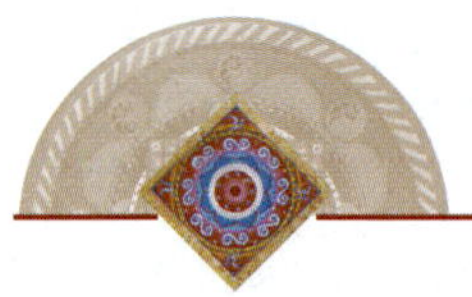

NCLEX-RN® REVIEW QUESTIONS

1. Which of the following is most congruent with the nursing process?
1. Social readjustment rating
2. General adaptation syndrome
3. Process of cognitive appraisal
4. Categorization of individuals as either "disease-prone" or "self-healing"

2. Your client, a survivor of Hurricane Katrina, now owns her own house and business. She describes herself as "successful and blessed." She reports difficulty falling asleep "nearly every night," and has had sleep deprivation for over 2 years. "I didn't have insomnia before the storm. I should be happy. I have more than I ever did before." Based on this information, your tentative nursing diagnosis is:
1. Insomnia related to anticipation of threat to basic needs and security.
2. Insomnia related to survivor guilt.
3. Alteration in self-concept related to survivor guilt.
4. Anxiety related to inevitability of future loss.

3. Which of the following scenarios depicts an individual using symbolic substitutes as a coping strategy?
1. Despite knowledge of the health consequences, a health care provider smokes one pack of cigarettes per day, and two packs every Monday. The individual reports smoking as "soothing."
2. Your client has been in recovery from alcohol and chemical dependence for 25 years. The client states, "When I don't know what else to do, I go to bed. I always feel better when I get out of bed."
3. Your coworker, a psychiatric–mental health nurse, does not believe psychotherapy would be effective for herself. "I'm into self-analysis. I usually get what I need as I meditate on the problem."
4. Your friend informs you that when she is stressed, she copes with massages, manicures, and cosmetic makeovers. "When my body looks better and feels better, it makes me feel emotionally grounded, like the outside mirrors the inside."

4. Everyday methods people use to cope and Antonovsky's generalized resistance resources (GRRs) are congruent with which of the following?
1. Resistance phase of the General Adaptation Syndrome
2. The client's score on the Social Readjustment Scale
3. Defense mechanisms
4. Lazarus's secondary appraisal results

5. A peer on a medical–surgical floor consults with you regarding a client admitted with an infection-induced delirium. Her family reports she has never discussed religion, but in her delirium, she appears fearful and she screams, "I repent here before the fires of Hell!" Your peer says, "Her family wants to know where that came from." The information you recommend for the family is based on your knowledge of which of the following defense mechanisms?
1. Repression
2. Introjection
3. Fantasy
4. Suppression

6. Which of the following statements is FALSE?
   1. Fantasy is a common defense mechanism of young children.
   2. Dissociation is functional for adults.
   3. Projection and reaction formation are associated with paranoid thinking.
   4. Rationalization is associated with rejection of personal responsibility.

7. Whenever you inquire about the circumstances of your client's admission to your inpatient psychiatric unit, your client responds, "I would rather not talk about that." As the client's discharge date approaches, which nursing intervention is most essential?
   1. Reiterate the need to deal with recent stressors, since discharge is imminent.
   2. Confront the client's denial.
   3. Review the police report and list some coping strategies for the client to utilize after discharge.
   4. Create a safe interpersonal environment so that the client can explore precipitating events.

8. Your client blames his family for the exacerbation of ulcerative colitis. You establish the foundation for a trusting relationship. The client reports "having rapport" with you. If your goal is to explore family relationships, which nursing strategy should you implement next?
   1. Gather data about family circumstances prior to the illness exacerbation.
   2. Matter-of-factly point out the need to accept responsibility for physical illness.
   3. Explore stressors and methods of coping that have been effective in the past.
   4. Connect the client's family with a chronic illness support group.

9. Your client has been hospitalized for the 17th time with chronic schizophrenia, paranoid type. For years, he has steadfastly denied having mental illness. During this hospitalization, you overhear him telling another client that he thinks he may have "this horrible disease." Which nursing intervention is most essential?
   1. Modify his priority nursing care plan problem from "Ineffective Denial" to "Spiritual Distress."
   2. Give him positive reinforcement for his insight.
   3. Gather more data regarding his mental status and suicidality.
   4. Reassure him that many clients with schizophrenia may lead productive lives.

10. Clients whose medical conditions are intensely influenced by psychological or behavioral factors:
    1. Have few dependence and aggression conflicts.
    2. Are excellent candidates for long-term psychotherapy.
    3. Display insight and interest in self-awareness and personal growth.
    4. Demonstrate involvement of the neurological, endocrine, and immunological systems.

See Appendix C for answers.

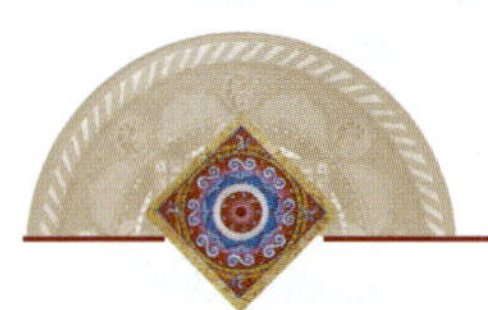

REFERENCES

Ah, D. V., Kang, D. H., & Carpenter, J. S. (2007). Stress, optimism, and social support: Impact on immune responses in breast cancer. *Research in Nursing & Health, 30*(1), 72–83.

American Psychiatric Association, (2000). *Diagnostic and statistical manual of mental disorders* (4th ed., Text Revision) (DSM-IV-TR). Washington, DC: Author.

Antonovsky, A. (1991). *Unraveling the mystery of health: How people manage stress.* Boston: Jossey-Bass.

Antonovsky, A. (1996). The sense of coherence: An historical and future perspective. *Israel Journal of Medical Sciences, 32*, 170–178.

Carlson, L. E., Speca, M., Patel, K. D., & Goodey, E. (2004). Mindfulness-based stress reduction in relation to quality of life, mood, symptoms of stress and levels of cortisol, dehydroepiandrosterone sulfate (DHEAS) and melatonin in breast and prostate cancer outpatients. *Psychoneuroendocrinology, 29*(4), 448–474.

Eriksson, M., & Lindstrom, B. (2006). Antonovsky's sense of coherence scale and the relation with health: A systematic review. *Journal of Epidemiology and Community Health, 60*(5), 376–381.

Ferris, P. A., Sinclair, C., & Kline, T. J. (2005). It takes two to tango: Personal and organizational resilience as predictors of strain and cardiovascular disease risk in a work sample. *Journal of Occupational Health Psychology, 10*(3), 225–238.

Fitzpatrick, J. J., & Wilke, P. A. (2001). *Psychiatric–mental health nursing digest.* New York: Springer.

Friedman, H., & VandenBos, G. (1992). Disease-prone and self-healing personalities. *Hospital and Community Psychiatry, 43*(12), 1177–1179.

Hart, K. E., Wilson, T. L., & Hittner, J. B. (2006). A psychosocial resilience model to account for medical well-being in relation to sense of coherence. *Journal of Health Psychology, 11*(6), 857–862.

Hellhammer, D., & Wade, S. (1993). Endocrine correlates of stress vulnerability. *Psychotherapy and Psychosomatics, 60*, 8–17.

Holmes, T. H., & Rahe, R. H. (1967). The social readjustment rating scale. *Journal of Psychosomatic Research, 11*, 213–218.

Kobasa, S. C. (1979). Stressful life events, personality, and health: An inquiry into hardiness. *Journal of Personality and Social Psychology, 37*, 1–11.

Kreitzer, M. J., Gross, C. R., Ye, X., Russas, V., & Treesak, C. (2005). Longitudinal impact of mindfulness meditation on illness burden in solid-organ transplant recipients. *Progress in Transplantation, 15*(2), 166–172.

Kunzendorf, S., Janischek, G., Straubinger, K., Heberlein, I., Homann, N., Ludwig, D., et al. (2007). The Luebeck interview for psychosocial screening in patients with inflammatory bowel disease. *Inflammatory Bowel Diseases, 13*(1), 33–41.

Lazarus, R. S., & Folkman, S. (1984). *Stress, appraisal, and coping.* New York: Springer.

Lützén, K., Cronqvist, A., Magnusson, A., & Andersson, L. (2003). Moral stress: Synthesis of a concept. *Nursing Ethics, 10*(3), 312–322.

McCaffery, J. M., Snieder, H., Dong, Y., & de Geus, E. (2007). Genetics in psychosomatic medicine: Research designs and statistical approaches. *Psychosomatic Medicine, 69*(2), 206–216.

Meisenhelder, J. B., & Chandler, E. N. (2000). Prayer and health outcomes in church members. *Alternative Therapies in Health and Medicine, 6*(4), 56–60.

Meyers, J. (1972). Life events and mental status. *Journal of Health and Human Behavior, 1*, 398–406.

Miller, T. Q., Smith, T. W., Turner, C. W., Guijarro, M. L., & Hallet, A. J. (1996). A meta-analytic review of research on hostility and physical health. *Psychological Bulletin, 119*, 322–348.

Monat, A., & Lazarus, R. S. (1991). *Stress and coping* (3rd ed.). New York: Columbia University Press.

Moore, T. (1994). *Care of the soul: A guide for cultivating depth and sacredness in everyday life.* New York: Harper Perennial.

Nickel, C., Lahmann, C., Muehlbacher, M., Pedrosa Gil, F., Kaplan, P., Buschmann, W., et al. (2006). Pregnant women with bronchial asthma benefit from progressive muscle relaxation: A randomized, prospective, controlled trial. *Psychotherapy & Psychosomatics, 75*(4), 237–243.

Picardi, A., Porcelli, P., Pasquini, P., Fassone, G., Mazzatti, E., Lega, I., et al. (2006). Integration of multiple criteria for psychosomatic assessment of dermatological patients. *Psychosomatics, 47*(2), 122–128.

Pilkington, F. B. (2007). Envisioning nursing in 2050 through the eyes of nurse theorists: Leininger and Watson. *Nursing Science Quarterly, 20*(1), 8.

Ringel, Y., & Drossman, D. A. (2001). Psychosocial aspects of Crohn's disease. *Surgical Clinics of North America, 81*(1), 231–252.

Schneider, G., Driesch, G., Kruse, A., Nehen, H. G., & Heuft, G. (2006). Old and ill and still feeling well? Determinants of subjective well-being in > or = 60 year olds: The role of the sense of coherence. *American Journal of Geriatric Psychiatry, 14*(10), 850–859.

Selye, H. (1956). *The stress of life*. New York: McGraw-Hill.

Sephton, S. E., Salmon, P., Weissbecker, I., Ulmer, C., Floyd, A., Hoover, K., et al. (2007). Mindfulness meditation alleviates depressive symptoms in women with fibromyalgia: Results of a randomized clinical trial. *Arthritis & Rheumatism, 57*(1), 77–85.

Shenefelt, P. D. (2005). Complementary psychocutaneous therapies in dermatology. *Dermatologic Clinics, 23*(4), 723–734.

Smith, J. C. (1993). *Understanding stress and coping.* New York: Macmillan.

Starkweather, A. R. (2007). The effects of exercise on perceived stress and IL-6 levels among older adults. *Biological Research for Nursing, 8*(3), 186–194.

Taché, Y., & Bonaz, B. (2007). Corticotropin-releasing receptors and stress-related alterations of gut motor function. *Journal of Clinical Investigation, 117*(1), 33–40.

Tosevski, D. L., & Milovancevic, M. P. (2006). Stressful life events and physical health. *Current Opinion in Psychiatry, 19*(2), 184–189.

Weaver, K. E., Liabre, M. M., Duran, R. E., Antoni, M. H., Ironson, G., Penedo, F. J., et al. (2005). A stress and coping model of medication adherence and viral load in HIV-positive men and women on highly active antiretroviral therapy (HAART). *Health Psychology, 24*(4), 385–392.

Weze, C., Leathard, H. L., Grange, J., Tiplady, P., & Stevens, G. (2007). Healing by gentle touch ameliorates stress and other symptoms in people suffering with mental health disorders or psychological stress. *Evidence-Based Complementary & Alternative Medicine, 4*(1), 115–123.

Wyman, P. A., Moynihan, J., Eberly, S., Cox, C., Cross, W., Jin, X, et al. (2007). Association of family stress with natural killer cell activity and the frequency of illnesses in children. *Archives of Pediatrics & Adolescent Medicine, 161*(3), 228–234.

ADDITIONAL REFERENCES

Bengtssen-Tops, A., & Hansson, L. (2001). The validity of Antonovsky's sense of coherence measure in a sample of schizophrenic patients living in the community. *Journal of Advanced Nursing, 33*(4), 432–438.

Landsverk, S. S., & Kane, C. F. (1998). Antonovsky's sense of coherence: Theoretical basis of psychoeducation in schizophrenia. *Issues in Mental Health Nursing, 19*(5), 419–431.

Rahe, R. H. (1979). Life change events and mental illness: An overview. *Journal of Human Stress, 5*, 2–10.

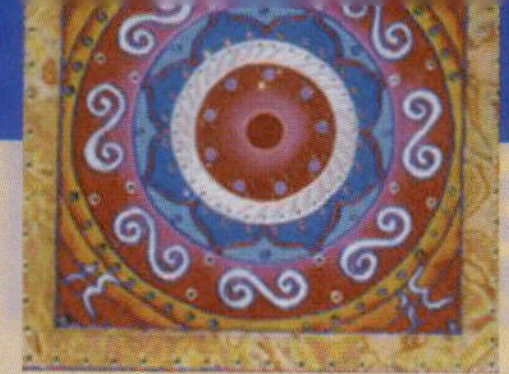

CHAPTER

9

Mental Health, Mental Disorder, and Cultural Competence

BETH MOSCATO

KEY TERMS

acculturation *171*
comorbidity *185*
cultural competence *168*
cultural sensitivity *168*
culture-bound syndrome *185*
culture brokering *171*
ethnicity *168*
ethnocentrism *168*
global burden of disease *169*
incidence rate *180*
nurse-as-culture-broker *172*
prevalence rate *180*
psychiatric epidemiology *180*
risk factor *181*

LEARNING OUTCOMES

After completing this chapter, you will be able to:

1. Explain what it means to be a culturally competent nurse.
2. Describe the role of the psychiatric–mental health nurse as culture broker.
3. Describe the personal strategies you can use to develop cultural competence in your work with specific cultural groups.
4. Identify the risk factors associated with mental disorders that affect the experience, expression, reporting, and evaluation of mental disorders among culturally diverse groups.
5. Explain the natural history of disorder, including its four stages.
6. Discuss when and how you would apply epidemiologic principles in your psychiatric–mental health nursing practice.

CRITICAL THINKING CHALLENGE

Janiece is a nurse in a psychiatric outpatient clinic in a downtown medical center of a large city near the Gulf of Mexico. Her clients come from a variety of backgrounds. Some are local people who have lived in and farmed in the surrounding towns or work in the tourist industry. Others are retirees who have moved from the North. Many are Central American immigrants who originally came to help out in reconstruction after a hurricane but now live and work there. There is also a large Czech community. Janiece meets with clients one–to–one or with clients and families in a group setting. Clients may or may not have a cultural background similar to hers. Even more complex relationships exist when groups of clients or family members from varied cultural backgrounds meet together with her in a psychoeducation group.

1. How might the clients' or family members' cultural beliefs, values, practices, and healing traditions influence the goals Janiece has set for their treatment?
2. Do such clients and families represent "what kind" and "how much" mental disorder is "out there" in the community?
3. Are you willing to expand your nursing skills by considering the community itself as a potential "client" for mental health assessment and services?
4. How can you apply principles of cultural competence and psychiatric epidemiology to your psychiatric–mental health nursing experiences with culturally diverse groups as well as individual clients?

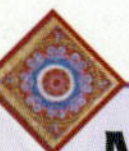

MEDIALINK 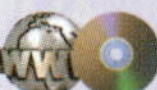 www.prenhall.com/kneisl

Go to the Pearson Health MediaLink CD-ROM and the Companion Website at www.prenhall.com/kneisl for interactive resources for this chapter.

To meet global needs and opportunities in the 21st century, nursing is addressing cultural diversity in a health care system in which multicultural individuals are both recipients of care and care providers. America is undergoing demographic shifts that include increasing numbers of diverse cultural groups. The population of the United States will continue to grow, but at a slower rate. Fifty-year projections (2000 to 2050) from the U.S. Bureau of the Census highlight increases in each of the major cultural groups (African-American, Native American, Eskimo and Aleut, Asian and Pacific Islander, and those with Hispanic origins) other than Caucasian. It is estimated that these diverse cultural groups will represent almost half (47%) of the population by 2050. Population trends reveal that Hispanics represented the largest minority group in 2005 and will comprise 25% of the population by 2050. Census information can be found on the Census Bureau website (www.census.gov) and accessed through the Companion Website for this book.

MediaLink U.S. Census Bureau

Culture shapes human behavior and assigns unique meanings to the world around us. Nurses need to be aware that these cultural forces are powerful determinants of health-related behaviors in any population. Thus, culture can influence the experience, expression, reporting, and evaluation of mental disorders. Symptoms related to major depression, as highlighted by the DSM-IV-TR, may illustrate this point. Depression may be experienced in somatic terms, rather than with sadness or guilt, in some cultures. People of Latino and Mediterranean cultures may complain of headaches and "nerves." People of Chinese and Asian cultures may emphasize weakness and tiredness. Middle Easterners may refer to problems of the "heart." The Hopi may express the depressive experience by being "heartbroken." Cultures may differ regarding the seriousness placed on symptoms and share distinctive culture-specific experiences (such as the feeling of being hexed). It is essential to identify those cultural factors that may facilitate, or deter, desired health-related behaviors.

As a nurse, you are called upon to participate in a health care system comprising individuals from different national, regional, ethnic, generational, socioeconomic, religious, and health status backgrounds. The range and variety of health care beliefs, rituals, traditions, and healing practices across cultures are staggering (see FIGURE 9-1 ■). It is your professional responsibility to understand, respect, and work with these cultural differences. Professional effectiveness in this multicultural health care environment requires the development of essential skills related to an understanding and integration of cultural phenomena in all aspects of your professional nursing care. Developing cultural competence is an important link to the reduction of mental health disparities (Mahoney, Carlson, & Engebretson, 2006). Several nursing organizations have taken the lead in reshaping health care policies to eliminate health care disparities. The American Academy of Nursing (Giger et al., 2007) is striving to ensure that measurable outcomes are achieved, and the International Society of Psychiatric Nurses (Yearwood, Hines-Martin, Dato, & Malone, 2006) has specifically challenged psychiatric nurses to support diversity and cultural competence. Thus, this chapter has two sections. The first section will emphasize the knowledge necessary for developing an understanding of cultural competence, especially in relation to nursing practice. The subsequent section will highlight psychiatric epidemiology in our culturally diverse society.

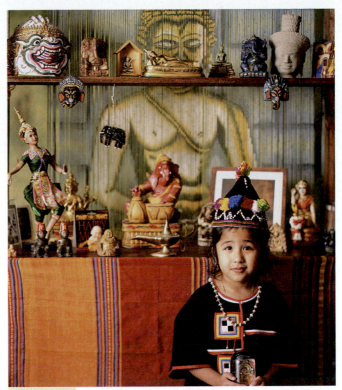

FIGURE 9-1 ■ This young American girl's parents were born in Thailand. Their home contains many cultural artifacts that help their daughter to understand and appreciate the rituals and traditions associated with her cultural heritage.

Source: Duane Rieder/Getty Images Inc.—Image Bank

Specific strategies for cultural competence are also integrated throughout this text. For example, Chapter 3 discusses the nurse's own sociocultural background and its influence on nursing practice. The chapters in Unit 4 discuss sociocultural theories that expand our understanding of specific mental disorders. Chapters 7 and 32 discuss psychotropic medications and how ethnicity or cultural background affect how specific medications work. Chapter 33 discusses a variety of complementary and alternative treatments that stem from non-Western traditions. Several special features in this chapter and throughout the text such as What Every Nurse Should Know, Your Self-Awareness, Your Assessment Approach, Your Intervention Strategies, Rx: Communication, and Partnering with Clients and Families also provide specific strategies for cultural competence.

DEVELOPING AN UNDERSTANDING OF CULTURAL COMPETENCE

In the Western biomedical model, illness is often reduced to a particular disease, pathophysiology is emphasized, and the focus is most often on the client's body rather than on the whole individual. (See Chapter 33 for a discussion of non-Western traditions.) To understand the client's experience of illness, you must attempt to enter the client's world, understand the client's beliefs about "what is wrong, what happened, and what should be done" to achieve well-being. Thus, the client's perceptions, understandings, and approaches to health and disease are an integral part of any nursing care plan activities.

Cultural Competence

Cultural competence refers to the capacity of nurses or health service delivery systems to effectively understand and plan for the needs of a culturally diverse client or group. Spector (2004) views cultural competence as a complex combination of knowledge, attitudes, and skills used by the health care provider to deliver services that attend to the total context of the client's situation across cultural boundaries. With cultural competence, you are able to move beyond a superficial analysis of cultural differences, having the capacity to understand and work with cultural nuances.

The concept of cultural competence may be applied to health service delivery systems as well. It embraces the notion that health care systems should be able to understand and plan for the health needs of a specific cultural group. Thus, agencies that acknowledge, accept, and work with cultural differences may be viewed as "culturally competent," whereas those agencies that ignore culture when delivering services are viewed as "culturally blind." The National Center for Cultural Competence assists health care and mental health organizations in promoting culturally competent values, policy, structures, and practices. The center's mission is to design, implement, and evaluate culturally and linguistically competent service delivery systems. Its website (www11.georgetown.edu/research/gucchd/nccc) can be accessed through the Companion Website for this book.

MEDIALINK National Center for Cultural Competence

Worldview

Simply put, cultural competence incorporates the client's worldview. A *worldview* is the way a group of people (culture or subculture) see their social world, symbolic system, and physical environment and their own place in each. Worldview is revealed in people's religion, art, language, values, and health care beliefs and practices. A people's worldview provides a sense of identity as a Native American, a Puerto Rican, or a Masai tribesman. It promotes a group's survival and gives members a generally useful picture of the universe.

Ethnicity and Ethnocentrism

Ethnicity refers to one's sense of identity, providing social belonging and loyalty to a particular reference group within society. This sense of identity may be based on common ancestry and religious, national, language, tribal, or cultural origins. In contrast, **ethnocentrism** is the belief that one's own cultural values and behaviors are superior and preferable to those of any other cultural group. The nurse may be unaware of personal ethnocentric behavior that can undermine establishment of a balanced and respectful partnership with a multicultural client or group.

The terms *culturally diverse, multicultural*, and *ethnic* are used throughout this chapter. Likewise, the terms *cross-cultural* and *transcultural* are used interchangeably.

Cultural Sensitivity

Related to cultural competence is the concept of **cultural sensitivity**, the process of increasing professional effectiveness through understanding, respecting, and appreciating the importance of cultural factors in the delivery of health services. These cultural factors may include health beliefs, values, practices, and healing traditions of a client or group from another culture. Refer to the What Every Adult Health Nurse Should Know feature to expand your knowledge as you develop cultural sensitivity.

It is also important to appreciate the subculture, or culture within a culture. Recently researchers have referred to the "culture" of the hospital, the operating room, or the nursing school and the "subculture" of the mentally ill, the physically handicapped, or the elderly. Anthropologists point out that simply sharing some common characteristics does not make people members of a culture or subculture. There must be considerably more homogeneity in the group for it to be considered a culture or a subculture. For example, the Choctaw Indians living on a reservation in Philadelphia, Mississippi, are a subculture because they share a language, values and beliefs, and behavioral patterns. They are part of the

WHAT EVERY ADULT HEALTH NURSE SHOULD KNOW

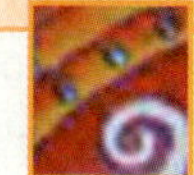

The "Hot and Cold" Healing Practice

Some cultures have widely held and sanctioned beliefs that might be considered unusual or unacceptable outside those cultures. Many cultures believe that health is the result of equilibrium between the vital elements of hot and cold—an imbalance between hot and cold causes illness. To cure the illness, the opposite element is given to restore balance in the body. For example, among Afghans and Afghan-Americans, a "hot" illness (such as a fever or infection) may be treated with a diet emphasizing cold foods and medicines. In contrast, a "cold illness" (such as arthritis) may be treated with hot foods and herbs.

Cultures that tend to embrace this hot and cold healing practice include Afghan, Puerto Rican, Mexican, Chinese, Filipino, Korean, and Vietnamese. Illnesses and treatments (foods, medications, and/or herbs) are all classified according to their hot or cold properties and vary from culture to culture. Chinese, Vietnamese, and Korean people may connect a person's internal balance to harmony with nature. Note that Koreans may believe that certain mental states are related to excessive cold (depressive and hypoactive) or excessive hot (hyperactive and irritable) imbalances.

larger Native American culture. In contrast, the physically handicapped are not a subculture because they have various disabilities, come from different socioeconomic levels, and may only rarely come into contact with other physically handicapped people.

A case can be made for viewing a hospital or part of it as a culture or subculture. The transient inhabitants of the hospital share a language, standards of acceptable behavior, and a similar worldview. This can be seen even more clearly in specialty units, such as intensive care or psychiatric units. People can be viewed as working within a hospital culture while living within the American culture. Applying the term *culture* or *subculture* to these environments may help us understand a hospital, an emergency room, a school, or a church. Some nurse anthropologists view nursing as a subculture (the health care providers subculture) and document its definite set of beliefs, practices, habits, rituals, and values, often stemming from dominant American cultural values.

Global Burden of Disease

Cultural competence and sensitivity are increasingly essential skills when addressing mental health in the global community. The **global burden of disease** (Murray & Lopez, 1996) represents comprehensive estimates of patterns of mortality and disability from diseases and injuries. Traditionally, a population's health status has been measured by number of deaths (i.e., "who's dying from what"). The goal of this study was to measure health status by measuring disease burden in years of life lost to premature death (i.e., "who dies sooner") and disability (i.e., "who's living with a disability of known severity and duration"). Here, disability plays a central, rather than invisible, role in determining the overall health status of a population. This extensive 5-year study provides information on disease burden by age, gender, cause, and region, including estimates for developing countries.

When looking at number of deaths alone, self-inflicted injuries rank among the top ten leading causes of death in developed countries. However, this study shows that the burden of psychiatric disorders has been heavily underestimated by traditional approaches that account for death but not disability. Psychiatric disorders emerge as a highly significant component of global disease burden. Of the ten leading causes of disability in the world in 1990, five were mental health conditions. These conditions, outlined in TABLE 9-1 ■, included unipolar depression, alcohol use, bipolar disorder, schizophrenia, and obsessive–compulsive disorder. In fact, unipolar depression was responsible for more than 1 in every 10 years of life lived with a disability globally. Depression was women's leading cause of disease burden worldwide.

This study also provides projections of disease burden to 2020. Unipolar depression, plus several types of injuries (including war, violence, and suicide) are likely to increase (see FIGURE 9-2 ■). Tobacco is expected to cause more premature death and disability than any single disease by 2020. These projections help to anticipate future mental health needs globally. The website of the World Health Organization (WHO) has extensive documentation of recent programs and resources related to the global burden of disease and can be accessed through the Companion Website for this book.

TABLE 9-1 ■ Leading Causes of Disability in the World: Documenting the Global Burden of Disease

All Causes	Percent of Total Disability
1. Unipolar major depression	10.7
2. Iron-deficiency anemia	4.7
3. Falls	4.6
4. Alcohol use	3.3
5. Chronic obstructive pulmonary disease	3.1
6. Bipolar disorder	3.0
7. Congenital anomalies	2.9
8. Osteoarthritis	2.8
9. Schizophrenia	2.6
10. Obsessive–compulsive disorders	2.2

Source: Adapted from Murray, C. J. L., & Lopez, A. D. (1996). *The global burden of disease: A comprehensive assessment of mortality and disability from diseases, injuries, and risk factors in 1990 and projected to 2020.* Cambridge, MA: Harvard University Press.

MEDIALINK World Health Organization

Many collaborators from around the world worked intensively to update and provide a more precise, comprehensive assessment of the global burden of disease and its causes. The latest text, *Global Burden of Disease and Risk Factors* (Lopez et al., 2006), is available for download at http://www.dcp2.org. WHO yearly reports are available at http://www.who.int/whr/en. For example, Prince et al. (2007) observed that about 14% of the global burden of disease is attributed to neuropsychiatric disorders, particularly due to the chronic disabling nature of depression, substance use disorders, and psychoses. They suggest that the burden of mental disorders is likely to be underestimated because of a lack of awareness of the connection between mental disorders and

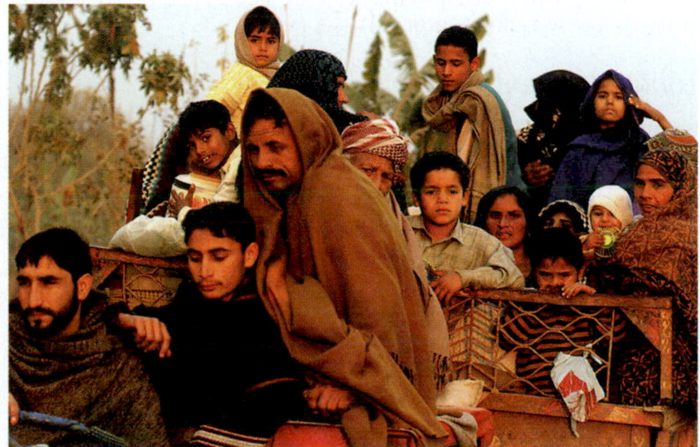

FIGURE 9-2 ■ Fleeing one's home to a refugee camp to avoid war or massacre presents many complex human problems—psychological, physiologic, political, and environmental.

Source: Peter Arnold, Inc., Sebastian Bolesch/Das Fotoarchiv.

other health conditions. Mental disorders may interact to increase risk for communicable diseases (e.g., alcohol and drugs for HIV/AIDS; see Chapter 25), noncommunicable diseases (e.g., depression and coronary heart disease), and intentional and unintentional injuries (e.g., alcohol as a risk factor in traffic accidents). Conversely, many health conditions may increase the risk of mental disorder (e.g., depression subsequent to debilitating chronic illness).

Cultural Values

Be aware that perceptions of health, disease, prevention, and treatment may differ among multicultural groups and that many interpretations of reality exist in the world. Acknowledging divergent values can be a significant first step toward improving one's cultural competence and sensitivity to differences, especially when the nurse is from the dominant culture (i.e., of white Anglo-American origin). TABLE 9-2 ■ highlights common values that may differ between dominant Anglo-American and nondominant cultural groups.

TABLE 9-2 ■ Common Values That May Differ Between Dominant and Nondominant Cultural Groups

Anglo-American (Dominant)	Other Cultural Groups (Nondominant)
Competition	Cooperation
Control over environment	Fate
Directness/honesty	Indirectness/"saving face"
Doing	Being
Efficiency	Idealism
Future orientation	Past or present orientation
Human equality	Hierarchy/ranking
Individualism	Group welfare
Informality	Formality
Mastery over nature	Harmony with nature
Materialism	Spiritualism
Self-help	Birthright inheritance
Time dominates	Personal interaction dominates
Youth	Elders

Source: Adapted from Huff, R. M., & Kline, M. V. (Eds.) (1999). *Promoting health in multicultural populations: A handbook for practitioners*. Thousand Oaks, CA: Sage Publications.

Cross-Cultural Communication

Consider the challenge of learning to communicate across cultures. The need to increase awareness of your own communication style is important in becoming competent and sensitive to cultural differences. For example, you may carefully choose a rate of speaking that promotes understanding and respect of the client. Other helpful techniques may be to speak in simple sentences and avoid use of slang, jargon, or technical words. Practical suggestions to improve cross-cultural communication skills may include:

- Attending multicultural events
- Reading about different cultural groups
- Talking to members of the cultural group
- Spending time in a particular ethnic community
- Learning another language

MEDIALINK Care Plan: Culture and Communication

In everyday practice, you may find yourself working with a client from a cultural background that is unfamiliar to you. Mirroring the client's communication style is one technique for effective cross-cultural communication. Mirroring is more fully discussed in Chapter 10.

Language and Dialect

You may need to determine the client's level of fluency in English and assess the degree to which another language is used as the primary language. Such language use may vary by age, gender, or generational level. In a given setting, language differences represent a serious barrier to all aspects of health care delivery. When you are unfamiliar with the client's language, great care must be taken to pay attention to nonverbal communication. The linguistically isolated client may look to your nonverbal behavior in an attempt to understand what is expected in an unfamiliar situation.

The use of a well-trained, effective interpreter is essential if the client does not speak the language or dialect of the dominant culture. Examples of people who may assist you in the delivery of linguistically appropriate services may include other health care workers familiar with the culture, a professional interpreter, a cultural consultant, multicultural community resources, or a nurse anthropologist. Family members may be helpful if their presence would not violate the client's confidentiality. In these instances, allow extra time for careful translation and back-translation.

Degree of Literacy

Determine the client's reading ability in English or other languages before using written materials related to health care. If the client cannot read English, then determine how best to provide appropriate translated materials that are culturally relevant in the particular setting.

Other Cultural Phenomena Affecting Health

In addition to cross-cultural communication, pay attention to the following five cultural phenomena that also affect health and health care among diverse cultural groups: environmental control, biological variations, social organization, space, and time orientation (Giger & Davidhizar, 2004). Attend to these factors during any cultural assessment, since each may influence health perceptions, beliefs, practices, and healing traditions.

Environmental Control

Environmental control refers to the ability to organize activities that attempt to control nature or environmental factors. Thus, a multicultural group may embrace specific health and illness beliefs, practices, use of folk healers, and healing traditions in attempts to intervene with the complex environment.

Biologic Variations

There may be distinct genetic and physical differences from one multicultural group to another. Examples of such differences include: nutritional habits and preferences, skin color, body build and structure, selective susceptibility to certain diseases, and variation in the metabolism of psychoactive medications (discussed in Chapter 7∞).

Social Organization

Social organization describes the type of family unit (e.g., extended, nuclear, or single-parent family) and type of social organizations (e.g., religious or multicultural) that shape the identity of a culturally diverse client or group. Socialization from one's early family life strongly contributes to cultural identification and development.

Space

How a person uses space may be defined and have different meanings based on one's particular culture. There may be different norms for intimacy as well as personal, social, and public distances among various cultural groups.

Time Orientation

Emphasis on the past, present, or future varies among culturally diverse groups. Note in the Partnering with Clients and Families feature on page 172 that nondominant cultural groups may value the past and present, whereas the dominant Anglo-American culture may emphasize the future.

Cultural Assessment

An appropriate cultural assessment is essential to culturally competent nursing care. This cultural assessment may be incorporated into routine assessment procedures as the first step of the nursing process when working with any client or group.

Degree of Acculturation

Assess the degree of acculturation for any client or group in a multicultural setting. **Acculturation** may be defined as the degree to which a particular client or group from another culture has adopted the values, attitudes, and behaviors of mainstream U.S. culture. Acculturation may be one of the most important factors that explain health status and risk behaviors.

One cannot assume that there is acculturation into the mainstream culture because a client or group from another culture is in the United States. There is likely to be a range of acculturation levels from the very traditional to the very acculturated. You are likely to find that the more traditional the client or group, the less likely it is for the client or group to be familiar with, understand, or practice Western approaches. It is important to assess the degree of acculturation in a multicultural setting because there may be a natural tendency on the part of many culturally diverse clients to resist acculturation. The measurement of acculturation is an important assessment activity. You can use a variety of scales, such as the assessment tool on page 174.

Heritage Assessment

The term *cultural care* incorporates professional health care that is culturally sensitive, culturally competent, and culturally appropriate. Within this framework, the Heritage Assessment Tool for the multicultural client in the Your Assessment Approach feature on page 174 represents a practical, useful way for you to investigate a client's (or your own) ethnic, cultural, and religious heritage. Such assessment may be used to understand a client's health traditions and reveal how deeply a client may identify with any particular tradition. It is important to emphasize that multicultural clients may embrace health beliefs and traditions from more than one culture, based on their unique heritage (Spector, 2004). A heritage assessment will help you to identify positive elements that can be reinforced to facilitate health promotion and disease prevention and anticipate rigid adherence to health beliefs and traditions that may conflict with effective Western practices.

Cultural assessment applies to agencies and health service delivery systems as well as to individuals or groups. Thus, you may have an opportunity to assess where a particular agency stands in terms of cultural competency and sensitivity.

Transcultural Care Planning

Begin to review the information that you have obtained thus far through your cultural assessment. Think about what additional information may be helpful as you prepare or revise your nursing care plan in everyday practice. A list of specific techniques for possible use in transcultural care planning is detailed in the Your Assessment Approach feature on page 175.

Culture Brokering

You are challenged to develop critical skills on behalf of clients, especially when clients and their families do not understand or accept biomedical interventions or treatments. This process, most useful when working with multicultural clients, is called culture brokering. **Culture brokering** is defined as the act of bridging, linking, or mediating between groups of people of different cultural systems to reduce conflict or produce change (Jezewski, 1995).

The Nurse-as-Culture-Broker

The term *culture broker* is used in many disciplines—nursing, medical anthropology, psychology, and social work in relation to numerous client populations, such as clients in hospitals and community settings, persons with disabilities, prisoners, and immigrants. Within nursing, the effective use of health care services may be thwarted by cultural, social, economic, political, and institutional constraints. Conflict in

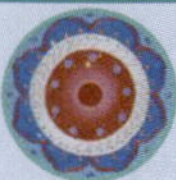

PARTNERING WITH CLIENTS AND FAMILIES

DEVELOPING CULTURAL COMPETENCE WITH SPECIFIC CULTURAL GROUPS

Use the information below to help you understand the health beliefs and practices of clients and families from cultural backgrounds that differ from yours. Think about incorporating the suggestions in your plan of care.

Cultural Groups/Nations of Origin	Health Beliefs and Practices	Suggestions to Consider
Hispanic (including Spain, Cuba, Puerto Rico, Mexico, Central and South America)	Belief in folk illnesses may characterize many traditional Hispanic groups. *Curanderismo* is the traditional health care system that may be used first, but not discussed, with a Western health care provider. Traditional folk healers may be the first health practitioners consulted. They are culturally acceptable, much less expensive than Western health care, and are willing to make house calls. *Fatalism* (i.e., the belief that an individual cannot control one's health) may be a common attitude among traditional groups. Health care decisions may involve the head of the household who decides what is best for the family.	Be aware that family and family support are very important core values. Respect is an extremely important factor in all relationships. Avoiding conflict and achieving harmony are strong cultural values.
African-American (including West Indian Islands, Haiti, Dominican Republic, Brazil, England, many West African countries)	Traditional explanations for disease and illness may involve natural causes (e.g., stress, poor eating habits) and unnatural causes from witchcraft practices (e.g., voodoo, bad spirits, other works of the devil). The Western health care system is generally well respected and used for serious illness, although folk healing traditions may also be utilized. Traditional folk healers may be the only health practitioners used by African-Americans of low income.	Be aware that there may be caution about using programs from inside and outside some black communities. Prior programs and services may have lost funding and personnel. African-Americans who have been trained "outside" the community may need to earn trust by demonstrating sincere interest in the community's particular needs and concerns. Churches often have been used as sites for health education and intervention.
Native American and Alaskan Native (including First Nation and indigenous American Indian Nations, Alaskan Aleuts and Eskimos)	Traditional ceremonies may be practiced among tribal groups to promote well-being and balance. Many tribal groups feel distrustful and exploited by Westerners. Medicine men, traditional healers, and herbal treatments are very important to some groups. Taboos and modesty are important in tribal life.	Be aware that every tribal group has its own unique history, traditions, and values. Become familiar with acceptable verbal and nonverbal communications of the group. Respect tribal sovereignty and work within the tribal group. Be aware that use of "talking circles" together with tribal stories have been useful for culturally appropriate educational interventions.

(continued on page 173)

interactions in health care settings between the "client seeking care" and the "provider giving care" is the most important antecedent to culture brokering. A conflict may arise when there are differences in values, beliefs, or behaviors between a client and provider concerning the appropriateness and feasibility of a treatment plan. The disadvantaged client may be in desperate need of intervention but politically, economically, or personally powerless to access health care.

The **nurse-as-culture-broker** serves as a bridge between the client and the providers in the health care system by "stepping in," or intervening, to facilitate the acquisition of effective heath care. You may act as a broker of information about

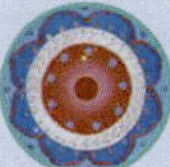

PARTNERING WITH CLIENTS AND FAMILIES *(continued)*

Cultural Groups/Nations of Origin	Health Beliefs and Practices	Suggestions to Consider
Asian-American (including Asian Indians, Chinese, Cambodians, Thais, Vietnamese, Laotians, Filipinos, Hmong, Koreans, Japanese)	A central concept of the traditional health care system is the need to attain a harmonious relationship with nature. This traditional health care system may be the first one used for any illness. There may be a tendency not to discuss this with a Western health care practitioner. Teachings of Buddhism, Confusianism, and Taoism may emphasize upholding a public presentation that avoids admission of physical or mental illness. Many Asians may prefer traditional forms of native medicine, seeking help from Chinatown "masters" who treat with traditional herbs and other methods. Asians may not use the Western health care system because of painful diagnostic tests and lack of information.	Be aware that balance or equilibrium and kinship solidarity are two beliefs that may be prominent among Asians. Kinship solidarity refers to the belief that an individual is subservient to the family or kinship-based group. Thus, separation from family members may be stressful. Respect for elders and male authority may determine decision-making practices regarding health care for recent immigrants. Use "active listening" and watch for nonverbal cues since some Asian groups may not disagree openly with health care providers. Likewise, conflicts are generally handled within the family and may not be shared with a health care provider unless trust is established. It is helpful if outreach workers are perceived as nonthreatening and nonintrusive.
Pacific Islander (including Guamanian, Samoan, Hawaiian, Pacific Islander–American)	Health beliefs and practices among these cultural groups may vary greatly. Thus, knowledge of the geographic location and particular ethnic group is essential. In general, indigenous illnesses may be treated with traditional healing practices, whereas Western illnesses may be treated with Western medical approaches. Taboos, modesty, and traditional healing practices are very important to these cultural groups.	Be aware that health data may not be available for the particular Pacific Islander group of interest. It may be helpful to involve women in all aspects of health care since many island cultures are matriarchal. Emphasize concepts of wholeness and interconnectedness, which are central features of several Pacific Islander groups. Culturally acceptable and appropriate strategies for health promotion may include use of "talk stories," role playing, pictures, and folk media (e.g., song, dance, music).
Anglo-American/European-American (including Germany, Ireland, England, Italy, the former Soviet Union, and all other European countries)	Often the dominant cultural group that influences the determination of health care needs, beliefs, practices, and programs in communities. Primary reliance on a "modern" or "Western" health care system, emphasizing use of technology and diagnostic tests. There may be reliance on traditional health beliefs and practices that may vary greatly, depending on the country of ancestry. There is a recent increased interest in complementary and alternative (CAM) practices which emphasize holistic, naturalistic healing. Judeo-Christian beliefs may influence health practices.	Individualism, materialism, and emphases on time and youth may be strong cultural values. Directness and efficiency may be factors in relationships with health care providers. Assess the utility of self-help literature and groups when planning health care interventions.

Sources: Adapted from Huff, R. M., & Kline, M. V. (Eds.). (1999). *Promoting health in multicultural populations: A handbook for practitioners*. Thousand Oaks, CA: Sage Publications; and Spector, R. E. (2004). *Cultural diversity in health & illness* (6th ed.). Upper Saddle River, NJ: Prentice Hall.

YOUR ASSESSMENT APPROACH
Heritage Assessment Tool

An assessment tool like the one below will help you structure your assessment to include the salient points that are important to cover. *Note*: The greater the number of positive responses, the greater the degree to which the person may identify with his or her traditional culture. The one exception to positive answers is the question about whether or not a person's name was changed.

1. Where was your mother born? _____
2. Where was your father born? _____
3. Where were your grandparents born?
   a. Your mother's mother? _____
   b. Your mother's father? _____
   c. Your father's mother? _____
   d. Your father's father? _____
4. How many brothers _____ and sisters _____ do you have?
5. What setting did you grow up in? Urban _____ Rural _____ Suburban _____
6. What country did your parents grow up in?
   Father _____
   Mother _____
7. How old were you when you came to the United States? _____
8. How old were your parents when they came to the United States?
   Mother _____ Father _____
9. When you were growing up, who lived with you? _____
10. Have you maintained contact with
    a. Aunts, uncles, cousins? (1) Yes _____ (2) No _____
    b. Brothers and sisters? (1) Yes _____ (2) No _____
    c. Parents? (1) Yes _____ (2) No _____
    d. Your own children? (1) Yes _____ (2) No _____
11. Did most of your aunts, uncles, cousins live near your home?
    (1) Yes _____ (2) No _____
12. Approximately how often did you visit your family members who lived outside your home?
    (1) Daily _____ (2) Weekly _____ (3) Monthly _____
    (4) Once a year or less _____ (5) Never _____
13. Was your original family name changed?
    (1) Yes _____ (2) No _____
14. What is your religious preference?
    (1) Catholic _____ (2) Jewish _____ (3) Protestant _____
    (4) Denomination _____ (5) Other _____ (6) None _____
15. Is your spouse the same religion as you?
    (1) Yes _____ (2) No _____
16. Is your spouse the same ethnic background as you?
    (1) Yes _____ (2) No _____
17. What kind of school did you go to?
    (1) Public _____ (2) Private _____ (3) Parochial _____
18. As an adult, do you live in a neighborhood where the neighbors are the same religion and ethnic background as yourself?
    (1) Yes _____ (2) No _____
19. Do you belong to a religious institution?
    (1) Yes _____ (2) No _____
20. Would you describe yourself as an active member?
    (1) Yes _____ (2) No _____
21. How often do you attend your religious institution?
    (1) More than once a week _____ (2) Weekly _____
    (3) Monthly _____ (4) Special holidays only _____
    (5) Never _____
22. Do you practice your religion at home?
    (1) Yes _____ (2) No _____
    (If yes, please specify)
    (3) Praying _____ (4) Bible reading _____
    (5) Diet _____ (6) Celebrating religious holidays _____
23. Do you prepare foods of your ethnic background?
    (1) Yes (2) No
24. Do you participate in ethnic activities?
    (1) Yes _____ (2) No _____
    (If yes, please verify)
    (3) Singing _____ (4) Holiday celebrations _____
    (5) Dancing _____ (6) Festivals _____
    (7) Costumes _____ (8) Other _____
25. Are your friends from the same religious background as you?
    (1) Yes _____ (2) No _____
26. Are your friends from the same ethnic background as you?
    (1) Yes _____ (2) No _____
27. What is your native language? _____
28. Do you speak this language?
    (1) Prefer _____ (2) Occasionally _____ (3) Rarely _____
29. Do you read your native language?
    (1) Yes _____ (2) No _____

Source: Spector, R. E. (2004). *Cultural diversity in health & illness* (6th ed.). Upper Saddle River, NJ: Prentice Hall, pp. 321–323.

regulations that control health benefits or facilitate a multicultural client's entry into various hospital departments. A skilled culture broker may develop and maintain working relationships with multicultural and bilingual professionals, staff, and members of the local community. When necessary, you may secure linguistically appropriate services by working with a professional medical interpreter when a client does not speak English or has limited English proficiency. You may act as a culture broker if conflict occurs in a culturally diverse staff. Finally, you may use culture brokering within your own profession to bridge the gap between disparate areas of nursing.

Culture Brokering Model

Jezewski (1993, 1995) is credited with the development of a culture brokering model evolved from health-related, anthropological, and business literature sources. This model of conflict resolution is based on several studies of clients displaying vulnerability from extreme circumstances that hin-

YOUR ASSESSMENT APPROACH
Transcultural Care Planning

Unique information may be useful in tailoring nursing care to a culturally unique client. Evaluate the information you obtained through cultural assessment as you prepare or revise the nursing care plan. Include the client's cultural preferences in your care plan where possible. Some specific and practical techniques to consider in transcultural care planning are:

- Describe any language barriers. Note what strengths or resources the client might have available to reduce any language barrier.
- When assessing religious beliefs, note any specific religious rituals or religious dietary requirements observed by the client.
- Note any lack of financial resources, including the ability to purchase prescription medicines or food for specific diets. Note whether any local agencies provide financial assistance to the client.
- Identify other barriers to care such as lack of transportation or lack of child care.
- Once barriers are identified, explore alternative resources available to the client's family and community.
- Assess any cultural demands that the client may face at home which may conflict with important health care needs.
- Describe any culturally generated feelings such as shame that may interfere with the client's willingness to embrace a health care plan.
- Note the multicultural client's concerns and address them in the care plan where possible.

Source: Muñoz, C., & Luckmann, J. (2005). *Transcultural communication in nursing* (2nd ed.). Clifton Park, NY: Thomson-Delmar Learning.

dered their autonomous use of the health care system. Jezewski's studies focused on clients who were politically and economically powerless (migrant farmers and homeless people) as well as critical care and oncology nurses working with clients experiencing life-threatening illness with the need to make informed Do Not Resuscitate decisions.

Conditions That Affect Brokering Several conditions may either enhance or hinder effective health care. Powerlessness of the client is a primary reason for brokering. Other conditions may include economics (the ability to pay for services), politics, and stigma associated with mental disorder. Two very important conditions in the culture brokering model are cultural background (including ethnicity) and cultural sensitivity. The nurse-as-culture-broker demonstrates cultural sensitivity by being aware of, and sensitive to, the needs of clients from backgrounds other than your own. Note that there may be an increased risk of breakdown or conflict in health care services when providers lack cultural sensitivity.

Stages of Culture Brokering The resolution of conflict or breakdown in the health care situation occurs in three stages: perception, intervention, and outcome. These stages briefly describe the process of facilitating care by maintaining a client's connectedness to the health care system. "Staying connected" is the overall dimension that involves linking the client to the health care system, as well as helping the client remain engaged to that health care system in a manner that meets the client's needs.

Stage 1: Perception (perceiving the need for brokering). Assess the impact of conflict or breakdown in health care interaction. Breakdowns in health care interactions are generally less serious than conflict. Assess the conditions that may enhance or hinder the resolution of conflict. Identify barriers to access and health care utilization.

Stage 2: Intervention (strategies to resolve conflict or breakdown). Establish rapport and trust with clients to foster and maintain connections between those clients and their providers. Facilitate links with personnel within and outside the health care setting, using strategies such as networking, negotiating, advocating, and innovating.

Stage 3: Outcome (evaluating strategies to resolve identified conflict or breakdown). Maintain connectedness across various systems. Evaluate connections between the client and the health care system. Evaluate whether conflicts or breakdowns are resolved. If they are not resolved, return to Stage 1 for further assessment or Stage 2 and try different strategies.

The Partnering with Clients and Families feature on page 176 invites you to explore the key components of culture brokering activities in a health care setting.

DEVELOPING CULTURAL COMPETENCE IN NURSING PRACTICE

Developing an understanding of cultural competence requires paying attention to considerations of global health, cultural values, cultural phenomena affecting health, and the importance of cultural assessment as part of the nursing process. Cultural competence in nursing practice requires practical strategies (general as well as specific to a particular cultural group), considerations of community-based health care promotion and disease prevention programs, and the need to advocate for cultural diversity in nursing practice, research, and education. At the same time, it is important to be aware that there are varying degrees of acculturation and individual differences—assessment of one Chinese person may be dramatically different than another and from one generation to another.

The Transcultural Nursing Society (TCNS) promotes knowledgeable culturally based care. You can obtain information about this organization through its website, which can be accessed through the Companion Website for this book. Certification as a transcultural nurse can also be obtained through TCNS.

MEDIALINK Transcultural Nursing Society

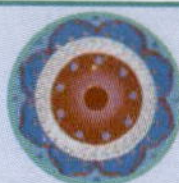

PARTNERING WITH CLIENTS AND FAMILIES

A CLIENT FROM ANOTHER CULTURE

Imagine that you are a psychiatric consultation-liaison nurse at a local medical center and are contacted by a frustrated family health nurse unable to communicate with an elderly Asian man. The man apparently arrived at the family-practice clinic alone that morning and did not appear to speak English. He would gently shake his head as if to indicate "yes" to any question, repeat the words "Laos" and "Mr. Phet" (pronounced "pet"), but refuse any attempt at physical examination to help determine a possible reason for his visit. Drawing on past experiences in culture-specific clinical nursing care, you recall several Laotian beliefs, values, practices, and healing traditions. You recall the intervention strategies used in other, similar situations, as past experiences may provide valuable working knowledge to guide your culture brokering activities in the present context. They are reviewed below.

Laotian Belief, Value, Practice, or Healing Tradition	General Intervention Strategies
"Saving face," i.e., the Laotian tendency to respond in a manner to please the inquirer. Not knowing an answer may be viewed as extremely embarrassing.	Create an environment in which the client is comfortable describing symptoms as well as answering questions. Find ways to help the client to demonstrate that he or she understands what is happening or what needs to be done.
Incomplete use of prescribed medication or unwillingness to refill a prescription.	Give a clear, simple description of how a particular medication works. Explore, if possible, the client's understanding of the illness and your role as provider in relation to the illness.
Possible misunderstanding about the use of vaccines. For example, a yearly flu vaccine may protect against bird flu.	Give a clear, simple description of how each particular vaccine works. Spell out specifically what a vaccine may or may not prevent.
May relate feeling ill in relation to the temperature inside the body. The need to ingest warm food (soups, hot water, etc.) when ill.	Try to incorporate this healing practice into any nursing care plan whenever possible. (Refer back to What Every Adult Health Nurse Should Know on page 168).
Belief that the top of the head is sacred but the feet are vulgar.	During physical examination, always ask permission to touch the client's head. When necessary, touch the head first and feet last during any physical assessment. *Never point your feet at someone.*

As a skilled culture broker, your crucial goals are to facilitate care by linking Mr. Phet to the health care system and by helping him "stay connected" to that system. There is a perceived need for brokering because the system has broken down—there is a gross lack of verbal communication in the health care interaction between Mr. Phet and the busy family health nurse. You quickly recognize Mr. Phet's position of powerlessness because of the language barrier. Based on your perception of Mr. Phet's powerlessness, you immediately implement several intervention strategies to resolve the breakdown.

- You negotiate with a family health nurse interested in developing cultural competence to participate in transcultural care planning and to volunteer as the designated client care coordinator.
- Since a professional medical interpreter is not available, you call on a bilingual Asian staff member to participate in information gathering for transcultural assessment and care planning.
- You identify as assessment priorities other conditions that may affect culture brokering such as the client's ability to pay and stigma associated with illness.
- You attempt to identify family members and community resources that might serve to alleviate the language barrier where possible.
- You network, if necessary, to locate a Laotian consultant in the community who may help to interpret Laotian cultural beliefs, values, practices, and healing traditions.
- You consider a referral to the local home health service to further assess Mr. Phet's basic needs in his home environment.
- During these initial culture brokering activities, you actively evaluate strategies to resolve the identified breakdown, helping to maintain connections across the various health systems that may work with Mr. Phet.

MEDIALINK Case Study: Culturally Sensitive Nursing

General Strategies for Developing Cultural Competence

An essential step toward developing cultural competence is to examine your own perceptions, prejudices, and stereotypes regarding the particular cultural group of interest. It is helpful to suspend personal judgments in favor of learning more about "who these people really are." Learn about the culture's history, migration, and immigration patterns. What specific cultural beliefs, values, practices, and healing traditions may relate to particular lifestyle habits (e.g., religion, gender, dietary patterns, use of alcohol and drugs, use of touch, use of time, etc.)? Be careful of your own ethnocentrism because culturally diverse groups may initially view you as foreign and uneducated regarding their proper forms of address, social customs, and appropriate methods for dealing with their concerns and health problems. If possi-

YOUR SELF-AWARENESS
Applying Principles of Cultural Competence and Sensitivity

Assess your ability to carry out these suggestions when working with a culturally diverse client or group. Which of these suggestions are most useful to you as you develop cultural competence and sensitivity in your particular setting?

- Learn about the culture of interest by making multiple visits to the community to become familiar with the community's way of life. Activities may include talking to community leaders and residents, eating at local restaurants, visiting cultural sites, and attending local events.
- Learn specifically about the culture's orientation to health, disease, health traditions, and traditional healing practices.
- Identify and learn about the traditional healers within the community. Note the healers' ease of access, medicines used, cultural acceptability, and cost of care.
- Be open and nonjudgmental regarding specific cultural practices that are not part of your cultural heritage.
- Add questions to your assessment tools that reflect these cultural beliefs, values, practices, and healing traditions.
- Practice cross-cultural communication skills.
- Learn how to work with a competent interpreter as necessary.
- Take time to explain Western concepts of health, disease, treatment, and prevention that are relevant and understandable to the culture of interest.
- Use educational materials that are culturally appropriate and relevant to this culture.
- Work with, and learn from, indigenous health care providers when addressing the needs of this culture.
- Learn how to work with peer educators from the community.
- Seek ways to improve access to services for multicultural groups with emphasis on availability, accessibility, and acceptability.

ble, attempt to identify issues related to access to health care for this cultural group as well. Such issues may include patterns of care, barriers to care (including accessibility, availability, and acceptability), and the use of social assistance services.

The Your Self-Awareness feature above outlines several helpful suggestions for working with culturally diverse clients and groups. Such strategies will help you to apply principles of cultural competence and sensitivity.

Developing Cultural Competence with Specific Cultural Groups

Summaries of cultural health beliefs and practices for five major cultural groups (Hispanic, African-American, Native American and Alaska Native, Asian-American, and Pacific Islander populations) are in the Partnering with Clients and Families feature on pages 172–173. Helpful suggestions to consider when working toward cultural competence are provided for each of these groups. It is advantageous to consult with family members, a professional interpreter, a cultural consultant, multicultural community resources, or a nurse anthropologist whenever possible to facilitate your development toward cultural competence with a particular cultural group. You may also wish to consult the bibliography at the end of this chapter for specific applications to clinical care (Lipson & Dibble, 2005) and transcultural assessment and intervention (Giger & Davidhizar, 2004).

Community-Based Health Care Promotion and Disease Prevention Programs

Nurses often may be able to plan, implement, and/or evaluate a program designed to meet the complex nursing needs of a specific cultural group. Examples of such community-based programs include:

- A community-level anger management program in an urban barrio to reach Mexican-Americans, using the media as part of a mental health campaign
- An HIV sexual-risk-reduction intervention among young adult African-American women
- A "talking circle" program with Native Americans to reduce alcohol-related injuries and alcoholism

A useful planning framework for health promotion and disease prevention programs in multicultural populations is provided in the Your Intervention Strategies feature on page 178. The first formal step of any program planning process is to involve those individuals affected by the problem. This principle of participation appears to be the most important component of any program development. Collaboration between planner and participants can be achieved only if there is respect for each other's values and for the agenda to be accomplished. As you become involved in any community-based program, remember to utilize the group's cultural uniqueness by incorporating how group members define health problems, identify proposed solutions, and select activities to be emphasized. Group members are invaluable participants in identifying how health-promoting behavioral changes, once achieved, can be sustained in that community.

Advocating Issues of Cultural Diversity in Nursing

Nurses need to make a conscious decision to acknowledge and value the diversity in others. Developing cultural competence and sensitivity needed for comprehensive care is based on new knowledge, personal self-assessment, supervised practice, mentoring experiences, experience in culturally diverse clinical practice settings, participation in discussions, and diversity training.

MediaLink Critical Thinking Exercise: Cultural Diversity in the Clinic

MEDIALINK Transcultural Nursing

YOUR INTERVENTION STRATEGIES
A Planning Framework for Health Promotion and Disease Prevention Programs Involving a Specific Cultural Group

When planning a program for a specific cultural group, use the therapeutic tasks and specific intervention strategies below as a basis for your plan.

Therapeutic Task	Intervention Strategies
1. Planning the program	Involve those affected by the problem.
	Assess the needs of the cultural community.
	Diagnose health-related concerns (problems and needs) in the community.
	Prioritize and select the target cultural group, problem, and setting.
	Assess the specific needs of your target cultural group.
	Develop appropriate target group goals and objectives.
	Select health promotion program intervention activities that consider the unique characteristics of the target group, health problem, and setting.
2. Implementing the program	Preimplementation preparation.
	Program implementation.
	Implementation administration and monitoring.
3. Evaluating the program	Assess the immediate impact of the program (impact evaluation).
	Assess the long-term target group health and social outcomes (outcome evaluation).
	Assess the quality of the program inputs during the development and implementation phases (process evaluation).

Source: Adapted from Huff, R. M., & Kline, M. V. (Eds.). (1999). *Promoting health in multicultural populations: A handbook for practitioners.* Thousand Oaks, CA: Sage Publications.

MEDIALINK Application: The Need for Cultural and Linguistic Competence

Nursing Practice

Nursing competencies must include the ability to actively and effectively work with culturally diverse clients. Look for opportunities for meaningful dialogue and relationship building across cultures. You may seek out practicing nurses of a particular cultural background to serve as resource consultants. You may mentor nurse colleagues from other cultures who work in your setting. You may seek information from transcultural health care nurses with experiences in developing countries, such as the nurses who sponsor www.culturediversity.org, which can be accessed through the Companion Website for this book.

You may read transcultural journals (e.g., *Journal of Transcultural Nursing, Journal of Cultural Diversity*, etc.) to familiarize yourself with critical culture-based issues and opportunities. You may become a member of an organization such as TCNS or a certified transcultural nurse. Make every attempt to openly discuss cultural conflicts in order to actively address suspicions and distortions. Avoiding conflict may result in chronic strained communication, insensitivity, and exclusion that thwart culturally competent care. Recognize the importance of fostering transcultural communication with other health care providers, and take into account the presence of a multicultural workforce (Muñoz & Luckmann, 2005).

Nursing Research

According to Gary, Sigsby, and Campbell (1998) nurses can use research training and development to seek collaboration, coalition, and compassion across cultures. Nursing research may define what knowledge is meaningful for a particular multicultural group. Through research, nurses can become informed regarding which interventions might be useful in specific community-based programs. Research may contribute to the development of more inclusive theories to account for behaviors observed in multicultural groups. Finally, research may better identify important health-related distinctions among numerous cultural groups that are currently classified into one category (e.g., various values and traditions of specific Native American Indian Nations such as the Cherokee, Navajo, and Sioux).

Nursing Education

Vinson (2000) advocates the development of an appreciation of how cultural identity influences health and illness as a professional education competency. Although the nursing profession remains a field dominated by white females, accrediting agencies are now encouraging nursing faculty to integrate content that emphasizes cultural diversity. Educators need to work within multicultural and multidisciplinary frameworks to tackle issues in the "real world." Yet, recruitment and re-

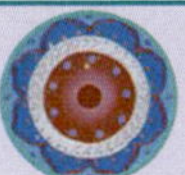

EVIDENCE-BASED PRACTICE

CULTURAL DIVERSITY IN NURSING

Juireith is a 24-year-old African-American female beginning the baccalaureate nursing program at your local university. She was born in Jamaica and then moved to the Bronx, New York, to live with extended family. She now lives alone in your town, determined to earn a university degree in nursing. She sits with the few other African-American nursing students in class. As a student interested in the development of cultural sensitivity in professional nursing education and practice, you understand that racial and ethnic minority students have high attrition rates in nursing school. Loneliness and isolation, peers' lack of understanding of cultural differences, and coping with insensitivity and discrimination are some of the experiences that racial and ethnic minority students may have in nursing school. You practice specific strategies, based on the following research studies, as a way of demonstrating the personal value you place upon diversity:

- Evaluate your assumptions, understand your attitudes, and learn about the differences in others to eliminate stereotyping.
- Listen to the concerns and issues of students from other cultures.
- Offer opportunities for participation in scholarly efforts to students from other cultures, thereby encouraging collaboration.
- Confront feelings of racism, as most individuals in mainstream U.S. culture may not be aware of passive racism. Using your culture brokering skills, emphasize that words or actions can be discussed and explained if misinterpreted.
- Acknowledge and appreciate cultural differences. Welcome and value change and a new approach.
- Contribute toward building a student learning environment that accommodates cultural differences.

Amaro, D. J., Abriam-Yago, K., & Yoder, M. (2006). Perceived barriers for ethnically diverse students in nursing programs. *Journal of Nursing Education, 45*(7), 247–254.

Gardner, J. (2005). Barriers influencing the success of racial and ethnic minority students in nursing programs. *Journal of Transcultural Nursing, 16*(2), 155–162.

CRITICAL THINKING APPLICATION

1. How would valuing cultural diversity enhance psychiatric–mental health nursing practice?
2. If someone from another culture comes to your school or your hometown, isn't it up to that person to adjust?
3. What specific actions could you take in a mental health setting that would show that you acknowledge and appreciate cultural differences?

tention of students from diverse cultures continue to be problems in schools of nursing. Educational institutions need to recruit and mentor students from diverse cultures to serve as clinicians, managers, faculty, and leaders who can then serve as role models for other students. One way to attract and educate a diverse student group is to practice diversity in faculty recruitment. When considering nursing curricula, it is important to note that knowledge of a foreign language will be essential as we strive to meet global needs in the 21st century. Nursing students themselves also have a responsibility to their classmates from diverse cultures. The Evidence-Based Practice feature suggests practical strategies you can use in your relationships with classmates from other cultures.

Finally, while it may be easy to discuss strategies, make recommendations, and pay lip service to the value of developing cultural competence and sensitivity, nurses need to step out of their personal frames of reference, confront their own stereotypes and biases, and be open to different worldviews. One practical way to enhance such culture brokering skills is through periodic workshops and seminars. Nurses also need to accept the challenge to incorporate cultural competence and sensitivity into all aspects of professional nursing care.

PSYCHIATRIC EPIDEMIOLOGY IN A CULTURALLY DIVERSE SOCIETY

Epidemiology represents an emerging specialty that focuses on human populations rather than on individual clients. *Epidemiology* consists of these three Greek word roots: *epi*, meaning "among"; *demos*, meaning "people"; and *logos*, meaning "doctrine"—the doctrine of what is among people or happening to people.

Epidemiologists often study the biopsychosocial factors that influence health status in populations. Epidemiologic information for the United States is available through the Centers for Disease Control and Prevention (www.cdc.gov) and for Canada through Health Canada (www.hc-sc.gc.ca) and can be accessed through the Companion Website for this book. The CDC also partners with other nations around the world. Epidemiologic principles and methods may be applied to determine the cause of a disorder (such as HIV), to assess risks associated with a harmful exposure (such as rape), to determine whether a particular treatment (such as behavior therapy) is effective, and to identify health service utilization needs and trends. Psychiatric epidemiology is particularly useful to the psychiatric–mental health nurse as the basic discipline for preventive and community psychiatry. Information about psychiatric epidemiologic studies is available through the National Institute of Mental Health (www.nimh.nih.gov) and can be accessed through the Companion Website for this book.

MEDIALINK Information on Psychiatric Epidemiology

Hundreds of millions of people worldwide in both developing and developed countries suffer from psychiatric disorders that cause personal suffering, social disruption, and economic losses. The worldwide occurrence of psychiatric disorders prompts nurses to address multicultural diversity as principles of psychiatric epidemiology are applied to various human populations. The United States represents a multicultural country consisting of numerous subgroups who have brought unique cultural traits with them from waves of immigration over the years.

An important premise of psychiatric epidemiology is that mental illness is not randomly distributed across populations. Not all people are at equal risk for developing mental disorders. One client may be depressed, another may be psychotic, while a third may suffer from debilitating physical illness. Such differences in the occurrence of mental disorders are of prime interest in epidemiology.

Definition of Psychiatric Epidemiology

Psychiatric epidemiology is the study of the distribution and determinants of mental disorders (or other health-related conditions or events) in human populations. Purposes include prevention, surveillance (monitoring), and the control of mental disorders. Epidemiology traditionally investigated the cause of disease. More recently, "disease" has been generalized to include a wide variety of mental disorders and health-related problems. Health-related conditions or events may include injuries; exposure to environmental pollutants, natural and man-made disasters, and traumatic or violent events; behavioral problems; and the nonuse or misuse of mental health services.

A psychiatric epidemiologist is an investigator who studies mental disorders or other health-related conditions or events in defined populations to develop a comprehensive picture of mental health problems and to evaluate interventions. An advanced professional degree (master's or Ph.D.) from a school of public health or similar institution is required. Epidemiologists ask, "Which characteristics among individuals (such as genetic) or their environment (such as exposure to stressful life events) explain differences in morbidity from specific mental disorders?" Nursing provides an excellent background for investigating disease occurrence and its relation to various characteristics of individuals or their environment.

Within the context of psychiatric epidemiology, cultural diversity refers to varied cultural and ethnic backgrounds that may influence the experience, expression, reporting, and evaluation of mental disorders. Depression is the basis for several examples in this chapter because depression is among the most common disorders in the United States today.

Uses of Psychiatric Epidemiology

Psychiatric epidemiology is used to do the following:

- Determine causative factors for specific disorders.
- Identify groups of people (populations) at high risk of developing specific disorders.
- Recognize changes in health problems, especially the emergence of new problems.
- Plan for current health needs and predict future needs.
- Evaluate preventive and therapeutic measures.

It is important to note that both the patterns of occurrence of mental disorders in a community and the patterns of delivery of psychiatric care are studied. The services offered influence, and are influenced by, the amount and nature of the disorders and changes in modes of therapy.

KEY EPIDEMIOLOGIC CONCEPTS

Several key concepts commonly used in epidemiology may serve as a foundation for applying epidemiologic principles to your work in psychiatric nursing. Knowledge of these terms is also useful when reviewing current medical literature.

Prevalence and Incidence

Prevalence rate refers to the *total number of active cases*, both old and new, present in a population during a specific period of time. Prevalence rates may be used for the following purposes:

- To express the burden of a disorder in the population
- To identify population subgroups (by age, sex, etc.) for prevention strategies
- To track changes in patterns of a disorder over time
- For the planning and evaluation of mental health services

A formula that illustrates the basic components in determining prevalence rate is in FIGURE 9-3 ■.

An **incidence rate** measures the *number of new cases* of a disease or disorder in a population over a specific period of time. Incidence is a direct measure of the rate at which individuals in a given population develop a disease or disorder. Thus, incidence is a direct measure of risk. Clues to the causes of a disorder may be obtained as new "incident" cases are studied. A formula that illustrates the basic components in determining an incidence rate is in Figure 9-3.

Studies of chronic diseases, such as schizophrenia, generally use prevalence measures; studies of acute disorders or events, such as rape, generally use incidence measures. One can examine prevalence or incidence rates by age, sex, race/ethnicity, and other biopsychosocial factors to determine which subgroups are at greatest risk for specific diseases. The identification of vulnerable subgroups may be the first step in the development of intervention strategies that target resources for people at greatest risk.

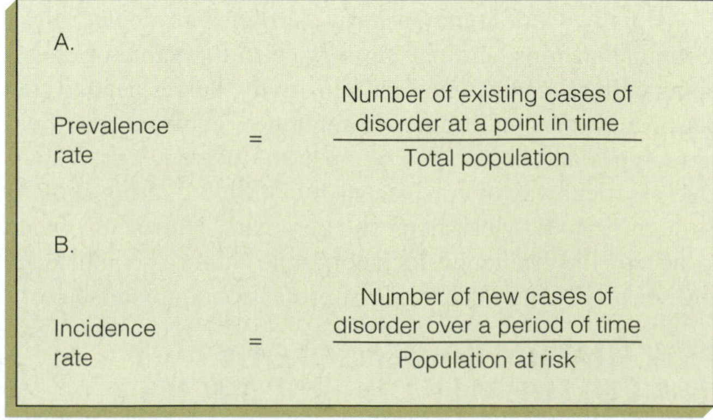

FIGURE 9-3 ■ A. Prevalence rate. B. Incidence rate.

Risk Factors

A critical issue related to cultural diversity in psychiatric epidemiology is that important factors reflecting varying cultures need to be assessed in clinical practice and research. Ethnicity, race, dietary patterns, the use of alcohol and drugs, health and healing practices, other lifestyle habits, religious or spiritual beliefs, the use of time, and migration patterns may differentially affect the experience, expression, reporting, and evaluation of mental disorders among culturally diverse groups. The field of research has been criticized in retrospect for studying white males and, to a lesser extent, white females, and then generalizing the results to all other groups.

The notion of biopsychosocial risk factors is common in psychiatric literature. A **risk factor** is a factor whose presence is associated with an increased chance or probability of mental disorder. Some risk factors, such as age, cannot be modified. Other risk factors, such as personal lifestyle habits regarding the use of alcohol and tobacco, are susceptible to change. A limited review of numerous risk factors associated with the occurrence of many psychiatric disorders as outlined by Bromet (1998) is given in the following sections.

Gender

Differences in rates between males and females are found for substance abuse, anxiety disorders, and depression. The male-to-female ratios are estimated at 6:1 for alcoholism, 1:2 for depression, and 1:2 for phobias.

Age

Age is associated with the occurrence of mental disorders. An important finding from the early Epidemiologic Catchment Area (ECA) studies, discussed further later in this chapter, was that young adults (age 25–44) had the highest prevalence estimates for most disorders (Bruce, Leaf, Rozal, Florio, & Hoff, 1994). Alcoholism is known to peak in the early forties. Heavy drinking associated with driving or fighting while intoxicated appears to peak in the early twenties.

Social Class

Lower social class status is associated with increased rates of depression, alcohol and other substance abuse, and antisocial personality disorder. Although risk factors vary among mental disorders, studies indicate that adults in poverty are at higher risk for an episode of at least one mental disorder compared with those not in poverty.

Ethnicity

Ethnicity appears to be indirectly associated with mental disorders because different ethnic groups share different social and physical environments. Again, the early ECA studies reported similar prevalence rates for most mental disorders between African-Americans and Caucasians (Bruce et al., 1994). For major depression, Caucasian men tended to have higher rates than African-American men, while African-American women had higher prevalence rates than Caucasian women. Caucasians of all ages have higher suicide rates than African-Americans, with Native American youth at increased risk for suicide.

WHY I BECAME A PSYCHIATRIC–MENTAL HEALTH NURSE

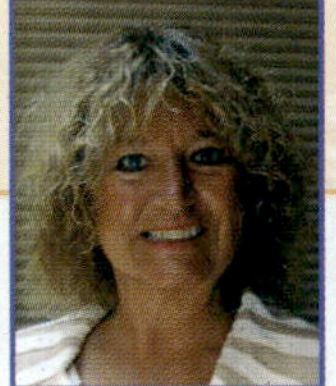

Beth Moscato, Contributor, Chapters 9 and 29

There is nothing more fascinating than human behavior. What people perceive, feel, say, and do never ceases to intrigue me. I am grateful for the unique opportunities I have had in psychiatric nursing in a federal hospital for the treatment of substance abusers, on a locked ward of an inpatient service, as an outpatient therapist in a state psychiatric facility, and as a psychotherapist and consultant in an interdisciplinary private practice group. Most recently, I challenged myself to expand the field of psychiatric epidemiology as a teacher of graduate students and as a researcher in the conduct of several international psychiatric studies. In addition, I am dedicated to volunteer international health projects in developing countries including Ecuador, British Guyana, and Ukraine.

For those of you who may start on a path in psychiatric nursing: Respect and reinforce resiliency. Keep your focus on the issues that really matter to you—the issues that you feel passionate about. Develop a global perspective. Realize that resources are not limitless. Look into the eyes of the underserved and reinforce their dignity. Seek mentors who can support and enrich you and your practice. Remember that clients will teach you more about who you are and who you can become. Enjoy the journey. Gandhi said that a majority of one is all that is needed. Be that one.

Marital Status

Marital status, especially being single, may be associated with psychiatric disorders such as schizophrenia. The highest rates of depression occur among those recently divorced or separated. Married women are more depressed than nonmarried women. In contrast, married men are less depressed than unmarried men.

Physical Health Status

The link between physical and mental health is noteworthy. Studies provide evidence that psychiatric clients may have an increased mortality rate. Medically hospitalized clients have increased rates of mental disorder as well. Major depression is associated with many chronic medical conditions and is predictive of shortened life expectancy.

Positive Family History

Depression and schizophrenia appear related to a history of such disorders in the family. Evidence points to a genetic vulnerability for developing alcoholism. There is some evidence that dementia of the Alzheimer's type may show a familial pattern. Bipolar disorder (manic depression) and anxiety disorders are being studied extensively with regard to family history. Recent developments in genetics may contribute to further understanding regarding the contribution of family history to the development of mental disorders.

Season of Birth

Seasonal variation is well studied in relation to stillbirths and neonatal deaths. Studies in some countries, including the United States, reveal that individuals with schizophrenia are more likely to be born during winter or spring.

Social Environment

Higher levels of stress associated with particular events in one's social environment may be associated with increased rates of mental disorder. Loss of life or property is a risk factor related to *natural disasters,* such as earthquakes, floods, and tornadoes. *Single traumatic events,* such as bereavement or unemployment, may produce adverse mental health consequences. The diagnosis of post-traumatic stress disorder (PTSD) represents a response to an unusual, intense stressor. *Adverse life events* are known to contribute to some forms of depression. A stressful family environment is an established risk factor for behavioral problems in children. The feature What Every Family Health Nurse Should Know highlights surprising cultural differences regarding possible causes of mental disorder.

Physical Environment

High-level *chemical exposures* to mercury, carbon monoxide, carbon disulfide, and lead are related to serious central nervous system disturbances. Environmental exposure to lead is related to deleterious effects on children. When considering *homelessness,* rates of mental disorder among homeless adults and children are remarkably high.

Note that the presence of one particular risk factor does not inevitably lead to the development of a mental disorder. Rather, a number of factors occurring in a defined time period may cause a disorder. *Multifactorial causation* is the term used to describe the requirement that a combination of causes or factors may be needed to produce the disorder.

Lifestyle Habits

It is important to reemphasize that culturally diverse lifestyle habits should be incorporated in any nursing assessment. Such habits may influence the experience, expression, reporting, and evaluation of mental disorders. Lifestyle habits may include dietary patterns, use of alcohol and drugs, health and healing practices, religious and spiritual beliefs, use of time, and migration patterns.

The Natural History of Disorder

Many disorders, especially chronic disorders, have a natural life history. The natural history of disorder refers to the course of disorder over time in the absence of intervention. Chronic

WHAT EVERY FAMILY HEALTH NURSE SHOULD KNOW

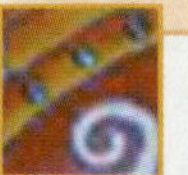

Cross-Cultural Attitudes Toward Mental Disorder

Clients and their families from certain cultures may seek medical or psychiatric care only as a last resort and when absolutely necessary after other cultural treatments have been tried. Various cultures have very divergent views of the causes of mental disorder that may be surprisingly different from the biopsychosocial framework of this textbook. Becoming familiar with the common beliefs of a culture contributes to your cultural competence in everyday practice.

Many cultures often attribute mental disorder to spiritual or supernatural origins. Examples include: disruption in the spiritual world (Filipinos, Koreans), supernatural influences (Central Americans), a curse or spell (Dominicans), or evil spirits (Ethiopians, Samoans). Haitians often believe in supernatural causes, (e.g., a hex or retaliation for not honoring protective spirits). Mexicans and Dominicans may view a mental disorder as a punishment for past misdeeds. Many East Indians and Pakistanis believe that psychosis may originate from an evil spirit or because of an enemy casting a spell. Perceived causes by Arabs may include sudden fearfulness, the devil's curse, God's wrath, or loss of country and family. It is common for Vietnamese to believe in possession by evil spirits, but bad karma from past mistakes (for Buddhists) and bad luck in family inheritance may also contribute to mental disorder. Causes of mental disorder among Native American groups may include loss of harmony with the environment, violation of taboos, and ghosts. It is important to assess both the client's and the particular tribe's degree of acculturation to determine how mental disorder is perceived. Families may seek spiritual advice first when the cause of disorder is perceived to be spiritual or supernatural in origin.

Family stigma and shame may accompany mental disorder. The client's family may fear stigmatization or actually be highly stigmatized when mental disorder is evident in a family member (Cubans, Puerto Ricans, West Indian/Caribbean islanders, Central Americans, Haitians, East Indians, Irish, Nigerians). Mental disorder in a family may be viewed as shameful (Greeks). In addition, seeking treatment may be perceived as bringing shame to the family (Arabs). In many cultures, the family may be concerned about the negative effect that mental disorder may have on matrimonial prospects. Some Colombians maintain that emotional problems in women result from love deceptions.

Several cultures associate the effects of war with the origins of mental disorder. Bosnians and Serbs seem familiar with post-traumatic stress disorder (PTSD) as a result of the devastating impact of events related to war in their country. Cambodians believe that emotional problems resulted from the Khmer Rouge brutalities, and that evil spirits or ancestors may cause mental disorder. Jewish Holocaust survivors may have experienced psychiatric effects because of war atrocities. The Hmong appear to accept those who have depression and PTSD because these conditions are common among those who experienced war.

Be aware that these insights are generalities and may not necessarily reflect the uniqueness of people within their own countries.

disorder may be viewed in a sequence of stages. Risk factors favoring the development of a disorder may be present early in life, preceding the appearance of symptoms by many years. It is important to note that we do not have a complete understanding of the natural history of many psychiatric disorders (Tsuang & Tohen, 2002). Every disorder has its own life history, but in general, disorders have these four basic stages: susceptibility, presymptomatic disorder, clinical disorder, and disability.

Stage of Susceptibility

During this stage, the groundwork has been laid by the presence of risk factors that favor the occurrence of disorder. The individual is susceptible to the disorder, but the disorder has not yet developed. Identification of those at high risk for developing a disorder is a major mental health care challenge. For example, the following risk factors may "set the stage," placing a woman at increased risk for depression: lack of a primary relationship, not employed outside the home, having three or more children under the age of 6, and having endured the loss of a parent in childhood.

Stage of Presymptomatic Disorder

During this stage, there is no apparent disorder, but pathological changes have started to occur. The disorder has begun but remains unrecognized because it may be asymptomatic. If signs of the disorder are present, they may be considered the ordinary discomforts of daily living. Mild depression serves as an example of this presymptomatic stage.

Stage of Clinical Disorder

This stage is characterized by recognizable signs and symptoms of disorder. For some disorders, people regularly come under nursing or medical care at some point over the course of an illness. These disorders are "high profile" because they cause such symptoms as peculiar behavior, failure to thrive, severe or chronic distress, or pain. Classification may be based on laboratory findings or on functional or therapeutic considerations. Cancer is usually classified by the location, extent, and type of tumor. The most current source of classification of psychiatric disorders is the American Psychiatric Association's *Diagnostic and Statistical Manual of Mental Disorders*, 4th edition, Text Revision, or DSM-IV-TR (American Psychiatric Association, 2000). DSM-IV-TR criteria for psychiatric disorders rely on a descriptive diagnostic classification scheme. It is important to note that "clinical disorder" describes a disorder that has come under nursing or medical care and is then treated in a variety of ways that may alter the subsequent course of events. The disorders according to DSM-IV-TR criteria are thoroughly described in the chapters in Unit 4.

Stage of Disability

Some disorders run their course and resolve completely, either spontaneously or in response to therapy. However, some disorders leave residual impairment or disability of short or long duration. While there is a substantial amount of disability associated with acute disorders, the extended disability resulting from chronic disorders is of greater significance to society.

These stages are illustrated in FIGURE 9-4 ■ on page 184.

Epidemiologic Studies Involving Culture

Two common types of studies that examine the distribution and determinants of mental disorders are descriptive studies and cross-sectional studies.

Descriptive Studies

Knowing about patterns of occurrence is a useful first step in identifying factors that may play a causative role or otherwise contribute to the development of a disorder. A descriptive study identifies the amount and distribution of a disorder within a population by answering the following questions related to person, place, and time:

- *Who* is affected? (person)
- *Where* do the cases occur? (place)
- *When* do cases occur? (time)

"*Who*" addresses important personal characteristics (such as age, gender, and ethnicity/race) to determine which of these characteristics differ in comparisons of disorder frequency across populations. Age is generally the most important personal characteristic associated with disorders. Gender is also a factor among disorders; depression, for example, shows male–female differences in patterns of disorder and death. Rates of depression are almost twice as high in women compared to men. Women also have a higher rate of attempted suicide, but completed suicides are more common in men.

Many disorders differ markedly in frequency and severity by racial group. Like race, ethnicity may influence the development of disorder. For example, cultural differences are believed to influence the use of alcohol among different groups, which may explain why alcoholism is less common among Jews compared to many other ethnic groups. Psychological stress among Hispanics may be related to *mal de ojo*, thought to be the result of a witch purposefully casting a spell by looking admiringly at a child. Native Americans may experience *pibloqtok* (active, convulsive hysterical seizures) or ghost sickness (confusion, dizziness, and fear). Some Asians express psychological disharmony through somatic complaints (headaches, stomachaches, and palpitations). These disorders are called *culture-bound syndromes* and are discussed later in this chapter.

"*Where*" addresses the geographic location where disorders are clustered. Variations in location can provide clues to factors associated with the occurrence of disorders. International comparisons are widely used to assess relative progress in the control of disorders. "Where" also may address political subdivisions, such as entire nations, states, counties, and towns. Location, such as a remote rural setting, may influence access to mental health services.

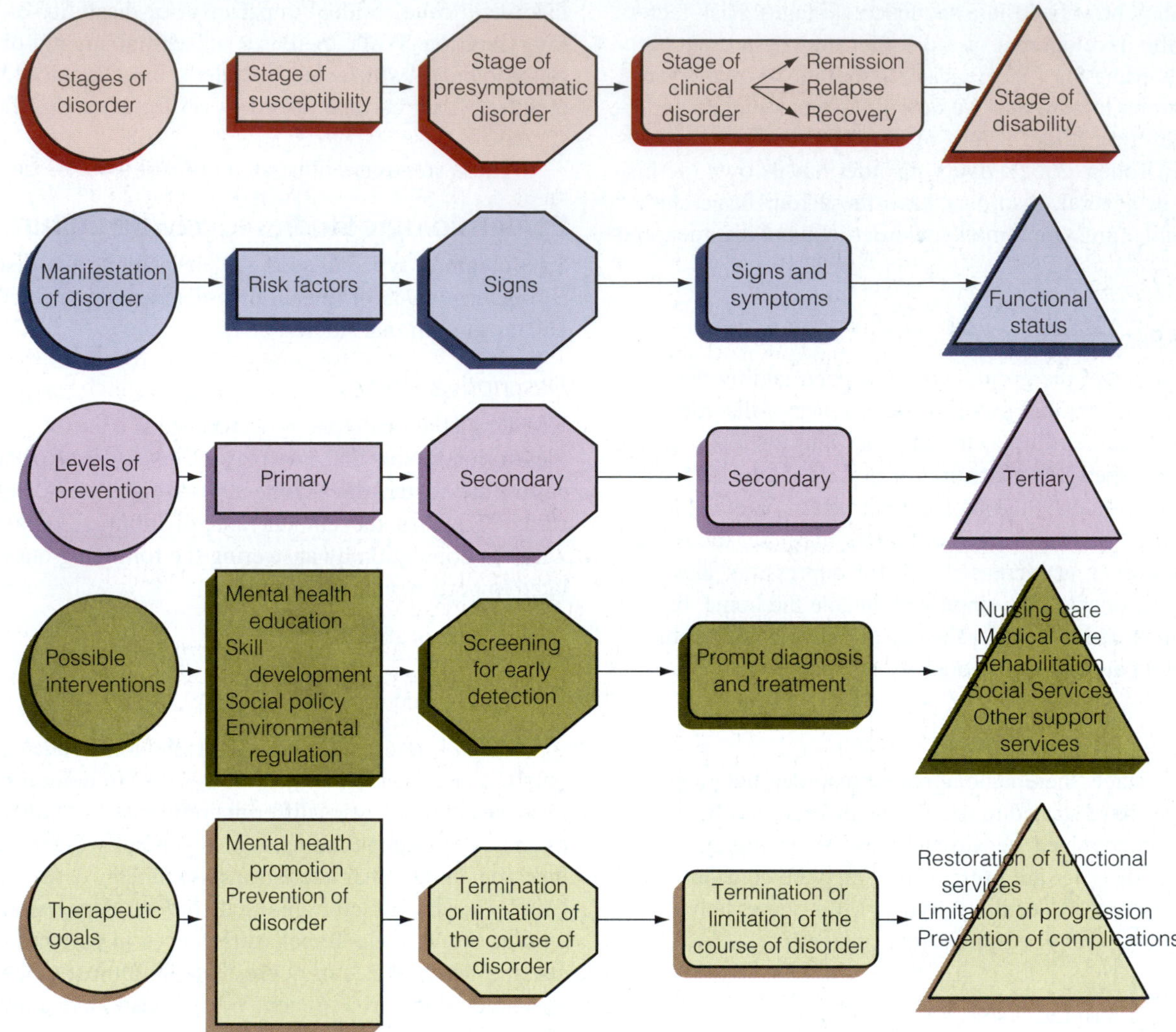

FIGURE 9-4 ■ Stages in the natural history of disorder.

"*When*" addresses the occurrence of disorders by time, which is usually expressed on an annual or lifetime basis. Prevalence rates are commonly presented in terms of lifetime and 1-year periods for various disorders. Incidence rates may be reported in terms of a 1-year time span. Seasonal fluctuations in the frequency of disorders may also be noted, such as the seasonal patterns associated with some mood disorders.

Cross-Sectional Studies

A cross-sectional study is conducted at one point in time. The prevalence of disorder is measured by surveying a group that consists of some people with and some without a disorder. These studies, often called prevalence studies, are relatively inexpensive, simple to carry out, and may provide clues to factors associated with disorder. The landmark National Comorbidity Survey (NCS), discussed later in this chapter, is an example of a cross-sectional (prevalence) study (Kessler, McGonagle, & Zhao, 1994). Cross-sectional studies are among the most common types of research designs reported in the psychiatric literature.

Often, the ideal population to be studied is either too large or too spread out over time, and there is a need to select a smaller group of individuals for study. A sample or representative portion of the population may actually participate in the study. A representative sample resembles the population in relation to important characteristics such as age and gender. If the study sample is truly representative of the larger population, then the results of the study can be safely extended to that population.

RECENT DEVELOPMENTS RELATED TO CULTURAL DIVERSITY

Several recent developments in psychiatric epidemiology are assessment and diagnostic advances in relation to cultural diversity, key findings from major recent studies, and patterns in the use of mental health services.

Using DSM-IV-TR for Cultural Assessment

In psychiatric epidemiology, a "case" is a person in the population or study group identified as having a particular mental disorder. The definition of a case in epidemiology is not necessarily the same as the ordinary clinical definition. Cases may be identified by clinical nursing diagnoses, by psychiatrists' clinical diagnoses, by clinical records, by surveys of the general population, and by population screening (Last, 2001).

Although discussions regarding the DSM-IV-TR are incorporated throughout this textbook, DSM-IV-TR features relating to cultural diversity deserve emphasis. DSM-IV-TR field trials were carried out in more than 70 diverse sites. Representative groups of subjects were selected from a range of sociocultural and ethnic backgrounds to test diagnostic categories as a whole, as well as specific items within each category. A DSM-IV-TR section for each disorder entitled "Specific Culture, Age, and Gender Features" systematically offers guidance concerning variations that may be attributable to one's cultural setting and provides information on differential prevalence rates related to culture. The section also provides information about differential prevalence rates related to culture. One cultural variation, amount of eye contact, is explored in the What Every Pediatric Nurse Should Know feature.

Guidelines for a detailed cultural assessment are offered in the DSM-IV-TR to provide a systematic review of the client's cultural and ethnic background and to identify ways in which the cultural context influences nursing care. The DSM's glossary of **culture-bound syndromes** describes locality-specific patterns of experience—localized folk diagnostic categories that explain repetitive and troubling behaviors to specific societies. Some of the more common culture-bound syndromes that you may encounter in North America are described in Box 9-1 on page 186. We encourage you to familiarize yourself with these specific culture-bound syndromes as you strive for cultural competence in your clinical work.

WHAT EVERY PEDIATRIC NURSE SHOULD KNOW

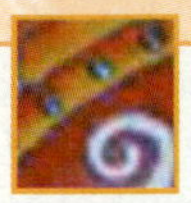

Eye Contact and Ethnicity

The extent, directness, and frequency of eye contact vary among cultures. A lack of eye contact may suggest possible emotional problems for an American child, whereas the same behavior may be culturally normal for an Asian child.

In the United States, avoidance of eye contact may indicate rudeness, a lack of attention, or be a sign of mental disturbance. Cultures that are comfortable with direct eye contact include most African-Americans and Mexican-Americans. In Cuba, looking away actually may be interpreted as a lack of respect or dishonesty.

In some cultures, gender-specific differences are noted. For example, in Arab, East Indian Hindu, and Amish cultures, men may maintain direct eye contact with each other when talking. However, traditional women may avoid eye contact with men or people they do not know. Looking downward may show respect when talking to a husband, father, or grandfather.

Several cultures avoid eye contact, especially with older people, authority figures, or strangers. Some Native American and Alaskan Natives may avoid eye contact as an outward sign of interpersonal respect. Several Asian groups (such as Chinese, Vietnamese, and Korean) avoid direct eye contact to emphasize formality, especially with older generation members. The Japanese culture is a relatively non–eye-contact culture. Japanese may value nonverbal communication, and nonverbal cues like facial expression that establish meaning, more than they value verbal communication. Other cultures that may avoid eye contact include Nigerians, Pakistanis, and East Indians.

How do you interpret a child's degree of eye contact in nonverbal communication? Avoidance of eye contact should not be interpreted as inattentiveness or evasiveness. Ask your cultural consultant, interpreter, or a multicultural community member if the client's behavior is acceptable within the culture or if the behavior is unique to this client.

Sources: Lipson, J. G., & Dibble, S. L. (Eds.) (2005). *Culture & clinical care.* San Francisco, CA: UCFS Nursing Press; Muñoz, C., & Luckmann, J. (2005). *Transcultural communication in nursing* (2nd ed.). Clifton Park, NY: Thomson-Delmar Learning.

Key Findings from Major Studies: A Historic Perspective

Key findings from major population-based studies on mental disorders are relevant to psychiatric–mental health nurses in these areas: mortality, morbidity and comorbidity, and the use of mental health services. This discussion is limited to highlights from the two most comprehensive and historic studies to date, namely the Epidemiologic Catchment Area (ECA) Studies and the National Comorbidity Survey (NCS), to provide background for your development of cultural competence.

Mortality

Information about mortality associated with psychiatric diagnoses is important for two reasons.

1. An increased risk of mortality represents a serious negative outcome that may contribute information about the natural history of disorder.
2. Information about mortality may be used to identify high-risk groups in community settings.

Researchers recently followed a community sample of adults who were first interviewed in 1980 as part of the ECA study in New Haven, Connecticut (Bruce et al., 1994). Nine years later, the researchers determined who was living or deceased. A key finding was the greater risk of mortality among adults with the following disorders: major depression, alcohol abuse or dependence, and schizophrenia. The high prevalence of depression and of alcohol-related disorders highlights the great impact these problems have on community health in general. Mental disorder is independently associated with a substantial excess in mortality risk based on results from numerous international studies (Prince et al., 2007).

Morbidity and Comorbidity

There is increasing awareness of the issue of comorbidity among people with mental disorders, particularly depression, anxiety, and alcohol and other substance abuse. **Comorbidity** is defined as the occurrence of two or more psychiatric disorders over an individual's life span.

Box 9-1 **Culture-Bound Syndromes**

- *Amok:* A dissociative episode characterized by a period of brooding followed by an outburst of violent, aggressive, or homicidal behavior directed toward objects or other people. May be found in Malaysia, Laos, the Philippines, Polynesia, Papua New Guinea, Puerto Rico, and among the Navajo.
- *Falling-out* (or blacking out): Occuring primarily in the southern United States and in Caribbean groups, these episodes are characterized by a sudden collapse. Although the person's eyes are open and the person can hear and understand what is occurring, the person feels powerless to move.
- *Ghost sickness:* Various symptoms such as nightmares, weakness, feelings of impending doom, fainting, hallucinations, loss of consciousness, and a sense of suffocation, among others, along with a preoccupation with death are associated with the deceased and sometimes with witchcraft.
- *Latah:* This syndrome is characterized by hypersensitivity to sudden fright, with the automatic repetition by imitation of the movements of another (echopraxia), the parrotlike repetition of a word or phrase just spoken by another (echolalia), command obedience, and trancelike or dissociative behavior. Originally of Malaysian or Indonesian origin, this condition has also been found in Siberian groups, Thailand, the Philippines, and Japan.
- *Mal de ojo:* This Spanish phrase means "evil eye." Common in other Mediterranean cultures, the evil eye can be a curse instituted by an enemy. Children are especially at risk; their symptoms include fitful sleep, crying without apparent cause, diarrhea, vomiting, and fever.
- *Nervois:* A term that means a distress of the nerves, common among Latinos in North America and Latin America. It includes a wide range of symptoms of emotional and somatic disturbance and refers to a general state of vulnerability to stressful life experiences. Other ethnic groups (such as *nevra* among the Greeks) have similar ideas about "nerves."
- *Shenkui:* In China and Taiwan, this folk label describes marked anxiety or panic symptoms accompanied by somatic complaints, frequent dreams, and sexual dysfunction (such as erectile dysfunction and premature ejaculation). It is attributed to excess semen loss through frequent intercourse, masturbation, and nocturnal emission. Excessive semen loss is feared because it represents the loss of vital essence and can be seen as life threatening.
- *Susto:* This folk illness is prevalent among some Latinos in the United States and among people in Mexico and Central and South America. Also known as "soul loss," it is thought to be caused by a frightening event that causes the soul to leave the body, resulting in unhappiness and sickness including appetite disturbances, feelings of sadness, lack of motivation, troubled sleep, feelings of diminished self-worth, headache, stomachache, and diarrhea.

The National Comorbidity Survey (NCS) The landmark National Comorbidity Survey, a congressionally mandated survey conducted with a representative national sample, remains the most extensive research regarding psychiatric disorders to date (Kessler et al., 1994). The goals of the NCS included:

- Carrying out a national survey to estimate the prevalence of psychiatric morbidity and comorbidity in the United States
- Investigating the implications of comorbidity for mental health service utilization and course of illness
- Investigating the risk factors for comorbidity

More specifically, this survey of the noninstitutionalized U.S. household population (age 15–54) reported on about 10,000 subjects using a study design that enabled investigation of seasonal variation in the prevalence of mental disorders. A structured psychiatric interview was used to generate DSM-III-R psychiatric diagnoses (the version in use at that time).

The prevalence of psychiatric disorders was greater than previously thought. Nearly half the subjects reported at least one mental disorder in their lifetime. The most common disorders were major depression and alcohol dependence. The following findings were consistent with previous research:

- Women had higher rates of affective and anxiety disorders.
- Men had higher rates of substance abuse disorders and antisocial personality disorder.
- Most disorders declined with age and with higher socioeconomic status.
- Fewer than 40% of those with a lifetime disorder had ever received professional treatment.

A most striking finding is that mental disorders are more highly concentrated than previously recognized in approximately one-sixth (14%) of the population who have had a history of three or more comorbid disorders. When severity is considered, this group also includes the great majority of those with severe disorders. Less than 50% of this highly comorbid group ever obtained specialty mental health treatment, despite the number and severity of their disorders. Findings point to the need for community-based preventive programs aimed at more outreach. There is also a need for more research on barriers, including cultural barriers, to mental health services.

Kessler and associates (2005) replicated the National Comorbidity Study (NCS Replication) to examine what changes, if any, had occurred in the prevalence of mental disorders over the previous decade. They conducted face-to-face interviews of people diagnosed with anxiety, mood, and substance use disorders during the 12 months prior to the interview and found that the prevalence of mental disorders had not changed during the decade. Their findings in relation to the rate of treatment are summarized later in this chapter.

The Epidemiologic Catchment Area (ECA) Studies Additional findings from the ECA studies provide information from community and institutional samples regarding the comorbidity of mental disorders related to alcohol and other drug abuse. Regier et al. (1990) reported that, in general, 37% of those with a mental disorder also had an alcohol abuse disorder. Among mental disorders associated with alcoholism, anxiety disorders were most prevalent (19%), followed by antisocial personality disorder (14%) and depressive disorder (13%). The relationship between mental disorder and drug abuse (other than alcohol) is also noteworthy: A comorbid mental disorder was found among more than half of those with drug (other than alcohol) abuse disorders.

Expressed in terms of risk, those having a mental disorder in their lifetime had more than twice the risk of having an alcohol abuse disorder and over four times the risk of having another drug abuse disorder. Individuals treated in specialty mental health and addictive disorder clinics were at significantly higher risk for having comorbid disorders. Issues related to comorbidity are receiving significant attention in psychiatric research.

Mental Health Care-Seeking Patterns Care-seeking patterns need to be especially addressed in the conduct of epidemiologic studies. The research on care-seeking patterns may be summarized as follows:

- Most people with mental disorders do not seek professional treatment.
- Comorbidity increases the likelihood that a person will seek treatment. Still less than half of the highly comorbid group identified in the NCS ever obtained specialty mental health treatment, despite the number and severity of their disorders.
- When seeking treatment, most people with mental disorders seek treatment from primary care physicians, who prescribe the majority of psychotropic medications. Yet, there is a current decrease in primary care physicians, especially in impoverished and rural areas.
- Individuals with chronic mental disorders comprise the majority of those who seek treatment. The NCS Replication (Kessler et al., 2005) also examined changes in the rate of treatment for mental disorders over the previous decade. Despite an observed increase in the rate of treatment, most clients with a mental disorder did not seek treatment.
- Psychiatrists tend to treat individuals with severe disorders, yet there is a current undersupply of psychiatrists in the United States.

Awareness of these care-seeking patterns is essential in order to address the nonuse or misuse of mental health services. Knowledge of such patterns is also useful in determining who are the most appropriate subjects for a given epidemiologic study. Pivotal issues are the availability, accessibility, cost, and quality of mental health services, especially since prognosis is affected by the duration of any mental disorder.

Cost is the most frequently addressed mental health topic in current literature on medical care organization. Financial incentives appear to drive the provision of services to those with mental disorders, and funding sources appear to drive the entire health care industry. Insurance coverage for mental health care appears to lag behind that for other medical care. Severely underserved groups in relation to mental health services include:

- Substance abusers
- Older adults (especially if minority)
- Uninsured persons
- Homeless persons

Unfortunately, mental health policy continues to be reactive rather than proactive, situational rather than long term and strategic, and rehabilitative rather than preventive.

Jacob and colleagues (2007) highlight three main obstacles to improved mental health:

1. Scarcity of resources
2. Inequities in the distribution of resources
3. Inefficiencies in the use of resources

These researchers assess the availability of resources in low-income and middle-income countries, where the poorest countries spend the lowest proportion of their overall health budgets on mental health. In these countries, current mental health care is institutionally based and human resources are very limited. Populations with the greatest need for mental health services appear to have the lowest access to care. In countries without protective legislation, people with mental disorders may be vulnerable to abuse of their human rights.

Many barriers to improvement of mental health services are identified for low- and middle-income countries. As outlined by Saraceno et al. (2007), these barriers include:

- The prevailing public health agenda and funding
- Resistance to decentralization of mental health services
- Difficulties in implementing mental health services in primary care settings
- Few workers trained and supervised in mental health care
- Lack of emphasis on public health by the mental health leaders

An example is the lack of political will in Sri Lanka in the district most severely affected by the tsunami in 2004.

To improve mental health services from a global perspective, the Lancet Global Mental Health Group (2007) offers the following five targeted strategies to improve the coverage of an evidence-based package of services for mental disorders, especially in low- and medium-income countries:

1. Make mental health a priority on the public health agenda.
2. Enhance the organization of mental health services.
3. Incorporate mental health into general health care.
4. Develop human resources for mental health.
5. Strengthen leadership in public mental health.

The financial requirement for a core package of mental health services is estimated to be $2 (U.S.) per person per year for low-income countries, and $3 to $4 (U.S.) per person per year for middle-income countries. This group of international authors issue a "call to action" from the global health community for immediate advocacy, political will, and solidarity to advance global mental health.

Implications for Psychiatric–Mental Health Nursing Practice

In general, epidemiologic principles extend nursing skills by considering the community itself as a potential "client" for mental health assessment and services. More specifically, epidemiologic principles may be applied to each step of the nursing process. Assessment may include collecting information on the natural history of disorder, potential risk factors, and the client's cultural and ethnic background. Nursing diagnoses may involve the use of one or more psychiatric instruments as part of diagnostic procedures. Epidemiologic findings may influence the planning, implementation, and evalation of nursing interventions, as well as determining outcome criteria. The following Your Self-Awareness feature suggests questions that you can ask yourself to determine your skill at applying the principles of psychiatric epidemiology.

Because most people with mental disorders never seek professional treatment, there is a need for more outreach to ensure availability, accessibility, reasonable cost, and quality of mental health services for all subgroups of the population. Psychiatric nurses may advocate for more outreach aimed at high-risk groups, such as the impoverished, the homeless, and those with comorbid conditions.

We encourage you to develop and expand your psychiatric–mental health nursing practice by continuing to familiarize yourself with global mental health issues. The websites suggested throughout this chapter and the references that follow will help you to do so. Some countries have progressed in developing their mental health services, despite a lack of funding. You can learn some valuable lessons by carefully scrutinizing what seems to work for them.

Implications for Psychiatric–Mental Health Nursing Research

The results from studies suggest that the causes and consequences of high comorbidity should be the focus of continued research. More research on potential barriers to professional care seeking is needed, including care-seeking patterns that consider ethnic and cultural differences.

The research contains gaps. There continues to be a lack of systematic, evaluative study aimed at determining which treatments are most effective for which disorders in which groups at any given time. Research into productivity and efficiency is important: Many clients, especially those with severe or persistent mental disorders, have found a fragmented, underfinanced, uncoordinated, and frequently inaccessible system of care.

Potential areas for future psychiatric–mental health nursing research include:

- Expanded cross-national comparisons, including how to assess and develop mental health systems in developing countries
- Studies across the life span, especially involving children, adolescents, and the elderly
- Use of various study designs, especially "first episode" clinical studies of those affected by a specific disorder
- Influence of environmental factors (e.g., physical illness, traumatic life events, lack of support)
- The development of preventive programs based on research of risk factors

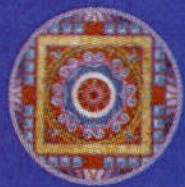

YOUR SELF-AWARENESS
Applying Principles of Psychiatric Epidemiology

Attempt to identify the following concerns regarding a particular population:

- Am I able to identify groups of people (such as children, elderly, or homeless) at high risk for the development of specific psychiatric disorders?
- Have I obtained information on any changes in health problems at this setting, especially the emergence of new problems?
- In what ways might I be involved in the identification of the current health needs of this population, and the prediction of the future needs of this population?
- Are there particular care-seeking patterns related to the use of mental health services (including nonuse or misuse of services) of which I need to be aware?
- How might I be involved in the evaluation of preventive and therapeutic measures aimed at this population?

Attempt to answer the following questions regarding a particular client:

- Have I assessed which risk factors associated with psychiatric disorders may relate to this client?
- Have I obtained information about this client's cultural identity as part of my psychiatric–mental health nursing assessment?
- Do I have an understanding of this client's lifestyle habits that may impact mental health care (such as health and healing practices, religious and spiritual beliefs, and use of alcohol and drugs)?
- Can I identify useful cultural resources for this client?

- Studies in health services research, especially to increase the proportion of people with mental disorders who receive treatment
- Advances in psychopharmacology, genetics, and neurobiology
- Treatment outcome studies, including pharmacologic effects
- Refinement of brief interview instruments for use in screening programs
- Studies on resiliency despite adversities (see information on resilience in Chapter 34)

Patel et al. (2007) emphasize that from a global mental health perspective, research is essential for ongoing mental health service reform and innovation.

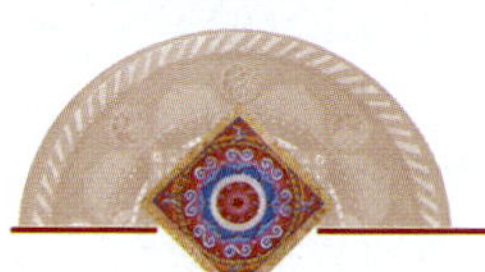

EXPLORE MEDIALINK

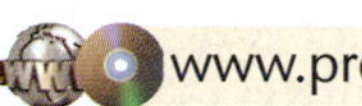

www.prenhall.com/kneisl

For NCLEX-RN® review questions, case studies, and other resources for this chapter see the Pearson Health MediaLink CD-ROM that accompanies this book and the Companion Website at www.prenhall.com/kneisl.

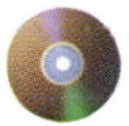

CD-ROM
Audio Glossary
NCLEX-RN® Review Questions

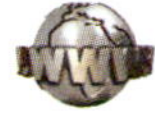

Companion Website
Audio Glossary
NCLEX-RN® Review Questions
Critical Thinking Exercise
- *Addressing Cultural Diversity in the Clinic*

Case Study
- *Culturally Sensitive Nursing*

Care Plan
- *Culture and Communication*

MediaLinks
MediaLink Application
- *The Compelling Need for Cultural and Linguistic Competence*

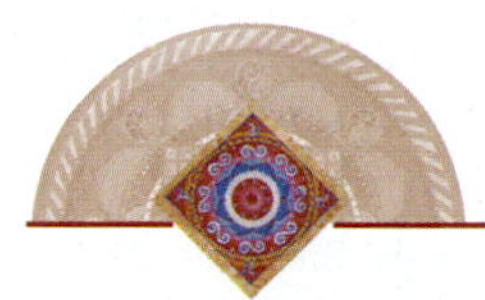

NCLEX-RN® REVIEW QUESTIONS

1. Characteristics of the presymptomatic stage of a disorder include:
1. Risk factors such as single parenting.
2. Chronic distress.
3. Lack of formal education.
4. Pathological changes.

2. Cultural sensitivity can best be described as:
1. The ability to understand and care for culturally diverse groups of clients.
2. Successful conflict resolution between different cultural systems.
3. Professional awareness of the significance of cultural factors in the delivery of health care.
4. The manner in which a subculture views their social environment.

3. The role of the nurse as a culture broker includes (select all that apply):
1. Disseminating information.
2. Conflict resolution with a culturally diverse nursing staff.
3. Providing hands-on nursing care.
4. Facilitating acquisition of health care for clients.
5. Planning care that reflects the cultural practices of the health care institution.

4. The nurse and client are developing a transcultural nursing care plan related to heart disease. The nurse will include in the plan:
1. Religious practices that are relevant to the client.
2. Educational material that is given to all clients with heart disease.
3. Nutritional teaching specific to a cardiac diet.
4. Contact information for a community support group.

5. Biopsychosocial risk factors associated with the incidence of mental disorders:
1. Have the same significance in all ethnic populations.
2. Address the cultural diversity of the different cultural groups.
3. Include individual lifestyle habits.
4. Do not influence treatment planning.

6. A combination of risk factors needed to produce a disorder is known as:
1. Comorbidity.
2. Prevalence rate.
3. Incidence rate.
4. Multifactorial causation.

7. The nurse is organizing a disease prevention program for a specific cultural group. To effectively meet the needs of this group the nurse will:
1. Assess the needs of the community in general.
2. Develop generalized goals and objectives for the program.
3. Assess the immediate impact of such a program.
4. Involve those affected by the problem in the planning process.

8. The most effective way for a nurse to enhance her understanding of a specific cultural group is to:
1. Treat all clients the same.
2. Use educational materials that are simplistic and have many pictures.
3. Learn about traditional healers within the community.
4. Educate the specific cultural group about Western concepts of health and illness.

9. Social belonging and loyalty to a particular reference group within society is known as:
1. Ethnocentrism.
2. Ethnicity.
3. Cultural sensitivity.
4. Acculturation.

10. A client expresses frustration in accessing health care. Which stage of cultural brokering will the nurse initially engage in to assist the client?
1. Intervention
2. Susceptibility
3. Presymptomatic
4. Perception

See Appendix C for answers.

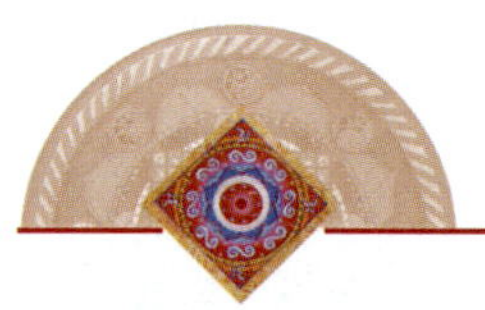

REFERENCES

Amaro, D. J., Abriam-Yago, K., & Yoder, M. (2006). Perceived barriers for ethnically diverse students in nursing programs. *Journal of Nursing Education, 45*(7), 246–254.

American Psychiatric Association. (2000). *Diagnostic and statistical manual of mental disorders* (4th ed., Text Revision). Washington, DC: Author.

Bromet, E. J. (1998). Psychiatric disorders. In R. B. Wallace (Ed.), *Maxcy–Rosenau–Last public health and preventive medicine* (14th ed.). Stamford, CT: Appleton & Lange.

Bruce, M., Leaf, P., Rozal, G., Florio, L., & Hoff, R. (1994). Psychiatric status and 9-year mortality data in the New Haven Epidemiologic Catchment Area Study. *American Journal of Psychiatry, 151*(5), 716–721.

Gardner, J. (2005). Barriers influencing the success of racial and ethnic minority students in nursing programs. *Journal of Transcultural Nursing, 16*(2), 155–162.

Gary, F. A., Sigsby, L. M., & Campbell, D. (1998). Preparing for the 21st century: Diversity in nursing education, research, and practice. *Journal of Professional Nursing, 14*(5), 272–279.

Giger, J. N., & Davidhizar, R. E. (2004). *Transcultural nursing: Assessment and intervention* (4th ed.). St. Louis, MO: Mosby.

Giger, J., Davidhizar, R. E., Purnell, L., Harden, J. T., Phillips, J., & Strickland, O. (2007). American Academy of Nursing Expert Panel Report: Developing cultural competence to eliminate health disparities in ethnic minorities and other vulnerable populations. *Journal of Transcultural Nursing, 18*(2), 95–102.

Huff, R. M., & Kline, M. V. (Eds.). (1999). *Promoting health in multicultural populations: A handbook for practitioners.* Thousand Oaks, CA: Sage Publications.

Jacob, K. S., Sharan, P., Mirza, I., Garrido-Cumbrera, M., Seedat, S., Mari, J. J., et al. (2007). Mental health systems in countries: Where are we now? *Lancet, 370*(9592), 1061–1077.

Jezewski, M. A. (1993). Culture brokering as a model for advocacy. *Nursing and Health Care, 14*(2), 78–85.

Jezewski, M. A. (1995). Evolution of a grounded theory: Conflict resolution through culture brokering. *Advances in Nursing Science, 17*(3), 14–30.

Kessler, R. C., Demler, O., Frank, R. G., Olfson, M., Pincus, H. A., Walters, E. E., et al. (2005). Prevalence and treatment of mental disorders, 1990 to 2003. *New England Journal of Medicine, 352*(24), 2515–2523.

Kessler, R., McGonagle, K., & Zhao, S. (1994). Lifetime and 12-month prevalence of DSM-III-R psychiatric disorders in the United States: Results from the National Comorbidity Survey. *Archives of General Psychiatry, 51*, 8–18.

Lancet Global Mental Health Group. (2007). Scale up services for mental disorders: A call for action. *Lancet, 370*(9594), 1241–1252.

Last, J. M. (2001). *A dictionary of epidemiology* (4th ed.). New York: Oxford University Press.

Lipson, J. G., & Dibble, S. L. (Eds.). (2005). *Culture & clinical care.* San Francisco, CA: UCFS Nursing Press.

Lopez, A. D., Mathers, C. D., Ezzati, M., Jamison, D. T., & Murray, C. J. L. (2006). *Global burden of disease and risk factors.* Washington, DC: World Bank Publications.

Mahoney, J. S., Carlson, E., & Engebretson, J. C. (2006). A framework for cultural competence in advanced practice psychiatric and mental health education. *Perspectives in Psychiatric Care, 42*(4), 227–237.

Muñoz, C., & Luckmann, J. (2005). *Transcultural communication in nursing* (2nd ed.). Clifton Park, NY: Thomson-Delmar Learning.

Murray, C. J. L., & Lopez, A. D. (1996). *The global burden of disease: A comprehensive assessment of mortality and disability from diseases, injuries, and risk factors in 1990 and projected to 2020.* Cambridge, MA: Harvard University Press.

Patel, V., Araya, R., Chatterjee, S., Chisholm, D., Cohen, A., DeSilva, M., et al. (2007). Treatment and prevention of mental disorders in low-income and middle-income countries. *Lancet, 370*(9591), 991–1005.

Prince, M., Patel, V., Saxena, S., Maj, M., Maselko, J., Phillips, M. R., et al. (2007). No health without mental health. *Lancet, 370*(9590), 859–877.

Regier, D., Farmer, M. E., Rae, D. S., Locke, B. Z., Keith, S. J., Judd, L. L., et al. (1990). Comorbidity of mental health disorders with alcohol and other drug abuse. *Journal of the American Medical Association, 264*, 2511–2518.

Saraceno, B., van Ommeren, M., Batniji, R., Cohen, A., Gureje, O., Mahoney, J., et al. (2007). Barriers to improvement of mental health services in low-income and middle-income countries. *Lancet, 370*(9593), 1164–1174.

Spector, R. E. (2004). *Cultural diversity in health & illness* (6th ed.). Upper Saddle River, NJ: Prentice Hall.

Tsuang, M. T., & Tohen, M. (2002). *Textbook in psychiatric epidemiology* (2nd ed.). New York: Wiley-Liss.

Vinson, J. A. (2000). Nursing's epistemology revisited in relation to professional education competencies. *Journal of Professional Nursing, 16*(1), 39–46.

Yearwood, E. L., Hines-Martin, V., Dato, C., & Malone, M. (2006). Creating an organizational diversity vision: Goals, outcomes, and future directions of the International Society of Psychiatric Nurses. *Archives of Psychiatric Nursing, 20*(3), 152–156.

ADDITIONAL REFERENCES

Eaton, W. W. (Ed.). (2006). *Medical and psychiatric comorbidity over the course of life*. Washington, DC: American Psychiatric Publishing.

Gordis, L. (2004). *Epidemiology* (3rd ed.). Philadelphia, PA: Elsevier Saunders.

Leininger, M. M., & McFarland, M. R. (Eds.). (2006). *Culture care diversity and universality: A worldwide nursing theory* (2nd ed.). Boston, MA: Jones and Bartlett Publishers.

Scrimshaw, Susan C. (2006). Culture, behavior, and health. In M. H. Merson, R. E. Black, & A. J. Mills (Eds.), *International public health: Diseases, programs, systems, and policies* (2nd ed.). Boston, MA: Jones and Bartlett Publishers.

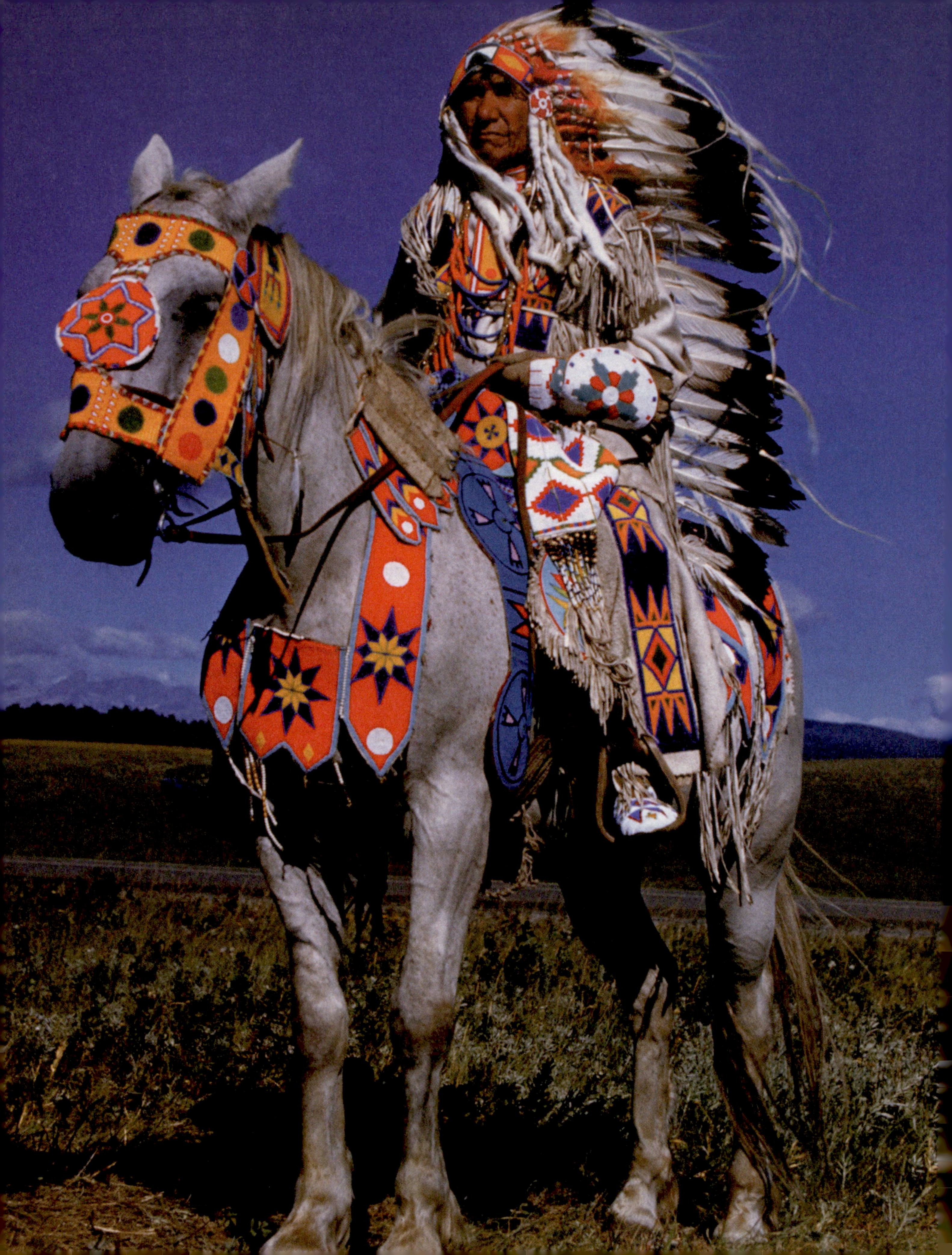

Unit 3

PSYCHIATRIC–MENTAL HEALTH NURSING PROCESSES

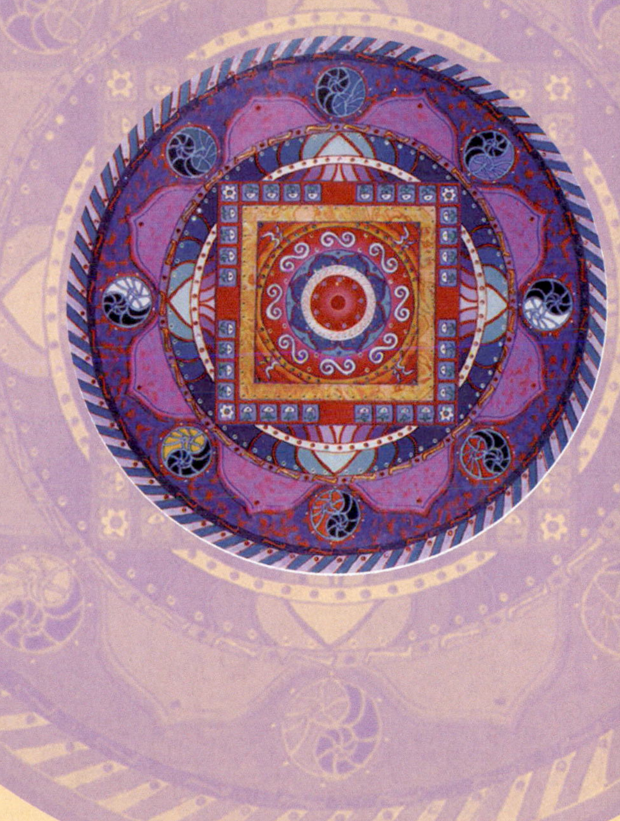

JOHN lives in northern Alberta, Canada. A member of the Cree First Nation people, John is dressed in ceremonial garb for the Cree Nation Powwow. This brotherhood of First Nation peoples spans a broad territory through six provinces of Canada, Montana, the Dakotas, and Minnesota, and through the Rocky Mountains to the Atlantic Ocean. In this particular population, illegal drug use, alcohol abuse, and suicide are a means of escape from hopelessness, despair, and deplorable socioeconomic conditions for those who have few alternative choices. The young people hunger for culture, identity, and a future. For them, these mental health problems are marks of shame and disgrace. In First Nation families or communities where cultural practices and traditions have been maintained or restored, there is less social disorganization and marginalization. The body, mind, and spirit, all important to First Nation people, can more easily align in harmony and connect on an everyday level when cultural factors—original languages, cultural traditions, spiritual orientation, and an interdependence with nature and the land—are intact or restored. A commitment to improve global mental health requires that we practice evolved, compassionate empathy.

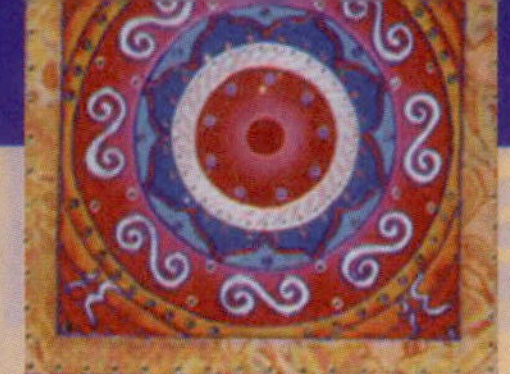

CHAPTER

10

Communicating and Relating

CAROL REN KNEISL

KEY TERMS

feedback *202*
illusion *195*
interpersonal communication *199*
intrapersonal communication *199*
mixed message *197*
neologism *197*
nonverbal communication *197*
overload *202*
perception *195*
subculture *196*
tangential reply *202*
underload *202*

LEARNING OUTCOMES

After completing this chapter, you will be able to:

1. Describe the factors that influence the process of human communication.
2. Explain why nonverbal communication is as important as verbal communication.
3. Incorporate the theories of human communication discussed here into interpersonal relationships with clients and their families.
4. Identify the principles of therapeutic communication and explain why they are essential ingredients of interpersonal relationships.
5. Employ the skills discussed here to foster relationships and communication in the psychiatric–mental health setting.
6. Explain how the skills discussed here foster relating and communicating in any health care setting.

CRITICAL THINKING CHALLENGE

You are about to embark on your first inpatient psychiatric nursing experience. You feel anxious because although you've read the therapeutic communication techniques described in this chapter, you feel uncomfortable about using them. They seem artificial, stilted, and "not you."

1. What can you do to decrease your discomfort and anxiety and help make your psychiatric–mental health nursing experience a positive learning experience for you as well as for your clients?
2. Are therapeutic communication techniques "written in stone," or is it appropriate to change them to match your own personal style?
3. What problems could you run into by overusing a communication technique?
4. How can therapeutic communication techniques be useful when communicating with classmates? Friends? Family members?

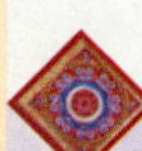

MEDIALINK 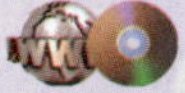 www.prenhall.com/kneisl

Go to the Pearson Health MediaLink CD-ROM and the Companion Website at www.prenhall.com/kneisl for interactive resources for this chapter.

When John Bowlby discovered in the 1950s that infants in foundling homes were literally dying for lack of contact and affection, the scientific community began to attach new importance to the old saying that "People need people." Today we recognize that the mechanism for establishing, maintaining, and improving human contacts is interpersonal communication. Communication is a very special process and the most significant of human behaviors. Moreover, it is the main method for implementing the nursing process.

When they tell "their story," clients explain themselves, the events of their lives, and the circumstances they face. Psychiatric–mental health nurses help clients tell their stories, help them explore the circumstances of their lives, and help them move in a more satisfying and mentally healthier direction.

We are instructed to engage in "therapeutic use of self." We are also told that our "relationship" with a client is the primary therapeutic tool, that we should demonstrate qualities of sensitivity and caring. Two other chapters correlate closely with this chapter. Chapter 3 discusses the nurse's personal characteristics that are a basis for therapeutic use of self. Chapter 29 discusses the actual structure and process of the one-to-one relationship such as the differences between formal and informal one-to-one relationships, the stages and strategies, and processes such as resistance, transference, and countertransference, among others. For many students, like the student in the clinical example that follows, the instruction to use oneself therapeutically is mysterious jargon quite unlike the clear-cut step-by-step procedures they learn for some physical treatments.

CLINICAL EXAMPLE

I found myself watching my instructors and the nurses on the unit closely when they talked with clients. Somehow I thought that by imitating things that they did or said I'd figure out what "being therapeutic" was supposed to mean. I knew it had something to do with things the nurse said or didn't say when she talked with clients. But it all got very fuzzy to me beyond that very elementary grasp of it. I used to latch on to ideas like "Agreeing is untherapeutic. So is giving advice or opinions." The only entries I felt safe putting down in my process recording were stiff-sounding reflections like "You sound angry."

Because the process of human communication is complex and has many dimensions, it cannot be reduced to a few simple steps that you can simply memorize and perform. However, there are some principles and techniques that we will teach you to use so that you can be comfortable and therapeutic at the same time. Effective communication is the cornerstone for all psychiatric–mental health nursing practice.

THE PROCESS OF HUMAN COMMUNICATION

As you will see in this chapter, communication is an ongoing, dynamic, and ever-changing series of events. Each event in the series affects and is affected by all the others. Some people mistakenly believe that communication is simply the transfer of information or meaning from one human being to another. The truth is that meaning cannot be transferred; it must be mutually negotiated, because meaning is influenced by a number of significant factors.

Role of Perception

A person's image or perception of the world is an essential element in communicating. The term **perception** refers to the experience of sensing, interpreting, and comprehending the world in which one lives. Perception is a highly personal and internal act.

People process through their senses all the information they have about the world around them. However, seeing is not always believing. Communication specialists have discovered that because of human physiologic limitations, the eye and brain are constantly being tricked into seeing things that are not really what they seem; these are called **illusions**. Before continuing to read, stare at FIGURE 10-1 ■ for 20 seconds. The illustration will appear to swing back and forth. You can verify that the movement is an illusion by checking your visual perception against your tactile sensations.

What people "see" or sense is strongly influenced by many factors. For example, past experiences have prepared us to see things, people, and events in particular ways.

Also, we tend to observe more carefully when a purpose guides the observation. The purposes or reasons for engaging in an observation also determine what we observe. The nurse in an intensive care unit observes a cardiac surgery client differently than a family member does.

Finally, when understandings differ, you and I can look at the same object and see different things. Mental set helps determine how and what a person perceives. Before you read any further, look at the picture of the young woman in FIGURE 10-2 ■ on page 196. Do you see the silhouette of a young woman? Do you also see the face of an elderly woman? Using the phrase "the picture of the young woman in Figure 10-2" encouraged

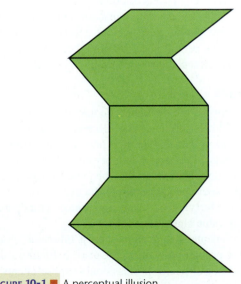

FIGURE 10-1 ■ A perceptual illusion.

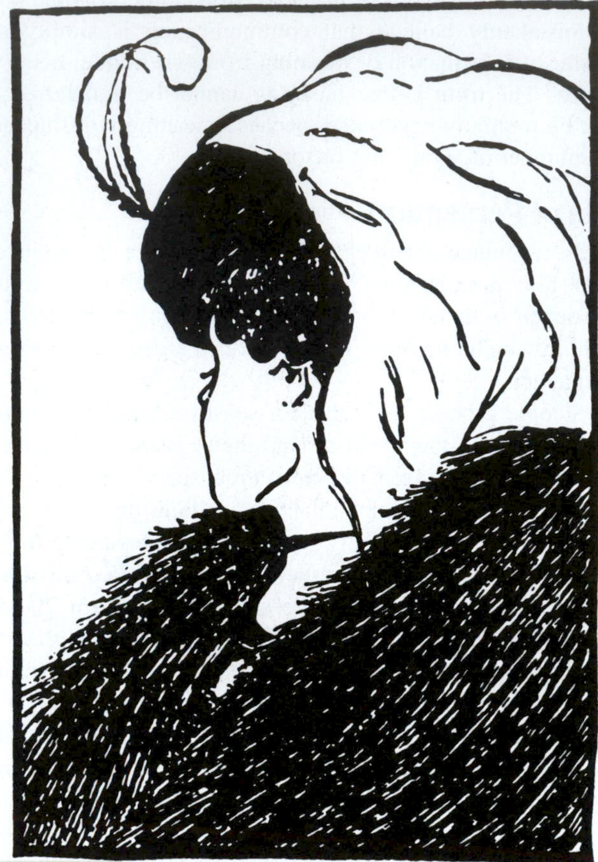

FIGURE 10-2 ■ The influence of mental set on perception.

you to perceive the illustration in a particular way. Now you should also be able to see the elderly woman in the illustration.

As the illustrations demonstrate, the old axiom might be better stated: "Believing is seeing." Because we tend to perceive in terms of past experiences, expectations, and goals, perceptions may be a prime obstacle to communication. No two individuals perceive the world in exactly the same way, and the meanings of events differ because people's perceptions of them differ. Perceptions of other human beings are of particular importance because human communication is inevitably affected by how we perceive one another. To see others at all as they are, people need to know themselves and to know how the self affects their perceptions of others.

Role of Values

Values are concepts of the desirable. People value what is of worth to them. Values influence the process of communication because people's values, like their perceptions, differ.

Value systems differ for a number of reasons. Age is one. Children's values shift when they become teenagers. The college or work experience generally influences values in yet other directions. Marrying or being a parent or grandparent may cause other value changes or shifts.

Psychiatric–mental health nurses must ultimately come to terms with the problem of values, because conflicting value systems among mental health professionals expose clients to uncertainty and confusion. Consider the following examples.

CLINICAL EXAMPLE

The parents of a 15-year-old girl were upset to find a small plastic bag of marijuana in her dresser drawer. She had been playing hooky from school and wore low-slung jeans that her parents considered too sexy. After a series of lengthy, angry discussions with her parents, she was confined to her room. During this period she refused to eat or drink. When the teenager was seen by a mental health treatment team, the members' opinions were divided. Some said that her behavior signaled an emotional disturbance. They labeled her antisocial, depressed, and anxious. Others believed the parents were old-fashioned and too rigid in attempting to force her to accept their values.

In another instance, a 35-year-old man was firmly committed to prayer. Most of his spare time involved church-related activities. Staff members at a mental health clinic where he sought counseling told him that he was resorting to an early infantile attitude about God as the magic worker.

Clearly, these staff members were influenced by their own values.

The daily roles people take also influence their values. In any one day a man may be a student, husband, father, nurse, citizen, speaker, artist, son, and teacher.

Role of Culture

Each culture provides its members with notions about how the world is structured and what it means. These preconceptions, learned at an early age, are so subtle that they often go unrecognized. They nonetheless set limits on communication and interaction with others. Relying on culturally determined generalizations or stereotypes can have profound effects on one's relationships with others.

Communication is culture-bound in a wide variety of ways. The culture and the **subculture** (the culture within the culture) teach people how to communicate through language, hand gestures, clothing, and even in the ways they use the space around them. If you do not know that "run it by me" means to explain something, that "getting jumped" is a fist-fight, or that "he's really PHAT" means that the person is Pretty Hot And Tempting, you may be confused by conversations with members of certain subcultures—adolescents and street people, for example. When you overhear two clients talking about "angel dust" you need to know that the term refers not to something religious, but to PCP—an animal tranquilizer. In some cultures, belching after dinner is a compliment to the host. In other cultures, belching may be considered uncouth or an insult. When Americans make a circle with thumb and forefinger and extend the other fingers, they mean "OK." To Brazilians, the same gesture is an obscene sign of contempt.

These examples make it obvious that communicating with meaning requires that the participants take culture well into account. How people communicate with others who do not share similar histories, heritages, or cultures is of critical importance in humanistic psychiatric–mental health nursing practice. Chapter 9 discusses the personal strategies you can use to develop cultural competence in your clinical work.

The Spoken Word

Verbal language, the ability to utter the spoken word, makes people human and distinguishes them from other animals. Yet problems arise when we discover that words mean different things to different people. That is, *words* do not "mean" something; *people* do.

If communication between yourself and the client is to be mutually negotiated in order to be understood by both of you, then you must understand the four concepts discussed next.

Denotation and Connotation

A *denotative meaning* is one that is in general use by most people who share a common language. A *connotative meaning* usually arises from a person's personal experience. While all Americans are likely to share the same general denotative meaning of the word *pig*, the word may have a completely different positive or negative connotation for a farmer, a consumer of meat, a person of the Moslem faith, an orthodox Jew, a prisoner, and a police officer. These positive and negative connotative meanings can evoke powerful emotions.

Private and Shared Meanings

For communication to take place, meaning must be shared. People can use private meanings to communicate with others only when the parties agree about what the word means. The private meaning then becomes a shared meaning. It is common for families, two friends, or members of larger social groups (military personnel, drug users, adolescents) to use language in highly personal and private ways. Problems arise when the assumption is made that people who are outside the group share these meanings.

People with schizophrenia (refer to Chapter 16) may use language in an idiosyncratic way or may use a private, unshared language referred to as **neologisms**. Such people are unaware that others don't share this use of language. People who use neologisms, such as the young man in the following clinical example, expect to be understood and may become upset when they are not.

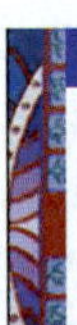

CLINICAL EXAMPLE

A young man who was hospitalized on a psychiatric unit complained to other clients and staff members that he had been odenated, and he became increasingly frustrated and anxious when it became apparent that he wasn't being understood. Rather than simply writing him off as confused or crazy, his primary nurse recognized that odenated most likely had a private meaning. With some help he was able to explain that he was upset about having been moved to a private room. The room was, he said, so dark and dingy that it looked like a cave. Animals live in caves that are called dens. In his view he had been o-den-ated—put into a cave.

In trying to make private meanings shared, make an effort to reach mutual understanding of the client's message. It is insufficient, and quite possibly inaccurate, to attach meaning based solely on your (or the client's) interpretation of an event, a word or phrase, or a gesture.

Nonverbal Messages

Most researchers agree that **nonverbal communication** channels carry more social meaning than verbal channels. There is a wide variety of nonverbal channels: body movements, including facial expressions and hand gestures; pitch, rate, and volume of the voice; the use of personal and social space; touch; and the use of cultural artifacts (such as clothing and cosmetics). Nonverbal cues help us judge the reliability of verbal messages more readily, especially in the presence of a **mixed message** (inconsistency between the verbal and nonverbal components).

Body Movement

The study of body movement as a form of nonverbal communication is called *kinesics*. Facial expressions, gestures, and eye movements are the most common categories.

Facial expressions are the single most important source of nonverbal communication. They generally communicate emotions. The silent-film comedians—blank-faced Buster Keaton and comic Charlie Chaplin—and the great mime Marcel Marceau communicate not only isolated acts but complete sequences of behavior with kinesics alone.

Body movements and gestures provide clues about people and about how they feel toward others. For example, hand gestures can communicate anxiety, indifference, and impatience, among other things. Foot shuffling and fidgeting may express the desire to escape.

Body position gives cues about how open one person is to another person, or how interesting and attractive one person is to another. People tend to position their bodies according to their feelings about the person with whom they are communicating. Choosing to stand or sit close to another usually indicates attraction, whereas creating greater physical distance may signify an attempt at interpersonal distance.

Eye contact is another very important cue in communicating. For example, proper sidewalk behavior among Americans is for passers-by to look at each other until they are about eight feet apart. At this distance, both parties look downward or away so they will not appear to be staring. Several common but unstated rules about eye contact are:

- Interaction is invited by staring at another person on the other side of the room. If the other person returns the gaze, the invitation to interact has been accepted. Averting the eyes signals a rejection of the looker's request.
- A person's frank gaze is widely interpreted as positive regard.
- Greater mutual eye contact occurs among friends.
- People who seek eye contact while speaking are usually perceived as believable and earnest.

MEDIALINK Case Study: Communication Skills

- If the usual short, intermittent gazes during a conversation are replaced by gazes of longer duration, the person looked at is likely to believe that the person gazing considers the relationship between the two people to be more important than the content of the conversation.

Keep in mind that nonverbal messages are often moderated by culture.

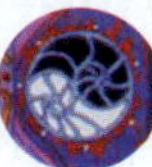

Voice Quality and Nonlanguage Sounds

Voice quality, such as pitch and range, and nonlanguage vocalizations, such as sobbing, laughing, or grunting—noises without linguistic structure—are components in addition to language itself.

Vocal cues can differentiate emotions. Who hasn't heard the injunction, "Don't speak to me in that tone of voice!" Sometimes people use vocal cues to make inferences about personality traits. For example, people who increase the loudness, pitch, timbre (overtones), and rate of their speech are often thought to be active and dynamic. Those who use greater intonation and volume and are fluent are thought to be persuasive. Status cues in speech are based on a combination of word choice, pronunciation, grammar, speech fluency, and articulation, among other factors.

Personal and Social Space

Proxemics is the study of space relationships maintained by people in social interaction. It includes the dimensions of *territoriality* (fixed and permanent territory that is somehow marked off and defended from intrusion) and *personal space* (a portable territory surrounding the self that others are expected not to invade). FIGURE 10-3 ■ illustrates the various relationships between intimacy and personal space.

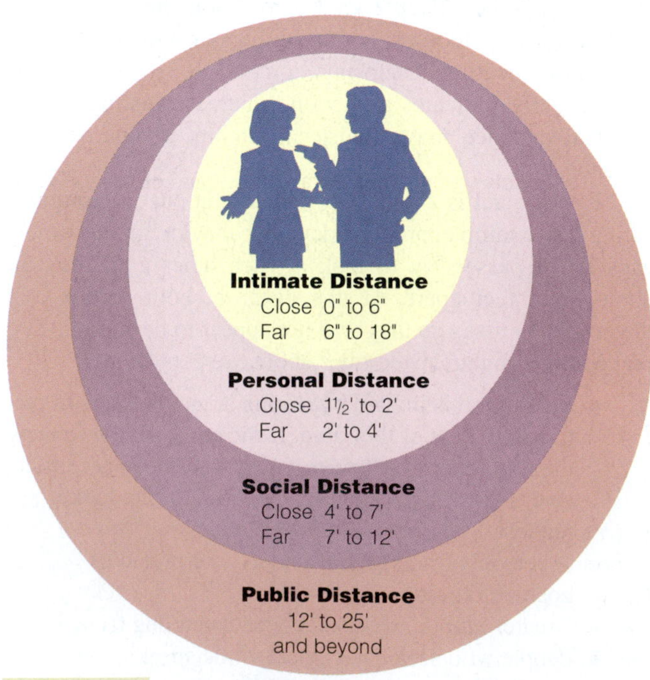

FIGURE 10-3 ■ Intimacy and personal space.

Knowing something about proxemics is useful, for example, in planning the physical space in which communication is to occur. You can arrange furniture to increase or decrease interpersonal distance. A cozy, open seating arrangement encourages interaction; chairs in a row that face the front of a room discourage interaction. It is important to be especially sensitive to the constraints imposed on communication by physical objects. An understanding of proxemics coupled with paying attention to how others use interpersonal space will enhance your ability to decipher verbal communication.

Touch

Touching behaviors, because they tend to personalize communication, are extremely important in emotional situations. In North American society, the use of touch is governed by strong social norms. Unwritten guidelines control who, when, why, and where people touch.

Most of the taboos against touching seem to stem from the sexual implications of touching behavior. However, although touching is a physical act, it may or may not be sexual in nature. A realization of the importance of touch and an understanding that touching is not necessarily a sexual behavior may make this channel of communication available to more people. It is equally important to be sensitive to the other person's disposition toward touching, so as not to alienate another by infringing on the person's right not to be touched. The use of touch in therapeutic work is discussed in Chapters 3, 29, and 33.

Cultural Artifacts

Artifacts are items in contact with interacting people that may function as nonverbal stimuli: clothes, cosmetics, perfume, deodorants, jewelry, eyeglasses, eyebrow and nose pierces, wigs and hairpieces, beards and mustaches, and so on.

Think about what information is communicated through artifacts such as a full-length mink coat, hair that is dyed purple, a gold band on the third finger of the left hand, a military uniform, or a Phi Beta Kappa key.

Verbal and Nonverbal Links

The verbal and nonverbal elements of human communication are inextricably linked. Six different ways in which verbal and nonverbal systems interrelate are discussed here.

1. A nonverbal cue may *repeat* a verbal cue but in a different way. The deep-sea fisherman who verbally describes the size of the sailfish he caught may also extend both hands to indicate its length. The gesture repeats the idea.
2. Nonverbal behavior may also *contradict* verbal behavior. Consider the woman who meets a college roommate she hasn't seen for some time. She says, "You haven't changed a bit," but her tone of voice and facial expression convey sarcasm. When verbal and nonverbal cues contradict one another, it is usually safer to put more faith in the nonverbal cues.

3. Nonverbal messages may *add to or modify* verbal messages. When a man says he is a "little" irritated about being kept waiting, his tone of voice and body actions may indicate a more profound anger.
4. Certain nonverbal cues *accent or emphasize* verbal cues. A woman shrugs her shoulders when she says she doesn't really care which movie she and her companion see. A master of ceremonies holds up his hand when he asks for quiet. These gestures and body movements emphasize the words.
5. Cues that *regulate*, such as those that tell people when to start talking or when to stop talking, are usually nonverbal. A woman who keeps opening and closing her mouth briefly while others are talking is indicating that she wants a turn too.
6. Sometimes nonverbal cues are used to *substitute* for words. A wave from a friend at a distance replaces "hello." Applause at the end of a play tells the actors that they have pleased the audience.

BIOPSYCHOSOCIAL THEORIES AND MODELS OF HUMAN COMMUNICATION

Communication takes place on at least three different levels: intrapersonal, interpersonal, and public (such as communication through the mass media or giving a public speech). Psychiatric–mental health nurses are more concerned with intrapersonal and interpersonal communication. **Intrapersonal communication** occurs when people communicate within themselves. When you walk into a client's room and think, "The first pint of blood is almost finished. I'd better get the next one ready for infusion," you are communicating intrapersonally.

Interpersonal communication, which this chapter discusses in depth, takes place in dyads (groups of two people) and small groups. This level of person-to-person communication is at the heart of psychiatric–mental health nursing.

One of the easiest ways to illustrate the nature of human communication and the elements of the process of human communication is through a model, or visual representation. People use models frequently for many purposes. They might use a map, which is a visual representation of a geographic location, to find their way to the community mental health center they plan to visit. Health professionals use electroencephalograms (EEGs) to see a visual representation of the electrical activity in the brain. However, models provide incomplete views—a map does not show all the trees, buildings, or park statues in the territory; an EEG tracing does not show the color, size, or blood supply of the brain. It is important to keep this in mind when looking at models. They sometimes make a process look simpler than it is.

Symbolic Interactionist Model

A symbolic interactionist model is based on a transactional perspective. It views human communication on the social–interpersonal level and accounts for the whole persons involved in the process. Communication is viewed as a process of simultaneous mutual influence, rather than as a turn-taking event. The participants are products of their social system and integral parts of it. In the communication, some events take place *within* the participants (they are intrapersonal), and some take place *between* the participants (they are interpersonal).

Participants are who they are in relationship to the other person with whom they are communicating. For example, in this dyadic (two-person) communication event between Jeff and Sarah, there are at least *six* perceptions involved:

1. Jeff's perception of himself
2. Jeff's perception of Sarah
3. Jeff's impression of the way Sarah sees him
4. Sarah's perception of herself
5. Sarah's perception of Jeff
6. Sarah's impression of the way Jeff sees her

Therefore, in addition to the content message, a relationship message also exists. Suppose Jeff passes Sarah in the corridor and Jeff says, "Hi, how are you?" Sarah answers, "Just fine, thanks," but moves down the corridor and away from Jeff as quickly as possible. Their subsequent communication will be affected by whether Jeff perceives Sarah as walking away because she wanted to get home before a rainstorm, or because he believes that Sarah is angry with him and her behavior is a comment on their relationship. The symbolic interactionist model helps explain what takes place between Jeff and Sarah.

A model constructed by Hulett (1966) according to symbolic interactionist principles, and adapted for this text, is shown in FIGURE 10-4 ■ on page 200. It shows five phases in each person's communication sequence: input, covert rehearsal, message generation, environmental event, and goal response.

During the phase of *input*, the person is motivated through some stimulus, either external or internal, toward some goal that requires engaging in a social interaction with another. Let's say that Jeff is attracted to Sarah and would like to get to know her better.

In the *covert rehearsal* phase, the person moves to make sense of the input received and develops and organizes a message *before* generating it. FIGURE 10-5 ■ on page 201 represents the covert rehearsal phase of human communication. The individual first scans the information about self and others (Jeff enjoys movies and remembers hearing Sarah tell a friend that she'd really like to see one particular movie) and then mentally rehearses possible actions to take (*role-playing*) and possible reactions of the other (*role-taking*). This gives Jeff the chance to think of four or five different ways to approach Sarah. This process is represented by the intrapersonal feedback loop.

The covert rehearsal phase is really the core of the communication process. In it, Jeff decides what to say, how to say it, and even whether to send the message to Sarah at all.

During *message generation*, the third phase, the instrumental act of giving a message is performed. (Jeff asks Sarah to the movie.) A message generated by one person serves as the input or the stimulus for another person. (Sarah thinks about Jeff's invitation, decides whether she wants to go to the movie with him, and considers what response to make to Jeff.) Once the second person completes the covert rehearsal

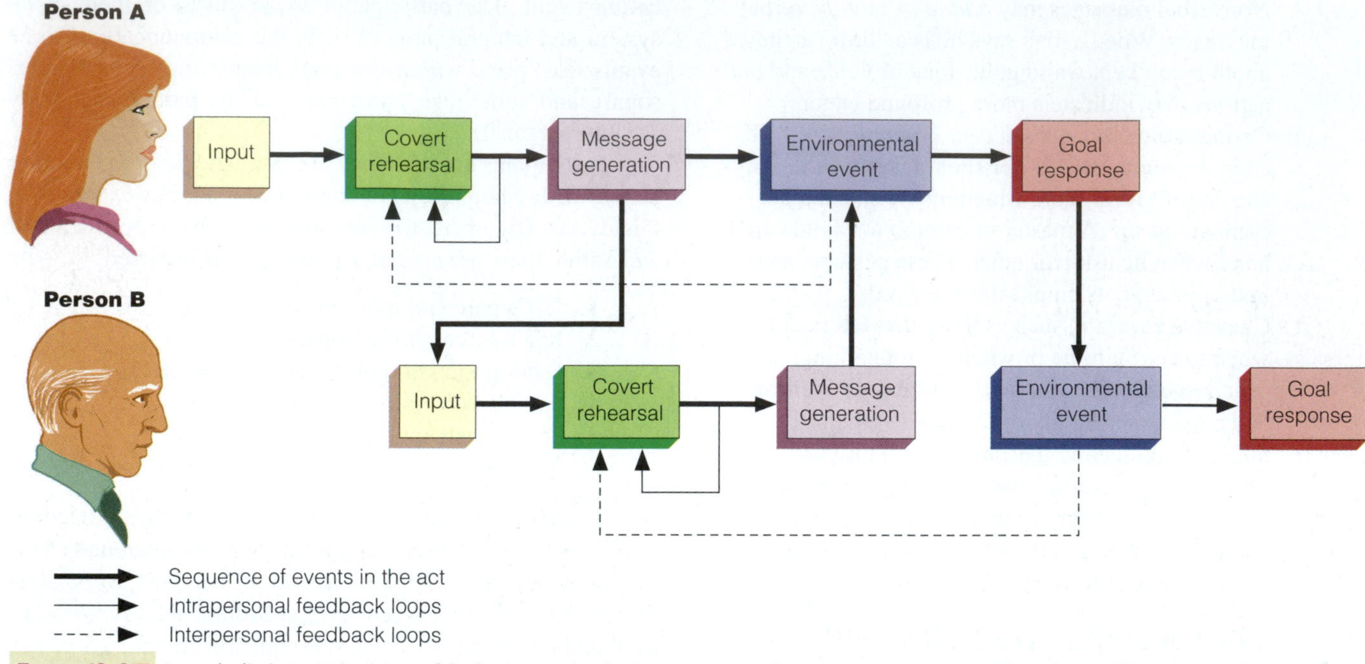

FIGURE 10-4 ■ A symbolic interactionist model of communication.

Source: Adapted from Hulett, J. E., Jr. (1966). A symbolic interactionist model of human communication. *AV Communication Review, 14,* 5–33. The Association for Educational Communications and Technology.

and generates a message, this message becomes an *environmental event* or stimulus for the first person. In our example, the environmental event is the fourth stage in the sequence for Jeff, whose *goal response* serves as an environmental event or stimulus for Sarah, and so on.

A second, or interpersonal, feedback loop connects the person's environmental event phase to the covert rehearsal stage. It allows the person an opportunity to determine whether he or she has made an error in the approach to the other and to make appropriate corrections by repeating the covert rehearsal and devising an altered message. (Jeff carefully considers Sarah's response. He listens to what she says and watches her behavior toward him. If her response is less than enthusiastic, he will try to determine what went wrong and how to correct it.)

In summary, the symbolic interactionist view of communication includes the following concepts:

- People run through a series of internal trials in the process of organizing a message.
- People select and transmit the message that will, in their view, have the highest probability of success.
- Success depends on the accuracy and completeness of the cognitive map and the accuracy and efficiency of the intrapersonal and interpersonal feedback loops.
- Communication is a dynamic (ever-changing) process that is unrepeatable and irreversible.
- Communication is complex.
- The meaning of messages is not transferred; it is mutually negotiated.

Communication is, at the very least, a very complicated process.

Neurobiologic Factors

Looking at communication in its broadest sense requires us to go beyond the spoken word, the written word, and motor activity to the molecular level. In this broad view, communication can also be thought of as the movement of neurotransmitters within a synapse between neurons (Restak, 2000). Neurobiology researchers believe that energy and movement at the molecular level may be the root of all brain functioning, including communication.

The neuron, the functional unit of the brain, differs from other cells in the body in that it is specialized for the function of information processing. The flow of information from one nerve cell to another involves the passage of electrically charged chemical particles—sodium, potassium, calcium, and chloride—across the cell membrane of the neuron. Neurotransmitters released by the presynaptic membrane of the axon cross the synaptic cleft and bind to their receptors on the postsynaptic membrane of the dendrite of the target cell. This process is more fully described in Chapter 6.

Therefore, brain activity can also be thought of in terms of messages and receptors. It makes sense to acknowledge that when communication is disrupted at one level—for example, when a crucial chemical in the brain undergoes an alteration—the end result can be felt at other, more obvious communication levels of the individual (such as verbal and nonverbal communication and intrapersonal and interpersonal communication). To put this into perspective, your understanding of the words on this page is related not only to your understanding of written English but also to the chloride ion channel activity on the membranes of millions of your brain cells.

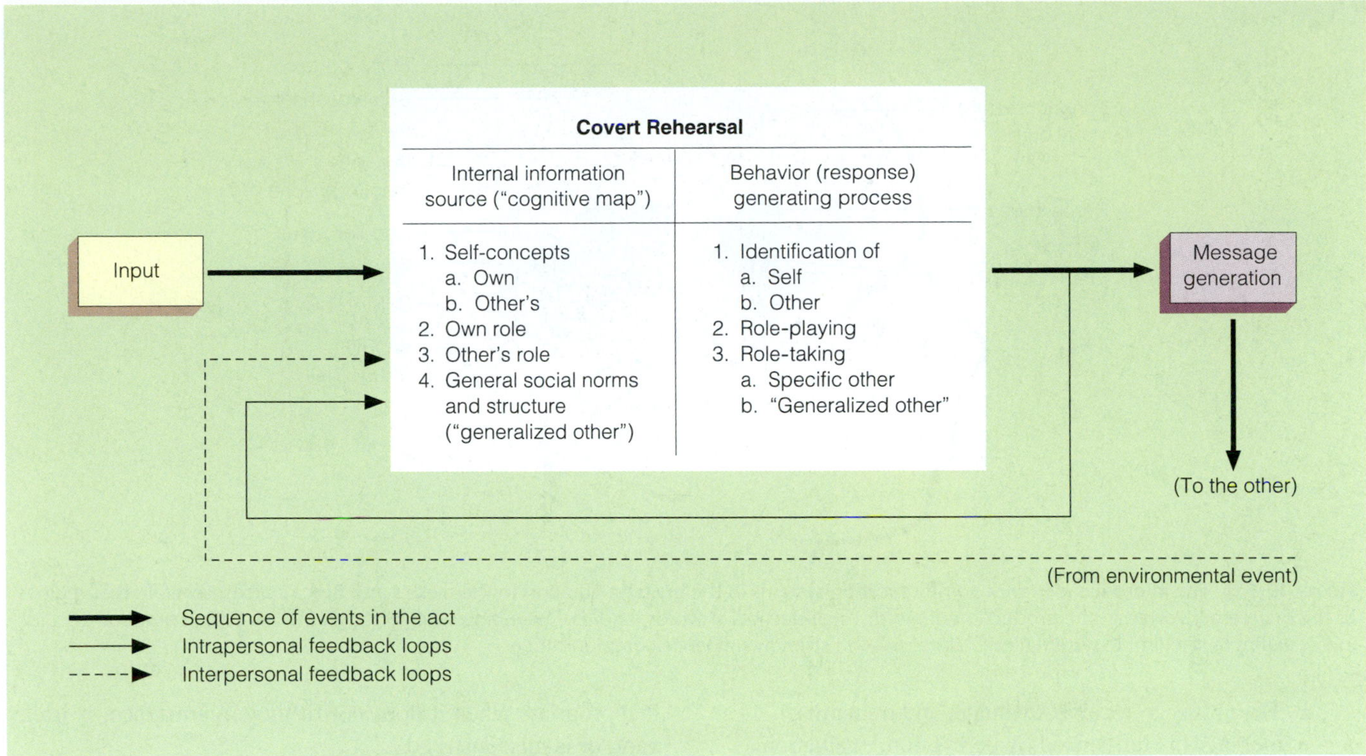

FIGURE 10-5 ■ The covert rehearsal phase of the symbolic interactionist model.

Source: Adapted from Hulett, J. E., Jr. (1966). A symbolic interactionist model of human communication. *AV Communication Review, 14*, 5–33. The Association for Educational Communications and Technology.

The neurobiology of human communication is very complex and not yet fully understood. For example, we know that there is a speech circuit in the brain between the auditory cortex on the left, which passes to Wernicke's area in the temporal cortex, and from there to Broca's area in the left frontal lobe via the arcuate fasciculus (a pathway composed mainly of axons that synapse with other neurons). This speech circuit is detailed in FIGURE 10-6 ■.

However, knowing about the speech circuit does not go far enough in explaining the complexities of the neurobiologic basis of human communication. Some elements of the communication process are distributed more widely in the brain than was previously believed. To add to the complexity, these areas are not the same in all of us. Therefore, there is no specific map of the brain that can locate specific communication functions with absolute certainty. Nor does it mean that damage in a specific region will necessarily cause a deficiency in a function thought to be contained in that region. FIGURE 10-7 ■ on page 202 illustrates the interdependence of various regions of the brain thought to influence communication.

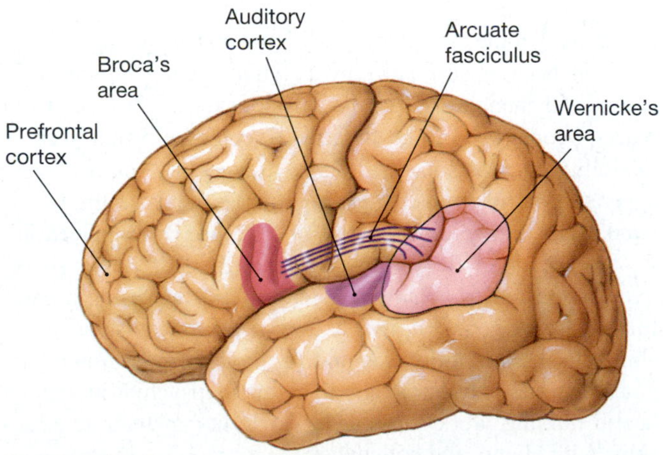

FIGURE 10-6 ■ The speech circuit.

Source: Smock, T. K. (1999). *Physiological psychology: A neuroscience approach.* Upper Saddle River, NJ: Prentice Hall.

Therapeutic Communication Theory

In the view of psychiatrist Jurgen Ruesch (1961), communication includes all the processes by which one human being influences another. Ruesch's theory takes into account the perceptions and interpretations that influence one person's view of the other. Further, Ruesch assumes that, to survive, the individual must communicate successfully.

According to Ruesch, communication is one of the most difficult human skills to master. It takes a long time to learn because it occurs in a series of steps, each building on the previous one. To communicate effectively requires decades of continuous practice. It is believed that interference hampers development and leaves an indelible mark.

Basic Concepts

The basic concepts of Ruesch's theory are as follows:

- Communication occurs in four different settings: intrapersonal, interpersonal, group, and societal.

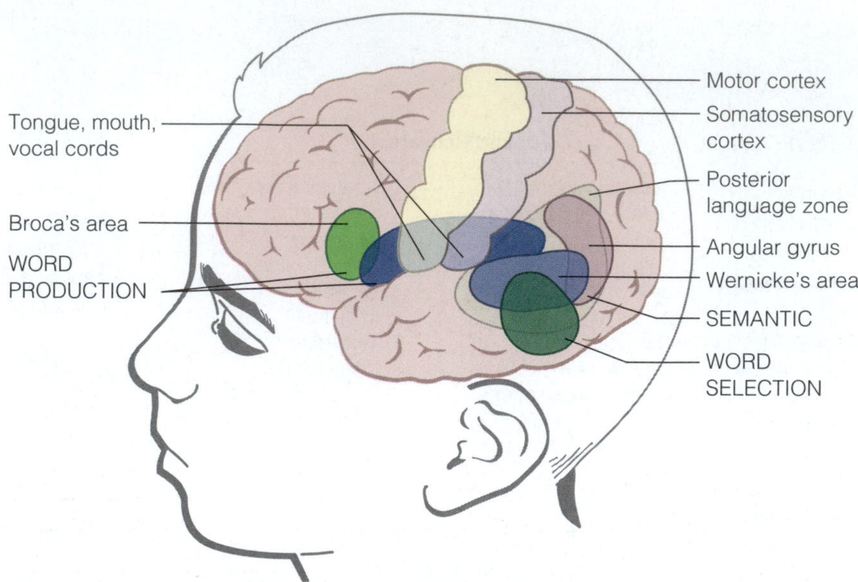

FIGURE 10-7 ■ The interdependency of communication systems in the brain. In addition to Wernicke's and Broca's areas, several other regions of the brain are involved in the production of words, the selection of words, and the meaning assigned to words. The brain's emotion circuits in, for example, the limbic system (see Chapter 6) strongly influence communication.

- The ability to receive, evaluate, and transmit messages is influenced by perception, evaluation (which involves memory, past experiences, and value systems), and the transmission quality of messages (amount, speed, efficacy, and distinctiveness).
- Messages achieve meaning when they are mutually validated or verified between the two parties.
- Correction through feedback is basic to adaptive, healthy behavior and successful communication.

Successful versus Disturbed Communication

The four formal criteria for successful communication are efficiency, appropriateness, flexibility, and feedback. When these criteria are not met, communication is disturbed (Ruesch & Bateson, 1968).

Efficiency Simplicity, clarity, and correct timing are all components of efficient messages. Psychiatric–mental health nurses and other mental health professionals may find themselves using complex and scientific words or professional mental health jargon to convey messages. Obscure or clumsy language and irrelevant or useless information may also prevent others from understanding a message.

Clear messages give a sense of order or structure and reduce ambiguity by narrowing the number of possible interpretations of meaning. Emphasizing the important ideas helps.

Proper timing is also important. It is best to give messages when the other person is able to "hear" them, when there are no intervening noises or inputs, and when the other person can interpret them without undue haste. Problems occur if the interval between the messages is either too short or too long.

Appropriateness Messages are appropriate when they are relevant to the situation at hand and when there is mutual fit of overall patterns and constituent parts. Communication is inappropriate when it does not fit the circumstance, is irrelevant, or is misconstrued.

Communication can also be inappropriate in amount. Since every individual has both high and low tolerance levels for stimulation, a person's ability to cope with ideas, make decisions, and act is affected by the amount and rate of sensory input received. Exceeding a tolerance level is called **overload**. A person who is overloaded by too many messages or by messages too closely spaced cannot handle incoming messages. **Underload** occurs when delay or lack of information interferes with a person's ability to comprehend the message of another.

The **tangential reply** is another example of inappropriateness. A tangential reply to a statement disregards the content of the message and is directed toward either an incidental aspect of the initial statement, the type of language used, the emotions of the sender, or another facet of the same topic.

Flexibility People cannot always be sure how a message will be received, because each person with whom they communicate is unique and changing. Since they cannot expect constancy from others, people need to be flexible. In communication, lack of flexibility manifests itself as either exaggerated control or exaggerated permissiveness. Both extremes increase the likelihood of frustrating, ungratifying, or disturbed communication.

Maintaining flexibility can be difficult if doing so requires a person to abandon or temporarily lay aside a carefully planned goal. To be flexible, a person must have the ability to set new priorities and to move to meet immediate goals. People who practice humanistic psychiatric–mental health nursing work to achieve flexibility in their relationships with clients and colleagues.

Feedback **Feedback** is the process by which performance is checked and malfunctions corrected. It performs a regulatory

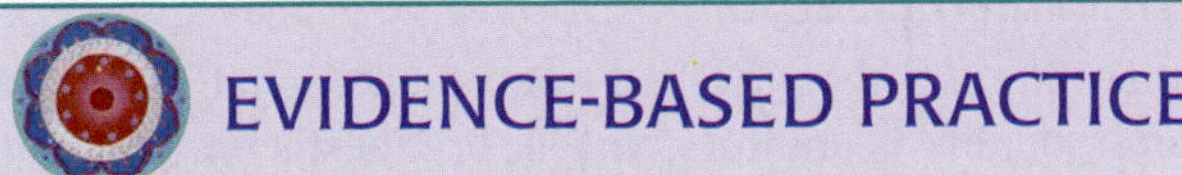

FEEDBACK HELPS CREATE A MORE HUMAN SETTING

Julie Rodriguez, a staff nurse in the psychiatric emergency department of a large metropolitan hospital, has been concerned because of the unfavorable evaluations left in the comment box by visitors to the emergency department. Although the waiting room has been newly remodeled and has comfortable seating, visitors to the department feel they are ignored for long periods of time while waiting to be seen. Their view of the staff is that staff members are very busy and seem to be working very hard. This doesn't seem to make up for the visitors' feelings that nurses and other staff are emotionally distant or "just there to do a job." The majority of visitors believe they have waited longer to be seen than what the documented records show; for them time seems to pass very slowly.

Julie believes the emergency department staff should be rated as highly as the physical environment. To achieve this goal, Julie has come up with the following plan, which she presented to her colleagues in their weekly meeting:

1. Provide a staff member presence at intermittent intervals—a nurse attuned to client needs and concerns related to their condition or to their care, and a volunteer to assist visitors with other questions or concerns such as those related to insurance, transportation, hospital admission, and so on.
2. Provide relaxing music, educational videos, books and puzzles, magazines and newspapers, and games for visitors' use. The volunteer would be responsible for maintaining these activities.

Julie's rationale for her proposal is that providing more than a physical presence in the waiting room avoids the perception that staff members are emotionally distant or just there to do a job and, in conjunction with the additional activities, transforms a technical, potentially impersonal setting into a more human place. Her rationale is based on knowledge she gained from several research articles, including:

Roper, J. M., & Manela, J. (2000). Psychiatric patients' perceptions of waiting time in the psychiatric emergency service. *Journal of Psychosocial Nursing and Mental Health Services, 38*(5), 18–27.

Snyder, M., Brandt, C. L., & Tseng, Y. (2000). Use of presence in the critical care unit. *AACN Clinical Issues, 11*(1), 27–33.

CRITICAL THINKING APPLICATION

1. What personal steps could busy nurses take to reduce emotional distance between themselves and clients or themselves and family members?
2. Clients and family members waiting to be seen in an emergency department often feel anxious. If anxiety is interpersonally communicated (see Chapter 8), what staff behaviors in this example could add to their anxiety?
3. Which verbal and nonverbal therapeutic communication skills are likely to help reduce their anxiety?

function in the communication process. One example of how feedback can help to correct a system malfunction is illustrated in the Evidence-Based Practice feature. Feedback allows people to decide which messages have been understood as intended. It requires the cooperation of two people—one to give it and one to receive it. Giving helpful feedback is discussed further later in this chapter.

Under certain circumstances of disturbed communication, feedback either fails or functions poorly. When messages do not get through or are distorted, appropriate replies cannot be obtained, and corrective feedback does not occur. Content that elicits anxiety, fear, shame, or any of several other strong emotions is likely to hamper feedback.

Behavioral Effects and Human Communication Theory

Watzlawick, Beavin, and Jackson (1967) base their theory of human communication on the assumption that communication is synonymous with interaction. These authors maintain that, in the presence of another, all behavior is communicative. This theory is concerned with the pragmatics, or the behavioral effects, of human interaction. What makes this theory particularly useful for this book is its conception of human communication as a reciprocal process.

Communication Levels

According to this theory, one cannot *not* communicate. Both activity and inactivity, verbalizations and silences, convey messages. This communication occurs on two levels. The *content level* of a communication is the report aspect, in which information is conveyed. The *relationship level* is communication about a communication.

All interchanges can be viewed as either *symmetric* (based on equality) or *complementary* (based on difference). In symmetric relationships, the partners usually mirror each other's behavior, thus minimizing difference. Complementary relationships, in contrast, maximize difference.

Communication Disturbances

Communication can be disturbed when a person attempts *not* to communicate. As an example, in this framework, the basic dilemma occurs when a person attempts not to communicate. However, because it is impossible not to communicate, the attempt to not communicate is a communication in itself.

Another disturbance occurs when a person communicates in a way that invalidates the messages sent to or received from the other person. Such communications, called *disqualifications,* include a wide range of behavior such as self-contradictions, inconsistencies, subject switches, incomplete sentences, and misunderstandings.

A person may communicate in a way that confirms, rejects, or *disconfirms* the other person's view of self. Confirmation of one person's self-view by another is thought to be the greatest single factor in ensuring mental development and stability. Rejection of the other's definition of self essentially conveys this message: "You're wrong." Disconfirmation, by contrast, conveys this message: "You don't exist." Disconfirmation questions the other's authenticity. Disconfirmation leads to alienation and has been found to occur with some regularity in the experiences of people with schizophrenia.

Although all relationships are necessarily either symmetric or complementary, *runaways* (exaggerations to the point of disturbance) may occur in either of the patterns. For example, the danger of competitiveness is ever-present in symmetric relationships. Symmetric interactions that lose their stability may enter a spiral in which each individual attempts to be just a little bit "more equal" than the other. Runaways are seen in quarrels between people or wars between nations, behaviors that are relatively open. Rejection of the other's self generally occurs when a symmetric relationship breaks down.

Breakdowns in complementary relationships, however, are generally characterized by disconfirmation of the other. For this reason, they are usually viewed as more serious (Watzlawick, 1993).

Neurolinguistic Programming Theory

Neurolinguistic programming (NLP) is a communication model developed in the early 1970s by Richard Bandler and John Grinder. The model is derived from theory in linguistics, neurophysiology, psychology, cybernetics, and psychiatry (Bandler, 1993).

Bandler and Grinder first observed psychotherapists who were known as expert communicators to discover what made them so effective as therapists (Dilts, Bandler, & Bandler, 1990). They concluded that people take in, or *access*, information in three sensory modalities:

1. Auditory
2. Visual
3. Kinesthetic

Further, each person prefers one mode over the others. Sounds may facilitate communication with one person, while touch or sight may be more effective with another person. In addition, people process information, or make sense out of it, according to the representational system (the NLP phrase for sensory modality) through which they receive it.

They also found that the expert communicators they observed were able to adapt themselves to match the client's representational system and to imitate the client in a natural and respectful way. Bandler and Grinder theorized that by tuning in to and then using the other person's preferred sensory mode, one could greatly enhance the ability to establish rapport. The most effective communicators, according to NLP theory, are those who can use all three modalities and easily move from one representational system to another.

Determining the Sensory Modality

To determine whether a client's representational system or sensory modality is auditory, visual, or kinesthetic, one identifies the client's:

- Preferred predicates (verbs, adjectives, adverbs that tell something about the subject)
- Eye-accessing cues
- Gross hand movements
- Breathing pattern
- Speech pattern and voice tones

Preferred Predicates A necessary first step before attempting to link words with nonverbal behavior is observing the client to see which set of predicates is preferred. Sample preferred predicates of the auditory, visual, and kinesthetic types are listed in the Your Assessment Approach feature.

Eye-Accessing Cues Eye-accessing cues correlate with an individual's thinking process. People who are visualizing generally turn their eyes upward or look straight ahead, focusing on nothing. Someone processing auditory information usually moves the eyes from side to side. A person engaging in intrapersonal communication usually focuses the eyes down in the direction of the nondominant hand. A person in the kinesthetic mode looks down toward the dominant hand when experiencing sensations or emotions.

Gross Hand Movements Gross hand movements also give clues to the client's sensory mode. People have a tendency to point toward or touch the sense organ that matches their cur-

YOUR ASSESSMENT APPROACH
Preferred Predicates

Auditory	Visual	Kinesthetic
Argue	Appear	Attach
Chant	Bright	Breathless
Debate	Colorful	Calm
Eavesdrop	Glimpse	Excite
Hassle	Image	Fondle
Hear	Observe	Hurt
Listen	Pretty	Rough
Overhear	Scan	Sharp
Praise	Sight	Soft
Quiet	Spy	Sore
Scream	Stare	Support
Silent	Ugly	Tension
Tell	View	Throw
Whine	Watch	Touch
Whisper	Wink	Warm

rent sensory mode. The person in a visual mode often points toward the eye, and the person in an auditory mode often points toward or touches the ear.

Breathing Pattern Assessing the breathing patterns helps the observer understand the client's representational model. Shallow, thoracic breathing is often associated with visual accessing. Even breathing or prolonged expiration is associated with auditory accessing, and deep abdominal breathing is associated with kinesthetic accessing.

Speech Pattern and Voice Tones Visual accessing often correlates with quick bursts of words that are high pitched, strained, or nasal. Auditory accessing is often associated with a clear, midrange voice tone or with a rhythmic tempo and clearly enunciated words. Kinesthetic accessing is associated with a slow voice and a low volume or deep tone, or with a breathy tone and long pauses.

Therapeutic Use of NLP

Using NLP theory in psychiatric–mental health nursing practice gives us yet another way to empathize with clients by "trying on" their style. People tend to be less anxious with the familiar. Those of us who mirror the client's sensory mode are likely to be experienced as more comfortable and safer to be with, conditions that facilitate rapport.

We can use mirroring to help the client follow our lead. For example, with an anxious client, we might begin by mirroring the behaviors that indicate the client's anxiety and then shift into a more relaxed posture and less anxious behaviors. It is easier to lead the client from a more anxious state to a less anxious state by employing the NLP principles discussed here.

An important benefit of the NLP approach is that it allows us to assess the client's style and preferred sensory mode and to communicate more effectively by using both verbal and nonverbal communication in the client's preferred mode. The following examples express the same nursing intervention with different predicates, depending on the client's preferred mode:

> Visual—"Yes, I can *see* that you are much better. You *look* good, your eyes are *clear*, your *appearance* has certainly changed."
>
> Auditory—"Yes, I can *hear* from the *sound* of your voice that you are better. *Talking* with you today is quite different from yesterday."
>
> Kinesthetic—"Yes, you do seem to be *feeling* much better today, you're *holding* your head up, and your *grasp* is certainly *firmer* than yesterday."

By expanding our abilities to communicate with clients in all three modes, we can become more effective communicators.

FACILITATING COMMUNICATION AND BUILDING A RELATIONSHIP

Therapeutic communication aims at initiating, building, and maintaining fulfilling and trusting relationships with other people. Communicating ideas and feelings with clarity, efficiency, and appropriateness helps a person be interpersonally effective. In reading the rest of this chapter, try to relate the therapeutic communication principles and practices discussed earlier to these ideas about facilitating communication.

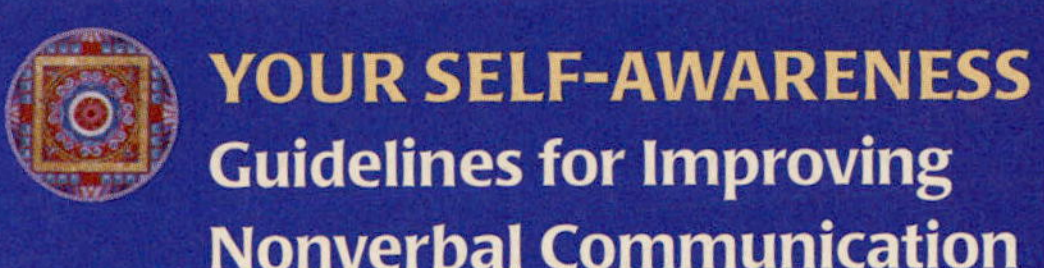

YOUR SELF-AWARENESS
Guidelines for Improving Nonverbal Communication

1. **Relax.** The simple act of relaxing makes it easier for others to be relaxed and more open. Remember, anxiety is interpersonally communicated (see Chapter 8). Take some deep breaths, do a quick body scan, and allow the tension to flow out of your body (see Chapter 33 for directions for these relaxation techniques).
2. **Use facial, hand, and body gestures judiciously.** Nonverbal gestures that are used indiscriminately lose their effectiveness. Overdoing a gesture—constantly smiling, constantly nodding your head—may become annoying to others and make it more difficult for them to talk with you.
3. **Get feedback on your nonverbal communication.** Your classmates and instructors are sources of feedback. Ask them to comment on the facial expressions and body gestures that you use when you converse with them. Consider being videotaped so that you can see for yourself any mannerisms or gestures that intrude on your ability to be an effective communicator.
4. **Practice.** Once you've identified any intrusive facial expressions or body gestures, practice blending your verbal message with appropriate nonverbal cues such as hand gestures, body posture, facial expression, and tone of voice. Then, role-play with your classmates and ask them to comment on your effectiveness.

Don't forget about using appropriate nonverbal skills. Your verbal and nonverbal messages should be consistent with one another. Nonverbal messages should enhance, not detract from, verbal messages. The Your Self-Awareness feature above presents some guidelines for you in achieving this goal.

Superficiality versus Intimacy

Most relationships between people begin at the level of social superficiality. In a nurse–client relationship, we try to develop facilitative intimacy, which differs from social intimacy. For example, the interdependence that characterizes the social relationship is greatly reduced. In social relationships, participants may "tell their stories" to one another. In relationships that have therapeutic goals, only the client is engaged in storytelling with the nurse. (If necessary, review the section on self-disclosure in Chapter 3.) The process is specifically focused. Clients not only explain themselves, the events of their lives, and the circumstances they face, they do so with a purpose in mind—understanding the circumstances through exploring them and moving to improve their lives.

Movement toward therapeutic intimacy may be difficult at first. For one thing, such intimacy violates certain social taboos. For example, at a party it may be socially incorrect to

MediaLink Care Plan: Developing the Nurse–Client Relationship

comment on a person's anxiety, stuttering, or facial tic. When communication has a therapeutic goal, all messages, including these nonverbal ones, are heeded and may be discussed.

Therapeutic intimacy also requires that the participants move beyond social "chitchat" into meaningful areas of concern for the client. Therapeutic intimacy requires high involvement and commitment.

Facilitating Intimacy

Several interpersonal principles and practices are essential to facilitating intimacy.

Responding with Empathy

Most theorists believe that empathy is the most important dimension in the helping process. Without a high level of empathic understanding, nurses have no real basis for helping. Empathy facilitates interpersonal exploration. A more complete discussion of empathy follows.

Responding with Respect

Responding with respect demonstrates that you value the integrity of the client and have faith in the client's ability to solve problems, given appropriate help. By encouraging clients to put forward possible plans of action, you convey respect for their ability to take charge of their own destiny. Giving advice, by contrast, conveys a directly opposite message.

Responding with Genuineness

Genuineness refers to the ability to be real or honest with another. To be effective, genuineness must be timed properly and based on a solid relationship. Honesty is not always the best policy, especially if it is brutal or if the client is not capable of dealing with it.

Clients who can experience your authenticity can risk greater genuineness and authenticity themselves. The nurse who is genuine is more likely to deal with and eventually help the client resolve all problems, rather than just those that are safe or socially acceptable.

Responding with Immediacy

Responding with immediacy means responding to what is happening between the client and yourself in the here-and-now. Because this dimension may involve the feelings of the client toward you, it can be one of the most difficult to achieve. For example, the client may confront you with overt or implied criticism of your role or competence. If you respond in a defensive or evasive way, the relationship may be threatened. If you are open, reasonable, and concerned, the relationship may be strengthened.

Responding with Warmth

Warmth is so closely linked with empathy and respect that it is seldom communicated as an independent dimension. It is important, however, to note some additional points about the expression of warmth. Effusive, chatty, "buddy-buddy" behavior should not be confused with warmth. Warmth is most often conveyed in communications of respect and empathy.

Be aware of and accept the client's right to maintain distance (refer back to Figure 10-3). Warmth and intimacy cannot be forced. Initially high levels of warmth can be counterproductive for clients who have received little warmth from others in their lives, are suspicious, or have been taken advantage of by others. Warmth alone is insufficient for building a relationship and solving problems.

THERAPEUTIC COMMUNICATION SKILLS

Think of the communication techniques presented here as having the potential to foster effective communication. You must make them your own and adapt them individually for each human encounter. Blend them with the understanding you have gained from the interpersonal communication principles and practices discussed earlier in this chapter and the dimensions of self-knowledge that you examined in Chapter 3∞.

Be aware that using a set of communication skills as a sort of relationship "magic" will probably doom you to failure. Relationships, and the people in them, are unique and much too complex to rely on a communication formula that can be applied to all people and all situations. Remember that a holistic approach is inconsistent with the rigid, inflexible application of communication techniques.

Speaking to the Hard of Hearing

Be considerate and respectful when a client is hard of hearing. Here are some suggestions based on the work of Dreher (2001) for communicating with a client who is hard of hearing:

1. Move close enough to the client so that you are speaking from a distance of 3 to 6 feet.
2. Determine if the client hears better through one ear than the other. If so, speak into the good ear.
3. Choose an environment that is free of competing noise and turn off television sets, radios, etc.
4. Place yourself so that the client can see you clearly, preferably with light on your face.
5. Make sure the client can see your lips and be careful not to obscure them with gestures or articles of clothing.
6. Speak at a natural rate. Since people comprehend faster than they speak, it is not necessary for you to slow down unless the client does not understand.

If you fail to recognize and compensate for a client's hearing problem, you risk miscommunication.

Empathizing

Psychiatric–mental health nursing students are taught the skills of active listening. But listening without *empathy* is not enough. Empathic understanding not only increases your grasp of the client's difficulties but also helps you offer feedback on how the client affects others. Empathy can best be understood as a process through which people feel with one another. They are able to sense the feelings of another because they have evoked in themselves the attitude of the person to whom they are relating (in other words, they have engaged in role-taking, discussed earlier in this chapter). Central to learn-

MEDIALINK Application: Communicating with Special Populations

ing the skill of emphathizing is embracing the idea that what the client has to say or what the client feels is important (to the client) and deserves acknowledgment. A recent study of what it means to individuals with mental illness to be understood revealed three predominant themes: "I was important," "It really made us connect," and "They got on my level" (Shatell, McAllister, Hogan, & Thomas, 2006). Being empathic helps to connect with clients and validates their importance.

The term *empathy* is often mistakenly used synonymously with *sympathy*. Empathy contains no elements of condolence, agreement, or pity. When nurses sympathize rather than empathize, they assume that there is a parallel between their feelings and those of the client. The perceived similarity makes professional judgment and objectivity difficult.

Empathic involvement with troubled clients can have a number of stressful consequences. Problems can arise at any phase in the empathy process. The obstacles to achieving an empathic concern for clients can be understood as a failure to cope with one of the four phases of achieving empathy. These four phases are discussed in Box 10-1. Be careful not to overidentify and lapse into sympathy for the client. By doing so, you may fail to incorporate the client's feelings and instead project personal ones. Bypassing the reverberation phase and substituting gut-level intuitions for rational problem solving can be another problem. Be sure to guard against overdistancing or burnout.

Sympathy can also be an appropriate response given the right circumstances. The What Every Nurse in Any Setting Should Know feature discusses how to respond appropriately with sympathy.

Mindful Listening

Most of us assume that we are good listeners. The truth is that *mindful listening* (also known as active listening) is more difficult than you might think. It is more than being quiet while the other person talks—it requires paying undivided attention to what the client says, does, and feels, and putting aside your own judgments and ideas long enough to really hear. Mindful listening requires intention—that is, when you intend to really hear what another is saying, and what that other person thinks, feels, and needs, the better you can understand that person and his or her needs. If you don't listen mindfully, you won't be able to comprehend the message. If you don't comprehend the message, you will not be able to effectively use the therapeutic communication techniques that follow.

There are several blocks to listening that may prevent you from hearing what the client is saying and convey the message that what he or she is saying is not very important:

1. Rehearsing: Being too busy planning what you are going to say next

Box 10-1 Four Phases of Therapeutic Empathizing

The process of empathic understanding has four phases:

1. *Identification.* Through the relaxation of conscious controls, we allow ourselves to become absorbed in contemplating the client and the client's experiences.
2. *Incorporation.* We take in the experiences of the client rather than attribute our own experiences and feelings to the client.
3. *Reverberation.* We interplay the internalized feelings of the client and our own experiences or fantasies. While fully absorbed in the identity of the client, we still experience ourselves as separate personalities.
4. *Detachment.* We withdraw from subjective involvement and totally resume our own identity. We use the insight gained from the reverberation phase as well as reason and objectivity to offer responses that are useful to the client.

WHAT EVERY NURSE IN ANY SETTING SHOULD KNOW

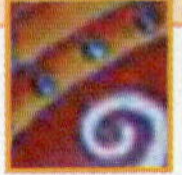

Expressing Sympathy to the Bereaved

Although empathizing is preferable to sympathizing when you are serving in a professional role, there are occasions in which sympathy is not only appropriate but helpful. One such example is when a client you are taking care of dies, or a friend, colleague, or acquaintance has just lost a loved one and you wish to reach out and offer support to the bereaved individual or family. Many people worry about finding the right words or worry that they will say the wrong thing. It is hard to go wrong if you are sincere in offering support. Remember that nonverbal messages enhance verbal messages and your sincerity when acknowledging the bereaved person's feelings will temper any words that are not quite perfect. Here are some suggestions for expressing sympathy in a therapeutic way:

- Celebrate the deceased person's life rather than dwell on the death. Not everyone gains comfort from hearing that a death "was a blessing" or that the deceased is "in a better place."
- Invite the bereaved person to talk, and listen carefully. Talking often helps the bereaved person feel better. Inviting the bereaved person to share stories about the deceased's life can be a healing experience.
- Share a good memory that you have about the deceased. Sharing memories, mementos, and photographs of the person who died may help spark happy memories.
- Be proactive in providing help. People in mourning may find making decisions taxing. Rather than asking if they would like help—making a dish, mowing the lawn, walking the dog, doing the food shopping—just go ahead and do it.
- Keep checking in. There is often a rush of support from people wanting to help, but typically, support wanes quickly. Keep in mind that holidays and anniversaries of the person's death can be especially difficult and make an effort to let the person know that you care.

Doing something to provide comfort is much preferable to doing nothing because you are unsure of what to say.

2. Being concerned with yourself—your intelligence, your level of competence, your feelings, or your accomplishments
3. Assuming: Thinking that you know what the client "really means" because of your assumptions and hunches
4. Judging: Framing what you hear or what you see in terms of your judgment of the client as being wrong, immature, anxious, paranoid, or depressed
5. Identifying: Focusing on your own similar experiences, feelings, or beliefs when what the client says triggers your own memories or concerns
6. Getting off track: Changing the subject or making light of it when you become uncomfortable, bored, or tired
7. Filtering: Tuning out certain topics or hearing only certain things, perhaps because of anxiety, regardless of what else is said

Mindful listening is best accomplished when environmental distractions are minimized. Consider finding a quiet place, turning off the television, or closing the door if it is appropriate and safe. Avoid taking extensive notes; they take your attention away from the client, and you will miss some of what is being said on the verbal level and done on the nonverbal level.

Face the client, use eye contact, show interest, and listen objectively while minimizing your own personal responses. Remaining silent while clients express themselves is a sign of respect and interest. Avoid interrupting the client because you feel the need to say or do something. Specific circumstances in which it is appropriate, for therapeutic reasons, to interrupt the client or steer the conversation in another direction are discussed in the chapters in Unit 3.

When listening, pay attention not only to what the client says (the verbal communication) but also to what the client does and how the client looks (the nonverbal communication). Nonverbal cues often shed light on what the client says. Although listening enables you to observe the client's nonverbal messages, it does not follow that you will necessarily interpret the nonverbal cues accurately. Nonverbal cues should be validated with your clients.

Using Silence

Do not feel obligated to respond after every statement a client makes. *Using silence* goes beyond mindful listening and can be a very effective therapeutic technique when it encourages the client to communicate, when it allows the client time to ponder what has been said or a connection the client has made, when it allows the client time to collect his or her thoughts, or when it allows the client time to consider alternatives. Looking interested while maintaining an open posture or a questioning look will encourage the client to use the time effectively.

Uncomfortable silences should be broken and analyzed. You would not want a client to become increasingly anxious or resistive. (See Chapters 8 and 18∞ for suggestions on handling anxiety and Chapter 29∞ for suggestions on handling resistance.)

Remember, silence is an effective communication technique only when it is used as an appropriate and purposeful therapeutic intervention. For example, clients who are depressed and feel pressured to interact benefit from your silent, undemanding presence. Nurses who are silent because they are uncomfortable or because they lack the knowledge or the skill to communicate effectively must seek an experienced clinical supervisor to help them analyze their own personal and professional growth needs.

Reflecting

Reflecting is repeating the client's verbal or nonverbal message for the client's benefit. It encourages the client to become more actively involved. Reflecting also actively acknowledges what you have heard or seen.

Reflecting Content

Reflecting the *content* of the message basically repeats the client's statement. This gives clients the opportunity to hear and mull over what they have told you.

- "You believe things will be better soon."
- "You think it would be better to take a part-time job."

Content reflection is perhaps one of the most misused and overused methods in mental health counseling. Use it judiciously. It loses its effectiveness when used for lack of other choices.

Reflecting Feelings

Reflecting *feelings* is verbalizing the implied feelings in the client's comment. Remember to respect the client's right to his or her opinion and feelings even when you may disagree with them.

- "Sounds like you're really angry at your brother."
- "You're feeling anxious about being discharged from the hospital."

In reflecting feelings, you attempt to identify latent and connotative meanings that may either clarify or distort the content. Reflection is useful because it encourages the client to make additional clarifying comments.

Imparting Information

Imparting information is helping the client by supplying additional data. This encourages further clarification based on new or additional input.

- "Group therapy will be held on Tuesday evening from 6:30 until 8:00."
- "I am a psychiatric nursing student."

It is not constructive to withhold useful information from the client or to reply "What do you think?" to a straightforward, information-seeking question. However, be careful not to cross the line between giving information and giving advice, or giving information as a way of avoiding an area of interpersonal difficulty. Also, by giving personal, social information you will likely move out of the realm of therapeutic intervention (see the discussion of self-disclosure in Chapter 3). Information that is important to disclose to the client to protect the client's rights includes your title and position. Resist the temptation to deny you are new to the field—it may only cause mistrust.

Remember that clients' participation in decision making begins when they take in and understand information about their own condition. The goal of imparting information should be to provide effective education that empowers clients and their families. Studies have shown that an educated, empowered client is more likely to achieve positive mental health outcomes and less likely to need admission or readmission to an acute care facility. You can help clients by using each teachable moment.

Avoiding Self-Disclosure

When the nurse chooses to avoid self-disclosure in a given instance (such as those discussed in the section on self-disclosure in Chapter 3), several communication techniques may be helpful. For instance, a client might ask the nurse to disclose marital status, home address, religious affiliation, or a pressing personal problem. Auvil and Silver (1984) offer these ways to deflect a request for self-disclosure:

- *Use honesty*. "I don't want to share my home address with you."
- *Use benign curiosity*. "I wonder why you're asking me this today?"
- *Use refocusing*. "You were talking about how your father treats you. I wonder why you changed the topic? You were saying that. . . ."
- *Use interpretation*. "I notice that every time you talk about your father, you change the subject and ask me a question." (pause)
- *Seek clarification*. "You keep asking me my home address. I wonder what concerns you might have about me today."
- *Respond with feedback and limit setting*. "I'm really uncomfortable when you ask me who pays my tuition. Talking about my finances isn't part of our agreement to work together." Adding "The last time we met, you were deciding if you were going to call your boss on the phone . . ." helps restructure the situation.

Use these communication techniques in the context of the therapeutic relationship, and assess and evaluate client responses in an ongoing manner with an instructor or clinical supervisor.

Clarifying

Sometimes, even though you've listened carefully, you're still not totally clear. In this situation, it is important to ask for clarification. *Clarifying* is an attempt to understand the basic nature of a client's statement.

- "I'm confused about exactly what is upsetting to you. Could you go over that again, please?"
- "You say you're feeling anxious now. What's that like for you?"

Asking the client to give an example to clarify a meaning helps you understand the client's intended message better. A person who describes a concrete incident is more likely to see the connections between it and similar occurrences. Illustrations or examples are also very useful qualifiers.

Paraphrasing

In *paraphrasing*, you assimilate and restate in your own words what the client has said.

- "In other words, you're fed up with being treated like a child."
- "I hear you saying that when people compliment you, you feel embarrassed. If they knew the real you, they'd stay away."

Paraphrasing gives you the opportunity to test your understanding of what a client is attempting to communicate. It is reflective in nature, in that it lets the client know what you heard and how you understand what has been said. It also gives the client the opportunity to clarify content or feelings.

Checking Perceptions

Checking perceptions means sharing how one person perceives and hears another. After sharing perceptions of the client's behaviors, thoughts, and feelings, ask the client to verify the perception.

- "Let me know if this is how you see it too."
- "I get the feeling that you're uncomfortable when we're silent. Does that seem to fit?"

You can use perception checks to make sure that you understand a client. An effective perception check conveys the message, "I want to understand. . . . " It gives the other person the opportunity to correct inaccurate perceptions. It also allows you to avoid actions based on false assumptions about the client.

Questioning

Questioning is a very direct way of speaking with clients. But when used to excess, questioning controls the nature and range of the client's responses. Questions can be useful when you are seeking specific information. When your intent is to engage the client in meaningful dialogue, however, questions should be limited.

When using questions, it is best to make them open-ended rather than closed. An *open-ended question* focuses the topic but allows freedom of response.

- "How were you feeling when your mother said that to you?"
- "What's your opinion about . . . ?"

The *closed-ended question* limits the client's choice of responses, generally to "yes" or "no" ("Were you feeling angry when your mother said that?"). Closed-ended questions limit therapeutic exploration. However, clients whose thinking is disorganized may need to be guided by closed-ended questions (e.g., questions on suicidal thoughts; see Chapter 23).

MediaLink Critical Thinking Exercise: Communicating in the Clinical Setting

"Why" questions usually have the same effect. They are often impossible to answer and rarely lead to a clearer understanding of the situation. However, "who," "what," "when," and "how" questions may be helpful when used judiciously.

Be careful when questioning not to steer the client to answer in a certain way. For example, "You don't drink alcohol to excess, do you?" suggests that the client should answer "no."

Structuring

Structuring is an attempt to create order or evolve guidelines. It helps the client become aware of problems and the order in which the client might deal with them.

- "You've mentioned that you want to improve your relationships with your wife, your sister, and your boss. Let's put them in order of priority."
- "No, I won't be giving you advice, but we can discuss some possible solutions together."

Structuring is particularly useful when clients introduce a number of concerns in a brief period and have little idea of where to begin. Use structuring not only to explore content but also to delimit the parameters of the nurse–client relationship and to identify how you will participate with the client in the problem-solving process.

Pinpointing

Pinpointing calls attention to certain kinds of statements and relationships. For example, you may point to inconsistencies among statements; to similarities and differences in the points of view, feelings, or actions of two or more people; or to differences between what one says and what one does.

- "So, you and your wife don't agree about how many children you want."
- "You say you're sad, but you're smiling."

Linking

In *linking*, you respond to the client in a way that ties together two events, experiences, feelings, or people. You can use linking to connect past experiences with current behaviors. Another example is linking the tension between two people with current life stress.

- "You felt depressed after the birth of both your children."
- "So, the arguments didn't really begin until after you got your promotion."

Giving Feedback

Giving *feedback* is telling the other person your reaction to what he or she has said. It helps clients become aware of how their behavior affects others and how others perceive their actions. Responding with feedback can be therapeutic self-disclosure on your part. It allows you to offer clients constructive information that makes them aware of their effect on others. However, total self-disclosure by the nurse (discussed in greater detail in Chapter 3∞) is inappropriate in the nurse–client relationship. It places a burden of interdependence on the client and limits the time and energy available to work on the client's concerns. Reciprocal self-disclosure is more appropriate in friend and colleague relationships.

Effective feedback should be immediate (given as soon as possible), honest (giving your true reaction), and supportive (given in ways that are tolerable to hear and not hurtful or brutal).

- "When you wring your hands, I feel your anxiety."
- "Sometimes when you turn your head away from me, I think you're angry."

It is important to give feedback in a way that does not threaten the client and result in increased defensiveness. The more defensive the client, the less likely the client will hear and understand the feedback. Clients may feel offended if they perceive you as rejecting them (Hem & Heggen, 2004). Feedback that is harsh, hurtful, or cruel, or appears to reject the client, creates boundaries between yourself and the client. You want to do your best to prevent the client from experiencing your feedback as a personal rejection. The Your Intervention Strategies feature in this section lists strategies and rationales for giving helpful, nonthreatening feedback.

Be aware that clients express not only information about themselves when they interact with you; but also information about how they perceive you. Cues about how your words and your behavior affect clients are there if you look for them. Be open and receptive to these unsolicited cues—the client's feedback to you—that can help you to become a more effective psychiatric–mental health nurse. The Your Self-Awareness feature in this section will help you to engage in self-reflection.

Confronting

Constructive confrontations often lead to productive change. *Confronting* is a deliberate invitation to examine some aspect of personal behavior that indicates a discrepancy between what the person says and what the person does. Confrontation requires careful attention to nonverbal communication and the discrepancies between nonverbal and verbal messages.

Confrontations may be informational or interpretive, and they may be directed toward both the resources and the limitations of the client. An *informational confrontation* describes the visible behavior of another person.

- "You say you're 'the dummy in the family,' yet none of your brothers or sisters made the honor roll like you did."

An *interpretive confrontation* expresses thoughts and feelings about the other's behavior and draws inferences about the meaning of the behavior.

- "Ever since Sally and Joe criticized the way you conducted the meeting, you haven't spoken to them. It looks like you're feeling angry."

Six skills to be incorporated in constructive confrontations are:

1. Use of personal statements with the words *I*, *my*, and *me*

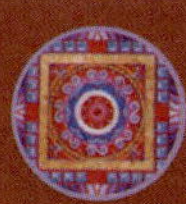

YOUR INTERVENTION STRATEGIES
Giving Helpful, Nonthreatening Feedback

Strategy	Rationale
■ Focus feedback on behavior rather than on client.	Refer to what client actually does rather than how you imagine client to be.
■ Focus feedback on observations rather than inferences.	Refer to what you actually see or hear client do; inferences refer to conclusions or assumptions you make about client.
■ Focus feedback on description rather than judgment.	Report what occurred rather than evaluating it in terms of good or bad, right or wrong.
■ Focus feedback on "more or less" rather than "either/or" descriptions of behavior.	"More or less" descriptions stress quantity rather than quality (which may be value-laden).
■ Focus feedback on here-and-now behavior rather than there-and-then behavior.	The most meaningful feedback is given as soon as it is appropriate to do so.
■ Focus feedback on sharing of information and ideas rather than advice.	Sharing ideas and information helps client make decisions about own well-being; giving advice takes away client's freedom to be self-determining.
■ Focus feedback on exploration of alternatives rather than answers or solutions.	Focusing on a variety of alternatives for accomplishing a particular goal prevents premature acceptance of answers or solutions that may not be appropriate.
■ Focus feedback on its value to the client rather than on catharsis it provides you.	Feedback should serve client's needs, not your own.
■ Limit feedback to amount of information client is able to use rather than amount you have available to give.	Overloading will decrease effectiveness of feedback.
■ Limit feedback to appropriate time and place.	Excellent feedback presented at an inappropriate time may be ineffective or harmful.
■ Focus feedback on what is said rather than why it is said.	Focusing on why things are said or done moves away from observations and toward motive or intent (which can only be assumed, unless verified).

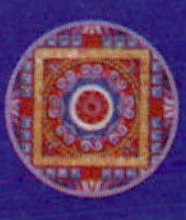

YOUR SELF-AWARENESS
Reflecting on Feedback from Your Clients

Input—both positive and negative—from clients, classmates, instructors, staff, and family members and friends can help you to become aware of your "blind spots," the characteristics about yourself that you ignore, deny, or defend. Protecting oneself through self-deception interferes with both relating and communicating. To become more self-aware, do the following:

- Think about a recent interaction with a client and how that client responded to you.
- Identify the positive/negative elements in the interaction.
- Try to determine what the client was telling you about yourself in this interaction, that is: What characteristic(s) do you have that enables clients to openly express their thoughts and feelings? What characteristic(s) do you have that prevents clients from openly expressing their thoughts and feelings?
- Discuss the interaction and your interpretation of it with an instructor.
- Ask for feedback on your behavior from others—family members, classmates, staff, friends.

2. Use of relationship statements expressing what you think or feel about the client in the here and now
3. Use of behavior descriptions (statements describing the visible behavior of the client)
4. Use of description of personal feelings, specifying the feeling by name
5. Use of responses aimed at understanding, such as paraphrasing and perception checking
6. Use of constructive feedback skills (see the Your Intervention Strategies box)

Summarizing

Summarizing is the highlighting of the main ideas expressed in an interaction. It shows the client that you understand. Both you and the client benefit from this review of the main themes of the conversation. Summarizing is also useful in focusing the client's thinking and aiding conscious learning.

- "The last time we were together you were concerned about. . . ."
- "You had three main concerns today."

You can use this technique appropriately at different times during an interaction. For example, it is useful to summarize the previous interaction in the first few minutes you and the client spend together. Early summarizing helps the client recall the areas discussed and gives the client the opportunity to see how you have synthesized the content of a previous session. Summarizing is useful because it keeps the participants directed toward a goal.

Injudicious use of summarizing is a common pitfall. You may rush to summarize despite other, more pressing and immediate client concerns. In this instance, summarizing is likely to meet your needs for structure but does nothing to address the client's here-and-now concerns.

Processing

Processing is a complex and sophisticated technique. Process comments direct attention to the interpersonal dynamics of the nurse–client experience—in the content, feelings, and behavior being expressed.

- "It seems that important things that need to be taken care of come up in the last five minutes we have together."
- "Today is the first day our time together has started out with silence. Last week it seemed there wouldn't be enough time."

As you can see, processing is an advanced skill. Processing is most useful when therapeutic intimacy has been achieved.

COMMON MISTAKES

When we are experiencing discomfort or strong negative feelings it becomes difficult to empathize and to communicate with clients in a therapeutic way. Some common mistakes to guard against are:

- *Giving advice.* Giving advice ("You should . . .", "Why don't you . . .", "It would be better if you . . .") carries the implicit message that the client is incapable of solving his or her own problem.
- *Minimizing or discounting feelings.* Telling a client that he or she is overreacting, that there is nothing to be afraid of, or not to worry are attempts at reassurance that minimize and discount the client's feelings.
- *Deflecting.* Hearing clients express their pain can be anxiety-provoking. Changing the subject or making a joke are attempts to move to something less painful. This is not a positive shift of focus—rather, it gives the client the message that you cannot or do not want to cope with the pain the client is feeling. Joking and humor are more fully discussed in Chapter 3.
- *Interrogating.* Asking a barrage of questions implies that you are more interested in gathering information than you are in listening to the client.
- *Sparring.* No matter what the client says, you know better. Debating or disagreeing with the client prevents you from listening to the client.

CIRCUMVENTING POTENTIAL CULTURAL BARRIERS TO COMMUNICATION

When English is not the client's primary language and you are a monolingual provider, it will help if you select the words you use carefully, avoiding buzz words, slang, and technical jargon. Show respect by speaking clearly and directly to the client, pacing yourself to be neither too fast nor too slow. Words that are slurred, have many syllables in them, or are too technical make communication more difficult. Speaking too fast may overload the client and make it difficult for the client to follow. Speaking too slowly may lose the client's attention.

Select the gestures you use with care, using your nonverbal behavior to underscore your words and your actions. The proper use of gestures can clarify a message, and drawings can sometimes be helpful. Be careful however; as discussed earlier in this chapter, not all gestures mean the same thing in all cultures and some body language may be offensive or misunderstood.

Listen to your client's words and watch your client's gestures carefully. Do your best to understand and validate the meaning they have for you. Listening carefully to the client helps you avoid focusing on what you will say or do next and demonstrates your genuine concern for the client's distress.

If the client attempts to speak English, his or her thoughts may appear distorted when language is the real problem. There have been a number of documented instances in which people have been diagnosed as mentally disordered and confined to a mental hospital because mental health professionals erroneously diagnosed a language problem or value difference as disordered thinking or psychosis. Use open-ended questions and rephrase them in several ways to obtain accurate information.

An interpreter may be necessary if language is a barrier. If the client does not have his or her own interpreter, you may be able to enlist the aid of a bilingual staff member. For the sake of confidentiality and the client's privacy and reputation, avoid using family members as interpreters. Clients may not want family members privy to personal information (Martin & Nakayama, 2006), for example, sexual preference, drug or alcohol use, or content of hallucinations (what the voices say). Health and social services departments, international institutes, college language departments, neighborhood houses, or cultural centers will often know of people who are willing to volunteer as interpreters. Remember to always speak directly to the client and not to the interpreter.

Being aware of cultural phenomena that affect etiquette will be appreciated by the client. Spector (2006) suggests the following strategies:

1. Use the proper form of address for a given culture.
2. Know the ways by which people from that culture welcome one another, that is, when a handshake or embrace is expected as well as when physical contact is prohibited.

3. Be aware of when smiling indicates friendliness or is taboo, and when eye contact is a sign of respect or aggression.
4. Remember that gestures do not have universal meaning.

Emphasizing similarities can help to form a therapeutic relationship. Differences may serve as topics for discussion. An open, ongoing dialogue is beneficial for both parties because it promotes understanding.

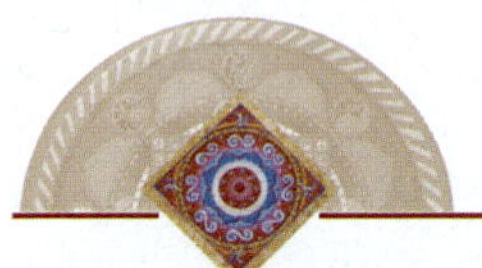

EXPLORE MEDIALINK

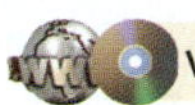 www.prenhall.com/kneisl

For NCLEX-RN® review questions, case studies, and other resources for this chapter see the Pearson Health MediaLink CD-ROM that accompanies this book and the Companion Website at www.prenhall.com/kneisl.

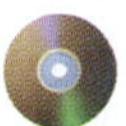

CD-ROM
Audio Glossary
NCLEX-RN® Review Questions

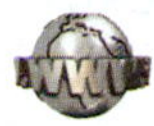

Companion Website
Audio Glossary
NCLEX-RN® Review Questions
Critical Thinking Exercise
- *Communicating in the Clinical Setting*

Case Study
- *Communication Skills*

Care Plan
- *Developing the Nurse–Client Relationship*

MediaLinks
MediaLink Application
- *Communicating with Special Populations*

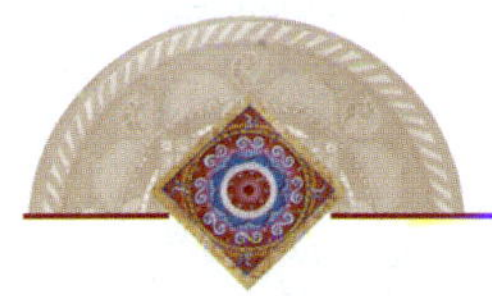

NCLEX-RN® REVIEW QUESTIONS

1. According to the therapeutic communication theory, what criteria must be met for successful communication?
1. The communication must be intrapersonal, interpersonal, group, or societal in nature.
2. The communication needs to be efficient, appropriate, flexible, and include feedback.
3. Nonverbal communication is consistent with verbal communication.
4. The individuals communicating with each other must share a similar perception of the conversation.

2. The nonverbal communication that expresses emotion is:
1. Body positioning.
2. Cultural artifacts.
3. Facial expressions.
4. Eye contact.

3. In the symbolic interactionist view of communication, how is the meaning of the message determined?
1. It is predetermined by the person initiating the interaction.
2. It is based on the recipient's perception and interpretation.
3. It is transferred from the sender to the receiver.
4. It is mutually negotiated between the individuals involved in the interaction.

4. The nurse is discussing problem-solving strategies with a client who recently experienced the death of a family member and the loss of a full-time job. The client says to the nurse, "I hear what you're saying to me, but it just isn't making any sense to me. I can't think straight now." The client is expressing feelings of:
1. Rejection.
2. Overload.
3. Disqualification.
4. Hostility.

5. The nurse is interacting with a client and observes the client's eyes moving from side to side prior to answering a question. The nurse interprets this behavior as:
1. The client responding to auditory hallucinations.
2. The client processing auditory information.
3. The client being bored with the interaction.
4. The client engaging in intrapersonal communication.

6. The nurse is caring for a client who is hard of hearing. To facilitate communication with the client, the nurse will:
1. Stand 5 to 8 feet from the client when speaking.
2. Speak slowly, using monosyllabic words whenever possible.

3. Ask closed-ended questions.
4. Make sure the client can see her lips move when she is speaking.

7. A client with a history of major depression tells the nurse "I wish I weren't alive. I have been a failure my entire life and I am totally useless to anyone." The most therapeutic response to the client is:
1. "You shouldn't talk like that. You're not a failure."
2. "Once the antidepressants start working you will feel better about yourself."
3. "Things could be worse. You should be grateful for what you have."
4. "You've been feeling like a failure your entire life?"

8. The nurse is completing the sexual history section of the admission assessment. The client tells the nurse "I don't want to talk about this. This is private between my spouse and me." Which nurse response reflects empathy?
1. "Yes, I know just how you feel."
2. "I understand this is difficult for you to talk about, but I have to complete the admission assessment."
3. "I know some of these questions are difficult for you."
4. "I am a professional nurse and I know what I am doing."

9. To provide effective feedback to a client, the nurse will focus on:
1. The client.
2. The present and not the past.
3. Providing solutions to the client.
4. Making inferences of the behaviors observed.

10. The use of facial expressions and gestures communicates:
1. Personality traits.
2. Interest in, and attraction to, another person.
3. Emotions.
4. Rejection.

See Appendix C for answers.

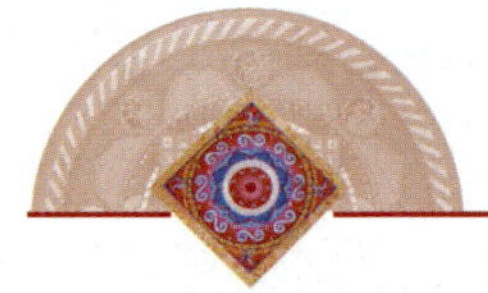

REFERENCES

Auvil, C. A., & Silver, B. W. (1984). Therapist self-disclosure: When is it appropriate? *Perspectives in Psychiatric Care, 22*, 57–61.

Bandler, R. (1993). *Time for a change*. Denver: Meta Publications.

Dilts, R., Bandler, R., & Bandler, L. C. (1990). *Neurolinguistic programming*. Denver: Meta Publications.

Dreher, B. B. (2001). *Communication skills for working with elders* (2nd ed.). New York: Springer.

Hem, M. H., & Heggen, K. (2004). Rejection: A neglected phenomenon in psychiatric nursing. *Journal of Psychiatric and Mental Health Nursing, 11*(1), 55–63.

Hulett, J. E., Jr. (1966). A symbolic interactionist model of human communication. *AV Communication Review, 14*, 5–33.

Martin, J. N., & Nakayama, T. K. (2006). *Intercultural communication in context* (4th ed.). Philadelphia: McGraw-Hill.

Restak, R. M. (2000). *Mysteries of the mind*. New York: National Geographic Society.

Roper, J. M., & Manela, J. (2000). Psychiatric patients' perceptions of waiting time in the psychiatiric emergency service. *Journal of Psychosocial Nursing and Mental Health Services, 38*(5), 18–27.

Ruesch, J. (1961). *Therapeutic communication*. New York: Norton.

Ruesch, J., & Bateson, G. (1968). *Communication: The social matrix of psychiatry*. New York: Norton.

Shatell, M. M., McAllister, S., Hogan, B., & Thomas, S. P. (2006). "She took the time to make sure she understood": Mental health patients' experiences of being understood. *Archives of Psychiatric Nursing, 20*(5), 234–241.

Snyder, M., Brandt, C. L., & Tseng, Y. (2000). Use of presence in the critical care unit. *AACN Clinical Issues, 11*(1), 27–33.

Spector, R. E. (2006). *Cultural care: Guide to heritage assessment and health traditions* (5th ed). Upper Saddle River, NJ: Prentice Hall.

Watzlawick, P. (1993). *The language of change: Elements of therapeutic communication*. New York: Norton.

Watzlawick, P., Beavin, J., & Jackson, D. (1967). *The pragmatics of human communication*. New York: Norton.

ADDITIONAL REFERENCES

Adler, R. B. (2006). *Interplay: The process of interpersonal communication*. New York: Oxford University Press.

Davis, M., Paleg, K., & Fanning, P. (2004). *How to communicate workbook*. New York: MJF Books.

Gregory, R. (2001). Listening. *Journal of Psychosocial Nursing and Mental Health Services, 39*(2), 48–51.

Klagsbrun, J. (2001). Listening and focusing: Holistic health care tools for nurses. *Nursing Clinics of North America, 36*(1), 115–130.

Northouse, P. G., & Northouse, L. L. (2007). *Health communication: Strategies for health professionals* (4th ed.). Upper Saddle River, NJ: Prentice-Hall.

Poss, J. E., & Beeman, T. (2000). Effective use of interpreters in health care: Guidelines for nurse managers and clinicians. *Seminar for Nurse Managers, 7*(4), 166–171.

Reynolds, W. J., & Scott, B. (2000). Do nurses and other professional helpers normally display much empathy? *Journal of Advances in Nursing, 31*(1), 226–234.

Reynolds, W., Scott, P. A., & Austin, W. (2000). Nursing, empathy, and perception of the moral. *Journal of Advances in Nursing, 32*(1), 235–242.

Ryan, M., Twibell, R., Brigham, C., & Bennett, P. (2000). Learning to care for clients in their world, not mine. *Journal of Nursing Education, 39*(9), 401–408.

Stein-Parbury, J. (2005). *Patient and person: Interpersonal skills in nursing* (3rd ed.). Sydney, Australia: Elsevier.

Tamparo, C. D., & Lindh, W. Q. (2007). *Therapeutic communications for health professionals* (3rd ed.). Albany, NY: Delmar.

Wood, J. T. (2006). *Interpersonal communication: Everyday encounters*. Belmont, CA: Wadsworth.

Assessing

CHAPTER

11

EILEEN TRIGOBOFF
CAROL REN KNEISL

LEARNING OUTCOMES

After completing this chapter, you will be able to:

1. Perform an ongoing psychiatric–mental health assessment of clients in your care.
2. Determine how and when to apply assessment principles in professional practice.
3. Describe the steps a psychiatric–mental health nurse would take to elicit a psychiatric history from a client and the client's family.
4. Describe the steps a psychiatric–mental health nurse would take to conduct a mental status examination on a client.
5. Explain how to use the Mental State Examination and the Mini-Mental State Exam.
6. Determine the circumstances in which the mental status examination would be used and the circumstances in which the Mini-Mental State exam would be used.
7. Differentiate among a physiologic assessment, neurological assessment, psychological testing, and psychosocial assessment.
8. Describe the DSM-IV-TR multiaxial system.
9. Demonstrate the DSM-IV-TR multiaxial system for making a psychiatric diagnosis.
10. Incorporate the results of a Global Assessment of Functioning Scale in the development of a nursing care plan.
11. Document the clinically relevant care given to the client as well as the client's response to that care.

CRITICAL THINKING CHALLENGE

You are responsible for an intake assessment with Jared, a 35-year-old male client. He is being admitted to inpatient care from an emergency room after driving his car off a freeway ramp into a building. His psychiatric diagnosis is major depression with psychotic features, and he has had prior hospitalizations for "suicidal gestures," as noted in his chart. Most guidelines for conducting a mental status intake examination emphasize the importance of a suicide assessment, which includes questions such as "Have you ever thought of ending it all?", "Have you ever considered suicide?", or "Do you plan to hurt yourself?"

Jared is single, unemployed, and has a problem with alcohol abuse. In your interview you ask if he is considering hurting himself again, and he says "no." He seems anxious and does express feelings of hopelessness. You also know he's been on the

(continued)

MEDIALINK 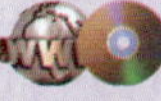 www.prenhall.com/kneisl

Go to the Pearson Health MediaLink CD-ROM and the Companion Website at www.prenhall.com/kneisl for interactive resources for this chapter.

KEY TERMS

Beck Depression Inventory *224*
Benton Visual Retention Test *225*
blocking *218*
circumstantiality *218*
compulsions *219*
confabulations *220*
daydreams *219*
delusions *219*
fantasies *219*
flat affect *218*
flight of ideas *218*
Global Assessment of Functioning (GAF) *228*
hallucinations *219*
intelligence tests *222*
Mental Status Examination (MSE) *217*
Millon Clinical Multiaxial Inventory–II (MCMI–II) *224*
Mini-Mental State Exam (MMSE) *220*
Minnesota Multiphasic Personality Inventory–2 (MMPI–2) *224*
mutism *218*
Nurses' Observation Scale for Inpatient Evaluation (NOSIE) *221*
objective personality tests *224*
obsessions *219*
perseveration *218*

(continued)

KEY TERMS *(continued)*

projective personality tests *224*
psychiatric history *216*
Raven's Progressive Matrices Test *225*
Rorschach Test *224*
Sentence Completion Test *225*
State–Trait Anxiety Inventory *224*
Thematic Apperception Test (TAT) *225*
Weschler Adult Intelligence Scale–III (WAIS–III) *225*

CRITICAL THINKING CHALLENGE *(continued)*

Internet and has been to the Hemlock Society website. He hopes to find a new life as a result of his hospitalization.

1. What recommendations would you make for Jared's first few days on the psychiatric inpatient unit, and why?
2. What would your purpose be in specifically asking Jared what he learned from the Hemlock Society website?
3. At what level of risk would you place Jared?

The systematic scientific approach known among nurses as the *nursing process* has evolved as the cornerstone of clinical practice. The nursing process begins with assessment for the purpose of collecting and analyzing objective and subjective data about the clients with whom nurses work.

In keeping with the professional responsibilities for assessment identified in *Psychiatric–Mental Health Nursing: Scope and Standards of Practice,* published jointly by the American Nurses Association [ANA], American Psychiatric Nurses Association, and International Society of Psychiatric–Mental Health Nurses (2007), the psychiatric–mental health registered nurse, designated as RN-PMH, who implements the following, meets the measurement criteria for the assessment standard:

- Collects data in a systematic and ongoing manner
- Involves the client, family, other health care providers, and others in the client's environment, as appropriate, in holistic data collection
- Demonstrates effective clinical interviewing skills that facilitate development of a therapeutic alliance
- Prioritizes data collection activities based on the client's immediate condition or anticipated needs of the client or situation
- Uses appropriate evidence-based assessment techniques and instruments in collecting pertinent data
- Uses analytical models and problem-solving techniques
- Ensures that appropriate consents, as determined by regulations and policies, are obtained to protect client confidentiality and support client rights in the process of data gathering
- Synthesizes available data, information, and knowledge relevant to the situation to identify patterns and variances
- Uses therapeutic principles to understand and make inferences about the client's emotions, thoughts, and behaviors
- Documents relevant data in a retrievable format

There are additional measurement criteria for the psychiatric–mental health advanced-practice registered nurse, designated the APRN-PMH.

A comprehensive assessment enables the nurse to make sound clinical judgments and plan appropriate interventions. The primary sources of client data in most instances are the clients themselves. Nurses' documentation, psychological evaluations and tests, physicians' orders, social workers' information, and other secondary data sources can enlarge, clarify, and substantiate data obtained directly from the client. A nurse's assessment skills are utilized throughout an individual client's care and are essential to the success of a treatment regimen.

PSYCHIATRIC EXAMINATION

Systems of data collection and assessment vary among mental health agencies. The psychiatric examination consists of two parts: the psychiatric history and the mental status exam. It is most often done during initial or early interactions with a client. The traditional psychiatric examination is discussed in this chapter because it is still used in settings where psychiatric nurses work and is considered the counterpart of the physical examination and history.

Psychiatric History

The **psychiatric history** gathers information about the client's current condition and previous diagnoses, interventions, and treatment, along with a family history.

Data Sources

Not all data gathered during psychiatric history taking are obtained from the client. There are several other sources. Family, friends, police, mental health personnel, and others may contribute data to the psychiatric history. When the sources are varied, the psychiatric history focuses on the perceptions of others: how they see the client and the circumstances of the client's life. The sources of the information to be included in the psychiatric history and their relationship to the client should always be clearly indicated. Information given by these collateral sources should be reviewed and understood in terms of that relationship.

The psychiatric history generally includes the following categories of data:

- *Complaint*—the main reason the client is having a psychiatric examination. The client may have personally initiated the psychiatric examination, or others (such as courts, hospital staff, family, referral from school or employer) may have initiated it. The "chief complaint" should be recorded verbatim and indicated as such with quotation marks ("I just don't want to live any longer" or "I know these are crazy thoughts but I can't stop them. They're too strong.").
- *Present symptoms*—the nature of the onset and the development of symptoms. These data are usually traced from the present back to the last period of adaptive functioning.
- *Previous hospitalizations and mental health treatment*
- *Family history*—generally, whether any family members have ever sought or received mental health treatment
- *Personal history*—the client's birth and development; past and recent illnesses; schooling and educational problems; occupation; sexual development, interests, and practices; marital history; the use of alcohol, drugs, caffeine, and tobacco; trauma history; and religious, spiritual, or cultural practices
- *Personality*—the client's relationships with others, moods, feelings, interests, and leisure activities

Input from family and friends can give a better perspective of the client you are interviewing as well as insight into the psychosocial aspects of the circumstances in which the client lives. This input includes perceptions of the client by others (how they see the client), how symptoms are expressed in that environment, and patterns of interaction. Keep in mind that family and friends have their own perspectives through which they filter events. All information from family and friends is treated as important data to be contributed to the whole assessment and not necessarily a total picture of the client.

The main purpose of history taking is to gather information, although it is often also effective in establishing rapport with a client. The information offered by the client will not likely emerge in the exact order of the forms to be completed. You can shape and guide the interview while allowing the client to provide information at a comfortable pace. You can also promote rapport by avoiding an interrogative approach and allowing the client's story to unfold naturally. For the most part, the assessment process involves inserting all collected data for documentation without maintaining a rigid structure.

Assessing for psychological symptoms is not substantially different for nurses in different specialty areas. It may be more demanding to be an Emergency Department nurse and have to assess for emergent physical situations in addition to psychological symptoms; however, the basics remain the same. See What Every Emergency Department Nurse Should Know for an example of adjusting to include assessing a mentally ill client.

WHAT EVERY EMERGENCY DEPARTMENT NURSE SHOULD KNOW

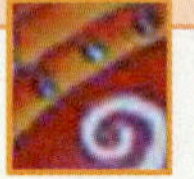

Assessing a Mentally Ill Client

People move quickly in the Emergency Department (ED). Lives hang in the balance; speed can make all the difference. Bringing a mentally ill client into this fast-paced environment requires adjustments in order to assess properly and provide good nursing care.

Verbal interactions are the main approaches appropriate for interacting with a mentally ill client in the ED, as opposed to the algorithms for physical care. Your assessment of a client with chronic psychiatric difficulties focuses on why the client is in the ED at this time. Something happened to make today different from yesterday, when the client was not in the ED. Ask questions about the current situation and what has changed for the client.

Other considerations for ED assessments of a mentally ill client include allowing for greater personal space than you would with someone receiving physical care. Physical contact may be interpreted entirely differently than usual, especially normally supportive gestures such as hand holding or shoulder touching.

Keep in mind that speed is not an asset under these circumstances (Stanton, 2007). People who have psychiatric illnesses likely have cognitive difficulties, cannot absorb information quickly, have trouble concentrating and remembering, and need a quieter environment to reduce distractions. Using your assessment skills can promote client safety and enhance the movement of the client through the system in a timely manner (referred to as *ED throughput*).

Mental Status Examination

The **Mental Status Examination (MSE)** is usually a standardized procedure in agencies that use it. The primary purpose of the MSE is to help the examiner gather more objective data to be used in determining etiology, diagnosis, prognosis, and treatment, and to deal immediately with any risk of violence or harm. The sections of the MSE that deal with sensorium and intellect are particularly important in establishing the existence of delirium, dementia, amnestic, and other cognitive disorders. The purpose of this examination differs from that of the psychiatric history in that it identifies the person's present mental status.

The mental status examiner generally seeks the following categories of information (not necessarily in the sequence presented here):

1. *General behavior, appearance, and attitude*—a complete and accurate description of the client's physical characteristics, apparent age, manner of dress, use of cosmetics, personal hygiene, and responses to the examiner. Postures, gait, gestures, facial expression, and mannerisms are included in the description. The examiner also notes the client's general activity level.

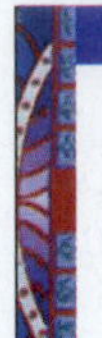

CLINICAL EXAMPLE

A 35-year-old white male, appears stated age, dressed in torn, disheveled jeans. Presents a blank facial expression, slouched posture, shuffling gait, generally low activity level, and sullen behavior.

Other descriptors that may be used include *frank, friendly, irritable, dramatic, evasive, indifferent,* and so forth. Details should be sufficient to identify and characterize the client.

2. *Characteristics of speech*—the form, rather than the content, of the client's speech. Speech is described in terms of loudness, flow, speed, quantity, level of coherence, and logic. A sample of the client's conversation with the examiner may be included in quotation marks. The goal is to describe the quantity and quality of speech to discern difficulties in thought processes. The following patterns, if present, should be particularly noted.
   a. **Mutism**—no verbal response despite indications that the client is aware of the examiner's questions
   b. **Circumstantiality**—cumbersome, convoluted, and unnecessary detail in response to the interviewer's questions
   c. **Perseveration**—a pattern of repeating the same words or movements despite apparent efforts to make a new response
   d. **Flight of ideas**—rapid, overly productive responses to questions that seem related only by chance associations between one sentence fragment and another; with flight of ideas you might hear rhyming, clang associations, punning, and evidence of distractibility
   e. **Blocking**—a pattern of sudden silence in the stream of conversation for no obvious reason but often thought to be associated with intrusion of delusional thoughts or hallucinations
3. *Emotional state*—the person's pervasive or dominant mood or affective reaction. Both subjective and objective data are included. Subjective data are obtained through the use of nonleading questions, for instance, "How are you feeling?" If the client replies with general terms, such as *nervous,* the interviewer should ask the client to describe how the nervousness shows itself and its effect, since such words may have different meanings to different individuals.

   The examiner should observe objective signs, such as facial expression, motor behavior, the presence of tears, flushing, sweating, tachycardia, tremors, respiratory irregularities, states of excitement, fear, and depression. The attitude of the client toward the examiner sometimes offers valuable clues. Hostility, suspiciousness, flirtatiousness, a desire for bodily contact, or outspoken criticism should be noted.

   The psychiatric client is apt to have a persistent emotional trend reflective of a particular emotional disorder, such as depression. If this is true, the examiner should probe further to discover the intensity and persistence of this reaction, in keeping with *Diagnostic and Statistical Manual of Mental Disorders,* 4th edition, Text Revision (DSM-IV-TR) criteria.

   It is desirable to record verbatim the replies to questions concerning the client's mood. The relationship between mood and the content of thought is particularly significant. There may be a wide divergence between what clients say or do and their emotional state as expressed by attitudes or facial expressions.

   Note whether intense emotional responses accompany discussion of specific topics. Shallowness or **flat affect** is indicated by an insufficiently intense emotional display in association with ideas or situations that ordinarily would call for a stronger response. *Dissociation* or *disharmony* is often indicated by an inappropriate emotional response, such as smiling or silly behavior, when the attitude should be one of concern, anxiety, or sadness. It is difficult to evaluate emotional reactions in clients who use *simulation* or play-acting. Clients who are trying to cover up a deep depression may feign cheerfulness and good spirits.

   The client's emotional reactions may be constant or may fluctuate during the examination. Try to specify the ease or readiness with which such changes occur in response to pleasant or unpleasant stimuli. The following terms can be used to describe intensity of response:
   - Composed, complacent, frank, friendly, playful, teasing, silly, cheerful, boastful, elated, grandiose, ecstatic
   - Tense, worried, anxious, pessimistic, sad, perplexed, bewildered, gloomy, depressed, frightened
   - Aloof, superior, disdainful, distant, defensive, suspicious
   - Irritable, resentful, hostile, sarcastic, angry, rageful, furious
   - Indifferent, resigned, apathetic, dull, affectless

   Pay attention to the influence of content on affect, and note especially disharmony between affect and content or thought. Also important is constancy or change in the emotional state.
4. *Content of thought: special preoccupations and experiences*—delusions, illusions, or hallucinations, depersonalizations, obsessions or compulsions,

MEDIALINK Case Study: Assessment Strategies

phobias, fantasies, and daydreams. You can elicit these data by asking such questions as "Do you have any difficulties?" or "Have you been troubled or ill in any way?"

Delusions are false beliefs. These beliefs are held even in the face of contradicting or no evidence. If the client has delusions of someone or something in the environment paying extra attention to him or her, some of the following questions might reveal them: "Do people like you?" "Have you ever been watched or spied on or singled out for special attention?" "Do others have it in for you?" Delusions of *alien control* (passivity) are feelings of being controlled or guided by external forces. If you suspect these delusions, ask the client such questions as "Do you ever feel your thoughts or actions are under any outside influences or control?" or "Are you able to influence others, to read their minds, or to put thoughts in their minds?" Chapter 16 discusses these psychotic symptoms in more detail. See the Rx Communication feature for examples and rationales for these interactions.

A client with *nihilistic delusions* more or less completely denies reality and existence. The client states that nothing exists, or that everything is lost. Statements such as "I have no head, no stomach," "I cannot die," or "I will live to eternity" suggest nihilistic delusions.

Delusions of *self-deprecation* are often seen in connection with severe depression. The client describes feeling unworthy, sinful, ugly, or foul smelling. *Delusions of grandeur* are associated with elated states such as great wealth, strength, power, intellect, sexual potency, or identification with a famous person or a god. *Somatic delusions* are focused on having physical problems such as cancer, obstructed bowels, leprosy, or some horrible disease. These are to be distinguished from a preoccupation with normal, visceral, or peripheral sensations.

Hallucinations are false sensory impressions with no external basis in fact. Hallucinations occur with the five senses of hearing, seeing, smelling, tasting, or touching. Try to elicit details of the experience—for example, the source of sounds or voices (from outside or inside the head), the clarity and distinctness of the perception, and the intensity. Be subtle when approaching the client for evidence of hallucinatory phenomena, unless the client is obviously hallucinating. In the case of obvious hallucinations, it is appropriate to ask direct questions.

Obsessions are insistent thoughts recognized as arising from the self. The client usually regards them as absurd and relatively meaningless, yet they persist despite endeavors to get rid of them.

Compulsions are repetitive acts performed through some inner need or drive but supposedly against the client's wishes; yet not performing them results in tension and anxiety.

Fantasies and **daydreams** are preoccupations that are often difficult to elicit from the client. The difficulty may be that the client is not sure what you want in terms of detail or is ashamed to discuss fantasies and daydreams because of their content.

5. *Orientation*—in terms of time, place, person, and self or purpose; helps determine the presence of confusion or clouding of consciousness. You may introduce such questions by asking, "Have you kept track of the time?" If so, "What is today's date?" Clients who say they don't know should be asked to estimate approximately or to guess at an answer. Many clinicians begin the MSE with these questions because disorientation should cause the examiner to question the validity and reliability of data obtained subsequently.
6 *Memory*—attention span and ability to retain or recall past experiences in both the recent and remote past. If memory loss exists, determine whether it is

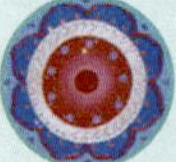

RX COMMUNICATION

ASSESSING YOUR CLIENT

CLIENT: "I don't trust you."

NURSE RESPONSE #1: "You're very uncomfortable, so let's get this done efficiently."	**NURSE RESPONSE #2:** "That tells me how hard this is for you, but let's put it into your words."
RATIONALE: Empathic reflection, redirection, guidance, and limit setting	***RATIONALE:*** Accurate empathy, therapeutic reframe

constant or variable and whether the loss is limited to a certain time period. Be alert to **confabulations**—memories invented to take the place of those the client cannot recall. It is useful to introduce questions relating to memory with some general question such as "Has your memory been good?" Then you can move on to more specific questions such as "Have you had difficulty remembering telephone numbers or appointments?"

a. *Recall of remote past experiences.* Ask for a review of the important events in the client's life. Then compare the response with information obtained from other sources during the history taking.
b. *Recall of recent past experiences.* These are events leading to the present seeking of treatment.
c. *Retention and recall of immediate impressions.* The examiner might ask the client to repeat a name, an address, or a set of objects—for example, rose, teacup, and battleship—immediately and again after 3 to 5 minutes. Another test is to have the client repeat three-digit numbers at a rate of one per second, or repeat a complicated sentence.
d. *General grasp and recall.* You might ask the client to read a story and then repeat the gist of the story to you with as many details as possible. In a classic, concise guide for conducting a psychiatric examination, Small (1980) includes the following story as an example:

CLINICAL EXAMPLE

A cowboy from Arizona went to San Francisco with his dog, which he left at a friend's while he purchased a new suit of clothes. Dressed in the new suit, he went back to the dog, whistled to him, called him by name, and patted him. The dog would have nothing to do with him in his new hat and coat, but gave a mournful howl. Coaxing had no effect, so the cowboy went away and donned his old garments. The dog immediately showed wild joy on seeing his master as he thought he ought to be.

7. *General intellectual level*—a nonstandardized evaluation of intelligence. The examiner explores the person's ability to use factual knowledge in a comprehensive way.
   a. *General grasp of information.* The client may be asked to name the five largest cities of the United States, the last four presidents, or the governor of the state.
   b. *Ability to calculate.* Tests of simple multiplication and addition are useful for this purpose. Another test consists of subtracting from one hundred by sevens until the person can go no further (serial sevens test).
   c. *Reasoning and judgment.* A common test of reasoning is to ask what the client might do with a gift of $10,000. Examiners must be particularly careful to correct for their own biases and values in assessing each client's answer.
8. *Abstract thinking*—making distinctions between such abstractions as poverty and misery or idleness and laziness. It is common to ask the client to interpret simple fables or proverbs such as "Don't cry over spilled milk."
9. *Insight evaluation*—whether clients recognize the significance of the present situation, whether they feel the need for treatment, and how they explain the symptoms. Often, it is helpful to ask clients for suggestions for their own treatment.
10. *Summary*—the important psychopathologic findings and a tentative diagnosis. Any pertinent facts from the medical history and/or physical examination should be added to the summary.

Mini-Mental State Exam

If there is not enough time to complete a full MSE, it is possible to fairly accurately assess and evaluate a client's functioning in a streamlined manner. The **Mini-Mental State Exam (MMSE)** (Folstein, Folstein, & McHugh, 1975) provides a framework for such an assessment. The main focus of the exam is cognitive functioning, although the client's mood can be ascertained in the process.

For the test to be efficient and valid, the questions must be asked in the order they are listed. Box 11-1 shows four sections of the MMSE and the general area of information the questions address. A total of 11 questions cover the scope of a client's thinking and reactions. Scores are assigned to each question, and the total score indicates the likelihood and level

Box 11-1 MMSE Sample Items

- Orientation to Time "What is the date?"
- Registration "Listen carefully, I am going to say three words. You say them back after I stop. Ready? Here they are: APPLE [pause], PENNY [pause], TABLE [pause]. Now repeat those words back to me." [Repeat up to 5 times, but score only the first trial.]
- Naming "What is this?" [Point to a pencil or pen.]
- Reading "Please read this and do what it says." [Show examinee the words on the stimulus form.

Source: Reproduced by special permission of the Publisher, Psychological Assessment Resources, Inc., 16204 North Florida Avenue, Lutz, Florida 33549, from the Mini-Mental State Examination, by Marshal Folstein and Susan Folstein, Copyright 1975, 1998, 2001 by Mini Mental LLC, Inc. Published 2001 by Psychological Assessment Resources, Inc. Further reproduction is prohibited without permission of PAR, Inc. The MMSE can be purchased from PAR, Inc. by calling (800) 331–8378 or (813) 968–3003.

of cognitive decline. The maximum score is 30 points, and the score is represented as a fraction with the actual points scored as the numerator and 30 points as the denominator (e.g., 28/30, 20/30, etc.).

It is important to note that there are limitations to using the MMSE with people who have certain disabilities with sight or motor movement related to writing. If a client is not able to perform one of the activities, it may be necessary to conduct a full MSE or to document the results of the relevant aspects of the MMSE without a score.

Nurses' Observation Scale for Inpatient Evaluations

An assessment tool designed specifically for use by inpatient nurses is the **Nurses' Observation Scale for Inpatient Evaluations (NOSIE)**. Developed and determined to be a valid and reliable tool in 1966 (Honigfeld, Gillis, & Klett, 1966), it has been useful in quickly assessing client functioning in six areas—three on positive features, three on negative features. The NOSIE comes in a long and short version. The assessment takes place within a specific time period, typically within three days of admission.

Scoring the NOSIE, after interrater reliability has been established, is convenient and can give valuable information regarding likelihood of particular behaviors and interactions while clients are in inpatient settings. Interrater reliability is the process of ensuring that all raters use similar scoring measures and techniques. These measures and techniques are usually established when all raters score the same client at the same time, or score a videotape of the same client and compare scores for consistency. If the NOSIE is incorporated into an inpatient setting as a regular feature of assessing client assets, routine interrater reliability checks need to take place. This assessment tool has remained useful across the decades. It reinforces the value of nursing determinations made when assessing behavior.

PHYSIOLOGIC ASSESSMENT

As the summary of the MSE suggests, nurses must carefully consider the possibility that a client's symptoms may have a physiologic, a biologic, or, in particular, a neurologic basis. In some reported instances, clients with brain tumors or bromide intoxication have been hospitalized on psychiatric units and treated exclusively for their apparent psychiatric symptoms. Such a critical oversight obviously delays and seriously hampers appropriate treatment of the correct biologic or neurologic problem. The value of careful assessment regarding general health issues and screening for biologic disorders cannot be overemphasized. In many community settings, psychiatric–mental health nurses are the only mental health care providers prepared to undertake a biologic and neurologic assessment and interpret the results.

The objectives of a biologic and neurologic assessment are:

1. Detection of underlying and perhaps unsuspected organic disease that may be responsible for psychiatric symptoms
2. Understanding of disease as a factor in the overall psychiatric disability
3. Appreciation of somatic symptoms that reflect primarily psychological rather than physiologic problems

Biologic History Taking

Taking the client's history is an important procedure among several that can contribute to a fuller understanding of the biologic aspects of psychiatric symptoms. Inquire into three primary areas of a client's biologic history:

1. Facts about known physical diseases and dysfunction
2. Information about specific physical complaints
3. General health history

Information about previous illnesses may provide essential clues. Clients with comorbidities of substance abuse and mental disorder are particularly challenging. For example, suppose a client's presenting symptoms include paranoid delusions and the client has a history of similar episodes. During each previous episode, the client responded to diverse forms of treatment and demonstrated no residual symptoms. This history suggests a strong possibility of amphetamine- or other drug-related psychosis, and a drug screen laboratory test may be indicated. An occupational history may provide information about exposure to inorganic mercury, leading to symptoms of psychosis, or exposure to lead, resulting in mental disorder.

The second area of emphasis in biologic history taking is eliciting information from the client about specific physical complaints. Again, it is crucial to consider symptoms in terms of both psychiatric conditions and physical diseases. Symptoms that are atypical of psychiatric disorders are particularly revealing clues. For example, suppose a client with hallucinations and delusions also complains of a severe headache at the onset of the symptoms. All symptoms together suggest possible brain disease and call for careful and repeated neurologic assessment and use of brain imaging techniques.

History taking should also include information about medications the client is currently taking. Digitalis intoxication may result in impairment. Reserpine may produce symptoms generally considered psychiatric in nature.

The third area is the general health history. As mentioned above, psychiatric nurses need to assess for a variety of general health problems and must therefore have medical–surgical nursing skills. During your assessment of any client, assess for medical problems as well as the psychiatric symptomatology. Keep in mind that some medical problems are masked by psychiatric symptoms and that psychiatric symptomatology can be the result of a medical disorder.

Observation

Observation also yields important data bearing on the possible presence of organic disorders.

- An unsteady gait may suggest diffuse brain disease or alcohol or drug intoxication.

- Asymmetry—dragging a leg or not swinging one arm—might be a sign of a focal brain lesion.
- Although inattention to proper hygiene and dress, particularly mismatched socks or shoes, is common in people with emotional disorders, it is also a hallmark of dementias.
- Frequent, quick, purposeless movements are characteristic of anxiety, but they are equally characteristic of chorea and hyperthyroidism.
- Tremors accompanied by anxiety may point to Parkinson's disease.
- Recent weight loss, although often encountered in depression and schizophrenia, may be due to gastrointestinal disease, carcinoma, Addison's disease, and many other physical disorders.

Observe skin color, pupillary changes, alertness and responsiveness, and quality of speech and word production, keeping in mind the possibility of delirium, dementia, substance intoxication, or other medical conditions.

NEUROLOGIC ASSESSMENT

A careful neurologic assessment is mandatory for each client suspected of having brain dysfunction. Its goal is to discover signs pointing to circumscribed, focal cerebral dysfunction or diffuse, bilateral cerebral disease.

Brain Imaging Techniques

As described in Chapter 6, a range of brain imaging techniques are now available for viewing the living brain to detect seizure activity; evaluate sleep disorders; detect disorders such as multiple sclerosis; detect tumors, trauma, and strokes; examine the blood flowing to the brain; and identify cerebral atrophy, cerebral hemorrhage, cerebral infarct, hematomas, and abscesses. All of these conditions may present as psychiatric or behavioral symptoms. The most frequently used brain imaging techniques are described in Box 6-1, "Tools of Psychobiology," in Chapter 6 (page 84). The positron-emission tomography (PET) scan brain image (see Figure 11-1) shows two scans of the same brain tumor (glioma) at different areas (levels) of the brain.

Authorities in mental health practice consistently remind clinicians of the need for thorough biologic and neurologic assessment of clients seen in psychiatric settings. The psychiatric literature abounds with accounts of clients whose symptoms were initially considered exclusively psychiatric but ultimately proved medical, especially neurologic. Assessment errors occurred not because the symptoms did not suggest medical disease but because such symptoms were given too little weight or were misinterpreted. Changes in the American Psychiatric Association's (APA's) DSM-IV-TR (2000) require that both medical condition and substance abuse be ruled out as conditions resulting in psychiatric symptoms.

PSYCHOLOGICAL TESTING

Clinical psychologists administer and interpret a wide variety of psychological tests. There are three basic types: those concerned with intelligence, those concerned with personality, and those concerned with cognitive function. Both intelligence and personality tests are typically included in a comprehensive psychological evaluation. The three types are summarized below and in Table 11-1.

Intelligence Tests

Intelligence tests may be useful particularly in evaluating the presence and degree of mental retardation and in assessing cognitive function. Commonly used intelligence tests are the Wechsler Adult Intelligence Scale–III, Stanford–Binet Test–IV, Wechsler Intelligence Scale for Children–III,

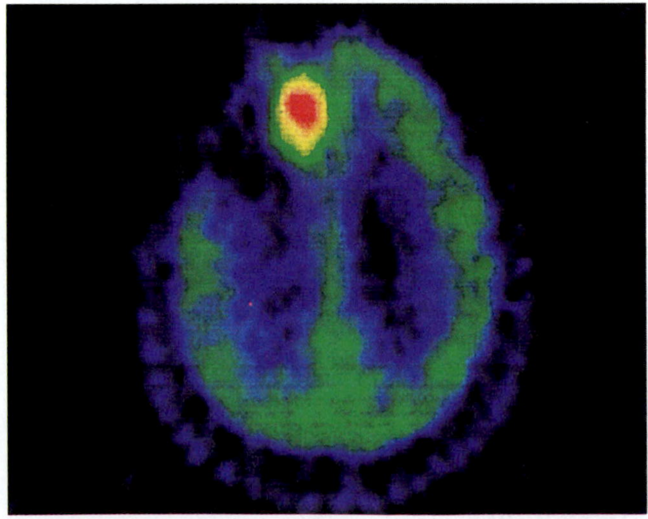
A

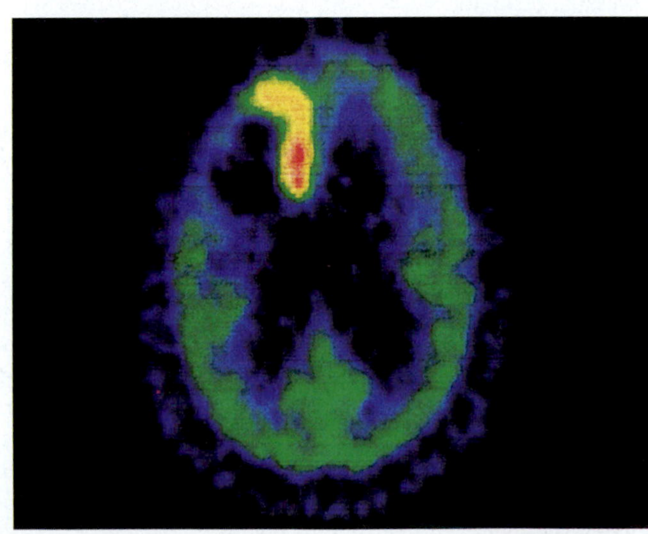
B

Figure 11-1 This frontal lobe glioblastoma multiforme, a primary tumor, is metabolically very hot. (A) Note the large red area of the tumor. (B) The same tumor at a different level in the brain.

Source: Courtesy of Dr. Giovanni DiChiro and Dr. Ramesh Raman of the Neuroimaging Branch, National Institute of Neurological Disorders and Stroke, National Institutes of Health.

TABLE 11-1 ■ Common Psychological Tests in Clinical Use

Name of Test	Description	Method
Objective Personality Tests		
Minnesota Multiphasic Personality Inventory–2 (MMPI–2)	A self-administered objective (as opposed to projective) personality test designed to yield a broad examination of personality functioning that is amenable to statistical interpretation, such as profiles of symptoms or psychopathology.	The client responds to 567 statements by indicating either "true" or "false." The client's personality profile is formulated using 10 major clinical scales and dozens of subscales.
State–Trait Anxiety Inventory	Measures state and trait anxiety. State anxiety is conceptualized as a transitory emotional state or condition; trait anxiety refers to relatively stable individual differences in vulnerability to anxiety.	This is a paper-and-pencil, self-report instrument.
Millon Clinical Multiaxial Inventory–II (MCMI–II)	Profiles the presence and intensity of personality traits consistent with the DSM-IV-TR Axis II personality types.	Like the MMPI–2, this test consists of true–false questions.
Beck Depression Inventory	Quick, reliable, and valid measure of the extent to which depression may be present.	The client is asked to rate the presence and intensity of various symptoms of depression.
Projective Personality Tests		
Rorschach Test	A projective test that is thought to reveal aspects of inner psychodynamic functioning. It reveals personality features and symptoms and is commonly used as a diagnostic tool.	The client responds to 10 cards, one at a time, consisting of black-and-white or colored standardized inkblots. Responses include the impressions, thoughts, and associations that come to mind while the client looks at the inkblot.
Thematic Apperception Test (TAT)	A projective test offering a standardized set of stimuli for exploring the client's emotional life. Themes and interpersonal problems emerge in the client's responses.	The client is shown a series of ambiguous pictures of people in various significant situations and is asked to describe what is happening in each picture and tell a story about it. Adaptations have been designed for use with children. In these, the central figure is a child or the pictures are cartoons of animals.
Sentence Completion Test	A projective test designed to elicit conscious associations to specific areas of functioning, thus illustrating the fears, preoccupations, ambitions, and idiosyncrasies of the client.	The client is asked to spontaneously complete sentences such as "I feel guilty about . . . ," "Sex is . . . ," "My mother . . . ," "Sometimes I wish . . ." Both mood and content are noted.
Cognitive Function Tests		
Stanford-Binet Intelligence Test	A general intelligence test based on an age-level concept from 2 years to about 15 years. It is particularly useful for testing children and evaluating mental retardation.	The client is asked to do a graded series of tasks designed to correlate with the abilities of children of a particular age group. Each set is more difficult than the one before it.
Wechsler Adult Intelligence Scale–III (WAIS–III)	A general intelligence test for people 16 and older. It is the most widely used and best standardized intelligence test.	The client completes 11 subtests that yield both verbal and performance scores as well as full-scale IQs. Subtest raw scores may also be compared to reveal variability in functioning. The subtests are: information, comprehension, arithmetic, similarities, memory for digits, vocabulary, digit symbol, picture completion, block design, picture arrangement, and object assembly.
Wechsler Intelligence Scale for Children–III (WISC–III)	A general intelligence test for children.	Similar to the WAIS-III for adults, this test asks the client to complete subtests that yield separate verbal, performance, and full-scale IQ scores.
Raven's Progressive Matrices Test	Designed to provide data on intellectual ability in a relatively culturally unbiased manner.	The client is asked to solve two-dimensional visual–spatial problems of increasing difficulty.

Raven's Progressive Matrices Test, and Wide Range Achievement Test–Revised (WRAT–R).

Personality Tests

There are objective and projective personality tests. **Objective personality tests** provide data on various aspects of the client's personality, which are scored or analyzed using empirically derived criteria. An example is the Minnesota Multiphasic Personality Inventory–2 (MMPI–2). **Projective personality tests** involve presenting the client with a somewhat ambiguous stimulus, often a visual one, to which the client responds with an idiosyncratic perception. For example, the client states what the stimulus looks like or makes up a story about it. It is thought that in this process the client projects something of herself or himself into the response. An example is the Rorschach Test.

Common Objective Personality Tests

Treatment can be consistently enhanced once the objective personality test data are incorporated. Common objective personality tests are discussed below.

Minnesota Multiphasic Personality Inventory–2 The **Minnesota Multiphasic Personality Inventory–2 (MMPI-2)** is a psychological test that consists of 567 items to which the test taker responds with "true" or "false." It is an actuarial test; the test taker's patterns of response to groups of items are compared to the response patterns generated by standardization samples of psychiatric clients with different diagnoses. A rigorous effort was made to incorporate cross-cultural considerations in the test's construction, including the use of ethnically and culturally diverse standardization samples. The test includes 10 major clinical scales that measure aspects of different psychopathologies (see TABLE 11-2 ■).

The test taker's item responses are scored according to complex formulas that permit the construction of a profile of scores on the 10 major clinical scales and on numerous subscales. This profile can then be interpreted, with the help of several different profile code books, and individual features of the profile can be closely examined to allow a comprehensive interpretation. This interpretation can include the following:

- A behavioral description of courses of action in which the test taker may engage
- Information about internal motivating factors, feelings, and symptoms
- Information concerning relationships with friends and with significant others
- Diagnostic formulation
- Treatment recommendations as needed

A large number of empirical studies support the use of the MMPI–2 in clinical settings. It may, in fact, be the most researched psychological test in existence today. Some other uses suggested for the MMPI–2 include personnel screening, employment screening, and prediction of response to medical and surgical treatment, as well as screening in colleges and universities, industry and business, and government agencies; however, its use in these contexts is not as well researched.

TABLE 11-2 ■ The 10 Major Clinical Scales Measured by the MMPI–2

The MMPI–2 measures aspects of different psychopathologies:

1. Hypochondriasis
2. Depression
3. Hysteria
4. Antisocial personality features
5. Comfort with sexual orientation
6. Paranoia
7. Anxiety
8. Schizophrenia
9. Mania
10. Social introversion

State–Trait Anxiety Inventory The **State–Trait Anxiety Inventory** is a paper-and-pencil self-report instrument that measures state and trait anxiety. *State anxiety* is conceptualized as a transitory emotional state or condition characterized by subjective and consciously perceived feelings of tension and apprehension, and heightened autonomic nervous system activity. *Trait anxiety* refers to relatively stable individual differences in vulnerability to anxiety (Spielberger, 1976).

Millon Clinical Multiaxial Inventory–II Like the MMPI–2, the **Millon Clinical Multiaxial Inventory–II (MCMI–II)** test consists of true–false questions. A profile based on the client's responses is developed, indicating the presence and intensity of personality traits consistent with the DSM-IV-TR Axis II personality types. This test can provide valuable assistance in clarifying underlying stable personality features that can strongly influence the way clients interact with, and present symptoms to, you and other health care providers.

Beck Depression Inventory The **Beck Depression Inventory** consists of questions that ask the client to rate the presence and intensity of various symptoms of depression. The score is then compared to empirically derived cutoff scores. This test is a quick but reliable and valid screening measure of the extent to which depression may be present.

Common Projective Personality Tests

Note how the following selected projective personality tests differ from the objective personality tests discussed earlier.

The Rorschach Test The **Rorschach Test** consists of 10 standardized inkblots in black and white (or color) on separate cards. The psychologist displays the cards one by one. Clients are asked to state what the inkblots look like to them, and why. Because each card contains only inkblots, clients' responses are thought to be *projections* of important aspects of their inner psychodynamic functioning. The examiner scores the responses according to:

- *Location.* The part of the blot area the client associates with the response is referred to as a *percept.*
- *Content.* What did the client see?
- *Determinant.* What characteristic of the blot prompted the response?
- *Form level.* How closely did the response correspond to the contour of the blot area used?
- *Originality.* How common a response is it?

Interpretation is based on a complicated system of scoring responses and analyzing content. In recent years, there have been efforts to develop empirically based systems of content analysis to enable greater standardization of Rorschach scoring and interpretation.

Thematic Apperception Test The **Thematic Apperception Test (TAT)** also consists of a series of cards shown by the psychologist to the client one by one. However, TAT cards are pictures of people in various situations. Clients are asked to describe what seems to be happening in the picture, what the people are feeling and thinking, and how the situation will be resolved. Because the pictures are ambiguous, the responses are thought to reveal aspects of the clients' own emotional lives. The TAT can reveal very important information about the client's emotional and interpersonal tendencies. The psychologist who scores and interprets the TAT looks for themes, threads, and patterns in the responses. Some adaptations of the TAT for use with children are available.

Sentence Completion Test The **Sentence Completion Test** asks clients to complete an extensive series of incomplete sentences with the first thoughts that come to mind. The sentences are designed to elicit responses concerning fantasies, fears, daydreams, and aspirations, among other things.

Cognitive Function Tests

Cognitive function tests generally measure how well, or how poorly, a person is able to think and process information. The information processed contributes to intellectual functioning and is counted as a gauge of intelligence.

Common Cognitive Function Tests

Common cognitive function tests are discussed below.

Wechsler Adult Intelligence Scale–III The **Wechsler Adult Intelligence Scale–III (WAIS–III)** consists of 14 subtests. Generally only the 11 subtests that are necessary for the derivation of intelligence quotient (IQ) scores are administered. These subtests are picture completion, vocabulary, digit symbol, similarities, block design, arithmetic, matrix reasoning, digit span, information, picture arrangement, and comprehension. In addition to providing information on the verbal and nonverbal (performance) abilities of the client, comparisons between individual subtest scores can be evaluated to yield data on the client's relative specific cognitive strengths and weaknesses.

Raven's Progressive Matrices Test The **Raven's Progressive Matrices Test** is designed to provide data on intellectual ability in a relatively culturally unbiased manner. Many other intelligence tests depend on knowledge and skills that are somewhat culturally bound. The Raven's Progressive Matrices Test asks the client to solve two-dimensional visual–spatial problems of increasing difficulty, problems that are relatively culturally unbiased. Scores on this test can be translated into empirically derived categories of intellectual ability.

Benton Visual Retention Test The **Benton Visual Retention Test** is an example of a neuropsychological assessment instrument that can yield valuable data on aspects of a person's cognitive functioning. It is sometimes used as a quick screening device to see if the test taker may be manifesting signs of cognitive dysfunction. It is generally used to provide details on the nature of cognitive dysfunction being manifested by someone who has already been determined to have a cognitive problem or difficulty. The test taker is asked to reproduce various geometric designs after examining the designs for a few seconds. The type and frequency of different kinds of errors, as well as the number of designs reproduced correctly, are compared with empirically based frequency tables to determine the extent to which cognitive dysfunction may be possible, probable, or strongly indicated. The test performance is strongly influenced by any difficulties in the test taker's visual processing, organization, memory, and visual–motor skills.

PSYCHIATRIC DIAGNOSTIC PRACTICE ACCORDING TO THE DSM-IV-TR

The American Psychiatric Association (APA) published the first edition of the *Diagnostic and Statistical Manual* in 1952. The second edition, DSM-II, published in 1968, attempted compatibility with the *International Classification of Diseases, Injuries, and Causes of Death* (ICD-9) published by the World Health Organization. The DSM-II was criticized for its low reliability and tendency to reflect an individual psychiatrist's philosophy. The APA published a third edition entitled the *Diagnostic and Statistical Manual of Mental Disorders III* in 1980 and a revised edition in 1987. Important features distinguished the DSM-III-R from its predecessors. It used specified diagnostic criteria to improve the reliability of diagnostic judgments and offered a multiaxial or multidimensional approach to clinical assessment of psychiatric clients in which five different classes of data are collected and assessed. The DSM-IV was published in 1994 and further clarified and codified psychiatric diagnostics.

The DSM-IV-TR (the "TR" stands for Text Revision), published in 2000, represents the current state of knowledge about diagnosing mental disorders. A code revision (CR) being planned for the DSM-IV has not yet been published. The continual evolution of this specialty area is represented in the changes made from the original DSM-IV. DSM-IV-TR

MEDIALINK Critical Thinking Exercise: Using the DSM-IV-TR

is composed of a list of all the official numeric codes and terms for all recognized mental disorders, along with a comprehensive description of each and specified diagnostic criteria that must be present in order to make each diagnosis. Highlights of the changes made in the DSM-IV-TR are listed and discussed in the manual's Appendix D. Updated information regarding numerous clinical issues such as prevalence and comorbidity, among others, have been incorporated in this latest edition. (For a complete list of codes and diagnoses according to the DSM-IV-TR, see this text's Appendix A.)

Basic Principles of the Multiaxial System

In the DSM-IV-TR multiaxial system, every person is evaluated on five axes, each dealing with a different class of information about the client. DSM-IV-TR's multiaxial assessment is congruent with holistic views of people, recognizes the role of environmental stress in influencing behavior, and requires that the clinician collect data about client adaptive strengths as well as about symptoms or problems. One of the most important features of the DSM-IV-TR is increased interclinician reliability resulting from the use of specified observable criteria that have been field tested for interrater reliability. Its multiaxial approach is of significance to psychiatric–mental health nursing because it expresses the multidimensionality of human responses to environment, one of the hallmarks of the nursing process.

The following example illustrates the principle behind a multiaxial system.

CLINICAL EXAMPLE

A 54-year-old woman came to an outpatient mental health clinic for evaluation and treatment of severe fear and avoidance of flying that amounted to a phobia. However, she also had a long-term personality disturbance and had noticeable eczema.

Suppose three different clinicians were asked to evaluate this woman. A biologically oriented clinician would certainly diagnose the eczema but might fail to notice the personality disturbance and make little of the phobia. A psychodynamically oriented clinician would be sure to diagnose the personality disorder but might overlook the eczema and the phobia, considering them to be merely manifestations of the underlying personality disturbance. Finally, a clinician who was behaviorally oriented would notice the phobia but might not diagnose the personality disturbance and the eczema. It is clear, then, that because of their differing theoretic orientations, these clinicians have a rather high likelihood of diagnostic disagreement.

Now suppose this same woman were presented to the same three colleagues, but this time the clinicians were required to evaluate her in each of three different areas of functioning: behavioral or psychological, personality, and physical functioning. In this case, all three clinicians would be much more likely to diagnose all three conditions and thus, their evaluations are much more likely to be congruent.

Box 11-2 DSM-IV-TR Axes

Axis I:	Adult and Child Clinical Disorders Conditions not attributable to a mental disorder that are a focus of clinical attention Additional codes
Axis II:	Personality Disorders Mental Retardation No diagnosis on Axis II (V codes)
Axis III:	General Medical Conditions
Axis IV:	Psychosocial and Environmental Problems
Axis V:	Global Assessment of Functioning (GAF)

Source: Reprinted with permission from the *Diagnostic and Statistical Manual of Mental Disorders,* Fourth Edition, Text Revision. (Copyright 2000). American Psychiatric Association.

The DSM-IV-TR multiaxial system includes the five axes listed in Box 11-2. Axes I and II include all the mental disorders in the DSM-IV-TR and therefore might be said to represent the intrapersonal or *psychological* area of functioning. Axis III is for recording general medical conditions related to understanding the cause of psychiatric symptoms and treating the individual and thus represents the area of *physical* functioning. Axes IV and V, for identifying psychosocial and environmental problems and the Global Assessment of Functioning (GAF) scale, include an assessment of social functioning. In this sense, the multiaxial system provides a comprehensive biopsychosocial approach to assessment.

Description of the Axes

The following are the components of the multiaxial system.

Axis I: Clinical Disorders Axis I includes all of the Adult and Child Clinical Disorders. Axis I also contains other conditions that may be a focus of clinical attention, but it is not universally agreed that these conditions actually constitute clinical syndromes. Nevertheless, the symptoms elucidated in these conditions are observed often enough to warrant their inclusion in the diagnostic array available to the clinician. These include psychological factors that would affect a physical condition, medication-induced movement disorders, relational problems, and others. More specific examples include such conditions as marital problems, occupational problems, and parent–child problems, in which the problem being evaluated or for which clinical care is sought is not due to a mental disorder.

A mental disorder is differentiated from other problems as a clinically significant behavioral or psychological syndrome or pattern that occurs in an individual. A mental disorder is associated with either a painful symptom (distress) or impairment in functioning (disability), or with an increased risk of suffering, death, pain, disability, or loss of freedom. Further, the distress or disability does not primarily reflect a sanctioned response to an event, deviant behavior, or conflict between an individual and society.

CLINICAL EXAMPLE

A man with bipolar disorder that has been in remission for many years develops marital difficulties for reasons unrelated to his psychiatric history or condition. He and his wife have been arguing about her intent to resume a career.

Both "marital problem" and "bipolar disorder in remission" could be recorded on Axis I. If, however, the bipolar disorder is not in complete remission, and marital conflict develops as a result of the client's changeable moods and other symptoms associated with the mental disorder, the marital problem would not be recorded in addition to the bipolar disorder, since the marital problem in this case is due to the client's mental disorder.

Axis II: Personality Disorders Axis II contains the personality disorders, usually diagnosed in adults, and developmental disorders including mental retardation, diagnosed in children and adolescents. Axis II is also used to report maladaptive personality traits. All the remaining mental disorders of adults and children and associated conditions are recorded on Axis I.

The classes of disorders on Axis II were given their own axis because their usually mild and chronic symptomatology is often overshadowed by a more florid Axis I condition. DSM-IV-TR clarifies the conceptual distinction between Axis I and Axis II by noting that Axis II conditions have an early onset and a stable, not episodic, course. Axis II also has options for describing the lack of a diagnosis or condition on the axis. Examples of evaluations using only Axes I and II are presented in Box 11-3.

Axis III: General Medical Conditions Clinicians use Axis III to record physical disorders and medical conditions that must be taken into account in planning treatment, or that are relevant to understanding the etiology or worsening of the mental disorder. A clinician might also want to record other significant physical findings, such as "soft" neurologic signs or even a single symptom (such as vomiting).

If there is a lack of information on Axis III, that fact should be stated: "No information," or "Diagnosis deferred—not evaluated," or "Referred to Dr. Smith for evaluation." In any event, *something* should be noted on this axis; omitting it for lack of information undermines the purpose of a holistic, multiaxial system. Of course, recent advances in psychobiologic knowledge make Axis III findings particularly important for psychiatric–mental health nursing. Box 11-4 provides an example of multiaxial evaluation on Axes I, II, and III.

Axis IV: Psychosocial and Environmental Problems Axis IV is used to identify psychosocial problems that may affect the diagnosis and treatment of mental disorders. General categories of psychosocial problems are listed in Box 11-5.

In addition to identifying the type of problem(s), evaluators should also note in their own words the specific problems they consider pertinent. Thus, a multiaxial evaluation, up through Axis IV, might look like the example in Box 11-6.

Box 11-3 Examples of DSM-IV-TR Multiaxial Evaluation on Axes I and II

Example 1

Axis I:	303.90	Alcohol dependence, in remission in a controlled environment
Axis II:	301.7	Antisocial personality disorder

Example 2

Axis I:	V71.09	No diagnosis
Axis II:	301.22	Schizotypal personality disorder

Box 11-4 Example of DSM-IV-TR Multiaxial Evaluation on Axes I, II, and III

Axis I:	312.8	Conduct disorder, moderate childhood-onset type
Axis II:	V71.09	No diagnosis
Axis III:		Diabetes

In this example, the client, a child in this case, will probably not be very compliant with the diabetes treatment regimen because of psychologic problems (conduct disorder, noted on Axis I).

Box 11-5 Axis IV: Psychosocial and Environmental Problems

- Problems with primary support group
- Problems related to the social environment
- Educational problems
- Occupational problems
- Housing problems
- Economic problems
- Problems with access to health care services
- Problems related to interaction with the legal system/crime
- Other psychosocial and environmental problems

Source: Reprinted with permission from the *Diagnostic and Statistical Manual of Mental Disorders*, Fourth Edition, Text Revision. (Copyright 2000). American Psychiatric Association.

Box 11-6 Example of a DSM-IV-TR Multiaxial Evaluation on Axes I, II, III, and IV

Axis I:	300.01	Panic disorder without agoraphobia
Axis II:	301.83	Borderline personality disorder
Axis III:		No diagnosis
Axis IV:		Unemployment

MEDIALINK Care Plan: Integrating the GAF to Plan Care

Box 11-7 Global Assessment of Functioning (GAF) Scale

Consider psychological, social, and occupational functioning on a hypothetical continuum of mental health–illness. Do not include impairment in functioning due to physical (or environmental) limitations.

Code	(Note: Use intermediate codes when appropriate, e.g., 45, 68, 72.)
100 ↓ 91	Superior functioning in a wide range of activities, life's problems never seem to get out of hand, is sought out by others because of his or her many positive qualities. No symptoms.
90 ↓ 81	Absent or minimal symptoms (e.g., mild anxiety before an exam), good functioning in all areas, interested and involved in a wide range of activities, socially effective, generally satisfied with life, no more than everyday problems or concerns (e.g., an occasional argument with family members).
80 ↓ 71	If symptoms are present, they are transient and expectable reactions to psychosocial stressors (e.g., difficulty concentrating after family argument); no more than slight impairment in social, occupational, or school functioning (e.g., temporarily falling behind in schoolwork).
70 ↓ 61	Some mild symptoms (e.g., depressed mood and mild insomnia) OR some difficulty in social, occupational, or school functioning (e.g., occasional truancy, or theft within the household), but generally functioning pretty well, has some meaningful interpersonal relationships.
60 ↓ 51	Moderate symptoms (e.g., flat affect and circumstantial speech, occasional panic attacks) OR moderate difficulty in social, occupational, or school functioning (e.g., few friends, conflicts with peers or coworkers).
50 ↓ 41	Serious symptoms (e.g., suicidal ideation, severe obsessional rituals, frequent shoplifting) OR any serious impairment in social, occupational, or school functioning (e.g., no friends, unable to keep a job).
40 ↓ 31	Some impairment in reality testing or communication (e.g., speech is at times illogical, obscure, or irrelevant) OR major impairment in several areas, such as work or school, family relations, judgment, thinking, or mood (e.g., depressed man avoids friends, neglects family, and is unable to work; child frequently beats up younger children, is defiant at home, and is failing at school).
30 ↓ 21	Behavior is considerably influenced by delusions or hallucinations OR serious impairment in communication or judgment (e.g., sometimes incoherent, acts grossly inappropriately, suicidal preoccupation) OR inability to function in almost all areas (e.g., stays in bed all day; no job, home, or friends).
20 ↓ 11	Some danger of hurting self or others (e.g., suicide attempts without clear expectation of death; frequently violent; manic excitement) OR occasionally fails to maintain minimal personal hygiene (e.g., smears feces) OR gross impairment in communication (e.g., largely incoherent or mute).
10 ↓ 1	Persistent danger of severely hurting self or others (e.g., recurrent violence) OR persistent inability to maintain minimal personal hygiene OR serious suicidal act with clear expectation of death.
0	Inadequate information

The rating of overall psychological functioning on a scale of 0–100 was operationalized by Luborsky in the Health-Sickness Rating Scale (Luborsky, L.: Clinicians' judgments of mental health. Archives of General Psychiatry *7:407–417, 1962). Spitzer and colleagues developed a revision of the Health-Sickness Rating Scale called the Global Assessment Scale (GAS) (Endicott, J., Spitzer, R. L., Fleiss, I. L., and Cohen, J.: The Global Assessment Scale: A procedure for measuring overall severity of psychiatric disturbance.* Archives of General Psychiatry 33*:766–771, 1976). A modified version of the GAS was included in* DSM-III-R *as the Global Assessment of Functioning (GAF) Scale.*

Source: Reprinted with permission from the *Diagnostic and Statistical Manual of Mental Disorders,* Fourth Edition, Text Revision. (Copyright 2000). American Psychiatric Association.

Axis V: Global Assessment of Functioning Axis V, the **Global Assessment of Functioning (GAF)**, reports on the client's overall level of functioning. This information is useful in planning treatment and measuring its impact, and in predicting outcomes. The reporting of overall functioning on Axis V can be performed using the Global Assessment of Functioning (GAF) Scale as shown in Box 11-7. The GAF Scale gives the clinician an opportunity to examine the overall impact of the client's circumstances on psychological, social, and occupational performance. The ratings on this scale fall within decile ranges and track both symptom severity and functional level. When symptoms and functioning are at different levels, the worse of the two is shown through the score. For example, if a client has moderate symptoms and severe problems functioning, the rating would demarcate the severe problems in functioning. If a client's functioning is basically unimpaired but the symptoms experienced are significant, the symptom level would be represented in the GAF rating. Generally, ratings on the GAF Scale reflect the client's current level of functioning, meaning the lowest level of functioning within the previous 7 days.

One of the most accurate indicators of clinical outcome is the individual's sustained level of premorbid functioning. For this reason, the GAF Scale can be used to rate the highest level of psychological, social, and occupational functioning that an individual was able to sustain for at least a few months during the previous year as well as at the time of evaluation.

PSYCHIATRIC–MENTAL HEALTH NURSING AND THE DSM SYSTEM

From the perspective of psychiatric–mental health nursing, the DSM-IV-TR represents some progress toward values that psychiatric–mental health nurses have espoused for decades. Our knowledge of the DSM allows us to communicate with colleagues from different disciplines using a common language and perform as intermediaries or translators for clients and their families on mental health issues. It also:

- Represents progress toward a more holistic view of mind–body relations
- Bases revisions on a series of formative evaluations
- Represents a collaborative achievement
- Provides for diagnostic uncertainty
- Incorporates biologic, psychologic, and social variables
- Achieves positive results in extensive field testing for validity and reliability
- Considers adaptive strength as well as problems
- Reflects a descriptive, phenomenologic perspective rather than any psychiatric theory

PSYCHOSOCIAL ASSESSMENT

Psychosocial assessment is a dynamic process. It begins during the initial contact with the client and continues throughout the nurse–client experience. Individual psychosocial assessments are an option, as are family or group psychosocial assessments. In every case, they begin with the identifying characteristics, such as name, gender, age, marital status, and ethnic and cultural origins. Problem identification and definition are also necessary phases in the assessment process. The method for assessing a client using an active problem-solving approach, within a person-centered framework, is a model that gathers the appropriate information while enhancing a therapeutic relationship (Knight, 2007).

Individual Assessment

During the individual assessment, consider the following factors:

1. *Physical and intellectual*
   a. Presence of physical illness and/or disability
   b. Appearance and energy level
   c. Current and potential levels of intellectual functioning
   d. How the client sees his or her personal world and translates events around self; client's perceptual abilities
   e. Cause-and-effect reasoning; ability to focus
2. *Socioeconomic factors*
   a. Economic factors—level of income and adequacy of subsistence, and their effect on lifestyle, sense of adequacy, and self-worth
   b. Employment and attitudes about it
   c. Racial, cultural, and ethnic identification; sense of identity and belonging
   d. Religious identification can be linked to significant value systems, norms, and spiritual practices. Spirituality and its meaning for the client are a part of the Psychosocial Assessment. Attachment to a system of meaning, whatever that system may be, can be an asset. (See the Caring for the Spirit feature on page 230 for sample questions that can be used during a spiritual health assessment.)
3. *Personal values and goals*
   a. Presence or absence of congruence between values and their expression in action; meaning of values to individual
   b. Congruence between the individual's values and goals and the immediate systems with which the client interacts
   c. Congruence between the individual's values and the assessor's values; how agreement or divergence regarding values impacts intervention
4. *Adaptive functioning and response to present involvement*
   a. Manner in which the individual presents self to others—grooming, appearance, posture
   b. Emotional tone and change or constancy of levels
   c. Style of communication—verbal and nonverbal; ability to express appropriate emotion, follow train of thought; factors of dissonance, confusion, uncertainty
   d. Symptoms or symptomatic behavior
   e. Quality of relationships the individual seeks to establish—direction, purposes, and uses of such relationships for the individual
   f. Perception of self
   g. Social roles that are assumed or ascribed; competence in fulfilling these roles
   h. Relational behavior:
      - Capacity for intimacy
      - Degree of dependence or independence on a continuum from one extreme to the other
      - Power and control conflicts
      - Exploitative nature
      - Openness
5. *Developmental factors*
   a. How role performance equates with life stage
   b. How developmental experiences have been interpreted and used
   c. How past conflicts, tasks, and problems have been handled
   d. Whether the present problem is unique in the person's life experience

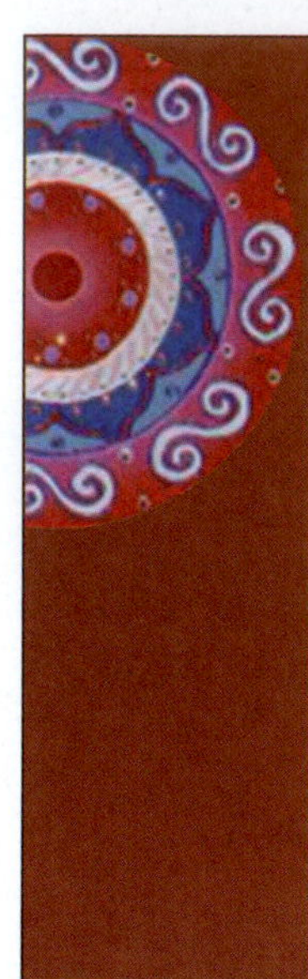

CARING FOR THE SPIRIT

Spiritual Health Assessment

For these first five statements, indicate whether you *never, sometimes, often,* or *nearly always* agree.

1. I trust myself.
2. I feel my life has meaning and purpose.
3. Other people give meaning to my life.
4. I trust other people.
5. I have close friends.
6. I have experienced the following in my life:
   Loss ___ Separation ___ Divorce ___
   Geographic moves ___ Rejection ___ Death ___
7. Do *religion* and *spirituality* mean the same thing to you? If not, what are the differences to you?
8. With 1 being the lowest and 10 the highest, place an X on the scale below to indicate your relationship with your higher power, and circle the place on the scale that you feel would be ideal for your relationship with your higher power. Explain why you chose each of these points.
   (no relationship) (turn only problems over) (turn total self over)
   1 2 3 4 5 6 7 8 9 10
9. My religious upbringing and background can be described as (check as many as apply):
   Nurturing ___ Helpful ___ Strict ___
   Conservative ___ Liberal ___
   Punishing ___ Negative ___ Had very little ___
   Had none ___

The Place of Assessment in Practice

Assessment is essential in clinical practice and serves several purposes:

- Identifying problems
- Identifying client motivations, strengths, and resources
- Identifying forces (both internal and external to the client) that may hinder the team's therapeutic plan
- Setting reasonable goals with the client, given who the client is at this time
- Determining appropriate intervention strategies
- Providing continuous evaluation of the process and indicating when the therapeutic plan should be changed

Assessment is an ongoing, dynamic process that utilizes all your senses and all your skills. Your observations, combined with all the information you receive from the client, interdisciplinary team members, and other collateral sources, provide an opportunity to engage in a partnership based on mutual definition of problems and goals. If a medically ill client says, "I'd be better off dead," you must assess the lethality risk (Bryant, 2007) and intervene to prioritize the client's safety. If you see physical signs of abuse such as bruises in various stages of healing without adequate explanation, your assessment warrants a private interview with the client during which you can ask, "Does anyone ever hurt you?" (Pullen, 2007).

MediaLink Application: Assessing Elders for Signs of Abuse

Assessment is the solid base upon which you build your practice and perform your interventions. See the Evidence-Based Practice feature for an example of how assessment is vital to good nursing care. Information and services that help nurses, physicians, consumers, other providers, and health plans navigate the complexity of the health care system can be found at WebMD, www.webmd.com, and can be accessed on the Companion Website for this book.

MediaLink WebMD

DOCUMENTATION

When recording client data, it is your responsibility to protect the client from identification and unwarranted exposure. The client's name should not be discussed out of the treatment area unless it is a secure environment and the discussion is among treatment providers for that client. Documentation is a legal and clinically relevant expression of care given to the client and the client's response to that care. The use of any of this information in other arenas must be in the context of delivering that care. For the client, the nurse's respect for the client's self-disclosures is one measure of the nurse's trustworthiness. See specific information on confidentiality in Chapter 13.

Nursing Care Plans

Nursing care plans are a means of providing nursing personnel with information about the needs and therapeutic plans for each client. They are of major importance when an agency uses source-oriented documentation, because they provide an ongoing, up-to-date record of goal-directed, individualized nursing care. When problem-oriented documentation is used, nursing care plans may be an outgrowth of that documentation.

Critical Pathways

Critical pathways are another way to represent a nursing plan of care. Their use varies geographically and with facility procedures. They are usually formatted in columns and emphasize client outcomes tied to target dates (see Figure 4-2 on pages 50–51). Critical pathways in general specify the following categories of information:

1. Daily client outcomes (short-term goals)
2. Assessments, tests, and treatments
3. Knowledge deficit (daily prescriptions for nursing interventions focused on client teaching)

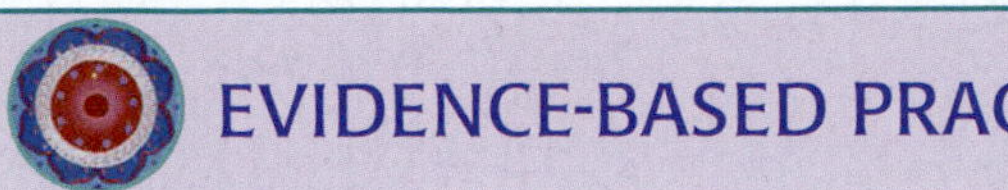

PHYSICAL AND PSYCHOSOCIAL ASSESSMENT OF A HOSPICE CLIENT AND HER FAMILY MEMBER

Jane is an 84-year-old woman who recently started receiving hospice services in her home for end-stage heart disease. Even though she voluntarily entered hospice care, Jane never told anyone that she believed she could live considerably longer than the few months caregivers suggested. Her sister has been taking care of her. Fatigue and shortness of breath have been the main symptoms Jane experiences, although she has been sad and feeling unsupported lately. Jane has not told anyone about these feelings.

Your assessment of Jane is based on current research results. Your research review highlights quality-of-life issues for end-of-life care and the role of perceived social support in the experience of physical symptoms. You have learned that Jane, and possibly her sister, will likely have psychosocial symptoms. A discussion with Jane and her sister may help both of them voice their feelings and consider the interplay of physical and emotional symptoms.

Assessing physical and psychosocial symptoms allows a complete picture of the status of a client and directs interventions.

The hospice treatment team discusses the information you gathered during your assessment. The plan is to incorporate feeling identification, support system structures, and ongoing assessment of symptoms of depression into the overall care that Jane receives. Intervening with Jane's caregiver is similarly important.

Action should be based on more than one study, but the following research would be helpful in this situation.

McMillan, S. C., Dunbar, S. B., & Zhang, W. (2007). The prevalence of symptoms in hospice patients with end-stage heart disease. *Journal of Hospice & Palliative Nursing, 9*(3), 124–131.

CRITICAL THINKING APPLICATION

1. How could you use the Global Assessment of Functioning Scale to develop a plan of care for Jane?
2. Why would you approach Jane and her sister to discuss these issues?
3. What specific communication techniques (based on the information in Chapter 10) would be helpful in obtaining an accurate assessment and encouraging Jane and her sister to talk with you about their concerns?

4. Diet (daily prescriptions)
5. Activity (daily prescriptions for nursing interventions)
6. Psychosocial considerations (daily prescriptions for nursing interventions)

The precise format for critical pathways may vary from setting to setting or may be based on the client's condition. As is the case with nursing care plans, critical pathways are not set in stone and must be modified based on changes in client assessment data. Furthermore, standardized critical pathways should always be individualized for individual clients.

Algorithms

Algorithms are behavioral steps, or step-by-step procedures, for the management of common problems. Algorithms have proved to be useful protocols, particularly in settings that employ large numbers of paraprofessionals. At intake points in community mental health settings, such as walk-in neighborhood clinics, mental health workers often make the initial psychosocial assessment and may plan and implement treatment strategies.

Clinical algorithms for common mental health problems provide the nonprofessional with structured, standardized guidelines for decision making. Professional nurses in nonpsychiatric settings find clinical algorithms particularly useful when assessing psychiatric symptoms. Algorithms for depression and suicidal lethality have been found to be reliable and valid in these circumstances.

QUALITY ASSURANCE

Quality Assurance is known by many names, including Performance Improvement (PI), Quality Management (QM), Continuous Improvement (CI), and Continuous Quality Improvement (CQI). (For our purposes we will use the term Quality Assurance [QA] in this text.) No matter what name is used, the basis of QA is to assure that quality is maintained through an ongoing effort to find new and better ways of doing things and achieving better results.

When QA is properly conducted, it involves the entire organization, whether a large bureaucratic hospital setting or a small private practice. All members of the workforce are involved in evaluating procedures, looking for ways to improve them, and then improving them. In fact, QA is best conducted by the people doing the work rather than by supervisors and administrators.

You will hear QA referred to as a process. This is because QA is evolving as it improves clinical practice. It is not a fixed or rigid plan. QA involves four basic steps—Plan, Do, Check, and Act—that are continuously in progress (see FIGURE 11-2 ■ on page 232). (Hence the word "continuous" in the terms *Continuous Improvement* and *Continuous Quality Improvement.*)

Quality assurance is about asking questions, using perception surveys and questionnaires, and listening carefully to both compliments and complaints from the people involved in the process. The recipient of your clinical services can be viewed as your customer, someone who can make choices to a certain extent about from whom they receive services. And

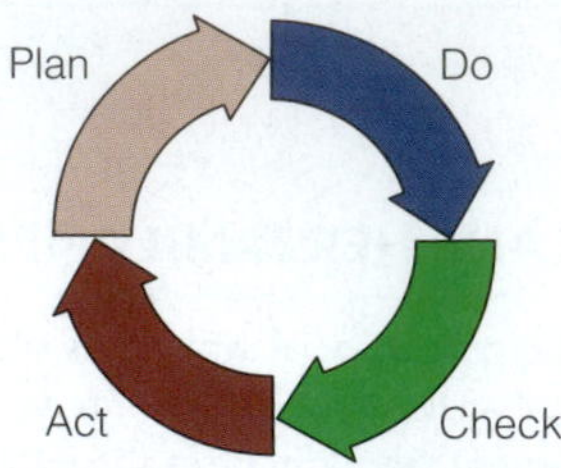

FIGURE 11-2 ■ The Quality Assurance Cycle of Activities. The four steps of Quality Assurance are labeled Plan, Do, Check, and Act and are performed in a cyclic fashion.

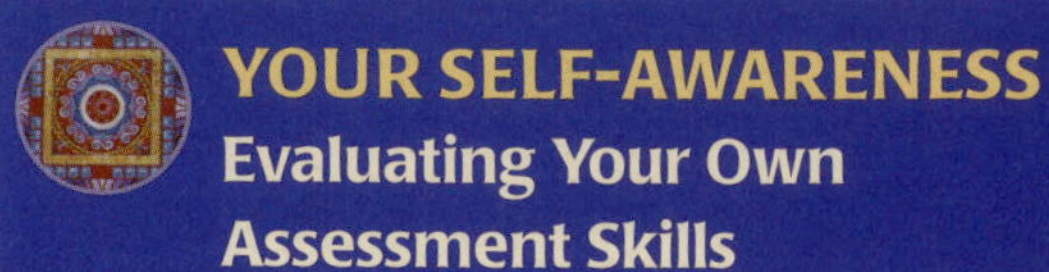

YOUR SELF-AWARENESS
Evaluating Your Own Assessment Skills

Evaluate your assessment skills by responding to the following:

1. Can you ask an open-ended question and not anticipate the answer?
2. Are you able to remain silent during an interview without being uncomfortable?
3. Do you accept information given to you without criticism or judgment?
4. Can you show empathy, not sympathy, for others' problems?
5. Gauge your tolerance for unusual or abnormal behavior.
6. Evaluate how aware you are of other cultures and their expressions of distress.
7. What is your skill level for understanding the content of what is said to you as well as the process (how things are said, not said, done, and not done)?
8. Do you have success getting your message across to others?
9. Have you been able to make necessary changes when you received feedback on your interactions?
10. Rate your skills for assessing someone accurately on a scale of 0 to 10, with 0 being the lowest level and 10 being the highest. (For example, use a brief interaction with a new colleague and then discuss your assessment with the colleague). Discover your weak assessment areas and work on improving them (and raising your score). Repeat regularly.

customers are the best judges of quality. They know best whether their needs and expectations are being met.

When you assess a client, are your procedures the best they can be? Have you utilized all possible and available resources to form the most comprehensive impression of this individual and how to approach treatment? One useful strategy for applying QA to assessment procedures is to compare the outcome of a clinical case with the assessment. Were the recommendations for treatment from the assessment helpful in treating the individual? The involvement of several clinicians in this effort can shape more and more advantageous procedures. If you follow a QA format when examining your practices, then you are more likely to be able to create a truly quality assessment.

The *psychiatric audit* is one way to evaluate the quality of mental health services that consumers receive. An audit consists of a review of the client's chart to compare criteria for quality care with actual practice. Problem-oriented documentation provides the descriptive documentation necessary for such QA programs. Although documentation may not always accurately indicate the quality of the care given, it is an important part of the process that keeps mental health care workers accountable to consumers of their services.

When QA is utilized in this way, it benefits everyone. Recipients and their families have an opportunity to receive a higher quality of care, which means better health and greater satisfaction with treatment. You and your coworkers find better ways to do things, which can lead to greater job satisfaction. The treatment setting benefits from QA as an ongoing focus on improving quality, which helps the facility fulfill its mission and do its job.

Accurate problem identification and intervention strategies often depend on the quality of the assessment. Mental health client information is gathered, assessed, and communicated through the various interdisciplinary assessments. The primary purpose of your assessment is to gather data to formulate a psychiatric diagnosis, prognosis, and treatment plan. If the assessment of a client is based on incomplete, misinterpreted, or inaccurate information, the psychiatric diagnosis, prognosis, and treatment plan may be faulty. Read the Your Self-Awareness feature to determine your ability to assess clients with minimal interference from your own cultural background and views.

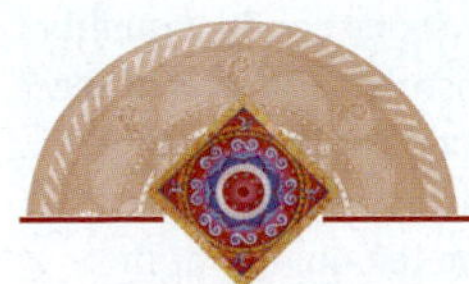

EXPLORE MEDIALINK

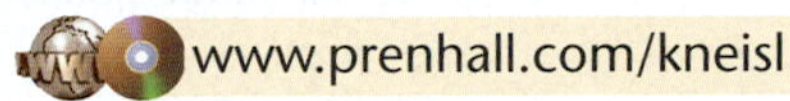

For NCLEX-RN® review questions, case studies, and other resources for this chapter see the Pearson Health MediaLink CD-ROM that accompanies this book and the Companion Website at www.prenhall.com/kneisl.

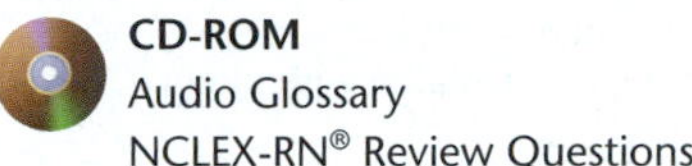

CD-ROM
Audio Glossary
NCLEX-RN® Review Questions

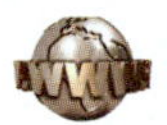

Companion Website
Audio Glossary
NCLEX-RN® Review Questions
Critical Thinking Exercise
- *Using the DSM-IV-TR*

Case Study
- *Assessment Strategies*

Care Plan
- *Integrating the GAF to Plan Care*

MediaLinks
MediaLink Applications
- *From the Outside Looking In: Assessing Elders for Signs of Abuse*

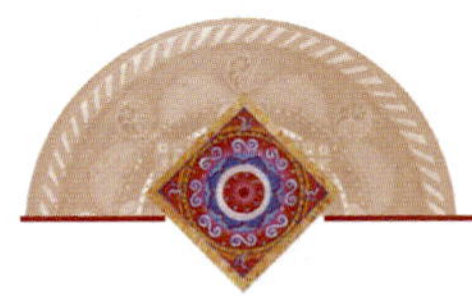

NCLEX-RN® REVIEW QUESTIONS

1. Which of the following principles assist the nurse in maintaining objectivity and validity in the psychiatric–mental health assessment? (Select all that apply.)
1. Maintain client confidentiality.
2. If data from different sources conflict, document all versions of the event(s), clearly identifying the sources of information.
3. Document, using the client's own words.
4. Identify the client's strengths.
5. Maintain self-awareness throughout the assessment process.

2. The psychiatric–mental health assessment most resembles:
1. The nursing process.
2. An admission history.
3. A battery of psychological tests.
4. The nursing admissions assessment.

3. Order the steps a psychiatric–mental health nurse would take for gathering a client's psychiatric history.
1. Meet with family members, noting relationships to client, and encourage them to share their stories and concerns.
2. Encourage the client to share his story.
3. Review the admission assessment form with the client and ask direct questions.
4. Document your findings.

4. Order the steps a psychiatric–mental health nurse would take to logically organize a mental status examination.
1. Content of thought
2. Characteristics of speech
3. General appearance and behavior
4. Orientation and memory

5. Which of the following statements accurately describes the Mental State Examination and the Mini-Mental State Exam?
1. The Mental State Examination and the Mini-Mental State Exam provide valid and reliable results for any cooperative client.
2. The Mini-Mental State Exam is a thorough, abbreviated version of the Mental State Examination.
3. The Mental State Examination assists the clinician in identifying risks for harm of self and others.
4. It is essential that the topics in both the Mental State Examination and the Mini-Mental State Exam be addressed in order.

6. Your colleague informs you, "I decided to do a Mini-Mental State Exam instead of a Mental State Examination." Which of the following do you predict is your colleague's rationale?
1. "I knew the order of the questions was less important in administering the Mini-Mental State Exam."
2. "I did not have time to complete a full Mental State Examination."
3. "I just needed to know about hallucinations and delusional thinking."
4. "The client was not cooperative and was unable to answer questions."

7. Health care history and examination are associated with which type of assessment?
1. Physiologic assessment
2. Neurological assessment
3. Psychological testing
4. Psychosocial assessment

8. Which of the following is associated with Axis IV?
1. Persistent traits
2. Functional grade from 1–100
3. External (nonpsychological) psychosocial stressors
4. Reason for treatment

9. In developing realistic, measurable outcome criteria for your client's ability to function, you review your client's previous health records, tracking changes on:
1. Axis I.
2. Axis II.
3. Axis III.
4. Axis V.

10. Many psychiatric–mental health organizations conduct quality assurance audits on 100% of client assessments. Which of the following statements provides the rationale for these audits?
1. The quality of treatment plans and the appropriateness of subsequent interventions depend upon the quality of the assessment.
2. Each clinician's assessments can be compared with those of his or her peers, providing a basis for peer review as necessary.
3. It is a high-frequency activity and it generates a lot of reliable statistics.
4. The quality of the assessment correlates with client satisfaction.

See Appendix C for answers.

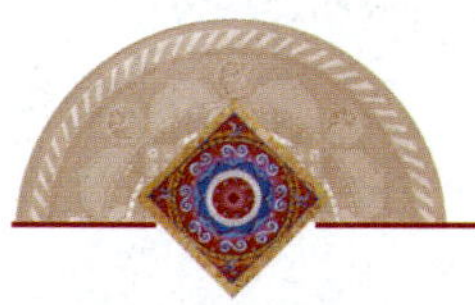

REFERENCES

American Nurses Association, American Psychiatric Nurses Association, and International Society of Psychiatric–Mental Health Nurses. (2007). *Psychiatric–mental health nursing: Scope and standards of practice.* Silver Spring, MD: American Nurses Association.

American Psychiatric Association. (2000). *Diagnostic and statistical manual of mental disorders* (4th ed., Text Revision). Washington DC: Author.

Bryant, S. (2007). Clinical queries. How do I respond to a chronically ill patient who's suicidal? *Nursing, 37*(2), 24.

Folstein, M., Folstein, S., & McHugh, P. (1975). Mini-mental state: A practical method for grading the cognitive state of patients for the clinician. *Journal of Psychiatric Residents, 12,* 189.

Honigfeld, G., Gillis, R. D., & Klett, C. J. (1966). NOSIE-30: A treatment-sensitive ward behavior scale. *Psychological Reports, 19,* 180–182.

Knight, T. A. (2007). Showing clients the doors: Active problem-solving in person-centered psychotherapy. *Journal of Psychotherapy Integration, 17*(1), 111–124.

McMillan, S. C., Dunbar, S. B., & Zhang, W. (2007). The prevalence of symptoms in hospice patients with end-stage heart disease. *Journal of Hospice & Palliative Nursing, 9*(3), 124–131.

Pullen, R, L., Jr. (2007). Clinical do's & don'ts. Screening for abuse and neglect. *Nursing, 37*(2), 69.

Small, S. M. (1980). *Outline for psychiatric evaluation.* New York: Sandoz/Novartis.

Spielberger, C. D. (1976). The nature and measurement of anxiety. In C. D. Spielberger & R. Diaz-Guerrero (Eds.), *Cross cultural anxiety* (pp. 3–12). Washington, DC: Hemisphere/Wiley.

Stanton, K. (2007). Emergency: Communicating with ED patients who have chronic mental illnesses. *American Journal of Nursing, 107*(2), 61–65.

ADDITIONAL REFERENCES

Bender, L. (1938). *A visual–motor gestalt test and its clinical use.* Research monograph 3. American Orthopsychiatric Association.

Bucher, G. M., Szczerba, P., & Curtin, P. M. (2007). A comprehensive fall prevention program for assessment, interventions and referral. *Home Healthcare Nurse, 25*(3), 174–183.

Covill, S. E. (2007). Nurses' knowledge in assessing depression in the palliative care patient. *Nursing News (New Hampshire), 31*(2), 17–20.

Murray, H. A. (1943). *Thematic apperception test.* Cambridge, MA: Harvard University Press.

Raichle, M. E. (1994, April). Visualizing the mind. *Scientific American,* 58–64.

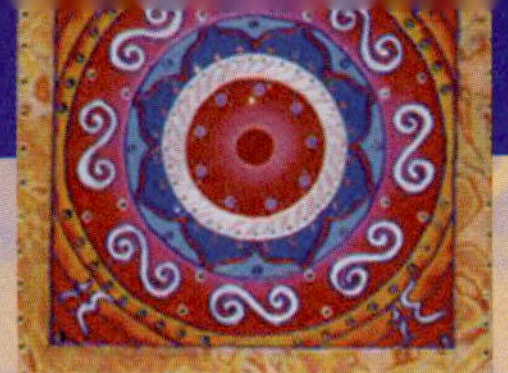

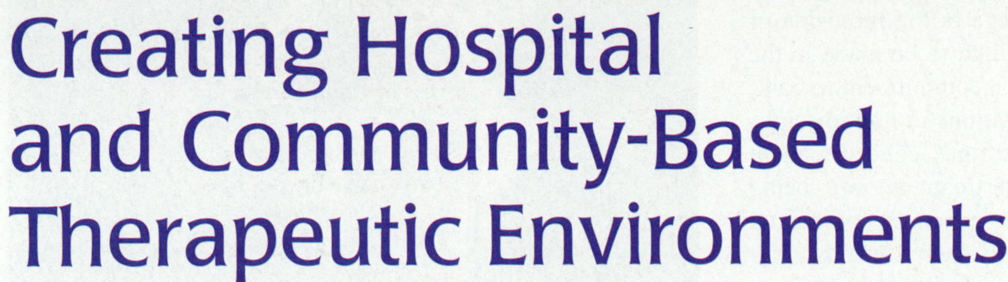

Creating Hospital and Community-Based Therapeutic Environments

CHAPTER 12

CAROL REN KNEISL

LEARNING OUTCOMES

After completing this chapter, you will be able to:

1. Identify the types of hospital-based and community-based settings in which psychiatric–mental health nurses practice.
2. Discuss the specific challenges that psychiatric home care nurses face.
3. Discuss the specific challenges that case managers face.
4. Explain how managed mental health care organizations influence psychiatric–mental health care.
5. Differentiate case management from other types of care.
6. Incorporate therapeutic environment principles in a plan of care for psychiatric–mental health clients.
7. Determine the adaptations in programming necessary to meet the needs of the severely and persistently mentally ill.
8. Discuss the challenges associated with caring for high-risk severely and persistently mentally ill clients.

KEY TERMS

case management *244*
client government *250*
deinstitutionalization *236*
National Alliance on Mental Illness (NAMI) *255*
psychiatric rehabilitation *255*
severe and persistent mental illness (SPMI) *252*
therapeutic environment *246*

CRITICAL THINKING CHALLENGE

At a nursing care conference, you and your nurse colleague, Sylvia, disagree about the future direction of mental health care for Tommy, a client at the outpatient clinic of the community mental health center where you both work. Tommy, now 53 years old, has been in and out of psychiatric hospitals since he was 18. Tommy now lives in an adult foster care home and visits the clinic monthly for follow-up purposes. Sylvia believes that the number-one nursing goal should be to provide support to Tommy so that he can maintain his current level of functioning. You believe that the number-one nursing goal should be for Tommy to achieve a more independent, higher level of functioning.

1. Can these two different stands be reconciled? How?
2. Do you see this issue as a matter of psychiatric nursing practice or as a question of moral beliefs? Why?
3. Is it possible to provide support for Tommy while helping him to become more independent at the same time?

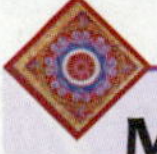

MEDIALINK 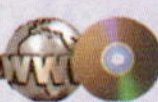 www.prenhall.com/kneisl

Go to the Pearson Health MediaLink CD-ROM and the Companion Website at www.prenhall.com/kneisl for interactive resources for this chapter.

Economic, political, technologic, legal, and demographic forces are propelling reform and change in the provision of mental health care. Great strides continue to be made in the treatment of mental illness along with a commitment to comprehensive service delivery and innovations in multidisciplinary approaches to care. At the same time, concerns about gaps in coverage for mental health treatment are being voiced. Continued high out-of-pocket expenses for mental health treatment may impede access to mental health treatment, especially for those who need more intense treatment (Zuvekas & Meyerhoefer, 2006).

Our clients and their care are increasingly located in the larger community of which they are a part. In fact, pockets of mentally ill in the community will not seek care within the confines of the four walls of a psychiatric hospital, a comprehensive community mental health center, or even a walk-in clinic in a storefront. Intensive outreach programs currently lead community mental health efforts. The shift away from institution-based care began with what is known as the community mental health movement.

This chapter discusses the wide variety of hospital- and community-based mental health treatment services and programs available today and the high-risk populations most likely to use them. Managed care and case management, psychiatric rehabilitation, and establishing therapeutic environments are discussed as processes by which the goals of services and programs are met. In addition to this chapter, each disorder chapter in Unit 4 of this text discusses home care, community-based care, and case management.

DEINSTITUTIONALIZATION AND THE COMMUNITY MENTAL HEALTH MOVEMENT

From the early 19th century until the 1950s, state and county mental hospitals constituted the major treatment resource for the mentally ill (see Figures 12-1 ■ and 12-2 ■). As it often turned out, these hospitals served as the mentally ill client's long-term, and sometimes permanent, residence.

Deinstitutionalization, bringing mental health clients out of the hospital and into the community, began in the post–World War II period, when large public mental hospitals were overcrowded, had fallen into disrepair, and were widely criticized among humanitarians for "warehousing" their residents.

With the development of psychotropic drugs in 1954 and the enactment of state statutes that restricted involuntary detainment in psychiatric facilities, the resident population of state and county mental hospitals declined. By the late 1970s, only one-third as many people were hospitalized in psychiatric hospitals. This phase-down of large bureaucratic institutions occurred within the context of a much broader movement for community mental health that reached its apex in the 1960s.

When federal funds became available in the 1960s for the construction of community mental health centers and the provision of acute care and ambulatory services in the community, it was assumed that equal access to all levels of mental

MediaLink Application: Deinstitutionalization

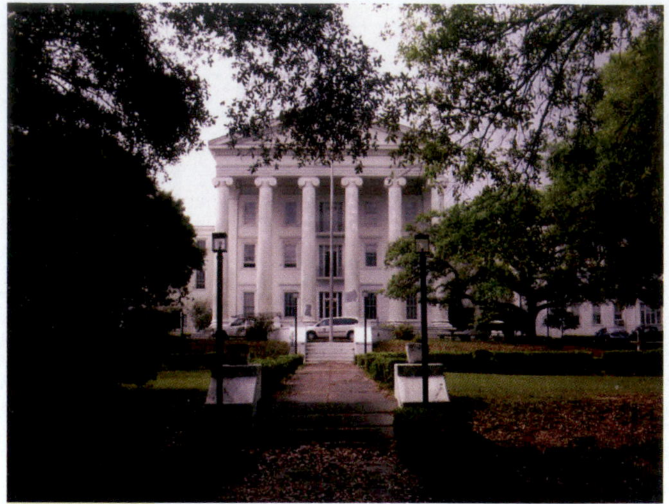

Figure 12-1 ■ One of the first 10 mental hospitals in the country, the Insane Asylum of the State of Louisiana (now East Louisiana State Hospital) was built in the 1840s. Once housing over 5,000 people before deinstitutionalization, this national historic landmark, an example of Greek Revival architecture, has a current hospital population of 260.

Source: Photo courtesy of Kay R. Hanks, RN, East Louisiana State Hospital, Jackson, Louisiana.

disorder prevention and treatment would exist. However, several disturbing trends cast this assumption into doubt. First of all, hospital care remained the main treatment modality for the severely mentally ill: Repeated readmissions replaced long-term institutional residence. New populations of the mentally ill in the community—the homeless, crack cocaine addicts, mentally ill criminal offenders—were unable or unwilling to use the provided services. It became apparent that aggressive outreach services were needed in order to make both hospital-based and community-based treatments and programs accessi-

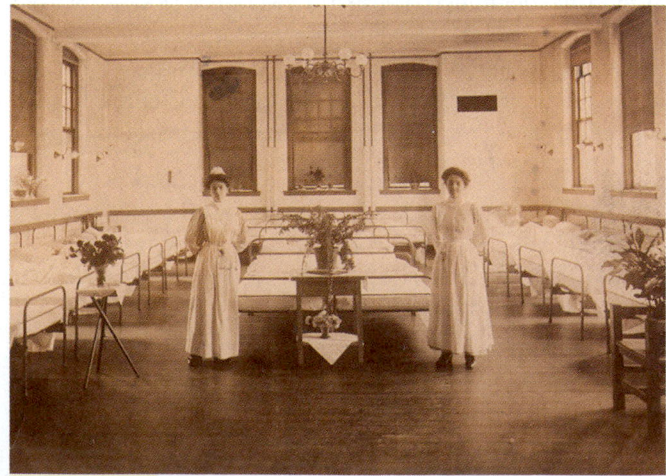

Figure 12-2 ■ Psychiatric nurses in 1901 in a typical ward at the Buffalo State Hospital (now the Buffalo Psychiatric Center). At this time, it was believed that architecture could influence the course of mental illness. For example, depressed persons were housed in wards with high ceilings such as this one to elevate their spirits.

Source: Photo courtesy of Buffalo Psychiatric Center, Buffalo, New York.

ble to those individuals who needed them. The greatest problems have been in creating adequate and accessible community resources (Lamb & Bachrach, 2001).

TYPES OF TREATMENT SERVICES AND PROGRAMS

Hospital-based inpatient treatment and community-based outpatient treatment constitute the two major umbrellas under which care is provided.

Hospital-Based Treatment

Clients admitted to inpatient settings, such as the one in FIGURE 12-3A, ■ must meet admission criteria. The admitting diagnosis is often one that is life threatening. Overall effectiveness of functioning using the DSM Axis V global assessment of functioning scale (GAF; see Box 11-7 on page 228 in Chapter 11) determines the acuity of the illness. In most instances impairment in functioning must be in the 10 to 50 range to qualify for admission. Clients experiencing this degree of discomfort require intense, skilled nursing care to provide for safety needs. For example, a GAF score of 30 indicates that behavior is strongly influenced by delusions or hallucinations, serious impairment in communication or judgment, or an inability to function in almost all areas. Some managed care organizations (MCOs) have designed their own criteria that require ratings of functioning, physical impairments, family support, and other elements as part of a preadmission assessment.

You can easily see how your role as a nurse in the inpatient psychiatric setting is similar to that of the critical care nurse in the general hospital. Clients who are admitted to the psychiatric unit with active suicidal ideation, who are psychotic, or who are experiencing withdrawal symptoms require intensive nursing care and case management.

Community-Based Treatment

There are a wide variety of community-based treatment settings. Box 12-1 on page 238 gives you several examples of settings in which psychiatric–mental health nurses practice, some of which are discussed next. Several others are discussed in other sections of this chapter.

Community Mental Health Centers

Community mental health centers (CMHCs) vary considerably in their appearance (see Figure 12-3) and in the services they offer. Services offered in CMHCs include:

- Emergency services
- Medication management clinics
- Psychoeducation groups
- Vocational rehabilitation
- Consultation services to hospitals, nursing homes, and primary care centers
- Other specialty services as determined by the population they serve (programs for the severely and persistently mentally ill, mental health clinics for the homeless, dual diagnosis services for chemically dependent mentally ill clients, elder services, etc.)

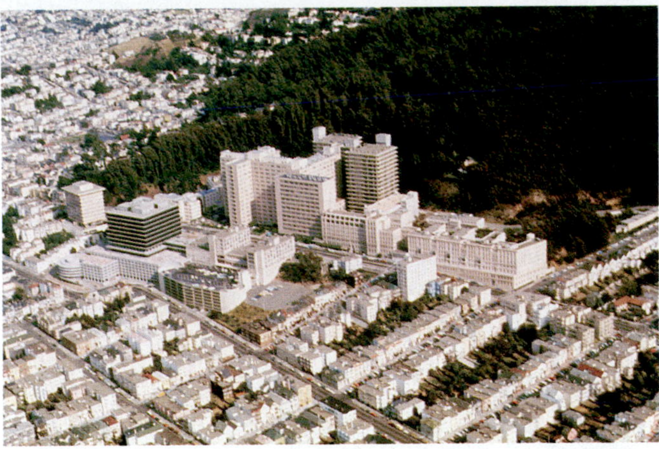

A

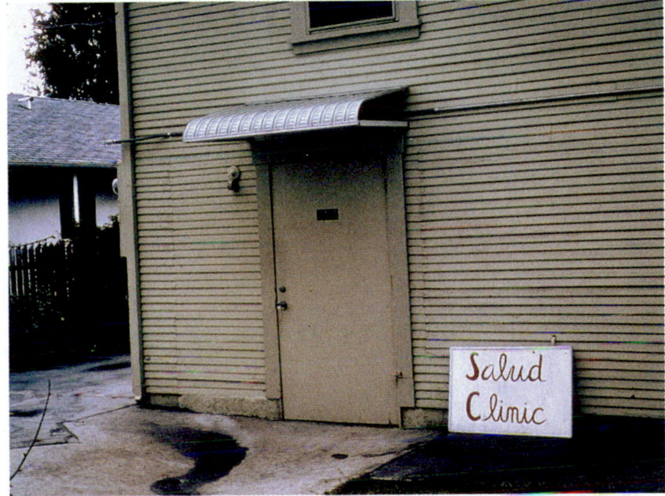

B

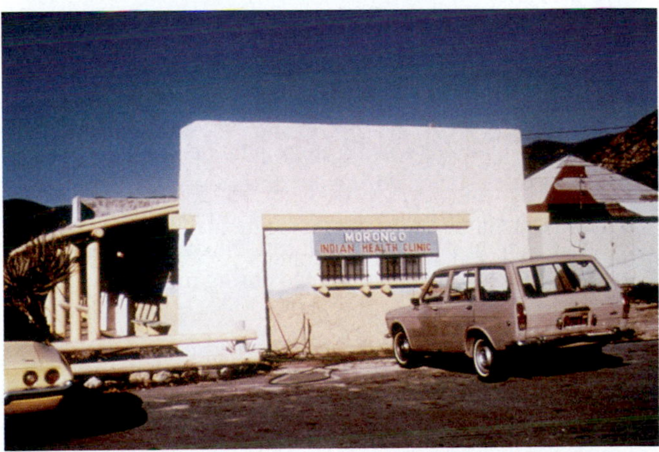

C

FIGURE 12-3 ■ A community mental health center is more a concept than a place. Community mental health centers cannot be recognized by appearance alone.
(A) A university-based medical center with a community mental health center and a neuropsychiatric inpatient unit.
(B) An inner-city mental health outreach clinic.
(C) A rural mental health outreach clinic and day treatment program.
Source: Holly Skodol Wilson, RN, PhD.

Box 12-1 Community Treatment Settings

- Adult day care settings
- AIDS support programs
- Assisted living facilities
- Child day care centers
- Client's own home
- Community mental health centers
- Correctional facilities (jails, prisons, detention centers)
- Courts (mental health evaluation, mentally ill offenders, victims of violence)
- Crisis services
- Day treatment centers
- Emergency departments of hospitals
- Ethnic cultural centers
- Foster care homes for adults and youths
- Group homes
- Halfway houses
- Hospices
- Houses of worship (churches, synagogues, mosques, temples)
- Immigrant centers
- Industry and business centers
- Mobile outreach teams
- Nursing homes
- Rural mental health clinics
- Partial hospitalization programs
- Primary care centers
- Private practice offices (psychiatric–mental health nurses, psychiatrists, psychologists, social workers)
- Residential facilities for cognitively impaired
- Schools
- Senior centers
- Sheltered workshops
- Shelters and residential services (battered women, homeless, youths, people in crisis)
- Substance abuse programs
- Youth centers
- YMCAs/YWCAs

A study in Australia (McCann, 2002) indicated that an important function of community mental health nurses is to uncover their clients' hope for the future. These community mental health nurses used two main strategies to enable the process of hopefulness:

1. Enhancing motivation
2. Developing pathways to wellness

These activities enhance the quality of the nurse–client relationship, and advance client self-determination, education, and planning for the future.

In large metropolitan areas, CMHCs often include:

- Inpatient hospital-based care
- Partial hospitalization programs:

1. Day care services for those who need supervision and assistance during daytime hours
2. Night treatment services for those who are able to maintain employment during the day but need supervision and assistance during nighttime hours

Mobile Outreach Units

Mobile treatment teams go out into the community by car or on foot to deliver services in whatever setting makes the client comfortable—a public place, a jail, a home, a shopping mall, a fast-food restaurant, under a bridge, or in an alley. Common treatment goals of mobile outreach units are:

- Bringing community-based treatment programs to homeless clients and to those who would not otherwise seek mental health services or have little or no access to mental health care
- Providing medication management prescribed by another mental health professional to clients who have problems in adhering to treatment by psychotropic medications
- Preventing relapse and hospitalization
- Identifying and assessing persons in the community in need of mental health care and facilitating their entry into a mental health service program
- Providing emergency intervention or crisis prevention services to mental health consumers, police, employers, landlords, business owners, and so on
- Satisfying the requirements of court-ordered treatment

Mobile treatment teams have also been able to reduce the need for hospitalization in many instances. Major mental health consumer characteristics that relate to the likelihood of hospitalization are:

1. Being young and homeless and experiencing acute problems
2. Having been referred by psychiatric hospitals, the legal system, or other treatment facilities
3. Showing signs of substance abuse, having no income, and being severely mentally disabled (Guo, Biegel, Johnsen, & Dyches, 2001)

Assertive Community Treatment (ACT)

Assertive programs have shown much promise in terms of service delivery to high-risk groups and are believed to prevent psychotic relapse and rehospitalization (Bustillo, Lauriello, Horan, & Keith, 2001) and reduce arrests, emergency room visits, and homelessness of clients with severe and persistent mental illness. These are expensive, sophisticated programs that are believed to be cost-effective because they offset still more expensive hospital episodes. Assertive programs are known by names other than ACT—Continuous Treatment Teams (CTTs), Intensive Case Management (ICM), and Programs for Assertive Community Treatment (PACT) are some of them.

These teams may include interdisciplinary groups of 7 to 12 staff members—nurses, psychiatrists, social workers, peer specialists who are mental health consumers, and mental health paraprofessionals—who deliver service in the client's own environment. Treatment teams not only provide a mobile outreach capacity, they also provide consumers with access to multidisciplinary providers and comprehensive services. It is believed that communities should provide enough ACT teams to serve approximately 50% of their populations of persons with severe mental illness (Cuddeback, Morrissey, & Meyer, 2006).

The team structure is believed to reduce stress and burnout of individual case managers by sharing the load of difficult clients. The client benefits from both reduced dependence on an individual clinician and the support of a large multidisciplinary group for backup during crisis. In addition, clients benefit because staff members in these teams must be clinically sophisticated and capable of managing acute care in the community. The Evidence-Based Practice feature below is an example of how a multidisciplinary team can assist clients in a crisis.

Concerns about coercion have arisen with ACT treatment programs. A major concern has been that ACT teams often become actively and directly involved in many areas of the client's life and may control access to resources such as housing and money in return for adherence to medication and treatment programs through outpatient commitment (Torrey & Zdanowicz, 2001). This paternalism interferes with the client's personal autonomy. Members of ACT teams must be sure to look for opportunities to enhance clients' quality of life through personal goal setting and decision making to the extent possible for each individual client.

Guidelines and standards developed by the National Alliance on Mental Illness (NAMI) and recommended for assertive community treatment teams are available at www.nami.org/about/pactstd.html and can be accessed through the Companion Website for this book.

MediaLink National Alliance on Mental Illness

Psychiatric Home Care

Psychiatric home care nursing has a long history in community mental health (Fagin, 2001). Some of the most successful programs for the severely mentally ill in the early years of community mental health employed visiting nurses to deliver home-based services. Today, there is growing demand for psychiatric home care nursing as a cost-effective alternative to hospitalization. Medicare, Medicaid, managed care organizations, and private health insurance all fund psychiatric home care at different levels and with different requirements for reimbursement.

MediaLink Case Study: Psychiatric Home Care

Clients with a primary psychiatric diagnosis should be cared for in the home by an experienced psychiatric–mental

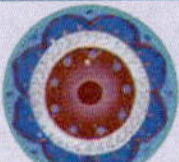

EVIDENCE-BASED PRACTICE

ASSERTIVE COMMUNITY TREATMENT

Angie is a 42-year-old woman who has been hospitalized several times for acute schizophrenic episodes. Each episode has been preceded by a period in which Angie stopped taking her medication. Angie usually becomes argumentative, hallucinates, fails to pay attention to her personal care, does not show up for her job, and withdraws from others, staying in her apartment in the dark. This time, Angie, who has a key to her boyfriend's apartment, entered his apartment when he wasn't there and locked herself in. She played a CD over and over at such a high volume that the neighbors next door and in the apartment below complained to the building superintendent.

When the building superintendent knocked on the door, Angie refused to let him in. His pleas with her to keep the noise down were met with increasing rage. Angie began throwing things in the apartment, broke a window, and damaged the walls. Fortunately, Angie's boyfriend arrived on the scene and called the mental health clinic where Angie was registered as a client. Soon after, the police arrived in response to calls from neighbors. Angie refused to open the door for them.

The mobile mental health team from the mental health clinic arrived on the scene and was able to persuade Angie to let them in the apartment. They negotiated an agreement among Angie, her boyfriend, the building superintendent, and the police that charges would not be filed against Angie, providing that she agreed to assertive community treatment that would involve involuntary outpatient commitment including medication management. Angie's boyfriend agreed to repair the window and any damaged walls. The goals were to avoid hospitalization for Angie, to avoid criminal charges, to help her adhere to a medication regimen, and to keep close contact with her and preempt future violent behavior. The mobile mental health team considered the following research studies in developing a plan of action for Angie:

Coldwell, C. M., & Bender, W. S. (2007). The effectiveness of assertive community treatment for homeless populations with severe mental illness: A meta-analysis. *American Journal of Psychiatry, 164*(3), 393–399.

Essock, S. M., Mueser, K. R., Drake, R. E., Covell, N. H., McHugo, G. J., Frisman, L. K., et al. (2006). Comparison of ACT and standard case management for delivering integrated treatment for co-occurring disorders. *Psychiatric Services, 57*(2), 185–196.

CRITICAL THINKING APPLICATION

1. Which actions of the mobile mental health team could be considered coercive?
2. Since Angie caused the damage, shouldn't she be the person financially responsible for repairing the damages to her boyfriend's apartment?
3. Does Angie's behavior warrant her arrest by the police to protect public safety?
4. Angie has stopped taking her medication. Does that warrant hospitalization?

health nurse. In fact, Medicare (which funds most psychiatric home care) requires this experience. Basic-level and advanced-level psychiatric–mental health nurses provide direct psychiatric care to mental health consumers through home care agencies. Advanced-level nurses may also provide direct psychiatric care or function as intensive case managers and consultants to staff as well as mental health consumers.

Other requirements for Medicare reimbursement are homebound status and the presence of a diagnosed psychiatric disorder. Homebound status for psychiatric home care would include clients who are immobilized by depression or anxiety attacks, clients who are disoriented or confused, clients with hallucinations or delusions that compromise their safety, or clients whose physical health prevents them from going to other locations where mental health services are offered.

Psychiatric home care is more likely to be used for clients recently discharged from a psychiatric hospital, the homebound elderly, persons with dementia, young adults with severe and persistent mental illness, or clients who have an associated medical condition such as neuropsychiatric problems as a result of infection with HIV (human immunodeficiency virus; see also Chapter 25).

As clients are discharged from hospitals more quickly, the nurse who is providing home care may be providing services that traditionally would have been delivered in a hospital setting. For example, the medication clozapine (Clozaril), used to alleviate symptoms of schizophrenia, requires frequent blood tests to monitor for side effects. The home care nurse draws the blood and monitors the medication protocol in the home setting. Alcohol-related complications such as diabetes may require extensive family teaching to enable family members to successfully manage a chronic alcoholic family member who is also diabetic.

You might encounter your clients in personal care homes or hospices. Clients with AIDS-related dementia often require extensive counseling and supportive services as they struggle with their illness. These types of clients are often quite medically ill, and you may collaborate with another nurse provider in meeting their needs.

In some personal care homes, you may be the only professional who visits an elderly client. In these instances, part of your teaching plan is to work with ancillary staff members who are responsible for running the personal care home. The importance of medication adherence for a severely, persistently mentally ill person cannot be overemphasized. Your method of ensuring that clients in personal care homes receive their medication as ordered is often to teach the managers of these facilities about the medication and its effects on behavior.

If you encounter your clients in retirement complexes, your teaching emphasis may be with an aging spouse. This person may not be able to carry out instructions and may require repetitive teaching plans and other aids to ensure that your client follows treatment protocols. In these instances, your skills in family systems will be useful aids in planning appropriate interventions (see Chapter 30).

WHAT EVERY PSYCHIATRIC HOME CARE NURSE SHOULD KNOW

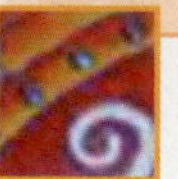

Challenges of Psychiatric Home Care

- Remember that you are a guest in the client's home and that the client has the right to refuse your admittance to that home.
- As a guest in the client's home, be aware of the client's cultural background and strive to be culturally sensitive. Incorporating the client's cultural beliefs into the care you give will not only enhance your relationship with the client and family, but will also positively influence the client's participation in the treatment process.
- Be sensitive to the factors that can influence a client's behavior, such as the physical environment, finances, or the presence of family and friends. For example, the presence of family and friends may raise concerns of confidentiality.
- Work collaboratively with the psychiatrist, other mental health professionals, or the client's primary medical care provider to provide in-depth psychiatric home care.
- Be sensitive to changes in the client's behavior that may indicate relapse or a worsening of symptoms.
- Remember to assess for medical problems that may compound or be compounded by the mental disorder.
- Provide psychoeducation, especially concerning psychotropic medications even for clients who have been on the same medication for years (medication nonadherence accounts for the majority of psychiatric hospital readmissions). Do not assume that clients received adequate instruction, or that they remember the instruction.
- Empower your clients and encourage increasing independence by involving them in the treatment plan.
- Be aware of any factors in the environment that threaten either the client's or your safety. Take a colleague with you on high-risk visits and leave the door open. Leave the client's home if your safety seems to be in question (see also Chapter 35) and inform family, caregivers, or other involved mental health professionals or community resources.

In some home care agencies, there has been a lack of psychiatric services, reluctance to address behavioral problems, a failure to identify undiagnosed disorders, and a bias against accepting individuals with primary psychiatric disorders (Zeltzer & Kohn, 2006). Clearly, such agencies fail to meet the needs of clients with psychiatric diagnoses or behavioral problems. Providing direct psychiatric home care services requires that you are sensitive to several factors. They are outlined in the What Every Psychiatric Home Care Nurse Should Know feature.

MANAGED MENTAL HEALTH CARE

Managed mental health care, a method for capping the rate of increase in the cost of mental health care while ensuring access to quality mental health care services, has become an increasingly important force in psychiatric–mental health nursing. As a service delivery system, managed mental health care creates a rich climate for nurses to become actively involved in primary prevention and education.

Managed Care Settings

Nursing is responding to pressures to use health care resources more efficiently. Clients are admitted to hospitals in later stages of disease or illness, or perhaps not admitted at all. Criteria for hospitalization are based on medical necessity. For instance, the once standard 28-day program for substance abuse treatment has given way to innovative and shorter models for detoxification services and outpatient treatment that meet the lifestyle needs of clients and their employers. Employer demands, coupled with cost containment, have created an entire range of ambulatory care services that at one time would have been considered ineffective. Substance-dependent clients may have options of day, evening, or weekend partial hospitalization programs. Some programs adhere to a Monday through Friday schedule of 4 to 6 hours per day or evening. Weekend programs are usually 8 hours on Saturday and 8 hours on Sunday.

Inpatient Settings

The admission criteria for inpatient care have been discussed earlier in this chapter. These goals are achieved through shorter, more intense hospital stays and the use of critical pathways and case management.

Shorter, More Intense Stays A focus on shorter, more intense stays came about through the emphasis in MCOs on the need to maximize value for the mental health consumer and to keep costs down through the judicious use of available resources. These goals are achieved through the use of critical pathways and case management. Case management is discussed in detail later in this chapter in the section on creating a therapeutic environment. Case management for clients with specific mental disorders is discussed in the nursing process sections of each chapter in Unit 4.

Critical Pathways Critical pathways, or road maps of expected outcomes described earlier in Chapter 11∞, are valuable tools for helping nurses deliver care within managed-care frameworks. When a client "falls off the map" or fails to meet the desired outcomes, this information can be fed to a quality-improvement program to avoid such deviations in the future. However, since critical pathways are the tools by which MCOs achieve their goals, they have become increasingly important.

Primary Care Centers

Alternatives to hospitalization and accelerated discharge to ambulatory care settings create a demand for sophisticated, comprehensive, and well-coordinated services in the primary care setting. Managed care sites can offer rich concentrations of primary care resources to meet client needs. Such a setting is conducive to delegating responsibility to the most cost-effective, medically appropriate provider. The ambulatory care facilities of MCOs are ideal settings for psychiatric–mental health nurses to function in the role of primary mental health care provider.

Generally, psychiatric–mental health nurses in MCOs perform mental health assessments, monitor chronic illness, provide direct care for acute problems, and facilitate health-promotion groups. Examples of some of the health-promotion activities nurses can initiate in primary care settings are stress management, parenting education, violence prevention, bereavement counseling, suicide prevention, and teen pregnancy prevention.

Triage Services

Psychiatric–mental health nurses provide effective *triage* services in the ambulatory care and primary care settings. Triage involves determining the severity of the illness and the need for immediate care in order to direct care and ensure the efficient use of medical and nursing staff and facilities. In the triage role, you often act as the *gatekeeper* of the system. You essentially decide who will use the system and at what level of care. The gatekeeping function is discussed in the case management section of this chapter.

Many factors need to be considered in the role of triage nurse. The common denominator in all instances is allocation of resources for ensuring quality and cost effectiveness. You may be performing face-to-face assessments or telephone triage. One of the most important required skills is good listening ability, coupled with an ability to collect information for making a decision about appropriate intervention. Information may be fragmented, and interviews with several people may be required to provide a comprehensive view of the client's presenting problem.

Triage clinicians in mental health care settings provide short-term, episodic intervention to members enrolled in the plan and simplify access to appropriate points of service in the system. FIGURE 12-4 ■ on page 242 depicts the triage process and the complexity of options available to clinicians in managed care. Collaboration and consultation are important processes nurses use when performing this first-point-of-contact service.

When triaging, you use a variety of nursing skills to evaluate the client's presenting problem. Using listening skills, you combine verbal and nonverbal data with information available in the client's medical record, as in the clinical example that follows.

CLINICAL EXAMPLE

Margaret, a 35-year-old woman, is referred after several visits for minor medical problems. You note from the record a pattern of medication refills for antianxiety medication from the primary care provider. You also notice she has been referred for mental health care on two other occasions but has failed to keep these appointments. This information is valuable as you begin your assessment.

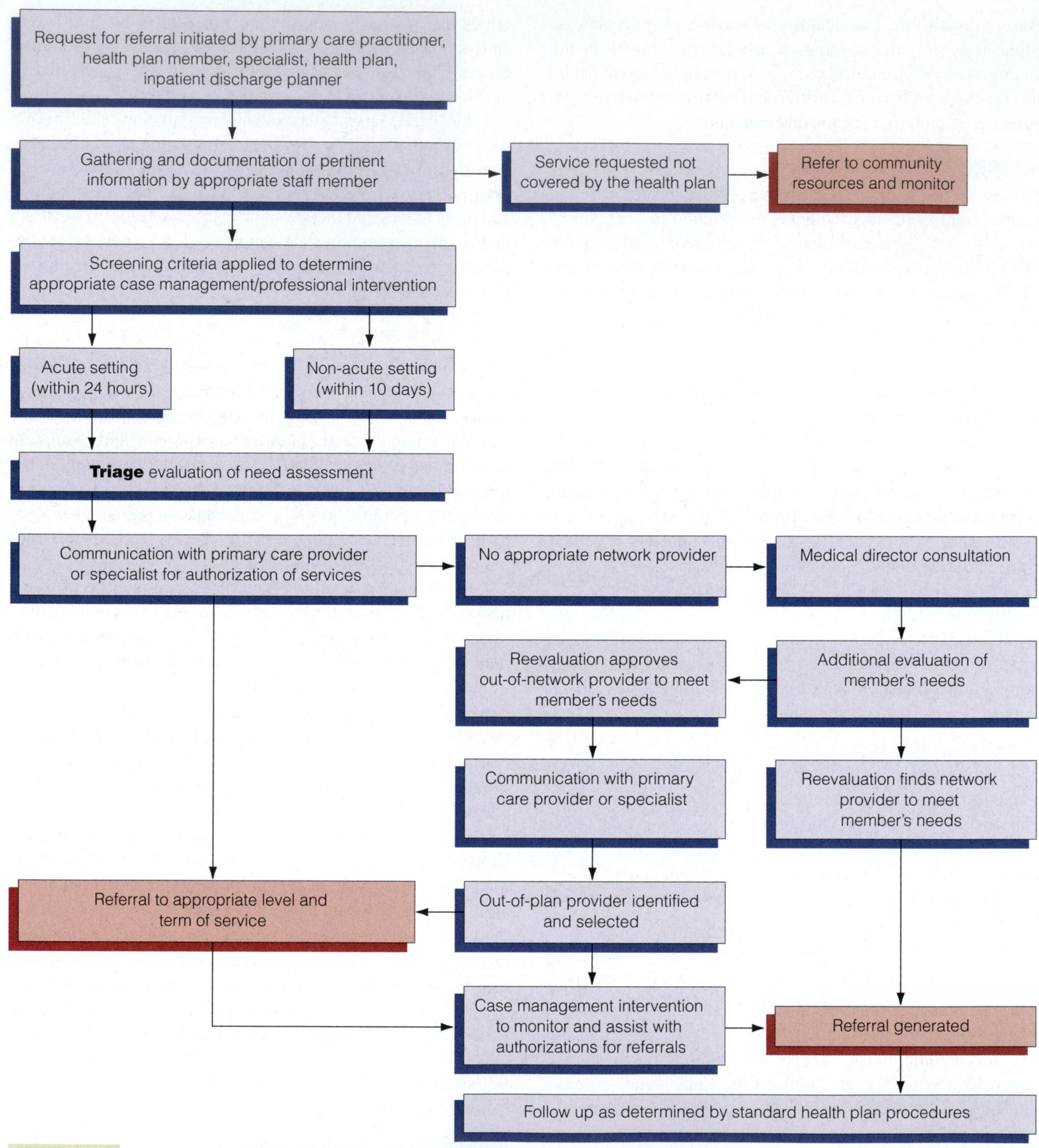

FIGURE 12-4 ■ Psychiatric–mental health nursing triage process.

After completing the assessment, your next step is to decide a course of action. Using the nursing process, you begin to plan appropriate interventions. Choices include no intervention, immediate intervention, intervention within 24 hours, or routine appointment. Your further options include referral to a private mental health provider's office, a public clinic, or a hospital emergency room.

Employer-Based Clinics

As managed health care continues to develop new models, employers are becoming increasingly sophisticated in developing systems to meet the needs of their employees. Employers may establish on-site clinics with an MCO. The office is staffed with MCO employees. Here the psychiatric–mental health nurse might be asked to serve as a consultant, counseling at the site a day or two per week, seeing clients referred through the primary care providers in the employer-based clinic.

MCOs as a Practice Environment

There are several other aspects of practicing in managed care settings in mental health that are unique to this delivery system. These include boundaries, legal issues, treatment and medication compliance, unrealistic member expectations, and continuity of care.

Boundaries

Boundaries are personal limits we use to differentiate between one event and another. Working as a clinician in the managed-care arena exposes one to demands, crises, time pressures, schedules, and other stressful events inherent in any health care delivery system. It is crucial for you to maintain adequate boundaries to prevent burnout, maintain objectivity, and be comfortable setting limits with consumers.

Psychiatric–mental health nurses working in MCOs need orientation to the structure, goals, and operating philosophy to become part of the culture of the practice setting. Nurses whose own values are congruent with the MCO will be less susceptible to burnout and able to feel satisfied in practice. Burnout prevention is discussed in Chapter 3∞.

Legal Issues

In traditional fee-for-service practice, when a judge mandates treatment, there is usually acceptance of the client into the system for service. Service is delivered on demand, and then a charge is issued to the client. In MCOs, court-ordered treatment is negotiated on a case-by-case basis. What this means is that not every person with a request for court-ordered treatment will automatically receive this service.

CLINICAL EXAMPLE

A transportation worker who has received his third DUI (driving under the influence) citation requests service. The member has already received two previous episodes of treatment and is not covered for services in the current calendar year.

A decision must then be made about how to respond to this request. These sometimes thorny and difficult legal cases are often referred for individual case review to the medical director.

A decision may be made to allow for a "flexing" of benefits or authorization of out-of-plan services. In flexing, an outpatient mental health care benefit may be converted to an inpatient benefit to allow for the needed hospitalization. The psychiatric–mental health nurse sometimes plays the role of client advocate, helping negotiate uncharted territory in these unusual circumstances.

Treatment Adherence

Issues of compliance or adherence (the term we use in this text) are more readily observed in MCOs, particularly in closed panel systems where appointment clerks, clinicians, and pharmacists may work side by side. Perhaps because services are prepaid, MCO consumers find it easier not to keep scheduled appointments. This is sometimes referred to as DNKA (did not keep appointment). In mental health care, this behavior has clinical and administrative significance. It is important to note that different MCOs deal with this problem in different ways. One alternative is to set strict limits and not allow future appointments to be scheduled until the client makes copayment for all missed appointments. Another is to require clients to wait their turn in line for the next available appointment. Finally, the DNKA must be handled as a therapeutic issue in the therapy.

Some MCOs "double-book" appointments, relying on no-shows to balance out the schedule. When these missed appointments occur following hospitalization for a major psychiatric episode of illness, the clinician must aggressively maintain contact with the client. The importance of adhering to an after-care plan to avoid relapse is crucial. Phone calls, letters, or catching clients while they are visiting another department in the facility are all useful interventions. Some MCOs have developed transportation systems such as a free bus to ensure that clients keep appointments and follow after-care plans.

Medication Adherence

Encouraging medication adherence follows many principles used in other settings. Nurses in MCOs often work in collaborative relationships with other providers to ensure adherence, especially when uncomfortable side effects are responsible for a client's failure to adhere. When medication copayments are low, appointments are available, and transportation is accessible, the likelihood of adherence is increased. In the MCO setting, the primary care provider is an ally of the mental health care team. Primary care providers who see clients for routine medical problems are in a position to reinforce the importance of staying on psychotropic drugs. Often a discussion of side effects eliminates confusion and increases understanding of the medicine's effect. When side effects are a problem, MCO nurses often contact the prescriber to arrange for a change in medication. Managed-care pharmacists can also help the mental health team ensure that clients adhere to their medication regimens.

Unrealistic Member Expectations

In a managed-care setting, you will be challenged to resolve unrealistic member expectations. Members' understanding of the managed care philosophy is crucial for effective and responsible health behaviors, including expectations of available services.

The member's entitlement expectations is the member's understanding of the care he or she expects to receive. Entitlement expectations often differ from the specific provisions of the health plan contract. Examples of excluded mental health services of several large MCO contracts appear in Box 12-2.

Health plan members often do not consider what type of mental health benefits they have purchased until they are in

Box 12-2 Mental Health Services Often Excluded from Typical Managed Care Plans

Following are some examples of mental health services that are not included in typical MCO plans:

- Psychiatric or substance abuse therapy on court order, unless plan-approved as medically necessary
- Psychological testing, except for diagnosis or treatment of a psychiatric disorder
- Marriage counseling or treatment for stress, except when connected to treatment for a DSM-IV-TR psychiatric disorder
- Smoking cessation, obesity treatment, weight reduction, aversion therapy, custodial care, V code conditions (non–DSM-IV-TR conditions that may be a focus of clinical attention such as noncompliance with treatment, malingering, age-related cognitive decline, etc., as discussed in Appendix A), autism, learning disabilities, mental retardation, congenital disorders
- Experimental treatment (psychosurgery, megavitamin therapy, codependence therapy, or treatment for sexual addiction)

MEDIALINK American Psychological Association

crisis. The memory of television commercials suggesting inpatient care as the only solution to adolescent adjustment problems is often the first point of reference for many parents. Your role as consumer educator is crucial to helping your clients understand how to use their managed-care plans in a manner that is satisfactory for all concerned.

Continuity of Care

Some MCOs are seamless delivery systems. In other words, consumers can move from one level of care to the next while remaining in the same delivery system. In this sense, members of an MCO can be considered to be in continuous therapy. This has clinical implications that require new conceptual frameworks for treatment. Primary care services tend to focus on the present impasse, while secondary care services are geared to examine the underlying obstacle. It is essential to the healing process that both are coordinated.

Ethics in Managed Mental Health Care

In effect, managed mental health care creates a situation in which the mental health professional no longer controls decisions about the type of treatment or the setting (inpatient versus outpatient). The autonomy and independent judgment of the nurse are limited in managed care environments (Smoyak, 2000). Instead, decisions—such as two therapy sessions each week or outpatient drug rehabilitation—are monitored by an agent employed by insurers. Therapists in managed mental health care settings speak of a culture clash between themselves and managed care companies (Cohen, Marecek, & Gillham, 2006). They feel that some practices undermine therapeutic work and the therapist–client relationship and violate their standard of care and professional ethics. Clearly, managed psychiatric care raises serious ethical issues related to client autonomy of choice (see Chapter 13) regarding therapist and site, the integrity of the nurse–client relationship, and the risk that nonadherent psychiatric clients may be denied access to additional treatment.

Four principles to guide you through the ethical dilemmas posed by managed mental health care systems are:

1. Recognize that as a clinician, you are dedicated to caring for clients in a relationship of fidelity and, at the same time, must act as a steward of society's scarce mental health care resources.
2. Recognize that it is ethically correct to recommend the least costly treatment unless you have evidence that a more costly intervention will yield a superior outcome.
3. Recognize that you need to advocate for the ethical principle of justice in managed mental health care situations so that cost savings with one client are used to meet the mental health care needs of another, not pay off an insurance company's debts.
4. Recognize that it is your responsibility to discuss the situation openly with your clients so that they understand the reimbursable parameters of their care and can act in their own interests.

A mental health consumer's bill of rights that also examines insurance coverage and managed care plans in light of the principles identified in the bill is located at http://www.apa.org/topics/rights and can be accessed through the Companion Website for this book.

There is an ongoing moral debate about the ethics of applying managed care to psychiatric clients. Be prepared to sharpen your ethical reasoning skills and tools.

CASE MANAGEMENT

Rapid changes in the health care system have contributed to client feelings of being overwhelmed and confused about how to use services effectively. In many systems, clients no longer rely on a single provider or institution to shepherd them through an episode of illness. **Case management** is one strategy that has evolved in response to the shift in focus from inpatient to community care (Hangan, 2006). The central element that differentiates case management from other types of care is the coordination of one episode of care across the multiple settings of the care continuum. Each chapter in Unit 4 discusses specific case management stretegies for each mental disorder.

The fundamental focus of case management is to integrate, coordinate, and advocate for individuals, families, and groups requiring extensive services. Like the nursing process, case management focuses on the following elements:

- Assessment and problem identification
- Planning
- Procurement, delivery, and coordination of service
- Monitoring to ensure that the multiple service needs of the client are met

The process of case management enhances quality by preventing unnecessary hospitalization, focusing treatment goals in least-restrictive settings, and preventing the duplication and fragmentation of services.

Case Manager Role

Nurses who perform the case manager role must be vested with the authority and accountability necessary to negotiate with complex systems and a wide diversity of providers and populations. Nurses are particularly prepared to function in this role by the very nature of the profession. This is especially evident in the managed care setting where clients from diverse backgrounds sometimes struggle to negotiate a new system of health care delivery. We know that race and poverty are factors that impede a client's access to mental health services and that race and ethnicity affect how clients use mental health services. Our racial diversity as a nation is increasing, and case management can help individuals and families who bring unique needs and cultural experiences to the managed care setting.

As case managers, nurses can provide physical assessment or illness-detection skills. An additional factor contributing to the natural fit between nurses and consumers is the increased emphasis on psychobiology and pharmacology in helping clients cope with alterations in their mental health.

Gatekeeping and Facilitating

The service you provide as a case manager is one of gatekeeping and facilitating. As gatekeeper, you serve as the client's initial contact for care and referrals, as in the clinical example that follows.

CLINICAL EXAMPLE

James, the case manager for Jerrod, a client with bipolar disorder, was contacted when Jerrod arrived at an emergency department in a manic state. Because James had knowledge of Jerrod's prior history and treatment, he was able to determine if inpatient care was required. James also had access to recent laboratory studies regarding Jerrod's lithium carbonate levels and also had an established relationship with family members.

In other words, case management helps clients and their caregivers make informed decisions, such as whether the client needs hospitalization, based on client needs, abilities, resources, and personal preferences.

In a case of recurring substance abuse, the nurse case manager can help a family make informed decisions, taking into consideration the client's health status and diagnosis, treatment plan, payment resources, and health care options. This facilitation aspect of case management assures that clients receive care that is appropriate, individualized, cost effective, and has optimal outcomes.

Client Advocacy

Agencies that provide client services must have clear statements regarding client rights and responsibilities. The case manager often refers to these in negotiating with both client and system regarding appropriate referrals and authorizations for treatment.

A statement of rights helps focus our awareness on the most fundamental aspect of the case manager role, that of being a client advocate. While there are many and varied models of case management, the nurse who defines this role as client advocate will have the greatest chance of success. When you carry out your role in this framework, you bring to the multidisciplinary team skills and knowledge that extend beyond biologic or pathologic aspects of care. You view the client through a holistic perspective. You piece together the fragmented pieces of the client's care. This cannot be done in the isolation of an office or simply by telephone. It requires active, on-site presence, interviews, meetings, attendance at treatment planning conferences, and appropriate documentation.

In the role of case manager the nurse may be caught in the middle of conflicting value systems. For example, clients with alcoholism or bulimia have been treated traditionally with intensive, extended inpatient treatment programs. Managed care plans may authorize this treatment only in an outpatient setting. The nurse must respond to clients' need for autonomy in making decisions regarding treatment as well as negotiate within the limitations of the managed care plan. Case managers must use creativity and flexibility in negotiating among the conflicting needs of several parties. Clients and families who are accustomed to specific treatment models for illnesses with relapse potential often feel confused and misunderstood when new treatment approaches are suggested that appear economically motivated.

Assessment Phase Challenges

Nurses who function as case managers must interact with all members of the health care team. Trust, mutual support, and clear communication among team members is necessary before case management services can be implemented. Meetings with administrative personnel and tactful systems-entry strategies must be employed while laying the groundwork for a case management program. Careful introduction of the case management role, which differentiates it from medical care management, is necessary in clarifying role responsibilities. Other members of the team may feel threatened by the addition of a case manager and view it as an indictment of their own role performance. When system administration can orient its members to the case manager's role, there is a higher level of acceptance of the service as augmenting client care rather than interfering with it.

Planning Phase Challenges

In this phase of care, the nurse can bring valuable information concerning benefits, limits, family resources, expectations, and other pertinent data to the treatment planning table. Using the formal and informal support systems, the treatment team is able to set mutually agreed-upon goals with desired outcomes and can begin to plan action steps using intended time frames or critical pathways as a guide.

MEDIALINK Critical Thinking Exercise: Case Manager Role

Implementation Phase Challenges

The next phase of the case management process is to ensure that the client gets needed care. In some systems the case manager may be asked to deliver care. However, this approach is not in the best interest of the client because the case manager's role is to remain the objective, internal consultant, looking at the whole picture. When pulled into delivering the care, the case manager loses perspective and may find important issues clouded. For example, a case management nurse who is asked to function as the client's primary therapist because the primary nurse is overloaded will sacrifice time and resources needed to monitor the quality of care delivered and perhaps lose objectivity.

Keep in mind during the implementation phase that your role involves conflict resolution. To set limits tactfully, arbitrate differences, and maintain successful outcomes for all, you need patience, maturity, and experience. The case manager is also called on to provide additional data or client/family education where a denial or extension of service is in question. As client advocate, you may identify gaps in care that require action in the community, in a treatment facility, or within the nursing system. Nurse case managers are among the best consultants to nursing departments for improving quality because they view problems in the system from the client's perspective.

Evaluation Phase Challenges

The case manager's role in evaluation consists of continuous monitoring of intervention responses and progress toward desired outcomes. This may include medication monitoring for dosage and adherence, as well as monitoring client response to other therapies. You may interview the client directly to gather this information, and then compare it with what is recorded in the medical record. Inconsistent data are always a red flag for intervention by the case manager. Perhaps the process is moving too slowly or the client is not an active participant in the care plan. Once outcomes are achieved and the client is discharged, there must be a mechanism for ongoing quality improvement based on recommended standards of nursing practice. Critical incidents and inconsistencies in the care must be communicated in an ongoing, systematic program of continuous quality improvement. This information is ultimately used to measure provider and facility performance for contract renewal decisions.

THE THERAPEUTIC ENVIRONMENT IN HOSPITAL-BASED CARE

The **therapeutic environment** is the purposeful use of people, resources, and events in the client's immediate environment to:

- Ensure safety.
- Promote optimal functioning in the activities of daily living.
- Develop or improve interpersonal skills.
- Enhance the capacity to live independently outside the institutional setting.
- Various terms such as *therapeutic milieu, therapeutic community*, and *milieu therapy* have been used to identify treatment environment philosophies. The terms are often used interchangeably and refer to the impact of the authority structure and the roles and relationships that affect decision making and client interactions.

In milieu therapy models, organizational hierarchy is flattened, therapeutic potential is seen in multiple relationships, and the client assumes personal responsibility for behavior. Originally, therapeutic milieu programs were at least several months long and had homogenous client populations. Today, we incorporate milieu therapy principles in all treatment settings.

A Unique Role for Nurses

Nursing's 24-hour daily contact with clients in inpatient treatment settings provides a unique opportunity for creating and managing the therapeutic environment as a special domain. No other discipline literally shares with clients the living space of the treatment unit. Nurses individually influence the environment through their presence. Nurses provide human contact, support, and direction; they share philosophy and values; and they establish collaborative work relationships. Nurses can indirectly influence client behavior by the assessment and manipulation of both the physical and social environments. These responsibilities make it increasingly important that you review and explore your attitudes about organizational rules and client autonomy and self-determination. The Your Self-Awareness feature that follows lists some questions that merit your thoughtful consideration.

While many milieu principles remain relevant in current treatment environments, trends such as short lengths of stay, high client acuity, and resurgence of the biomedical model require reexamination of the relevance of the assumptions of the therapeutic community in acute inpatient care. The emergence of subacute treatment settings and community-based rehabilitation programs also offers new arenas to implement therapeutic environment principles. A continuing challenge of psychiatric–mental health nursing is to synthesize a new model that includes the best aspects of both the psychobiologic and therapeutic milieu models.

External Factors

A variety of external factors, discussed in Box 12-3, affect the therapeutic environment. These issues have an impact on the treatment environment in several ways. It is more difficult to develop group cohesiveness and involvement with other clients' progress when group membership changes frequently. Symptom acuity may also limit a client's ability to be actively involved with the treatment issues of others. Staff roles may be more traditional and typical of medical care settings, and this may create more hierarchical relationships. In actual practice, these factors will be influenced by the program's attitude toward privacy, autonomy, safety, and group well-being.

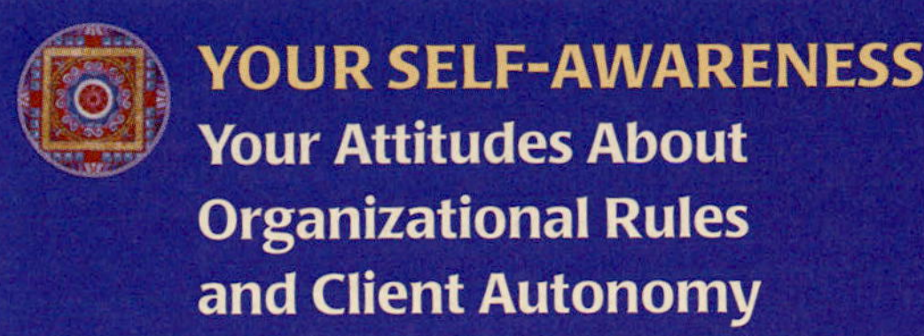

YOUR SELF-AWARENESS
Your Attitudes About Organizational Rules and Client Autonomy

To increase self-awareness of your own attitudes about organizational rules in a treatment setting, ask yourself the following questions:

- What kinds of client behaviors make me uncomfortable or angry?
- What unit rules are most important?
- How do I feel when a client breaks a unit rule?
- What do I do in response to a client who breaks a unit rule?

To increase self-awareness of your own attitudes about client autonomy and self-determination, ask yourself the following questions:

- Am I comfortable with clients deciding what the program's schedule, activities, or rules will be?
- Am I comfortable with clients deciding their own treatment goals?
- How do I feel when a client chooses a treatment goal that is not the same as the one I would have selected or that I do not think is in the client's "best interest"?
- Should clients be allowed to comment on each other's behavior or treatment goals?

Privacy

Individuals routinely vary their patterns of contact with and withdrawal from others, as well as the information they share about themselves. The very nature of psychiatric hospitalization conflicts with the need for privacy. Intimate personal details are examined and discussed, and there may be no opportunity to escape staff surveillance or social contact. Nurses must respect a client's privacy by keeping surveillance and monitoring to the minimum necessary for client safety, honoring the confidentiality of personal information, and maintaining routine social practices such as knocking on the door and waiting for an answer before entering a bedroom or bathroom.

Autonomy

The rules and schedules that characterize psychiatric–mental health treatment settings usually promote the management of groups of people and may interfere with the personal decision making and autonomy of the individual client. Although the ability of clients with mental disorders to carry out age-appropriate roles may be significantly impaired, the therapeutic environment provides opportunities for normal functioning according to each client's abilities.

Safety

Mentally disordered clients may pose significant safety hazards to themselves or others because of suicidal or assaultive behaviors, poor judgment, or confusion. Efforts to maintain client safety may deprive clients of privacy and autonomy. For example, clients requiring close surveillance have little or no privacy; nurses may intervene to override decisions made by clients whose judgment is impaired.

Group Well-Being

A client's behavior may be disruptive or detrimental to the overall well-being of other clients. Nurses may need to monitor or manage certain clients to maximize the common good. As with the concept of safety, the individual's privacy and autonomy may be violated when group well-being is considered primary. (Some philosophers, however, consider that the group's well-being enhances the individual's autonomy.) Individual autonomy, individual well-being, and group well-being are often conflicting issues. Nurses must be sensitive to situations in which clashes occur.

Therapeutic Environment Principles

Some of the current ideas about the therapeutic environment, particularly the philosophic values, do not easily lend themselves to quick evaluation or manipulation. Staff must

Box 12-3 External Factors That Affect the Therapeutic Environment

- Client groups are not homogenous.
- Clients frequently have dual diagnoses, such as psychiatric and substance abuse problems or psychiatric and medical problems.
- Managed mental health care organizations increasingly limit access to inpatient care to those who are a danger to themselves or others.
- The length of inpatient stays has decreased to an average of about 7 days.
- Treatment is closely monitored to determine the need for medication, seclusion, restraint, or other intensive supervision.
- Case managers quickly assess discharge planning needs and obstacles and coordinate access to other levels of services.
- There has been a resurgence of the biologic model of care as psychopharmacology (see Chapters 7 and 32) and other somatic treatments such as ECT (see Chapter 17) and transcranial magnetic stimulation (see Chapters 7 and 33) offer specialized treatment approaches to symptom reduction.
- Clients with multiple medical problems and dementias may also require more traditional medical interventions.
- Staff members now have diverse and specialized training and are expected to work as multidisciplinary teams to address individualized treatment goals.
- Regulatory agencies, client rights groups, and professional practice standards establish criteria for the therapeutic environment.

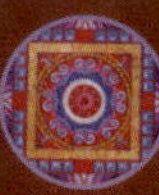

YOUR INTERVENTION STRATEGIES
Guidelines for Working with Clients in the Therapeutic Environment

Strategy	Rationale
Safety and the Structural Environment	
■ Assess appropriate structural security, including locked doors, nonbreakable glass, seclusion room, silent alarms, and devices such as concave nonbreakable mirrors to view blind spots.	■ Security must be appropriate to client acuity and type of treatment program.
■ Provide unit rules and staff policy related to acceptable conduct.	■ Rules should be clearly stated.
■ Implement procedures and training for use of time-outs, seclusion, restraint, special precautions, and search and management of client personal belongings such as razors.	■ Staff training promotes consistency and safe implementation of security and client management techniques.
Structure	
■ Orient client to behavior expectations through multiple sources, including handbook, bulletin boards, community meeting, and identification of a primary nurse.	■ Clients are unfamiliar with expectations; new information may need to be repeated.
■ Delineate program schedule and expectations for client participation.	■ Clear expectations and written schedule promote client independence.
Support	
■ Guide and monitor client activities by being visible and available.	■ Demonstrates role-modeling skills and provides an opportunity for informal assessment and interaction.
■ Implement least restrictive interventions such as confirming messages, calming, personal control, setting limits, and medication to minimize the need for more restrictive behavior management.	■ Least restrictive interventions promote client autonomy and demonstrate respect.
■ Enhance normality of the environment through use of clocks, calendars, and furniture.	■ Reduces the institutional qualities of environment.
■ Promote opportunities for self-care decision making, and activities that prepare for return to community.	■ Reduces dependence on hospital; promotes positive transition to community.
■ Integrate client's existing social supports, including family and spiritual support system to reinforce goals and interventions.	■ Promotes family involvement and empowerment; extends opportunities for positive outcome by involving social supports.
■ Monitor and discuss staff concerns to promote communication, identify parallel issues, and ensure a positive social climate.	■ Staff interactions affect the general atmosphere and capacity for therapeutic interventions.
■ Support cultural diversity and staff self-awareness related to issues of client rights and social control.	■ Demonstrates respect and supports client autonomy and independence.
Socialization	
■ Orient client and family to the steps and process of psychiatric treatment.	■ Clients and family may be unfamiliar with psychiatric treatment; may have misinformation.
■ Identify fears and stereotypes client/family may have about "brain surgery, shock treatment, or padded cells," as well as concerns about how psychotherapy works.	■ Reduces fear and encourages engaging in treatment.
■ Educate client/family about legal rights of psychiatric clients and confidentiality of information.	■ Engages client and family in treatment process.
■ Encourage client participation in determining and evaluating treatment goals.	■ Promotes involvement and empowerment.
Self-Understanding	
■ Encourage formal and informal group participation.	■ Provides opportunities to gain social skills.
■ Emphasize commonalities of experience.	■ Reduces sense of isolation and hopelessness.
■ Identify skills gained through hospital experience.	■ Offers hope and focuses on the future.
■ Instill hope and social connectedness.	■ Reduces isolation.
■ Encourage client feedback about satisfaction with treatment and hospital experience.	■ Promotes empowerment.

consider the clients' levels of functioning as well as the discrete features of the structural environment. What is suitable for one group of clients may be too strict or too lenient for another. Some general guidelines for incorporating therapeutic environment principles in your work with clients are in the Your Intervention Strategies feature on page 248. Selected guidelines are discussed later in this chapter.

Restrictiveness

The restrictiveness of the treatment environment is characterized according to physical, psychologic, and social dimensions. The physical environment includes the nature of the setting, such as location in the community, security, and options for behavior control (e.g., seclusion). The psychological environment is composed of staff and client backgrounds, behavior, attitudes, and values. The social environment consists of the rules and regulations that govern the operation of the setting as well as the treatment standards for managing client behavior.

The importance of evaluating a program's restrictiveness stems from mental health legislation mandating care according to the least restrictive alternative. This concept is heavily influenced by ethical and legal theories that hold individual autonomy paramount. Thus, program rules or staff attitudes that interfere with a client's autonomy would be considered more restrictive than a program that supported autonomy and self-determination. (See Chapter 13 ∞.)

A facility's physical structure is a major focus of attention in pursuing the least restrictive alternatives for treatment. Physical restrictiveness is ranked according to the degree of interference with client independence. The physical structure of many institutions—such as locked doors, communal living arrangements, and limited access to community resources—interferes with client freedom of movement and individuality. Thus, facilities located in huge hospital complexes, which do not interface with the community's shopping, religious, or entertainment activities or provide for client privacy, have a more restrictive environment than community-based settings.

Orienting Client and Family

Clients and their families or significant others need to be informed about all aspects of the therapeutic environment. Encourage them to relate their concerns and questions about what to expect during the treatment experience. Be sure to accomplish the following:

1. Orient and educate client, family, and significant others about hospitalization and treatment by reviewing the clinical problems, treatments, and behavioral outcomes that are the focus of hospitalization or treatment in a community facility.
2. Engage clients, family, and significant others in the treatment process by encouraging them to identify personal goals and participate in evaluating the course of treatment.

The Partnering with Clients and Families feature below lists questions they may ask. Be sure to include information on all unasked questions in your health teaching orientation activities.

Safety and the Structural Environment

Although building features are beyond your ability to influence, other aspects of the physical structure are open to your interventions. As the nurse, you should:

1. Evaluate whether security is sufficient.
2. Assess the advantages and necessity of the security.
3. Assess whether the security has any detrimental impact.
4. Consider whether the security advantages could be accomplished through some other intervention that does not have a detrimental impact.
5. Reevaluate structural controls implemented for specific reasons to determine whether they are no longer relevant and should be discontinued.

The following clinical example illustrates a structural control based on an unclear rationale.

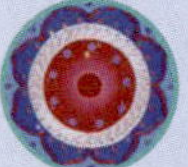

PARTNERING WITH CLIENTS AND FAMILIES

TEACHING ABOUT LEGAL RIGHTS

When you orient clients and their families to the therapeutic environment, be prepared to answer their questions. Answers to the questions following should be individualized to reflect each unit's treatment philosophy and the specific legal rights of the client according to the state in which you practice.

1. What psychiatric treatment can I expect to receive?
2. Will I receive medications? Do I have to take the medications?
3. Do I have to share a room with someone else?
4. Will I have to tell other clients about my problems?
5. Will you write down information that I tell you about myself or my family?
6. Is this unit a safe place for me?
7. Can I leave the unit on passes?
8. What happens if I no longer want to be a client in this hospital?
9. What happens if I have a disagreement with someone?
10. Who are the staff here? Who can I talk to if I have questions?
11. Can I smoke?
12. When is bedtime?
13. What time are the meals? Can I keep my own snacks?
14. Is there a way for me to wash my own clothes?
15. Is there a telephone I can use?
16. When are the visiting hours?
17. Can I write letters and get mail?
18. Can I keep my money with me? Is my personal property safe?
19. Are religious services available?

MediaLink Care Plan: Therapeutic Environment

CLINICAL EXAMPLE

A 15-bed unit in an inpatient setting had laundry facilities for clients to care for their own clothes. A psychotic and confused client put a potted plant through a wash cycle, causing major damage to the washing machine. Staff members locked the laundry facilities to prevent future damage to the machines. The doors remained locked even after the client was discharged, preventing any independent client access to the facilities. Preventing possible future damage to machines became a predominant staff concern.

While locking laundry room doors was intended as a short-term structural solution to avoid further environmental damage, the solution itself created a new problem of interference with self-care performance by more independent clients.

Seclusion and restraint are interventions that use structure to control client behavior in order to implement safety measures. Because seclusion and restraint are highly restrictive interventions that interfere with client autonomy and freedom of movement, it is important to implement alternative steps whenever possible. Chapter 13 discusses the ethical and legal facets of seclusion and restraint, and Chapter 35 discusses how and why seclusion and restraint may be used in clinical settings.

The structural environment should not dehumanize its inhabitants; moreover, it should actively contribute to their improved functioning and comfort. Reality-oriented resources such as the following contribute to a sense of normality:

1. Clocks and calendars to promote time orientation
2. Newspapers to encourage an awareness of social events
3. Ramps and rails to facilitate mobility and movement
4. Furniture arranged to promote interpersonal interaction

Healthy people may take these for granted, but they are critical resources to the impaired client.

Program Structure

Program structure, another aspect of the therapeutic environment, is composed of the schedule and expectations for client treatment and participation. Nurses have a number of opportunities to communicate expectations and to address issues that arise. How expectations are communicated and issues assessed and addressed are strongly influenced by the individual nurse's attitudes toward organization rules in a treatment setting (refer back to the Your Self-Awareness feature on page 247).

Program Rules All clients should be given the regulations of the setting either before or as soon after admission as possible. Although written expectations do not automatically ensure that clients pay attention to the program rules, they provide a clear baseline, serve as reminders, and provide structure for clients. These rules reinforce the staff's commitment to basic safety and specify obligations for all members of the setting. Written expectations may be presented to clients at the time of admission, discussed in community meetings, and used as a reference if a client violates a rule. In some instances, individualized behavioral contracts with specific clients may be necessary. Individualized behavioral contracts are discussed in Chapter 31.

While all programs have a set of rules and regulations, not all use community meetings or client government as an integral part of the program. The latter are more likely to be seen in settings that subscribe to the therapeutic milieu philosophy. These are more likely to be therapeutic communities for children and adolescents or those with eating disorders or substance abuse.

Community Meetings Groups provide an opportunity for clients to solve problems of conflicting interests, experience cooperation with others, share responsibility, and experience leadership in the group. The most common milieu-oriented group in long-term facilities is the community meeting. Its functions include:

- Welcoming new members
- Identifying and discussing unit rules (expectations)
- Discussing aspects of the unit environment such as cleanliness, privacy, radio and television use, or other interpersonal problems that may interfere with the quality of life for the group
- Planning activities

Clients usually chair the community meeting and report on assignments, such as checking for cleanliness of areas of responsibility (e.g., the kitchen or bedrooms). The community meeting is also used to solve problems related to living with a large group of people or living in the hospital unit.

CLINICAL EXAMPLE

Clients on a 25-bed unlocked unit had access to two pay telephones. Both telephones, however, were near the nurses' station, and conversations could be overheard easily. Clients complained in community meeting of the lack of privacy, and a nurse intervened to help them write a letter to the hospital administration. The administration purchased a new cordless telephone that allowed clients to make and receive calls in any area of the unit.

Client Government Some client community groups also grant clients privileges for demonstrating certain behaviors in the community living groups. Clients are expected to take responsibility for themselves and each other and to learn the consequences of their actions. Involving clients in the management of the unit and in therapeutic activities with one another allow opportunities for participation, corrective learning experiences, and the development of new behavior patterns. Feedback is an essential technique for increasing insight and promoting learning. This type of community group, known as **client government**, may be most suitable to intermediate and long-term care settings, where the client group is stable and a group culture evolves over time.

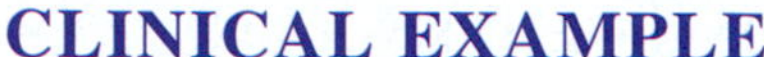

CLINICAL EXAMPLE

The community meeting group of a 20-bed adolescent program bases recommendations for weekend passes on members' requests and the individual's functioning in the client community. Lisa, 14 years old, has a history of running away from home, lying, drug and alcohol abuse, prostitution, and suicide threats. She requested a Saturday day pass, although she did not have specific plans for how she would spend the time. Other clients commented that Lisa had not completed her ward job of checking the cleanliness of the kitchen, and the staff noted that she continued to withdraw from social contacts. The group agreed that Lisa should not receive a pass until she could demonstrate some improved ability to structure her time and interact with others.

Supportive Social Climate

The multiple influences on individual and group behavior may come from external sources such as professional practice standards, regulatory agencies, and laws. The client's attitudes, beliefs, and behaviors, as well as styles of interaction between people, also have an impact on the therapeutic environment.

Nursing routines that limit client self-care can be detrimental to the unit atmosphere, signaling overinvolvement and loss of client autonomy.

CLINICAL EXAMPLE

Acutely psychotic and chronically mentally ill men and women are admitted to a 20-bed locked unit in a large county hospital. Nurses on this unit seem rushed and complain of having no time to discuss nursing care issues or write nursing care plans. A nurse consultant observed work patterns for several days and noted that the staff were involved (frequently unnecessarily) in intimate details of the clients' daily activities. This involvement extended to lighting matches for cigarettes and squeezing toothpaste onto toothbrushes. Simple routines that interfered with client autonomy also controlled the staff by preventing professional performance and relationships.

The nurse consultant in the clinical example assessed that the staff's involvement in the daily details of client activities actually created self-care deficits for clients. The consultant recommended that the staff promote clients' self-care skills in accordance with their actual ability. This resulted in greater client independence and improved staff performance and morale.

Spirituality

Nurses can use the spiritual beliefs of clients to enhance the therapeutic environment. Specific assessment of a client's spiritual beliefs and practices provides the nurse an opportunity to understand their clinical impact and to use spiritual resources available to the client to enhance wellness and coping. Of 48 persons in a psychosocial rehabilitation program, 20 participated in an optional spirituality group, while the other 28 did not. Within 6 months, 100% of the spirituality group participants attained their treatment goals, and 57% in the control group did not (Wong-McDonald, 2007). In another study, 71% of the study population participating in a psychiatric rehabilitation program reported that their spiritual life played a significant role in their recovery (Bussema & Bussema, 2007). The Caring for the Spirit feature on page 252 lists some specific strategies you can use to incorporate spirituality into the therapeutic environment.

Discussion of beliefs enables the nurse to reassure clients who fear that their beliefs will be challenged or minimized in a psychiatric environment. Finally, acknowledging the significant influence of spirituality in American life encourages nurses to recognize and explore their own beliefs in order to minimize the impact of bias in their client interactions.

Remember also that clients come from various cultural backgrounds and their beliefs about spirituality or religion may vary from culture to culture and will be influenced by the degree of cultural assimilation. Strive to provide spiritual resources that are both culturally congruent and culturally competent.

Encouraging a Partnership with Clients and Families

It is important to recognize that, in addition to educating the client and family about the client's illness and treatment, you also have a responsibility to teach them how to implement the principles of the therapeutic environment outside the treatment setting. The goal is to partner with the client and family to reach a mutually agreeable plan for a safe, secure, and supportive living arrangement that meets their needs.

Establishing a Daily Schedule A routine helps clients keep on track and organize their thinking as well as their activities. Suggest that clients:

- Have a routine for waking up, eating, accomplishing daily activities, and resting
- Identify specific tasks that need to be accomplished that day, or skills that need to be performed
- Complete tasks in small, manageable increments
- Take medications as prescribed

Using Positive Communication Skills Misunderstandings and resentments between clients and their family members often result from inadequate, incomplete, or negative communication. Suggest to family members that misunderstandings and resentments can often be eliminated or reduced by following these guidelines as well as those presented in Chapter 10∞:

- Give instructions or directions at the level of the client's ability. This may include verbal prompting along with physical assistance, verbal prompting alone, and, especially, praise for independent performance.

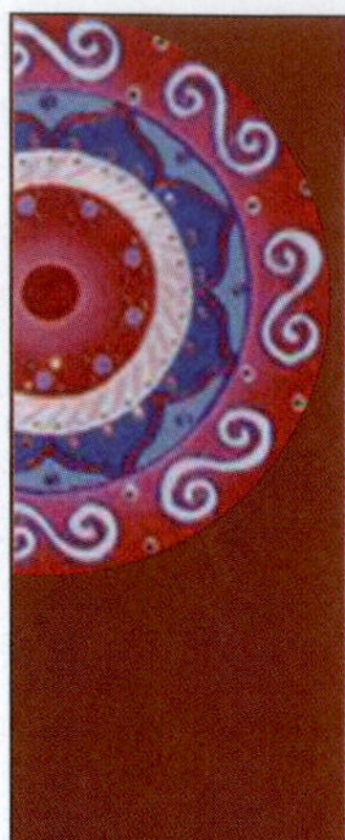

CARING FOR THE SPIRIT

Incorporating Spirituality into the Therapeutic Environment

Incorporate spirituality into the therapeutic environment by:

- Providing opportunities for ceremonies, such as weekly services or holiday celebrations
- Facilitating group discussions based on sharing religious or spiritual beliefs
- Demonstrating tolerance and acceptance of differing beliefs and rituals
- Encouraging the social support that can be provided by acceptance in a community that shares similar beliefs
- Being aware of how one's own beliefs may influence client interactions
- Defining a negative life event in terms of an opportunity for spiritual growth
- Using spiritual music or ceremonies to promote relaxation and reduce anxiety
- Collaborating with clergy or a representative of the client's faith who is accepted by the client to (a) correct misinterpretations of spiritual information that the client may be using maladaptively; (b) translate to clinicians spiritual aspects of a client's decision making; or (c) identify options and alternatives consistent with the faith that support adaptive resolution

- Avoid criticism, argument, and negative reinforcement (see Chapter 31 ∞ for a discussion of negative reinforcement).
- Be empathic by putting yourself in the client's shoes.

Identifying and Participating in Support Groups Support groups help both clients and families to cope (see also Chapter 30 ∞). Families need to recognize signs of family stress and have a plan for respite, perhaps by trading off responsibilities with other family members or significant others, or arranging for client day care or respite care. Families need to take the following steps:

1. Gather information about resources for the client and the family, including social, health care, and long-term financial resources.
2. Choose mental health care workers on the basis of their abilities and the degree of comfort in relating to them.
3. Evaluate the client's options for living arrangements and rehabilitation.

Recognizing Illness Relapse or Exacerbation Clients' symptoms can return (relapse) or worsen (exacerbate). Clients and their families should have:

- A plan for managing symptoms. This might include reducing schedule demands and/or contacting the mental health team or case manager for assistance.
- A plan for emergency behavior management for possible instances of suicide or violence (see Chapters 23 and 35 ∞).

TREATMENT SETTINGS AND PROGRAMS FOR SEVERE AND PERSISTENT MENTAL ILLNESS

The term **severe and persistent mental illness (SPMI)**, or serious mental illness (SMI), came into use because it avoids some of the more undesirable features of its predecessor term used to describe clients, the *chronically mentally ill*. There is no common course for SPMI. This is a clinically diverse population, with different diagnoses and varied patterns of illness. This population also needs a variety of treatment programs.

Psychiatric Disability

The core feature of a severe and persistent disorder is not diagnosis or prognosis, but the experience of *psychiatric disability*. Whether mild or severe, whether ongoing, recurring, or remitting, these disorders require services that go beyond the limits of an acute disease model. Severely and persistently mentally ill individuals have psychiatric disorders that disrupt major role functioning over time, involving some level of disability.

Schizophrenic disorders provide the prototype for SPMI; they are typically disabling, on an intermittent or ongoing basis (see Chapter 16 ∞). However, even schizophrenic disorders vary considerably in terms of symptom profile, pattern of relapse or acute exacerbations, and quality of long-term functioning. Bipolar disorders, recurrent depressions, and severe personality disorders can be just as disabling as some forms of schizophrenia.

In 1980, the World Health Organization (WHO) developed and published a classification system for the phases of a long-term illness. As FIGURE 12-5 ■ shows, the etiology of the disorder, known or unknown, gives rise to changes in structure or functioning, manifested as signs and symptoms and collectively known as *impairment*. If the impairment alters functional performance or behavior, it produces *disability*. When the impairment or disability places the person at a disadvantage within the community, a *handicap* occurs.

The profile that emerges of people with SPMI is that of a highly vulnerable subgroup in our mental health care system, one of the groups least likely to access social resources to protect that vulnerability. This subgroup of our population accounts for the majority of persons being treated in hospital-based systems and in many community programs. They are at risk for developing secondary or concurrent psychiatric problems and for problems associated with socioeconomic status. They account for a significant percentage of homeless persons in our communities. These multiple, interacting problems require complex approaches to services.

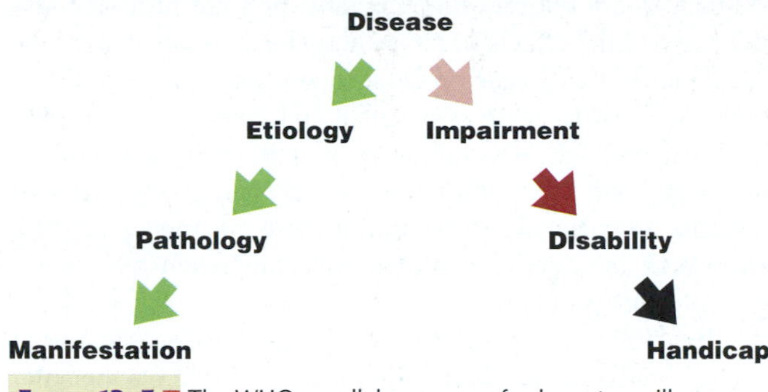

FIGURE 12–5 ■ The WHO parallel sequence for long-term illness.

Community Support Programs for SPMI

Community support programs offer a range of treatment and rehabilitation services, with a case management component to assess needs, coordinate care, and monitor outcomes.

Case Management

Case management is the linchpin for community support programs. The case manager remains a consistent figure in the treatment plan. This avoids duplication and overlap of services. It also avoids shunting vulnerable clients between services because of fluctuations in their clinical status.

Case managers often find that they are fulfilling many roles for their clients that have not been satisfied by other clinical resources, including a sense of social support. High-risk groups such as clients with dual diagnoses, the homeless mentally ill, and frequently hospitalized clients may receive more intensive and clinically sophisticated forms of case management to address their unique service requirements. The case management philosophy has generated enthusiasm in systems for the psychiatrically disabled, because it acknowledges the pervasive nature of their problems, their need for multiple services, and the oscillating or unpredictable course of illness.

Support for Basic Needs

Community mental health programs generally emphasize the importance of self-support and gainful employment whenever possible. However, surveys of the severely mentally ill indicate generally low rates of competitive employment. This situation reflects general economic conditions as well as work disability. In times of high unemployment, people with psychiatric disabilities may be pushed out of jobs that can be performed by competing groups in the labor force. Certainly many mentally ill individuals without "gainful" employment are meaningfully occupied in supported employment and/or volunteer work. However, low rates of competitive employment among members of this population underscore their dependence on income assistance programs such as Supplemental Security Income (SSI).

A community support system helps ensure the severely mentally ill both access to and linkage with appropriate services to secure income and obtain other entitlements (such as health benefits) and basic resources such as food, clothing, and transportation. This may be a more complex task than it appears because accessing financial resources may mean helping the client through difficult applications procedures and even appeals. It may also involve providing money management services to help severely mentally ill individuals who cannot budget their monthly income independently.

Residential Services

Recent reports continue to document the lack of affordable and decent housing options for many of the severely mentally ill and their consequent concentration in what may be marginal or unsafe areas. Many of the severely and persistently mentally ill live with families, but those who live alone frequently depend on residential hotels and boarding homes. It is difficult to generalize about the quality of these housing options because they vary a great deal. For example, some boarding arrangements encourage autonomy and provide a warm, stable environment for residents. Other arrangements, however, fall far below standards that should be applied to living environments for the chronically disabled.

The question of housing satisfaction can also be highly subjective. Some people prefer the privacy of a hotel, despite what may be other negative features, such as location or small living space. Other people prefer a more cozy, homelike environment such as the one in FIGURE 12-6 ■. Programs with an active treatment component may be attractive to some people, but others appreciate a fairly calm and nondemanding environment despite its monotony. For this reason, a community support system focuses not only on accessing some form of acceptable housing but on evaluating the quality of that housing for the individual, working with the client to find "a good fit."

Medication Management

Medication regimens are the mainstay of treatment programs for the severely and persistently mentally ill. Research on the efficacy of medication, particularly neuroleptic regimens for schizophrenia, demonstrates that these agents reduce rates of relapse and hospital readmission. However, they have not been problem-free. Medication regimens demand adherence, tolerance of temporary

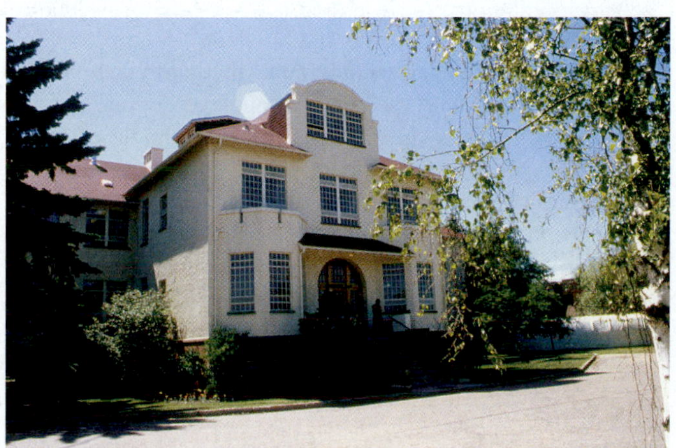

FIGURE 12-6 ■ A halfway house for transitional care after discharge from a hospital-based unit.
Source: Holly Skodol Wilson, RN, PhD.

side effects, and acceptance of the risk of long-term problems such as tardive dyskinesia. Secondary effects of medications can be uncomfortable and embarrassingly visible (e.g., tongue thrusting).

Medication services for the severely and persistently mentally ill should address the impact of medications on quality of life and should promote collaboration with clients to develop a regimen that is tolerable and beneficial. *Depot medication therapy*, usually consisting of an injection every 2 to 4 weeks, does not require the client to take medications several times a day and is a valuable strategy for some people. Current advances in psychopharmacology have produced new classes of medications that may prove less uncomfortable and socially limiting than standard treatments and may help people who have been resistant to medication, or nonadherent, in the past. The introduction of newer therapies makes the medication component of community care all the more important.

CLINICAL EXAMPLE

Ms. Linnea is a 57-year-old widow who came into the medication clinic for her monthly injection, accompanied by her case manager. Ms. Linnea has carried a diagnosis of schizophrenia, paranoid type, for many years but she was maintained well with outpatient care and medications, requiring only brief crisis intervention and two short hospital stays by the time she was 50.

After her husband died, Ms. Linnea had a severe decompensation, experiencing frightening hallucinations and delusions, and was threatening her neighbors. Police were called and she was hospitalized. Ms. Linnea was stabilized on depot medications and was referred to a community-support program for assistance with both housing and rehabilitation. A case manager helped Ms. Linnea apply for SSI, arranged for a shared apartment, facilitated medication and clinic appointments, visited her weekly, and encouraged regular participation in a social rehabilitation program. Ms. Linnea has not required hospitalization in six years. Although she still "hears voices," she is able to monitor her symptoms and advises her son or her case manager when her symptoms increase.

Outpatient Treatment

Traditional outpatient psychotherapies that address *problems in living* may not meet the needs of all severely and persistently mentally ill persons because disabled people often require a broader range of support services to function well in the community. Many of the severely mentally ill also require rehabilitation interventions that address their specific functional deficits and treatment goals, rather than insight-oriented therapies. Nevertheless, these clients need individual, family, and group treatments that are sensitive to their particular problems and needs.

Crisis Stabilization

The severely and persistently mentally ill are at risk for acute exacerbations of an illness. This may be particularly true during times of stress or transition. But in some cases, acute exacerbations are entirely unpredictable and are probably less indicative of the effects of environmental stressors than of the fluctuations of a disease process. In any case, this population requires access to acute assessment and treatment services as part of a package of community support including 24-hour emergency and crisis units and outreach programs. Nursing expertise is extremely important in these emergency settings because of the need for skilled and comprehensive assessment of acute problems.

In addition to the need for crisis stabilization because of acute exacerbation of psychiatric illness, the severely mentally ill are also frequent victims of violent crime. More than one-fourth of people with severe mental illness were the victims of violent crime in the 1-year period of a study that compared the incidence of victimization of severely mentally ill persons with the general population rate in the National Crime Victimization Survey (Teplin, McClelland, Abram, & Weiner, 2005). Crisis stabilization is often required in these situations as well.

General Health Care

The severely mentally ill are a medically underserved group in the community, with needs in the areas of primary health care, dental care, and vision care. Health needs are most pronounced in such subgroups as substance-abusing clients and the elderly mentally ill, who have concurrent physical disorders. However, many of the severely mentally ill are to some extent at risk from lifestyle factors (problematic housing or nutrition) or from the consequences of psychiatric treatment (problematic medication side effects or medication interactions). Any person with a serious psychiatric diagnosis risks underdiagnosis of medical illness by both primary care and psychiatric providers.

In psychiatric services, many clinicians focus on mental disorders with inadequate attention to the total person. Only a small proportion of medical problems are diagnosed in physical assessments. Those most likely to be underdiagnosed are substance abusers, elderly clients, and women. Community support and case management interventions can help the severely mentally ill obtain services despite these problems of "falling between the cracks" in systems that are poorly organized to meet the needs of clients with multiple diagnoses.

Vocational Programs

When the severely mentally ill are surveyed about their preferences, they usually indicate a strong desire to work. Work not only provides income, it also helps create a sense of self-worth and social belonging. However, psychiatric disability limits access to employment by its impact on healthy functioning and because of the stigma attached to mental disorders. Vocational services address this problem by providing training and protected alternatives to the competitive workplace.

Vocational training may occur in specialized programs, or it may be integrated into other mental health modalities such as day treatment. It provides assessment of work capacities and preferences, technical preparation, and social skills training to prepare people for the workplace. However, not all people with psychiatric disabilities enter the competitive workplace. Many, by desire or by necessity, work within protected environments. Sheltered workshop programs have a long history of offering work in a low-stress, low-demand environment. Transitional vocational programs also provide a low-stress environment but emphasize the development of skills for movement to the competitive workplace.

Supported employment is an approach that provides training and support in the place of employment. For example, a job coach might accompany a group of psychiatrically disabled workers to a place of employment where the coach learns the same job as the team, provides on-the-job training, and provides daily backup and support. Urban-based randomized clinical trials have found that supported employment has double the employment rates of adults with severe mental illness as compared to traditional vocational rehabilitation (Gold et al., 2006). This approach is based on the principle that the mentally ill learn skills best in the environment where they will be practiced. Supported employment models may become increasingly prominent because the Americans with Disabilities Act (ADA) guarantees people with psychiatric disabilities the right to reasonable accommodation in the workplace. To learn how the ADA applies to people with psychiatric disabilities, use the Companion Website for this book to access the policy guidelines of the Equal Employment Opportunity Commission at www.eeoc.gov.

Day Programs

Day treatment and partial hospitalization programs provide continuity of care between the hospital and the outpatient sector in a less restrictive setting. These programs can also provide an alternative to hospital care for individuals who need complex treatment monitoring.

Day treatment programs offer groups and activities that provide for recreation and socialization and that help people function in the community. They may be used on a short-term basis for specific goals or on a long-term basis for relapse prevention. Day programs are increasingly incorporating a rehabilitation philosophy that maximizes opportunities for meaningful activities in environments that are as "normal" as possible, focusing on strengths rather than on pathology.

Family and Network Support

Family support interventions are directed at reducing stress in the client's interpersonal environment and minimizing the burden of care for family members. If clients have little contact with families, interventions may target the people in their networks that provide them with support: friends, landlords, service providers.

With this emphasis on support to the supporters, interventions include:

- Psychoeducational activities that increase knowledge about the disorder and reduce family stress
- Practical assistance with information about homemaking or legal services
- Respite services (short-term placements to relieve the family of the burden of care)

Such services have been widely recommended as a way to reduce the family's burden and enhance the quality of life of both client and family for the long term (Beebe, 2007).

Nurses working with families of the severely and persistently mentally ill need to become attuned to their concerns. Families may express ambivalence about care giving. For example, they may want to promote the client's autonomy yet feel discomfort or guilt about the type of living situation the client is able to maintain independently. Clear information and nonjudgmental attitudes from you and other providers can do much to alleviate a family's distress and assure them that there may not be a single ideal solution to their problems.

Advocacy

Many of the difficulties the severely mentally ill experience in the community reflect a poor understanding of psychiatric illness among the general population and inadequate resources for their needs. For example, access to housing is a function of resources and community acceptance. Attention to housing is futile if no residential resources exist; vocational programs require access to employers. For this reason, one component of community support for the severely mentally ill is advocacy, or activities increasing access to resources. Advocacy can occur on an individual basis; for example, a case manager might intervene with a landlord to help a client obtain housing. Advocacy activities also occur at the level of the community, such as in programs for community education or outreach to employers.

Families of the severely and persistently mentally ill have also assumed a much greater advocacy role than in the past. Family advocacy arose in response to problems accompanying the deinstitutionalization process that placed an enormous burden of care on families. It also developed in reaction to the stigmatization of parents by people who attributed serious mental disorders to child-rearing practices. The major family organization for people with severe and persistent mental disorders is the **National Alliance on Mental Illness (NAMI)**. The national and local chapters of NAMI have grown tremendously over the past 25 years and have become a recognized force in mental health policy development. Chapter 30 ∞ discusses NAMI in greater detail.

Psychiatric Rehabilitation

Although the components of community support models provide the structure for services to the severely and persistently mentally ill, their effectiveness depends on the content of these component services. **Psychiatric rehabilitation**, an emphasis on the prevention or reduction of impairment or handicap as opposed to the treatment of disease, serves as a guide for the content of practice at many levels of care, and it includes an overall treatment philosophy as well as specific interventions and programs.

Psychiatric Rehabilitation Philosophy

Psychiatric rehabilitation has its roots in theory about physical disabilities (Anthony, Cohen, Farkas, & Gagne, 2006) and separates the treatment of disease from the prevention or

MEDIALINK Equal Employment Opportunity Commission

reduction of impairment and handicap. Research in schizophrenia and related severe mental illness suggests that psychiatric rehabilitation facilitates recovery of psychosocial functioning (Peer & Spaulding, 2007). Treatment addresses the disease process and its consequent symptoms. Rehabilitation approaches emphasize specific interventions to address targeted areas of functioning. Rehabilitation approaches are also strongly grounded in beliefs about empowerment of clients, emphasizing client feelings of control and worth.

Rehabilitation-oriented services begin with functional assessment and identification of highly individualized goals. A plan is developed to meet objectives by behavioral interventions that target specific functional deficits, or by environmental interventions that enable functioning with an existing deficit. From a rehabilitation perspective, it is important to extend support as long as possible. Support is not necessarily withdrawn because a client improves. For example, clients doing well in supported employment programs would not be expected to necessarily "graduate" to independent employment and thereby forfeit the support.

Rehabilitation philosophy is entirely consistent with self-care and symptom management interventions developed by psychiatric–mental health nurses. In fact, rehabilitation theory and conceptual models in nursing share a common focus on functional adaptation in supportive environments.

Psychosocial Rehabilitation Centers/Clubhouses

Although a rehabilitation philosophy can inform and enhance many treatment modalities, some specific rehabilitation programs make a unique contribution to service systems. One of the most important types of psychiatric rehabilitation programs is psychosocial rehabilitation centers, modeled after clubs formed by former psychiatric hospital clients to provide mutual support and assistance (Anthony et al., 2006). Under a community support system structure, psychosocial rehabilitation centers or clubhouses would fall at the level of day programming, but may be very different in program content from "maintenance" day treatment centers, which do not apply a rehabilitation perspective. These evolved into service centers providing multiple services such as group activities, successful supported employment (Macias et al., 2006), and housing. Psychosocial centers emphasize a collaborative relationship between staff and members, and provide experiences in a supportive but realistic milieu for the development of abilities for functioning in the real world.

Vocational Rehabilitation

While all mental health programs have some emphasis on vocational rehabilitation, not all vocational programs conform to a psychiatric rehabilitation model. Supported employment models reflect a rehabilitation perspective because of their emphasis on adding support to the normal environment. This model delineates basic competencies that are necessary for employment and offers classes that prepare the client to set goals and choose a job focus. Once clients are placed, they are supported by job coaches who serve as role models, provide feedback, and act as liaisons to employers.

Social Skills Training

Social skills training methods are based on principles of social learning and use behavioral techniques such as role-playing, practicing, and reinforcement to promote the learning of instrumental role behavior as well as problem-solving abilities and interpersonal skills. Social skills training techniques may be incorporated into individual, group, and family treatment modalities (see Chapter 30 for examples), where they may add measurable benefits.

High-Risk SPMI Clients

Subgroups of the severely and persistently mentally ill are at particularly high risk for poor outcomes and are also extraordinarily difficult to serve in conventional programs. These subgroups include:

- Substance-related problems
- Homelessness
- Frequent readmissions to acute care
- Frequent criminal justice system involvement

The interrelationships among these problems are complex, making it difficult to separate them or to distinguish root problems from their consequences. For example, substance use may exacerbate symptoms and lead to rehospitalization. This in turn may disrupt stability of residence, increasing the possibility of arrest and reducing the likelihood of medication adherence. In other words, if individuals belong to one subgroup at risk, it is likely that they belong to several, thus increasing their overall vulnerability.

Concurrent Substance-Related Disorders

Psychiatric illness greatly increases the odds of having a substance-related disorder. Alcohol has typically been the drug of choice with the severely mentally ill, perhaps because it is relatively inexpensive and easily accessible. Psychostimulant use has also increased among this population, a phenomenon partially attributed to the emergence of crack cocaine as a major drug of abuse. Concurrent substance-related disorders are probably the most consistent predictor of readmission to psychiatric hospitals.

Substance use contributes to a host of undesirable outcomes, which are thoroughly discussed in Chapter 15. It is highly correlated with homelessness and criminal justice system involvement (Zweben, 2000). It is also a cause of concurrent medical morbidity, including exposure to HIV (see Chapter 25). Several hospital surveys indicate a high rate of seropositivity among severely mentally ill adults. Triple-diagnosis clients—such as those with HIV disorders, substance-related disorders, and psychiatric disorders—require a complex and demanding range of services.

For a variety of reasons involving different funding streams and different treatment philosophies, substance abuse services and psychiatric care are often poorly integrated. In mental health care systems, the dually diagnosed client encounters little specific expertise related to drug or alcohol use. The severely mentally ill sometimes do poorly in substance abuse programs stressing confrontation or demanding sobriety as a precondition to treatment. Integrated programs for the dually diagnosed mentally ill include inpatient programs and some of the assertive treatment models discussed on pages 238–239. Adjusting the psychotropic medications for these clients may help them deal with problems such as dysphoria and anxiety that lead to self-medication with drugs and alcohol.

Homeless and Mentally Ill

Homelessness is at an all-time high among psychiatric clients (Booth, 2006). Various estimates of the extent of homelessness among the mentally ill range from 25% to more than 50%. Whichever numbers are more accurate, it is clear that the mentally ill constitute a prominent subgroup among the homeless. Unfortunately, discharge from the hospital to no fixed address (a shelter or the street) is not uncommon (Forchuk, Russel, Kingston-Macclure, Turner, & Dill, 2006).

The goal of providing acceptable and long-term housing for the mentally ill remains elusive, particularly in urban centers. While the proportion of the mentally ill in the community who are permanently homeless is thought to be relatively small, a large and heterogeneous group experiences spells of residential instability.

CLINICAL EXAMPLE

Rob is a 29-year-old man who was referred to an intensive case management team after his third hospital admission within one year. Rob has a diagnosis of schizoaffective disorder, but it is unclear whether his diagnosis accounts for his frequent acute episodes or whether the episodes are precipitated by his use of stimulants and alcohol. Rob has no stable place of residence and has stayed in shelters over the past few years. He describes himself as too preoccupied with his survival needs to seek treatment between emergency episodes. He claims that alcohol helps him manage his anxiety and his "voices" when he is on the streets. The case management team will first address Rob's need for safe housing. The team will then work with Rob to help him acknowledge that alcohol and drugs can increase his discomfort, and to support his use of psychotropic medication. When Rob is stabilized, he will work with the team and consider other treatment goals.

Whether these periods of homelessness involve movement between transient accommodations or actual street dwelling, they impose very harsh living conditions on people who are highly vulnerable. Homelessness interferes with the ability to use services, including the use of psychotropic medications. It increases the risk of trauma, substance abuse, infectious disease exposure, and victimization. Homelessness also makes conventional services unworkable, since the undomiciled can rarely store medication and use regular outpatient services. A study of previously homeless mentally ill adults in New York City who now have independent housing found that such factors as constancy, daily routines, privacy, and having a secure base in which to construct one's identity helped them become capable of living independently in the community (Padgett, 2007). A nursing study of the housing preferences of psychiatric clients identified the need for housing that makes one feel comfortable and secure (Forchuk, Nelson, & Hall, 2006). Despite this and other recent evidence that favors a "housing first" approach, in many geographic locations a dominant "treatment first" approach persists in which individuals must meet a hierarchy of program requirements before becoming eligible for an apartment of their own.

Services to the homeless include supported housing models with case management components, shelter-based rehabilitation and substance abuse services, and mobile outreach teams to identify cases and link them with services. Case management services are particularly important (Bhui, Shanahan, & Harding, 2006). Clients who formed a positive alliance with their case manager had significantly fewer days of homelessness (Chinman, Rosenheck, & Lam, 2000). While shelters and emergency programs serve a critical short-term need, they also contribute to instability. It is preferable, by far, to develop permanent housing for people with psychiatric disabilities. The Homelessness Resource Center specifically focuses on the delivery of services to people who are homeless and have serious mental illnesses. Its website, www.nrchmi.samhsa.gov, can be accessed through the Companion Website for this book.

MEDIALINK Homelessness Resource Center

Frequent Readmissions and Relapse

Recidivism, or frequent readmission, in acute psychiatric settings is a problem for several reasons:

1. It represents a considerable expense.
2. It is a signal of relapse, indicating severe difficulties for the individual.
3. It suggests a failure of the community system to link the client between acute episodes and to institute the type of treatment and monitoring that might manage symptomatic shifts without hospitalization.

Virtually all severe and persistent disorders will involve some kind of relapse at some time; more than one or two admissions in 12 months exceeds norms.

Client-based factors that contribute to recidivism include substance abuse, which may be the best predictor of readmission. Cycling through emergency and acute care has been attributed to a "chronic crisis" style among some diagnostic groups, particularly those with severe DSM Axis II disorders. However, many younger clients with schizophrenia and bipolar disorder use alcohol and drugs to combat boredom and medication side effects, and to self-medicate or treat symptoms in what they consider a "normal" way.

On a systems level, readmission may reflect a failure to link the client with services that the client considers meaningful and accessible. The system as a whole may respond best to clients who "fit" into programs and benefit from treatment alone. Those with more social needs or less acceptance of their illness may not consider ambulatory services relevant to their needs and may require assertive outreach to link with appropriate outpatient providers.

Frequent Criminal Justice System Involvement

Prevalence rates of major psychiatric disorders in the jails have increased gradually but continuously, at least in part because of deinstitutionalization policies. Society has a low tolerance for disordered behavior, and the lack of services for the severely and persistently mentally ill in the mental health care system may lead to a funneling into the criminal justice system. According to the Bazelon Center for Mental Health Law (2007), mentally ill persons have a 64% greater chance of being arrested than those who are not mentally ill but have committed the same crime. Four fact sheets offering specific information for advocates on combating the criminalization of people with mental illness can be found at www.bazelon.org/decrim.html and accessed through the Companion Website for this book.

MediaLink Bazelon Center for Mental Health Law

Unemployment, homelessness, and substance abuse contribute to the profile of the severely mentally ill forensic client. Many forensic inpatient services are filled to capacity. Most mentally ill offenders end up in county jails rather than forensic mental hospitals; they rarely become connected with local mental health networks and are frequently counted among the homeless because they have no fixed address. Psychiatric–mental health nurses provide valuable case management and advocacy services for this specific population as well as for high-risk SPMI clients in general.

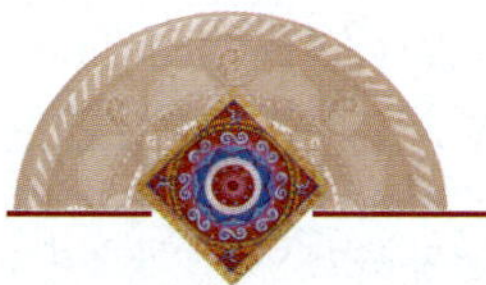

EXPLORE MediaLink

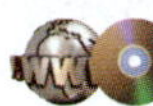

www.prenhall.com/kneisl

For NCLEX-RN® review questions, case studies, and other resources for this chapter see the Pearson Health MediaLink CD-ROM that accompanies this book and the Companion Website at www.prenhall.com/kneisl.

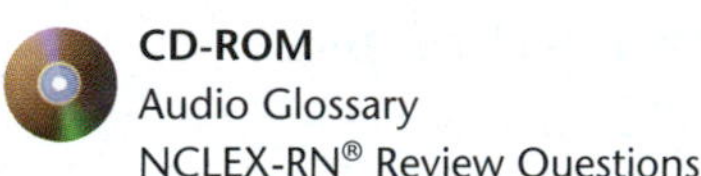

CD-ROM
Audio Glossary
NCLEX-RN® Review Questions

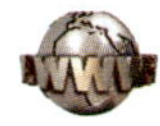

Companion Website
Audio Glossary
NCLEX-RN® Review Questions
Critical Thinking Exercise
- *Case Manager Role*

Case Study
- *Psychiatric Home Care*

Care Plan
- *Therapeutic Environment*

MediaLinks
MediaLink Applications
- *Deinstitutionalization*

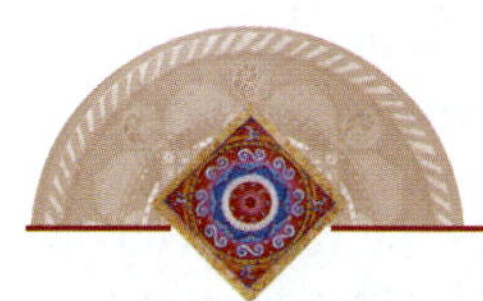

NCLEX-RN® REVIEW QUESTIONS

1. A nurse and a nurse's aide share a van, visiting locations where homeless, mentally ill individuals congregate, offering food, showers, clean clothing, and medication needs assessment. Which of the following descriptors best characterizes this setting?
1. Private outpatient services
2. Managed care organization
3. Assertive community mental health outreach
4. Community hospital intake and triage

2. During your multidisciplinary treatment team meeting, the case manager states, "This client has been refusing to let the medication aide into his apartment, so we do not know if he has been taking his medications. We may need to tell him that his housing is contingent upon cooperating with all aspects of the treatment plan." Which of the following describes the ethical conflict? (Select all that apply.)
1. Autonomy versus beneficence
2. Justice versus beneficence/nonmaleficence
3. Privacy versus veracity
4. Fidelity versus autonomy
5. Veracity versus beneficence

3. Identify a concern of psychiatric–mental health nurses that other home care nurses do not have to face as often.
1. The client's ambivalence about in-home assessment
2. Reliance on individuals other than the client for history
3. Delegation to nonprofessional caregivers
4. Decreased control of the treatment environment

4. Your community mental health center is considering reorganization, with implementation of interdisciplinary treatment teams. Your colleague tells you, "It will be difficult to coordinate team meetings. I'd rather continue as a case manager with my own caseload." Based on your knowledge, what is your most accurate response?
1. "The clients may be more likely to cooperate if a united team presents a treatment plan to them."
2. "It will be harder for clients to have to deal with a whole group of people."
3. "You might experience more professional autonomy as a case manager in a managed care organization."
4. "It may present a challenge, but it is a change in the best interest of both the clients and the mental health center staff."

5. You are currently employed in a community mental health center as a psychiatric–mental health triage nurse. You are considering employment as a case manager at a managed mental health care organization. What changes can you expect?
1. Decreased role as gatekeeper
2. Increased continuity of care between inpatient and outpatient services
3. Coordination of resources with client's entitlement expectations
4. Application of different criteria for hospital admission

6. At a managed care organization, you coordinate a "flexing" of terms for the inpatient client to include the following: 1) the exchange of 5 inpatient benefit days to 5 weeks of home visits (Monday, Wednesday, and Friday); and 2) the modification of client outcomes from "return to 40 hours/week employment within 2 months" to "return to 32 hours/week employment within 6 weeks." If you were not in a position to authorize this "flexing," which of the following describes your role? (Select all that apply.)
1. Director of out-of-plan services
2. Case manager
3. Gatekeeper
4. Client advocate
5. Utilization review manager

7. Which characteristic distinguishes managed care organization case management from inpatient case management?
1. Coordination of inpatient care using critical pathways
2. Responsibility to recommend termination of ineffective therapies
3. Ethical conflicts between organizational needs and the individual needs of the client
4. The potential for blurring of professional boundaries as the case manager provides social support

8. Which of the following nurse's statements best reflects understanding of therapeutic milieu?
1. "We provide the least restrictive safe environment. Clients participate in their treatment and aftercare planning."
2. "Our unit has a schedule and a strict routine. Clients are informed of the rules upon admission."
3. "At first, the staff makes decisions for the client. As the client demonstrates improvement, the staff provides the client with more choices."
4. "Our unit balances group well-being with client autonomy."

9. Flexibility and individualization of treatment planning are essential for clients with severe and persistent mental illness because:
1. Prognosis is poor despite diagnostic homogeneity.
2. The only commonality in this population is the presence of psychiatric disability.
3. This population often has Axis II diagnoses.
4. Disease models are not useful in designing services.

10. Which of the following are challenges associated with caring for high-risk severely and persistently mentally ill clients?
1. Readmission is equated with failure of the current treatment intervention(s).
2. Clients with multiple diagnoses are perceived to be more likely to benefit from treatment plans than clients with a single diagnosis.
3. High-risk severely and persistently mentally ill clients are more adherent with their treatment.
4. Health care provider–client relationships based on trust are less difficult to establish with these clients.

See Appendix C for answers.

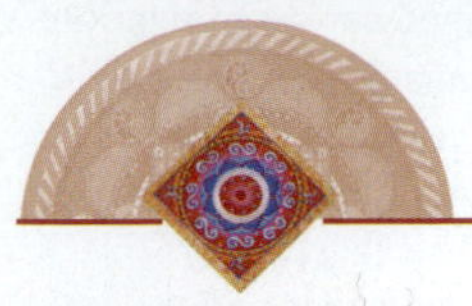

REFERENCES

Anthony, W. A., Cohen, M., Farkas, M., & Gagne, C. (2006). *Psychiatric rehabilitation* (3rd ed.). Boston: Boston University Center for Psychiatric Rehabilitation.

Bazelon Center for Mental Health Law. (2007). Ending the criminalization of people with mental illness. Retrieved June 7, 2007, from www.bazelon.org/decrim.html.

Beebe, L. H. (2007). Beyond the prescription pad: Psychosocial treatments for individuals with schizophrenia. *Journal of Psychosocial Nursing and Mental Health Services, 45*(3), 35–43.

Bhui, K., Shanahan, L., & Harding, G. (2006). Homelessness and mental illness: A literature review and a qualitative study of the perceptions of the adequacy of care. *International Journal of Social Psychiatry, 52*(2), 152–165.

Booth, R. G. (2006). Using electronic patient records in mental health care to capture housing and homelessness information of psychiatric consumers. *Issues in Mental Health Nursing, 27*(10), 1066–1077.

Bussema, E. F., & Bussema, K. E. (2007). Gilead revisited: Faith and recovery. *Psychiatric Rehabilitation Journal, 30*(4), 301–305.

Bustillo, J., Lauriello, J., Horan, W., & Keith, S. (2001). The psychosocial treatment of schizophrenia: An update. *American Journal of Psychiatry, 158*(2), 163–175.

Chinman, M. J., Rosenheck, R., & Lam, J. A. (2000). The case management relationship and outcomes of homeless persons with serious mental illness. *Psychiatric Services, 51*(9), 1142–1147.

Cohen, J., Marecek, J., & Gillham, J. (2006). Is three a crowd? Clients, clinicians, and managed care. *American Journal of Orthopsychiatry, 76*(2), 251–259.

Coldwell, C. M., & Bender, W. S. (2007). The effectiveness of assertive community treatment for homeless populations with severe mental illness: A meta-analysis. *American Journal of Psychiatry, 164*(3), 393–399.

Cuddeback, G. S., Morrissey, J. P., & Meyer, P. S. (2006). How many assertive community treatment teams do we need? *Psychiatric Services, 57*(12), 1803–1806.

Essock, S. M., Mueser, K. T., Drake, R. E., Covell, N. H., McHugo, G. J., Frisman, L. K., et al. (2006). Comparison of ACT and standard case management for delivering integrated treatment for co-occurring disorders. *Psychiatric Services, 57*(2), 185–196.

Fagin, C. M. (2001). Revisiting treatment in the home. *Archives of Psychiatric Nursing, 15*(1), 3–9.

Forchuk, C., Nelson, G., & Hall, G. B. (2006). "It's important to be proud of the place you live in." Housing problems and preferences of psychiatric survivors. *Perspectives in Psychiatric Care, 42*(1), 42–52.

Forchuk, C., Russel, G., Kingston-Macclure, S., Turner, K., & Dill, S. (2006). From psychiatric ward to the streets and shelters. *Journal of Psychiatric Mental Health Nursing, 13*(3), 301–308.

Gold, P. B., Meisler, N., Santos, A. B., Carnemolla, M. A., Williams, O. H., & Keleher, J. (2006). Randomized trial of supported employment integrated with assertive community treatment for rural adults with severe mental illness. *Schizophrenia Bulletin, 32*(2), 378–395.

Guo, S., Biegel, D. E., Johnsen, A., & Dyches, H. (2001). Assessing the impact of community-based mobile crisis services on previous hospitalizations. *Psychiatric Services, 52*(2), 223–228.

Hangan, C. (2006). Introduction of an intensive case management style of delivery for a new mental health service. *International Journal of Mental Health Nursing, 15*(3), 157–162.

Lamb, H. R., & Bachrach, L. (2001). Some perspectives on deinstitutionalization. *Psychiatric Services, 52*(8), 1039–1045.

Macias, C., Rodican, F. F., Hargreaves, W. A., Jones, D. R., Barreira, P. J., & Wang, Q. (2006). Supported employment outcomes of a randomized controlled trial of ACT and clubhouse models. *Psychiatric Services, 57*(10), 1406–1415.

McCann, T. V. (2002). Uncovering hope with clients who have psychotic illness. *Journal of Holistic Nursing, 20*(1), 81–99.

Padgett, D. K. (2007). There's no place like (a) home: Ontological security among persons with serious mental illness in the United States. *Social Science and Medicine, 64*(9), 1925–1936.

Peer, J. E., & Spaulding, W. D. (2007). Heterogeneity in recovery of psychosocial functioning during psychiatric rehabilitation: An exploratory study using latent growth mixture modeling. *Schizophrenia Research, 93*(1–3), 186–193.

Smoyak, S. (2000). The history, economics, and financing of mental health care. Part 3: The present. *Journal of Psychosocial Nursing and Mental Health Services, 38*(11), 32–38.

Teplin, L. A., McClelland, G. M., Abram, K. M., & Weiner, D. A. (2005). Crime victimization in adults with severe mental illness: Comparison with the National Crime Victimization Survey. *Archives of General Psychiatry, 62*(8), 911–921.

Torrey, E. F., & Zdanowicz, M. (2001). Outpatient commitment: What, why, and for whom. *Psychiatric Services, 52*(3), 337–341.

Wong-McDonald, A. (2007). Spirituality and psychosocial rehabilitation: Empowering persons with serious psychiatric disabilities at an inner-city community program. *Psychiatric Rehabilitation Journal, 30*(4), 295–300.

Zeltzer, B. B., & Kohn, R. (2006). Mental health services for homebound elders from home health nursing agencies and home care agencies. *Psychiatric Services, 57*(4), 567–569.

Zuvekas, S. H., & Meyerhoefer, C. D. (2006). Coverage for mental health treatment: Do the gaps still persist? *Journal of Mental Health Policy Economics, 9*(3), 155–163.

Zweben, J. E. (2000). Severely and persistently mentally ill substance abusers: Clinical and policy issues. *Journal of Psychoactive Drugs, 32*(4), 383–389.

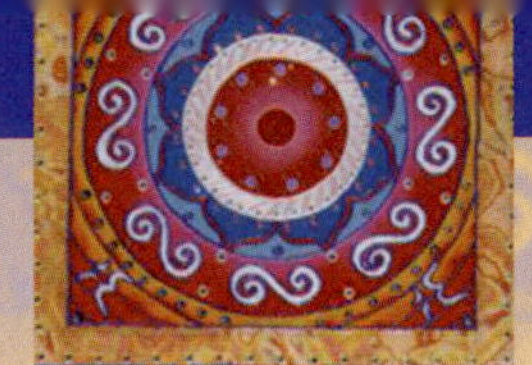

Ethics, Clients' Rights, and Legal and Forensic Issues

CHAPTER 13

CAROL REN KNEISL

LEARNING OUTCOMES

After completing this chapter, you will be able to:

1. Relate the six principles of bioethics to the practice of psychiatric–mental health nursing.
2. Discuss how ethical guidelines can be applied in reconciling crucial ethical dilemmas.
3. Describe how psychiatric–mental health nurses can avoid indirectly contributing to the stereotypes associated with psychiatric diagnostic categories.
4. Explain why psychiatric–mental health nurses need to be knowledgeable about the mental health statutes and regulations in the state in which they practice.
5. Compare admission and release procedures for voluntary admission and involuntary commitment.
6. Differentiate between psychiatric forensic nursing and correctional mental health nursing roles.
7. Deliver psychiatric–mental health nursing care in a manner that preserves and protects client rights, dignity, and autonomy.
8. Partner with clients and their families in developing psychiatric advance directives.
9. Identify the acts for which psychiatric–mental health nurses can be held legally liable.
10. Serve as a client advocate while assisting clients and families to develop skills for self–advocacy.

KEY TERMS

competency *276*
diminished capacity *272*
expert witness *274*
habeas corpus *285*
informed consent *276*
involuntary commitment *268*
least restrictive setting *281*
legal sanity *270*
malpractice *287*
negligence *286*
privileged communication *283*
psychiatric advance directives (PADs) *275*
psychiatric forensic nursing *272*
voluntary admission *268*

CRITICAL THINKING CHALLENGE

Sue Aberdeen is a client of a mental health outreach clinic. She was diagnosed with bipolar disorder more than 20 years ago. At one time or another during this period, various mental health care providers have prescribed several different medications for Sue. Most have been only slightly helpful or ineffective. Most recently, Sue has been taking lithium, which seems to be the most helpful. Her long-time friend brought Sue to the clinic because Sue has not been taking her medication. She has been unable to sleep and is distracted and agitated. Sue has been to a different bar every night this week, and has gone home with and had sex with a different man each night. The nurse assigned to

(continued)

MEDIALINK 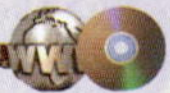 www.prenhall.com/kneisl

Go to the Pearson Health MediaLink CD-ROM and the Companion Website at www.prenhall.com/kneisl for interactive resources for this chapter.

CRITICAL THINKING CHALLENGE *(continued)*

her case has been attempting to persuade Sue to take her lithium. Sue has continued to refuse, and the nurse has continued to explain and cajole. Finally, Sue shouted: "You just don't get it, do you? Buzz off, you bitch!" and stomped out of the clinic.

1. How can you reconcile the desire and duty to help with a client's refusal for treatment?
2. When do you think it is acceptable for a client to refuse to be treated?
3. How do you think refusal to cooperate with treatment should be handled?

Ethical, judicial, legislative, political, and economic decisions profoundly influence mental health practice. Many factors bring about changes in the understanding and practice of mental health intervention. These changes challenge the psychiatric–mental health nurse to examine central issues, such as:

- How does one balance the common and the individual "good" in health care?
- How does one define mental health?
- What are nurses', mental health consumers', and society's rights, liability, and accountability?

An examination of these issues generally improves care, but it often confuses the boundaries of ethical behavior, mental health practice, and the law. This confusion entraps mental health care professionals, mental health consumers, families, lawyers, and the public in a muddle of conflicting policies and procedures. In addition, a client's right to privacy, to receive and refuse treatment, and to define happiness and growth pivot on society's values.

This chapter will bring some clarity to the ever-changing relationship between ethics, the law, and mental health services so that psychiatric–mental health nurses can not only practice ethically and with confidence, but also exercise their power as citizens, professionals, and advocates to influence the direction of mental health care.

ETHICS

You may find yourself having to identify alternative courses of action and decide what to do when there is a conflict of rights and obligations between clients and families, between yourself and other mental health care workers, or between the client's good and the community or social good. *Ethics* is a branch of philosophy that deals with the values that are related to human conduct, the rightness or wrongness of actions, the goodness and badness of one's motives, and the goodness and badness of the results of one's actions. *Bioethics* is a field that applies ethical reasoning to issues and dilemmas in the area of health care.

The predominant character of ethical conflicts is, according to Redman and Fry (2000), disagreement with the quality of care given to clients:

- Differences in the definition of adequacy of care among professionals, the institution, and society
- Differences in the philosophical orientations of nurses, physicians, and other health care professionals involved in the care of clients
- A lack of respect for the knowledge and expertise of nurses
- Difficulty in carrying out the nurse's advocacy role for clients

These conflicts involve complex ethical issues and dilemmas that are tempered by the need to provide culturally congruent care.

Ethical Analysis

One of the major difficulties in ethical analysis is that there are no definite, clear-cut solutions to ethical dilemmas. For centuries moral philosophers—beginning with Socrates, Plato, and Aristotle—have struggled with two main ethical questions: What is the meaning of right or good? and What should I do? To identify, clarify, define, and defend a stand on an ethical issue, we must engage in a process of ethical reasoning. Six critical questions set out in the Your Assessment Approach feature below will help you to gather data to use in the process of ethical reasoning.

Taking a stand on an ethical issue involves much more than merely accepting the moral position or personal values of another. It requires an understanding of the principles of bioethics.

Principles of Bioethics

The six principles of bioethics discussed here are autonomy, beneficence, fidelity, justice, nonmaleficence, and veracity.

Autonomy

Autonomy is the freedom to choose a course of action, to act on that choice, and to live with the consequences of that

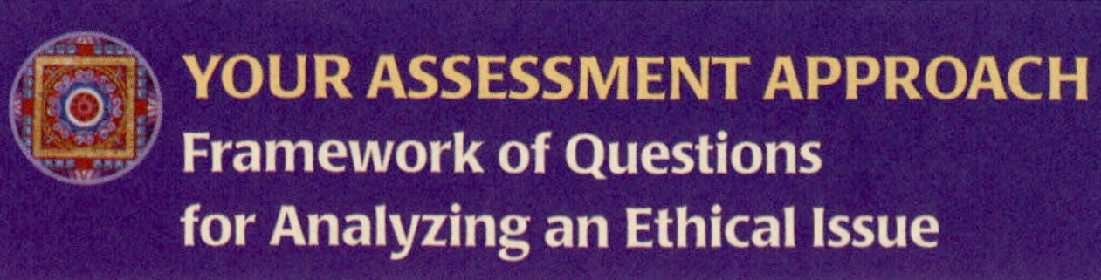

YOUR ASSESSMENT APPROACH
Framework of Questions
for Analyzing an Ethical Issue

1. Who are the relevant actors in the situation?
2. What is the required action?
3. What are the probable and possible consequences of the action?
4. What is the range of alternative actions or choices?
5. What is the intent or purpose of the action?
6. What is the context of the action?

choice. Helping clients, their families, and their significant others make choices fosters autonomy. You help clients by providing them with the information they need in order to choose, helping them to understand and sort through the information, and supporting their choice, even when that choice is one that you may not have made. Professional autonomy for you, as a psychiatric–mental health nurse, means having to account for and accept the consequence of professional decisions and actions. Professionals must balance the goal of greater autonomy in nursing with efforts to achieve what providers and consumers determine are the common and the individual good in health care.

Beneficence

Beneficence is the principle of attempting to do things that benefit others or promote the good of others. You operate under the principle of beneficence whenever you help clients who cannot decide for themselves or are incapacitated or incompetent. Protecting clients from harming themselves because of thoughts, feelings, or behaviors that lead to self-harm is done in a spirit of beneficence.

Fidelity

Fidelity means that you maintain loyalty and commitment to your clients and are faithful to your promises, duties, and obligations. Fidelity is crucial to establishing trusting relationships with clients, their families, and other mental health workers.

Justice

Justice is the principle of treating others fairly and equally. It is the fair and equitable distribution of burdens and benefits. The principle of justice has always been a cornerstone of bioethics and has become even more important when considered in issues related to health care reform and managed care. The principle of justice raises questions such as:

- Should indigent persons receive electroconvulsive therapy (ECT) to treat depression, but those who can afford it be treated with newer and costly psychotropic drugs?
- Is insurance coverage for psychiatric–mental health services a basic service or a luxury?
- Should mental health care be given to those who need it or only to those who can pay for it?

Nonmaleficence

Nonmaleficence is the intention to do no wrong. Your motives for actions should be in the direction of helpfulness based on sound knowledge of psychiatric–mental health theory. Nonmaleficence requires you to be self-aware and is the principle behind the Your Self-Awareness features throughout this text.

Veracity

Veracity is the intention to tell the truth. Veracity is critical to establishing trust with clients, their families, and other mental health care workers. If you cannot be trusted to do what you say you will do or to tell the truth, you cannot be depended on; what you do and what you say will be open to suspicion. Veracity means that you do not lie to clients to "humor" them.

Neuroethics, an Emerging Field

The field of neuroethics is emerging from a 21st-century partnership between bioethics and neuroscience. Rapid advances in neuroscience, brought about by brain research, have raised critical ethical, social, and legal issues about neuroimaging, psychopharmacology, deep-brain stimulation (discussed in Chapter 33∞), and psychosurgery (discussed later in this chapter). The critical questions revolve around the prediction of disease (including mental disorders in certain instances); questions of privacy and confidentiality; concerns about the effects on an individual's autonomy; and the influences of neuroimaging, psychopharmacology, deep-brain stimulation, brain implants, and psychosurgery on an individual's concept of self and personal identity (Illes & Racine, 2005; Fuchs, 2006).

Despite the myriad of new neuroscience information, the brain remains the most complex and least understood of all the organs in the human body. Mapping the neural correlates of the mind through brain scans and altering these correlates through surgery, stimulation, or psychopharmacological interventions can affect people in both positive and negative ways (Glannon, 2006). The potential benefits of these knowledges and technologies have to be carefully weighed against their potential harm and actively debated by neuroscientists and mental health professionals.

Ethical Guidelines for Psychiatric–Mental Health Nurses

Most professions develop guidelines for the behavior of their members. Ethical guidelines for psychiatric–mental health nurses stem from two sources. The first source is the standards for psychiatric–mental health nursing practice published by the American Nurses Association (ANA) (2007). (These standards are reproduced and discussed in detail in Chapter 2∞.) The standard of professional performance that deals specifically with ethics for psychiatric–mental health nurses, Standard 12, is reproduced in Box 13-1 on page 264. You are most likely familiar with the second source from your nursing fundamentals course—the general code of ethics for nurses, also developed by the ANA (2001). If you need to refresh yourself on the ANA Code of Ethics, refer to a nursing fundamentals text. Use these sources to make clinical judgments and to engage in ethical reasoning. You may also find ANA's online journal of issues in nursing (OJIN) helpful in your practice. The journal can be accessed through the Companion Website for this book.

MediaLink American Nurses Association

Clinical Judgment and Ethical Reasoning

Nursing is frequently faced with two goals:

1. Responding to the therapeutic needs of individuals
2. Serving society by preserving social order

Often these two goals are in conflict, and nurses must face the dilemma of placing one above the other. The only way to

Box 13-1 **ANA Psychiatric–Mental Health Nursing Standards of Professional Performance**

Standard 12. Ethics

The Psychiatric–Mental Health Registered Nurse integrates ethical improvisions in all areas of practice.

Measurement Criteria

The Psychiatric–Mental Health Registered Nurse (RN-PMH):

- Uses *Code of Ethics for Nurses with Interpretive Statements (ANA, 2001)* to guide practice.
- Delivers care in a manner that preserves and protects patient autonomy, dignity, and rights.
- Is aware of and avoids using the power inherent in the therapeutic relationship to influence the patient in ways not related to the treatment goals.
- Maintains patient confidentiality within legal and regulatory parameters.
- Serves as a patient advocate protecting patient's rights and assisting patients in developing skills for self-advocacy.
- Maintains a therapeutic and professional patient–nurse relationship with appropriate professional role boundaries.
- Demonstrates a commitment to practicing self-care, managing stress, and connecting with self and others.
- Contributes to resolving ethical issues of patients, colleagues, or systems as evidenced in such activities as participating on ethics committees.
- Reports illegal, incompetent, or impaired practices.

Additional Management Criteria for the Psychiatric–Mental Health Advanced Practice Nurse

The APRN-PMH:

- Informs the patients of the risks, benefits, and outcomes of health care regimens.
- Participates in interdisciplinary teams that address ethical risks, benefits, and outcomes.
- Promotes and maintains a system and climate that is conducive to providing ethical care.

Source: Reprinted with permission from American Nurses Association, American Psychiatric–Mental Health Nurses Association and International Society of Psychiatric–Mental Health Nurses. (2007). *Psychiatric–mental health nursing: Scope and standards of practice* (p. 51), Silver Spring, MD: Nursesbooks.org.

resolve the conflict is for us to clarify our own values through a process of ethical reasoning.

Nurses are necessarily guided in therapeutic work by a belief system—some vision of what kinds of changes would improve a client's life. Nurses are further guided by some moral principles that limit the extent to which they will help a client obtain happiness at the expense of others, and the extent to which they will participate in the oppression of an individual in the interests of societal control. Laws represent yet another source of limits. They are discussed later in this chapter in the section on clients' rights.

Situations that involve ethical dilemmas require you to understand the concept of *moral claims*. Ethical reasoning is the process you can use when there is a conflict of claims and you have to make a choice favoring one claim over another. Anyone who is responsible for moral choices is obliged to recognize the reason, virtue, ideal, rule, or principle on which he or she makes a decision. Such a virtue-based helping relationship is characterized by moral compassion, moral judgement, and moral wisdom (Armstrong, 2006).

Ethical Dilemmas in Psychiatric–Mental Health Nursing

Ultimately, nurses must reconcile a number of crucial ethical dilemmas with their personal and professional values. Among these issues are:

- The potential stigma of psychiatric diagnostic labels
- Psychiatry's right to control individual freedom
- The justification for involuntary treatment
- The use of restrictive treatment interventions
- The client's right to suicide
- The client's right to privacy

Practicing psychiatric–mental health nursing requires ethical responsibility. The quality of a nurse's moral commitment is a measure of professional excellence. However, problems arise when there is conflict about the ground rules for behavior, whether the conflict is between client and social group, nurse and profession, or nurse and agency. These problems are phrased in the ethical language of right and wrong. Circumstances likely to give rise to such problems include the following:

- The professional and the client are from different social classes and may have different cultural values.

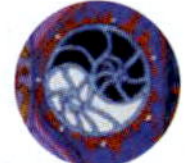

- The voluntary nature of the client's participation is compromised.
- The client's competence to enter into an agreement about intervention is questionable, or the client does not realize that certain interventions are being implemented.
- External factors (lack of time, lack of staff, high demands) prevent the professional from doing what is best for the client.

It has been suggested that having moral insight, virtue, and ethics in nursing can be taught through appropriate experience, habitual practice, and good role models (Begley, 2006). Look for a nurse mentor who can provide the experience, supervise your ethical practice, and serve as a good role model.

Every nursing relationship begins with an unusual burden of ethical responsibility. The following sections explore some of these moral issues.

Stigma of Psychiatric Diagnoses

The list of stereotypes associated with psychiatric diagnostic categories is well known to most nurses. Equally familiar are the consequences to people with these diagnoses. As Chapter 1 points out, people labeled as drug addicts, alcoholics, convicts, paranoids, and so on acquire a discredited social identity because of the character flaws often associated with the labels. To much of society, the labels used in psychiatry suggest decadence, immorality, and wanton disregard for society's values. It is important to consider how and when psychiatric–mental health nurses, while advocating humane treatment for clients, indirectly contribute to discrediting a client's social identity by participating in the arbitrary use of oppressive labels. Keep this in mind while you review the Your Self-Awareness feature below.

Need for Diagnostic Labels Diagnosis has considerable value in psychiatric practice, as Chapter 11 points out. Putting clients into diagnostic categories makes it easy for health care professionals to communicate with each other about the client. The diagnosis often dictates a particular course of treatment and enables the mental health team to prognosticate about a client's recovery. Diagnostic categories enable nurses to plan comprehensively for client care and to conduct research.

Nurse's Moral Stance on Diagnoses Take time to consider carefully how you would answer the following questions:

- Does labeling with psychiatric diagnoses merely provide psychiatric professionals with some additional sense of control in their dealings with clients?
- Is it true that a diagnosis gives staff members an increased sense of being able to predict client behavior and a way of calmly viewing what might otherwise be upsetting behavior: "That's just her hysterical personality coming out," or "Those complaints are just paranoid delusions."

The consequences of psychiatric labels for clients and their families, however, raise moral questions about their legitimacy when they are used arbitrarily or without current knowledge of diagnostic criteria.

Nurses have a moral responsibility to question practices that exact a price from clients far in excess of the benefits. Every moment of moral injustice takes its toll on us, as well as our clients. Every moment of moral responsibility strengthens our own, as well as our clients', sense of personal integrity.

Controlling Individual Freedom

Involuntary hospitalization and treatment of psychiatric clients are usually considered humanitarian efforts. Yet, any practice that directly and coercively deprives a person of freedom has political implications. In some states clients have no guarantee that they will ever be released from the hospital. This ethical issue is further complicated by the fact that psychiatric professionals can no longer argue that involuntary hospitalization is necessary to restore mental health. Instead, the confinement must be justified as necessary to protect the client or others from harm.

Violence Against Others Psychiatric–mental health nurses are faced with the dilemma of trying to be both healer-helpers and agents of social control. In dealing with violently destructive clients, they must balance the value of life against the value of liberty. A thorough discussion of violence in the psychiatric setting is in Chapter 35.

Suicide Traditionally, nurses have felt that they should do everything possible to preserve life. We have relied on this imperative to justify intervention in suicide attempts as well as heroic technical measures to avert impending deaths. Psychiatry, in general, rejects the notion of rational suicide and assumes that suicidal ideation is an irrational belief resulting from mental disorder (Hewitt & Edwards, 2006). Further, we assume that a person without a mental disorder would not choose suicide. Thus, we seek to prevent suicide on the basis that this is what the client would choose if the client were mentally capable of choosing. In this, as well as in many areas of psychiatric–mental health nursing practice, there are contested matters and areas of differing opinion (Cutcliffe, Stevenson, Jackson, & Smith, 2006).

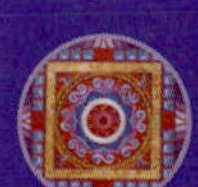

YOUR SELF-AWARENESS
Does Standardized Terminology Conflict with Individualized Client Care?

This textbook challenges psychiatric–mental health nurses to engage in reflective and creative responses to complex mind–body–spirit problems. We are challenged to face issues of global mental health with intelligence, stamina, creativity, and moral courage. The word *courage* is rooted in a French word meaning "heart." In many of the chapters in this book, you are presented with a vocabulary of standardized language including NANDA, NIC, NOC, and DSM-IV-TR. As you know, language and symbols are critical in creating the assumptions, emotional climate, and behavioral norms that define people and their environments and what is possible within them. Reflect on your own ideas about the following questions:

- Do you believe that any standardized vocabulary dismisses the unique stories of clients and their families?
- What do you think are the advantages and disadvantages of using an accepted language or vocabulary when working as a mental health team member?
- When evaluating the categories and language in NANDA, NIC, NOC, and DSM-IV-TR, do you think they adequately portray the diversity of people's lived experience and contribute to a nurse's ability to plan effective care?
- Do you think that standardized language systems are compatible with bringing "heart" to psychiatric–mental health nursing?

The treatment given to dying clients is often in conflict with the treatment they desire. For example, a physician may disregard a client's protests against treatment. The physician may assert that the client's medical condition is causing the client to behave irrationally. There is not necessarily an ethical difference between clients dying of physical deterioration and clients dying of emotional or mental deterioration. Many of the same ethical questions emerge about the suicidal client:

- How is *quality of life* defined?
- Is the definition limited to physical factors?
- Who should have the right to make the definition?
- How is rationality to be measured?
- Are people always in conscious control of their choices?

A thorough discussion of suicide is in Chapter 23∞.

An individual's right to choose when and how to die is a complex biomedical issue. The thoughtful professional nurse needs to clarify the issues, give them careful consideration, and search for a personal position. There are many ways in which people can deliberately shorten or end their own lives. They can destroy themselves quickly with a gun, or slowly through the chronic use of drugs such as tobacco or alcohol. When is coercive intervention by psychiatric practitioners justified?

Psychosurgery The most dramatic of restrictive measures is *psychosurgery*, the surgical removal or destruction of brain tissue with the intent of altering behavior even though there may be no direct evidence of structural disease or damage in the brain. Psychosurgery has become the subject of marked controversy on ethical grounds. Advocates claim that it is done to restore rather than destroy individual freedom. They argue that before psychosurgery, the client is crippled by mental illness and individual autonomy is compromised by the client's bizarre behavior or internal psychologic state. After the surgery, clients supposedly are more autonomous than before, by their own and others' criteria. Advocates of the selective use of psychosurgery, even against the client's will, outline three conditions that must be met to justify it:

1. The illness being treated is seriously disabling and untreatable by nonsurgical means such as medication or psychotherapy.
2. The treatment is undertaken with some sort of systematic investigative protocol; it is accompanied by evaluation research.
3. The treatment occurs in settings with as many safeguards as possible to arrive at informed consent, if possible, perhaps using a client advocate during the procedure.

The most common psychosurgery in the mid-1900s was prefrontal lobotomy (severing of the prefrontal tracts in the cortex) to treat schizophrenia. Although prefrontal lobotomy has been discredited after having been found to be ineffective in treating schizophrenia, there are older mental health clients who still must contend with the untoward aftereffects—memory loss, personality changes, the absence of emotional responses—of this treatment.

Today, the case for psychosurgery is most likely to be made in instances of severe and resistant depression (Malhi & Bartlett, 2000), or when obsessive–compulsive disorder is not helped by behavior therapy or psychotropic medications and is severely disabling (Jenike, 2001). In this instance, cingulotomy, a surgical procedure in which small, precisely pinpointed regions of the brain are selectively destroyed, may be employed. Another procedure, stereotactic amygdalotomy, the purposeful production of lesions in the amygdala, has been performed for the treatment of severe aggressive behavior disturbances (Fountas & Smith, 2007) and for self-mutilation disorder refractory to treatment (Fountas, Smith, & Lee, 2007). Although these procedures are not as destructive as prefrontal lobotomy, they cause irreversible brain damage.

Psychotropic Medications The discovery that certain medications can radically alter the expression of human emotions has had an enormous impact on psychiatry. The mental hospital is no longer seen as a "warehouse" for storing society's deviants; it is now a "clearinghouse" where clients are sorted, renovated, and dispatched back into their communities with symptomatic behavior under control through one or another of the current psychiatric medications.

Mental health professionals have associated the advent of psychotropic medications with a new optimism and less fear about working with people labeled mentally ill. Conceivably, the impact of the drugs on the attitudes of nurses may increase the amount of humane contact clients are given while in a treatment setting. Furthermore, it might be argued that the drugs have helped keep people out of the hospital and have decreased the need for other more dramatic measures, such as electroshock treatment.

Medications that make people feel better, however, can lessen their motivation to confront an oppressive situation. This can have serious implications for the political and moral climate of society. It is conceivable that pills could be developed to keep a person quietly enslaved. Suppose drugs were coercively given to anyone whose unhappiness was rooted in social oppression?

The cautious and judicious use of drugs with the client's consent can be helpful. Used irresponsibly, they can close off moral and political confrontations. Decisions about the use of drugs must be made in the context of the social situation and environment.

In hospital settings, medications are regularly used to reduce symptoms and make client behavior more manageable. Most staff members justify their use of chemical controls by defining violent or bizarre behavior as an indirect request for limits, as in the clinical example that follows. By assigning this meaning to the use of drugs, practitioners can feel that their actions to suppress symptoms are based on the needs of the client rather than on the staff's management motives. The process of justifying coercion allows one to retain a self-image of a "good" nurse (Vuckovich & Artinian, 2005).

CLINICAL EXAMPLE

After pacing angrily up and down the hall in front of the nurses' station for 20 minutes or so, Carlotta kicks over some mops in a bucket. A male staff member shouts to the nurse to get her PRN medication ready and strides into the hall telling the client to stop it. Carlotta cries and shouts, and they begin struggling. Several other staff members rush over to assist. They drag and carry Carlotta into her room, where she is given 10 mg of haloperidol (Haldol). She continues fighting and screaming. Staff members continue to wrestle with her in her room. Finally they decide to transfer her to the unit downstairs, where she can be put into a seclusion room. In a report, a staff member describes the incident as: "Carlotta blew up and needed controls."

It is possible that all these controls would not have been necessary had a staff member responded to the nonverbal cues of mounting tension (see Chapter 35∞) before the client kicked over the mops.

Restraints Even the physical characteristics of psychiatric inpatient settings convey the notion that clients are not expected to be capable of self-control and that staff members have the responsibility for providing it. Many clients view these interventions as forms of abuse, while the staff sees them as "helping people who can't take care of themselves."

All the judgments that must be made about restraining clients involve moral decisions such as:

- What other techniques have been tried?
- Is the client obviously out of control?
- How does the nurse decide?
- Is the client cognitively compromised?
- What will be the effects on the client of such a dramatic intervention?
- What are the effects on others in the milieu?

Legal factors that influence judgments about restraints are discussed later in this chapter.

Client Privacy and Confidentiality

When people seek psychiatric help, they must usually reveal highly personal, possibly embarrassing, and potentially damaging information about themselves. Almost all modes of therapeutic intervention rely on the client's willingness to talk openly and honestly about personal concerns, feelings, or problems. The solo therapist in private practice with voluntary clients is usually able to avoid compromising the client's right to confidentiality. In fact, many private therapists view themselves as vigilant protectors of their clients' privacy. You, however, may encounter a serious ethical conflict in being both the confidante of the client and the employee of the organization. Nurses have dual allegiances—to the client and to the agency.

Clients usually assume that health care professionals have no other purpose than to help them. They lose sight of the fact that nurses are often asked to collect data about them that might be highly influential in determining their medications, their disposition, and even their civil rights. While it is often the psychiatrist who makes final pronouncements about a client's mental health status, diagnosis, prognosis, and the like, such pronouncements rest on information collected and communicated to the physician by nurses. This information-gathering process merits serious scrutiny.

Information gathering and sharing are part of your role. Thoughtful handling of client confidentiality is facilitated by three safeguards:

1. Conveying to clients the limit of confidentiality in your exchanges—that is, what you do with the information a client shares
2. Attempting to portray accurately to others the reliability, validity, and representativeness of the data you communicate about a client
3. Recognizing that strict confidentiality may have to be violated when an innocent third party is endangered

Confidentiality is discussed further in this chapter in the section on client rights.

LEGISLATION, COMMITMENT, AND HOSPITALIZATION ISSUES

In the last 30 years, the courts have had significant impact on the direction of mental health legislation and state statutes. As a review of history tells us, the courts have traditionally been concerned with the possibility of wrongful commitment. Little attention was paid to the restrictions placed on the legal and civil rights of an individual once hospitalized. In recent years, however, the courts have become more concerned with the substantive rights of psychiatric clients whether hospitalized or not, including the right to treatment, the right not to perform institutional labor, and retention of civil rights such as the rights to communication, visitation, religious activities, and medical self-determination. This is reflected in many state statutes, along with an emphasis on procedural safeguards.

A review of mental health laws and judicial decisions underscores the fact that there is *great variability from state to state*; thus an exploration of the mental health laws of each and every state is beyond the scope of this chapter. Because of this variability, it is critical to safe practice that you are knowledgeable about the mental health statutes and regulations in the state in which you practice. Most mental health agencies and psychiatric facilities maintain copies of these statutes, as do local law libraries. You may also refer to the agency in your state that oversees mental health care.

Admission and Commitment Categories

The two major categories of hospitalization are voluntary admission and involuntary commitment. Admission and release procedures differ accordingly. They are described in the following section and compared in TABLE 13-1 ■ on page 268.

Table 13-1 ■ Voluntary Admission and Involuntary Commitment Compared

	Voluntary Admission			*Involuntary Commitment*		
	Informal	**Voluntary**	**Emergency**	**Temporary**	**Extended**	**Outpatient**
Release	Anytime	Usually conditional	Average after 3–5 days	48 hours to 6 months	After 60–180 days or an indeterminate time	Can be indeterminate
Use	Limited	Increasing	Increasing	Increasing	Decreasing	Increasing
Criteria for admission	Client request	Client request	Usually client dangerousness	Client dangerousness or need of care and treatment	Client dangerousness or need of care and treatment	Client condition deteriorating or client in need of treatment

Voluntary Admission

Voluntary admission comes about by written application for admission by prospective clients, or someone acting in their behalf, such as a parent or guardian, a partner, or a mental health agent appointed through a psychiatric advance directive (discussed in a later section of this chapter). As the word *voluntary* implies, the client has a right to demand and obtain release. Depending on the state, the client agrees to give notice, usually in writing, of the intention to leave during a grace period from 24 hours to 15 days. It is justified on the grounds that the hospital staff needs time to examine the client to determine whether a change to involuntary status is indicated. The extra time also gives family and staff the opportunity to persuade the client to remain voluntarily. This "conditional provision" is seen by some as a covert form of involuntary hospitalization. In most states there are now statutory assurances that voluntary clients must be adequately informed of their rights and status.

Informal voluntary admission, an alternative to the structure and personal concessions required in voluntary admission, is an option in several states. This procedure is similar to that required in a medical admission. The prospective inpatient verbally requests admission and is free to leave the institution at any time. Informal voluntary admission procedures are more likely to be an option in general hospital psychiatric units and private facilities than in state institutions, and they account for a small percentage of all admissions in states that have this provision.

MediaLink Case Study: Involuntary Admission

Involuntary Commitment

Involuntary commitment can come about if the designated body, such as a court, an administrative tribunal, or the required number of physicians find that the prospective client's mental state meets the statutory criteria for involuntary commitment. The state's ability to hospitalize or commit an individual involuntarily is sanctioned by one of two state powers:

1. Police power enables the state to hospitalize people who are considered dangerous to others because of their illness.
2. *Parens patriae* power enables the state to take on the role of protector and assume reponsibility for people considered dangerous to themselves or unable to care for themselves in a potentially dangerous situation because of a mental disability.

Most states provide for more than one involuntary hospitalization procedure. The criteria vary from state to state according to the type of involuntary hospitalization. However, all state involuntary commitment statutes can be expected to include one or more of the following criteria:

- Dangerous to self or others
- Unable to provide for basic needs
- Mentally ill

In an increasing number of states, involuntary commitment is justified only if the individual is dangerous to self or others because of a mental disorder. The remaining states augment this by stating that the client's need for care and treatment may also justify commitment. There is a growing movement for involuntary treatment for drug and alcohol dependence because the availability of third-party funding for the voluntary treatment of individuals with substance use disorders has decreased (Nace et al., 2007).

Involuntary commitment can be divided into four categories:

- Emergency
- Temporary or observational
- Extended or indeterminate
- Outpatient commitment

Emergency Emergency involuntary hospitalization is available in almost all states. It is a temporary measure with limited, short-range goals, and it deals largely with the prevention of behavior likely to create a "clear and present" danger to the client or others. Under common law, any official or private person has the right to detain a dangerous mentally disordered person.

Some formal application is required to initiate emergency detention. In some states, any citizen may make the application. In others, it is limited to police officers, health officers, and physicians. Because this type of involuntary admission is an emergency measure and is warranted only until the appropriate legal steps can be taken, the statutes limit the amount of time an individual can be detained. The usual practice is to allow detention for 3 to 5 days, although some states set a limit of 24 hours.

Temporary or Observational Temporary or observational involuntary hospitalization is the involuntary commitment of an allegedly mentally disordered individual for a specified period of time to allow for adequate observation so that a diagnosis can be made and treatment instituted. The actual time period can vary from 48 hours to as long as 6 months.

In some states, any citizen can make an application for the temporary hospitalization of a person in need of aid. Others require a family member or guardian, a health or welfare officer, or a physician to apply. Temporary hospitalization may be brought about by the medical certification of one or two physicians, or it may require further approval by a judge, justice, or district attorney in some jurisdictions.

At the end of the observation period, several options are available. The treating physician may (a) discharge the client, (b) encourage the client to stay voluntarily, or (c) file an application for extended hospitalization. In some states, observational hospitalization is mandatory before a court ruling may be made in favor of extended hospitalization.

Extended or Indeterminate Extended or indeterminate involuntary hospitalization can come about through either judicial or nonjudicial procedures. Judicial hospitalization procedures require that a judge or jury determine whether the person is mentally ill to a degree that requires extended hospitalization. If so, the court orders the client hospitalized for an extended period (60 to 180 days) or an indeterminate time.

Proceedings are usually initiated by an application for hospitalization of an allegedly mentally ill person. About half the states permit any responsible person or citizen to make or swear to the application. Others allow only one or more of the following groups: relatives, public officers, physicians, and hospital superintendents. Supporting medical evidence may or may not be required at the time of application.

Most states having judicial hospitalization procedures make some provision for a prehearing medical examination in addition to the medical certification required to support the application. In all jurisdictions having judicial hospitalization procedures, it is mandatory to notify the person proposed to be hospitalized of the hearing. Most states also require notice to the client's attorney, family, or guardian.

A hearing is mandatory in most states, although a few states leave it to the client to request it. While the client's presence is required at the hearing in a few states, most states merely permit attendance if it is not thought to be harmful to the client's condition or if the client in fact demands it. Few states require the hearing to be held in a courtroom. Most say the choice of site is entirely discretionary. Jury trials are no longer mandatory in any state, although a few states still have provisions for the use of a jury to decide the question of hospitalization.

Nonjudicial hospitalization procedures for extended or indeterminate involuntary hospitalization include both administrative and medical certification, but such procedures are now much less prominent on the statute books. Extended hospitalization brought about by an administrative board follows the same procedure used in judicial hospitalization.

Involuntary hospitalization by medical certification, an alternative to the more traditional judicial commitment, is usually advocated for clients who are incapable of consenting to voluntary treatment, although they do not protest hospitalization. The need for hospitalization is usually determined by an examination by one or more physicians and documented by a medical certificate. All states having medical certification provide either for judicial proceedings (if the client contests the hospitalization at any time after certification), or for expanded habeas corpus proceedings, described later in this chapter in the section on client rights.

Involuntary Outpatient Commitment

In response to several highly publicized and dramatic instances of violent acts by mentally disordered persons, most states have modified their statutes and regulations to allow for court-ordered outpatient treatment. In most states allowing for involuntary outpatient commitment (IOC), the criteria are similar to that necessary for inpatient commitment: proof of mental illness and dangerousness. A few states have passed statutes permitting preventive commitment. In these instances, IOC is used to avert a further deterioration of the person's mental health that would require inpatient hospitalization (Segal & Burgess, 2006). IOC has also been used to ensure that mentally ill offenders follow through with outpatient treatment once they are released from prison. Conditional release, a concept related to IOC, is discussed later in this chapter.

Thought to be a way to ensure adherence to a medication regimen, the ethicality of IOC has been questioned because of its coercive nature (Wales & Hiday, 2006). Its effectiveness has been questioned on the basis that it may actually accomplish the opposite, that is, drive people away from treatment (Allen & Smith, 2001). IOC may also be vulnerable to legal challenge on the basis of constitutional standards.

MEDIALINK Critical Thinking Exercise: A Client's Rights

Ethical Dilemmas

Involuntary hospitalization is an exercise of power, and like all forms of power, it can be abused. Because of this potential for abuse, commitment criteria are important. In this country, a person's loss of liberty can be justified only under certain circumstances.

As the review of mental health statutes shows, a degree of "dangerousness" is the favored justification for loss of liberty by involuntary hospitalization. The "dangerousness" criterion is not without its inherent problems. Some of these are considered to be the following:

- Definitions of "dangerousness" vary from state to state.
- It is impossible to predict dangerous behavior reliably.
- In the absence of other criteria, "dangerousness" will be overused to justify admission.

- The stigma of *dangerous* will be added to that of *mentally ill.*
- The stereotype of *mentally disabled* will be reinforced and thus will work against the development of community programs.
- The media will be encouraged to continue selective reporting of instances in which mental illness and criminal behavior appear to be linked.
- Clinical practice shows that "dangerous" individuals are often not treatable, while the most treatable individuals are not dangerous.

Discharge or Separation Categories

A client can separate from a mental institution in one of three ways: discharge, transfer, and escape.

Discharge

Like admission, discharge from a mental hospital can have various layers of complexity. Discharges occur in one of two ways—conditionally or absolutely.

Conditional As implied by the word *conditional*, complete discharge in this situation depends on whether the person fulfills certain conditions over a specified period of time, usually 6 months to 1 year. Adherence to outpatient care, demonstrated ability and willingness to take medications, and the ability to meet the needs of daily living are a few of the many possible prerequisites.

A person who is unable to meet the specified conditions can be reinstitutionalized without going through any legal admission procedure. An individual committed for an extended or indeterminate time is more likely to be a candidate for conditional, rather than absolute, discharge.

Absolute The legal relationship between the institution and the client is terminated by an absolute discharge. If the client should require readmission to the hospital at any time, even a few hours after discharge, a new hospitalization proceeding would be required.

An absolute discharge can be achieved in three ways:

1. An administrative discharge is issued by hospital officials.
2. A judicial discharge is ordered by the courts.
3. A writ of habeas corpus is ordered by the courts on the client's application.

As a rule, the authority for discharging involuntary clients rests in the hands of the hospital director, and these clients are given administrative discharges. However, a few statutes extend this power to the central agency responsible for supervising mental institutions in the state, such as the Department of Mental Health. The client has no formal method of initiating an administrative discharge.

The majority of states have provisions for judicial discharge, which is initiated by an application to the court by the client, the client's family, or any citizen who is in disagreement with hospital authorities over the client's need to be hospitalized. A few states require the application to be accompanied by a medical certificate supporting the idea that the client is ready for discharge. In many states, judicial discharge does not depend on complete recovery. A degree of improvement may be sufficient. Some states guard against frequent applications for discharge by the same clients by imposing a 3-month to 1-year waiting period between requests.

Transfer

Transfers account for a small number of separations from a mental health care facility. Most are transfers within state and county mental health systems. A smaller number are transfers from state to federal facilities or from one state to another.

Escape

A client may take the initiative and decide to terminate the relationship with the institution by informally leaving the hospital grounds. This is commonly referred to as escape, elopement, or being AWOL (absent without leave). Voluntary clients cannot generally be returned to the hospital against their will. However, involuntarily committed clients may be brought back to the hospital against their will with the assistance of the police, if necessary.

PSYCHIATRY AND CRIMINAL LAW

Our legal system in the United States is based on the assumption that the majority of criminal offenders choose to commit crimes for rational reasons, of their own free will, and deserve to be punished for their acts. However, some offenders are mentally disturbed, irrational, or unable to control their behavior. Only a minority of criminal offenders are mentally disturbed—fewer than 4% pursue a defense of legal insanity, and even fewer, 1%, are eventually acquitted by reason of insanity (Bazelon Center for Mental Health Law, 2007).

Determining Legal Sanity

Legal sanity differs from *clinical sanity,* which is the absence of a major mental disorder. **Legal sanity** is defined as an individual's ability to know right from wrong with reference to the act charged, the capacity to know the nature and quality of the act charged, and the capacity to form the intent to commit the crime. Legal sanity is determined for the specific time of the act, as determined by the court order. It may be the brief period of a physical assault or the length of a crime spree over several days.

In most states, the presence of a major mental disorder is a prerequisite for a finding of legal insanity. State insanity laws may have wording variations, but will cite the "presence of mental disorder or defect." Either can be used toward a finding of legal insanity. The term *mental disorder* usually refers to a major mental illness, such as that described in the clinical example that follows; while *mental defect* usually refers to developmental disability or some physiologic condition affecting cognition, such as a head injury, brain tumor, or dementia.

CLINICAL EXAMPLE

Carolyn has a 12-year history of bipolar disorder and had not been taking her medication since being discharged from a psychiatric hospital. Two weeks prior to the alleged offense, Carolyn began having difficulty sleeping, her behavior became erratic, and she spent most nights walking up and down the streets in her neighborhood. Two nights ago, neighbors called the police after they saw her removing items from garages and painting driveways with colorful rainbows. Carolyn was arrested and charged with burglary and malicious mischief.

The burden of proving legal insanity has shifted to the defense as a result of the Hinckley case (John Hinckley is the person who shot President Ronald Reagan in 1981). In the Hinckley trial, the prosection failed to prove that Hinckley was sane beyond a reasonable doubt (the practice at that time in the federal courts). Most states now place the burden of proof on the defense. In federal courts the defense now must prove a defendant's insanity rather than the prosecution having to prove that the defendant is sane (American Bar Association, 1995).

Proof of criminal guilt must be determined "beyond a reasonable doubt" (i.e., it is about 90% to 95% likely that the defendant committed the act). The need for civil commitment in mental health law is based on "clear, cogent, and convincing" evidence (somewhere between 51% and 90%, usually around 75%). Legal insanity is determined by "a preponderance of the evidence" (at least 51%). The situations in which a legal insanity defense is usually raised are listed in Box 13-2.

In criminal cases in which the question of legal sanity is raised, the possibility of malingering a mental disorder will also be raised. Malingering a mental illness (intentionally producing false or exaggerated psychological symptoms) is not uncommon. The *Diagnostic and Statistical Manual of Mental Disorders,* published by the American Psychiatric Association (APA), states that facing a forensic evaluation is a strong indicator for suspecting the malingering of a mental illness (APA, 2000). Malingering is discussed in Chapter 18.

The legal standards most commonly used to determine legal sanity are discussed in the following section.

M'Naghten Rule

In most jurisdictions, the determination of legal sanity is based on the *M'Naghten Rule,* which was the result of a famous case in England.

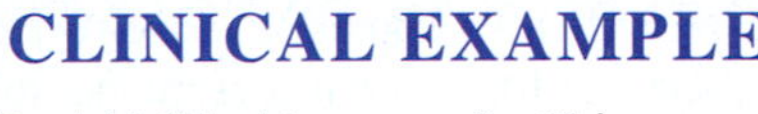

CLINICAL EXAMPLE

Daniel M'Naghten was a Scottish carpenter who believed that Jesuits and Tories were tormenting him. He told his family that spies for the government were following him and laughing at him. He was evicted from his boardinghouse because of his bizarre behavior. In 1843 he stalked Prime Minister Sir Robert Peel, eventually shot Peel's secretary, and was charged with the death. Nine physicians who were experienced in the care of persons with mental disorders testified at the trial (three for the defense, three for the prosecution, and three who listened to the evidence and observed M'Naghten's behavior in the courtroom). All nine agreed M'Naghten suffered from monomania (probably paranoid schizophrenia today) and was not legally sane, according to the legal tests at the time. The jury huddled in the courtroom for two minutes and then found him to be legally insane. He was sent to the local mental institution, Bethlehem Hospital. The public was outraged, believing hospitalization to be too lenient. The queen ordered a task force in the House of Lords to review the case and come up with a new legal standard.

Although the M'Naghten Rule was not applied in this famous case, it was a result of its conclusion. The M'Naghten Rule established the "right from wrong" principle for determining insanity. That is, if a mental disease or defect prevents a criminal from knowing the wrongfulness of his or her actions, the criminal can be found to be "not guilty by reason of insanity" (NGRI). Subsequent developments first broadened, then later narrowed, the grounds for determining legal sanity.

Irresistible Impulse

A volitional component was added to the cognitive component of the M'Naghten Rule in 1929. This became known as the Irresistible Impulse test, which holds that a defendant is exculpated (freed from blame) even if the defendant knew the criminal act was wrong but could not restrain his conduct because of mental disease or defect. A modern interpretation of the standard is known as *The Policeman at the Elbow Test.* That is, would the defendant have committed the act had he known he was being observed by a police officer?

American Law Institute Model Penal Code

The Model Penal Code was approved in 1962 to serve as a guide for states wishing to reform their criminal law. It suggests

Box 13-2 Reasons for Raising an Insanity Defense

A legal insanity defense is raised most often because of:

- Presence of or history of mental disorder
- Depression with suicidality
- Developmental disability
- Sexual deviance
- Amnesia and dissociative states, including a claim of multiple personality
- Medical issues such as brain tumor or other conditions that affect behavior
- Factitious disorder by proxy (formerly known as Munchausen syndrome by proxy)
- Medications that affect behavior
- Personality disorder
- Substance addiction

that a person is not responsible for criminal conduct if, at the time of such conduct, the person, because of mental disease or mental defect, lacked substantial capacity either to appreciate the criminality (wrongfulness) of his conduct or to conform his conduct to the requirements of the law. The code specifies that the terms *mental disease* and *mental defect* do not include abnormal thinking that is manifested by only repeated criminal or otherwise antisocial conduct. The intent of the wording was to preclude the use of personality or character disorders in an insanity defense, especially antisocial personality disorder.

Guilty but Mentally Ill

The insanity defense periodically comes under fire from a public who believes that it is too lenient a response to violence. Some states have opted to use another option—guilty but mentally ill (GBMI)—in an attempt to reform the insanity defense (American Bar Association, 1995). Defendants can be found GBMI if they are guilty of the crime and were mentally ill but not legally insane at the time the crime was committed. The defendant's psychotic state is acknowledged, the defendant is sentenced in the same manner as any criminal, and the defendant receives court-ordered treatment for the mental disorder as well. Once stable, the defendant is transferred to a prison for the remainder of the sentence.

Diminished Capacity

Diminished capacity is an element of the insanity law that refers to an individual's capacity to form the intent to commit a specific act. There are four levels of intent—purposely, knowingly, recklessly, or negligently—and a court may order an evaluation specific to one level, depending on the degree of crime charged. A finding of diminished capacity is based on legal criteria in each state. For example, in some states, the cause of the inability to form intent must be a mental disorder, not amounting to insanity, and not emotions like jealousy, fear, anger, or hatred. The mental disorder must be causally connected to the lack of specific intent, not just reduced perception, awareness, understanding, or overreaction.

Competence to Stand Trial

No person may be tried if he is incompetent. The conviction of an incompetent defendant is a violation of the Fourteenth Amendment—the right to due process. Therefore, a court will remand the incompetent defendant to a "suitable facility" (usually a locked unit in a mental hospital) for treatment to regain competency. Since courts have held that defendants cannot be hospitalized or incarcerated indefinitely, court orders stipulate a specific period of time in which the defendant is given treatment.

While legal insanity is a test of culpability, competence to stand trial is an issue of ability to stand trial. It is defined as having the capacity to understand the proceedings and to assist one's attorney. The presence of a developmental disability, symptoms of a mental disorder, or a history of mental disorder does not necessarily preclude one's competence to stand trial. For example, the presence of delusions may or may not have an impact. It depends on whether the delusion is related to the courtroom, the crime, or the proceedings. The specific content of the delusion, and the degree to which the symptoms affect the abilities and skills needed to be competent, are the important factors. National standards for determining competence to proceed, such as the McGarry Checklist, are available for assessing competence.

PSYCHIATRIC FORENSIC NURSING

Psychiatric forensic nursing can be defined as the psychiatric nursing assessment, evaluation, and treatment of individuals pending a criminal hearing or trial. The defendant is the client, and the client's thinking and behavior prior to, and during, the commission of the crime are the primary focus of the nurse–client relationship.

Psychiatric forensic nursing as an expanded role is evolving into an advanced practice role. However, some role functions can be undertaken by nurses at the generalist level, usually those who work in correctional mental health settings in a jail, a prison's psychiatric unit, or in a forensic psychiatric hospital's long-term unit where persons who are not guilty by reason of insanity are treated. TABLE 13-2 ■ differentiates forensic psychiatric nursing from correctional mental health nursing.

Dimensions of Practice

The dimensions of practice in psychiatric forensic nursing are affected both by the nature of the client and the client's current involvement with the criminal justice system. While the core of practice is psychiatric–mental health nursing, the relationship between nurse and client is markedly different from that in a psychiatric–mental health nursing role because of the alternative social context of the situation that precipitates their interaction. In addition, the setting—a crime scene, a courtroom, a forensic treatment setting, or a correctional facility—influences the forensic nurse's practice.

Role Credibility

The psychiatric forensic nurse must be highly skilled in interpersonal relations and communication. Developing collegial relationships with other disciplines is central to the role because of the intersections of practice that overlap with the domain of other disciplines (forensic science, criminal science). The prerequisite to this expanded role is educational preparation—a graduate degree in forensic nursing or a graduate degree in psychiatric–mental health nursing with additional training in forensic nursing. Several colleges and universities offer degree programs as well as certificate courses in forensic subspecialties.

The International Association of Forensic Nurses (IAFN) is at work on certification examinations for forensic nurses, including advanced practice certification. To date, testing has been developed for sexual assault nurse examiner certification only. You can check on the status of the development of other certification programs through the IAFN website, www.iafn.org, which can be accessed on the Companion Website for this book. Credibility is substantiated by membership or certification in such organizations as the

MEDIALINK International Association of Forensic Nurses

TABLE 13-2 ■ Differentiating Psychiatric Forensic Nursing and Correctional Mental Health Nursing

Variables	Correctional Mental Health Nursing	Psychiatric Forensic Nursing
Who is the client?	Jail/prison inmate Client committed to forensic hospital following "not guilty by reason of insanity" plea	Attorney The court
Mindset of nurse	Supportive Accepting Empathic	Objective Neutral Detached
Focus of the nurse–client relationship	Inmate or client's current and future needs with eye to reintegration into community	Defendant's behavior and thinking at time of crime
Location	Psychiatric unit within a jail/prison Long-term unit within a forensic hospital	Community Jail or prison Hospital ward
Primary purpose of relationship	Psychiatric nursing care of client's (inmate's) present mental health needs	Pretrial completion of court-ordered sanity/competency evaluation
Examples of nursing role functions	Medication teaching Therapeutic groups One-to-one counseling	Evidence collection Report to court Court testimony
Timing	Length of court-ordered commitment, after adjudication	Pretrial

IAFN, the American Academy of Forensic Sciences (www.aafs.org), and the American College of Forensic Examiners (www.acfei.org), which has a board of forensic nurse examiners. Information on these memberships and certifications can be found on the Companion Website for this text. Psychiatric forensic nurses are guided by the standards of forensic nursing practice developed by the American Nurses Association and the International Association of Forensic Nurses (1997). This set of standards is currently undergoing revision.

Roles and Functions

Psychiatric forensic nursing combines elements of nursing science, forensic science, and criminal justice. Psychiatric forensic nursing appeals to a particular type of nurse, male or female, who thrives on the opportunity to work in a stimulating intellectual environment, and who seeks out the opportunity to apply clinical skills to complex legal problems.

Psychiatric forensic nurses work as forensic examiners, competency therapists, expert witnesses, and consultants to law enforcement, attorneys, or the criminal justice system. The wide range of possible psychiatric forensic nursing role functions are listed in Box 13-3.

Forensic Examiner

The forensic examiner conducts court-ordered evaluations of legal sanity or competency to proceed, answers any specific medicolegal questions as directed by the court, and renders an expert opinion in a written report or courtroom testimony. Court-ordered sanity or competency evaluations can be requested by the defense, the prosecution, or the court. They are usually initiated because of the defendant's history or behavior at the scene, in jail, or in the courtroom. A thorough and complete forensic examination includes face-to-face interviews, review of police reports, and thorough psychosocial history.

The ethical forensic examiner's expert opinion is based on the scientific processing of:

- Collected pertinent clinical data
- Observed client behavior
- Forensic evidence in police reports and laboratory reports
- Results of psychological testing
- Thorough psychosocial history

As a forensic examiner, you must be able to verbalize an exceptional understanding of major mental illnesses and personality disorders. You must keep abreast of theories being developed on social deviancy and interpersonal violence, and

Box 13-3 Psychiatric Forensic Nursing Roles

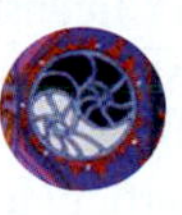

- Forensic evaluation for legal sanity or competence to proceed at trial
- Assessment of capacity to formulate intent
- Assessment of potential for violence or to reoffend
- Parole/probation considerations
- Assessment of racial/cultural factors during crime
- Consultation on countermeasures to violence
- Assisting in jury selection
- Investigation of criminal history
- Sexual predator screening and assessment
- Courtroom consultation to attorneys
- Competency therapy
- Formal written reports to court
- Expert witness services
- Police training
- Review of police reports
- On-scene consultation to law enforcement

MEDIALINK Forensic Nursing

keep current on social trends (for example, changes in drug use, growth of gang activity, or cult participation) both nationally and in your own jurisdiction.

The successful forensic examiner is able to:

- Separate personal opinion from professional opinion. *Personal opinion is based on your background, upbringing, education, and values. Professional opinion is based on scientific principle, advanced education in a specific field of endeavor, and the unbiased standards set by research in that area.*
- Isolate personal feelings in dealing with cases of criminal violence. *Sexual deviance, ethnic norms, or cultural behaviors that may not reflect your own personal value system may be integral to the questioning.*

Competency Therapist

Traditionally, treatment for incompetence meant little more than the prescribing of antipsychotic or other medications. With registered nurses moving into this role, a more holistic approach is being taken—one that encompasses the client's physical, emotional, and spiritual needs. Psychiatric forensic nursing role functions for the competency therapist include:

- Administration of assessment tools
- Assessment of competence and mental disorder
- Forensic interview
- Documentation of the client's progress toward competence
- Completion of formal reports to the court
- Expert witness testimony

Competency therapists work with defendants on one-to-one and group levels. It is important that the competency therapist retains objectivity and does not confuse competency therapy with psychotherapy. Competency therapy is education/training-based. The focus of the relationship is on the defendant's thinking and behavior at the time of the crime, not, for instance, on the defendant's history of abuse or failed interpersonal relationships. The client of the competency therapist is the court, not the defendant, and the goal is a competent defendant and completed report.

Expert Witness

By license, any registered nurse can be subpoenaed to court as a *fact witness*. In this role, you testify as to what you personally saw, heard, performed, or documented related to a particular client's care. You are questioned as to these first-hand experiences, and then excused from the courtroom.

An **expert witness** is recognized by the court as having a high level of skill or expertise in a designated area in order to render an opinion on a legal matter in court. As an expert witness, you will be subpoenaed to court to testify on your involvement with the defendant. You will testify as to the role functions you performed and to your documentation. At this point, the court will allow you to give additional testimony in the form of your professional opinion, based on your conclusions, as to the defendant's legal sanity, competence to proceed, future dangerousness, or likelihood of committing future felonious acts.

To establish credibility as an expert and to have one's opinion given equal weight in court opposite a psychiatrist, the forensic nurse specialist must have:

1. *Expertise.* Expertise is established by your credentials.
2. *Trustworthiness.* Trustworthiness is the degree of honesty exuded in your demeanor and opinion, as perceived by the judge or jury.
3. *Presentation style.* Presentation style is how you come across to others. You may be credible, trustworthy, and an authority in a specialty area, but without the ability to communicate in a concise and convincing fashion, the value of your testimony is limited.

Consultant to Attorneys

Psychiatric forensic nurses may be called on as a resource for education and information about mental illness by either side of the courtroom. Or you may be asked to attend the hearing as a courtroom observer who listens to other witness testimony for the purpose of guiding further cross-examination. You may also be asked to assist in preparation for trial by giving information about mental illness, personality disorders, or paraphilias, give suggestions for cross-examining a defendant, or evaluate potential jurors. You may be asked to testify regarding mental health treatment options, medications, and community resources.

Consultant to Law Enforcement

Interagency cooperation between mental health agencies and law enforcement has increased over the last decades, partly due to community need caused by deinstitutionalization. The mental health personnel summoned in those situations function as advocates for the defendant, whose well-being is the focus of the interaction that may result in civil detention and admission to a hospital. Community mental health nurses have traditionally acted in this role.

Psychiatric forensic nurses are expanding their scope of practice by working as consultants to law enforcement in hostage negotiation and criminal profiling. In addition to giving suggestions on how to interview a subject, psychiatric forensic nurses may be involved in actual hostage negotiation or criminal profiling. These roles differ from that described earlier in purpose and philosophy.

Hostage Negotiation In the late 1970s, the Federal Bureau of Investigation began expanding hostage negotiation team structure by recommending the use of consultants who could address the mental state of the perpetrator and recommend appropriate negotiation strategies. In the next decade, local police agencies began to develop specialized teams and use consultants. Over half of all hostage incidents involve hostage-takers who are classified in law enforcement as mentally disturbed. Police agencies that used a consultant in hostage incidents reported significantly more negotiated surrenders, significantly fewer incidents ending with tactical team assaults, and fewer incidents in which the perpetrator killed or seriously injured a hostage (Slatkin, 2000).

When functioning as a behavioral sciences expert, the role of the psychiatric forensic nurse on a hostage negotiation team differs markedly from that of the community mental health nurse. You are not an advocate of the perpetrator, but of the process of hostage negotiation. This may involve being on 24-hour call for a Special Weapons and Tactics Team (SWAT) or patrol officers on the scene, assessing the perpetrator's mental status, liaising with mental health agencies, assessing released hostages, assessing hostage negotiator stress, participating in postincident critiques, and providing communication skill training to law enforcement officers. The psychiatric forensic nurse hostage negotiator should receive the same negotiator training as law enforcement officers.

Criminal Profiling Psychiatric forensic nurses working with law enforcement may be asked to participate in the part of an investigation now formally known as Criminal Investigative Analysis. This will occur only after you have established your credibility as a forensic practitioner in your specialty area. Formerly known as criminal profiling, it is no substitute for a thorough and well-planned investigation and is only one tool among many that law enforcement uses to eliminate suspects or to narrow leads. Criminal profiling is an educated attempt to provide law enforcement with specific information on the type of individual who would have committed a certain crime after studying behavioral and psychological indicators left at a violent crime scene.

Profilers come from a variety of backgrounds—law enforcement, psychology, psychiatry, criminal justice, sociology, and now, forensic psychiatric nursing. A background in behavioral science, an understanding of psychopathology, and investigative experience are fundamental to this role.

The profiler collects all of the data, attempts to reconstruct the situation, formulates a hypothesis, develops a profile, tests it, and checks for results. As you can see, the method of developing a profile is similar to the nursing process. In testing the hypothesis, skilled profilers isolate their own emotions and attempt to reconstruct the crime using the criminal's reasoning process (Fintzy, 2000). If you attempt to analyze the situation based on your own values or logic, you will misinterpret the criminal's behavior. A skilled profiler is patient. By not jumping to conclusions, the skilled profiler's opinion is slowly formed based on an examination of the data.

Correctional Mental Health Nursing

Correctional mental health nurses care for inmates housed in a jail or prison's psychiatric unit, or in a forensic psychiatric hospital's long-term ward where persons adjudicated as "not guilty by reason of insanity" are treated. However, the nature of their relationship with the client remains focused on the client's present needs rather than on his or her thinking or behavior in the past (at the time of the crime). Correctional mental health nurses perform psychiatric nursing skills rather than forensic nursing skills. Refer back to Table 13-2, which illustrates the differences in forensic psychiatric nursing and correctional mental health nursing.

Correctional mental health nurses make substantial and valued contributions to the care, treatment, rehabilitation, and management of individuals in secure facilities who are deemed legally insane. It is a difficult and challenging client population to work with (Rayel, 2000), and personal safety is an issue during every shift. The dedication of correctional mental health nurses has significantly increased the quality of care for their clients. There are high expectations for this specialized area of practice that continues to contribute to the growing fund of nursing knowledge. Correctional mental health nurses are guided by the standards of nursing practice in correctional facilities developed by the American Nurses Association (2007).

CLIENT RIGHTS

The current concern for client rights did not develop overnight. It actually has been evolving since the 1960s, when there was an increased interest in underrepresented minority groups, the poor, women, and the mentally disabled.

In 1980, the United States Congress passed the Mental Health Systems Act, which included a model mental health client's bill of rights. This piece of legislation can be thought of as a set of recommendations; it is not a requirement that individual states follow them. In 1990, the American Hospital Association published a Patient's Bill of Rights that many health care settings throughout the United States have adopted. Consumer groups and professional organizations have, at various times, published their own versions of a bill of rights. A mental health consumer's bill of rights has been developed and supported by 15 professional organizations, including nursing, for those seeking mental health and substance abuse treatment. This particular bill of rights can be found on www.apa.org/pubinfo/rights/rights.html and accessed through the Companion Website for this book.

However, there is no one standard mental health client bill of rights at the national level, and the variability among states is great. Some states guarantee several important rights, while some states guarantee only a few. In other words, there is no consistency among states. The rights that mental health consumers should have in practice and that you should consider when planning your interventions are outlined in the Your Intervention Strategies feature on page 276. A discussion of several of these important rights follows later in this chapter. One means of helping clients protect some of their rights is through the execution of a psychiatric advance directive.

MEDIALINK Mental Health Patient's Bill of Rights

Psychiatric Advance Directives

Psychiatric advance directives (PADs) are modeled after advance directives for end-of-life care. They are legal instruments that allow competent persons to document their preferences regarding mental health treatment. Any person can prepare a PAD as a contingency plan to put in place should the person be incapacitated, found to be incompetent, or unable to make reliable decisions about psychiatric care. Some people *expect to become incapacitated* in the future—for example, a person with symptoms of early Alzheimer's or Pick's disease

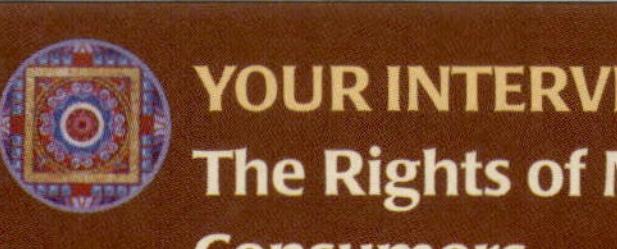

YOUR INTERVENTION STRATEGIES
The Rights of Mental Health Consumers

Keep the following rights in mind when planning and implementing nursing interventions:

- Right to informed consent
- Right to treatment
- Right to refuse treatment
- Right to treatment in the least restrictive setting
- Right to communicate with others
- Right not to be subjected to unnecessary mechanical restraints
- Right to privacy
- Right to periodic review of status
- Right to independent psychiatric examination
- Right to participate in legal matters including making a valid contract, executing a will, marrying or divorcing, voting, driving a motor vehicle, practicing a profession, suing or being sued, managing or disposing of property
- Right to habeas corpus
- Right to legal representation
- Right to keep clothing and personal effects
- Right to religious freedom
- Right to education
- Right to civil service status

MEDIALINK Psychiatric Advance Directives

(see Chapter 14). Others may simply *anticipate the possibility of becoming incapacitated* in the future—for example, a person with a family history of Alzheimer's or Pick's disease. Still others have experienced an episode of mental disorder—perhaps depression requiring a period of hospitalization during which they received ECT—and wish to register their preferences for any future psychiatric intervention.

A written PAD allows a person to:

1. Register refusal of certain psychiatric interventions such as ECT, psychotropic medications, psychosurgery, and the like.
2. Register consent and desire for certain psychiatric interventions.
3. Specify the conditions under which these interventions are acceptable.
4. Appoint a trusted surrogate decision maker, a person(s) authorized to give consent on the person's behalf.
5. Register whether the person is willing or unwilling to participate in psychiatric research studies.
6. Improve communication between the person and the mental health care provider.
7. Possibly shorten a hospital stay (Bazelon Center for Mental Health Law, 2007).

Increasing numbers of mental health professionals favor PADs because in addition to guiding family members, significant others, and professionals, they respect the client's autonomy. Advance directives become even more important when the surrogate decision maker is other than the client's next of kin (see the accompanying Evidence-Based Practice feature). In this instance, a PAD can also reduce the use of court proceedings.

While PADs are becoming more popular (they first came into existence in the 1990s), they are still not in common use. A survey of 1,011 psychiatric outpatients in five U.S. cities indicated that only 4% to 13% of participants had completed a PAD, but between 66% and 77% reported wanting to complete one if given assistance (Swanson, Swartz, Ferron, Elbogen, & Van Dorn, 2006). Some 22 states have created specific forms for PADs. They can be accessed through a resource center created in 2006, the National Resource Center on Psychiatric Advance Directives (NRC-PAD), which can be accessed through the Companion Website for this text or at www.nrc-pad.org. Persons in states that do not have a specific PAD form can use the Bazelon Center for Mental Health Law template at www.bazelon.org. All states have a provision for a durable power of attorney for health care to which a PAD can be attached.

Mental health consumers who are now using these documents find that a PAD is a tool for empowerment and self-determination. At the same time that mental health consumers anticipate the likelihood that mental health care providers, hospitals, and judges honor their choices, they are concerned about the limited knowledge of PADS among mental health service providers (Kim et al., 2007). An advance directive such as a PAD provides written direction for ethically sensitive judgment on the part of professionals and surrogates even in states in which they are not legally recognized. FIGURE 13-1 ■ on page 278 illustrates the elements that comprise a PAD and a step-by-step process that you can use to help a client develop and implement a PAD.

Right to Informed Consent

A client has the right to understand the treatment process prior to consenting to treatment. This is called **informed consent** and is required by all states. The main purpose of the doctrine of informed consent is to encourage individual autonomy and sound decision making. Client self-determination is the basic principle of informed consent.

Key elements of informed consent are **competency**, information, and voluntariness. Being competent means that a client must be cognitively able to understand the situation and the implications of treatment. If a client's competency is in question, a mental status examination may be necessary. The medication record may need to be reviewed to determine if the client received medication that might interfere with cognitive ability. Any deficits in the client's reception and processing of information need to be taken into account. The client must be competent to understand the problem, along with the negative and positive effects from the proposed treatment, and the likely outcome with and without treatment.

Many illnesses impair the ability to acquire new information. In some cases this is a response to the biologic com-

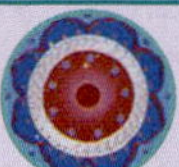

EVIDENCE-BASED PRACTICE

ACTING AS A CLIENT ADVOCATE

Heather Adams is a neighbor in your apartment building. On weekends, the two of you sometimes get together for morning coffee. Last weekend, Heather shared with you a concern that has been troubling her for a few weeks. She is 31 years old, unmarried, and lives alone. Her father died 3 years ago in a construction accident. Since that time, Heather's mother has become increasingly incapacitated with Alzheimer's disease and is now a resident in a long-term care facility for the cognitively impaired. When she was in her early 20s, Heather was hospitalized and treated for depression. Heather's next of kin is her brother, Ed, from whom she has been estranged for 5 years. Her fear is that, should she become incapacitated again with depression, the brother whom she actively dislikes and with whom she does not get along will make treatment decisions as next-of-kin.

You have decided to invite Heather for coffee on Saturday. Because Heather seems to be a person who would benefit from a formal PAD, you intend to educate her about her choices. You plan to use Figure 13-1 on page 278 as the basis for a discussion with Heather and to help her formalize her wishes concerning any possible future psychiatric treatment such as medication and ECT, treatment setting, the selection of a trusted surrogate, and whether or not she is willing to participate in psychiatric research studies. The next step is to obtain a sample PAD from the Bazelon Center for Mental Health Law (see the References at the end of this chapter) for Heather to review. This way, as suggested in the following studies, you can serve as an active resource for Heather.

Kim, M. M., Van Dorn, R. A., Scheyett, A. M., Elbogen, E. E., Swanson, J. W., Swartz, M. S., & McDaniel, L. A. (2007). Understanding the personal and clinical utility of psychiatric advance directives: A qualitative perspective. *Psychiatry, 70*(1), 19–29.

Swanson, J., Swartz, M., Ferron, J., Elbogen, E., & Van Dorn, R. (2006). Psychiatric advance directives among public mental health consumers in five U.S. cities: Prevalence, demand, and correlates. *Journal of the American Academy of Psychiatry and the Law, 34*(1), 43–57.

CRITICAL THINKING APPLICATION

1. On what basis do you act as an advocate for Heather?
2. Is it ethical for you to serve as the surrogate decision maker?
3. Why might some mental health professionals have negative attitudes about PADs?

ponents of the illness or the effects of medication. In other cases there may be an educational deficit. For some long-term clients, the presence of a mental illness may have affected the educational experience. This does not mean that intelligence is affected, but that reading and writing skills may not be consistent with chronological age. Developing plans for offering information that would be needed in the decision-making process helps to ensure a client's right to informed consent. It may be necessary to present information in small pieces using simple language and pictures. Several short presentations may be required, with some mechanism to assess learning to determine whether the client understands the proposed treatment.

All clients must be offered choices and given the advantages and disadvantages of each. While members of the mental health team can offer suggestions, it must be clear to the client that there is no self-serving bias on the part of the treatment team for one choice or another. The client must have the opportunity to ask questions or gain a second opinion. The client should not be rushed or coerced into giving consent.

Informed consent must be documented in writing through the use of a specific form signed by the client, or by an entry into the client's medical record. While written documentation of informed consent will likely fulfill the legal obligation, it is helpful to think of informed consent as more of a recurring process. While hospitalized, clients should be offered many chances to participate in their own care.

At times, it may become clear that the client lacks the ability to offer consent. In this case, it is important to interact with legal counsel to determine what should be done. Some states allow legal relatives to participate for a client who cannot consent. Other states demand that the client have an advocate appointed to serve as decision maker. For a summary of informed consent requirements, see the Your Assessment Approach feature below.

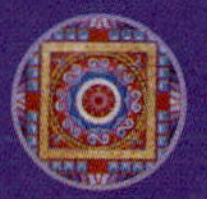

YOUR ASSESSMENT APPROACH
Informed Consent Requirements

In assessing whether informed consent has been obtained, you must determine whether the client:

- Is of the age of consent
- Is deemed mentally competent
- Can state that he or she is acting voluntarily
- Can repeat the elements of the condition
- Can repeat the treatment options
- Can repeat the benefits and consequences of each treatment
- Can repeat the consequences of inaction
- Is not impaired by alcohol or other drugs
- Can complete specific written forms such as consent forms, treatment plans, and discharge plans

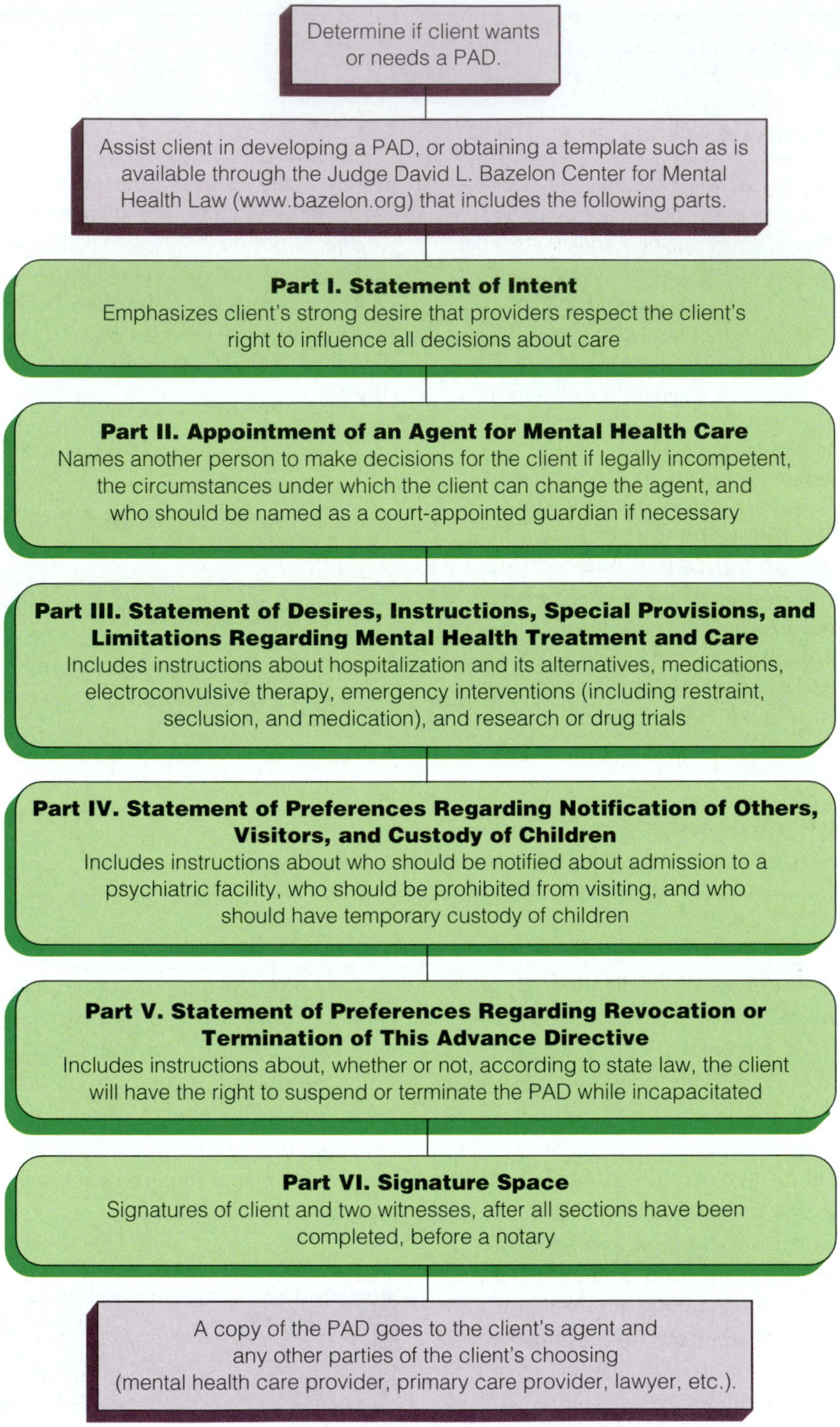

Determine if client wants or needs a PAD.

Assist client in developing a PAD, or obtaining a template such as is available through the Judge David L. Bazelon Center for Mental Health Law (www.bazelon.org) that includes the following parts.

Part I. Statement of Intent
Emphasizes client's strong desire that providers respect the client's right to influence all decisions about care

Part II. Appointment of an Agent for Mental Health Care
Names another person to make decisions for the client if legally incompetent, the circumstances under which the client can change the agent, and who should be named as a court-appointed guardian if necessary

Part III. Statement of Desires, Instructions, Special Provisions, and Limitations Regarding Mental Health Treatment and Care
Includes instructions about hospitalization and its alternatives, medications, electroconvulsive therapy, emergency interventions (including restraint, seclusion, and medication), and research or drug trials

Part IV. Statement of Preferences Regarding Notification of Others, Visitors, and Custody of Children
Includes instructions about who should be notified about admission to a psychiatric facility, who should be prohibited from visiting, and who should have temporary custody of children

Part V. Statement of Preferences Regarding Revocation or Termination of This Advance Directive
Includes instructions about, whether or not, according to state law, the client will have the right to suspend or terminate the PAD while incapacitated

Part VI. Signature Space
Signatures of client and two witnesses, after all sections have been completed, before a notary

A copy of the PAD goes to the client's agent and any other parties of the client's choosing (mental health care provider, primary care provider, lawyer, etc.).

FIGURE 13-1 ■ Helping a client develop and implement a psychiatric advance directive.

Right to Treatment

The first argument for a right to treatment for involuntarily committed individuals came from Morton Birnbaum, a lawyer and physician, in an article published in 1960. However, the groundbreaking cases did not come from the familiar circles of civil commitment but from people who had been sidetracked from the prison system into hospitals.

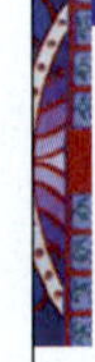

CLINICAL EXAMPLE

Instead of being convicted for carrying a dangerous weapon and receiving a maximum sentence of 1 year, a man in Washington, D.C., who pleaded "not guilty by reason of insanity," was sent to the maximum security unit of a federal psychiatric hospital for treatment on an involuntary commitment basis.

Four years later, he questioned his detention on the basis of not having received any psychiatric treatment.

A man indicted for murder was sent to a Massachusetts state hospital after having been found incompetent to stand trial. He requested transfer to another facility on the grounds that he was not receiving adequate treatment. Through the testimony of experts, his attorneys were able to show that he was simply receiving custodial care.

An involuntary client in a Florida mental hospital for over 14 years brought suit against the hospital director, claiming that he had been deprived of his constitutional right to liberty. At trial, the jury found that (a) he had received not merely inadequate treatment but no treatment at all; (b) he was not dangerous; (c) acceptable community alternatives were available; and (d) because the hospital director knew all this, he had "maliciously" deprived him of liberty.

In these instances, the courts found a constitutional rationale for treatment. Depriving a citizen of liberty on the altruistic theory that the loss of liberty is for the purpose of therapy, and then failing to provide adequate therapy, violates the rights of citizens guaranteed by the Constitution.

Right-to-treatment issues also have to do with inappropriate releases, or passes to leave a hospital when prudent care would indicate that freedom was inappropriate.

CLINICAL EXAMPLE

Eight days after admission to a New Orleans hospital for severe depression, a client was given a weekend pass, during which she attempted suicide. She sued the hospital and psychotherapists for allowing her to leave the hospital when she was not in a fit mental condition.

In Washington, D.C., a client who had been committed to a hospital after being acquitted of murder by reason of insanity left the hospital grounds and stabbed his wife. The hospital was found liable based on its failure to take reasonable measures to ensure that the client did not leave the hospital grounds.

The concept of right to treatment is an outgrowth of the philosophic point of view that the deprivation of liberty, whether voluntary or involuntary, must have an overriding purpose. A review of court cases indicates that the right to treatment came about because there was no overriding purpose: Because of overcrowded conditions, inadequate staffing, financial and programmatic deficiencies, there were not enough resources to deliver the bare minimum of treatment. "Right to treatment" ensures that clients are not in a treatment setting for custodial purposes only. The necessary elements in a treatment-oriented program are listed in the Your Intervention Strategies feature that follows.

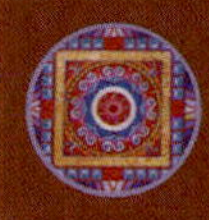

YOUR INTERVENTION STRATEGIES The Necessary Elements in a Treatment-Oriented Program

Be sure that your facility's program includes the following:

- Physical examination and psychosocial assessment on admission and then as indicated
- Treatment plans with clear objectives and interventions
- Evidence of client participation in treatment planning and consent for all treatment methods
- Up-to-date medical records
- Treatment in as normal an environment as possible
- Staff in adequate numbers and with sufficient training to provide quality care
- Availability of treatment that meets client needs as identified in the treatment plan
- Necessary support services such as dental, speech, physical, and rehabilitation therapy
- Ongoing treatment plan evaluations
- Programs to help clients develop skills needed for independent versus institutional living
- Adequate planning for discharge to a less restrictive setting, according to client needs

Right to Refuse Treatment

At some time in their lives, all people experience the kind of excessive stress that makes them feel miserable or even desperate. But some people communicate these feelings in ways that are inappropriate, troublesome, unreasonable, or frightening to others. A young woman who in times of stress mutilates her body by burning it repeatedly with cigarettes; a teenager who breaks everything in sight during violent, destructive outbursts; and a belligerent man who initiates physical fights with anyone and everyone without provocation—all usually become candidates for *symptomatic treatments,* behavioral control measures often used against a person's will. However, all clients have the right to refuse treatment. The clinical example that follows demonstrates how the right to refuse treatment has been upheld by the courts.

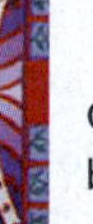

CLINICAL EXAMPLE

One of the first cases against restrictive treatment was brought in Minnesota in 1976. In this case, ECT was felt to be an "intrusive" treatment and was not allowed to be given against a competent client's wishes.

An involuntarily committed client at a New Jersey state hospital claimed that forcibly administering medications violated his constitutional rights. He objected to the side effects produced by chlorpromazine (Thorazine) and lithium carbonate. The judge ruled in the client's favor, noting that a person subjected to the harsh side effects of psychotropic drugs should have control over their administration.

Clients at a Massachusetts state hospital initiated a class action suit contending that their constitutional rights were being violated by the hospital's practice of using forced seclusion and medication in nonemergency situations. The court granted competent clients and guardians of incompetent clients an absolute right to refuse medication in nonemergency situations.

An issue that captured public attention was the notorious case of a homeless New York woman forcibly removed from the streets because of her self-neglect and provocative behavior. She was judged competent, however, to refuse medication despite her status as an involuntary patient.

In another case, the court found that a nurse who forcibly administered medication to a competent adult client had committed an intentional tort (a wrongful act). The client was involuntarily committed to a mental hospital. She was a practicing Christian Scientist and refused medication. The court held that medication could be given over the client's religious objections only if she were harmful to herself or others. The court allowed her damages for assault and battery.

A more recent trend in some states is toward assisted outpatient treatment (AOT), spurred by New York's Kendra's Law.

CLINICAL EXAMPLE

Kendra was a young woman pushed to her death from a subway platform by a man with schizophrenia who had a documented history of assaults and failed to follow prescribed medication regimens. Kendra's parents and other advocates pushed for a statewide law in New York to ensure that persons who are deemed a danger to themselves and others are given assistance in adhering to prescribed medication regimens.

Less than 10 years have passed since Kendra was pushed to her death, yet 42 states now have some form of statewide AOT that is court ordered for medication nonadherence. Securing the common good is undoubtedly the basis for this form of legislation.

In almost all states, ECT is closely regulated by statute. Most state statutes specify that ECT can be administered only if informed consent is obtained from the client. In the case of an incompetent client, consent must be obtained from the guardian or next of kin. The client's right to refuse ECT is specifically mentioned in many state statutes.

Psychosurgery, referred to in various state statutes as "brain surgery," "lobotomy," or "experimental" or "hazardous" procedures, is also closely regulated by state statute. Most state statutes specify that psychosurgery can be performed only if informed consent is obtained from the client. In several states, psychosurgery can be performed only upon a court order if the client is incompetent. The client's right to refuse psychosurgery is also specifically mentioned in many state statutes.

If written consent is withheld by a client already declared "legally incompetent" by the court or certified "functionally incompetent" by a treating psychiatrist, the decision to medicate forcibly would be referred to a client advocate. It would be up to the client advocate's discretion to request a hearing before an independent psychiatrist. In the case of a competent though involuntarily hos-

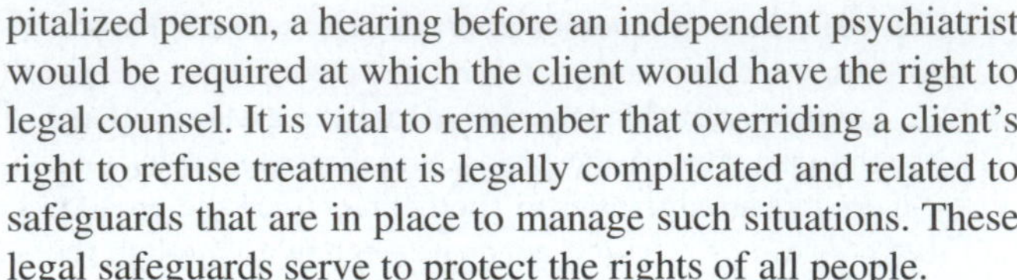

pitalized person, a hearing before an independent psychiatrist would be required at which the client would have the right to legal counsel. It is vital to remember that overriding a client's right to refuse treatment is legally complicated and related to safeguards that are in place to manage such situations. These legal safeguards serve to protect the rights of all people.

Ethical Dilemmas

There are a number of areas of judicial disagreement in the right to refuse treatment that can create dilemmas for the mental health care professional. For example, there is no common definition of the term *psychiatric emergency.* The traditional definition of *emergency* refers to an overt and immediate threat to a person's life. The contemporary definition focuses on the immediate, impending, and significant deterioration of the client's condition.

Another area of controversy is: At what point can the state override an involuntarily committed client's right to refuse psychotropic medication in a nonemergency? Is it only when a person has been judged incompetent, or does danger to self or others provide a legitimate reason under the state's police power to administer treatment?

In the case of an incompetent individual, there is disagreement over who should decide for the person and what standard should be used. Is it to be a guardian, the hospital staff, or the judiciary? Is the standard what the best interests of the client seem to be, as judged by an informed outsider, or is it what the client would want if competent to make the choice?

Here are some criteria a court is likely to use in ruling on a case involving the right to refuse treatment:

- *Client competency.* If the client is competent, informed consent is possible.
- *Intrusiveness of treatment.* As the intrusiveness increases, so does the court's scrutiny.
- *Permanence of treatment effect.* If side effects are adverse and permanent, the court is less likely to override refusal.
- *Experimental nature of treatment.* The treatment must have scientific merit, and the client must give informed consent.
- *Risk–benefit ratio.* The benefits of treatment must outweigh the risk.
- *Motivation for treatment.* The treatment cannot be used to punish or "quiet" the client for the staff's benefit.
- *Motivation for refusal.* Religious objections are usually upheld.

Despite the difficulties and issues raised by the client's right to refuse treatment, some very real positive outcomes are these:

- Clients must be involved in treatment choices, process, and outcome.
- Clients must be informed of choices and offered alternatives.
- Staff members must acquire a second opinion on potentially harmful procedures.

YOUR SELF-AWARENESS
Right to Refuse Treatment

To increase self-awareness of your own opinions about a client's right to refuse treatment, think about the following questions:

- How do I feel when a client's legal right to leave a treatment setting is deemed more important than the client's need for treatment?
- Should clients whose behavior disrupts and frightens other clients be allowed to refuse treatment even when interventions such as medication would definitely reduce their symptoms?
- In the case of a client judged to be mentally incompetent, what standard should be used to make decisions about treatment? Should it be what the hospital staff wants? What a guardian wants? The best interests of the client? What the client would want if competent to make the choice?
- Does society have an obligation to care for a seriously mentally ill person even if this requires limiting that person's freedom to refuse treatment?
- Do we need to protect rights vigorously or is the duty to treat a greater obligation?
- Should a person on the street who is gesturing and talking to herself and carrying a few belongings in a plastic bag be allowed to continue living on the street or be mandated into outpatient commitment?

Consider the other dilemmas outlined in the Your Self-Awareness feature above.

Right to Treatment in the Least Restrictive Setting

The idea of least restrictive setting or least restrictive alternative has become an important component of both the deinstitutionalization and client rights movements. The term **least restrictive setting** generally refers to the placement of clients in the therapeutic setting that will provide care while allowing maximum freedom. By extension, it also means providing for the least amount of limitation or interference in an individual's thought and decision making, physical activity, and sense of self as necessary to provide for safety.

CLINICAL EXAMPLE

A 61-year-old District of Columbia woman had difficulty caring for herself because of confusion secondary to arteriosclerotic brain disease. While not considered a danger to others, she did wander when confused and was subsequently admitted to the federal psychiatric hospital. The court ruled that she did not need 24-hour psychiatric supervision and that a less restrictive form of treatment should be found. Today, such clients can be supervised in assisted living facilities for the cognitively impaired.

The American Nurses Association's standards of psychiatric–mental health nursing practice (2007) direct the nurse to choose the least restrictive limit and use it only for as long as it is necessary for the safety of the client and others.

Treatment Setting

A treatment setting is evaluated on such criteria as the limitations it places on physical freedom (locked or unlocked), choice of activities, and the presence of "adult status" as shown by locked bedrooms and the unsupervised use of private bathroom facilities. In this scheme, inpatient psychiatric settings would be considered the most restrictive, halfway houses less so, and family or independent living the least.

Institutional Policy

Institutional policy is the degree of restriction imposed by the rules and regulations necessary to run the treatment setting. Criteria to evaluate a setting would include such items as the amount of supervision in daily living tasks, the amount of client involvement in treatment planning, and the priority of activities that increase the client's autonomy.

Enforcement

The enforcement dimension includes the methods sanctioned to enforce the treatment setting's rules. Is coercion or threat of punishment used? Is the standard for socially acceptable behavior higher in the treatment setting than it would be in the client's own environment? How readily and to what extent is the client's autonomy compromised to meet organizational needs?

Treatment

The treatment dimension has to do with the intrusiveness of the treatment used. Psychosurgery and ECT would be considered more intrusive than medication. Long-acting medication such as fluphenazine decanoate would be considered more intrusive than oral medication. The clarity of treatment goals is also a consideration. Nebulous or nonexistent goals increase restrictiveness.

Client Characteristics

The client's illness characteristics are seen by some as restricting behavior to a much greater degree than any locked door. Some believe it is simplistic to think that moving a client from an inpatient setting to the community will automatically result in less restriction. Without effective community-based treatment, including safe housing, many chronically ill clients frequently end up on the streets (see Chapter 12).

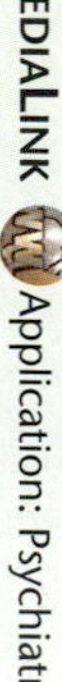

MEDIALINK Guidelines for the Use of Restraint and Seclusion

Right to Communicate with Others

The basis for laws granting communication rights is that such communication can expose cases of wrongful hospitalization. Generally, communication is unrestricted or guaranteed to named public officials or the central hospital agency for the state. Most states extend this guarantee to include correspondence with attorneys. Most states also require that any correspondence limitation be part of the client's clinical record. Approximately half the states require the client to have reasonable access to writing materials and postage.

Most states have some statutory provisions concerning visitation. However, hospital authorities are generally given broad discretionary powers to curtail this right. Before implementing any restriction in communication or visitation, you should ask: Is it fair and reasonable? Could I defend it to a noninvolved professional?

Right Not to Be Subjected to Unnecessary Mechanical Restraints

Though improvements in treatment have decreased the use of mechanical or physical restraints, such restraints still play a role in some treatment programs. Most states have attempted to regulate their use by statute through specifying that restraints can be used only in emergency situations, and only as a measure of last resort, when the client presents a risk of harm to self or others. In those states not having statutory provisions regarding restraints, the procedures to be followed are usually found in the administrative regulations.

Many states and mental health facilities have statutes or protocols that relate to manual restraint. Manual restraint includes holding or restraining an individual against his or her will, regardless of the intent or purpose. For example, holding a person's arm or hand while the person receives an injection or has blood drawn can be considered manual restraint against the person's will unless the person requests physical contact or accepts it when it is offered.

Half the states have laws relating to seclusion. Prevention of harm to self or others is the most common criterion, followed by treatment or therapeutic reasons. The use of either restraints or seclusion must be documented in the client's medical record. Nursing organizations such as the American Psychiatric Nurses Association (APNA) (2007) and mental health consumer advocacy groups such as the National Alliance on Mental Illness (NAMI) have developed position statements on the use of seclusion and restraint. The position statements are available at the APNA website at http://www.apna.org/i4a/pages/index.cfm?pageid=3504, and at www.nami.org, the website for NAMI. Both websites can be accessed through the Companion Website for this book. See also Chapter 35∞.

It has become clear that changes in a unit's philosophy can reduce the incidence of the use of seclusion and restraint. A unit with a culture of structure, calmness, negotiation, and collaboration (Delaney & Johnson, 2006) in which staff assess early changes with clients and intervene early with less restrictive measures—verbal and nonverbal communication, reducing stimulation, active listening, diversionary techniques, limit setting, and the judicious use of prn medication (Johnson & Delaney, 2007)—more clearly safeguard the rights of clients.

Right to Privacy

Almost all states have a specific statute regarding the mental health consumer's right to keep personal information secret, and the specific steps to be taken for release of that information. The confidential nature of the client information is also cited in the American Nurses Association Code of Ethics—maintaining client confidentiality within ethical, legal, and regulatory parameters—as it is in most professional codes (refer to Box 13-1 on page 264).

The goal of confidentiality is to ensure the client's privacy. A significant amount of stigma is attached to being the recipient of psychiatric treatment. Though professionals may argue that this is unfair, it is a fact. Because of this, it is important that clients are the ones to give out this information about themselves. Instructors, students, supervisors, or team members who receive information about a client in the course of supervision or in providing treatment for the client are also obligated to treat this material as confidential.

In order for the disclosure of information to occur, a client must sign a release form. To be a valid release, the client must be told as specifically as possible what information is to be released. The client should know the following prior to signing:

- What information is going to be released?
- Who needs it?
- Why do they need it?
- When will they need it?
- How will it be used?

Certain situations require signed consents. FIGURE 13-2 ■ illustrates situations in which signed consents are necessary.

Emergency situations may arise. For example, a client may be in a car accident or take an overdose and require treatment in a hospital emergency room. In these situations, the

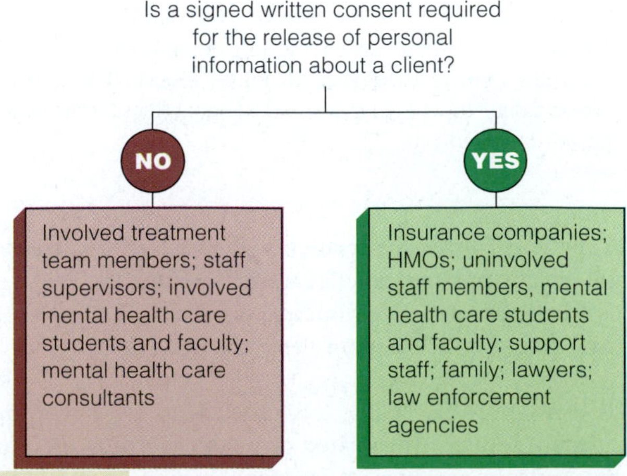

FIGURE 13-2 ■ When a written consent from a mental health consumer is required for release of personal information.

release of information can occur without the client's approval. It is important to document such a breach of confidentiality.

Confidentiality of information is not easy to maintain. Medical records are generally kept not in locked files, but at an easy access point in the nurses' station. Medical files usually travel all over the hospital with the client and are often available for the perusal of others not directly involved in the client's treatment. The increased use of computers for communication and data storage, along with the information requested by the government, third-party payers, and employers, often poses a threat to a client's privacy. More mundane, but equally serious, incidents of breaches of confidentiality occur when staff members talk about clients in the halls, elevator, and cafeteria.

Privileged Communication

Privileged communication is a narrower concept than confidentiality. It is established by state statute to protect possibly incriminating disclosures made by the client to specified professionals.

CLINICAL EXAMPLE

A minister brought suit because his former psychiatrist disclosed confidential information about him to his clerical superiors. The court held that unless a client poses a serious threat to himself or to others, the psychiatrist owes a duty of confidentiality. The client was able to recover damages for lost earnings, harm to his reputation, and emotional distress.

Privileged communication has traditionally existed between husband and wife, attorney and client, clergy and church member, and physician and client. In some states, communication between psychologist and client is also accorded privileged status. Only a few states recognize privileged communication between nurse and client. Be sure that you are informed about the law in your state. The privilege is the client's and can be claimed only if a therapeutic relationship exists. The professional can reveal the information at the client's request.

Each state that grants a privilege also specifies exceptions to that privilege. Instances in which the right to privacy can be breached are discussed in the Your Intervention Strategies feature that follows.

Disclosure to Safeguard Others

An exception to confidentiality and privilege that has developed from a California Supreme Court decision illustrates the competition between two responsibilities of the mental health care professional: (1) confidentiality to the client, and (2) protection of the public from the "violent" client. The court's ruling underlines the mental health care professional's responsibility to balance confidentiality with the "duty to warn" and the "duty to protect." The classic case is discussed in the clinical example that follows.

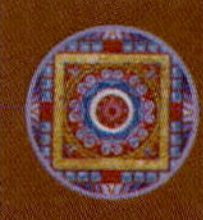

YOUR INTERVENTION STRATEGIES When the Right to Privacy Can Be Breached

The release of information without the client's consent can be made under the following conditions:

- When acting in the client's best interests in an emergency situation
- When acting to protect third parties
- During commitment proceedings
- When making a court-ordered evaluation or report
- When a client is incompetent and consent is given by a guardian, or when the guardian is not available
- When reporting child abuse, gunshot wounds, or contagious diseases, as required by state law
- During criminal proceedings
- In child custody disputes
- During child abuse proceedings
- When a client introduced a defense of mental illness into litigation proceedings

CLINICAL EXAMPLE

The parents of a young woman successfully sued the University of California, claiming that a psychotherapist from the student counseling center had a responsibility to warn their daughter that his client had threatened to kill her. At the time, the psychologist did notify campus security officers that he believed his client was dangerous and should be involuntarily committed for observation and treatment. However, the man appeared rational to the police and promised them he would stay away from the young woman. He then terminated treatment, and two months later killed her. The California Supreme Court said that, despite the unsuccessful attempt to confine the client, the therapist knew that he was at large and dangerous and had a duty to warn the young woman of the danger. The court recognized the client's right to confidentiality but said this must be weighed against the public's need for safety against violent assault, especially when an individual in danger can be identified.

In a number of cases, therapists were held liable for not taking some action to protect potential unidentified victims. The Your Intervention Strategies feature on page 284 shows a model to help mental health caregivers decide on a course of action in implementing the duty to warn or protect.

The duty to warn has stirred up controversy in the mental health community. There is a concern that clients with aggression problems will drop out of therapy, not use it effectively, or be less likely to seek treatment for fear of being betrayed. Remember also that no mental health care professional can reliably predict the future violence of a mentally disordered person.

MEDIALINK Care Plan: Duty to Warn

YOUR INTERVENTION STRATEGIES
A Model for Implementing the Duty to Warn or Protect

Action	Implementation
Assess dangerousness.	Compare data to factors believed to correlate with dangerous behavior such as increasing use of drugs and/or alcohol, current and past threats of violence and/or assaultive behavior, and presence of command hallucinations. Be sure to review past and current treatment records. Interview client, family, and significant others. Ask: Is the threat serious? Are the threats repeated? Are the means to carry out the threat available? Can the victim be identified? Is the victim accessible?
Select a course of action to protect the victim.	Consider either voluntary hospitalization, or, if necessary, initiate involuntary commitment. If the client is already hospitalized, is a more secure unit needed to prevent escape? If the client is an outpatient, is medication needed? Are more frequent visits needed? Is a more intensive outpatient care needed, such as a day program? Because threats often involve family members, is intensive, systems-oriented therapy indicated to include the intended victim? If containment or control is not possible, contact the identified victim. Consider also alerting the police.
Implement decision.	Continue to monitor: If initial course of action fails, take other measures. Be sure to document this decision-making process in the client's record.

Right to Periodic Review

Most states have some provision for periodic review of involuntary clients. Periodic review provides some protection for the individual against spending more time than necessary in the hospital. Review is required every 30 days in some states, every year in others. A few states require review "as frequently as necessary," or "from time to time." The actual scope of the review is usually not governed by statute. The trend in recent years has been away from hospitalization for indeterminate periods of time. In New York and California, short-term commitment is the rule, and court review is necessary to extend commitment for another short period.

Right to Independent Psychiatric Examination

Mental health consumers have the right to an independent psychiatric assessment by a physician of their own choosing. The client must be released if the physician determines the client is not mentally ill.

Right to Participate in Legal Matters

Mental health consumers have rights to participate as citizens in legal matters.

Contracts

Clients committed to a mental hospital generally maintain their right to make a valid contract, unless they have also been judged incompetent. In most states, commitment proceedings are separate from those for competence. Therefore, an individual who is "legally incompetent" is not necessarily subject to commitment, and an individual committed to an institution is not automatically legally incompetent. Even though the issue of contracts may seem clear-cut, in reality a client's right to contract may be restricted by the administrative regulations of hospitals and state mental health agencies. A contested contract would most likely be a matter for the court to decide.

Wills

To make a valid will, a person must:

- Be aware of making a will.
- Be familiar with the property being disposed of.
- Know the names, identities, and relationships of the people named in the will.

A person with a psychiatric diagnosis, whether in or out of the hospital, can make a valid will as long as these requirements are met. Psychosis with accompanying delusions does not by itself negate a valid will. The delusions have to produce a significant distortion of the person's perception of the property, family, or personal relationships to invalidate the will.

Marriage and Divorce

According to statute and common law, a valid marriage contract hinges on the individual's possession of sufficient mental capacity to give consent. Sufficient mental capacity implies that the person:

- Understands the nature of the marriage relationship
- Knows the duties and obligations involved

The statutes of a small number of states prohibit marriage by mentally disordered people because they are believed to be incapable of making a contract. More states, however, prohibit marriage by the mentally disordered on the grounds that they are "insane" or "of unsound mind," without specifically defining these terms. Despite these prohibiting statutes, few states even try to enforce the prohibition outside mental institutions.

Most states have provisions for annulment or divorce on the grounds of prenuptial mental disability. Within the last 25 years, divorce on the grounds of postnuptial mental disability has been incorporated in the statutes of most states.

Voting

Most states do not actually prohibit hospitalized people from voting. In fact, some specifically preserve this right by legislation. The hospitalized client's right to vote is probably more restricted by caretaker and community apathy than it is by statute.

Right to Drive

Statutes on driving privileges are difficult to interpret. Most states do not issue a driver's license to mentally disturbed people. In some states this restriction also applies to people with seizure disorders or substance abuse problems. Several states suspend a driver's license as soon as the individual enters a mental institution. Other jurisdictions limit the restriction to those admitted involuntarily, while still others base suspension on legal competency.

Right to Practice a Profession

The ability of a hospitalized client to practice a profession is usually impaired simply by the physical confinement. However, most states have some statutes prohibiting the practice of a profession by a mentally disturbed person. The vagueness of the statutes often makes it difficult to know when they are applicable. As a rule, it is up to the professional licensing board to suspend or revoke the license of a member who is believed to be too mentally incapacitated to practice a profession safely, even though not hospitalized.

Right to Habeas Corpus

Mental health consumers in all states have the protection of the constitutional right of **habeas corpus**. Habeas corpus requires the speedy release of any person who has been illegally detained. Any client can petition for release on the grounds of being sane. If found sane in a hearing, the client must be discharged.

Rights of Children or Minors

The rights of children have been the subject of judicial and legislative action over the last 20 years. In most states, an individual is considered a minor or juvenile if younger than 18 years of age. As a minor the person is considered legally incompetent. Legal consent for medical treatment must come from parents or a guardian. There are, however, a number of exceptions to this general rule of presumed legal incompetency in some state statutes. These include the rights to:

- Seek treatment for drug abuse.
- Consent to contraception.
- Seek psychiatric treatment.

Other factors, such as military service, marriage, emancipation, pregnancy, and parenthood, may also affect the age at which a minor may be considered competent.

The most controversial issue of a minor's role in the mental health system involves involuntary commitment. Like adults, minors can be committed to a mental hospital against their will. But, unlike adult admissions, the admission of a minor who objects is considered "voluntary" if the parents have authorized it. Because of the realization that parents may not always be acting in the best interests of the child, a number of lawsuits challenging this practice were filed. It was argued that the "voluntary" admission of minors without procedural safeguards was unconstitutional, and that a court hearing should always be held to determine if commitment is warranted. The United States Supreme Court upheld the rights of parents to admit their children to psychiatric facilities as long as a "neutral factfinder" (physician) believes medical standards for admission have been met.

The trend for inclusion of procedural safeguards continues as an increasing number of states have modified their "voluntary" parental commitment statute by one or more of the following factors:

- Lowering the age of required consent: the majority of states specify age 16 to 18
- Requiring the consent of the child
- Providing for a court hearing if the child protests
- Providing for self-initiated institutionalization for minors

LIABILITY AND THE PSYCHIATRIC–MENTAL HEALTH NURSE

Criminal and civil are the two main classes of law. *Criminal law* pertains to behavior considered to be a threat to the order of society as a whole, such as murder, assault, and robbery. *Civil law* is concerned with the legal rights and duties of private parties. Most legal actions against nurses are civil actions.

An important division of civil law is known as *tort law*. A tort is a wrongful act resulting in injury for which the injured party files a civil suit requesting legal redress, usually in the form of monetary damages. Torts may be intentional, as in assault, battery, defamation of character, invasion of privacy, false imprisonment, fraud, and misrepresentation; or unintentional, as in negligence. Under tort law, nurses can be held responsible for their own actions. Therefore, all nurses should carry their own malpractice insurance.

Negligence

The concepts of duty and responsibility permeate human relationships. In healthy relationships, expectations are negotiated between individuals that delineate the responsibilities of each person. People who experience times of stress and illness may have difficulty forming realistic expectations, accepting responsibility for actions, and understanding the roles and limits of those who would like to help.

There are times when two people may experience problems understanding and meeting the duties and responsibilities of the relationship. The resolution of such problems is often a therapeutic issue. At times, however, the legal system may become involved. This is particularly true if the client, or the client's family, perceives that the nurse failed to provide the quality of care expected.

All nurses are responsible for determining the quality of care as experienced by their clients. If lapses in the quality of care occur, they should be addressed. The term **negligence** is used whenever a nurse fails to act in a manner in which most reasonable and prudent people would act or when a nurse acts in a way that a reasonably prudent person would not act under similar circumstances. How does one determine what is reasonable and prudent? First, you are accountable to external legal authorities such as the nurse practice acts of the state in which you practice, as well as civil and criminal codes. You are also accountable to maintain the standards of psychiatric–mental health nursing practice (2007) published by the American Nurses Association, and to the employing agency or hospital. You are also accountable for familiarizing yourself with current journal and textbook information related to the care of mental health clients.

Conditions for Establishing Negligence

A simple breach in the quality of care does not necessarily mean that a nurse was negligent (Lee, 2000). Certain conditions must be met to determine negligence and hold the nurse accountable. These conditions are discussed in the following section and summarized in Box 13-4.

Contract for Care A contract for care must have been established between the nurse and the client. A nurse may also begin this contract by accepting a client assignment, having a discussion with the client, offering information or education, providing treatment, serving as a group leader, accepting a client into an activity, or supervising the activities of a mental health worker. It is important to note that entering into a therapeutic relationship creates a legally binding contract between the nurse and the client.

Duty of Care There must be identifiable, explicit, and manifest duty of care in which the intentions of the nurse are to help the client. This intention to help is termed *good faith*. One example is the "good faith" use of the nursing process, including pertinent and timely assessment, planning, outcome identification, intervention, and evaluation of the client. Another example is a nursing care policy that indicates a course of action. A policy of a given mental health agency might state that each nurse must perform an assessment that includes information related to the emotional, physical, and social health of each client. Failure to use the nursing process and to follow the procedure to provide such an assessment (and take actions based upon this assessment) might be grounds for a charge of negligence.

Ignorance of a policy or procedure is not an acceptable rationale for not following a policy or procedure. For example, all nurses are expected to assess clients for the potential to commit suicide. All reasonable, prudent nurses perform an assessment for suicide potential. The nurse must act to safeguard the life of the client within the limits of the law. Failure to perform such an assessment or take actions to protect the client might be deemed negligent, if harm is present.

Presence of Harm The client must suffer harm that can be directly linked to the failure of the nurse to act in a reasonable and prudent manner. A nurse who fails to assess for suicide potential, thus failing to protect the client, can be held negligent only if the client suffers harm in a suicide attempt or dies as a result of self-inflicted action.

Common Practice There may be no written policy or procedure, nor a law to guide a practitioner in acting, but there is strong indication for action based on what is generally considered *common practice*. Consider a client who lacks any contact with reality. The client cannot perform activities of daily living such as eating, bathing, toileting, or making decisions about safety. It is common practice, in this situation, to perform the activities of daily living for the client. Conversely, it is common practice to encourage clients to do as much for themselves as possible.

Boundary Violation Another example concerns the boundaries of personal relationships between clients and mental health care professionals. Some states fail to define the boundaries of personal relationships between clients and mental health care professionals. In these cases, each nurse must define the nature of the nurse–client relationship. Nurses do not form social relationships with mental health clients with whom there is or has been a professional relationship. This implies that nurses do not date nor engage in sexual activity with a client. Any suggestion or promise that the relationship might be personal can be considered negligence—the failure to explain the limits of the relationship to the client and to act within the boundaries of that relationship.

Acting Against the Nurse's Advice Clients sometimes contribute to the harm they suffer. A client may be informed of the dangers of certain actions and yet may decide to act against the advice of the nurse. Each client maintains the civil rights of freedom of speech, movement, and action unless

Box 13-4 Determining Negligence

- Did a contract for care exist?
- Was the care reasonable and prudent?
- Did the care follow guidelines suggested by external sources such as nurse practice acts, the ANA Code of Ethics, the ANA Standards for Psychiatric–Mental Health Nursing, and the state Mental Health Act?
- Was the care consistent with internal sources such as policies and procedures of the agency or physician orders?
- Was there evidence of thorough assessment of the client, including old records and interviews with family members?
- Did the action taken reveal appropriate ongoing monitoring of the client's condition?
- Did harm result to the client?
- Was the harm due to violation of the duty to care?

there are grounds to curtail these rights, as in the case of harm to self and others. Consider the following clinical example.

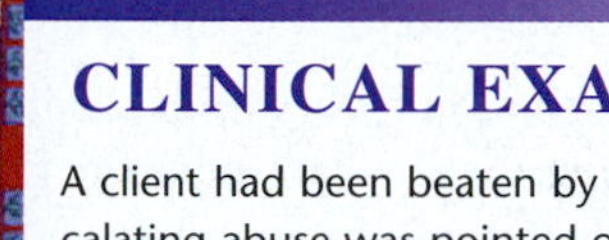

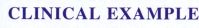

CLINICAL EXAMPLE

A client had been beaten by her boyfriend. The pattern of escalating abuse was pointed out to her, and she was given the phone numbers of agencies that were available on a 24-hour basis, encouraged to form a safe plan, and offered alternative living arrangements. She decided to return to her boyfriend and suffered paralysis from another beating. She claimed the staff did not act to protect her.

Refer back to Box 13-4 to consider whether the staff was negligent in this case.

Malpractice

Malpractice refers to the negligent acts of health care professionals when they fail to act in a responsible and prudent manner in carrying out their professional duties. The most common sources of liability in psychiatric–mental health services are identified in Box 13-5.

Need to Document

The following cases illustrate a breach of the ANA's standards of psychiatric–mental health nursing practice and emphasize the importance of written communication between nurse and physician.

CLINICAL EXAMPLE

A man was admitted to a hospital after becoming increasingly depressed and suicidal secondary to the medication used to treat his hypertension. As a new client, he was not allowed to leave the unit. Four days later the nursing staff assumed without a verifying written medical order (later a verbal order would be claimed) that he was allowed to leave the unit, unescorted, to attend Mass with permission of the nurse on duty. The following morning he was allowed to go to breakfast unescorted. This time, however, he committed suicide by jumping from a seventh-floor window. The court ruled that the nurse involved with his care breached the standard of care due under Alaska law. The nurse failed to exercise reasonable care to protect a suicidal client against foreseeable harm to himself.

Box 13-5 Common Sources of Liability in Psychiatric–Mental Health Services

1. Client suicide
2. Improper treatment
3. Misuse of psychotropic medications
4. Breach of confidentiality
5. False imprisonment
6. Injuries or problems related to ECT
7. Sexual contact with a client
8. Failure to obtain informed consent
9. Failure to report abuse
10. Failure to warn potential victims

Another case shows the importance of nursing observation and documentation, even though in this case it did not prevent a tragedy.

CLINICAL EXAMPLE

Distraught with problems and a pending divorce, a 35-year-old man was voluntarily admitted to a psychiatric hospital. During this admission he expressed thoughts of suicide and also thoughts of killing his wife and her mother. Three weeks after his discharge, he was readmitted voluntarily after a suicide attempt. Nurses' notes revealed his repeated homicidal threats. Three weeks after his second admission, he was given a pass. He subsequently secured a gun and shot and killed his wife and her friend. He was tried and convicted on two counts of murder. The children brought a wrongful death action against the hospital, seeking damages for the murder of their mother by their father. The court granted substantial damages to the children. No liability was attributed to the nurses involved, but the physician was judged negligent.

It is important to remember the nature and purpose of hospital records and to follow prudent, appropriate, and ethical procedures in record maintenance. Records that have been changed for whatever reason need to include the date, the reason for the change, and the signature of the person making the change. A dishonest change could result in the charge of fraud or misrepresentation, as occurred in the next example.

CLINICAL EXAMPLE

A 23-year-old woman was admitted with a diagnosis of schizophrenia. She spent three days in a bare, quiet room for safety reasons. On the fourth day the bed was returned to the room, but no rationale was noted in the chart. A few days later, an order on the client's chart for an antipsychotic medication was not noted, and the client was without medication for three days. The client was later found in a semicomatose condition with her head lodged between the side rails and mattress. Subsequently, the nursing director ordered the nursing staff to "rewrite" the nursing notes. The substituted record clearly conflicted with other records and staff testimony. A $3.6 million verdict against the hospital was upheld.

Many factors contribute to the initiation of a malpractice suit by a client. As long as you are involved in practice, lawsuits are a possibility.

CLIENT ADVOCACY

Despite the prevalence of mental disorder in the United States, mental health services remain poorly funded, mental illness remains misunderstood, and individuals with recurring

MEDIALINK Bazelon Center for Mental Health Law

mental illness live lives characterized by isolation, underemployment, stigma, and denial of rights (Kelly, 2006).

The gap between the rights clients have in theory and in practice may be the result of a knowledge deficit on the part of treatment providers. If so, the remedy is simple: Educate the treatment providers so that they in turn can educate their clients. Another possibility that may not be so amenable to an easy solution is that direct care providers are threatened by the expansion of client rights. Mental health staff have been heard to say that new regulations not only hampered treatment but made their job both more difficult and more dangerous.

The federal government has encouraged states to develop ombudsmen (persons who speak for or champion the cause of others) or advocacy programs. These state advocacy programs have the authority to investigate reported incidents of neglect and abuse to the mentally ill in public or private mental health treatment settings, research facilities, and nursing homes. Private advocacy organizations such as the Bazelon Center for Mental Health Law (www.bazelon.org), developed by Judge David Bazelon, can be accessed through the Companion Website for this book.

Two recent pieces of federal legislation have implications for the rights of clients. In 1990, the Americans with Disabilities Act (ADA) extended federal protection to individuals with physical and/or mental health disabilities for access to public services, employment, and benefits. In an effort to increase the involvement of individuals in directing their own medical care, the Patient Self-Determination Act (PSDA) of 1991 was ratified by Congress as part of the Omnibus Budget Reconciliation Act. The PSDA was designed to inform competent patients at the time of their admission to a hospital of their rights to accept or reject aspects of their medical care.

Although laws can protect certain aspects of human rights, there is a far greater area that laws cannot protect. Laws rarely have a direct effect on a person's beliefs, values, and attitudes, which to a great extent determine whether the letter or the spirit of the law will be carried out. Remember that while the letter of the law may require reading clients their rights on admission, the spirit of the law may not necessarily be satisfied. Clients may not understand the information, remember it, or be able to take it in because anxiety may be causing selective inattention (see Chapter 8 ∞). Wariness of staff may also cause client discomfort, such as occurred in a study of adult clients with PADs who experienced psychiatric crises. Some clients revealed their discomfort in acknowledging that they had a PAD because they feared a negative response from staff or even involuntary treatment (Kim et al., 2007). Psychiatric–mental health nurses practicing from a humanistic perspective are often in a position to advocate both the letter of the law and the spirit of clients' rights.

Physical and Psychological Abuse of Clients

Clients are particularly vulnerable to both physical and psychological abuse and often do not have the ability or power to defend themselves. There is little actual information on how much client abuse exists in treatment settings. One advocate group ranked client abuse as the most frequent rights-violation complaint. Another ranked it third. These are the types of abuse reported to occur with some frequency:

- Supplying clients with drugs or alcohol in return for favors
- Making privileges contingent on favors from clients
- Slapping and kicking clients when staff members felt frustrated
- Using restraints when other less intrusive alternatives were available
- Verbal harassment, including threats, sarcasm, and other "put-downs"
- General threats of harm if clients do not behave "appropriately" or as they are told
- Inhumane physical facilities

Sexual misconduct with clients is also a form of abuse.

Advocacy Interventions

Psychiatric–mental health nursing advocacy interventions would be directed at some of the identifying causes that may lead to client abuse, including:

- Unsuitability of certain staff members who do not have the patience or understanding to work with clients having trouble with control
- A buildup of stresses that have reduced both the staff's patience and ability to problem-solve (burnout)
- An actual lack of knowledge of other means of interacting with clients in a high-stress situation

Other areas of advocacy include:

- Educating clients and their families about their legal rights
- Monitoring treatment planning and delivery of service for the abuse of client rights
- Evaluating policies and procedures regarding client rights infringement
- Making sure clients have the necessary information to make an informed decision or give informed consent
- Questioning other health care professionals when their care is based more on stereotypic ideas than on an assessment of the client's needs
- Speaking out for safe practice conditions when threatened by budget cutbacks
- Supporting an organization such as the Bazelon Center for Mental Health Law that defends the rights of children and adults with mental disabilities through policy advocacy

Duty to Intervene

In medical–surgical nursing, it is often very easy to determine when and how to help clients. If a client has low blood sugar, you offer food to increase the blood sugar level. In psychiatric–mental health nursing, it is often difficult to determine when and how to intervene in particular situations. What is my responsibility? What should be done? Who should do it? What are the appropriate legal choices? What is an appropriate ethical response? Am I going to get sued for doing this? Am I going to get sued if I don't?

Contract for Care

A contract for care implies that the client has a need for help and that the nurse has agreed to act in good faith for the interest of the client. Nurses form this contract when they accept the duty to care for a client during the process of working on a mental health unit. This contract focuses on the nurse's professional perception that there is an issue that requires management.

Notice that the client may not have asked for help. There are many times when the client is so ill that asking for help is not a reasonable expectation. When working with mental health clients, one general rule applies: Once a situation has come to your awareness, it is important that you take all reasonable and prudent actions to intervene to be helpful to the client.

The process of admission should prepare a client for the actions that will be taken given certain situations such as suicidal threats or acts of violence. Most mental health units have a list of client rights and administrative policies and procedures. For example, material that is confidential is explained and material that must be shared is discussed. At times, clients may attempt to use the mental health unit as a shield against facing legal charges. In these instances, relevant policies must be made explicit to the client.

Assessment

All interventions must follow a thorough assessment. The client must be informed that staff members will perform ongoing assessments to facilitate care. When clients are unable to cooperate with assessments because of cognitive impairment, it is vital to obtain information from other sources including records from previous hospitalizations, family members, or community therapists (with client permission). The staff may need to review lab work to explore the level of reliability in the information presented by clients with respect to drug or alcohol use, for example.

Lying on the part of the client has several aspects with legal implications. A client may deliberately mislead the staff member by telling stories that the client knows are not true. This is best dealt with through respectful confrontation. A client may not actually lie but may frame a situation so that the client is viewed as a victim, without including details pertinent to a full understanding of the situation. In this case, it may be helpful to walk through the situation several times, with more than one interviewer, and ask for further details.

Some mental disorders affect the perception and memory of events so profoundly that only a third party such as a family member can offer an accurate view. Nurses must make a good faith effort to perform a full assessment of a client before intervening. This information must be recorded in the chart with statements not only related to information the nurse was able to obtain but also actions the nurse took to obtain information. Failure to assess the client and the situation may result in errors in judgment. It is essential to take the time to collect information essential for decision making. This process requires expert communication skills not only with the client but with others involved in the client's care.

Responsibility to Communicate and Collaborate

The duty to intervene requires that information be communicated clearly to others, particularly those who participate in the decision-making process. The nurse is responsible for informing all individuals involved in the care of a client of the results of the assessment and of the considerations for the intervention phase.

Providing optimal care to clients requires cooperation and collaboration with others. No one professional can make decisions without consultation with others. Each psychiatric–mental health nurse must be able to communicate effectively within the established protocols of the agency of employment. These policies and procedures are often called the *chain of command*. The chain of command is the expected pattern of communication surrounding the care of clients. Several aspects of the chain of command are important to remember.

1. Nurses are often responsible for the care provided by others. The nurse may work with several nursing assistants or mental health technicians. The nurse must make clear to nonprofessionals the situations that demand immediate attention. The paraprofessionals working on a psychiatric–mental health nursing unit must be able to recognize situations that should be immediately reported.
2. The nurse often serves as a liaison to other departments. The nurse practice act in the state of employment will determine the dependent, independent, and interdependent roles of the nurse. Often these roles need to be explained to other professionals.
3. The ANA's standards for psychiatric–mental health nursing practice (2007) provide standards of care. Many professionals do not know that the psychiatric nurse must judge her or his practice based on these guidelines. The hospital or mental health agency will provide guidelines for notification and decision making that must be followed. It is vital to know the policies of the institution.

These three elements form a framework for actions that need to be taken. Once an event has occurred, you must notify team members who may not be present on the unit. Usually, the nurse manager or supervisor, physician, psychologist, social worker, security department, and at times the family, a person who has been threatened, or the police must all be notified.

Formulating a Plan to Intervene

It is vital to formulate a plan before making a decision to intervene. Nurses often complain of not having "think time," time to consider all options before acting. Many nurses indicate that they respond based on past experience or intuition. While this may work for many expert nurses, beginning

A 34-year-old female client who is admitted with borderline personality disorder states that a male peer raped her. She alleges the incident occurred last night and insists that the male client be arrested. The unit has a "no sex policy" stating that each offending member must be transferred or discharged from the unit.

You notify the nurse manager, the nursing supervisor, the physician, the therapist, the social worker, the risk manager, and security. The hospital's legal counsel is called to help determine options for the client and the man identified as the rapist.

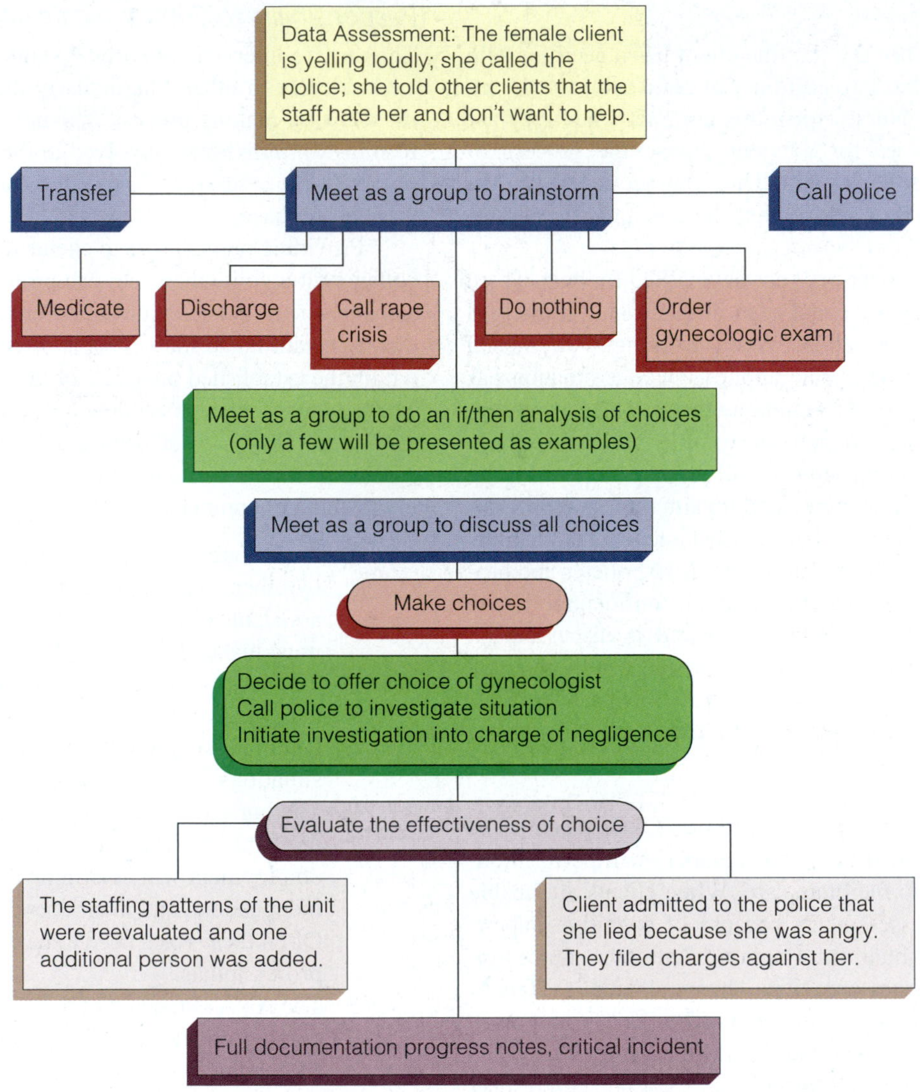

FIGURE 13-3A ■ "If/then" analysis as a model in decision making.

nurses need to carefully think through options and learn to assess the clinical and legal implications of actions in a methodical fashion. FIGURE 13-3A ■ illustrates a model that might be helpful in decision making. FIGURE 13-3B ■ illustrates possible options and potential results of individual interventions.

Illegal, Immoral, or Unethical Activities of Professionals

At times, the nurse may notice that peers are engaging in illegal activities. It is vital that every nurse understand the legal mandate that requires a response from any professional who has knowledge of illegal, immoral, or unethical activities. Normally, this response is to report the activity to others in the agency, using the chain of command. At other times, the nurse may need to seek the guidance of the State Board of Nursing or the American Nurses Association.

Nurse impairment is perhaps the most common situation encountered by professional staff. A nurse may be impaired through addiction to alcohol or narcotics, or through an event of personal experience with emotional illness. This

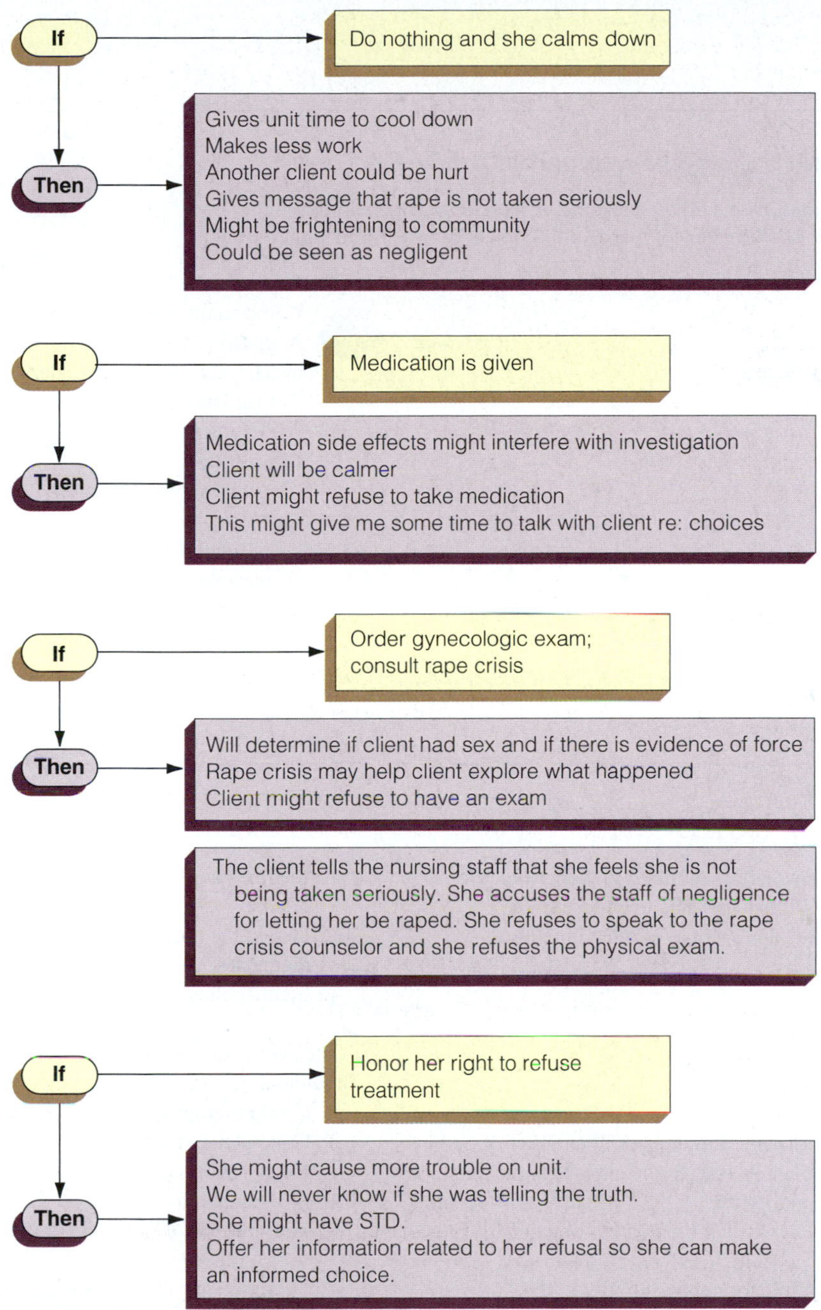

If
Do nothing and she calms down
Then
Gives unit time to cool down
Makes less work
Another client could be hurt
Gives message that rape is not taken seriously
Might be frightening to community
Could be seen as negligent
If
Medication is given
Then
Medication side effects might interfere with investigation
Client will be calmer
Client might refuse to take medication
This might give me some time to talk with client re: choices
If
Order gynecologic exam; consult rape crisis
Then
Will determine if client had sex and if there is evidence of force
Rape crisis may help client explore what happened
Client might refuse to have an exam
The client tells the nursing staff that she feels she is not being taken seriously. She accuses the staff of negligence for letting her be raped. She refuses to speak to the rape crisis counselor and she refuses the physical exam.
If
Honor her right to refuse treatment
Then
She might cause more trouble on unit.
We will never know if she was telling the truth.
She might have STD.
Offer her information related to her refusal so she can make an informed choice.

FIGURE 13-3B ■ Possible options and potential results of interventions.

impairment may be linked with other illegal acts such as theft of drugs or a client's personal property. Each nurse is first responsible to the client and must report such impairment to an immediate supervisor in a reasonable, prudent, and timely manner. Although some nurses erroneously view this intervention as an invasion of privacy or "tattling," prompt, efficient action may safeguard the client from harm while offering the impaired nurse a chance at recovery. Most hospitals have programs to assist impaired nurses to recover. Many state nursing boards or state professional associations have programs to assist the nurse addict or emotionally impaired nurse.

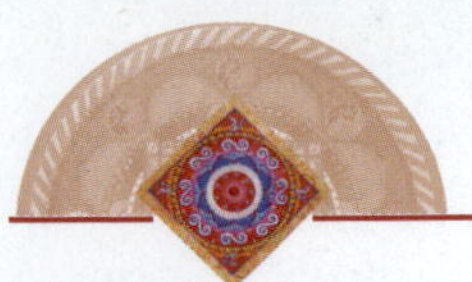

EXPLORE MEDIALINK 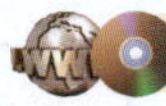 www.prenhall.com/kneisl

For NCLEX-RN® review questions, case studies, and other resources for this chapter see the Pearson Health MediaLink CD-ROM that accompanies this book and the Companion Website at www.prenhall.com/kneisl.

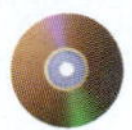

CD-ROM
Audio Glossary
NCLEX-RN® Review Questions

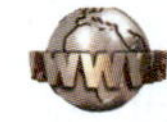

Companion Website
Audio Glossary
NCLEX-RN® Review Questions
Critical Thinking Exercise
- *A Client's Rights*

Case Study
- *Involuntary Admission*

Care Plan
- *Duty to Warn*

MediaLinks
MediaLink Application
- *Psychiatric Hospital Bans Smoking*

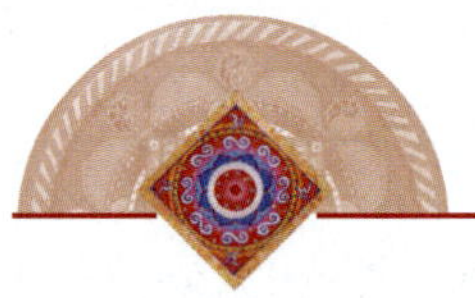

NCLEX-RN® REVIEW QUESTIONS

1. The client is being involuntarily committed to the psychiatric unit after threatening to kill his spouse and children. The involuntary commitment is an example of what bioethical principle?
1. Fidelity
2. Beneficence
3. Veracity
4. Autonomy

2. A client expressed concern regarding the confidentiality of her medical information. The nurse assures the client that the nurse maintains client confidentiality by:
1. Sharing the information with all members of the health care team.
2. Explaining the exact limits of confidentiality in the exchanges between the client and the nurse.
3. Summarizing the information the client provides during assessments and documenting this summary in the chart.
4. Limiting discussion about clients to the group room and hallways.

3. Which of the following criteria must be met for an involuntary mental health commitment?
1. The client requests admission to the hospital.
2. The client reports a history of depression.
3. The client is unable to provide for basic needs.
4. The client is homeless.

4. When caring for clients with psychiatric diagnoses, the nurse recalls that the purpose of psychiatric diagnoses or psychiatric labeling is to:
1. Enable the client's treatment team to plan appropriate and comprehensive care.
2. Identify those individuals who are at risk for harming others.
3. Define the nursing care for individuals with similar diagnoses.
4. Identify those individuals in need of more specialized care.

5. The role of the psychiatric forensic nurse includes (select all that apply):
1. Group therapist.
2. Competency therapist.
3. Expert witness.
4. Individual client therapy.
5. Group leader for a group of clients.

6. A benefit to a psychiatric advance directive (PAD) is that it:
1. Provides the health care team with general consent to treat the client.
2. Eliminates the need for involuntary hospitalizations.
3. Provides clients with some control over their treatment and empowers them.
4. Identifies individuals who are at high risk for becoming incapacitated in the future.

7. The physician asks the nurse to obtain written consent from the client for electroconvulsive therapy. The client was medicated with lorazepam (Ativan) 30 minutes ago and is currently sleeping. In order to obtain an informed consent the nurse knows that:
1. The client cannot receive any medication 15 minutes prior to signing the consent form.
2. The client cannot have a diagnosed mental disorder or illness.

3. The client cannot be under the influence of medication that may alter cognition.
4. The client has to have a high school education.

8. The nurse restrains a client in a locked room for 3 hours until the client acknowledges who started a fight in the group room last evening. The nurse's behavior constitutes:
1. Standard of care practice.
2. False imprisonment.
3. Duty of care.
4. Contract of care.

9. The day staff nurse suspects that clients are more frequently restrained on the night shift when a particular nurse is scheduled. What is the day nurse's responsibility?
1. Monitor the situation for 1 month to try to establish a pattern of behavior.
2. Review the records of restrained clients to determine if the restraints were warranted.
3. Discuss her concerns with the nurse manager.
4. Discuss her concerns with the clients who were restrained.

10. A client is admitted to a psychiatric–mental health unit on an emergency involuntary status. What is the minimum length of time the client will remain hospitalized?
1. 12 hours
2. 3 to 5 days
3. 48 hours
4. 60 days

See Appendix C for answers.

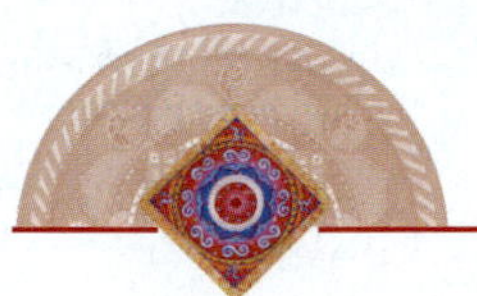

REFERENCES

Allen, M., & Smith, V. F. (2001). Opening Pandora's box: The practical and legal dangers of involuntary outpatient commitment. *Psychiatric Services, 52*(3), 342–346.

American Bar Association. (1995). *Mental disability law* (5th ed.). Washington, DC: Author.

American Nurses Association. (2001). *Code of ethics for nurses with interpretive statements.* Washington, DC: Author.

American Nurses Association. (2007). *Corrections nursing: Scope and standards of practice*. Silver Spring, MD: Nursesbooks.org.

American Nurses Association, American Psychiatric–Mental Health Nurses Association, and International Society of Psychiatric–Mental Health Nurses. (2007). *Psychiatric–mental health nursing: Scope and standards of practice*. Silver Spring, MD: Nursesbooks.org.

American Nurses Association & International Association of Forensic Nurses. (1997). *Scope and standards of forensic nursing practice*. Washington, DC: Author.

American Psychiatric Association. (2000). *Diagnostic and statistical manual of mental disorders* (4th ed., Text Revision). Washington, DC: Author.

American Psychiatric Nurses Association. (2007). *Position statement on seclusion and restraint.* Retrieved August 6, 2007, from http://www.apna.org.

Armstrong, A. E. (2006). Towards a strong virtue ethics for nursing practice. *Nursing Philosophy, 7*(3), 110–124.

Bazelon Center for Mental Health Law. (2007). *Psychiatric advance directive.* Washington, DC: Bazelon Center.

Begley, A. M. (2006). Facilitating the development of moral insight in practice: Teaching ethics and teaching virtue. *Nursing Philosophy, 7*(4), 257–265.

Cutcliffe, J. R., Stevenson, C., Jackson, S., & Smith, P. (2006). A modified grounded theory study of how psychiatric nurses work with suicidal people. *International Journal of Nursing Studies, 43*(7), 791–802.

Delaney, K. R., & Johnson, M. E. (2006). Keeping the unit safe: Mapping psychiatric nursing skills. *Journal of the American Psychiatric Nurses Association, 12*(4), 1–10.

Fintzy, R. T. (2000). Clinical profiling: An introduction to behavioral evidence analysis. *American Journal of Psychiatry, 157*(9), 1532–1555.

Fountas, K. N., & Smith, J. R. (2007). Historical evolution of stereotactic amygdelotomy for the management of severe aggression. *Journal of Neurosurgery, 106*(4), 710–713.

Fountas, K. N., Smith, J. R., & Lee, G. P. (2007). Bilateral stereotactic amygdalotomy for self-mutilation disorder. Case report and review of the literature. *Stereotactic Functional Neurosurgery, 85*(2-3), 121–128.

Fuchs, T. (2006). Ethical issues in neuroscience. *Current Opinions in Psychiatry, 19*(6), 600–607.

Glannon, W. (2006). Neuroethics. *Bioethics, 20*(1), 37–52.

Hewitt, J. L., & Edwards, S. D. (2006). Moral perspectives on the prevention of suicide in mental health settings. *Journal of Psychiatric and Mental Health Nursing, 13*(6), 665–672.

Illes, J., & Racine, E. (2005). Imaging or imagining? A neuroethics challenge informed by genetics. *American Journal of Bioethics, 5*(2), 5–18.

Jenike, M. A. (2001). An update on obsessive–compulsive disorder. *Bulletin of the Menninger Clinic, 65*(1), 4–25.

Johnson, M. E., & Delaney, K. R. (2007). Keeping the unit safe: The anatomy of escalation. *Journal of the American Psychiatric Nurses Association, 13*(1), 42–52.

Kelly, B. D. (2006). The power gap: Freedom, power and mental illness. *Social Science and Medicine, 63*(8), 2118–2128.

Kim, M. M., Van Dorn, R. A., Scheyett, A. M., Elbogen, E. E., Swanson, J. W., Swartz, M. S., et al. (2007). Understanding the personal and clinical utility of psychiatric advance directives: A qualitative perspective. *Psychiatry, 70*(1), 19–29.

Lee, N. G. (2000). Proving nursing negligence. *American Journal of Nursing, 100*(11), 55–56.

Malhi, G. S., & Bartlett, J. R. (2000). Depression: A role for neurosurgery? *British Journal of Neurosurgery, 14*(5), 415–422.

Nace, E. P., Birkmayer, F., Sullivan, M. A., Galanter, M., Fromson, J. A., Frances, R. J., et al. (2007). Socially sanctioned coercion mechanisms for addiction treatment. *American Journal of Addictions, 16*(1), 15–23.

Rayel, M. G. (2000). Clinical and demographic characteristics of elderly offenders at a maximum-security forensic hospital. *Journal of Forensic Sciences, 45*(6), 1193–1196.

Redman, B. K., & Fry, S. T. (2000). Nurses' ethical conflicts: What is really known about them? *Nursing Ethics, 7*(4), 360–366.

Segal, S. P., & Burgess, P. M. (2006). The utility of extended outpatient civil commitment. *International Journal of Law and Psychiatry, 29*(6), 525–534.

Slatkin, A. A. (2000). The role of the mental health consultant in hostage negotiations: Questions to ask during the incident phase. *The Police Chief, 67*(7), 64.

Swanson, J., Swartz, M., Ferron, J., Elbogen, E., & Van Dorn, R. (2006). Psychiatric advance directives among public mental health consumers in five U.S. cities: Prevalence, demand, and correlates. *Journal of the American Academy of Psychiatry and the Law, 34*(1), 43–57.

Vuckovich, P. K., & Artinian, B. M. (2005). Justifying coercion. *Nursing Ethics, 12*(4), 370–380.

Wales, H. W., & Hiday, V. A. (2006). Is outpatient commitment the answer? *International Journal of Law and Psychiatry, 29*(6), 451–468.

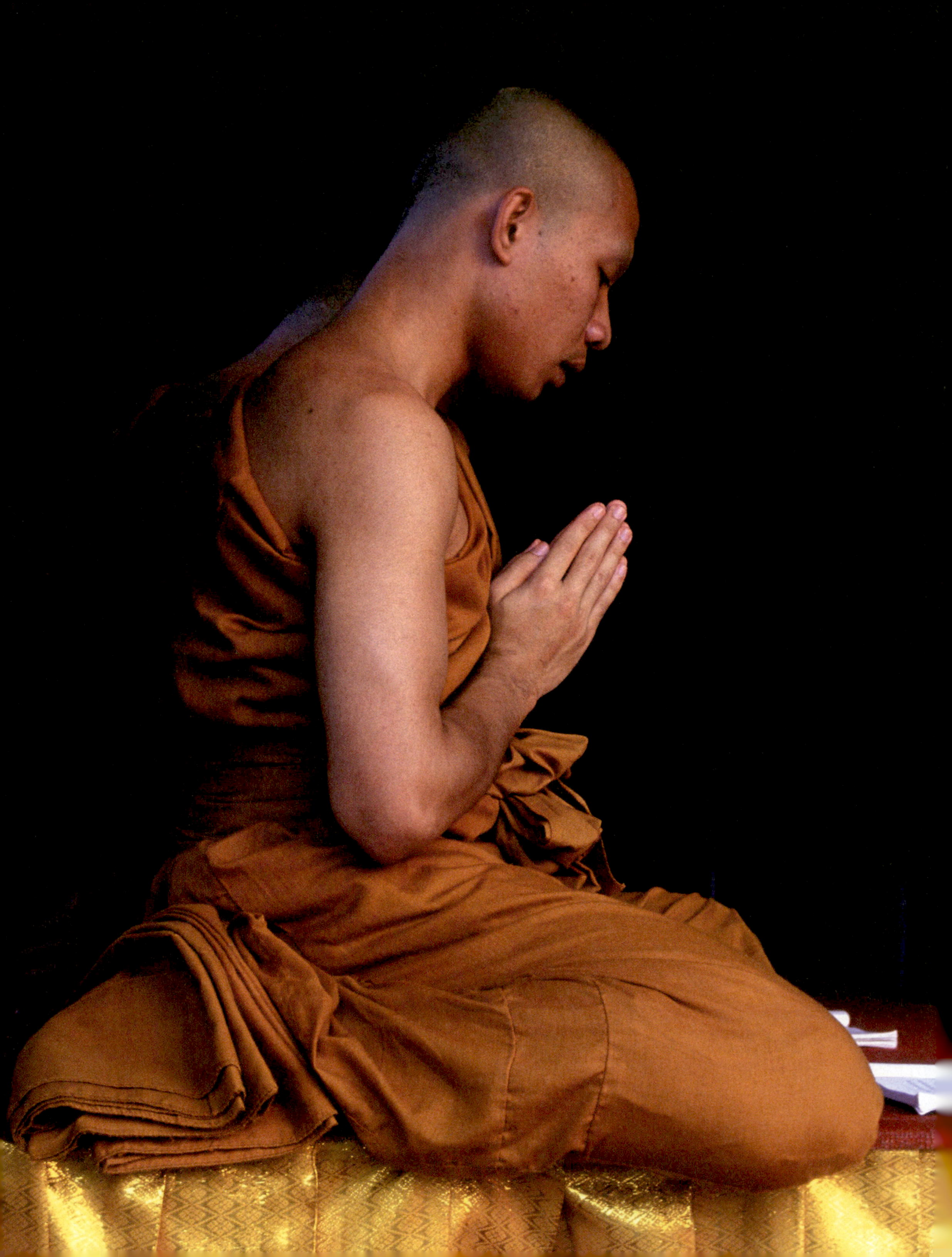

Chapter 14 • Cognitive Disorders
Chapter 15 • Substance-Related Disorders
Chapter 16 • Schizophrenia and Other Psychotic Disorders
Chapter 17 • Mood Disorders
Chapter 18 • Anxiety and Dissociative Disorders
Chapter 19 • Somatoform and Sleep Disorders
Chapter 20 • Gender Identity and Sexual Disorders
Chapter 21 • Eating Disorders
Chapter 22 • Personality Disorders

Unit 4

CLIENTS WITH MENTAL DISORDERS

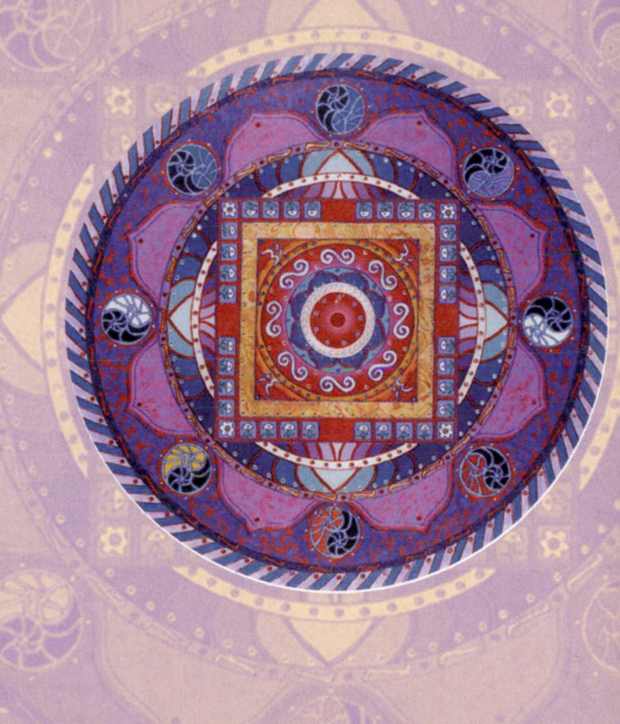

THANET, a Buddhist monk, meditates in the late afternoon heat in the Wat Chiang Man, a temple inside the old city quadrangle of Chiang Mai, Thailand. His morning alms rounds took him through winding, narrow lanes past noodle vendors, housewives hanging out their laundry, and backpacking tourists searching for a guesthouse. Even though mental health services are available through the government, the *wats* (temples), which are centers of communal life, still play dominant roles. In Thailand, mental illness is considered *karma* (fate or destiny based on all the words and acts of one's life) and is taken care of by the family and the temple. The wat provides health services, particularly traditional medicine, to the people of Chiang Mai. Some provide services to drug addicts and people with AIDS. The people of Chiang Mai cope with major mental health problems such as narcotics addiction, a sharp rise in methamphetamine use, a sharp rise in HIV-associated dementia, intimate partner violence, and communication disorders in children, including autism. Our responsibility in a diverse world is a commitment to care for the spirit of our clients, to engage with them, and to support the transcendent, spiritual domain.

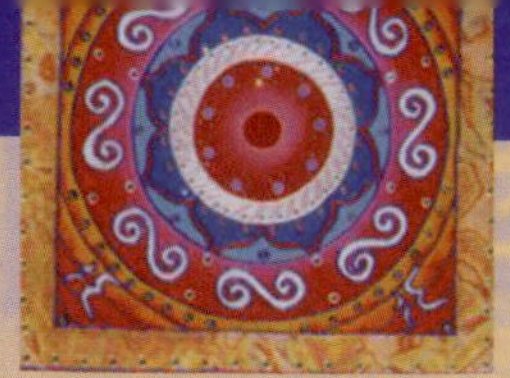

CHAPTER

14

Cognitive Disorders

EILEEN TRIGOBOFF

KEY TERMS

amnestic disorder *306*
aphasia, expressive *310*
aphasia, receptive *310*
Creutzfeldt–Jakob disease *305*
delirium *297*
dementia *299*
dementia of the Alzheimer's type (DAT) or Alzheimer's dementia (AD) *301*
Huntington's disease *304*
new variant Creutzfeldt–Jakob disease (nvCJD) *305*
Parkinson's disease *304*
Pick's disease *305*
pseudodementia *305*
sundowning *311*
vascular dementia *304*

LEARNING OUTCOMES

After completing this chapter, you will be able to:

1. Discuss the biopsychosocial theories that explain delirium, dementia, amnestic disorders, and other cognitive disorders.
2. Differentiate among the various types of cognitive disorders.
3. Explain the differences between delirium, dementia, and depression.
4. Compare possible assessment findings in delirium and dementia.
5. Compare and contrast the nursing interventions and their rationales for clients with delirium and dementia.
6. Incorporate psychiatric–mental health nursing strategies that support optimal memory and cognitive functioning in the care of clients with cognitive disorders.
7. Identify the difficulties caregivers may face when working with clients who have cognitive disorders.
8. Discuss the personal feelings and attitudes that are likely to interfere with the psychiatric–mental health nurse's ability to care for cognitively impaired clients.

CRITICAL THINKING CHALLENGE

You are the community mental health nurse for Mrs. Downston, an elderly widow with dementia of the Alzheimer's type (DAT). This client has lived with her daughter Dolores, her son-in-law Don, and their two teenage daughters in their suburban home for the past three years. You have been involved with this case throughout this set of circumstances. It is notable how the stress of Mrs. Downston's deterioration is affecting the entire family. Dolores and Don have been rearranging and strictly limiting their social activities to make sure Mrs. Downston is supervised. The load of physical care is increasing, and they both have physical problems that will soon make rendering this care difficult, if not impossible. Because Mrs. Downston is frightened by newcomers and screams in terror, her teenage granddaughters have been unable to invite their friends to the house.

Psychiatric practitioners frequently advocate institutionalizing clients with DAT. Family caregivers, on the other hand, often have difficulty with this decision and may even take offense at this suggestion despite feeling mentally and physically exhausted.

1. What suggestions or alternatives would you propose to Mrs. Downston's family?
2. At what point, if ever, should a professional exert pressure on family caregivers to institutionalize their loved one?

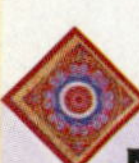

MEDIALINK 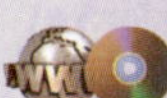 www.prenhall.com/kneisl

Go to the Pearson Health MediaLink CD-ROM and the Companion Website at www.prenhall.com/kneisl for interactive resources for this chapter.

As a result of the aging of the U.S. population, psychiatric–mental health nurses are increasingly in contact with clients who have delirium, dementia, amnestic disorder, and other cognitive disorders. Clients with these disorders provide a special challenge because they may perceive themselves and their environment differently than we do and often have problems in communication reception and expression. These are similar to challenges psychiatric–mental health nurses face when communicating with a client who has a florid psychosis. Discovering how to communicate, how to assess how they feel, and how to care for them are vital nursing skills.

In addition to family caregivers, nurses are the most logical advocates for these clients. Frequently, we are in charge of day treatment centers or nursing homes, or we facilitate support groups. Families look to us for suggestions to ease their burdens, for strategies to cope with difficult behavioral symptoms, for education to explain unpredictable behavior, and for resources that might alleviate their situation.

Your knowledge of psychobiology and your holistic approach to client care are unique assets essential to providing quality care for clients with cognitive disorders. Before the 20th century, all organic brain disorders of older adults were categorized as senile dementia. At the turn of the 20th century, neuropathologists doing autopsy work distinguished senile dementia from arteriosclerotic conditions and neurosyphilis. Arteriosclerotic brain disease was then considered the primary cause of confusional states in older adults and the result of diseased cerebral vessels.

By the middle of the 20th century, a new category, organic brain disease (OBD), was added. This category was broader, allowing for a defect both in the vessels and in the brain itself. The category organic brain syndrome (OBS) then followed, which recognized the need for a diagnosis that included symptoms without a known cause. A few years ago, the term *organic mental syndrome* (OMS) referred to a group of psychological or behavioral signs of unknown or unclear etiology, while *organic mental disorder* (OMD) referred to a particular syndrome whose etiology was known or presumed. The term is no longer used; the term *cognitive disorder* is preferred.

DELIRIUM

Older adults, especially those with dementia, are prone to transient cognitive disorders usually referred to as either delirium or acute confusional state. There is a wide range (11% to 89%) to the estimation of how many older general medical clients experience a life-threatening acute confusional state (Skrobik, 2007). If hospitalized, they remain in the hospital twice as long as clients without delirium, and one-fourth of these older adults with delirium die within one month of admission. Residents over 75 years of age in long-term care facilities are at particular risk and significant numbers may be delirious at any time.

Delirium is an abrupt-onset type of confusional state that is marked by:

1. Prominent disorientation
2. Disorders of perception
3. Terrifying hallucinations and vivid dreams
4. A kaleidoscopic array of strange and absurd fantasies and delusions
5. Agitated behavior
6. Inability to sleep
7. Tendency to convulse
8. Intense emotional disturbances (Macleod, 2006; Meagher et al., 2007)

Additional elements include impaired attention and concentration and diminution of all mental activity. Rage, depression, fear, apathy, and incontinence are common.

Differentiating delirium from dementia can be a difficult process for nurses and physicians; however, failure to recognize delirium in clients can delay appropriate treatment, with serious health consequences. See the DSM-IV-TR Diagnostic Criteria feature on page 298 for the taxonomy of delirium.

Signs of Delirium

Detecting delirium involves examining how the person thinks (cognition), as well as the ability to pay attention, degree of wakefulness, and psychomotor behavior.

Cognition

The three components of cognition—perception, thinking, and memory—are all disrupted in delirium:

1. *Perception.* The person shows a reduced ability to distinguish and integrate sensory information and to differentiate it from hallucinations, dreams, illusions, and imagery.
2. *Thinking.* The thinking process is fragmented and disorganized to the extent that the person is unable to reason, judge, abstract, or solve problems.
3. *Memory.* Memory is impaired in all three aspects; the person is unable to form memories or store and retrieve (register, retain, or recall) information.

Attention and Wakefulness

Attention is impaired in all three areas. The person has difficulty with:

- Alertness, or maintaining vigilance
- Selectiveness, or the ability to focus and filter out or selectively attend to stimuli at will
- Directiveness, or the ability to pull oneself back to a task or direct and focus one's mental processes

Wakefulness is usually reduced during the day, leading to drowsiness and naps. The person often experiences sleeplessness, restlessness, and agitation at night. There is a disturbed

DSM-IV-TR Diagnostic Criteria for Cognitive Disorders

Diagnostic Criteria for Delirium Due to . . . [Indicate the General Medical Condition]

A. Disturbance of consciousness (i.e., reduced clarity of awareness of the environment) with reduced ability to focus, sustain, or shift attention.
B. A change in cognition (such as memory deficit, disorientation, language disturbance) or the development of a perceptual disturbance that is not better accounted for by a preexisting, established, or evolving dementia.
C. The disturbance develops over a short period of time (usually hours to days) and tends to fluctuate during the course of the day.
D. There is evidence from the history, physical examination, or laboratory findings that the disturbance is caused by the direct physiological consequences of a general medical condition.

Diagnostic Criteria for Dementia of the Alzheimer's Type (DAT)

A. The development of multiple cognitive deficits manifested by both
   1. memory impairment (impaired ability to learn new information or to recall previously learned information)
   2. one (or more) of the following cognitive disturbances:
      a. aphasia (language disturbance)
      b. apraxia (impaired ability to carry out motor activities despite intact motor function)
      c. agnosia (failure to recognize or identify objects despite intact sensory function)
      d. disturbance in executive functioning (i.e., planning, organizing, sequencing, abstracting)
B. The cognitive deficits in Criteria A1 and A2 each cause significant impairment in social or occupational functioning and represent a significant decline from a previous level of functioning.
C. The course is characterized by gradual onset and continuing cognitive decline.
D. The cognitive deficits in Criteria A1 and A2 are not due to any of the following:
   1. other central nervous system conditions that cause progressive deficits in memory and cognition (e.g., cerebrovascular disease, Parkinson's disease, Huntington's disease, subdural hematoma, normal-pressure hydrocephalus, brain tumor)
   2. systemic conditions that are known to cause dementia (e.g., hypothyroidism, vitamin B_{12} or folic acid deficiency, niacin deficiency, hypercalcemia, neurosyphilis, HIV infection)
   3. substance-induced conditions
E. The deficits do not occur exclusively during the course of a delirium.
F. The disturbance is not better accounted for by another Axis I disorder (e.g., major depressive disorder, schizophrenia).

Source: Reprinted with permission from the *Diagnostic and Statistical Manual of Mental Disorders,* Fourth Edition, Text Revision. (Copyright 2000). American Psychiatric Association.

Using DSM-IV-TR

Health care providers often use language unfamiliar to clients and their families. Explain the term *cognitive deficit* to make it easier for your clients and their family members to understand.

sleep–wake cycle, with hour-to-hour variation. Interestingly, delirium and dreaming are both characterized by the same electroencephalographic (EEG) changes. The person with delirium is then caught between dreaming and hallucinating, sleeping and wakefulness.

Psychomotor Behavior

The delirious client is either hyperactive or hypoactive, often alternating between the two extremes. Speech may be slurred and disjointed, with aimless vocalizations and repetitions. Tremors and irregular spasmodic (choreiform) movements may be present, as illustrated in the following clinical examples of delirium.

CLINICAL EXAMPLE

Mr. Robio, an 80-year-old bachelor with bilateral cataracts, lived alone in a small midwestern town with his pet cat Suzy. Mr. Robio was admitted to the community hospital for a hernia repair that he had been putting off for several months. Never hospitalized before, he was extremely anxious on admission and became more so with each preoperative procedure that day. At 10:00 that evening, Mr. Robio was found wandering in the hallway, looking and calling for Suzy. The nurse assisted him to return to his room. Three hours later he was again found wandering, this time he was nude and more disoriented than before. He was sedated with a nonbenzodiazepine and confined to bed with a vest and soft wrist restraints. By morning, Mr. Robio was so disoriented and agitated that the surgery was canceled. Mr. Robio's physician then ordered the client confined to bed. Within one week, Mr. Robio's behavior had deteriorated to the extent that he required institutionalization. He was transferred to a local nursing home for permanent care.

A 55-year-old man, Mr. Bruener, was in the midst of a difficult divorce and went drinking with his friends. He drank numerous "straight shots" and shortly thereafter began screaming, crying, and acting aggressively toward others in the bar. At one point he tried to choke a man, and later picked up a chair and threw it. The police took him to jail and, when he began to convulse, to the hospital.

Mrs. Weinstein, a 65-year-old woman, was in the hospital with renal problems. Although previously alert, she rapidly became agitated and confused about where she was. She was unresponsive to the nurse's efforts to orient her and refused to cooperate during her morning care. Within hours after this extreme agitation, she lapsed into a stupor and then a coma.

DIFFERENTIATING DELIRIUM FROM DEMENTIA

Several criteria distinguish delirium from dementia (Tschanz et al., 2006):

- *State of consciousness.* People with delirium have fluctuating consciousness, but people with dementia are as attentive as they can be and do not have clouded consciousness until terminal stages.
- *Stability.* In clients with delirium, the ability to pay attention and respond changes from hour to hour. Clients with dementia pay attention and respond at a particular level in a relatively stable manner.
- *Duration.* Delirium is short lived; dementia is prolonged.
- *Rate of onset.* Delirium develops rapidly, whereas dementia is usually an insidious, gradual process.
- *Cause.* Delirium may be traced to a recent source, whereas dementia cannot be linked to another cause.

For a summary of the characteristics of delirium and dementia, and the differentiation between them and depression, see Table 14-1 ■ on page 300. Depression is discussed in Chapter 17∞.

DEMENTIA

The prevalence of dementia is 1.5% to 2% starting at 65 years of age and doubles every 10 years. Dementia of the Alzheimer's type (DAT) alone affects as many as 25 million people worldwide (Schutte & Holston, 2006). This number is 10 times greater than at the turn of the last century, and it is likely to double by 2030. Nurses in all clinical settings should be alert for the presence of symptoms that could indicate an early form of dementia. The What Every Community Health Nurse Should Know feature gives an example that may pique your interest.

WHAT EVERY COMMUNITY HEALTH NURSE SHOULD KNOW

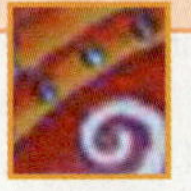

A Family Member's Cognitive Skills

As a community health nurse you will have contact with a number of people who are aged but still living independently in their own community living situations. When you make a home visit to an elderly couple to treat the husband's surgical incision site, you also notice that his wife is having some difficulty. Her shoelaces are not tied and when you mention it, she looks down and pushes them into the inside of her shoes instead of tying them. Her emotions seem blunted, she has been neglecting her personal hygiene, and her husband is worried about her decreased energy and motivation and lack of initiative. This, in combination with her problem understanding some of your conversation with her about her husband's bandages, leads you to believe she may be having some cognitive problems. Under these circumstances, an assessment of the wife is warranted.

Over 60% of people in nursing homes have been diagnosed with dementia. A now common clinical syndrome, dementia is marked by the following:

- Global cognitive impairment extending to the areas of abstract thinking, judgment, insight, complex capabilities (language, tasks, recognition), and personality change
- Memory impairment
- Decline in intellectual function
- Altered judgment, in awake and alert states
- Altered affect
- Spatial disorientation

Dementia is a mental disorder involving functional declines in multiple cognitive areas, including memory, along with behavioral and psychological symptoms. Symptoms related to specific areas of brain damage are shown in Figure 14-1 ■ on page 301. The DSM-IV-TR further differentiates dementia as "sufficiently severe to cause impairment in occupational or social functioning" (American Psychiatric Association [APA], 2000, p. 148).

Dementias are classified according to either the cause or the area of neurologic damage (such as cortical or subcortical). Dementia of the Alzheimer's type (DAT) is the classic cortical dementia, whereas Huntington's disease and Parkinson's disease are common subcortical types. The cortical and subcortical types are quite similar. People with subcortical dementias, however, have a higher order of functioning.

Some sources suggest that as many as 5% of dementias evaluated in clinical settings may be attributable to reversible causes. Some of these causes include metabolic abnormalities (e.g., hypothyroidism), nutritional deficiencies (e.g., vitamin B_{12} or folate deficiencies), or dementia syndrome due to

MediaLink Application: Dementia: It's Not Always Alzheimer's Disease

TABLE 14-1 ■ **Comparing Delirium, Dementia, and Depression**

	Delirium	Dementia	Depression
Diagnostic Features	Disturbance of consciousness accompanied by a change in cognition unaccounted for by a preexisting or evolving dementia. Reduced clarity of awareness of the environment. Impaired ability to focus, sustain, or shift attention. Change in cognition may include memory impairment, disorientation to time and/or place, or language disturbance such as rambling, irrelevant, or pressured and incoherent speech. Simple or complex perceptual disturbances may include misinterpretations, illusions, or hallucinations.	Multiple cognitive deficits, including memory impairment and either aphasia, apraxia, or agnosia; or a disturbance in executive functioning (the ability to think abstractly, to plan, initiate, sequence, monitor, and stop complex behavior). Impairment in occupational or social functioning that represents a decline from earlier level of functioning.	Dysphoric mood, loss of interest or pleasure in usual activities and pastimes, appetite disturbance, change in weight, sleep disturbance, psychomotor agitation or retardation, decreased energy, feelings of worthlessness or guilt, difficulty concentrating or thinking, thoughts of death or suicide or suicide attempts.
Associated Features	Emotional disturbance: fear, anxiety, irritability, anger, euphoria, apathy. Disturbance in sleep–wake cycle with daytime sleepiness or nighttime agitation and difficulty falling asleep. Disturbed psychomotor behavior including groping or picking at bedclothes, sudden movements, or sluggishness and lethargy. Possible extremes of psychomotor activity during the day.	Spatial disorientation, poor judgment, poor insight, violence, suicidal behavior, disinhibited behavior, slurred speech, anxiety, mood and sleep disturbances, delusions, hallucinations, vulnerability to physical and psychosocial stressors.	Depressed appearance, tearfulness, feelings of anxiety, irritability, fear, brooding, excessive concern with physical health, panic attacks, phobias. Delusions or hallucinations may be present. In older adults, symptoms suggesting dementia (e.g., disorientation, memory loss, distractibility, apathy, difficulty in concentration, inattentiveness).
Onset	May begin abruptly. Relatively rapid: over hours. Short period of time: a few days. Especially common in children and after the age of 60.	Depends on underlying etiology. May be rather sudden (e.g., head trauma) or insidious in onset and slow, but progress is relentless over several years (e.g., primary degenerative dementia).	Usually able to date onset with some precision. Onset is variable; symptoms usually develop over a period of days to weeks but may be sudden. In some instances, prodromal symptoms may occur over several months.
Course	Fluctuates; symptoms usually worse at night; lucid intervals usually in the morning.	Depends on underlying etiology. May be progressive, static, or remitting.	Often not recognized or misdiagnosed in older adults. Need to differentiate from dementia.
Duration	May resolve in a few hours or a few weeks.	May progress to death over several years. May be slowed.	Self-limiting. Median time period is 8 months; may last up to 2 years.
Outcome	Recovery if underlying disease is corrected or self-limiting. If disorder persists, shift to another, more stable organic brain syndrome. May cause death.	Generally irreversible. Slowing of deterioration depends on underlying pathology, timely diagnosis, and treatment. The more widespread the structural damage to the brain, the less likely the clinical improvement.	Can be successfully treated. Spontaneous recovery is expected. Severe depression may end in suicide.
Etiologic Factors	Systemic infections. Metabolic disorders (hepatic or renal disease, hypoxia, hypercapnia, hypoglycemia, ionic imbalances, thiamine deficiency). Postoperative states. Substance intoxication and withdrawal. Head trauma. Lesions of the right parietal lobe and occipital lobe. Toxin exposure. Anticholinergic effects of medication.	Primary degenerative dementia, Alzheimer type. Infections of central nervous system. Brain trauma. Virus (e.g., AIDS, Creutzfeldt–Jakob disease). Toxic metabolic disturbance. Vascular disease (e.g., vascular dementia). Normal pressure hydrocephalus. Neurologic conditions such as Huntington's disease, multiple sclerosis, Parkinson's disease. Postanoxic or posthypoglycemic states.	Situational: bereavement, loss of health, major catastrophic event in person's life, trauma.

Source: Blazer, D., Hughes, D. C., & George, L. K. (1987). The epidemiology of depression in an elderly community population. *The Gerontologist, 27,* 281–287.

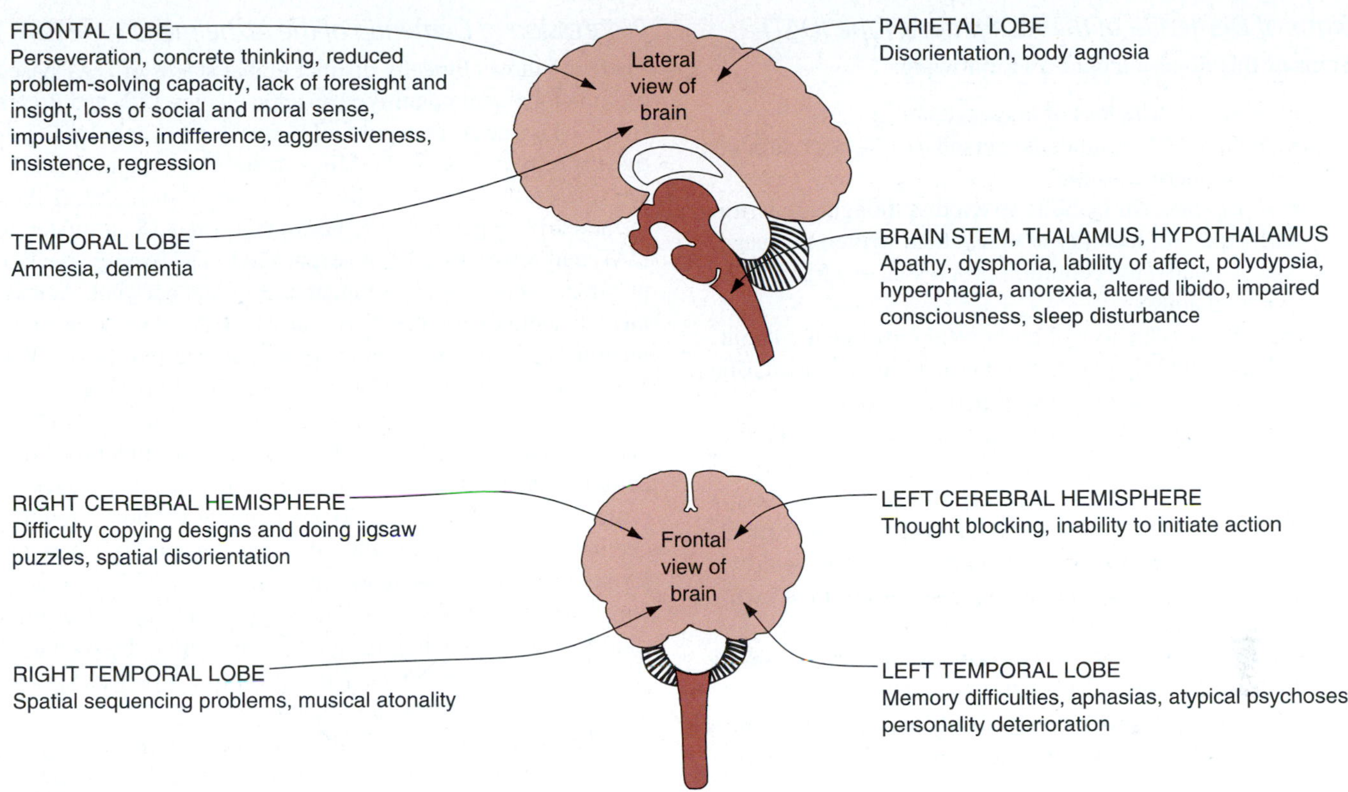

FIGURE 14-1 ■ Behavioral changes related to specific areas of brain damage. Damage to each part of the brain results in specific alterations and deficits in client behaviors and skills.

depression (Goroll & Mulley, 2007). How dementia affects function depends on the area of the brain involved in the disease. There will be different behavioral, neurologic, psychiatric, and cognitive symptoms depending on the type of dementia. An added frequent complication is the presence of mixed dementias. With such a broad array of dementias, establishing a clear diagnosis is complex, difficult, and time consuming but worth the effort in order to determine appropriate psychiatric treatment.

Dementia of the Alzheimer's Type (DAT)

Dementia of the Alzheimer's type (DAT), also known as *Alzheimer's disease* or *Alzheimer's dementia (AD)*, a chronic progressive disorder, is the most common form of dementia among older adults. (See the Diagnostic Criteria for Cognitive Disorders on page 298.) Reference to this disease with either abbreviation—DAT or AD—is accepted; however, to keep the distinction clear that this is one type of dementia, and to prevent confusion with the abbreviation AD used to refer to anxiety disorder, it will be referred to as DAT throughout this chapter.

Today, 5 million Americans have DAT. Unless a cure or prevention is found, that number will jump to 16 million by the year 2050. In addition to the quality-of-life issues for the clients involved, there are financial realities that affect the individual, the family, the community, and our health care system in general. DAT costs the U.S. economy over $250 billion a year for long-term care. Additional data can be accessed through links to DAT resources through the Companion Website for this book.

Alois Alzheimer first recognized the features of what would come to be called dementia of the Alzheimer's type (DAT) in 1907 while conducting an autopsy on a 51-year-old woman with a 4 1/2-year history of dementia. He discovered senile plaques in the brain and other pathologic lesions that he called neurofibrillary tangles. Neurofibrillary tangles are illustrated in FIGURE 14-2 ■. These are now referred to as Alzheimer-type changes. This disease may also destroy the neurons that secrete the neurotransmitter acetylcholine, which plays a role in memory and learning.

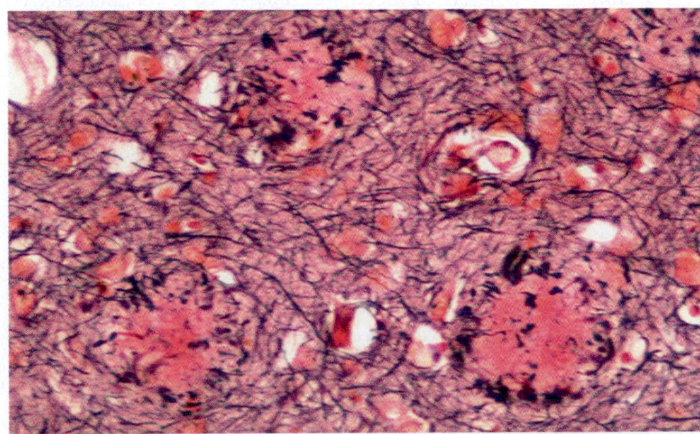

FIGURE 14-2 ■ Neurofibrillary tangles. Characteristic senile plaques and neurofibrillary tangles are seen in this microphotograph using a silver stain of the hippocampal cortex in a client with DAT.

Source: Smock, T. K. (1999). *Physiological psychology: A neuroscience approach.* Upper Saddle River, NJ: Prentice Hall.

Source: Phototake NYC, Martin Rotker.

MEDIALINK Dementia of the Alzheimer's Type

Signs of Dementia of the Alzheimer's Type (DAT)

Signs of this disease include the following:

- *Aphasia:* The loss of language ability
- *Anomia:* Over time, the person experiences difficulty remembering words
- *Agraphia:* An inability to express thoughts in writing
- *Alexia:* An inability to understand written language (eventually, the condition progresses to a loss of all verbal ability)
- *Apraxia:* The loss of purposeful movement without loss of muscle power or coordination in general. The ability to conceptualize or perform motor tasks deteriorates. People with apraxia may have difficulty carrying out complex tasks.
- *Agnosia:* The loss of sensory ability to recognize objects. Initially, the person has difficulty recognizing everyday objects. In the later stages, people with agnosia recognize neither loved ones nor their own body parts.
- *Mnemonic disturbances:* Memory loss. The inability to remember recent events, especially in new or changing environments, extends to profound memory loss of both recent and past events (Goroll & Mulley, 2007).

Frequently, symptoms of DAT occur insidiously. Hallucinations, more often visual than auditory, can be quite disturbing to the unsuspecting client. Behaviors can become agitated and will run counter to the client's usual personality and interactional style. Spending time in a health care facility for physical reasons such as rehabilitation or surgery can bring some of the symptoms to the attention of health care providers. The following is a clinical example of dementia.

CLINICAL EXAMPLE

Therese Thomas, an 81-year-old retired piano teacher, is recuperating from knee replacement surgery at a rehabilitation center. Nursing staff noticed slight changes in her interactions over the past two weeks, including refusing to use silverware during meals, a significant difference from her typically fastidious habits. During an assessment interview, Ms. Thomas was asked how her vision and hearing have been lately, because seeing well and hearing well frequently become issues with older adults. She replied that she has been seeing and hearing just fine. These questions can be asked or stated in such a way as to seem more a physical set of questions than an emotional or psychiatric-focused set of questions (e.g., "Sometimes people may not hear as well as others and words are missed."). Ms. Thomas denied she was having a problem with her hearing. Then the question was asked, "Sometimes your hearing may be such that you are hearing things that other people don't hear. Does that ever happen to you?" Ms. Thomas admitted she did hear things to which other people were not reacting. When asked to elaborate, Ms. Thomas stated that her silverware had begun speaking to her. When the nurse asked what was being said, Ms. Thomas replied, "Nothing good."

Progression of Dementia of the Alzheimer's Type (DAT)

There are three clinically distinct global stages of DAT based on functional and cognitive capacity: Stages 1, 2, and 3 (see Box 14-1). One assessment tool useful in assessing the cognitive capacity in DAT is the Mini-Mental State Exam (MMSE, see Chapter 11). Usually, a score of 18 or higher is seen in the early stages of DAT, between 12 and 18 in moderate DAT, and lower than 12 in severe DAT. The average decline in MMSE scores is approximately 3 points per year. Assessment guidelines for the three stages of the disease are outlined in the Your Assessment Approach feature on page 304. Functional disability can be assessed grossly through determining competence with activities of daily living (ADLs). When you assess a client for DAT, observe for functional disabilities. There is a correspondence between the stages of central nervous system (CNS) aging and DAT. Note cognitive decline and the corresponding functional disability when you formulate your assessments. In as many as 20% of clients with dementia of the Alzheimer's type you can expect mild rigidity and a slowing of movement, called bradykinesia (Dale & Federman, 2007). This will affect how quickly and how well they will be able to function.

The available treatment choices for a person with dementia of the Alzheimer's type include pharmacologic interventions. The target symptoms are agitation, aggression, and psychosis. Medications called cholinesterase inhibitors, or acetylcholinesterase inhibitors, slow progression of the symptoms but do not treat the disease. They cause elevated acetylcholine levels in the cortex, which slow the neuronal degradation that occurs in DAT. Cholinesterase inhibitors are indicated for the treatment of mild to moderate dementia of the Alzheimer's type. Medication treatment issues are discussed in more detail in Chapters 7 and 32. Controlled studies looking at behavior as an outcome measure suggest that cholinesterase inhibitors used in moderate dementia may improve anxiety, apathy, and possibly aggression, irritability, and disinhibition (Goroll & Mulley, 2007). Most frequently, clients with Alzheimer's disease are already taking cholinesterase inhibitors when they become agitated. At that point, adjunctive therapy with another cholinesterase inhibitor or an atypical antipsychotic can be clinically effective.

Dementia with Lewy Bodies

Dementia with Lewy bodies (DLB) is the second most common late-onset dementia after dementia of the Alzheimer's type, accounting for 15% to 20% of the neurodegenerative dementias. It is also known as Lewy body disease, diffuse Lewy body disease, cortical Lewy body disease, and Lewy body dementia. The name of this dementia subtype comes from the pathologic feature of Lewy body inclusions. Lewy bodies are abnormal concentrations of protein that develop inside nerve cells. Lewy bodies appear as spherical masses that displace other cell components. There are two shapes—classical and cortical. A classical Lewy body is a dense core surrounded by a halo of radiating fibrils. The cortical Lewy body is less well-defined and lacks the halo.

Box 14-1 Behavioral Changes of Dementia of the Alzheimer's Type (DAT)

DAT has an average course of 5 to 10 years, with a range of 2 to 20 years. Early onset often leads to very rapid deterioration.

Stage 1 (2–4 Years)

Changes in behaviors include the following:

- Complex tasks become more difficult, related to a recent decline in memory.
- Concentration decreases while distractibility increases.
- Making accurate judgments becomes difficult.
- Disorientation about time occurs, but memory about people and places remains.
- Personal appearance may decline and the person needs help in selecting appropriate clothing.
- Planning in general is seriously limited, so incomplete verbal or written reports are common at work sites.
- Verbal skills decline and word-finding and object-naming become difficult. Speech in noisy, distracting environments is too difficult.
- Client may accuse others of wrongdoing because of transitory delusions of persecution ("You hid my keys"). People recognize their own confusion and are frightened by it. They cover up and rationalize symptoms.
- Poor driving skills because of misperceptions and errors in judgment can lead to accidents.
- *Hypertonia* (an increase in muscle tone) can happen with dementia and may result in muscle twitching.
- Anxiety and depression are common, as are frustration, helplessness, apathy, and shame.
- Psychotic symptoms are common.
- Depression worsens the symptoms of dementia and should be treated.

Stage 2 (Several Years)

Changes in behavior include the following:

- Progressive recent and remote memory loss are characteristic.
- New information cannot be retained.
- Failure to recognize family members or past significant events signals loss of remote memory.
- Behavior deteriorates rapidly and is often socially unacceptable.
- Poor impulse control leads to outbursts and tantrums.
- Emotional lability is common—the mood quickly shifts from a flat affect to marked irritability.
- Comprehension of language, interactions, and significance of objects is greatly diminished.
- Disorientation occurs to the three spheres of person, place, and time.
- Wandering occurs.
- The person has difficulty tracking the sequence of events especially for bathing, dressing, and toileting.
- Psychotic symptoms are common.
- *Misidentification syndrome* frequently occurs, in which familiar people are seen as unfamiliar and vice versa.
- Sleep cycle is impaired, with a decrease in total sleep time and frequent awakenings.
- Accidents are common, especially falls and injuries because of difficulty in using sharp objects.

Stage 3 (1–2 Years)

Changes in behavior include the following:

- Hyperorality (placing everything within reach into the mouth) and periodic binge eating occur.
- Hypermetamorphosis occurs (the need to compulsively touch and examine every object in the environment).
- Motor skills seriously deteriorate.
- Emotional responses dwindle to nonresponsiveness.

DLB has only recently been the subject of intense consideration and scrutiny, and there is more information available now than just 5 years ago. There is a distinct presentation of the dementia with parkinsonism (symptoms that resemble Parkinson's disease resulting from effects on the extrapyramidal tracts of the CNS), fluctuating confusion, disturbances of consciousness, falls, and psychiatric symptoms.

One of the main concerns regarding DLB is making the diagnosis before pharmacologic treatment is initiated. This is important because neuroleptics typically used in dementia can cause a severe and even fatal sensitivity to the extrapyramidal side effects in DLB clients. People who have DLB are unusually sensitive to many antipsychotic medications. In response to the traditional antipsychotics (such as haloperidol), these clients are at much higher risk of developing side effects such as tardive dyskinesia or neuroleptic malignant syndrome. Although the newer atypical antipsychotic agents are generally less likely to provoke side effects in clients overall, DLB clients can be at unacceptably high risk. Quetiapine (Seroquel), however, is an atypical antipsychotic that has a relatively low risk of provoking these side effects and clients with DLB are often better able to tolerate quetiapine than other antipsychotics. There is an unlabeled use of cholinesterase inhibitors (used to treat DAT) in the treatment of the behavioral effects of dementia with Lewy bodies (Wilson, Shannon, Shields, & Stang, 2008).

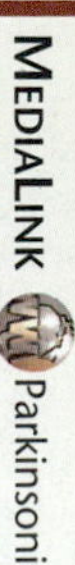

The three core diagnostic features of DLB were defined by McKeith et al. (1996):

1. Spontaneous parkinsonism or extrapyramidal signs
2. Persistent or recurrent visual hallucinations
3. Fluctuating cognition

Clients who have DLB alone are much less common than those who have a concomitant DAT. Neuropathologic studies have found that 20% to 30% of older adult clients with degenerative dementia have an overlap of both DAT and DLB. It is also difficult to differentiate DLB that is comorbid with DAT as a unique clinical syndrome from DAT alone. It is also

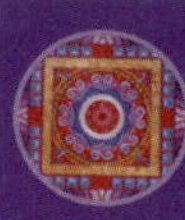

YOUR ASSESSMENT APPROACH
Early, Middle, and Late Stages of Dementia of the Alzheimer's Type (DAT)

Early Stage

- Client complains of forgetfulness, as in remembering names and appointments.
- Client covers up forgetfulness.
- Client may blame others for forgetfulness.
- Client acts confused, becomes irritable or quiet. Emotional lability is common.
- Client begins to have problems in family, work, and social life.
- Client notices trouble finding the right word.
- Client cannot manage demands.
- Client experiences a noticeable decrease in knowledge of current events and recent events.
- Client experiences concentration difficulties.
- Client has problems with any process involving multiple steps, such as finances or preparing a meal.

Middle Stage

- Memory problems become more pronounced. Recall of recent events is minimal.
- Client is unable to remember a major relevant part of his or her life (address, phone number, names of close family members).
- Activities of daily living, including cooking, eating, bathing, and dressing, become increasingly problematic. Family and friends begin to take over for client.
- Client has difficulty with orientation and concentration.
- Client may become restless at night and may sleep only a few hours off and on throughout the day.
- Client may become aggressive, even violent, when frustrated or when family attempts to help client.
- Client may exhibit wandering and may call out and search for children or loved ones.
- Client has increased aphasia, agnosia, and apraxia.
- Hypertonia and unsteady gait are common.
- Client may have insatiable appetite, yet lose weight.
- Social habits are forgotten. Client may be socially inappropriate.

Late Stage

- Client exhibits severe disorientation including delusions, hallucinations, and paranoid ideation.
- Client may perseverate or echo sounds.
- Speech ability becomes limited to a few words others can understand.
- Intelligible vocabulary may become limited to a single word.
- Client needs help with the steps and mechanics of toileting (wiping, flushing, redressing)
- Client needs to be fed.
- Client experiences incontinence of urine and stool.
- Client may lose all speech.
- Client may touch self and objects frequently.
- Client becomes bedridden, emaciated, and completely helpless.
- Client loses abilities for ambulation, sitting up, smiling, holding up head.

difficult to distinguish these clients from those with a Parkinson's Disease (PD)–Alzheimer's disease blended syndrome.

An action tremor may precede other parkinsonian features, and dementia is often heralded by levodopa-induced sedation, myoclonus, and hallucinations. Early on, the response to treatment with levodopa can be substantial, making it difficult to differentiate Lewy body dementia from Parkinson's disease. The progression of symptoms of DLB appears to be intermediate, as compared with the progression of symptoms in the PD and PD–Alzheimer's disease subgroups (Dale & Federman, 2007).

In addition to parkinsonian features, dementia, and a frequent tendency to episodic delirium, the syndrome may be clinically indistinguishable from dementia of the Alzheimer's type. On autopsy, there will be diffuse involvement of cortical neurons with Lewy body inclusions and an absence of, or inconspicuous number of, neurofibrillary tangles and senile plaques.

Vascular Dementia

Vascular dementia, also known as ischemic vascular dementia (IVD) and formerly known in DSM-IV as multi-infarct dementia, accounts for about 19% of the dementias. Unlike Alzheimer's disease, vascular dementia is abrupt in onset and episodic, with multiple remissions. The client also demonstrates focal neurologic signs, such as one-sided weakness, emotional outbursts, and a stepwise rather than progressive decline in intellectual functioning, and has a history of hypertension, diabetes, or cardiovascular disease affecting other organs.

In vascular dementia the brain tissue is destroyed by intermittent emboli that can range from a few to over a dozen. Individual infarcts may vary by 1 cm in diameter. Symptoms are commonly absent until 100–200 cc of brain tissue have been destroyed.

Parkinson's Disease

The association between **Parkinson's disease** and dementia has deepened over the years. A minority of clients with dementia have Parkinson's disease. A subset of clients has both Parkinson's disease and DAT, and this diagnosis may be difficult to determine. There are several varieties of Parkinson's disease, and the cause of classic Parkinson's disease is unknown. Another type, postencephalitic, has been linked to previous viral infection in the brain. An interesting feature of this type is the presence of neurofibrillary tangles similar to those found in clients with DAT (Dale & Federman, 2007).

Huntington's Disease

Huntington's disease is a genetic, progressive, degenerative disorder characterized by both motor and cognitive changes, chorea, and dementia. This disease, one of the more frequently observed types of hereditary nervous system diseases, usually begins between the ages of 40 and 50. By the time of diagnosis, the client has usually reproduced, passing this inherited disease to another generation. The movement disorder is thought to be caused by vulnerability to damage and subsequent loss of nerve cells in the brain.

Movement abnormalities slowly increase until all muscle groups are involved (Bourne, Clayton, Murch, & Grant, 2006). The motor dysfunction is characterized by *chorea:* quick, jerky, purposeless, involuntary movements. The average life span after an initial diagnosis is 15 years. Mood disturbances, especially depression, are common early in the disease, followed by deterioration of cognitive function.

Supplementing with coenzyme Q10 (CoQ10) has been known to replace deficient levels of the enzyme in muscle and decrease cerebellar-based ataxia. Treatment with CoQ10 to see if the enzyme could have an impact on the disease's progression (Kieburtz, 2006) has yielded promising results. There is some evidence of a trend toward a slower decline. Interestingly, the CoQ10 was tolerated very well, while other treatments were associated with several adverse effects. Rigorous research is required to explore this issue further. Associated concerns are the cost (from $60 to $150 per month) and the fact that as a nutritional supplement, CoQ10 may not have the quality and control guarantees of a pharmaceutical-grade product.

Pick's Disease

Pick's disease is a rare disorder in which cerebral atrophy is present in the frontal and/or temporal lobes. These circumscribed pathologic changes are different from DAT, in which atrophy is mild and diffuse.

The two patterns of behavior evident in Pick's disease represent the temporal and frontal types of the disease. People with the temporal type are talkative, lighthearted, joyous, anxious, and hyperattentive. People with the frontal type are locked into inertia, emotional dullness, and lack of initiative. As the disease progresses, the deterioration becomes more global, affecting memory and language. There is profound atrophy of the frontal and/or temporal lobes. Pick's disease worsens rapidly.

CLINICAL EXAMPLE

Marlene was a respected member of the faculty at a large state university. Three years after she first stated her concern about forgetting things—where she put her keys, frequently used phone numbers, the occasional word to describe an object or person—she became a resident in a skilled nursing facility. Marlene became unable to feed or bathe herself or to recognize friends and family.

The expected life span after the original diagnosis is 7 years. A higher incidence is seen in some families, suggesting a genetic predisposition. Attending to the behavioral messages of clients with Pick's disease may minimize their discomfort (Ito, Takahashi, & Liehr, 2007).

Creutzfeldt–Jakob Disease

Creutzfeldt–Jakob disease is an infectious, transmissible degenerative dementia affecting the cerebral cortex through cell destruction and overgrowth. It is marked clinically by a very rapid onset and involuntary movements. This profound dementia is evidenced by cerebellar ataxia, diffuse myoclonic jerks, and other visual and neurologic abnormalities. There are distinctive electroencephalographic changes with this disease. The infection is presumed to be caused by a *prion*, a small proteinaceous particle that is resistant to treatment and sterilization procedures. There may be a genetic susceptibility to infection; however, the only definitive spreading mechanism is iatrogenic as seen after corneal transplantation and after the injection of human growth hormone derived from the pituitary gland of cadavers with the disease. Repeating lumbar punctures to detect elevated levels of brain-derived proteins in the cerebrospinal fluid (CSF)—even when the first test is negative—may be a valuable diagnostic practice (Sanchez-Juan et al., 2006).

New Variant Creutzfeldt–Jakob Disease

Once the disease known as mad cow disease (bovine spongiform encephalopathy [BSE]) became widespread, an unusual presentation of Creutzfeldt–Jakob disease was noted and since 1996 has been identified as **new variant Creutzfeldt–Jakob disease (nvCJD)**. It appears to be caused by the same agent as BSE, although it is unclear how transmission to humans takes place. There is no blood or tissue test for nvCJD. Studies showing that nvCJD can be transmitted through blood transfusion, and fears that persons with nvCJD may remain asymptomatic for a decade or more are still public health concerns (Samson, 2006). There is evidence suggesting that nvCJD in Europe is linked to eating contaminated beef. Usually, Creutzfeldt–Jakob disease occurs in older clients and begins as dementia. This new variation can occur in younger clients and includes unusual spongiform changes in the cerebellum. nvCJD is currently more of a problem in Europe than in North America due to varying health codes and standards.

Pseudodementia

Affective disorders, particularly depression, can be masked by symptoms suggestive of dementia. Clinical symptoms may include impaired attention and memory, apathy, self-neglect, and no complaints of depression. The term **pseudodementia** has been used to describe the reversible cognitive impairments seen in depression. It is essential to detect pseudodementia in clients because, with appropriate treatment, they can recover. Pseudodementia should be suspected when the onset is abrupt, the clinical course is rapid, and the client complains about cognitive failures (Rubin, 2006). Clients with dementia often fail to perceive, or attempt to cover up, their deficits. Evidence of these deficits can be seen, such as in the clinical example that follows.

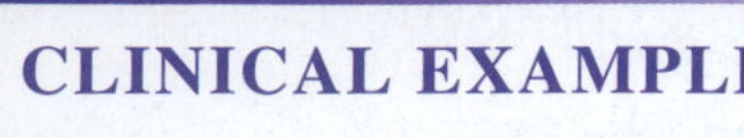

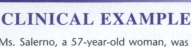

CLINICAL EXAMPLE

Ms. Salerno, a 57-year-old woman, was having problems selecting the words she wanted to use and putting her thoughts on paper. She began to miss appointments and her scheduled workdays, and she could no longer handle her daily responsibilities.

Mr. Jorgensen, a 45-year-old man, was in the hospital in the final stages of AIDS. He would forget what day it was and whether or not his family had visited. Occasionally he had visual hallucinations and on one occasion seemed to think he was at summer camp.

AMNESTIC DISORDER

Amnestic disorder, a relatively uncommon cognitive disorder, is characterized by short- and long-term memory deficits, an inability to recall previously learned information or past events, an inability to learn new material, confabulation, apathy, and a bland affect. Impairment ranges from moderate to severe. Possible causes include head trauma, hypoxia, encephalitis, thiamine deficiency, and substance abuse. These causes shape the three main types of amnestic disorder, which are briefly described here: those due to (1) a medical condition, (2) a substance, or (3) other causes.

Traumatic brain injury (TBI) is frequently associated with amnesia (Hirtz et al., 2007). The cause of the trauma creates a connection between the general medical condition (which includes physical trauma), and the amnestic disorder when this type is diagnosed. The diagnosis of amnestic disorder is supported by the timing of the onset of amnesia (the amnesia is coordinated with physical trauma), an atypical presentation of a memory problem, and the ruling out of other explanations for the disorder.

Substance-induced amnesia persists beyond the immediate effects of the substance and the duration of intoxication or withdrawal from the substance. Deficits can worsen over the years despite abstinence from the substance.

Amnestic disorder not otherwise specified (NOS) is the diagnosis used when the criteria are not met for the two other types described earlier, or when there is not enough supporting evidence to link a cause to the amnesia.

BIOPSYCHOSOCIAL THEORIES

Theories about the causes of cognitive disorders are as varied as the disorders themselves. Genetics, infection, and vascular insufficiency are all believed to be causative factors. Because delirium is usually caused by an underlying systemic illness, a prompt search is essential for treatable conditions such as dehydration, diabetes, hyponatremia, hypercalcemia, thyroid crisis, infection, silent myocardial infarction, drug intoxication, or liver or renal failure (Meagher et al., 2007). If the cause is removed quickly, complete recovery from delirium can be achieved.

The actual cause of dementia of the Alzheimer's type remains unknown, but several factors are believed to play a role. DAT has been correlated with the loss of specific groups of nerve cells and the disruption of communication between nerve cells from acetylcholine and serotonin deficits. Researchers are working to identify a slow-acting, virus-like causative agent. This work has been prompted by the findings of just such an agent in Creutzfeldt–Jakob disease.

To date, advanced age, family history of the illness, Down's syndrome, and a history of head trauma are risk factors for DAT (APA, 2000; White & Cummings, 1997). There are linkages between genetic markers and DAT on a number of chromosomes, namely chromosomes 1, 14, and 21, and one or both alleles coding for the E4 variant of apolipoprotein on chromosome 19 (called apo E4). People with DAT have four times the family incidence of dementia. Yet in identical and fraternal twins, in only 40% of cases do both get DAT, suggesting that DAT cannot be due to a single autosomal dominant gene. The disease also appears in twins and in various family members at different times, making it difficult to interpret the markers found in genetic studies.

Other possible risk factors are environmental toxins, stroke, thyroid disorder, lower educational status, and female gender (Tschanz et al., 2006). Ongoing research focuses on causes and medication treatment that can either protect or restore neurons, thereby combating memory loss. Additional medication studies focus on ameliorating behavioral symptoms. Vitamin B_{12} deficiency has been identified as a condition that mimics DAT, as explained in the Caring for the Spirit box.

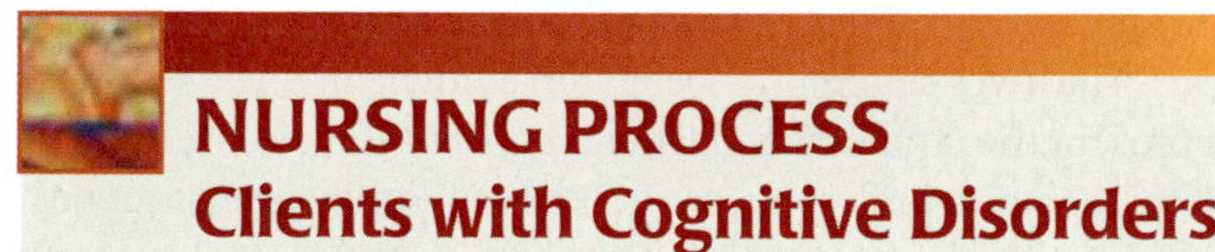

NURSING PROCESS
Clients with Cognitive Disorders

The nursing process with all cognitive disorders revolves around the principles of care used in dementia.

Assessment

Your skills in assessing clients with these disorders are important for developing and delivering competent client care. Use this information in each subsequent step of the nursing process.

Subjective Data

It is often difficult to gather data about clients with delirium, dementia, amnestic disorder, and other cognitive disorders. They are sometimes anxious, defensive, and confused, and give unreliable histories. Often there is no dependable secondary source of information. To maximize your efforts, gather all data in a setting that is free from distraction and discomfort:

- Decibel levels of ambient (surrounding) noise must be low.
- Light should be sufficient to dispel shadows.
- Room temperature should be comfortable for the client.

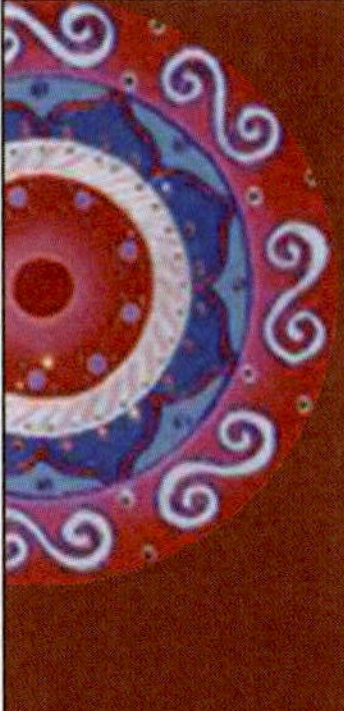

CARING FOR THE SPIRIT

Is It Alzheimer's Disease or Vitamin B_{12} Deficiency?

Imagine what it must feel like to sense the deterioration of your cognitive abilities and the slow but steady loss of your sense of self. But what if your distress could have been prevented?

A deficiency of vitamin B_{12} can easily be mistaken for dementia of the Alzheimer's type. Vitamin B_{12} depletion is common among older adults because of age-induced changes in the gastrointestinal tract. Many nursing and medical textbooks state that a lack of vitamin B_{12} first causes pernicious anemia, and clinicians look for a drop in hemoglobin and a variety of other hematologic markers. The same texts explain that, with time, anemia is accompanied by neurologic signs and symptoms, including diminished vibration and position senses and dementia. Unfortunately, it is rare for a clinician to suspect B_{12}-induced dementia when a client's complete blood count is normal. Older clients can suffer the psychiatric effects of vitamin B_{12} deficiency *without* developing anemia.

A few words of caution, however, are in order about B_{12} screening: Recognizing a deficiency in its early stage is possible but requires astute assessment skills and a willingness to act as a strong client advocate, even in the face of resistance from other health professionals. Special effort is needed because some health care providers may not know how to interpret the diagnostic markers used to pinpoint the disorder. Clinicians' ability to detect this common dietary disorder can prevent a great deal of misery and spiritual distress among older adult clients.

When you ask questions, pace the questions slowly to allow the client time to answer comfortably. Aging people can normally process information after receiving it but may have difficulty taking in information. Placing the client in a situation that interferes with an already compromised sensory apparatus only heightens the client's anxiety and seriously compromises your attempts to evaluate.

Health History When completing the client's health history, include all past and present medical conditions, paying special attention to chronic conditions for which the client is being treated and any recent changes in health status. Ask the client: "Are you seeing a health care provider at this time?" "Why did you seek medical help?" "What does your health care provider say is the problem?" Infections may present as confusion and other symptoms of dementia before any change in temperature, pulse, and respirations is noted. The Your Assessment Approach features that follow here and on page 308 suggest instruments or tests that can be used to evaluate people with possible dementia or delirium.

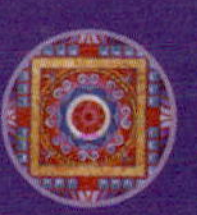

YOUR ASSESSMENT APPROACH
Assessment Instruments for Dementia

Cognitive

- Brief Cognitive Rating Scale
- Clinical Dementia Rating Scale
- Clock Completion Test
- Hamilton Depression Scale
- NINCDS/ADRDA Criteria (National Institute of Neurological and Communication Disorders and Stroke; Alzheimer's Disease and Related Disorders Association)
- SET Test
- Short Portable Mental Status Questionnaire
- Wechsler Adult Intelligence Scale
- Mini-Mental State Exam (MMSE)

Memory

- Blessed Orientation, Memory Concentration Test
- The Story Retell
- Procedural Memory Task
- Wechsler Memory Scale

Language

- Token Test
- Figural Fluency
- Proteus Mazes
- Verbal Fluency Task
- Wepman Aphasia Screening Test
- Western Aphasia Battery

Motor

- Manual Apraxia Battery
- Specific Activity Scale

Functional Level (Activities of Daily Living)

- Performance Test of Activities of Daily Living
- Physical Self-Maintenance Scale
- Refined ADL Assessment Scale (RADL)

For more information on dementia, visit the websites of the National Institute of Neurological Disorders and Stroke (http://www.ninds.nin.gov) and the Alzheimer's Association (http://www.alz.org).

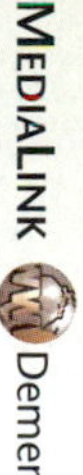

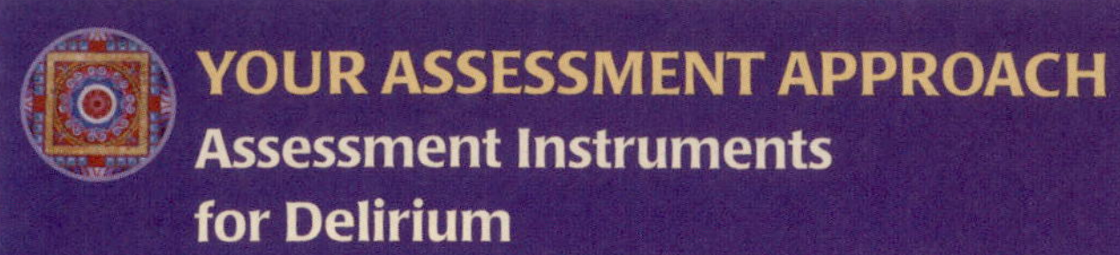

YOUR ASSESSMENT APPROACH
Assessment Instruments for Delirium

- Delirium Symptom Interview (DSI)
- Confusion Rating Scale
- Clinical Assessment of Confusion—A NEECHAM Confusion Scale
- Visual Analogue Scale for Confusion

Sensory Impairment Older adults are particularly sensitive to the confusion associated with sensory deprivation. Physiologic changes in their sensory apparatus may be directly related to aging or to pathologic processes. Both diminish sensory receptive ability. The changes in sensory apparatus, however, are not clear-cut. The older adult may have difficulty hearing high-frequency sounds, such as consonants. Turning up the volume on the radio may help the person hear one range of sounds but may also cause sensory overload because the rest of the sounds are too loud. The overall result is deprivation and distortion.

Try to ascertain any possible sensory problems, especially in hearing and vision. To test hearing, stand so that the client cannot see your face, and ask a question in a normal tone of voice. The question should require more than a yes or no answer. Test vision with pictures that the client will easily recognize. See Chapter 10 on communicating with a hearing-impaired person.

Dietary History When possible, obtain an estimate of the client's food intake. "What do you usually eat for breakfast? Lunch? Dinner?" Make special note of protein and vitamin intake. Avitaminosis, pellagra, anemia, and hypoglycemia have all been associated with reversible brain syndromes. Hydration is also an important factor, easily noted in the client's physical state (adequate hydration is indicated by a saliva pool below the tongue). Dehydration can also cause confusion. Anticholinergic side effects from any number of typically prescribed medications and over-the-counter (OTC) drugs can cause dehydration and confusion.

Head Trauma Falls are common among older adults. Misjudging distances and not being aware of obstructions also contribute to injuries. Cerebral contusions, midbrain hemorrhage, and subdural hematoma may result from a fall. Confusion may be the result of any of these conditions.

Medication Older adults are prone to adverse drug reactions as a result of age-related bodily changes. These factors are compounded by high consumption of many different medications: one third of all drugs are consumed by the 15% of the population who are older clients. Older adults are particularly susceptible to medications with anticholinergic properties (major tranquilizers, antidepressants, barbiturates, adrenal steroids, atropine, antiparkinsonians, antihistamines, antihypertensives, and diuretics). Question the client about both prescription and over-the-counter medications: "Are you now taking any medicines that your doctor prescribed?" "Do you take laxatives, cold pills, or other medicines that you buy at your drugstore without a prescription?" "Have you tried some of the health foods, herbs, supplements, or remedies they have at some of these stores?"

Alcohol Consumption Ask the client about alcohol consumption. Beyond being another source of dehydration, alcohol is a CNS depressant, and intoxication may mimic symptoms of cognitive disorders. Alcohol also compromises nutritional status and may cause withdrawal effects. Ask questions such as "What is your favorite drink?" "How much alcohol do you drink in one day/week?" and "Have you ever had periods of not remembering after you have been drinking?" Beer, wine coolers, and hard lemonade are sold in grocery stores with advertising and packaging that may be perceived as nonalcoholic or not "counting" as alcohol consumption. Questions about these substances could be asked separately from alcohol consumption questions, possibly when discussing diet and eating habits.

Psychosocial History

The psychosocial history should include an assessment of the client, the client's family, and their joint coping styles and level of intimacy. Some assessment of the client's functioning in the community should be included. Unlike cognitive testing, assessing an individual's actual functioning in the community shows what clients are doing rather than what they might do or should do.

Family History The families of impaired older adults can be a major source of information and support. In the United States, the majority of older adults have seen one or more relatives the previous week, and many live within 30 minutes of their nearest child. Common living arrangements include living with a spouse, child, or sibling. Family assessment should include the following:

- Living arrangements
- Care arrangements for the client (e.g., shopping assistance, daily visits, telephone calls)
- Family knowledge of the current illness
- Family expectations for the future
- Special family concerns about client care
- Family style of coping with stress (e.g., death of a relative, illness)
- The identified spokesperson for the family
- The family's perception of the client's coping abilities

Throughout the interview, note the interactions between family members and the client. Do family members support the client and respect what the client says? Do people listen to one another? What is the atmosphere in the family group? What is the level of intimacy between family members? Do they relate to each other with warmth and affection? Chapter 30 includes an expanded family assessment.

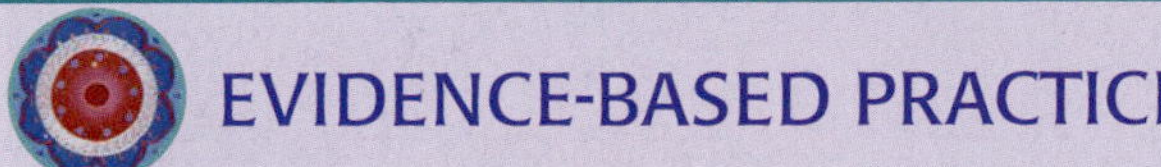

DEVELOPING A SENSITIVE AND HUMANE BATHING PROTOCOL FOR A COGNITIVELY IMPAIRED CLIENT

You are a nurse in a treatment setting that combines long-term community care and short-term respite care. Abe, a 76-year-old client with dementia who owned his own business for years, is being treated at the long-term care section of the center. His daughter Esther is his caregiver and has been involved in both her father's care and in some program development at the clinic. Bathing has become an issue with Abe—it seems to frighten and embarrass him. Discussions with his daughter revealed this to be a new problem.

The first difficulty arose when staff members entered Abe's room with bathing equipment and announced it was time to wash up. This time, what had been a usual routine was not received well. Abe grabbed a female staff member and murmured that there was no way she was going to see what he needed to keep private, nor could she squeeze the life out of him with "that stuff." Calm explanations of the staff's intentions did not dissuade Abe. He was determined not to allow bathing.

You recognize that Abe needs some control over the situation, and that bathing routines can be designed to be pleasant and comfortable for clients. Letting Abe have a say in when he bathes ("Not now" is an acceptable response) and what gets cleaned (wash his hair first, last, or not at all) has immediate positive results. Keep in mind that older skin can be dry, bathing can cause further drying (soybean oil-based no-rinse cleansers promote healthier skin), and arthritis and other conditions make movement painful. This also helps make bathing more pleasant, more comfortable, and safer. Embarrassment can be alleviated if Abe is washed under a bath blanket or a towel of sufficient size to adequately cover him.

Action should be based on more than one study, but the following was helpful in developing this bathing protocol:

Rader, J., Barrick, A., Hoeffer, B., Sloane, P. D., McKenzie, D., Talerico, K. A., et al. (2006). The bathing of older adults with dementia. *American Journal of Nursing, 106*(4), 40–48.

CRITICAL THINKING APPLICATION

1. What are the physical and emotional benefits to clients of altering a general routine to meet their specific needs?
2. Staff members derive benefits also. How can altering Abe's bathing routine help the staff?

Activities of Daily Living Assess the client carefully for level of self-care. This is often called a functional assessment. What activities of daily living can the client do without help? For which activities is help required? What type of help is needed? As cognitive deficits increase, the client becomes more dependent on others for assistance. For a study about the ADL needs of clients with DAT, see the Evidence-Based Practice feature.

Community Functioning The Comprehensive Functional Assessment (CFA) tool measures the ability to sustain oneself in the community. It covers the basic skills of living, working, relating to others, and recreating in community settings. Assess not only the ability to live independently in the community but also the degree of social involvement. Does the client belong to any clubs or groups? Do friends visit the client at home? Does the client belong to a particular church or temple? Ask about attendance at senior citizen programs and the level of participation in activities involving others.

Objective Data

Evaluating older adults with mental impairment is usually organized into three areas: physical assessment, laboratory assessment, and imaging techniques.

Physical Assessment A thorough assessment, including a complete neurologic exam (evaluation of cranial nerves, motor and sensory systems, and reflexes) and a psychiatric consultation for possible psychiatric illness, is important for all older adults with mental impairment. Because older adults with organic illness frequently manifest confusion and depression, clinicians work from the assumption that reversible illness is present. Chest x-ray films and an electrocardiogram are taken.

Laboratory Assessment The following tests are routinely ordered for older clients:

- Complete blood count, including folic acid and vitamin B_{12} levels to detect anemia
- Erythrocyte sedimentation rate (ESR) to detect infection
- SMA (Sequential Multiple Analyzer) to detect electrolyte imbalances
- Syphilis tests (Venereal Disease Research Laboratory [VDRL])
- Thyroid function studies
- Serum levels of barbiturates, bromides, and digitalis
- Liver function studies
- Human immunodeficiency virus (HIV)
- Serology
- Heavy metals
- Toxicology
- Urinalysis

Imaging Techniques Views of the brain's structure and function can be provided through a computed axial tomographic brain scan (CAT scan) or computed tomographic brain scan (CT scan), positron emission tomography (PET), and single-photon emission computed tomography (SPECT). FIGURE 14-3 ■ on page 310 presents PET scan brain images. These tests can be ordered for clients at high risk, that is, those having acute deterioration in cognitive functioning of recent onset. Acute deterioration is often associated with focal lesions and hydrocephalus.

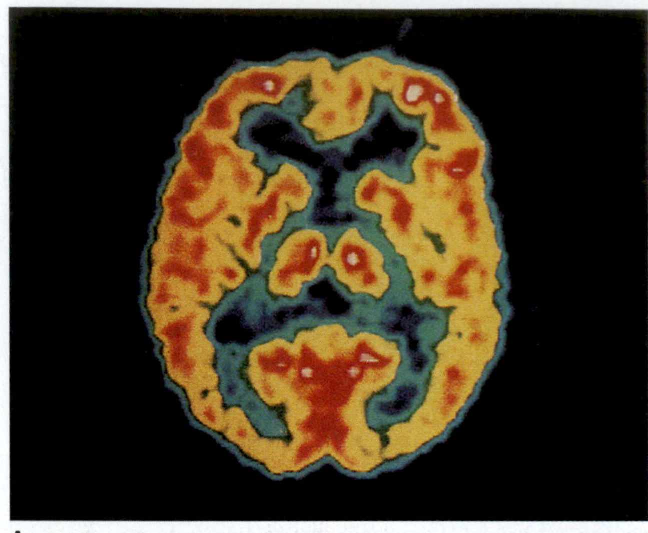
A

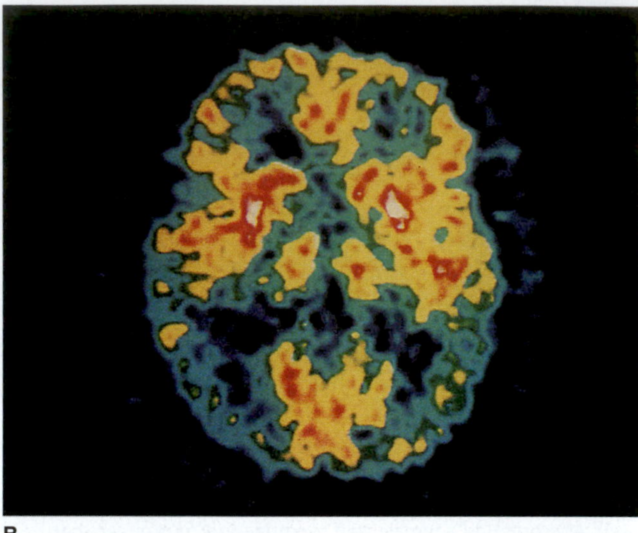
B

FIGURE 14-3 ■ PET scan brain images in dementia of the Alzheimer's type. Compare a normal brain scan (A) with the brain of a person with Alzheimer's disease (B). (A) The red and yellow areas indicate normal metabolic rates. (B) Note the blue areas indicating abnormally low metabolism in the parietal and temporal lobes.

A number of other diagnostic procedures may be used. Because of their intrusive nature or their cost, their use should be limited unless indicated. These are:

- Lumbar puncture
- Skull x-ray films
- Electroencephalography (EEG)
- Magnetic resonance imaging (MRI)
- Cerebral angiography
- Isotope cisternography

Cognitive Functioning

MEDIALINK PET/SPECT Dementia Animation

Cognitive functioning includes memory, reasoning, abstraction, calculation ability, and judgment. Refer back to Box 14-1 on page 303 for detailed information on cognitive functioning during the various stages of DAT. Clients will not respond effectively unless they feel that the information requested is relevant, they see some purpose in the interview, and they are interested in the material. Choose testing materials carefully, and keep the endurance of the client in mind at all times. When assessing cognitive functioning, pay particular attention to the following clinical manifestations.

Appearance Clients who appear disheveled, dirty, or unkempt may be experiencing problems with poor memory or a shortened attention span. This diminished ability to perform self-care may not be apparent if the client has a caregiver who helps with grooming.

Manner and Attitude Some clients may exaggerate mannerisms to compensate for a perceived decline in functioning. For example, clients who have compulsive tendencies may become more set in their ways. An attitude of defensiveness, withdrawal, or paranoia may be a response to increasing anxiety about diminished abilities.

Communication Assess communication in the areas of speech, gestures, facial expression, and writing. Difficulty in finding words and naming objects may suggest **expressive aphasia**. Difficulty grasping complex concepts may suggest **receptive aphasia**. Assess the client's ability to use gestures and facial expressions to compensate for verbal aphasia. Not using facial expressions and gestures and speaking in a monotone may indicate depression. Also test written communication and reading ability, and assess the individual's language ability. Older individuals whose primary language is not English may revert to their native language; therefore, arrangements should be made for a translator.

Perception Perception is the client's ability to recognize and integrate sensory information, including the conscious recognition of oneself in relation to the environment. Clients with asymmetric brain involvement of DAT may neglect one side of their body. These clients may also have difficulty recognizing objects (agnosia). Clients with perceptual difficulty may distort sensory information, with resulting hallucinations and delusions.

Attention and Wakefulness Attention refers to alertness and the ability to attend selectively to stimuli and to direct one's focus. Can the client sustain or pay attention to the interview process, or is he or she easily distracted by the environment? Attention can be assessed by asking the client to spell a word backwards. Wakeful states range from hyperalertness to stupor. Stupor can be the result of medication intoxication or an acute systemic disease.

Motor Activity Lethargy is often a symptom of depression, but it can also be the result of such medications as tranquilizers, antihypertensives, antidepressants, and antihistamines. Combinations of medications can also cause lethargy even when one of the medications alone may not be sedating. Lethargy can be caused by a number of disease processes, such as urinary tract infection, anemia, and meningitis. A shift between hypermotor and hypomotor activity is a sign of delirium. Agitation and physical striking out are occasionally demonstrated.

Mood and Affect Depression may accompany the earlier stages of dementia. The more serious the dementia, however, the less depressed the client. Clients with organic disease of the cerebral area are emotionally labile. Ask the client about any changes in eating or sleeping habits, and inquire about a recent loss of energy and interest in usual activities. If depression is suspected, evaluate the client for risk of suicide (see Chapter 23 ∞). Thoughts about dying, plans regarding self-harm, or self-neglect to the point of harm or death need to be explored. Ask questions about suicide in a matter-of-fact manner, without hesitation, and record the findings carefully in the assessment notes.

Orientation Disorientation to time, place, and person must be measured in an environment where the client has easy access to the information. Days in a hospital are all the same to clients housed without calendars and seasonal cues. Acute disorientation in all spheres is commonly found in people having toxic states and traumatic brain disease. Disorientation to place and person usually indicates a degenerative disorder.

Memory People with dementias have difficulty acquiring recent memory or learning; this symptom may be a key to the early detection of dementia. At present there is no set of tests that can adequately measure the memory capacity of clients with dementia. Most tests measure *episodic memory*: the processing and storage of information, like recalling the events of the day. This type of memory is impaired in most clients with cognitive disorders, depression, and drug or alcohol intoxication. *Semantic memory*, or knowledge memory, is the ability to synthesize and think about events. It is used in language, abstraction, and logical operations. People with DAT have difficulty with semantic memory; however, depressed clients do not.

Test episodic memory by asking the client to repeat a series of words or recall a recent event, such as a meal. Test semantic memory by asking the client to develop a scenario, such as describing the events from dinner until bedtime. Episodic memory is also tested in relation to time and is usually divided into three spheres: recent, remote, and past.

Abstract Reasoning Proverbs are the most common way of testing abstract reasoning. You might ask: "What does it mean when we say, 'People who live in glass houses shouldn't throw stones'?" or "What does 'A stitch in time saves nine' mean to you?" Clients with DAT often interpret these proverbs quite literally or concretely, for example replying to your question about the latter proverb with a statement such as "If you sew a single stitch you won't have to sew nine."

Calculation Ability The most common test of calculation ability is the serial sevens test: The person subtracts 7 from 100 and continues to subtract 7 from the answer. This is a difficult process for the client with dementia or delirium. The test measures the client's ability to concentrate and focus thought. It may also be a measure of educational level.

Judgment The test for judgment should predict whether a person will behave in a socially accepted manner, including the planning and carrying out of activities that require the client to discriminate reality from unrealistic situations. You might ask the client, "If you needed help during the night, how would you get it?" or "If you lost your wallet while doing errands, what would you do?"

Nursing Diagnoses: NANDA

A discussion of several nursing diagnoses common to clients with cognitive disorders follows.

Impaired Physical Mobility

Gait changes due to neurologic involvement are seen in people with a number of the dementias. These include DAT, Huntington's disease, Parkinson's disease, and Creutzfeldt–Jakob disease. Restlessness in the client with delirium is reflected in hyperactive behavior. The client usually alternates between hyperactivity and hypoactivity.

Self-Care Deficit: Bathing/Hygiene, Dressing/Grooming, Feeding, Toileting

Clients with delirium are unable to perceive, organize, or carry out the activities of daily living (e.g., bathing/hygiene, dressing/grooming, feeding, toileting). They are far too distracted by stimuli and unable to focus. The DAT client has a distinct problem: apraxia, the loss of ability to perform formerly known skills. In the late stages of all the dementias, total care is a necessity as the client moves toward brain failure.

Readiness for Enhanced Sleep

Also called *sundowner syndrome*, **sundowning** is commonly understood as confused behavior when environmental stimulation is low. It can be seen in clients with delirium and dementia. The client catnaps during the day and wanders at night. Poor sensory processing can also occur in clients who wander at night. The client with DAT may not sleep for several days, moving about in a confused state. The client becomes increasingly agitated, disoriented, or even aggressive/paranoid or impulsive and emotional later in the day and at night.

Disturbed Thought Processes

Altered thought processes can occur as a variety of experiences. Clients behave differently depending on their ability to think as a result of these alterations.

Agnosia Agnosia, the failure to recognize familiar objects, is a progressive problem that eventually renders the person unable to recognize or remember loved ones. Overall, in both delirium and dementia, the client's ability to use information in making judgments may be seriously impaired.

Memory Episodic short-term memory is affected by delirium, dementia, and mood disorders. Long-term memory is diminished in the later stages of DAT and acute delirium. See FIGURE 14-4 ■ on page 312 for a diagram of how short-term and long-term memory is established.

Orientation Disorientation is seen in clients with both dementia and delirium. In the former it is related to progressive cerebral changes; in the latter, to an acute, usually identifiable causal agent.

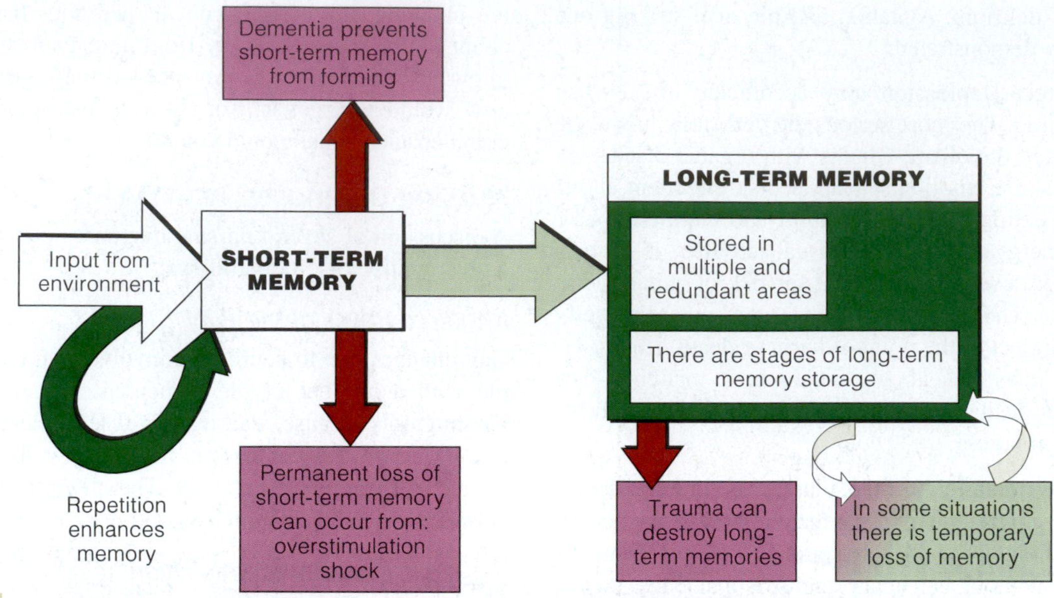

FIGURE 14-4 ■ The path to short-term memory, whether short-term memory is created, and the conversion of short-term to long-term memory.

Impaired Verbal Communication

Aphasia, both receptive and expressive, is one of the hallmarks of DAT. In the late stage of the illness, the client is completely mute. Confabulation is a common defense used by clients who cannot remember required information and therefore use fantasy to fill in the memory gaps. Confusion and paranoid ideation require that you interact with the client in a nonthreatening manner. The Rx Communication feature (Client with Dementia) describes interactions with this in mind.

Risk for Self-Directed Violence and Risk for Other-Directed Violence

In clients with DAT and most of the other dementias, there is a gradual decline in the social acceptability of their behavior. Overstating distress and making threats are common, especially if this was the mode of coping when the client was more intact. See the Rx Communication feature (Client with Dementia at Risk for Self-Harm) for an example of an interaction with a client making threats. High risk for violence is linked with impulsivity and unpredictability in these clients (see also Chapter 35 ∞). The client may also strike out at others while hallucinating or in a hyperactive phase. These behaviors are also seen in delirious clients, who are similarly unpredictable.

Ineffective Role Performance

As a result of decreasing intellectual competence, the client with dementia moves from the role of spouse, parent, employee, and community member to that of a dependent, regressed family member. The role loss and role change are anxiety provoking and at times overwhelming for the client and family. Characteristically, the family members experience a period of acute grief after receiving the diagnosis. Their level of depression should be assessed. Feelings of isolation and being overwhelmed are also common.

Disturbed Sensory Perception

The inability to attend and focus concentration is a hallmark of delirium. Decreased attention is also seen in the later stages of the dementias when the client loses the ability to encode. Delirium alters perception by reducing the client's ability to distinguish and integrate sensory information. As a

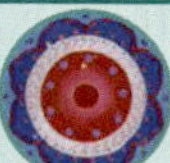

RX COMMUNICATION

CLIENT WITH DEMENTIA

CLIENT: "What are you doing here?"

NURSE RESPONSE 1: "Hello, my name is Betty and I would like to talk to you."

RATIONALE: This response helps you make contact with the client, establish what you are going to do to allay fears, and give an opportunity to interact in a nonthreatening manner.

NURSE RESPONSE 2: "I'd like to talk with you. Can you tell me if anything is hurting you?"

RATIONALE: Many clients find it easier to talk about physical pain than to articulate complex notions such as feelings and desires.

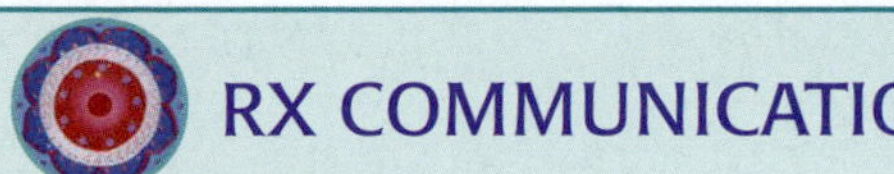

RX COMMUNICATION

CLIENT WITH DEMENTIA AT RISK FOR SELF-HARM

CLIENT: "I'm going to walk outside and get hit by a truck."

NURSE RESPONSE 1: "Tell me about why you are so upset."

RATIONALE: Client ventilates feelings in more constructive ways when discussing feeling states with the nurse.

NURSE RESPONSE 2: "Let's take a walk together."

RATIONALE: Client has the opportunity to use physical energy constructively by being distracted with empathic and supportive social interaction.

result, the client has difficulty discriminating reality from hallucinations, dreams, illusions, and imagery. In the later stages of dementia, clients also experience hallucinations and delusions, which complicate delivery of care. The client is prone to hallucinations and delusions as a result of a reduced ability to distinguish and integrate sensory information. The accompanying Rx Communication feature (Client with Dementia and Hallucinations) shows an interaction with a client who experiences hallucinations.

Risk for Situational Low Self-Esteem

During the first stage of DAT and other dementias, the client is acutely aware of cognitive failure. This awareness and the resulting anxiety can be damaging to the self-esteem of a person living in a culture that does not tolerate or provide for dependence.

Functional Urinary Incontinence, Bowel Incontinence

Incontinence of urine or feces is usually the result of confusion and difficulty finding or using the bathroom facilities. In the later stages of dementia, clients lose cortical control, but physiologic function remains. It is essential to ensure proper hygiene for clients; poor hygiene will result in infections and skin breakdown.

Imbalanced Nutrition, Less Than Body Requirements

Poor nutrition and some metabolic disorders can be the direct cause of confusion in older adult clients. The reverse can also be true; confusion and cerebral change can cause nutritional deficits. Without supervision, many older clients are not capable of preparing or ingesting adequate amounts of food. Clients who are in the later stages of DAT have symptoms of bulimia followed by total loss of appetite.

Outcome Identification: NOC

Clients with these disorders have varying outcomes; delirium in many cases is reversible, while dementia is not. Specific outcomes for clients experiencing cognitive disorders are listed in the nursing care plans. Clients' abilities to return to their previous lifestyles remain somewhat intact when disorders are reversible. However, in the deterioration of dementing conditions, the expectations for outcomes must be carefully scrutinized. Family members and the client must have information about the illness and how it will change lifestyle. Maximizing the quality of life can be an outcome for clients who have dementia.

Planning and Implementation: NIC

Nursing interventions for clients with cognitive disorders can be divided into two broad groups: interventions for (1) clients with dementia and (2) clients with delirium. A sample nursing care plan for a client with delirium is presented at the end of this chapter. A case study for the client with dementia of the Alzheimer's type (DAT) can be accessed on the Companion Website for this text.

With few exceptions, the interventions are similar, although the overall goals are different as noted earlier in the Outcome Identification. The goal with the dementia client is to minimize the loss of self-care capacity. Although functional loss is progressive, at every stage of the illness the nurse must assess and support the client's self-care capacity. Family members must also learn how to work with the client.

MEDIALINK Case Study: Needs of the Client with Dementia of the Alzheimer's Type

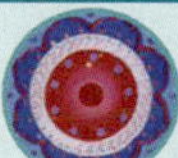

RX COMMUNICATION

CLIENT WITH DEMENTIA AND HALLUCINATIONS

CLIENT: "Get those women out of here!"

NURSE RESPONSE 1: "Come with me. We'll go down the hall."

RATIONALE: Distracting the client from the internal stimuli, which may be transient, calms and addresses the emotional component of the client's experience.

NURSE RESPONSE 2: "You must be very nervous. Let's get you something to help you feel better."

RATIONALE: Client may need interventions (nonpharmacologic or pharmacologic) to control breakthrough symptomatology.

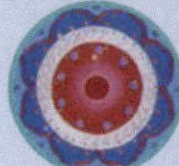

PARTNERING WITH CLIENTS AND FAMILIES

SUGGESTIONS FOR FAMILIES WHO HAVE JUST HAD A FAMILY MEMBER DIAGNOSED WITH DAT

- Have a family meeting and discuss strategies to care for the client at the present time and in the future, based on family responsibilities and resources.
- Contact the Alzheimer's Disease and Related Disorders Association (ADRDA) and request information. View their videotapes and read the available written material.
- Go to a support group for family caregivers.
- Contact an attorney and make decisions about power of attorney and the control and distribution of client/family assets.
- Consider developing a psychiatric advance directive (discussed in Chapter 13).
- Familiarize yourself with community resources such as day care treatment centers, nursing homes, and respite care for DAT clients.
- Purchase a bracelet for the client identifying her/him as having DAT.

See the Partnering with Clients and Families feature for suggestions for families. With delirious clients, the overall goal for nursing intervention is to support existing sensory perception until their cognitive function can return to previous levels of functioning. Of course, in both conditions, keeping the client safe is the first priority.

Promoting Normal Motor Behavior

Because of impaired coordination in dementia, falls become a safety concern. Living areas must be well lit and furniture must remain in the same place. Remove any loose rugs and ensure that clients are wearing properly fitting shoes with a strap. Evaluate the client for visual and balance disturbances. Safety bars should be installed near toilets, showers, and tubs. Teach clients who need assistance the safe use of walkers and wheelchairs. Evaluate all clients using tranquilizers and antidepressants for postural hypotension. A difference in blood pressures (BPs) taken supine and standing, wherein the standing BP is lower than the supine BP, is an indication of postural hypotension. Restlessness and wandering can be dealt with by allowing the client to wander in a safe, enclosed environment. Avoid crowds or large open spaces without boundaries.

Hyperactivity in clients with delirium can be decreased by controlling environmental stimuli. If this does not help, medications can be used judiciously. Take vital signs one hour before and after the administration of any medication, and observe the client carefully for signs of stupor. Interrupt prolonged periods of hypoactivity with range-of-motion exercises, frequent turning, and having the client stand up at the bedside, as tolerated. During periods of fluctuating motor behavior, there is always concern for the client's safety. A staff member should be present at all times; keep the bed lowered and the side rails up. In DAT, wandering is a common and troublesome behavioral symptom. See the Your Intervention Strategies feature in this section for guidelines for working with the wandering client.

Maintaining Self-Care

Allow the client to do as much as possible unassisted. The more the client can effectively control the daily routine, the less anxiety the client will experience. Remind the client about daily grooming and personal hygiene, and repeat instructions. If the client resists oral hygiene, use mouth swabs with dilute hydrogen peroxide. If the client resists this as well, having the client eat an apple may help to clean the

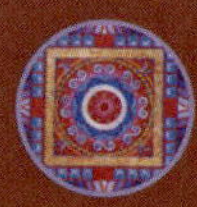

YOUR INTERVENTION STRATEGIES
Guidelines for Working with the Wandering Client

Strategy	Rationale
■ Stay with the client, or be sure the client is in a safe, enclosed area.	■ Wandering clients can get hurt. Safety is the first priority.
■ Maintain a calm demeanor.	■ Clients notice the feelings of others.
■ Approach the client slowly and give her or him space. Use touch only if the client responds positively to it.	■ The aim is to prevent aggressiveness, fear, and anxiety. Each client is different in response to touch, and with specific people.
■ Determine why the client is wandering. Is she or he upset? Thirsty? Hungry? Searching for family?	■ When we understand why the client wanders, we can plan client-specific interventions.
■ Meet the client's needs. If the client is searching, be supportive: "You are looking for X. . . ." "You must miss X . . ."	■ Support decreases anxiety, fear, and hostility.
■ Attempt to engage the client in a repetitive activity such as rolling yarn or folding towels.	■ Repetitive activities use energy and can be diversional.

mouth. If the client resists any routine procedures, wait a few moments and try again. The client often forgets to offer new resistance. Clients who are acutely delirious or in the last stages of dementia need total bed care.

Promoting Adequate Sleep

Clients with dementia and delirium respond poorly to hypnotics, which increase confusion and aggravate the disorientation that may be experienced in lowered light in older adults. A small amount of beer or wine at bedtime may produce enough relaxation without side effects. The most helpful measure may be to allow sleepless clients to wander in a confined area until they are tired. If the client is disoriented at night, make sure the room is light and without shadows. Possibly leave a radio on to provide more stimulation. Low doses of risperidone or an antianxiety agent may be prescribed. (Antianxiety medications should be used with caution and reevaluated regularly if used on a nightly basis.)

In some instances it may be necessary to use mechanical restraints to protect the client from injury or prevent the client from disrupting necessary medical treatments (e.g., a delirious client repeatedly tries to bear weight on a damaged limb or attempts to remove IV tubing or bandages). Use mechanical restraints only as a last resort and according to established policy (refer to the American Psychiatric Nurses Association position statement on the use of restraints in Chapter 13 ∞). Before using restraints, apply effective and imaginative alternatives. If restraints are deemed unavoidable, remember to evaluate their use and replace them with less restrictive alternatives. Reassure clients who have been restrained that they are safe and that the restraints are there to protect and help them. See Chapter 35 ∞ for guidelines in the use of restraining techniques.

Supporting Knowledge Processes

The same interventions that are used to support memory and orientation are applied to the support of knowledge processes. Family education is imperative and can take the form of professional help and/or self-help groups. For a listing of professional help and/or self-help groups, refer to the Companion Website.

Supporting Optimal Memory Functioning

Gently orient the client. To allay anxiety, do not argue with the client about verbal discrepancies. Rather, direct the client toward areas of interest that are familiar and pleasurable. The environment should support whatever memory functions are still intact. Do not test the client for episodic memory unless it is absolutely necessary. If the client uses confabulation to fill in the memory gap, do not argue; remember that it is an ego-protective mechanism. Other strength-enhancing behavioral and psychotherapeutic treatment reminders are summarized in the Your Intervention Strategies feature below.

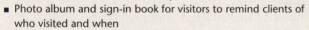

MEDIALINK Education on DAT

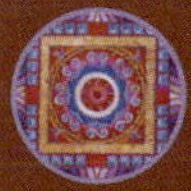

YOUR INTERVENTION STRATEGIES
Guidelines for Supporting Optimal Memory Functioning

Behavioral and Psychotherapeutic Reminders

- Calendars or other concrete reminders of what is going on by day of the week, date, and time
- Objects or wall hangings that mirror the current season or holiday events; pictures that reflect seasonal events and people's actions and behaviors around those events (remember to be culturally sensitive)
- Photo album and sign-in book for visitors to remind clients of who visited and when
- If the client is very attached to a family member who visits, prominently display a large photo of that family member in the client's room.
- Discover a client's preferred hobbies and interests to add cues to the environment, which will be positively received (e.g., a team schedule for a sports fan).

Reminiscence

- Clients often need to talk, even repetitively, about important prior experiences, which encourages the process of resolving feelings about these experiences as well as the difficulties the client has in recalling them.
- Encourage discussion of likely social and historical contexts operative during earlier phases of the client's life (e.g., The Great Depression of the 1930s, World War II, and important events of the 1950s).

Adaptive Functioning and Cognitive Preservation

Careful evaluation of remaining cognitive strengths through:

- Observation
- Psychological testing
- Diagnostic interviewing

When areas of strength are diagnosed:

- Provide opportunities for the client to exercise them.
- Give positive reinforcements such as praise, a pleasant experience such as listening to music, or a caring interaction when the client is exercising his or her better preserved abilities.

When areas of deficit are diagnosed:

- Assist the client in coping with deficits (e.g., training and encouragement to use written reminders to compensate for failing memory).
- Give the client positive reinforcement for using such strategies.

YOUR SELF-AWARENESS
Triggering Semantic Memory

DAT clients experience episodic memory loss; therefore, interactions may not be retained, and repetition is necessary. Answer the following questions about your skill level at triggering semantic memory.

1. In this leading technique, a combination of words and nonverbal cues are used. Are your words and nonverbal cues:

   Precise? ☐ Yes ☐ No

   Concise? ☐ Yes ☐ No

   Clear? ☐ Yes ☐ No

2. Constant repetition in a kind, firm manner is necessary. When you have to repeat yourself a number of times, are the following interaction impacts present?

   Is your tone on the third repetition identical to your tone the first time you said this? ☐ Yes ☐ No

   Is your affect kind the fourth time you've repeated yourself? ☐ Yes ☐ No

   Do your movements remain the same even though you have to repeat them? ☐ Yes ☐ No

   Are you consistent? ☐ Yes ☐ No

   If you answered "Yes," you are using this technique effectively and your communication with clients who have these disorders is more likely to be successful. If any of these areas has a "No" response, you may need to improve the connection between your verbal and nonverbal cues and evaluate your personal reaction (action, emotion, attitude) to the need to repeat basic instructions.

Because of their episodic memory loss, DAT clients do not respond well to reality orientation classes. However, you can trigger semantic memory by initiating a procedure the client can then complete. In this leading technique, a combination of words and nonverbal cues are used. For instance, while handing the client a toothbrush and pointing toward the mouth with a brushing motion, say, "Brush your teeth." Constant repetition in a kind, firm manner is often necessary. See the Your Self-Awareness feature in this section to evaluate your skills in this area. Music therapy may also trigger past associations, aid the client's long-term memory, and help a normally aphasic client participate in a group.

Promoting Optimal Medication Management

Medication therapy has also been proposed to assist the client in the early stages of DAT to maintain memory and orientation (see Chapter 7 ∞). Galantamine (Reminyl), donepezil (Aricept), rivastigmine (Exelon), and tacrine (Cognex), all potent acetylcholinesterase inhibitors, are available to treat DAT. Clinical trials and treatment outcome information for these medications have resulted in both positive and negative results. The problems in demonstrating overall efficacy are believed to be due to the heterogeneity in DAT clients and the fact that these medications provide mild to moderate improvement. Memantine (Namenda) is the first DAT medication to work by targeting glutamate rather than acetylcholine. This medication is for moderate to severe disease treatment and expands the choices in the psychopharmacologic management of the disease.

Medication management with this group of disorders has a variety of purposes and options. Examples of these options are included in Table 14-2 ■.

Promoting Optimal Orientation

Structure the client's environment to support cognitive functions. The client should be wearing whatever aids (hearing, vision) are necessary to prevent sensory loss or distortion. Familiar objects from home, such as slippers, robe, and photographs, may also help orient the client. Easily read clocks, orientation boards, and a consistent daily routine that includes physical activity and socialization without sensory overload will also help orient the client. Verbally orient the client during conversation. Do not quiz the client about discrepancies.

Supporting Optimal Verbal Expression

As communication skills decrease, the client's nonverbal communication becomes more important. Clients respond physically to the environment, especially if they feel threat-

Table 14-2 ■ Common Medications Used to Treat Certain Cognitive Disorders

Cognitive Disorder	Common Medications (generic and trade names)	Use
Dementia of the Alzheimer's type (DAT)	donepezil (Aricept)	Slow the rate of cognitive decline
Dementia with Lewy bodies	escitalopram (Lexipro)	Reduce symptoms of depression when present
Pick's disease	valproic acid (Depakote)	Reduce problematic mood swings and agitated behavior
Vascular dementia with psychosis	quetiapine (Seroquel)	Reduce or eliminate delusions and hallucinations

ened. Call the client by name, approach in clear view, and give simple directions.

Supporting Appropriate Conduct/Impulse Control

The client may strike out in response to hallucinations or delusions. All measures used to support perception and orientation are imperative here because clients function best in an environment where stimulation is controlled and sensory overload prevented. All changes, whether environmental or personal, need to be made slowly. Always approach the client in full view, calling his or her name, and refrain from touching the client. Requests should be simple and nondemanding.

Supporting Optimal Role Performance

To promote functioning in the family, the client must be viewed as an active member. Most clients with dementia remain at home until the caregiver can no longer manage the client's needs. The family needs support throughout this time, such as home visits, day care, respite care, and support groups.

If the client is institutionalized, the family should be an integral part of the client's daily routine. Family members need extra emotional support as the rewards for maintaining involvement diminish. For the client with dementia, role maintenance involves supporting the client's need to be oriented.

Maintaining Optimal Attention Span

Repeat requests as needed. Speak in simple phrases, loud enough to be heard, and reinforce meaning with gestures. To decrease distractibility and hyperalertness, keep environmental stimulation at a minimum. Every effort should be made to lower the client's anxiety level by moving slowly, speaking clearly, and providing new information slowly.

Promoting Optimal Self-Concept/Self-Esteem

During the early stages of dementia, every effort should be made to maintain clients' self-esteem as they struggle with the personal awareness of cognitive loss. Encourage clients to express their fears and concerns, and listen attentively. Allow for the expression of anger and sadness.

Manipulate the environment to help the client with a failing memory. Helpful measures include labeling the bathroom and bedroom, posting notes to remind the client to turn off the stove and lock the door, and labeling the contents of drawers. Gently remind the client of forgotten events, and do not confront confabulations. Encourage the family to maintain the client as a productive member of this important group.

Supporting Optimal Perceptual Functioning

A quiet environment with soft music prevents the client from experiencing sensory overload. When speaking with the client, stand or sit so that you are in direct view. Use touch with caution. First give a verbal warning before touching the client's shoulder or hand, and slowly and clearly explain all procedures. Sometimes even a very soothing touch can overexcite the client, who may respond by striking out. Make sure that the client is wearing hearing aids and eyeglasses if necessary.

In responding to hallucinations, simply state that you understand that these sensations can be very powerful and even disturbing. Do not argue or ask the client to elaborate. Take care of the emotional response (e.g., if the client is frightened, reassure) in your interactions. Give reassurance that these thoughts will go away. Say, "You are in a safe place." Do not leave the client alone or in an isolated room without some stimulation to help the client block out the hallucinations and support reality testing. The room should be well lit and without shadows or glare. If the client becomes combative, briefly intervene to redirect and prevent harm to self or others. Then attempt to distract, reassuring the client, "You are in a safe place."

Promoting Optimal Patterns of Elimination

A regular toileting schedule helps clients with dementia control bowel and urinary incontinence. Clients are often not able to let the nurse know when they have to use the toilet or have soiled themselves. Use clothing that is easy to remove and clean.

During the early stage of dementia, a toileting routine is essential. It helps confused clients to place a large sign on the bathroom door labeled, "Toilet." As the disease progresses, the client no longer recognizes a toilet or its purpose. Such a client may resist sitting on the toilet. Forcing the client will only produce agitation and combativeness. Distract and try again. If all efforts at maintaining a routine fail, use disposable pants or diapers. The use of catheters and external drains is not recommended because of the possibility of infection and their certain removal by a confused client.

Promoting Optimal Nutritional Status

Monitor the client's food and fluid intake. Give hyperactive clients a diet high in protein and carbohydrates, in finger-food form. Some clients may need double portions. Clients who chew constantly need to be reminded to swallow. Depending on the client's level of perception and motor activity, supervision and assistance at mealtimes may be necessary. Weigh the client routinely, and increase caloric intake as needed. In the final stages of the disease, the client loses all interest in food and may receive nasogastric, gastrostomy, or intravenous feedings.

Evaluation

Assess both the effectiveness of all interventions and the client's response to them. For guidance on self-assessment, see the Your Self-Awareness feature on page 318.

Delirium Evaluation Criteria

The evaluation of nursing care for clients with delirium is based on the premise that clients are capable of returning to their previous level of functioning. During that process the goal is to help the client maintain optimal levels of sensory perception, participate in activities of daily living, and maintain physiologic homeostasis.

Dementia Evaluation Criteria

Dementia entails progressive intellectual, behavioral, and physiologic deterioration. The goal of nursing care is not to

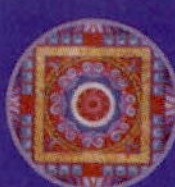

YOUR SELF-AWARENESS
An Inventory for Nurses Who Care for Clients with Cognitive Disorders

Caring for clients with cognitive disorders can be difficult and frustrating at times. The self-awareness information you gather by thoughtfully considering your responses to the following questions will help you to become more successful in working with cognitively impaired clients and their families.

- How do I feel about working with clients with cognitive disorders?
- What do I like about working with them?
- What frustrates me about working with them?
- What behavioral symptoms (e.g., wandering, agitation, hallucinations, delusions, hostility, eating problems, etc.) do I feel most competent to deal with? Least competent?
- What strategies have I used with clients that have been successful? Unsuccessful?
- Who are my favorite clients? Why? My least favorite clients? Why?
- What can I do to become more knowledgeable and/or skilled in dealing with clients with cognitive disorders?

effect a cure but rather to sustain the client at the optimal level of self-care. Help the family sustain a personally rewarding relationship with their loved one throughout this terminal process.

CASE MANAGEMENT

Case management of the client with dementia involves developing and organizing a program to address the symptoms present. It must be a flexible system to respond to the changing needs of the client as deterioration progresses. There is a great deal of contact with the caregiver(s). Provide regular monitoring and supervise the following:

- Regular physical examinations with a primary care provider
- Prescription medications
- Nutrition
- Over-the-counter medications
- Finances
- Interpersonal relationships

COMMUNITY-BASED CARE

Community-based care for the client with dementia could involve appointments in a clinic setting, a day program designed for the current level of difficulties in functioning, medication clinic appointments, a supportive group, or some combination. Frequently, a family member or caregiver is involved, especially due to the need for transportation.

Counseling and face-to-face contacts are a way to decrease the social isolation inherent in a client with dementia. Psychotherapy can be useful to help clients with mild to moderate dementia cope with the loss of cognitive functions. The features of counseling or therapy would include:

- Empathic listening
- Support
- Working on coping methods
- Providing the client with outlets for distress that might otherwise exacerbate disturbed behavior (e.g., talking over fears rather than acting out behaviorally)

HOME CARE

The most effective treatment for the client with dementia is a balance between stimulation/environmental demand and whatever internal resources remain for the client. The home would need to be evaluated to determine if it will meet the changing needs of the client. Some revisions are usually necessary so that safe wandering is possible, dangers are minimized through safety devices, and activity can be controlled. A cycle of stimulation and rest is best so the client's abilities are engaged but not overwhelmed.

Supportive counseling is frequently helpful when providing home care for clients with dementia. You must understand the premorbid personality and developmental history of someone with dementia because the dementing process is superimposed on the preexisting personality. Determine what role anxiety played in clients' lives, their previous self-view, and how conscious they were of themselves and the impact of their actions on others. Once the client's anxiety is reduced, the tendency toward better functioning will ensue.

The focus of treatment for clients with dementia expands to include caregivers. Whether the caregivers are relatives, friends, or health care providers, they may require explanations of symptoms and help in designing behavioral interventions. Caregivers working with severely demented clients may require help in coping with stress, discouragement, and a sense of hopelessness.

MEDIALINK Critical Thinking Exercise: Caregiver Support

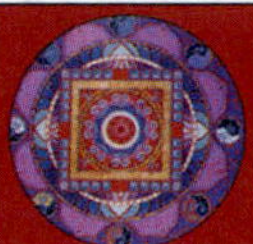

NURSING CARE PLAN: CLIENT WITH DELIRIUM

Behavioral Changes of Dementia of the Alzheimer's Type (DAT)

Identifying Information

Mr. Hennessey is a 50-year-old married man who entered the hospital to have colon surgery. He is a physically fit man in a physically demanding job, typically jogging several miles a week for exercise. This is his first serious physical problem. His wife of 25 years is extremely devoted and stayed with him following his surgery. While still in the ICU, Mr. Hennessey became disoriented. Staff members were careful to check his electrolyte balances, which were within normal limits. Within 2 days he began hallucinating. He cried out that the hovering bats he saw in the corners of the room were trying to kill him. He has had other hallucinations and believes that his life is at great risk. When his wife offered him a newspaper, he whispered that she should give him the bucket of pills he'd been hiding under his bed. He lashed out at his wife following this exchange and ripped out his IV and nasogastric tube.

History

Mr. Hennessey has no prior psychiatric history, nor are there any family members with major psychiatric problems. His wife and two grown children, who live nearby, are concerned about his well-being. All are attentive to Mr. Hennessey, love him, and are willing to help with his care.

Mr. Hennessey is a contractor and owns his own business. He and his wife have many friends and activities. He was diagnosed with a colon tumor one month ago and had a colon resection. The pathology report was positive for cancer. Mr. Hennessey had been healthy all his life until he noticed rectal bleeding a month ago. He has had regular physicals and responded immediately when symptoms of a problem arose.

Current Mental Status

Mr. Hennessey is disoriented the majority of time, and he is often aggressive. He has been having frightening visual hallucinations, especially at night. He is delusional that people are trying to hurt him.

Other Subjective or Objective Clinical Data

Mr. Hennessey is on morphine for pain management.

Nursing Diagnosis: High Risk for Violence related to confusion and fear inherent in delirium

Expected Outcome: Mr. Hennessey does not attempt to harm self or others.

Short-Term Goals	Interventions	Rationales
Mr. Hennessey will have decreased symptoms of persecutory delusions.	▪ Directly address the fear he is feeling (i.e., "I understand how frightening this all is, and we will make sure you are safe").	Talking about the feelings is more reassuring and shifts interactions from argumentation.
	▪ Prevent overstimulation and understimulation.	ICUs can be overwhelming in certain sensory areas while not providing enough cues to the outside world (such as windows).
Mr. Hennessey displays considerably less agitation and fear.	▪ Orient Mr. Hennessey whenever he is confused. ▪ Promote relaxation in both active and soothing modes. ▪ Move slowly, speak clearly, and explain all procedures. ▪ Make sure only one person is speaking to Mr. Hennessy at a time. ▪ Following clearance on neurologic examination, medicate Mr. Hennessey with a low-dose antipsychotic. ▪ Explain to family about ICU psychosis and the temporary nature of it.	Decrease the stimuli that can exacerbate symptoms or confusion.

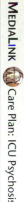

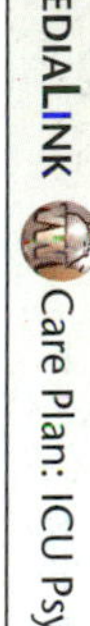

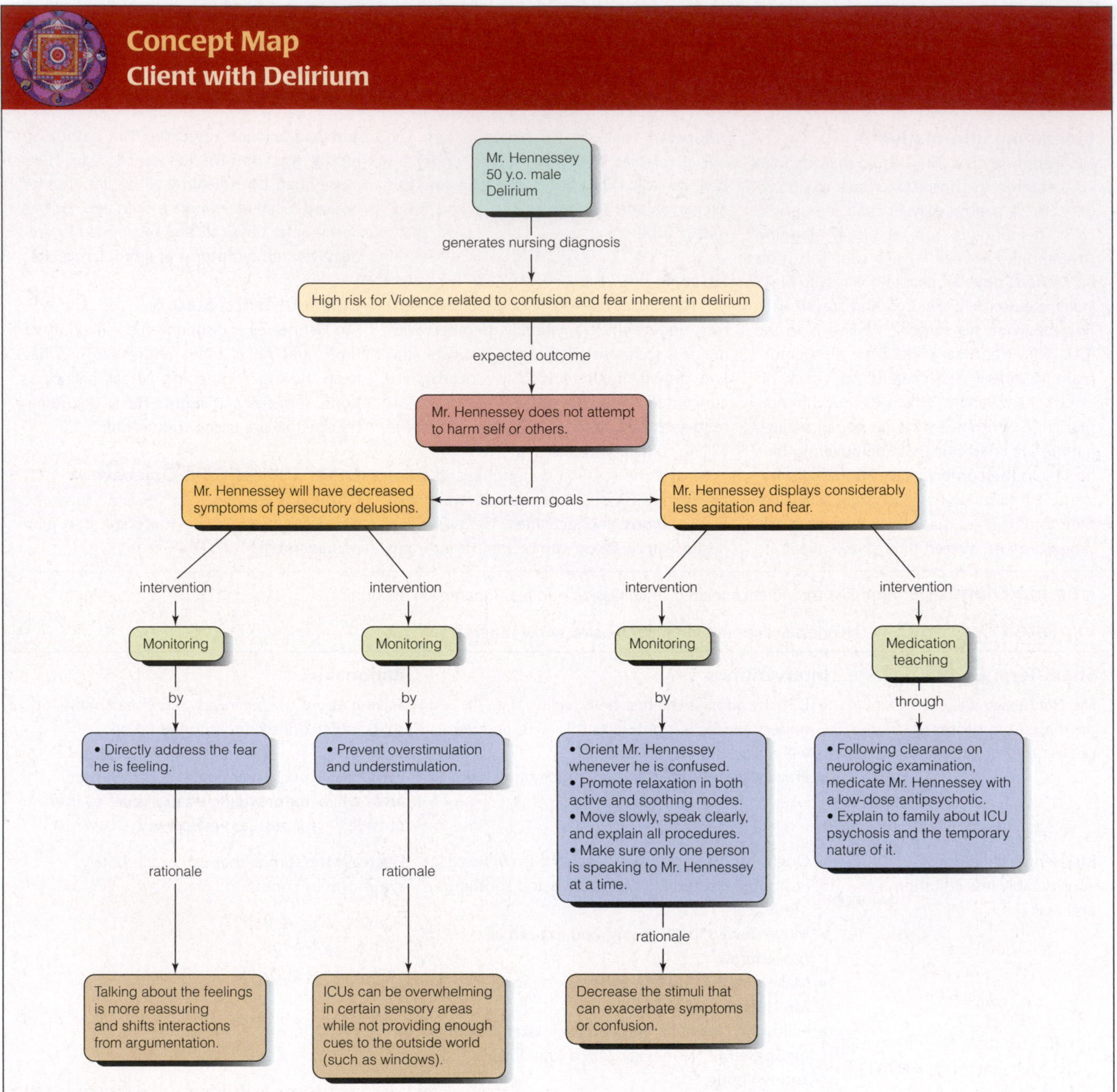
Concept Map
Client with Delirium
Mr. Hennessey 50 y.o. male Delirium
generates nursing diagnosis
High risk for Violence related to confusion and fear inherent in delirium
expected outcome
Mr. Hennessey does not attempt to harm self or others.
short-term goals
Mr. Hennessey will have decreased symptoms of persecutory delusions.
Mr. Hennessey displays considerably less agitation and fear.
intervention
intervention
intervention
intervention
Monitoring
Monitoring
Monitoring
Medication teaching
by
by
by
through
• Directly address the fear he is feeling.
• Prevent overstimulation and understimulation.
• Orient Mr. Hennessey whenever he is confused.
• Promote relaxation in both active and soothing modes.
• Move slowly, speak clearly, and explain all procedures.
• Make sure only one person is speaking to Mr. Hennessey at a time.
• Following clearance on neurologic examination, medicate Mr. Hennessey with a low-dose antipsychotic.
• Explain to family about ICU psychosis and the temporary nature of it.
rationale
rationale
rationale
Talking about the feelings is more reassuring and shifts interactions from argumentation.
ICUs can be overwhelming in certain sensory areas while not providing enough cues to the outside world (such as windows).
Decrease the stimuli that can exacerbate symptoms or confusion.

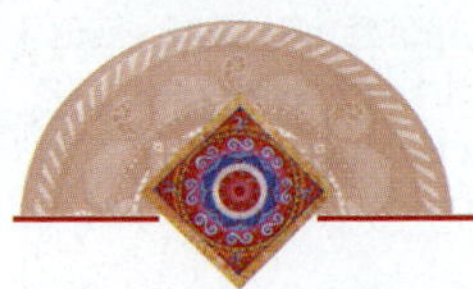

EXPLORE MEDIALINK

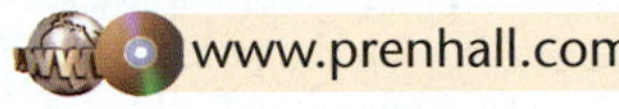

For NCLEX-RN® review questions, case studies, and other resources for this chapter see the Pearson Health MediaLink CD-ROM that accompanies this book and the Companion Website at www.prenhall.com/kneisl.

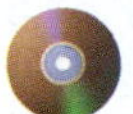

CD-ROM
Audio Glossary
NCLEX-RN® Review Questions
Videos and Animations
- *PET/SPECT Dementia*
- *Hands & Arms Tremor*
- *Grasping Tremor*
- *Lateral Tremor*
- *Akinesia & Pill Rolling*
- *Parkinsonism*

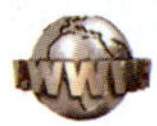

Companion Website
Audio Glossary
NCLEX-RN® Review Questions
Critical Thinking Exercise
- *Caregiver Support*

Case Study
- *Needs of the Client with Dementia of the Alzheimer's Type*

Care Plan
- *ICU Psychosis*

MediaLinks
MediaLink Application
- *Dementia: It's Not Always Alzheimer's Disease*

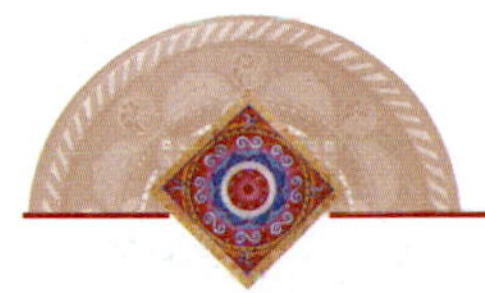

NCLEX-RN® REVIEW QUESTIONS

1. The client presents in the emergency room with hallucinations, insomnia, disorientation, and extreme agitation. A family member reports the symptoms started abruptly 2 days ago after the client was diagnosed with a urinary tract infection. The client is presenting with symptoms associated with:
1. Dementia.
2. Delirium.
3. Vascular dementia.
4. Huntington's disease.

2. Which of the following symptoms is *not* seen in dementia of the Alzheimer's type (DAT)?
1. Alexia
2. Agnosia
3. Agoraphobia
4. Apraxia

3. A graduate nurse is assigned to work on a unit with clients who have cognitive impairments. Which of the following statements by the nurse is reason for concern?
1. "I need to learn more about cognitive disorders so I can better care for the clients."
2. "I don't feel safe around clients who hallucinate."
3. "These clients do not have any idea what is going on."
4. "I will ask other staff for suggestions on therapeutic interventions with the clients."

4. The community health nurse is teaching a family whose father is experiencing memory lapses associated with early-onset DAT how to adapt to memory problems. The nurse knows the family member understands when the individual states:
1. "I will rearrange the furniture so my father does not fall."
2. "I will put notes on the different rooms of the house so my father remembers what room he is in."
3. "If Dad forgets things, I will make sure I notify the nursing staff immediately."
4. "I will keep Dad in the house so he does not get lost on the streets."

5. One of the differences between delirium and dementia is that clients with delirium:
1. Are very attentive to their environment.
2. Experience a slow, insidious onset of symptoms.
3. Have fluctuating consciousness.
4. Respond to questions appropriately and correctly.

6. The relevant events that can be associated with delirium are:
1. An infection.
2. Old age.
3. History of acting-out behavior.
4. Depression.

7. A priority nursing diagnosis for the client experiencing altered perception, extreme agitation, and acute confusion is:
1. Risk for Injury.
2. Altered Role Performance.
3. Impaired Verbal Communication.
4. Disturbed Sensory Perception.

8. What is the drug of choice to improve cognitive functioning in a client with dementia of the Alzheimer's type?
1. Lorazepam (Ativan)
2. Alprazolam (Xanax)
3. Quetiapine (Seroquel)
4. Donepezil (Aricept)

9. The actual cause of dementia associated with dementia of the Alzheimer's type is:
1. Diabetes.
2. Infection.
3. Unknown.
4. Drug intoxication.

10. The community health nurse is instructing a family who cares for a client with DAT about safety measures to protect the client. An appropriate safety measure would include:
1. Putting locks on the outside of doors so the client cannot leave the room or house.
2. Purchasing a MedicAlert® bracelet that identifies the client as having DAT.
3. Chemically restraining the client to prevent agitation and confusion.
4. Restraining the client in a chair or bed to prevent falls.

See Appendix C for answers.

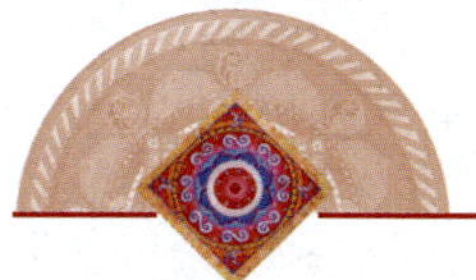

REFERENCES

Alzheimer, A. (1907). Uber eine eigenartige Erkraukung der Hirwrinde. *Allegmeine Zeitschrift für Psychiatrie, 64*, 146–148.

American Psychiatric Association. (2000). *Diagnostic and statistical manual of mental disorders* (4th ed., Text Revision) (DSM-IV-TR). Washington, DC: Author.

Bourne, C., Clayton, C., Murch, A., & Grant, J. (2006). Cognitive impairment and behavioural difficulties in patients with Huntington's disease. *Nursing Standard, 20*(35), 41–44.

Dale, D. C., & Federman, D. D. (2007). *ACP Medicine* (2007 Edition). WebMD Inc. Professional Publishing.

Goroll, A. H., & Mulley, A. G. (2007). *Primary care medicine* (5th ed.). Baltimore: Lippincott Williams & Wilkins.

Hirtz, D., Thurman, D. J., Gwinn-Hardy, K., Mohamed, M., Chaudhuri, A. R., & Zalutsky, R. (2007). How common are the "common" neurologic disorders? *Neurology, 68*(5), 326–337.

Ito, M., Takahashi, R., & Liehr, P. (2007). Heeding the behavioral message of elders with dementia in day care. *Holistic Nursing Practice, 21*(1), 12–18.

Kieburtz, K. (2006). Issues in neuroprotection clinical trials in Parkinson's disease. *Neurology, 66*(10) (Suppl. 4), S50–S57.

Macleod, A. (2006). The management of terminal delirium. *Indian Journal of Palliative Care, 12*(1), 22–28.

McKeith, I. G., Galasko, D., Kosaka, K., Perry, E. K., Dickson, D. W., Hansen, L. A., et al. (1996). Consensus guidelines for the clinical and pathologic diagnosis of dementia with Lewy bodies (DLB): Report of the consortium on DLB international workshop. *Neurology, 47,* 1113-1124.

Meagher, D. J., Moran, M., Raju, B., Gibbons, D., Donnelley, S., Saunders, J., et al. (2007). Phenomenology of delirium: Assessment of 100 adult cases using standardised measures. *British Journal of Psychiatry, 190*(2), 135–141.

Rader, J., Barrick, A., Hoeffer, B., Sloane, P. D., McKenzie, D., Talerico, K. A., et al. (2006). The bathing of older adults with dementia. *American Journal of Nursing, 106*(4), 40–48.

Rubin, C. D. (2006). The primary care of Alzheimer disease. *American Journal of the Medical Sciences, 332*(6), 314–333.

Samson, K. (2006). Is cutting funds for mad cow disease research justified? *Neurology Today, 6*(3), 39–40.

Sanchez-Juan, P., Green, A., Ladogana, A., Cuadrado-Corrales, N., Saanchez-Valle, R., Mitrovaa, E., et al. (2006). CSF tests in the differential diagnosis of Creutzfeldt–Jakob disease. *Neurology, 67*(4), 637–643.

Schutte, D. L., & Holston, E. C. (2006). Chronic dementing conditions, genomics, and new opportunities for nursing interventions. *Journal of Nursing Scholarship, 38(4)*, 328–334.

Skrobik, Y. (2007). Delirium as destiny: Clinical precision and genetic risk. *Critical Care Medicine, 35*(1), 304–305.

Tschanz, J. T., Welsh-Bohmer, K. A., Lyketsos, C. G., Corcoran, C., Green, R. C., Hayden, K., et al. (2006). Cache County Investigators. Conversion to dementia from mild cognitive disorder: The Cache County Study. *Neurology, 67*(2), 229–234.

White, K. T., & Cummings, J. L. (1997). Neuropsychiatric aspects of Alzheimer's disease and other dementing illnesses. In S. C. Yudofsky & R. E. Hales (Eds.), *Textbook of neuropsychiatry* (3rd ed., pp. 823–854). Washington, DC: American Psychiatric Press.

Wilson, B. A., Shannon, M., Shields, K., & Stang, C. L. (2008). *Prentice Hall nurse's drug guide 2008.* Upper Saddle River, NJ: Prentice Hall.

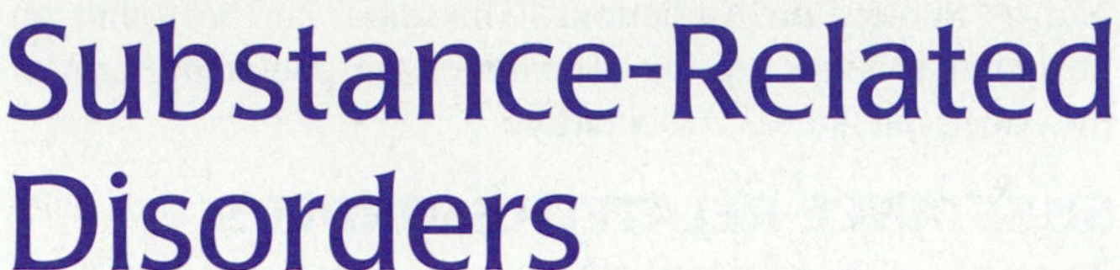

Substance-Related Disorders

CHAPTER

15

EILEEN TRIGOBOFF

LEARNING OUTCOMES

After completing this chapter, you will be able to:

1. Discuss the major theoretic explanations for substance-related disorders.
2. Describe the populations at risk for substance-related disorders.
3. Explain how the physical, psychological, and withdrawal effects of the major categories of substances manifest themselves.
4. Identify treatment approaches for the major categories of abused substances.
5. Discuss how the presence of both a substance-related disorder and a major mental disorder (such as schizophrenia) complicates nursing care.
6. Compare and contrast the short-term and long-term nursing intervention strategies for clients with substance-related disorders.
7. Identify the strategies for helping a client avoid relapse.
8. Discuss outcome criteria for clients who have substance-related disorders.
9. Assess your own feelings and attitudes about clients with substance-related disorders and how they may affect professional practice.

CRITICAL THINKING CHALLENGE

Billie is a 19-year-old homeless African-American woman pregnant with her third child and addicted to crack cocaine. When she appeared at your hospital's Family Practice Clinic for prenatal care one month before her delivery, she was referred to your team for assessment and treatment for her addiction. Billie is concerned about losing her children if she enters a drug treatment program, and she is fearful that her unborn baby is already damaged. She shuns Alcoholics Anonymous (AA) and Narcotics Anonymous (NA) because admitting "powerlessness" and "turning her life over to God the Father" is unacceptable to her; as a marginalized poor black woman, she's had it with powerlessness and would rather empower her daughters so that they "don't turn their lives over to men." Others on your treatment team refuse to accept her as an outpatient because she will not promise complete abstinence and is reluctant to commit to attending one NA or AA meeting per day.

1. Under what conditions does the treatment team have the right to refuse outpatient treatment for Billie?
2. What are some other options for Billie's care?
3. Should Billie lose her children?

KEY TERMS

alcohol-induced persisting amnestic disorder (Korsakoff's syndrome) *333*
alcoholic encephalopathy (Wernicke's encephalopathy) *333*
blackouts *332*
codependency *327*
delirium tremens (DTs) *331*
enabling *328*
fetal alcohol syndrome (FAS) *333*
substance abuse *325*
substance dependence *325*
substance intoxication *325*
substance withdrawal *325*
substance withdrawal syndrome *325*
tolerance *325*
withdrawal *325*

MEDIALINK 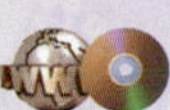 www.prenhall.com/kneisl

Go to the Pearson Health MediaLink CD-ROM and the Companion Website at www.prenhall.com/kneisl for interactive resources for this chapter.

Drug and alcohol abuse, already a widespread problem, is rapidly escalating. Substance abuse is a psychosocial and a biologic problem. Television and radio advertisements entice viewers with the hope of relief from pain and problems; they demonstrate that a life without stress is possible. The values portrayed are clear: Discomfort should be erased; drinking is vital to a stress-free life; drugs are acceptable mediators of emotions.

Substance abuse is a complex public health issue with grave ramifications. It increases the crime rate, auto accident deaths, number of teenage pregnancies, and the suicide rate. Individuals and families are destroyed. Every part of a substance abuser's life—social life, family life, work productivity and relationships, physical health—is affected. Substance abuse in the work environment increases accidents, workers' compensation claims, absenteeism, and theft while decreasing the quality of life for other workers and potentially decreasing the quality of the work performed overall.

This chapter is a biopsychosocial exploration, applying the nursing process to clients who have substance-related disorders. Be aware of the need to keep up-to-date on the trends, fads, and activities related to substance abuse, because they change quickly. The importance of having a knowledge base on this topic, developing caring attitudes, and developing skilled therapeutic interventions are discussed in the standards of addiction nursing, jointly written by the American Nurses Association and the International Nurses Society on Addictions. This data can be found on http://nursesbooks.org, the website of the publishing arm of the American Nurses Association.

SUBSTANCE-RELATED DISORDERS

According to the DSM-IV-TR (American Psychiatric Association [APA], 2000), substance-related disorders are disorders that are: (1) a consequence of abusing a drug (such as alcohol), (2) the side effects of a medication (such as antihistamines), or (3) related to exposure to a toxin (fuel, paint, or other inhalants). Substance-related disorders are divided into two groups:

1. Substance use disorders that include substance dependence and substance abuse
2. Substance-induced disorders (including substance intoxication and substance withdrawal as well as other substance-induced disorders such as substance-induced cognitive disorders, mood disorders, and the like)

This chapter focuses on substance dependence and substance abuse, including the intoxication and withdrawal issues for those classes of substances that have traditionally been called psychoactive drugs. The DSM-IV-TR diagnostic criteria for substance abuse and substance dependence are listed in the diagnostic criteria feature.

DSM-IV-TR Diagnostic Criteria for Substance Abuse vs. Substance Dependence

Diagnostic Criteria for Substance Abuse

A. A maladaptive pattern of substance use leading to clinically significant impairment or distress, as manifested by one (or more) of the following, occurring within a 12-month period:
   1. recurrent substance use resulting in a failure to fulfill major role obligations at work, school, or home
   2. recurrent substance use in situations in which it is physically hazardous
   3. recurrent substance-related legal problems
   4. continued substance use despite having persistent or recurrent social or interpersonal problems caused or exacerbated by the effects of the substance

B. The symptoms have never met the criteria for substance dependence for this class of substance.

Diagnostic Criteria for Substance Dependence

A maladaptive pattern of substance use, leading to clinically significant impairment or distress, as manifested by three (or more) of the following, occurring at any time in the same 12-month period:

1. tolerance
2. withdrawal
3. the substance is often taken in larger amounts or over a longer period than was intended
4. there is a persistent desire or unsuccessful efforts to cut down or control substance use
5. a great deal of time is spent in activities necessary to obtain the substance
6. important social, occupational, or recreational activities are given up or reduced
7. the substance use is continued despite knowledge of having a persistent or recurrent physical or psychological problem that is likely to have been caused or exacerbated by the substance

Source: Reprinted with permission from the *Diagnostic and Statistical Manual of Mental Disorders,* Fourth Edition, Text Revision. (Copyright 2000). American Psychiatric Association.

USING DSM-IV-TR

Health care providers often use language unfamiliar to clients and their families. Explain abuse and dependence in such a way that clients and family members can understand the difference.

SUBSTANCE DEPENDENCE

Substance dependence is defined as a maladaptive pattern of substance use leading to clinically significant impairment or distress. The hallmarks of this pattern are:

- **Tolerance**, which is needing increased amounts of a substance to achieve the desired effect
- **Withdrawal**, which is the uncomfortable and maladaptive physiologic and cognitive behavioral changes that are associated with lowered blood or tissue concentrations of a substance after an individual has been a heavy user
- Compulsive use
- Needing larger amounts of the substance than intended
- Making unsuccessful efforts to cut down or regulate substance use
- Devoting a great deal of time to trying to obtain the substance
- Using the substance or recovering from the effects of the substance
- Continuing to use the substance despite the recognition of associated adverse effects and difficulties

This diagnosis can be made for every class of substance except caffeine. The latest information on substance abuse can be found at the Substance Abuse & Mental Health Services Administration (SAMHSA) website at www.samhsa.gov/.

SUBSTANCE ABUSE

Substance abuse is characterized by a pattern of repeated use of substances that is maladaptive in that significant adverse consequences occur. Examples include the failure to fulfill major role obligations, using substances in physically hazardous situations, and recurrent social and relationship problems. The DSM-IV-TR diagnostic criteria for substance abuse are also listed in the diagnostic criteria feature on page 324.

SUBSTANCE INTOXICATION

Substance intoxication refers to a reversible syndrome of maladaptive physiologic and behavioral changes that are due to the effects of a substance on a person's central nervous system (CNS). The syndrome includes disturbances of mood (such as belligerence or mood lability), perception, the sleep–wake cycle, attention, thinking, judgment, and psychomotor as well as interpersonal behavior. The DSM-IV-TR diagnostic criteria for substance intoxication are listed in the feature that follows.

SUBSTANCE WITHDRAWAL

Substance withdrawal refers to the development of maladaptive physiologic, behavioral, and cognitive changes that are the result of reducing or stopping the heavy and regular use of a substance. **Substance withdrawal syndrome** is associated with distress and/or impairment in important areas of social functioning. The clinical example below describes the difficulties of withdrawing from the long-term use of a substance. See the diagnostic criteria for substance withdrawal in the box below.

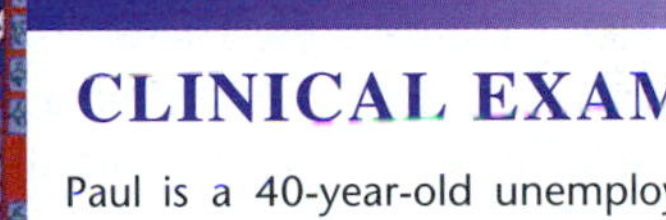

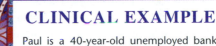

CLINICAL EXAMPLE

Paul is a 40-year-old unemployed banker with a history of daily alcohol consumption that has gradually exceeded a quart of vodka per day over the past 25 years. He is estranged from his ex-wife and their two teenage children. He has tried unsuccessfully to cut back on his drinking on numerous occasions. His attempts to quit were particularly motivated when it became clear he would lose his job because of his declining

MEDIALINK SAMHSA

DSM-IV-TR Diagnostic Criteria for Substance Intoxication and Withdrawal

Diagnostic Criteria for Substance Intoxication

A. The development of a reversible substance-specific syndrome due to recent ingestion of (or exposure to) a substance. **Note:** Different substances may produce similar or identical syndromes.

B. Clinically significant maladaptive behavioral or psychological changes that are due to the effect of the substance on the central nervous system (e.g., belligerence, mood lability, cognitive impairment, impaired judgment, impaired social or occupational functioning) and develop during or shortly after use of the substance.

C. The symptoms are not due to a general medical condition and are not better accounted for by another mental disorder.

Diagnostic Criteria for Substance Withdrawal

A. The development of a substance-specific syndrome due to the cessation of or reduction in substance use that has been heavy and prolonged.

B. The substance-specific syndrome causes clinically significant distress or impairment in social, occupational, or other important areas of functioning.

C. The symptoms are not due to a general medical condition and are not better accounted for by another mental disorder.

Source: Reprinted with permission from the *Diagnostic and Statistical Manual of Mental Disorders,* Fourth Edition, Text Revision. (Copyright 2000). American Psychiatric Association.

USING DSM-IV-TR

Health care providers often use language unfamiliar to clients and their families. Explain "impaired judgment" using language and examples that clients and family members can easily understand.

performance and when he received a second arrest for driving while intoxicated. He is brought into the community crisis unit for medical detoxification and referral to Alcoholics Anonymous (AA) meetings and a mandatory outpatient recovery group program. He smokes at least a pack of cigarettes each day and drinks six cups of strong coffee as well. His physical exam reveals hypertension that is not responsive to medication, elevated liver enzymes, and ascites. He complains of dull abdominal pain, dry skin, diarrhea, and indigestion. He is sweaty, shaking, and irritable. He has been requesting that the physician write a prescription for pain medications to ease his current discomfort.

MEDIALINK Application: The Science of Addiction

BIOPSYCHOSOCIAL THEORIES

The theoretical frameworks for understanding substance problems include biologic/genetic, psychological, sociocultural, and family systems theories.

Biologic/Genetic Theories

The biologic explanation of alcoholism has assumed a great deal of importance in the last few years. Research to determine a genetic predisposition to alcoholism continues. Following are some examples of research that contributes to our evidence-based practices.

- Classical research by Jellinek during the 1940s, 1950s, and 1960s, described as the Disease Model of Alcoholism, revealed that alcoholics proceed through phases, including the prealcoholic symptomatic phase, the prodromal phase, the crucial phase, and the chronic phase (Jellinek, 1946). He recognized "loss of control" in addictive alcoholics and hypothesized that it may have a biochemical basis. Building on this early work, current research examines biochemical differences in these clients such as lower levels of dopamine (DA) neurotransmission, increased density of dopaminergic D2 receptors in the brain, and early relapse in alcohol-dependent clients.
- Pharmacologic management of addictions, as opposed to psychosocial interventions, includes the use of standard and new compounds.
  1. Disulfiram (Antabuse), an agonist medication, inhibits acetaldehyde metabolism. Acetaldehyde, which is highly toxic, accumulates in the bloodstream if the client who takes disulfiram consumes alcohol. It produces nausea, vomiting, dizziness, and other uncomfortable and sometimes potentially dangerous symptoms when the person drinks alcohol, and is used to discourage the use of alcohol.
  2. Naltrexone (ReVia, Trexan) was developed in 1984 for the treatment of heroin abuse, and approved in January 1994 for blocking the craving for alcohol and the pleasure derived from drinking it.
  3. Acamprosate (Campral) Delayed-Release Tablets were approved by the U.S. Food and Drug Administration (FDA) in 2004. Acamprosate is indicated for the maintenance of abstinence from alcohol in clients with alcohol dependence who are abstinent at treatment initiation. This compound alleviates the physiological and psychological distress during the postacute withdrawal period, making it easier not to drink. Its mechanism of action is not completely understood; however, recent evidence suggests the main interaction is with the glutamate system (Saitz et al., 2007).
- Advances in neuroimaging and anatomical discoveries help explain substance abuse in terms of changes in the limbic area of the brain (Heimer & Van Hoesen, 2006). Other studies propose biological explanations of substance abuse such as how genes affect the functioning of differential biochemical systems (Serretti et al., 2006), a consistent relationship between genotypes and substance abuse problems (Prescott et al., 2006), and the role of family genetics in the development of substance-use disorders (Vieten et al., 2004).
- Substance abuse prior to conception and pregnancy has grave consequences for fetuses. In both males and females, it has been validated as damaging to the genetic makeup of the child (Muthen, Asparouhov, & Rebollo, 2006). Research demonstrates that children of alcoholics are at four times the risk of becoming alcoholics. Even if adopted by different families at birth, identical twins of alcoholic parents have more than a 60% chance of becoming alcoholics; fraternal twins have just under a 30% chance.
- Individuals who have biological relatives with substance problems have an increased risk for developing problems with substance abuse or dependence due to their inherited vulnerability. However, vulnerability to the development of substance abuse or dependence does not guarantee that either will occur. Environment and experience have an enormous influence on whether the individual with inherited vulnerability will develop a substance abuse problem (Dick & Bierut, 2006). Adolescents who are helped to cope with the impacts of both biology and experience are often better prepared to resist developing substance abuse and dependence problems. Substance use and abuse is not a simple formula with a simple ingredient; it results from a complex layering and melding of experiences and susceptibilities.
- Drug use affects human development on the genetic level because drug use negatively affects sperm and egg health. Each partner contributes to the negative effect when a male uses a substance and subsequently impregnates a woman, when a woman uses drugs prior to pregnancy, and when a woman uses substances during pregnancy. Birth defects are more commonly linked with paternal DNA damage than

with maternal DNA damage (National Drug Intelligence Center, 2006). In other words, there are a number of physiological consequences for the offspring in addition to an increased risk for substance abuse itself.

- Adult alcoholism develops as a result of the considerable role genetics play when a person's gene pool has alcoholics in it. However, it is acknowledged that family environmental factors significantly influence whether the addiction is asserted or not (Doweiko, 2006). Similarly, adult substance abuse has been examined in those who were adopted and had birth parents with substance abuse. Again, the research supports that having the genes for substance abuse does not, in and of itself, guarantee an addicted adult. The environment must interact with the genetics to create the development of highest risk (Dick & Bierut, 2006).
- Alcoholics may have neurophysiologic defects. They may be vulnerable to intense sensory input and use alcohol as a protection from this heightened sensitivity.
- Neurobiologic studies clearly attest that biologic factors such as genetics underpin one's vulnerability to substance-related disorders. Neurobiologic studies also indicate that medications with anxiolytic and antidepressant effects are being used effectively in both detoxification and relapse-prevention treatment (Brunelle, Barrett, & Pihl, 2006).

Psychological Theories

From the psychologic perspective, the substance abuser is viewed as regressed and fixated at pregenital, oral levels of psychosexual development. Some writers relate the pattern of drug taking to parental inconsistency, self-centeredness, and inner dishonesty. The following personality traits are often associated with disruptive drug abuse:

- Dominant and critical behavior with underlying self-doubts and passivity
- Overt extroversion
- Tendency to describe one's own parents as self-reliant and efficient but not emotionally warm
- Personal insecurity, with low self-esteem and self-criticism
- Problems with sexual identification
- Rebellious attitudes toward authority
- Tendency to use defense mechanisms that are primarily escapist or sensation seeking
- Difficulty with intimacy
- Absence of a strong and efficient superego
- Marked narcissistic trends
- Difficulty with impulse control and feelings

There is no real agreement about whether certain personality traits are sufficient to account for drug dependence, because the personality traits in question are studied after the diagnosis of substance abuse is made.

Sociocultural Theories

Sociocultural models of substance abuse emphasize social forces, role models, and adaptive responses to stress in the sociocultural environment. Life's harsh realities come in many forms: the hopelessness and defeat of urban poverty, the academic and social pressures generated by upper-middle-class families, the adolescent's feeling of impotence and alienation, the peer group pressure to join in and share experiences, the social vacuum of unloving families in which meaningful attachments are dissolved or dissolving. All of these social conditions and contexts help create and sustain substance abuse. Another sociocultural aspect is situational—people who become addicts or alcoholics tend to live in environments where access to chemicals is easy and initiation into their use is widespread. Such an environment might include a neighborhood where abandoned houses become places to sell, buy, and use substances.

Substance abusers describe in interviews how they learned to drink or use drugs at school, in social circumstances with their peers, or at home by watching their families. They recognized chemicals as a social lubricant, an escape, or a remedy for psychic and physical pain.

Studies clearly show that substance abuse is present in all cultures; however, which substance people abuse is often culturally determined. In Western culture, alcohol is the drug of choice. In Moslem countries, marijuana use is a problem because Islam prohibits alcohol use. Opium is used in China and other Eastern countries, while people in India and Africa use native herbs and chemicals. Native Americans use peyote (a cactus button with hallucinogenic properties) and alcohol more than other drugs.

Family Systems Theories

A family systems explanation for substance abuse has gained increasing acceptance among health care professionals. When assessing substance abuse and the psychological impacts, ask yourself, "Could the addiction be serving a purpose in this family?" The addiction may serve to:

- Shift the family's focus
- Give them a purpose or a challenge to distract them from other issues
- Relieve one family member of a burden or provide a needed burden to one or several members
- Provide a cohesive cause in which all family members can involve themselves

The family systems perspective includes the phenomenon of codependence. **Codependency** involves being preoccupied with controlling another person's behavior. Codependency can be seen when a family member both rescues and blames (persecutes) the addict.

Although Alcoholics Anonymous (AA), a support group for alcoholics, does not openly endorse the family systems theory, it does recognize clearly that alcoholism is a family disease. Al-Anon and Ala-Teen are groups for spouses, parents, friends, coworkers, and teenage children of alcoholics. The focus is on helping these nonalcoholics learn to live and work effectively with alcoholics.

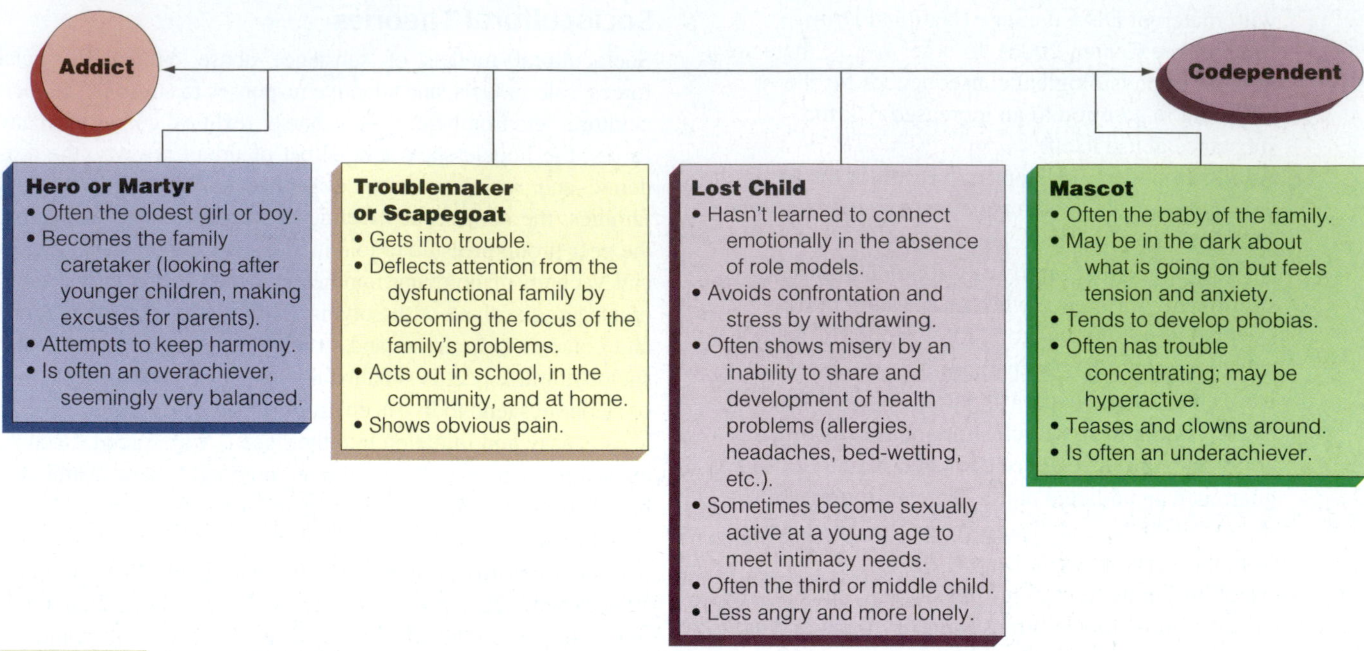

Addict
Codependent
Hero or Martyr
• Often the oldest girl or boy.
• Becomes the family caretaker (looking after younger children, making excuses for parents).
• Attempts to keep harmony.
• Is often an overachiever, seemingly very balanced.
Troublemaker or Scapegoat
• Gets into trouble.
• Deflects attention from the dysfunctional family by becoming the focus of the family's problems.
• Acts out in school, in the community, and at home.
• Shows obvious pain.
Lost Child
• Hasn't learned to connect emotionally in the absence of role models.
• Avoids confrontation and stress by withdrawing.
• Often shows misery by an inability to share and development of health problems (allergies, headaches, bed-wetting, etc.).
• Sometimes become sexually active at a young age to meet intimacy needs.
• Often the third or middle child.
• Less angry and more lonely.
Mascot
• Often the baby of the family.
• May be in the dark about what is going on but feels tension and anxiety.
• Tends to develop phobias.
• Often has trouble concentrating; may be hyperactive.
• Teases and clowns around.
• Is often an underachiever.

FIGURE 15-1 ■ Dysfunctional family roles in the presence of addiction–codependency.

The underlying belief, as the following clinical example illustrates, is that other people often assume the role where **enabling**, or co-alcoholic behavior, perpetuates the alcoholic's drinking patterns.

CLINICAL EXAMPLE

Louise has been drinking for many years. She works full-time as a secretary in a financial office setting. Adrienne, Louise's coworker for many years, routinely does Louise's work when Louise is too tired, confused, or otherwise unable to perform her duties. Adrienne believes she is helping Louise keep her job and her self-esteem. In reality, Adrienne is enabling Louise to continue to drink and not suffer the consequences of her drinking.

A cycle begins when people who enable do what they think is best in the situation. They begin to cover for the addict, such as by saying that he or she has a cold, is bruised because of stumbling in the dark, is asleep because of fatigue. Protected by the enabling behavior, the addict is spared the consequences of his or her behavior and continues drinking or using drugs. The person who is enabling, believing that the addict is coping with family, marital, or work problems "the best way he can," denies the disease of addiction. The addict blames the person who is enabling; the person who is enabling feels guilty and then attempts to control family life and the behaviors of the alcoholic/addict by throwing out liquor or taking the car keys. Of course this behavior does not work. Enabling behavior was employed to protect, rescue, control, and blame, but none of these behaviors is effective in altering the course of the disease. Consequently, those who enable feel worthless and helpless because they are unsuccessful in terminating the addiction. Intervention and confrontation are necessary to break the cycle. Chapter 30∞ details family features.

Dysfunctional Family Roles

When a family includes one parent whose role consists of addictive behavior and who is incapable of being emotionally present and adequately fulfilling the parenting role; and one parent whose role involves codependency or enabling, whose attempts to fix addictive behaviors prevail, children may be forced into dysfunctional family roles. Such children are consumed with meeting family needs and miss out on nurturing. Children's roles may consist of:

- The Hero or Martyr
- The Troublemaker or Scapegoat
- The Lost Child
- The Mascot

These defensive personalities represent survival strategies for children living in what they perceive to be a frightening family environment. Behaviors associated with each of these dysfunctional family roles appear in FIGURE 15-1 ■. Adult personalities are partially imprinted during childhood, and the roles that children take in order to cope in a family burdened by addiction can continue into adulthood if appropriate treatment is not provided.

ALCOHOL

Alcohol is a common, accessible substance that has just as much destructive power as any other substance of abuse. According to the World Health Organization, alcohol is one of the most widely used and abused substances in the world and causes as much, if not more, death and disability as measles, malaria, tobacco, or illegal drugs. It is a liquid recreational drug that happens to be legal. Characteristic features of abuse of this drug are seen in the clinical example that follows.

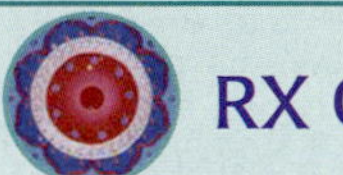

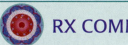

RX COMMUNICATION

CLIENT WITH ALCOHOLISM WHO IS INTOXICATED

CLIENT: "I'm so sorry I'm such a burden to you. You're such a good nurse, and I never want to be the type of person who. . . ."

NURSE RESPONSE 1: "I'm going to take your vital signs and then you will have some time to yourself."

RATIONALE: This interaction treats the event as an illness in which there are physical consequences to the behavior as well as set limits on the interaction.

NURSE RESPONSE 2: "We will talk later when you are able to concentrate."

RATIONALE: An intoxicated client is not able to benefit from a detailed discussion.

CLINICAL EXAMPLE

Colleen, a 48-year-old woman, arrived at the hospital to be admitted for the fifth time. Her gait was unsteady and her speech slurred. Even though she was drunk, she avoided eye contact, appeared embarrassed, and apologized profusely for "getting into this mess again." She said, "I really don't need to be here. I can handle this." Then Colleen burst into tears, began to say something, got distracted, and argued repetitively with staff. Blackouts were evident; Colleen had no memory of how she got to the hospital (she had, in fact, driven herself and parked her car on the front lawn of the hospital).

Interacting with someone who is intoxicated from alcohol requires implementing a set of guidelines and understanding the processes at work. See the Rx Communication feature on interacting with an alcohol-intoxicated individual.

Because of the increasing incidence of alcoholism and the highway carnage attributed to alcohol use, alcoholism is now the focus of magazine articles and radio and television programs. Media attention heightens awareness of the devastating effects of chronic alcoholism: depression; loss of self-respect; alienation from family, friends, and coworkers; malnutrition; infections; and damaging physiologic effects to most body systems. The physical effects of chronic alcoholism are listed in Box 15-1.

Box 15-1 Physical Effects of Chronic Alcoholism

Hepatic System

- Alcoholic fatty liver syndrome
- Alcoholic hepatitis
- Laënnec's cirrhosis

Neurologic System

- Wernicke–Korsakoff syndrome (related to thiamine deficiency)
- Peripheral neuropathy (related to vitamin B deficiency)
- Marchiafava-Bignami syndrome or disease*
- Central pontine myelinosis*
- Cerebellar degeneration*
- Alcoholic amblyopia*

Cardiovascular System

- Alcoholic cardiomyopathy
- Hypokalemia
- Hypomagnesemia
- Hyperlipidemia
- Altered fluid balance
- Beriberi heart disease (related to thiamine deficiency)
- Hematologic abnormalities

Musculoskeletal System

- Acute alcoholic myopathy
- Subclinical alcoholic myopathy
- Chronic alcoholic myopathy

Gastrointestinal System

- Gastritis
- Esophagitis
- Mallory–Weiss syndrome
- Boerhaave's syndrome
- Pancreatitis
- Nutritional deficiency diseases
- Nausea
- Abdominal pain
- Erratic bowel function (constipation and diarrhea)
- Gastrointestinal hemorrhage
- Jaundice
- High incidence of digestive tract cancers
- Glucose intolerance

Reproductive System

- Impotence
- Sterility
- Gynecomastia
- Anorgasmy (women)
- FAS

**Very rare*

Although alcoholism was historically viewed as a moral problem, increased awareness played a part in the redefinition of alcoholism as a disease. As research about its biochemical aspects became known, earlier beliefs were challenged. The social stigma attached to alcoholism is decreasing, and more people are seeking help. Professionals, laypeople, alcoholics, and nonalcoholics are attending workshops and seminars on alcoholism; college courses at the undergraduate and graduate levels are offered. Recovery programs are reported widely in the popular media. The latest research related to the treatment of alcoholism and other drug abuse can be accessed at the website for the National Institute on Drug Abuse (NIDA) at www.nida.nih.gov/.

MEDIALINK National Institute on Drug Abuse

The Effects of Alcohol

A sedative anesthetic (CNS depressant), alcohol is absorbed in the mouth, stomach, and small intestine. Approximately 95% of alcohol is broken down by the liver; the rest is excreted through the lungs, kidneys, and skin. Generally, a person can metabolize 10 mL of alcohol (1 oz of whiskey) every 90 minutes. The rate of absorption varies based on many factors, such as weight, intake of food, and liver function. If taken in exceedingly high doses, alcohol can depress respiration and cause death. Intoxication occurs when a person's blood alcohol level (BAL) is 0.10% or more. This blood alcohol level is the legal definition of inebriation in most states, although 0.08% is the drunk driving limit in all 50 states and represents definite impairment in coordination and judgment. FIGURE 15-2 ■ illustrates the amount of alcohol that results in a BAL of 0.10 percent. The Your Assessment Approach feature compares BALs and the behaviors exhibited at various levels.

YOUR ASSESSMENT APPROACH
Blood Alcohol Level (BAL) and Behaviors

Blood Alcohol Level (BAL)	Behavior
0.05 to 0.15 g/dL	Initial euphoria
	Mood lability
	Cognitive disturbances, including:
	■ Decreased concentration
	■ Impaired judgment
	■ Sexual disinhibition
0.15 to 0.25 g/dL	Mood lability with outbursts
	Slurred speech
	Staggered gait or ataxia
	Diplopia
	Drowsiness
0.3 g/dL	Aggressive behavior
	Incoherent speech
	Labored breathing
	Vomiting
	Stupor
0.4 g/dL	Coma
0.5 g/dL	Severe respiratory depression
	Death

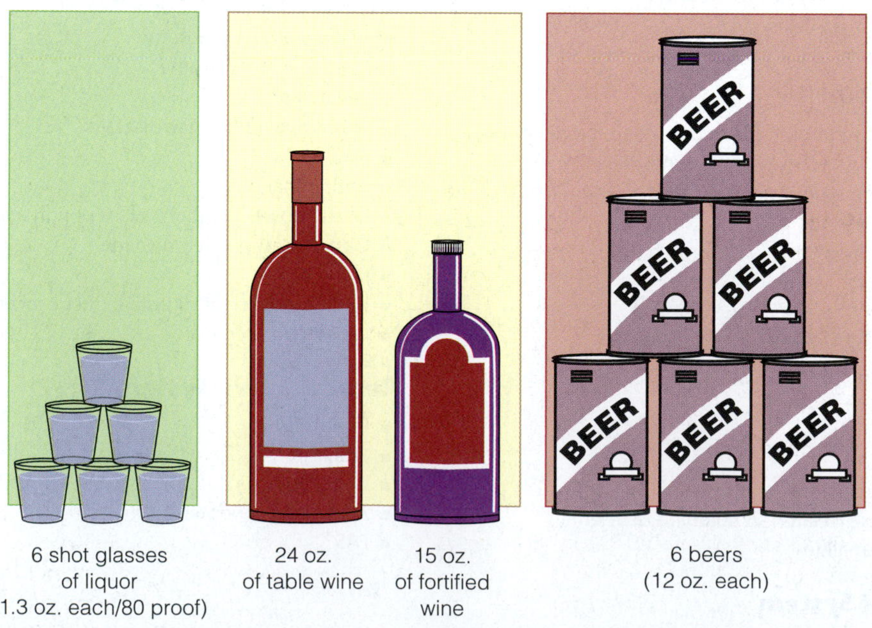
BEER
6 shot glasses of liquor (1.3 oz. each/80 proof)
24 oz. of table wine
15 oz. of fortified wine
6 beers (12 oz. each)

FIGURE 15-2 ■ Intoxication. These amounts of alcoholic beverages, when consumed within a 2-hour period, will give a 160-pound person a BAL of 0.10.

Patterns of Use

Alcoholics manifest one of three patterns of use: regular daily intake of large amounts of alcohol, regular heavy drinking limited to weekends, or long periods of sobriety interspersed with binges of heavy drinking lasting for weeks or months. Regardless of the preferred pattern, people who drink excessively experience numerous negative physiologic and psychological symptoms.

Alcohol Withdrawal Syndrome

Alcohol withdrawal often includes the symptoms described in the following section.

Hangover

The term *hangover* is used to describe the unpleasant symptoms of mild alcohol withdrawal occurring approximately 4 to 6 hours after alcohol ingestion. These symptoms include:

- Nausea and vomiting
- Gastritis
- Headache
- Fatigue
- Sweating and thirst
- Restlessness
- Irritability
- The "shakes"
- Vasomotor instability

The cause of the symptoms is unclear, but they are attributed to dehydration, hypoglycemia, and the accumulation of lactic acid and acetaldehyde in the blood.

Alcoholic Hallucinosis

Alcoholic hallucinosis refers to auditory hallucinations reported by clients with alcohol dependence. The hallucinations occur approximately 24 to 48 hours after heavy drinking and may be vivid and frightening to the client.

Generalized Seizures

Generalized seizures (also known colloquially as "rum fits") may occur 2 to 3 days after the person stops drinking. They can be prevented in a well-monitored medical withdrawal program.

Delirium Tremens

Delirium tremens (DTs), one symptom of withdrawal, is a condition of severe memory disturbance, agitation, anorexia, and hallucinations. The symptoms are described more thoroughly in the section on withdrawal that follows.

Generally, DTs begin a few days after drinking stops and end within 1 to 5 days. They may, however, appear as late as the second week, especially when there is cross-addiction to other drugs. Additional medical illnesses may be present, such as pneumonia, pancreatitis, and hepatic decompensation.

Withdrawal from Alcohol and Medical Treatment

Alcohol withdrawal occurs after the addicted individual stops drinking. This syndrome is composed of a constellation of physiologic and behavioral symptoms that occur when the alcohol level drops. Medical treatment of alcoholism involves the management of withdrawal symptoms and the use of medication to deter the alcoholic from drinking.

Minor Withdrawal

A *minor withdrawal* from alcohol can occur within 6 to 12 hours after the alcoholic's last drink. Early symptoms include anxiety, agitation, and irritability. As the syndrome progresses, other symptoms occur. These include tremor, tachycardia, hypertension, diaphoresis, and hallucinations. Gastrointestinal symptoms of nausea, vomiting, diarrhea, and anorexia may also be present. These symptoms may last 48 to 72 hours. The appearance of hallucinations (visual, auditory, olfactory, or tactile) and seizures marks the onset of a *major withdrawal.* See the stages of withdrawal from alcohol in the Your Assessment Approach feature on page 332.

Major Withdrawal

A major withdrawal is the most advanced, potentially life-threatening stage of alcohol withdrawal. Major withdrawal symptoms appear within 2–3 days following the last drink and may last 3–5 days. Symptoms associated with DTs usually develop 72 hours after the last drink. Physical symptoms of impending DTs include elevated temperature, severe diaphoresis, hypertension, and tachycardia. Behavioral symptoms include confusion and disorientation, agitation, tremors, and alterations in sensory perception (auditory and visual hallucinations).

Treatment of Withdrawal

The best treatment for major alcohol withdrawal involves early detection. Medical treatment for withdrawal includes:

1. Monitoring the client's fluid status. Although some clients are overhydrated, many are dehydrated or have the potential for developing a fluid volume deficit. Fluids should be encouraged, up to 3,000 mL/day if no evidence exists to contraindicate this. If the client is unable to take fluids by mouth, fluids may be administered intravenously.
2. Administering magnesium sulfate to decrease the irritability caused by low magnesium levels and to prevent seizures.
3. Administering vitamins, especially thiamine (vitamin B_1) because alcohol interferes with the absorption of B vitamins.
4. Prescribing benzodiazepines, such as diazepam (Valium) or chlordiazepoxide (Librium), to help prevent DTs. Seizures may be treated with IV diazepam, and the client may be placed on phenytoin (Dilantin).

YOUR ASSESSMENT APPROACH
Stages of Withdrawal from Alcohol

State	Peak Time of Onset After Last Drink	Symptoms	Potential Duration of Symptoms
Tremulousness	24 hours	At rest: slight tremors; during activities: gross and irregular tremors	1 week
		Diaphoresis	3–4 days
		Anorexia, nausea, vomiting	3–4 days
		Increased vital signs	3–4 days
		Sense of agitation and inner shakiness	2 weeks
		Insomnia with nightmares of seemingly real events	2 weeks or longer
Tremors and transitory hallucinosis	24 hours	Tremors plus visual hallucinations of events (e.g., having an accident while driving drunk)	3 days
Alcoholic hallucinosis	24 hours	Cues of tremulousness state plus vivid persecutory and auditory hallucinations, agitation, increased suicide, preassaultive potential	3 days–2 weeks
Delirium tremens	24–48 hours	Cues of tremulousness state plus delirium, generalized seizures, disorientation for time and place, visual hallucinations, agitation, panic level of anxiety	3–5 days
Rum fits	24–48 hours	2–6 generalized seizures; cues of delirium tremens	3–5 days

5. Prescribing disulfiram (Antabuse, an agonist medication). The use of disulfiram may be prescribed in the treatment of alcoholic clients, although it is not used as often as it used to be. Recall that disulfiram inhibits acetaldehyde dehydrogenase, which normally metabolizes acetaldehyde. As a result, acetaldehyde accumulates if alcohol is consumed. Acetaldehyde is highly toxic. If the client uses alcohol, a powerful *disulfiram reaction* may occur and last for up to 2 weeks. Reaction symptoms include nausea, vomiting, flushing, dizziness, tachycardia, and hypotension. Hypotension may lead to shock and can be fatal. Because of the potential danger involved, instruct the client orally and in writing not to use alcohol in any form, including alcohol-based cough syrups or cold remedies such as those listed in TABLE 15-1 ■ when taking disulfiram.
6. Prescribing naltrexone (ReVia, Trexan). Rather than making the alcoholic sick, naltrexone blocks the need to ingest alcohol and thus may help prevent relapse when it is combined with long-term support groups and individual counseling. It has had more treatment success than disulfiram.

Withdrawal from alcohol, or any chemical substance, should include and emphasize the principle of controlling the physical discomfort of withdrawal while minimizing intoxication with the withdrawal agent(s).

Blackouts

Having **blackouts** is frequently confused with passing out. In fact, passing out refers to unconsciousness, whereas a blackout is anterograde amnesia: loss of short-term memories with retention of remote memories. A person can function effectively for up to several days—talking on the telephone, working, and shopping—yet have absolutely no memory of doing so. To others, the alcoholic may appear normal or "high." Interestingly, alcoholics appear unconcerned about the blackouts and eventually learn to cover them up. This appearance of unconcern may, in part, be due to euphoric recall: The al-

TABLE 15-1 ■ Alcohol Content of Selected Over-the-Counter Cough and Cold Mixtures and Mouthwashes

Preparation	Amount of Alcohol (%)
Cough and Cold Mixtures	
Benylin Cough Syrup	5
Halls Mentho-Lyptus Decongestant Cough Formula	22
Nyquil Nighttime Cold Medicine	25
Robitussin Night Relief Cold Formula	25
Sudafed Cough Syrup	2.4
Vicks Formula 44 Cough Mixture	10
Mouthwashes	
ACT Fluoride	7
Cepacol	14
Listerine	26.9
Scope	18.5

coholic recalls feeling good but does not recall his or her behavior. Reality is distorted. Some clients find blackouts very disturbing and seek treatment at that point.

Blackouts appearing later in the disease process may be indicative of physical dependence and are not related to the amount of alcohol consumed. They are unpredictable, and exactly how or why they occur is not clear. Some authorities believe blackouts are an acute syndrome caused by dehydration of brain tissue. When assessing an alcoholic client, determine whether blackouts are part of the symptoms. See the Nursing Care Plan for chronic alcoholism at the end of this chapter, which addresses alcohol abuse.

Alcohol-Induced Persisting Amnestic Disorder

Alcohol-induced persisting amnestic disorder (Korsakoff's syndrome) is a disturbance of short-term memory that occurs in people who have been drinking alcohol heavily for many years and have a thiamine deficiency. Korsakoff's syndrome is the result of damage to the hippocampus and surrounding tissue from heavy alcohol ingestion.

If treated early, Korsakoff's syndrome may be avoided. Once this disorder is established, however, it has a chronic irreversible course, and impairment can become severe. It often follows an acute episode of alcoholic encephalopathy.

Alcoholic Encephalopathy

Alcoholic encephalopathy (Wernicke's encephalopathy) is a neurologic disease associated with chronic alcoholism and is characterized by ataxia, sixth cranial nerve palsy, nystagmus, and confusion. Wernicke's encephalopathy may clear spontaneously in a few days or weeks and responds rapidly to large doses of parenteral thiamine in its acute, early stage. Both Korsakoff's syndrome and Wernicke's encephalopathy are covered in Chapter 14.

Fetal Alcohol Syndrome

Nurses need to be aware of the harmful effects of alcohol on pregnant women and unborn children. **Fetal alcohol syndrome (FAS)** is found in children of women who engage in heavy drinking of alcohol during pregnancy. Approximately 100 babies are born daily with alcohol-related defects. It is considered the most common nonhereditary form of mental retardation.

Physical and mental defects of FAS include severe growth deficiency, heart defects, malformed facial features, mental retardation, low birth weight, learning problems, and hyperactivity. The characteristic physical features of a child with FAS are seen in FIGURE 15-3 ■. If a child has one or two of these characteristics, the condition is called fetal alcohol effects. FAS affects 1 in 750 babies born in the United States. A baby born to an alcoholic mother may need to be withdrawn gradually from alcohol immediately after birth. Even brief exposure to very small amounts of alcohol may kill fetal brain cells and cause peripheral nerve damage as well. Further research is needed to explore this sensitivity (Olney, 2004).

There is hope as a result of ongoing FAS research at the National Institute of Child Health and Human Development. Animal studies show that pretreating mothers with a substance called activity-dependent neurotrophic factor-12 prevents alcohol-induced fetal death and developmental learning abnormalities (Endres et al., 2005). Further studies using the active peptides from two brain proteins known to protect nerve cells against a variety of toxins also protect—at least in the animal models. For up-to-date information about FAS, see the link to the National Organization on Fetal Alcohol Syndrome on the Companion Website for this text.

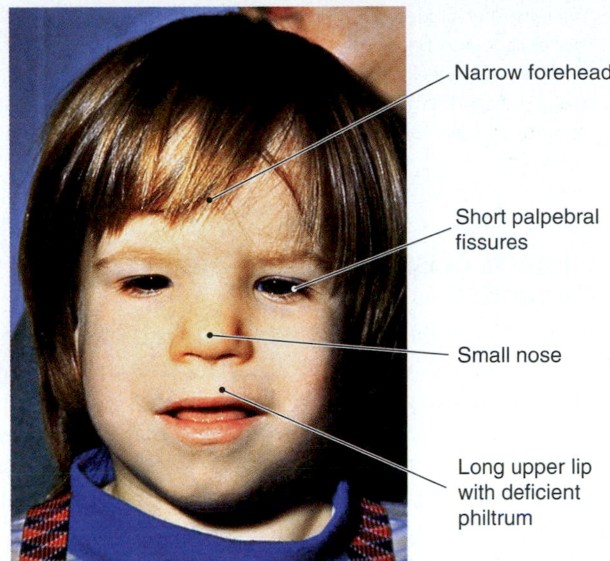

FIGURE 15-3 ■ Fetal alcohol syndrome is the result of alcohol consumption during pregnancy, and it can have many severe effects on the child, including physical malformations such as those shown here: narrow forehead, short palpebral fissures, small nose, and long upper lip with deficient philtrum.

Source: Fetal Alcohol & Drug Unit (FAS).

Suicide and Alcoholism

Be alert to the possibility of suicide attempts by alcoholics. Of the roughly 30,000 suicides committed in the United States each year, 1% are completed by the general population and 15% by alcoholics. Watch for self-destructive behavior and for events in a client's life that represent a loss such as work, family, health, or legal problems. Such behavior and events put people in a high-risk category. Suicide is thoroughly discussed in Chapter 23.

MEDIALINK National Organization on Fetal Alcohol Syndrome

BARBITURATES OR SIMILARLY ACTING SEDATIVES OR HYPNOTICS

Barbiturates are overprescribed for anxiety, stress, and sleep difficulties because health care practitioners treat the symptoms of anxiety, stress, or insomnia without first determining the cause, as in the clinical example that follows.

CLINICAL EXAMPLE

Elizabeth, a 45-year-old housewife, has been depressed and irritable over an impending divorce. Her physician prescribed diazepam (Valium) 5 mg for sleep and for anxiety (every 6 hours as needed). Because this dosage was not helping decrease her anxiety as much as she wanted, she increased her dosage and began taking 50 to 100 mg a day over a period of a few weeks. This evening, Elizabeth's estranged husband found her mumbling incoherently. Her speech was slurred, she was bumping into furniture, and she was quite drowsy.

MediaLink Case Study: Prescription Substance Abuse

The Effects of Barbiturates, Sedatives, or Hypnotics

Barbiturates are highly addictive drugs that cause people to feel euphoric, yet relaxed. They are frequently prescribed to relieve pain, reduce anxiety (sedative effects), and induce sleep (hypnotic effects). Barbiturates were the first drugs used to treat anxiety and insomnia. They were considered dangerous because of their ability to cause significant CNS depression and their lethality upon overdose.

Anxiolytic drugs, the benzodiazepines (BZDs), began to be widely used because of their ability to reduce anxiety without causing significant CNS depression. However, they also have the drawbacks of producing dependence and withdrawal syndromes. BZDs include many widely prescribed drugs, including diazepam (Valium), clorazepate (Tranxene), lorazepam (Ativan), and alprazolam (Xanax). These drugs are thought to modify anxiety by altering the balance of neurotransmitters, especially norepinephrine (NE) and gamma-aminobutyric acid (GABA) in the brain's limbic system. The limbic system is involved in the regulation of emotion. These drugs have a high risk for abuse and physical dependence. When the drug stops working and tolerance builds up, people tend to increase the dosage just "to cope." Even the nonbenzodiazepines such as zolpidem (Ambien) and zaleplon (Sonata) can be used to excess and have dependence issues associated with their use (see Chapter 7).

MediaLink Animation: Morphine Drug Mechanism in Action

Patterns of Use

In party situations, some teenagers and young adults take high doses of barbiturates, often in combination with alcohol, to get "high." The resultant CNS depression makes this practice especially dangerous. "Speed freaks" (amphetamine abusers) use barbiturates to "come down" from a high. Dependence, tolerance, and cross-tolerance to other depressant drugs develop rapidly.

Action

Barbiturates are metabolized in phases by the liver. When taken orally, they are initially absorbed and partially metabolized. However, the unmetabolized parts become active metabolites that are stored in the fatty tissues. Consequently, taking these drugs over a period of time results in a cumulative effect, unsuspected dependence, and possible overdose. Nurses in other specialty areas also need to be aware of the frequency of substance abuse among their clients and its impact. See the What Every Emergency Department Nurse Should Know feature that follows for further information.

More Americans die from barbiturate overdose than from opioid addiction. Many take alcohol and barbiturates together. While judgment is impaired they take more pills, thereby unintentionally overdosing. Because alcohol and barbiturates are synergistic, an overdose can occur quickly. Barbiturates are often used in suicide attempts.

> **WHAT EVERY EMERGENCY DEPARTMENT NURSE SHOULD KNOW**
>
> 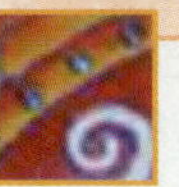
>
> **The Substance-Abusing Client**
>
> In an emergency situation the substance-abusing client may be unable to answer key questions like these:
>
> - What did you take?
> - How much did you take?
> - When did you take it?
> - What have you taken in the last 24 hours? In the last week?
>
> When this happens, you must rely on family or friends as data sources, and then corroborate what you learn with the client once he or she is alert.

Withdrawal

Barbiturate withdrawal is unpleasant and life threatening. A deep sleep is followed by decreased respiration, coma, and sometimes death. Babies born to mothers addicted to barbiturates are physically dependent and need to be helped through withdrawal.

Withdrawal from BZDs may produce symptoms similar to those of barbiturate withdrawal. Symptoms include autonomic hyperactivity (alterations in vital signs and diaphoresis), marked anxiety, agitation, insomnia, depression, and seizures. Medically supervised detoxification treatment can prevent a potentially serious emergency during withdrawal.

OPIOIDS

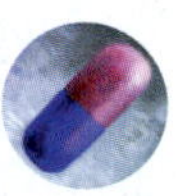

The opioids include heroin and morphine, derived from the poppy plant, and synthetic drugs, such as oxycodone (OxyContin), meperidine (Demerol), codeine, methadone, and others.

The Effects of Opioids

Opioids have analgesic qualities and are prescribed after surgery. They are quite potent and have the ability to remove painful stimuli. Depending on the person, the drugs may produce a euphoric high, as in drug addicts, but they generally cause people to feel drowsy and out of touch with the world. Postoperative nurses, for example, need to be knowledgeable about the use of opioids as a substance of abuse. See the following What Every Postoperative Nurse Should Know feature.

Heroin addiction by itself is not inherently dangerous. Unless there is an accidental overdose, heroin alone as a substance will not harm the individual. The ancillary issues

WHAT EVERY POSTOPERATIVE NURSE SHOULD KNOW

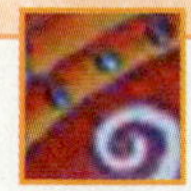

Pain Medication Use and Overuse

There are special circumstances in which it is important to pay attention to the proper use of pain medications to prevent the establishment of chronic pain pathways and responses, while at the same time being careful not to promote inadvertent or deliberate overuse of pain medications. This is especially true for nurses in the postsurgical areas. There will be times when people electively choose repeated surgeries. Under these circumstances it is important to evaluate the client's intent and the follow-up behaviors for the surgeries. Assess for substance dependence in the form of prescription pain medication overuse or dependence. Use the assessment skills described in this chapter to ensure healthy recoveries and intervene appropriately.

of possibly contaminated diluting agents, needle cleanliness, and exposure to transmissible diseases such as hepatitis C, tuberculosis, and HIV, along with typically criminal behaviors necessary to support the addiction, put the individual at great risk and make the addicted individual of concern to others. Methadone as a treatment option for these clients has been successful to a certain extent, but is controversial ethically and economically and is viewed as a public health concern.

Patterns of Use

In 1898, heroin became widely available and initially was not believed to be addictive. Within a short time, its addictive properties became known, and the government intervened (Harrison Narcotics Act of 1914). Addiction to opiates has increased through the years. Because most opioid abusers take the drugs intravenously, they are at high risk for HIV/AIDS and hepatitis C. Overdose, malnutrition, and infections spread by dirty drugs and needles are dangers. Dealers often add impurities to "cut" the heroin, thus increasing the quantity and their own profit. The impurities may cause poisoning and other problems.

Overdose

Constricted pupils, euphoria, psychomotor retardation, slurred speech, and/or drowsiness indicate opioid intoxication.

CLINICAL EXAMPLE

Steven, a 20-year-old male, arrived at the hospital in an ambulance. He was unconscious. His respirations were slow, and his pupils were pinpoints. "Tracks" were visible on his arms and behind his knees. A source said Steven had just "shot up" heroin.

If a client overdoses, naloxone (Narcan) (0.4 to 2.0 mg IV repeated in 2 to 3 minutes) is given. It is a fast-acting narcotic antagonist that counteracts respiratory depression. Abdominal cramps, rhinorrhea, and lacrimation may be treated with belladonna alkaloids or with phenobarbital.

MediaLink Animation: Overdose

Withdrawal

Because opioids are physically addictive, withdrawal is a threat. People who use high doses of a drug and who "shoot up" or "mainline" (use the drug intravenously) are at high risk for severe withdrawal symptoms. Withdrawal symptoms are usually evident within 12 hours after the last dose. The person experiences the most severe withdrawal within 36 to 48 hours, with the symptoms decreasing gradually over 2 weeks. During this stressful time, the person craves the drug and may terminate treatment against advice of health professionals.

Babies born to addicted mothers must be treated for opioid withdrawal. These babies are irritable and have high-pitched crying, increased respirations, fever, sneezing, yawning, and tremors.

Treatment

In 1964, methadone was introduced to treat opiate addiction. By the late 1960s and early 1970s, when federal governments allocated money for treatment, methadone maintenance programs mushroomed all over North America. Methadone, a synthetic narcotic, was dispensed daily at clinics to narcotic addicts.

Although addictive, methadone does not produce the "rush" (ecstatic feeling) associated with heroin. Methadone alleviates the addict's craving for narcotics and, therefore, was expected to decrease the illicit drug trafficking, theft, prostitution, and crime necessary to obtain money for the drugs, thereby allowing addicts to lead productive lives. Also, methadone therapy is far less expensive than residential programs or jail. Today, methadone maintenance programs remain a major treatment for opioid addicts.

Clients who are assessed to be not at risk for complications of the drug are first stabilized on methadone (3 to 5 days). Within 1 to 3 days after the methadone is discontinued, opiate withdrawal symptoms often appear. At this time, clonidine (Catapres) is administered and given in increasing doses, until withdrawal symptoms are alleviated (up to 14 days). Clonidine blocks the withdrawal symptoms, making the detoxification process less painful and more rapid than with methadone. Psychologically, the client feels less anxious and depressed.

The effectiveness of Schedule III, IV, and V controlled substances, including buprenorphine (Buprenex), makes them alternatives to methadone. Buprenorphine is an opioid mixed agonist and potent analgesic. The advantages of buprenorphine include low abuse potential and high availability for office-based treatment. Disadvantages include its high cost and possible lack of effectiveness in clients who require high methadone doses (Donaher & Welsh, 2006). Buprenorphine is also being investigated for its effectiveness in treating cocaine abuse. Office-based treatment of opiate addictions is discussed in the Evidence-Based Practice feature on page 336.

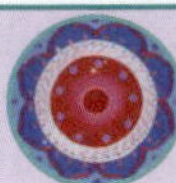

EVIDENCE-BASED PRACTICE

OFFICE-BASED TREATMENTS FOR SUBSTANCE ABUSE

Sekov is a 33-year-old native of Macedonia who has been in the United States since high school. Although bright and active in sports in high school, he began socializing with a group using alcohol and marijuana regularly and cocaine and heroin on occasion. After high school his activities dwindled and his opportunities shrank as he spent more and more time with these friends. Within a few years he was marginally functional and lived solely to obtain heroin. Five years ago, Sekov agreed to enter a treatment program on the insistence and with the help of his large extended family.

A significant barrier to Sekov's treatment and subsequent recovery has been the lack of available treatment slots at methadone clinics. You are involved as the nurse in an office-based buprenorphine treatment program that incorporates psychosocial treatments and education. Research shows that selected clients do well in this type of program in an office setting.

As part of your role, you present information about access to these types of office-based programs at various community centers. It was at one of these presentations that you met Sekov and his mother. As a result, you were able to assess his circumstances, noting that they paralleled the research successes. You provided Sekov with the access to treatment that may allow his recovery to proceed unimpeded.

Action should be based on more than one study, but the following is a study that would be helpful in this situation.

Ison, J., Day, E., Fisher, K., Pratt, M., Hull, M., & Copello A. (2006). Self-detoxification from opioid drugs. *Journal of Substance Use, 11*(2), 81–88.

CRITICAL THINKING APPLICATION

1. What factors do you believe will increase the likelihood that Sekov will benefit from a methadone treatment program?
2. What factors do you believe will decrease this likelihood?
3. How can Sekov's mother be helpful to him?

AMPHETAMINES OR SIMILARLY ACTING SYMPATHOMIMETICS

Amphetamines belong to a group of compounds called sympathomimetics that is also referred to colloquially as "speed." This group of compounds contains synthetic drugs derived from ephedrine that stimulate the release of adrenaline and do speed up the user's system—hence the common name. The following clinical example shows how the best intentions can lead to dire and unexpected consequences.

CLINICAL EXAMPLE

Laura, a 16-year-old high school girl, was on a diet so she could get into her favorite bathing suit. Her friend's brother, a pharmacist, gave her some Dexedrine "just until you lose the weight." Laura's mother initially noticed her rather unusual hyperactivity, her euphoria, and the fact that she refused dinner. Over a period of a few weeks, Laura's behavior changed. She appeared suspicious and irritable and continued to speak and move rapidly, and her grades dropped significantly. Laura was rushed to the hospital after being found unconscious in the girls' locker room at school.

The Effects of Amphetamines

In small doses, amphetamines cause a person to feel energetic, euphoric, and "turned on" to life. Users take these CNS stimulants to feel good. A growing number of people take amphetamines (uppers) to counteract the effects of barbiturates (downers) in a cyclic fashion. Amphetamines are dangerous because they alter judgment and obscure feelings. Taken in high doses or intravenously, amphetamines can have dangerous side effects. Tolerance develops rapidly, and chronic abusers may suffer a toxic psychosis characterized by the symptoms of paranoid schizophrenia. Argumentativeness, delusions, hallucinations, stereotypic compulsive behavior, increased libido, interpersonal sensitivity, panic, and violence may occur (APA, 2000).

Amphetamines act by mimicking two of the brain's most important neurotransmitters, dopamine (DA) and norepinephrine (NE). A drug must be able to act on a receptor site or on a number of receptor sites to have an impact. The body may not have a specific amphetamine or cocaine receptor site, so amphetamine and cocaine will take what is called illegal control at the existing receptor sites. Dopamine and dopamine receptor sites are intricately involved in the effects substances of abuse have on the nervous systems of clients. (The specific ways in which morphine, amphetamine, and cocaine are involved in this process are shown in FIGURE 15-4 ■.) Chronic use of methamphetamines changes the way a person thinks and behaves because the brain's cortex is no longer activated during decision making. This change in the ability of the brain to transport dopamine to any significant degree creates the clinical characteristics of severe psychiatric symptoms (Kim et al., 2006).

Patterns of Use

Amphetamine was first synthesized in 1887, and experimental medical use began in the 1920s (McGuinness, 2006). In the 1950s and 1960s, amphetamines were heralded as won-

MEDIALINK Animation: How a Substance of Abuse Occupies a Receptor Site

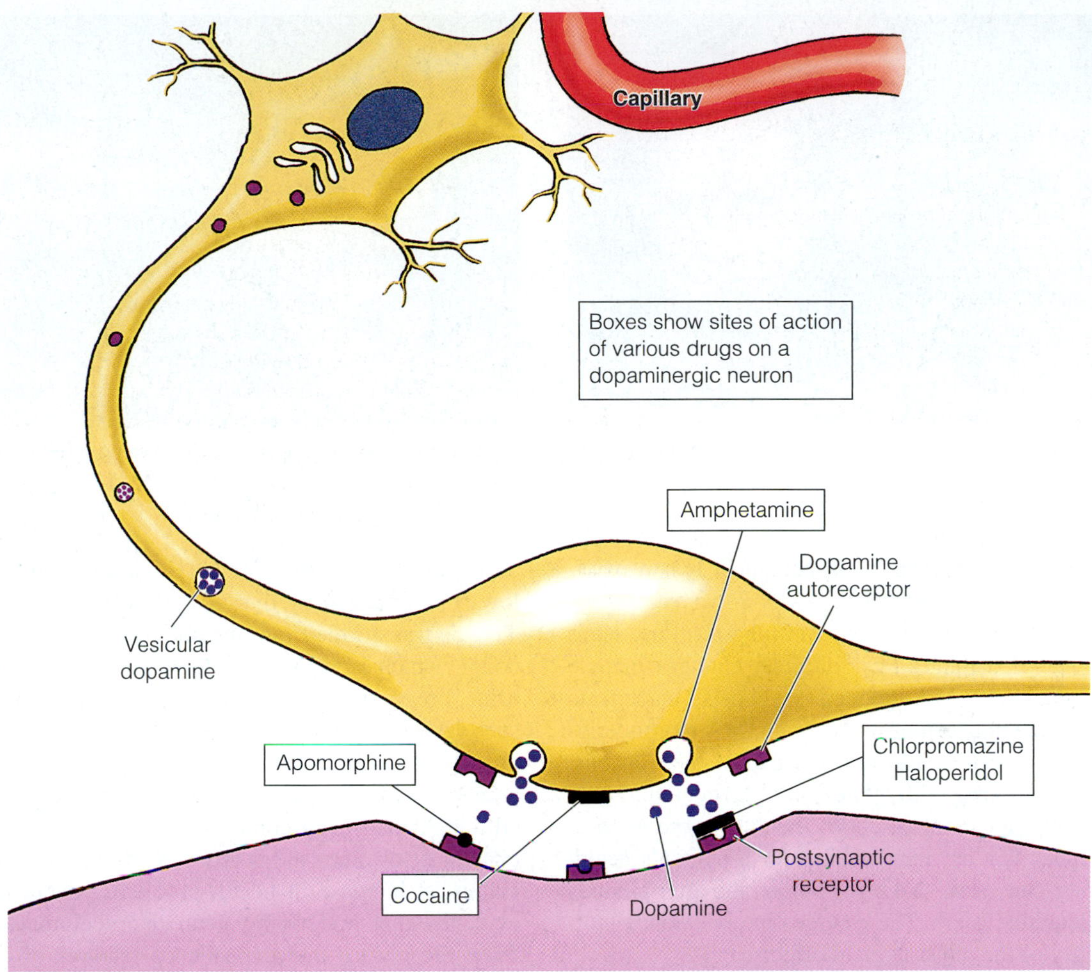

FIGURE 15-4 ■ Action of Drugs on Dopaminergic Neurons. Note how apomorphine can take the place of dopamine in the receptor and cocaine can block reception of a neurotransmitter instead of an antipsychotic.

Source: Smock, T. K. (1999). *Physiological psychology: A neuroscience approach.* Upper Saddle River, NJ: Prentice Hall.

der drugs for depression, management of obesity, and exhaustion. By the 1970s their dangers became known and today they are prescribed less frequently because alternative compounds are available to safely and effectively treat those symptoms. Amphetamines are still used to control appetite and treat depression, narcolepsy, minimal brain dysfunctions, and attention deficit disorders in children. Amphetamine abusers are usually teenagers or young adults who are looking for a good time. The uninformed—truck drivers on long road trips, students studying for exams, and athletes—hoping for alertness and improved performance can be lured into the "speed trap."

Amphetamine abusers crave these drugs and require higher and higher dosages. Abusers are rowdy, paranoid, and irritable. A "crash" (depression), often with suicidal symptoms, may last for several weeks. It is so uncomfortable that the user ingests more amphetamines in an attempt to feel better and develops a cyclical pattern of using and crashing.

Physiologically, the overuse of speed has been tied to stroke and death. Diazepam given intravenously decreases tachycardia and the chance of convulsions. Depression, anxiety, and increased stress symptoms are the most common psychological pitfalls in recovering from the use of speed. Changes in neurotransmitter activity increase the client's sensitivity to stress and may contribute to the spontaneous recurrence of amphetamine and methamphetamine psychosis, called flashbacks. Recurrent flashbacks contribute to recurrent major mood disorders (Barr et al., 2006).

Methamphetamine

The most hypercharged form of speed is methamphetamine (MA). It is less expensive than cocaine and has similar CNS stimulant characteristics. Recently methamphetamine use has become an enormous public health/substance abuse issue. Recipes for manufacturing MA in home drug labs using everyday ingredients (over-the-counter pseudoephedrine, starter fluids, and drain cleaner) are widely available and have influenced how these products are sold. For example, as a result of the Combat Methamphetamine Epidemic Act of 2005, pseudoephedrine is now stocked behind the pharmacist's counter and buyers, especially those who purchase pseudoephedrine frequently or in large quantities, can be tracked and reported. Lower-quality MA is called "speed" or "crank"; higher-quality MA is sold in small chunks as "glass"

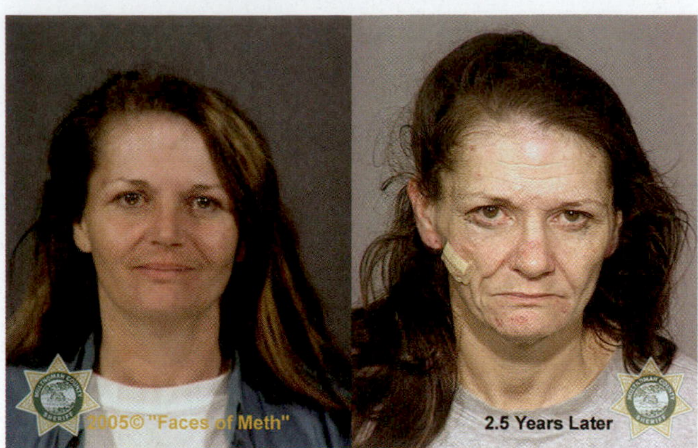

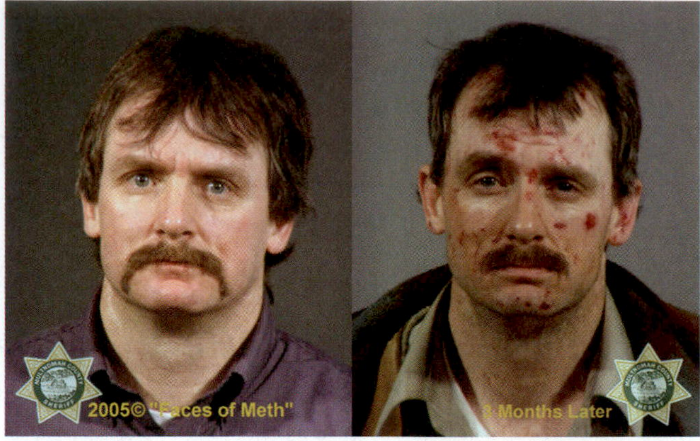

FIGURE 15-5 ■ Weight loss, apparent stress, and opportunistic infections are some of the visible consequences of using methamphetamine.
Source: Faces of Meth? Program.

or "ice" because of its crystalline appearance. It is a maximum stimulant with maximum risks.

Exposure to MA is neurotoxic, and long-term use leads to extensive neural damage. Physiological changes include cognitive impairments, MA-induced psychosis, inadequate perfusion, and ischemic lesions of the brain. MA morphologically changes the corpus callosum and causes skin lesions, perinatal complications, and hypertension (Arria et al., 2006; Barr et al., 2006; McGuinness, 2006). Each of these impacts has consequences that are far-reaching for a person's health and functioning. See FIGURE 15-5 ■ for before and after pictures of methamphetamine users. The changes in appearance indicate the severity of the physiological effects.

The National Survey on Drug Use and Health (NSDUH) Report (2007) on Methamphetamine Use is available online at www.oas.samhsa.gov/nhsda.htm and on the Companion Website for this text. Methamphetamine use is an enormous public health problem; however, its use among the civilian, noninstitutionalized population aged 12 or older declined overall between the 2002 and 2006 statistics. This is not a statistically significant decrease, but the trend is in the right direction.

MEDIALINK NSDUH Report

Withdrawal

Chlorpromazine (Thorazine) combats the physiologic effects of amphetamines. Diazepam (Valium), given intravenously, decreases tachycardia and the chance of convulsions. Depression and anxiety are the most common psychological pitfalls in recovering from the use of speed. Physiologically, the overuse of speed has been tied to stroke and even death.

CANNABIS

Marijuana arrived in North America in the early 1900s. Although it has been illegal in the United States since 1937, marijuana is used more than any other chemical except tobacco, alcohol, and caffeine.

The Effects of Cannabis

Derived from an Indian hemp plant (*Cannabis sativa*), marijuana contains the psychoactive substance delta 6-3,4-tetrahydrocannabinol (THC). THC is found in the sticky yellow resin secreted by the tops and leaves of the ripe plants. THC is transformed into metabolites in the body. Unlike alcohol, which is water-soluble and leaves the body through urine, breath, and perspiration, THC is stored in the fatty tissues (especially the brain and reproductive system). Consequently, it can be detected in the body for up to 6 weeks. The potency of marijuana has steadily increased over the years. Although marijuana contains over 400 chemicals, the THC content determines the potency. With an increase in potency comes an increase in health problems. There is compelling evidence that underlying neurochemical mechanisms reinforce the reward and dependence features of this drug and contribute to addiction (Fride et al., 2006).

Researchers have found that marijuana produces a significant analgesic effect and is modestly effective against the nausea and vomiting associated with chemotherapy. Medicinal applications of both THC and cannabidiol (a derivative) on pain have been examined, showing significant pain relief (Buttarelli et al., 2004; Trossman, 2006). Dronabinol is a synthetic delta 9-tetrahydrocannabinol or delta-9-THC that contains standardized THC content in an FDA-approved pharmaceutical. It is mainly used to treat weight loss, nausea, and vomiting associated with a number of medical conditions.

As of this writing, despite a Supreme Court ruling to the contrary, the federal Drug Enforcement Administration considers marijuana illegal and opposes its use for medical purposes. There remain legal conflicts regarding medical marijuana: a 1996 California law legalized some medical use of it, a federal law prohibits distribution or use of marijuana regardless of state law, and health care providers in seven states are allowed to discuss medical marijuana for pain relief without risking loss of license. The use of medical marijuana is a subject of continuing social and medical debate.

Patterns of Use

Marijuana smoking is prevalent among teenagers and young adults. Long-term marijuana use has been associated with both physical and emotional changes, as in the following clinical example.

CLINICAL EXAMPLE

Joe, a 35-year-old captain of a rescue squad, was having trouble at his job. He paid less and less attention to the accuracy of his client reports; he was often late for work; he forgot to repair and replace his equipment, causing his unit to be unsafe and ill equipped. Joe told an emergency room nurse that he felt all the marijuana he was smoking was beginning to affect him. He revealed that he'd been a daily smoker for 5 years. At first, he felt there were no long-term effects, but lately he was concerned because "I never feel like doing anything." He has trouble concentrating, forgets what he is talking about in midsentence, and is unmotivated to make any positive changes in his life.

Because marijuana smoking is so prevalent among teenagers and because its dangers are becoming increasingly known (see Box 15-2), some health care professionals advocate urine screening when teenagers have a checkup by a family doctor. Chemical dependence takes 10 to 15 years to develop in adults and only a few years to develop in a child. Only 25% of children in drug rehabilitation succeed, compared with 75% of adults. Because of this danger, pediatricians should initiate educational and treatment programs on drug and alcohol abuse. Likewise, psychiatric–mental health nurses need to respond to this vital public health issue.

For information on efforts to prevent and treat youth drug abuse, see the Center for Treatment Research on Adolescent Drug Abuse (CTRADA) website via the Companion Website for this book.

Box 15-2 Dangers of Marijuana

- Marijuana appears to lower testosterone levels in boys.
- In girls, hormone levels remain normal, but marijuana's chemicals may accumulate in the ovaries.
- Marijuana smoke has 50% more tar than regular cigarette smoke.
- Marijuana tar contains 70% more benzopyrene, a major cancer-causing chemical.
- Marijuana smoke produces greater cellular changes in the lungs than does tobacco smoke.
- Marijuana may cause emphysema 20 times faster than tobacco.
- Marijuana smoke increases airway resistance 25% under laboratory conditions in which a similar amount of tobacco smoke produces no significant increase in airway resistance.
- Brain wave tests show that teenagers who get high twice a week or more often have evidence of diffuse brain impairment for up to 2 months after the last time they use the drug. They experience disruptions in learning, short-term memory loss, problems concentrating, and amotivation syndrome (confusion, declining performance, and difficulty finishing tasks).
- After a person smokes marijuana, THC can be found in the blood and urine for up to 2 weeks; if the THC is radioactively labeled, it can be detected for up to a month.

Marijuana use is endemic in the teenage culture. Therefore, nurses who work with teenagers must be knowledgeable about marijuana and its effects. When admitting a teenager to a psychiatric unit or interviewing a teenager as an outpatient, be aware of a variety of indicators of marijuana use. Parents need to be knowledgeable about marijuana use and alert to indications that it is being used:

- Marijuana smells like hemp or burning rope.
- Teenagers often burn incense or use perfumed sprays to mask its pungent odor.
- Teenagers may use eyedrops (Murine) so that their eyes will not be red, and they may cough a lot. Conjunctival redness and coughing can occur with marijuana use.
- A teenager who uses marijuana may have smoking paraphernalia—plastic baggies filled with dried leaves, rolling papers, and "roach" clips (clips that hold the marijuana cigarette once it becomes too small to handle).

COCAINE

Since cocaine abuse has been recognized as a widespread problem, government agencies have spent significant amounts of money trying to block cocaine shipments from South America. Planes, boats, and "mules" (people who transport cocaine) have been seized, and tons of cocaine have been confiscated and destroyed. Yet, it remains plentiful and is purer today than ever before. The cocaine industry is a multibillion-dollar enterprise involving bribery, corruption, and murder.

MEDIALINK CTRADA

The Effects of Cocaine

Cocaine is a stimulant extracted from the leaves of the coca plant, found in Bolivia and Peru. It has long been known and used. For hundreds of years, South American Indians have chewed coca leaves, enjoying the effects of decreased appetite and increased ability to work at high altitudes. Slaves became more productive when given cocaine. Freud experimented with cocaine. It was an ingredient in Coca-Cola before federal regulations prohibited it in 1903. Today, cocaine is used as a local anesthetic in ear, nose, and throat surgery. When inhaled or injected, cocaine produces alertness and energy and makes users feel sociable, confident, and "in control." The drug blocks appetite and erases fatigue, which makes it appear to be an ideal performance booster.

MEDIALINK Animation: Cocaine Drug Mechanism in Action

Although cocaine is not believed to be physically addicting, it is psychologically addicting. Those who use cocaine heavily or regularly frequently encounter great difficulty in discontinuing its use. Cocaine addicts develop a tolerance to the drug, using amounts that would previously have been lethal to them. Euphoria diminishes with tolerance. The development of new dendrites (branches of the nerve cells) to aid the uptake of the increased amount of DA accounts for the tolerance. Ultimately, the cocaine no longer produces pleasure, but not taking it feels even worse. Dopamine is eventually depleted, and the user becomes chronically fatigued, irritable, and anxious, even mentally confused and paranoid, as in the clinical example that follows.

CLINICAL EXAMPLE

Will, a 32-year-old male, was brought to the hospital by his father. He was talkative and jumpy, and his eyes darted around the examining room. He repeatedly wiped his nose with his finger and rubbed the bottom of his face. He acted suspicious and kept saying someone was after him. His family stated he had a $400-a-day cocaine habit. He began casually snorting a few lines once in a while when he needed a sense of control over his full load of graduate school courses and full-time job. His cocaine use increased to every day, then every few hours.

Suicide attempts, accidents, and overdoses are common. The only effect of cocaine that is increased as tolerance develops is its ability to induce a convulsion or seizure. Be sure to carefully assess clients to differentiate the symptoms of cocaine use from the symptoms of bipolar disorder and chronic anxiety. Figure 15-6 ■ illustrates the cocaine use cycle.

Cocaine Intoxication

Interestingly, the symptoms of low-level cocaine intoxication are similar to those of alcohol withdrawal: sweating, dilated pupils, psychomotor agitation, and increased blood pressure/heart rate. With higher doses of cocaine, a person becomes increasingly intoxicated. Symptoms include high fever, cardiac arrhythmia, seizures, hallucinations, and a paranoid schizophrenic syndrome. Hallucinations typically involve "cocaine bugs," which feel like bugs under the skin. The client may scratch furiously in an attempt to get rid of them. Haloperidol (Haldol) is used to combat the psychotic symptoms; phenothiazines should not be used because they may decrease the seizure threshold.

The strength of the physiologic effects of cocaine is revealed in animal research. Monkeys work harder at pressing a bar to receive cocaine intravenously than to get any other drug. Even when starving to death or when confronted with a sexually receptive female, monkeys continue pressing the bar. Receiving an electric shock every time they touch the bar does not alter their behavior. Research with cocaine users indicates that the medication bromocriptine mesylate (Parlodel), a DA receptor agonist, eliminates the craving that users feel after they stop using cocaine. Cocaine initially increases DA neurotransmission. Over time, however, cocaine abuse depletes DA in the brain, and this depletion may be the basis for craving.

The "Post-Coke" Blues

It has not been proven that cocaine is physically addictive, but its ability to cause psychological dependence is clear (recall that cocaine users crave the drug). After a brief post-use euphoria (lasting approximately 5 to 10 minutes), they experience a strong desire to repeat the high. This high is followed by a crash—a terrible letdown called the "post-coke blues," or cocaine abstinence syndrome. Anxiety, depression, and fatigue are part of this syndrome. The cocaine crash, lasting approximately 30–60 minutes, results from depletion of DA, the neurotransmitter responsible for feelings of pleasure and well-being. The addict responds to the crash by feeling irritable, depressed, and tired. Although the brain needs to synthesize more DA (because of chemical misprogramming resulting from the addiction) it craves more cocaine, which offers immediate relief. The crash intensity appears to be related to the amount of cocaine used. In an attempt to feel better and reduce these uncomfortable symptoms, addicts often use other drugs, such as alcohol, marijuana, or sleeping pills, during the crash.

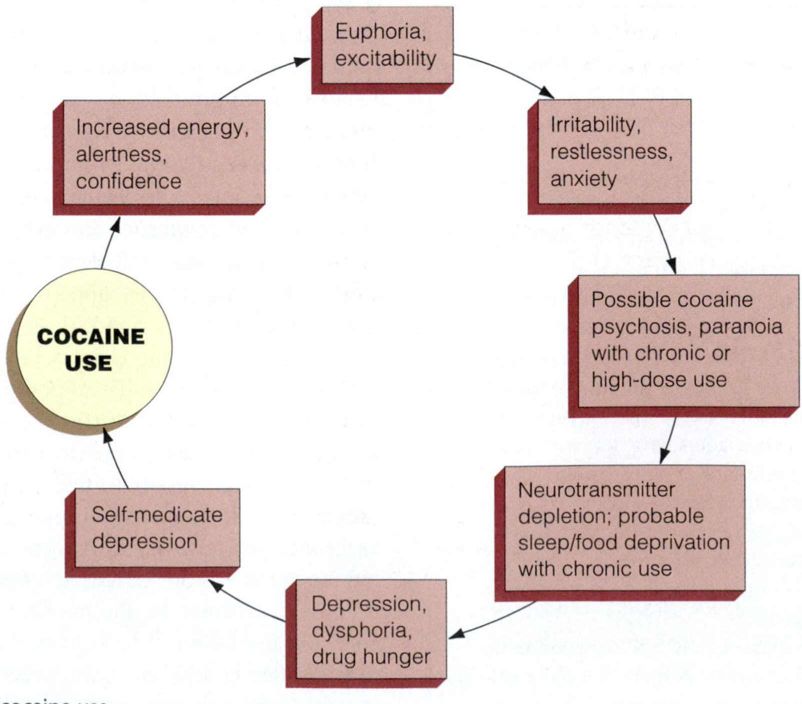

Figure 15-6 ■ The cycle of cocaine use.

Source: Reprinted with permission from Mim Landry, Danya International, Silver Spring, MD.

One addict described the post-coke blues as "pure hell, the most painful depression I have ever felt. I wanted to die from the pain." This painful depression, along with the memory of the cocaine high, causes people to want to use cocaine again and again to recapture the momentary ecstasy. The period of agitation, anxiety, and insomnia usually ceases within 2 weeks.

Patterns of Use

Cocaine is no longer just the chic, expensive drug of choice (the champagne of drugs) of young upwardly mobile professionals and celebrities. Smokable forms that have an effect similar to that of the injectable drug are in great demand. With the advent of cheaper rock cocaine, cocaine is now available to people in all cultural and socioeconomic groups.

For some years cocaine was believed to produce euphoria without addictive potential and without negative side effects. Lately, the horrors of cocaine abuse have been described in both lay and professional literature. Intranasal cocaine users place themselves at risk for hepatitis C. Those who inject cocaine place themselves at risk for HIV/AIDS as well as hepatitis C.

Treatment

Detoxification for cocaine abusers depends on the client's symptoms. In some treatment centers, the procedure is detoxification by going "cold turkey"; no medications are used to ease withdrawal symptoms. In some treatment centers 1–20 mg of diazepam is administered intravenously at a slow rate (not more than 5 mg/min). In other centers, cocaine abusers are treated with a diazepam protocol that lasts approximately 4 days; diazepam is decreased from 10 mg q4hr PO/IM to 5 mg q8hr PO/IM, with additional doses as needed if the client has withdrawal symptoms. Yet other centers have PRN diazepam protocols only. Another protocol involves the use of phenobarbital in decreasing doses and imipramine hydrochloride (Tofranil).

Because the depression is so great, Tofranil or other tricyclic antidepressants (TCAs) may be given for several weeks after detoxification. TCAs build up existing levels of neurotransmitters and make them available for transmission. Beta-adrenergic blockers such as propranolol (Inderal) may be used to counteract the tachycardia and hypertension that accompany acute cocaine intoxication, but their use may result in paroxysmal hypertension due to unopposed alpha-adrenergic stimulation. Therefore, they should be used cautiously and with constant blood pressure monitoring.

Using TCAs to increase the number of neurotransmitters in the synapse is called synaptic treatment. Postsynaptic treatment for cocaine withdrawal and dependence includes the use of medications such as bromocriptine (Parlodel) or amantadine (Symmetrel), which increase dopaminergic activity in the synapse and enhance the effects of DA on the postsynaptic receptors. Presynaptic treatment with amino acids such as tryptophan was used until 1989, when tryptophan was removed from the market because of several deaths associated with its use. These amino acids were prescribed because the body converted them to neurotransmitters, which had been depleted by cocaine abuse.

Crack

Crack, or "rock" cocaine, recently labeled "the most addictive drug known to man," is a potent form of hydrochloride cocaine that is mixed with baking soda and water, heated, allowed to harden, and then broken or "cracked" into little pieces and smoked in cigarettes or glass water pipes. Crack is more insidious, addictive, and toxic than cocaine. One user said, "I am worse in 3 weeks of using crack than in 6 years of using cocaine."

Crack is cheap and easily bought on the street or in special crack houses where people congregate to smoke. A crack high has a rapid onset and is intensely euphoric, followed by a dramatic crash. Within seconds after "coming down," users feel compelled to smoke more crack. Because addiction is so rapid, many people are "hooked" and seek help when they can no longer support their habit. Crack users are flooding treatment centers, many of which have long waiting lists. Recidivism is estimated at over 90%. See the Your Self-Awareness feature on page 342 for guidance in dealing with the frustration and discouragement common in work with substance-abusing clients.

Symptoms of Crack Use

Symptoms of crack use include irritability, paranoia, depression, and physical symptoms that accompany the smoking of a toxic chemical, such as wheezing and coughing blood and black phlegm. Cardiac dysrhythmias caused by crack use may lead to death.

The number of babies being born to mothers who use crack is growing. These babies are more likely to be premature or have low birth weights. They are irritable and exhibit tremors and muscle rigidity.

Freebase

Freebase is a purified form of cocaine made by applying solvents to ordinary cocaine. Melting the cocaine with small butane torches helps in the purifying and delivery process. This action alone is dangerous due to the hazard of the solvent exploding. The effects of freebase are brief but intense, and the short euphoria (3 to 5 minutes) immediately becomes a restless desire for more "base."

PHENCYCLIDINE (PCP)

PCP was originally used as an anesthetic for humans and as a tranquilizer for animals. Because of its dangerous side effects, it was removed from the market except for veterinary use. However, by the mid-1960s, PCP was readily available as a street drug. PCP is inexpensive and easily synthesized by home chemists, making a ready supply always available.

The Effects of PCP

People who use PCP frequently arrive at the emergency room in a psychotic, violent, and agitated state. The agitation and sensations generate incredible power and strength in the user

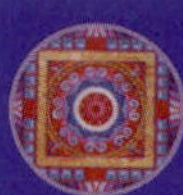

YOUR SELF-AWARENESS
Maintaining Therapeutic Optimism

- **Realize that both mental illness and substance disorders are chronic, relapsing conditions.** *Understand that progress may be slow and setbacks inevitable despite your best efforts and those of the client. Appreciate small steps forward and reframe setbacks as learning opportunities.*
- **Understand that even if a client is not currently making much effort toward better management of his or her disorders, the development of a trusting relationship with you is helping to set the stage for movement toward recovery in the future.** *A positive, valued relationship with a mental health professional is one of the factors that prompt mental health clients to move toward sobriety.*
- **Talk to people who are in recovery.** *Hearing about how these individuals overcame challenges to become happier and more stable will give you more confidence that clients who are currently struggling with similar obstacles can also overcome them.*
- **Don't be afraid to talk to clients about spirituality.** *Mental health providers often underestimate how important spiritual concerns are in the lives of clients with substance disorders. Ask clients about their spiritual beliefs and practices, and be flexible in helping clients find support for their spirituality. Access to these inner resources is especially important when clients lack external support.*
- **Find mentors who are successful in working with clients with substance disorders.** *Seek their help in dealing with situations you find difficult or frustrating.*
- **Take good care of your own physical, mental, and spiritual health.** *You can role-model healthy behavior for clients (never underestimate the power of a good example!), and renewing your own energy means you have more to give in your relationships with clients.*

so that even a small, slight person is capable of breaking heavy glass or fighting several people.

CLINICAL EXAMPLE

Pete, an 18-year-old college student, was offered marijuana at a fraternity party. After smoking several joints, he was driving home with a friend when he became severely agitated. He insisted his friend stop the car near a pay phone; he jumped out and attempted to call the police, believing someone was trying to kill him. When the police arrived because of the disturbance he was causing (by then he was shouting and hallucinating), he rushed them, kicking at a passerby and shooting at them as if he had a gun. During an assessment interview, the friend confessed to putting PCP in the marijuana.

Some users fluctuate between coma and violence. Hallucinations are common. A differential diagnosis is important but difficult because the symptoms are similar to those of schizophrenia. It is believed that schizophrenics are particularly sensitive to PCP and that PCP may aggravate symptoms of schizophrenia.

A PCP high appears about 5 minutes after a person takes the drug and lasts 4 to 6 hours. Effects may last up to 48 hours. PCP may be recovered from the blood and urine for 7 to 10 days. While using PCP, a person experiences a wide variety of feelings ranging from euphoria and utter peace to violence, confusion, and disorganization. Distorted sensory perceptions are common. During a bad "trip," anxiety, fear, and paranoia predominate. The dramatic physical and emotional effects of PCP may last for several weeks. Users may suffer from depression, fatigue, memory loss, concentration difficulty, and poor impulse control.

A substance very similar to PCP is ketamine, also known as Special K, K, Vitamin K, and Cat Valium, among other names. Distorted perceptions of sight and sound and feelings of detachment—dissociation—from the environment and self are mind-altering but not hallucinations. PCP and ketamine are therefore more properly known as "dissociative anesthetics." Dextromethorphan, a widely available cough suppressant, when taken in high doses can produce effects similar to those of PCP and ketamine. Dissociative drugs act by altering distribution of the neurotransmitter glutamate throughout the brain. Glutamate is involved in perception of pain, responses to the environment, and memory. PCP is considered the typical dissociative drug, and the description of PCP's actions and effects largely applies to ketamine and dextromethorphan as well (Lofwall, Griffiths, & Mintzer, 2006).

Ketamine has a much shorter duration of action than PCP and is used recreationally because of its sedative and hallucinogenic properties. It can cause delirium, amnesia, tachycardia, anxiety, and high blood pressure. Ketamine use increases every year, as does the use of the club drug GHB and Rohypnol (the date rape drug, discussed later in this chapter and in Chapter 24∞). More young people are discovering these dangerous drugs.

A vital problem with PCP is the question of its purity and concentration. Because it is generally manufactured illegally, users never really know what they are buying. Adulterants used in street drugs are often toxic to humans, causing a wide variety of responses, including death. Originally called the "peace pill," PCP is now recognized for its potential to cause violence, especially when the drug is taken in high dosages.

Treatment

Treatment of acute PCP intoxication may include the use of diazepam (Valium) for muscle spasms, seizures, and agitation. Risperidone (Risperdal) or haloperidol (Haldol) may be used for severe psychotic behavior, but phenothiazines should not be used because PCP is anticholinergic. The combined anticholinergia of phenothiazines and PCP creates a number of severe side effects, including hallucinations. Calcium channel blockers such as verapamil may be given. These drugs are thought to prevent or reverse PCP-induced vasospasm, thereby decreasing the hallucinogenic effects of PCP. This treatment is controversial, however, because some clinicians believe that the use of verapamil may potentiate the effects of PCP.

Treatment during the acute phase of PCP intoxication should focus also on protecting the client and others from injury and reorienting the client to reality. Providing a quiet, safe environment and addressing the client in a calm, reassuring manner are important.

HALLUCINOGENS

Hallucinogens are synthetic and natural drugs that cause hallucinations and unusual sensory experiences. Developed in 1938 for scientific research, LSD (lysergic acid diethylamide) became popular in the 1960s when Timothy Leary, a Harvard psychologist, described how it stimulated great insight and increased awareness. In the 1960s and 1970s, the U.S. Army experimented with LSD by giving it without informed consent to unsuspecting army employees. One dramatic and much-publicized event concerned an army officer who leapt to his death from a window after unknowingly ingesting LSD. Once the danger of LSD use was publicized, the unethical research became public knowledge. Physician researchers also were interested in experimenting with the uses of LSD in the treatment of a variety of diseases; however, in 1966 LSD became illegal and could no longer be used in human research.

Peyote, the active hallucinogen in cactus buttons, is still an integral part of religious rituals of Native Americans in the southwestern United States and Mexico. Psilocybin is the active hallucinogen in certain mushrooms, sometimes called "magic mushrooms."

The Effects of Hallucinogens

After a lull in use, LSD ("acid") is again being used by teenagers because it is cheap ($2 to $5 a "hit") and causes an intense high that lasts 6 to 12 hours. It is typically delivered orally, usually on absorbent blotter paper (FIGURE 15-7 ■), a sugar cube, or gelatin. Teenagers today are unacquainted with the LSD horror stories of the 1960s. Today, people use LSD predominantly to get high rather than to expand consciousness. Psychological and physical dependence are unlikely because each experience with a hallucinogen is different.

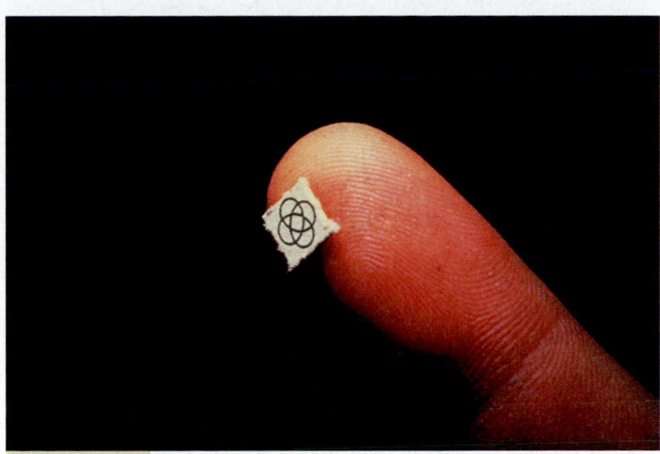

FIGURE 15-7 ■ Blotter LSD. Both LSD and the psilocybin in "magic mushrooms" induce psychedelic effects; however, LSD is much more potent than psilocybin (a product of various kinds of mushrooms).

Source: Custom Medical Stock Photo, Inc.

CLINICAL EXAMPLE

Two high school seniors decided to take LSD. After 8 hours, one student was enjoying music, describing the varied colors he saw as the music changed in tempo. The other student was sweating profusely. His pupils were dilated, and he was trembling. He saw brightly colored dogs with huge teeth and claws changing into cats, snakes, and lions. He said he felt his gallbladder working with his liver and stomach. He eventually became so out of control that the other student took him to the emergency room.

Increased creativity and brilliant personality revelations, presumed effects of the drugs, are short-lived at best.

Treatment

The dangers of hallucinogens include "bad trips" and flashbacks.

Bad Trips

Users who experience *bad trips* may appear psychotic and extremely fearful. Reassuring the person and pointing out reality are helpful; occasionally, tranquilizers or antipsychotics are given. The symptoms usually disappear within 12 hours but may persist for months. People who are mentally ill or emotionally conflicted are more likely to have bad trips and flashbacks and to require hospitalization than are ordinary users.

Flashbacks

Flashbacks are a spontaneous reliving of the experiences the person felt while under the influence of the drug, although the person is drug free. The experience may involve perceptual distortions, a variety of physical feelings, and strong emotions such as fear and pleasure. Flashbacks are generally brief, and they occur less frequently over time. Flashbacks may be induced by stress, fatigue, and drug or alcohol ingestion.

Some authorities believe hallucinogens pose a particular danger to adolescents in that they may precipitate a psychosis. Because teenagers' egos and defenses are weak, they may be especially susceptible to the effects of hallucinogens.

INHALANTS

Inhalants—glue, fuels, paints, aerosols, air fresheners, the substance used to resole shoes, hairspray, and the propellants in canned whipped cream—are popular among school-age children because they are cheap and easy to obtain. An unusual new development in preferences for inhalants has recently been noted: embalming fluid.

The Effects of Inhalants

The abuse of inhalants is increasing at a frightening rate. Inhalants are inexpensive, easily available, and often legal. Their use causes euphoria, light-headedness, and excitement. Children are the most frequent users.

> **CLINICAL EXAMPLE**
>
> Carlos is an 11-year-old homeless child from Brazil living on the streets in Miami, Florida. He came to the attention of the clinic because he had been arrested for purse snatching. On clinical examination, Carlos appears giddy, dirty, disheveled, confused, and belligerent. His speech is slurred, he has an unsteady gait, and he smells like glue. His eyes are red and tearing, he is coughing, and he is nauseated. He has avoided attending school and has received no health care.

Adult users often have a long history of polydrug abuse.

Patterns of Use

Inhalants are sniffed or inhaled (called "huffing") in a variety of ways, such as from a rag soaked with the inhalant and placed in a plastic bag. Gas is frequently inhaled directly from a tank. Amyl and butyl nitrate (called "poppers") can be easily concealed and passed around a classroom, and paint thinner can be concealed in a soft drink can. Use of these inhalants and solvents can cause ventricular fibrillation, decreased cardiac output, serious brain damage, and sudden death.

Treatment

Although withdrawal must be managed as with the other substances covered in this chapter, careful assessment, early identification, detoxification, education, and prevention are particularly critical because so many inhalant abusers are children under the age of 12. Nurses need to be aware of the programs and resources available and should support legislation to make it more difficult for minors to obtain glue and paint products.

NICOTINE

Nicotine is the psychoactive stimulating substance found in tobacco. The behavioral and physiological effects of nicotine frequently lead to addiction. Access to this legal drug for adults endangers those under the legal smoking age. Populations with psychiatric conditions and substance abuse problems have higher rates of smoking and show a lack of responsiveness to smoking cessation treatments (Ranney et al., 2006).

The Effects of Nicotine

Nicotine is a stimulant that acts in the central and peripheral nervous systems at cells that are normally acted upon by the neurotransmitter acetylcholine. In the CNS, nicotine occupies the receptors for acetylcholine in both dopamine and serotonin neural pathways. This causes the release of both dopamine and norepinephrine. The stimulant nicotine initially increases alertness and cognitive ability, and then has a depressant effect.

Research suggests that dopaminergic processes have a role in regulating the reinforcing effects of nicotine, making cessation of use more difficult. Dopamine blockers can alter smoking behavior for a limited time, but people compensate for this by smoking more (Glover, 2006). The usual effect of increased dopamine turnover in the system is the reduction of hunger impulses. Once someone tries to quit smoking and dopamine is reduced, hunger impulses return and the person may gain weight.

Although smoking rates in the general population have fallen over the past 25 years from 34% in 1980 to close to 22% in 2005 (Hoeppner et al., 2006; Ranney et al., 2006), smoking is still of concern given its negative physiological impact. Nicotine is associated with cancer, heart disease, emphysema, hypertension, and death.

Patterns of Use

Smoking cigarettes is an extremely common addiction and is seen routinely despite smoke-free environments and restrictions on cigarette access. Approximately 46 million adults and 4.5 million adolescents in the United States smoke. There are also socioeconomic differences in smoking rates; the highest rates are among those living below the poverty line. Cigarette and cigar smoking is more common among unemployed adults aged 18 or older than among adults who are working full-time or part-time. This is especially true with psychiatric–mental health clients. Their work activities may be dictated by their symptom level and they frequently experience unemployment.

Typically, people begin smoking at a young age, because of peer pressure, or during times of stress. Use of tobacco products can be interrupted briefly during respiratory illnesses, hospitalizations, pregnancy, and following health care providers' advice on smoking cessation. Return to tobacco use after a brief time is all too common; smokers find it very difficult to quit smoking successfully. Long-term quit rates range from 10% to 25%, including pharmacological cessation

TABLE 15-2 ■ The Transtheoretical Model (TTM) of Behavior Change

TTM explains the stages and processes of change. Knowing how change occurs throughout the stages, how decisional balance impacts the process of change, an individual's vision of self-efficacy, and how temptation is likely to be handled, make this perspective a useful one for promoting change.

Stage	Processes and Principles
1. Precontemplation	The client does not intend to change the health behavior in the near future, usually a 6-month period of time.
	The client avoids communication designed to help change occur.
2. Contemplation	The client does intend to change the health behavior in the next 6 months.
	There is awareness of the benefits of change, but the barriers to change are being attended to and ambivalence is potent.
3. Preparation	The client intends to make the change in the next month.
	A plan of action is developed with small, important steps taken toward change.
4. Action	The client overtly modifies risky behavior and makes the change.
	Considerable time and energy are necessary in order to resist reverting to previous risky behaviors.
5. Maintenance	The client works to prevent relapse.
	Temptation gradually recedes over 6 months to 5 years. This stage is meant to extend through the client's life.

support (nicotine replacement systems, psychopharmacology) (Evans et al., 2006; Killen et al., 2006). Evidence indicates that smoke-free environments only protect people from the force of secondhand smoke but do not reduce actual smoking. Smokers practice anticipatory smoking to assure their desired level of nicotine is maintained (Doweiko, 2006).

Treatment

The most commonly used approach for treating nicotine dependence is nicotine replacement therapies (patch, inhaler, lozenge, gum), which reduce craving by maintaining the blood level of nicotine. Bupropion (Zyban), an antidepressant, has demonstrated effectiveness in shorter-term abstinence. Support in a variety of forms is also useful in assisting clients with this difficult addiction. Office-based nursing and centralized telephone counseling services with an emphasis on relapse prevention have demonstrated long-term abstinence effectiveness (Hoeppner et al., 2006). Educational programs designed to enhance the smoking cessation knowledge base of health care providers in prenatal, pediatric, and community health are needed to promote effective treatment of nicotine dependence (Klesges et al., 2006). There are some newer treatments for nicotine addiction (including the use of laser, auricular acupuncture, and magnets) that have not been rigorously researched yet, but there is reason to believe that results are promising.

Every person trying to make a change in behavior must go through transitional stages before, during, and after the change is made. The transtheoretical model of behavior change (TTM) has been applied successfully in the treatment of substance abuse as well as to co-occurring disorders (Finnell & Osborne, 2006). TTM describes a continuum of five stages of behavior change and the processes of movement from stage to stage. The stages, processes, and principles that undergird the theory are described in TABLE 15-2 ■. You will find that the transtheoretical model can help you to understand health care behaviors in other clinical areas throughout your nursing career.

CAFFEINE

Caffeine is available in a number of products: coffee, tea, chocolate, and some pain relievers. It is a common substance totally integrated into our social and occupational lives. In the United States more than half the population over the age of 10 drinks coffee. As with most other foodstuffs, an excessive intake of caffeine is not recommended; around 300 mg per day is safe for most people. Over 600 mg per day is considered excessive.

Coffee has variable amounts of caffeine, depending on its preparation method; there are 64 mg of caffeine in a cup of instant coffee and 150 mg in a cup of filter coffee. A cup of coffee contains two or three times more caffeine than a cup of tea or chocolate. The amount of caffeine in tea varies according to the plant variety and how long the tea is brewed—the longer it is brewed, the higher the caffeine level—but on average a 6-ounce cup of tea contains 40 mg of caffeine. The average amount of caffeine ingested by a coffee-drinking adult each day is around 360 to 450 mg (Iso et al., 2006). TABLE 15-3 ■ on page 346 lists the caffeine content of selected beverages and drugs.

The Effects of Caffeine

Caffeine acts as a stimulant, increasing the heart rate and stimulating the CNS. It is also a diuretic. There is evidence that a relationship exists between the amount of coffee consumption, total cholesterol, and low-density lipoprotein (LDL) cholesterol levels (Lopez-Garcia et al., 2006). The greater the amount of caffeine ingested, the higher the total

TABLE 15-3 ■ Caffeine Content of Certain Beverages and Drugs

Source	Approximate Caffeine Content per 5 oz/dose
Beverages	
Drip coffee	56–176 mg (average 112)
Percolated coffee	39–168 (average 74)
Instant coffee	29–117 (average 66)
Decaffeinated coffee	1–8 mg (average 3)
Tea (bag or leaf)	30–91 mg (average 27)
Cocoa	2–7 mg (average 4)
Cola drinks (12 oz)	30–46 mg
Jolt (12 oz)	71.2 mg
Red Bull (8.2 oz)	80 mg
Over-the-Counter Drugs	
Analgesics	
Aspirin (plain)	0 mg
Anacin, Bromo Seltzer, Cope, Empirin Compound, Midol	32 mg
Excedrin	65 mg
Vanquish	33 mg
Diuretics	
Aqua-Ban	100 mg
Stimulants	
NoDoz	100 mg
Vivarin	200 mg
Caffedrine	250 mg
Weight Control Aids	
Dexatrim	200 mg
Dietac	200 mg

cholesterol and LDL cholesterol levels. Peak concentrations of caffeine are achieved 30 to 60 minutes after ingestion, and it takes around 3 hours to clear the system.

If coffee is withdrawn suddenly from people who drink large quantities of filtered coffee (six or more cups a day), they may become irritable and can even suffer from headaches. Strong coffee is capable of causing palpitations. Given the stimulant effect of caffeine, it makes sense to advise those who complain of insomnia to switch to decaffeinated coffee or to have their last cup of coffee at least 3 hours before going to bed. Since tea has much less caffeine per cup than coffee, it does not have such a strong stimulating effect. However, if there is a complaint of insomnia, it is worth not drinking large quantities of tea just before going to bed to address that problem. Because of its stimulant properties, very young children should not drink coffee.

The negative physiologic effects of caffeine, especially those related to cardiac risks, are of grave concern. There have been variable research outcomes in this regard; however, it has become clear that some of the difficulty results from the use of both coffee and nicotine. The risk of congestive heart failure and death is much more competently explained by smoking and high serum-cholesterol levels in combination with caffeine use than with caffeine ingestion alone (Lopez-Garcia et al., 2006).

Patterns of Use

People who use caffeine use it for its stimulant properties. It is typically taken upon awakening, during times of low energy or fatigue, and when an external source of comfort is required. Once a pattern of use has been established, individuals continue to use caffeine in order to avoid withdrawal symptoms. Smokers also continue to smoke to avoid the symptoms of nicotine withdrawal.

Treatment

Reduction-of-harm modes of caffeine ingestion have been successful. The individual decreases the overall intake of the substance vehicle (such as coffee or tea), begins using decaffeinated mixtures in increasing proportions, then completes the effort by ceasing to ingest caffeine. This process weans the individual from the substance without causing, or by at least minimizing, jarring and uncomfortable withdrawal symptoms. Treatment facilities frequently limit or restrict access to caffeinated beverages so that interference from their stimulating effects does not complicate psychiatric treatment. Advance planning for alternatives to caffeine in social and occupational situations is helpful.

POLYDRUG USE

Most substance abusers today are polydrug users, that is, they abuse more than one drug. This fact complicates diagnosis and treatment and increases the hazards associated with abuse. The impact of these multiple drugs on each other and on our clients occurs in a variety of ways:

- *Synergistic or potentiating effects* are possible where the effects of two or more drugs taken together are greater than the singular effects of each drug.
- *Additive effects* occur when two drugs that have similar effects are used together.
- *Paradoxical effects* occur if a drug causes a reaction opposite to that expected. Paradoxical effects may occur when only one drug is taken or when several drugs are taken.
- A *pathologic reaction* may also result from the ingestion of only one or several drugs; it is an unexpected and dramatic response to the drug. For example, the combination of alcohol and marijuana is especially dangerous because THC suppresses the nausea that results from an overdose of alcohol. Consequently, the person may continue to drink, risking respiratory depression, coma, and death.

Cocaine and alcohol are frequently used together; the cocaine gives the user a brief high, and the alcohol masks the ensuing depression. When the cocaine wears off, the person is intoxicated and unable to drive safely. Prescription drugs and alcohol are also a common combination. For up-to-date information on drugs of abuse, prevention, and treatment, see the resources and links listed in the Companion Website for this text.

As illustrated in the clinical example on PCP on page 342, polydrug use can be inadvertent. Marijuana is often laced with PCP. In recent years dealers have also been putting heroin in marijuana. When heroin is smoked, it becomes a hidden addiction. The individual smokes more marijuana, increasing the amount of heroin needed to get the same high. The move from marijuana use to heroin use is then completed.

DESIGNER DRUGS

According to the Controlled Substance Act of 1970, controlled substances (federally regulated substances) are classified from I (most regulated) through V, according to the potential for abuse and the current accepted medical use. As new information is made available, drugs may be reclassified. Designer drugs, also called "club drugs," are chemical derivatives of controlled drugs. They are called analog drugs because they retain properties of controlled drugs but one molecule is changed, making them initially not classifiable as controlled.

Produced by underground and cottage industry chemists, analog drugs are initially legal until the government has them analyzed and researched by chemists. Once a dangerous pattern of use is determined (often 3 to 6 months after police discover the drug), the drug may be classified as a controlled substance.

Fentanyl citrate (Sublimaze), a synthetic anesthetic agent, is similar chemically to some designer drugs. Fentanyl is 100 times as strong as morphine and 20 to 40 times as strong as heroin. It provides a fast rush and an extraordinary high. A person can become addicted after one shot of fentanyl.

Methylenedioxymethamphetamine, also called Ecstasy, X, MDMA, Adam, XTC, Clarity, and Lover's Speed, has recently been classified as a Schedule I narcotic because research demonstrates that it causes structural damage to the brain. It is an amphetamine with hallucinogenic properties with effects lasting 3 to 6 hours. Currently, Ecstasy is the drug of choice for adolescents. It is easily and readily accessible. In high doses, MDMA has been associated with malignant hyperthermia and rhabdomyolysis.

MTPT (China white), an analog of meperidine (Demerol), has an adverse reaction similar to the rigidity caused by Parkinson's disease.

Flunitrazepam, also known as Rohypnol, Roofies, Rophies, the Date-Rape Pill, and the Forget-Me Pill, is a fast-acting benzodiazepine that causes anterograde amnesia (memory loss of events occurring while under the influence of the drug) and is tasteless, colorless, and odorless. Because it can be used to sexually victimize women when mixed into drinks, it is the modern-day version of a Mickey Finn (alcohol and chloral hydrate). Another date-rape substance is gamma-hydroxybutyrate (called GHB, G, Liquid Ecstasy, Grievous Bodily Harm, and Georgia Home Boy). It produces euphoria and disinhibition, is used by body builders because of its anabolic properties, and is available on the Internet and in health food stores (Wu, Schlenger, & Galvin, 2007).

GROUPS AT RISK FOR SUBSTANCE ABUSE

People in a number of different circumstances can use and abuse a substance. However, there are those who are at greater risk for substance problems than others.

Teenagers

Drug abuse among teenagers is pervasive in our society. Although many adolescents experiment with drugs for only a brief time, many more who do so become addicted. Susceptibility to addiction seems to depend on several variables:

- Form and potency of the drug
- Dosage
- Frequency of use
- Pattern of use
- Stress
- Personality and genetic makeup of the user
- Family culture

People use drugs that initially produce good feelings to escape from the stress and strain of life. A teenager who relies on a quick "fix" (a drug) to ease mental pain does not learn healthy coping skills. If teenagers do not learn healthy coping skills or work through the pains and mood swings associated with living, they fail to complete a necessary developmental stage. Consequently, they remain fixated at a dependent level of development. They enter a dangerous cycle that is unlikely to be interrupted without professional intervention. Drug use, regardless of what drug is used, inevitably affects all areas of a teenager's life: school, work, social and family relationships, and sense of self-worth. (See Chapter 27 ∞ for an assessment of teenage drug use.)

Adolescent drug users manifest more psychopathologic conditions than nonusing adolescents do. Symptoms include feelings of depression, inadequacy, frustration, helplessness, and self-alienation. These teenagers also have ego structure deficiencies and poor impulse control. The earlier a child begins using a dependence-producing drug, the more likely the child is to use other dependence-producing drugs. Teenagers who use alcohol and drugs are likely to continue to use them in adulthood (Wu, Schlenger, & Galvin, 2006).

Psychiatric Clients with Coexisting Substance Abuse Disorders

Nurses need to be alert to possible, and very likely, substance abuse by psychiatric clients. Problems may occur if clients take a combination of substances, and treatment is hindered if clients are under the influence of drugs or alcohol. There are a number of different ways to refer to psychiatric clients who use substances. *Mentally ill chemical abusers (MICAs), chemically abusing mentally ill (CAMI), co-occurring mental and substance use disorders,* and *dual diagnosis* (referring to both a mental illness and substance abuse diagnosis), among others, are terms that try to explain the coexistence of two or more demanding and divergent disorders. The numerous

MediaLink Information on Polydrug Use

MediaLink Critical Thinking Exercise: Substance Abuse in a Vulnerable Population

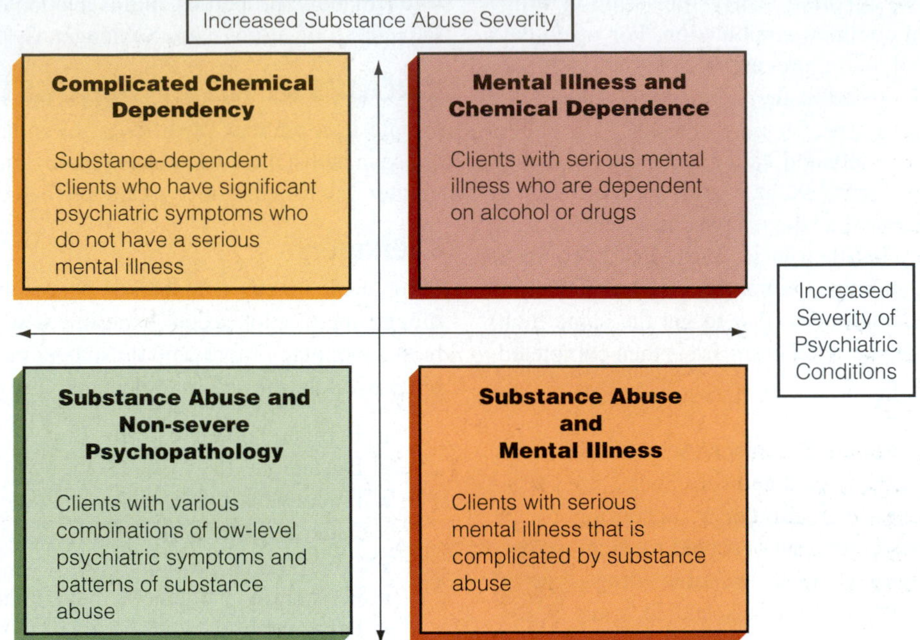

FIGURE 15-8 ■ Characteristics of clients with coexisting disorders.

problems facing psychiatric–mental health clients make them susceptible to both substance use and targeting by drug dealers. Poor coping mechanisms, heightened stress, economic factors, and challenging and demoralizing illnesses influence a client's ability to steer clear of the escapism drugs offer. The characteristics of clients who have coexisting disorders are discussed in FIGURE 15-8 ■.

It is estimated that between 16% and 60% of psychiatric clients have a substance use or abuse issue. In the United States, integrated substance abuse/mental health treatment is lacking (Liddie & Rowe, 2006). Both types of disorders are chronic, and clients tend to relapse. You should ask clients directly if they are taking drugs. In most psychiatric hospitals, urine is routinely tested for the presence of drugs if there is suspicion of use. Drug screening is usually carried out on admission and when the client returns from a pass. Close observation of teenagers and their visitors is also useful.

Treatment programs for clients with psychiatric and substance use/abuse problems are best constructed with a reduction-of-harm perspective and built-in extensive psychosocial supports. Because this combination creates consequences (see Box 15-3) of which people may not be aware, it is important to educate yourself and your clients. Staff members with credentials in psychiatry and substance treatment and rehabilitation work collaboratively with the client to manage the numerous chaotic upheavals characteristic of either one of the disorders at any time. When a client with these problems is treated in a setting designed for one or the other disorder, not both, the client is not likely to receive the specialized care for his or her condition.

The same demographic factors that are associated with substance use disorders in the general population affect people with mental illness. Being male, unmarried, young adult, and poor are associated with a higher risk of substance abuse.

Box 15-3 Consequences of Using Substances When Having a Serious Mental Illness

- Increased psychiatric symptoms
- Poor treatment adherence
- Increased need for, and use of, emergency health care services
- Poor response to psychiatric medications
- Unstable clinical course
- Increased frequency and length of hospitalization
- Chronic threats to health
- Increased risk of tardive dyskinesia
- Behavioral problems
- Suicide
- Homelessness
- Violence

CLINICAL EXAMPLE

Ian is a 25-year-old man who was diagnosed with schizophrenia 6 years ago, when he was a student at a local junior college. After becoming ill, Ian lost most of his friends because he was preoccupied with a delusional relationship with a radio talk-show host and spent most of his time alone in his room. He dropped out of college because his mental disorganization and frequent psychiatric hospitalizations interfered with his ability to attend classes. He has tried several times to work, but has not been able to keep a job.

After Ian's most recent hospitalization, he moved into a supervised residence for psychiatric clients and began receiving biweekly injections of a long-acting neuroleptic medication. He became much less delusional and started making friends. Several months ago, Ian and two of his male friends from the halfway house moved into an apartment in a neighborhood known for its high incidence of crack cocaine use.

Ian's case manager believes Ian is using crack. He has lost weight, become aggressive and paranoid, and has been threatened with eviction for failing to pay his rent. Ian was brought to psychiatric emergency services by the police after becoming agitated and threatening the cashier in a convenience store. Ian's urine toxicology screening was positive for cocaine.

People with coexisting disorders display a wide range of clinical characteristics and service needs, depending on the nature and severity of their psychiatric and substance-related problems (Kessler et al., 2005).

Gender Differences

Since men and women have different rates of substance use disorders and different rates of some psychiatric disorders, gender differences in the range of coexisting psychiatric and substance use disorders also exist. Women have a lower prevalence of all types of substance use disorders when compared to men; however, women—across ethnic groups—often have more serious and disabling medical complications from alcohol dependence.

Women are more likely to have preexisting mood and/or anxiety disorders than men. They are also reported to link their substance abuse with specific past traumas such as physical or sexual abuse much more often than men do. Women are much less likely to have antisocial personality disorder, which is a significant risk factor for substance use disorders.

Women tend to undergo treatment earlier, possibly due to their increased comfort with socialization and accessing help systems, or perhaps because of more rapid escalation of medical and social consequences. Women often have different motivations for entering treatment, such as child custody concerns.

Biologic Aspects

Biologic, as well as psychological, factors are thought to contribute to the use of drugs and alcohol to self-medicate the symptoms of mental illness. Some substances of abuse may stimulate neurotransmitter systems in the brain that have been altered both by the disease and by some of the agents used to treat schizophrenia. Animal studies indicate that addictive agents increase activity in brain systems dependent on dopamine (DA), a neurotransmitter whose functioning is altered in schizophrenia. The use of stimulants by people with schizophrenia may be seen as an attempt to "normalize" certain brain functions that have been impaired by the disease. In addition, nicotine relieves problems with sensory processing caused by schizophrenia and counteracts side effects of psychotropic medication, which may help to explain the extremely high frequency of smoking in this group (Evans et al., 2006).

Although substance use may produce symptom relief, it is often true that this decrease in symptoms is short lived and likely to be followed by an exacerbation of symptoms. It is also true that the same substance may relieve some psychiatric symptoms and worsen others—for example, stimulants may briefly elevate depressed mood and increase energy, but exacerbate anxiety and psychotic symptoms.

Women

Although alcoholism is a greater stigma for women than men, more women than ever before are drinking today. Many of these women are also using other drugs. Women respond to alcohol somewhat differently than men do because they metabolize alcohol less effectively than men. The vast majority of studies on substance abuse used male participants, creating gaps in our understanding of the neuropsychological effects of substances on women (Medina, Shear, & Schafer, 2006). Research on women and alcohol makes it clear that treatment programs should be geared to women's needs. Such programs might include women-only groups, lesbian-only groups, female therapists, meetings with recovered women alcoholics/addicts, and help for the client families.

General Hospital Clients

Nurses who work in general hospitals must be alert to the possibility that clients with physical illnesses may be substance abusers and may be in danger of withdrawal. If you see symptoms that do not mesh with the condition under treatment, you may want to keep in mind that you may be seeing symptoms of substance withdrawal. Be alert and sensitive if physical assessment reveals any of the following:

- Debilitation out of proportion to the presenting health problem
- Physical findings that do not correlate to the chief complaint
- Unsteady gait, slurring of speech, dilated pupils, night sweats, chills, blackouts, tremors, skin tracks, abscesses, nasal septum perforation, or jaundice
- Weight loss, poor hygiene, and poor nutrition
- Symptoms of substance withdrawal
- Failure to attain pain relief with the usual and customary dosage of medication

Alert the primary health care provider and suggest appropriate laboratory studies (such as liver function tests). A nursing assessment may include questions about a client's drinking habits. If alcoholism is suspected, a helpful, matter-of-fact, but nonjudgmental stance will facilitate the client's acceptance of treatment for possible withdrawal symptoms. Even among obviously intoxicated clients, however, responses to such direct questions may be angry and defensive.

Older Adults

Older clients who are being treated for several chronic illnesses by different health care providers are at risk for drug problems from drug interactions and/or for drug dependence. For this reason, you should obtain a good history from the client, including a list of all the drugs taken, frequency of use, dosage, and duration of use. It is often useful to ask the family of an older client to bring all drugs to the hospital for review rather than relying on memory. Frequently, the confusion seen in older clients is a direct consequence of drug interactions or malabsorption.

In addition, substance abuse (especially alcoholism) is less likely to be detected and treated in older adults than in younger clients. It often goes unrecognized because the signs of substance abuse are difficult to distinguish from the changes associated with normal aging or degenerative brain disease. Heavy drinking declines with age; when medical illnesses, uncomfortable physical symptoms, increased medication use, and acute health events become more common. There is a higher likelihood of abstinence with aging. However, we also know that an overall health burden predicts subsequent problematic drinking behavior (Christensen, Low, & Anstey, 2006). Therefore, it is likely that problematic drinking behaviors are likely to increase with the future graying of America. Early- and late-onset older adult alcoholics have reported loneliness, losses, depression, and meager social support networks as antecedents of their alcohol abuse.

Adult Children of Alcoholics

Adult children of alcoholics (ACOA) are at great risk for becoming alcoholics. This type of alcoholism has been labeled *familial*. Research on familial alcoholism has shown that:

- A family history of alcoholism is present.
- Alcoholism develops early, usually by the time the person is in his or her late twenties.
- The alcoholism is generally severe and usually requires treatment.
- The risk of alcoholism is increased, but not the risk of other psychiatric disorders.

However, research also indicates that resiliency (the power to rebound, resist, or recover readily) typically overtakes the expression of genetic predisposition with alcoholism. ACOAs' resiliency levels are similar to those of non-ACOAs. Self-help exposure increases resiliency when compared to ACOAs who have not had self-help exposure. There does not appear to be validity to the idea that there are universal ACOA personality traits (Hill et al., 2007; Powell, 2006).

Health Care Providers

Many factors place health care providers at risk for developing chemical dependence. Healthcare providers in general work under a great deal of stress and have easy access to drugs. Every day, they give people medication to relieve pain. It is an easy leap to self-medication. However, such behavior is a violation of state practice acts and ethical standards of practice and, depending on the drug and method of obtaining it, may be a criminal offense. It is estimated that approximately 10% to 15% of all health care professionals will misuse drugs or alcohol at some time during their career (Baldisseri, 2007).

Colleagues of chemically dependent health care workers need to be alert to behavior that suggests a problem. They should attempt to talk with the professional who is having difficulty before documenting and reporting such behavior to a supervisor. It is very common for colleagues to cover up for one another. Shielding a chemically dependent health care provider—whatever the professional discipline—puts clients, the health care provider, and the profession at risk and violates professional practice, the code of ethics, and the law in many states. Nurses, however, need to understand that their chemically dependent colleagues suffer from a disease, not a moral problem. This understanding empowers us to work together to help one another. Warning signs of behavior by health care providers that suggest chemical dependency are in the Your Assessment Approach feature.

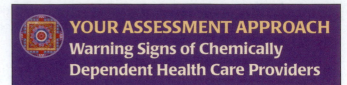

YOUR ASSESSMENT APPROACH
Warning Signs of Chemically Dependent Health Care Providers

Be alert for the following behaviors that suggest a colleague may have a problem with chemical dependency:

- Frequent absenteeism before and after days off; always working (in order to obtain a supply)
- Irritability
- Abrupt mood changes; inappropriate affect
- Sloppy charting and client care
- Problems with record keeping of drugs or drug inventory (missing drugs, frequent "wasting" of drugs, inaccurate records)
- Frequent errors in judgment
- Alcohol (stale or fresh) on breath
- Frequent disappearance from the assigned area
- Offering to give medication to clients who do not request or do not seem to need it
- Frequent night shift work
- Having clients who complain of little or no pain relief after the health care provider has administered the medication

NURSING PROCESS
Clients with Substance-Related Disorders

As substance abuse becomes a greater problem in society, more clients will be admitted to hospitals and clinics for help with intoxication and withdrawal. Substance abuse is a disease and not a weakness or flaw. A moralistic attitude always alienates the client and is not scientifically sound. It may be true that some health care providers have negative biases regarding addicts, labeling their behaviors as selfish and self-destructive. Some may question whether the substance abuse client has a right to health care resources.

It is always important for the health care provider to maintain an objective, clinical perspective that does not lapse into personal bias or prejudice, particularly in ways that sabotage the delivery of quality health care to the recipient. Rec-

YOUR SELF-AWARENESS
Your Stress Response and Susceptibility to Substance Use

Examine who you are when you are stressed by answering the following questions. Attend to what your answers suggest about your coping mechanisms and your susceptibility to substance use.

Check the substances you choose to use when you seek comfort from stress:

- ❑ Food (carbohydrates)
- ❑ Food (noncarbohydrates)
- ❑ Cigarettes
- ❑ Coffee
- ❑ Wine
- ❑ Beer
- ❑ Liquor
- ❑ Chocolate
- ❑ Tea
- ❑ Pain relievers (ASA, acetaminophen, ibuprofen, other)
- ❑ Marijuana
- ❑ Recreational drugs

At what rate do you use any of the above?

- ❑ More than five times a day
- ❑ More than two times a day
- ❑ Daily
- ❑ Only at work/school
- ❑ Only on the weekends
- ❑ Only at dinner
- ❑ Only at parties
- ❑ Monthly
- ❑ Occasionally

At what rate would you use these substances if you had the money, time off, no weight concerns, or other release from responsibility?

- ❑ More than five times a day
- ❑ More than two times a day
- ❑ Daily
- ❑ Only at work/school
- ❑ Only on the weekends
- ❑ Only at dinner
- ❑ Only at parties
- ❑ Monthly
- ❑ Occasionally

ognizing and accepting that the disease is chronic, often with remissions and exacerbations, should keep you from succumbing to the frustration felt by many who treat substance abusers who relapse. At stressful times in life, anyone may develop a dependence on drugs or alcohol; however, certain people seem to be predisposed to the illness. Your expertise in the stages of the nursing process is vital to the care of clients with substance abuse problems. Your focus should be on helping clients work toward self-awareness, good health, and good interpersonal relationships so that they can lead productive, fulfilling, happy lives.

Drugs change rapidly, and nurses must keep up with the "drug scene" to assess and treat clients. Along with the knowledge acquired from reading, continuing education programs, and seminars, nurses need self-knowledge to be good therapists with substance abusers. Ongoing critical self-analysis of your own susceptibility to substance use is useful. See the Your Self-Awareness feature above for a list of questions to guide this self-analysis.

Assessment

Carry out an accurate assessment of the substances used and abused to anticipate potential toxic and withdrawal effects and to make nursing care plans as specific and relevant as possible. For example, a methamphetamine user who is malnourished, exhausted, and depressed needs immediate diet regulation, rest, and gradual involvement in a treatment program. See the Nursing Care Plan for the Client with Methamphetamine Intoxication at the end of this chapter. Cocaine or crack abusers are likely to be resistant to treatment and need active staff intervention and a structured program to involve them in treatment. They should not be left alone or purposefully isolated, as might be done with an alcoholic.

Subjective Data

As part of the mental status exam and the psychiatric history, conduct a thorough, nonjudgmental substance use assessment. Include the following interview questions:

1. How many packs of cigarettes do you smoke?
2. Do you take any prescription drugs now?
3. Do you drink alcohol each day? If yes, do you drink a pint or about a quart? (Let the client correct you on your overstatement rather than fear shocking you with the truth.)
4. Do you drink a pint or quart of alcohol or more on occasion? When was your last drink?
5. When did you last drink more than you wanted to?
6. Do you have a drug habit?
7. What drugs do you use, and what is your daily cost?

Simply asking, "How many drinks do you have at a time?" can be misleading and can minimize the problem if each drink exceeds standard bar amounts of about 2 ounces. The CAGE questions discussed in the Your Assessment Approach feature on page 352 are also helpful.

Accurate responses to these questions are most likely when they are part of an interview that includes general lifestyle inquiries about cigarette smoking, coffee consumption,

MEDIALINK CASA Columbia

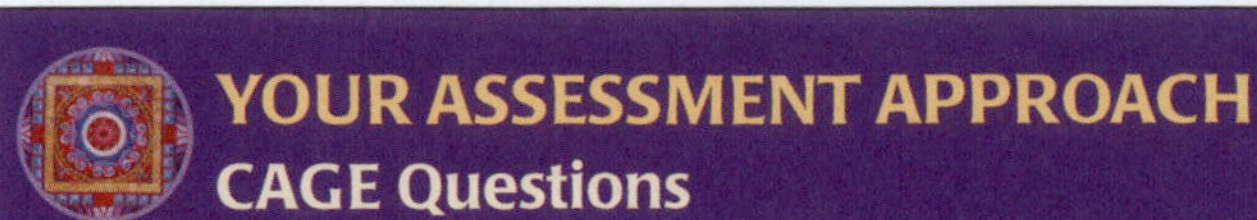

YOUR ASSESSMENT APPROACH CAGE Questions

The CAGE is most frequently used for the detection of alcoholism in clinical settings. CAGE is a mnemonic for these four questions:

1. Have you ever felt like you should **C**ut down on your drinking?
2. Have people **A**nnoyed you by criticizing your drinking?
3. Have you ever felt bad or **G**uilty about your drinking?
4. Have you ever had a drink in the morning as an **E**ye-opener to get rid of a hangover?

Source: Ewing, J. A. (1999). Screening for alcoholism using CAGE. *Journal of the American Medical Association, 281*(7), 611. Reprinted with permission from the American Medical Association.

and exercise habits. Experts agree that skillful assessment interviewing of clients and their family members remains the best source of data.

Common Defense Mechanisms in Client Responses Denial, rationalization, and projection are three defense mechanisms common to substance abusers. These defense mechanisms, along with other behaviors—conning, bargaining, feigning illness or an injury—complicate the assessment.

Alcoholics and other drug abusers tend to deny that they have a problem or minimize the problem: "I drink/use drugs every day, but it rarely interferes with my work." Rationalization is common: "I know I shouldn't drink, and I'll stop as soon as I get through this problem. Drinking keeps me calm enough to function." Projecting the problem onto others is also common: "You are so uptight that perfectly normal social drinking bothers you for no good reason. It's your issue, not mine."

A detailed assessment, along with family/coworker interviews, reveals that the problem is generally worse than the client says. Cocaine users tend to project and blame their difficulties on others, often a spouse. For instance, a man may bring up the issue of his wife's drinking and give a dozen reasons why he does not need treatment.

Substance abusers sometimes "con" (manipulate) people to get drugs. Drug-seeking behaviors (DSB), a term used in some treatment centers, refers to feigning illness or an injury to get a drug. Clients also bargain with themselves and staff members to get what they want. An alcoholic/drug abuser is likely to think, "I know I shouldn't hang out with B and P since we all get loaded together, but I like them. I'll just be with them, I won't drink/use." Later on, the person may think, "I'll only use a gram of cocaine"; later, "I'll just do an eight-ball." This client might tell the nurse, "I'll be glad to go to group therapy next week; just let me rest for a few days." Of course, substance abusers always con themselves first.

Motivation for Treatment Nurses need to consider some important psychosocial issues when clients come for treatment. Clients may enter a treatment program voluntarily. This situation is best, because they are internally motivated and therefore have a better chance of success. However, they may be coerced by family, friends, physicians, or the police to undergo treatment. See the website for the National Center on Addiction and Substance Abuse at Columbia University, www.casacolumbia.org/, for information on every form of substance abuse.

Coerced treatment inevitably causes anger and resentment. These clients may lash out at people, blame them (including you, the nurse), and demonstrate resistant or arrogant behavior. In these difficult situations, you must remain detached and nonjudgmental to avoid both power struggles and taking the role of persecutor or rescuer. At this time, you function as a data gatherer: "I know you are [uncomfortable, anxious, afraid, angry] now. To help you feel better, I need to ask you some questions about your drug use." A judgmental question is, "Don't you know that if you don't get help now you will only get worse?" Such questions prevent rapport and alienate the client.

The Importance of Language Knowing the language of the drug world is important in obtaining an accurate nursing assessment of a substance abuser. Drug users have a language all their own; to understand them and the extent and nature of their habit, you need to be familiar with this language. For example, "basing and balling" refer to freebasing (using ether to purify cocaine and make it more potent) and speed-balling (combining heroin and cocaine); "copping an eight-ball" means acquiring one-eighth ounce of cocaine; a "mission" is several days' use of crack; "drug of choice" is the client's favorite drug. Often, the clients themselves or a recovering addict can teach you this language.

Mental Status Abnormal mental status findings are seen in substance-induced disorders but are not specific to them.

- Confusion, disorientation, and agitation are often seen in intoxicated individuals, but can also indicate other problems, such as dementia, head injury, or metabolic abnormalities.
- Paranoia is common in stimulant abuse but can also indicate paranoid schizophrenia.
- Hallucinations can be caused by hallucinogens, withdrawal from alcohol, or psychotic illnesses.
- Signs of impaired thinking, such as loose associations, are unlikely to be caused by substance use and are more likely to be due to schizophrenia.

Objective Data

In addition to assessing subjective data, you should include a thorough consideration of relevant objective data. An assessment of behavioral changes can cue you to drug use.

Physical Findings Less dramatic physical findings may include dry skin, hangnails, malnutrition, ascites, elevated blood pressure, and the smell of alcohol or an inhalant on the client's breath. As alcoholism progresses, be alert to signs and symptoms of liver cirrhosis (see the Your Assessment Approach feature on page 353).

YOUR ASSESSMENT APPROACH
Signs and Symptoms of Liver Cirrhosis

- *Skin.* Extremely dry skin; severe pruritus; abnormal pigmentation; spider angiomas on the face, neck, arms, and trunk; telangiectasis on the cheeks; prominent abdominal vessels; ecchymosis; palmar erythema; jaundice
- *Gastrointestinal.* Abnormal nutrient absorption; anorexia; indigestion; nausea and vomiting; diarrhea or constipation; hemorrhoids; dull, aching abdominal pain; musty breath; ascites
- *Central nervous system.* Lethargy; slurred speech; asterixis (flapping tremor of the hands); peripheral neuritis; confusion; coma
- *Hematologic.* Bleeding tendencies (frequent nosebleeds, easy bruising, bleeding gums); anemia
- *Hepatic.* Hepatomegaly. Replacement of lobules with fibrous tissue. In the early stages of cirrhosis, the liver feels large and firm, with a sharp edge. Eventually it shrinks, and the edge feels nodular. There may also be pain in the right upper quadrant that intensifies when the client leans forward.

Standardized, Structured Questionnaires and Scales The list of standardized, structured interviews; questionnaires; and scales used to assess substance abuse is long and includes the following, which are among the best known:

- DSM-IV-TR Structured Clinical Interview (SCID)
- Addiction Severity Index
- Chemical Use, Abuse, and Dependence Scale (CUAD)
- Millon Clinical Multiaxial Inventory
- Drinking Problems Index
- CAGE Questionnaire (see page 352)

Laboratory Tests For years, researchers and clinicians have been searching for an objective biologic marker that will reflect problem drinking and make assessment less challenging. Common laboratory tests in which elevated values are associated with excessive alcohol intake are:

- Blood alcohol concentration
- Gamma-glutamyl transferase (GGT)
- Alanine aminotransferase (ALT, formerly SGPT)
- Aspartate aminotransferase (AST, formerly SGOT)
- Lactate dehydrogenase
- Alkaline phosphatase
- Total bilirubin
- Cholesterol
- Triglycerides
- Uric acid
- Mean corpuscular volume (MCV)

Elevated laboratory test values are only one of the alerting factors for problem drinking. No single test or combination of tests alone is appropriate for clinical screening. Confirmation of the excessive use of alcohol in a sensitively conducted assessment interview remains the preferred assessment approach and is considered a prerequisite for successful intervention.

Nursing Diagnoses: NANDA

Because substance-related disorders are associated with biologic, psychosocial, and even spiritual distress, a wide variety of nursing diagnoses is likely to be fundamental to planning comprehensive care. Nursing diagnoses for clients with substance-related disorders may include, among others:

- Ineffective Coping
- Dysfunctional Family Processes
- Fear
- Imbalanced Nutrition: Less Than Body Requirements
- Decisional Conflict
- Chronic Pain
- Disturbed Sensory Perception
- Impaired Social Interaction
- Disturbed Thought Processes

Outcome Identification: NOC

When designing care for clients who have substance abuse disorders, outcomes must be specifically delineated. While the outcome of total and permanent abstinence may be achievable for some clients, for others it may be an unattainable goal. Reducing the harm of substance use may be an intermediate step that is attainable for some. This is referred to as harm reduction. Harm reduction as a philosophy is discussed in Chapter 25 ∞. Each situation must be assessed individually. Make sure your outcomes can be measured so both you and your client are aware of progress and relapse. Outcome criteria for substance abusers that relate to sobriety, abstinence from drugs and alcohol, and "being clean" include:

- Coping
- Decision making
- Impulse control

Further outcomes include risk reduction; improvement of work, family, and social relationships; and lifestyle changes that may include a growing sense of spirituality. Clients become more effective in using new attitudes and behaviors. As a result, clients feel better about themselves. Although the fear of relapse is always present, over time the craving for chemicals diminishes, and the client establishes a new, healthy lifestyle.

Ask yourself, "Is the outcome one this client can relate to and invest energy into?" None of the addictions or abuse situations discussed in this chapter are easy for a client to abandon as a lifestyle. Imagine a habit you have that is not in your best interests (we all have such habits to one extent or another). Then, imagine how you would best be able to work with a nurse to change that habit or eradicate it completely.

Planning and Implementation: NIC

Your role may be slightly different in each of the following settings, depending on the client's stage of illness and presenting symptoms.

General Hospital Care

Substance abusers who are suicidal or acutely ill with DTs, hepatic coma, respiratory depression, or cardiac dysrhythmias are often treated in the medical–surgical unit of a general hospital. Life-threatening physiologic symptoms are attended to first. In this setting, nurses:

- Monitor vital signs and respiratory and cardiovascular support.
- Administer prescribed medications.
- Apply ice packs for fever, such as fever caused by amphetamine intoxication or following cocaine use.
- Decrease stimulation; provide a darkened, quiet room.
- Point out reality: "I know you are seeing things, and I know you are frightened. You are in the hospital, and we are caring for you. There are no bugs or monsters here. You are safe and will feel better soon."
- Make sure that clients receive adequate nutrition and fluids (they are disoriented and generally forget to eat and drink).
- Assess changes in level of consciousness.
- Monitor fluid intake and output.
- Protect skin integrity.
- Offer emotional support and encouragement to the client and family.
- Refer clients to community resources for recovery programs.

When the client is out of danger, then the alcoholism or drug addiction issues are addressed.

Specialty Hospital Care

Specialty hospital care is given in inpatient hospital units that are geared specifically for the treatment of substance abuse. If the hospital is equipped with trained personnel and appropriate resources, acutely ill clients, including those who are intoxicated, may be admitted. The physical environment is modified to handle problems with substance abusers. For example, rooms devoid of furniture and potentially harmful materials offer a quiet, unstimulating environment that prevents convulsions and decreases anxiety.

A primary nurse may be assigned to decrease confusion and stimulation. Members of the staff are experts in detoxification, education, and treatment. Clients also receive treatment for coexisting medical and psychiatric problems. Staff efforts are geared toward stabilization.

Residential Rehabilitation

Residential rehabilitation facilities offer inpatients expert care for substance abuse, but in some cases staff members are not skilled in treating medical or psychiatric problems.

Extended Residential Care

Extended-care facilities provide services for people with physical impairments and a home for recovering alcoholics or drug addicts who have been rejected by their families. Apartments for independent living, a relatively new concept, are useful for these clients.

Outpatient Care

Outpatient care may consist of daily, weekly, or monthly individual, group, or family therapy in a variety of treatment centers. Daily care is usually given only in intensive programs of limited duration, usually 3–4 weeks. Employee assistance programs (EAPs) are now common in many industries and are one example of outpatient care given not in a clinic but in the workplace. Substance abuse outreach counselors work with chemically dependent employees.

Remember when you work with clients with substance-related disorders in any of these settings that addiction is a chronic, progressive disease. Each treatment setting calls for different skills. For example, in general or specialty hospitals, nurses need psychosocial skills along with technical skills to assess and monitor the physiologic components of abuse and withdrawal. In residential rehabilitation and extended residential care centers, nurses may educate clients about the disease, help clients reenter the community as much as possible, and facilitate or lead support groups. At a student counseling center in a university or college, nurses are involved in treating the college student who has difficulty with drugs or alcohol (see FIGURE 15-9 ■).

Self-Help Groups

In self-help groups, also called mutual help groups, people with similar problems help one another. Groups composed of peers share experiences and knowledge of the problem to support and educate one another.

Twelve-Step Programs In contrast to the previously described treatment programs, twelve-step programs such as Alcoholics Anonymous (AA) and Narcotics Anonymous (NA) are not specifically treatment programs. They are spiritual programs based on the fellowship among its members. Both are successful self-help groups that meet daily or more often in different parts of large cities and weekly in smaller towns. Meetings are held in places of worship, schools, town halls, and various mental health treatment facilities. Anyone with a desire to stop drinking or taking drugs is welcome. This belief pervades both organizations: "Once an alcoholic/addict, always an alcoholic/

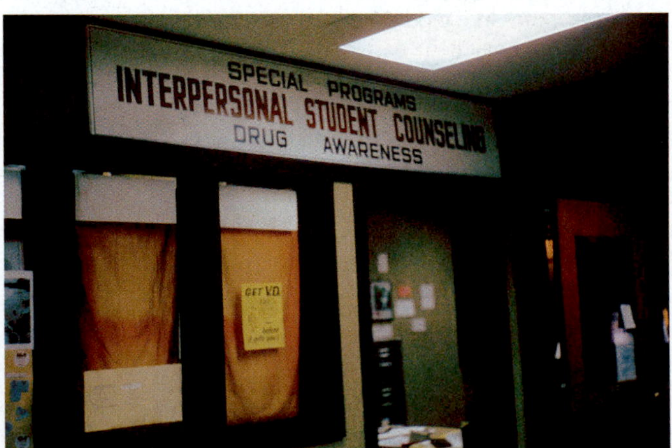

FIGURE 15-9 ■ Entrance to a student counseling center in a university or college.

Source: Holly Skodol Wilson, RN, PhD.

Box 15-4 The Twelve Steps of Alcoholics Anonymous

1. We admitted we were powerless over alcohol—that our lives had become unmanageable.
2. Came to believe that a Power greater than ourselves could restore us to sanity.
3. Made a decision to turn our will and our lives over to the care of God, as we understood Him.
4. Made a searching and fearless moral inventory of ourselves.
5. Admitted to God, to ourselves, and to another human being the exact nature of our wrongs.
6. Were entirely ready to have God remove all these defects of character.
7. Humbly asked Him to remove our shortcomings.
8. Made a list of all people we had harmed, and became willing to make amends to them all.
9. Made direct amends to such people wherever possible, except when to do so would injure them or others.
10. Continued to take personal inventory and when we were wrong, promptly admitted it.
11. Sought through prayer and meditation to improve our conscious contact with God, as we understood Him, praying only for knowledge of His will for us and the power to carry that out.
12. Having had a spiritual awakening as the result of these steps, we tried to carry this message to alcoholics, and to practice these principles in all our affairs.

Source: The Twelve Steps are reprinted with permission of Alcoholics Anonymous World Services, Inc. (AAWS). Permission to reprint the Twelve Steps does not mean that AAWS has reviewed or approved the contents of this publication, or that AAWS necessarily agrees with the views expressed herein. AA is a program of recovery from alcoholism *only*—use of the Twelve Steps in connection with programs and activities which are patterned after AA, but which address other problems, or in any other non–AA context, does not imply otherwise.

addict." Members admit they are powerless over chemicals, live "one day at a time," recite the serenity prayer, and believe in "a power greater than man." Members learn to turn their problems over to "the God of my understanding." Their philosophy is revealed in part through their key slogans, "First things first," "Easy does it," and "Let go and let God." Members of both organizations learn the "twelve steps." The twelve steps of AA are reproduced in Box 15-4. Jellinek's work is thought to be the basis for the contemporary view of alcohol addiction as a disease and the foundation upon which twelve-step programs are based (1946).

Through AA/NA, people learn to change negative attitudes and behaviors into positive ones. A key concept of AA/NA is that total abstinence is essential to recovery. As members become sober or drug free, they begin "sponsoring" (helping) other substance abusers. This offering of support is believed to be vital to recovery, as is regular attendance at AA/NA meetings. Twelve-step recovery programs also emphasize spirituality through meditation and prayer rather than willpower as the means to recovery.

Recognize that AA's twelve steps were written in the 1930s by and for white Christian males and may not be culturally relevant for all people. Adapting the language to a less patriarchal, less traditionally Christian, approach that is spiritual yet culturally relevant to diverse groups of people makes the twelve-step principles available to people who might otherwise discount them. The Caring for the Spirit feature on page 356 includes adaptations that are spiritually focused and culturally relevant.

AA and NA, while excellent for clients with substance abuse problems, may cause some difficulties for the psychiatric client with a coexisting abuse or use problem. The AA/NA philosophy of complete abstinence from substances has been said to include psychiatric medications. This requirement causes a rift between what clients are told by their psychiatric–mental health nurses and the path toward wellness according to AA/NA. Programs designed to provide the most effective treatment for the psychobiologic underpinnings of psychiatric disorders and accommodate the added stress of substances of abuse work best.

Women for Sobriety Women for Sobriety (WFS) is another self-help group. Unlike AA/NA, WFS is not based on a spiritual philosophy; instead, the program is based on abstinence. WFS's 13 acceptance statements focus members on new ways of thinking. The women learn to cope and, over time, to change their daily lives. The group recognizes the differences of alcoholism in males and females. For example, women become inebriated faster than men.

Rational Recovery (RR) Alcoholics Anonymous is the most popular mutual-help recovery organization in the world, but it is not the only one. Alcoholics and addicts who failed to find a comfortable home in AA but were nevertheless determined to become sober have founded at least one other major organization to help others become clean and sober. This group, Rational Recovery (RR), rejects the spiritual approach of AA.

In addition, RR rejects the notion that alcoholics and addicts are powerless to stop their addictions, suggesting instead that until now they simply have not chosen to do so. Instead of reliance on a higher power (which RR considers another form of dependence), RR members are urged to build on strengths within themselves; the movement inspires independence whenever humanly possible. A constant theme is "Think yourself sober."

In RR, there are no steps, sponsors, moral inventories, making amends to others, or even caring about what others think of you. According to rational emotive therapy, on which RR is based, human beings should love themselves because they are human beings and not because others think well of them. The concept of staying sober one day at a time is rejected in favor of a decision to never drink or use again, period. Sobriety is not supposed to become the cornerstone of one's life. The goal is for members to wean themselves from dependence on alcohol, then from dependence on people, and finally from dependence on the group.

Meetings take place only twice a week, and most people attend for only one year, after which they may be considered

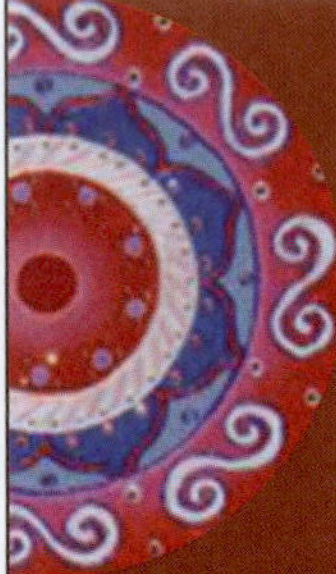

CARING FOR THE SPIRIT

A Culturally Broadened Twelve-Step Recovery

The twelve steps are grouped here into four categories: Surrender, Acceptance, Fellowship, and Bliss of Living. Each step is given a one-word description to indicate how the step works in the recovery process.

Surrender Steps

Step One: Honesty
Step Two: Hope
Step Three: Faith

Because many view surrender as a negative activity, using the words *honesty*, *hope*, and *faith* to describe each of the steps in the first category gives new meaning to the purpose of these steps. When seen from a patriarchal hierarchical view, the first step may appear to be a command. However, when it is a call to "get honest" with oneself, the step takes on new meaning without rewriting it or discounting the value it has had in helping others find recovery.

When seen as a way to expand one's spirituality through meditation and contemplation, the second step takes on new meaning as well. Hope comes from observing others who have given up the need to control and be self-centered and have found peace as a result of that action. The "came to believe" part of this step occurs over time as the client hears similar stories from multiple sources who share at twelve-step meetings. This is in part why a new member is urged to "Keep coming back so more can be revealed."

The faith that results from taking the third step allows the client to move from ego-centered thinking to belief in a power greater than self, permitting that power to work on his or her behalf.

Acceptance Steps

Step Four: Courage
Step Five: Integrity
Step Six: Willingness

The next three steps follow from the change of attitude in the first three steps. These are action steps.

In the fourth step, clients use newly discovered courage to examine the specific aspects of their character that they need to nurture and develop, as well as those character aspects that need to be eliminated because they are responsible for the client's current discomfort and distress.

The fifth step works to restore integrity to the client's life and may be responsible for the euphoria reported by many during early recovery. The client may feel a growing spiritual connection, and the nurse may be in a position to support the client's awareness of how the steps have contributed to his or her improved condition.

The sixth step is a willingness activity in which clients must decide how to convert their growing spirituality into a change of behavior.

Fellowship Steps

Step Seven: Humility
Step Eight: Forgiveness
Step Nine: Discipline

The fellowship steps help clients progress in their spiritual awareness and recovery by developing qualities of humility, forgiveness, and discipline in their personal relationships and public lives.

Bliss of Living Steps

Step Ten: Perseverance
Step Eleven: Love of self
Step Twelve: Gratitude

The bliss of living steps bring clients back to a life with meaning. By developing perseverance, clients gain a freedom from worry about when the accumulation of undesirable behavior will be discovered and how it will lead back to the pain of the past. In the eleventh step, clients learn through prayer and meditation the love of self, love of others, and love of life. They come to feel that they are not in charge of the world and that trusting in a higher power who is in charge is "OK." In the twelfth step, recovering addicts and alcoholics express their gratitude for what they have achieved and learn to value reaching out to other sufferers to share the hope of step two, the courage of step four, and the love of step eleven.

Nurses have the opportunity to assist with the unfolding of the process of twelve-step recovery. Clients do the work supported by their spiritual beliefs. Nurses can nourish the process of learning to live life in a new way.

"recovered." They can, however, return to meetings whenever the need arises. Discussions at meetings focus on the here and now rather than past history, and interactive discussion is encouraged.

Whereas AA relies totally on nonprofessionals helping one another, professional coordinators lead RR, and each group has volunteer professional advisors available for advice and input. This is necessary because, unlike AA, there are no old-timers around to help newcomers. Advisors attend meetings only occasionally. RR, like AA, offers written materials, the core of which is *Rational Recovery from Alcoholism: The Small Book* (meant to contrast with the *Big Book* of AA).

Looking within oneself for strength and direction is a major focus in RR. We all have within us an inner voice, RR believes, that challenges us to go wrong. It is this voice, nicknamed "Beast," that urges one to drink or use drugs, takes

Box 15-5 BEAST Acronym

- **B** is for Boozing Opportunities (weddings, parties, trips, etc.). Rational Recovery (RR) cautions to be aware of the pitfalls but not necessarily avoid them. You are not powerless in the face of temptations, and you can choose not to succumb.
- **E** is for Enemy Recognition. Recognize as the Enemy (Beast) those thoughts that are positive about booze or drugs.
- **A** is for Accuse the Beast of Malice. You can be angry at the Beast for its evil deeds (trying to tempt you), or you can laugh at it. Either way, make clear to the Beast that you have the upper hand and you won't relinquish it.
- **S** is for Self-Control and Self-Worth Reminders. Find ways of showing the Beast that you have self-control (like moving your hands in front of your face and holding them there, totally in your control, until the Beast backs down). Find ways of telling yourself that you are a worthwhile person. Choose not to drink for the same reason you drank: to feel good about yourself.
- **T** is for Treasuring Your Sobriety. Focus on the pleasures of life that are attainable only in sobriety (a concept similar to that in AA).

over during blackouts, encourages one to do terrible things, and speaks louder than one's rational self. It is the voice that tells one "You can stop anytime (but not now)" or "You're not really addicted (you just like the taste)" and that tears angrily into those who criticize or try to help. BEAST is an acronym used to help RR members avoid taking another drink or drug. The BEAST acronym is outlined in Box 15-5.

Relapse

Relapse is common among substance abusers, and it seriously complicates treatment. Authorities in the field of alcoholism estimate that 60% to 75% of those who complete treatment programs drink again within the first 90 days. Data suggest that only 10% to 20% of alcoholics remain abstinent for one year following treatment, and that only 35% of these are abstinent five years later. In fact, recidivism rates are notoriously high across the spectrum of addictive behaviors.

Stages of Recovery Several common stages of the recovery process are:

1. Commitment to recovery and motivation for abstinence
2. Initiating change
3. Maintaining change

As a result of a successful initial change, the person experiences perceived control while remaining abstinent.

Stages of Relapse The feeling of perceived control continues until the person encounters a high-risk situation involving negative emotional states, interpersonal conflict, or social pressure. The Partnering with Clients and Families feature on page 358 includes a checklist of symptoms leading to relapse. The person can avoid relapse by using effective coping responses in the high-risk situation. (See the Rx Communication box for an example of how you might discuss these issues with a client dependent on substances but not currently using them.)

If, however, the individual cannot cope successfully, an initial "lapse" occurs in which he or she resorts to the use of a chemical to control stress. The person then feels less able to exert control and develops a tendency to "give in" to the situation ("It's no use, I can't handle this"). In subsequent high-risk situations, the individual again resorts to the use of chemicals to relieve stress. Repeated lapses set the stage for a return to uncontrolled use (relapse).

Relapse Prevention Many treatment centers incorporate the concept of relapse prevention into their treatment programs. This concept is designed to teach clients how to anticipate relapse. By learning skills to use in high-risk situations, clients gain confidence and the expectation of being able to cope successfully, thus decreasing the probability of relapse. Research indicates that participation in a twelve-step program with a focus on the individual being "in recovery" and maintaining sobriety, as opposed to having recovered or being cured, can prevent relapse.

General Treatment Approaches

A number of general interventions for substance abuse that have been found to be useful are discussed in the next section.

MediaLink Care Plan: Potential for Relapse

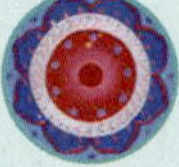

RX COMMUNICATION

CLIENT DEPENDENT ON SUBSTANCES BUT NOT CURRENTLY USING THEM

CLIENT: "I don't need to spend a lot of time talking to you about this stuff. I'm not going to take it anymore and you can bet on that."

NURSE RESPONSE 1: "I hear that you have no intention to use again, and that's good. I also want to make sure you have every support available to you when that time comes when your resolve gets shaky."

RATIONALE: This interaction provides direction around the eventual difficulties that face everyone dependent on a substance—temptation and relapse.

NURSE RESPONSE 2: "We don't have to do a lot of talking, but you have to make the changes in what you do and who you do it with."

RATIONALE: Clear statements about how the client is responsible for his or her behavior and for making necessary changes interfere with urges to shift blame.

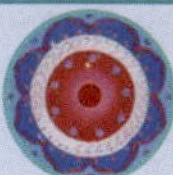

PARTNERING WITH CLIENTS AND FAMILIES

TEACHING ABOUT RELAPSE

A Checklist of Symptoms Leading to Relapse

1. **Exhaustion.** Don't allow yourself to become overly tired or to have poor health. Many chemically dependent people are also prone to work addictions. Perhaps they are in a hurry to make up for lost time or are overworking to compensate for feelings of guilt or personal inadequacy. Good health and enough rest are essential to recovery. Good feelings of physical well-being are associated with a healthy, optimistic mental outlook. Fatigue and feelings of physical illness often induce negative thinking and a pessimistic attitude. You may begin to think a drug or drink would help you return to a positive frame of mind.
2. **Dishonesty.** This symptom begins with a pattern of unnecessary little lies and deceits with fellow workers, friends, and family. Then come important lies to yourself. This is called rationalizing—making excuses for not doing what you do not want to do, or for doing what you know you should not do.
3. **Impatience.** Things are not happening fast enough; others are not doing what they should or what you want them to.
4. **Argumentativeness.** Arguing about small and ridiculous points of view indicates a need to always be right. Chemically dependent people need to learn an attitude of acceptance of their disease and the value of the tools of recovery.
5. **Depression.** Unreasonable and unaccountable melancholy and despair may occur from time to time as a *natural part of recovering* from chemical dependence. Periods of depression are times when the risk of relapse is very high. Deal with your negative feelings; talk about them.
6. **Frustration.** Remember, not everything is going to be just the way you want it.
7. **Self-pity.** "Why do these things happen to me?" "Why must I be chemically dependent?" "Nobody appreciates what I'm doing for them."
8. **Cockiness.** "I've got this problem licked; I have nothing to fear from drugs or booze." This dangerous attitude may lead to going into situations where friends are drinking and using drugs to prove to others that you don't have a problem. Do this often enough and your defenses against relapse will wear down. Don't *test* your recovery. You may lose!
9. **Complacency.** It is dangerous to let up on discipline because everything seems to be going so well. Always having a little fear is a good thing when it comes to maintaining abstinence. *More relapses occur when things are going well than when things are going badly.*
10. **Expecting too much from others.** "I've changed—why hasn't everybody else?" It's a plus if they do, but be prepared to deal with disappointment in your expectations of others. They may not trust you yet or they may be looking for more evidence of your improved physical and mental health. You may be setting yourself up for a lot of frustration and other negative feelings if you expect others to change their lifestyle just because you have.
11. **Letting up on discipline.** Continue with prayer, meditation, daily inventory, and twelve-step meeting attendance. This attitude may stem from complacency or from boredom. No chemically dependent person can afford to be bored with his or her recovery. The cost of relapse is too great.
12. **Wanting too much.** Do not set goals you cannot reach with normal efforts.
13. **Forgetting gratitude.** You may be looking negatively on your life, concentrating on problems that still are not totally corrected. It is important to remember where you started from and how much better life is now.
14. **"It can't happen to me."** This kind of thinking is very dangerous. Almost anything can happen to you and is all the more likely to happen if you become careless with your recovery. Remember that you have a progressive disease and will be in even worse shape if you relapse.
15. **Omnipotence.** This is a feeling that results from a combination of many of the above attitudes. You may come to believe you have all the answers for yourself and for others. No one can tell you anything new. You may begin to ignore suggestions or advice from others. Relapse is probably imminent unless drastic change takes place.

Source: Anonymous.

Using Confrontation Strategies. For many years, it was believed that alcoholics and drug abusers needed to "hit bottom" before they could accept their problem and request help. Today, most people believe that intervention can occur as soon as the problem is identified. Group intervention/confrontation is one strategy that aims to break down the substance abuser's denial. Nurses are often "intervention specialists" and leaders in the process.

Several family members, friends, employers, coworkers, and an alcohol/drug intervention specialist confront the substance abuser in a private meeting. They list the evidence by going around the group, one by one. The family/friends/employer, following the leader's cues, speak calmly and slowly with minimal emotion, presenting the facts, the objective evidence, to the alcoholic/drug abuser. Shouting, blaming, and haranguing are avoided because the alcoholic/drug abuser inevitably responds by denying the behavior or making excuses for it. However, confrontation by several people who really care and who persistently present the facts can break through the denial. Examples of confrontation strategies are given in the Partnering with Clients and Families feature that follows.

The next step in group intervention/confrontation requires the family/friends/employer to make clear and direct statements to the alcoholic/drug abuser about the consequences of his or her behavior:

- "Either you get help now or you will have to leave your job."
- "Either you enter a treatment program now or I will move out with the kids."

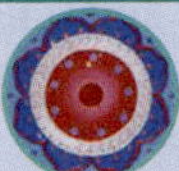

PARTNERING WITH CLIENTS AND FAMILIES

HOW TO INTERACT DURING A GROUP INTERVENTION

Use this series of steps to educate family or friends on how to interact with the substance-abusing client during a group intervention. Encourage family members to integrate the tone and style cues described in the chapter text.

Presentation of Facts

"You had slurred speech and didn't even respond when I told you I had to be hospitalized for surgery."
"You have not made your daughter's dinner all week. And you forgot to pick her up from school."
"You missed work for 3 days, and you have been late 8 days in the past month."
"You have alcohol on your breath (or needle marks on your arms)."
"I found two bottles (a syringe and empty vial) hidden in the bathroom."

Consequences

"Either you get help now or you will have to leave your job."
"Either you enter a treatment program now or I will move out with the kids."

If the client agrees to treatment, the caring people agree to remain involved.

Educating Videotapes and talks by recovered substance abusers or experts in the effects of substance abuse are helpful. Education may take place in or out of the hospital, in one comprehensive session or several sessions over time. Nurse educators should focus on the types of abused substances and their physical, psychological, and social effects. Families are often involved in these sessions because substance abuse is a family problem. The belief underlying such education is that knowledge and awareness may be useful in decreasing self-destructive behavior. But knowledge alone is never enough. Culturally sensitive and relevant educational resources should be used.

Referral and Self-Help Groups Support and self-help groups are extremely useful in helping clients feel better about themselves and acquire new attitudes and behaviors. Merely being with many people who are suffering in similar ways is beneficial. By observing people who have been sober or drug free for long periods, clients can begin to learn similar behaviors. They can see that there is hope and that recovery is possible. Self-help groups also provide new friends, generally with healthy lifestyles. Clients may choose to attend support groups for the rest of their lives. Some clients who experiment with drugs or alcohol during one period of their lives (for example, during a crisis) may choose to attend only during the crisis once they succeed in discontinuing their drug or alcohol use.

Lifestyle Change An emphasis on the requirement for a total lifestyle change is necessary. You can help clients discuss ways to alter their destructive habits by suggesting different coping strategies and by encouraging clients to discover new interests and capabilities within themselves. You and your clients can role-play new responses to old situations. Recognizing that relapse is always a threat, you may set up contracts with clients. For example, clients may agree to contact the nurse or an AA/NA sponsor if and when they feel the urge to drink or do drugs. This agreement represents new behaviors that are necessary for a lifestyle change.

Clients must realize that spending time with friends who are substance abusers or hanging out at places where they used to take drugs or alcohol is not helpful. The mere sight or smell of paraphernalia or the desired substance is often enough to trigger a relapse. Old ties must be broken; new friends and activities must be pursued.

Helping the Family

Substance abuse affects not only the client but also the entire family system. Family members often engage in behaviors that enable clients to continue their substance abuse by protecting them from its consequences. Helping family members includes clarifying the problem and presenting possible solutions (treatment) and creating a support system for family members. Referring family members to Al-Anon can be a very helpful strategy.

In dysfunctional families, the substance abuser often becomes the "identified patient," focusing attention on that individual and away from the other problems in the family. Treatment for the substance abuser may require some type of family therapy. Family members may need treatment for codependence through group or individual therapy or involvement in a twelve-step program such as Al-Anon or Codependents Anonymous (CODA). The Adult Children of Alcoholics (ACOA) support groups are also helpful.

Evaluation

Evaluating the recovery process requires an evaluation of the client's ability to change. Is there evidence that the client is being honest, open, and willing to take responsibility for his or her own actions? Regardless of the substance of abuse, once a client stops blaming others for his or her use/abuse, treatment has made a positive impact. Another criterion is the amount of substance the client is placing in his or her body. Has it decreased? Other indications of positive treatment outcome are increased job stability, improvement in interpersonal relationships, and improved problem-solving techniques. Evaluating clients for emotional maturity and the ability to make lifestyle changes that include people, places, and things are critical for victory over substance dependence. Improvement in these areas is a good indication that the client is well on the road to recovery.

CASE MANAGEMENT

Case management services for clients with addictions has the potential to cover many areas. At any time, for any client, you would be involved in:

- Arranging for services at clinics
- Responding to emergent and chronic health care needs
- Designing access to educational resources
- Monitoring the client's living situation and residential movements
- Revamping recreational options

In fact, there are as many different case management needs as there are different substance abuse clients. See the Nursing Care Plan for the Client with Methamphetamine Intoxication at the end of this chapter for examples of the variety of case management needs a client may have.

Perhaps the most important task of the nurse case manager for a substance abuse client is availability and flexibility in response to client needs. These clients can experience a plethora of difficulties in their social, occupational, living, and familial/relationship arrangements. Any one of these has the potential to serve as a trigger for relapse into substance abuse or dependence. Assist the client in managing difficulties in these areas to lower the risk of a relapse. This must be done in a manner that does not breach interpersonal boundaries and maintains the client's responsibility for self care.

COMMUNITY-BASED CARE

In an outpatient treatment center, where the nurse functions in a community-based care environment, you may take the role of a counselor or a therapist. In all cases, the nurse must have psychosocial, physiologic, and spiritual skills. Such skills include interviewing, teaching clients about the disease process and alternative coping strategies, referring clients to appropriate sources and community support systems, and knowing how to conduct individual, group, or family therapy (for advanced-practice nurses). You cannot give quality care without an in-depth understanding of the disease process—from the varying theoretic explanations to the varying methods of treatment at different stages.

Another feature of community-based care for substance abuse is that of court-mandated treatment. Addicts often exhibit poor judgment. For example, alcoholic clients may continue to drive while intoxicated. In most states, driving under the influence of alcohol or drugs is considered a crime for which the driver will face legal penalties. The law enforcement system may interact with the mental health system to force treatment on those found guilty of driving while intoxicated. A psychiatric–mental health nurse may care for those clients who have been mandated for treatment.

Clients with poor judgment mandated to treatment may initially respond with minimal or superficial cooperation, although many clients do make positive changes as a result of mandated therapy. All clients mandated for treatment must be informed in writing of all policies related to the treatment process and the court mandate. Often, this mandate will include written evidence of participation in one-to-one therapy, family therapy, educational programming, and attendance at 12-step meetings. At times, random drug testing may be court-ordered.

Clients may attempt to manipulate you into withholding information from the court. Allowing the client to manipulate you will jeopardize the treatment process. Successful manipulation may decrease the client's feeling of responsibility for recovery. At no time can you consider violating the court mandate. The law enforcement system has the right to file charges against a nurse who fails to cooperate fully with court mandates.

When state laws clearly mandate a treatment course, you must work within legal mandates. It is much more difficult to decide what to do when public opinion and legal mandate are less clear, or when the mandates seem to interfere with prudent treatment. For example, pregnant women who suffer from substance addiction potentially face conflict between the legal system and basic prenatal care. States vary in their approach to the pregnant addict. Some states seek to incarcerate pregnant women who continue to use illegal drugs, and others mandate that health care workers report all women who have tested positive for drugs, determining such behavior to be child abuse.

At times you may need to interact with the legal system during mandated treatment. You may serve as an advocate who will facilitate treatment for the addict and her baby. This process of intervention can be complex. For example, it is difficult to identify active addiction, secondary use, and recreational use. While any drug use is potentially hazardous, regular use seen in addiction may be more damaging to mother and baby.

HOME CARE

Home care can revolve around a physiologic event resulting from substance use or abuse. Cerebral vascular accident from crack use, injury from driving while intoxicated, or brain damage from inhalant abuse are all likely scenarios requiring nursing home care services. In these circumstances, recovery from the physiologic threat is coupled with treatment for substance abuse.

One aspect of treatment for substance abuse that can be accomplished in the home is helping the client to develop drink- or drug-refusal skills. In many cases substance abuse clients who are sober relapse into using substances when they encounter stressful events in their home lives with which they are poorly equipped to cope. Often, these events can lead to situations that include the offer of alcohol or drugs for personal use. A home-based training component can help clients develop the interactional and social skills needed to successfully negotiate refusals of these offers. You can play an instrumental role in designing and implementing this training.

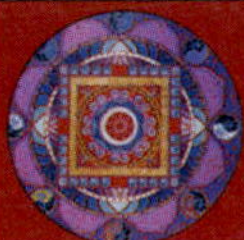

NURSING CARE PLAN
Client with Chronic Alcoholism

Identifying Information

John Mills is a 54-year-old married civil servant. He is Catholic, has a high school education, and was referred from the Care Unit (a specialty hospital) where he has been for the last 28 days.

John states, "I've had a drinking problem for 35 years. My wife and boss told me if I don't shape up they'll kick me out of my home and my job. I want to feel better. It's been a living hell. But, I'm not sure I can stop drinking; I've tried before." He describes his drinking as a way "to cope with my problems for most of my life." He "wants to stay dry." Fifteen years ago, his social drinking escalated and he began binge-drinking on the weekends. Then he began drinking throughout the week. He has been drinking daily for most of the last 3 years. He drank "enough to keep a buzz on" and occasionally "enough to pass out." John's problems with work include tardiness, absenteeism, and errors on the job. Marital problems are described as "she either yells at me or takes care of me." He gives as examples his wife pouring out his hidden liquor and calling his boss to say John had the flu when he was really "hung over."

History

John has been in and out of AA groups and has seen three psychiatrists. He has been hospitalized three times for car accidents and injuries due to drinking (broken leg and ribs, contusions, concussion). After the last general hospital admission, he was admitted to the Care Unit for a 28-day alcohol treatment program.

Both of John's parents are deceased and both were alcoholics. His sister, age 58, is a recovering alcoholic (has been "dry" for 10 years). The family has never been close. John feels he was "never allowed to be a normal, active kid." His sister cared for him when he was young and functioned as a surrogate mother.

John developed normally but always "felt different." He worked every summer and took a full-time job after high school graduation. He enjoyed being with his "drinking buddies" from work, but has never had a close friend on whom he could depend. He smokes one pack of cigarettes daily and uses no other drugs. He spends his leisure time watching TV and at bars with friends.

John has cirrhosis of the liver. He is malnourished from chronic alcoholism and has a long history of insomnia.

Current Mental Status

John is well groomed, clean, and alert. His sensorium is within normal limits; affect appropriate yet apathetic. He appears depressed and expresses feelings of self-reproach and guilt for his years of drinking and its effect on others. Speech is slow and spontaneous. Motor behavior, thought content, and thought processes are within normal limits. Insight is questionable.

Other Subjective or Objective Clinical Data

Multivitamins qd; no indications of suicide or violence potential.

Nursing Diagnosis: Ineffective Coping related to alcohol abuse

Expected Outcome: Reduction of ineffective and self-destructive coping through alcohol abuse and regular use of more effective coping styles.

Short-Term Goal	Interventions	Rationale
Identification of two effective coping mechanisms	■ John inventories those situations that challenge his ability to cope. ■ John recognizes the automatic mechanisms involved in habitually responding to stress with alcohol.	Revision of coping styles requires identification of the situations that place him at risk, typical problematic responses, and acknowledgment of the need to learn new coping styles.
	■ John rehearses various coping strategies to prepare to select two for regular use. ■ John begins to substitute effective coping for alcohol use when stressed.	Rehearsing new behaviors and thoughts incorporates them into a repertoire.

Nursing Diagnosis: Insomnia related to alcohol abuse

Expected Outcome: John will use sleep-inducing strategies nightly and report satisfaction with his quality of sleep.

Short-Term Goal	Interventions	Rationale
John will sleep a total of 6 hours per night.	■ Assess current pattern and effective strategies. ■ Respond to awakening with sleep hygiene: warm milk, reading, relaxation strategies. ■ Employ effective strategies regularly.	Reestablish a consistently healthy sleep routine.

(continued)

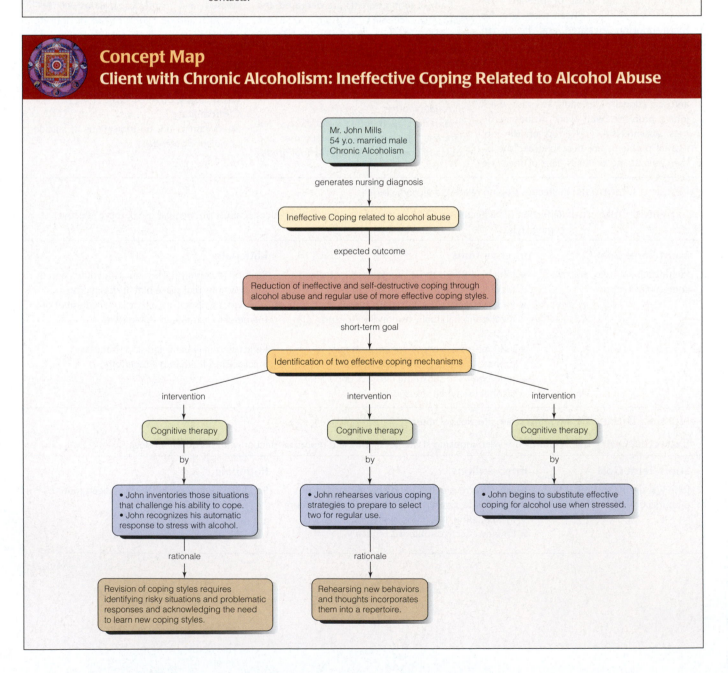

NURSING CARE PLAN
Client with Chronic Alcoholism *(continued)*

Nursing Diagnosis: Imbalanced Nutrition: Less than Body Requirements, related to alcohol abuse

Expected Outcome: John eats three meals every day plus snacks and takes a multivitamin as recommended.

Short-Term Goal	Interventions	Rationale
John identifies the relationship between alcoholism and malnutrition.	▪ Monitor intake of meals and snacks.	Malnutrition from chronic alcoholism can be addressed with a comprehensive nutrition program.
John gains weight through a balanced diet.	▪ Initiate dietary consult.	
	▪ Investigate dietary preferences to maximize John's abilities to expand his intake appropriately.	John is more likely to eat food he prefers, as part of a balanced diet.
	▪ Educate regarding the impact of chronic alcohol ingestion on the digestive tract, metabolism, and overall health.	Alcohol impairs the ability of the digestive tract to absorb nutrients.
	▪ Offer frequent food and fluids throughout contacts.	

Concept Map
Client with Chronic Alcoholism: Ineffective Coping Related to Alcohol Abuse

Mr. John Mills
54 y.o. married male
Chronic Alcoholism

generates nursing diagnosis

Ineffective Coping related to alcohol abuse

expected outcome

Reduction of ineffective and self-destructive coping through alcohol abuse and regular use of more effective coping styles.

short-term goal

Identification of two effective coping mechanisms

intervention → Cognitive therapy → by → • John inventories those situations that challenge his ability to cope. • John recognizes his automatic response to stress with alcohol. → rationale → Revision of coping styles requires identifying risky situations and problematic responses and acknowledging the need to learn new coping styles.

intervention → Cognitive therapy → by → • John rehearses various coping strategies to prepare to select two for regular use. → rationale → Rehearsing new behaviors and thoughts incorporates them into a repertoire.

intervention → Cognitive therapy → by → • John begins to substitute effective coping for alcohol use when stressed.

Concept Map
Client with Chronic Alcoholism: Insomnia Related to Alcohol Abuse

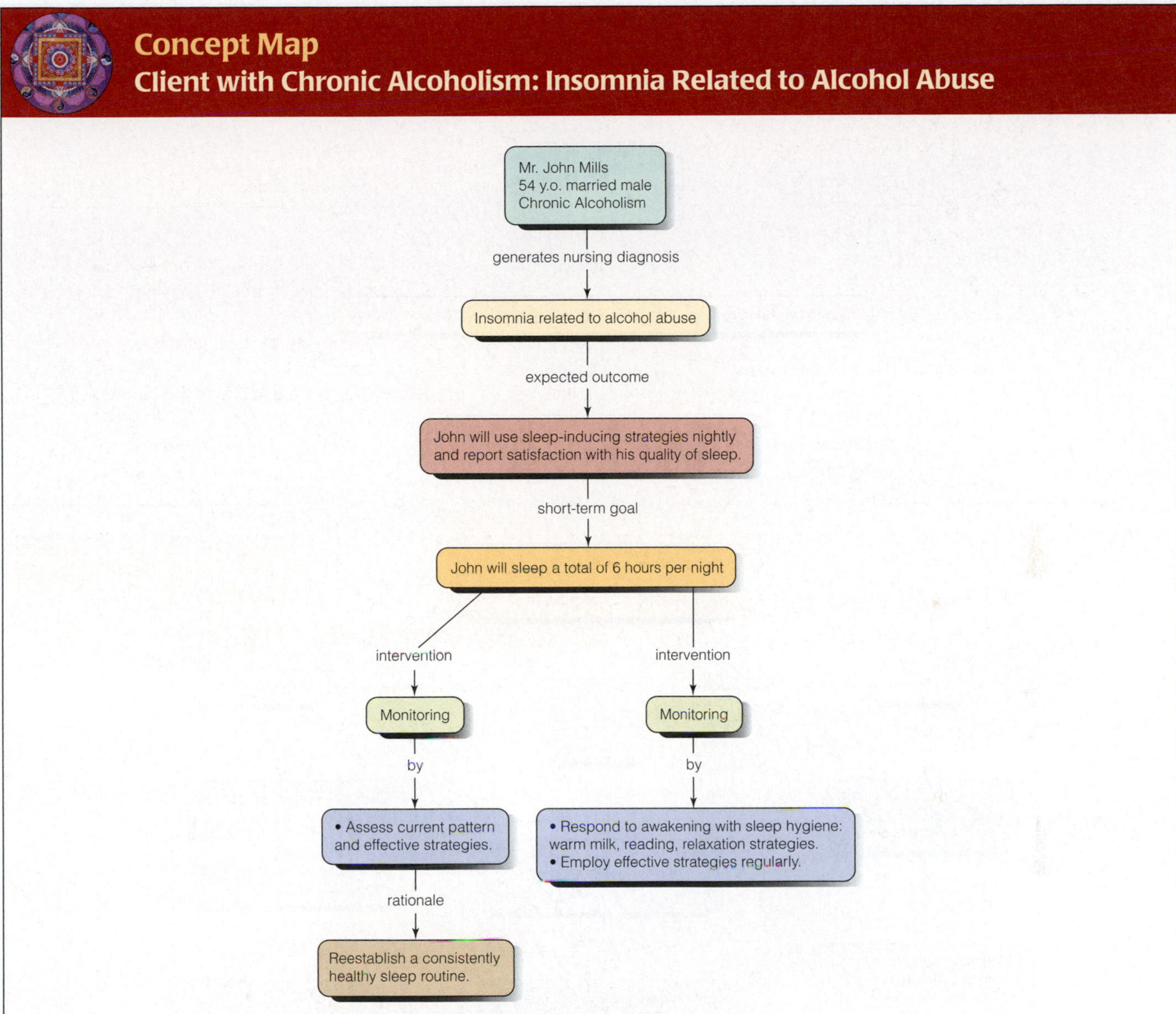
Mr. John Mills
54 y.o. married male
Chronic Alcoholism
generates nursing diagnosis
Insomnia related to alcohol abuse
expected outcome
John will use sleep-inducing strategies nightly and report satisfaction with his quality of sleep.
short-term goal
John will sleep a total of 6 hours per night
intervention
Monitoring
by
• Assess current pattern and effective strategies.
rationale
Reestablish a consistently healthy sleep routine.
intervention
Monitoring
by
• Respond to awakening with sleep hygiene: warm milk, reading, relaxation strategies.
• Employ effective strategies regularly.

Concept Map
Client with Chronic Alcoholism: Imbalanced Nutrition

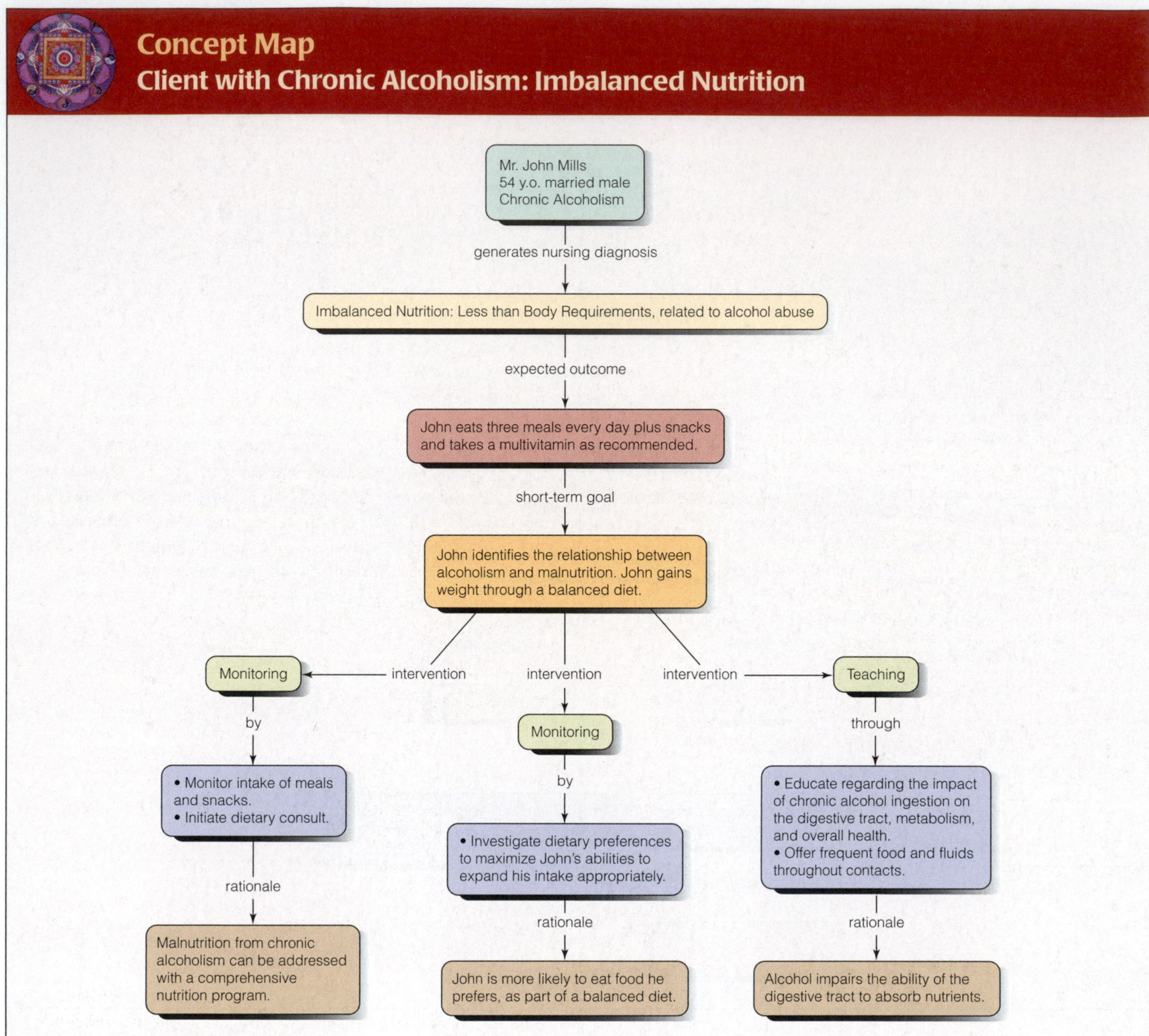

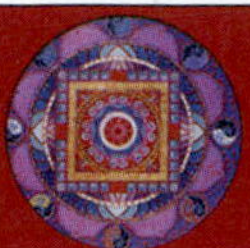

NURSING CARE PLAN
Client with Methamphetamine Intoxication

Identifying Information
Brianna is a 29-year-old married woman. Her husband brought her to the hospital. Brianna was an advertising executive with a large local firm prior to being recently fired. She has an MBA in marketing. She is not now, and has never been, in treatment or therapy.

Brianna does not believe she needs to be hospitalized, especially as she needs to find work. She asserts she is extremely creative and productive and needs "to get my ideas down on paper before someone steals them as their own." She is agitated, aggressive, elated, loud, and occasionally incoherent during the interview. Her only complaint is increased libido "that my husband can't keep up with." Brianna admits to "working very hard at working very hard," but does not believe she needs treatment right now. She feels she can handle this herself.

She has been using methamphetamine for one year, spending most of her salary on it. For the last five days she has used methamphetamine two to three times a day. Prior to that, her use was once or twice weekly. Brianna explains her recent increase in use as "helping me work harder and faster to find a job somewhere in this town. I feel more productive." She is having trouble sitting still and she is perspiring visibly. Brianna states she has been feeling nauseous for several days. Brianna's husband and one female friend are her main support system.

History
Brianna has no prior psychiatric history. Her parents are both living and work together in their own business (retail shoe store). Her younger brother is a college senior. Although close and loving, Brianna's family is 2,000 miles away and they seldom see each other. Brianna's father is an alcoholic who has not been actively drinking for five years.

Brianna is a competitive woman who has always excelled at academics and at work. She "likes being number one." Brianna has few close friends and socialized with acquaintances from work who have not been accessible to her since her firing. Smoking cigarettes since age 17, Brianna admits to "moderate" drinking with occasional weekend alcohol bingeing. She has experimented with a variety of recreational drugs but states "meth really works for me." Brianna describes herself as "the best kind of hard-driving, career-focused woman" but enjoys reading and tennis when time permits.

Brianna has no current or past medical problems. She states she is in good health despite "feeling horrible now." BP 140/90, AP 110.

Current Mental Status
Brianna is attractive, disheveled, agitated, hyperalert, alternatively compliant and hostile, and occasionally incoherent. Sensorium is impaired. Oriented to time, place, and person. Judgment is impaired. Affect is labile; mood swings are evident. Motor behavior is notable for rapid and frequent movements. Thought content is grandiose. Delusions are present. Brianna reports seeing "signs" on billboards that are messages to her that she should "move onward and upward to take over a company." Thought processes are occasionally incoherent, tangential, with difficulty concentrating and easy distraction. There is limited insight: "I can take care of myself. I have a great deal of innate skill and knowledge. I know what I'm doing."

Other Clinical Data
Brianna is not taking any medications; suicide/violence potential is minimal.

Nursing Diagnosis: Ineffective Coping related to methamphetamine abuse

Expected Outcome: Client will complete detox program and will remain free of methamphetamine.

Short-Term Goals	Interventions	Rationale
Meets with staff and attends group meetings according to schedule without prompting.	■ Individual meetings with Brianna regarding consequences of drug use in work, home, social, and physical arena.	Improve Brianna's awareness of her behaviors, reduce denial, and educate about the addictions process.
"Clean" urine 72 hr after last use.	■ Convey agreement to work with Brianna on her problem areas.	Monitor drug-seeking behavior as an inevitable aspect of her problem.
Brianna discusses problems created by methamphetamine use.	■ Assign Brianna to daily individual and group therapy.	
Replaces destructive coping with two effective individual coping options.	■ Observe every half hour. When drug-seeking behavior commences, encourage Brianna to express feelings, educate about cravings and time frames for resolution.	
	■ Assist Brianna in recognizing the automatic mechanisms involved in turning to methamphetamine.	Revision of coping styles requires learning and practice.
	■ Encourage Brianna to rehearse various coping strategies and select two for regular use.	
	■ Explore with Brianna how to substitute effective coping for methamphetamine use.	

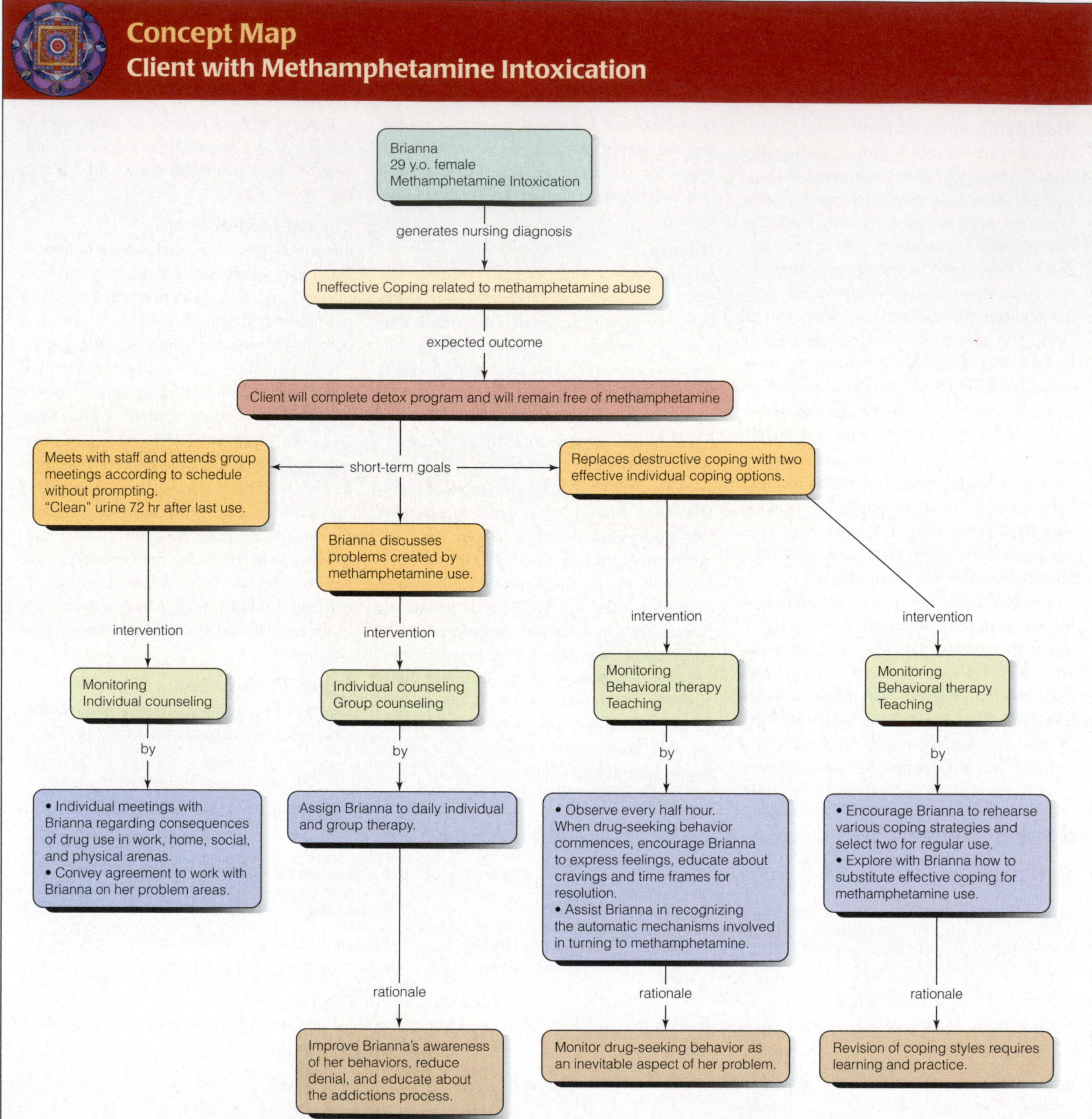
Concept Map
Client with Methamphetamine Intoxication
Brianna
29 y.o. female
Methamphetamine Intoxication
generates nursing diagnosis
Ineffective Coping related to methamphetamine abuse
expected outcome
Client will complete detox program and will remain free of methamphetamine
short-term goals
Meets with staff and attends group meetings according to schedule without prompting.
"Clean" urine 72 hr after last use.
Brianna discusses problems created by methamphetamine use.
Replaces destructive coping with two effective individual coping options.
intervention
Monitoring
Individual counseling
by
• Individual meetings with Brianna regarding consequences of drug use in work, home, social, and physical arenas.
• Convey agreement to work with Brianna on her problem areas.
intervention
Individual counseling
Group counseling
by
Assign Brianna to daily individual and group therapy.
rationale
Improve Brianna's awareness of her behaviors, reduce denial, and educate about the addictions process.
intervention
Monitoring
Behavioral therapy
Teaching
by
• Observe every half hour. When drug-seeking behavior commences, encourage Brianna to express feelings, educate about cravings and time frames for resolution.
• Assist Brianna in recognizing the automatic mechanisms involved in turning to methamphetamine.
rationale
Monitor drug-seeking behavior as an inevitable aspect of her problem.
intervention
Monitoring
Behavioral therapy
Teaching
by
• Encourage Brianna to rehearse various coping strategies and select two for regular use.
• Explore with Brianna how to substitute effective coping for methamphetamine use.
rationale
Revision of coping styles requires learning and practice.

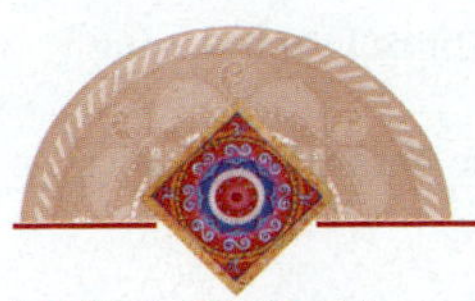

EXPLORE MEDIALINK

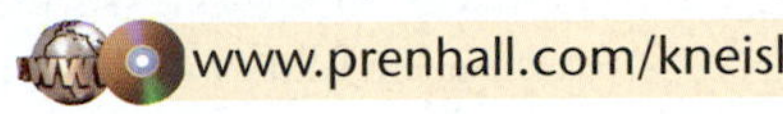

For NCLEX-RN® review questions, case studies, and other resources for this chapter see the Pearson Health MediaLink CD-ROM that accompanies this book and the Companion Website at www.prenhall.com/kneisl.

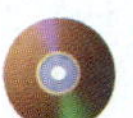

CD-ROM
Audio Glossary
NCLEX-RN® Review Questions
Animations
- *How a Substance of Abuse Occupies a Receptor Site for a Neurotransmitter*
- *Morphine (Astramorph PF, Duramorph, and Other Opioids) Drug Mechanism in Action*
- *Cocaine Drug Mechanism in Action*
- *Overdose*

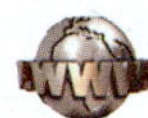

Companion Website
Audio Glossary
NCLEX-RN® Review Questions
Critical Thinking Exercise
- *Substance Abuse in a Vulnerable Population*

Case Study
- *Prescription Substance Abuse*

Care Plan:
- *Potential for Relapse*

MediaLinks
MediaLink Application
- *The Science of Addiction*

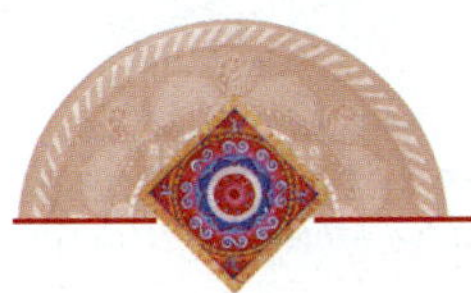

NCLEX-RN® REVIEW QUESTIONS

1. According to psychological theorists, personality traits associated with drug abuse include (select all that apply):
1. Low self-esteem.
2. Difficulty dealing with intimacy.
3. Introverted personality.
4. Poor impulse control.
5. Narcissistic behaviors.

2. The nurse is assessing a client who has a current history of alcohol dependence for signs of major withdrawal. What findings would the nurse expect to find?
1. Hypotension, bradycardia
2. Cold, clammy skin, decreased body temperature
3. Tachycardia, severe diaphoresis
4. Anxiety and increased appetite

3. A priority nursing diagnosis for the client experiencing delirium tremens is:
1. Ineffective Coping related to alcohol abuse.
2. Altered Nutrition: Less than Body Requirements.
3. Risk for Injury.
4. Fluid Volume Excess.

4. The client presents in the emergency room with constricted pupils, slurred speech, drowsiness, and respirations of 8/min. The person who accompanied the client to the emergency room reports the client had taken an unknown quantity of meperidine (Demerol) tablets 30 minutes earlier. Which medication should the nurse anticipate giving the client?
1. Diazepam (Valium)
2. Phenytoin (Dilantin)
3. Naloxone (Narcan)
4. Methadone

5. A graduate nurse is assigned to work on a unit with mentally ill chemically abusing (MICA) clients. Which of the following statements by the nurse is reason for concern?
1. "These clients have more excuses for their problems than anyone I know."
2. "I never really understood what the clients were going through until I attended a counseling group session."
3. "The client should be complimented for maintaining 1 week of sobriety."
4. "It must be very frightening for the client who experiences hallucinations while withdrawing from using alcohol."

6. Which factor does not increase the risk of a teenager developing a drug dependence?
1. Dosage
2. Family culture
3. Frequency of use
4. High school graduate

7. The nurse is completing an admission assessment for a client admitted to the medical unit with a diagnosis of Acute Alcohol Intoxication. When asked to describe his drinking pattern and amount, the client states, "I only drink when I am under a lot of stress." The client's response indicates what defense mechanism?
1. Denial
2. Rationalization
3. Projection
4. Regression

8. Treatment interventions to assist the client with a current history of drug and alcohol abuse and prevent relapse include (select all that apply):
1. Individual therapy.
2. Self-help groups.
3. Twelve-step program.
4. Lifestyle changes.
5. Support from established friendships.

9. Which of the following statements by the client participating in group therapy for meperidine (Demerol) abuse indicates that the client is making progress in treatment?
1. "I would not have to use as much Demerol if my nerves were not shot."
2. "I cannot get addicted to Demerol. You have to take twice as much Demerol as I do to get addicted."
3. "I have not used Demerol in 2 days since I started using relaxation exercises."
4. "I'm trying to work a full day but the boss keeps sending me home."

10. The client with paranoid schizophrenia and cocaine abuse is at risk for:
1. Decreased tardive dyskinesia.
2. Increased psychiatric symptoms.
3. Increased response to psychiatric medications.
4. Decreased frequency and length of psychiatric hospitalizations.

See Appendix C for answers.

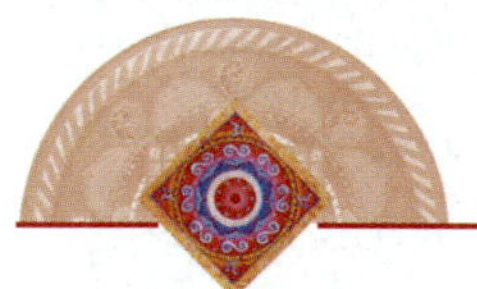

REFERENCES

American Psychiatric Association. (2000). *Diagnostic and statistical manual of mental disorders* (4th ed., Text Revision). Washington, DC: Author.

American Nurses Association & International Nurses Society on Addictions. (2004). *Scope and standards of addictions nursing practice.* Silver Spring, MD: American Nurses Association.

Arria, A. M., Derauf, C., LaGasse, L. L., Grant, P., Shah, R., Smith, L. et al. (2006). Methamphetamine and other substance use during pregnancy: Preliminary estimates from the infant development, environment, and lifestyle (IDEAL) study. *Maternal & Child Health Journal, 10*(3), 293–302.

Baldisseri, M. R. (2007). Impaired health care professional. *Critical Care Medicine. Organizational and Management Ethics in the Intensive Care Unit, 35*(2) S106–S116.

Barr, A. M., Panenka, W. J., MacEwan, G. W., Thornton, A. E., Lang, D. J., Honer, W. G., et al. (2006). The need for speed: An update on methamphetamine addiction. *Journal of Psychiatry & Neuroscience, 31*(5), 301–313.

Brunelle, C., Barrett, S. P., & Pihl, R. O. (2006). Psychostimulant users are sensitive to the stimulant properties of alcohol as indexed by alcohol-induced cardiac reactivity. *Psychology of Addictive Behaviors, 20*(4), 478–483.

Buttarelli, F. R., Patacchioli, F. R., Palladini, G., Brunetti, E., & Pontieri, F. E. (2004). Neuropharmacology of cannabinoid system: From basic science to clinical applications. *Current Neuropharmacology, 2*(1), 1–7.

Christensen, H., Low, L., & Anstey, K. J. (2006). Prevalence, risk factors and treatment for substance abuse in older adults. *Current Opinion in Psychiatry, 19*(6), 587–592.

Dick, D. M., & Bierut, L. J. (2006). The genetics of alcohol dependence. *Current Psychiatry Reports. 8*(2), 151–157.

Donaher, P. A., & Welsh, C. (2006). Managing opioid addiction with buprenorphine. *American Family Physician, 73*(9), 1573–1578, 1580, 1509–1511.

Doweiko, H. F. (2006). *Concepts of chemical dependency* (2nd ed.). Washington, DC: American Psychological Association.

Endres, M., Toso, L., Roberson, R., Park, J., Abebe, D., Poggi, S., et al. (2005). Prevention of alcohol-induced developmental delays and learning abnormalities in a model of fetal alcohol syndrome. *American Journal of Obstetrics & Gynecology, 193*(3) 1028–1034.

Evans, S. E., Blank, M., Sams, C., Weaver, M. F., & Eissenberg, T. (2006). Transdermal nicotine-induced tobacco abstinence symptom suppression: nicotine dose and smokers' gender. *Experimental and Clinical Psychopharmacology, 14*(2), 121–135.

Ewing, J. A. (1999). Screening for alcoholism using CAGE. Cut down, Annoyed, Guilty, Eye opener. *JAMA, 281*(7), 611.

Finnell, D. S., & Osborne, F. H. (2006). Stages of change for psychotropic medication adherence and substance cessation. *Archives of Psychiatric Nursing, 20*(4), 166–174.

Fride, E., Perchuk, A., Hall, F. S., Uhl, G. R., & Onaivi, E. S. (2006). Behavioral methods in cannabinoid research. *Methods in Molecular Medicine, 123,* 269–290.

Glover, E. D. (2006). Successfully treating nicotine dependence. *American Journal of Health Education, 37*(1), 6–14.

Heimer, L., & Van Hoesen, G. W. (2006). The limbic lobe and its output channels: Implications for emotional functions and adaptive behavior. *Neuroscience & Biobehavioral Reviews, 30*(2), 126–147.

Hill, S. Y., Muddasani, S., Prasad, K., Nutche, J., Steinhauer, S. R., Scanlon, J., et al. (2007). Cerebellar volume in offspring from multiplex alcohol dependence families. *Biological Psychiatry, 61*(1), 41–47.

Hoeppner, B. B., Velicer, W. F., Redding, C. A., Rossi, J. S., Prochaska, J. O., Pallonen, U. E., et al. (2006). Psychometric evaluation of the smoking cessation Processes of Change scale in an adolescent sample. *Addictive Behaviors, 31*(8), 1363–1372.

Iso, H., Date, C., Wakai, K., Fukui, M., Tamakoshi, A., & JACC Study Group. (2006). The relationship between green tea and total caffeine intake and risk for self-reported type 2 diabetes among Japanese adults. *Annals of Internal Medicine, 144*(8), 554–562.

Ison, J., Day, E., Fisher, K., Pratt, M., Hull, M., & Copello, A. (2006). Self-detoxification from opioid drugs. *Journal of Substance Use, 11*(2), 81–88.

Jellinek, E. (1946). *Phases in the drinking history of alcoholics.* New Haven, CT: Hillhouse Press.

Kessler, R. C., Chiu, W. T., Demler, O., & Walters, E. E. (2005). Prevalence, severity, and comorbidity of twelve-month DSM-IV disorders in the National Comorbidity Survey Replication (NCS-R). *Archives of General Psychiatry, 62*(6), 617–627.

Killen, J. D., Fortmann, S. P., Murphy, G. M. Jr., Hayward, C., Arredondo, C., Cromp, D., et al. (2006). Extended treatment with bupropion SR for cigarette smoking cessation. *Journal of Consulting and Clinical Psychology, 74*(2), 286–294.

Kim, S. J., Lyoo, I. K., Hwang, J., Chung, A., Hoon Sung, Y., Kim, J., et al. (2006). Prefrontal grey matter changes in short-term and long-term abstinent methamphetamine abusers. *International Journal of Neuropsychopharmacology, 9*(2), 221–228.

Klesges, R. C., DeBon, M., Vander Weg, M. W., Haddock, C. K., Lando, H. A., Relyea, G. E., et al. (2006). Efficacy of a tailored tobacco control program on long-term use in a population of U.S. military troops. *Journal of Consulting and Clinical Psychology, 74*(2), 295–306.

Liddie, H. A., & Rowe, C. L. (2006). *Adolescent substance abuse: Research and clinical advances.* Washington, DC: American Public Health Association.

Lofwall, M. R., Griffiths, R. R., & Mintzer, M. Z. (2006). Cognitive and subjective acute dose effects of intramuscular ketamine in healthy adults. *Experimental and Clinical Psychopharmacology, 14*(4), 439–449.

Lopez-Garcia, E., van Dam, R. M., Willett, W. C., Rimm, E. B., Manson, J. E., Stampfer, M. J., et al. (2006). Coffee consumption and coronary heart disease in men and women: A prospective cohort study. *Circulation, 113*(17), 2045–2053.

McGuinness, T. (2006). Methamphetamine abuse. *American Journal of Nursing, 106*(12), 54–59.

Medina, K. L., Shear, P. K., & Schafer, J. (2006). Memory functioning in polysubstance dependent women. *Drug and Alcohol Dependence, 84*(3), 248–255.

Muthen, B., Asparouhov, T., & Rebollo, I. (2006). Advances in behavioral genetics modeling using Mplus: Applications of factor mixture modeling to twin data. *Twin Research & Human Genetics, 9*(3), 313–324.

National Drug Intelligence Center. (2006). Johnstown, PA: US Department of Justice; Product No. 2006-Q0317-01. http://www.DEA.gov/concern/18862/18862p.pdf.

Olney, J. W. (2004). Fetal alcohol syndrome at the cellular level. *Addiction Biology, 9*(2), 137–149.

Powell, L. S. (2006). Effects of self-help discourse upon adult children of alcoholics' resiliency levels as measured by self perception of problem solving and quality of life. *Dissertation Abstracts International, 67*(4-B), 2283.

Prescott, C. A., Sullivan, P. F., Kuo, P. H., Webb, B. T., Vittum, J., Patterson, D. G., et al. (2006). Genomewide linkage study in the Irish affected sib pair study of alcohol dependence: Evidence for a susceptibility region for symptoms of alcohol dependence on chromosome 4. *Molecular Psychiatry, 11*(6), 603–611.

Ranney, L., Melvin, C., Lux, L., McClain, E., Morgan, L., & Lohr, K. (2006). *Evidence report on tobacco use: Prevention, cessation, and control.* Evidence report/Technology Assessment no. 140. Prepared by RTI-UNC Evidence-based Practice Center under Contract No. 290-02-0016. Rockville MD: Agency for Health Care Research and Quality. AHRQ Publication 06-E 015.

Saitz, R., Palfai, T. P., Cheng, D. M., Horton, N. J., Freedner, N., Dukes, K., et al. (2007). Brief intervention for medical inpatients with unhealthy alcohol use: A randomized, controlled trial. *Annals of Internal Medicine, 146*(3), 167–176.

Serretti, A., Liappas, I., Mandelli, L., Albani, D., Forloni, G., Malitas, P., et al. (2006). Interleukin-1 alpha and beta, TNF-alpha and HTTLPR gene variants study on alcohol toxicity and detoxification outcome. *Neuroscience Letters, 406*(1–2), 107–112.

Trossman, S. (2006). Issues update. Rx for medical marijuana? Promoting research on and acceptance of this treatment option for patients. *American Journal of Nursing, 106*(4), 77–79.

Vieten, C., Seaton, K. L., Feiler, H. S., & Wilhelmsen, K. C. (2004). The University of California, San Francisco family alcoholism study. I. Design, methods, and demographics. *Alcoholism: Clinical and Experimental Research, 28*(10), 1509–1516.

Wu, L., Schlenger, W., & Galvin, D. M. (2006). Concurrent use of methamphetamine, MDMA, LSD, ketamine, GHB, and flunitrazepam among American youths. *Drug and Alcohol Dependence, 84*(1), 102–113.

Wu, L., Schlenger, W., & Galvin, D. M. (2007). Concurrent use of methamphetamine, MDMA, LSD, ketamine, GHB, and flunitrazepam among American youths. *Drug and Alcohol Dependence, 86*(2–3), 301.

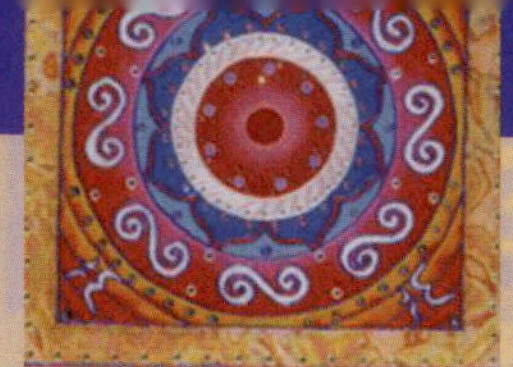

CHAPTER

16

Schizophrenia and Other Psychotic Disorders

EILEEN TRIGOBOFF

KEY TERMS

LEARNING OUTCOMES

After completing this chapter, you will be able to:

1. Describe the central features of schizophrenia.
2. Distinguish among the subtypes of schizophrenia.
3. Compare and contrast the various biopsychosocial theories that address the possible causes of schizophrenia.
4. Explain how psychological and social pressures can influence the course of schizophrenia.
5. Discuss the major nursing implications in caring for clients with difficult and chronic illnesses such as schizophrenia.
6. Discuss the major nursing implications in supporting the families of persons with schizophrenia.
7. Describe methods to prevent or minimize relapses in schizophrenia.
8. Identify the personal characteristics you bring to the care of clients with schizophrenia that might cause you to distance yourself or fail to understand their experience and difficulties.

CRITICAL THINKING CHALLENGE

Like most individuals with schizophrenia, Alicia is extremely sensitive to her environment. When stressed, she often runs the risk that her symptoms will worsen. In the course of living in usual ways, everyone experiences stress related to conducting day-to-day activities. Alicia's nurse at the mental health clinic has been preparing her to cope with working at a local store. Specific environmental features, such as noise and visual distractions, are particularly difficult for Alicia to deal with.

1. Why do mental health care providers advocate that people with schizophrenia interact with the larger community in treatment programs, jobs, and living in the community?
2. Would people with schizophrenia be better off in protected environments such as semistructured group homes or structured and sheltered workshops?
3. How would you help Alicia deal with noise and visual distractions?
4. How do most working people create an environment that suits their strengths and weaknesses? Can these methods be useful for Alicia?

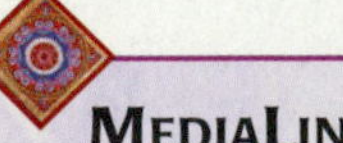

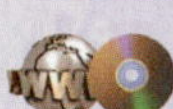

MEDIALINK www.prenhall.com/kneisl

Go to the Pearson Health MediaLink CD-ROM and the Companion Website at www.prenhall.com/kneisl for interactive resources for this chapter.

Schizophrenia is a complex disorder with an extremely varied presentation of symptoms. It affects cognitive, emotional, and behavioral areas of functioning. According to the National Institute of Mental Health the prevalence rate for schizophrenia is approximately 1.1% of the population over the age of 18. The age of onset is typically between the late teens and mid-thirties, although there are cases outside that range. For example, there is a rarely seen childhood schizophrenia as well as a late-onset schizophrenia (referred to as LOS) that is diagnosed after age 45 and seen more often in women. The illness is diagnosed most frequently in the early twenties for men and late twenties for women. The progression of the disease is as variable as its presentation. In some cases, the disease progresses through exacerbations and remissions; in other cases, it takes a chronic, stable course; while in still others, a chronic, progressively deteriorating course evolves. The National Institute of Mental Health website on schizophrenia (www.nlm.nih.gov/medlineplus/schizophrenia.html), which can be accessed through a direct link on the Companion Website for this book, will also serve as a resource on schizophrenia for you, your clients, and their families.

SYMPTOMS OF SCHIZOPHRENIA

The diagnosis of schizophrenia requires not only the presence of distinct symptoms but also the persistence of those symptoms over time. Symptoms must be present for at least 6 months, and active-phase symptoms (called Criterion A symptoms in the DSM-IV-TR) must be present for at least 1 month during that time, before schizophrenia can be diagnosed. The diagnostic criteria for schizophrenia are presented in the DSM-IV-TR feature below.

The symptoms of schizophrenia are conceptually separated into **positive symptoms**, which represent an excess or distortion of normal functioning, or an aberrant response; and **negative symptoms**, which represent a deficit in functioning.

Positive Symptoms

Positive symptoms include the three most pronounced outward signs of the disorder: hallucinations, delusions, and disorganization in speech and behavior.

Hallucinations

Hallucinations are the most extreme and yet the most common perceptual disturbance in schizophrenia. A **hallucination** is a

MEDIALINK National Institute of Mental Health

DSM-IV-TR Diagnostic Criteria for Schizophrenia

A. *Characteristic symptoms:* Two (or more) of the following, each present for a significant portion of time during a 1-month period (or less if successfully treated):
   1. delusions
   2. hallucinations
   3. disorganized speech (e.g., frequent derailment or incoherence)
   4. grossly disorganized or catatonic behavior
   5. negative symptoms (i.e., affective flattening, alogia, or avolition)

   Note: Only one Criterion A symptom is required if delusions are bizarre or hallucinations consist of a voice keeping up a running commentary on the person's behavior or thoughts, or two or more voices conversing with each other.

B. *Social/occupational dysfunction:* For a significant portion of the time since the onset of the disturbance, one or more major areas of functioning such as work, interpersonal relations, or self-care are markedly below the level achieved prior to the onset (or when the onset is in childhood or adolescence, failure to achieve expected level of interpersonal, academic, or occupational achievement).

C. *Duration:* Continuous signs of the disturbance persist for at least 6 months. This 6-month period must include at least 1 month of symptoms (or less if successfully treated) that may meet Criterion A (i.e., active-phase symptoms) and may include periods of prodromal or residual symptoms. During these prodromal or residual periods, the signs of the disturbance may be manifested by only negative symptoms or two or more symptoms listed in Criterion A present in an attenuated form (e.g., odd beliefs, unusual perceptual experiences).

D. *Schizoaffective and Mood Disorder exclusion:* Schizoaffective Disorder and Mood Disorder with psychotic features have been ruled out because either (1) no Major Depressive, Manic, or Mixed Episodes have occurred concurrently with the active-phase symptoms; or (2) if mood episodes have occurred during active-phase symptoms, their total duration has been brief relative to the duration of the active and residual periods.

E. *Substance/general medical condition exclusion:* The disturbance is not due to the direct physiological effects of a substance (e.g., a drug of abuse, a medication) or a general medical condition.

F. *Relationship to a Pervasive Developmental Disorder:* If there is a history of Autistic Disorder or another Pervasive Developmental Disorder, the additional diagnosis of Schizophrenia is made only if prominent delusions or hallucinations are also present for at least a month (or less if successfully treated).

Source: Reprinted with permission from the *Diagnostic and Statistical Manual of Mental Disorders,* Fourth Edition, Text Revision. (Copyright 2000). American Psychiatric Association.

USING DSM-IV-TR

Health care providers often use language unfamiliar to clients and their families. Reword this DSM statement to make it easier for clients and family members to understand: "Two (or more) of the following, each present for a significant portion of time during a 1-month period (or less if successfully treated): delusions, hallucinations, disorganized speech, grossly disorganized or catatonic behavior, or negative symptoms."

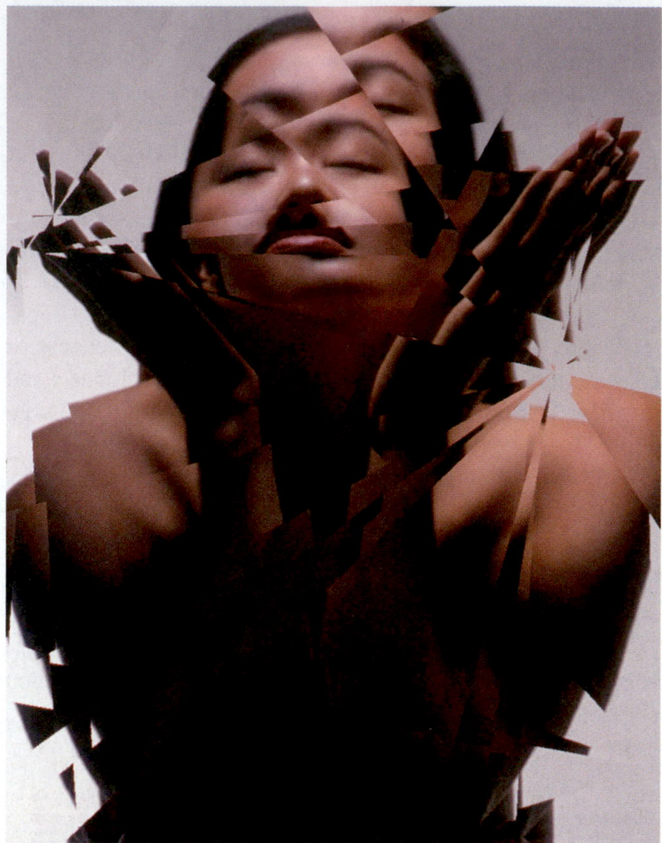

FIGURE 16-1 ■ Distorted perceptions. The distorted visual perceptions indicated by this figure exemplify what is experienced by someone during visual hallucinations.

Source: Photo Researchers, Inc., Dennis D. Potokar.

subjective sensory experience that is not actually caused by external sensory stimuli. One or more of the five senses are involved in hallucinations. Hallucinations may be auditory (heard), visual (seen), olfactory (smelled), gustatory (tasted), or tactile (touched). FIGURE 16-1 ■ represents how someone with visual hallucinations may distort a scene.

The most common form of hallucination in schizophrenia, at least in the western hemisphere, is hearing voices or sounds that are distinct from the person's own thoughts. If a voice is heard, it (or they) may be friendly or hostile and threatening. It is particularly characteristic of schizophrenia if the person hears two or more voices conversing with each other, or hears a voice that provides continuous comments on the train of thought.

Having auditory hallucinations does not necessarily mean that the individual hears human speech. As you will see in Table 16-3 on page 373, several other sounds made by clocks, animals, insects, and so on may be hallucinated. Do not confuse hallucinatory experiences with *synesthesia*, which is the experience of having multiple senses involved in a single event; synesthesia is not a disease or disorder. Distinguishing between synesthesia and hallucinations can be accomplished by ensuring that there is no external stimulation to the sensations. Examples of synesthesia include seeing sounds, seeing colors when in pain, and hearing

TABLE 16-1 ■ **Types of Hallucinations**

Perceptual Disturbance	Commonly Associated Disease Process
Auditory	Schizophrenia
Visual	Dementia
Tactile*	Acute alcohol withdrawal
Somatic*	Schizophrenia
Olfactory*	Seizure disorders
Gustatory*	Seizure disorders

*Also referred to as "proprioceptive hallucinations," associated with infections and tumors.

smells. This knowledge must, necessarily, influence the way you gather information during assessment.

Hallucinations also occur in several other illnesses besides schizophrenia. Dementia (Chapter 14∞), substance abuse (Chapter 15∞), and depression (Chapter 17∞) are some of them. TABLE 16-1 ■ links hallucinations with commonly associated disease processes. Hallucinations can also be experienced under extreme physiologic stress or as a side effect of medications.

Delusions

Delusions are mistaken or false beliefs about the self or the environment that are firmly held even in the face of disconfirming evidence. Delusions may take many forms. In *delusions of persecution*, the person may think that others are following him, spying on him, trying to damage or take something of value like a reputation, or trying to torment him (e.g., "They have misters in my apartment that spray LSD onto me when I walk around."). In another common form, *delusions of reference*, the person thinks that public expressions, like a story on the television or a newspaper article, are specifically addressed to him or her or that the event occurred because of his or her thoughts or actions (e.g., "When the newscaster wears navy blue, she is speaking my thoughts to the world."). Specific delusions are discussed in TABLE 16-2 ■ on page 373.

Disordered Speech and Behavior

Other positive symptoms represent excesses of language or behavior. Disorganized speech is the outward sign of disordered thoughts and may range from less severe forms (the person moves rapidly from one topic to another), to severe forms (the person's speech cannot be logically understood). Positive symptoms include low-level behavioral responses to the environment characterized by such disorganized behavior as agitated, nonpurposeful, or random movements, and waxy flexibility (discussed and defined later in this chapter). The positive symptoms of schizophrenia are discussed in TABLE 16-3 ■ on pages 373–374.

TABLE 16-2 ■ Types of Delusions

Disturbances in Thinking	Definition	Example
Delusions of persecution	Belief that others are hostile or trying to harm the individual	A woman notices a man looking at her and believes that he is trying to follow her.
Delusions of reference	False belief that public events or people are directly related to the individual	A man hears a story on the evening news and believes it is about him.
Somatic delusions	Belief that one's body is altered from normal structure or function	An elderly woman believes that her bowel is filled with cement and refuses to eat.
Thought broadcasting	Belief that one's unspoken thoughts can be heard	A young client believes that everyone around him knows he's attracted to a nurse although he has said nothing.
Delusions of control	Belief that one's actions or thoughts are controlled by an external person or force	A woman believes that her neighbor controls her thoughts by means of his home computer.

TABLE 16-3 ■ Positive Symptoms

Positive Symptom	Examples	
Hallucinations		
Auditory	Human speech (speaking clearly, mumbling, whispering, singing, yelling, screaming, one voice, several voices, voice speaking to client, voices speaking to each other, male, female, both, indistinguishable, imitating nonhuman sounds) Mechanical sounds (clocks, metal clanging, clicking) Music Animal sounds Insect sounds Wind through the trees Grating sounds made by walking on sand Crinkling sound from plastic or aluminum wraps The sound of the earth moving or heaving as during an earthquake	
Visual	Blood Animals Distortions of everyday sights	People Movement of large objects Auras
Olfactory	Green peppers Fumes Garlic Semen Sulfur	Blood Burning materials Urine or feces Rotting meat
Gustatory	Metallic flavor Urine or feces	Blood Semen
Tactile	Being pregnant Being beaten Being raped Grease on hands Internal movements	Giving birth Electrocution Band around head Moving tumors
Delusions		
Persecutory	"I cannot leave my apartment more than once a month. I have to have this cardboard in my pockets when I go out so the CIA can't take pictures of me."	
Referential	"I didn't mean to do it. I was just thinking what would happen if the train derailed. I'm sorry I killed all those people."	

(continued)

TABLE 16-3 ■ Positive Symptoms *(continued)*

Positive Symptom	Examples	
Delusions—*Continued*		
Somatic	"I am going to be hemorrhaging, bleeding to death through my mouth." Or: "I have an alien gestating in my belly. When he is mature he'll drip from my palms like sweat."	
Religious	"My daughter is the devil, saturated with evil, because her age of ascendancy is 666 (June 6, 2006)."	
Substitution	"It looks just like my wife but it's really a robot."	
Thought insertion	"These thoughts are being put in my head by the alien conspiracy." Or: "When I get angry it's because the NSA is altering my brain waves."	
Nihilistic	"Everything is falling apart. My insides are rotting away and so is everything else."	
Grandiose	"I made $7 million from a software program I developed and they're keeping it from me until I tell them my secret programming wizardry." Or: "I am not who you think I am. I work midnights at all the top law firms so I can get all their work done for them."	
Disorganized Speech		
Loose associations	"I came here by bus, but bussing is kissing, I wasn't kissing but if you keep it simple that is a business tenet for KISS. That was a great group that played on and on, but I'm not playing with you. You are youthful looking. Look out for yourself too."	
Word salad	"Wimple sitting purple which the twilighted cheshire, for then frames of silver ticking bubble and."	
Clanging	"I want to eat neat treat seat beat." "I'm fine it's a sign fine whine wine pine dine."	
Echolalia	Client repeats pieces of what is said or entire phrases: Nurse asks, "How are you today?" and the client states, "You today." Or client states, "I love smelling roses. I love smelling roses."	
Behavior		
Disorganized	Client walks around aimlessly picking up everything available to him and touching all objects and surfaces.	
Catatonic	Excited catatonia: A client in the ER is repeatedly assaultive, hyperactive, or cannot sit still. Waxy flexibility: Client maintains a rigid position, allows another to move him or her into new positions and maintains the new position.	
Thinking		
Lack of planning skills	Indecisiveness	Lack of problem-solving skills
Concrete thinking	Blocking	Difficulty initiating tasks

Negative Symptoms

Negative symptoms of schizophrenia are less dramatic but just as debilitating as positive symptoms. TABLE 16-4 ■ on page 375 gives examples of negative symptoms of schizophrenia. Negative symptoms include the "four As" of schizophrenia:

1. Flat *a*ffect and apathy
2. *A*logia
3. *A*volition
4. *A*nhedonia

Flat Affect

People with schizophrenia often appear to have unemotional or very restricted emotional responses to their experiences. **Flat affect** "is the absence or near absence of any signs of affective expression" as well as poor eye contact (American Psychiatric Association [APA], 2000). To see how flat affect differs from a normal range of affect, imagine someone responding to winning a prize ("This is great! I'm so happy!"). Now imagine that same person with much less emotion in her response and no emotion showing on her face ("Oh."). The difference between the two responses is the flattening of affect.

Alogia

Brief, empty verbal responses are known as *alogia*. Rather than saying a few sentences in response to a question, clients with alogia reply with a single word or a very limited number of words. This **poverty of speech** is thought to be symptomatic of diminished thoughts and is different from a refusal

Table 16-4 ■ Negative Symptoms

Negative Symptom	Examples
Flat Affect	The client maintains the same emotional tone when told his mother has died as when told it is time to attend programs. "OK."
Apathy	The client has feelings of indifference toward people, events, activities, and learning.
Avolition	The client does not get to the job he really wanted because he couldn't get up and take the bus.
Anhedonia	The client apparently derives no pleasure from bowling when, prior to getting sick, he used to enjoy it.
Alogia	Rather than using a series of sentences or several words, the client, when asked about his day, speaks sparsely in a limited, stilted manner: "Fine."

to speak. Under these circumstances, the client does not use many words to express experiences or thoughts.

Avolition

A symptom that is frequently misunderstood by families and members of the larger community is **avolition**, an inability to pursue and persist in goal-directed activities. You may see evidence of this negative symptom when a client fails to go for a job interview or fails to become involved in an easily available activity. The schizophrenic person's experience of avolition is often misinterpreted as laziness or an unwillingness to support him- or herself, rather than as a symptom of this chronic disorder. This misunderstanding often affects the ability of family members and friends to stay involved in relationships with the client. They may feel frustrated, as if their efforts have been wasted, or personally rejected because their suggestions have gone unheeded.

Anhedonia

Anhedonia, the inability to experience pleasure, is an important symptom that challenges many nurses. It is difficult to imagine, and even more arduous to empathize with, someone who cannot seem to enjoy even small aspects of life. It is important to remember that people who have schizophrenia cannot enjoy experiences because of a physiologic reason over which they have no control.

Negative symptoms of schizophrenia are difficult to assess because they differ in degree, but not in form, from everyday experience. While few of us have experienced true hallucinations, many of us know what it is like to have a day without the energy to pursue goal-directed activities. Another difficulty in recognizing the presence of negative symptoms stems from the fact that people with schizophrenia often live in difficult situations that may lead to restricted emotional expression and disturbed goal-directed activities. Living in poverty or in unsettled circumstances—homelessness, for example—can induce feelings of desperation or despair, which may mimic the negative symptoms of schizophrenia. It is important to try to separate environmental influences on experience from the disease process, and to note the persistence of the symptoms over time across a variety of circumstances. For example, if a client is living in a rooming house where others around him are likely to steal, that client will not be safe talking excitedly about having received a gift from his parents. If, however, the client is not excited when in his own home in front of his parents and trusted others, the presence of a negative symptom of schizophrenia is likely.

Another important criterion for recognizing schizophrenia is detecting an impaired ability to perform and complete social and work obligations. It is diagnostic of schizophrenia when the person has difficulty performing in one or more areas of life including work, school, social relationships, and the maintenance of everyday activities such as dressing and providing food for oneself.

SUBTYPES OF SCHIZOPHRENIA

Subtypes of schizophrenia are used to designate which symptoms are prominent. The subtypes are discussed below and in the DSM-IV-TR Diagnostic Criteria feature on page 376.

Paranoid Type

Prominent hallucinations and delusions are present in the **paranoid type** of schizophrenia. Delusions are often persecutory or grandiose, and they often connect into a somewhat organized story. Delusions may also be varied and include somatic or religious delusions. Hallucinations often link with the delusions, although this is not necessary. For example, a person who believes he is being monitored by the FBI may hear the voices of people he identifies as FBI agents laughing at him or talking to him.

Disorganized Type

The central features present in the **disorganized type** of schizophrenia are disorganized speech and behavior and flat or inappropriate affect. The client appears disorganized and unkempt because basic everyday tasks like dressing oneself cannot be accomplished. The client may have all the necessary clothing on, but the order of putting on each item of clothing or the steps required to accomplish dressing (e.g., buttoning, zipping, tying) may be too much to handle. Emotional expression may be either inappropriate to the content of what the client is saying (e.g., laughing when discussing being thrown out of the house by roommates) or restricted and flat. Hallucinations and delusions are typically more fragmentary and disorganized than in the paranoid type. This subtype has been referred to as potentially being the most severe form of the disease.

Catatonic Type

Although not seen frequently in the United States, the **catatonic type** of schizophrenia is a distinctive type characterized by extreme psychomotor disruption. The client may display substantially reduced movement to the point of stupor, accompanied by negativism and resistance to any intervention. A client could display a type of posturing known as **waxy flexibility**, a feature of catatonic motor behavior in

MediaLink Application: About Mental Illness: Schizophrenia

DSM-IV-TR Diagnostic Criteria for Schizophrenia Subtypes

PARANOID TYPE

A type of Schizophrenia in which the following criteria are met:

A. Preoccupation with one or more delusions or frequent auditory hallucinations.

B. None of the following is prominent: disorganized speech, disorganized or catatonic behavior, or flat or inappropriate affect.

DISORGANIZED TYPE

A type of Schizophrenia in which the following criteria are met:

A. All of the following are prominent:
   1. disorganized speech
   2. disorganized behavior
   3. flat or inappropriate affect

B. The criteria are not met for Catatonic Type.

CATATONIC TYPE

A type of Schizophrenia in which the clinical picture is dominated by at least two of the following:

1. motoric immobility as evidenced by catalepsy (including waxy flexibility) or stupor
2. excessive motor activity (that is apparently purposeless and not influenced by external stimuli)
3. extreme negativism (an apparently motiveless resistance to all instructions or maintenance of a rigid posture against attempts to be moved) or mutism
4. peculiarities of voluntary movement as evidenced by posturing (voluntary assumption of inappropriate or bizarre postures), stereotyped movements, prominent mannerisms, or prominent grimacing
5. echolalia or echopraxia

UNDIFFERENTIATED TYPE

A type of Schizophrenia in which symptoms that meet Criterion A are present, but the criteria are not met for the Paranoid, Disorganized, or Catatonic Type.

RESIDUAL TYPE

A type of Schizophrenia in which the following criteria are met:

A. Absence of prominent delusions, hallucinations, disorganized speech, and grossly disorganized or catatonic behavior.

B. There is continuing evidence of the disturbance, as indicated by the presence of negative symptoms or two or more symptoms listed in Criterion A for Schizophrenia, present in an attenuated form (e.g., odd beliefs, unusual perceptual experiences).

Source: Reprinted with permission from the *Diagnostic and Statistical Manual of Mental Disorders,* Fourth Edition, Text Revision. (Copyright 2000). American Psychiatric Association.

USING DSM-IV-TR

Health care providers often use language unfamiliar to clients and their families. Reword this DSM statement to make it easier for clients and family members to understand: "Preoccupation with one or more delusions or frequent auditory hallucinations."

which, when clients are placed in peculiar positions, they remain almost completely immobile in the same position for long stretches of time. Alternatively, extremely active and purposeless movement (excitement) that is not influenced by what is going on around the person may be present. Additional signs of the catatonic type of schizophrenia are repeating what others say or mimicking their movements.

Undifferentiated Type

When a client is in an active psychotic state, meaning that Criterion A symptoms for schizophrenia are met and the client does not have prominent symptoms that match any of the prior subtypes, then **undifferentiated type** is diagnosed. Remember that a client's diagnosis may also change over the years as symptoms form and re-form. The particular subtype diagnosed at one point in time may not match what is currently happening to a client. The subtype of schizophrenia may have shifted, with the undifferentiated subtype now most representative of the course of the disease.

Residual Type

The **residual type** of schizophrenia is a subtype diagnosis reserved for a client who has had at least one documented episode of schizophrenia but now has no prominent positive symptoms of the illness. Negative symptoms such as flat affect and inability to work are present, but prominent hallucinations, delusions, and disorganized thoughts and behavior are not. When a client has these characteristics, the client is considered to have residual features of the illness and receives this subtype diagnosis.

SOMATIC TREATMENTS

Prior to the 1950s—which is referred to as the pre-neuroleptic age—insulin coma, drug or electrically induced shock treatments, and psychosurgery, including prefrontal lobotomies, were used to treat schizophrenia. The impact of these extreme somatic treatments did make a difference, for a time, in symptomatology but were not durable or beneficial and often not ethical. Many hoped these treatments were the long-sought-after cure for schizophrenia because they were relatively quick and inexpensive compared to lengthy and costly analytic therapies. This hope was not realized.

Contemporary psychosurgery has been refined from a gross assault on cranial tissue (the lobotomy of decades past) to procedures in which specific involved areas of the brain are delicately shaped to reduce repetitive and destructive behaviors (amygdalotomy, cingulotomy). Electroconvulsive therapy (ECT) has been improved upon and crafted to an impressive degree in the last 20 years. Effective treatment with minimal risks has been offered mostly for mood-disordered clients.

The introduction of psychoactive drugs in the 1950s provided new alternatives for the treatment of schizophrenia. Psychotropic medications, which influence the thoughts, mood, and behavior of clients, made previously uncontrolled symptoms manageable. In the period following the introduction of psychotropic medications, the use of seclusion and restraints declined dramatically, as did the duration of hospital stays and numbers of clients in state mental hospitals.

A new optimism arose regarding the possible outcomes of mental illness. Because they controlled the most difficult symptoms of psychosis, psychotropic medications made psychosocial or behavioral treatments possible for a much greater percentage of psychiatric clients. The major tranquilizers did not live up to their promise of providing a cure for schizophrenia and other chronic psychiatric illnesses. However, these drugs relieved the most debilitating symptoms for many clients and were the first step toward recovery or a higher level of functioning.

Refer to Chapters 5, 6, 7, and 32 for more details on the history and the science behind somatic treatments. Ethical and legal aspects of somatic treatments are discussed in Chapter 13.

RELAPSE

A client with schizophrenia is vulnerable after a period of stability, however brief or extended, partial or complete, to a return of symptoms. This is referred to as a **relapse**, and the disease itself has a pattern of relapse and recovery. As a chronic disorder, schizophrenia is characterized by relapses alternating with periods of full or partial remission.

Although antipsychotic medication is effective in reducing relapse rates, 30% to 40% of clients relapse within 1 year after hospital discharge even if they are receiving maintenance medication. This is a tremendous difficulty for the client to overcome; therefore, acknowledge the sense of demoralization likely with such a recurrent and debilitating course that cannot be altered significantly. The current hope is that the relapse rate will be reduced from around 35% to about 15% to 20%. The need to improve methods for relapse prevention is clear (van Meijel et al., 2006). The following clinical examples detail how relapses can occur under certain circumstances.

CLINICAL EXAMPLE

Daryl, a 26-year-old with a diagnosis of paranoid schizophrenia, decided to stop taking his quetiapine (Seroquel) because he didn't think he needed it anymore. Within a few days of stopping the medication, he was unable to leave the house for fear of someone harming him. Although he liked his job at the local cannery and knew that he had the chance to earn more money in the near future, he refused to go to work for fear that he would be hit by a bus on his way there. He was eventually fired because of poor attendance. The loss of a structured schedule furthered his deterioration and Daryl relapsed, requiring hospitalization.

In this instance, a decrease in medication increased Daryl's biologic vulnerability, with marked behavioral, and eventually environmental, consequences. His relapse began with a medication issue and could have been prevented.

CLINICAL EXAMPLE

Jeanne, 22, lived with her divorced mother and younger sister Maura since her release from the hospital after her second psychotic episode. She found living alone too frightening and was more comfortable staying in her old room at home. When Maura began preparing to leave home for college, Jeanne became increasingly anxious, demanding to sleep in Maura's room at night and hiding Maura's belongings. As Maura's departure grew near, Jeanne began actively hallucinating and withdrew to her room, refusing to talk to her mother or sister.

In this case, the client did not have sufficient coping skills to deal with her sister's departure from the household, and her psychosis reemerged. Jeanne's relapse may have been averted had she been taught coping skills and had the opportunity to practice them. However, learning is unfavorably affected by schizophrenia, motivation and energy are problems, and even a competent program of teaching cannot remove all the negative consequences in response to life stress.

OTHER PSYCHOTIC DISORDERS

Psychosis occurs in a number of disorders in addition to schizophrenia. The problems with symptoms can be short-lived or may extend into significant periods of time with disability.

Schizophreniform Disorder

Schizophreniform disorder is very similar to schizophrenia except the person has not been ill for very long. The diagnostic criteria are the same as the Criterion A symptoms for schizophrenia. The main difference is that the client has experienced the symptoms for at least 1 month and either recovered from the symptoms before 6 months, or 6 months have not yet elapsed since the original symptoms began. Under the latter set of circumstances, the diagnosis of schizophreniform disorder is provisional until the 6 months have elapsed and then a diagnosis is set. A second difference, besides duration, is that the client may show no impairment in social and work functioning.

Schizophreniform disorder may occur just prior to the onset of schizophrenia (i.e., be prodromal to [precede] schizophrenia), yet approximately one third of clients diagnosed with this disorder recover. The other two thirds go on to have either schizophrenia or schizoaffective disorder.

MEDIALINK 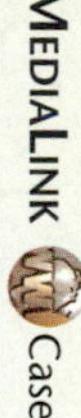 Case Study: The Client with Schizoaffective Disorder

Schizoaffective Disorder

In **schizoaffective disorder**, two sets of symptoms—psychotic and mood symptoms—are present concurrently in the same period of illness episode: Criterion A symptoms of schizophrenia and symptoms of a mood disorder (either a major depressive or manic disorder; see Chapter 17). Schizoaffective disorder is less common than, and has a slightly better prognosis than, schizophrenia, but it has a substantially worse prognosis than mood disorders. Interacting with a client who has schizoaffective disorder may require the same skills you would employ with a client

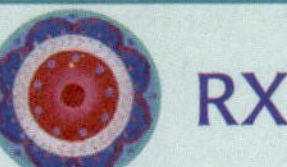

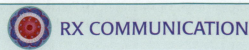

RX COMMUNICATION

CLIENT WITH CLANG ASSOCIATIONS

CLIENT: "The dining room lining trying to eat forever."

NURSE RESPONSE 1: "Jack, are you having a problem getting your food?" *RATIONALE:* Direct question allows the client with clang associations to answer with a "yes" or "no" response, models how the communication can be stated, and labels the situation as a problem.	**NURSE RESPONSE 2:** "Come with me and let's get you set up." *RATIONALE:* This response reinforces the appropriateness of the client's coming to the nurse with a problem and concretely shows the client how to resolve the problem.

who has schizophrenia. Disorganized speech may be an expression of this client's psychosis. The Rx Communication box above provides examples of therapeutic communication with a client with the clang association form of disorganized speech.

One of the defining characteristics of schizoaffective disorder is when the hallucination or delusion occurs. A person who has schizoaffective disorder is likely to have hallucinations or delusions regardless of mood state. In other words, if the person were delusional only when he or she had extreme problems with mood (mania or depression), it is likely the diagnosis would be mood disorder with psychotic features rather than schizoaffective disorder.

Delusional Disorder

Delusional disorder is diagnosed when the client holds one or more nonbizarre delusions for a period of at least 1 month. The client must never have met the Criterion A symptoms for schizophrenia. Although it is sometimes difficult to differentiate bizarre from nonbizarre delusions, the key is that the nonbizarre delusions could conceivably arise in everyday life. A nonbizarre delusion is the focus of the clinical example that follows.

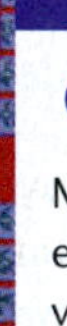

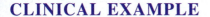

CLINICAL EXAMPLE

Martin holds the delusional belief that the police are trying to entrap him. He goes to extremes to protect his home with surveillance and security equipment. At the same time, he believes that the police won't bother him at work because his boss, with whom he gets along well, is the son of a policeman.

People with delusional disorders may function quite well in areas of their life not affected by the delusion, yet behave oddly in activities touched by the delusion. Delusional disorders are not common and arise predominantly during middle and late adulthood.

A subtype of delusional disorder, the erotomanic type, occurs when clients believe that another person is in love with them. Typically this other person has no relationship whatsoever to the client, or the relationship is superficial at best. Contacting the person, stalking the person, and displays to impress the imagined lover have involved celebrities, politicians, and even the man or woman next door.

Brief Psychotic Disorder

In a brief psychotic disorder, at least one of the Criterion A symptoms for schizophrenia are present (hallucinations, delusions, disorganized speech or behavior) for at least 1 day, but for less than 1 month. Upon remission of these symptoms, clients return to their level of functioning prior to the onset of the illness. This disorder may be brought on by a particular stressful event in the person's life, including childbirth. In other instances, a stressful life event cannot be specifically identified. Brief psychotic disorder is an unusual and seldom-seen phenomenon.

Additional Psychotic Disorders

Several additional psychotic disorders are specified in the DSM-IV-TR:

- Shared psychotic disorder
- Psychotic disorder due to a general medical condition
- Substance-induced psychotic disorder
- Psychotic disorder not otherwise specified (NOS)

Consult the DSM-IV-TR for diagnostic criteria for these disorders. However, in diagnosing any psychotic disorder, the diagnostician must explore the alternative explanation that symptoms may be caused by an underlying medical disorder or by substance use.

BIOPSYCHOSOCIAL THEORIES

Beliefs about the causes of schizophrenia have changed over the centuries since schizophrenia was equated with early senility. Theories about the treatment for schizophrenia have also undergone change. For example, at one point it was erroneously believed (based on the writings of Sigmund Freud) that people with schizophrenia could not be treated because they were unable to form a therapeutic relationship with a psychoanalyst. At another point, a now discredited theory pointed to the behavior of parents, especially mothers, causing schizophrenia in their offspring. It is likely that several factors interrelate to cause schizophrenia and several forces influence the effectiveness of treatment. A multifactorial cause and a varied approach to treatment, responsive to the individual's needs, seem to be most accurate and effective.

Biologic Theories

It is unlikely that schizophrenia is caused by one specific biologic abnormality. Scientists have searched unsuccessfully for a unique biologic marker consistently present in people with schizophrenia but absent in healthy people. At the same time, evidence suggests that the disorder is not merely psychological and that biologic alterations are present. Particularly convincing is the fact that the symptoms associated with schizophrenia, such as delusions or hallucinations, are found in healthy people only when they are in a state of metabolic imbalance or suffer from organic diseases. Individuals who have brain tumors, have infections, or have ingested certain drugs, for example, may experience hallucinations.

Genetic Theories

People with schizophrenia inherit a genetic predisposition to the disease rather than inheriting the disease itself. What supports this theory is the fact that relatives of people with schizophrenia have a greater chance of developing the disease than do members of the general population. While 1.1% of the population develops schizophrenia, 10% of the first-degree relatives (parents, siblings, children) of persons with schizophrenia are diagnosed with the disease during their lifetimes (Brookes et al., 2006; Karayiorgou & Gogos, 2006; Kessler, Chiu, Demler, & Walters, 2005). The risk of developing schizophrenia increases with the closeness of one's relationship to a diagnosed person. Siblings have a greater risk of developing the disease than do half-siblings or grandchildren, and these have a greater risk than more distant relatives, such as cousins.

There is no clear genetic marker for schizophrenia at this time, although several research projects are involved in the search for susceptibility genes. The most promising development has been the Human Genome Project. The Project's completion of the sequence of the human genome has been guiding the study of the genetic variations implicated in human disease. The quest for the schizophrenia gene is exciting news for psychiatric–mental health nurses. On the other hand, Joseph and Leo (2006) make a strong argument that much of what we have assumed is genetic can also be explained by environmental factors. The risk of susceptibility may remain the same, but the notion that there is one specific schizophrenia gene may have weaker support than previously thought.

In fact, it is becoming obvious that a single gene is not responsible for schizophrenia (Paz et al., 2006; Riley & Kendler, 2006). This illness resists easy genetic codification due to its complexity and its variety of forms. It has been suggested that schizophrenia may be a collection of disorders rather than a single disease entity. The current front-runner among possible susceptibility genes for schizophrenia is neuregulin 1 (NRG1), a very complex gene (Harrison & Law, 2006). It has six known types but only two may be relevant to schizophrenia.

Research examining the occurrence of schizophrenia in twins indicates that both environmental and genetic factors are important. Rates of concordance (in which both twins either express or do not express the trait) for schizophrenia are consistently higher for monozygotic twins than for dizygotic twins. Interestingly, monozygotic, or identical, twins need not both have schizophrenia, but the chance of both twins having schizophrenia is 25% to 39%. This finding supports the hypothesis of some level of genetic transmission. The fact that both twins are not always affected when they are genetically identical, however, indicates that environment plays a large part in the expression of the illness. If the disease were solely genetically determined, the concordance rates in this group would be close to 100%. (See also pages 89–92 and 100 in Chapter 6 for another discussion of genetics in schizophrenia.)

Brain Structure Abnormalities

As a group, people with schizophrenia differ in their brain structure from people who do not have schizophrenia. People with chronic schizophrenia show changes to their frontotemporal cortical gray matter, among other areas. Magnetic resonance imaging (MRI) studies show hippocampal structural differences between people who have schizophrenia and those who do not. When the hippocampus is formed, brain-derived neurotrophic factor (BDNF) is involved. Checking for abnormalities in BDNF may be able to tell us who is at risk for developing schizophrenia (Szeszko et al., 2005).

Altered brain structures may be genetically based and could represent a marker of vulnerability to schizophrenia that precedes any other symptomatology. How the brain structure abnormalities influence the progress of the disease is not well understood and requires further study. An example of PET scan differences between identical twins where one has schizophrenia and the other is unaffected is seen in FIGURE 16-2 ■.

Biochemical Theories

The biochemical basis of schizophrenia is captured in the **dopamine hypothesis**, which states that schizophrenic symptoms may be related to overactive neuronal activity that is dependent on dopamine (DA). In other words, positive psychotic symptoms are associated with excessive DA transmission.

The hypothesis was supported by numerous studies demonstrating that DA blockers, which are medications that decrease DA activity, alleviate symptoms. The traditional antipsychotic medications were shown to be effective because of their ability to antagonize DA receptors; however, this causes undesirable side effects such as extrapyramidal symptoms. The relief of positive symptoms with these traditional agents was not complete, and the negative symptoms of the disorder were much less responsive to DA blockers. See FIGURE 16-3 ■ for a graphic representation of this concept.

Research suggests that the relationships between DA activity and schizophrenic symptoms are much more complex than originally hypothesized. It is now known that there are multiple types of DA receptors, and different types of receptors are concentrated in different regions of the brain. Another feature of this theory is catechol-O-methyltransferase (COMT), a catecholamine-metabolizing enzyme involved in dopamine flux and the dopaminergic regulation problems seen in schizophrenia (Meyer-Lindenberg et al., 2006; Tunbridge, Weinberger, & Harrison, 2006). The regulation of DA activity

MediaLink PET/SPECT Schizophrenia Animation

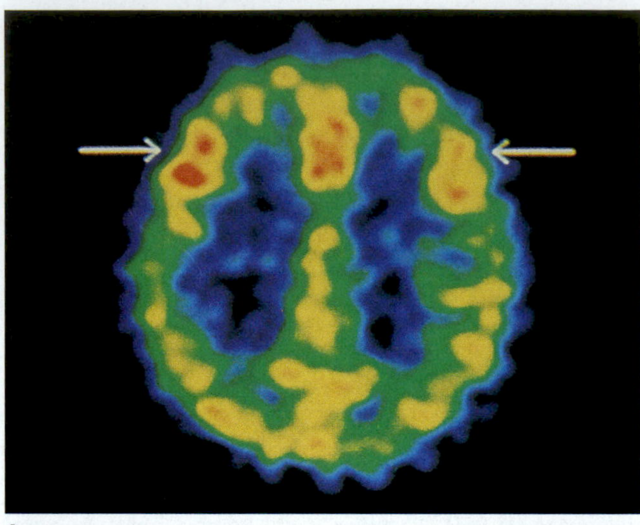

A

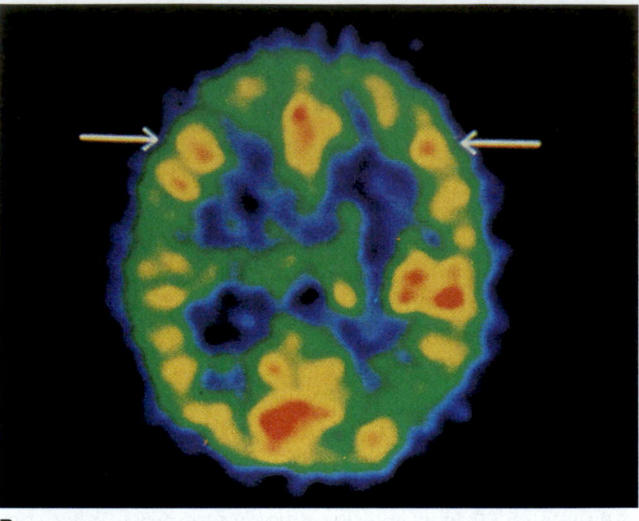

B

FIGURE 16-2 ■ Schizophrenia scans. PET scans of discordant monozygotic twins taken during a test to provoke activity and measure regional cerebral blood flow. (A) Arrows indicate areas of normal blood flow and brain activity in the unaffected twin. (B) Arrows indicate areas of lower blood flow and brain activity in the twin with schizophrenia.

Source: Courtesy of Dr. Karen F. Berman, *Clinical Brain Disorders Branch,* National Institute of Mental Health.

continues to be thoroughly studied, as DA dysregulation from every source is recognized as being inherently involved in the pathology of schizophrenia (Eastwood & Harrison, 2006).

Further evidence that supports a biochemical theory is the physical impact that atypical antipsychotic agents have on clients with schizophrenia (Kelly & Conley, 2006; Kelly et al., 2006). These medications block DA as well as serotonin. This may help lessen extrapyramidal side effects such as dystonia and akathisia (uncomfortable or painful side effects, explained in detail in Chapter 32), and may be the reason they are so useful in reducing negative symptoms.

MEDIALINK Extrapyramidal Side Effects Videos

Psychological Theories

Most psychological theories focus on the processing of information as well as attention and arousal states in schizophrenia.

Information Processing

Many clients with schizophrenia have information-processing deficits. Two central types of information processing have been identified:

1. Automatic processing
2. Controlled or effortful processing

Automatic processing occurs when you take information in unintentionally. Automatic processing can occur without your being aware of it and does not interfere with conscious thought processes that occur at the same time. An example of automatic information processing is being aware of the physical features of a new environment, such as a room being large and spacious as opposed to small and confined.

People with schizophrenia are deficient in controlled information processing (Lee, Lee, Lee, & Kim, 2007; Nicode-

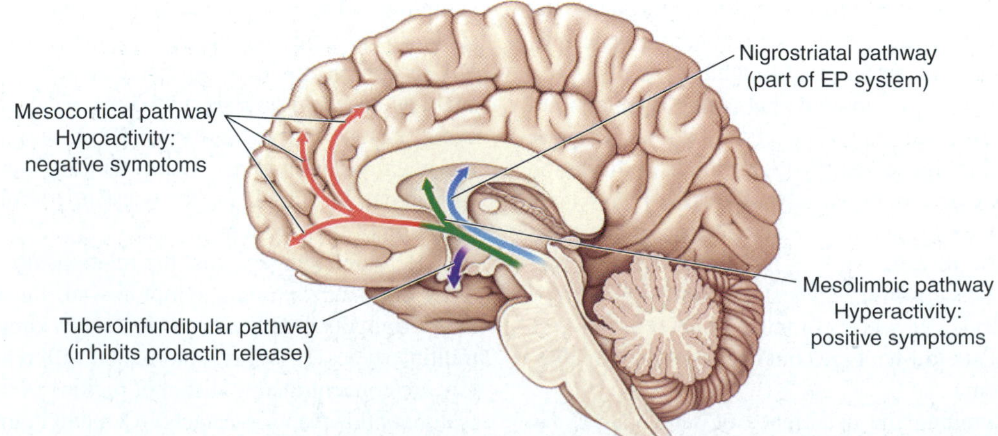

FIGURE 16-3 ■ The dopamine hypothesis of schizophrenia holds that the amount of dopamine in various areas of the brain creates the various symptoms of the disease. Note how too much dopamine in the mesolimbic area (the middle of the limbic system) is thought to cause positive symptoms, while too little dopamine in the mesocortical area (the middle of the cortex of the brain) is thought to cause the negative symptoms of schizophrenia.

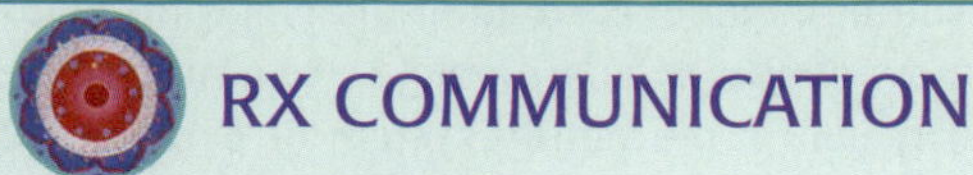

UNFOCUSED CLIENT

CLIENT: "I went to the ballgame and I had great seats and I saw the whole game and I saw all the home runs and all the hits and all the strikeouts and I saw the pitcher throw all the pitches, fast ball, curve ball, change up, and. . . ."

NURSE RESPONSE 1: "Keith, tell me about this more slowly so I can keep up with you."

RATIONALE: This response is structured to be brief, focused, and to direct the client's attention to the speed with which he speaks.

NURSE RESPONSE 2: "How about if I ask you some questions about the game? If you give me a chance to ask questions I'll have a better idea of what you saw."

RATIONALE: This response defines the special skills required for a conversation.

mus et al., 2006). Their ability to perform directed, conscious, sequential thinking—for example, making comparisons between two stimuli or organizing a set of stimuli—is consistently inferior to that of people who do not have schizophrenia. Someone with schizophrenia would not easily be able to perform the series of steps necessary to organize a classroom debate. Any level of cognitive dysfunction creates ripple effects in treatment and quality of life. See the Rx Communication feature for an example of an interaction with a client who is unfocused and having a problem processing information.

We do not know whether the inability of a person with schizophrenia to sustain conscious, directed thought is the primary problem or the result of a primary deficit in automatic thinking. If the primary deficit is in automatic processes, then the person is forced to complete automatic tasks at the conscious level, inhibiting and slowing controlled information processing. There is research support for the presence of attention and cognitive impairments (Donohoe et al., 2006) and the presence of negative impacts on working memory in the current literature. Sufficient evidence to resolve this question is not yet available.

Attention and Arousal

Attention and arousal are measured by physiologic states and alterations, such as galvanic skin response, heart rate, blood pressure, skin temperature, and pupillary response. Physiologic studies of attention and arousal in clients with schizophrenia show promise in identifying clinically significant subgroups.

One subgroup of clients exhibits abnormally low response levels to novel, or different, stimuli. This finding suggests that these clients are less adept than healthy people at attending to and responding to novel situations. An example of this state can be seen when a client with schizophrenia does not register that a ball is being thrown at him during a game of catch. The ball may even strike him, drop to the ground, and roll away before the client looks at it.

A second group of clients with schizophrenia demonstrates a state of hyperarousal evidenced by elevated electrodermal activity, heart rate, and blood pressure. Hyperarousal has been noted during both symptomatic and nonsymptomatic periods. These clients demonstrate symptoms of irritability, excitement, and anxiety rather than apathy and withdrawal. An example of this state occurs when a client with schizophrenia angrily and loudly criticizes someone for using incorrect grammar in a sentence.

Family Theories

Numerous theories implicating family interaction alone as a cause of schizophrenia have been proposed and unsupported. Research has failed to support the theory that dysfunctional family interaction alone causes the illness.

Suggestions have been supported that disordered family communication (the inability to focus on and clearly share an observation or thought) causes schizophrenia only in the presence of a genetic predisposition to the disease. For example, the communication taking place at the dinner table may be chaotic and constant. No one finishes a sentence and nothing is discussed to its logical conclusion. Living with this pattern of family communication during early development is thought to impair the ability of the person with schizophrenia to perceive the environment and communicate with others about it. People with schizophrenia are more likely to show symptoms of thought disorder when they are raised by people who have dysfunctional communication.

Individuals with schizophrenia who are raised by adoptive parents, who themselves showed elevated levels of communication deviance, demonstrate as much thought disorder as those raised in birth families. In contrast, adoptees who were raised by adoptive parents with more functional communication were less likely to show thought disorder. In one study, this pattern was not evident in control adoptees—there was no discernible relationship between thought disorder in the adoptees and communication deviance in the adoptive parents. In other words, these findings did not detect the presence of a "schizophrenogenic" environment for individuals without a preexisting genetic liability. These examples support the view that genetic factors alone do not explain the development of schizophrenia, and that interactions with the environment are important. Individuals who live in aversive environments tend to have higher rates of schizophrenia, suggesting there may be a neighborhood and social context to development of the disease (Allardyce & Boydell, 2006).

A second theory is that the family's emotional tone can influence the course of schizophrenia over time. Researchers

MEDIALINK NARSAD

found that individuals with schizophrenia from families who are highly critical, hostile, overprotective, or overinvolved tend to relapse more often. Families exhibiting such characteristics have been described as having high **expressed emotion (EE)**. There is some evidence that family expressed emotion, life events, and biological factors combine with the individual's genetic liability to the disorder to cause schizophrenia. In other words, the disorder is responsive to psychosocial attributes such as the emotional climate of the family (Kymalainen, Weisman, Rosales, & Armesto, 2006). Recent research on schizophrenia can be found on the website for NARSAD at www.narsad.org and through a direct link on the Companion Website for this book.

Humanistic–Interactional Theories

An interactional model of schizophrenia integrates many of the biologic and psychosocial theories already discussed. In this view, schizophrenia is due to the interaction of a genetic predisposition or biologic vulnerability, stress or change in the environment, and the individual's social skills and supports. In an interactional model, the influences are multidimensional. A biologic vulnerability may inhibit the individual's capacity to cope with even minor stressors such as the loss of a primary source of support. Similarly, the symptoms of schizophrenia may worsen upon entering an environment that demands coping skills the person with schizophrenia may not have developed.

A precursor to present-day interactional theories is the enduring interpersonal-psychiatric theory of Harry Stack Sullivan (discussed in detail in Chapter 5). Sullivan, a psychiatrist, emphasized modes of interaction and the role of anxiety as the real focus of psychiatric inquiry in his work with people with schizophrenia. Hildegard Peplau (known as the "mother" of psychiatric nursing) based her interpersonal psychiatric nursing approach on the work of Sullivan. However, Peplau had more to say than Sullivan about the social and cultural conditions that influence behavior. The ideas of Sullivan and Peplau continue to influence our practice with clients who are schizophrenic.

MEDIALINK The Influence of Stressors on Schizophrenia

Stress–Vulnerability Model

An interactional model for understanding schizophrenia that has received wide acceptance is the stress–vulnerability model, which suggests that people with schizophrenia have a genetically based, biologically mediated vulnerability to personal, family, and environmental stress. In this model, risk factors and protective factors interact in any of three ways:

1. Stressors, risk, and vulnerability factors combine and potentiate each other.
2. As long as stress is not excessive, it enhances competence.
3. Protective factors modulate or buffer the impact of stressors by improving coping and adaptation.

People with schizophrenia have a potentially increased vulnerability to stress. High-EE relatives may cause them great stress, resulting in an exacerbation of symptoms and/or a relapse. It is now almost standard practice to aim to reduce high EE and criticism in the family system of persons with schizophrenia. However, as one study indicates, while some families are identified by researchers as having a critical home environment, the clients themselves do not necessarily perceive their relatives as critical (Weisman, Rosales, Kymalainen, & Armesto, 2006).

As we know, the stressors a client with schizophrenia experiences can overwhelm the resources available, and symptoms result. Psychobiologic stressors include the stress of living with schizophrenia itself. Altered attention and perception, as well as problems with motivation and energy, create stresses for people with schizophrenia. Environmental and interpersonal stressors include those we all encounter; however, a person with schizophrenia is particularly sensitive to them. These include stressful life events, environments that are highly demanding or stimulating, and family or living environments that are highly negative.

It is not unusual for clients to make statements that point to the validity of the stress–vulnerability concept, especially the protective qualities. One client said, "I'm not saying it [referring to an antipsychotic medication] is a perfect solution. It's not. There are painful side effects. But I know I can count on it when the going gets rough. If things get stressful it will help me through it." A second client said: "I feel raw inside and out when I'm off it [referring to an antipsychotic medication]. Everything bothers me. So it cushions the blows that are my life."

Resources That Moderate Stress

Resources that can moderate stress (and are thought to affect the development of symptoms in schizophrenia) include:

- Skill in symptom recognition and management
- Social support
- Antipsychotic medication

The capacities to self-monitor the waxing and waning of schizophrenia and to develop coping strategies to influence symptoms at the first sign of trouble show promise in influencing the longer-term course of the illness. An example of how you can help a client to self-monitor symptoms and develop coping strategies is in the Evidence-Based Practice feature on page 383. This capacity to detect prodromal symptoms and acute symptoms and institute self-care before completely decompensating is a resource that may work to mediate the stress that occurs in the person, family, or environment.

Social support has proven helpful in moderating stress for general populations and for people with schizophrenia in particular. Supportive others who provide empathy, interpersonal contact, financial aid, problem solving, and other forms of support help to mitigate the difficulties of schizophrenia (Montgomery, Tompkins, Forchuk, & French, 2006). Finally, antipsychotic medications moderate some, and sometimes most, symptoms of the disease, and thus some of the stressors induced by the disease.

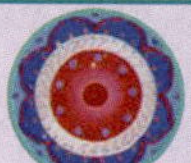

EVIDENCE-BASED PRACTICE

ASSESSING THE PARENTING SKILLS OF A CLIENT WITH SCHIZOPHRENIA

Jane is a 33-year-old female, mother of two small children, who has paranoid schizophrenia. She is one of the people with whom you work in an outpatient clinic for moderately ill people who have schizophrenia. Your education and experience have taught you that schizophrenia is a complex illness that requires more than just medications to address it adequately.

Jane typically hides her illness from her children. She wants to protect them from the stress and stigma of a mentally ill mother, and she wants her role as mother to be unsullied by illness and incapacitation. In order to achieve this, she watches what she says and masks her troubles. Jane has appointments at the clinic only when her children are otherwise occupied. They do not know she is in therapy or takes medications. What happens as a result is that Jane gets very symptomatic from the stress of pretending she is not ill.

This situation suggests the need to be sensitive to mothers who have a serious mental illness. Carefully and accurately assess and reassess the mothering skills needed to make sure the children are nurtured, their relationship is healthy, and the mother receives the care she needs. Action should be based on more than one study, but the following is a study that would be helpful in this situation.

Montgomery, P., Tompkins, C., Forchuk, C., & French, S. (2006). Keeping close: Mothering with serious mental illness. *Journal of Advanced Nursing, 54*(1), 20–28.

CRITICAL THINKING APPLICATION

1. Is it possible for Jane to truly hide her illness from her children?
2. How will you know if Jane's relationship with her children is a nurturing one?

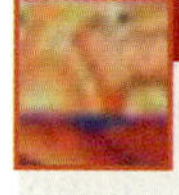

NURSING PROCESS
Clients with Schizophrenia

Schizophrenia is a difficult and chronic illness requiring understanding and competent care in every facet of the client's life. In addition to the discussion that follows, a nursing care plan for the client with schizophrenia is presented at the end of the chapter.

Assessment

Assessing clients who have schizophrenia occurs at individual, family, and environmental levels. Be aware of the client's status and of changes in the client's personal life, family situation, and environment in order to plan care and intervene effectively. In addition, care that addresses multiple levels of the client's life is consistent with the interactional theory of schizophrenia because it is assumed that changes in any aspect of the client's environment influence all other aspects of the personal environmental balance.

Subjective Data

These data describe the client's inner experience of schizophrenia.

Perceptual Changes The perceptions of clients with schizophrenia may be either heightened or blunted. These changes may occur in all the senses or in just one or two. For example, a client may see colors as brighter than normal or may be acutely sensitive to sounds. Another may have a heightened sense of touch and therefore be extremely sensitive to any physical contact. **Illusions** occur when the client misperceives or exaggerates stimuli in the external environment. A client with schizophrenia may mistake a chair for a person or perceive that the walls of a hallway are closing in. The perceptual changes are sufficient to cause the client to mistake the stimulus for something else (see the example of an illusion in Figure 10-1 on page 195). Hallucinations are the most extreme and yet the most common perceptual disturbance in schizophrenia. Auditory hallucinations are the most common form of hallucination. Although hallucinations are a hallmark of schizophrenia, their presence alone does not establish the presence of the disorder. Refer back to Table 16-1 on page 372, which lists various types of hallucinations.

Assess perceptual disturbances by asking the client about the experience and by observing for behaviors that indicate the client is frightened or attending to internal stimuli. Ask the client, "What are you seeing and hearing?" Note the degree to which this description differs from your perceptions of the environment.

Clients may be reluctant to discuss the extreme perceptual disturbance of hallucinations. One of the ways you can introduce the topic is to discuss physical symptoms such as pain or discomfort. Then ask about hearing and vision skills. From there it is a smooth transition to asking about unusual experiences with hearing and seeing.

A classic sign of auditory hallucinations is placing the hands over the ears when clients are frightened by the voices and attempt to block them out. Less obvious signs of hallucinations are inappropriate laughing or smiling, difficulty following a conversation, and difficulty attending to what is happening at the moment. Fleeting, rapid changes of expression that are not precipitated by events in the real world can be another sign. The degree to which clients believe the hallucinatory experience is real and their ability to verify the reality of the experience by checking with others have important implications for interventions. Note the client's emotional response to hallucinations. Some clients experience depression or despair about the continued presence of voices; others may be comforted or kept company by their voices. Client coping

MEDIALINK Schizophrenia Interview Video

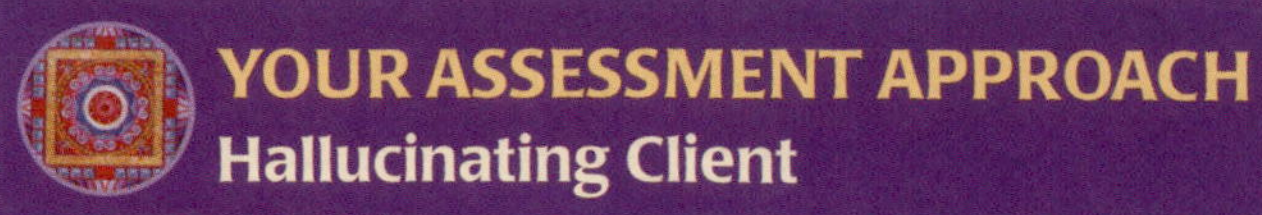

YOUR ASSESSMENT APPROACH
Hallucinating Client

A complete assessment of hallucinations should identify the following:

- Whether the hallucinations are solely auditory or include other senses
- How long the client has experienced the hallucinations, what the initial hallucinations were like, and whether they have changed
- Which situations are most likely to trigger hallucinations, and which times of day they occur most frequently
- What the hallucinations are about (Are they just sounds, or voices? If the client hears voices, what do they say?)
- How strongly the client believes in the reality of the hallucinations
- Whether the hallucinations command the client to do something, and if so, how potentially destructive the commands are
- Whether the client hears other voices contradicting commands received in hallucinations
- How the client feels about the hallucinations
- Which strategies the client has used to cope with the hallucinations and how effective the strategies were

strategies, and their effectiveness or ineffectiveness, are also an important aspect of assessment. Finally, clients may talk to themselves, presumably in answer to the voices they hear. Specific guidelines for assessing hallucinations are given in the Your Assessment Approach feature.

Objective Data

These data are the observable symptoms and manifestations of schizophrenia that you, as a nurse, will assess.

Disturbances in Thought and Expression Clients with schizophrenia find that their thinking is muddled or unclear. Their thoughts are disconnected or disjointed, and the connections between one thought and another are vague.

The clarity of the client's communication often reflects the level of thought disorganization. Client responses may be simply inappropriate to the situation or conversation. They may have difficulty responding or stop in midsentence, as if they are stuck, a sign of **thought blocking**.

Note the rate and quality of the client's speech. Is it unusually loud, insistent, and continuous? Does the client wander from topic to topic or have *tangential communication* (communication with only a slight or tenuous connection to the topic)? An example is, "You want to know how I came here? I came here by bus, but bussing is kissing, I wasn't kissing but if you keep it simple that is a business tenet for KISS. That was a great group that played on and on but I'm not playing with you." Does the client bring up minute details that are irrelevant or unimportant to the topic at hand (*circumstantial communication*)? An example is, "You want to know how I came here? I came here on a blue and yellow bus with a lady bus driver. There were three teenage kids and a blind man with a seeing-eye dog on the bus. It didn't have to make a stop at the corner of Main and 9th." Are the client's responses slow and hesitant, reflecting difficulty in taking in stimuli and responding to them?

Clients with schizophrenia also have difficulty thinking abstractly. Their responses may be inappropriate because they interpret words literally rather than abstractly. For example, when told to prepare to have his blood drawn, a young man readied some paper and marking pens. You can assess abstract thinking by asking clients the meaning of proverbs, a test requiring the client to abstract a general meaning from a specific or metaphysical statement, for example, "People who live in glass houses shouldn't throw stones." Clients with schizophrenia are more likely to give concrete ("If you throw a stone the glass will break") rather than abstract ("Don't criticize someone else if you behave the same way") responses.

Disruptions in Emotional Responses Tone of voice, rate of speech, content of speech, expressions, postures, and body movements indicate emotional tone. Many individuals with schizophrenia demonstrate inappropriate affect—emotional responses that are inappropriate to the situation. For example, a client may smile or laugh while relating a history of having been abused as a child. Or, a client may become angry or anxious when asked to join a group of other clients for dinner. The degree to which a client's emotions are inappropriate is a prognostic indicator. Clients whose emotional response is preserved and generally appropriate have a more favorable prognosis than clients who demonstrate inappropriate affect.

A marked decrease in the variation or intensity of emotional expression is called **blunted affect**. The client may express joy, sorrow, or anger, but with little intensity. In flat affect, there is a total lack of emotional expression in verbal and nonverbal behavior; the face is impassive, and voice rate and tone are regular and monotonous. The absence of emotion and the presence of anhedonia are also often indicative of schizophrenia.

Motor Behavior Changes Disruptions seen in schizophrenia include disorganized behavior and catatonia. Disorganized behavior lacks a coherent goal, is aimless, or is disruptive. Catatonic behavior is manifested by unusual body movement or lack of movement. This activity disturbance includes *catatonic excitement* (the client moves excitedly but not in response to environmental influences), *catatonic posturing* (the client holds bizarre postures for periods of time), and *stupor* (the client holds the body still and is unresponsive to the environment).

Changes in Role Functioning An important factor in predicting the course of schizophrenia is the client's level of functioning before the symptoms of the disease became pronounced. Assessment should therefore include a complete history of the client's success at completing developmental tasks. The prognosis is best if the client functioned at a high level prior to the onset of schizophrenic disturbance. Assess how well the client fulfilled role responsibilities in the family, in school, in relation to peers, and in work. Obtain a history of the rate of decline in these various roles. The onset of schizophrenia may be relatively acute, or degeneration may be slow.

Drug Use Clients with drug toxicity or withdrawal may have behavior disturbances similar to those seen in clients with schizophrenia. They may have auditory or visual hallucinations and may be confused, illogical, and highly anxious. For this reason, it is essential to obtain a detailed drug history. Assess both long-term and recent use of chemical substances. If the client is not a reliable historian, interview family or friends. In addition, both blood and urine should be tested for drugs if reliable information cannot be obtained.

Family Health History Part of a thorough and complete assessment is noting any history of mental disorder in the client's family (Chafetz, White, Collins-Bride, Nickens, & Cooper, 2006). Of particular interest is a history of schizophrenia or any thought disorder, mood disorders (such as cyclical highs or depressions), or alcoholism in any family member. Note any report that family members had "nervous breakdowns" or any other colloquial descriptions of mental or emotional disorders.

Family Cohesion and Emotion In families of people with schizophrenia, enmeshment (see Chapter 30), combined with a negative emotional tone, is thought to be detrimental to the ill member's well-being. However, the presence of acquaintances and family members showing emotional warmth in low expressed emotion (EE) situations can have a protective function.

Much of the nursing assessment of family cohesion and emotion can be carried out unobtrusively. Chapter 30 has specific guidelines for assessment of these and other family dynamics. The nursing staff, in conjunction with the interdisciplinary team, can also arrange formal family assessment interviews (also discussed in Chapter 30). When you are observing interactions, note signs of dysfunction.

Family Overinvolvement and Negativity At present there are no clear-cut clinical determinants of exactly how much overinvolvement and negative emotion in families is problematic. Note families who seem excessively bonded emotionally. The inability of family members to maintain emotional, social, or physical separateness is a clear sign of this problem. Also assess for the presence of a high level of criticism among family members. Discuss families that seem seriously enmeshed or hypercritical with the treatment team.

Family Communication Problems Unclear or incomplete communication is frequent in families of people with schizophrenia. This area requires nursing assessment. Unclear communication may result from continual interaction with the ill member or may contribute to the disorder. Clinicians must evaluate how effectively the family communicates to determine the potential need for intervention.

Assess these aspects of family communication:

- Ability to focus on a topic
- Ability to discuss a topic in a meaningful way with other family members
- Ability to maintain the discussion without wandering from the subject or becoming distracted
- Use of language and explanations that are generally understandable (not peculiar to that family alone)

Also note who in the family seems to do the talking, who talks to whom, and whether members talk for, or interrupt, one another. Communication problems that commonly occur with the diagnosis of schizophrenia and interfere with interpersonal relationships, especially family communication, are discussed in Box 16-1.

Family Burden Most families of individuals with schizophrenia report that caring for the ill member places a burden on the family unit. Ask about the challenges the family is facing so that you can determine the information and support needs to be met. See Chapter 30 for examples of common family burdens.

Environment Assess the availability of support and services beyond the bounds of the family, including extended family and friends, as well as community groups and organizations that support people with schizophrenia. Assess also the availability of mental health programs that address the specific mental health needs of people with schizophrenia.

Nursing Diagnosis: NANDA

Nursing diagnoses with clients with schizophrenia focus on alterations in the patterns of activity, cognition, emotional processes, interpersonal processes, and perception. Alterations in ecologic, physiologic, and valuation processes are assessed

Box 16-1 Problematic Communication Patterns Common in Schizophrenia

Blocking

The client has trouble expressing a response or stops in midsentence, as if stranded without a thought.

Clang Associations

Words that rhyme or sound alike are distributed throughout conversations without necessarily making sense.

Echolalia

Phrases, sentences, or entire conversations said to the client are repeated back by the client.

Neologisms

Words or meanings are invented by the client. This can include multisyllabic, pseudo-scientific words or simple words.

Perseveration

The client maintains a particular idea regardless of the topic being discussed or attempts to change the subject.

Word Salad

An incoherent medley of words is emitted in conversation as if it was a sensible and articulate phrase.

as well; however, the central nursing problems relate to the former five processes.

Impaired Communication

Schizophrenia interferes with the ability to communicate, a complex and demanding function.

Verbal Clients with schizophrenia may communicate in a disorganized, sometimes incomprehensible fashion. Some clients, because their thinking is disorganized, speak very little (alogia, or poverty of speech). Also note there may be a poverty of content in speech, in that the client converses but actually says very little.

Often, clients with schizophrenia communicate in ways that are overly concrete (a sign of an inability to think and communicate abstractly) or overly symbolic (a sign of preoccupation with unreal or delusional material). The symbols are usually difficult to decipher because their meanings are idiosyncratic to that particular individual.

Nonverbal The facial and bodily expressions that accompany the verbal communication of people with schizophrenia frequently do not match the content of the verbal message. This lack of congruence is primarily due to the blunting of emotions found in schizophrenia. Expected facial expressions—smiles, looks of concern or disgust—may not accompany the client's statements. In addition, clients with motor or behavioral abnormalities—posturing, unusual movements, or grimacing—convey a confusing mix of verbal and nonverbal messages.

Self-Care Deficits

People with schizophrenia frequently appear indifferent to their personal appearance. They may neglect to bathe, change clothes, or attend to minor grooming tasks such as combing their hair. Some show little awareness of current fashion styles, and many wear clothing that makes them look out of place. Of greater concern are those who wear clothing that is inappropriate to the current season and weather conditions.

Although lack of attention to grooming might be a simple annoyance to those who must live in close proximity to the person with schizophrenia, health risks related to prolonged poor hygiene can arise. Assess immediate problems, such as inadequate nutrition, fluid intake, and elimination, as well as long-term problems, such as dental caries and increased susceptibility to infections.

Disregard for appearance and hygiene may extend to the client's environment. The client may fail to maintain a clean and safe living space. He or she may not take good care of personal belongings and may misplace them. Self-care deficiencies may result from consistently disturbed thought and perceptual processes. For example, a client whose chronic hallucinations are only partly relieved by medication may have difficulty concentrating for long periods and paying attention to grooming.

Activity Intolerance

The emotional disturbances of ambivalence and apathy, common in schizophrenic disorders, can result in lack of interest and inactivity. Inactivity induced by ambivalence is associated with higher levels of emotion. Anxious about choosing one course of action and rejecting another, the client is immobilized. The following clinical examples describe the experience of intolerance to activity.

CLINICAL EXAMPLE

Jim is ambivalent about taking a pass to go out alone from the inpatient unit for the first time. He is undecided about taking the risk of leaving the hospital setting without a staff member, yet yearns for the freedom of walking the streets alone. Indecision leaves him standing, immobilized, by the doorway to the unit.

Extreme ambivalence can manifest itself in even the most automatic of behaviors.

CLINICAL EXAMPLE

Melissa cannot eat because of ambivalence about where to sit or what to eat. She stands in the center of the dining room, turning first to one chair and then another, unable to choose where to sit so that she can begin eating.

Clients who are inactive because of apathy demonstrate little emotional tone. Such clients may spend long hours lying in bed staring into space or listening to music. Often, but not always, apathetic individuals prefer isolation. You might find several clients sitting in the same room, engaged in no apparent activities, and interacting with one another only when absolutely necessary.

Social Isolation

Extreme anxiety about relating to others often leads clients with schizophrenia to withdraw from interaction and to isolate themselves. Some clients tolerate only a few moments of direct communication, whereas others can manage extended periods of contact. Assess the client's tolerance of brief periods of contact with staff and other clients. Document patterns of relating and withdrawal, also noting in which activities the client engages when in contact with others and which activities the client undertakes when alone. Nurses who work in skilled nursing facilities also need to be able to diagnose social isolation as a symptom of schizophrenia (see the What Every Skilled Facility Nurse Should Know feature on page 387).

Decisional Conflict

Decisional conflict in schizophrenia is probably due to biochemical alterations in the brain that make it difficult for clients to take in, synthesize, and respond to information. Decisional conflict may be evident both in the mundane activities of daily life (e.g., selecting one's diet) and in major life decisions. This can be frustrating for caregivers and for clients. The following clinical example shows how decisional conflict can remove what is a pleasant aspect of life from the client.

CLINICAL EXAMPLE

Murray refuses to take medications, even though not taking them means that he will be evicted from the residential treatment program he likes.

Disturbed Sensory Perception

Alterations in the five senses (sound, sight, smell, taste, touch) create an altered perception of the world.

Hallucinations Hallucinations are both a clinical diagnostic sign of schizophrenia and a focus for nursing care. You need to know the extent and nature of clients' hallucinations so that you can document the hallucinatory experience. Discuss with the client, if the client is able to, the details of his or her symptoms. Look for major themes in the content of the hallucinations, particularly whether the hallucinations command the client to take action. *Command hallucinations* such as "Jump up and down. Jump up and down. Don't look at her, she has cancer and you'll catch it," can be difficult for the client to cope with and can affect the client's behavior. The client may not be able to withstand pressured commands to say things or perform acts that could include violence or a refusal to remain in a housing situation (which could lead to homelessness).

Illusions Illusions make the client vulnerable to emotional and physical injury. The level of misperception may vary from day to day and even throughout the day. Misperceptions of the social environment make the client vulnerable to inappropriate responses that may be ridiculed by others. Misperceptions of the physical environment, such as misjudging the speed of an oncoming car, may lead to physical harm.

WHAT EVERY SKILLED NURSING FACILITY NURSE SHOULD KNOW

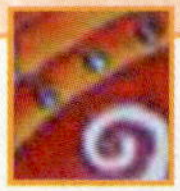

Primary Symptoms of Schizophrenia

A skilled nursing facility (SNF) nurse needs to be familiar with the primary symptoms of schizophrenia—delusions, hallucinations, agitation, and general decompensation. There are two reasons SNF nurses should be familiar with these symptoms:

1. These symptoms are part of a disease process that require treatment.
2. The presence of these symptoms can distort or mask the presentation of symptoms of physical illnesses, and severe psychiatric distress can impair healing from medical and surgical procedures and injuries.

When an SNF resident represents symptoms that appear to include behavioral and psychiatric features, the SNF nurse should be prepared and able to document, classify, and report these symptoms correctly, and to help ensure the resident receives necessary treatment. Knowing the interventions, pharmacological and nonpharmacological, can speed stabilization and improve the quality of life the residents experience.

Disturbed Body Image

A body image disturbance is common in people with schizophrenia. Clients may lose the sense of where their bodies leave off and where inanimate objects begin. They may become dissociated from various body parts and believe, for example, that their arms and legs belong to someone else. They may worry about the normalcy of their sexual organs. Clients often verbalize this altered sense of self directly, saying "I don't feel like myself" or "I feel like I am looking at my body from somewhere else in the room."

Excess Fluid Volume

Excess fluid intake, or water intoxication, is a problem that is observed primarily in clients who reside in institutions such as state mental hospitals. This physiologic state is brought on by excessive drinking, characterized by hyponatremia, confusion, and disorientation, and progresses to apathy and lethargy. In severe cases, seizures and death may result. This behavior can lead to irreversible brain damage. Polydipsia appears to be significantly associated with male gender, smoking, celibacy, and psychiatric chronicity. Polydipsia in schizophrenia has been treated effectively with clozapine (Margetic, Aukst-Margetic, & Zarkovic-Palijan, 2006). For clients suspected to be at risk because of frequent drinking, preventive measures include regular measures of urine specific gravity, and regular weights designed to screen for increases in the body's fluid volume.

Disturbed Thought Processes

Schizophrenia changes the way thoughts are processed by distorting logic and organization.

Delusions Clients express delusional thinking in direct interactions and, to a lesser extent, through behaviors. When asked, many clients willingly describe their delusional beliefs in detail. They seldom withhold this information because they believe firmly in the validity of the delusion, no matter how bizarre it seems to others. Clients' actions reflect the fixedness of their beliefs.

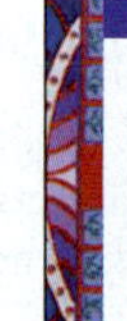

CLINICAL EXAMPLE

Gerry has the somatic delusion that her body is riddled with holes. She flatly refuses to drink, convinced that the fluid will flow directly out of the holes and soil her dress.

The content of delusions varies: delusions of persecution, reference, and so on (see Table 16-3). Reality-based delusions may seem plausible because they could, under some circumstances, actually occur. Bizarre delusions, more common among clients with schizophrenia, have no possible basis in reality. On the other hand, the false belief that one's husband is having an affair with a neighbor has a possible basis in reality, and is called a reality-based delusion. In contrast, the belief that one's thoughts are directed by a television announcer, or that one's unspoken thoughts can be heard by others, are known as bizarre delusions.

Delusions often reflect the client's fears, particularly about personal inadequacies. For example, a man's grandiose delusion that he is the mayor of New York City could be a defense against feelings of inferiority. Similarly, persecutory delusions defend against the person's own feelings of aggression. Aggressive feelings are projected onto a person or organization—for example, the police, whom the client then fears.

Magical Thinking Magical thinking is the belief that events can happen simply because one wishes them to. Some people with schizophrenia claim they can exert their will to make people take certain actions or make specific events occur, like winning the lottery.

Thought Insertion, Withdrawal, and Broadcasting Hallmarks of schizophrenic thought are the beliefs that others can put ideas into one's head (*thought insertion*) or take thoughts out of one's head (*thought withdrawal*). In addition, some clients believe that their thoughts are transmitted to others via radio, television, or other means but not directly by the client. This belief is known as *thought broadcasting*.

Dysfunctional Family Processes

When a family has a member with a significant illness, regardless of whether it is a mental or physical illness, that family's functioning and dynamics change. The operations of the family must change to accommodate the ill family member as well as how the rest of the family deals with the illness. The symptoms of the illness may be alien to family members, and they may not know how they should respond. See the Partnering with Clients and Families feature for guidelines on how to teach families about the negative symptoms of schizophrenia.

Interrupted Family Processes

Families burdened with the long-term responsibility of caring for a relative with schizophrenia may suffer disruptions in their household routine, work, social interactions, and physical well-being. The household may be disrupted by the client's insistence that the family act on and accommodate delusional beliefs. The family may bend to the client's wish, fearing an increase in the client's anxiety and possible fighting or shouting if they do not comply.

CLINICAL EXAMPLE

The Walker family built an extra bathroom rather than fight with Tim, their son with schizophrenia, who spends hours in the bath completing elaborate washing rituals.

The Sherman family must eat out several times a week because Suzanne, their daughter with schizophrenia, refuses to allow anyone in the room when she eats.

The family social life may be disrupted. For instance, the family may fear leaving the ill person alone, or they may fear that the ill person will embarrass visitors if friends are invited in. Some families are willing to be open about the adjustments they make in living with a loved one with schizophrenia, whereas others choose to live isolated lives.

Family members' work can suffer because of the emotional strain of living with an ill member. They must take time off to accompany the schizophrenic person to doctors' appointments, make hospital visits, and help during interviews with social agencies or the police. Family health may suffer because of general inattention or because of prolonged stresses within the home.

Outcome Identification: NOC

The outcome criteria established for a client with schizophrenia need to be flexible and include the option to acknowledge a partial behavior change as success. For example, the out-

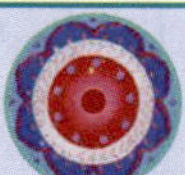

PARTNERING WITH CLIENTS AND FAMILIES

TEACHING ABOUT THE NEGATIVE SYMPTOMS OF SCHIZOPHRENIA

Families and caregivers have a difficult time understanding that symptoms of an illness include not just those experiences that are unusual and extra, such as hallucinations and delusions, but also those aspects of being human that are missing, such as enjoyment and motivation. You need to evaluate the family's current level of awareness of negative symptoms and provide important information.

Suggestions	Rationale
Discuss how not having motivation and not seeming to care about surroundings are part of the illness.	Families may be comforted to know that their loved one is not choosing to behave in this way.
Inform the family members about how these symptoms look and feel to the client.	Frequently, family members may blame medication for causing the client to be "zoned out" or "just sitting and staring."
Help families identify their responses to the negative symptoms.	Families often misinterpret negative symptoms as laziness or refusing to cooperate, and communicate this to the client. This increases the negativity to which the client is exposed.
Talk about when and how negative symptoms respond to medications.	The time frame of 18–24 months before negative symptoms respond to atypical antipsychotics may seem a long time to family members, and they will need support so their expectations are realistic.

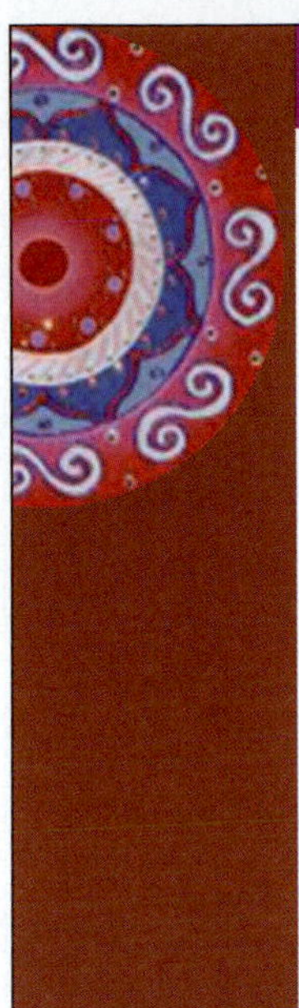

CARING FOR THE SPIRIT

Can Culturally Adapted Interventions Make a Difference in Outcome?

Schizophrenia is a difficult illness with many presentations. The distress people experience during symptom exacerbation motivates the search for treatments that are effective and useful in fulfilling the needs of the client. The search for answers has taken a variety of pathways, including the realm of spirituality and cultural sensitivity.

The quality of mental health services available to people who have schizophrenia are greatly enhanced when the relevant content of both psychoeducational and mental health interventions are culturally linked. Think about the last time you spoke with somebody about a problem you were having. If that person had an understanding of both your culture and your value system, such as spirituality, you probably had an easier time explaining your problem. Now think about a time when you spoke with somebody about a problem you were having and that person had no idea what you were talking about. How would you describe that experience? As you can imagine, this happens quite often with people who have schizophrenia when their symptoms are unusual or they are not able to articulate them clearly.

Culture, spirituality, and a value system are intricately interwoven. They form the fabric for a system of meaning. Symptom expression, stressors, coping mechanisms, and interactions with others arise from this system. Keeping the cultural and spiritual context of a client's experience in mind while interacting around psychiatric symptoms and treatment reduces the client's frustrations and increases the effectiveness of your communication.

come for Body Image Distortion may include (a) recognizes symptom regularly, (b) speaks often with important other person regarding body feelings, and (c) manages to function despite symptomatology much of the time. Setting realistic goals and continually reevaluating expectations based on your client's current desires and status is imperative with outcomes development. Other issues for outcomes with this population are an awareness of the client's multiple functional deficits, your personal response to working with this population, cultural differences, and lethality factors (Griner & Smith, 2006; Muñoz & Hilgenberg, 2006; Netto, 2006). See the Caring for the Spirit box above for cultural awareness contributions to outcomes.

Planning and Implementation: NIC

Nursing interventions are most effective when they focus on the needs and wants of the client to maximize functioning. In order to accomplish this, you must attend to the issues that are important to the client. The client's perspective is the most valuable tool you have to create competent and meaningful treatment interventions. Box 16-2 discusses the issues most important to the client with schizophrenia, from the unique perspective of the client.

When planning care for any client with a chronic illness, nurses must be careful to set realistic goals for client change. Particular care must be taken with clients who are schizophrenic because they are extremely sensitive to change and failure. Deterioration in all aspects of functioning is characteristic of the disease. Focus on the most troublesome areas of client functioning and set incremental, short-term goals that pave the way for successes in achieving long-term goals. Answering the questions in the Your Self-Awareness: Working with Clients Who Have Schizophrenia feature will increase your effectiveness in working with a psychotic client.

Preventing Relapse

Combining maintenance antipsychotic medication therapy with psychosocial approaches has been found to be more effective than pharmacotherapy alone in delaying or preventing relapse. It has been suggested that early intervention would be effective in preventing relapse in clients with schizophrenia. This could be accomplished through close clinical or family monitoring for the client's particular *prodromal symptoms* (those symptoms that occur early in the relapse process for that client). Once identi-

Box 16-2 Important Issues for the Client with Schizophrenia

People who have schizophrenia have to deal with an illness different from any other disease. The symptoms are unlike anything else, and anosognia (unawareness of the illness) can further complicate their lives. Imagine not knowing you have an illness and not, therefore, needing help. It makes accepting treatment and staying in treatment particularly challenging. Developing meaningful treatment and conducting effective interventions incorporate these vital aspects into effective nursing care:

- Personal power and efficacy
- Interpersonal relationships
- Social expectations
- Differences between what one hoped for oneself and what one has now
- Connecting with people
- Personal growth
- Stability
- Coping with relapses
- Expression of spirituality
- Understanding the symptoms of the illness

fied, prompt clinical intervention with antipsychotic medication may reduce the overall frequency of the relapse event.

Programs for relapse prevention typically combine standard doses of maintenance antipsychotic medication with psychosocial treatment and result in lower relapse rates. Weekly group therapy for clients is an opportunity to monitor prodromal symptoms. Such clinical scrutiny may prevent or minimize relapse and rehospitalization. A multi-family group component is helpful to support and educate the families as well as provide peer contacts and here-and-now experiences.

For clients residing with their families, educational and supportive family interventions have an important effect on relapse prevention. Those clients who live more independently and experience relapses could benefit from a community treatment contact. Prevention is more effective when clients and their families understand the likely relapse triggers, as outlined in TABLE 16-5 ■.

Other aspects of relapse prevention have been implemented clinically with good results. Clients with a psychosis that is not responsive to pharmacotherapy may benefit from specific cognitive–behavioral therapies (see Chapter 31), while persons with persistent negative symptoms and limited social competence may find social skills training useful. In addition, new programs of supported employment may enable some clients to maintain competitive employment. The impacts of regularly scheduled employment and improved skills can be

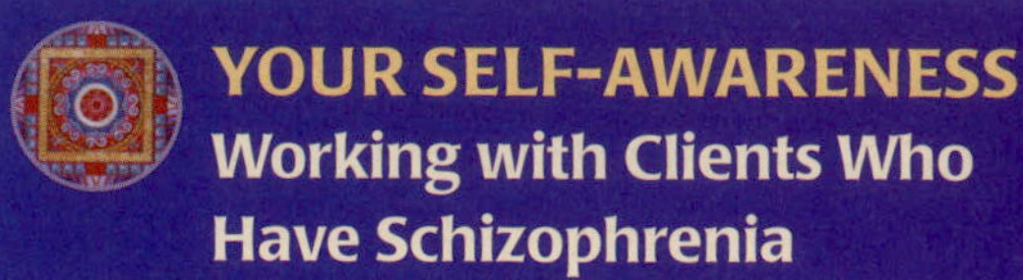

YOUR SELF-AWARENESS
Working with Clients Who Have Schizophrenia

To increase self-awareness about working with a person with active psychosis, ask yourself:

- How do I feel about approaching a person who is having hallucinations?
- How do I feel about talking to someone who has delusions that frighten him?
- Have I ever encountered someone in public who was psychotic?
- Do I fear that I might do something that might make the person's illness worse?
- What kinds of understanding and knowledge do I need to feel comfortable working with clients with psychosis?

To increase self-awareness about working with clients with disrupted ability to care for themselves, ask yourself:

- Do I react negatively when I think about someone my age who has never worked?
- What goes through my mind when I see someone who is disheveled, unclean, or oddly dressed?
- How can I find a point of connection between myself and someone whose life is so dramatically different from my own?

TABLE 16-5 ■ Relapse Triggers in Schizophrenia

Physiological Stressors	
Infection	Pain
Acute illness	Fatigue
Chronic illness	Side effects of medications
Dehydration	Appetite changes
Insomnia	Injury
Rape	Surgery
Personal Stressors	
Exacerbation/relapse of illness	Financial difficulties
Depression	An increase in responsibility
Negative symptoms of schizophrenia	A decrease in access to resources
Spiritual distress	Recreational activity choice/access
Pet loss/illness/aging	Maturational/developmental changes
Interpersonal Stressors	
Perceived rejection/abandonment	Loss of job or status within a job
Conflict, anger	Altered contact with another or others
Relationship changes (family, intimate relationships, friendships, etc.)	High expressed emotion
Community Stressors	
Difficulties making living arrangements	Disruption of living situation
Roommate/family stressors	Transportation
Community disruption	

a helpful distracter from the onslaught of psychosis if it does not tax the client's coping abilities.

Promoting Adequate Communication

Clients with schizophrenia try to communicate, even though their statements may be difficult to understand. Close attention to what the client is saying and honest attempts to understand the real and symbolic aspects of the message are important. The client will perceive nuances of your behavior. Therefore, one of the most direct and successful ways to demonstrate caring and respect is to attend seriously to the client (this is discussed in depth in Chapter 10).

Clients make valid observations about their environment, needs, and concerns. Some, if not all, of their observations and sensations exist in reality and are not to be treated as if they are all totally psychotic symptoms. The sensitivity to the environment that can overwhelm someone with schizophrenia also clues him or her into aspects to which others may not have access. A client may make observations about events or situations that are beyond your awareness. For example, take seriously a client's statement about another client's drug use or suicidal threats. If a client complains of a physical symptom such as stomach distress, consider the symptom as real until there is evidence otherwise. It is easy to dismiss a client's statements, particularly those of a delusional client. Doing so, however, shows lack of respect for the client's intact capacities to see and respond to what is happening in the environment.

Promoting Adherence with Medication Regimen

Psychotropic medications play an important part in the treatment of schizophrenic disorders. Drugs that diminish focal symptoms (hallucinations and delusions) and yet produce relatively few untoward effects are now available. Complying with treatment, which for schizophrenia means medications, is a complex demand. You will need to be creative and ever-mindful of your client's specific barriers to learning and maintaining specific behaviors. The disease itself causes difficulty in adhering to a treatment regimen when a client lacks the ability to recognize the illness. This is called poor insight and can be compared to the unawareness or lack of insight into neurological deficits following a stroke. Recognize that individuals respond to their illness, their circumstances, and their medications in different ways.

The idea of adherence can be expressed through a number of terms such as treatment adherence, role reliability, collaboration for health behaviors, and cooperation. Interviews and clinical contacts tell us that clients are able to participate in the treatment if they are included and made an integral part of the design of their care (Haynes et al., 2006; Isherwood, Burns, & Rigby, 2006; Rosenberg & Rosenberg, 2006). See Box 16-3 for a description of the barriers and challenges to treatment adherence.

Consistent adherence in taking medications as prescribed is not common among this client population. Researchers estimate that as few as 68% of psychiatric clients adhere to medication regimens while in the hospital (Uko-Ekpenyong, 2006). When these clients return to the community, 37% or fewer adhere to drug regimens. Clients may stop taking their medications for these reasons:

- They don't understand the administration instructions.
- They are too disorganized to follow the instructions.
- The side effects of major tranquilizers are too uncomfortable.
- They do not wish to be stigmatized as having schizophrenia so they reject treatment.
- They begin to feel better and believe the medication is no longer necessary.
- They don't have easy access to pharmacies because of transportation, financial, or interpersonal difficulties.

Clients who do not take medications are more vulnerable to stressors and risk more frequent relapse of symptoms. Efforts to educate clients about their medications and to have them practice self-medication prior to discharge have increased the rate of adherence only marginally. Client attitudes toward the medications prescribed also influence their willingness to comply. You must be an active participant in assessing adherence and fostering a positive attitude toward medications. Commonly used antipsychotic medications and side effects are presented in Chapter 32.

Clients are often ambivalent about taking medications. Maintaining adequate blood levels of therapeutic medications is important for clients with schizophrenia. To help them overcome ambivalence, give them time to think about taking the medications. Set a time limit. For an inpatient who fails to comply, come back later and try again. Two useful strategies are reminding clients of the positive effects of the medication and framing the action as a way for them to help themselves get better. The Your Intervention Strategies feature on page 392 is a compendium for increasing treatment adherence for clients with schizophrenia.

Box 16-3 Challenges to Adherence

- Difficulties with prescribed psychotropic medications
- Severe level of symptomatology
- Cognitive difficulties secondary to thought disorder
- Motivational problems secondary to negative symptoms
- Motivational problems secondary to flight into health (wanting to be "normal")
- Unpleasant side effects
- Persistence of positive symptoms (delusions) mitigating against adherence
- Financial issues
- Misperceptions and misunderstanding of the information presented in medication teaching
- Cursory or minimal medication teaching that lacks relevance to all areas of the client's life
- Unresolved issues with treatment providers
- Cultural impacts

YOUR INTERVENTION STRATEGIES
Increasing Medication Adherence for Clients with Schizophrenia

- Involve the client as a partner in medication-based treatment planning decisions.
- Change to another medication with a different neurotransmitter action with lower or different side effects that may be more tolerable. Atypical antipsychotic medications have a lower side-effect profile and can increase adherence because they're not so hard to take.
- Teach the client how to report side effects, including their severity (from dry mouth to priapism). This may require role-playing or assertiveness training.
- Teach the client how to manage the side effects he does get—if possible, with such solutions as hard candy and a rubber pillow case liner. It may make it tolerable to continue on the medication.
- Instruct, educate, and arrange for reminders well before discharge (especially with geriatric recipients) to maximize both knowledge and adherence (knowledge can be the number-one factor determining adherence).
- Simplify the medication regimen.
- Match the medication dosing strategy to the client's schedule, preferences, work situation, and recreational pursuits.
- Discuss the client's expectations of the medication—are they realistic?
- Take cultural impacts into account during comprehensive treatment planning.
- Use concrete educators. The tried-and-true cognition enhancers are: pamphlets, booklets, handbooks, workbooks, sheets, cards, videos, audiotapes, posters, magnets, logs, journals, etc.
- Assess the client's perception of control over the treatment regimen.
- Assess the client's self-administration of medications.
- Help the client take action to prevent untoward effects, such as maintaining fluid intake to avoid postural hypotension.
- Teach coping efforts involving problem solving, which increases adherence.
- Peer support is important. Hearing from *peers* how a new medication could help with symptoms, and asking the prescriber to consider it, improves adherence.
- Give hope—it pays to be well. It takes all the small steps to recovery in addition to medications to get better.
- Repetition—say the same thing over and over, with patience, especially if clients have schizophrenia or depression.
- Develop reminders, cues to remembering (visual cues—when I see this I need to take my pills, when I eat lunch I take my pills, rubber band on wrist, calendars, to-do lists; auditory cues—alarm clocks or watches).
- Depot medications given weekly, biweekly, or monthly can contribute to adherence because the client does not have to remember to take pills. The marketing of an atypical antipsychotic in depot form (risperidone) adds to the choices.
- Pill boxes—come in many shapes, sizes, and organizational styles (multiple daily doses, layers for time of day, Braille markings, timer with small alarm clock feature that opens compartment). If the medication can't be taken out of its original container without affecting the potency, place a small button or candy in the pill box to serve as a reminder.
- Keep all medications and information about them in one dry, cool place. Use plastic products such as containers and bags—*not* in the bathroom or by a dishwasher in the kitchen.
- Involve the family.
- Match the degree of client autonomy in treatment to the needs of the individual client.
- Financial assistance might be available.
- Have clients teach about their medications (after they have learned sufficiently) to other recipients or to significant others. Nothing speeds learning as much as teaching others.

Assisting with Grooming and Hygiene

Helping clients establish and maintain personal care habits is a complex process. If the client clearly lacks the skills, then teach the skills. If, however, the client has learned grooming skills but does not practice them, focus on ways to motivate the client. Intervention begins by establishing clear expectations about essential grooming habits. The frequency and timing of all aspects of grooming—including bathing, dressing, hair care, oral hygiene, and room care—can be specified in writing if that would be a useful learning device for your client.

Formal training programs for helping chronically mentally ill clients improve their grooming skills can be applied in inpatient as well as outpatient settings. These programs are well developed and tested. They systematically help clients in all steps of personal grooming, including collecting grooming supplies, moving to the grooming area (a bathroom or bedroom with sink and mirror), completing each grooming step, completing appropriate dressing, and storing grooming materials. Nursing interventions at each step can progress from simple verbal coaching, to modeling, to gentle physical guidance. Acknowledge client efforts during each phase with realistic encouragement and praise. The success of these programs probably depends on daily staff attention to the client's training, along with consistent, meaningful rewards. Avoid power struggles regarding the completion of tasks. If initial prompts don't work, leave the client alone for a short period.

Promoting Organized Behavior

Clients whose behavior is disorganized require direction and limits to make their actions more effective and goal-directed.

In working with a disorganized client, proceed slowly and remain calm. The client's perception of the environment may be distorted, but your calmness can help calm the client. Try to direct the client in simple, safe activities. Nursing goals and interventions for a disorganized client must focus on manageable steps. A clinical example of one such intervention follows.

CLINICAL EXAMPLE

George is moving quickly yet aimlessly from the refrigerator to the cupboard. He pulls a box of cereal from the cupboard, opens it, and then wanders away. Next he goes to the refrigerator, opens the door, peers in, and closes the door. Rummaging through all his pockets, he locates a comb, combs through his hair, sets the comb on the counter, and wanders back to the cupboard. This effortful yet unproductive behavior continues for several minutes when the nurse enters.

Nurse: George, are you trying to get some cereal for yourself?

George: Sort of. I was going to . . . brush . . . no . . . comb. . . no . . . eat something. Yeah, I wanted something to eat.

Nurse: Try to concentrate on one thing. First, put the comb back in your pocket. (He does so.) Now, come over here and get the cereal box. Here's a bowl. Here's a spoon. (She hands him the utensils.) Why don't you sit right here? (She seats him so that he has his back to the rest of the activity in the room.) Can you sit still for a bit?

George: I think so.

Nurse: Pour yourself some cereal. I'll get the milk for you. (She does so.)

George begins to eat his cereal quietly. The nurse stays with him for a few minutes and directs him to continue eating each time he becomes distracted by others who come into the room.

Promoting Social Interaction and Activity

The client's efforts to withdraw from social contact stem from past relationship failures and fear of rejection. Clients often find their internal world less risky and therefore more attractive than a world that requires interpersonal relating. When making efforts to help the client become less withdrawn, respect the client's sometimes overwhelming anxiety about human contact.

After establishing a basic level of trust, encourage the client to try out new behaviors within the relationship. The goal is to have the client experience success; therefore, encourage even small increments of change. If, for example, the client has difficulty initiating conversation, encourage the client to practice this skill once a day. Similarly, if the client avoids any activity in the environment because of fear of relating to groups, structure an activity involving the client, yourself, and one other client. Reinforce the client when he or she approaches you to communicate, even if that communication contains problematic patterns (refer back to the Rx Communication features on pages 378 and 381).

Promoting Social Skills and Activities

Address social skills that are essential to functioning in the environment: introducing oneself, starting a conversation, ending a conversation, saying no, asking for assistance, and listening. Staff members can model these skills and help clients role-play each skill. Focus discussion on situations in which clients might need the skill. If they see its applicability to dilemmas in their personal lives, they will be motivated to learn the skill. Praise and, if available, material rewards can also motivate clients. Social skills training can also be done in small groups (see Chapter 30).

Schizophrenia can disturb a person's will and capacity to accomplish meaningful activity. Clients with distorted perceptions and thinking expend considerable energy merely taking in and interpreting their immediate worlds. In addition, major tranquilizers, which control the positive symptoms of the disease, can further inhibit a client's active involvement and interest in activities. Be aware of how much work it takes to cope with schizophrenic symptoms. Do not assume that periods of quiet or inactivity are due to laziness or lack of interest. Rather, assess each individual's need for quiet periods in which to organize perceptions and thoughts.

At the same time, clients with schizophrenia live in a culture in which action and accomplishment are highly prized and rewarded. They are not immune to the pressure for personal productivity as a measure of personal worth (Thomas, Seebohm, Henderson, Munn-Giddings, & Yasmeen, 2006). For this reason, they feel better about themselves when they are involved in meaningful activities. Your task is to help clients find activities that are intrinsically rewarding or that bring some social or tangible reward, yet are within their capacities.

Learning clients' personal interests is a first step. Providing opportunities for the client to actively engage in an activity of interest (by providing records, books, craft materials, or access to newspapers and television) is the next intervention. In addition, activities within the therapeutic milieu, such as attending groups and completing unit "jobs," can provide the external rewards of praise from staff and peers (Connor & Wilson, 2006). These activities give clients confidence and develop and promote their work habits. Success in these activities can lead to success in volunteer or paid work in the community after discharge.

MEDIALINK Care Plan: Social Isolation and Schizophrenia

Intervening with Hallucinations and Delusions

Delusions or hallucinations often frighten clients. You can intervene by:

- Reassuring clients that they are safe
- Protecting them from physical harm as they respond to their altered perceptions
- Validating the feelings they are having in response to their experience
- Validating reality
- Helping them distinguish what is real from what is a hallucination or a delusion

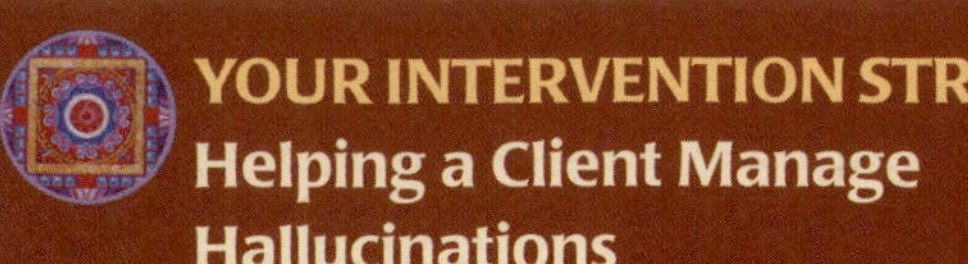

YOUR INTERVENTION STRATEGIES Helping a Client Manage Hallucinations

- Determine the kind of hallucinations (auditory, visual, etc.).
- Can the symptom be managed with current coping?
- Access resources (advocacy groups, peers, staff, literature) for fresh ideas, better management techniques.
- Discuss options and success rate with professionals.
- Select options for coping with the stimuli:
  Distraction
  Resisting
  Calming
  Treatment (such as medication)
- Practice using an option to cope.
- Use a technique based on the success you have with it.
- Be ready to replace coping styles when they don't work anymore.

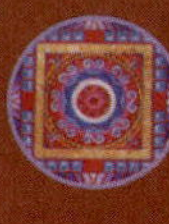

YOUR INTERVENTION STRATEGIES Helping a Client Manage Delusions

- Determine if the client can tell the difference between the delusion ("I don't drink the water because it's poisoned") and a personal preference ("I'm not drinking water because I prefer orange juice").
- Work with advocacy groups, peers, and professional staff to clearly demarcate what constitutes delusional thinking.
- Suggest options to cope with delusional thoughts:
  Support from others
  Concrete tasks
  Caretaking activities
  Refocusing thoughts
  Determined efforts to steer thinking in another direction
- Make sure client understands how important it is to be surrounded by people who reinforce the client's efforts.
- Encourage clients to self-validate the struggle they are in and any level of effectiveness they achieve at coping.

Hallucinations are especially frightening if the client has never experienced them before or if their content is threatening or angry. Attempt to alleviate this anxiety by describing your perception of the frightened behavior and asking clients to discuss what they are experiencing. Make simple reassuring remarks, such as "I hear what you're telling me. This sounds very frightening. No one means to harm you." See the Your Intervention Strategies feature above for intervention strategies that help a client manage hallucinations.

Protect clients from harm and reassure them about safety. A client may take impulsive action to escape the frightening experience or to obey voices in the hallucination. Prevent this by:

- Closely observing client behavior during active hallucinations
- Using calming techniques and one–to–one interactions to shape and guide the situation
- Reducing excess noise and distractions. One person speaks to the client at a time.
- Intervening quickly by giving additional doses of psychotropic medications or placing the client in a quiet room

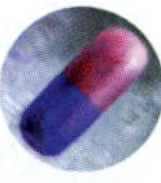

- If necessary, securing the unit so that the client cannot leave and take self-destructive or impulsive action

Make every effort to help the client attend to real rather than internal stimuli, orient the client to the real situation, and encourage the client to focus on you rather than on the hallucination (England, 2006; Grant, 2006). "George, listen to me rather than to the sounds you hear. Remember, you are in the hospital and I am your nurse. I will help you find your shoes. Come with me." Active involvement in some activity, such as finding shoes, will help the client maintain a focus on real events and perceptions.

General guidelines for working with delusional individuals are to avoid arguing with their false beliefs, to focus on the reality-based aspects of their communication, and to protect them from acting on their delusions in a way that might harm themselves or others (Hunt et al., 2006). It may also be important to teach clients that sharing their delusional content directly with others in community settings such as the workplace or the social club may frighten others and lead to stigmatization. Keeping delusional content to oneself in these situations can improve interpersonal relationships. See the Your Intervention Strategies feature above for suggested nursing interventions that contain or manage delusions.

Promoting Congruent Emotional Responses

Working with clients who display blunted or flat affect can be confusing for nurses who are accustomed to reading emotional responses that fall within a more normal range. Be aware that these clients have feelings about events around them, including their interaction with you and other staff members, yet may have difficulty expressing those feelings.

Note any lack of congruence between the person's affect and the content of the message. If your relationship with the client is well established, you might comment on the incongruity and explore it with the client. ("Malcolm, what you are telling me is sad but you are laughing. What shall I pay attention to?") Modeling clear, congruent communication is helpful. Little can be done to change the client's anhedonia, yet empathic listening might comfort the client.

Ambivalence, the simultaneous experience of contradictory feelings about a person, object, or action, can trouble clients with schizophrenia. Ambivalence can become great enough to immobilize a client. Such clients cannot express

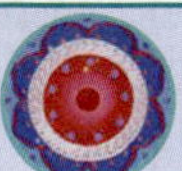

PARTNERING WITH CLIENTS AND FAMILIES

TEACHING ABOUT SCHIZOPHRENIA

To assist families, you need to evaluate the family's current responses to living with and caring for a family member with schizophrenia. The following suggestions apply to the time period shortly after the disorder has been diagnosed.

Suggestions	Rationale
Discuss the basic nature of the disorder: Schizophrenia is a disease of the brain, like any other biologic disease.	Families misunderstand mental illness to be a personal failing and are comforted by the fact that it has a biologic basis.
Help families identify their responses to the early ambiguous signs of the illness and notice how their responses have changed now that the diagnosis has been made.	Families often misinterpret early signs of the disorder as acting out or developmentally appropriate behavior. On learning that these signs are part of the illness, they feel guilty for not seeking help sooner.
Reinforce families for supporting the ill member in seeking treatment.	Stigma about mental illness persists, and families need support for taking action and engaging with treatment systems.
Refer families to structured educational or psychoeducational programs in which they can learn about the disease and its treatment, as well as receive support.	Schizophrenia is extremely complex, and its treatment is multifaceted. Families can benefit from structured classes. Programs that offer support to families in addition to education have proven efficacy in improving the illness course for the ill member.
Inform families about how to reach the local branch of the National Alliance on Mental Illness (NAMI). Hand out fliers that provide telephone numbers and people to contact.	NAMI is a nationwide family support organization that provides peer support, education, and advocacy for the seriously mentally ill and their families.

Provide families with access to information such as:

Mueser, K. T., & Gingerich, S. (1994). *Schizophrenia: A guide for families*. New York: Harbinger.

Torrey, E. F. (1995). *Surviving schizophrenia: A manual for families, consumers, and providers* (3rd ed.). New York: Harper Collins.

one emotion or the other, or choose one action over the other. You may be able to partially alleviate the client's unease by identifying aloud the emotions the client may be experiencing. ("Lily, I think you might be feeling both very happy to see your father and at the same time very angry.") Naming the conflicting emotions gives the client the opportunity to talk about them, although many times he or she may not be able to do so.

Immobility due to ambivalence is extremely uncomfortable. One way of intervening is to limit the number of choices the indecisive client has to make. For example, a man may be immobilized by his inability to decide whether to go out alone for the first time. You can help by telling him that it seems too soon for him to go out alone and that, for today, he must be accompanied. Another example is a young woman who is undecided about where to sit. You can remove extra chairs at the table in the dining room so that she has only one choice.

Promoting Family Understanding and Involvement

When a person with schizophrenia is hospitalized, encourage the family and help them remain involved in the client's care. Except for unusual circumstances, share information on the client's status, treatment program, and future treatment plans, including discharge plans. Nurses may need to be active advocates for families' rights to information about, and involvement in, the care of their loved one with schizophrenia. Of course, nurses need to comply with the client's wishes and with the laws governing disclosure of information, which vary by state and by institution.

Referral to Psychoeducation Programs If assessment suggests that family members need information about the disease and treatment, refer the family to education programs, if they are available. Family psychoeducation programs are preferable to direct teaching because they often combine education with mutual support. In such groups, families can meet others who share their life difficulties. These peers can provide informal support and information to help the family deal with the tasks that lie ahead. You can reinforce the formal teaching that occurs in such programs when you meet with individual families. See the Partnering with Clients and Families: Teaching about Schizophrenia feature above.

Referral to NAMI Without exception, families should know about a national family support group with many local and state affiliates. The National Alliance on Mental Illness (NAMI) serves families through educational programs, local support groups, and political activism. Most local organizations are listed in telephone directories or can be reached through the local community mental health agency responsible for information and referral. For a resource link to NAMI, go to the Companion Website for this book.

MEDIALINK National Alliance on Mental Illness

CLINICAL EXAMPLE

The Oldstads were worried about their daughter's failing grades at college for the last semester and were surprised to learn that she had ended a relationship with her boyfriend. When she came home for spring break, she seemed disinterested and uncommunicative and wouldn't eat or socialize with the family. Her parents found her burning incense and chanting to herself in the mirror at 3:00 A.M. In a panic, they took her to the local emergency room. After a complete workup, they were shocked to learn that the probable diagnosis was schizophrenia. Furthermore, the physician wanted their daughter to begin taking medication.

The rapidity of the decline in their daughter's functioning, and the fact that she had hidden many of her symptoms from them, left the Oldstads feeling guilty, sad, and disbelieving. They could not fathom how this had happened to their beautiful daughter. A nurse at the emergency room had given them the number of a local NAMI support group and hotline. In their anguish, they called and were able to speak with other parents, who helped them begin to deal with their emotions and directed them to helpful books that explained schizophrenia and its treatment.

The importance of NAMI to families and the NAMI education program are discussed in detail in Chapter 30∞.

Promoting Community Contacts

An awareness of a client's community supports and potential treatment programs can guide nurses in preparing clients for discharge. For example, the client's most important peer support group might be the clientele at a local day treatment program or social club. If so, several visits prior to discharge will help the client make the transition back to the community.

Preparing clients for the residence they will enter after hospital discharge is a central nursing task. Often, placement depends on how the client functions in the hospital (Stroup et al., 2006). If the client is able to manage medications, participate in a variety of groups, and live cooperatively with other clients, then placement in a residential care facility that supports independent functioning is appropriate. In contrast, clients who need assistance with structuring free time, resist taking medications, or cannot be responsible for self-care require a more structured and supervised environment (Wilson, 2006).

Nurses work with clients to help them achieve their highest level of functioning. They document clients' abilities to perform various tasks and make recommendations to the treatment team about appropriate placements.

Evaluation

To complete the nursing process, nurses evaluate changes in client status and behavior in response to nursing interventions. Evaluation criteria are linked to nursing goals and reflect an understanding of the limitations of clients with schizophrenia. However, you must keep the concept of recovery in mind, as every client can improve and recover to a certain extent. The National Library of Medicine MEDLINEplus website offers search options on schizophrenia and other topics and can be accessed via the Companion Website for this text.

Communication

Clients will, with greater regularity, express their thoughts clearly and congruently. They will feel sufficient trust to talk to the nurse about troublesome symptoms or experiences. Because clients will probably continue to experience some symptoms even after medications have taken effect, this trust allows them to express what has changed and what is still troublesome.

Self-Care

Clients will consistently appear clean and well groomed and will independently manage personal grooming and hygiene. Clients will have clean and reasonably appropriate clothes, in terms of both fashion and season. Individual styles of dress, which are the client's way of expressing or presenting the self, will be supported by nurses. The means for maintaining self-care after discharge from acute care are identified.

Activity Intolerance

Clients will participate in goal-directed activities with minimal intervention. Clients will complete the activities they begin. Clients will demonstrate a broader range of interest and activities than they did on admission.

Social Isolation

Clients will demonstrate the capacity to interact, at least for brief periods, with nursing staff, with other clients, and in small groups. They will consistently demonstrate socially required interactions, such as greeting and starting a conversation with a stranger, asking for assistance, saying no, and listening to another's conversation. Clients will be inactive for shorter periods and spend more time engaged in interesting or meaningful activity. They will demonstrate the capacity to function outside the protective environment of acute or sheltered care.

Sensory/Perceptual Alterations

Clients will have fewer episodes of attending to internal stimuli. If hallucinations or delusions persist, clients will begin to identify stressors or situations that precipitate them. Clients will identify and practice personal coping strategies that decrease the hallucinations, delusions, or their effects, such as going to a quiet room, engaging in social activities, and performing activities that demand concentration.

Thought Processes

Clients will engage in reality-based discussions. If delusions persist, clients will not act on delusions in ways that are harmful or detrimental to themselves or others. They will also identify significant others in their current living environment who can help them limit their hallucinations via distraction or social contact.

Emotional Responses

Clients will have increased awareness that their emotional expressions at times do not match their verbal communications. They will monitor others' responses to them to learn cues about how they are varying their emotional expressions. Clients will experience fewer episodes of extreme discomfort due to ambivalence about people, events, or actions.

Family Functioning

Families will be involved in all aspects of client care, including assessment, planning and carrying out interventions, inpatient treatment choices, and planning for discharge. Family understanding of the illness trajectory and the client's capacities and limits will improve (Segrin, 2006). Family difficulties in caring for clients will be considered in treatment and discharge planning, and adequate resources will be identified to support family needs. Families will report that their questions about the schizophrenic disease process, and about varying modes of treatment for the disorder, have been answered.

CASE MANAGEMENT

Knowledge of the impact schizophrenia has on the way an individual thinks and functions is the underpinning of a competent case management program. In order to carry out any particular task, an individual with this illness must have specific duties coupled with realistic expectations. The case management strategies that work best with schizophrenia and other psychotic disorders include:

1. Tasks broken into manageable steps
2. Concrete actions
3. Structured environment
4. Routines and schedules
5. Dependable professionals
6. Flexibility to accommodate the shifts of the illness

Intensive Case Management (ICM) assists people with schizophrenia in outpatient settings (discussed in Chapter 12). With a smaller caseload, you have greater involvement with clients who require more supervision and care. You would orchestrate appointments and daily functioning issues to enhance the client's abilities to remain in the community and to foster a more independent lifestyle. Whether your assignment involves case management or intensive case management, the difficulties with thought processing and communication mentioned earlier in the chapter will shape your management of the case.

COMMUNITY-BASED CARE

People who have schizophrenia can have repetitive inpatient hospitalizations. The transition from an inpatient unit back to the community setting must begin prior to the client's discharge from the inpatient setting, forming a bridge from inpatient to outpatient care.

There are a number of services necessary and available in the community to maximize both quality of life and more independent functioning for people with schizophrenia and other psychotic disorders. Examples are:

1. Continuing day treatment programs
2. Independent living centers
3. Day hospitals
4. Community mental health centers
5. Social clubs
6. Wellness centers

These various settings are described in Chapter 12.

Counseling, psychotherapy, medication management, and other treatments are part of the care delivered in the community. In addition, remember that recreation is a quality-of-life issue. Community-based care can be instrumental in providing the guidance needed for clients to integrate into community living with an illness that can be debilitating and difficult.

HOME CARE

You may conduct different roles in delivering clinical services and care to clients with schizophrenia in a home setting. For example, you may function as a case manager and make home visits. This can be particularly important for clients with schizophrenia who often have great difficulty successfully meeting daily responsibilities and maintaining independence in a healthy home environment.

An important function of the nurse, whether or not you are a case manager, is to assist clients who have schizophrenia with medication adherence. Clients with schizophrenia are at high risk for relapse because they may stop taking their antipsychotic medications. This can happen because of side effects (those reported and not reported to the prescriber), confusion about medication administration schedules, environmental factors that do not encourage adherence to a medication regimen, or any number of other factors. You can play an important role in reducing the likelihood of relapse during home care visits. The home will shape adherence practices because the home is the environment in which most doses of their medications are taken.

Home interventions by nurses, however, are not limited to case management or medication adherence issues. Some people with schizophrenia can benefit from supportive psychotherapeutic interventions delivered by you in the client's home. These interventions can help generalize what they have learned beyond the confines of the nurse's office or the clinic. When people who have schizophrenia live with significant others, it is sometimes possible for you to deliver psychoeducational interventions for everyone living together as a unit. This allows the significant others and the client the opportunity to increase their skills in living together and coping with this serious illness in a way that lowers the probability of client relapse.

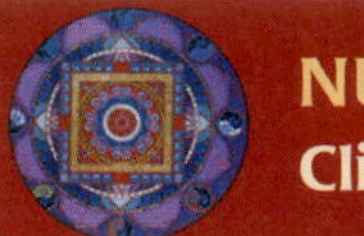

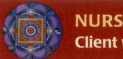

NURSING CARE PLAN
Client with Schizophrenia

Identifying Information

Jack May is a 24-year-old single male who lives with his mother and supports himself with SSI. He is brought to the psychiatric emergency service by his mother. He currently attends a structured work program 5 days a week, but stopped attending 8 days ago.

Jack says that he does not need to be hospitalized and that his mother is the one with the problem. He wants to be left alone to work on his computer projects. He admits that he has been hearing multiple voices in his head for the past week. For the past 2 weeks, Jack has been increasingly isolated, working on his personal computer in his room. He will not tell anyone what the work is about, but his mother has seen printouts that suggest it is a plan to soundproof and secure his room. Jack stopped attending his work program a week ago, saying that he had "more important work" to do at home. He refuses to eat or talk with his mother. His mother believes he stopped taking his medications. An identifiable stressor is that 2 weeks ago his father announced plans to remarry in the near future.

Symptom History

Two years ago, Jack had a serious psychosis precipitated by his move to a college out of state. He was diagnosed with schizophrenia, paranoid type. He was hospitalized for 2 weeks, stabilized on Haldol, and discharged home. Persecutory delusions that shift with news events are always present at a low level. He has lived with his mother since diagnosis, attending day treatment and, for the last 8 months, a structured work program. He occasionally attends client support network meetings. His work attendance has been sporadic, and he has been on and off probation for nonattendance in this structured work environment. He receives medications and follow-up treatment at the community mental health center.

Family History

The Mays are both living and well. They were separated 3 years ago and divorced 2 years ago. Jack's father is an attorney, and Jack sees him approximately once a month. Their relationship is pleasant but not close. His mother runs her own crafts store and is agreeable to having Jack live with her. There are no other children.

Psychosocial History

Jack has completed high school and a few courses at the local community college. He was an above-average student and was always involved in school and extracurricular activities, until about 9 months before his first psychotic episode. Since that time, he has socialized primarily with his mother and rarely with a few acquaintances from the client support group. He smokes a pack of cigarettes a day and drinks beer occasionally. He denies any illicit drug use. Jack has a keen interest in computers. He took extensive coursework in computers in school and has collected considerable equipment and software, primarily gifts from his father. Other pastimes are listening to rock music and watching television.

Medical History

No notable medical problems.

Current Mental Status

Jack is a healthy-looking 24-year-old who is anxious, somewhat guarded, but cooperative in the interview. He is oriented to person, time, and place, and demonstrates good memory and recall. Judgment is impaired. His affect is anxious. Speech is rapid, pressured, tangential. He is hyperalert to his environment and is notably startled by a siren outside. Persecutory delusions about people trying to take over his home and work are present, and he has hallucinations of unrecognizable voices and the voice of his father. No command hallucinations. Some loosening of associations present. Abstractions are concrete and self-referential. Insight poor; believes that his mother is "sick" and that she should not impede him in his important projects.

Other Clinical Data

Evidence that Jack may have stopped taking medications approximately 2 weeks ago. Suicide/violence potential minimal.

Nursing Diagnosis: Disturbed Thought Processes

Expected Outcome: Client will demonstrate the ability to cope competently with delusions.

Short-Term Goals	Interventions	Rationales
Client able to function in a variety of settings without intrusive delusional thought content.	▪ Make frequent, supportive, and brief contacts. ▪ Allow description of delusional thoughts and acknowledge emotional impact of same. ▪ Focus discussions on the client's feeling level concerning the delusions, and not the content.	Some contacts can be overwhelming for a client with schizophrenia and need to be of a manageable length.
	▪ Teach client how to cope with delusional thinking through engagement in activities for distraction, active self-talk promoting his efforts, support from others, treatment. ▪ Reinforce adaptive efforts.	The client must be taught how to cope with the symptoms of the illness in an effective manner.

Nursing Diagnosis: Anxiety related to delusions

Expected Outcome: Client will demonstrate decreased anxiety.

Short-Term Goals	Interventions	Rationales
Client able to describe a reduction in his anxiety. Client participates in his treatment.	▪ Make frequent, supportive, and brief contacts.	Some contacts can be overwhelming for a client with schizophrenia and need to be of a manageable length.
	▪ Reassure client verbally, with a structured routine, and by giving explanations congruent with client's ability to understand.	People with schizophrenia often do not have their feelings acknowledged. Reassurance validates their feelings.
	▪ Prompt client to interact with others when able to reduce feelings of isolation and alienation.	
	▪ Provide an array of coping skills client may use when anxious.	You must teach a variety of coping skills to suit various situations.

Concept Map
Client with Schizophrenia: Disturbed Thought Processes

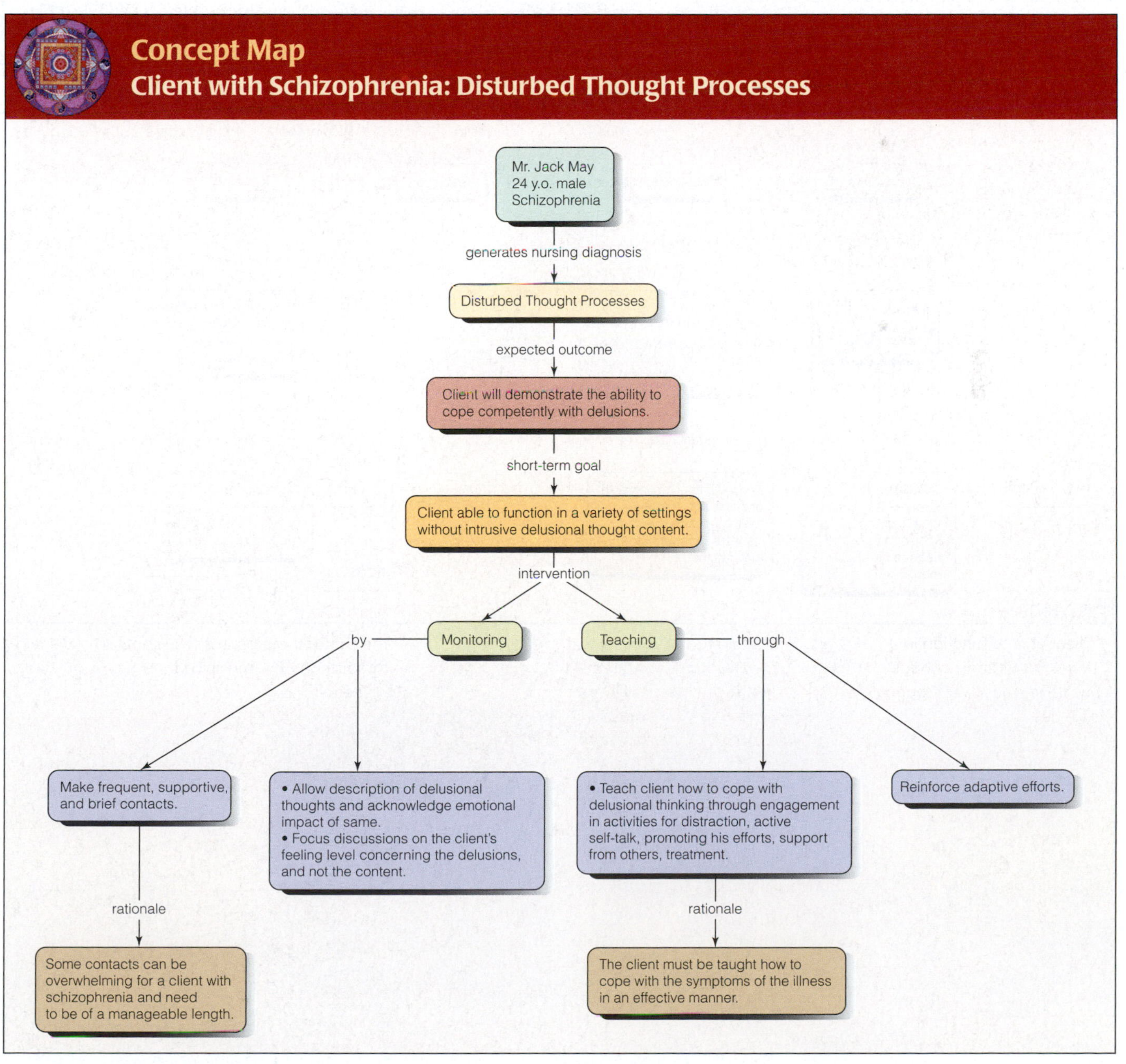
Mr. Jack May
24 y.o. male
Schizophrenia
generates nursing diagnosis
Disturbed Thought Processes
expected outcome
Client will demonstrate the ability to cope competently with delusions.
short-term goal
Client able to function in a variety of settings without intrusive delusional thought content.
intervention
Monitoring
Teaching
by
through
Make frequent, supportive, and brief contacts.
• Allow description of delusional thoughts and acknowledge emotional impact of same.
• Focus discussions on the client's feeling level concerning the delusions, and not the content.
• Teach client how to cope with delusional thinking through engagement in activities for distraction, active self-talk, promoting his efforts, support from others, treatment.
Reinforce adaptive efforts.
rationale
Some contacts can be overwhelming for a client with schizophrenia and need to be of a manageable length.
rationale
The client must be taught how to cope with the symptoms of the illness in an effective manner.

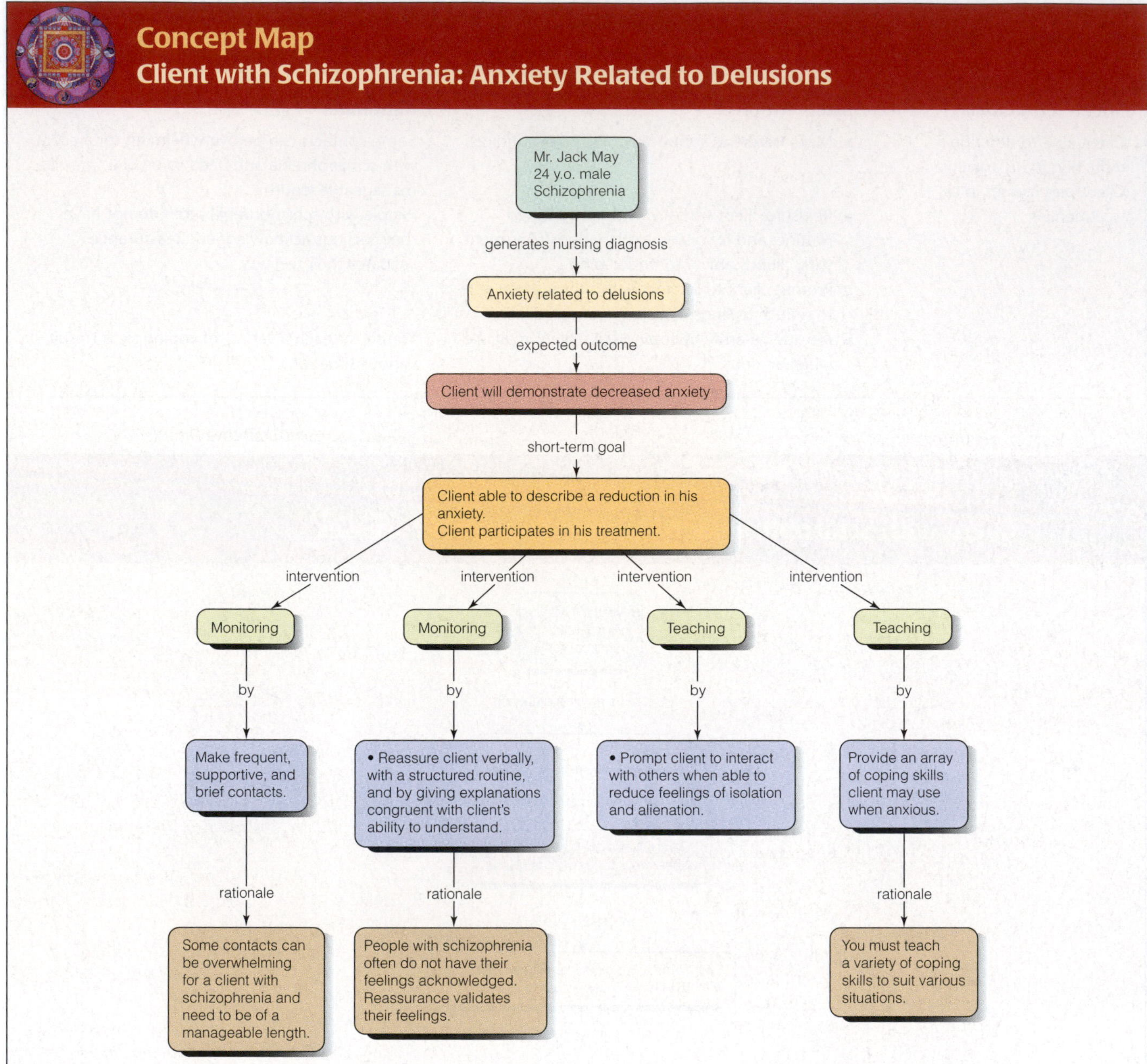
Concept Map
Client with Schizophrenia: Anxiety Related to Delusions
Mr. Jack May
24 y.o. male
Schizophrenia
generates nursing diagnosis
Anxiety related to delusions
expected outcome
Client will demonstrate decreased anxiety
short-term goal
Client able to describe a reduction in his anxiety.
Client participates in his treatment.
intervention
intervention
intervention
intervention
Monitoring
Monitoring
Teaching
Teaching
by
by
by
by
Make frequent, supportive, and brief contacts.
• Reassure client verbally, with a structured routine, and by giving explanations congruent with client's ability to understand.
• Prompt client to interact with others when able to reduce feelings of isolation and alienation.
Provide an array of coping skills client may use when anxious.
rationale
rationale
rationale
Some contacts can be overwhelming for a client with schizophrenia and need to be of a manageable length.
People with schizophrenia often do not have their feelings acknowledged. Reassurance validates their feelings.
You must teach a variety of coping skills to suit various situations.

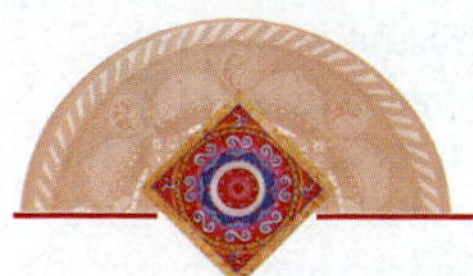

EXPLORE MEDIALINK

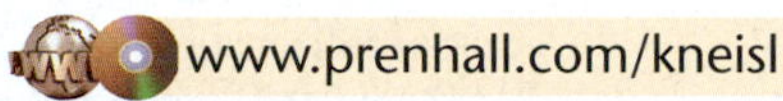

For NCLEX-RN® review questions, case studies, and other resources for this chapter see the Pearson Health MediaLink CD-ROM that accompanies this book and the Companion Website at www.prenhall.com/kneisl.

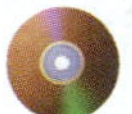

CD-ROM
Audio Glossary
NCLEX-RN® Review Questions
Videos and Animations
- *PET/SPECT Schizophrenia*
- *Dystonia (Blepharospasm, Cervical Torticollis)*
- *Bradykinesia (Shuffling Gait)*
- *Akathisia (Legs)*
- *Akinesia & Pill Rolling*
- *Tardive Dyskinesia (Mouth, Trunk, Ambulation)*
- *Schizophrenia Interview*

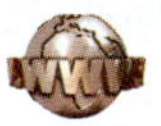

Companion Website
Audio Glossary
NCLEX-RN® Review Questions
Critical Thinking Exercise
- *The Influence of Stressors on the Client with Schizophrenia*

Case Study
- *The Client with Schizoaffective Disorder*

Care Plan
- *Social Isolation and Schizophrenia*

MediaLinks
MediaLink Application
- *About Mental Illness: Schizophrenia*

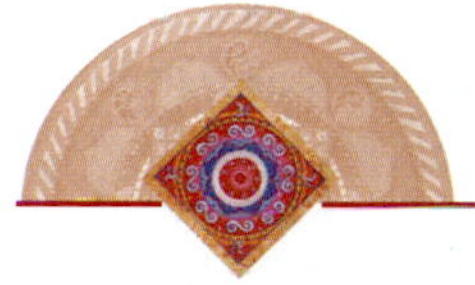

NCLEX-RN® REVIEW QUESTIONS

1. Which of the following client statements demonstrates the major symptoms of schizophrenia?
1. "I've been depressed ever since our house was destroyed by fire."
2. "You can read my mind. This light of mine will shine, fine; blinding world will end at nine."
3. "I had too much to drink last night, started feeling all-powerful, and stupidly drove my truck into a tree."
4. " 'A stitch in time saves nine' means that prevention is easier than fixing a real problem."

2. A family member asks you, "Since both of my siblings have schizophrenia, why are my brother's symptoms so different from my sister's? He withdraws when there's a change in his environment or routine. She starts cursing and yelling about the Mafia and the CIA when I do something that's less than perfect." Based on your knowledge, your response should address:
1. The many differences in the presentation of schizophrenia.
2. The typical progression of symptoms within an individual over time.
3. The effect of gender on clinical presentation in schizophrenia.
4. The significance of paranoid content in the differential diagnosis of paranoid schizophrenia.

3. Which family member statements demonstrate recognition of the effects of social pressures associated with schizophrenia? (Select all that apply.)
1. "I'm going to help my family member figure out what to tell other family members, friends, and business associates about why he's been on medical leave."
2. "If my family member would just move in with me, it would be a lot easier for me to maintain my household and care for my children."
3. "I used to protect my family member from a lot of the big interpersonal conflicts in the family, but we need to express our emotions more openly."
4. "I'll attend a support group, but I'm afraid my family member will not go . . . s/he would rather try to 'pass' as not mentally ill."
5. "It would be great if my family member could identify somebody to trust and believe when that person says, 'Your symptoms are worse. Let's go to the psychiatrist.' "

4. Which client statements demonstrate acknowledgment of the effects of psychological pressures associated with schizophrenia? (Select all that apply.)
1. "Next month, my sister and I are going to write a grant proposal for a psychiatric day treatment/social center."
2. "I'm going to look for a job where I can use my college degree but have less day-to-day stress."

3. "I just want to get back to what I was doing and put this whole episode behind me."
4. "If I can't stand the side effects, how will I ask my prescriber to change my medication?"
5. "I have designed a weekly schedule so that I can get tasks done and have planned time to relax."

5. You have presented your client with written aftercare medication directions: "Take one capsule three times per day." Your client informs you that s/he has reviewed the material. Which response specifically addresses your concerns about adherence?
1. "This medication really works best if you take one capsule three times per day."
2. "If you forget one dose, you can double the next one."
3. "What might get in the way of your taking your medications?"
4. "Do you understand everything?"

6. The client with schizophrenia is preparing for discharge. To minimize relapse, what is the most important feature of planning the client's aftercare?
1. An accurate description of the medication regimen with a specific plan for obtaining refills
2. Identification of three new methods of spending leisure time
3. Ensuring that the client lists three potential sources of social support
4. Identification of two new ways to bolster self-esteem

7. While you are employed as a charge nurse on an inpatient psychiatric unit, you recognize that you are choosing to spend less time interacting with the clients with schizophrenia. Your first action is:
1. Forcing yourself to interact with the clients with schizophrenia.
2. Reflecting on your behavior.
3. Discussing your observation with your clinical supervisor.
4. Requesting a transfer to another unit.

8. A peer approaches you and shares her frustration with her older brother, who has had multiple hospitalizations with schizophrenia. "He used to show interest in me, but since his discharge 5 days ago, he just stares into space. I cannot get a reaction out of him." Which of the following statements impart accurate information? (Select all that apply.)
1. "He may be demonstrating flattening of affect and anhedonia."
2. "Have you confronted him with this?"
3. "Maybe he's depressed about having a chronic illness."
4. "It's sad when a loved one does not have any feelings."
5. "He may have sedation or masked facial expressions from his medications."

9. A nurse is designing a relapse-prevention inpatient group for clients with schizophrenia. Which statement addresses a main category of nursing activities?
1. "We will go around the room and each person will state a personal goal for today."
2. "We're going to discuss current events."
3. "Let's go around the room and have each person say something positive about our group."
4. "If you can increase your self-assessment skills, you'll be able to tell when you're getting more stressed."

10. You overhear a family member discussing medication adherence with your client. Which of the following statements do you want to encourage the family member to reiterate?
1. "Your support group encourages you to make healthy choices. Taking your meds is a healthy thing you can do every day, just like brushing your teeth."
2. "Your children are getting tired of watching you get sick every time you stop your meds."
3. "If you stop taking your medication, I'll take custody of your children."
4. "You should let these health care providers get you well. Why do you fight that?"

See Appendix C for answers.

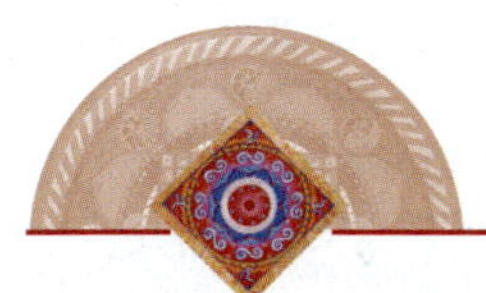

REFERENCES

Allardyce, J., & Boydell, J. (2006). Review: The wider social environment and schizophrenia. *Schizophrenia Bulletin, 32*(4), 592–598.

American Psychiatric Association. (2000). *Diagnostic and statistical manual of mental disorders* (4th ed., Text Revision). Washington, DC: Author.

Brookes, K., Xu, X., Chen, W., Zhou, K., Neale, B., Lowe, N., et al. (2006). The analysis of 51 genes in DSM-IV combined type attention deficit hyperactivity disorder: Association signals in DRD4, DAT1 and 16 other genes. *Molecular Psychiatry, 11*(10), 935–953.

Chafetz, L., White, M. C., Collins-Bride, G., Nickens, J., & Cooper, B. A. (2006). Predictors of physical functioning among adults with severe mental illness. *Psychiatric Services, 57*(2), 225–231.

Connor, S., & Wilson, R. (2006). It's important that they learn from us for mental health to progress. *Journal of Mental Health, 15*(4), 461–474.

Donohoe, G., Clarke, S., Morris, D., Nangle, J. M., Schwaiger, S., Gill, M., et al. (2006). Are deficits in executive sub-processes simply reflecting more general cognitive decline in schizophrenia? *Schizophrenia Research, 85*(1-3), 168–173.

Eastwood, S. L., & Harrison, P. J. (2006). Cellular basis of reduced cortical reelin expression in schizophrenia. *American Journal of Psychiatry, 163*(3), 540–542.

England, M. (2006). Cognitive intervention for voice hearers. *Issues in Mental Health Nursing, 27*(7), 735–751.

Grant, A. (2006). Cognitive remediation therapy for schizophrenia: Theory & practice. *Journal of Mental Health, 15*(2), 259.

Griner, D., & Smith, T. B. (2006). Culturally adapted mental health intervention: A meta-analytic review. *Psychotherapy: Theory, Research, Practice, Training, 43*(4), 531–548.

Harrison, P. J., & Law, A. J. (2006). Neuregulin 1 and schizophrenia: Genetics, gene expression, and neurobiology. *Biological Psychiatry, 60*(2), 132–140.

Haynes, R. B., Yao, X., Degani, A., Kripalani, S., Garg, A., & McDonald, H. P. (2006). Interventions for enhancing medication adherence. *The Cochrane Library,* 4–163.

Hunt, I. M., Kapur, N., Windfuhr, K., Robinson, J., Bickley, H., Flynn, S., et al. (2006). Suicide in schizophrenia: Findings from a national clinical survey. *Journal of Psychiatric Practice, 12*(3), 139–147.

Isherwood, T., Burns, M., & Rigby, G. (2006). A qualitative analysis of the 'management of schizophrenia' within a medium-secure service for men with learning disabilities. *Journal of Psychiatric & Mental Health Nursing, 13*(2), 148–156.

Joseph, J., & Leo, J. (2006). Genetic relatedness and the lifetime risk for being diagnosed with schizophrenia: Gottesman's 1991 figure 10 reconsidered. *Journal of Mind and Behavior, 27*(1), 73–90.

Karayiorgou, M., & Gogos, J. A. (2006). Schizophrenia genetics: Uncovering positional candidate genes. *European Journal of Human Genetics, 14*(5), 512–519.

Kelly, D. L., & Conley, R. R. (2006). A randomized double-blind 12-week study of quetiapine, risperidone or fluphenazine on sexual functioning in people with schizophrenia. *Psychoneuroendocrinology, 31*(3), 340–346.

Kelly, D. L., Dixon, L. B., Kreyenbuhl, J. A., Medoff, D., Lehman, A. F., Love, R. C., et al. (2006). Clozapine utilization and outcomes by race in a public mental health system: 1994-2000. *Journal of Clinical Psychiatry, 67*(9), 1404–1411.

Kessler, R. C., Chiu, W. T., Demler, O., & Walters, E. E. (2005). Prevalence, severity, and comorbidity of twelve-month DSM-IV disorders in the National Comorbidity Survey Replication (NCS-R). *Archives of General Psychiatry, 62*(6), 617–627.

Kymalainen, J. A., Weisman, A. G., Rosales, G. A., & Armesto, J. C. (2006). Ethnicity, expressed emotion, and communication deviance in family members of patients with schizophrenia. *Journal of Nervous & Mental Disease, 194*(6), 391–396.

Lee, S., Lee, J., Lee, B., & Kim, Y. H. (2007). A 12-week, double-blind, placebo-controlled trial of galantamine adjunctive treatment to conventional antipsychotics for the cognitive impairments in chronic schizophrenia. *International Clinical Psychopharmacology, 22*(2), 63–68.

Margetic, B., Aukst-Margetic, B., & Zarkovic-Palijan, T. (2006). Successful treatment of polydipsia, water intoxication, and delusional jealousy in an alcohol dependent patient with clozapine. *Progress in Neuro-Psychopharmacology & Biological Psychiatry, 30*(7), 1347–1349.

Meyer-Lindenberg, A., Nichols, T., Callicott, J. H., Ding, J., Kolachana, B., Buckholtz, J., et al. (2006). Impact of complex genetic variation in COMT on human brain function. *Molecular Psychiatry, 11*(9), 867–877.

Montgomery, P., Tompkins, C., Forchuk, C., & French, S. (2006). Keeping close: Mothering with serious mental illness. *Journal of Advanced Nursing, 54*(1), 20–28.

Muñoz, C., & Hilgenberg, C. (2006). Ethnopharmacology: Understanding how ethnicity can affect drug response is essential to providing culturally competent care. *Holistic Nursing Practice, 20*(5), 227–234.

Netto, G. (2006). Creating a suitable space: A qualitative study of the cultural sensitivity of counselling provision in the voluntary sector in the UK. *Journal of Mental Health, 15*(5), 593–604.

Nicodemus, K. K., Luna, A., Vakkalanka, R., Goldberg, T., Egan, M., Straub, R. E., et al. (2006). Further evidence for association between ErbB4 and schizophrenia and influence on cognitive intermediate phenotypes in healthy controls. *Molecular Psychiatry, 11*(12), 1062–1065.

Paz, R. D., Andreasen, N. C., Daoud, S. Z., Conley, R., Roberts, R., Bustillo, J., et al. (2006). Increased expression of activity-dependent genes in cerebellar glutamatergic neurons of patients with schizophrenia. *American Journal of Psychiatry, 163*(10), 1829–1831.

Riley, B., & Kendler, K. S. (2006). Molecular genetic studies of schizophrenia. *European Journal of Human Genetics, 14*(6), 669–680.

Rosenberg, J., & Rosenberg, S. (Eds.). (2006). *Community mental health: Challenges for the 21st century.* New York: Routledge.

Segrin, C. (2006). Family interactions and well-being: Integrative perspectives. *Journal of Family Communication, 6*(1), 3–21.

Stroup, T. S., Lieberman, J. A., McEnvoy, J. P., Swartz, M. S., Davis, S. M., Rosenheck, R. A., et al. (2006). Effectiveness of olanzapine, quetiapine, risperidone, and ziprasidone in patients with chronic schizophrenia following discontinuation of the previous atypical antipsychotic. *American Journal of Psychiatry, 163*(4), 611–622.

Szeszko, P. R., Lipsky, R., Mentschel, C., Robinson, D., Gunduz-Bruce, H., Sevy, S., et al. (2005). Brain-derived neurotrophic factor val66met polymorphism and volume of the hippocampal formation. *Molecular Psychiatry, 10*(7), 631–636.

Thomas, P., Seebohm, P., Henderson, P., Munn-Giddings, C., & Yasmeen, S. (2006). Tackling race inequalities: Community development, mental health and diversity. *Journal of Public Mental Health, 5*(2), 13–19.

Tunbridge, E. M., Weinberger, D. R., & Harrison, P. J. (2006). A novel protein isoform of catechol O-methyltransferase (COMT): Brain expression analysis in schizophrenia and bipolar disorder and effect of Valsuperscript 1-sup-5-sup-8Met genotype. *Molecular Psychiatry, 11*(2), 116–117.

Uko-Ekpenyong, G. (2006). Improving medication adherence with orally disintegrating tablets. *Nursing, 36*(9), 20–21.

van Meijel, B., Kruitwagen, C., van der Gaag, M., Kahn, R. S., & Grypdonck, M. H. F. (2006). An intervention study to prevent relapse in patients with schizophrenia. *Journal of Nursing Scholarship, 38*(1), 42–49.

Weisman, A. G., Rosales, G. A., Kymalainen, J. A., & Armesto, J. C. (2006). Ethnicity, expressed emotion, and schizophrenia patients' perceptions of their family members' criticism. *Journal of Nervous & Mental Disease, 194*(9), 644–649.

Wilson, W. H. (2006). Neuropsychiatric perspectives for community mental health theory and practice. In J. Rosenberg & S. Rosenberg (Eds.), *Community mental health: Challenges for the 21st century* (pp. 83–100). New York: Routledge.

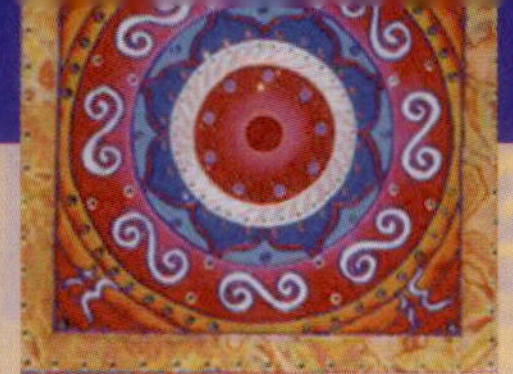

CHAPTER

17

Mood Disorders

EILEEN TRIGOBOFF
KAY K. CHITTY

KEY TERMS

affect *405*
anergy or anergia *407*
anhedonia *405*
bereavement *412*
bipolar disorders *408*
circadian rhythms *415*
cyclothymic disorder *411*
dysfunctional grieving *413*
dysthymic disorder *407*
electroconvulsive therapy (ECT) *422*
flight of ideas *409*
generalized seizure *424*
grandiosity *409*
grief *413*
hypersomnia *407*
hypomania *409*
insomnia *405*
major depressive disorder *405*
major depressive episode *405*
mania *409*
monoamine oxidase inhibitors (MAOIs) *422*
postpartum mood episode *412*
psychomotor retardation *407*

(continued)

LEARNING OUTCOMES

After completing this chapter, you will be able to:

1. Compare and contrast the similarities and differences between major depressive disorder and bipolar disorder.
2. Differentiate between bereavement and dysfunctional grieving.
3. Describe the elements of the biopsychosocial theories discussed here that contribute most to the current understanding of mood disorders.
4. Explain the principles upon which the various biologic therapies for clients with mood disorders are based.
5. Systematically conduct a nursing assessment of a client with a mood disorder.
6. Implement an understanding of suicide prevention and safety promotion in the plan of care for clients with mood disorders.
7. Design a plan of care to reduce negative thinking and promote improved self-esteem.
8. Educate clients and their families about biologic treatment for mood disorders such as antidepresessant medications and electroconvulsive therapy.
9. Assess personal feelings, values, and attitudes toward clients with mood disorders that may provide challenges to professional practice.

CRITICAL THINKING CHALLENGE

Consuela R. is a 38-year-old woman with severe mania who has not responded to psychopharmacologic interventions. The treatment team on her inpatient psychiatric unit has recommended electroconvulsive therapy (ECT) to Consuela and her family. Consuela is quite fearful of this procedure and believes that it will enable others to control her mind. She is adamantly opposed to it.

1. What are the rights of severely ill psychiatric clients in determining their own treatment? Do they differ from those of other clients with physiologic disorders who now enjoy almost complete self-determination if they choose to exercise it?
2. At what point does a client's right to autonomy and self-determination end?
3. How might a treatment facility's philosophy on this issue be implemented to ensure consistency of care?

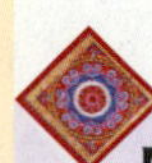

MEDIALINK 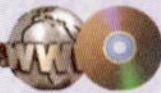 www.prenhall.com/kneisl

Go to the Pearson Health MediaLink CD-ROM and the Companion Website at www.prenhall.com/kneisl for interactive resources.

KEY TERMS *(continued)*

relapse 425
seasonal affective disorder (SAD) 408
selective serotonin reuptake inhibitors (SSRIs) 422
serotonin and norepinephrine reuptake inhibitors (SNRIs) 422
tricyclic antidepressants (TCAs) 422
tyramine 422
vegetative symptoms 405

Approximately 12% of Americans suffer from the wide spectrum of mood disorders. Mood disorders are a group of psychiatric diagnoses characterized by disturbances in physical, emotional, and behavioral response patterns. These patterns of **affect** (mood) range from extreme elation and agitation to extreme depression with a serious potential for suicide. They are the most common of all mental disorders, largely due to the prevalence of depression. Other mood disorders that occur less frequently than depression, but can be severely incapacitating, include dysthymic disorder and the bipolar disorders. The spectrum of bipolarity in the community, estimated at 6.4%, is of great public health significance (McIntyre et al., 2007).

The symptoms of mood disorders—poor memory and concentration, fatigue, apathy, indecisiveness, and loss of self-confidence in depressed clients and grandiosity and unrealistic overconfidence in those with mania—reduce the capacity to work and maintain the activities of daily living. Some mental health authorities believe that major depression is more disabling than many medical disorders, such as chronic lung disease, arthritis, and diabetes. It is the leading cause of lost workdays and diminished productivity on the job.

Many people with mood disorders are never seen for treatment in psychiatric settings because:

1. Some people may not realize they have a problem.
2. Other people do not realize they have a treatable illness.
3. Physical complaints brought to primary health care providers may be determined to require medical, or surgical, treatment instead of mental health care.
4. Health care policy and insurance coverage for mental disorders may be nonexistent or meager.

Nearly two thirds of depressed people in this country go undiagnosed and untreated.

As a nurse and a citizen, you are in an excellent position to identify early signs of mood disorders and initiate action leading to early treatment.

MAJOR DEPRESSIVE EPISODE/DISORDER

A **major depressive episode** is characterized by a change in several aspects of a person's life and emotional state consistently throughout at least 14 days. Of prime importance is the client's mood state. Be aware that clients do not always describe their mood as "depressed." Instead, they may say they are sad, discouraged, "down in the dumps," or say that they feel helpless. Or, they may complain of having no feelings at all or of feeling "blah." In other cases, vague somatic complaints such as aches and pains are reported, while other clients report increased anger, frustration, and irritability, with uncharacteristic outbursts over minor matters. It is not difficult to imagine that someone who looks and feels sad or empty is depressed. A diagnosis of depression is more likely to be missed when a person simply seems anxious or irritable.

Major depressive disorder may consist of a single episode or may recur as recurrent major depression at various points in life. The description of the diagnostic criteria for single-episode and recurrent major depression is found in the DSM-IV-TR Diagnostic Criteria for Depressive Disorders box. Key facts about major depression are in Box 17-1.

Individuals with a history of a manic or hypomanic episode (discussed later in this chapter) are considered to have a bipolar disorder and are not classified under these categories.

When a person experiences a major depressive disorder, activities that previously gave pleasure, such as socializing, hobbies, sports, and sexual activities, often are no longer enjoyed. This condition is known as **anhedonia**. Changes in physiologic functioning during depression are called **vegetative symptoms**. Changes in appetite, usually experienced as a reduction or loss of interest in food, are often seen, although increased appetite and cravings are also reported.

Sleep disturbances are also common, particularly **insomnia** (the inability to fall asleep or stay asleep, or awakening early in the morning). Two types of insomnia are most often

MEDIALINK Case Study: Depressive Mood Disorder

Box 17-1 Key Facts About Major Depression

- The average age of onset is the mid-twenties, although major depressive disorder can begin at any age and seems to be occurring in younger and younger people.
- The risk of developing major depressive disorder during one's lifetime ranges from 15% to 25% for females and from 8% to 15% for males, making depression twice as likely for women as for men.
- First-degree biologic relatives (parents or siblings) of people with major depressive disorder are up to three times as likely to develop depression as are members of the general population (APA, 2000).
- Symptoms usually develop over a period of time. The person may experience anxiety and mild depression for several days, weeks, or months before the onset of a full major depressive episode.
- If untreated, major depression lasts 6 or more months. In about 20% to 30% of cases, some depressive symptoms persist for longer periods, ranging from months to years. This is considered a partial remission and thought to be predictive of later depressive episodes and the development of chronic depression.

DSM-IV-TR Diagnostic Criteria for Depressive Disorders

Major Depressive Episode

A. Five (or more) of the following symptoms have been present during the same 2-week period and represent a change from previous functioning; at least one of the symptoms is either (1) depressed mood or (2) loss of interest or pleasure. **Note:** Do not include symptoms that are clearly due to a general medical condition, or mood-incongruent delusions or hallucinations.
   1. depressed mood most of the day, nearly every day, as indicated by either subjective report (e.g., feels sad or empty) or observation made by others (e.g., appears tearful). Note: In children and adolescents, can be irritable mood.
   2. markedly diminished interest or pleasure in all, or almost all, activities most of the day, nearly every day (as indicated by either subjective account or observation made by others)
   3. significant weight loss when not dieting or weight gain (e.g., a change of more than 5% of body weight in a month), or decrease or increase in appetite nearly every day. Note: In children, consider failure to make expected weight gains.
   4. insomnia or hypersomnia nearly every day
   5. psychomotor agitation or retardation nearly every day (observable by others, not merely subjective feelings of restlessness or being slowed down)
   6. fatigue or loss of energy nearly every day
   7. feelings of worthlessness or excessive or inappropriate guilt (which may be delusional) nearly every day (not merely self-reproach or guilt about being sick)
   8. diminished ability to think or concentrate, or indecisiveness, nearly every day (either by subjective account or as observed by others)
   9. recurrent thoughts of death (not just fear of dying), recurrent suicidal ideation without a specific plan, or a suicide attempt or a specific plan for committing suicide

B. The symptoms do not meet criteria for a Mixed Episode.

C. The symptoms cause clinically significant distress or impairment in social, occupational, or other important areas of functioning.

D. The symptoms are not due to the direct physiological effects of a substance (e.g., a drug of abuse, a medication) or a general medical condition (e.g., hypothyroidism).

E. The symptoms are not better accounted for by bereavement (i.e., after the loss of a loved one), the symptoms persist for longer than 2 months or are characterized by marked functional impairment, morbid preoccupation with worthlessness, suicidal ideation, psychotic symptoms, or psychomotor retardation.

Major Depressive Disorder, Single Episode

A. Presence of a single Major Depressive Episode.

B. The Major Depressive Episode is not better accounted for by Schizoaffective Disorder and is not superimposed on Schizophrenia, Schizophreniform Disorder, Delusional Disorder, or Psychotic Disorder Not Otherwise Specified.

C. There has never been a Manic Episode, a Mixed Episode, or a Hypomanic Episode. **Note:** This exclusion does not apply if all of the manic-like, mixed-like, or hypomanic-like episodes are substance or treatment induced or are due to the direct physiological effects of a general medical condition.

Major Depressive Disorder, Recurrent

A. Presence of two or more Major Depressive Episodes. **Note:** To be considered separate episodes, there must be an interval of at least 2 consecutive months in which criteria are not met for a Major Depressive Episode.

B. The Major Depressive Episodes are not better accounted for by Schizoaffective Disorder and are not superimposed on Schizophrenia, Schizophreniform Disorder, Delusional Disorder, or Psychotic Disorder Not Otherwise Specified.

C. There has never been a Manic Episode, a Mixed Episode, or a Hypomanic Episode. **Note:** This exclusion does not apply if all of the manic-like, mixed-like, or hypomanic-like episodes are substance or treatment induced or are due to the direct physiological effects of a general medical condition.

DYSTHYMIC DISORDER

A. Depressed mood for most of the day, for more days than not, as indicated either by subjective account or observation by others, for at least 2 years. **Note:** In children and adolescents, mood can be irritable and duration must be at least 1 year.

B. Presence, while depressed, of two (or more) of the following:
   1. poor appetite or overeating
   2. insomnia or hypersomnia
   3. low energy or fatigue
   4. low self-esteem
   5. poor concentration or difficulty making decisions
   6. feelings of hopelessness

C. During the 2-year period (1 year for children or adolescents) of the disturbance, the person has never been without the symptoms in Criteria A and B for more than 2 months at a time.

D. No Major Depressive Episode has been present during the first 2 years of the disturbance (1 year for children and adolescents) (i.e., the disturbance is not better accounted for by chronic Major Depressive Disorder, or Major Depressive Disorder, in Partial Remission). **Note:** There may have been a previous Major Depressive Episode provided there was a full remission (no significant signs or symptoms for 2 months) before development of the Dysthymic Disorder. In addition, after the initial 2 years (1 year in children or adolescents) of Dysthymic Disorder, there may be superimposed episodes of Major Depressive Disorder, in which case both diagnoses may be given when the criteria are met for a Major Depressive Episode.

E. There has never been a Manic Episode, a Mixed Episode, or a Hypomanic Episode, and criteria have never been met for Cyclothymic Disorder.

F. The disturbance does not occur exclusively during the course of a chronic Psychotic Disorder, such as Schizophrenia or Delusional Disorder.

G. The symptoms are not due to the direct physiological effects of a substance (e.g., a drug of abuse, a medication) or a general medical condition (e.g., hypothyroidism).

H. The symptoms cause clinically significant distress or impairment in social, occupational, or other important areas of functioning.

(continued)

DSM-IV-TR Diagnostic Criteria for Depressive Disorders *(continued)*

Seasonal Pattern Specifier

Specify if:

With Seasonal Pattern (can be applied to the pattern of Major Depressive Episodes in Bipolar I Disorder, Bipolar II Disorder, or Major Depressive Disorder, Recurrent)

A. There has been a regular temporal relationship between the onset of Major Depressive Episodes in Bipolar I or Bipolar II Disorder or Major Depressive Disorder, Recurrent, and a particular time of the year (e.g., regular appearance of the Major Depressive Episode in the fall or winter).

Note: Do not include cases in which there is an obvious effect of seasonal-related psychosocial stressors (e.g., regularly being unemployed every winter).

B. Full remissions (or a change from depression to mania or hypomania) also occur at a characteristic time of the year (e.g., depression disappears in the spring).

C. In the last 2 years, two Major Depressive Episodes have occurred that demonstrate the temporal seasonal relationships defined in Criteria A and B, and no nonseasonal Major Depressive Episodes have occurred during that same period.

D. Seasonal Major Depressive Episodes (as described previously) substantially outnumber the nonseasonal Major Depressive Episodes that may have occurred over the individual's lifetime.

Source: Reprinted with permission from the *Diagnostic and Statistical Manual of Mental Disorders*, Fourth Edition, Text Revision. (Copyright 2000). American Psychiatric Association.

USING DSM-IV-TR

Health care providers often use language unfamiliar to clients and their families. To help clients and families understand the symptoms of a major depressive episode, reword the DSM statement that symptoms may be characterized by "psychomotor retardation."

experienced by people having a major depressive episode. *Middle insomnia* refers to waking up during the night and having difficulty falling asleep again. *Terminal insomnia* refers to waking at the end of the night and being unable to return to sleep. Also reported is **hypersomnia**, in which the person sleeps for prolonged nighttime periods as well as during the day, but still wakes up tired or fatigued. These sleep disturbances are discussed at length in Chapter 19.

Fatigue and decreased energy are characteristic symptoms of depression, a condition known as **anergy** or **anergia**. Individuals report being tired upon awakening, regardless of how long they have slept. Even the smallest task seems insurmountable, and routine activities require substantial effort and take longer to accomplish. Decreased energy may be manifested in **psychomotor retardation**, in which thinking and body movements are noticeably slowed and speech is slowed or absent. Psychomotor agitation also may occur, in which the person cannot sit still, paces, wrings the hands, and picks at the fingernails, skin, clothing, bedclothes, or other objects. Psychomotor retardation is a prominent symptom in the clinical example that follows.

CLINICAL EXAMPLE

Becky is a 26-year-old insurance underwriter who visited a local Planned Parenthood clinic for a yearly checkup and Pap test. During the examination by the family planning nurse, Becky asked whether she might be anemic because she was "just exhausted all the time." Becky revealed that for the past month she had had difficulty getting out of bed in the morning. Getting dressed and ready for work left her drained. She described standing in front of her closet for long periods, unable to decide what to wear. Becky was also having extreme difficulty calling potential clients. Whereas she was normally an assertive salesperson who called on perfect strangers with ease, she now described sitting at her desk for hours, trying to work up the motivation to pick up the phone. Coworkers, including her boss, had commented on her 15-pound weight gain, and these comments precipitated several uncharacteristic angry and tearful outbursts at work.

Other common symptoms in significantly depressed individuals include guilt or a sense of worthlessness, self-blame, impaired concentration and decision-making ability, even about trivial things, and suicidal ideation. The characteristics of a major depressive episode are illustrated in FIGURE 17-1.

MEDIALINK Depression Video

DYSTHYMIC DISORDER

The term **dysthymic disorder** describes chronic depression for the majority of most days for at least 2 years (1 year for children and adolescents). Throughout those 2 years, no more than 2 months can be described as symptom-free. In general the symptoms of dysthymic disorder, while distressing, tend to be less severe than those in major depressive disorder, with fewer physiologic symptoms. The diagnostic criteria for dysthymic disorder are given on page 406. Dysthymic disorder tends to predispose people to the development of major depressive disorder. According to the DSM-IV-TR, 10% to 25% of individuals diagnosed with dysthymic disorder will develop major depressive disorder within the next year (American Psychiatric Association [APA], 2000).

Dysthymic disorder often occurs in childhood, adolescence, or early adulthood and tends to be chronic. While both females and males are equally affected as children, there are two to three times as many adult females as males with dysthymic disorder. The lifetime risk of developing dysthymic disorder is approximately 6% in the general population.

The symptoms of dysthymic disorder are similar to those of chronic major depressive disorder. This similarity makes it difficult, even for experienced clinicians, to make an accurate

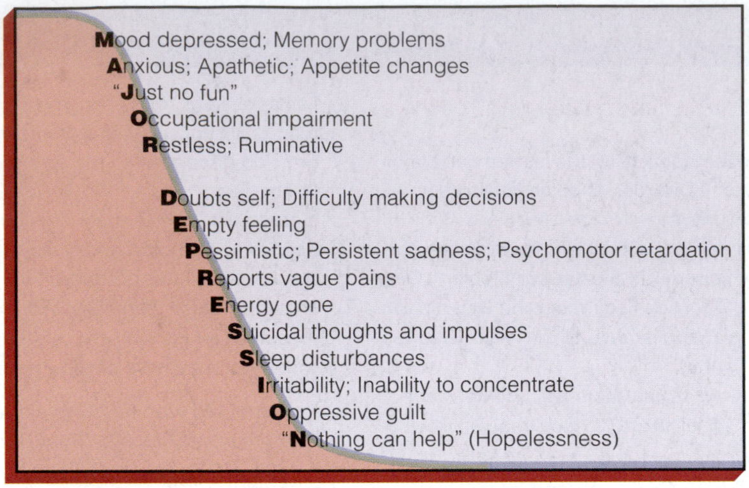

Mood depressed; Memory problems
Anxious; Apathetic; Appetite changes
"Just no fun"
Occupational impairment
Restless; Ruminative

Doubts self; Difficulty making decisions
Empty feeling
Pessimistic; Persistent sadness; Psychomotor retardation
Reports vague pains
Energy gone
Suicidal thoughts and impulses
Sleep disturbances
Irritability; Inability to concentrate
Oppressive guilt
"Nothing can help" (Hopelessness)

FIGURE 17-1 Characteristics of major depression.

differential diagnosis. In clinical practice, nursing care of the dysthymic client is similar to that of depressed clients. The clinical example included here describes such a case.

CLINICAL EXAMPLE

Gregory G. is a 14-year-old who was brought to a nurse psychotherapist by his mother on the suggestion of the guidance counselor in his private school. In the letter of referral, the counselor stated that she was concerned because of Gregory's "persistent pessimistic outlook on life."

According to Mrs. G., who was interviewed alone, Gregory has always been a cranky and irritable child. Since starting kindergarten, he has had difficulty relating to other children and is often left out of activities and social invitations. At home, he stays in his room much of the time, where he plays computer games and writes poetry. He does not do well in school, although testing has shown him to be far above average in intelligence. Despite their best efforts, his parents have never been able to interest him in scouting, sports, or other activities they deem appropriate for a boy his age. His parents reported that Gregory's weight, eating habits, and sleeping patterns were unchanged.

When Gregory was interviewed, he responded in monosyllables, made poor eye contact with the therapist, and sat slumped in his chair with no facial expression. He stated that he knew his parents were "disappointed" in him.

SEASONAL AFFECTIVE DISORDER

MEDIALINK SAD Treatment

Natural light is frequently taken for granted, and most people may be unaware of how it influences the human experience. As early as the days of Hippocrates, observers of human behavior noticed that some people suffer mood changes as the seasons change.

The relationships between light, biological rhythms, and mood are the subject of robust and thorough scientific study. This research focuses on the use of light in the treatment of **seasonal affective disorder (SAD)**, a depressive disorder that occurs in relation to the seasons, usually during winter months. Natural light may help modulate daily rhythms that influence sleep and activity patterns, neuroendocrine functions, and brain chemical systems. The criteria for specifying the occurrence of SAD are listed in the Diagnostic Criteria box.

Many antidepressants are typically used to treat the depressive features of SAD, but only one currently is indicated for this diagnosis by the Food and Drug Administration (FDA). Bupropion extended-release (Wellbutrin ER) may prevent major depressive episodes in people with SAD. Treatment for SAD has entered areas well beyond therapy and medication. Researchers are exploring the application of different forms of light to the skin and eyes at different times of day, and the results indicate a reduction of fatigue and depression as well as improved alertness (Joseph, 2006). The exact relationship between SAD and light, biologic rhythms, and events at the cellular level has not yet been determined. Information on SAD and the clinical application of light therapy is available through the Society for Light Treatment and Biological Rhythms (www.sltbr.org) and the Seasonal Affective Disorder Association (www.sada.org.uk) and can be accessed through the Companion Website for this book.

BIPOLAR DISORDERS

The **bipolar disorders** are a group of mood disorders that include manic episodes, hypomanic episodes, mixed episodes, depressed episodes, and cyclothymic disorder. The DSM-IV-TR diagnostic criteria for these disorders are listed on pages 410–411.

A *bipolar I disorder* consists of one or more manic or mixed episodes, and the course of illness can be accompanied by major depressive episodes. A *bipolar II disorder* consists of one or more major depressive episodes accompanied by at least one hypomanic episode.

Bipolar disorders tend to be recurrent, and have the unusual tendency to increase in frequency as the individual ages. The majority of bipolar I disorder clients do not have the chance to experience a baseline mood—called euthymic—because a major depressive episode may quickly follow. Many clients return to normal functioning during remissions, but approximately 20% to 30% have residual mood symptoms and as many as 60% have continuing interpersonal and occupational difficulties. Five to 10% of clients with bipolar II disorder have four or more mood episodes in a given year, and approximately 15% experience continuing mood lability and interpersonal and occupational difficulties (APA, 2000).

Manic and Hypomanic Episodes

Mania is characterized by an abnormal and persistently elevated, expansive, or irritable mood lasting at least one week, significantly impairing social or occupational functioning, and generally requiring hospitalization. This disturbance in mood must be accompanied by at least three additional symptoms such as "inflated self-esteem or **grandiosity**, decreased need for sleep, pressure of speech, **flight of ideas** (rapidly changing, fragmentary thoughts), distractibility, increased involvement in goal-directed activities or psychomotor agitation, and excessive involvement in pleasurable activities with a high potential for painful consequences" (APA, 2000, p. 362). Psychotic symptoms, such as delusions or hallucinations, may be a feature of severe mania. The DSM-IV-TR diagnostic criteria for a manic episode are listed in the box on the next page.

Hypomania is a less extreme form of mania that is not severe enough to markedly impair functioning or require hospitalization. Individuals experiencing hypomania feel wonderful, "on top of the world," and do not recognize changes in themselves. Those who know them well, however, are aware of the changes in mood and behavior. There are no psychotic features in hypomania.

The onset of manic episodes is usually in the early twenties but may begin at any time. It often follows a severe disappointment, embarrassment, or other psychic stressor. The mood of clients experiencing a manic episode is euphoric or "high." Their behavior is excessive and out of bounds. It is characterized by overly enthusiastic involvement in projects of an interpersonal, political, religious, or occupational nature. When someone or something gets in the way or appears to put a snag in their way, they become irritable. Moods alternate between euphoria and irritability. Increased sexual behaviors are often seen, including flirting, making sexual overtures, having inappropriate sexual relationships, and feeling compelled to seduce and be seduced. Women may dress in an uncharacteristically flashy or seductive manner and wear garish makeup. Speech is pressured, and racing thoughts or flight of ideas are often present. Grandiosity can reach delusional proportions. Clients with mania rarely believe they are sick, even when they are in financial or legal trouble, and may vehemently protest the need for treatment. The characteristics of a manic episode are described in the following clinical example and illustrated in FIGURE 17-2 ■.

MEDIALINK Bipolar Disorder Video

CLINICAL EXAMPLE

Mr. Grey, a 52-year-old engineer, was brought to the emergency psychiatric clinic by two adult sons at 2:00 A.M. Their mother had called them to come help with their father, who had not slept in three days. When they arrived at their parents' home, they found their father working in the backyard on a large landscaping project involving stonework, a waterfall, a fish pond, and extensive plantings of trees, shrubs, and flowers.

According to the sons, Mr. Grey had three prior episodes of manic behavior, beginning when he was in the Army many years earlier. He was stabilized on lithium carbonate for years, but stopped taking it about a year ago because he felt so good. The current episode began about one week ago after he was passed over for a promotion at work. He then took a leave of absence from his job to create what he called "the world's first home-based theme park." Any attempt by his wife to talk him out of the project was met with anger and renewed resolve. Mr. Grey angrily told the admitting nurse, "I don't know why these boys brought me here. I need to get back to work! I'm going to get millions for this franchise."

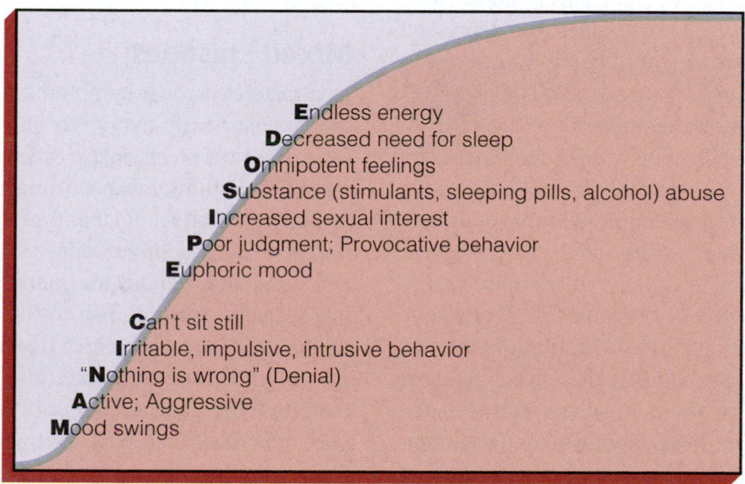

Endless energy
Decreased need for sleep
Omnipotent feelings
Substance (stimulants, sleeping pills, alcohol) abuse
Increased sexual interest
Poor judgment; Provocative behavior
Euphoric mood
Can't sit still
Irritable, impulsive, intrusive behavior
"Nothing is wrong" (Denial)
Active; Aggressive
Mood swings

FIGURE 17-2 ■ Characteristics of a manic episode.

DSM-IV-TR Diagnostic Criteria for Bipolar Disorders

Manic Episode

A. A distinct period of abnormally and persistently elevated, expansive, or irritable mood, lasting at least 1 week (or any duration if hospitalization is necessary).

B. During the period of mood disturbance, three (or more) of the following symptoms have persisted (four if the mood is only irritable) and have been present to a significant degree:
   1. inflated self-esteem or grandiosity
   2. decreased need for sleep (e.g., feels rested after only 3 hours of sleep)
   3. more talkative than usual or pressure to keep talking
   4. flight of ideas or subjective experience that thoughts are racing
   5. distractibility (i.e., attention too easily drawn to unimportant or irrelevant external stimuli)
   6. increase in goal-directed activity (either socially, at work or school, or sexually) or psychomotor agitation
   7. excessive involvement in pleasurable activities that have a high potential for painful consequences (e.g., engaging in unrestrained buying sprees, sexual indiscretions, or foolish business investments)

C. The symptoms do not meet criteria for a Mixed Episode.

D. The mood disturbance is sufficiently severe to cause marked impairment in occupational functioning or in usual social activities or relationships with others, or to necessitate hospitalization to prevent harm to self or others, or there are psychotic features.

E. The symptoms are not due to the direct physiological effects of a substance (e.g., a drug of abuse, a medication, or other treatment) or a general medical condition (e.g., hyperthyroidism).
   Note: Manic-like episodes that are clearly caused by somatic antidepressant treatment (e.g., medication, electroconvulsive therapy, light therapy) should not count toward a diagnosis of Bipolar I Disorder.

Hypomanic Episode

A. A distinct period of persistently elevated, expansive, or irritable mood, lasting throughout at least 4 days, that is clearly different from the usual nondepressed mood.

B. During the period of mood disturbance, three (or more) of the following symptoms have persisted (four if the mood is only irritable) and have been present to a significant degree:
   1. inflated self-esteem or grandiosity
   2. decreased need for sleep (e.g., feels rested after only 3 hours of sleep)
   3. more talkative than usual or pressure to keep talking
   4. flight of ideas or subjective experience that thoughts are racing
   5. distractibility (i.e., attention too easily drawn to unimportant or irrelevant external stimuli)
   6. increase in goal-directed activity (either socially, at work or school, or sexually) or psychomotor agitation
   7. excessive involvement in pleasurable activities that have a high potential for painful consequences (e.g., the person engages in unrestrained buying sprees, sexual indiscretions, or foolish business investments)

C. The episode is associated with an unequivocal change in functioning that is uncharacteristic of the person when not symptomatic.

D. The disturbance in mood and the change in functioning are observable by others.

E. The episode is not severe enough to cause marked impairment in social or occupational functioning, or to necessitate hospitalization, and there are no psychotic features.

(continued)

Depressed Episodes

A diagnosis of bipolar disorder does not always mean that manic or hypomanic behaviors will be manifested in the current illness. There are several types of bipolar disorders in which manic or hypomanic episodes have occurred in the past, but the features of the current episode are purely depressive. This is termed a *depressed episode*. Treatment of depressed bipolar disorders is similar to treatment of depression, with the exception that pharmacologic treatment adds a mood stabilizer to antidepressant treatment.

Recent studies explain what many clinicians have been struggling with when treating people who are not responsive to antidepressant pharmacotherapy. People who have already been diagnosed with major depression and have these five features—anxiety, experiencing people as unfriendly, family history of bipolar disorder, a recent diagnosis of depression, and legal problems—may very well have bipolar disorder as opposed to depression. The probability that these features predict bipolar disorder risk in those unsuccessfully treated with antidepressants is high (Perlis, Brown, Baker, & Nierenberg, 2006). Previous research has shown that nearly half of all people who have bipolar disorder are first diagnosed with major depression.

Many clients with bipolar disorder are not correctly diagnosed in a timely manner. This can mean that an individual loses years of his or her life to an illness that could have been successfully managed if correctly diagnosed and treated.

Mixed Episodes

In a *mixed episode*, symptoms of both mania and depression are present nearly every day in rapidly alternating succession over a period of at least a week. These clients are often agitated, are suffering from insomnia and appetite disturbances, and may exhibit suicidal and psychotic thinking. The presentation also can resemble depression, with a great deal of energy and animation behind the sadness. Clients may have recently had a manic episode or a major depressive episode, although this is not always the case. Because depressive symptoms are part of the clinical picture, clients suffer more psychic pain than do individuals who are in a state of mania, and they may seek help more readily. The clinical example that follows illustrates one type of presentation of a mixed episode.

DSM-IV-TR Diagnostic Criteria for Bipolar Disorders *(continued)*

F. The symptoms are not due to the direct physiological effects of a substance (e.g., a drug of abuse, a medication, or other treatment) or a general medical condition (e.g., hyperthyroidism). **Note:** Hypomanic-like episodes that are clearly caused by somatic antidepressant treatment (e.g., medication, electroconvulsive therapy, light therapy) should not count toward a diagnosis of Bipolar II Disorder.

Mixed Episode

A. The criteria are met both for a Manic Episode and for a Major Depressive Episode (except for duration) nearly every day during at least a 1-week period.
B. The mood disturbance is sufficiently severe to cause marked impairment in occupational functioning or in usual social activities or relationships with others, or to necessitate hospitalization to prevent harm to self or others, or there are psychotic features.
C. The symptoms are not due to the direct physiological effects of a substance (e.g., a drug of abuse, a medication, or other treatment) or a general medical condition (e.g., hyperthyroidism). **Note:** Mixed-like episodes that are clearly caused by somatic antidepressant treatment (e.g., medication, electroconvulsive therapy, light therapy) should not count toward a diagnosis of Bipolar I Disorder.

Cyclothymic Disorder

A. For at least 2 years, the presence of numerous periods with hypomanic symptoms and numerous periods with depressive symptoms that do not meet criteria for a Major Depressive Episode. **Note:** In children and adolescents, the duration must be at least 1 year.
B. During the above 2-year period (1 year in children and adolescents), the person has not been without the symptoms in Criterion A for more than 2 months at a time.
C. No Major Depressive Episode, Manic Episode, or Mixed Episode has been present during the first 2 years of the disturbance. **Note:** After the initial 2 years (1 year in children and adolescents) of Cyclothymic Disorder, there may be superimposed Manic or Mixed Episodes (in which case both Bipolar I Disorder and Cyclothymic Disorder may be diagnosed) or Major Depressive Episodes (in which case both Bipolar II Disorder and Cyclothymic Disorder may be diagnosed).
D. The symptoms in Criterion A are not better accounted for by Schizoaffective Disorder and are not superimposed on Schizophrenia, Schizophreniform Disorder, Delusional Disorder, or Psychotic Disorder Not Otherwise Specified.
E. The symptoms are not due to the direct physiological effects of a substance (e.g., a drug of abuse, a medication) or a general medical condition (e.g., hyperthyroidism).
F. The symptoms cause clinically significant distress or impairment in social, occupational, or other important areas of functioning.

Source: Reprinted with permission from the *Diagnostic and Statistical Manual of Mental Disorders,* Fourth Edition, Text Revision. (Copyright 2000). American Psychiatric Association.

USING DSM-IV-TR

Health care providers often use language unfamiliar to clients and their families. To help clients and family members understand manic episode, explain "flight of ideas," one possible symptom.

CLINICAL EXAMPLE

Mrs. Kent is a 32-year-old high school teacher who was readmitted to the psychiatric unit 2 weeks after she was discharged following treatment for a major depressive episode. Her husband described her recent behavior as extremely unstable, with a strange mix of moods. "She is driving herself and me crazy, crying and talking about killing herself because her life is so sad and she is so depressed, but every action is so full of energy. She tried to go back to work right after she got out of the hospital the first time, but the principal put her on a leave of absence until the end of the year. He said she made wildly gesticulating movements while describing how miserable she was to some of her students."

Cyclothymic Disorder

When clients have suffered for at least 2 years from "chronic, fluctuating mood disturbances involving numerous periods of hypomanic symptoms and numerous periods of depressive symptoms," they are diagnosed with **cyclothymic disorder** (APA, 2000, p. 398). They must be free of severe symptoms that qualify for the diagnosis of manic disorder or major depressive disorder. These individuals are often considered to be moody, unpredictable, or temperamental, and they may go on to develop an overlay of symptoms that are of major depressive or manic intensity. FIGURE 17-3 ■ compares mood in major depressive disorder, bipolar disorders, dysthymia, and cyclothymia.

Cyclothymic disorder begins early, usually in adolescence or early adulthood. Although not common, with a lifetime risk of only 0.4% to 1% of the general population, it is thought to predispose the person to other mood disorders. The incidence is approximately equal between males and females.

MOOD DISORDERS DUE TO OTHER CONDITIONS

It is widely recognized that mood disorders may be manifestations of physiologic conditions such as hepatitis or thyrotoxicosis. Mood disorders may also be induced by substance abuse, such as cocaine or amphetamines; prescribed medications, such as antihypertensives or oral contraceptives; or toxins, such as lead or carbon monoxide. Mood disorders may also be precipitated by withdrawal from substance intoxication or abuse. Chapter 15 ∞ has

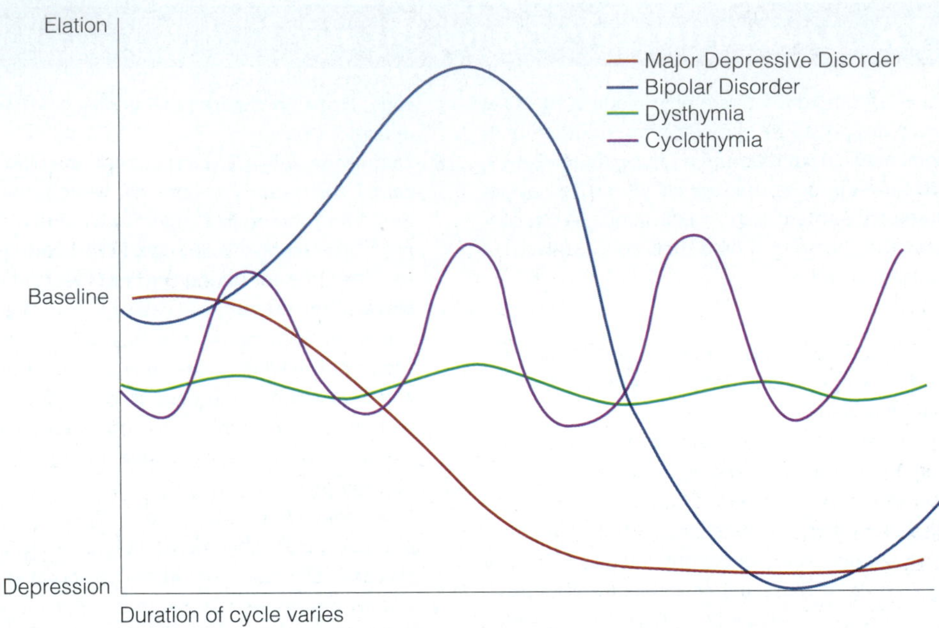

FIGURE 17-3 ■ Comparison of affect (mood) in major depressive disorder, bipolar disorder, dysthymia, and cyclothymia.

MEDIALINK Application: Depression During and After Pregnancy

MEDIALINK Postpartum Support International

details on this phenomenon. The general medical condition of clients should be carefully evaluated before making a diagnosis of mood disorder.

POSTPARTUM MOOD EPISODES

Almost 70% of women experience the "baby blues"—transient mood changes, usually depression, that do not impair functioning—in the 10-day period after the birth of a baby (APA, 2000). However, when the symptoms meet the criteria for any of the mood disorder categories discussed earlier in this chapter, the client is diagnosed as having a mood disorder with postpartum onset or **postpartum mood episode**. This rate is set conservatively at 13% to 19%. The onset of a mood disorder with postpartum onset occurs within 4 weeks of giving birth but may occur anytime in the first year following childbirth (Horowitz & Cousins, 2006).

The symptoms the client experiences are no different from the symptoms of other mood disorders except for a major one—preoccupation with infant well-being. This preoccupation can range from overconcern for the safety of the infant to severe ruminations about the infant's safety. Sometimes, but not always, psychotic features are evident. For example, the woman may have delusional thoughts about her infant (the infant is possessed by an evil presence) or command hallucinations (to kill or injure the infant). The following clinical example describes the illness.

CLINICAL EXAMPLE

A woman drowned her five children, ages 2 months through 7 years old, believing that they were evil and that she was saving them from hell. Each of the five births, all within a period of 7 years, was characterized by a postpartum mood episode, some with psychotic features that required hospitalization and psychotropic medications. She had attempted suicide at least twice during a mood episode. Despite the severity of her postpartum mood episodes, which occurred after each pregnancy, the couple did not modify their dream to have a large family.

The risk for a postpartum mood episode with psychotic features is increased in women who have had a prior mood disorder (especially bipolar I disorder) or a previous postpartum episode with psychotic features, or in women with no history of a prior mood disorder but with a family history of bipolar disorders. The risk for recurrence with a subsequent delivery is between 30% and 50% (APA, 2000).

You can refer depressed postpartum women to Postpartum Support International for a postpartum self-assessment test and help in locating a support group. Their website, www.postpartum.net/, can be accessed through the Companion Website for this book.

BEREAVEMENT

Bereavement is a term that refers to the state of loss. We all have losses that have to be dealt with, and how we cope affects not only us but our loved ones. Bereavement is a natural process and not a mental illness. Certainly, people may have significant difficulties at some point; however, this is a transient state. Overall, bereavement is a process that everyone handles in a slightly different manner. Although we might wish for a logical and firm set of rules, there is no lock-step progression of bereavement or grieving through routinized categories, but rather an ebb and flow.

You will notice in your work with depressed clients that many episodes of major depressive disorder are preceded by a major loss of some kind. One prospective study (Harris, 2006) set up a befriending intervention to contribute to and maximize resilience and prevent depression. The positive effects of this action should be taken into account when intervening with bereaved individuals.

Grief is a multifaceted reaction to loss. It has emotional components as well as physical, cognitive, behavioral, social, spiritual, and philosophical dimensions. Caring about someone or something and having a real relationship means putting yourself at risk for intense feelings of grief. People do not grieve for losses that are unimportant to them. The term "grief struck" is an apt one, for many people are shocked by the jarring impact of the loss. Grieving is a personal process that is best supported by others who understand and care.

Dysfunctional Grieving

Dysfunctional grieving is a term that describes the failure of an individual to follow the course of normal grieving to a point of resolution. When normal grieving deviates from the norm, the individual becomes overwhelmed and resorts to maladaptive coping. The Yale Bereavement Study (Johnson, Zhang, Greer, & Prigerson, 2007) examined the development of severe grief symptoms following bereavement, in which the individual exhibits symptoms of complicated grief. Dependency on a deceased spouse contributed to dysfunctional grieving as an emotional state following the bereavement. This clinical example is of a dysfunctional grief reaction.

CLINICAL EXAMPLE

Jacki was particularly close to her father all of her life. As she matured into adulthood, she developed healthy relationships with others, including friendships, marriage, and motherhood. Through it all she maintained a very close relationship with her father. When he died suddenly when she was 50, Jacki reacted strongly, as everyone expected she would. She accused other family members of not caring and was estranged from some for months following his death. As the months, then years, went by, Jacki exhibited tearful and grief-stricken reactions especially on her father's birthday and the anniversary of his death.

In telephone conversations with her siblings she would ask, sobbing, "Do you know what today is?" When her siblings did not recognize the date as being significant, Jacki would yell and accuse them of never loving their father because they failed to note that this was the day he usually held the first barbecue of the year (or some other fairly insignificant activity). Ten years following her father's death Jacki is still highly emotional, erratic, and not functioning well interpersonally. She is having a dysfunctional grief reaction.

Treatment for dysfunctional grieving can resemble treatment for depression, including cognitive-behavioral therapy, other talk therapies, and antidepressants. Group therapy composed of people all of whom were experiencing complicated or dysfunctional grief reactions had better outcomes when participants had a history of relatively mature relationships (Piper, Ogrodniczuk, Joyce, Weideman, & Rosie, 2007). Focusing on competent relationships and receiving support from capable others have been shown to treat or prevent emotional lives that can become problematic.

Grief experienced by health care providers is not typically addressed at the worksite. A "grief team," as suggested by Brosche (2007), can be assembled to intervene with staff to prevent or reduce compassion fatigue and eventual dysfunction. Such a measure can be nurturing as well as cost effective.

BIOPSYCHOSOCIAL THEORIES

People with certain personality types or temperaments are more prone than others to develop depressive and elated behaviors. Significant efforts have been devoted to identifying a single psychologic factor, trait, or mechanism that is unique to the development of mood disorders.

Research exploring the causative factors of mood disorders has focused on reactions to early separation from parents or parental loss, early mother–child relationships, errors in thinking, inherited tendencies, biologic factors, and other aspects of human development and experience. To date, no single personality type, biologic or psychological trait, or constellation of experiences has been established to account for all forms of mood disorders. Multiple complex factors contribute to the development of mood disorders.

Psychoanalytic Theory

The psychoanalytic theory of depression was originally formulated by Freud and later refined by others. It focuses on an unsatisfactory early mother–infant relationship as the primary factor predisposing individuals to later depression. If an infant's needs go unmet, a sense of loss occurs. Unresolved grief over the loss results in anger turned inward and the development of self-hate. The child's ego development is thereby adversely affected, resulting in a weak ego and an overdeveloped, punitive superego.

The psychoanalytic school of thought suggests a different etiology for bipolar disorder. This theory holds that the mother/primary caregiver derives pleasure from the infant's early dependence but feels threatened by increasing autonomy as the child develops. Independent behaviors are considered "bad," and the child must suppress his or her needs in order to sustain parental affection. Ambivalence resulting from the coexisting desires to please the parents and become more autonomous causes resentment and leads to a love–hate relationship with the parenting figures. Again, a weak ego and punitive superego create depression. Mania is seen as the denial of depression taken to the extreme.

Contemporary theorists and researchers criticize psychoanalytic theory for its tendency to blame mothers while ignoring biologic factors.

Cognitive Theory

Cognitive theorists such as Clark and Beck (1999) believe that depression results from impaired cognition, or distorted thinking processes. People who think negative thoughts evaluate themselves critically and interpret stressful events as having a powerful, global impact on them. They feel guilty, inadequate, and hopeless about the future. Recent models of cognitive vulnerability to depression theorize that negative thoughts alone are not sufficient to cause depression unless the individual already suffers from a mildly depressed mood. In these instances, the combination of adverse life events (or the perception of adverse life events) and mildly depressed mood combine to create a downward spiral into depression. Current data (Oei, Bullbeck, & Campbell, 2006) do not support this direction of thinking and emotion. Instead, the data indicate that reduced depressive symptoms contributed to the reduced generation of depressive thoughts and dysfunctional attitudes, not the reverse.

The Beck Depression Inventory is a clinical assessment tool. It asks clients to rate themselves on 21 groups of questions designed to detect negative thinking. Cognitive therapy seeks to teach individuals how to stop negative thinking and replace it with more positive self-appraisals. Cognitive therapies are discussed in detail in Chapter 31.

The theory of *learned helplessness* is a cognitive theory that proposes that learning plays an instrumental role in the development of depression. This theory holds that depression is based on the person's belief that he or she has no control over life situations. This conclusion is drawn from repeated failures, either real or perceived, to control life events. The result is that the individual gives up, stops trying to control, becomes dependent on others, and is thereby predisposed to depression (McDermott, 1995).

Object Loss Theory

In Bowlby's (1973) object loss theory of depression, the forced, often traumatic separation from, or abandonment of an infant by, the primary caregiver during the first 6 months of life plays a major role. Separation interrupts the bonding process essential to the later development of relationships, and the child withdraws from other people and the environment. This establishes a pattern of anxiety, grief, helplessness, and hopelessness. Once the pattern is established, the individual uses these behaviors to deal with all subsequent losses, whether of major or minor magnitude. Such people feel helpless to cope with the normal ups and downs of life and assume a hopeless, depressed attitude.

Biologic Theories

Promising findings are emerging from studies of biologic factors that alter brain function. Research on the physiologic basis for depression has been under way for more than 50 years and has generated a variety of hypotheses. Because mood disorders vary widely, it is unlikely that any single biologic causative factor can be isolated. This has led to research on how the various biologic factors already identified relate to one another, how they affect behavior, and how they respond to different therapies. In searching for biologic changes in mood disorders, it is important to remember that although a biologic abnormality may coexist with a mood disorder, it is not necessarily a causative factor. It could be a cause, a coexisting factor, or a consequence. The Your Assessment Approach feature lists some abnormal findings on laboratory tests that may indicate the presence of a mood disorder.

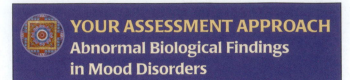

YOUR ASSESSMENT APPROACH
Abnormal Biological Findings in Mood Disorders

While there are no laboratory studies that definitively diagnose mood disorders, some abnormal findings are noted more often in mood-disordered individuals when symptoms are present than in control subjects. These are:

- Sleep abnormalities in 40% to 60% of outpatients and up to 90% of inpatients with major depressive episode and in 25% to 50% of adults with dysthymic disorder; decreased need for sleep and abnormal polysomnographic findings in people with manic episode (sleep abnormalities may precede the onset of a mood disorder and may persist in the absence of other symptoms)
- Neurotransmitter and neuropeptide dysregulation in major depressive episode and manic episode
- Hormonal disturbances (blunted growth hormone and thyroid-stimulating hormone); elevated urinary free cortisol; dexamethasone nonsuppression of prolactin; elevated plasma cortisol
- Brain imaging studies may show increased blood flow in limbic and paralimbic regions and decreased blood flow in the lateral prefrontal cortex in depression; increased rates of right hemispheric lesions, or bilateral subcortical or preventricular lesions in persons with bipolar I disorder
- Preventricular vascular changes when depression begins in late life
- Urine and blood drug screens may indicate a substance-induced mood disorder

Gender

Women are more prone to major depression and dysthymia than are men. This is true across cultures. Endocrine and reproductive cycles may play a role, although menopause alone, contrary to popular belief, does not appear to be a risk factor for depression in women. It is also unclear whether prenatal and postpartum depression are hormonal in nature, result from the increased stress of motherhood, or represent an interaction of these and other factors. It is clear, however, that of all population groups, those at greatest risk for depression are rural elderly with very few close friends, some financial strain, and a recent emergency department visit (Friedman, Conwell, & Delavan, 2007).

Gender is important given the propensity of women to succumb to depression more than men. However, environment and life experiences play a major role in the development of depression in both men and women.

Genetic Theories

Numerous studies have concentrated on the role heredity plays in depressive illness. Interest in this field of research was stimulated by the observation that the incidence of depression is higher among relatives of depressed individuals than in the general population. Studies of illness rates within and between generations of families, of monozygotic and dizygotic twins, and of the general population, and those using known genetic markers such as blood type or color blindness all validate the increased incidence of depression in relatives of depressed individuals.

Studies have demonstrated that bipolar disorder is also increased among first-degree relatives of individuals with that disorder. Studies of identical twins report an 80% concordance rate in bipolar disorder. This means that if one twin has the disorder, there is an 80% chance that the other twin will also develop it.

The role of genetics in the development of major mood disorders is complicated by the familiar question: Which plays the more important role, genes or environment? People who are biologically related tend to spend time together and influence one another's thinking. They share similar values and beliefs and are subjected to similar stressors, such as poverty or death of loved ones. It is therefore difficult to determine the relative weight of genetics, thinking patterns, family relationships, and learning in the development of mood disorders.

Depression and the most effective treatments for it can now be tested. Following the recent FDA approval of a test to predict differences in the cytochrome P_{450} (CYP450) gene, clinicians and clients must decide whether using genetic tests to select a specific antidepressant medication from the class known as selective serotonin reuptake inhibitor (SSRI) might improve the response to treatment for depression. New research on gene-based tests intended to personalize the dose of SSRIs to improve outcomes, or aid in treatment decisions in the clinical setting, have not been well supported by the evidence thus far (Matchar & Thakur, 2007). Diet and other medical conditions may have had a more robust impact on the outcome of treatment for depression. However, the studies completed to date included flaws such as testing after only one dose of an SSRI, or testing people who did not have depression. This type of genetic research is still in a very early stage.

Biochemical Theories

Early biochemical studies established that an error in metabolism results in an electrolyte imbalance that seems to play a role in depression. The studies demonstrated that sodium and potassium were transposed in the neurons of depressed individuals. This transposition alters the sensitivity of the neuronal cell membranes. Alterations in sensitivity of neuronal receptors are likely to lead to alterations in behavior. This may account for the efficacy of medications, such as lithium carbonate and antidepressants, in the treatment of mood disorders.

Since then, scientific research has focused on the role of certain chemicals, the neurotransmitters, in the central nervous system. These are chemicals that transmit nervous impulses along neuronal pathways in the limbic area of the brain. Levels of certain monoamine neurotransmitters—norepinephrine, serotonin, epinephrine, and dopamine—were found to be deficient in many depressed people. Until the 1980s scientists believed that major depression resulted from norepinephrine or serotonin deficiencies, and the early antidepressants were formulated accordingly.

The monoamine hypothesis prevailed for years until it was found insufficient to explain fully the etiology of a complex disorder such as depression. Deficient levels of monoamine neurotransmitters have not been consistently found in depressed people and have not been able to relieve symptoms reliably. It is now believed that monoamine deficiencies are only one manifestation of depression. Many pharmacologic agents successfully used to treat depression and mania, however, do enhance monoamine activity. For example, study of the metabolism of serotonin and the discovery of the dysfunction of certain serotonergic neurons in depressed individuals led to the development of the SSRIs and subsequent generations of these useful antidepressants.

Much current biochemical research focuses on the role of psychosocial stress in the pathophysiology of depression. The damaging effects of chronic stress, including its impact on limbic activity, are under extensive study. Current research indicates that the underlying biochemical process involves the neurotransmitters dopamine, norepinephrine, serotonin, and gamma-aminobutyric acid (GABA) (Murphy, 2006). Interferences with the smooth transmission of impulses from one neuron to another, associated with depressive and manic phases of bipolar disorder, can be explained by inadequate release of neurotransmitters or faulty storage mechanisms. It is expected that interactive hypotheses of depression—that is, those that take into consideration a variety of biologic and psychosocial factors—are likely to be most useful in the future understanding of these complex disorders.

Biologic Rhythms

It is widely recognized that we have self-sustained internal physiologic cycles that occur every 24 hours. These **circadian rhythms**, which include body temperature, sleep, and appetite, are activated, controlled, and integrated by the hypothalamus in the brain. The central controlling pacemaker is commonly known as the biological clock. A biological clock cell animation can be accessed through the Companion Website for this book.

Diurnal variations in mood, rest and activity cycles, EEG patterns, and neuroendocrine secretions have been clinically demonstrated, and you have no doubt seen the impact of many of these variations yourself. Circadian rhythm dysfunction can explain a number of mood disorder symptoms, such as insomnia, hypersomnia, early morning awakening, and variations in appetite, rest, and activity cycles. Animal studies have demonstrated that alcohol and antimanic medications, such as lithium, slow the biological clock, while estrogen and tricyclic antidepressants accelerate it or restore normal rhythms. The precise role biological rhythms play in mood disorders is yet to be determined. The role of circadian rhythms in sleep disorders is discussed in Chapter 19∞.

The presence of physical problems has also been thought to play a role in mood disorders. Certain somatic problems, such as chronic or disabling headaches in women, have been linked with major depressive disorder (Tietjen, Brandes, &

MediaLink HHMI BioInteractive

Digre, 2007). There may be a common factor at work with certain illnesses in which both depression and another physical problem are present. It is interesting to note that in order to make a diagnosis of mood disorder, the diagnostician must rule out infections, chemical imbalances, environmental toxins, alcohol abuse, and other biological processes (Noonan, Warren, & White, 2007). All of these physical problems may present in such a way as to look like depression.

Psychological Factors

Regardless of temperament and personality patterns, people can and do become depressed. Mild depression is widely acknowledged as a part of the human experience.

Although most of us have had "the blues" from time to time, it has been established that certain people are more prone to developing true depression than others. Individuals who exhibit certain attitudes and beliefs—such as low self-esteem; lack of personal goals and direction; the tendency to avoid difficult situations rather than facing them directly; dependence and passivity in interpersonal relationships; acting and reacting impulsively; a limited ability to form enduring, mature relationships; and internalization of blame—are thought to be at risk for the development of depressive disorders.

Sociocultural Factors

Most clinical investigators believe that life events and environmental stress play a role in mood disorders. There is less agreement, however, as to whether life events play a primary role or merely contribute to the onset of an inevitable episode of a mood disorder. Certain events, such as the death of a loved one, divorce, and other losses, are widely recognized by both mental health professionals and the general public as precipitating events for depression. The impact of stress reactions and stress hormones on mood has been established. The unremitting stresses of living in poverty, and society's devaluation of the disadvantaged, also seem to predispose people to developing depression.

Predictors of bipolar mood disorder episodes, for the most part, include stressful life events, increased number of previous bipolar episodes, decreased interval between bipolar episodes, and persistence of the effect of symptoms on functioning (Altman et al., 2006). Having longer periods between episodes is typically associated with active involvement in psychotherapy, adhering to a medication regimen, and having a strong support system. Unfortunately, the presence of substance abuse interferes with any semblance of stability, and the prevalence of substance abuse in this population is notably high.

Culture exerts a powerful influence on how individuals experience and communicate psychic distress. Spiritual or religious concerns such as guilt may predominate and mask the underlying mood disorders. Some cultures experience depression largely in somatic terms. Be alert to complaints of headaches or "nerves" in Hispanic clients, of weakness or "imbalance" in Asian clients, and of body metaphors involving the heart in Middle Eastern and certain Native American clients (see Chapter 9 for a discussion of culture-bound syndromes). These may be culturally determined ways of expressing depression.

Active problem-solving styles, including general coping, are associated with healthier emotional outcomes. Fewer symptoms of mood disorders resulted from a combination of high acculturation and high intercultural competence in a sample of Hispanic participants (Torres & Rollock, 2007). Contact with the mainstream culture, and then consistently developing the ability to acculturate, acted as a potential buffer against negative mental health consequences such as mood disorders.

Be aware of the unique needs of clients who are likely to perceive the meaning and severity of psychiatric symptoms in relation to the norms of their cultural reference group. They include new immigrants to this country, individuals who are still heavily involved in the culture of origin, those who do not speak English, and those whose entire network of social and religious support remains embedded in the culture of origin.

Differences in culture and social status of clients and caregivers can create problems in diagnosis and treatment. Language differences, for example, create barriers in forming therapeutic relationships in talk therapies and in other treatment settings such as day treatment. Barriers, as well as ease, in therapeutic pathways can also result from transference issues (Evans, 2007). Cultural differences in the expression of symptoms make it difficult to determine whether a behavior is normal or pathological, and the culture itself may dictate or affect clients' attitudes toward and adherence to treatment. The influence of culture on clients' attitudes toward treatment and beliefs about healing are discussed in Chapter 9.

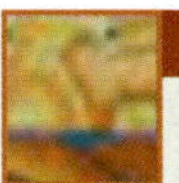

NURSING PROCESS
Clients with Major Depressive Disorder

Nursing care of clients with mood disorders follows a problem-solving model you are already accustomed to using, the nursing process.

Assessment

As already discussed, depression is characterized by low mood, often related to a loss. The loss may be concrete, such as the loss of a loved one or a job, or perceived, such as the loss of a cherished wish or disillusionment with a respected role model.

Subjective Data

Clients with depressive disorders may express some of the following:

- Feelings of sadness
- Fatigue
- Lack of interest in relationships and activities that were previously pleasurable

MEDIALINK Care Plan: Assessing the Client with Mood Disorder

- Feelings of worthlessness
- Impaired concentration
- Impaired decision-making ability
- Sleep disturbances
- Appetite changes; weight loss or weight gain
- Excessive sleep

Clients will often describe how long it takes them to complete activities that formerly were easily accomplished, such as preparing a simple meal. Tearfulness and emotional outbursts may also be a part of their description of the problem. They may or may not mention a loss or disappointment that they relate to the feelings.

Somatic Concerns Somatic concerns are often the presenting complaint. Depressed clients may complain of abdominal pains, headaches, and vague bodily aches. A problem with sexual functioning or lack of desire may also be a presenting complaint. Constipation is a common result of the general slowing of metabolism due to inactivity. Some cultures more easily express symptoms of depression through complaints about body function and discomfort. See the feature What Every Medical Office Nurse Should Know for information on how depression evidenced by somatic concerns can be detected in other settings.

Suicide Assessment All clients who describe depressive symptoms should be assessed for suicide risk by direct questioning. Ask about suicidal thinking, history of suicide attempts, and whether the client has a specific suicide plan. This aspect of assessment is reassuring, not alarming, to clients. Ask these questions in a direct fashion. You might ask, for example, "Tell me how you plan to kill yourself. Do you have or can you get the gun/pills/poison?" It is important to know whether the client has actually planned the suicide or if it is a vaguely formed thought. The more organized the plan is, the more concern it generates, particularly if the client has access to a lethal weapon, chemical, or other means of self-injury.

Other aspects of suicide will be discussed more fully later in this chapter under the heading "Preventing Suicide and Promoting Safety." Suicide lethality assessment is thoroughly discussed in Chapter 23.

WHAT EVERY MEDICAL OFFICE NURSE SHOULD KNOW

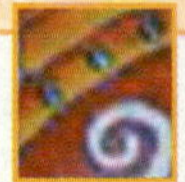

Physical Complaints and Depression

Frequently, people will feel aches and pains more acutely when they are depressed. The natural reaction to pain is to seek help from one's primary medical health care provider. One out of every six people going to a medical office is depressed. Only one out of every six of those people are diagnosed and treated for depression. It is important for people who are suffering from depression to talk to their health care providers about other experiences and symptoms over their lifetime. As a medical office nurse, be aware that in some cultures, people express depression through body systems—headaches, stomachaches, muscle spasms, and visual problems, among others. When you assess people from these cultures, consider the possibility that they may be depressed. A discussion of culture and depression is integrated throughout Chapter 9.

People seldom self-diagnose depression. They are much more likely to assume that not enjoying their usual activities, experiencing changes in eating or sleeping habits, and feeling bad in one way or another are caused by a medical problem. Ferreting out the real cause of distress will ensure effective responses to treatment.

Objective Data

Depressed clients are most likely to be females under the age of 40. They often have had prior episodes of depression and a family history of depression or bipolar disorder. A history of a recent stressful event and the lack of social support are also common features.

Objective Signs Objective signs and symptoms of depression are few. Psychomotor agitation or retardation may be observable if it is profound or if the nurse is familiar with the client's usual level of functioning. Family members may report observations of the client's agitation or apathy and lack of pleasure in usual activities. They may describe a pattern of social withdrawal and lack of social participation, combined with an intense preoccupation with the client's own feelings. Be alert to a change in behavior.

Checklist Depression Inventories During assessment, many clinicians find it useful to provide a list of symptoms and ask clients to check the ones they are experiencing. A widely used and highly regarded self-reporting instrument designed to assess mood state is the Beck Depression Inventory, mentioned earlier in the chapter. It has been in use for over 35 years and has been revised several times based on clinical research. This inventory is useful for detecting depression, anxiety, apathy, and irritability. Several different types of Beck inventories are now available (Beck, Steer, & Brown, 1996).

Medical Illnesses Other objective information to obtain during the nursing assessment includes concurrent general medical illnesses. Autoimmune, neurologic, metabolic, oncologic, and endocrine disorders often trigger depression. For example, hypothyroidism may be accompanied by depressive symptoms due to the underlying medical disease, while a client with AIDS or cancer may become depressed as a result of the diagnosis, prognosis, or disability connected with the disease.

Substance Use and Abuse Alcohol, which is a CNS depressant, and certain legal and illegal drugs can cause or complicate depression. A complete list of all substances and medications used by the client should be obtained through matter-of-fact questioning. A few prescription medications have depression as a side effect, and these should not be overlooked in the complete assessment. Birth control pills, sedatives, reserpine, glucocorticoids, and anabolic steroids have all been associated with the development of depression.

Laboratory Tests There are currently no laboratory tests specific for depression, but abnormal findings on several tests were discussed earlier in this chapter in the Your Assessment Approach feature on page 414.

Nursing Diagnosis: NANDA

The following sections discuss the implications of several nursing diagnoses commonly seen in depressed clients.

Risk for Self-Directed Violence

Thoughts about and impulses toward self-harm are related to feelings of worthlessness, feelings of guilt, repeated failure experiences, feelings of helplessness and hopelessness, or psychotic thinking. Suicidal clients should be hospitalized on either a general or a specialized hospital unit. Regardless of setting, whenever a client is at high risk for self-harm, that becomes *the* priority nursing diagnosis, and client safety becomes the most important aspect of nursing care.

Situational Low Self-Esteem or Chronic Low Self-Esteem

Depressed clients often express, either directly or indirectly, negative feelings about themselves and their abilities. Reduced self-esteem may be related to a variety of factors, including feeling abandoned by loved ones, experiencing repeated failures or losses, lacking positive feedback from others, thinking negative thoughts, engaging in negative "self-talk," or feeling guilty over real or perceived transgressions.

Evidence of low self-esteem is seen in clients who withdraw from social interaction; have difficulty accepting compliments or positive feedback; are harshly critical of themselves or others; are reluctant to try new activities because of fear of failure; express feelings of inferiority, worthlessness, and pessimism about the future; are overly sensitive to criticism; see social slights where none are intended; or set unrealistic goals and engage in grandiose thinking (denial of low self-esteem).

Hopelessness

Individuals who lead lives characterized by hopelessness believe that their own actions cannot significantly influence an outcome. They believe there is no solution to their problems. They come to doubt their own abilities and are passive in response to others.

Evidence of hopelessness is seen in the behavior of clients who lack energy and initiative, refuse to engage in self-care, do not participate in decision making, verbally express a lack of control and doubts about their abilities, are reluctant to express feelings, avoid eye contact, generally lack involvement, and exhibit decreased affect.

Social Isolation

Low self-esteem and doubts about abilities lead many depressed clients to withdraw socially. Because inadequate social skills and self-absorption create impediments to positive interpersonal relationships, clients with low self-esteem frequently *are* avoided by others. This further reinforces their fears of undesirability and increases their social isolation. Evidence of social isolation and impaired social interaction is seen in behaviors such as spending inordinate amounts of time in bed, lack of verbalization, lack of eye contact, dull or monosyllabic responses to others' attempts at conversation, a preference for being alone, turning away or closing the eyes, and exhibiting discomfort in the presence of others.

Outcome Identification: NOC

Suggested outcomes for each NANDA diagnosis presented in the previous section are discussed in the following section.

Risk for Self-Directed Violence

NOC outcomes have not yet been identified for this nursing diagnosis. Appropriate potential choices for depressed clients include Impulse Control: Ability to restrain compulsive or impulsive behavior, and Suicide Self-Restraint: Ability to refrain from gestures and attempts at killing self.

Situational Low Self-Esteem or Chronic Low Self-Esteem

The suggested NOC outcome for depressed clients with this nursing diagnosis is Self-Esteem: Personal judgment of self-worth.

Hopelessness

Several NOC outcomes are relevant to depressed clients with this nursing diagnosis. They include Decision Making: Ability to choose between two or more alternatives; Hope: Presence of internal state of optimism that is personally satisfying and life supporting; Mood Equilibrium: Appropriate adjustment of prevailing emotional tone in response to circumstances; and Quality of Life: expressed satisfaction with current life circumstances.

Social Isolation

The depressed client with this nursing diagnosis has several potentially appropriate NOC outcomes. These outcomes include Loneliness: The extent of emotional, social, or existential isolation response; Social Interaction Skills: Use of effective interaction behaviors; Social Involvement: Frequency of social interactions with persons, groups, or organizations; and Social Support: Perceived availability and actual provision of reliable assistance from other persons.

Planning and Implementation: NIC

When planning and implementing interventions designed to help depressed clients, keep two general principles in mind:

1. It is impossible to make depressed people feel better by being cheerful. In fact, an overly cheerful attitude tends to make them feel even worse because it trivializes or minimizes the impact of their feelings. Try to adopt a more emotionally neutral attitude while maintaining confidence that they will feel better.
2. Recognize that working with depressed people may eventually lower your mood and make you feel

Box 17-2 A Sample Process Recording with a Client Who Is Depressed

Client	Nurse	Process
"I don't think I can take this anymore – it's too much for me."	"You sound so overwhelmed.	Validating
	How long have you felt this way?"	Exploring
"It's been like this for as long as I can remember. It just never ends."	"How have you handled these feelings over the long time you've had them?"	Opening the topic of client's successes in managing
"I just put one foot in front of the other. It doesn't make it better, though."	"It does seem to work to some extent. You've made it through this long."	Reframing the effort as a success
"I guess. I just don't know how I can keep doing it."	"It can be tiring. Keep in mind you're not alone in this effort. You have people who support you and care about you."	Validation Reinforcing the social supports in place
"As long as I have some help."	"There is help you can depend on."	Reassurance

"down" yourself. This is called emotional contagion. Stay in touch with your own feelings. If you find yourself feeling down, assert yourself by asking to be assigned to a different type of client for a time.

Examine and learn from your interventions by processing your interactions with depressed clients. The process recording method will help you to structure your examination. A process recording usually consists of three columns—one for the nurse's statements, one for the client's, and one that identifies the process or action taking place. A sample process recording of an interaction between a nurse and a depressed client is in Box 17-2.

Preventing Suicide and Promoting Safety

There are few times when "always" and "never" are applicable. Client safety, however, *always* takes priority over other nursing care concerns. When the risk for self-directed violence is high, a number of actions call for immediate intervention. These actions are discussed in the Your Intervention Strategies box at right. *Be aware that the risk of suicide increases as the severest stage of depression is alleviated, because clients then have sufficient energy and cognitive ability to plan and successfully implement a suicide plan.*

Encourage discussing all feelings. Clients need to know that all feelings are valid and that it benefits them to express their emotions, particularly anger and hopelessness, rather than act them out through maladaptive behaviors. Having the feeling is always accepted. Acting on the feeling, however, may be problematic. What counts in the long run is what one decides to do about the feeling. Assist in the transition from hospital to home by helping clients identify people in their usual environments to whom they can express feelings candidly without being judged.

Use a calm, reassuring approach and teach calming measures, such as time-outs and controlled breathing. Provide safe physical outlets for expression of anger or increasing tension. Specific nursing interventions for anger are discussed in Chapters 22 and 35.

Collaborate with clients to identify community resources to which they can turn if suicidal thoughts recur outside the treatment setting. Almost all communities have access to hotlines that are staffed around the clock with trained volunteers or professionals who are available to discuss feelings before they reach crisis proportions. Refer to Chapter 23 for specific information on suicide and suicide prevention.

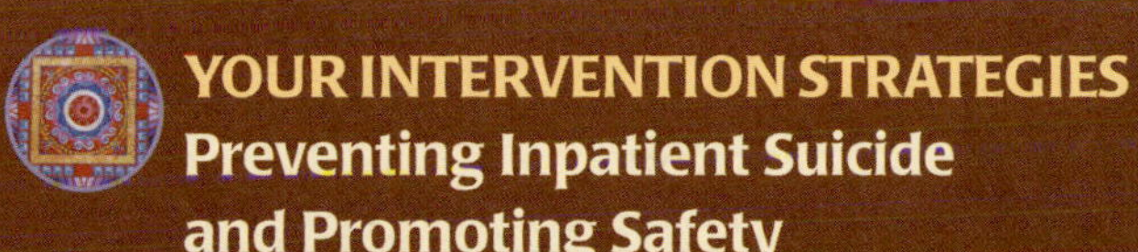

YOUR INTERVENTION STRATEGIES
Preventing Inpatient Suicide and Promoting Safety

Be sure to check the policy and procedures of the individual inpatient treatment facility and implement those guidelines as well.

- Evaluate the level of suicide intent regularly, and institute the appropriate level of staff supervision following unit protocol.
- Suicidal clients need to know that the environment is safe for them. Reassure them by removing sharp objects, razors, breakable glass items, mirrors, matches, and straps or belts, and explain why these objects are being removed. Monitor the use of scissors, razors, and other potential weapons.
- Place suicidal clients in a centrally located room near the nurses' station to facilitate ease of observation.
- Avoid establishing a predictable pattern of observation during the day and especially at night.
- Be particularly alert during change of shifts and on holidays or other times when staffing is limited, and during times of distraction, such as mealtimes and visiting hours.
- Examine items brought by visitors and monitor for safety.
- The no-suicide contract, discussed in detail in Chapter 23, is a useful intervention.

Encourage clients to seek you or another staff member when bothered by suicidal thoughts or impulses. Discussing these thoughts and impulses may be sufficient to diminish them and prevent a suicidal crisis from occurring. Avoid discussing suicidal ruminations in repetitious detail, as this may reinforce maladaptive behavior.

Promoting Self-Esteem

While low self-esteem is a chronic problem, there are a number of actions you can take to reduce negative thinking, thereby promoting improved self-esteem.

- Provide distraction from self-absorption by involving the client in recreational activities and pleasant pastimes. Simple conversation with a staff member or another client helps interrupt the pattern of negative thoughts. Use care to select activities that are not too complex for the client's current level of functioning. Experiences of success, not more failures, are needed. Increase the complexity of activities as the client progresses.
- Dispel the notion clients often have that, *when* they feel better, they will want to engage in activities. Explain that they must begin doing things *in order* to feel better. Being active promotes a more balanced feeling state. Be sure to acknowledge that it takes self-discipline and energy to do something when one doesn't really feel like it.
- Recognize accomplishment; do not use flattery or excessive praise. Give positive, matter-of-fact reinforcement, such as "I notice that you combed your hair," rather than overly enthusiastic compliments, such as "What a great hairstyle!" Appropriate recognition will increase the likelihood that the client will continue the positive behavior, while insincerity can be perceived as ridicule or infantilizing.
- Help clients identify their personal strengths. It may be useful to write these down. Recognize that it often takes some time for clients with low self-esteem to realize that they have any strengths. Avoid the temptation to point out the characteristics you have noticed. It is far more useful to support their ability to recognize their own positive qualities.
- Be accepting of clients' negative feelings, but set limits on the amount of time you will listen to accounts of past failures. Be alert for opportunities to interrupt the negative conversational patterns with more neutral ones.
- Teach assertiveness techniques, such as the ability to say no to protect one's own rights while respecting the rights of others. Clients with low self-esteem often allow others to take advantage of them. Defining passive, aggressive, and assertive behavior and giving examples of each are also helpful when teaching assertiveness (the Partnering with Clients and Families feature has a description). Encourage clients and their family members to practice the new techniques in their relationship with you, so that you can give feedback on how it feels to the recipient of an assertive communication or action.

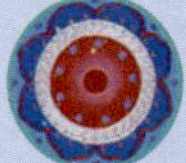

PARTNERING WITH CLIENTS AND FAMILIES

TEACHING ABOUT AGGRESSIVE, PASSIVE, AND ASSERTIVE BEHAVIORS

Assertiveness is a learned behavior. Everyone has assertiveness potential, but we aren't born knowing how to be assertive. Children learn patterns of communicating from the adults around them. You can unlearn communication patterns if they aren't working and learn new ones, and that is what assertiveness training is all about. The goal is to help people express themselves without fear of disapproval from others. Being assertive does not guarantee that others will always agree with you, but you do have the satisfaction of giving your opinion.

Definitions

Aggressive behavior is directed toward getting what one wants without considering the feelings of others. Aggressive communicators want to get their own way at any cost. They want others to "back off" and use intimidation to convey this message. An example of aggressive behavior is insisting on going to a certain movie even though you know your companion does not enjoy that type of movie. The outcome of aggressive behavior is that although you may get what you want in the short run, others feel discredited and tend to avoid you.

Passive behavior consists of avoiding conflict at any cost, even at the expense of one's own happiness. An example of passive behavior is agreeing to go to a movie you don't want to see because your friend pressures you to go. Passive communicators hold their feelings in and allow anger to build up. Anger can come out suddenly in an explosion or can be expressed in what is known as passive–aggressive behavior. An example of passive–aggressive behavior is taking a long time to get ready to go out while your friend is waiting because you are angry at him for insisting on seeing a movie you don't want to see. The outcome is that the passive person gives up control and is left with resentment, which usually emerges in other ways that damage relationships.

Assertive behavior consists of expressing one's wishes and opinions, or taking care of oneself, but not at the expense of others. An example of assertive communication is saying, "I really don't care for violent movies. Let's look at the movie listings and see if there is something playing that we can both enjoy." The outcome of assertive behavior is self-confidence and self-esteem. Clients and family members can learn about assertiveness in other ways as well. Share with them the helpful hints in the feature Partnering with Clients and Families: Teaching About Assertiveness on page 39 of Chapter 3∞. Also refer them to books that can be obtained through your local library or bookseller: *The Assertiveness Handbook: Overcoming Common Problems,* by Mary Hartley, 2007; *Peace at Any Price: How to Overcome the Please Disease,* by Deborah Day Poor, 2005; and *Civilized Assertiveness for Women: Communication with Backbone...Not Bite,* by Judith Selee, 2007.

Instilling Hope

Assisting depressed clients to develop a positive outlook is a priority nursing intervention. Clients who feel hopeless tend to form dependent relationships. Be aware of this tendency, and work from the first contact to minimize the likelihood that maladaptive dependence occurs in your nurse–client relationship. The list in the Your Self-Awareness feature below will give you direction on minimizing maladaptive dependence.

Provide clients choices in the planning of their own care and encourage them to assume some responsibility for that care. For example, allow a client to choose whether to bathe in the morning or at night, or to choose from a short list of activities to attend.

Encourage clients to set their own goals that identify what they hope to achieve during hospitalization or outpatient therapy. Remember that unrealistically optimistic goals will ensure another failure experience and reinforce the client's sense of powerlessness. Make sure that goals are attainable.

Clients who feel hopeless also need help in identifying how they can gain a sense of control in their relationships and lives outside the hospital. Collaborate with clients to identify changes they wish to make and action steps toward achieving them. Make the steps small and manageable. Accomplishing even small steps leads to a sense of mastery and optimism.

Teach clients coping measures such as problem-solving techniques, and encourage them to use them when confronting life situations. For example, if a client has difficulty paying the rent, help him or her identify options, such as moving to a less expensive apartment or taking in a roommate. Explore the pros and cons of each option and their possible consequences. Emphasize confidence in the client's ability to identify, select, and carry out problem-solving activities that will result in a greater sense of involvement in his or her life.

Equally important is to help clients identify the aspects of their lives that are not within their control. The ability to accept what *cannot* be changed is just as essential as developing the ability to bring about positive change.

Planning for discharge should begin with the first client contact and is particularly important with hopeless, dependent clients. Help them and their families and significant others to identify resources in the community and to build support systems. Support groups, therapy groups, and social groups can all help clients separate from caregivers more readily when the time comes to end therapy.

YOUR SELF-AWARENESS
Minimizing Maladaptive Dependence

Be aware of the tendency of hopeless clients to form dependent relationships and work from the first contact to minimize the likelihood that maladaptive dependence occurs in the nurse–client relationship.

- Emphasizing the short-term nature of the relationship is essential.
- If the client singles out one staff member exclusively and refuses to relate to others, this is a clue that undue dependence is developing.
- Avoid giving dependent clients the hope that the nurse–client relationship can continue after the end of the therapy.
- Kindly, but firmly, refuse requests for your address or telephone number.
- Remind clients that social contact will not be allowed.
- If you find yourself wanting to continue relationships with certain clients, discuss these feelings with your instructor (if you are a student), or your supervisor or a respected professional peer (if you are a practicing nurse). It is essential that you separate your professional life from your social life.

Enhancing Socialization

When designing interventions for promoting social interactions, realize that both the quality and the quantity of a client's social behavior may be impaired. Early in the nurse–client relationship, make brief but frequent contacts with withdrawn clients, without making any demands. Your interest can increase a client's self-worth.

With extremely uncommunicative clients, simply spending time sitting quietly without any demand for interaction may be helpful. This approach communicates your belief that they are worth the investment of time. If you find it difficult to be comfortable with silence, you may communicate that discomfort to clients. Remember that silence conveys acceptance and is a useful therapeutic communication technique. Using silence therapeutically is discussed in Chapter 10∞.

When clients express feelings or cry, remember to be nonjudgmental. Avoid showing surprise or disapproval. Two examples of how you can do this are in the Rx Communication feature that follows. Recognize that ventilating feelings may provide temporary relief, particularly if anger is expressed. If clients are unable to verbalize feelings, they sometimes can act them out in safe and appropriate ways, such as tearing up an old magazine or beating on a pillow or bed. Provide privacy during these times.

Encourage both verbal and nonverbal expressions of feelings by teaching clients that these are healthy behaviors. This intervention reinforces your acceptance of clients as unique and valuable individuals. Avoid disagreeing with, or otherwise belittling, a client's feelings by using overly cheerful reassurances like, "Now, now, Mrs. Hamilton. You're feeling down right now but you'll feel better after a good night's sleep."

Once clients are comfortable interacting with one person, encourage group activities. Although this step may be difficult and frightening for clients, you can minimize their discomfort by attending activities with them at first. If their anxiety becomes too uncomfortable, let them know that they can leave the situation without losing your approval. Give recognition for even small steps, gradually removing yourself and allowing them to stay in groups on their own.

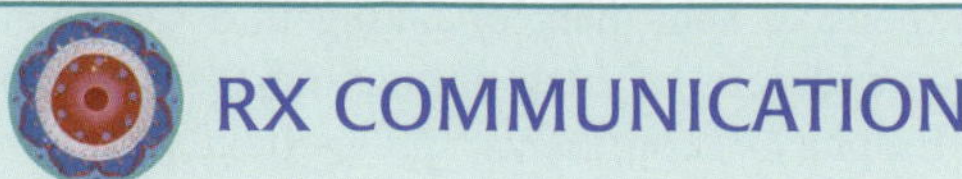

RX COMMUNICATION

CLIENT WITH MAJOR DEPRESSION

CLIENT: "I am upset and irritated all the time. All I do is yell at my kids and snap at my husband."

NURSE RESPONSE 1: "What can you tell me about feeling so upset?"

RATIONALE: Open-ended questions elicit the client's perception of the problem and allow her to begin to explore her feelings where she can. Accepts the client where she is now without judging her.

NURSE RESPONSE 2: "It sounds like you are feeling out of control right now."

RATIONALE: Shows empathy and acceptance. By reflecting her expression of feelings, you validate the accuracy of your understanding and lay the groundwork for further exploration.

Sometimes clients avoid social situations because they lack social skills and self-confidence. Create opportunities for clients to learn social skills and practice them in a protected environment. For example, teach them to read the newspaper or see a movie and select several items of interest to use in making "small talk." Demonstrate making small talk, and encourage them to practice with you. Give feedback on their progress. Make sure this is an enjoyable and nonthreatening activity.

Individuals who are either extremely passive or too aggressive in their social interactions are often avoided by others. Teaching such clients how to use assertive behavior can improve their interpersonal relationships. Use role-playing to help them become comfortable with new skills. (Refer again to the Partnering with Clients and Families feature on page 39 in Chapter 3.)

WHY I BECAME A PSYCHIATRIC–MENTAL HEALTH NURSE

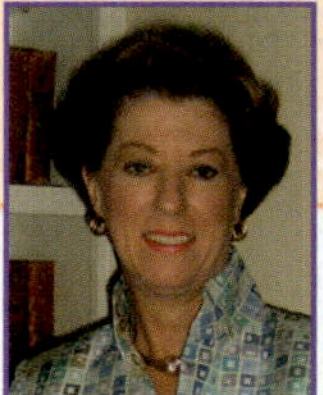

Kay K. Chitty
Contributor, Chapters 17 and 21

My first psychiatric nursing course when I was a junior in college included a practicum in the locked psychiatric ward of a huge public hospital in Atlanta. I was petrified! My only previous exposure to psychiatric clients took place when my Girl Scout troop toured the back wards of the state hospital in my hometown. Although I never lost my initial anxiety about stepping off the elevator onto "the unit," I emerged from that semester with the realization that I had found my niche in nursing, and I have never looked back.

Psychiatric nursing has been good to me. I have had a wonderfully varied career, ranging from staff nurse in a New York City psychiatric hospital to independent practice in North Carolina. I have practiced, written about, and taught psychiatric nursing for 40 years in several states and never once considered changing to another field. Every day is different and none is predictable. Working with people who have emotional problems is, to me, the most challenging field in nursing. There have been many times when I felt inadequate—it goes with the territory. But additional study, further experience, and supervision by more experienced nurses gradually molded me into a competent (I'd like to think excellent) psychiatric nurse. I love sharing my knowledge with students and I never forget how they feel when they embark on their first course in psychiatric nursing!

Administering Medications

The main types of antidepressants nurses will administer to depressed clients are **tricyclic antidepressants (TCAs)**, **monoamine oxidase inhibitors (MAOIs)**, **selective serotonin reuptake inhibitors (SSRIs), serotonin and norepinephrine reuptake inhibitors (SNRIs)**, and atypical antidepressants such as bupropion. See Chapter 7 for detailed discussions of these medications.

The intended action of all antidepressants is to exert positive effects on mood and behavior. Because some are sedating and others are energizing, the individual client's symptoms guide the choice of medication. The use of antidepressants during pregnancy may be necessary and is weighed against both the dangers to the fetus of an untreated, unstable mother and the risk of birth defects. Current clinical practice is to treat the mood disorder to protect both the mother and the baby.

Antidepressants are generally effective in alleviating most clients' symptoms and are helpful adjuncts to treatment. Because they do nothing to affect underlying psychosocial conflicts, they should not be used as the single treatment modality for depressed clients but should be used in conjunction with individual, family, and/or group therapy.

Responsibility for correct administration, monitoring for effects, and client education rests with nurses. Specific information such as maintaining a low-tyramine diet (**tyramine** is an amino acid) while on MAOIs is an educational point that must be discussed with clients and families. Both the Partnering with Clients and Families feature on page 423 and Chapter 32 have additional information about antidepressant therapy and related nursing responsibilities.

Monitoring Electroconvulsive Therapy

Electroconvulsive therapy (ECT), a treatment procedure during which an electric current is passed through the brain, is useful to clients with severe depression, acute mania, some psychotic conditions, and those who are acutely suicidal. It is

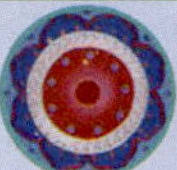

PARTNERING WITH CLIENTS AND FAMILIES

TEACHING ABOUT ANTIDEPRESSANT THERAPY

Proper client education enhances the effectiveness of medication therapy and can help make the difference between client adherence and nonadherence with the medication regimen. Client education begins when medication therapy begins and is repeated during the course of the client's hospitalization. Give instructions orally and in writing. Include family members or significant others if they will supervise home administration. See also Chapter 32.

Initiating Antidepressant Therapy

- Make sure the client knows the name and dose of the medication(s) being taken. *(Rationale: This is basic information every client should know.)*
- Advise the client to arise slowly from a sitting or lying position, and to sit on the side of the bed before standing up. *(Rationale: This allows the body time to compensate for medications that have postural hypotension as a side effect.)*
- Encourage the use of ice chips, gum, hard candy, and increased fluids. *(Rationale: Alleviates dryness of mouth.)*
- Advise both client and family that it may take 2 to 4 weeks to see a therapeutic response to antidepressant therapy. *(Rationale: Prevents discouragement and impatience.)*
- Monitor for urinary retention or constipation, and take necessary actions. *(Rationale: These conditions may result from the anticholinergic effects of some antidepressants.)*
- Give medication early in the day if insomnia occurs as a side effect. *(Rationale: Some antidepressants have a stimulating effect.)*
- Give medication later in the evening if sedation occurs as a side effect. *(Rationale: Some antidepressants have sedating side effects.)*
- Monitor and record sleep patterns. *(Rationale: Normalization of sleep patterns should occur.)*
- Avoid giving TCAs or SSRIs and MAOIs concurrently. *(Rationale: To avoid hypertensive crisis, give 2 to 3 weeks apart.)*
- Observe the client for skin rashes, photosensitivity, weight gain, and signs of infection. *(Rationale: These are adverse side effects and should be evaluated.)*
- Advise the client that drowsiness, blurred vision, dry mouth, and jittery feelings will diminish after a few days on the medication. *(Rationale: Sedation and anticholinergic effects [except dry mouth] usually diminish over time. They will recur when dosage is raised, however.)*
- Monitor the client for suicide risk, particularly as depression begins to lift. *(Rationale: Profoundly depressed clients lack the energy to plan and implement suicide. As they begin to improve and energize but are still profoundly depressed, risk increases.)*
- Observe clients on high doses of TCAs closely for seizures. *(Rationale: High-dose tricyclics lower the seizure threshold.)*

Clients on MAOIs

- Supervise the client's intake, and make sure no tyramine-rich agents are offered. *(Rationale: Tyramine may precipitate hypertensive crisis.)*
- Monitor the client closely for headaches and elevated blood pressure. Withhold medication, and report these signs to the prescribing professional immediately. *(Rationale: These may be early signs of hypertensive crisis.)*
- Keep phentolamine mesylate (Regitine) on hand for treating hypertensive crisis. *(Rationale: This is an alpha-adrenergic blocker and potent antihypertensive agent.)*
- Observe diabetic clients closely for hypoglycemia. *(Rationale: MAOIs promote hypoglycemia.)*

Prior to Discharge

- In collaboration with the client, work out a time schedule that fits the client's lifestyle. *(Rationale: This will increase the likelihood that the client will actually take the medication.)*
- Advise the client to take the medication as ordered and to avoid using alcohol or other central nervous system depressants during therapy. *(Rationale: Varying the dosage impairs the maintenance of therapeutic blood levels. Alcohol and other central nervous system depressants have a potentiating effect on antidepressants and may cause stupor or coma.)*
- Teach the client and family about possible adverse reactions and measures to initiate if they occur. *(Rationale: Ensures maximum comfort and safety.)*
- Caution the client not to operate dangerous equipment, drive a car, or engage in tasks requiring mental alertness if drowsiness persists. *(Rationale: Ensures safety.)*
- Teach the client not to discontinue the medication abruptly. *(Rationale: Antidepressant dosage should be gradually decreased to avoid withdrawal symptoms of nausea, dizziness, insomnia, and headache.)*
- For clients on MAOIs, provide a list of tyramine-containing substances (see Chapter 32) and make sure the client and family understand the consequences of consuming tyramine. *(Rationale: Ensures client safety.)*
- Record accurately and completely what medication education the client and family have received. *(Rationale: Documenting client education provides legal protection for the nurse and institution in the event of an adverse reaction.)*

usually given several times a week until a course of 12 treatments is completed. Caution is advised when ECT is administered to clients with increased intracranial pressure and those who have had recent myocardial infarctions. Guidelines for working with clients receiving ECT are discussed in the Your Intervention Strategies box on page 424.

During a course of ECT, a transient short-term memory loss is expected. This is distressing to some clients, and they need to be reassured that memory is usually completely restored. Because ECT is not curative, ongoing psychotherapy and pharmacotherapy are often continued to prevent *relapse*. For a complete explanation of this treatment modality, considered the treatment of choice for treatment-resistant depression, see Chapter 6. The practical issues of ECT treatment and how the treatment is conducted are described in the following clinical example.

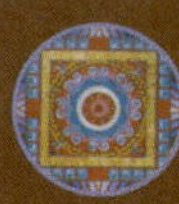

YOUR INTERVENTION STRATEGIES
Working with Clients Receiving ECT

- Prepare the client by explaining the procedure and answering all questions as fully as possible.
- A separate consent for treatment must be signed because ECT requires the administration of anesthesia. While informing clients and obtaining consent forms is legally a medical responsibility, in practice it is often shared by nurses.
- Clients are kept NPO for at least 4 hours before treatment.
- Just prior to treatment, request that the client void and remove contact lenses, jewelry, hairpins, and dentures.
- Assess vital signs.
- The anesthetic preparation usually consists of the following:
  1. Generally, an atropine-like medication, such as glycopyrrolate (Robinul), is given to decrease secretions and block cardiac vagal reflexes during the seizure.
  2. A short-acting anesthetic, such as methohexital sodium (Brevital), is administered intravenously.
  3. Following induction, a skeletal muscle relaxant, such as succinylcholine chloride (Anectine), is administered to prevent injuries during the seizure.
  4. The client must be artificially ventilated until the muscle relaxant is fully metabolized, usually in 2 to 3 minutes. Oxygen is administered with a rubber bite block in place. If necessary, oxygen may be administered by positive pressure.
- An electrical current is passed through the brain by means of unilateral or bilateral electrodes placed on the temples. This causes a **generalized** (or tonic–clonic) **seizure**, the effects of which are masked by the muscle relaxant. Often the only observable signs of seizure are a fluttering of the eyelids and carpopedal spasms.
- Clients are recovered in the lateral recumbent position to facilitate drainage and prevent aspiration. Upon awakening they will be confused and somewhat disoriented. After they are fully recovered and have been reoriented by the nurse, they may eat breakfast.

CLINICAL EXAMPLE

Barry has been depressed for a number of months after having been accused of unfair practices at work. His feelings of guilt and worthlessness are far out of proportion to reality. Although he believes he has a successful defense against these charges, many people at work see it differently. His prescriber has tried several different antidepressants with him, but his symptoms of depression continue to worsen. Barry developed severe depressive symptoms such as suicidal thinking, psychomotor retardation, and weight loss because he believes that he does not deserve to eat.

Barry's psychiatrist has recommended a course of ECT for his treatment-resistant depression. Barry is concerned because he has heard many rumors about the negative effects of ECT. The prescriber has explained that it is a safe and effective treatment about which there are several negative and inaccurate myths. After several discussions, Barry agreed to try ECT. He was given a course of six ECT treatments over 2 weeks and experienced a significant improvement in his mood. He is no longer suicidal or delusional, and no longer has psychomotor retardation. It has become possible for him to function more effectively at work, including defending himself against what he declares are unfounded charges. Due to advances in ECT techniques Barry had no discomfort during or after any of the ECT treatments. He is relieved that ECT has been an effective treatment for his depression.

Evaluation

Specific client behaviors indicate that nursing interventions have been successful. Evaluation criteria answer the question, "How do we know that the depressed client's condition has improved?"

Impulse Control and Suicide Self-Restraint

The risk for self-directed violence is lessened when the client reports a decrease in suicidal thoughts and impulses and commits no acts of self-violence. Clients who are not suicidal can vent negative feelings appropriately and avoid high-risk environments or situations. They become more adept at identifying alternative ways of coping with problems and no longer depend on suicide as their primary coping skill.

Self-Esteem

Clients who have improved self-esteem can verbalize self-acceptance and identify positive characteristics of themselves. They can speak about increased feelings of self-worth. Their behaviors are consistent with increased self-esteem; for example, their posture is erect, and they groom and dress themselves with some care. They are able to accept a compliment, to express feelings directly and openly, and to communicate assertively with others, including maintaining eye contact. They express some optimism and hope for the future. Clients demonstrate self-esteem when they evaluate their own strengths realistically; set realistic, attainable goals for themselves; and work toward reaching them. See the Evidence-Based Practice feature on page 425 for more information on depression and self-esteem.

Hopelessness

Depressed clients demonstrate progress toward eliminating hopelessness by consistently weighing and choosing among alternatives and by expressing faith, the will to live, reasons to live, meaning in life, optimism, and belief in self or others. They can identify their own personal strengths, show interest in achieving life goals, and demonstrate satisfaction with life conditions or work to change them.

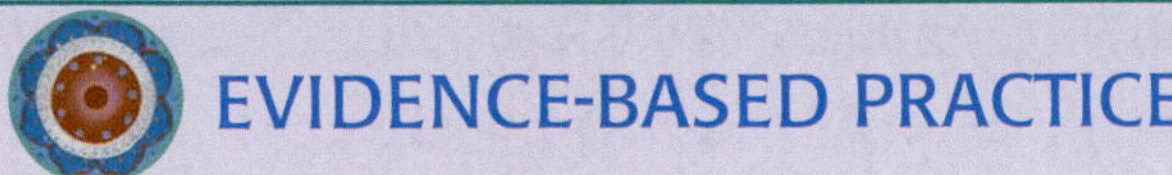

ADOLESCENT ACTING OUT

Brent is a large, muscular 13-year-old who was admitted to the crisis unit in your community after his parents called the police. He had been shouting obscenities at his mother, pushed his father to the floor, and broke the windows of neighbors' cars parked along the street as he ran from his home. Within an hour of his arrival on the unit, he began breaking light fixtures in the hall and in other clients' rooms with a broom he found in a closet. Other clients were visibly distressed and frightened by his fury.

Your plan for intervention options is based on current research results. For example, in your review of studies of cognitive–behavioral therapy and anger management, you consider the possibility that Brent will more quickly and effectively gain self-control of his behavior if you work with him on specific techniques in private. Consequently, you set limits on his free activity on the unit and insist that he take a "time-out" in his room before you talk with him privately about the incident.

Your initial nursing assessment reveals that Brent's low self-esteem and guilt make it difficult for him to talk openly and freely with adults about his anger. Because of this finding and research literature on group work with adolescents, you also ask him to talk about the circumstances around his admission and the incident on the unit with his peers at the next morning's group session.

Finally, given the goal/task phase for Brent's family treatment, you decide to confront him about his behavior in the impending family therapy sessions scheduled before his discharge from the unit.

Action should be based on more than one study, but the following research was helpful in developing this set of multiple intervention strategies:

Valente, S., & Nemec, C. (2006). An evidence-based project to improve depression and alcohol use screening. *Journal of Nursing Care Quality, 21*(1), 93–98.

CRITICAL THINKING APPLICATION

1. What elements would you take into consideration when planning to confront Brent?
2. How can Brent and his family benefit from psychoeducation?
3. What topics would be considered priorities for this family?

Social Involvement

Improved social involvement is apparent when clients communicate and socialize with others. Voluntarily attending group activities is a measure of success. They can initiate interaction with another person appropriately and assume responsibility for dealing with feelings, including finding others with whom to talk. Clients can identify their own personal characteristics or behaviors that contribute to social isolation and accept responsibility for them. They report fewer experiences of feeling excluded.

For additional information about working with depressed clients, see the Nursing Care Plan at the end of this chapter. Clients plan for discharge by establishing or maintaining relationships, a social life, and a support system outside the hospital, and by participating in leisure activities.

CASE MANAGEMENT

Case management with depressed clients attempts to ensure that they receive needed services in a timely, flexible, cost-effective manner. This requires that the case manager understands risk factors and possible complicating factors of major depression, recognizes prodromal/recurrence/relapse symptoms early, anticipates possible complications, and understands effective case management outcomes. Depending on his or her educational preparation and experience, the case manager may or may not deliver direct psychotherapeutic care to depressed clients.

Risk factors for recurrence or **relapse** (a return of symptoms after a period of time with no or very few symptoms) of depression include female gender, family history of depression, previous depression, lack of family/social support, stressful life events or losses, and substance abuse. Suicide attempts, substance abuse continuance or increase, having a personality disorder, having a coexisting medical or psychiatric condition, resistance to treatment, and/or failure to respond to treatment complicate the course of a depressive episode. While recurrence of depressive symptoms is of concern, the length of time it takes to recover from depressive symptoms affects longer-term planning and case management services. One study (Posternak et al., 2006) found that recovery time depended on whether or not the person sought treatment. Recovery took as long as 23 weeks when people sought treatment. People who did not seek treatment, or were on a long waiting list for treatment, recovered from depressive symptoms in about 13 weeks. This difference most likely indicated a different intensity of symptoms (i.e., those who sought treatment had more severe symptoms). Recognizing depressive symptoms, and treating them, earlier in the process can be an effective tool in reducing the long-term impacts of the illness.

Symptoms that would alert the case manager to evaluate a client's need for treatment for major depression are enumerated in the DSM-IV-TR diagnostic criteria box on pages 406–407. Case management interventions would respond to suicidal thoughts, suicide plans, or suicide attempts, prior self-destructive violence, concurrent chronic or severe acute medical problems, prior medication-resistant depression, social withdrawal, and decline in work productivity. Teach clients and family members to also be alert for symptoms that indicate the need for treatment.

Clients and families may find the following websites helpful:

- National Institute for Mental Health: http://www.nimh.nih.gov/publicat/depression.cfm (information presented in both English and Spanish)
- International Foundation for Research and Education on Depression (iFRED): http://www.ifred.org/

These sites can be accessed through the Companion Website for this book.

MediaLink Resources for Depression

Desired case management outcomes include symptom remission; improvement in social, family, and occupational functioning; reduced risk of self-harm; and either avoidance of hospitalization or shortened hospital stay. Clients who lack financial resources and family, social, and employer support, and who resist or respond poorly to treatment, represent greater challenges for the case manager. The ultimate case management goal is the earliest possible detection of symptoms, effective symptom reduction, and a rapid return to maximal premorbid functioning.

COMMUNITY-BASED CARE

A number of depressed clients can be effectively treated in community-based settings such as mental health centers, schools, occupational health settings, doctors' offices, hospices, skilled nursing facilities, and rehabilitation centers, among others. Nurses in community settings play a major role in recognizing symptoms of depression, providing screening and assessment, providing emotional support and information, monitoring antidepressant therapy, and educating family members and significant others about depression. Severely depressed and/or suicidal clients, however, should be referred to inpatient treatment to ensure their safety. The What Every Hospice Nurse Should Know feature presents information on depression for nurses in this specialty area as well as for nurses in skilled nursing facilities and rehabilitation centers.

Nurses working in community health settings may not be educationally prepared as psychiatric–mental health nurses. However, with minimal continuing education focused on the detection and treatment of depression, they can play a valuable role in the recovery of depressed clients while enabling them to remain in the community while in treatment.

HOME CARE

Nurses functioning in the home serve as bridges between hospital, home, and community. Home care may substitute for inpatient care in carefully selected cases, or it may precede or follow the client's inpatient treatment. Home care aims to maximize the client's ability to stay in the family context and overlaps somewhat with the case management model discussed earlier. The APRN psychiatric–mental health nurse, however, is prepared to provide psychotherapeutic interventions directly to depressed clients and their families.

Working with depressed clients in the home and family contexts allows the nurse to observe the family dynamics and their impact on the family members, including the depressed client. These nurses provide education to client and family about medications, side effects, desired effects, adverse effects, and possible medication and/or food interactions. In addition, home care nurses educate clients and families about the nature of depression, the usual course of depression, what to expect, and when to seek help. They assist clients and families in establishing realistic goals, both short and long term. They collaborate with other professionals such as physicians, psychologists, psychiatrists, social workers, and others to improve communication and prevent gaps and overlaps in services. They also serve as client advocates, ensuring that depressed clients receive comprehensive, cost-effective care in the home setting.

WHAT EVERY HOSPICE NURSE SHOULD KNOW

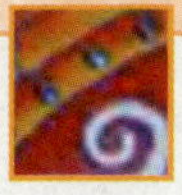

Grief and Depression

Depression is thought to be the natural reaction when people have been diagnosed with a terminal illness. When people know that their life is coming to an end, there is sadness and grieving. However, depression is much more than that. Symptoms of depression that last for 14 days or more are not a necessary emotional state. The final months of someone's life, while sad, can be made more comfortable, functional, and potentially satisfying when depression is treated. Nurses working in hospice settings interact with people whose lives will end in a few short months. Spending those months in an emotionally healthy setting is the priority.

Differentiating between normal sadness and grieving and the state called depression is done in clinical interviews and through observations. Statements such as, "I never should have sold the house. That house is where my children grew up and I took all their memories away when I sold it," represent irrational guilt more than legitimate regret. Similarly, taking more responsibility than is reasonable, interpreting interactions in morbid ways, not being able to enjoy any aspect of their current life, and drastic changes in appetite and sleeping pattern that are not related to their medical condition are all signs of depression. Make arrangements for a psychological consult when you detect depressive symptoms as a hospice nurse. Consultations of this nature are performed by advanced practice psychiatric–mental health nurses, psychologists, or psychiatrists.

Effective treatment of depressive symptoms, even during the final stages of life, is not only a possibility but a responsibility. Talk therapy and/or medications can have an impact within a matter of days or weeks, allowing clients to say goodbye and face this transition positively and peacefully.

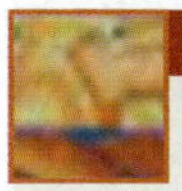

NURSING PROCESS
Clients with Bipolar Disorders

Because the nursing care of clients experiencing depressive symptoms is the same whether the diagnosis is major depressive disorder, dysthymic disorder, or depressed episode bipolar disorder, this section will focus on hypomania and mania, which constitute the other half of the bipolar continuum of behaviors.

Assessment

The onset of a hypomanic or manic episode may be gradual or dramatic. Affect is euphoric or elated, but can change quickly to irritability or hostility if the person is confronted with limits or is otherwise frustrated. The signs and symptoms range in severity from mild (in hypomania) to extreme (in a frank manic episode).

Subjective Data

Clients who experience mania have changes in their thought processes, sometimes stating that their "thoughts are racing." They often experience inflated self-esteem, sometimes to the extent of having delusions of grandeur. Delusions of persecution also may be a feature. They ignore fatigue and hunger, being too involved in activity to focus on physiologic sensations. Suffering from an inability to concentrate, they are easily distracted by the slightest stimulus in the environment. They may experience hallucinations. Hypomanic individuals and those early in manic episodes feel wonderful and do not understand why people are upset with their behavior.

Objective Data

Clients who are experiencing mania are most likely to be young people in their twenties, although adolescents are sometimes affected. Although bipolar disorder appears to have little gender specificity, the initial episode is likely to be manic in males and depressive in females (APA, 2000). To date, there is no documented evidence of the effect of race or ethnicity on bipolar disorder.

The hallmark of mania is constant motor activity. During a manic episode, clients will not stop to eat. They do not rest, have disordered sleep patterns, and may go for days without sleep. Bruises and other injuries sometimes result from the constantly agitated behavior.

Flight of ideas is manifested in the manic communications, and pressured speech is an obvious symptom. Family members often report that they exhibit poor judgment, such as going on spending sprees and committing sexual and other indiscretions that are completely out of character with their usual behavior. Appearance may be unusual, such as inappropriate dress and garish makeup or being disheveled and unkempt. Just as they fail to settle down long enough to eat and sleep, they also neglect bathing. In time, the absence of personal hygiene alienates them from other people.

Impairment in occupational functioning may result in work layoff or being placed on a leave of absence because the behavior is disruptive in the workplace. People who have mania cause interpersonal chaos with their manipulative behavior, testing of limits, and playing off one person against another. If their manipulation attempts fail, they become irritable or hostile, and such behavior further alienates others.

There are no laboratory findings specific for the diagnosis of mania. Abnormal biologic findings were discussed earlier in this chapter in the Your Assessment Approach feature on page 414. Individuals experiencing manic episodes have been noted to have abnormal cortisol levels as well as abnormalities in neurotransmitter systems, but it is not known whether these abnormalities are a cause of or result from the disorder.

Clients who have mania are not usually able to cooperate fully in the assessment process. In many cases, you will find it necessary to rely on your own assessment skills and secondary sources, such as family members, to obtain essential assessment data. Family members can often provide detailed information about the onset and progression of symptoms, as well as information about previous episodes, if any.

MediaLink Critical Thinking Exercise: Bipolar Disorder

Nursing Diagnosis: NANDA

Several nursing diagnoses are common in the care of clients who have mania.

Risk for Injury

Individuals with mania are at risk for injury because their usual adaptive and defensive abilities are impaired. Because of their hyperactivity and agitation, they often lose control of their movements and bump into objects, fall, and otherwise injure themselves.

Their impulsivity, poor judgment, and propensity toward hostile outbursts also place them at risk for injury. Other clients are often extremely annoyed by inappropriate or unacceptable social behavior and may attack clients who are manic. As with self-directed violence, preventing injury becomes the nursing priority.

Disturbed Thought Processes

Clients with mania experience disruption of their usual cognitive processes. This may be related to a variety of factors, including:

- Biochemical alteration
- Genetic predisposition
- Sleep deprivation
- A severe blow to self-esteem
- Massive denial of depression

Evidence of altered thought processes is seen in clients who cannot concentrate, have short attention spans, are easily distracted, and have impaired problem-solving abilities. They exhibit unwarranted optimism and poor judgment due to inaccurate interpretations of the environment. Delusional belief systems held by clients indicate a severe impairment of thought processes, as do hallucinations. Pressured speech, tangentiality, and flight of ideas are ample evidence of disrupted cognitive operations.

Impaired Social Interaction

Unlike depressed clients who may isolate themselves and avoid social interaction, most clients with mania are extremely gregarious and excessively social. But their social interactions are highly dysfunctional. Manipulating other people to meet their own wishes and needs is a major impediment to positive social interactions. Egocentrism, impulsiveness, lack of interest in the needs and concerns of others, and an unwillingness to accept responsibility for the effect of their behavior on others all make clients with mania difficult to tolerate. Poor personal hygiene aggravates the situation.

Nurses often have difficulty dealing with the challenging and unreasonable behavior of clients with mania. The Your Self-Awareness feature that follows will help you determine how you may be affected by these behaviors.

Self-Care Deficit

Clients experiencing a manic episode have an impaired ability to perform the self-care activities of feeding, bathing, toileting, dressing, and grooming. This is related to hyperactivity, the inability to make accurate judgments about personal needs, alterations in thought processes, lack of awareness of personal needs, and fatigue. Self-care deficit is evidenced by inadequate food and fluid intake, an inability or refusal to bathe, a lack of interest in grooming and appropriateness of appearance, and an inability or unwillingness to toilet without assistance.

Sleep Deprivation

The sleep pattern of clients in a manic episode is so disrupted that exhaustion and even death can result. Disrupted sleep is related to hyperactivity, agitation, and possibly to biochemical alterations. Sleep pattern disturbance includes the inability to fall asleep, roaming or pacing the halls during the night, awakening frequently during the night, and sleeping only for short naps with long periods of hyperactive, restless behavior in between.

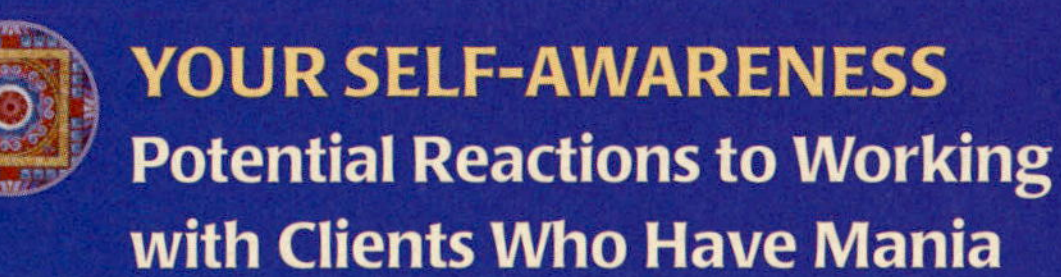

YOUR SELF-AWARENESS
Potential Reactions to Working with Clients Who Have Mania

Working with clients who have mania will challenge your maturity, self-control, and professionalism. Following are some common reactions. When you work with clients who have mania, you may experience some of these feelings. Think about and discuss with classmates and your instructor how you might handle each of these reactions in order to maintain a positive nurse–client relationship.

- I feel annoyed by the client's demanding behavior.
- I feel outsmarted and outmaneuvered; I question whether my judgments and actions are appropriate.
- I develop rescue fantasies in response to a client's flattery and think I am the only one who understands this client.
- I become defensive and angry when colleagues point out a client's manipulative behavior.
- I feel anxious and insecure when a client turns on me, saying, "I'm not progressing because you're cold and mean."
- I have difficulty being objective about clients who have manic symptoms.
- I disagree emphatically with colleagues about how to handle a client's manipulative behavior; the client sits back and watches nurses fight with each other.
- I become angry and unsure of my judgment when a client consistently exceeds established limits.
- I withdraw and avoid clients who have mania to prevent feeling embarrassed and experiencing self-doubt.

Outcome Identification: NOC

Outcomes for mood disorders include the expectation of a return to premorbid functioning. Suggested outcomes for each NANDA diagnosis presented in the previous section are discussed in this section.

Risk for Injury

NOC outcomes appropriate for the client with mania include Risk Control: Actions to reduce or eliminate actual, potential, and modifiable health threats; and Safety Behavior: Fall prevention: Individual or caregiver actions to minimize risk factors that might precipitate falls.

Disturbed Thought Processes

Outcomes that address the client's altered thought processes include Cognitive Orientation: Ability to identify person, place, and time; Concentration: Ability to focus on a specific stimulus; Decision Making: Ability to choose between two or more alternatives; and Distorted Thought Control: Ability to self-restrain disruptions in perception, thought processes, and thought content.

Impaired Social Interaction

Nursing outcomes relevant to the client's impaired social interaction include Social Interaction Skills: An individual's use of effective interaction behaviors; and Social Involvement: Frequency of an individual's social interactions with persons, groups, or organizations.

Self-Care Deficit

Clients' self-care deficits are addressed in the outcomes related to Self-Care: Feeding, bathing, toileting, dressing, and grooming. Some or all of these outcomes may be appropriate for a particular client.

Sleep Deprivation

Outcomes that address the client's tendency to physical and mental exhaustion include Rest: Extent and pattern of diminished activity for mental and physical rejuvenation; and Sleep: Extent and pattern of sleep for mental and physical rejuvenation.

Planning and Implementation: NIC

With clients who are manic, your demeanor should be calm and relaxed but firm and matter-of-fact, particularly when communicating limits. Your own behavior serves as a model and is reassuring to out-of-control clients. As with all clients, building a trusting relationship is important. Therefore, make promises only when you are certain you can keep them.

Promoting Client Safety

Taking steps to ensure the safety of clients and others in the environment is a priority.

Providing a Safe Environment Provide a safe environment for clients in a manic episode by reducing environmental stimuli. For inpatients this means providing a simply furnished private room that has had all unnecessary items removed. It should be in a quiet location to reduce noise stimulation. Low lighting can also be calming to the hyperactive client. Some hospitals have "quiet units." From there, clients can be transferred to milieu units when they are better able to deal with the distractions of community living.

Because clients experiencing mania have difficulty interacting appropriately with others, their participation in group activities should be limited until they are less agitated. Group settings tend to overstimulate these clients, and their behavior may antagonize others.

Smoking materials are particularly hazardous in the hands of agitated clients. They may burn themselves or leave burning cigarettes lying around when they become distracted by other stimuli. While not an issue in most institutions, allow the client who is experiencing mania to smoke only under supervision.

Monitoring Activities Scheduling a program of appropriate activity, interspersed with rest periods, helps provide an outlet for tension while protecting clients from exhaustion. Appropriate activities include walks, exercising or dancing with the supervision of an activity therapist, and supervised vacuuming or sweeping chores. Avoid highly competitive activities that bring out hostility and overtly aggressive behaviors.

Setting and Enforcing Limits Set and enforce limits on unsafe or socially inappropriate behavior when clients are unable to control their impulses. Matter-of-fact intervention rather than angry scolding is the most effective approach. Clients may respond to verbal reminders, or you can use their distractibility to redirect them into safer and more appropriate activities. Remember to reward appropriate behavior with positive reinforcement such as, "I enjoyed our walk today because you were able to walk with me rather than running ahead."

Administering Medications

Hyperactive and agitated behavior usually responds fairly rapidly to antipsychotic mood stabilizers such as risperidone (Risperdal) and olanzapine (Zyprexa). The atypical antipsychotics, effective as mood-stabilizing medications, are often given in conjunction with anticonvulsive mood stabilizers. Atypical antipsychotics are used to help manage the symptoms of mania when individuals have started on lithium carbonate therapy, since lithium takes 1 to 3 weeks to become effective.

Nursing interventions include monitoring clients for adverse side effects of antipsychotic medications. Side effects include sedation, agitation, postural hypotension, dizziness, dry mouth, and blurry vision (see Chapter 32). Several psychopharmacologic agents have proven effective in the long-term treatment of mania. One effective and widely used agent is lithium carbonate.

Lithium Carbonate Lithium carbonate is a potentially dangerous alkali metal that has been used in the treatment and prevention of acute manic episodes since the 1960s. It is now used in preventing the recurrence of bipolar disorder as well.

Lithium alters neurotransmission in the central nervous system. It is thought to interfere with the ionic pump mechanism in brain cells, but its exact mode of action is unknown. Its use is not recommended during pregnancy and breastfeeding or in clients with impaired renal function, congestive heart failure, sodium-restricted diets, organic brain disease, and impaired central nervous system functioning.

Administered orally, the onset of action ranges from 1 to 3 weeks. The dosage is gradually increased until the recommended therapeutic blood level of 1.0 to 1.5 mEq/L is achieved. Once the desired effect is achieved, the dosage is adjusted downward to the maintenance blood level of 0.6 to 1.2 mEq/L. There are cultural considerations to the therapeutic blood level: persons of Asian descent may have toxic reactions at dosages as low as 0.6 mEq/L. Monitor therapeutic effect as well as side effects.

Toxic symptoms begin appearing at blood levels above 1.5 mEq/L. Because there is such a narrow margin of safety, serum concentrations must be closely monitored until stabilized. The need for close monitoring means that clients are often hospitalized when lithium therapy is initiated. Before discharge, both clients and families must learn how to continue lithium therapy safely at home.

Include the following instructions in your teaching plan:

- The diet must include adequate salt and fluid intake, and the client should not take diuretics at any time.
- Regular testing of serum levels must be done, and the client's prescriber should be notified of any illness, especially if vomiting and diarrhea occur.
- The client should not vary the dosage and should continue to take the medicine even when feeling well because discontinuing lithium therapy often precipitates a manic episode.
- If symptoms of lithium toxicity occur, such as nausea, vomiting, diarrhea, polyuria, muscle weakness, fine hand tremors, headache, blurred vision, slurred speech, dizziness, sluggishness, abdominal cramping, and tinnitus, the client should immediately discontinue the medication and contact the prescriber.

The main agents used in mania therapy are the anticonvulsants valproic acid (Depakote, Depakene), lamotrigine (Lamictal), topiramate (Topamax), and carbamazepine

(Tegretol). These medications also cannot be discontinued abruptly. Abrupt discontinuance may precipitate a seizure. Additional information about the pharmacotherapy of mood disorders is found in Chapter 7.

Promoting Reality-Based Thinking

Present reality by spending time with clients; identify yourself, the time and day, location, and other orienting information as needed. Engage clients in reality-based, somewhat concrete activities, such as discussing a current event.

Consistency is reassuring to clients with altered thought processes. Establish consistency by having a schedule so clients understand what is expected of them. Consistency is also enhanced by assigning the same caregivers to work with the client whenever possible.

When dealing with delusional or hallucinating clients, communicate your acceptance of their need for false beliefs, while clearly stating that you do not share their perceptions. A statement such as, "I understand that you believe you are the owner of this facility, but I see it differently," conveys acceptance without supporting delusional thinking.

It is nontherapeutic to argue or try to reason with delusional clients. This often serves to harden the belief system and can impair the development of trust. Instead, use statements such as, "I find that hard to believe" or "That is extremely unusual," to instill reasonable doubt as a therapeutic intervention.

When clients communicate altered reality perceptions, reflect their statements back to them for validation. For example, "Are you saying that your husband is trying to poison you with monosodium glutamate?" can help a client understand how her perceptions sound to others. You will recognize that clients are becoming less delusional when they make statements such as, "I know this sounds bizarre, but. . . ." Remember to give positive reinforcement when clients begin to focus on reality.

Enhancing Socialization

Nursing activities are designed to facilitate the ability of the client to interact with others by identifying specific needed behavior changes and assigning tasks that will improve the client's interactions with others. This may require mediating between the client and others when the client exhibits negative behavior. Nursing actions should encourage and demonstrate honesty and respect for others' rights.

A maladaptive behavior of clients who are manic that significantly impairs social interactions is manipulation, an indirect way of getting their needs met. This may take a simple form, such as borrowing money from other clients rather than using their own. Or it may be highly complex, such as pitting staff members against one another, as in the Rx Communication feature below, by giving them false information about each other.

Manipulation meets a need for the client. It serves the purpose of increasing a client's sense of control and interpersonal power (the mania can be frightening as it spins out of control). Nursing interventions, such as setting limits, promote client security and often enable clients to curb their manipulative behavior or give it up entirely. Be aware of your own control needs, and provide opportunities for clients to be in control when appropriate. Forming a therapeutic alliance with the client, discovering his or her expectations, and providing opportunities for interpersonal interactions has been linked with positive long-term outcomes for people with bipolar disorder (Gaudiano & Miller, 2006).

Setting Limits Out-of-control, manipulative behavior requires setting limits. All staff members must agree upon the established limits and must enforce them consistently. Violations of limits must have established consequences, also agreed upon by all staff. Clients must know what behaviors are expected and what consequences will result if limits are exceeded. Inconsistent application of consequences will cause failure in the efforts to decrease manipulative behavior.

You can expect clients to give charming explanations of why they had to exceed this or that limit, but do not be disarmed by these explanations. They are another form of manipulative behavior. Matter-of-fact limit enforcement and the

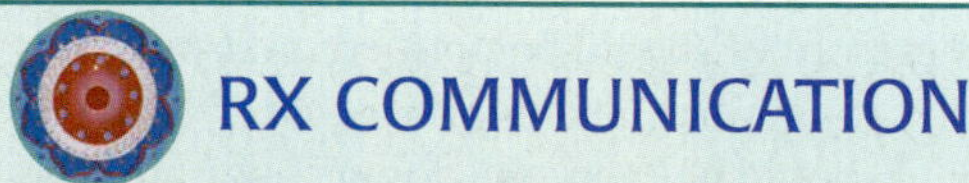

RX COMMUNICATION

CLIENT WITH BIPOLAR DISORDER

CLIENT: "I can't go to community group today! I'm expecting some top-level government officials to visit. The other nurse told me I didn't have to go."

NURSE RESPONSE 1: "I understand, Francis, but it is time for community group now and we expect everyone to attend. Let's walk over together."

RATIONALE: Acknowledges his need for the false belief without reinforcing or arguing with it. Maintains a consistent, routine schedule wherein this delusional client can feel safe. Clearly articulates what is expected of the client. Offers self.

NURSE RESPONSE 2: "All clients and staff members attend these meetings, Francis. You made some constructive comments last week. Let's go so we can get a good seat."

RATIONALE: Sets limits on manipulative behavior. Matter-of-fact enforcement of rules and expectations without allowing the client to involve you in a dispute with another staff member defuses the manipulative behavior and provides positive reinforcement of adaptive behavior.

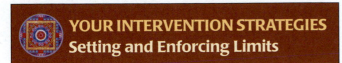

YOUR INTERVENTION STRATEGIES
Setting and Enforcing Limits

Effective limit setting requires that all members of the mental health team participate in establishing limits and determining and enforcing the consequences of exceeding them.

1. Establish limits only when and where there is a clear need. Limits must help client growth.
2. Establish reasonable and enforceable consequences for exceeding limits.
3. Explain the limits and consequences to clients in language they can understand. Explain why the limits are necessary, and allow clients to express their feelings about them.
4. Enforce the limits consistently. Written care plans help ensure consistency.
5. Evaluate the continued need for limits frequently. Turn control over to clients as soon as the client's behavior indicates the ability to exercise self-control.
6. Keep the client's dignity in mind at all times. Limit setting is not a punishment but a part of therapy.

consistent application of consequences are essential in promoting adaptive behaviors. The Your Intervention Strategies box above provides an overview of how to effectively set and enforce limits. (See also Chapter 22.)

Promoting Improved Self-Care

Well-being is compromised when clients do not receive sufficient nourishment and fluids for extended periods of time, particularly during periods of hyperactivity. Monitoring intake and output is an important nursing activity. Frequent small snacks that can be eaten "on the go" are most likely to be consumed by the hyperactive client who is unable to sit down to eat. Work with a dietitian to ensure that high-calorie finger foods and nutritious liquids are available on the nursing unit until the client is able to attend regular meals.

A minimal level of personal hygiene is needed to ensure health, self-esteem, and healthy social interactions. Assist hyperactive clients who are unwilling or unable to bathe, brush their teeth, shave, wash their hair, change clothes, or use the toilet. Autonomy is desirable, so allow clients to do as much for themselves as possible with verbal encouragement. Reinforce any attempts at self-care with recognition, for example, "I see you shaved today, Mr. Adams."

Incontinence of urine or feces is occasionally seen in severely regressed clients during mania. This can be very disturbing to other clients and staff and insults the dignity of the client who is experiencing incontinence. Nursing activities include establishing a schedule of frequent, regular toileting. Accompany the client to the bathroom every hour or half hour until "accidents" no longer occur.

A more common elimination problem is constipation. Hyperactive clients suppress the urge to defecate and may become severely constipated. The anticholinergic effect of some medications may also exacerbate constipation. Frequent fluid intake and a high-fiber diet can reduce constipation.

Enhancing Rest and Sleep

Clients in the manic phase of bipolar disorder appear deceptively energetic when they may actually be nearing the point of exhaustion. Design nursing activities to facilitate regular sleep–wake cycles. Monitor clients closely for signs of fatigue, and make provisions for rest periods. Promote nighttime sleeping by limiting extended daytime naps. Sleep may promote the rapid resolution of first episodes of mania. Prior to bedtime, decrease light and noise and encourage quiet activities and presleep routines, such as listening to soothing music. A warm bath and snack may aid relaxation, as may a backrub. Administer medications that do not suppress REM sleep such as zolpidem tartrate (Ambien) as prescribed.

If clients experience extended nighttime wakefulness, avoid engaging them in long conversations or otherwise stimulating or giving extra attention during the night. Firmly encourage clients to stay in their darkened rooms with the expectation that they will fall asleep. If they will not stay in their rooms, assign a monotonous, repetitive task, such as folding towels or sorting papers to encourage drowsiness.

When clients are able to sleep, avoid waking them for nonessential care or activities. Allow for sleep cycles of at least 90 minutes.

Evaluation

Specific client behaviors indicate that nursing interventions have been successful. Evaluation and outcome criteria answer the question, "How do we know that the client's condition has improved?"

Risk for Injury

If nursing interventions have been successful in promoting safety, clients will be free of accidental injuries. They will not engage in agitated or impulsive behaviors that can endanger them. Their social behaviors will no longer irritate or enrage other people, so they will no longer risk attacks from others. Clients will be able to enumerate safe ways of relieving excess tension when it occurs, such as verbal expression of feelings, writing feelings down in a diary or journal, or other adaptive methods. Clients will name their medications, understand the proper dosages, describe adverse effects, and explain lab monitoring needed, if any.

Cognitive Orientation and Reality-Based Thinking

Clients who base their thinking on reality will be oriented to time, place, and person. They will no longer experience delusional thinking or hallucinations. They will be able to establish trust relationships. Their attention spans will be increased. Their speech will be less pressured and will reflect diminished flight of ideas and tangentiality. Clients will recognize and verbalize errors in perception when they occur.

Their thought processes and perceptions of environmental stimuli will be accurate and can be validated by others. They demonstrate logical, organized thought processes.

Social Interaction Skills

Improvements in social interaction skills will be demonstrated when clients can recognize and describe which of their interactions are successful and which are unsuccessful, and acknowledge the effect of their own behavior on social interactions. They demonstrate behaviors that may increase or improve social interactions. Clients acquire or improve skills such as cooperation, sensitivity, genuineness, and compromise. The absence of, or dramatic decrease in, the use of manipulation as a method of meeting their own needs also will signal improvement in social interaction. They now accept responsibility for their own behavior.

Other signs of improved social interaction include nondisruptive participation in activities, reestablishment of a social life, and identification of individuals with whom they can develop a social and support network.

Self-Care

Clients who have reestablished self-care will demonstrate this ability by performing the activities of daily living autonomously and willingly. This includes adequately bathing and grooming themselves, selecting appropriate clothing and makeup, establishing and maintaining adequate nutrition and fluid intake, and establishing and maintaining patterns of elimination without reminders or assistance.

Rest and Sleep

The need for uninterrupted sleep varies from person to person depending on age, activity level, and usual pattern of sleep. Generally, clients who are able to sleep 6 or more hours per night without sleeping medication and awaken feeling refreshed will have demonstrated healthy sleep patterns. Being able to fall asleep within 30 minutes or less is another indicator. Recognizing fatigue and voluntarily resting or napping appropriately also indicates that clients are attending to their bodily sensations once again.

MEDIALINK Mood Disorders Resources

CASE MANAGEMENT, COMMUNITY-BASED CARE, AND HOME CARE

Case management and community-based care for clients with depressed phase bipolar disorders were described earlier in the nursing process section discussing the care of depressed clients. Clients in the manic phase of bipolar disorders, however, often require hospitalization until stabilized on medication or through ECT.

Following discharge, goals for clients who have mania are the same as for others—high-quality, cost-effective treatment aimed at returning the client to full functioning as soon as feasible. Communication with family members, mental health professionals, employers, social workers, and others involved in the client's case is essential.

Monitoring the client's lithium level is an important aspect of the community-based nurse's role for the treatment of mania. Additional client and family teaching are often required to reinforce the information they received in the inpatient setting. ECT is increasingly used as an outpatient procedure, again calling on the community- and home-based nurse's teaching skills and sensitivity to concerns about safety, memory loss, and effectiveness.

Nurses in case management, community settings, and home care must be alert for "red flags" that signal exacerbation of the client's manic symptoms. These include nonadherence with treatment including refusal to take medications as ordered, escalating activity level that may include psychomotor excitement/agitation, spending sprees, shortened attention span, impaired occupational functioning, and grandiosity. Early recognition of red flags and mobilization of the treatment team can ward off rehospitalization and enable the client to stay at home while being treated and maintained in a community setting. Be sure that family members are also aware of behaviors that signal exacerbation of the client's symptoms.

Clients and their family members will find help from Continuing Medical Education (www.cmellc.com/topics/bdfaq.html). A self-help resource for bipolar disorder and other mood disorders can be located at www.mentalhealthrecovery.com. Both websites can be accessed through the Companion Website for this book.

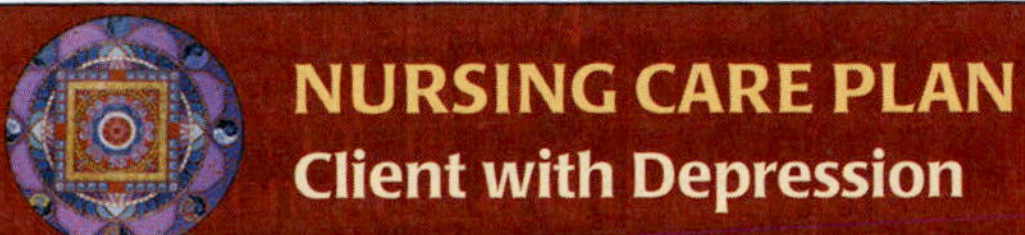

NURSING CARE PLAN
Client with Depression

Identifying Information

Margaret M. is a 59-year-old, unmarried legal assistant who was admitted to the psychiatric unit following a gastric lavage in the emergency department. She had ingested 30 antidepressant tablets in a suicide attempt. Margaret stated that she had been home alone for 2 days, became increasingly depressed and hopeless, and took the antidepressants that her family doctor had prescribed for depression a few weeks ago. She became frightened almost immediately thereafter, was unable to make herself vomit, and called 911. Margaret stated, "I just don't have anything to look forward to anymore. No one would care if I died."

History

Margaret is the eldest of seven children from a small rural community. She had to leave school after the seventh grade to stay home and help with the younger children. At the age of 22 she returned to school and became a legal assistant. She moved to a large city over 100 miles from her home and built her life around her work. She never married. Because she works long hours in a large metropolitan law firm, she has virtually no social life and, except for a few coworkers, no friends. She stopped going to church recently, stating, "I just don't fit in anywhere and I never have."

Margaret reports that she has been concerned about her impending retirement at age 65 and her elderly mother's declining health. About a month ago, the health of her 86-year-old mother, who still lives in their small town, began to deteriorate. Margaret now fears that she will have to go care for her mother, with whom she has never gotten along. Her siblings are pressuring her to move back home, live with their mother, and serve as her caregiver. She fears that because she has no family of her own and no family ties in the city, she will eventually have to give in to their pressure.

She has no prior psychiatric history and no significant health problems. Vital signs: T, 98.4; P, 88; R, 18; Ht, 5′3″; Wt. 157 lb; BP, 138/78.

Current Mental Status

Margaret is somewhat disheveled and weeps occasionally during the interview. She is cooperative with the interviewer, even eager to talk. She reports being "exhausted" for the past 3 weeks. She has not slept well, has lost weight, had crying spells, has been irritable with coworkers, and had difficulty concentrating at work. She reports having had suicidal thoughts but did not have a specific plan until the weekend after the firm's senior partner told her to take a few days off to "get yourself together." She fears being fired, in which case she will have no reason to resist her siblings' pleas to "come take care of Mama."

Margaret is alert, responsive, and well oriented. There is no sign of a thought disorder, confusion, or impairment. She weeps as she discusses her situation, stating, "I have always been unattractive and nobody has ever loved me. If I died, all my family would lose is a nursemaid for Mama."

Other Clinical Data

Margaret reports being in good health, although she is somewhat overweight. She has mild arthritis in her knees, which she treats symptomatically with aspirin. Until she began taking antidepressants, she took no other medicine.

Nursing Diagnosis: Risk for Self-Directed Violence related to recent suicide attempt

Expected Outcome: Impulse Control: Ability to restrain compulsive or impulsive behavior.
Suicide Self-Restraint: Ability to refrain from gestures and attempts at killing self.

Short-Term Goals	Interventions	Rationales
Client will not harm self during hospitalization.	■ Remove all dangerous articles from client's environment.	Client's safety is ensured.
	■ Observe client closely, using irregular schedule.	Irregular schedule prevents her from predicting when she will be alone.
	■ Adopt neutral, matter-of-fact attitude.	A neutral attitude prevents client dependency.
	■ Evaluate suicidal intention at every shift and institute appropriate level of supervision.	Suicidal thoughts and impulses may change rapidly.
	■ Establish no-suicide contract.	Nurse–client collaboration promotes self-responsibility.
	■ Encourage client to seek nurse out when bothered by suicidal thoughts or impulses.	Client learns to substitute talking it out for acting it out.
	■ Limit repetitive discussion of suicidal ruminations.	Repetition reinforces preoccupation with self-directed violence.
Client will demonstrate alternative ways of dealing with stress, such as talking, exercise, relaxation techniques.	■ Assist client to verbalize at least one reason for living.	Identifying reasons for living counteracts negative thinking.
	■ Encourage the expression of feelings in one–to–one and group activities.	Self-expression decreases isolation and elicits peer support.
	■ Assist client to identify and practice alternative ways of dealing with stress.	Client's coping behaviors are expanded.

(continued)

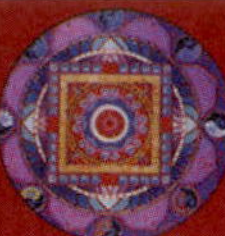

NURSING CARE PLAN
Client with Depression *(continued)*

Short-Term Goals	Interventions	Rationales
Client will identify resources where she can seek help if suicidal thoughts recur following discharge, such as crisis line, minister.	▪ Help client identify community resources and supports.	Client becomes more aware of social supports available to her.
Client will verbalize safe uses of antidepressant medication and describe potential drug/food interactions.	▪ Teach client safe use of antidepressant medication.	This is information every client should know.

Nursing Diagnosis: Self-Esteem Disturbance related to impaired cognition, fostering negative view of self

Expected Outcome: Self-Esteem: Personal judgment of self-worth

Short-Term Goals	Interventions	Rationales
Client will sit and walk erectly; comb hair neatly; wear clean, matching clothes.	▪ Help client with hygiene and grooming as needed.	Competant self-care increases feelings of self-worth.
Client will participate in unit activities.	▪ Teach client that activity helps decrease depression.	This is information all depressed clients should know.
	▪ Involve client in simple, noncompetitive recreational activities.	Cooperative recreation allows client to experience success.
	▪ Increase the complexity of activities as client progresses.	Client's growth and self-regard are enhanced by appropriate challenges.
Client will verbalize positive aspects of self and increased feelings of self-worth.	▪ Set limits on time spent reviewing past failures.	
	▪ Help client enumerate her own personal strengths.	Focusing on personal strengths counteracts negative self-view and increases self-worth.
Client will communicate assertively with others; will explain to siblings that she will not give up her career to come home to care for mother.	▪ Teach client assertiveness techniques.	Learning assertiveness validates client's right to take care of herself.
	▪ Practice (role-play) client's direct expression of feelings.	Role-playing promotes confidence in asserting herself.
	▪ Stay with client during difficult interactions, if desired.	
	▪ Give positive recognition when progress is shown.	Encouragement and recognition support healthy behaviors.

Nursing Diagnosis: Hopelessness related to inability to make and carry out decisions on her own behalf

Expected Outcome: Decision Making: Ability to choose between two or more alternatives
Hope: Presence of internal state of optimism that is personally satisfying and life supporting
Mood Equilibrium: Appropriate adjustment of prevailing emotional tone in response to circumstances
Quality of Life: Expresses satisfaction with current life circumstances

Short-Term Goals	Interventions	Rationales
Client will verbalize feelings about situations over which she has no control; will realize that siblings' expectations do not control her responses.	▪ Assist client to identify situations over which she has no control.	
	▪ Assist client to identify situations over which she can attain control.	A realistic appraisal of her situation allows client to focus on areas in which she can effect change.

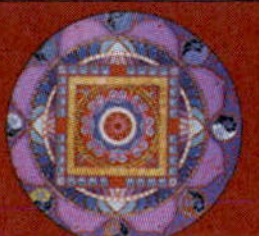

NURSING CARE PLAN
Client with Depression *(continued)*

Short-Term Goals	Interventions	Rationales
Client will set realistic goals for self and work toward them.	■ Engage client in goal setting for self.	Setting goals is a crucial step toward self-determination.
	■ Provide options when possible.	Options help client understand the concept of choice.
Client will demonstrate a problem-solving system that she has used successfully.	■ Explore problem-solving models with client and encourage her to select one.	
	■ Practice problem-solving with small daily problems.	Information and practice help build client's confidence.
Client will verbalize plans to attain control over life situations; works with siblings to find appropriate caretaker for mother.	■ Role-play possible situations with siblings.	Role-playing increases client's confidence and resourcefulness.
	■ Assist client to prepare for siblings' potential untoward responses.	
Client expresses some hope for the future.	■ Assist client to plan for retirement.	
	■ Identify community resources that assist individuals toward fulfilling retirement (e.g., AARP).	Planning for the future decreases fears of the unknown and introduces new sources of support.
	■ Involve client in identifying enjoyable leisure pastimes.	Positive use of leisure time is promoted.

Nursing Diagnosis: Social Isolation related to fear of rejection

Expected Outcome: Social Interaction Skills: Use of effective interaction behavior
Social Involvement: Social interactions with persons, groups, or organizations
Social Support: Perception of availability of reliable assistance from other persons

Short-Term Goals	Interventions	Rationales
Client will communicate with nursing staff and socialize with other clients on the unit.	■ Make brief, frequent contacts with client.	Frequent contact demonstrates your availability and interest.
	■ Spend time with client with no demands.	
	■ Use nonjudgmental attitude.	A nonjudgemental approach demonstrates acceptance.
	■ Encourage client to ventilate verbally or through activity.	Appropriate self-expression decreases internal tension and increases sociability.
Client voluntarily attends group activities.	■ Accompany client to group activities initially, withdrawing as tolerated.	Providing support as needed fosters gradual independence.
	■ Teach social skills and assist client to practice them.	Practice increases client's self-confidence in social situations.
Client assumes responsibility for dealing with feelings, including seeking others out; identifies key individuals outside hospital and initiates contact to renew relationships; makes concrete plans to go to church again.	■ Teach assertive communication.	Learning assertiveness helps client take care of herself.
	■ Encourage role-playing of phone calls, other contacts, anticipating others' possible responses.	Role-playing decreases social anxiety and builds resourcefulness and flexibility.
	■ Give positive feedback for all signs of progress.	Positive feedback validates client's efforts and reinforces growth.

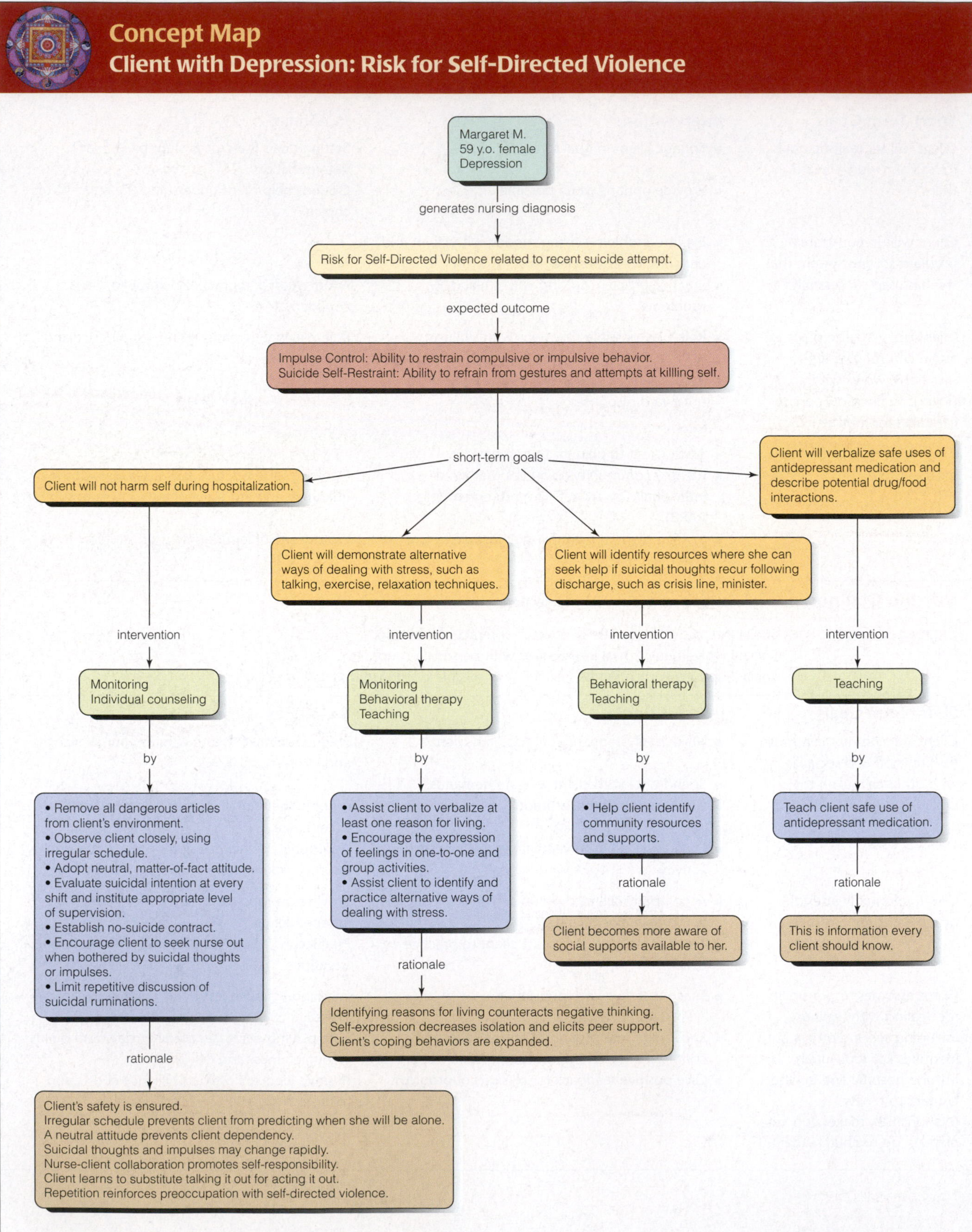
Concept Map
Client with Depression: Risk for Self-Directed Violence
Margaret M.
59 y.o. female
Depression
generates nursing diagnosis
Risk for Self-Directed Violence related to recent suicide attempt.
expected outcome
Impulse Control: Ability to restrain compulsive or impulsive behavior.
Suicide Self-Restraint: Ability to refrain from gestures and attempts at killling self.
short-term goals
Client will not harm self during hospitalization.
Client will demonstrate alternative ways of dealing with stress, such as talking, exercise, relaxation techniques.
Client will identify resources where she can seek help if suicidal thoughts recur following discharge, such as crisis line, minister.
Client will verbalize safe uses of antidepressant medication and describe potential drug/food interactions.
intervention
Monitoring
Individual counseling
intervention
Monitoring
Behavioral therapy
Teaching
intervention
Behavioral therapy
Teaching
intervention
Teaching
by
• Remove all dangerous articles from client's environment.
• Observe client closely, using irregular schedule.
• Adopt neutral, matter-of-fact attitude.
• Evaluate suicidal intention at every shift and institute appropriate level of supervision.
• Establish no-suicide contract.
• Encourage client to seek nurse out when bothered by suicidal thoughts or impulses.
• Limit repetitive discussion of suicidal ruminations.
by
• Assist client to verbalize at least one reason for living.
• Encourage the expression of feelings in one-to-one and group activities.
• Assist client to identify and practice alternative ways of dealing with stress.
by
• Help client identify community resources and supports.
by
Teach client safe use of antidepressant medication.
rationale
Client becomes more aware of social supports available to her.
rationale
This is information every client should know.
rationale
Identifying reasons for living counteracts negative thinking.
Self-expression decreases isolation and elicits peer support.
Client's coping behaviors are expanded.
rationale
Client's safety is ensured.
Irregular schedule prevents client from predicting when she will be alone.
A neutral attitude prevents client dependency.
Suicidal thoughts and impulses may change rapidly.
Nurse-client collaboration promotes self-responsibility.
Client learns to substitute talking it out for acting it out.
Repetition reinforces preoccupation with self-directed violence.

Concept Map
Client with Depression: Self-Esteem Disturbance

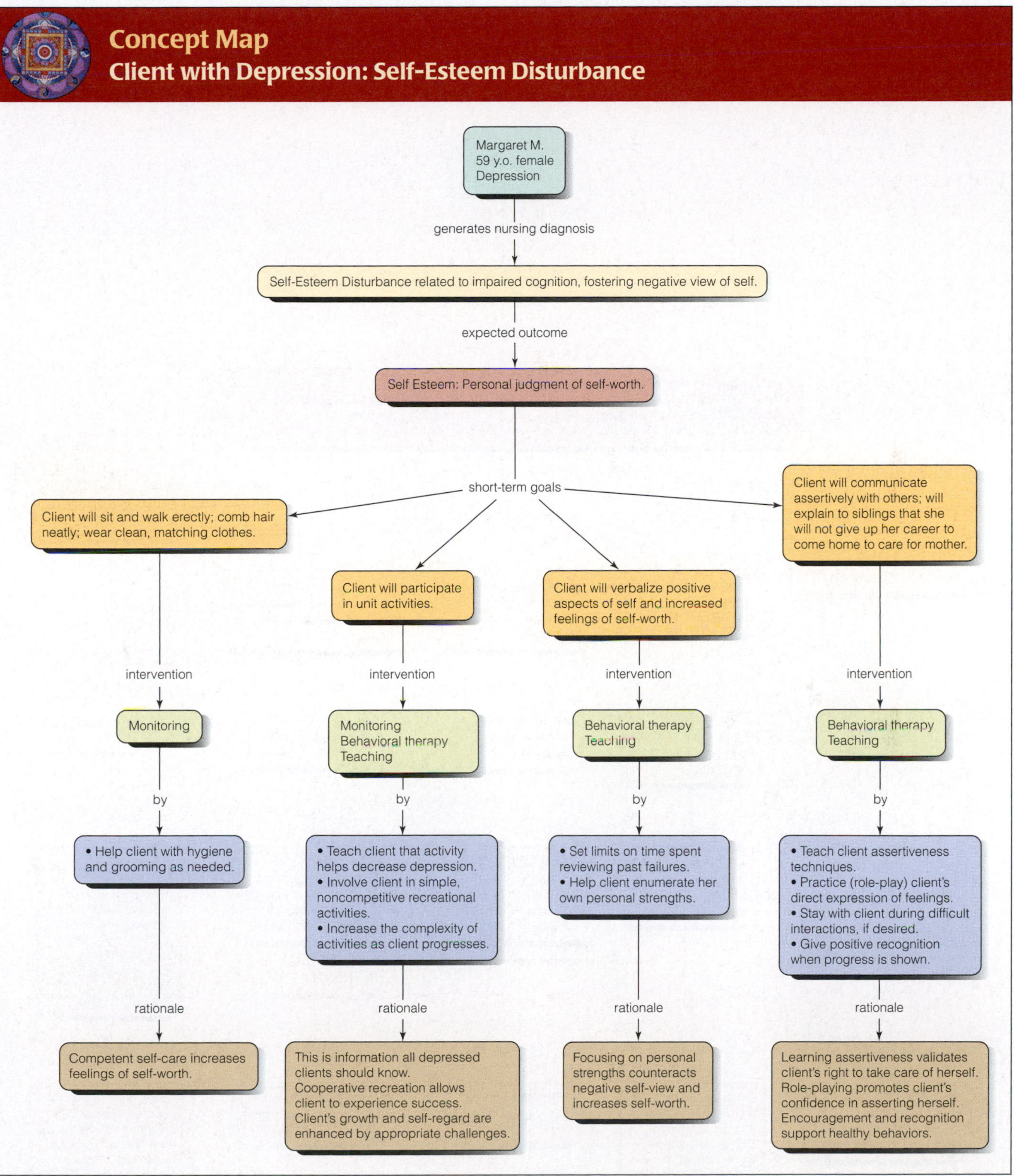
Margaret M.
59 y.o. female
Depression
generates nursing diagnosis
Self-Esteem Disturbance related to impaired cognition, fostering negative view of self.
expected outcome
Self Esteem: Personal judgment of self-worth.
short-term goals
Client will sit and walk erectly; comb hair neatly; wear clean, matching clothes.
Client will participate in unit activities.
Client will verbalize positive aspects of self and increased feelings of self-worth.
Client will communicate assertively with others; will explain to siblings that she will not give up her career to come home to care for mother.
intervention
Monitoring
Monitoring
Behavioral therapy
Teaching
Behavioral therapy
Teaching
Behavioral therapy
Teaching
by
• Help client with hygiene and grooming as needed.
• Teach client that activity helps decrease depression.
• Involve client in simple, noncompetitive recreational activities.
• Increase the complexity of activities as client progresses.
• Set limits on time spent reviewing past failures.
• Help client enumerate her own personal strengths.
• Teach client assertiveness techniques.
• Practice (role-play) client's direct expression of feelings.
• Stay with client during difficult interactions, if desired.
• Give positive recognition when progress is shown.
rationale
Competent self-care increases feelings of self-worth.
This is information all depressed clients should know. Cooperative recreation allows client to experience success. Client's growth and self-regard are enhanced by appropriate challenges.
Focusing on personal strengths counteracts negative self-view and increases self-worth.
Learning assertiveness validates client's right to take care of herself. Role-playing promotes client's confidence in asserting herself. Encouragement and recognition support healthy behaviors.

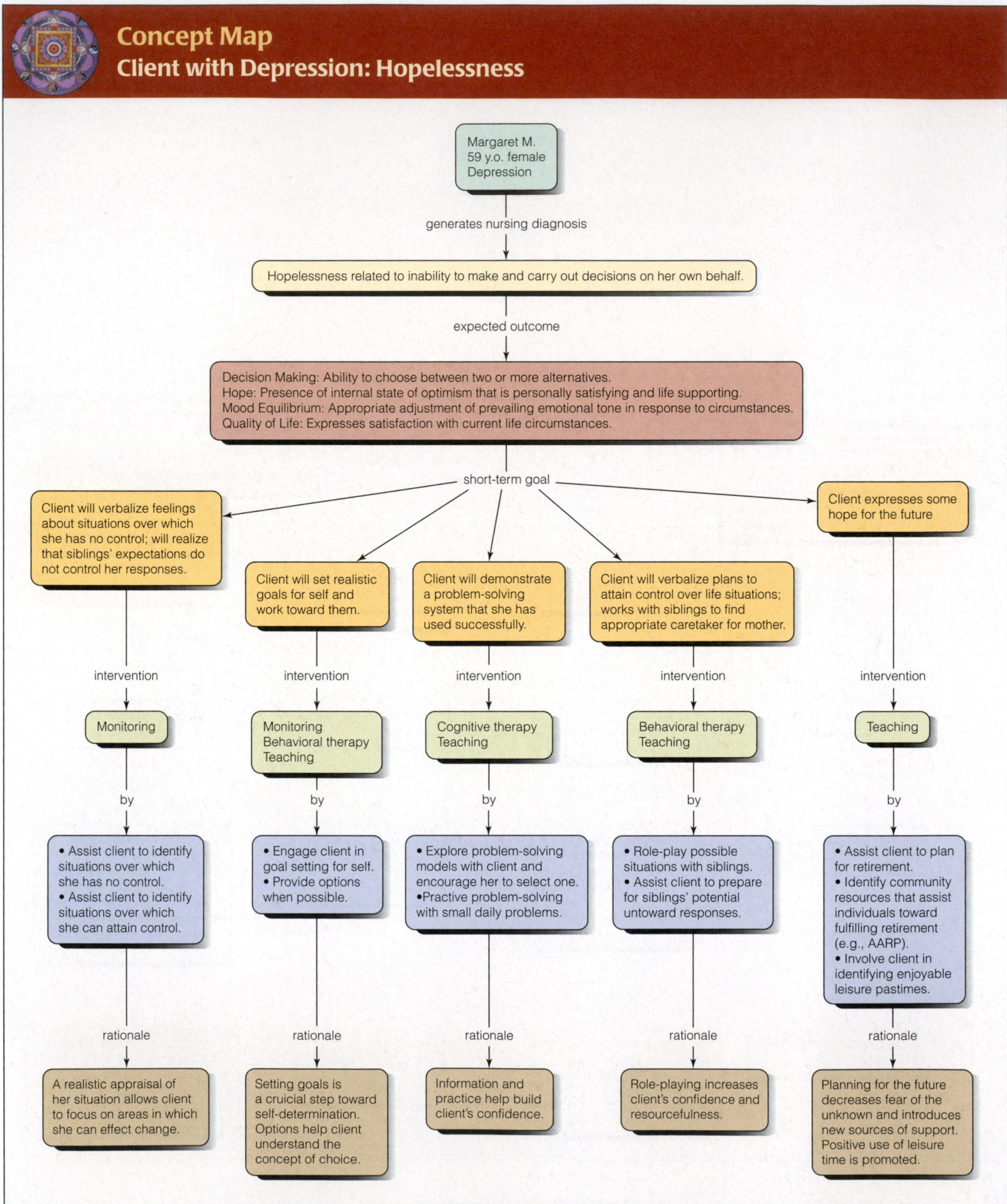
Concept Map
Client with Depression: Hopelessness
Margaret M.
59 y.o. female
Depression
generates nursing diagnosis
Hopelessness related to inability to make and carry out decisions on her own behalf.
expected outcome
Decision Making: Ability to choose between two or more alternatives.
Hope: Presence of internal state of optimism that is personally satisfying and life supporting.
Mood Equilibrium: Appropriate adjustment of prevailing emotional tone in response to circumstances.
Quality of Life: Expresses satisfaction with current life circumstances.
short-term goal
Client will verbalize feelings about situations over which she has no control; will realize that siblings' expectations do not control her responses.
Client will set realistic goals for self and work toward them.
Client will demonstrate a problem-solving system that she has used successfully.
Client will verbalize plans to attain control over life situations; works with siblings to find appropriate caretaker for mother.
Client expresses some hope for the future
intervention
Monitoring
Monitoring
Behavioral therapy
Teaching
Cognitive therapy
Teaching
Behavioral therapy
Teaching
Teaching
by
• Assist client to identify situations over which she has no control.
• Assist client to identify situations over which she can attain control.
• Engage client in goal setting for self.
• Provide options when possible.
• Explore problem-solving models with client and encourage her to select one.
•Practive problem-solving with small daily problems.
• Role-play possible situations with siblings.
• Assist client to prepare for siblings' potential untoward responses.
• Assist client to plan for retirement.
• Identify community resources that assist individuals toward fulfilling retirement (e.g., AARP).
• Involve client in identifying enjoyable leisure pastimes.
rationale
A realistic appraisal of her situation allows client to focus on areas in which she can effect change.
Setting goals is a crucial step toward self-determination. Options help client understand the concept of choice.
Information and practice help build client's confidence.
Role-playing increases client's confidence and resourcefulness.
Planning for the future decreases fear of the unknown and introduces new sources of support. Positive use of leisure time is promoted.

Concept Map
Client with Depression: Social Isolation

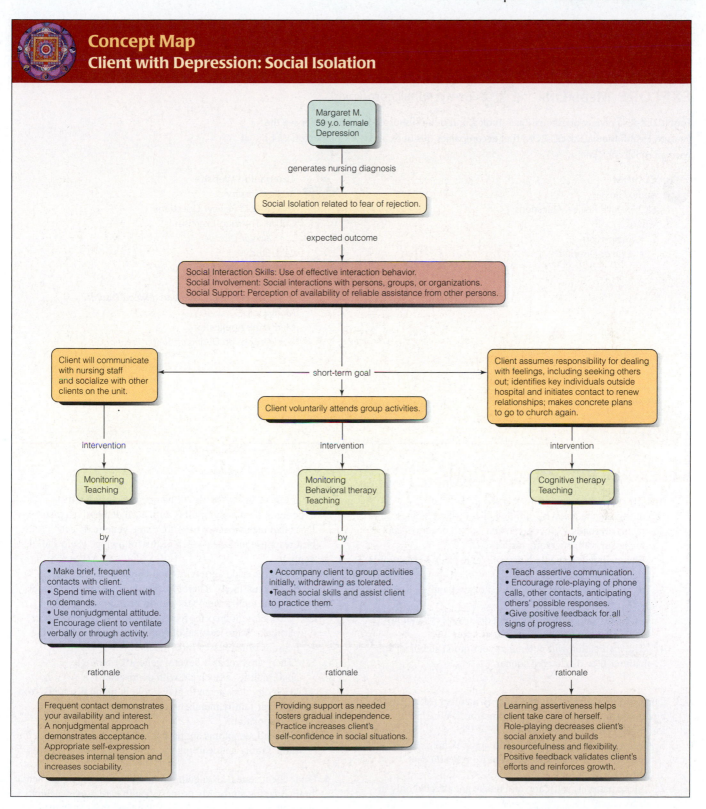

Margaret M.
59 y.o. female
Depression

generates nursing diagnosis

Social Isolation related to fear of rejection.

expected outcome

Social Interaction Skills: Use of effective interaction behavior.
Social Involvement: Social interactions with persons, groups, or organizations.
Social Support: Perception of availability of reliable assistance from other persons.

short-term goal

Client will communicate with nursing staff and socialize with other clients on the unit.

Client voluntarily attends group activities.

Client assumes responsibility for dealing with feelings, including seeking others out; identifies key individuals outside hospital and initiates contact to renew relationships; makes concrete plans to go to church again.

Left branch

intervention

Monitoring
Teaching

by

- Make brief, frequent contacts with client.
- Spend time with client with no demands.
- Use nonjudgmental attitude.
- Encourage client to ventilate verbally or through activity.

rationale

Frequent contact demonstrates your availability and interest. A nonjudgmental approach demonstrates acceptance. Appropriate self-expression decreases internal tension and increases sociability.

Center branch

intervention

Monitoring
Behavioral therapy
Teaching

by

- Accompany client to group activities initially, withdrawing as tolerated.
- Teach social skills and assist client to practice them.

rationale

Providing support as needed fosters gradual independence. Practice increases client's self-confidence in social situations.

Right branch

intervention

Cognitive therapy
Teaching

by

- Teach assertive communication.
- Encourage role-playing of phone calls, other contacts, anticipating others' possible responses.
- Give positive feedback for all signs of progress.

rationale

Learning assertiveness helps client take care of herself. Role-playing decreases client's social anxiety and builds resourcefulness and flexibility. Positive feedback validates client's efforts and reinforces growth.

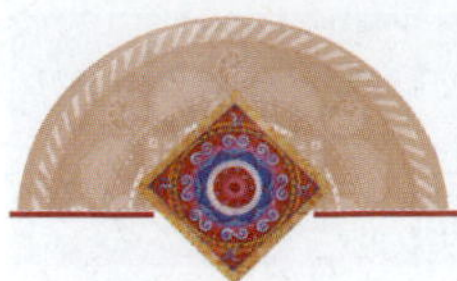

EXPLORE MEDIALINK

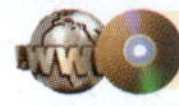 www.prenhall.com/kneisl

For NCLEX-RN® review questions, case studies, and other resources for this chapter see the Pearson Health MediaLink CD-ROM that accompanies this book and the Companion Website at www.prenhall.com/kneisl.

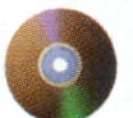

CD-ROM

Audio Glossary

NCLEX-RN® Review Questions

Videos

- *Depression*
- *Bipolar Disorder*

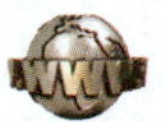

Companion Website

Audio Glossary

NCLEX-RN® Review Questions

Critical Thinking Exercise

- *Bipolar Disorder*

Case Study

- *Depressive Mood Disorder*

Care Plan

- *Assessing the Client with a Mood Disorder*

MediaLinks

MediaLink Application

- *Depression During and After Pregnancy*

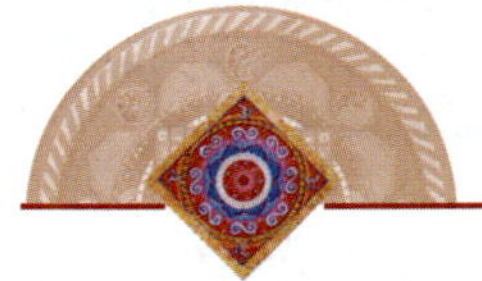

NCLEX-RN® REVIEW QUESTIONS

1. At 10:00 P.M., the nurse offers trazodone (Desyrel) 150 milligrams to a newly admitted client experiencing mania. The client responds, "I feel great, and I don't need to sleep." The nurse's most therapeutic response is:

1. "The medication should help you get to sleep so that you're at your best tomorrow."
2. "Remember that unit rules are to be quiet with lights out by 11:00 P.M."
3. "You and your family stated you did not sleep at all last night. That can be tough on your system."
4. "The medication will potentiate your mood stabilizer so that you'll be discharged sooner."

2. During family support group, a family member asks: "How is bipolar disorder different from depression?" Which of the following is the best response?

1. "People with bipolar disorder do not seek help. People with depression readily seek treatment from health care providers."
2. "Sleep patterns, self-care, and intake are affected only in depression."
3. "Individuals with bipolar disorder start out happy enough, but they eventually develop irritability."
4. "Often, individuals with bipolar disorder can feel elated, are productive, and do not think there is anything wrong when they have manic feelings."

3. Your client states, "Many of the people in my family experience similar symptoms with each depressive episode. Does that mean that we have the same genetic defect?" Your best response includes which of the following? (Select all that apply.)

1. "With the wide variety of mood disorders, a biological basis is not likely. Therefore, pharmacological treatments for your family members should be individualized."
2. "Most current theories focus on electrolyte disturbances, particularly the reversal of sodium and potassium in the neurons of depressed individuals."
3. "There are probably several genetic or biologic abnormalities associated with depression."
4. "Heredity does seem to play a role in mood disorders. You and your family members may have the same biologic predisposition."
5. "Related symptoms are probably due to being raised in the same family and learning the same behavioral responses."

4. Your client states, "I'm going to participate in an experimental brain imaging study. My primary health care provider thinks I have bipolar I disorder. Are there lab tests that can help diagnose mood disorders?" Your first response is:

1. "Although some abnormal results are found in individuals with mood disorders, there are no diagnostic lab tests specific to mood disorders at this time."

2. "There's the dexamethasone suppression test, but we don't know whether mood disorder causes the nonsuppression or whether the nonsuppression causes the disorder."
3. "You should probably ask your primary health care provider."
4. "Are you hoping for diagnosis based on the imaging study?"

5. You administer the first dose of an antidepressant to your inpatient client with major depression. The client asks, "Is this medicine going to fix my depression?" Your accurate response includes which of the following? (Select all that apply.)
1. "The medication will decrease the available dopamine, which is associated with psychotic thinking in major depression."
2. "In addition, we are going to assist you in regulating your circadian rhythms, which should improve your depression."
3. "It should help your depression, and you should feel the full therapeutic effect in 2 to 3 weeks."
4. "This medication should increase the availability of neurotransmitters in your brain."
5. "This medication should increase the production of serotonin in your brain."

6. Based on your knowledge of circadian rhythms, discharge teaching for clients with mood disorders should include which of the following?
1. Nonprescription medications and dietary supplements do not alter activity and rest cycles.
2. Antidepressants and mood stabilizers can help restore circadian rhythms.
3. Disruption of the client's usual diurnal pattern does not influence the course of illness.
4. Particularly during times of decreased stress, the client should do everything possible to maintain similar routines.

7. You are the triage nurse in an emergency room. Your initial assessment indicates that depression may be part of the client's problem. Which of the following nursing actions is essential?
1. Ask about depression and suicidal ideation directly.
2. Within 1 week, telephone the client to ensure that the client's mood has improved.
3. Redirect the client to discuss the stated reason for the visit.
4. Explore the client's perceptions regarding the severity of the stated reason for the visit.

8. Your client with intense suicidal ideation has been hospitalized for 1 week, during which time he has received a selective serotonin reuptake inhibitor (SSRI). He reports "no change" in suicidal ideation, although he demonstrates a wider range of affect and takes more initiative in self-care. The health care team is considering his imminent discharge. It is essential to consider which of the following factors?
1. The client will continue to improve because the medication has not yet exerted full therapeutic effect.
2. The health care team has to plan for discharge from the day of admission.
3. The client may have enough energy to plan and complete a suicide attempt.
4. For 1 week of pharmacotherapy, the client has been free of untoward side effects.

9. A colleague expresses frustration with a client with bipolar disorder on his seventh admission within 2 years. "I wish he would try taking his medication. Instead he keeps stopping the medicine and coming back here." Your best initial response is:
1. "Maybe you would rather work in the NICU, where all of your clients adhere to the prescribed treatment regimen."
2. "He stays on his meds. He is a rapid cycler and he has more episodes anyway."
3. "Get control of your anger so that you do not take it out on the client."
4. "It can be frustrating to care for chronically ill clients."

10. Frequent countertransference reactions in caring for clients with mood disorders include (select all that apply):
1. Emotional contagion.
2. Frustration with continued depression.
3. Indifference in response to the client's criticisms.
4. Rescue fantasy with a depressed client.
5. Anger at help-rejecting behavior.

See Appendix C for answers.

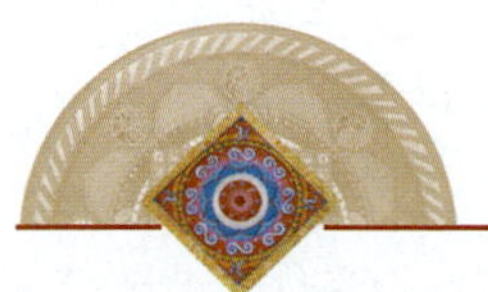

REFERENCES

Altman, S., Haeri, S., Cohen, L. J., Ten, A., Barron, E., Galynker, I., et al. (2006). Predictors of relapse in bipolar disorder: A review. *Journal of Psychiatric Practice, 12*(5), 269–282.

American Psychiatric Association. (2000). *Diagnostic and statistical manual of mental disorders* (4th ed., Text Revision). Washington, DC: Author.

Beck, A. T., Steer, R. A., & Brown, G. K. (1996). *Manual for the Beck depression inventory-II.* San Antonio, Texas: Psychological Corporation.

Bowlby, J. (1973). *Attachment and loss: Separation, anxiety, and anger.* New York: Basic Books.

Brosche, T. A. (2007). A grief team within a healthcare system. *Dimensions of Critical Care Nursing, 26*(1), 21–28.

Clark, D. A., & Beck, A. T. (1999). *Scientific foundations of cognitive theory and therapy of depression.* New York: John Wiley & Sons.

Evans, A. M. (2007). Transference in the nurse-patient relationship. *Journal of Psychiatric and Mental Health Nursing, 14*(2), 189–195.

Friedman, B., Conwell, Y., & Delavan, R. L. (2007). Correlates of late-life major depression: A comparison of urban and rural primary care patients. *American Journal of Geriatric Psychiatry, 15*(1), 28-41.

Gaudiano, B. A., & Miller, I. W. (2006). Patients' expectancies, the alliance in pharmacotherapy, and treatment outcomes in bipolar disorder. *Journal of Consulting and Clinical Psychology, 74*(4), 671–676.

Harris, T. (2006). Volunteer befriending as an intervention for depression: Implications for bereavement care. *Bereavement Care, 25*(2), 27–30.

Horowitz, J. A., & Cousins, A. (2006). Postpartum depression treatment rates for at-risk women. *Nursing Research, 55*(2), Supplement 1, S23–S27.

Johnson, J. G., Zhang, B., Greer, J. A., & Prigerson, H. G. (2007). Parental control, partner dependency, and complicated grief among widowed adults in the community. *Journal of Nervous & Mental Disease, 195*(1), 26–30.

Joseph, A. (2006). *The impact of light on outcomes in healthcare settings.* Concord California Center for Health Design, Issue Paper #2.

Matchar, D., & Thakur, M. (2007). Testing for CYP450 polymorphisms in adults wth non-psychotic depression treated with SSRIs. *Agency for Healthcare Research and Quality Publication* No. 07–E002.

McDermott, M. A. N. (1995). Learned helplessness: A more discriminating nursing diagnosis. *Classification of nursing diagnoses: Proceedings of the eleventh conference, North American Nursing Diagnosis Association* (Rantz, M. J. et al.). Cinahl Information Systems. (Glendale, CA), 212–213.

McIntyre, R. S., Soczynska, J. K., Beyer, J. L., Woldeyohannes, H. O., Law, C. W. Y., Miranda, A., et al. (2007). Medical comorbidity in bipolar disorder: Reprioritizing unmet needs. *Current Opinion in Psychiatry, 20*(4), 406–416.

Murphy, K. (2006). Managing the ups and downs of bipolar disorder. *Nursing 2006, 36*(10), 58–64.

Noonan, P., Warren, B. J., & White, D. (2007). Diagnosis and pharmacologic treatment of bipolar disorder: A roundtable discussion. *Psychiatric Nurse Counseling Points,* American Psychiatric Nurses Association, 1(4).

Oei, T. P., Bullbeck, K., & Campbell, J. M. (2006). Cognitive change process during group cognitive behaviour therapy for depression. *Journal of Affective Disorders, 92*(2–3), 231–241.

Perlis, R. H., Brown, E., Baker, R. W., & Nierenberg, A. A. (2006). Clinical features of bipolar depression versus major depressive disorder in large multicenter trials. *American Journal of Psychiatry, 163*(2), 225–231.

Piper, W. E., Ogrodniczuk, J. S., Joyce, A. S., Weideman, R., & Rosie, J. S. (2007). Group composition and group therapy for complicated grief. *Journal of Consulting and Clinical Psychology, 75*(1), 116–125.

Posternak, M. A., Solomon, D. A., Leon, A. C., Mueller, T. I., Shea, M. T., Endicott, J., et al. (2006). The naturalistic course of unipolar major depression in the absence of somatic therapy. *Journal of Nervous & Mental Disease, 194*(5), 324–329.

Tietjen, G. E., Brandes, J. L., & Digre, K. B. (2007). High prevalence of somatic symptoms and depression in women with disabling chronic headache. *Neurology, 68*, 134–140.

Torres, L., & Rollock, D. (2007). Acculturation and depression among Hispanics: The moderating effect of intercultural competence. *Cultural Diversity & Ethnic Minority Psychology, 13*(1), 10–17.

Valente, S., & Nemec, C. (2006). An evidence-based project to improve depression and alcohol use screening. *Journal of Nursing Care Quality, 21*(1), 93–98.

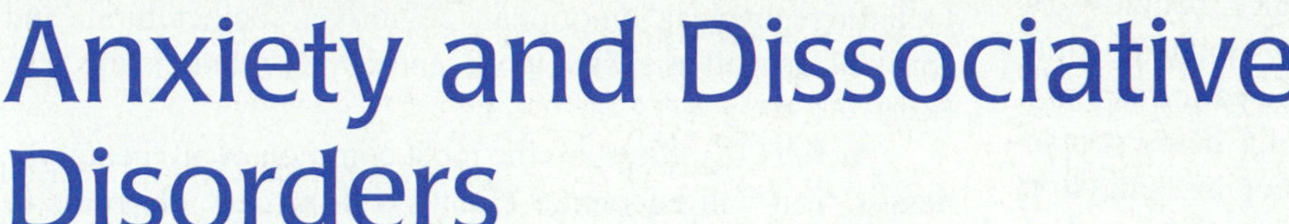

Anxiety and Dissociative Disorders

CHAPTER 18

SUE C. DELAUNE

LEARNING OUTCOMES

After completing this chapter, you will be able to:

1. Describe the theories that are helpful in understanding anxiety disorders and dissociative disorders.
2. Explain the concept of anxiety and how it relates to anxiety disorders and dissociative disorders.
3. Compare and contrast both the common themes and distinctive characteristics of anxiety disorders with dissociative disorders.
4. Incorporate an understanding of how dissociation serves as a defense mechanism for some individuals experiencing trauma into the care of clients with dissociative disorders.
5. Conduct a thorough and comprehensive assessment in the care of clients with anxiety and dissociative disorders.
6. Design a plan of care for intervening into mild, moderate, severe, and panic levels of anxiety.
7. Educate clients and their families about pharmacologic and nonpharmacologic measures for anxiety disorders and dissociative disorders.
8. Identify the possible personal challenges in caring for clients with anxiety disorders and dissociative disorders.

CRITICAL THINKING CHALLENGE

Barbara, a 32-year-old female diagnosed with dissociative identity disorder, has been admitted to the emergency department for attempting suicide by slashing her wrists. This is Barbara's fourth admission for self-inflicted wounds. You, the RN on duty, overhear another staff member referring to Barbara as someone who is "faking" her illness in order to gain attention. The other staff person says he does not believe in the existence of dissociative disorders and that "those people who say they have multiple personalities are making up their symptoms just to get some sympathy, just like those people who claim to suddenly remember sexual abuse from their childhood."

1. Is this staff member's assessment an accurate one?
2. Identify the elements you would consider in formulating a response to the staff member.
3. Should recovered memories of childhood sexual abuse be taken seriously?

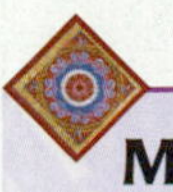

MEDIALINK 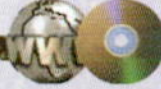 www.prenhall.com/kneisl

Go to the Pearson Health MediaLink CD-ROM and the Companion Website at www.prenhall.com/kneisl for interactive resources for this chapter.

KEY TERMS

acute stress disorder (ASD) *450*
agoraphobia *445*
alter *465*
anxiety disorders *444*
behavior modification *453*
compulsion *448*
depersonalization disorder *465*
dissociative amnesia *464*
dissociative disorders *464*
dissociative fugue *465*
dissociative identity disorder (DID) *465*
ego-dystonic *465*
free-floating anxiety *445*
generalized anxiety disorder (GAD) *447*
obsession *448*
obsessive–compulsive disorder (OCD) *448*
panic disorder *445*
pediatric autoimmune neuropsychiatric disorders associated with streptococci (PANDAS) *449*
phobia *445*
post-traumatic stress disorder (PTSD) *450*
social phobia *447*
specific phobia *447*
systematic desensitization *453*

Although anxiety is a universal experience, people vary in their ability to tolerate anxiety and anxiety-producing situations. Anxiety, a subjective feeling experienced in response to stressors, is a normal response that usually helps people cope with threatening situations. Common coping behaviors include withdrawal, acting out, avoidance, somatization, and problem solving. See Chapter 8 for a thorough discussion of the effects of anxiety and stress on individuals and levels of anxiety. This chapter examines the experience of individuals with anxiety disorders and dissociative disorders. People with these disorders have one thing in common: anxiety so disabling that their functioning is adversely affected.

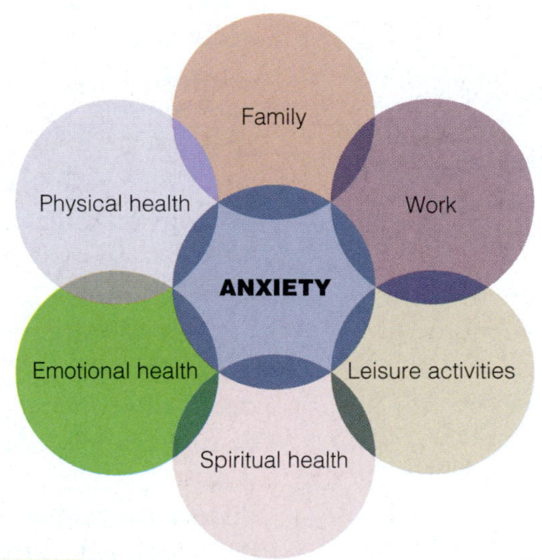

FIGURE 18-1 ■ The holistic impact of anxiety.

The functional disabilities may affect all dimensions of life, including physical, emotional, cognitive, sociocultural, and spiritual, as well as social, work, and family relationships (see FIGURE 18-1 ■).

Anxiety disorders are the most common of all mental illnesses. You will encounter clients with anxiety disorders in every clinical practice setting including primary care and general hospital settings, not just mental health facilities, and in your own community. What you learn about anxiety disorders in this chapter can be readily applied to your clinical work in any area in which you choose to work.

During their lifetimes, approximately 25% of Americans have an anxiety disorder (Antai-Otong, 2006). Anxiety disorders affect people of every socioeconomic status. It is also relatively common for a person to have one anxiety disorder coexisting with another.

ANXIETY DISORDERS

Anxiety disorders are characterized by a mixture of physiologic, psychological, behavioral, and cognitive symptoms. The types of anxiety disorders and their prevalence rates are listed in TABLE 18-1 ■. Anxiety disorders affect individuals of all ages, from childhood to senescence, and are one of the most common forms of mental disorders affecting adolescents (Farrugia & Hudson, 2006). Each anxiety disorder has its own distinct characteristics, but they all have the common theme of excessive, irrational fear and dread.

In anxiety disorders, anxiety is either the predominant disturbance, as in generalized anxiety disorder, or anxiety is experienced as avoidance behavior when the person attempts to master the symptoms, as in confronting the dreaded object

TABLE 18-1 ■ **Anxiety Disorders: Types and Prevalence**

Anxiety Disorder	Description	Prevalence
Acute stress disorder	A condition similar to post-traumatic stress disorder with a quicker onset and shorter duration	No long-term statistics available
Generalized anxiety disorder (GAD)	Persistent, pervasive, and exaggerated sense of worry and anxiety	3.1% (6.8 million)
Obsessive–compulsive disorder (OCD)	A combination of intrusive, irrational thoughts and stereotypical behavioral rituals performed to dispel the unwanted thoughts	1% (2.2 million)
Panic disorder	Feelings of extreme fear that occur for no apparent reason and are accompanied by intense physical symptoms	2.7% (2.4 million)
Phobias	Social phobia—fear of extreme embarrassment	6.8% (15 million)
	Agoraphobia—intense fear and avoidance of any situation in which escape might be difficult or help is unavailable	0.8% (1.8 million)
	Specific phobia—marked and persistent fear and compulsion to avoid the feared object or situation	8.7% (19.2 million)
Post-traumatic stress disorder (PTSD)	A reaction to a terrifying event; characterized by reexperiencing, avoidance/numbing, and hyperarousal	3.5% (7.7 million)

Note that percentages and numbers refer to the estimated incidence of occurrences in American adults within a given year.

Source: National Institute of Mental Health. (2006). *The numbers count: Mental disorders in America.* Retrieved January 2007 from http://www.nimh.nih.gov.

or situation in a phobic disorder. When anxiety is not related to a specific stimulus, it may be called **free-floating anxiety**.

People in anxiety states experience anxiety both as a subjective emotion and as a variety of physical symptoms resulting from muscular tension and autonomic nervous system activity. When acute, the anxiety drives the individual to seek help. When chronic, anxiety can lead to a number of somatic discomforts or disabilities (e.g., heartburn, epigastric distress, diarrhea, and constipation). Chronic muscular tension can lead to a variety of musculoskeletal aches and pains.

Onset of anxiety may be sudden or gradual. Some people experience an unexpected, incapacitating outbreak of acute anxiety, as in panic disorder. In other people (especially those with generalized anxiety disorder), anxiety may express itself through relatively mild somatic symptoms in which the existence of underlying anxiety is overlooked. Therefore, it is necessary to specifically assess the client's level of anxiety.

Panic Disorder

A common disorder, **panic disorder**, is characterized by recurrent attacks of severe anxiety lasting a few moments to an hour. These attacks are not associated with a stimulus but instead seem to occur suddenly and spontaneously. They may, however, become associated with certain situations, such as going to a shopping mall or driving a car. The person usually experiences physical symptoms such as palpitations, nausea, diarrhea, dyspnea, rapid pulse, and a feeling of choking or suffocation. The pupils are dilated, and the face is flushed. The person may feel dizzy or faint and often has a sense of impending doom or death. Restlessness is acute, and the person may make pleading, apprehensive appeals for help.

In its most advanced state, panic may create a group of symptoms that mimic myocardial infarction and mitral valve prolapse. Thus, the diagnosis of panic disorder is often not made until expensive medical procedures fail to provide a correct diagnosis. The following clinical example describes Loretta, who is experiencing a panic attack.

CLINICAL EXAMPLE

Loretta has been to her primary care physician on two different occasions convinced that she was having a heart attack. Both times, she was told that she was healthy. However, Loretta continued to experience palpitations, rapid pulse, and dizziness. Fearful that she would be labeled a hypochondriac, Loretta was reluctant to visit her physician again.

When panic attacks occur frequently and interfere with the person's functional abilities at work, school, or in the family, the condition is called panic disorder. People who have repeated attacks, or persistently worry about having another attack, are diagnosed with panic disorder. Anticipatory fear of helplessness or of losing control during a panic attack is a common occurrence. The individual frequently avoids situations that induce the fear, sometimes developing a phobic avoidance reaction. The next clinical example shows the impact of panic attacks on a person's functional abilities.

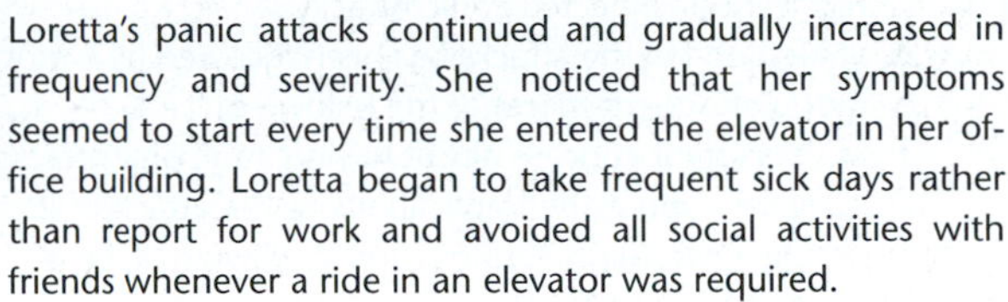

CLINICAL EXAMPLE

Loretta's panic attacks continued and gradually increased in frequency and severity. She noticed that her symptoms seemed to start every time she entered the elevator in her office building. Loretta began to take frequent sick days rather than report for work and avoided all social activities with friends whenever a ride in an elevator was required.

Agoraphobia, the marked fear of being in public places from which escape might be difficult or in which help might not be available (which often leads to the fear of being alone), is secondary to panic attacks. The DSM-IV-TR states that a diagnosis of panic disorder with agoraphobia is appropriate for an individual who experiences panic attacks and has phobic avoidance. In the absence of phobic avoidance, the condition is termed panic disorder without agoraphobia. Agoraphobia without panic attacks is uncommon. Agoraphobia with symptoms of panic attack is now treatable with some medications (e.g., antidepressants). See the DSM-IV-TR diagnostic criteria for panic disorder with and without agoraphobia.

Panic disorder is usually first noted in late adolescence or early adulthood. It is estimated to be one of the most frequently occurring psychiatric problems (Zwanzger & Rupprecht, 2005). It may be limited to a single brief period lasting several weeks or months, recur several times, or become chronic. Panic disorder is diagnosed much more frequently in women than in men, and may be related to sudden object loss and separation anxiety in childhood. Physical disorders such as hypoglycemia, hyperthyroidism, and amphetamine or caffeine intoxication must be ruled out before a diagnosis of panic disorder can be made. The ways in which hypoglycemia mimics a panic attack are discussed in the Caring for the Spirit feature.

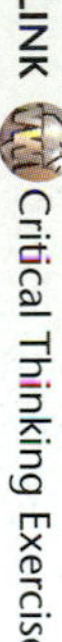

MediaLink Critical Thinking Exercise: Panic Attack

Phobic Disorders

A **phobia** is a persistent and irrational fear of a specific object, activity, or situation that results in a compelling desire to avoid the dreaded object or situation. Nearly all phobic individuals experience panic when in contact with the phobic situation. The fear is recognized by adults or adolescents as unreasonable in proportion to the actual danger. However, children do not always identify their fears as unrealistic.

In the development of phobia, fear arises through a process of displacing an unconscious conflict onto an external object symbolically related to the conflict. Thus, in becoming phobic, the individual fears a specific external object rather than an unknown internal source of distress. The phobic person can then control the intensity of the anxiety by avoiding the object with which the anxiety is associated.

MediaLink Panic Disorder Video

A diagnosis of phobic disorder is generally made when the avoidance behavior becomes extreme or the problem so

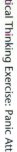

DSM-IV-TR Diagnostic Criteria for Panic Disorder

Diagnostic Criteria for Panic Disorder Without Agoraphobia and Panic Disorder With Agoraphobia

A. Both 1 and 2:
   1. recurrent unexpected Panic Attacks
   2. at least one of the attacks has been followed by 1 month (or more) of one (or more) of the following:
      a. persistent concern about having additional attacks
      b. worry about the implications of the attack or its consequences (e.g., losing control, having a heart attack, "going crazy")
      c. a significant change in behavior related to the attacks

B. The presence of Agoraphobia (for 300.21 Panic Disorder With Agoraphobia)
   OR
   The absence of Agoraphobia (for 300.01 Panic Disorder Without Agoraphobia)

C. The Panic Attacks are not due to the direct physiological effects of a substance (e.g., a drug of abuse, a medication) or a general medical condition (e.g., hyperthyroidism).

D. The Panic Attacks are not better accounted for by another mental disorder, such as Social Phobia (e.g., occurring on exposure to feared social situations), Specific Phobia (e.g., on exposure to a specific phobic situation), Obsessive–Compulsive Disorder (e.g., on exposure to dirt in someone with an obsession about contamination), Post-traumatic Stress Disorder (e.g., in response to stimuli associated with a severe stressor), or Separation Anxiety Disorder (e.g., in response to being away from home or close relatives).

Source: Reprinted with permission from the *Diagnostic and Statistical Manual of Mental Disorders,* Fourth Edition, Text Revision. (Copyright 2000). American Psychiatric Association.

USING DSM-IV-TR

Health care providers often use language unfamiliar to clients and their families. Define *agoraphobia* in terms that a client and family members can easily understand.

pervasive that it interferes with the person's normal functional ability. Phobic disorders are classified into three main types:

1. Agoraphobia: Fear of being alone or in public places from which escape might be difficult or help might not be available
2. Social phobia: Fear of situations in which the individual may be exposed to scrutiny by others or that may be humiliating or embarrassing
3. Specific phobia: Fear of specific objects

Agoraphobia

Individuals with agoraphobia often fear leaving the safety of home, worrying that they might develop an incapacitating symptom, such as dizziness, loss of bowel or bladder control, or cardiac distress. Normal activities are increasingly curtailed as the fears dominate the person's life. Agoraphobic people often limit travel and need a companion when away from home. Those who endure the phobic situation experience intense anxiety.

Agoraphobia without panic attacks is relatively rare. More commonly, people with agoraphobia have spontaneous panic attacks. Most people with agoraphobia have a history of generalized anxiety or anxiety attacks at the onset of the phobic behavior. Onset of this disorder usually occurs in the middle to late twenties. Agoraphobia is more frequently diagnosed in women than in men. Separation anxiety in childhood and sudden object loss appear to be predisposing factors. Depression, anxiety, rituals, minor "checking" compulsions, and rumination are frequently associated features of agoraphobia.

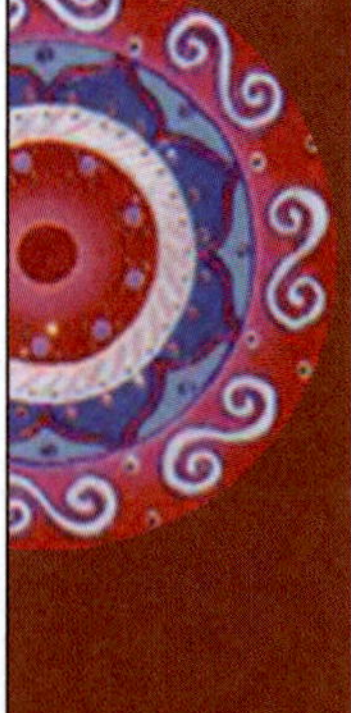

CARING FOR THE SPIRIT

Can Hypoglycemia Mimic an Anxiety Attack?

Much has been written in the lay press about the dangers of low blood sugar. Some popular authors claim it is a major scourge that afflicts millions of Americans, causing severe psychologic harm.

Postprandial hypoglycemia is a drop in plasma glucose following a carbohydrate load. It can occur after gastric surgery or in the very early stages of diabetes. However, when it has no clear-cut organic cause, it is called functional hypoglycemia.

Functional low blood sugar occurs in two major ways. Epinephrine-like signs and symptoms include nervousness, faintness, weakness, tremulousness, palpitations, sweating, and hunger. Central nervous system signs and symptoms include headache, confusion, visual disturbances, muscle weakness, ataxia, and marked personality changes.

Although there is little controlled clinical research to support the popular media view, psychiatric–mental health nurses should not dismiss hypoglycemia as a hypochondriac's invention. Negating a client's symptoms is akin to accusing the client of lying. Such insults wound the soul by dehumanizing the person. As holistic healers, nurses tend to the spirit by actively listening to the client and demonstrating support in all domains—physical, emotional, cognitive, and spiritual.

The prognoses for people with agoraphobia are variable. Some less severely disturbed individuals experience intermittent symptoms and may have periods of remission. Those who are more severely impaired may suffer lifelong disability.

Social Phobia

Social phobia (also referred to as social anxiety disorder) is characterized by persistent fear and avoidance of situations in which the person may be exposed to scrutiny by others. The person especially fears being humiliated or embarrassed. Examples of social phobias are extreme fear of performing or speaking in public, making complaints, or writing or eating in front of others. Other common phobias include fear of interacting with members of the opposite sex, superiors, or aggressive individuals. Usually a person has only one social phobia. This disorder is characterized by overwhelming anxiety and excessive self-consciousness in everyday situations.

According to the DSM-IV-TR, 10% to 20% of people who have anxiety disorders are also affected by social phobias. Generalized anxiety, agoraphobia, or specific phobia may also coexist with social phobia. Often appearing in late childhood or early adolescence, social phobia usually progresses to a chronic course. Although symptoms may decrease in middle age, the disorder is usually lifelong with only occasional remissions. Familial pattern and predisposing factors are unknown and the incidence is evenly distributed between men and women.

Specific Phobia

More common than any other type of phobic disorder, a **specific phobia** is an isolated fear focused on one situation or object, such as darkness, heights, or animals. This category of phobic disorders encompasses all phobias not included in agoraphobia or social phobia. Many specific phobias begin in childhood and subsequently disappear. Those that persist into adulthood rarely go away without treatment. Specific phobia is more often diagnosed in females than in males. One specific phobia in children that is often overlooked is school phobia, a serious problem that affects approximately 5% of elementary and middle school children (Tyrell, 2005). When not detected early and treated appropriately, the consequences may be academic failure, impaired social relationships, and self-esteem problems.

Specific phobias generally cause minimal impairment if the phobic object is rarely encountered and easily avoided; for example, a fear of snakes does not seriously impair an individual living in a high-rise condominium. The phobia can, however, be incapacitating if the phobic situation is frequently encountered and not easily avoided. A fear of heights or elevators would seriously incapacitate a person living in a high-rise condominium. A specific phobia may lead to lifestyle restrictions that vary in severity according to the degree of anxiety. A list of common, uncommon, and curious specific phobias appears in Table 18-2 ■.

The object or situation avoided determines the subtype of specific phobia. The DSM-IV-TR identifies these subtypes as:

- Animal type: Fear related to animals, birds, or insects
- Natural environment type: Fear triggered by elements of nature, such as water or weather
- Blood–injection–injury type: Fear caused by the sight of blood or injury, or by receiving invasive medical procedures, such as an injection. The vasovagal response often occurs with this type of phobic reaction. There is a strong familial pattern with this subtype.
- Situational type: Fear resulting from contact with enclosed places, bridges, and/or public transportation

Table 18-2 ■ Common, Uncommon, and Curious Phobias

Name of Phobia	Specific Fear
Acrophobia	Heights
Agoraphobia	Open spaces or crowds
Algophobia	Pain
Androphobia	Men
Arachnophobia	Spiders
Astraphobia	Thunder and lightning
Astrophobia	Stars and celestial space
Aviophobia	Flying
Claustrophobia	Enclosed places
Coprophobia	Excrement
Cynophobia	Dogs
Entomophobia	Insects
Erythrophobia	Blushing
Hematophobia	Blood
Hydrophobia	Water
Iatrophobia	Doctors
Lalophobia	Speaking
Necrophobia	Dead bodies
Nyctophobia	Darkness, night
Odynophobia	Pain
Ophidiphobia	Snakes
Pathophobia	Disease
Peccatophobia	Committing a sin
Phonophobia	Speaking aloud
Pyrophobia	Fire
Sitophobia	Food, eating
Taphophobia	Being buried alive
Thanatophobia	Death
Toxophobia	Being poisoned
Xenophobia	Strangers
Zoophobia	Animals

Generalized Anxiety Disorder

Generalized anxiety disorder (GAD) is considered less specific and less debilitating than panic disorder and phobic disorder. GAD is characterized by pervasive, persistent anxiety of at least 6 months' duration but without phobias, panic attacks, or obsessions and compulsions. The person experiences chronic feelings of nervousness and apprehension for no apparent reason and is unable to control the worry. The worry is greatly exaggerated in relation to the probability that the event will actually occur.

People with GAD are unable to stop worrying, even though they realize that their anxiety is more intense than the situation warrants. Overall, those with GAD are unable to relax. The excessive worries usually lead to insomnia and are associated with physical symptoms such as muscle tension, headaches, sweating, hot flashes, headaches, shortness of breath, and dizziness. Irritability is a common psychological manifestation of GAD. Autonomic symptoms may be less frequent or less severe than in panic attacks. In order to accurately diagnose GAD, a thorough physical examination must be done to determine the presence of any medical conditions that lead to anxiety. Some medical conditions that may contribute to the development of anxiety are thyroid imbalances, endocrine problems, and cardiovascular disease.

There is little generally accepted information about age of onset, predisposing factors, cause of illness, prevalence, familial pattern, or sex ratio, although there appears to be a more equal sex ratio than in panic disorder. Associated mild depressive symptoms are not uncommon in individuals with GAD. Although impairment in social or occupational functioning is rarely more than mild, the abuse of alcohol or other drugs may be a serious complication that interferes with effective motivation for treatment.

MEDIALINK Care Plan: Obsessive–Compulsive Behavior

Obsessive–Compulsive Disorder

Obsessive–compulsive disorder (OCD) is classified as an anxiety disorder because of the anxiety symptoms that develop when an individual tries to resist an obsession or compulsion. An **obsession** is a recurring thought that cannot be dismissed from consciousness. These intrusive thoughts are sometimes trivial or ridiculous, often morbid or fearful, and always distressing and anxiety provoking. Other common obsessive thoughts have to do with violence or contamination. The following clinical example compares an innocuous obsession to a serious one.

MEDIALINK Obsessive–Compulsive Disorder Video

CLINICAL EXAMPLE

Ernesto's inability to get the nursery rhyme "snips and snails and puppy dog tails" out of his mind is an example of a strange but trivial obsession. Even though Ernesto tried to distract himself with activities, he found the rhyme running through his mind at work and at home, especially when he was trying to sleep at night.

Melinda's obsession was much more ominous. She could not stop thinking that she must kill her children in order to prevent a worldwide race war.

A **compulsion** is an uncontrollable, persistent urge to perform certain acts or behaviors in order to relieve an otherwise unbearable tension. Most compulsive acts are attempts to control or modify obsessions because the compulsive person either fears the consequences or is afraid he or she will not be able to control the primary impulse. Although compulsions are attempts to reduce tension, they eventually increase tension because the individual becomes increasingly agitated, unable to decide whether to stop or continue the compulsive actions.

Typical compulsive acts are endless hand washing, checking and rechecking doors to see if they have been locked, and elaborate dressing and undressing rituals. Such compulsive acts are defenses used to contain, neutralize, or ward off the anxiety related to the primary impulse. Compulsive acts such as counting and elaborately checking routine duties are frequently associated with the fear of failing or making a mistake, or with the need to be perfect. The following clinical example describes the progression of obsessive thoughts to compulsive behaviors.

CLINICAL EXAMPLE

Ernesto, the young man who could not dismiss the rhyme from his mind, developed a compulsion that involved ritualistic washing of his genitals to ward off the anxiety generated by his apparently silly obsession.

Melinda, obsessed with thoughts about killing her children, engaged in symbolic rituals of touching religious objects to repel evil influences through magical interventions by the saints.

The DSM-IV-TR feature on pae 449 lists the diagnostic criteria for obsessive–compulsive disorder.

People with OCD usually fear that they will harm someone or something. They rely heavily on avoidance and are best understood in terms of their control needs. Individuals who develop obsessive–compulsive symptoms have a great need to control themselves, others, and their environment. Obsessions and compulsions have the following features in common:

- An idea or impulse persistently intrudes into the person's awareness.
- A feeling of anxious dread accompanies the primary manifestation and often leads the person to take countermeasures against the forbidden thought or impulse.
- Both the obsessions and the compulsion are ego-alien—foreign to one's self-perception.
- No matter how compelling the obsession or compulsion, the person has enough insight to recognize it as irrational and experience it as a significant source of distress.

TABLE 18-3 ■ on page 449 lists some common obsessions and compulsions.

Many of the personality traits associated with obsession and compulsion are highly valued in American culture. Success in several professions and occupations demands cautiousness, deliberateness, and rationality. These traits are usually associated with the tendency toward obsession or compulsion. When these personality traits are car-

DSM-IV-TR Diagnostic Criteria for Obsessive–Compulsive Disorder

A. Either obsessions or compulsions:

Obsessions as defined by 1, 2, 3, and 4:

1. recurrent and persistent thoughts, impulses, or images that are experienced, at some time during the disturbance, as intrusive and inappropriate and that cause marked anxiety or distress
2. the thoughts, impulses, or images are not simply excessive worries about real-life problems
3. the person attempts to ignore or suppress such thoughts, impulses, or images, or to neutralize them with some other thought or action
4. the person recognizes that the obsessional thoughts, impulses, or images are a product of his or her own mind (not imposed from without as in thought insertion)

Compulsions as defined by 1 and 2:

1. repetitive behaviors (e.g., hand washing, ordering, checking) or mental acts (e.g., praying, counting, repeating words silently) that the person feels driven to perform in response to an obsession, or according to rules that must be applied rigidly
2. the behaviors or mental acts are aimed at preventing or reducing distress or preventing some dreaded event or situation; however, these behaviors or mental acts either are not connected in a realistic way with what they are designed to neutralize or prevent or are clearly excessive

B. At some point during the course of the disorder, the person has recognized that the obsessions or compulsions are excessive or unreasonable. **Note:** This does not apply to children.

C. The obsessions or compulsions cause marked distress, are time consuming (take more than 1 hour a day); or significantly interfere with the person's normal routine, occupational (or academic) functioning, or usual social activities or relationships.

D. If another Axis I disorder is present, the content of the obsessions or compulsions is not restricted to it (e.g., preoccupation with food in the presence of an Eating Disorder; hair pulling in the presence of Trichotillomania; concern with appearance in the presence of Body Dysmorphic Disorder; preoccupation with drugs in the presence of a Substance Use Disorder; preoccupation with having a serious illness in the presence of Hypochondriasis; preoccupation with sexual urges or fantasies in the presence of a Paraphilia; or guilty ruminations in the presence of Major Depressive Disorder).

E. The disturbance is not due to the direct physiological effects of a substance (e.g., a drug of abuse, a medication) or a general medical condition.

Specify if:

With Poor Insight: if, for most of the time during the current episode, the person does not recognize that the obsessions and compulsions are excessive or unreasonable

Source: Reprinted with permission from the *Diagnostic and Statistical Manual of Mental Disorders,* Fourth Edition, Text Revision. (Copyright 2000). American Psychiatric Association.

USING DSM-IV-TR

Health care providers often use language unfamiliar to clients and their families. Explain obsession and compulsion in such a way that clients and family members can understand the difference.

ried to an extreme, or when the balance between control and impulse expression leads to paralysis, they become a liability.

OCD is equally common in both men and women. For many years, it was believed that OCD was extremely rare. Recent reports show that OCD is the 10th leading cause of disability of all medical conditions in the industrialized world (Eisen et al., 2006).

Children with Obsessive–Compulsive Disorder

Although OCD is usually diagnosed in older adolescents or young adults, children may also be affected by the disorder. Recent studies (Kirvan, Swedo, Snider, & Cunningham, 2006; Storch et al., 2006) have examined **pediatric autoimmune neuropsychiatric disorders associated with streptococci (PANDAS)**. The term *PANDAS* is used to describe a

TABLE 18-3 ■ Common Obsessive–Compulsive Behaviors

Behavior	Related Compulsion	Related Obsession
Repetitious hand washing	Urge to wash, scrub, or clean	Fear of disease or contamination
Returning home often to make sure appliances are turned off	Need to recheck related to self-doubt	Fear of disaster
Hoarding junk mail, receipts, and all types of papers	Need to keep everything	Fear of losing things
Ritualistic counting of number of stairs climbed	Urge to count repeatedly	Belief that counting will yield control and thus prevent making mistakes
Avoiding stepping on seams of tiles, carpets, sidewalks	Need for order and routine	Belief that order and routine will negate all anxiety

subset of children who have OCD and/or tic disorders, such as Tourette's syndrome, and in whom symptoms have exacerbated following streptococcal infections, such as strep throat. (Tic disorders are discussed in Chapter 26.) It is theorized that an antibody against strep throat bacteria mistakenly acts on a brain enzyme and disrupts communication between neurons. Children with PANDAS seem to have dramatic fluctuations in OCD and/or tic severity; that is, the children have "good days" and "bad days." OCD does occur in children without PANDAS. However, when a child has a very episodic course of OCD/tic symptoms and has had strep throat prior to or during a dramatic worsening of the symptoms, the possibility of PANDAS should be considered.

Post-Traumatic Stress Disorder

Post-traumatic stress disorder (PTSD) is the experience of a significant stressor or trauma, outside the range of usual experience, that is followed by recurrent subjective reexperiencing of the trauma. The types of trauma that precipitate PTSD are varied, including military combat, criminal attack (i.e., assault, rape), child abuse (especially incest), terrorist attack (i.e., bombing, skyjacking), and natural catastrophes (i.e., earthquakes, tornadoes, hurricanes). Children who have witnessed violence in their families, schools, or communities are also vulnerable to developing PTSD.

The psychological effects of trauma affect individuals throughout their lifetimes. As Moller and Rice tell us, "Despite the human capacity to survive and adapt, traumatic experiences can cause alterations in health, attitudes and behaviors, environmental and interpersonal functioning, and spiritual balance such that the memory of an event or a set of events taints all other experiences" (Moller & Rice, 2006, p. 22). The violence associated with rape, whether experienced or witnessed, is severe enough to precipitate the onset of PTSD. For further discussion of PTSD as it relates to the experience of rape or incest, see Chapter 24. For further discussion of PTSD as it relates to the experience of a natural or man-made disaster, see Chapter 34. The following clinical example provides a description of combat-related PTSD.

CLINICAL EXAMPLE

Bill and Joe, who are veterans of military action in Afghanistan and Iraq, are enrolled in a PTSD program at a veterans' hospital outpatient clinic. Upon returning home from combat, they essentially relived their experiences through recurrent nightmares about intermittent explosive devices. They both experienced insomnia and a loss of pleasure in previously enjoyed activities. Both men had trouble concentrating. Bill felt guilty about surviving when other men in his unit did not. Joe felt guilty about the actions he had to take in order to survive.

A common manifestation in individuals with PTSD is hyperarousal when reexperiencing the traumatic event. As a result, the person is unable to relax; hypervigilance occurs and the person is always "on edge." Another common feature of PTSD is dissociation, in which emotions about the traumatic event are blocked. The individual becomes emotionally numb and experiences impaired social relationships.

People with PTSD avoid the stimuli associated with the traumatic event. For example, a woman who is raped in an elevator may avoid using any elevator—an example of how PTSD can restrict daily functioning. A significant complicating problem is the person's use of alcohol or other substances in an attempt to maintain control and soothe emotions. The DSM-IV-TR diagnostic criteria for PTSD are listed in the DSM box on page 451.

The course of PTSD is variable. Most people who have suffered a significant stressor tend to have an acute reaction from which they recover spontaneously. In others, however, the reaction may be delayed or prolonged and eventually become chronic. PTSD is characterized by high rates of chronicity and comorbidity. PTSD is divided into categories according to onset and duration of symptoms:

- Acute: Symptoms last less than 3 months
- Chronic: Symptoms last 3 months or more
- Delayed onset: At least 6 months have elapsed between the trauma and the occurrence of symptoms

PTSD can occur in people of any age, including children and elders. According to Crane and Clements (2005), postdisaster assessment for children and adolescents must include psychological, as well as physical, domains. Since traumatic events can have a long-lasting effect on a person's well-being, it is important that you assess older adult clients for indicators of the disorder (Murray, 2005). Across the lifespan, associated symptoms of depression, anxiety, and increased irritability are common, sometimes leading to unpredictable explosions of hostility with little or no provocation.

Acute Stress Disorder

Acute stress disorder (ASD) is the development of anxiety and dissociative symptoms that occur within 1 month of an extremely traumatic event. The precipitating stressors of ASD are similar to those of PTSD. They include exposure to a trauma in which the individual experienced or witnessed event(s) that involved actual or threatened injury or death and were accompanied by feelings of intense helplessness, fear, or horror (see Chapter 34). As in PTSD, the precipitating event must be a trauma that is outside the usual human experience. The traumatic event may be a natural disaster or human-induced event (e.g., rape, terrorist bombing). One type of trauma that often triggers ASD is disasters, which may disrupt the normal functioning of a community and overwhelm personal and community resources (Mitchell, Sakraida, & Zalice, 2005). Individuals feel overwhelmed as a result of the trauma and are unable to cope effectively.

Although it is similar to PTSD, ASD can be differentiated in the following ways:

- The duration is shorter.
- The interval from the trauma to the development of symptoms is shorter.

DSM-IV-TR Diagnostic Criteria for Post-Traumatic Stress Disorder

A. The person has been exposed to a traumatic event in which both the following were present:
   1. the person experienced, witnessed, or was confronted with an event or events that involved actual or threatened death or serious injury, or a threat to the physical integrity of self or other
   2. the person's response involved intense fear, helplessness, or horror

   Note: In children, this may be expressed instead by disorganized or agitated behavior.

B. The traumatic event is persistently reexperienced in one (or more) of the following ways:
   1. recurrent and intrusive distressing recollections of the event, including images, thoughts, or perceptions

   Note: In young children, repetitive play may occur in which themes or aspects of the trauma are expressed.

   2. recurrent distressing dreams of the event

   Note: In children, there may be frightening dreams without recognizable content.

   3. acting or feeling as if the traumatic event were recurring (includes a sense of reliving the experience, illusions, hallucinations, and dissociative flashback episodes, including those that occur on awakening or when intoxicated)

   Note: In young children, trauma-specific reenactment may occur.

   4. intense psychological distress at exposure to internal or external cues that symbolize or resemble an aspect of the traumatic event
   5. physiological reactivity on exposure to internal or external cues that symbolize or resemble an aspect of the traumatic event

C. Persistent avoidance of stimuli associated with the trauma and numbing of general responsiveness (not present before the trauma), as indicated by three (or more) of the following:
   1. efforts to avoid thoughts, feelings, or conversations associated with the trauma
   2. efforts to avoid activities, places, or people that arouse recollections of the trauma
   3. inability to recall an important aspect of the trauma
   4. markedly diminished interest or participation in significant activities
   5. feeling of detachment or estrangement from others
   6. restricted range of affect (e.g., unable to have loving feelings)
   7. sense of a foreshortened future (e.g., does not expect to have a career, marriage, children, or a normal life span)

D. Persistent symptoms of increased arousal (not present before the trauma), as indicated by two (or more) of the following:
   1. difficulty falling or staying asleep
   2. irritability or outbursts of anger
   3. difficulty concentrating
   4. hypervigilance
   5. exaggerated startle response

E. Duration of the disturbance (symptoms in Criteria B, C, and D) is more than 1 month.

F. The disturbance causes clinically significant distress or impairment in social, occupational, or other important areas of functioning.

Specify if:

Acute: if duration of symptoms is less than 3 months

Chronic: if duration of symptoms is 3 months or more

Specify if:

With Delayed Onset: if onset of symptoms is at least 6 months after the stressor.

Source: Reprinted with permission from the *Diagnostic and Statistical Manual of Mental Disorders,* Fourth Edition, Text Revision. (Copyright 2000). American Psychiatric Association.

USING DSM-IV-TR

Health care providers often use language unfamiliar to clients and their families. Reword this DSM description to make it easier for clients and family members to understand: "recurrent and intrusive distressing recollections of the event."

- The person has at least three of these dissociative manifestations: sense of detachment or numbing, depersonalization, derealization, dissociative amnesia, decreased awareness of surroundings (being in a "daze").
- The dissociative symptoms interfere with effective coping.

Dissociation is a common experience for individuals with ASD, just as in those with PTSD. Severity of the ASD, according to Moulds and Bryant (2005), is associated with impoverished memory for trauma-related material.

Individuals with ASD may experience depression accompanied by despair and helplessness. Thus, there is a very real danger of suicide (refer to the thorough discussion of suicide in Chapter 23 ∞). The individuals may feel they are responsible for the outcome of the trauma. For example, if another person was killed in the traumatic event, survival guilt frequently occurs. People affected by ASD often neglect safety precautions and basic needs for daily living. The next clinical example describes the onset of ASD as a response to a natural disaster.

CLINICAL EXAMPLE

William was living in New Orleans when Hurricane Katrina caused devastating flooding of the city. He was unable to evacuate prior to the storm and had to be rescued from his rooftop by a Coast Guard helicopter crew. William and his family were stranded on the roof for 3 days before rescue. On the second day, William's 82-year-old mother fell off the roof and drowned. Even though William desperately tried to save her, she was swept away by the water. William also saw several neighbors drown in the floodwaters. William's symptoms of acute stress disorder began 1 week after the traumatic event.

BIOPSYCHOSOCIAL THEORIES

There are several schools of thought regarding the causes of anxiety disorders.

Biological Factors

Refresh your understanding of the biologic basis of anxiety disorders by referring to FIGURE 18-2 ■, which illustrates the physiologic responses in anxiety disorders in relationship to the sympathetic and parasympathetic divisions of the central nervous system. Notice that they are the same as the fight-or-flight response described in Chapter 8. A major research question that remains unanswered is: Are the physiologic imbalances a *cause* or a *result* of the anxiety disorder?

Recent research findings point to biologic changes in the brains of individuals experiencing anxiety disorders. Some of those findings are:

- The noradrenergic system in the brain is especially sensitive to the neurotransmitter norepinephrine (NE). One section of the noradrenergic system, called the locus ceruleus (located in the brain stem), appears to be involved in precipitating panic attacks. Drugs that increase the activity of the locus ceruleus have been found to cause panic attacks; drugs that inhibit the activity of the locus ceruleus block panic attacks (see Figure 18-2). Tricyclic antidepressant medications stabilize the locus ceruleus and noradrenergic system; thus, they are sometimes useful in alleviating the symptoms associated with panic attack (Sadock & Sadock, 2005).
- The dopamine system is involved in the pathophysiology of OCD in males who develop the disorder at an early age (Denys, Van Nieuwerburgh, Deforce, & Westenberg, 2006).
- The brain's benzodiazepine (BZD) receptor system is especially sensitive to BZDs. The BZDs enhance the action of gamma-aminobutyric acid (GABA), an inhibitory neurotransmitter. With the administration of GABA, or medications that potentiate GABA, anxiety is reduced. On the other hand, medications that inhibit the activity of GABA increase anxiety (Sadock & Sadock, 2005). GABA may have a slight tranquilizing effect (Bourne, 2005).
- Dysfunction of GABA receptors significantly affects the development of panic disorder (Zwanzger & Rupprecht, 2005).
- Abnormal control of glutamate (an excitatory amino acid) plays a role in anxiety disorders. In one study, a medication (riluzole) used in the treatment of amyotrophic lateral sclerosis (ALS, or Lou Gehrig disease) curbed anxiety by inhibiting the release of glutamate (Mathew, Amkiel, & Coplan, 2005).
- Hormonal changes experienced during pregnancy may affect the onset, duration, and intensity of certain anxiety disorders. For example, some women with panic disorder have a reduction in their symptoms during pregnancy as a result of increased levels of progesterone. The metabolism of progesterone results in byproducts that exert BZD-like effects, thus calming the panicked woman (Anxiety Disorders Association of America, 2007).
- Some pregnant women experience OCD symptoms for the first time after conception. This is theorized to be a result of hormonal changes (Anxiety Disorders Association of America, 2007).
- Lactic acid levels are higher in some individuals experiencing panic attack. Lactic acid may actually precipitate anxiety in some people (Bourne, 2005).
- Many substances increase anxiety levels. Caffeine stimulates the central nervous system (CNS) and increases NE production. In fact, caffeine produces the same physiologic arousal response experienced with exposure to stress. The result is increased sympathetic nervous system activity and a release of adrenalin. Caffeine causes some people to remain in a chronically tense, aroused condition and may trigger panic attacks.
- Nicotine is another substance that is a suspected trigger for panic attacks. Nicotine, which is a strong stimulant, results in increased physiologic arousal, vasoconstriction, and increased blood pressure. Nicotine consumers tend to sleep less well than nonsmokers.

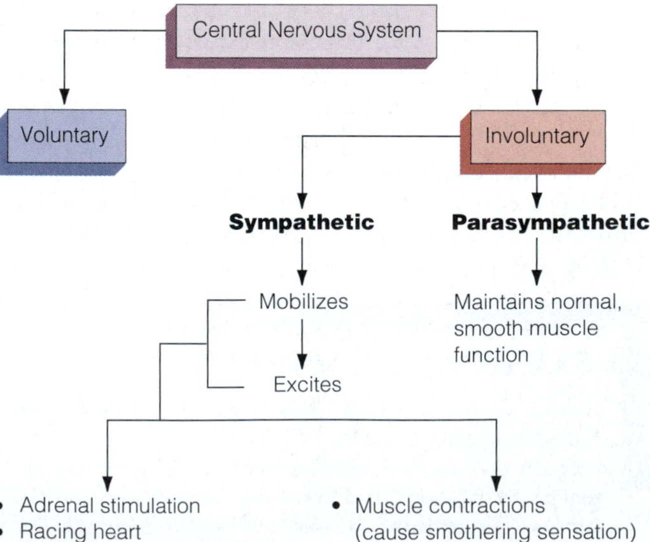

FIGURE 18-2 ■ Physiologic responses in anxiety disorders.

Genetic Theories

Research evidence indicates that a familial predisposition for anxiety disorders may exist. According to twin studies, there is a genetic factor in OCD and panic disorder (APA, 2000). First-degree relatives of people with panic disorder are four to seven times more likely to develop panic disorder (APA, 2000). In approximately 25% of individuals with GAD, there is a family history of the disorder (Sadock & Sadock, 2005).

Strong research evidence suggests that the transmission of certain genes contributes to the development of OCD. One example is the development of early-onset OCD. There is an alteration in serotonin synthesis in the brains of children and adolescents who develop OCD (Mossner et al, 2006). Another study (Arnold, Sicard, Burroughs, Richter, & Kennedy, 2006) identifies a genetic marker that predisposes some males to develop OCD.

Psychosocial Theories

Psychoanalytic theory views anxiety as a sign of psychologic conflict resulting from the threatened emergence into consciousness of forbidden or repressed ideas and/or emotions. The individual fears expressing the forbidden impulses; anxiety is an outcome of repressing such impulses. Other analytic views, sometimes referred to as neo-Freudian, evolved from the work of Freud and differ on the nature of anxiety. Rank (1952) believed that anxiety can be traced back to birth trauma. Sullivan (1953) stressed the importance of the early relationship between the mother and the child and the transmission of the mother's anxiety to the child.

According to the psychoanalytic model, the unconscious conflict must be brought into conscious awareness so that the real source of anxiety can be discovered and resolved. Treatment takes the form of analysis or the less time-consuming psychodynamic psychotherapy.

Behavioral Theories

Behaviorists (learning theorists) view anxiety as a learned response that can be unlearned. For example, behaviorists believe that the cause of phobias is traumatic exposure to the avoided object, situation, or activity. According to this theory, during the development of obsessions, an original neutral obsessive thought evokes anxiety because it becomes associated with an anxiety-provoking stimulus. In compulsions, a person discovers that a certain action relieves anxiety associated with the obsessive thought. The person repeats the action to achieve relief until eventually the act becomes a learned pattern of behavior. Compulsive behavior is viewed as a maladaptive attempt to alleviate anxiety.

Behavior modification is a treatment approach that teaches clients new ways to behave. "Conditioning" techniques—using positive and negative reinforcements—are examples of modification techniques. One behavior modification technique is **systematic desensitization**, a process in which a client builds up tolerance to anxiety through gradual exposure to a series of anxiety-provoking stimuli. The client is taught relaxation techniques that are to be used whenever the anxiety increases.

Behavioral approaches are often effective in the treatment of anxiety and are widely used for modifying symptoms in phobic disorder and obsessive–compulsive disorder (see Chapter 31 ∞). Behavioral therapists believe it is unnecessary to use insight-oriented psychotherapy to help clients cope with the anxiety. Instead, clients need only face the anxiety repeatedly until it becomes manageable. Behavioral treatment approaches are often used in treating phobias because the methods are more efficient, less costly, and less time consuming than insight-oriented psychotherapy treatment. Like some psychodynamically and psychoanalytically oriented therapists, behavioral therapists tend to avoid the use of medication because they believe it may interfere with the client's ability to learn more appropriate behaviors.

Humanistic Theories

The humanistic perspective is particularly important in understanding anxiety disorders. Environmental stressors, biologic factors, and intrapsychic fears or conflicts cannot be adequately dealt with separately but only as they interact with one another. For example, clients suffering from a phobic disorder experience shame and helplessness as they attempt to cope with fears of annihilation in the presence of the dreaded object or situation. The result may be interpersonal withdrawal and functional impairment, which create long-lasting disability.

This perspective has given rise to a multifaceted approach to the care of clients with anxiety disorders. Humanistic treatment approaches are integrative and may include a range of psychotherapeutic interventions, including psychotherapy (cognitive, behavioral, and/or dynamic), measures to develop effective social support systems, measures to reduce environmental stress, and psychopharmacologic treatment.

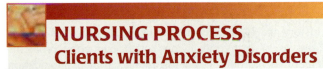

NURSING PROCESS
Clients with Anxiety Disorders

Chapter 8 ∞ covers concepts of anxiety, stress, and coping that are relevant to the care of clients with anxiety disorders; it also covers the general anxiety continuum and the need to identify the client's level of anxiety. The subject of this section is the nurse's role with clients whose anxiety is severe enough to be classified as an anxiety disorder. A nursing care plan for a client with Panic Disorder with Agoraphobia is at the end of this chapter.

MediaLink: Anxiety Disorders Association of America

Assessment

Clients with anxiety disorders have impaired psychosocial and physiologic function. The emotional disturbances and physical and intellectual changes that take place as a result of extreme or chronic anxiety affect the client's work, school, and social functioning and frequently impair or threaten previously meaningful interpersonal relationships. The clinical manifestations are listed in the Your Assessment Approach feature on page 454. Clients can also review a variety of self-tests for GAD, OCD, PTSD, and other anxiety disorders on www.adaa.org. You can also access these self-tests through the Companion Website for this book.

The occurrence of acute anxiety and its related symptoms is common to a number of physical conditions and acute medical emergencies. Therefore, a careful evaluation should

MEDIALINK Case Study: Assessing the Client with Anxiety

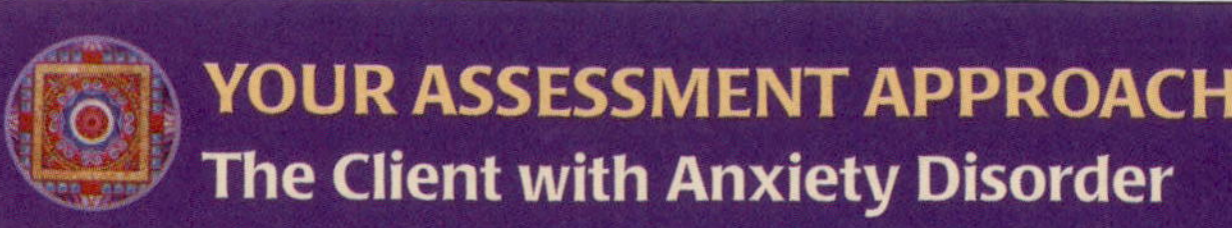

YOUR ASSESSMENT APPROACH
The Client with Anxiety Disorder

Use the questions that follow as guidelines for assessing clients with anxiety disorders.

Physiologic Assessment

- How often do you experience palpitations (heart pounding)?
- Do you have difficulty breathing?
- Do you experience muscle tightness? If so, where, and how long does it last?
- How often do you experience changes in bladder or bowel function?
- How do your symptoms affect your sleep?

Psychological Assessment

- Do you feel sad and/or hopeless?
- How often do you lose your temper?
- Do you enjoy being with other people?
- How often do you criticize yourself?

Cognitive Assessment

- Do you think about the same things over and over?
- Do you frequently have trouble concentrating on important activities?
- How often do you worry about the past or the future?
- Do you still enjoy activities that were pleasurable for you in the past?

YOUR ASSESSMENT APPROACH
The Client with Panic Attack

To determine the psychological effects of panic on your client, ask:	To determine the somatic effects of panic on your client, ask:
■ How do you feel right now? ■ When did you start feeling this way? ■ Did this feeling start gradually or all at once? ■ How well are you able to concentrate? ■ How do you feel about the future? ■ Do you sometimes feel out of control?	■ Are you having chest pains or shortness of breath? ■ Have you felt dizzy or faint? ■ Can you hold your hands steady, or do they shake?

always be conducted to initiate appropriate treatment quickly. A history and physical examination should rule out such conditions as hyperthyroidism and other endocrine problems, Ménière's syndrome, brain disorders, caffeine intoxication, mitral valve prolapse, and medical emergencies (such as myocardial infarction).

Differentiation from other psychiatric diagnoses is difficult when anxiety and depression are mixed. The question of which one predominates can puzzle many practitioners and necessitates ongoing thorough assessment. Some ways to differentiate anxiety and depression are listed in Table 18-4 ■. Anxiety is part of many other clinical syndromes, such as schizophrenia and mood disorders. The medical diagnosis may be made on the basis of the dominant, most debilitating symptom.

During assessment, determine not only whether the client is anxious (and, if so, to what extent) but also the possible source of the anxiety. Knowing the source will help you plan and implement effective care. It is important to assess the client's perception of threat; the greater the perceived threat, the more intense the anxiety. For extremely anxious clients, suspend formal data gathering in favor of immediate, direct action to reduce anxiety. Common features of panic attack are listed in the Your Assessment Approach feature above.

Subjective Data

Clients with an anxiety disorder may report a variety of physical and emotional symptoms. It is important to encourage clients to describe symptoms in their own words and to explain how the symptoms affect their daily activities. They may report emotional distress, cognitive and perceptual changes, somatic discomforts, and/or role impairments.

Emotional Distress Clients with anxiety disorders may reveal a number of distressing emotional feelings:

- "I feel like something terrible is going to happen."
- "I feel helpless, vulnerable, for no reason at all!"
- "I just can't seem to enjoy life—everything bothers me."

Anger, guilt, feelings of worthlessness, and anguish frequently accompany anxiety. When the anxiety is acute or ex-

Table 18-4 ■ Comparison of Anxiety and Depression

Clinical Manifestations	Anxiety	Depression
Affect	Fear and/or dread	Sadness, despair, helplessness, and/or hopelessness
Insomnia	Initial difficulty in falling asleep	Early morning awakening followed by difficulty returning to sleep
Motor activity	Agitation	Retardation (slowing)
Negativism	Limited to specific areas	Global

treme, as in panic disorder or PTSD, the client feels in immediate danger and may seek protection and reassurance from others. If the anxiety is too severe, however, clients may become immobilized and unable to report their terrifying feelings at all, or they may refuse assistance and run away or become physically aggressive.

Sometimes clients with anxiety disorders may deny the existence of anxious feelings. They try to protect themselves by dissociating these feelings. It is important to recognize clients' anxiety despite their denials. In such instances, assessment requires an especially careful observation of objective data.

Cognitive and Perceptual Changes Anxious clients frequently have difficulty concentrating and making decisions. Some clients report feeling as if they are "going in circles," unable to think through a problem in order to make an effective decision. They may worry about their effectiveness at work and fear job loss as a result of attention and judgment problems. In the clinical situation, clients may ask staff members to make decisions for them. At the same time, however, they may express difficulty following through with suggestions, finding many loopholes or possible problems with the plan of action. Other clients become forgetful or misinterpret what they hear.

In extreme anxiety, as in a panic attack, the client is unable to assess a situation accurately and realistically. The client needs immediate attention from, and orientation by, you. The client may later report having had a frightening feeling of personality disintegration.

Somatic Discomfort Clients with anxiety disorders may complain of nausea, indigestion, headache, decreased appetite, a constant feeling of fatigue, or other somatic problems. They may relate these somatic disturbances to having "bad nerves," or they may be unaware of any psychologic component of their discomfort.

Clients with OCD who engage in repetitive activity, such as compulsive hand washing or hair pulling, may report special health problems (tissue breakdown or hair loss) as a result. You must compare the psychological benefits to the physical consequences of the client's compulsive rituals when determining your appropriate interventions with these clients.

Clients with PTSD may report fitful sleep, terrifying nightmares, and a fear of returning to sleep. The subsequent sleep loss becomes an additional physiological stressor. Be sure to assess the sleep pattern of clients with PTSD. Common features of PTSD are listed in the Your Assessment Approach box.

Role Impairment Clients may be aware of the impact that emotional, cognitive/perceptual, and somatic changes have on their social, family, and work roles. They report worry about losing their jobs or being unable to continue caring for their families. This worry only exacerbates the underlying anxiety and sets up a vicious cycle of worry compounding anxiety which adds to the worry. The next clinical example describes two people who are experiencing interpersonal difficulties as a result of anxiety.

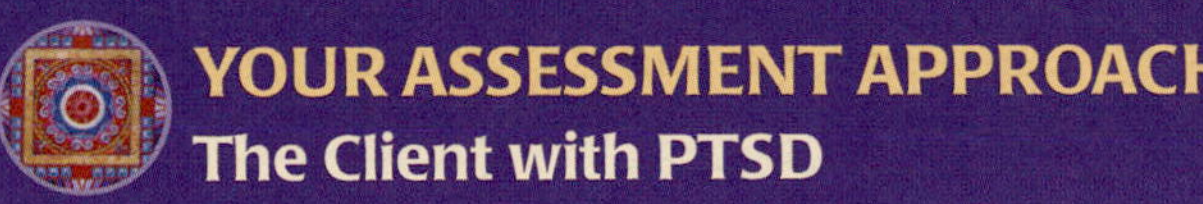

YOUR ASSESSMENT APPROACH
The Client with PTSD

The questions that follow will help you to assess PTSD.

- When was the last time you struck out in anger?
- Are you able to laugh and cry at appropriate times/situations?
- How would you describe your mood right now? Happy? Sad? Depressed?
- How much time do you spend thinking the same thing over and over?
- Are you able to relax?
- When was the last time you lost your temper? Or said something without thinking first?
- How do you sleep at night? Any nightmares or repetitive dreams?
- How is your memory?
- Are you able to finish tasks?

CLINICAL EXAMPLE

Gisela despairs that she is unable to take her daughter out to the playground because her phobias prevent her from leaving the house.

Abe, a middle-aged accountant, obsessed about tallying his firm's financial data, is unable to put his job aside for the weekend and misses his son's football game. He experiences anger, guilt, and self-recrimination as a result.

Objective Data

In addition to noting general signs and symptoms of anxiety as discussed in Chapter 8, other specific physical, emotional, cognitive, and role performance changes may be observed in very anxious clients.

Physical Findings

Clients with acute or extreme anxiety—clients with PTSD or panic disorder, and clients with phobic disorder who cannot avoid the phobic situation—may experience a panic reaction and show extreme discomfort. Look for acute physical changes, such as breathing difficulty, sweating, trembling, and/or vomiting, during these incidents. The client may be unable to verbalize, or verbalizations may be confused and incoherent. During a panic episode, clients may be so frightened that they refuse help at the moment and may require firm reassurance and protection until the episode subsides.

The client with an anxiety disorder may develop long-term physiologic effects, such as susceptibility to viral infections or the development of ulcers, hypertension, or asthma. Substance abuse may develop when clients try to alleviate anxiety through chemical means and can become a serious complicating problem. Substance abuse (discussed in Chapter 15), which frequently occurs in individuals experiencing PTSD, may be the client's attempt to avoid traumatic memories. Other physical findings may be the effects of ritualistic or compulsive activity—skin lesions in a client who obsessively picks at the skin, for example.

Emotional Changes Family and friends of a client with PTSD may report personality changes in the client, including increased irritability, suspiciousness, angry outbursts, and a tendency to blame others and to withdraw emotionally. Remember to pay attention to your own feelings when interacting with highly anxious clients. Because anxiety can be transmitted interpersonally, use self-awareness to determine the source of your own anxiety when interacting with anxious clients.

Individuals with phobic disorder and obsessive–compulsive disorder show a lack of emotional distress as long as the phobic object or situation is avoided or alleviated with activity. There may be little spontaneity or active involvement by the client during assessment as rigid, stereotyped behavior patterns are common.

Cognitive Deficits Unrealistic or distorted perception of a situation is common in anxiety states. During panic attacks, clients may distort or exaggerate details. They may complain about some seemingly insignificant detail. Clients may lose their ability to take in other pertinent data, and thus make errors in judgment. In assessment interviews, clients with anxiety disorders are often forgetful and unable to concentrate or attend to details. Errors in calculation and grammar are also common.

Impact on Role Function The symptoms of anxiety disorder affect social, work, and family relationships (refer back to Figure 18-1 on page 444). It is important to understand the possible effects of anxiety symptoms on interpersonal relationships. Obsessive–compulsive acts, for instance, may become so pervasive that they take the place of relating to other people. Sometimes, clients may use obsessions and compulsions to negotiate social interactions and social roles. Nurses who plan intervention strategies for clients with anxiety disorders should first assess the impact of the symptoms on the family system. In the following clinical example, the client knows that her compulsive cleaning is irrational but is unable to stop the behavior. Vanessa does not connect the excessive need for cleaning to an attempt to negate her sense of decreased control over her family members.

CLINICAL EXAMPLE

Vanessa's house is so clean and orderly that you could literally "eat off the floor." Vanessa spends a large amount of her time after work and on weekends making sure that the house is sparkling clean. She prepares to-do cleaning lists for her young adult children to follow when they visit. When Vanessa's husband comes home after traveling on business, he is often met with his own to-do list. Family social activities are put on hold until Vanessa's lists have been accomplished. Vanessa's husband and children complain about having to clean an already clean house. Vanessa is upset that her children are visiting less often and that her husband seems to be spending more and more time traveling on business.

Reports from the client and/or family that the client is having trouble at work are additional evidence of role impairment. The client may be in jeopardy of losing a job because of poor performance. A person with PTSD, for example, may be fired for absences, drug or alcohol abuse, or outbursts of temper.

Nursing Diagnosis: NANDA

It is impractical to try to identify all the nursing diagnoses that apply to clients experiencing anxiety disorders. However, there are three fundamental nursing diagnoses pertinent to these clients:

1. Fear—a response to a threat that is recognized as a danger
2. Anxiety—a vague feeling of dread accompanied by an autonomic response; a feeling of apprehension in anticipation of danger
3. Ineffective coping—an inability to form a reality-based appraisal of the stressors, inadequate selection of responses, and/or inability to use available adaptive resources

Following is a discussion of the three primary nursing diagnoses and other diagnoses that may apply to clients with anxiety disorders.

Fear

Fearful responses to anxiety can occur on a continuum ranging from slight apprehension to paralyzing terror. One anxious person may state, "I'm scared," whereas another may be filled with alarm and unable to verbalize feelings of panic. In extreme cases of anxiety, panic is communicated through behavioral responses rather than verbalizations. Behaviors such as being immobilized with fear or striking out at others are often exhibited by individuals experiencing panic.

Anxiety

Apprehension and tension are emotional experiences common to clients with anxiety disorders. Clients may worry excessively, ruminating about what might go wrong in the future. They may express anxiety through worry about their physical well-being; somatic preoccupation or hypochondriasis may develop. Sexual drive or behavior may also be inhibited by anxiety. The potential for substance abuse is high, and suicidal potential is increased.

Ineffective Coping

Excessive anxiety can cause alterations in conduct and impulse control. Some clients, such as those with PTSD or panic disorder, manifest unpredictable behaviors in an attempt to cope with their overwhelming fears. Individuals with OCD are unable to alter behavior, even though they may recognize it as harmful or irrational. In an attempt to cope, clients with anxiety may turn to substance abuse, which results in disordered conduct and impaired impulse control.

Ineffective Role Performance

Anxiety disorders impair performance in the family, at school, and at work. Anxious clients may become less efficient and accurate at work or school because of distractibility or other perceptual and cognitive difficulties. Clients may withdraw emotionally from formerly important and meaningful relationships, or they may become overly dependent on others for help. They may isolate themselves and avoid previously enjoyed activities and recreation. Excessive need for reassurance, decreased productivity, reduced creativity, impaired hygiene, and impaired home maintenance are all possible outcomes for the client with anxiety disorder.

Impaired Verbal Communication

Clients with anxiety disorders often have difficulty communicating. They may speak too quickly or too loudly, may overelaborate, or may talk about too many subjects at once. Easily distracted, anxious people may have trouble understanding explanations or retaining information. A client with severe anxiety may be incoherent, making verbal communication impossible. Written communication may also be impaired.

Risk for Trauma

Impairments in motor behavior are often related to hyperactivity and restlessness, which may place the client at risk for accidental injury. Wringing of the hands, poor coordination, and startle reaction are motor behaviors associated with anxiety disorders. Clients with OCD may perform bizarre repetitive acts, such as repeatedly washing the hands or counting, checking, and rechecking activity. These ritualistic acts often result in self-injury.

Disturbed Thought Processes and Disturbed Sensory Perception

Anxiety disorders affect perception and cognition and reduce the client's ability to solve problems. Judgment, concentration, abstract thinking, and attention are impaired. The client is indecisive but at the same time may make decisions impulsively in an attempt to relieve tension. In panic disorder, the client may become disoriented, misinterpret reality, and distort the meaning of situations or events. Loss of self-esteem and a lowered self-concept often result as the client is unable to use skills that were previously helpful in coping.

Ineffective Tissue Perfusion

Alterations in circulation and elimination may occur as a result of stimulation of the autonomic nervous system. The client may experience increased blood pressure, rapid heart rate, dizziness, and palpitations as well as dry mouth, cold or clammy hands, sweating, shortness of breath, and a bad taste in the mouth. Diarrhea, enuresis, and slowed digestion may occur.

With extreme anxiety or panic, these symptoms are intensified, and the client may faint or vomit. A medical emergency may arise if the client has a coexisting physical problem, such as cardiovascular disease.

Insomnia

Insomnia is a frequent response to anxiety. Nearly all clients with anxiety disorders complain of trouble sleeping. Sleep may be further disturbed by nightmares or night terrors, as experienced by people with PTSD. See Chapter 19 for more information on sleep impairments.

Outcome Identification: NOC

In order to determine client progress and the effectiveness of nursing interventions, expected client outcomes must be clearly identified. When developing client outcomes, you must specifically state the outcomes in behavioral terms. For example, the statement "Mr. Atkins will be less anxious" is ambiguous and not easily measured. However, the statement "Mr. Atkins will participate in one relaxation session per day" is observable and measurable. Outcome identification is individualized according to the client's clinical manifestations and needs. Listed below are some outcomes that generally apply to clients experiencing anxiety disorders:

- Client will demonstrate absence of physical manifestations of anxiety.
- Client will identify indicators of own anxiety.
- Client will verbalize feelings of anxiety appropriately.
- Client will demonstrate the use of new coping skills.

Planning and Implementation: NIC

Planning and implementing care for anxious clients depends on a thorough assessment and determining the appropriate nursing diagnoses. Anxiety, which is communicated interpersonally, often affects the client's family and friends, other clients, and staff members as well. Refer to the Your Self-Awareness feature for help in reading your own bodily cues of anxiety.

Most mental health care professionals believe that clients who cope with the stress of anxiety disorders can grow and change with therapeutic intervention. Nursing interventions for clients with anxiety disorders should be geared toward

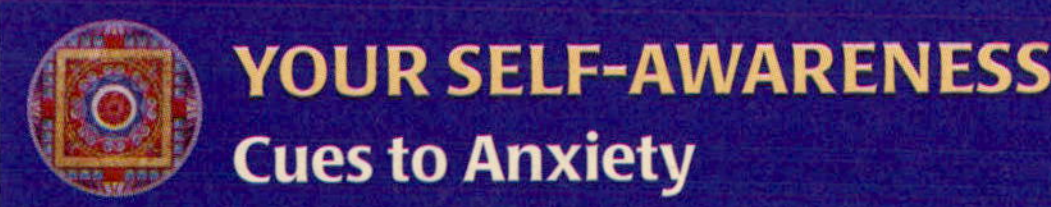

YOUR SELF-AWARENESS
Cues to Anxiety

Since anxiety is communicated interpersonally, it is imperative that you are able to read your own somatic clues that indicate increasing anxiety. Read the list below and identify the cues that you commonly experience when anxious.

Physical Cues	Emotional Cues	Behavioral Cues
Dry mouth	Irritability	Forgetfulness
Profuse sweating	Fearfulness	Short attention span
Urinary frequency	Suspiciousness	Pacing and fidgeting
Nausea ("butterflies" in stomach)	Sadness	Withdrawal

Take a few minutes and reflect on a time when you were very anxious. How did you feel both physically and emotionally? What were your behaviors? If you feel comfortable doing so, share your responses with others and ask for feedback. Are their perceptions of your responses to anxiety-provoking situations similar to yours?

effective coping. Refer to the Nursing Care Plan on panic disorder with agoraphobia at the end of this chapter.

Reducing Fear

Fear and anxiety usually coexist in that a person who is fearful is generally anxious as well. The clinical manifestations of fear and anxiety are very similar. Thus, when dealing with a client who is afraid, nursing interventions for reducing anxiety are appropriate (see the following).

Reducing Anxiety

Because anxiety is such an uncomfortable feeling, we learn early in life to reduce it or diminish its effects as soon as possible. Although individuals use a variety of behaviors, the most common automatic responses to anxiety are anger, withdrawal, and somatization. Automatic responses are limiting, rigid, and inflexible and, therefore, prevent a creative response to the stressor.

Intervening with Clients Experiencing Panic Clients who are extremely anxious or in a panic state require immediate, direct, and structured intervention. During an acute panic attack, perception and personality are disrupted to such a degree that the client cannot solve problems or discuss the source of anxiety. The first priority is to reduce the anxiety to more tolerable levels. The interventions for clients in panic listed in the following Your Intervention Strategies box can help to alleviate the client's panic.

Your goal is to reduce the client's immediate anxiety to more moderate and manageable levels. The family of the anxious person needs counseling about how to respond therapeutically because they are often present during a panic episode.

Intervening in Less Severe Anxiety You can frequently detect subtle indications of increasing anxiety and intervene early to prevent escalation. Some clients are adept at covering up their anxiety, even though their behavior usually transmits cues to the sensitive observer. Often your own feeling of increased tension is a useful cue that the source of anxiety is in the client. Anxiety may make people excessively demanding. Your response to the demands must take into account the consequences for the course of the client's anxiety. In some cases, it may be reassuring to set limits and deny the request. In other cases, such a response may place further stress on the client.

You must know how to treat clients who suffer from prolonged anxiety. The intervention strategies are intended to help clients use their anxiety to learn about themselves and their coping strategies. This requires the client to endure the anxiety while searching out its causes. The client must then develop more effective and satisfying coping strategies to replace the old ones. To help clients learn to cope more effectively with anxiety, first detect the anxiety and then make thoughtful observations and responses that facilitate learning. Refer to the Your Intervention Strategies feature below for the client experiencing anxiety.

YOUR INTERVENTION STRATEGIES
The Client in Panic

Strategy	Rationale
Stay with the client.	Being left alone may further increase the anxiety.
Maintain a calm, serene manner.	Knowing that you are calm and in control may be calming to the client.
Use short, simple sentences.	Disruption of the perceptual field causes difficulty in focusing.
Use a firm and authoritative voice.	Conveys your ability to provide external controls.
Place client in a quieter, smaller, less stimulating environment.	Prevents further disruption of the perceptual field by sensory stimuli.
Focus the client's diffuse energy on a repetitive or physically tiring task.	Repetitive tasks or physical exercise can help drain off excess energy.
Administer antianxiety medications if ordered.	Antianxiety medications may help reduce anxiety by altering brain chemistry.

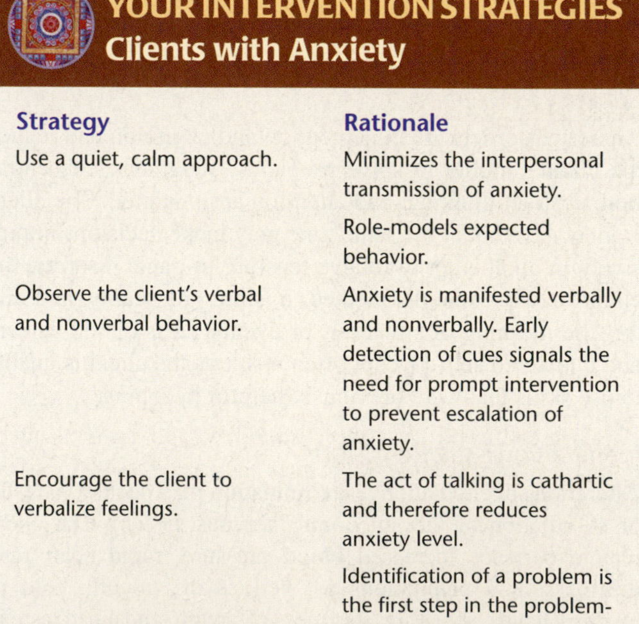

YOUR INTERVENTION STRATEGIES
Clients with Anxiety

Strategy	Rationale
Use a quiet, calm approach.	Minimizes the interpersonal transmission of anxiety. Role-models expected behavior.
Observe the client's verbal and nonverbal behavior.	Anxiety is manifested verbally and nonverbally. Early detection of cues signals the need for prompt intervention to prevent escalation of anxiety.
Encourage the client to verbalize feelings.	The act of talking is cathartic and therefore reduces anxiety level. Identification of a problem is the first step in the problem-solving process.
Teach relaxation techniques when the client's anxiety is at a mild level.	Clients with moderate, severe, or panic-level anxiety are unable to process new information. Maximum learning is possible at the mild anxiety level.
Encourage the client to use relaxation techniques as needed.	The relaxation response counters hyperarousal of anxiety states.

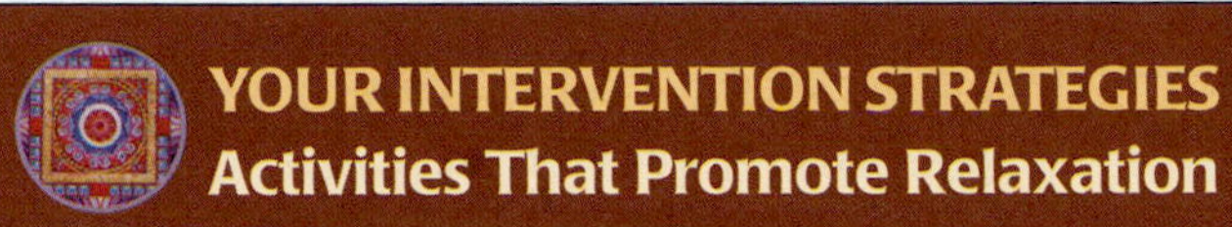

YOUR INTERVENTION STRATEGIES
Activities That Promote Relaxation

Passive Behaviors	Active Behaviors
■ Soak in a warm bath.	■ Take a long walk.
■ Listen to soothing music.	■ Ride a bicycle.
■ Have a back rub or massage.	■ Phone a friend and discuss your feelings.
■ Perform progressive muscle relaxation.	■ Organize your desk, pantry, or closet.
■ Take slow deep breaths, to counter the effects of hyperventilation.	■ Garden or mow the lawn.
	■ Paint a picture, or a house.

It is important that you avoid reinforcing clients' justifications for their usual coping patterns. Often, clients try to give plausible explanations for their ineffective anger, withdrawal, or somatization. However, these rationalizations do not explain the relief in terms of the factors that caused the anxiety. The relief afforded by the usual coping patterns does not last long because the needs or expectations that originally caused the symptoms still exist. The underlying needs may even become more intense. Clients can begin to change disturbed coping patterns only when they understand what their unmet needs are, what they did instead of fulfilling these needs, and their subsequent feelings.

Anxious clients have two alternatives. They can change their hopes and expectations, or they can try new tactics or resources to get their needs met. Discuss these options with the client, and negotiate a contract to work on one or both goals. Acting on either option involves problem solving. Simple physical activities often help reduce anxiety to more tolerable levels. Encourage adaptive mechanisms that work, such as those in the Your Intervention Strategies feature above.

You can use a variety of techniques and skills in intervening with clients who experience anxiety. Cognitive–behavioral therapy helps individuals face their fears in order to cope. Progressive muscle relaxation, meditation, thought-stopping techniques, autogenic training, and guided imagery may help clients learn new ways to reduce the disturbing affect. (Chapter 32 ∞ discusses several of these approaches.) Another way you can help clients relax is to encourage meditation in which the client repeats a word or phrase (Bormann et al, 2005). This technique activates the relaxation response. Other methods include helping clients test reality, because their sense of danger is often out of proportion to actual danger. Developing goal-oriented contracts may help reduce a client's sense of inner chaos by providing structure and direction. The use of contracts also actively involves clients in their own healing process. This involvement increases their sense of control, thereby alleviating feelings of powerlessness.

Teaching Clients about Medications

Educating clients about the use of medications is one of your essential responsibilities. Clients should be aware of the major medications used to manage acute anxiety and their limitations and possible side effects. Anxiety that is secondary to major medical illness or acute trauma (such as the death of a child) requires a different dosage than that prescribed for the treatment of primary anxiety. A guide to medications for anxiety is offered by the Anxiety Disorders Association of America (www.adaa.org) and can be accessed on the Companion Website for this book.

Antianxiety medication should be used cautiously and sparingly. Certain antianxiety medications (diazepam, for one) are among the most overprescribed and abused drugs in the United States and Canada. Older adults are particularly sensitive to the effects of CNS depression associated with diazepam. If a BZD is necessary for an older person, lorazepam (Ativan) or oxazepam (Serax) are safer because the risk of toxicity is lower than with longer-acting BZDs such as diazepam (Valium). The toxicity risk is lower due to the short elimination half-life and also because they are not active metabolites and are not metabolized actively in the liver (Flint, 2005).

Benzodiazepines have proved effective and relatively safe in controlling situational anxiety for periods of 4 to 8 weeks. Antianxiety agents such as diazepam and alprazolam (Xanax), or adrenergic blocking agents such as propranolol (Inderal) are sometimes used.

Selective serotonin reuptake inhibitors (SSRIs) are the class of medications of choice for treating anxiety disorders (Davidson, 2006). The primary reason that SSRIs are used most often in treating anxiety disorders is that they cause fewer side effects than other medications. Other types of medications that can be used effectively in treating anxiety disorders include tricyclic antidepressants (TCAs), BZDs, beta-blockers, atypical antipsychotic agents, and buspirone (BuSpar), which often helps clients cope with a moderate level of anxiety. Note that some antipsychotic medications may have a paradoxical effect and trigger the development of anxiety disorders. This is especially true of clozapine (Clozaril) as a precipitant to OCD in some individuals. When used to treat anxiety disorders, medications are started at a low dosage level and gradually increased until a therapeutic level is achieved. Inform clients that it may take up to 2 to 4 weeks before they begin to feel better. This information is crucial in helping clients continue to take the medication. These medications are discussed more fully in Chapters 7 and 32 ∞.

Although medications may alleviate the symptoms of anxiety, they do nothing to help clients understand the source of their anxiety. Ideally, these medications should be used for the short-term treatment of anxiety—days, weeks, or months instead of years. However, some clients may require longer-term treatment, depending on the degree of anxiety relief. Thus, you see it is necessary to closely monitor each client's anxiety level to determine the efficacy of medication. You will be providing medication education to all clients; see the Partnering with Clients and Families box for some specific teaching guidelines for anxiolytic and antidepressant medications.

MEDIALINK Anxiety Disorders Association of America

MEDIALINK Application: Managing Anxious Patients

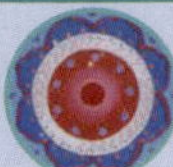

PARTNERING WITH CLIENTS AND FAMILIES

TEACHING ABOUT MEDICATIONS FOR ANXIETY DISORDER

- Drowsiness is a common side effect. Avoid driving until you know how the medication will affect you.
- Do not consume alcohol while taking this medication. Check labels on over-the-counter drugs and toiletries (e.g., mouthwash) as many contain alcohol.
- Drinking caffeine decreases the effect of your medication, so use decaffeinated beverages.
- Do not take other medications without first discussing with your health care provider. Many drugs interact negatively with others.
- Do not increase the dosage or stop taking the medication without checking with your health care provider.

Promoting Effective Coping

Coping skills can be taught to clients with every type of anxiety disorder. In addition to anxiety alleviation, there are other therapeutic benefits to using previously learned coping skills, such as increased self-esteem, improved self-efficacy, and more effective problem-solving. You need to demonstrate patience in order to project a sense of calm presence when working with anxious clients.

Obsessive–Compulsive Disorder Clients with OCD avoid anxiety by engaging in compulsive acts and rigid thinking. Regardless of your practice setting, you will likely encounter an obsessive–compulsive client whose problem is severe enough to require hospitalization. See the What Every Emergency Department Nurse Should Know feature. It is essential that you establish a therapeutic alliance with your clients. One way to foster a therapeutic bond is to let clients know that although their thoughts are irrational, they are individuals worthy of respect.

Clients with OCD use compulsive rituals to control anxiety. Therefore, schedule your intervention to avoid increasing the client's anxiety. It is usually countertherapeutic to interfere prematurely with a ritual unless it is life-threatening. Generally, the client needs plenty of time to complete the ritual. When the client is interrupted during or prohibited from performing the compulsive behavior, anxiety escalates. It is best to time therapeutic activities to occur immediately following the ritual because the client's anxiety level is lowered by performing the compulsive behavior.

Clients with OCD often have a strong tendency toward negativism, which may cause them to become more firmly entrenched in their defenses if modifications are introduced prematurely or hurriedly. Attempt to develop an affirming, dependable relationship before suggesting that clients change their behavior patterns, gradually introducing a substitute behavior. Balance the value of intervening in behavior that protects clients from mental anguish against the need to prevent physical deterioration caused by the behavior.

Post-Traumatic Stress Disorder Clients with PTSD frequently experience behavioral disturbances as a result of the intense anxiety triggered by reexperiencing the trauma. Alcohol or other drugs, when used to relieve anxiety, may contribute to destructive and impulsive acts. Clients often experience disordered family relationships, physical disability, social and recreational disruptions, and impaired ability to work or attend school. They may experience symptoms and attitudes of demoralization that further hamper their functional abilities. In the acute stage, crisis counseling is essential. Because of the chronic course of PTSD and the many psychosocial problems associated with it, a comprehensive treatment approach is needed.

When planning care for the client with PTSD, determine the type and duration of trauma experienced. Was the trauma a single, brief incident? Several ongoing incidents? A human-induced trauma (combat or rape)? A natural trauma (hurricane or earthquake)? Natural disasters and human-induced traumatic events can have very different effects on an individual. For example, a survivor of human-induced trauma (such as rape) frequently experiences more guilt and humiliation. After a natural disaster, a person may experience feelings of survivor guilt. Clients with PTSD verbalize feelings of no longer being safe and will often exhibit passive dependent behaviors.

WHAT EVERY EMERGENCY DEPARTMENT NURSE SHOULD KNOW

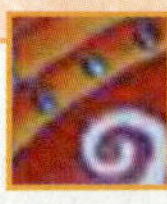

Anxiety

- When clients enter your emergency department, it is important to assess their level of anxiety, just as you assess every client's vital signs and pain level.
- Knowing how anxious your client is will help determine your next action.
- Approach each client with a calm, reassuring manner; this will help the client feel less threatened and more secure.
- Involve clients in their own care as much as possible. This will increase their sense of control, which helps keep anxiety in check.
- Protect the safety of the client whose anxiety is escalating as well as the safety of other clients and yourself.
- Call for help immediately if your interventions have not de-escalated the client's anxiety.

The goal of therapy in treating clients with PTSD is to desensitize them to the memories of the traumatic event so that they are able to cope with the anxiety. The techniques listed in the Your Intervention Strategies feature may be used singly or in combination to help alleviate anxiety.

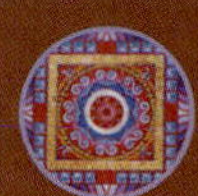

YOUR INTERVENTION STRATEGIES Clients with PTSD

- **Abreaction:** Focuses on exploring and reliving painful repressed experiences.
- **Cognitive restructuring:** Provides new, less threatening interpretations of events. Includes techniques such as thought stopping and thought substitution (see Chapter 31 for specific cognitive therapies).
- **Education:** Provides an explanation of the dynamics of the disability and of treatment modalities.
- **Exercise and nutrition:** Strengthens the body's adaptive efforts.
- **Family conferences:** Provides support to the client by encouraging the family to work on resolving the many psychosocial effects evoked by the trauma.
- **Group therapy:** Provides support and reinforces new coping skills.
- **Hypnosis:** Brings repressed material to conscious awareness so it can be integrated into the ego structure. (Note: You must have extra training such as graduate education or certification in order to practice hypnosis.)
- **Individual therapy:** Provides important ego-supportive and/or cathartic benefits.
- **Relaxation training:** Focuses on developing new skills that the client may use when faced with memories of the traumatic event.

Recent advances in psychopharmacology have led to the use of medication as an adjunct to the psychologic treatment of PTSD. As is true for the other anxiety disorders, however, you must be aware of the heightened potential for chemical abuse among extremely anxious clients. The desire for immediate, total relief is powerful and may foster chemical abuse and dependence.

BZDs, TCAs, SSRIs, lithium, beta blockers, alpha-adrenergic antagonists, and neuroleptics have all been reported to relieve PTSD symptoms. During the initial stage (4 to 8 weeks), the use of benzodiazepines may be helpful in the treatment of anxiety, insomnia, and nightmares.

Sleeplessness, another common feature of PTSD, is best treated with a behavioral approach such as relaxation techniques, guided imagery, muscle relaxation, and exclusion of daytime naps. Sedatives are discouraged except for very brief use. Your goal is to help the client reestablish the ability to sleep naturally and cope more effectively without relying on the use of drugs.

Phobic Disorders Clients with phobic disorders attempt to avoid anxiety by symbolically binding it to a specific object or situation. It is essential to recognize that forcing clients to come into contact with the feared object or the basic source of their anxiety can create an intense, disorganizing flood of panic.

Many clinicians agree that clients with phobic coping patterns are highly resistant to most insight-oriented therapies. Such therapies require clients to confront and, at least temporarily, experience some of their originating anxiety. It is not surprising that insight-oriented therapists are ineffective with phobic clients, since avoidance is a major dynamic in phobias. Some symptomatic improvements have been made using techniques derived from behaviorist theory. The most commonly used interventions are desensitization, reciprocal inhibition, and cognitive restructuring. They are discussed in TABLE 18-5 ■ and in Chapter 31. Read the Evidence-Based Practice feature for an example of planning care for a client with social phobia.

TABLE 18-5 ■ **Cognitive Behavioral Techniques for Treating Phobias**

Technique	Description	Example
Systematic desensitization (exposure therapy)	A client is exposed to a series of increasingly anxiety-provoking situations, beginning with the least threatening. The client gradually becomes desensitized to each stimulus in the series until the stimulus that induced the most anxiety is no longer threatening.	A man who is terrified of earthworms might first talk about earthworms until the topic no longer evokes the same level of anxiety. Then he might be shown pictures of earthworms until he masters that level of closeness. Over time, he will progress to holding a live earthworm in his hand without experiencing severe or panic-level anxiety.
Reciprocal inhibition	The anxiety-provoking stimulus is paired with another stimulus associated with an opposite feeling strong enough to suppress the anxiety.	Through the use of meditation, yoga, biofeedback training, hypnosis, or antianxiety medications, clients learn how to induce a calm state.
Cognitive restructuring	This intervention is based on the belief that anxiety stems from erroneous interpretations of situations. The client learns to reframe (or relabel) a frightening situation, object, activity, or event so that it becomes less threatening.	A woman who fears she is going to die if she leaves her apartment learns to change her perception to one that is more reality based by saying, "I may feel uncomfortable but I will not die. I can do this."

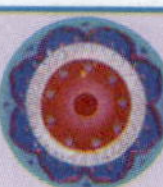

EVIDENCE-BASED PRACTICE

INTEGRATIVE THERAPY FOR ANXIETY

Charlene is a 19-year-old female client at a community mental health center. During her initial session, she tells you, the admitting nurse, her story: "I couldn't go on dates or to parties. For a while, I couldn't even go to class. My freshman year of college, I had to come home for a semester. My fear would happen in any social situation. I would be anxious before I even left the house, and it would escalate as I got closer to class, a party, or whatever. I would feel sick to my stomach—it almost felt like I had the flu. My heart would pound, my palms would get sweaty, and I would get this feeling of being removed from myself and from everybody else. When I would walk into a room full of people, I'd turn red and it would feel like everybody's eyes were on me. I was too embarrassed to stand off in a corner by myself, but I couldn't think of anything to say to anybody. I felt so clumsy, I couldn't wait to get out."

Your plan for intervention options is based on current research results. For example, in your review of cognitive-behavioral therapy (CBT) and social phobia, you understand that Charlene will likely experience positive long-lasting effects by participating in CBT groups.

After further sessions with Charlene, you determine that she has negative perceptions of her ability to interact with groups of peers at her college. Because of your understanding of current research findings, you decide to use the technique of cognitive restructuring with Charlene.

The multidisciplinary treatment team working with Charlene understands that current research shows the efficacy of BZDs and antidepressants in the treatment of social phobia. Therefore, Charlene is prescribed paroxetine (Paxil), an SSRI antidepressant, as an adjunct to the CBT group sessions and cognitive restructuring techniques.

This set of multiple intervention strategies is based on the following research:

Choi, Y. H., & Park, K. H. (2006). Therapeutic factors of cognitive behavioral group treatment for social phobia. *Journal of Korean Medical Science, 21*(2), 333–336.

Garcia-Lopez, L. J., Olivares, J., Beidel, D., Albano, A.M., Turner, S., & Rosa, A. I. (2006). Efficacy of three treatment protocols for adolescents with social anxiety disorder: A 5-year follow-up assessment. *Journal of Anxiety Disorders, 20*(2), 175–191.

CRITICAL THINKING APPLICATION

1. Why would cognitive restructuring be helpful to Charlene?
2. How do SSRIs help individuals with anxiety disorders?
3. Is it realistic for Charlene to expect total remission?

Promoting Effective Communication

Nursing interventions that reduce anxiety are important measures to promote more effective communication and behavior. Often, simply offering the opportunity to acknowledge and discuss feelings of anxiety helps the client regain control. At this point, clients are more likely to share their concerns because you have already taken the first steps in demonstrating genuine interest and concern. See the following Rx Communication feature for the client with social phobia.

After encouraging the client to express feelings, be sure to listen attentively. Clients may express fear, anger, sadness, disappointment, or alienation, and it may be difficult for you to hear about the client's pain. Some nurses feel helpless in the face of their client's catharsis and think they should be able to provide ready answers. Instead, ready answers are more likely to interfere with and thwart the client's communication. Genuine, concerned listening without judgment or giving advice is an effective intervention in itself.

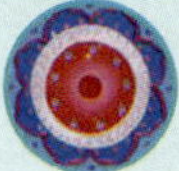

RX COMMUNICATION

THE CLIENT WITH SOCIAL PHOBIA

CLIENT: "I just had to get out of that room. I couldn't stand it with all those people looking at me. I thought I was going to die!"

NURSE RESPONSE 1: "That sounds very frightening. Tell me more about it."

RATIONALE: This response demonstrates reflection of the client's affect and encourages the client to verbalize more feelings.

NURSE RESPONSE 2: "Think of other times when you've felt that way. What helped you feel less frightened?"

RATIONALE: This response asks the client to identify specific coping methods that were helpful in a similar situation. Such methods can then be used in anticipatory planning for future anxiety-provoking situations.

Explanations should be simple, clear, and concise. Be careful not to overload severely anxious people with more information than they can handle. If anxiety has contributed to knowledge deficit, reduce the anxiety before trying to teach about health or provide information. If the client's perceptual field (see Chapter 8) is narrow or disrupted, the client will be unable to assimilate information.

Clients with OCD require patience and an unhurried attitude, especially in regard to details and ruminations. If you use the techniques of paraphrasing and reflecting, these clients will say you did not get the details right. They will then go on to correct, qualify, and clarify. This striving for accuracy produces greater vagueness and confusion. It is as if parallel conversations are going on simultaneously. Clients hear only themselves repeating and correcting insignificant details and completely lose the overall meaning of the message. Developing patience in listening and skill in providing well-timed, simple direction is crucial to working effectively with clients with OCD.

Promoting Safety

Lack of coordination, tremors, and impaired concentration make anxious clients prone to accidents. Counsel clients not to perform potentially dangerous activities, such as driving a car, when anxiety is high. Advise them to move more slowly or to repeat instructions carefully when they undertake new tasks or use tools and/or equipment that are potentially dangerous.

Promoting Optimal Tissue Perfusion

Tissue perfusion improves when anxiety is reduced. Focus on proper nutrition and adequate activity, because clients with anxiety frequently overlook self-care and their health needs. Walking, participating in sports, and/or developing new hobbies and interests promote healthy physiologic functioning and should be part of a comprehensive treatment plan for anxious clients.

Promoting Effective Sensory Perception and Thought Processes

To function more effectively and independently, the client needs to know about normal anxiety and anxiety disorders. Providing accurate information at the right time and in an appropriate manner is an essential nursing responsibility. Other strategies to promote effective perception and cognition include the following:

- Use adjuncts to verbal communication, such as visual aids or role-playing, to enhance the retention of information.
- Practice problem-solving vignettes to improve judgment and insight.
- Identify misperceptions that clients hold as a result of a narrowed perceptual field. Begin with comments such as "I wonder if you've considered this possibility?" or "Perhaps if we tried. . . ."
- Help clients reality-test, that is, explore their opinions in the light of validated experience rather than emotional needs that block accurate perception.

Promoting Sleep

Nonpharmacologic nursing measures to promote sleep should be used before medications. Such measures may include a variety of relaxation techniques. One effective method is the use of music that promotes a relaxing atmosphere; listening to the sounds of nature is soothing and sleep-promoting to some people.

Suggest that the client read a boring book in bed, drink warm decaffeinated liquids, or take a warm tub bath before retiring. A client with PTSD may fear going to sleep because of nightmares. Having another member of the family nearby and aware of the client's fear may be reassuring. (Chapter 19 discusses other ways of promoting sleep.)

Evaluation

Evaluation is used to determine the client's response to interventions. In other words, is the client demonstrating progress? Are the anxiety-related symptoms decreasing? Does the client use coping skills effectively? In addition to these questions, it is also important to evaluate clients in the following areas: anxiety, coping ability, role performance, communication, safety, thought processes, perception, tissue perfusion, and sleep.

Anxiety

Specific client outcomes indicative of decreased anxiety levels are described in this section. Clients will show no evidence of acute or intense anxiety and be able to perform activities of daily living independently when appropriate. Clients will verbalize feeling less anxious, and they will have fewer somatic complaints. They will state they feel more comfortable.

Clients will have fewer symptoms of physiologic distress, such as racing pulse, diaphoresis, and/or hyperventilation. Clients will be without signs of increased psychomotor activity. They will no longer complain of tearfulness, feelings of rage, or impatience. When appropriate, they will more readily engage in interactions with others. Phobic clients will tolerate the presence of the feared object, activity, or situation without experiencing panic or the need to flee.

Individual Coping

Clients will demonstrate the ability to continue with necessary activities even though some anxiety is present. They will be less likely to panic or flee. Family members will report that clients are "more like their old selves" and appear less agitated, driven, or explosive in conduct. The client with OCD will limit or cease performing compulsive rituals; for example, a client with a hand-washing compulsion will wash hands no more than four times a day.

Role Performance

The client will attend work or school on a regular basis. Family members will report that relationships at home have improved and that the client is once again participating in family activities. Clients will report engaging in recreational or social activity and independently performing self-care. They will express feeling more comfortable about their performance at home, work, or school. Phobic clients will perform daily activities with less restriction or interference from any feared object, activity, or situation.

Communication and Safety

Clients will state satisfaction with their communication; they feel heard and understood. There will be open lines of communication between client and nurse and client and family. Clients will report no tremors and will not have accidents due to poor motor coordination or concentration difficulties. They will report being able to perform usual small motor tasks, such as writing, in a competent manner.

Thought Processes and Sensory Perception

Clients will recall information taught by the nurse. They will begin to make decisions about their health care and ask questions about anxiety. Clients will describe what led to their anxiety and what happened after they felt anxious. They will verbalize techniques to reduce anxiety. Clients will correctly verbalize the use, side effects, and results of taking their medications. They will verbalize increased awareness of their environment.

Tissue Perfusion

Clients will report feeling energetic. Somatic complaints will decrease, and clients will report engaging in daily physical activity. Vital signs will be normal, and weight will be stable.

Sleep

Clients will sleep through the night without medication or with appropriately prescribed medication. They will have fewer nightmares and wake less frequently during the night. Clients will demonstrate energy during the day as a result of restful sleep during the previous night.

MEDIALINK Dissociative Disorders Video

CASE MANAGEMENT

The case manager plays an essential role in collaborating with clients, families, and significant others by providing information on when and where to seek help. The case manager also monitors clients for adherence to the aftercare plan, including the client's medication usage. Issues to be considered during outpatient therapy include: identifying personal strengths, establishing realistic time frames for outcomes, identifying and strengthening support systems, and locating community support services.

COMMUNITY-BASED CARE

Individuals with anxiety disorders are usually aware that their behaviors are problematic to themselves and others. However, insight alone does not necessarily result in behavioral changes. Or, when change does occur, it is a very gradual process. As a result, people with anxiety disorders are often treated in the community—in mental health clinics, crisis centers, and therapists' offices.

HOME CARE

Nurses who provide psychiatric–mental health care in the home are playing a significant role in helping clients with anxiety disorders improve their social interactions and shape behavior. The following interventions are especially helpful for homebound clients experiencing anxiety disorders:

- Meet with the client and family member or significant other to discuss realistic expectations for the client.
- Teach the client home management skills necessary for independent living.
- Determine with the client if testing, placement services, or job skill retraining are desired.
- Refer the client and family to community agencies as needed.

DISSOCIATIVE DISORDERS

Dissociative disorders have, as their common denominator, the defense mechanism of dissociation, in which the client strips an idea, object, or situation of its emotional significance and affective content. (Dissociation and other defense mechanisms are explored in Chapter 8∞.) Dissociation is a defense against trauma that separates emotions from behaviors. Consciousness, memory, identity, or perception of the environment are impaired in these disorders.

Dissociative disorders are complex and are usually difficult to distinguish from one another; see TABLE 18-6 ■ on page 465 for a comparison of the disorders. In every dissociative disorder, a cluster of related mental events is beyond the client's power of recall but can return spontaneously to conscious awareness. Dissociative disorders are not attributable to mental disorders that have an organic basis, such as dementia. Dissociation is a possible response to extreme trauma, especially trauma experienced during childhood. See Chapter 20∞ for a discussion of dissociation and recovered memory in childhood sexual abuse as well as the Caring for the Spirit feature in Chapter 8∞ on page 151.

Dissociative Amnesia

People with **dissociative amnesia** have one or more episodes of memory loss of important personal information. They suddenly become aware that they have a total loss of memory for events that occurred during a period that may range from a few hours to a whole lifetime. In localized amnesia, the most common form, a person forgets only specific and related past times, usually surrounding a disturbing event. Selective amnesia for some, but not all, of the events is less common. Least common are generalized amnesia, which encompasses the person's entire life, and continuous amnesia, in which the person cannot recall events up to a specific time, including the present. Systematized amnesia is the loss of memory for certain categories of information,

Table 18-6 ■ Comparison of Symptoms in Dissociative Disorders

Dissociative Amnesia	Dissociative Fugue	Dissociative Identity Disorder	Depersonalization Disorder
Abrupt memory loss Awareness of memory loss Mental status: alert	Wandering away from home Amnesia for past experiences Unaware of memory loss Assumption of new identity During fugue, acts "normal"	Presence of more than one distinct personality state (alter) Unable to remember blocks of time Alter assumes control of thoughts and actions Abrupt switch from one alter to another Amnesia for other alters	Sense of unreality about self and body Intact reality testing Ego-dystonic

Adapted from: Sadock, B. J., & Sadock, V. A. (2005). *Kaplan & Sadock's pocket handbook of clinical psychiatry* (4th ed.). Philadelphia: Lippincott Williams & Wilkins.

such as all memories related to one's occupation, or all memories related to one's family.

Dissociative Fugue

A person with **dissociative fugue** wanders, usually far from home and for days, perhaps even weeks or months, at a time. During this period, clients completely forget their past life and associations; but unlike people with amnesia, they are unaware of having forgotten anything. When they return to their former consciousness, they do not remember the period of fugue. Clients experiencing dissociative fugue are generally reclusive and quiet, so their behavior rarely attracts attention. During this period, they appear to function unremarkably, but may behave in a manner inconsistent with their usual pattern of functioning. They may assume a completely new and apparently well-integrated identity during the fugue state.

Dissociative Identity Disorder

Formerly known as multiple personality disorder, **dissociative identity disorder (DID)** is the presence of two or more distinct personalities within one individual. Each personality, at some time, takes full control of the person's behavior. Usually, one identity state, also called an **alter**, described later in this chapter, is unaware of the others' existence.

There is much controversy about dissociative identity disorder. Many professionals are skeptical that such a phenomenon exists. However, clinical evidence of the existence of DID abounds. Refer to the website for the International Society for the Study of Trauma and Dissociation (www.isst-d.org), which can be accessed through the Companion Website for this book.

Depersonalization Disorder

The central feature of **depersonalization disorder** is one or more episodes of feeling detached from oneself so that the usual sense of personal reality is temporarily lost or changed. The individual feels mechanical. Clyde's experience with depersonalization disorder is recounted in the following clinical example.

CLINICAL EXAMPLE

Clyde feels as if he is living in a dream or a movie. It seems to him as if he can observe his own life. He explains his experiences by saying, "I don't feel real anymore. It's like I can watch my life as if it's a TV show. I'm afraid I'm going crazy."

The feelings experienced by people with depersonalization disorder are **ego-dystonic**, meaning they are unacceptable to the person's sense of self. The client has intact reality testing; in other words, the client is not experiencing hallucinations or delusions.

BIOPSYCHOSOCIAL THEORIES

Although biologic and genetic factors are being studied, psychosocial theories are used most often to explain dissociative disorders.

Biological Factors

Physiological and neurobiological functions play a significant role in the development of amnesia. For example, the neurotransmitter serotonin affects recall of information. The formation and retrieval of memories relies on intact function of the hippocampus and the limbic system.

- Research suggests that the limbic system may be impaired in individuals who have experienced traumatic experiences in childhood (Sadock & Sadock, 2005).
- In DID, the various alters may have different cardiovascular and cerebral activation patterns when exposed to stressors (Reinders et al., 2006).
- Physical illnesses (such as brain tumors, epilepsy, and migraine headaches) may lead to symptoms indicative of depersonalization disorder. Certain drugs (e.g., alcohol, barbiturates, benzodiazepines, and hallucinogens) may cause some people to experience depersonalization symptoms (Sadock & Sadock, 2005).

MediaLink International Society for the Study of Trauma and Dissociation

- Studies performed with EEG have shown that various personality states in DID have different activity in the frontal and temporal lobes (Lapointe, Crayton, DeVito, Fichtner, & Konopka, 2006)
- A sleep study with EEG suggested that alterations in alpha and theta brain waves may help explain why dissociative symptoms are accompanied by deficits in attention and memory (Girsbrecht, Jorgen, Smelders, & Merckelbach, 2006).

Genetic Theories

According to the DSM-IV-TR, dissociative identity disorder occurs more often in first-degree biologic relatives of people with the disorder (APA, 2000).

Psychosocial Theories

Pierre Janet (1859–1947) was the first to develop the concept of the "splitting off," or dissociation, of a part of consciousness. He believed that the individual needed a normal amount of "mental energy" to maintain integrative mental processes. When the level of energy was high, integration was maintained. When it became low, however, the personality might cease to function as a unit and split or dissociate.

Freud, in contrast, proposed the concept of repression to explain the loss of conscious awareness in dissociation. He then introduced the notion of the dynamic unconscious, a part of the mind in which emotions or ideas that were unacceptable to a person were pushed from awareness. Freud and other early analytic theorists accepted the basic concept of psychologic dissociation.

Current explanations of dissociation are based on Freud's dynamic concepts. The repression of ideas that leads to amnesia and other forms of dissociation is conceived as a way of protecting the individual from emotional pain. External circumstances or internal psychologic conflicts are viewed as precipitating factors. A dissociative reaction may be viewed as a flight from crisis or danger—a major psychologic route of escape from anxiety. Sometimes, as in states of dissociative fugue and dissociative identity disorder, the dissociated area temporarily assumes direction and control of the entire personality. During such times, the person may appear to be functioning well.

Dissociative identity disorder originates in childhood as a result of chronic trauma, usually child abuse. The trauma may be physical, psychological, or both. The major form of child abuse that contributes to the development of DID is sexual abuse. In attempts to cope with the horror of reality, the child's ego splits through the dissociative process. Each trauma-induced dissociative experience shapes the development of alternate (**alter**) personalities. Each alter has a unique identity, holds different feelings and memories, and performs different functions. Chronic abuse leads to a fixation of the dissociated ego splits. Through dissociation, the child may see the abuse as if it were occurring to someone else, as in a movie. This ability to remove the self from the abuse is a defense mechanism that allows the individual to survive. The development of dissociative identity disorder is illustrated in FIGURE 18-3 ■.

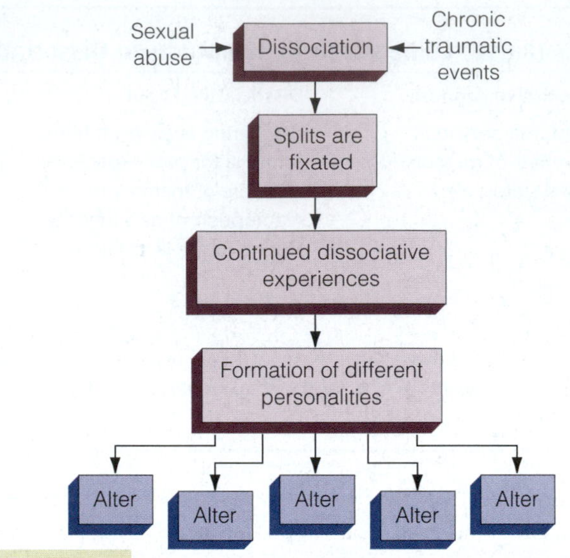

FIGURE 18-3 ■ The development of dissociative identity disorder.

Additional dynamic considerations relevant to dissociative disorders include the following ideas. In dissociative amnesia, the pattern is similar to conversion disorder except that the individual does not avoid some unpleasant situation by getting sick. Instead, the person does so by forgetting (repressing) certain traumatic events or stresses. In DID, there appears to be a deep-seated conflict between contradictory impulses and beliefs. A resolution is achieved by separating the conflicting parts and developing each into an autonomous personality (alter).

Behavioral Theories

Behavioral theorists explain the development of dissociative disorders as learned behaviors. An individual learns that avoidance behavior provides protection from a painful experience. After repeated experiences, this avoidance pattern is reinforced.

Humanistic Theories

Individuals with dissociative disorders have experienced intense psychological trauma during early childhood. As nurses, we take a holistic approach in dealing with these clients by accepting the fact that the dissociation was used as a defense mechanism that kept the abused child intact. Humanistic theories view the individual as a composite of life experiences, psychobiological factors, and interpersonal interactions. Individuals are also viewed within the context of their culture.

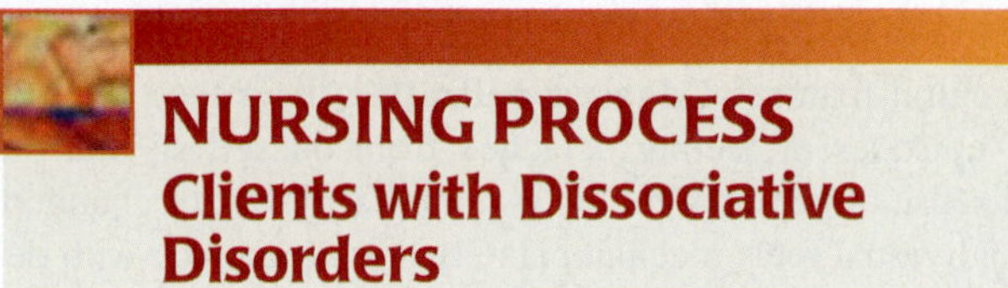

NURSING PROCESS
Clients with Dissociative Disorders

The nursing process is the framework for providing care to clients experiencing dissociative disorders. When caring for clients with dissociative symptoms, you must use a systematic approach in order to provide holistic, compassionate care. Most clients with dissociative disorders are treated in community rather than inpatient settings.

Assessment

It can become extremely challenging when you begin to gather data on a client with dissociative symptoms. For example, the client's amnesia will certainly be problematic when you are collecting a health history. The major areas to focus on during assessment are identity, memory, and consciousness.

Subjective Data

Clients with dissociative disorders often report a sudden loss of memory of events. Clients may report, for example, that they cannot recall certain important personal events or information. They may not recall important aspects of their own identity, such as their age and where they reside. As you interview clients, listen to their pronoun usage. If the client uses "we" when speaking, this may indicate the presence of alters.

Sometimes amnesia is only partial, and clients remain conscious of what happened, although they report that they feel no control over it. In cases of complete amnesia, the "lost" memories can be recovered under certain therapeutic circumstances (e.g., hypnosis), or they may return spontaneously. Clients who have sustained a loss of their own reality may have adopted a new identity.

If motor behavior is affected in dissociative disorders, clients or their families may report episodes during which clients physically traveled away from home. In clients with DID, the original personality typically is not aware of the existence of the secondary personalities. However, the secondary personalities may be aware of the original personality as well as of each other and may report this awareness to the staff. Clients with depersonalization disorder may report fears that they are going crazy and experience resulting anxiety. See the following Your Assessment Approach feature for assessment guidelines for clients with depersonalization disorder.

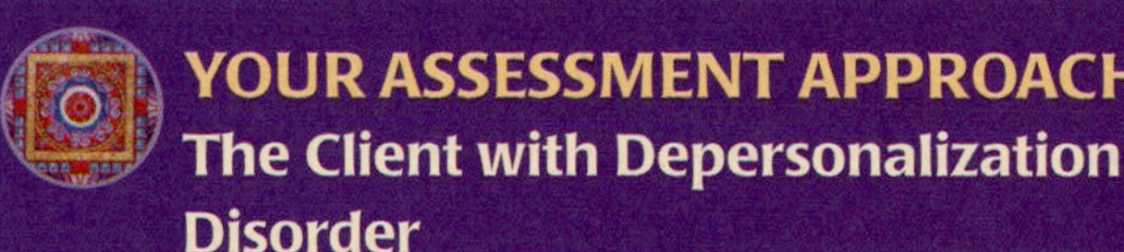

YOUR ASSESSMENT APPROACH
The Client with Depersonalization Disorder

To determine feelings of unreality, listen for the following client statements:

- "I just feel weird."
- "I'm not myself."
- "I feel like I'm floating away."

To determine altered bodily perceptions, listen for the following client statements:

- "My body doesn't feel real."
- "I looked at my arm and saw that it looked like a piece of wood."
- "When I was looking in the mirror, it was like the image was looking back at me."

To determine impaired behavioral perceptions, listen for the following client statements:

- "I feel like I'm on automatic pilot."
- "I'm walking through life like a zombie."
- "I feel like I'm a machine or a robot."

To determine altered external perceptions, listen for the following client statements:

- "Everything feels different . . . like I'm in a dream while I'm awake."
- "Everyone seems unreal."

Objective Data

Conduct a careful assessment of the client's physical condition to rule out the possibility of organic causes, such as a brain tumor. Many of the behaviors of clients with dissociative disorders resemble behaviors associated with organic conditions, including postconcussional amnesia and temporal lobe epilepsy. Your observations of the character, duration, frequency, and context of the dissociative disorder are crucial data. Physical examinations are not continued as part of the long-term intervention program, however, because they reinforce the symptoms and provide secondary gain. Therefore, the completeness and accuracy of the initial physical assessment are of the utmost importance.

A psychosocial assessment is conducted to discover the fundamental source of the anxiety as early as possible. Although many episodes of dissociation appear to occur spontaneously, there may be a history of a specific emotional trauma or a situation charged with painful emotions and psychological conflict. Family or friends may provide clues to the client's conflict and should be included in the psychosocial data gathering. When assessing for the presence of DID, consider the clinical manifestations listed in the Your Assessment Approach feature on page 468.

Events associated with the trauma can trigger memories that have been repressed; these stimuli can precipitate a switch of alters. When interacting with the client, be alert for evidence of forgetfulness and fluctuations of voice tone, speech, and mannerisms. Notice from session to session if there are uncharacteristic changes in behavior. Are there differences in hairstyles, adornment, mannerisms, or dress?

To assess for amnesia, ask if the client has ever had blackouts, blank spells, memory gaps, or has lost time. To assess for dissociation, question whether the client ever "spaces out" or is unable to remember periods of time or events. Ask others who know the client about episodes of uncharacteristic behavior that the client does not recall.

Nursing Diagnosis: NANDA

Several nursing diagnoses may be applicable to clients with dissociative disorders, depending on the client's specific needs. Dissociation is manifested by disturbances in sensory and thought processes. Dissociative disorders markedly interfere with the client's ability to perform role expectations.

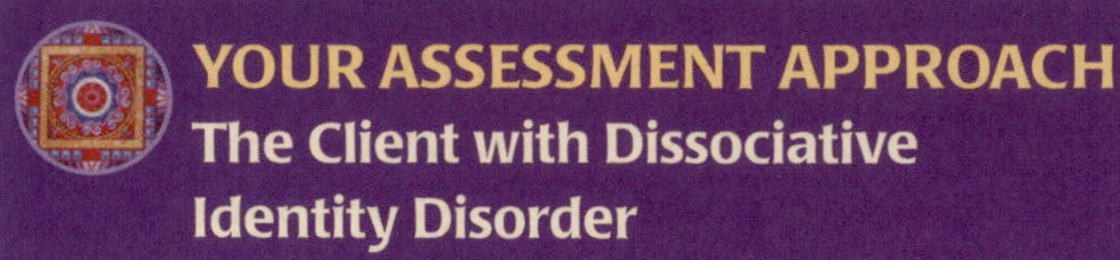

YOUR ASSESSMENT APPROACH
The Client with Dissociative Identity Disorder

- Are there blocks of time you are unable to remember?
- Have you ever awakened not knowing your name or where you were at that time?
- Do other people accuse you of being untruthful?
- Have you ever discovered unfamiliar objects, like clothing, in your home and not known how they got there?
- Do you have headaches? If so, how often? How intense are they?
- How often do you have sleeping problems?
- Do you ever have nightmares?
- As a child, were you hurt or abused by others?

Disturbed Sensory Perception and Disturbed Thought Processes

Clients with dissociative disorders may experience sudden memory loss, disorientation, loss of personal identity, and alteration in state of consciousness. Clients with dissociative amnesia have a partial or total inability to recall or identify past experiences. In clients with depersonalization disorder, feelings of unreality and estrangement can affect their perception of the physical and psychologic self and of the world around them. Parts of the body or the entire body may seem foreign, and dizziness, anxiety, and distortion of time and space are common.

Ineffective Role Performance

Unexplained disappearances, absences from work, unreliability, and unpredictability are common manifestations of dissociative disorders. Thus, the social or occupational functioning of the client is adversely affected.

Symptoms of depersonalization lead to limited or superficial involvement with others and to withdrawal or disengagement in work or social pursuits. As expected, relationships become highly complicated and disorganized when a client has multiple personalities.

Ineffective Coping

In addition to amnesia, a fugue state may occur in clients with dissociative disorders. In this state, clients defend against perceived danger by active flight. They may wander away from home and community. Days, weeks, or sometimes even years later they may suddenly find themselves in a strange place, not knowing how they got there. There is complete amnesia for the period of the fugue. Clients experiencing dissociative fugue may adopt a new identity and life pattern.

Outcome Identification: NOC

When developing expected outcomes, it is important to individualize plans for each client. For example, a client experiencing a dissociative identity disorder will probably need assistance in resolving issues related to self-concept. When planning outcomes, remember that they should be realistic and achievable. Some appropriate expected outcomes would include:

- The client will engage in a therapeutic alliance.
- The client will verbalize awareness of personality alters.

Following are some outcomes—written in NOC terminology (Johnson et al., 2005)—for clients experiencing ineffective coping. The client will:

- Seek information about illness and treatment
- Use stress-reduction behaviors
- Report decrease in negative feelings
- Demonstrate impulse control by consistently maintaining self-control without supervision

Planning and Implementation: NIC

In choosing intervention strategies for clients with dissociative disorders, the treatment team must decide whether to alleviate the troublesome symptoms or reintegrate the anxiety-producing conflict. Some teams emphasize the disruptions in day-to-day functioning precipitated by dissociative disorders. These include unexplained disappearances, absences from work, unreliability, and unpredictability. The dread associated with them justifies intervention strategies designed to change the disruptive behavior pattern. Others believe that new problems are created by removing the dissociative symptoms without considering how they help the client control internal anxiety and maintain some balance in external social life.

Keep in mind that although clients may complain about the difficulties associated with their symptoms, the symptoms often form the basis of relationships with other significant people in their lives. Clients' roles in social groups are likewise built around their coping styles. Anyone who tries to change these coping styles must offer clients more effective and satisfying ways to handle anxiety and get support in their social network. Such a task usually requires long-term psychotherapy. However, behavior modification strategies can alleviate some of the problematic behaviors. When planning care for a client with DID, remember that trust is a major issue. The basic building blocks of therapy with the dissociative individual are trust, safety, and acceptance.

For many individuals, receiving a diagnosis of DID actually provides a sense of relief. For years, they have been misdiagnosed and treated incorrectly. However, other individuals may be distressed by the diagnosis; learning the diagnosis may trigger the switching of alters. Thus, a safe, supportive environment is essential when informing the client of the diagnosis. The focus of treatment is to form a therapeutic alliance and work through the issues of each alternate identity.

The goal of integrating the alternate identities into one fused identity is difficult to achieve—but it is feasible. Integration occurs when there is no further need for separateness between identities. The integration process can be very painful for the client, as memories of previous trauma surface. However, it is important for the client to recall painful memories in order to work through unresolved conflicts. When planning care for clients with DID, remember to trust them to express their needs. You also need to actively listen to each identity state and provide support, especially when the client is struggling to accept the realization that he or she has DID.

Promoting Improved Sensory Perception and Thought Processes

Strategies for identifying the underlying source of anxiety include those for recovering unconscious content, such as free association or dream description. At times, more active strategies are used. These may include projective psychometric tests (Rorschach, Thematic Apperception Test) and hypnosis, with or without intravenous administration of thiopental sodium (Pentothal). These strategies require advanced and specialized training.

Supportive insight therapy may be used by the psychotherapist with the goal of surfacing and integrating traumatic experiences in order to learn new ways of coping with future anxiety. This is especially relevant for clients in whom dissociation arises primarily against a background of intrapsychic conflict.

Promoting Effective Role Performance

It is important to work with the client's family in order to help everyone in the family unit to adjust to role performance alterations. Including family members in a therapeutic counseling relationship helps them learn new ways of dealing with the client. As stated earlier, considerable secondary gain is often associated with dissociative behavior: Some clients may use the illness to escape responsibility and get special treatment. Families often need support in learning to avoid reinforcing dissociative behavior by acting as the source of secondary gain.

Environmental manipulation may be an indicated intervention. For example, it may be necessary to assist the client in problem solving with the goal of minimizing other stressful aspects of the environment. In learning to confront and become desensitized to the underlying conflict, the client will experience some anxiety and discomfort. This anxiety must be kept within manageable limits. Therefore, obvious stressors should be minimized.

Promoting Effective Coping

Psychotherapy, environmental manipulation, and behavior modification help the client cope more effectively with impairments of conduct and impulse, as evidenced by unpredictable and bizarre behavior. Treatment may prove to be long-term, and progress may be slow. Establishing a supportive therapeutic alliance with the client and the family is crucial in helping the family and client understand the periodic occurrence of symptoms and in supporting improved behaviors. See the following Rx Communication feature for clients with depersonalization disorder.

Evaluation

Evaluating the effectiveness of nursing interventions is essential, although it may be difficult with clients who are experiencing episodes of amnesia.

Sensory Perception and Thought Processes

Clients will no longer experience sudden memory loss, disorientation, loss of identity, or alteration in state of consciousness, or they will experience it less frequently. They will correctly recall and identify past experiences.

Role Performance

Clients will experience increased satisfaction with family and work relationships. Involvement with others will occur more often and will be more fulfilling. Clients will attend work or school regularly, without unexplained absences due to dissociative episodes.

Individual Coping

Clients will no longer exhibit bizarre or unpredictable behaviors, or they will experience them less frequently. For example, incidents of being missing from home without explanation will occur less frequently or not at all.

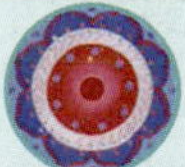

RX COMMUNICATION

THE CLIENT WITH DEPERSONALIZATION DISORDER

CLIENT: "I don't feel like myself. In fact, I don't even feel real."

NURSE RESPONSE 1: "You sound as if you're afraid when those unreal episodes occur."

RATIONALE: This response demonstrates empathy and reassures the client that it is appropriate to discuss her feelings.

NURSE RESPONSE 2: "When you are feeling this way, you look more anxious. We're here to help you learn to cope better with the anxiety."

RATIONALE: This response provides feedback on the congruence between the client's feelings and behavior. It also reassures the client that she can learn methods to decrease the anxiety associated with depersonalization.

CASE MANAGEMENT

Case management services for clients experiencing dissociative disorders usually involve extensive tracking of records for previous hospitalizations, especially for clients with DID. Clients with DID may often be disabled as a result of the seriousness of the disorder. The case manager must maintain ongoing communication with the client, family members, mental health professionals, other health care providers, and third-party reimbursers. Medication management is a major issue for many clients with dissociative disorders.

COMMUNITY-BASED CARE

Clients with dissociative disorders are not psychotic and, therefore, are often treated in the community instead of the hospital setting. The community setting includes mental health clinics, crisis centers, and therapists' offices. However, for those clients who are hospitalized, discharge goals seem straightforward but present a challenge: to provide quality, cost-effective care that allows the client to return to full functioning as soon as possible. Community care must focus on the client's safety in light of possible continued memory impairments.

HOME CARE

Some individuals with dissociative disorders are able to live independently. Others, however, may need to live in group homes or halfway houses in order to promote safety and functional ability. The client's ability to live at home is, after all, based on his or her functional abilities. Some individuals with DID need very close supervision, especially if they rapidly switch alters.

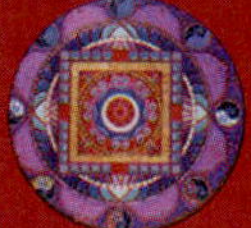

NURSING CARE PLAN
A Client with Panic Disorder with Agoraphobia

Identifying Information

Mrs. Randolph is 43 years old, married, and the mother of four daughters in their late teens and early twenties. She was referred to the psychiatric outpatient clinic for follow-up counseling by the emergency department of the local general hospital, where she had been rushed in acute distress the prior evening with symptoms of a panic attack.

Client's Description of the Problem

At the time of the panic attack, Mrs. Randolph believed she was having a heart attack and feared she was dying. She reported racing heartbeat, sweating, and feeling faint. She could not identify any events, thoughts, or feelings that precipitated the incident; it seemed to her to occur "out of the blue." She felt unable to cope with the severity of the symptoms of the attack: "I tried to talk myself out of it; to tell myself it would go away, but it only got worse."

Mrs. Randolph reported she had had similar attacks over the years and that she had always been reassured of her medical and cardiac health, but when these attacks occurred, she "feared the worst" and "lost all perspective." The previous attacks had lasted from 2 minutes to 2 hours. Her daily routine had become quite restricted, as she now sought to have one of her daughters or her husband with her when she went out of the home due to fear of an attack. She did not feel comfortable when alone in her home and could not go to sleep if the other family members were not home. She felt ashamed and angry about her growing disability and often tried to cover up her fears to friends and family.

By interviewing the family, the nurse was able to gather information about a number of significant recent life events preceding the panic episode:

- Recent major surgery: A hysterectomy 4 weeks earlier.
- Loss of employment due to her hospitalization: She was abruptly terminated from her position at a new job because of too many absences.
- The upcoming anniversary of her father's sudden death from a heart attack.

History

Mrs. Randolph had never been hospitalized for a psychiatric condition, although she had been to the emergency room on three prior occasions with symptoms of panic attack. She had seen a therapist years ago when the attacks first occurred, "about the time I left home to marry." She did not follow up with the therapist, however, saying she felt ashamed ("I've always been a strong and effective person!"), that the episodes were not so severe then, and that she found relief from panic attacks after she had the children.

Both Mrs. Randolph's parents died within the past 6 years. She was especially close to her father, and the second anniversary of his death was approaching. Mrs. Randolph's mother was considered a "homebody"; she rarely left the house and took part in social activities only if they occurred at the family home. Mrs. Randolph wondered if her mother had "these fears" too.

She reported she had begun to curtail social and recreational activities, preferring to stay at home where she was most comfortable.

She described her relationship with her husband as emotionally warm and supportive. Although she sometimes resented his being away from her, she recognized this as part of her "problem" with being alone. Her primary relationships had been with her husband and children. She talked of facing the "empty nest" as her daughters, one by one, left for work or college.

With the exception of chronic gynecologic problems leading to the recent hysterectomy, Mrs. Randolph reported a history of good health. She had no allergies or other chronic illnesses. Her only other hospitalizations were to have her children. The recent hospitalization had been more physically taxing than she expected, and the fact that she was not allowed to return to work after her recovery came as a blow.

Current Mental Status

Mrs. Randolph is an attractive, carefully groomed woman who looks her stated age. She sits erect in the office chair, appearing

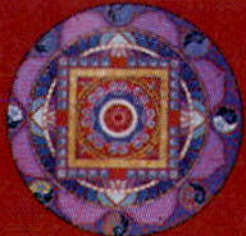

NURSING CARE PLAN
A Client with Panic Disorder with Agoraphobia *(continued)*

somewhat tense. She answers questions cooperatively, but at times with some hesitation and as if expecting criticism or judgment from the interviewer.

She is oriented to time, place, and person. Her memory is intact and her recall good. She has no difficulty with calculations. Her judgment is unimpaired. During times of panic, however, sensory and perceptive awareness are greatly impaired.

Affect appears normal, with occasional evidence of anger in the form of irritability and light sarcasm. Mood is within normal limits.

Speech is normal in flow and volume. It appears pressured at times when she attempts to correct an impression she believes the interviewer holds. Posture is at times rigid, but she relaxes as she becomes more comfortable with the interview.

There are no delusions, ideas of reference, or hallucinations. Obsessive worry about the occurrence of panic episodes and of her safety is present. Embarrassment and shame over her symptoms are apparent. Suicidal or homicidal thoughts are denied. Associations and abstractions are appropriate, and there is no evidence of thought process disorder or difficulty in concentration, except during acute panic, at which times concentration is impaired and thought processes are disorganized. Some guardedness toward the interviewer is noted. Insight into the meaning of the current situation is minimal.

Other Clinical Data

Mrs. Randolph is considering the use of antianxiety medication, despite "hating the idea" of medication.

Nursing Diagnosis: Ineffective Role Performance related to fear and anxiety level

Expected Outcome: Client will demonstrate role performance as evidenced by: ability to meet role expectations, knowledge of role transition periods, and reported strategies for role changes.

Short-Term Goals	Interventions	Rationales
Describe specific changes in role function.	■ Maintain a calm manner.	A calm approach prevents escalation of anxiety.
	■ Stay with the client.	Client's panic is alleviated.
	■ Use short, simple sentences.	Simple language facilitates anxious client's ability to concentrate and follow direction.
	■ Direct client's attention to repetitive or physical task.	Distraction serves as an outlet for anxious energy.
	■ Administer antianxiety medication.	Medication reduces anxiety by altering brain chemistry.

Nursing Diagnosis: Disturbed Thought Processes related to high level of anxiety

Expected Outcome: Client will demonstrate ability to choose between two or more alternatives.

Short-Term Goals	Interventions	Rationales
Demonstrate appropriate decision making.	■ Teach relaxation exercises.	Anxiety impairs the ability to concentrate and solve problems.
	■ Encourage client to identify previous coping skills.	Use of previously learned skills can reduce anxiety level.

Nursing Diagnosis: Ineffective Coping related to overwhelming fears

Expected Outcome: Client uses actions to manage stressors that tax personal resources.

Short-Term Goals	Interventions	Rationales
Demonstrate effective coping as evidenced by employing behaviors to reduce stress and reporting decreased negative feelings.	■ Help client identify coping resources (including social supports).	Client becomes aware of existing resources.
	■ Teach client relaxation techniques.	Relaxation counters the stress response.
	■ Encourage client to verbalize feelings.	Verbalization reduces stress through process of catharsis.

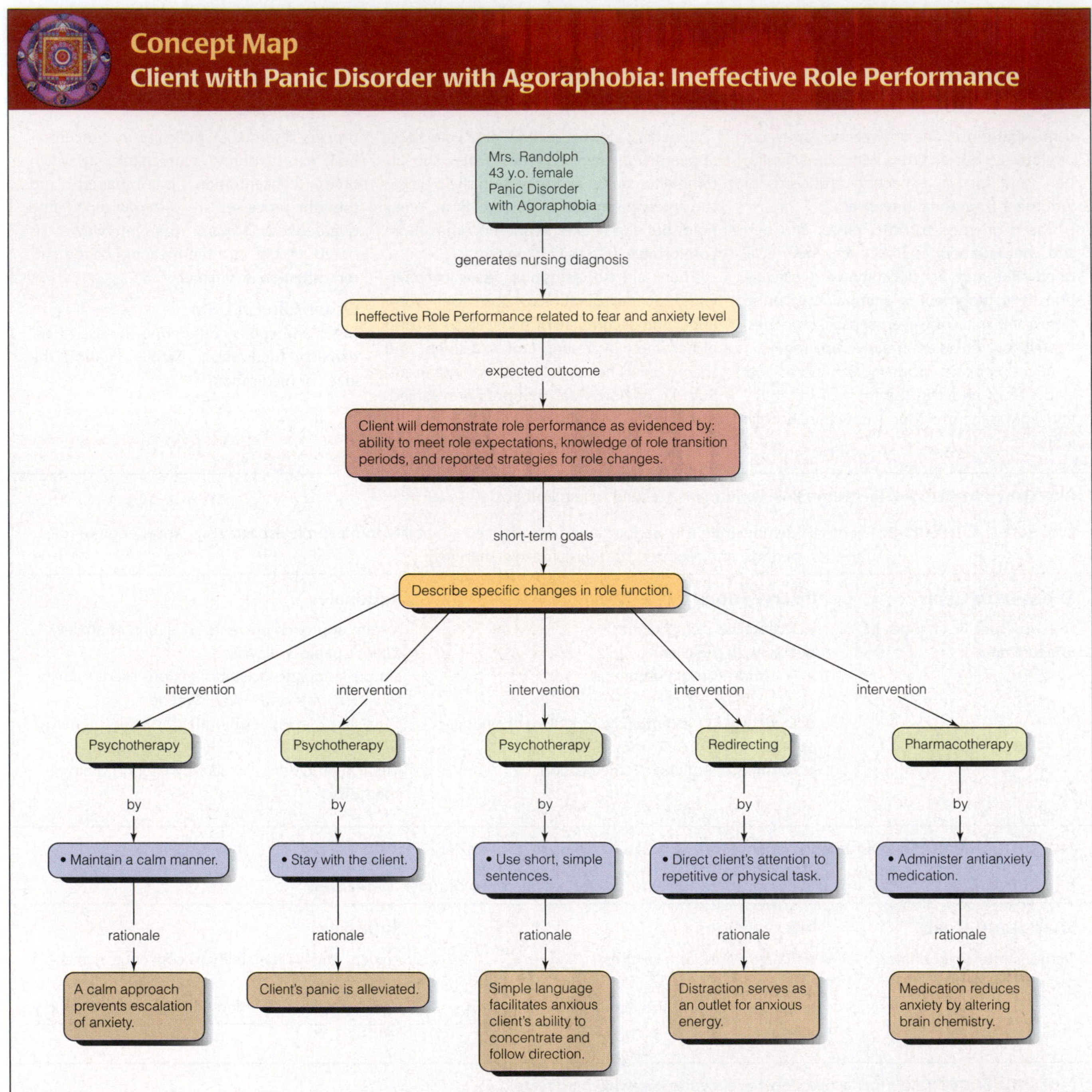
Concept Map
Client with Panic Disorder with Agoraphobia: Ineffective Role Performance
Mrs. Randolph
43 y.o. female
Panic Disorder
with Agoraphobia
generates nursing diagnosis
Ineffective Role Performance related to fear and anxiety level
expected outcome
Client will demonstrate role performance as evidenced by: ability to meet role expectations, knowledge of role transition periods, and reported strategies for role changes.
short-term goals
Describe specific changes in role function.
intervention
Psychotherapy
by
• Maintain a calm manner.
rationale
A calm approach prevents escalation of anxiety.
intervention
Psychotherapy
by
• Stay with the client.
rationale
Client's panic is alleviated.
intervention
Psychotherapy
by
• Use short, simple sentences.
rationale
Simple language facilitates anxious client's ability to concentrate and follow direction.
intervention
Redirecting
by
• Direct client's attention to repetitive or physical task.
rationale
Distraction serves as an outlet for anxious energy.
intervention
Pharmacotherapy
by
• Administer antianxiety medication.
rationale
Medication reduces anxiety by altering brain chemistry.

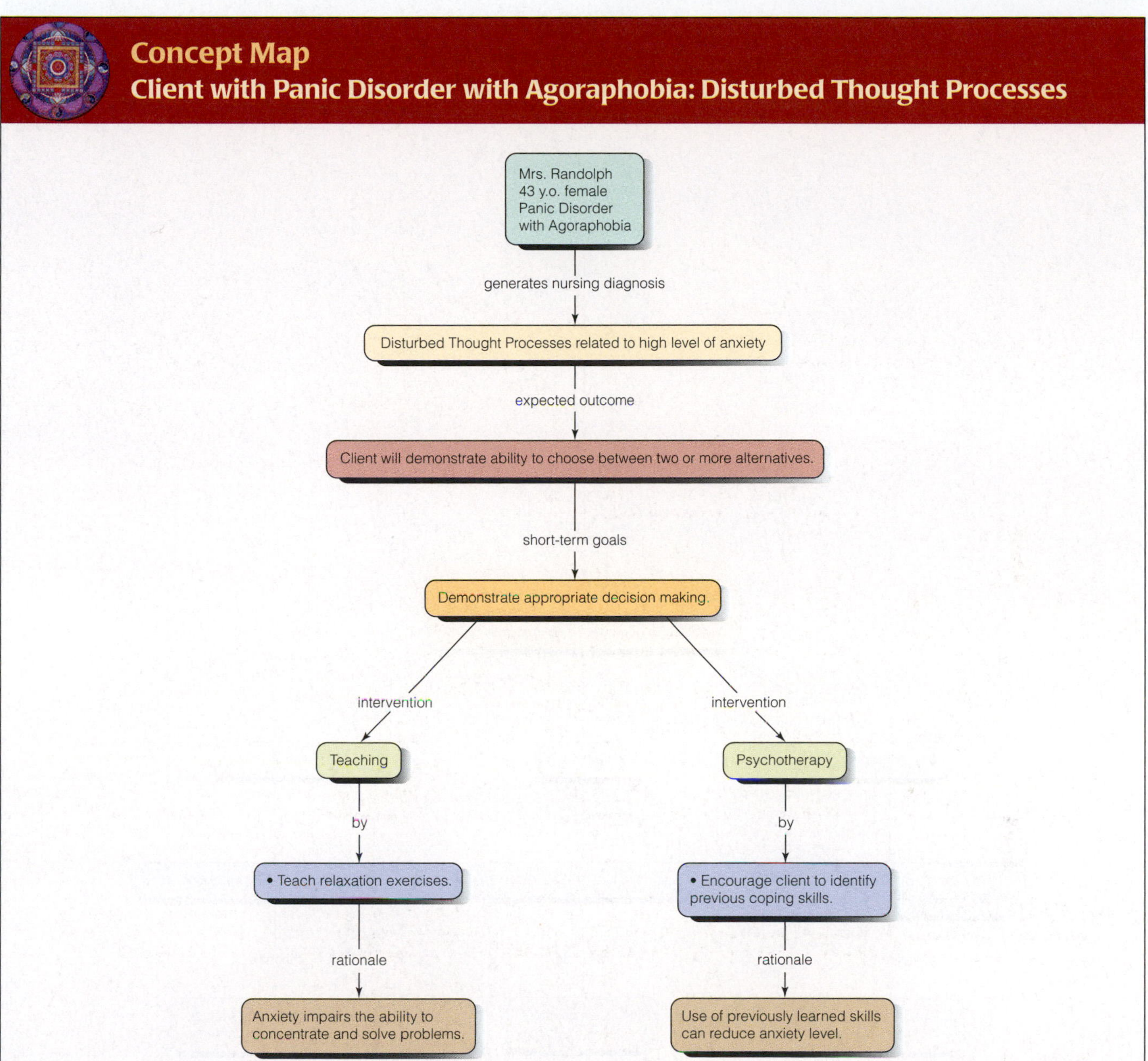
Concept Map
Client with Panic Disorder with Agoraphobia: Disturbed Thought Processes
Mrs. Randolph
43 y.o. female
Panic Disorder
with Agoraphobia
generates nursing diagnosis
Disturbed Thought Processes related to high level of anxiety
expected outcome
Client will demonstrate ability to choose between two or more alternatives.
short-term goals
Demonstrate appropriate decision making.
intervention
intervention
Teaching
Psychotherapy
by
by
• Teach relaxation exercises.
• Encourage client to identify previous coping skills.
rationale
rationale
Anxiety impairs the ability to concentrate and solve problems.
Use of previously learned skills can reduce anxiety level.

Concept Map
Client with Panic Disorder with Agoraphobia: Ineffective Coping

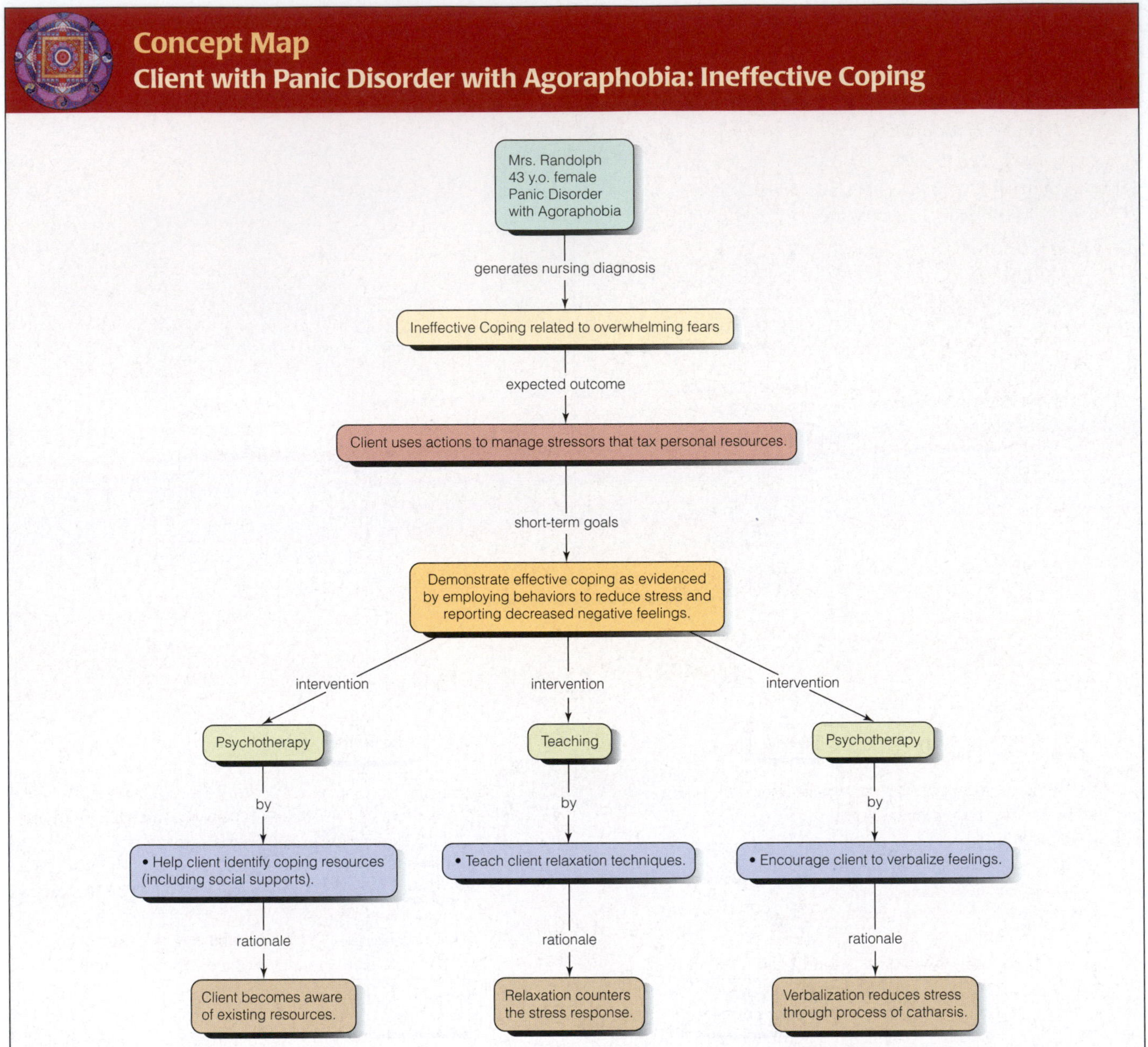
Mrs. Randolph
43 y.o. female
Panic Disorder
with Agoraphobia
generates nursing diagnosis
Ineffective Coping related to overwhelming fears
expected outcome
Client uses actions to manage stressors that tax personal resources.
short-term goals
Demonstrate effective coping as evidenced by employing behaviors to reduce stress and reporting decreased negative feelings.
intervention
intervention
intervention
Psychotherapy
Teaching
Psychotherapy
by
by
by
• Help client identify coping resources (including social supports).
• Teach client relaxation techniques.
• Encourage client to verbalize feelings.
rationale
rationale
rationale
Client becomes aware of existing resources.
Relaxation counters the stress response.
Verbalization reduces stress through process of catharsis.

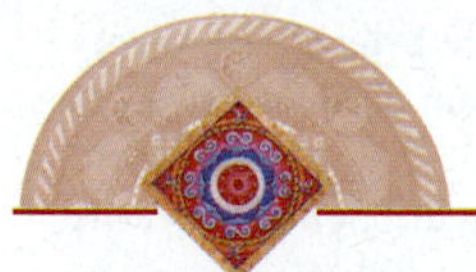

EXPLORE MEDIALINK

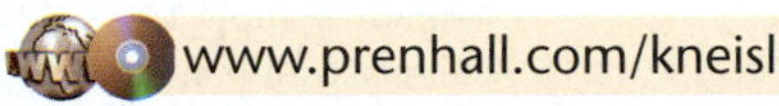
www.prenhall.com/kneisl

For NCLEX-RN® review questions, case studies, and other resources for this chapter see the Pearson Health MediaLink CD-ROM that accompanies this book and the Companion Website at www.prenhall.com/kneisl.

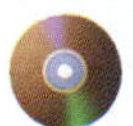

CD-ROM
Audio Glossary
NCLEX-RN® Review Questions
Videos
- *Panic Disorder*
- *Obsessive–Compulsive Disorder*
- *Dissociative Disorders*

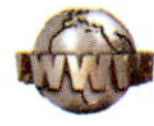

Companion Website
Audio Glossary
NCLEX-RN® Review Questions
Critical Thinking Exercise
- *Panic Attack*

Case Study
- *Assessing the Client with Anxiety*

Care Plan
- *Obsessive–Compulsive Behavior*

MediaLinks
MediaLink Application
- *Managing Anxious Patients*

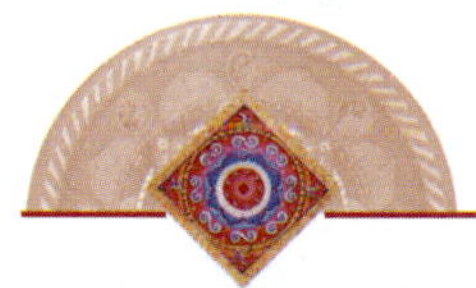

NCLEX-RN® REVIEW QUESTIONS

1. An alteration in serotonin synthesis is associated with which of the following anxiety disorders?
   a. Panic attacks
   b. Specific phobia
   c. Agoraphobia
   d. Childhood obsessive–compulsive disorder

2. A client's husband informs you, "She's had GAD for years, and we figured it would get worse during pregnancy, but instead, she seems more relaxed than ever before in her adult life." Based on your knowledge of neurobiological theory, your best response is:
   1. "She may be getting her psychosocial needs met with the frequent prenatal visits."
   2. "It is possible that progesterone metabolites are actually helping her to relax."
   3. "You are probably seeing the effect of less nicotine and caffeine."
   4. "Do you know if she is self-medicating?"

3. During family support group, a family member states, "I have an anxiety disorder, but I never experienced anything like my sister's dissociative disorder." Your best response is:
   1. "Anxiety disrupts your ability to function. It's the same for your loved one, who defends against anxiety by separating thoughts from feelings."
   2. "Do you know of any physical abuse in your sister's childhood? That is often part of a dissociative client's history."
   3. "Some people believe that clients who say they have multiple personalities are trying to elicit sympathy. Is that what you think?"
   4. "It may be that she has awareness of something you've repressed."

4. Which of the following are characteristic of dissociative disorders but not characteristic of anxiety disorders? (Select all that apply.)
   1. Markedly different presentations over time
   2. Hopelessness and powerlessness with suicidal ideation
   3. Need for long-term treatment with guarded prognosis
   4. Psychosocial history with "missing" blocks of time
   5. Absence of observable signs of anxiety

5. A client asks, "What makes dissociative episodes different from panic attacks?" Your most accurate response is:
1. "They are not very different."
2. "Panic attacks are associated with guilt, shame, or impending doom."
3. "There are physiological changes with dissociative episodes, but not with panic attacks."
4. "In dissociative disorders, an unconscious memory spontaneously enters conscious awareness, triggering the development of dissociation."

6. Which outcome is most realistic and appropriate in planning care for any newly diagnosed client with anxiety or dissociative disorder?
1. Within 2 months, the client will discuss the reasons for episodes with significant others.
2. Within 2 months, the client will be episode-free.
3. Within 1 month, the client will experience decreased frequency of episodes.
4. Within 2 months, the client will establish two new social relationships.

7. A family asks you why their loved one dissociates in response to trauma. Which of the following is your most accurate response?
1. "Dissociation helps decrease anxiety by isolating the thoughts from the feelings about the experience and keeps the person from being completely overwhelmed."
2. "It provides the individual with a 'witness' experience rather than a 'victim' experience, and it is less traumatic for the individual to witness trauma than it is to experience it oneself."
3. "It is not clearly understood, but it seems to have a definite biochemical basis."
4. "When we find out what happened in the months she cannot remember, we will have an explanation about why she dissociates."

8. Which of the following statements highlight the rationale for a thorough and comprehensive assessment for anxiety? (Select all that apply.)
1. Comorbidity with other anxiety disorders
2. Anxiety disorders are the least common of all mental illnesses and may present in a client whose chief complaint is not related to anxiety.
3. Individuals who succeed in avoidance behavior may not demonstrate anxiety despite significant disabling effects on occupational and social functioning.
4. Anxiety may express itself indirectly through nonspecific somatic symptoms.
5. Clients with panic disorder often appear asymptomatic.

9. Which of the following caregiver statements highlights the challenges associated with assessment of the client with a dissociative disorder?
1. "After dissociative clients are admitted, within 24 hours they show significant improvement in their symptoms and behavior."
2. "I know many survivors of physical and sexual abuse, and I can always tell when they dissociate."
3. "Anyone I have ever cared for with a dissociative disorder is a pathological liar."
4. "Clients with dissociative disorder consistently and accurately recall their histories from one hospitalization to the next."

10. Which nurse's statement indicates that she has reflected upon the personal challenges of caring for clients with anxiety and dissociative disorders?
1. "I'm not sure I believe there is such a thing as dissociative identity disorder, but I can certainly think of these clients as having immobilizing anxiety."
2. "Whenever a client starts causing me stress, I take some slow, deep breaths."
3. "Most of my clients with OCD find fault with something, but they appear less anxious if you give them some choices."
4. "When all the emergency room tests come back as unremarkable, we give the clients a brochure about panic disorder. It discusses the disorder as a legitimate medical disorder and gives them hope for recovery with treatment."
5. "If the client criticizes me, I gently remind the client that the critiquing is part of the pathology."

See Appendix C for answers.

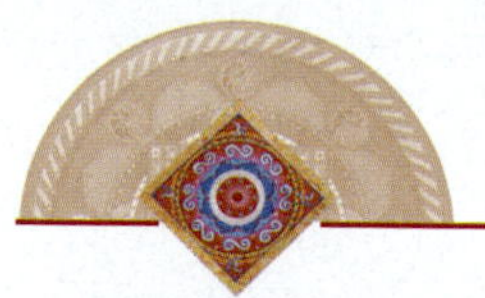

REFERENCES

American Psychiatric Association. (2000). *Diagnostic and statistical manual of mental disorders* (4th ed., Text Revision). Washington, DC: Author.

Antai-Otong, D. (2006). Anxiety disorders. *Nursing 2006, 36*(3), 48–49.

Anxiety Disorders Association of America. (2007). January monthly feature: anxiety disorders and pregnancy. Retrieved January 2007 from http://www.adaa.org/GettingHelp/MonthlyFeatures.asp.

Arnold, P. D., Sicard, T., Burroughs, E., Richter, M. A., & Kennedy, J. L. (2006). Glutamate transporter gene SLC1A1 associated with obsessive-compulsive disorder. *Archives of General Psychiatry, 63*(7), 769–776.

Bormann, J. E., Smith, T. L., Becker, S., Gershwin, M., Pada, L., Grudzinski, A. H., et al. (2005). Efficacy of frequent mantram repetition on stress, quality of life, and spiritual well-being in veterans: A pilot study. *Journal of Holistic Nursing, 23*(4), 395–414.

Bourne, E. J. (2005). *The anxiety and relaxation workbook* (4th ed.). Oakland, CA: New Harbinger Publications.

Choi, Y. H., & Park, K. H. (2006). Therapeutic factors of cognitive behavioral group treatment for social phobia. *Journal of Korean Medical Science, 21*(2), 333–336.

Crane, P. A., & Clements, P. A. (2005). Psychological response to disasters: Focus on adolescents. *Journal of Psychosocial Nursing & Mental Health Services, 43*(8), 31–38.

Davidson, J. R. (2006). Pharmacologic treatment of acute and chronic stress following trauma: 2006. *Journal of Clinical Psychiatry, 67*(Suppl 2), 34–39.

Denys, D., Van Nieuwerburgh, F., Deforce, D., & Westenberg, H. (2006). Association between the dopamine D_2 receptor TaqI A2 allele and low activity COMT allele with obsessive-compulsive disorder in males. *European Neuropsychopharmacology, 16*(6), 446–450.

Eisen, J. L., Mancebo, M. A., Pinto, A., Coles, M. E., Pagano, M. E., Stout, R., et al. (2006). Impact of obsessive-compulsive disorder on quality of life. *Comprehensive Psychiatry, 47*(4), 270–275.

Farrugia, S., & Hudson, J. (2006). Anxiety in adolescents with Asperger Syndrome: Negative thoughts, behavioral problems, and life interference. *Focus on Autism and Other Developmental Disabilities, 21*(1), 25–35.

Flint, A. J. (2005). Generalised anxiety disorder in elderly patients: Epidemiology, diagnosis and treatment options. *Drugs in Aging: 2005, 22*(2), 101–114.

Garcia-Lopez, L. J., Olivares, J., Beidel, D., Albano, A. M., Turner, S., & Rosa, A. I. (2006). Efficacy of three treatment protocols for adolescents with social anxiety disorder: A 5-year follow-up assessment. *Journal of Anxiety Disorders, 20*(2), 175–191.

Girsbrecht, T., Jorgen, E. M., Smelders, F. T., & Merckelbach, H. (2006). Dissociative resting EEG and subjective sleep experiences in undergraduates. *Journal of Nervous & Mental Disorders, 194*(5), 362–368.

Johnson, M., Bulecheck, G., Butcher, H., Moorhead, S., Maas, M., Dochtermann, J., et al. (2005). *NANDA, NOC, & NIC linkages: Nursing diagnoses, outcomes, and interventions.* St. Louis, MO: Elsevier Health Sciences.

Kirvan, C. A., Swedo, S. E., Snider, L. A., & Cunningham, M. W. (2006). Antibody-mediated neuronal cell signaling in behavior and movement disorders. *Journal of Neuroimmunology, 179* (1–2), 173–179.

Lapointe, A. R., Crayton, J. W., DeVito, R., Fichtner, C. G., & Konopka, L. M. (2006). Similar or disparate brain patterns? The intra-personal EEG variability of three women with multiple personality disorder. *Clinical EEG Neuroscience, 37*(3), 235–242.

Mathew, S. J., Amkiel, J. M., & Coplan, J. D. (2005). Open-label trial of riluzole in generalized anxiety disorder. *American Journal of Psychiatry, 162*, 2379–2381.

Mitchell, A. M., Sakraida, T. J., & Zalice, K. K. (2005). Disaster care: Psychological considerations. *Nursing Clinics of North America, 50*(3), 535–550.

Moller, M. D., & Rice, M. J. (2006). The BE SMART trauma reframing psychoeducation program. *Archives of Psychiatric Nursing, 20*(1), 21–31.

Mossner, R., Walitza, S., Geller, F., Scherag, A., Gutknecht, L, Jacob, C., et al. (2006). Transmission disequilibrium of polymorphic variants in the tryptophan hydroxylase-2 gene in children and adolescents with obsessive-compulsive disorder. *The International Journal of Neuropsychopharmacology, 9*(4), 437–442.

Moulds, M. L., & Bryant, R. A. (2005). An investigation of retrieval inhibition in acute stress disorder. *Journal of Traumatic Stress, 18*(3), 233–236.

Murray, A. (2005). Recurrence of post traumatic stress disorder. *Nursing older people, 17*(6), 24–30.

National Institute of Mental Health. (2006). *The numbers count: Mental disorders in America.* Retrieved January 2007 from http://www.nimh.nih.gov.

Rank, O. (1952). *The trauma of birth.* Philadelphia: Robert Brunner.

Reinders, A. A., Nijenhuis, E. R., Quak, J., Korf, J., Haaksua, J., Prans, A. M., et al. (2006). Psychobiological characteristics of Dissociative Identity Disorder: A symptom provocation study. *Biological Psychiatry, 60*(7), 730–740.

Sadock, B. J., & Sadock, V. A. (2005). *Kaplan & Sadock's pocket handbook of clinical psychiatry* (4th ed.). Philadelphia: Lippincott Williams & Wilkins.

Storch, E. A., Murphy, T. K., Geffken, G. R., Mann, G., Adkins, J., Merlo, L. J., et al. (2006). Cognitive-behavioral therapy for PANDAS-related obsessive-compulsive disorder: Findings from a preliminary waitlist controlled open trial. *Journal of the American Academy of Child and Adolescent Psychiatry, 45*(10), 1171–1178.

Sullivan, H. S. (1953). *The interpersonal theory of psychiatry.* New York: Norton.

Tyrell, M. (2005). School phobia. *Journal of Nursing Scholarship, 21*(3), 147–151.

Zwanzger, P., & Rupprecht, R. (2005). Selective GABAergic treatment for panic? Investigations in experimental panic induction and panic disorder. *Journal of Psychiatry Neuroscience, 30*(3), 167–175.

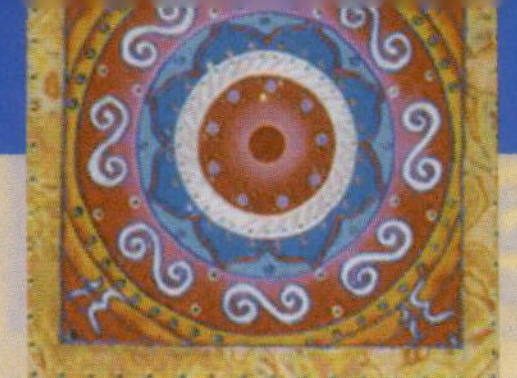

CHAPTER

19

Somatoform and Sleep Disorders

SUE C. DELAUNE AND CAROL REN KNEISL

KEY TERMS

body dysmorphic disorder (BDD) *481*
cataplexy *498*
circadian rhythm sleep disorders *498*
conversion disorder *479*
dyssomnias *495*
factitious disorder *483*
factitious disorder by proxy *484*
hypnagogic hallucination *498*
hypochondriasis *481*
la belle indifférence *481*
malingering *483*
Munchausen by proxy syndrome *484*
Munchausen syndrome *484*
narcolepsy *498*
nightmare disorder *501*
pain disorder *481*
parasomnias *500*
periodic limb movements disorder *500*
primary gain *479*
primary hypersomnia *497*
primary insomnia *495*
polysomnogram *495*
REM rebound *493*
restless legs syndrome *500*

(continued)

LEARNING OUTCOMES

After completing this chapter, you will be able to:

1. Compare and contrast the biopsychosocial characteristics of various somatoform disorders.
2. Describe theories that aid in the understanding of somatoform disorders.
3. Distinguish between somatoform disorders, factitious disorders, and malingering.
4. Explain the importance of performing a thorough and comprehensive assessment of clients with somatoform disorders.
5. Discuss possible personal challenges to professional practice when caring for clients with somatoform disorders.
6. Describe theories that aid in the understanding of sleep disorders.
7. Describe the sleep patterns most commonly associated with major depressive disorder, manic episodes in bipolar disorder, schizophrenia, and substance abuse.
8. Describe three key assessments that are pertinent to each of the major symptoms of sleep disorders.
9. Compare and contrast the guidelines for good sleep hygiene with those for dealing with insomnia.

CRITICAL THINKING CHALLENGE

Jackie DeJong, a 24-year-old student being seen in the university counseling center, tells you that she has not slept well in the last 2 months. She states, "The night I went to the sleep lab was particularly bad—I hardly slept a wink." However, you have read the sleep lab report on her health record. The polysomnogram showed a typical distribution of sleep stages for someone her age, with sleep onset 15 minutes after lights out and three brief awakenings in a 7-hour period.

1. How can you reconcile Jackie's subjective report with the objective evidence?
2. How might alternative explanations alter how you would apply the nursing process? Is any one view more correct than the other?

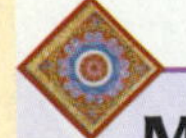

MEDIALINK 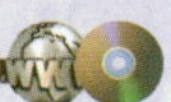 www.prenhall.com/kneisl

Go to the Pearson Health MediaLink CD-ROM and the Companion Website at www.prenhall.com/kneisl for interactive resources for this chapter.

KEY TERMS *(continued)*

secondary gain *479*
sleep apnea *497*
sleep paralysis *498*
sleep terror disorder *501*
sleepwalking disorder *502*
somatization disorder *479*
somatoform disorders *479*
substance-induced sleep disorder *504*
undifferentiated somatoform disorder *483*

As you know, individuals respond to stress in a variety of ways. Some individuals have a maladaptive response to stress in which they unconsciously transform their emotions into physical symptoms. Remember that this is not a deliberate process used by clients experiencing somatoform disorders. In order to work effectively and compassionately with clients with these disorders, you need to know that pain of psychogenic origin is as hurtful as pain with a biological basis.

Individuals also respond to stress, both physical and mental, with disruptions in sleep. Sleep is a basic human need. It affects mental health and, conversely, is affected by mental health. It is so much a part of the normal rhythm of our lives that we tend to take sleep for granted until it is disrupted. Disrupted sleep is a particularly important consideration in mental health and illness because of its subtle but pervasive effects on mood, performance, and physical functioning. Lack of sleep tends to decrease our ability to cope, to deal with ambiguity, to make decisions, and to feel confident. Sleep pattern disturbance is often an early symptom of mental illness. For example, a change in sleep patterns is among the diagnostic criteria for major depressive disorder, manic episode, and dysthymic disorder.

SOMATOFORM DISORDERS

The essential features of **somatoform disorders** are physical symptoms suggesting physical disorders for which there is no evidence of organic or physiologic causes. Somatoform disorders, formerly referred to as psychosomatic disorders, are sometimes confused with physical disorders because the predominant symptoms are physical. Client and family educational information about somatoform disorders is available on www.psyweb.com and can be accessed through the Companion Website for this book.

Somatization Disorder

The diagnosis of **somatization disorder** applies to clients who, like Sonya in the clinical example that follows, have sought medical attention for recurrent and multiple somatic complaints over a duration of several years.

CLINICAL EXAMPLE

Sonya has appointments with a gastroenterologist, a gynecologist, a cardiologist, and her primary care physician, all in the same month. Now 54 years old, Sonya has had multiple somatic complaints of nausea, bloating, constipation, heart palpitations, and dizziness for almost 30 years. Although several gastrointestinal X-rays, heart studies, and physical examinations have not indicated the presence of disease, Sonya is convinced her disorders are real. She changes physicians regularly.

Historically, somatization disorder has been referred to as "hysteria," "hysterical reaction," and "Briquet's syndrome." This problem usually begins before the age of 30, has a chronic course, and is often accompanied by anxiety and depressed mood. Clients believe they have been ill for a good part of their lives and report lengthy lists of symptoms, including blindness, paralysis, convulsions, dysmenorrhea, nausea, and other gastrointestinal difficulties. These symptoms are not caused intentionally, nor are they feigned (faked). The pain experienced by individuals with somatization disorder is real. A list of diagnostic criteria for somatization disorder is in the DSM-IV-TR Diagnostic Criteria feature on page 480.

Even though somatization is common in children, somatization disorder is rarely diagnosed in children and adolescents. Children who are diagnosed with somatization disorder tend to have caregivers who consistently overreact to the child's somatic complaints, thus reinforcing the complaints.

Conversion Disorder

In **conversion disorder,** clients report impaired physical function that is related to the expression of a psychologic conflict. The following clinical example illustrates what takes place in conversion disorder.

CLINICAL EXAMPLE

Ronald is the 17-year-old eldest son of a Baptist minister in a rural community. His father expects his family to be pillars of the community and to serve as wholesome examples for the congregation. Ronald has recently developed a paralysis of his right hand, for which no physical basis has been found. Unknown to others, Ronald has been masturbating almost daily since he was 13 years old. He finds masturbation pleasurable, but feels anxiety and guilt at the same time.

The loss of functional ability is due to psychological, not biological, problems. However, the symptoms in conversion disorder are not consciously produced. The diagnostic criteria for conversion disorder are listed in the DSM-IV-TR Diagnostic Criteria feature on page 480.

Two mechanisms are thought to explain what a person "gets" from having a conversion disorder. The first, **primary gain**, helps the person keep the psychologic need or conflict out of conscious awareness. For example, a woman may become blind to avoid acknowledging a traumatic event she has seen. In this instance, the symptom is a partial solution to the underlying conflict (not having to acknowledge witnessing the traumatic event because she has suddenly become sightless). The second mechanism, **secondary gain**, helps the person

MediaLink PSYweb.com

DSM-IV-TR Diagnostic Criteria for Somatization Disorder

A. A history of many physical complaints beginning before age 30 years that occur over a period of several years and result in treatment being sought or significant impairment in social, occupational, or other important areas of functioning.

B. Each of the following criteria must have been met, with individual symptoms occurring at any time during the course of the disturbance:

1. *four pain symptoms:* a history of pain related to at least four different sites or functions (e.g., head, abdomen, back, joints, extremities, chest, rectum, during menstruation, during sexual intercourse, or during urination)
2. *two gastrointestinal symptoms:* a history of at least two gastrointestinal symptoms other than pain (e.g., nausea, bloating, vomiting other than during pregnancy, diarrhea, or intolerance of several different foods)
3. *one sexual symptom:* a history of at least one sexual or reproductive symptom other than pain (e.g., sexual indifference, erectile or ejaculatory dysfunction, irregular menses, excessive menstrual bleeding, vomiting throughout pregnancy)
4. *one pseudoneurological symptom:* a history of at least one symptom or deficit suggesting a neurological condition not limited to pain (conversion symptoms such as impaired coordination or balance, paralysis or localized weakness, difficulty swallowing or lump in throat, aphonia, urinary retention, hallucinations, loss of touch or pain sensation, double vision, blindness, deafness, seizures; dissociative symptoms such as amnesia; or loss of consciousness other than fainting)

C. Either (1) or (2):

1. after appropriate investigation, each of the symptoms in Criterion B cannot be fully explained by a known general medical condition or the direct effects of a substance (e.g., a drug of abuse, a medication)
2. when there is a related general medical condition, the physical complaints or resulting social or occupational impairment are in excess of what would be expected from the history, physical examination, or laboratory findings

D. The symptoms are not intentionally produced or feigned (as in Factitious Disorder or Malingering)

Source: Reprinted with permission from the *Diagnostic and Statistical Manual of Mental Disorders,* Fourth Edition, Text Revision. (Copyright 2000). American Psychiatric Association.

USING DSM-IV-TR

Health care providers often use language unfamiliar to clients and their families. Explain *somatization* in such a way that clients and family members can understand its meaning.

avoid a distressing, uncomfortable, or repugnant activity while at the same time receiving support from others. For example, a soldier with a paralyzed arm could hardly be expected to fire a gun and is also likely to receive sympathy because of his paralysis. Unlike malingering and factitious disorder, discussed later in the chapter, the symptoms are not deliberately produced to obtain benefits.

Common characteristics associated with conversion disorder clients are:

1. Self-dramatization
2. Exhibitionism
3. Narcissism
4. Emotionalism
5. Seductiveness
6. Dependence
7. Manipulativeness
8. Childishness
9. Suggestibility

DSM-IV-TR Diagnostic Criteria for Conversion Disorder

A. One or more symptoms or deficits affecting voluntary motor or sensory function that suggest a neurological or other general medical condition.

B. Psychological factors are judged to be associated with the symptom or deficit because the initiation or exacerbation of the symptoms or deficit is preceded by conflicts or other stressors.

C. The symptom or deficit is not intentionally produced or feigned (as in Factitious Disorder or Malingering).

D. The symptom or deficit cannot, after appropriate investigation, be fully explained by a general medical condition, or by the direct effects of a substance, or as a culturally sanctioned behavior or experience.

E. The symptom or deficit causes clinically significant distress or impairment in social, occupational, or other important areas of functioning or warrants medical evaluation.

F. The symptom or deficit is not limited to pain or sexual dysfunction, does not occur exclusively during the course of Somatization Disorder, and is not better accounted for by another mental disorder.

Source: Reprinted with permission from the *Diagnostic and Statistical Manual of Mental Disorders,* Fourth Edition, Text Revision. (Copyright 2000). American Psychiatric Association.

USING DSM-IV-TR

Health care providers often use language unfamiliar to clients and their families. Explain *conversion disorder* in such a way that clients and family members can readily understand the difference between it and an actual medical condition.

Another frequent symptom characteristic of clients with conversion disorder, although not necessarily present in all instances, is **la belle indifférence**, an inappropriate lack of concern about a disability. Tom, in the clinical example that follows, demonstrates la belle indifférence.

CLINICAL EXAMPLE

Tom is experiencing a conversion disorder that has led to his inability to walk. Although Tom stated, "I woke up this morning with no feeling in my legs; for some reason they won't move," he seems totally unconcerned about his problem despite its severity.

The person is actually calmer as a result of the somatic symptom. This problem usually begins in adolescence or early adulthood, although a conversion disorder may appear at any time of life. Regardless of the time of onset, a conversion disorder can seriously impede normal life activities. Functional impairments may affect the individual's ability to function at work, at home, or in social situations.

Pain Disorder

In **pain disorder**, clients experience pain for which there is no physiologic basis and often have accompanying psychological factors. The pain is usually severe enough to disrupt several functional areas. As a result of this dysfunction, the client often experiences unemployment, disability, and/or family problems. A person with pain disorder is often convinced that somewhere there is a health care provider who can "cure" the pain. Thus, the person may spend much time, money, and energy needlessly in pursuit of a "cure." The pain becomes the central issue of one's life; pain takes control of one's ability to function. A list of diagnostic criteria for pain disorder is in the DSM-IV-TR Diagnostic Criteria feature below.

Hypochondriasis

Clients with **hypochondriasis** are preoccupied with the fear or belief that they have a serious disease, which, on physical evaluation, is not present. The preoccupation may be built around any of the following:

- Bodily functions (peristalsis, heartbeat)
- Minor physical problems (an occasional headache, a slight cough)
- Ambiguous, vague physical feelings ("tired ovaries" or "aching veins")

The unrealistic fear or belief persists for a period of at least 6 months despite medical reassurance that no illness is present. This fear impairs the client's social and/or occupational functioning.

CLINICAL EXAMPLE

Reading the newspaper and watching the news on television have become anxiety-provoking experiences for Lena. Lena has been worried about AIDS, avian flu, contaminated spinach and bean sprouts, and even head lice. She attributes any symptom she has—an itch, a runny nose, a loose bowel movement—to any one of a number of possible medical conditions. If her worries have not been relieved by her research on the Internet, Lena calls in sick to work and makes an appointment to see her primary physician or a nurse practitioner.

The diagnostic criteria for hypochondriasis are listed in the DSM-IV-TR Diagnostic Criteria feature on page 482.

Body Dysmorphic Disorder

Clients with **body dysmorphic disorder (BDD)** are preoccupied with some imagined defect in their physical appearance. The preoccupation is out of proportion to any actual abnormality.

DSM-IV-TR Diagnostic Criteria for Pain Disorder

A. Pain in one or more anatomical sites is the predominant focus of the clinical presentation and is of sufficient severity to warrant clinical attention.
B. The pain causes clinically significant distress or impairment in social, occupational, or other important areas of functioning.
C. Psychological factors are judged to have an important role in the onset, severity, exacerbation, or maintenance of the pain.
D. The symptom or deficit is not intentionally produced or feigned (as in Factitious Disorder or Malingering).
E. The pain is not better accounted for by a Mood, Anxiety, or Psychotic Disorder and does not meet criteria for Dyspareunia.

Source: Reprinted with permission from the *Diagnostic and Statistical Manual of Mental Disorders,* Fourth Edition, Text Revision. (Copyright 2000). American Psychiatric Association.

USING DSM-IV-TR

Health care providers often use language unfamiliar to clients and their families. Explain how psychological factors can affect pain in such a way that clients and family members can understand the basis for pain disorder.

DSM-IV-TR Diagnostic Criteria for Hypochondriasis

A. Preoccupation with fears of having, or the idea that one has, a serious disease based on the person's misinterpretation of bodily symptoms.
B. The preoccupation persists despite appropriate medical evaluation and reassurance.
C. The belief in Criterion A is not of delusional intensity (as in Delusional Disorder, Somatic Type) and is not restricted to a circumscribed concern about appearance (as in Body Dysmorphic Disorder).
D. The preoccupation causes clinically significant distress or impairment in social, occupational, or other important areas of functioning.
E. The duration of the disturbance is at least 6 months.
F. The preoccupation is not better accounted for by Generalized Anxiety Disorder, Obsessive-Compulsive Disorder, Panic Disorder, a Major Depressive Episode, Separation Anxiety, or another Somatoform Disorder.

Source: Reprinted with permission from the *Diagnostic and Statistical Manual of Mental Disorders,* Fourth Edition, Text Revision. (Copyright 2000). American Psychiatric Association.

USING DSM-IV-TR

Health care providers often use language unfamiliar to clients and their families. In terms that clients and family members can readily understand, explain how an individual can misinterpret his or her bodily symptoms.

CLINICAL EXAMPLE

Joanna is very worried about the size of her nose despite reassurances that her nose is normal. She spends an inordinate amount of time in front of the mirror using cosmetics designed to shadow or minimize her nose. Joanna recently turned down a job promotion that would have put her in charge of the entire human resources department at the company at which she works. The job involves training human resources staff at locations in ten other cities. Joanna cannot bear the thought that trainees will have to look at her nose all day.

This belief, even though it may be extreme, is not of delusional proportion. The majority of people with BDD have very little insight into the origins of their symptoms. In fact, the greater the perceived defects, the lower the degree of insight (Marazzita et al., 2006). See the following DSM-IV-TR Diagnostic Criteria feature for a description of the diagnostic criteria for BDD.

People with BDD often use avoidance, such as Joanna does, to cope with their perceived defect(s). Such avoidance may result in extreme social isolation. For example, a man who tries to camouflage his "defect" of imaginary hair loss may leave his home only at night, and then only with a hat covering the "defective" part. The preoccupation with one's appearance is very time consuming; thus, it restricts activities. In some cases, clients seek out cosmetic surgery to "cure" the imagined defect. In some people, BDD "interferes with their judgment and can lead them to make poor choices when considering cosmetic procedures" (Ritvo, Melnick, Marcus, & Glick, 2006, p. 194). This is a major reason why plastic and cosmetic surgeons should do careful screenings before performing cosmetic or reconstructive surgery.

DSM-IV-TR Diagnostic Criteria for Body Dysmorphic Disorder

A. Preoccupation with an imagined defect in appearance. If a slight physical anomaly is present, the person's concern is markedly excessive.
B. The preoccupation causes clinically significant distress or impairment in social, occupational, or other important areas of functioning.
C. The preoccupation is not better accounted for by another mental disorder (e.g., dissatisfaction with body shape and size in Anorexia Nervosa).

Source: Reprinted with permission from the *Diagnostic and Statistical Manual of Mental Disorders,* Fourth Edition, Text Revision. (Copyright 2000). American Psychiatric Association.

USING DSM-IV-TR

Health care providers often use language unfamiliar to clients and their families. Explain what it means to be preoccupied with an imaginary defect in such a way that clients and family members can understand the basis for body dysmorphic disorder.

DSM-IV-TR Diagnostic Criteria for Undifferentiated Somatoform Disorder

A. One or more physical complaints (e.g., fatigue, loss of appetite, gastrointestinal or urinary complaints).

B. Either (1) or (2):

1. after appropriate investigation, the symptoms cannot be fully explained by a known general medical condition or the direct effects of a substance (e.g., a drug of abuse, a medication)
2. when there is a related general medical condition, the physical complaints or resulting social or occupational impairment is in excess of what would be expected from the history, physical examination, or laboratory findings

C. The symptoms cause clinically significant distress or impairment in social, occupational, or other important areas of functioning.

D. The duration of the disturbance is at least 6 months.

E. The disturbance is not better accounted for by another mental disorder (e.g., another Somatoform Disorder, Sexual Dysfunction, Mood Disorder, Anxiety Disorder, Sleep Disorder, or Psychotic Disorder).

F. The symptom is not intentionally produced or feigned (as in Factitious Disorder or Malingering).

Source: Reprinted with permission from the *Diagnostic and Statistical Manual of Mental Disorders,* Fourth Edition, Text Revision. (Copyright 2000). American Psychiatric Association.

USING DSM-IV-TR

Health care providers often use language unfamiliar to clients and their families. Explain the difference between a general medical condition and a somatoform disorder in terms that clients and family members can understand.

Undifferentiated Somatoform Disorder

In **undifferentiated somatoform disorder**, clients have multiple physical complaints of at least 6 months' duration; extensive evaluation reveals no organic problem. When the client does have an organic disease, the complaints or impairments are grossly excessive. Remember that the symptoms experienced by an individual with this disorder are not intentionally produced. The pain, which is psychogenic in nature, is real to the client. The DSM-IV-TR Diagnostic Criteria feature above lists the diagnostic criteria for undifferentiated somatoform disorder.

MALINGERING

Malingering occurs when a person deliberately fakes symptoms in order to benefit. It is not considered a psychiatric disorder because it involves deliberate falsification of illness. Malingering is consciously motivated and usually results in secondary gain, which may be in the form of extra attention, relief from responsibilities, or financial rewards, as shown in the following clinical example.

CLINICAL EXAMPLE

Joyce is a police officer. She fakes episodes of back pain in order to avoid street patrol. Whenever she is assigned to this duty, Joyce claims to be in too much pain to work.

Malingering often occurs in young adulthood, and according to Peebles, Sabella, Franco, and Goldfarb (2005), about 5% or less of clients treated by primary care providers are either malingering or have factitious disorders such as those described in the next section. Malingering often occurs in the following situations: personal injury and workers' compensation litigation; military service; and criminal cases.

FACTITIOUS DISORDER

Malingering and somatoform disorders are sometimes mistakenly confused with **factitious disorder**, in which clients intentionally produce or feign physical or psychological symptoms (American Psychiatric Association [APA], 2000). The major difference between factitious disorder and malingering is that a person with a factitious disorder has a psychological need to assume the sick role. Unlike malingering, external incentives for the behavior are absent. According to Savino and Fordtran (2006), the self-induction of disease is a conscious act but the underlying motivation is usually unconscious. The course of factitious disorder usually consists of intermittent episodes.

Factitious disorder may occur on a continuum of mild (giving a verbal list of symptoms) to moderate (simulating physical symptoms) to severe (inflicting injury). Dermatologic manifestations are very common; however, physical symptoms can include almost any disease state (Peebles, Sabella, Franco, & Goldfarb, 2005). Thelma is an example of an individual with factitious disorder.

CLINICAL EXAMPLE

Thelma has been admitted to the hospital after being seen in an acute care walk-in clinic with blood in her urine. The admitting physician has ordered several invasive procedures—catheterization, blood work, and cystoscopy among others. The physician does not know that Thelma has been taking anticoagulants to produce blood in her urine.

Clients with factitious disorders deliberately give false medical histories that can be quite elaborate. It can be difficult to detect a factitious disorder because clients may use

DSM-IV-TR Diagnostic Criteria for Factitious Disorder

A. Intentional production or feigning of physical or psychological signs or symptoms.
B. The motivation for the behavior is to assume the sick role.
C. External incentives for the behavior (such as economic gain, avoiding legal responsibility, or improving physical well-being, as in Malingering) are absent.

Source: Reprinted with permission from the *Diagnostic and Statistical Manual of Mental Disorders,* Fourth Edition, Text Revision. (Copyright 2000). American Psychiatric Association.

USING DSM-IV-TR

Health care providers often use language unfamiliar to clients and their families. Explain what it means to be motivated "to assume the sick role" in such a way that clients and family members can understand.

several different names and usually seek treatment in several agencies to avoid detection or recognition by someone who has encountered the client during a previous hospitalization or office or clinic visit.

The fabricated symptoms—e.g., fever, anemia, hematuria—are indeed symptoms of "real" diseases; however, there is no organic reason for the appearance of the symptoms. The client provides an untruthful account of symptoms and fakes signs of illness in an attempt to receive medical treatment. Uncontrollable lying is the hallmark characteristic of individuals with factitious disorder; stories are fabricated in order to capture the attention of others. Even though symptoms are explained in very dramatic terms, it is difficult to gather specific information about their onset and duration (Malatack, Consolini, Mann, & Raab, 2006). Individuals with factitious disorder are usually very knowledgeable about medicine. Being knowledgeable, imaginative, and sophisticated about medical systems, medical terminology, and the routines of hospitals and other treatment facilities allows them to convincingly fake a constellation of symptoms. The diagnostic criteria for factitious disorder are given in the following DSM-IV-TR feature.

When the disorder is severe, chronic, and unremitting—involving repeated hospitalizations, traveling between health care providers and health care facilities, and pathological lying of an intriguing and fantastic nature (termed *pseudologica fantastica*)—it is often referred to as **Munchausen syndrome**. Ron is an example of such a person.

CLINICAL EXAMPLE

Ron is lying on a treatment table in the emergency department. He is in acute pain with a dislocated shoulder. This hospital is located 20 miles from the city in which Ron lives. What the emergency physician does not know is that Ron has been to several different physicians in his city and has had multiple prior hospitalizations for factitious symptoms—pain, fevers of undetermined origin, rashes, and dizziness. All physical assessments proved negative. Ron usually berates the physician, the nurse, or the X-ray technician for being unable to find the cause of his problem and signs himself out against medical advice. The emergency physician also does not know that Ron has dislocated his own shoulder.

As this clinical example demonstrates, Munchausen syndrome can become a lifelong pattern. TABLE 19-1 ■ identifies the distinctions between somatoform disorder, factitious disorder, and malingering.

Factitious Disorder by Proxy

Factitious disorder by proxy, sometimes called **Munchausen by proxy syndrome**, occurs when parents or caregivers deliberately induce signs of an illness in another person, usually their own child. It is difficult for health care providers to deal with situations in which a caregiver or parent deliberately injures the person under their care. In these

TABLE 19-1 ■ Comparison of Somatoform Disorder, Factitious Disorder, and Malingering

Somatoform Disorders	Factitious Disorders	Malingering
Symptoms are not under voluntary control.	Symptoms are deliberately produced.	Symptoms are feigned (consciously produced).
Unconscious motivation.	Motivation to assume sick role in order to gain attention and/or obtain medical treatment.	Various motivations, including financial gain, relief of duties, obtaining drugs.
Primary gain: reduction of anxiety.	No obvious secondary gain.	Obvious secondary gain(s).

situations, health care providers should seek clinical supervision or a consultant to help them to cope with their personal responses.

Unlike factitious disorder, factitious disorder by proxy is not yet recognized in the DSM multiaxial coding system because of insufficient information to warrant inclusion. It warrants further study for possible inclusion in a future edition of the DSM.

In factitious disorder by proxy, caregivers deliberately injure their victims in order to gain sympathy or attention for themselves. The victim is usually a preschool child, but could be of any age including adulthood through old age. The individual with this syndrome has an insatiable need for attention, even though the person's behavior is harmful to others. The child (or other victim) is viewed by the perpetrator not as a target but rather as a means of obtaining attention (Malatack et al., 2006). The following clinical example discusses a woman with factitious disorder by proxy.

CLINICAL EXAMPLE

A mother has been regularly and deliberately administering large doses of laxatives to her 15-month-old toddler over a period of several months. When the child has episodes of cramping, flatulence, and bloody diarrhea, the mother, appearing to be very concerned, takes her to the emergency department of a local hospital. Diagnostic studies show no medical reason for the toddler's symptoms.

It is wise to suspect the presence of factitious disorder by proxy if certain indicators are present. These indicators are identified in the What Every Pediatric Nurse Should Know feature.

WHAT EVERY PEDIATRIC NURSE SHOULD KNOW

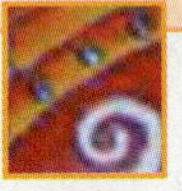

Factitious Disorder by Proxy

Factitious disorder by proxy is a potentially fatal form of child abuse. Not only is the child's life disrupted, the child is usually subjected to frequent hospitalizations and invasive medical procedures. Therefore, the child's safety is of the utmost concern.

An evaluation by an interdisciplinary team that includes health experts is called for whenever this syndrome is suspected. It requires the collection of evidence and the development of a plan to provide appropriate care for the hospitalized child, involve the appropriate authorities (such as child protective services), and obtain help for the child's parent or caretaker.

Child health care providers should be suspicious of situations in which:

- A child has unexplained, recurrent, or rare symptoms.
- The parent denies knowing the cause of the illness.
- When the caretaker is present, so are the symptoms; however, when the child is separated from the caretaker, the symptoms resolve.
- The illness is unresponsive to treatment.
- The clinical findings are inconsistent.
- There is a history of several hospital visits for treatment.

BIOPSYCHOSOCIAL THEORIES

Biologic, genetic, and psychosocial theories help to understand somatoform disorders. The following section presents current research findings about the etiology of somatoform disorders.

Biologic Factors

In somatoform disorders, physical symptoms are present but evidence of physiologic disease is not. The symptoms are thought to be linked to psychologic factors or emotional conflict. However, there is some evidence that brain abnormalities may lead to altered pain perception (Bourne, 2005; Sadock & Sadock, 2007). Biochemical imbalances, such as decreased amounts of endorphins and serotonin, may cause some people to experience pain more intensely than those with normal brain chemistry. Following are the results of other current studies that support a biological basis for somatoform disorders.

- Perceptual disturbances occur with a high frequency among individuals with somatoform pain disorder. In this study, subjects with pain disorder were unable to distinguish tactile stimuli that were self-produced from external stimuli (Karst et al., 2005).
- The positive response of clients to treatment with amitriptyline (Elavil) supports the belief that a biochemical imbalance is present in somatoform pain disorder (Ikawa, Yamada, & Ikeuchi, 2006).

Genetic Theories

Somatization disorder occurs in 10% to 20% of female first-degree biologic relatives of women with somatization disorder (APA, 2000). The results of adoption studies indicate that both genetic and environmental factors contribute to the risk for somatization disorder (APA, 2000). Other studies with identical twins have shown an increased occurrence of hypochondriasis (Sadock & Sadock, 2007).

Psychosocial Theories

Communication theorists believe that manifestations of somatization are nonverbal body language intended to communicate a message to significant others. Sometimes the message is as general as "pay attention to me" or "take care of me." At other times the *conversion of anxiety* actually symbolizes the nature of the specific underlying conflict. For example, a woman who wants to strike her children may develop a paralysis of her arm. A girl who feels guilty about reading erotic books may become blind. Both experience the primary gain of protection from the anxiety-provoking impulses, and both get secondary gains of attention and sympathy. Such behavior patterns are most likely to occur among clients who lack appropriate coping skills.

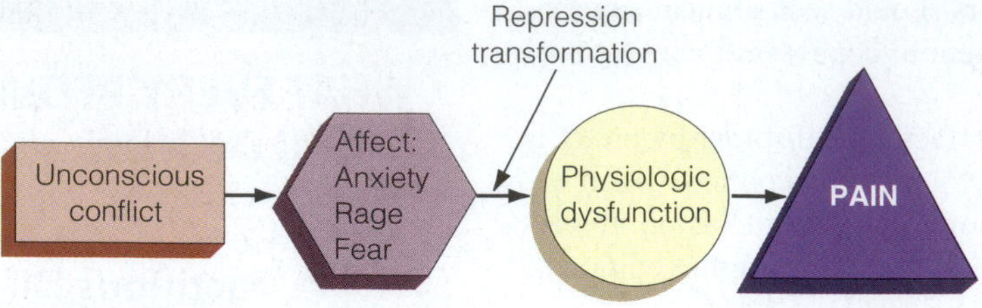

FIGURE 19-1 ■ The mechanism of idiopathic pain.

Many individuals who engage in somatization were reared in chaotic families. The family dysfunction was usually marital discord, substance abuse, and/or personality disorders. For whatever reason, the child received inadequate nurturing. Many adults with somatoform disorders experienced physical or sexual abuse as children. Clients who deal with anxiety by converting it to physical symptoms usually show no other psychological symptoms, such as disturbed thoughts or depressed moods.

Pain is associated with a great many disease processes, including some of the organ-specific somatoform disorders. Pain can be adaptive or maladaptive in that it often indicates real danger but sometimes it interferes with functioning. Consciousness, attention, perception, and cognition are all necessary for the experience of pain. According to modern theories of pain perception, humans have a control system over pain that operates as a "gate." Pain stimuli can be "allowed in" or "shut out" from the cerebral cortex, depending essentially on the meaning the person attaches to the stimulus. This underscores the importance of meaning, symbol, and affect in the experience of pain sensation. FIGURE 19-1 ■ shows the basic mechanism for so-called idiopathic pain (pain of unknown origin).

In psychoanalytic concepts, the unconscious conflicts are a result of traumatic or frustrating childhood experiences that are reawakened in adult life by a similar stress or frustration. According to this theory, the person cannot express the affect because of feelings of guilt, fear of loss of love, or fear of retribution. The affect is therefore repressed and transformed into physiologic correlates, such as pain.

Humanistic Theories

It is important to consider clients with somatoform disorders in the context of what is happening in their lives. Stress related to relationships and work may be the precipitants for somatic symptoms. One study on clients with conversion disorder states that instead of looking for a single cause we should consider "multifactorial stress models" (Roelofs, Spinhoven, Sandijck, Moene, & Hoogduin, 2005, p. 514).

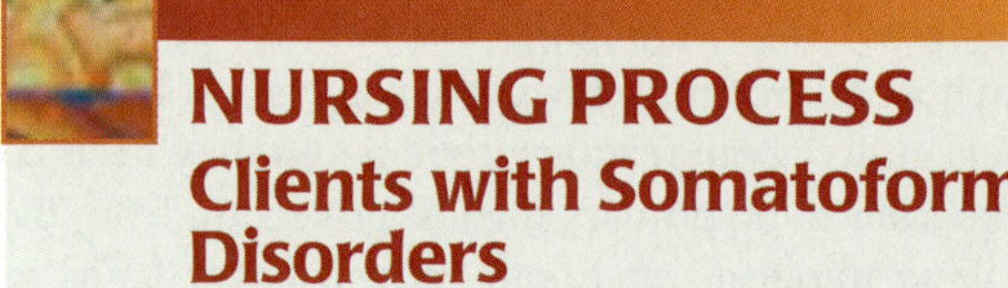

NURSING PROCESS
Clients with Somatoform Disorders

When you work with clients experiencing somatoform disorders, you will be challenged by multiple complex problems. The nursing process provides a systematic method for delivering care to clients affected by somatoform disorders. Your values and beliefs will influence how well you implement the nursing process. If you are unaware of your values and beliefs, you are likely to express them nonverbally to clients and family members. Therefore, it is imperative that you increase your self-awareness in order to be more effective when working with clients with somatoform disorders. The Your Self-Awareness feature below is designed to help you to become more self-aware.

Assessment

Assessment of clients with somatoform disorders is often difficult because of the many psychobiologic factors involved. Careful and thorough assessment—subjective as well as objective—to rule out the possibility of a physical problem is crucial, as shown in the following clinical example.

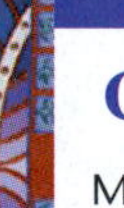

CLINICAL EXAMPLE

Magda was referred for treatment to a local mental health clinic by her primary care physician. She had weakness and numbness of her right arm. When her primary care physician could find no physiologic reason for Magda's symptoms, he diagnosed her problem as a conversion disorder and referred her to the mental health clinic. The nurse who admitted

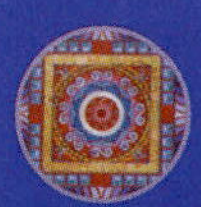

YOUR SELF-AWARENESS
Exploring Your Feelings Toward Clients with Somatoform Disorders

Focus on your feelings when you are caring for clients with somatoform disorders. Ask yourself the following questions and then evaluate the relationship between your answers and your reactions to clients with somatoform disorders.

- How well do you handle frustration?
- How do you respond to the expression of anger, either passive or aggressive, by others?
- How patient are you? Are you able to be satisfied with small successes?
- Can you tell when you are becoming defensive?
- How can you tell if another person is experiencing "real" pain?

Magda to the clinic performed a thorough physical assessment and history. The medical history revealed that Magda had surgery on her left kidney 3 months ago. The nurse made the connection between the surgical position (on her right side) necessary to perform Magda's surgery and Magda's symptoms. The numbness and weakness were actually caused by pressure on the brachial plexus in her right arm during surgery. Magda was discharged from the mental health clinic and referred for physical rehabilitation.

In this clinical example, a complete and accurate assessment of all factors identified the appropriate course of action for Magda and spared her from a stigmatizing psychiatric diagnosis. Some sample questions useful in determining the presence of this disorder are given in the following Your Assessment Approach feature.

Subjective Data

Clients with somatoform disorders report physical symptoms for which there is no positive evidence of organic or physiologic cause. For example, clients with hypochondriasis may return many times to the outpatient clinic or emergency department demanding to be reexamined or retested. They feel they are suffering from some major illness that has been undetected. They are not reassured by the lack of physical findings and may go from physician to physician in an attempt to find someone who will validate their fears. This "doctor shopping" may lead to fragmented care and misuse of medication. Because the person is usually a poor historian, a complete medical history (including medications taken) is not always obtained. Although individuals with somatoform disorder usually describe their condition with colorful, exaggerated language, you may find it is difficult to obtain specific facts about previous medical and surgical treatments. In conversion disorder, the individual has loss of or an alteration in function.

A nonchalant attitude toward physical problems (la belle indifférence) indicates that the symptom is providing primary gain; that is, the anxiety is alleviated through the conversion process.

In contrast, clients with somatization disorder or hypochondriasis are overly dramatic and emotional in telling about their symptoms and pain. They report the history in vivid detail and colorful language but often pay more attention to how the symptoms have affected relationships in their lives than to giving a careful description of the nature, character, location, onset, and duration of the symptoms.

Clients with body dysmorphic disorder may request unnecessary operations—for example, demanding cosmetic surgery for an imagined or greatly magnified defect in appearance. Societal expectations may pressure women with BDD into seeking unnecessary surgical procedures.

Careful interviewing frequently reveals a stressful life situation with which the client is failing to cope, suggesting that the preoccupation with somatic disorder is a way of avoiding underlying conflict. Helping the client identify and express feelings is a crucial beginning to psychotherapeutic intervention.

Objective Data

Physical examination reveals no organic evidence for the client's symptoms. Likewise, laboratory findings do not substantiate organic or physiologic disorder. Despite this, the client may have undergone many exploratory diagnostic and/or surgical procedures without diagnosis or relief.

Family members often report that the client is moody, self-centered, or demanding. They feel alienated from the client and are frustrated with the client's chronic preoccupation with physical symptoms.

In a health care setting, these clients often create scenes that bring them attention without regard for the needs of either fellow clients or staff. You may find it difficult to be kind, understanding, and nonjudgmental with such clients. If you do not cope with your reactions, you will be unable to effectively work with them. Recognizing the client's somatization as part of the illness will help you to avoid personalizing the behavior. It may help to remind yourself that these clients do not intentionally produce their symptoms, nor do they understand the effects of their behavior on others. When you understand the psychopathology of the disorder, you are more likely to have empathy for the client's coping style. The What Every Medical–Surgical Nurse Should Know feature on page 488 will help you apply these understandings in nonpsychiatric settings.

Nursing Diagnosis: NANDA

Clients with somatoform disorders experience a multitude of problems; therefore, several nursing diagnoses are likely to be appropriate. The following section discusses five major nursing diagnoses applicable to individuals with somatoform disorders.

Impaired Verbal Communication

Clients with somatoform disorders have an impaired ability to communicate their needs. Although they may be highly verbal, you need to listen carefully for gaps, oversimplifications,

YOUR ASSESSMENT APPROACH
Client with Somatoform Disorder

Listed below are some sample questions to help determine the presence of somatoform disorder:

- Have you ever felt as if you were smothering, or couldn't breathe easily?
- Have you ever had problems swallowing or felt as if you were choking? If so, how long did the episode(s) last?
- Have you ever had burning sensations in your mouth or throat?
- Do you ever experience painful menstrual periods?
- Do you have pain in your joints? If so, how often?
- Have you seen many doctors who have told you that nothing is wrong with you?

WHAT EVERY MEDICAL-SURGICAL NURSE SHOULD KNOW

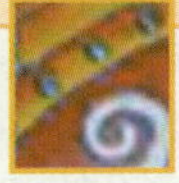

Somatoform Disorders

- Be careful not to rush to judge that "it's all in his/her head" when a client with a somatoform disorder is admitted to your unit. Even individuals with somatoform disorders can be ill or in pain.
- Pain and illness of psychogenic origin is as hurtful as pain of biologic origin.
- Be aware that hypochondriasis, conversion disorder, and other somatoform disorders are maladaptive responses to stress.
- Remember that unconscious (not deliberate) processes are at work, except for instances of malingering or factitious disorder.
- Be alert for signs of secondary gain and avoid reinforcing.
- Use a matter-of-fact approach when the client discusses somatic symptoms.
- Use a calm, patient approach in order to decrease the client's anxiety level.
- Decrease stimuli in order to promote relaxation.
- Anticipate the client's needs before somatization increases.
- Reward appropriate behavior.

overdramatizations, and overgeneralizations in the clients' stories. Somatoform symptoms are considered to be nonverbal substitutes for the expression of underlying conflicts.

Ineffective Role Performance and Compromised Family Coping

The manipulative and dependent behaviors of the client with a somatoform disorder lead to impairments in social, work, and family relationships and to diminished performance in these roles. Friends and relatives eventually tire of the demands and become less available for support. Clients become emotionally isolated because their self-absorption makes them unable to respond appropriately to the needs of others.

Work performance may suffer from frequent absences due to imagined illness. Preoccupation with health status uses up creative energy that could otherwise be directed toward work-related activities. When this occurs, the individual usually experiences negative consequences in the workplace.

Ineffective Coping

Clients with somatoform disorders generally experience anxiety, anger, and feelings of helplessness. They may feel these emotions acutely and demonstrate these feelings excessively, as in somatization disorder and hypochondriasis. Paradoxically, they may show an uncanny lack of feeling, as in the nonchalant reaction to loss of physical function that often occurs in conversion disorder.

The client's emotions become increasingly restricted. The focus of emotional experience becomes somatic concerns, and clients no longer experience meaningful emotional connections with other people, activities, and events. The range of emotional expression may be limited to making demands, manipulation, and symbolic manifestations of anxiety.

Disturbed Thought Processes and Disturbed Sensory Perception

Clients with somatoform disorders show selective inattention; that is, they filter out stimuli in response to anxiety. In a further effort to prove their ideas, they distort reality and tend to ramble. Judgment is often impaired and it is evident that conclusions are not logical. Clients may also distort memory and show selective memory.

Clients with somatoform disorders have body image disturbances and often sense that they are weak or vulnerable physically. They perceive sensory data incorrectly; for example, they may perceive abdominal discomfort as cancer rather than indigestion.

Outcome Identification: NOC

Expected outcomes are individualized for each client according to personal needs and the situation. However, some expected outcomes that are fairly common to those experiencing somatoform disorders are:

- Demonstrate the ability to cope with anxiety through the use of a new stress management skill (i.e., deep breathing).
- Verbalize feelings instead of expressing them symbolically through physical symptoms.
- Express an increased degree of comfort regarding each physical symptom.

It is essential that you and the client work together in establishing expected outcomes. Significant others should also be included in the planning process in order to help the client in achieving the goals.

Planning and Implementation: NIC

In order to intervene effectively, you need to recognize and understand the life problem or adjustment the client is facing. It is also important that you do the following:

- Recognize and understand the client's self-perception as an inability to cope.
- Help the client identify and learn more effective ways of adapting.

These goals may be accomplished by insight-oriented or supportive psychotherapy, behavior modification, hypnosis, or any of several other psychologic, as well as some physical, therapies. No one therapeutic modality can claim superior effectiveness, and new approaches and techniques are indicated when traditional ones prove inadequate. It is important to recognize that many clients with somatoform disorders are highly resistant to change. Thus, progress may be slow and

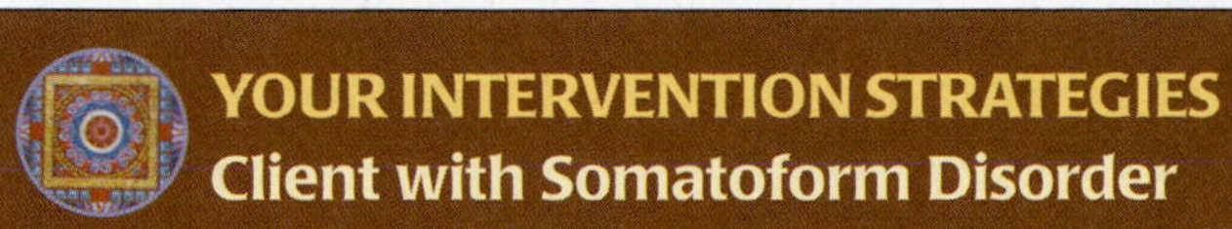

YOUR INTERVENTION STRATEGIES Client with Somatoform Disorder

Intervention	Rationale
Establish a trusting relationship.	Promotes client's psychologic safety.
Establish a daily routine.	Decreases client's anxiety.
Encourage verbalization of feelings.	Verbalization is healthier than somatization.
Assist client to relate stress to onset of physical symptoms.	Pointing out a cause-and-effect relationship helps eliminate triggers.
Encourage client to journal.	Increases personal insight.
Limit time for discussing physical symptoms.	Frees up time for problem-solving activities; decreases reinforcement of secondary gain(s).

recovery partial. Specific interventions and rationales are discussed in the Your Intervention Strategies feature.

Recall that you may also meet clients with somatoform disorders in general medical–surgical settings. Refer to the feature What Every Medical–Surgical Nurse Should Know on page 488 for specific interventions for medical–surgical settings.

Promoting Effective Communication

After assessing the meaning behind the client's communication patterns, plan intervention strategies such as encouraging exploration and demonstrating empathy that enhance the client's verbal communication and self-esteem to the point where the client feels ready to face problems. The Rx Communication feature gives examples of verbal communication strategies.

Establishing a trusting relationship is key to effective therapy with a somatizing client. It is usually necessary to help clients tone down their characteristic extravagances. Express respectful skepticism regarding oversimplifications and overdramatizations. The group setting provides clients the opportunity to receive feedback about the effect of their behavior on others.

Promoting Improved Role Performance and Family Coping

Working with the family is especially important for clients with somatoform disorders. The Partnering with Clients and Families feature on page 490 discusses educating the family and the client about the disorder, stressing the importance of avoiding unnecessary surgical or medical procedures.

Encourage independent functioning and reduce the possibility of secondary gain by not focusing on physical symptoms. Assume a matter-of-fact, supportive attitude, with the optimistic expectation that the client will regain functional abilities in work, family, and social roles.

Promoting Effective Coping

The goal of counseling clients with somatoform disorders is to help them express their conflicts verbally rather than acting them out through symptomatic behaviors. The aim of long-term (insight) therapy is to promote effective emotional expression by exploring the sources of anxiety. You will likely be challenged to help clients with somatoform disorders acknowledge the effects of psychosocial stress on symptoms. Supportive therapy seeks to improve self-esteem, perhaps through such measures as expanding clients' interest in their environment.

In general, try to avoid reinforcing the client's symptoms. A well-known psychiatric axiom applies to clients in this general category: *Ignore the symptom but never the client.* Concentrating on the physical symptom by trying to get a paralyzed client to walk or a blind client to see again is giving the symptom more importance than it merits, thus increasing the secondary gain associated with it. Ultimately, this makes it more difficult for the client to relinquish the symptom.

Promoting Improved Perception and Thought Processes

Help clients improve their capacity for perception and thinking by supporting general measures to reduce anxiety (see the Evidence-Based Practice feature on page 490). Maintain a calm, unhurried attitude toward the client, listen carefully, and maintain an objective, undistorted view of reality. Avoid a

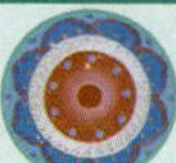

RX COMMUNICATION

CLIENT WITH SOMATOFORM DISORDER

CLIENT: "How can they help me get better if they can't even figure out what's wrong with me? I know I'm really sick."

NURSE RESPONSE 1: "It sounds as if you are feeling hopeless."

RATIONALE: This response focuses on the client's feelings and encourages further exploration. It also is a way to determine suicidal ideation that may be related to the client's hopelessness.

NURSE RESPONSE 2: "It must be very frustrating for you. All the exams and tests show no physical cause for your symptoms."

RATIONALE: This response demonstrates empathy while at the same time presenting reality. Reassurance that no organic pathology has been found helps dispute the client's unrealistic belief.

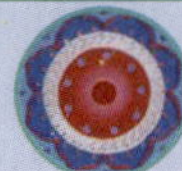

PARTNERING WITH CLIENTS AND FAMILIES

TEACHING ABOUT SOMATOFORM DISORDERS

- Provide information about the specific disorder.
- Teach about the relationship between stress and physical symptoms.
- Teach relaxation techniques (e.g., progressive muscle relaxation, guided imagery).
- Provide health promotion education (e.g., healthy diet, balance between exercise and rest, healthy sleep patterns).
- Teach the proper use of medications, including: target symptoms, side effects and adverse drug reactions, contraindications, and when to call for help.
- Teach the indicators for emergency treatment.
- Emphasize the need for continued treatment, including follow-up appointments.

premature challenge to the client's symptoms and complaints. As clients gradually relinquish their defenses, propose other ways of understanding the condition, such as by suggesting a psychologic explanation for a physical complaint.

Evaluation

Consider communication, role performance, coping, perception, and thought processes when evaluating clients with somatoform disorder. When evaluating these areas, it is important that you look for evidence of client progress. Expect that progress will be gradual and encourage the client and family to do the same.

Communication

Clients will express feelings and conflicts verbally and they will have fewer somatic symptoms. Your conversations with the client will "flow," with fewer monologues by the client and more natural dialogue between the client and you. In other words, the client's communication will become more spontaneous.

Role Performance and Family Coping

Clients will attend work regularly without frequent absences due to illness or worry about physical health status. They will be more interested in outside activities and may begin to

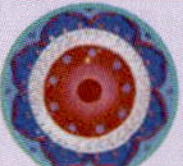

EVIDENCE-BASED PRACTICE

CONVERSION DISORDER

Alfred is a 22-year-old soldier. Even though he voluntarily joined the Army, Alfred never told anyone that he believed that killing under any circumstance is murder. After he finished military basic training, Alfred was deployed to Iraq. When on a routine patrol, Alfred's unit was attacked by enemy forces. While aiming his assault rifle at an Iraqi soldier, Alfred suddenly lost his vision. All medical tests show no physical basis for Alfred's blindness.

Your plan for intervention options is based on current research results. You have learned that Alfred will likely respond to cognitive–behavioral therapy (CBT) techniques such as those discussed in Chapter 31 ∞. Therefore, you teach Alfred the techniques of thought stopping and reframing. Your research review also shows that Alfred is likely to respond to the use of antidepressant medication as an adjunctive therapy to CBT and talk therapy.

The treatment team also decides to focus on establishing a therapeutic relationship with Alfred that includes an open, honest discussion of his disorder. Knowing that somatization may be triggered by stress, you will also demonstrate empathy and support to Alfred without reinforcing his symptoms.

This set of interventions is based on the following research:

Arnold, I. A., de Waal, M. W., Eekhof, J. A., & van Hemert, A. M. (2006). Somatoform disorder in primary care: Course and the need for cognitive–behavioral treatment. *Psychomatics, 47*(6), 498–503.

Fink, P., Toft, T., Hansen, M. S., Ornbol, E., & Olesen, F. (2007). Symptoms and syndromes of bodily distress: An exploratory study of 978 internal medical, neurological, and primary care patients. *Psychosomatic Medicine, 69*(1), 30–39.

Griffiths, R. F., & Ellis, P. M. (2007). Visual conversion disorder in a harbor pilot leading to sudden loss of control of a large vessel. *Aviation, Space, & Environmental Medicine, 78*(1), 59–62.

Jackson, J. L., O'Malley, P. G., & Kroenke, K. (2006). Antidepressants and cognitive–behavioral therapy for symptom syndromes. *CNS Spectrum, 11*(3), 212–222.

CRITICAL THINKING APPLICATION

1. How would you demonstrate empathy to clients with a conversion disorder without reinforcing the client's symptoms?
2. In what ways would it be useful to determine the underlying meaning of the client's symptoms?
3. How would thought stopping and reframing help someone with conversion disorder?
4. Why is antidepressant medication likely to be helpful?
5. What would be the purpose of talk therapy?

engage in socialization and recreation. Family members and friends will report being more satisfied with their relationship with the client and will be more willing to interact with the client.

Coping

Clients will be less demanding, manipulative, and attention-seeking in interactions with others. They will appear less anxious and will talk about subjects other than their physical status. They will appear less helpless and more able to participate in and make responsible decisions about their health care. For example, they may carry out a plan of treatment without voicing innumerable objections or worries. They will appear more interested and involved in the activities and attitudes of others and be more aware of the impact of their own behavior.

Perception and Thought Processes

The client will distort and misinterpret reality less frequently. Judgment, insight, and memory will improve as a result of reduced defensiveness in perception and cognition. Clients may report feeling more positive about their bodies. They will be more assertive in physical activities because they no longer tend to feel so vulnerable.

CASE MANAGEMENT

Case management for clients with somatoform disorders must focus on occupational functioning, which is usually significantly impaired by the disorder. Provision of job-search skills and communication techniques (e.g., how to listen actively to others) will enhance the client's career opportunities. Rehabilitative agencies can also be called upon to provide specific job-skills training. The case manager will often need to refer significant others to agencies that provide respite care and/or support to family members.

COMMUNITY-BASED CARE

Clients and family members usually need ongoing support for managing in the community setting. One organization that is designed to provide such support is the National Alliance on Mental Illness (NAMI). The website for this organization is www.NAMI.org. In addition to informing clients and families about NAMI, you can also encourage the client to adhere to medication therapy through education about the specific medications. Community mental health centers are very useful in helping clients obtain medications and adhere to the prescribed therapies.

HOME CARE

Home health nurses have a unique opportunity to support clients and help them maintain independence in activities of daily living. Home visits are done to provide support and education and to evaluate the client's need for continued treatment. Some tools that are especially useful in the home setting are cognitive behavioral therapy (discussed in Chapter 31) and relaxation skills (discussed in Chapter 33).

SLEEP DISORDERS

Sleep has been described as a neurobiologic window into the pathophysiology of psychiatric disorders (Kryger, Roth, & Dement, 2005). An association between depression and the chronic inability to get to sleep or to remain asleep during the usual sleep period was observed as long ago as the time of Hippocrates.

Two similar sets of diagnostic codes are used to categorize sleep disorders. In psychiatric–mental health settings, the DSM-IV-TR coding scheme for sleep disorders is used. However, you should also be aware of the more comprehensive International Classification of Sleep Disorders (ICSD) (AASM, 2005) used in sleep centers and medical–surgical settings.

Sleep disorders fall into four main categories: the primary sleep disorders, sleep disorder related to another mental disorder, sleep disorder due to a general medical condition, and substance-induced sleep disorder. The primary sleep disorders are further divided into dyssomnias and parasomnias. Understanding sleep disorders is based on an understanding of normal sleep, the basic anatomy of sleep, sleep pattern variations, and healthy sleep behaviors.

Normal Sleep

What does "normal sleep" mean? Several key points that are central to a basic understanding of normal sleep patterns are as follows:

- There is a wide range of sleep patterns among "good sleepers."
- Changes in sleep patterns normally occur as individuals progress through the life span.
- Humans have considerable capacity to adapt to variations in sleep patterns.
- The functions of sleep are still poorly understood.

Basic Anatomy of Sleep

We know that the "sleep switch" is located in the hypothalamus of the brain; the front regulates sleep, the back is the wakefulness center. However, a variety of other structures in the brain—ranging from the brain stem to the cerebral hemispheres—are involved in sleep and wakefulness. Neurons within these regions interact with one another, helping the body to sustain a sleep–wake balance, a homeostatic drive to sleep.

Working in tandem with these structures is the circadian clock (discussed later in this chapter). The circadian clock is regulated by a specific group of brain cells in the hypothalamus. It works in sync with the external environment to coordinate sleep and wakefulness. The circadian clock and our homeostatic drive to sleep tell our bodies when to sleep and when to wake up. Sleep disorders arise when there is confusion or disruption of the circuit.

A hormone, melatonin, is secreted by the pineal gland—a small, pea-sized protuberance situated at the back of the brain above the brain stem—and promotes sleep in lower light. Melatonin excretion occurs when it is dark; daylight

MediaLink National Alliance on Mental Illness

suppresses melatonin. The neurotransmitter serotonin is converted into melatonin in the pineal gland; therefore, medications that affect the synthesis of serotonin will also affect melatonin synthesis. Melatonin is further discussed in the section on circadian rhythm disorders.

Stages of Sleep

The discovery of rapid eye movement (REM) sleep by Kleitman and Aserinsky in the early 1950s was a major breakthrough in the effort to understand the relationship between the mind and the body. Until that time, sleep had been seen as a quiet state. However, in REM sleep, the stage in which most dreaming occurs, brain waves show a level of cognitive activity comparable to the waking state, and physiologic functions are also in a heightened state of activity, which usually constitutes 75% to 80% of sleep time.

A sleep period begins with NREM (non-REM) sleep.

- *Stage 1* of NREM sleep occurs right after the awake stage, comprises 4% to 5% of total sleep time, and is considered to be light sleep. In this stage there may be slow, rolling eye movements.
- *Stage 2* of NREM sleep is also considered to be light sleep and accounts for 45% to 50% of total sleep time.
- *Stage 3* of NREM sleep is deeper sleep and comprises 4% to 6% of total sleep time and is known as slow wave sleep or delta sleep. Eye movement activity is typically absent during this stage.
- *Stage 4* of NREM sleep is the deepest sleep of the four NREM stages. It usually comprises 12% to 15% of total sleep time (Thorpy & Yager, 2006). It is during this stage that sleep terror disorder or sleepwalking disorder (discussed later in this chapter) may occur. It is often combined with stage 3 because the two stages are so similar.

REM sleep is the time when we do almost all of our dreaming. It is characterized by rapid eye movement and loss of muscle tone. The major difference between REM sleep and the awake state and NREM sleep is the almost total paralysis of skeletal muscle during REM sleep, a factor that essentially prevents the acting out of dream states. More recent progress in the development of antidepressant medications has led to advances in our understanding of the physiologic aspects of sleep–wake states. A breakdown in the boundaries between the awake, NREM, and REM states is believed to be the cause of several sleep disorders.

A good sleeper most likely has recurrent sleep cycles about every 90 minutes, more slow-wave sleep (stages 3 and 4 of non-REM sleep) during the first part of the night combined with brief REM periods, changing to a greater percentage of REM sleep toward the end of the sleeping period. Cycles of sleep are illustrated in FIGURE 19-2 ■.

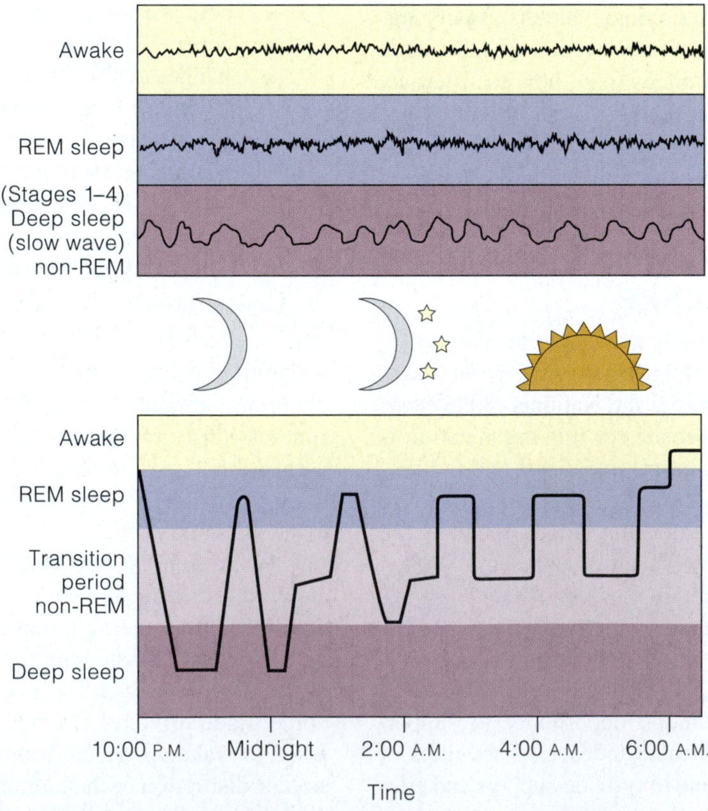

FIGURE 19-2 ■ Cycles of sleep. During sleep, we move in cycles among several stages of non-REM sleep, ranging from light (stages 1 and 2) to deep sleep (stages 3 and 4). Approximately every 90 minutes we move from non-REM to REM sleep for a short time. REM sleep is also known as paradoxical sleep because the brain wave patterns resemble those of a wakeful or drowsy state.

Source: Smock, T. K. (1999). *Physiological psychology: A neuroscience approach* (p. 308). Upper Saddle River, NJ: Prentice Hall.

Sleep Pattern Variations

The average amount of sleep required to feel rested varies widely from person to person. Requiring an average of 7 to 8 hours sleep per night is most common for adults. However, a small percentage of the population are short sleepers, requiring an average of 6 hours or less. Another small percentage are long sleepers, requiring an average of 9 or more hours each night (American Academy of Sleep Medicine, 2005).

The distinction between average hours needed and average hours obtained is important. Short or long sleepers by definition are good sleepers; that is, they habitually feel rested and alert after their normal sleep time. However, they may experience social pressure and/or even receive inappropriate pharmacologic intervention because they do not seem to conform to the norms of their family or peer group. More commonly, though, shortened sleep time is habitual, associated with the pressures of modern society.

There is growing concern that whole populations in developed countries are becoming chronically sleep deprived. As students, you are coping with pressures to study, to prepare for clinical experiences, and to complete assignments, as well as performing other roles that are important to you. Take the quiz in the Your Self-Awareness feature to see whether you are getting enough sleep.

Behavioral Factors

You may also know of individuals who increase their habitual sleep time (or at least their total time in bed) as avoidance. In your psychiatric–mental health nursing practice, you may encounter clients who report the need for long periods of sleep and rest, often in association with depression. To distinguish normally long sleepers from clients who are trying to cope by spending more time in bed, it is useful to inquire about previous sleep patterns.

Situational and Developmental Factors

Sleep requirements also vary in relation to situational and developmental factors. With increased physical work, exercise, mental stress, or exposure to adverse weather conditions, total sleep requirements tend to increase. Specific needs for REM sleep increase in relation to periods of intense learning or other psychological stimuli.

Developmental changes in sleep patterns and requirements across the life span are not emphasized here because they are discussed in most fundamental nursing textbooks. The important point for the psychiatric–mental health nurse is to include a consideration of the client's developmental stage as part of sleep pattern assessment. For example, approximately 15 million American children are affected by inadequate sleep associated with health, school, and family factors (Smaldone, Honig, & Byrne, 2007). Another example is the tendency of adolescents to sleep late and of older adults to go to sleep earlier in the evening and get up earlier in the morning (Wolkove, Elkholy, Baltzan, & Palayew, 2007), which appears to have some physiologic basis from age-related shifts in circadian rhythms. The number of arousals tends to increase as adults get older. This change is often greeted with concern that something is wrong. However, if clients are able to get back to sleep without much distress, or the awakenings are mainly associated with the need to void, you can help them to see the change as normal and to make minor adjustments such as reducing fluid intake after the evening meal.

Physiologic Factors

We physiologically prioritize among types of sleep. Following periods of acute or chronic sleep deprivation, a rebound phenomenon occurs in which the recovery of REM sleep is given priority. You may have noticed how you seem to dream more after several nights of interrupted sleep. (Dreams can occur during non-REM as well as REM sleep, but dreams in non-REM sleep are usually more fragmentary and mundane, without much of a story line.)

Clients who discontinue taking medications or other substances that suppress REM sleep (tricyclic antidepressants, short-acting benzodiazepines) may notice increased dreaming. Through anticipatory teaching, you can help clients understand that this catching up on REM sleep, known as **REM rebound**, is a normal and passing experience. Such support is important because clients who have been relying on medication or other substances to induce sleep often interpret the reduced quality of their sleep as evidence that they should go back on the medication.

Recognition of the REM rebound phenomenon can be important with regard to physiologic function as well. Vital signs fluctuate during REM sleep, possibly putting added stress on weakened cardiovascular and respiratory systems. There is reduced stimulus to breathe, and ventilatory movement is limited to the diaphragm (because of very low skeletal muscle tone). Thus, clients who are already compromised (as from drug overdose, sleep apnea, chronic obstructive lung disease, or major trauma) may become hypoxic during REM sleep in the first night or two after REM-suppressing medications are withdrawn (Thorpy & Yager, 2006).

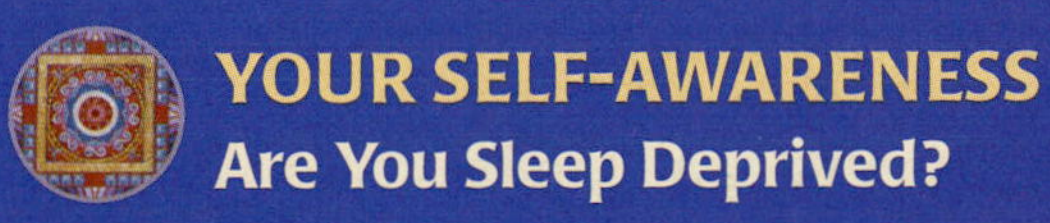

YOUR SELF-AWARENESS
Are You Sleep Deprived?

Ask yourself the following questions:

- Do you usually fall asleep within 5 minutes after you turn off the lights?
- Do you struggle to stay awake in lectures?
- Do you "get by" all week and then try to catch up by sleeping in on the weekend?
- Do you do shift work?
- Do you often wake up with a headache?
- Do you have trouble getting going in the morning?
- Do you push yourself to keep going?

If you answered yes to more than two of these questions, you may not be getting as much sleep as you need.

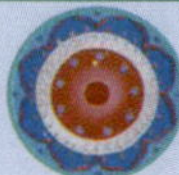

PARTNERING WITH CLIENTS AND FAMILIES

TEACHING ABOUT SLEEP HYGIENE

1. Maintain regularity in the sleep–wake schedule.
   - Avoid staying up too late or sleeping in too long on days off.
   - Enjoy an occasional nap, but stop taking naps if you notice that it is harder to get to sleep at night.
   - Be consistent in the time you get up, even if you have had less than usual sleep.
2. Go to bed only when you are reasonably sleepy and relaxed.
   - For a half-hour or so before you go to bed, engage in activities that are relaxing to you, even if you feel some pressure about things needing to be done.
   - If you are not drowsy when it is time to go to bed, engage in some activity that usually makes you drowsy, like reading something light.
   - Learn relaxation exercises (but practice them at other times of the day first).
   - Increase the physical exercise that you get during the day.
3. Maintain some sleep rituals as part of getting ready for bed.
   - Bring your day to a close with prayer or meditation if that is meaningful to you. Make this a time to focus on the good things that have happened and the accomplishments of the day, no matter how minor they may seem.
   - Get into a routine (brushing your teeth, winding the clock, opening the window, etc.).
4. Avoid the intake of stimulants or other substances that affect sleep patterns.
   - Instead of an alcoholic drink to induce sleep and relaxation, try a warm bath.
   - Experiment with decreasing the amount of coffee you drink, especially later in the day.
5. Enjoy what sleep you do get rather than thinking about what you think you need.
   - Move the clock so you cannot see what time it is every time you look in that direction.
   - Snuggle under the covers and think how nice it is that you can be resting in bed. If you are starting to feel restless or your mind is racing, get up and do some quiet activity such as reading until you feel drowsy again.

Healthy Sleep Behaviors

It is important to all clients, regardless of setting, that you create opportunities for teaching or reinforcing healthy sleep behaviors. Healthy sleep behaviors, sometimes referred to as sleep hygiene, are discussed in the Partnering with Clients and Families feature above.

There has been a tendency to be overprescriptive in terms of healthy sleep behaviors. For example, magazine and news articles often recommend a snack before bedtime as a means of encouraging sleep. A snack, however, is more likely to help people who generally snack before bedtime and not so likely to help those who usually do not snack. Likewise, guidelines intended for people with insomnia are often generalized to the rest of the population. For example, napping is not recommended for people with insomnia.

ASSESSMENT OF SLEEP PATTERNS

A "good sleeper" can be identified in any of three ways: self-defined, behaviorally defined, or sleep-study defined. Most people have a definite opinion about their sleep. Self-defined good sleepers generally describe themselves as getting enough sleep to feel refreshed in the morning, to have energy for the day, to fall asleep fairly quickly, and to wake up only briefly, if at all, during the night. To hypothesize that a client is a good sleeper from a subjective point of view, you would want to pay close attention to what he or she says about the quality of sleep.

For a behavioral assessment, observe alertness during sedentary, repetitive activity such as watching television or driving. You would note the ability to fall asleep in 10 to 30 minutes under usual circumstances, and final wakening at the habitual rising time, with or without an alarm clock. Photographic serializing of movement during sleep is another form of behavioral sleep assessment.

Assessment of sleep patterns should become part of your regular assessment with all clients, not only those with sleep disorders. The elements of a basic sleep pattern assessment are listed in the following Your Assessment Approach feature. The depth with which you pursue potential problems will vary according to the presenting problems and context of care. For example, clients with sleep apnea or narcolepsy are likely to have comprehensive sleep studies, while most people with insomnia need a detailed sleep and medical history, not necessarily an overnight sleep study. Specific assessment activities for clients with sleep disorders are discussed in the Nursing Process section later in this chapter.

Comprehensive Sleep Studies

Comprehensive sleep studies are conducted in sleep labs that may be located in hospitals or outpatient clinics. The two most common sleep studies are the polysomnogram and the multiple sleep latency test, discussed next.

Comprehensive sleep studies are also individualized and often include video recordings, a sleep scale such as the Epworth Sleepiness Scale (in which the client rates how likely he or she is to fall asleep in certain situations), the Fatigue Severity Scale (the impact of fatigue on how a person functions), and the Beck Depression Inventory (which screens for depression, often present in sleep complaints). Continuous positive airway pressure (CPAP) testing may also be done if indicated. In addition, clients are often asked to keep a sleep log or a sleep diary for a week or two, or even longer.

YOUR ASSESSMENT APPROACH
Basic Sleep Pattern Assessment

Sample questions for assessing a client's basic sleep patterns are given below.

Sleep–Wake Schedule

What time do you usually go to bed?

How long does it usually take you to fall asleep after you have turned off the light?

What time do you usually wake up?

What is different about your sleep–wake schedule on the weekend/days off?

How often do you take naps? (Be alert here for cultural influence, such as taking siestas, or occupational influence.) Under what circumstances?

Getting to Sleep

What helps you get to sleep?

What makes it difficult for you to get to sleep?

Staying Asleep

On average, how many times do you wake up during the night?

What seems to waken you?

How long does it usually take to get back to sleep?

What do you do if you are having trouble getting back to sleep?

Waking Up

How difficult is it for you to wake up?

How soon after waking up do you usually get up?

How do you feel when you first get up?

Daytime Functioning

At what time of day do you usually feel most energetic?

At what time of day do you feel most sleepy?

Would you call yourself a "morning person" or an "evening person"?

Satisfaction with Sleep; Potential Problems

How satisfied are you with the sleep you usually get?

Do you think you get enough sleep on average? How do you know?

How has your sleep been during the past 2 weeks in comparison to what is normal for you?

Are you concerned about any of the following things?

- Getting to sleep
- Waking up too many times during the night
- Waking up too early
- Having to fight sleepiness during the day
- Snoring, restlessness, talking or walking in your sleep
- Bad dreams
- Drinking too much coffee (or other caffeine/nicotine sources)

When do you enjoy sleep the most?

Polysomnogram

Conducted during an overnight stay in a sleep lab, a **polysomnogram** is the simultaneous recording of several physical parameters during sleep, including brain wave activity, eye movements, muscle tone, heart rate and rhythm, oxygen saturation, respiration, body position, and the absence or presence of snoring. The technique is useful in determining the type and stages of sleep, as well as number of arousals and total sleep time. In addition, since sleep disorders often affect several organ systems, it is vital to determine whether some of the measurements indicate the client is in danger.

Multiple Sleep Latency Test

The *multiple sleep latency test*, or MSLT, usually takes place approximately two hours after awakening from the overnight sleep study. Essentially, sleep latency is the period of time it takes one to fall asleep after awakening. The MSLT consists of a series of five 20-minute nap trials that take place at 2-hour intervals. The MSLT measures the presence and severity of excessive daytime sleepiness as occurs in narcolepsy (discussed later in this chapter). Electrodes placed on the head measure brain waves and eye movements and indicate how deeply the client sleeps during nap trials. Those who fall asleep in 5 minutes or less display signs of severe, excessive daytime sleepiness.

However, having a nap is common in some cultures, such as in countries where the siesta is part of the daily routine, in some farming communities, and among many retired people and older adults. Humans are biphasic, having a natural tendency for two sleep periods per 24-hour day, one major sleep period (commonly at night), and another shorter one (midafternoon).

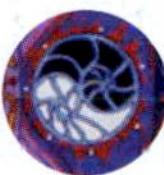

SLEEP DYSSOMNIAS

Dyssomnias are sleep disorders characterized by difficulty initiating or maintaining sleep, or excessive sleepiness. The diagnostic criteria for sleep dyssomnias are listed in the DSM-IV-TR Diagnostic Criteria feature on page 496.

Primary Insomnia

Insomnia, difficulty falling asleep or maintaining sleep, is a major public health problem affecting millions of individuals, along with their families and communities (National Institutes of Health, 2005). Up to 30% of adults report having insomnia—15% report severe or frequent insomnia, and another 15% report occasional episodes (APA, 2000). Depending on which statistic you read, the number is often higher.

Insomnia is not always a sleep disorder. Transitory insomnia, commonly associated with a change in environmental or situational stressors, is not a sleep disorder. Stress has a major impact on quality and duration of sleep.

Primary insomnia is the term used in the DSM-IV-TR to describe difficulty initiating or maintaining sleep, or nonrestorative sleep that lasts for at least a month and does not occur exclusively in association with another sleep disorder or mental disorder. The most common type of insomnia is a pattern of delayed sleep onset and/or broken sleep that can be

DSM-IV-TR Diagnostic Criteria for Sleep Dyssomnias

Primary Insomnia

A. The predominant complaint is difficulty initiating or maintaining sleep, or nonrestorative sleep, for at least 1 month.
B. The sleep disturbance (or associated daytime fatigue) causes clinically significant distress or impairment in social, occupational, or other important areas of functioning.
C. The sleep disturbance does not occur exclusively during the course of Narcolepsy, Breathing-Related Sleep Disorder, Circadian Rhythm Sleep Disorder, or a Parasomnia.
D. The disturbance does not occur exclusively during the course of another mental disorder (e.g., Major Depressive Disorder, Generalized Anxiety Disorder, a delirium).
E. The disturbance is not due to the direct physiological effects of a substance (e.g., a drug of abuse, a medication) or a general medical condition.

Primary Hypersomnia

A. The predominant complaint is excessive sleepiness for at least 1 month (or less if recurrent) as evidenced by either prolonged sleep episodes or daytime sleep episodes that occur almost daily.
B. The excessive sleepiness causes clinically significant distress or impairment in social, occupational, or other important areas of functioning.
C. The excessive sleepiness is not better accounted for by insomnia and does not occur exclusively during the course of another Sleep Disorder (e.g., Narcolepsy, Breathing-Related Sleep Disorder, Circadian Rhythm Sleep Disorder, or a Parasomnia) and cannot be accounted for by an inadequate amount of sleep.
D. The disturbance does not occur exclusively during the course of another mental disorder.
E. The disturbance is not due to the direct physiological effects of a substance (e.g., a drug of abuse, a medication) or a general medical condition.

Breathing-Related Sleep Disorder

A. Sleep disruption, leading to excessive sleepiness or insomnia, that is judged to be due to a sleep-related breathing condition (e.g., obstructive or central sleep apnea syndrome or central alveolar hypoventilation syndrome).
B. The disturbance is not better accounted for by another mental disorder and is not due to the direct physiological effects of a substance (e.g., a drug of abuse, a medication) or another general medical condition (other than a breathing-related disorder).

Narcolepsy

A. Irresistible attacks of refreshing sleep that occur daily over at least 3 months.
B. The presence of one or both of the following:
   1. cataplexy (i.e., brief episodes of sudden bilateral loss of muscle tone, most often in association with intense emotion)
   2. recurrent intrusions of elements of rapid eye movement (REM) sleep into the transition between sleep and wakefulness, as manifested by either hypnopompic or hypnagogic hallucinations or sleep paralysis at the beginning or end of sleep episodes
C. The disturbance is not due to the direct physiological effects of a substance (e.g., a drug of abuse, a medication) or another general medical condition.

Circadian Rhythm Sleep Disorder

A. A persistent or recurrent pattern of sleep disruption leading to excessive sleepiness or insomnia that is due to a mismatch between the sleep–wake schedule required by a person's environment and his or her circadian sleep–wake pattern.
B. The sleep disturbance causes clinically significant distress or impairment in social, occupational, or other important areas of functioning.
C. The disturbance does not occur exclusively during the course of another Sleep Disorder or other mental disorder.
D. The disturbance is not due to the direct physiological effects of a substance (e.g., a drug of abuse, a medication) or a general medical condition.

Specify type:

Delayed Sleep Phase Type: a persistent pattern of late sleep onset and late awakening times, with an inability to fall asleep and awaken at a desired earlier time.

Jet Lag Type: sleepiness and alertness that occur at inappropriate time of day relative to local time, occurring after repeated travel across more than one time zone.

Shift Work Type: insomnia during the major sleep period or excessive sleepiness during the major awake period associated with night shift work or frequently changing shift work.

Unspecified Type

Source: Reprinted with permission from the *Diagnostic and Statistical Manual of Mental Disorders,* Fourth Edition, Text Revision. (Copyright 2000). American Psychiatric Association.

USING DSM-IV-TR

Health care providers often use language unfamiliar to clients and their families. Explain *circadian rhythm* in terms that clients and family members can readily understand.

verified by polysomnography and that is perpetuated by an interaction between physically manifested tension (increased arousal) and learned associations that prevent sleep (negative conditioning). A careful history often identifies the onset of insomnia at the time of acute stress: The initial stressful event subsided, but the associations of frustration in trying to get to sleep persisted. A clinical example of a primary insomnia follows.

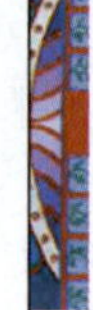

CLINICAL EXAMPLE

Peter Jacobi introduced himself to the other members of the insomnia group as someone who has always been a light sleeper. He has been having a lot more difficulty with sleeping, however, since he started working as a salesman about 3 months ago. He likes his job but finds it stressful, with lots of late nights entertaining customers. He denies excessive alcohol intake but admits he feels he has to be sociable with the guys and is usually one of the last to leave the bar. On weekends he tries to catch up on sleep. He drinks 5 to 7 cups of coffee a day but never after dinner. He comments that for some reason he can usually sleep better when he is on out-of-town trips.

This clinical example illustrates a fairly typical situation of what is sometimes termed *psychophysiological insomnia* (Kryger et al., 2005). Peter's history as a light sleeper suggests that he may have been predisposed to insomnia. The anxiety and change of lifestyle associated with his new job may have precipitated this episode. Perpetuating factors would include an irregular schedule, frequent alcohol and caffeine intake, and a learned association of his bedroom with the inability to sleep. See the Your Assessment Approach feature on page 508 for a structured exploration of insomnia's contributing factors.

Although sleep medications can be useful for transient insomnia, cognitive behavioral therapy (CBT) has been shown to be superior to pharmacologic therapy. A review of the research conducted by a task force of the American Academy of Sleep Medicine (AASM) (Morin et al., 2006) found that behavioral therapies are superior in the treatment of persistent insomnia. These therapies are stimulus control therapy, relaxation, and sleep restriction. CBT is also superior to sleep medications for the short- and long-term management of insomnia in older adults (Sivertsen et al., 2006).

Primary Hypersomnia

Hypersomnia refers to prolonged sleep and excessive sleepiness so severe as to interfere with function. **Primary hypersomnia** is that which is not better explained by another sleep disorder (e.g., breathing-related sleep disorder or narcolepsy, which also cause hypersomnia) or a mental disorder (e.g., depression). Such idiopathic hypersomnia is relatively uncommon, but the symptoms of hypersomnia are frequently seen in clients experiencing mental health challenges, and therefore the nursing process section will focus on the symptom more specifically.

Breathing-Related Sleep Disorder

The most common form of breathing-related sleep disorder is **sleep apnea**. Apnea is the absence of breathing. The most common form of sleep apnea is the obstructive type, in which the upper airway partially or totally collapses despite repeated respiratory effort. Opening of the airway requires a partial arousal. With polysomnography, up to 200 to 300 arousals per night may be observed, even though the client may say he or she slept soundly (Kryger et al., 2005). The outcome of the numerous arousals preceded by drops in oxygen saturation is hypersomnia, or excessive sleepiness. Clients with obstructive sleep apnea may report difficulty staying awake, even in social situations, at work, or driving despite a normal or longer nighttime sleep period, in addition to dozing off regularly when watching television.

People with obstructive sleep apnea are often obese middle-aged males with thick necks and a history of severe snoring. The loudness of the snoring, irregularity of nocturnal breathing, irritability, and constant sleepiness of the affected partner add strain to the interpersonal relationship. Bed partners often report that they, too, have a sleep pattern disturbance related to environmental noise and/or vigilance about breathing.

Women may also develop obstructive sleep apnea, with the incidence increasing after menopause. By age 50, women represent about the same number of new sleep apnea cases as men (Kryger, 2004). Older adult clients with obstructive sleep apnea may have insomnia rather than hypersomnia. The explanation may be that they have more difficulty getting back to sleep after their frequent arousals.

Clients suspected of sleep apnea should be seen by a sleep specialist. Overnight sleep monitoring is important for diagnosis and treatment. These clients often experience significant REM rebound when first treated.

The principle underlying the treatment of obstructive sleep apnea is reduction or removal of the obstruction. Conservative measures include weight loss, avoidance of alcohol and other central nervous system (CNS) depressants (which reduce muscle tone in the upper airway), and a change in habitual sleep positions (such as wearing something like a backpack to bed to prevent sleeping supine). Continuous positive airway pressure (CPAP) by nasal mask is the most common form of treatment. Surgical treatment includes removal of a portion of the soft palate, uvula, and residual tonsillar tissue. Dental splints are a form of treatment for reducing apnea and the associated snoring.

MediaLink National Sleep Foundation

In central sleep apnea, the airway remains open but the stimulus to breathe is missing or abnormal. This type of breathing-related sleep disorder is less common, except after some neurologic insults (such as brain stem lesions). Clients may have hypersomnia or insomnia or be asymptomatic. It is not unusual to observe some central apneas mixed with obstructive episodes. Rather than actual apneas, there may be prolonged hypoventilation resulting in low oxygen saturation, a condition called central alveolar hypoventilation syndrome. The National Sleep Foundation site at www.sleepfoundation.org provides interesting information about these issues and has ample links to other sleep-related sites.

MediaLink Critical Thinking Exercise: Sleep Apnea

As a psychiatric–mental health nurse, be vigilant for sleep apnea for several reasons. Clients may be unaware of a breathing-related sleep disorder and yet be concerned about hypersomnia, disrupted interpersonal relationships, or poor work performance. Depression secondary to obstructive sleep apnea is not uncommon. Other symptoms of mood disturbances, irritability, memory loss, and impaired concentration are similar to the presenting symptoms of various mental disorders. Furthermore, sleep apnea increases with aging, and is significantly associated with cognitive impairment and dementia, as well as cardio- and cerebrovascular disease (Wolkove et al., 2007). Thus, it is important to assess nocturnal breathing patterns in clients with dementia. Do not assume that their sleep pattern disturbance is the phenomenon called sundowning—increased restlessness and agitation during the evening and night hours.

Narcolepsy

Narcolepsy is a condition in which there is an almost irresistible urge to sleep followed by brief episodes of deep sleep. But unlike sleep apnea, the sleep is followed by a sense of refreshment. The causes of narcolepsy and how to prevent it are not yet clear. Recent research indicates that narcolepsy is likely caused by environmental exposures that destroy cells in the lateral hypothalamus in genetically susceptible individuals (Longstreth, Koepsell, Ton, Hendrickson, & van Belle, 2007).

Narcolepsy is associated with other symptoms such as cataplexy, sleep paralysis, and hypnagogic hallucinations. **Cataplexy**, which refers to the sudden collapse of muscle tone usually associated with intense emotion, occurs in about 70% of individuals with narcolepsy (APA, 2000). **Sleep paralysis**, a sense of being totally unable to move for a brief period after wakening or at sleep onset, occurs in 30% to 50% of those with narcolepsy. It may also occur occasionally in people who do not have narcolepsy or any other sleep disorder. **Hypnagogic hallucinations** are vivid dreamlike images that appear just before sleep onset and are reported by 20% to 40% of individuals with narcolepsy. All these symptoms are thought to be related to the recurrent intrusion of REM-like mechanisms into waking or the waking–sleep transition (APA, 2000). Polysomnography in the form of a multiple sleep latency test (MSLT), preceded by an all-night sleep study, will confirm the diagnosis.

About 40% of people with narcolepsy also have a concurrent or prior-onset mental disorder. With onset typically occurring in adolescence, often exacerbated by an acute psychosocial stressor, these clients have experienced a life-changing and poorly accepted chronic illness during an important developmental stage. The frequency of daytime sleeping and cataplexy attacks is embarrassing and disruptive in relation to occupational and social activities. Various theories have been offered about the association between narcolepsy and mental disorders, but no clear cause-and-effect explanation has been found.

It is likely that people with narcolepsy will have to be on medication for the rest of their lives. A stimulant, modafinil (Provigil in the United States, Alertec in Canada), is the most commonly prescribed medication for excessive daytime sleepiness. It promotes wakefulness and must be customized to the individual's specific degree of daytime sleepiness. When taken at night, sodium oxybate (Xyrem) reduces cataplexy the following day. There are tight controls on the use of this drug since the active chemical, gammahydroxybutyrate, has been used as a date rape drug. Sodium oxybate can reduce cataplexy by up to 85% (Robinson & Keating, 2007). Selective serotonin reuptake inhibitors (SSRIs) and tricyclic antidepressants (TCAs) have also been used to control the associated symptoms of cataplexy, sleep paralysis, and hypnagogic hallucinations. In addition, some lifestyle changes may be called for. These strategies include taking scheduled naps every day; avoiding stress, which may precipitate cataplexy; and maintaining a structured lifestyle.

Circadian Rhythm Sleep Disorders

The **circadian rhythm sleep disorders** are those disorders in which the 24-hour sleep–wake schedule is disturbed through internal cues (e.g., phase delay is more common in teenagers and young adults; phase advance is more common in young children and older adults) or external cues (e.g., shift work, travel across time zones). The 24-hour cycle of human biologic rhythms (as seen in FIGURE 19-3 ■) determines much of our mammalian activity level.

Jet Lag Type

Jet lag was unknown until the middle of the 20th century when large numbers of people began flying long distances in high-speed aircraft. Many people have noticed that their body clocks become disoriented and confused when they cross sev-

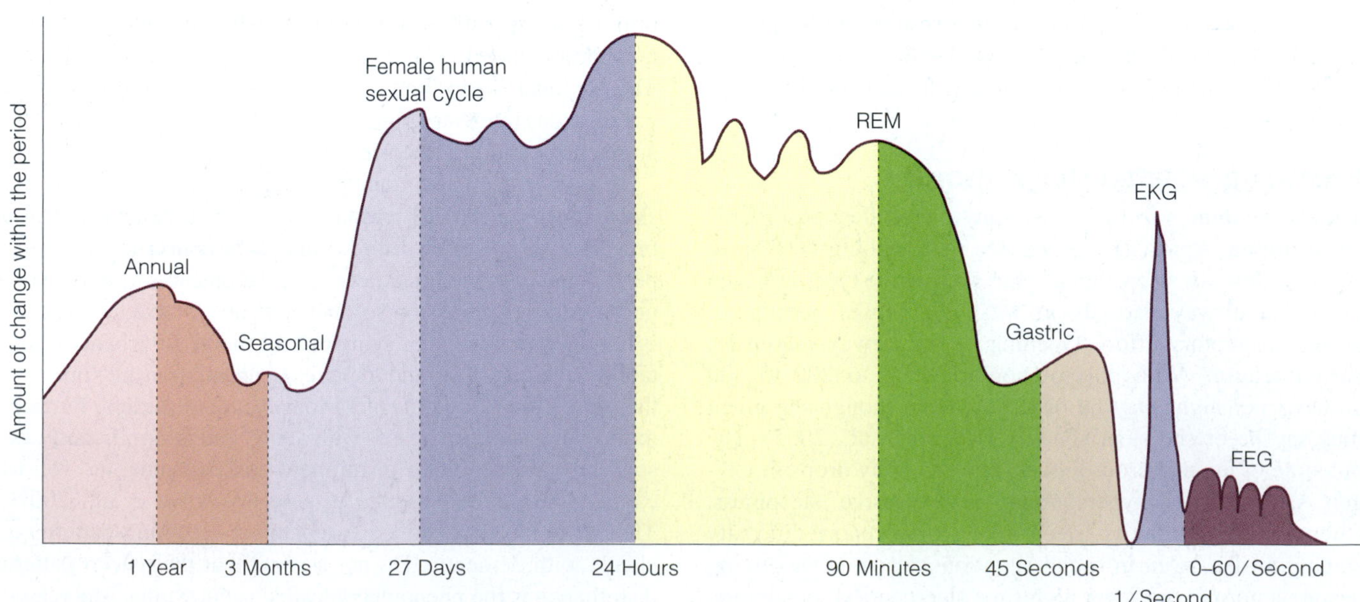

FIGURE 19-3 ■ Continuum of human biologic rhythms.

From New York

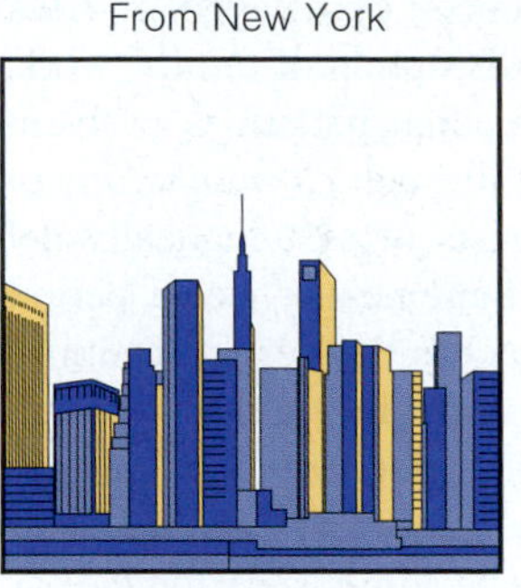

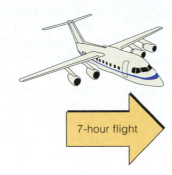

When you leave New York, it is 9:30 PM, and your body thinks it is 9:30 PM

7-hour flight

To Paris

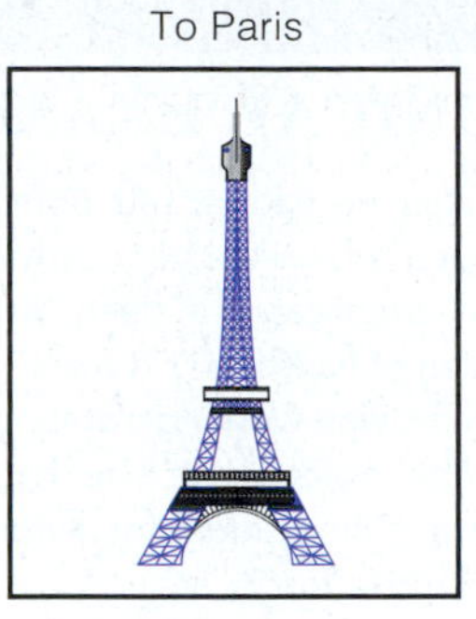

When you arrive in Paris, it is 10:30 AM (Paris time) but your body thinks it is 4:30 AM

FIGURE 19-4 ■ Flying east.

eral time zones. The impact on a passenger depends on the direction flown (east or west) and the number of time zones crossed. The impact on a passenger of flying east is illustrated in FIGURE 19-4 ■, and the impact of flying west in FIGURE 19-5 ■.

Sleeping pills are not recommended for trips of 8 hours or less. The medication may still have an effect if one has slept for only 4 or 5 hours, and individuals have been known to be disoriented or have memory problems or amnesia for several hours following the flight. For long-haul flights, a sleeping pill may help passengers fall asleep and keep airplane distractions from waking them up.

In a client with bipolar disorder, jet lag and the associated sleep deprivation may further exacerbate a manic phase.

CLINICAL EXAMPLE

Mr. Bernstein traveled from the United States to the Middle East on business. Upon his return to the United States, he made a series of irrational business decisions that he blamed on the stress of jet lag. However, it was subsequently determined that Mr. Bernstein had bipolar disorder.

Jet lag, a known stressor, may have precipitated Mr. Bernstein's first manic episode. The stressor may have also contributed to sleep deprivation, such as that experienced by travelers flying across several time zones. However, the body clock can be adjusted by both pharmacologic and behavioral interventions (Waterhouse, Reilly, Atkinson, & Edwards, 2007). Pharmacologic and behavioral interventions for circadian rhythm disorders are discussed in the relevant Nursing Process section later in this chapter. Two Internet resources that provide information on preventing or reducing jet lag are www.circadian.com and www.goodsleep.com.

MEDIALINK Reducing Jet Lag

Shift Work Type

More than 6 million Americans (Schwartz & Roth, 2006)—such as nurses, bakers, pilots, train conductors, truck drivers, police officers, firefighters, factory workers, gambling casino employees—work night shifts on a regular or rotating basis. As you might expect, shift work is a major source of circadian rhythm disruption, as demonstrated in the clinical example that follows.

To Tokyo

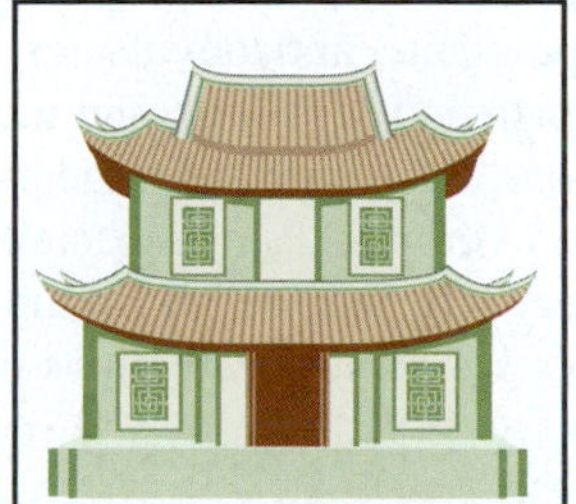

When you arrive in Tokyo 12 hours later, it is 4 PM (Tokyo time), but your body thinks it is midnight.

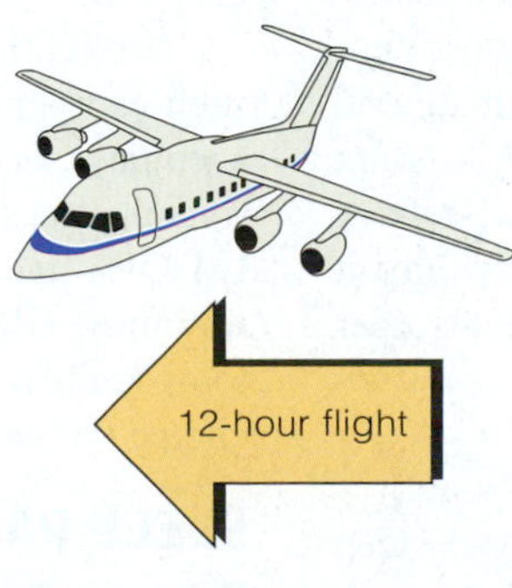

From Los Angeles, California

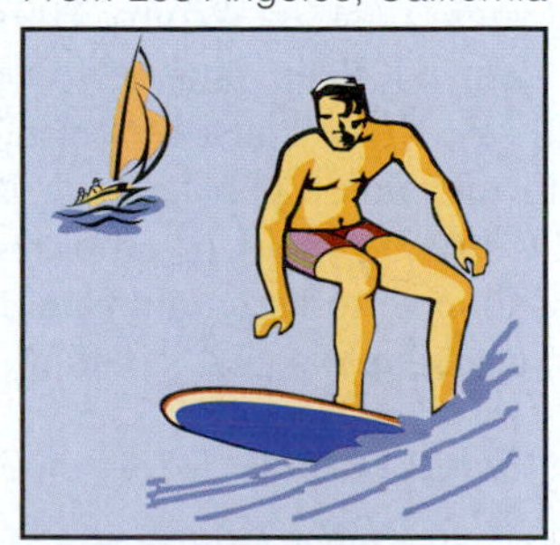

When you leave Los Angeles at 12 noon, your body thinks it is 12 noon.

FIGURE 19-5 ■ Flying west.

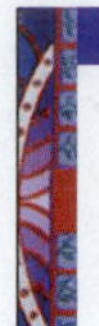

CLINICAL EXAMPLE

Years after he had retired from his bakery business, Yürgen continued to awaken very early in the morning. This pattern further complicated a sleep disorder related to his medical condition of Parkinson's disease.

Jane was working rotating shifts in an intensive care unit. She noted that she had worsening insomnia and feared that her judgment would be affected by increasing sleep deprivation.

If you choose hospital nursing, you may be concerned about this disorder for yourself as well as for your clients.

MEDIALINK Goodsleep.com

Chronobiology (the scientific study of the impact of time on the body) is rapidly expanding and has implications for coping with shift work. Inquiries about shift work should be a routine part of sleep assessment because the impact on sleep patterns and sleep disturbance often extends beyond the period of shift work. Specific suggestions for obtaining a good sleep despite a night-shift work schedule can be found on www.goodsleep.com. Although studies in sleep labs indicate that light exposure, melatonin, hypnotic agents, caffeine, and central nervous system stimulants are helpful, these measures have not yet been evaluated in persons with shift work disorder. Modafinil (Provigil) and armodafinil (Nuvigil) have been shown to be helpful in randomized, double-blind clinical studies (Schwartz & Roth, 2006; Valentino & Foldvary-Schaefer, 2007).

Delayed Sleep Phase Type

An abnormality in sleep phase can contribute to what may appear to be socially inappropriate or uncooperative behavior. Clients with the circadian rhythm disorder known as *delayed sleep phase type* seem programmed to stay up late and sleep in late. This syndrome should not be confused with normal tendencies to be either a "night owl" or "morning lark." Delayed sleep phase syndrome is a persistent problem that is resistant to standard attempts to get up earlier.

Treatment measures include chronotherapies to change the delayed sleep circadian rhythm, such as morning bright light exposure, the administration of melatonin, and behavioral strategies (Lack & Wright, 2007). However, most people with delayed sleep phase type do not seek treatment. Many will say, "That's just how I'm programmed." It is not unusual to encounter people with this disorder who have adapted by seeking types of employment and entertainment that are conducive to late nights and late rising. The disorder can also contribute to social isolation.

Advanced Sleep Phase Type

Advanced sleep phase type is the reverse of delayed sleep phase type in that early evening sleepiness regularly accompanies early wakening. A mildly advanced sleep phase is common among older adults and should not be confused with the early wakening associated with depression. With depression, other symptoms and sleep changes are evident.

The main consequences of delayed or advanced sleep phase syndrome are the disruption of family, work, and/or social activities. If the circadian pattern is problematic, phase shifting can be modified through *chronotherapy* or light therapy. Chronotherapy consists of systematically delaying bedtime, usually in 3-hour increments, over a period of several weeks until the client reaches the desired bedtime hour, after which the new schedule must be carefully maintained. Light therapy is timed to coincide with the time of day that sleepiness should be reduced. For people with advanced sleep phase syndrome, light therapy may be administered in the early evening.

Other Dyssomnias

There are other forms of dyssomnia that do not meet any other specified criteria. Two that you might encounter are periodic limb movements and restless legs syndrome.

Periodic Limb Movements

Periodic limb movements disorder is a condition that usually involves the legs, which repeatedly move in a jerking, stereotypic manner during sleep, often causing partial arousals. This disorder can contribute to excessive sleepiness, unrefreshing sleep, and multiple awakenings. Prevalence tends to increase with age; it occurs in up to 34% of individuals over age 60 (AASM, 2005). Benzodiazepines and dopaminergic agents such as pramipexole (Mirapex) provide some relief.

It is important to know that TCAs and monoamine oxidase inhibitors (MAOIs) can trigger or worsen the disorder (AASM, 2005). Withdrawal of anticonvulsants, benzodiazepines, and other hypnotic medications can also exacerbate the condition.

Restless Legs Syndrome

Periodic limb movements disorder should be distinguished from **restless legs syndrome**, which may occur prior to sleep and is characterized by disagreeable crawling, itching, and tickling sensations in the legs, most often in the calf, foot, and thigh, that are relieved only by movement. Persons with RLS usually have periodic limb movements as well, but periodic limb movements are not necessarily associated with restless legs syndrome. A positive family history is present in more than 50% of clients with RLS (Kushida, 2007).

Relief of the discomfort is available through medications such as hypnotics, antidepressants, anticonvulsants, benzodiazepines (such as clonazepam and trizolam), and narcotic derivatives such as oxycodone. Dopaminergic agents such as L-DOPA and pramipexole (Mirapex), and especially ropinirole (Requip), are very effective, relieve symptoms readily, and are now considered medications of choice (Hening, 2007).

SLEEP PARASOMNIAS

Parasomnias are abnormal sleep disorders that intrude into sleep, including disorders of arousal and sleep stage transition. The more common parasomnias include nightmare disorder, sleep terror disorder, and sleepwalking disorder. They are characterized by CNS activation, including autonomic

DSM-IV-TR Diagnostic Criteria for Sleep Parasomnias

Sleepwalking Disorder

A. Repeated episodes of rising from bed during sleep and walking about, usually occurring during the first third of the major sleep episode.
B. While sleepwalking, the person has a blank, staring face, is relatively unresponsive to the efforts of others to communicate with him or her, and can be awakened only with great difficulty.
C. On awakening (either from the sleepwalking episode or the next morning), the person has amnesia for the episode.
D. Within several minutes after awakening from the sleepwalking episode, there is no impairment in mental activity or behavior (although there may initially be a short period of confusion or disorientation).
E. The sleepwalking causes clinically significant distress or impairment in social, occupational, or other important areas of functioning.
F. The disturbance is not due to the direct physiological effects of a substance (e.g., a drug of abuse, a medication) or a general medical condition.

Sleep Terror Disorder

A. Recurrent episodes of abrupt wakening from sleep, usually occurring during the first third of the major sleep episode and beginning with a panicky scream.
B. Intense fear and signs of autonomic arousal, such as tachycardia, rapid breathing, and sweating, during each episode.
C. Relative unresponsiveness to efforts of others to comfort the person during the episode.
D. No detailed dream is recalled and there is amnesia for the episode.
E. The episodes cause clinically significant distress or impairment in social, occupational, or other important functioning.
F. The disturbance is not due to the direct physiological effects of a substance (e.g., a drug of abuse, a medication) or a general medical condition.

Nightmare Disorder

A. Repeated awakenings from the major sleep period or naps with detailed recall of extended and extremely frightening dreams, usually involving threats to survival, security, or self-esteem. The awakenings generally occur during the second half of the sleep period.
B. On awakening from the frightening dreams, the person rapidly becomes oriented and alert (in contrast to the confusion and disorientation seen in Sleep Terror Disorder and some forms of epilepsy).
C. The dream experience, or the sleep disturbance resulting from the awakening, causes clinically significant distress or impairment in social, occupational, or other important areas of functioning.
D. The nightmares do not occur exclusively during the course of another mental disorder (e.g., Delirium, Post-Traumatic Stress Disorder) and are not due to the direct physiological effects of a substance (e.g., a drug of abuse, a medication) or a general medical condition.

Source: Reprinted with permission from the *Diagnostic and Statistical Manual of Mental Disorders,* Fourth Edition, Text Revision. (Copyright 2000). American Psychiatric Association.

USING DSM-IV-TR

Health care providers often use language unfamiliar to clients and their families. Explain *amnesia for a sleepwalking episode* in terms that clients and family members can readily understand.

nervous system changes and skeletal muscle activity (AASM, 2005). The DSM-IV-TR diagnostic criteria for these disorders are listed in the Diagnostic Criteria feature above. Other less specific and less common parasomnias not discussed in this chapter are REM sleep behavior disorder (characterized by violent motor behavior usually associated with vivid dream recall) and sleep paralysis (defined on page 498).

Nightmare Disorder

Repeated occurrence of frightening dreams (during REM sleep) that lead to distressed awakening from sleep is called **nightmare disorder**. Between 10% and 50% of children between the ages of three and five have intense nightmares (APA, 2000). The diagnosis of nightmare disorder in children is most commonly associated with children under grave psychosocial stress. About 50% of all adults report at least an occasional nightmare (APA, 2000). In children, as well as adults, the diagnosis of nightmare disorder is not made unless there is persistent and significant distress or impairment.

Several medications that affect the autonomic nervous system—dopaminergic antagonists, antihypertensive medications, stimulants such as amphetamine and cocaine, antidepressants—can precipitate nightmares. Also, withdrawal of REM-suppressing agents—antidepressants, alcohol—may lead to REM sleep rebound accompanied by nightmares.

Sleep Terror Disorder

Sleep terror disorder, also known as night terrors, is characterized by the repeated occurrence of sudden arousal from slow-wave (non-REM) sleep, associated with intense autonomic and behavioral reactions characterized by fear. It is most common in children between the ages of 4 and 12, and resolves during adolescence, although it can occur in adults, particularly at times of intense stress.

The individual usually sits bolt upright in bed screaming or crying, with a frightened expression and obvious signs of anxiety. The individual is usually unresponsive to efforts by others to awaken and comfort him or her, and unlike nightmares, which occur in REM sleep, there is little or no memory of the frightening episode. With awakening there is usually confusion and disorientation for several minutes before the person returns to sleep.

Sleepwalking Disorder

Another sleep parasomnia that occurs during slow-wave (non-REM) sleep is sleepwalking, or somnambulism. **Sleepwalking disorder** is characterized by repeated episodes of rising from bed and walking about while asleep. While sleepwalking, the individual is often unresponsive to the communication of others or efforts to be awakened and has a blank stare and reduced alertness. Some people can respond to others while sleepwalking, use the bathroom, eat, leave the house, and even operate machinery.

Although sleepwalking is relatively common in children (between 10% and 30% have had at least one episode of sleepwalking), the prevalence of sleepwalking disorder is actually much lower, in the range of 1% to 5% (APA, 2000). Adults with sleepwalking disorder usually have a history of sleepwalking during childhood. If there is no such history, an adult should be assessed for a neurological condition or substance abuse. Certain medications used for psychiatric disorders, such as lithium (Lithane), desipramine (Norpramin), and thioridazine (Mellaril), may exacerbate or induce sleepwalking, as can fever or sleep deprivation (AASM, 2005).

SLEEP DISORDER RELATED TO ANOTHER MENTAL DISORDER

The sleep disorders discussed prior to this point are those that any individual, with or without a mental disorder, may have. Sleep disorders are so common that you can expect that some of your psychiatric–mental health clients will have a sleep disorder. In fact, insomnia is a primary symptom in 30% to 90% of psychiatric disorders (Becker, 2006).

A psychiatric illness or its treatment may cause a sleep pattern disturbance or have an interactive effect on a preexisting sleep pattern disturbance. Sleep disturbances that are symptomatic of underlying psychiatric illness are troublesome to clients. These symptoms are an important part of the experience of mental illness for clients, even though they may not be a predominant complaint.

Sleep disturbances that are secondary to psychiatric disorders are generally related to mood disorders and anxiety disorders, which account for 40% to 50% of all cases of chronic insomnia (Becker, 2006). Sleep disturbances can also be related to schizophrenia, alcohol use or abuse, and dementia and other cerebral degenerative disorders. While recognizing that a cyclical relationship is usually involved, it is helpful to try to differentiate primary sleep disorders from those that are secondary to a psychiatric disorder. Such differentiation can be particularly important for clients with depression, anxiety, and/or dementia. Sleep deprivation can lead to restlessness, reduced concentration, and, if prolonged, hallucinations and delusions. Likewise, chronic sleep deprivation may exacerbate dementia behaviors, as in the clinical example that follows.

CLINICAL EXAMPLE

Ellen, an older adult, was recently hospitalized for management of a medical condition. She was known to have early dementia of the Alzheimer's type but had been managing alone in her apartment up to this point. Over a period of several days, she became increasingly agitated, demanding cigarettes from nursing staff, other clients, and visitors. Attempts at distraction or providing unsolicited attention were unsuccessful.

A nursing student began questioning how much sleep this client had been getting. At that point the nurse's only cue was Ellen's lack of success with other interventions, but the nurse also knew that sundowning is common in clients with dementia. The brief chart notes made by the night staff offered little information. From a neighbor who came to visit, the nurse found out that prior to the hospitalization, Ellen had been phoning the neighbor during the night in an agitated state. The night staff agreed to observe and record the amount of time that Ellen spent sleeping, and the day staff did the same. With this additional data it was soon apparent that Ellen was averaging no more than 4 hours of sleep per 24-hour period. Meanwhile, her agitated behavior was increasing.

After a client conference in which the nursing student offered her nursing diagnosis hypothesis of Sleep Deprivation, the physician agreed to try a mild short-acting hypnotic for the next three nights. Nursing staff continued to monitor Ellen's sleep patterns and behavior. By the end of the three nights, during which she did appear to sleep for longer periods, the agitated behavior and demands for cigarettes subsided considerably.

The use of hypnotics was not a long-term solution for the client in the above example, but it broke the escalating cycle of increasing agitation and decreasing sleep. Recognizing the role of sleep deprivation in contributing to a daytime behavior problem can facilitate effective short-term intervention and create a context for more comprehensive assessment of possible contributing factors, such as fear, relocation stress, powerlessness, or sensory and/or perceptual alterations.

Differentiating sleep disorder secondary to psychiatric disorder from primary sleep disorder is a complex process that requires collaboration among clients, families, and health professionals. The sequence of onset may provide a clue. Many persons with unipolar depressive disorder initially see primary care practitioners or sleep clinics because of insomnia. As in the example of Ellen, it may take trying an intervention known to be effective for one or the other type of disorder to help clarify the primary diagnosis.

You need to be vigilant for the potential effects of a mismatched primary diagnosis and intervention. A depressed client misdiagnosed as having a primary sleep disorder of insomnia may be at risk of suicide if given a usual supply of hypnotic medication; likewise, obstructive sleep apnea with modest ingestion of alcohol can be mislabeled as alcohol abuse. As in any area of nursing practice, all components of the nursing process must be carefully and critically used. The DSM-IV-TR

DSM-IV-TR Diagnostic Criteria for Sleep Disorders Related to Another Mental Disorder

Insomnia Related to Another Mental Disorder

A. The predominant complaint is difficulty initiating or maintaining sleep or nonrestorative sleep, for at least 1 month that is associated with daytime fatigue or impaired daytime functioning.

B. The sleep disturbance (or daytime sequelae) causes clinically significant distress or impairment in social, occupational, or other important areas of functioning.

C. The insomnia is judged to be related to another Axis I or Axis II disorder (e.g., Major Depressive Disorder, Generalized Anxiety Disorder, Adjustment Disorder with Anxiety), but is sufficiently severe to warrant independent clinical attention.

D. The disturbance is not better accounted for by another Sleep Disorder (e.g., Narcolepsy, Breathing-Related Sleep Disorder, a Parasomnia).

E. The disturbance is not due to the direct physiological effects of a substance (e.g., a drug of abuse, a medication) or a general medical condition.

Hypersomnia Related to Another Mental Disorder

A. The predominant complaint is excessive sleepiness for at least 1 month as evidenced by either prolonged sleep episodes or daytime sleep episodes that occur almost daily.

B. The excessive sleepiness causes clinically significant distress or impairment in social, occupational, or other important areas of functioning.

C. The hypersomnia is judged to be related to another Axis I or Axis II disorder (e.g., Major Depressive Disorder, Dysthmic Disorder), but is sufficiently severe to warrant independent clinical attention.

D. The disturbance is not better accounted for by another Sleep Disorder (e.g., Narcolepsy, Breathing-Related Sleep Disorder, a Parasomnia) or by an inadequate amount of sleep.

E. The disturbance is not due to the direct physiological effects of a substance (e.g., a drug of abuse, a medication) or a general medical condition.

Source: Reprinted with permission from the *Diagnostic and Statistical Manual of Mental Disorders,* Fourth Edition, Text Revision. (Copyright 2000). American Psychiatric Association.

USING DSM-IV-TR

Health care providers often use language unfamiliar to clients and their families. Explain *nonrestorative sleep* in terms that clients and family members can easily understand.

diagnostic criteria for sleep disorders due to another mental disorder are listed in the following Diagnostic Criteria feature.

Schizophrenia

Significant sleep disruption often occurs in conjunction with an exacerbation of schizophrenia (AASM, 2005). Great difficulty in getting to sleep may accompany extreme anxiety and concern about delusional and hallucinatory phenomena. (Schizophrenia is discussed in detail in Chapter 16.) The overall circadian cycle may also be disrupted. Clients with schizophrenia have reduced REM sleep and do not experience REM rebound. Deficit of slow-wave sleep, particularly stage 4, has been found in acute and chronic schizophrenia (Kryger et al., 2005). A link with serotonin, a neurotransmitter associated with non-REM sleep, has been hypothesized. Depressed, alcoholic, and older adult clients also have reduced stage 4 sleep. Low nighttime levels of melatonin have been observed in persons with schizophrenia. A recent study (Suresh Kumar, Andrade, Bhakta, & Singh, 2007) of stable schizophrenic outpatients with insomnia concluded that melatonin may be a useful short-term hypnotic for clients in whom conventional hypnotic medication therapy or higher sedative antipsychotic medication doses may be problematic.

A careful sleep history should be undertaken for clients with schizophrenia whose psychosis is refractory (fails to respond) to antipsychotic medications, or only partially responds to antipsychotic medications. Karanti and Landen (2007) relate an instance in which a woman diagnosed with schizophrenia developed treatment-resistant auditory hallucinations along with extreme daytime fatigue and obesity. A careful sleep history led to a diagnosis of obesity-hypoventilation syndrome relieved by CPAP and followed by the complete remission of hallucinations.

Mood Disorders

As you learned in Chapter 17, insomnia of the maintenance or early wakening type commonly occurs in major depressive episodes. Insomnia is also among the most commonly reported residual symptoms (17–26%) after remission from depression (Carney, Segal, Edinger, & Krystal, 2007), suggesting that treatment to address insomnia after remission from depression is needed.

The sleep pattern disturbance may actually precede other symptoms of depression and likewise may respond to antidepressant medication more rapidly than the depression (AASM, 2005). Partial sleep deprivation, particularly of REM sleep, has been associated with modest improvement in depression, but the mechanism for this process is not well understood. Most antidepressants suppress REM sleep and lengthen latency to the first REM period.

Seasonal affective disorder (SAD) is related to fluctuations in melatonin levels by variation in the hours of sunlight. The positive response of SAD to light therapy lends strength to the argument that its development is related to weakened circadian rhythmicity.

In the manic phase of bipolar disorder, sleep time is significantly reduced but clients do not complain of insomnia. They have reduced slow-wave sleep and reduced REM latency. During the depressive phase, these clients may experience excessive sleepiness, similar to that of clients with SAD (AASM, 2005).

Anxiety Disorders

Sleep onset or maintenance insomnia is commonly associated with heightened anxiety. The proportion of stages 1 and 2 non-REM sleep tends to increase as part of the overall state of hyperarousal. Panic episodes may be associated with sudden awakenings, after which clients may find it very difficult to return to sleep. Sleep-associated panic episodes are most likely to occur during non-REM sleep, particularly stage 2. Current research and information about these problems can be found at the National Center on Sleep Disorders Research website at www.nhlbi.nih.gov/about/ncsdr/. See Chapter 18 for a complete discussion of anxiety disorders.

MEDIALINK National Center on Sleep Disorders Research

SLEEP DISORDER RELATED TO A GENERAL MEDICAL CONDITION

Many general medical conditions disturb sleep to some degree because of pain, discomfort, reduced mobility, itching, or gastrointestinal symptoms. However, in some cases the disturbance is so severe as to warrant identification as a sleep disorder. The symptoms may be those of insomnia, hypersomnia, parasomnia, or some combination thereof. A community-based cross-sectional study of 772 men and women aged 20 to 98 years old (Taylor et al., 2007) found that people with the following medical problems reported more chronic insomnia than did those without the medical problems: heart disease (44.1% vs. 22.8%), cancer (41.4% vs. 24.6%), hypertension (44.0% vs.19.3%), neurologic disease (66.7% vs. 24.3%), breathing problems (59.6% vs. 21.4%), urinary problems (41.5% vs. 23.3%), chronic pain (48.6% vs. 17.2%), and gastrointestinal problems (54.4% vs. 20.0%). This study demonstrated significant overlap between insomnia and multiple medical problems.

Dementia and Other Cerebral Degenerative Conditions

It has been suggested that sundowning may be the most common trigger for the institutionalization of clients with dementia because of the additional demands on caregivers. In an exploratory nursing study, activity patterns of clients with dementia were found to increase between 4:00 and 6:00 PM; whereas cognitively healthy clients had decreased activity at that time, corresponding to general population norms. The most common causal assumption has been a temporal relationship to conditions of decreased light and other environmental stimulation. Apparent deterioration of circadian patterns may be associated with deterioration of the suprachiasmatic nucleus in the brain (Kryger et al., 2005). Frequent arousals from sleep apnea, incontinence, or caregiver checks have also been implicated.

This population is particularly difficult to study because with increasing dementia, there is less and less tolerance of polysomnography. Other cerebral degenerative diseases that involve neurotransmitter imbalance, such as Parkinson's disease and Huntington's chorea, are also characterized by increasingly fragmented sleep. The DSM-IV-TR diagnostic criteria for sleep disorders due to a general medical condition are in the following Diagnostic Criteria feature. Cognitive disorders are discussed in Chapter 14.

SUBSTANCE-INDUCED SLEEP DISORDER

Substances of abuse or by prescription (e.g., alcohol, cocaine, opioids, hypnotics, anxiolytics) may cause a severe sleep disorder during intoxication or withdrawal. Even after prolonged abstinence, the abuse of some substances such as alcohol and hallucinogens may affect sleep architecture.

Substance-induced sleep disorder is characterized by sustained use of stimulants for staying awake, or of alcohol to induce sleep. You will probably work with many clients who use stimulants or alcohol periodically for their effect on sleep. For example, the use of stimulants is not uncommon among long-distance truck drivers, and alcohol is and has been one of the most frequently used hypnotics. While a drink at bedtime reduces sleep latency, it usually induces wakening later in the night.

A wide range of biochemical substances can contribute to this sleep disorder by their presence in sufficient quantities (such as caffeine and prescription drugs), their unaccustomed absence (alcohol), or their abuse (street drugs). Clients with psychiatric disorders, especially schizophrenia or mania, or clients with a history of traumatic brain injury are particularly vulnerable to sleep disorders due to chemical imbalances.

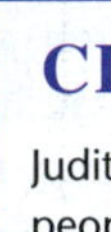

CLINICAL EXAMPLE

Judith and Karina participate in a maintenance program for people with schizophrenia. They often meet for a drink together at the conclusion of a meeting. Although they consume similar amounts of alcohol, Karina, who also has a history of minor brain injury, experiences greater disordered sleep.

The vulnerability may be twofold: direct effects of biochemical imbalance plus the use of alcohol or drugs as an attempt to cope with a psychiatric disorder.

With acute alcohol intoxication, there is increased sleepiness for 3 to 4 hours. Sleep may be deep (increased stages 3 and 4) with REM suppression. However, after that, sleep tends to be fragmented, restless, and often accompanied by bizarre dreaming. During alcohol withdrawal, sleep tends to be very fragmented, with REM rebound. The vivid dreaming may be associated with alcohol withdrawal delirium (APA, 2000). Sleep pattern disturbances persist even after a year or more of abstention.

Other abused drugs follow a similar pattern of exacerbation of their usual effect (sedation or stimulation) after exces-

DSM-IV-TR Diagnostic Criteria for Other Sleep Disorders

Diagnostic Criteria for Sleep Disorder Due to a General Medical Condition

A. A prominent disturbance in sleep that is sufficiently severe to warrant independent clinical attention.
B. There is evidence from the history, physical examination, or laboratory findings that the sleep disturbance is the direct physiological consequence of a general medical condition.
C. The disturbance is not better accounted for by another mental disorder (e.g., an Adjustment Disorder in which the stressor is a serious medical illness).
D. The disturbance does not occur exclusively during the course of a delirium.
E. The disturbance does not meet the criteria for Breathing-Related Sleep Disorder or Narcolepsy.
F. The sleep disturbance causes clinically significant distress or impairment in social, occupational, or other important areas of functioning.

Diagnostic Criteria for Substance-Induced Sleep Disorder

A. A prominent disturbance in sleep that is sufficiently severe to warrant independent clinical attention.
B. There is evidence from the history, physical examination, or laboratory findings of either (1) or (2):
   1. the symptoms in Criterion A developed during, or within a month of, Substance Intoxication or Withdrawal
   2. medication use is etiologically related to the sleep disturbance
C. The disturbance is not better accounted for by a Sleep Disorder that is not substance induced. Evidence that the symptoms are better accounted for by a Sleep Disorder that is not substance induced might include the following: the symptoms precede the onset of the substance use (or medication use); the symptoms persist for a substantial period of time (e.g., about a month) after the cessation of acute withdrawal or severe intoxication or are substantially in excess of what would be expected given the type or amount of the substance used or the duration of use; or there is other evidence that suggests the existence of an independent non–substance-induced Sleep Disorder (e.g., a history of recurrent non–substance-related episodes).
D. The disturbance does not occur exclusively during the course of a delirium.
E. The sleep disturbance causes clinically significant distress or impairment in social, occupational, or other important areas of functioning.

Source: Reprinted with permission from the *Diagnostic and Statistical Manual of Mental Disorders,* Fourth Edition, Text Revision. (Copyright 2000). American Psychiatric Association.

USING DSM-IV-TR

Health care providers often use language unfamiliar to clients and their families. Explain how medication use can be related to sleep disturbance in such a way that clients and family members can readily understand.

sive intake, along with rebound effects upon withdrawal (see Chapter 15). The DSM-IV-TR diagnostic criteria for substance-induced sleep disorders are in the Diagnostic Criteria feature above. Substance-related disorders are discussed in Chapter 15.

BIOPSYCHOSOCIAL THEORIES

Sleep is commonly believed to be restorative, but the evidence is actually quite conflicting. Arguments for sleep as a time of body restitution are based on the common observation that rest seems to promote healing; that growth hormone, which is anabolic, has its peak release during slow-wave sleep, whereas catabolic hormones such as the corticosteroids are at their lowest point of release during the night; and that conditions seem optimum for protein synthesis. However, protein synthesis is stimulated by amino acid absorption, little of which occurs during the nighttime fast; there is no sleep-related change in insulin release, a requirement for cell growth; and the release of growth hormone changes immediately with a change in sleep time, whereas change in corticosteroid release requires up to 2 weeks after a change in the sleep period.

Alternative theories about the function of sleep range from protective (there are fewer admissions to hospital emergency departments during the night) to adaptive (you cannot do much without light), from energy conservation to sleep being somewhat optional. Proponents of the latter view suggest that there is a core amount of required sleep but that the excess sleep time is not really required. There is more agreement on the role REM sleep plays in memory storage, consolidation of experience, and learning.

The important point is that although the functions of sleep are still poorly understood, client beliefs about the functions of sleep are important in psychiatric–mental health nursing practice. Through recognition and an exploration of client beliefs about sleep, you may be able to reinforce healthy attitudes and offer alternative perspectives based on your knowledge of sleep and its disorders.

Insomnia has been associated with increased physiologic arousal, emotional arousal, cognitive arousal, and conditioning. Current theory suggests that primary insomnia occurs in the presence of a combination of predisposing, precipitating, and perpetuating factors.

Physiologic Factors

The evidence for a physiologic basis for insomnia comes from studies that have shown that people with chronic insomnia are more likely to have a higher core body temperature and increased vasoconstriction at bedtime than those without symptoms of insomnia (Kryger et al., 2005). Poor sleepers also tend to have a higher and more variable heart rate and a higher metabolic rate. A family history of being light sleepers or being predisposed to depression suggests a possible genetic link to depression, but this has not been confirmed. Heightened physiologic arousal is most frequently a predisposing factor. It could become a precipitating or perpetuating factor in the context of regularly increased core body temperature (e.g., with heavy regular exercise immediately before bedtime) or regular intake of stimulants (e.g., prescription or nonprescription medication). For examples of sleep-inducing and arousal-inducing substances, see TABLE 19-2 ■.

Genetic Factors

Genetic analyses of circadian rhythm sleep disorders has revealed a relationship between variations in clock genes and diurnal change in human behaviors and suggest that further, as yet unidentified, gene variations are involved in human circadian activity (Ebisawa, 2007). Genetic susceptibility has also been proposed as influential in the development of narcolepsy (Longstreth et al., 2007). Predisposition to sleepwalking disorder is based on genetic susceptibility and has a familial pattern, although other predisposing factors such as sleep deprivation, alcohol, medications, situational stress, and fever are thought to trigger the sleepwalking episode (Pressman, 2007).

MEDIALINK Care Plan: Insomnia

Psychosocial Factors

Emotional arousal, as in anxiety, or cognitive arousal, as in worry and racing thoughts, can precipitate or perpetuate insomnia. There is some evidence to suggest that people who prefer a high degree of control or tend to internalize emotion may be more predisposed to insomnia. Grief and loss, as through death or divorce, may precipitate an episode of insomnia. Some clients report the onset of insomnia after the birth of their first baby because of their sense of needing to be more vigilant and adjusting to the new responsibilities.

Environmental Conditioning

Association of the sleeping room with lying awake may become a powerful perpetuating factor. Other clients may associate the bedroom with marital discord and thus also be conditioned to have increased arousal in that environment.

TABLE 19-2 ■ Substances Involved in Sleep and Wakefulness

Sleep-Inducing Substances	Arousal-Inducing Substances
1. Adenosine	Acetylcholine (ACh)
2. Antihistamines	Caffeine
3. Certain herbs (such as chamomile and valerian)	Dopamine (DA)
4. Endogenous melatonin (only that produced by the body's pineal gland)	Histamine
5. Free calcium (as found in warm milk)	Nicotine
6. Serotonin (5-HT)	Norepinephrine (NE)

MEDIALINK National Sleep Foundation

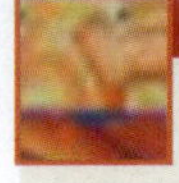

NURSING PROCESS
Clients with Primary Insomnia

The common nature of insomnia will likely mean it will coexist with many other aspects of psychiatric–mental health nursing care and overall medical–surgical nursing care. Many medications affect sleep. They are discussed in the following feature, What Every Medical–Surgical Nurse Should Know.

Assessment

Assessment is primarily subjective unless there are symptoms suggestive of other disorders. Building from the basic sleep pattern assessment in the Your Assessment Approach feature on page 495, it is particularly useful to follow up on a history of onset of insomnia, and possible contributing factors. Specific assessment guidelines for insomnia are given in the Your Assessment Approach feature on page 508. An ability to sleep better away from the usual bedroom suggests a conditioned response to that setting from many sleepless nights. Explore potential environmental factors, from condition of the mattress to sounds heard from outside the personal dwelling. Inquiring into the client's thought processes while trying to go to sleep may help detect fears, anxiety, or work/family/financial pressures. Listen for evidence of a perceived need for increased vigilance, either currently or at the time the problem developed. Explore beliefs about sleep and its importance. Particularly among individuals with a history of mental or physical disorders, there may be associated fears about death, disturbing dreams, or vulnerability to external threat. Encourage the client to discuss and describe the difficulty using the Rx Communication feature on page 508 as a guideline.

Nursing Diagnosis: NANDA

Specify Insomnia as the type of sleep pattern disturbance; further identify it as sleep onset, maintenance, or early wakening as appropriate. If the insomnia seems secondary to a mental disorder, that can be specified; but even for those clients, it is helpful to include other contributing factors. Even if environmental factors were not contributory initially, the client may begin to associate them with sleeplessness and/or they may become disturbing because of chronic hyperarousal.

Outcome Identification: NOC

The outcome expected from treatment of insomnia is improved sleep quality as reported by the client. Decreased sleep latency (time to fall asleep after lights out), fewer wakenings after sleep onset, and shorter time to get back to sleep after wakening can be estimated by the client through the use of a sleep diary such as the National Sleep Foundation Sleepiness Diary, which can be obtained through www.sleepfoundation.org.

Planning and Implementation: NIC

A few basic interventions for insomnia will be discussed in this section, but the overall treatment may be quite complex,

WHAT EVERY MEDICAL–SURGICAL NURSE SHOULD KNOW

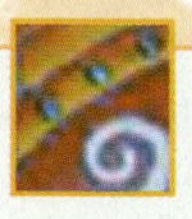

Medications that Affect Sleep

Type	Examples	Comments
Antidepressants	Tricyclic antidepressants such as amitriptyline (Elavil)	Induce drowsiness to varying degrees; effect on insomnia associated with depression usually occurs earlier than antidepressant effect. Suppress REM.
	Selective serotonin reuptake inhibitors such as fluoxetine (Prozac)	Generally decrease total sleep time, increase wakefulness, may induce vivid dreaming.
Antiepileptics	Phenytoin (Dilantin) and phenobarbital	Sedation common, less so with newer seizure control medications.
Antihistamines	Chlorpheniramine (Chlor-Trimeton) and pseudoephedrine compounds (Benylin cold capsules)	Induce drowsiness to varying degrees. Sometimes used as sleep-promoting agents because of their availability over the counter.
Antimanic medications	Lithium (Lithane)	Improves sleep but may cause daytime sleepiness initially.
Antiparkinson medications	Levodopa–carbidopa combinations (Sinemet)	Low doses may improve sleep, but generally persons on medication for Parkinson's have poor sleep with insomnia, vivid dreaming.
Antipsychotics	Traditional antipsychotics such as chlorpromazine (Thorazine) and haloperidol (Haldol)	Chlorpromazine very sedating, haloperidol less so.
	Atypical antipsychotics such as clozapine (Clozaril), risperidone (Risperdal)	High incidence of sedation with clozapine, less so with risperidone.
Anxiolytics	Benzodiazepines such as temazepam (Restoril)	May be used as hypnotics to induce and sustain sleep (note differences between short- and long-acting types).
	Buspirone (BuSpar)	Little effect on sleep and alertness.
Caffeine	Additive to some pain and headache remedies, coffee, tea, colas	Increases wakefulness, effects may last 8–14 hours.
Cardiovascular medications	Antihypertensives such as propranolol (Inderal), clonidine (Catapres), captopril (Capoten)	Insomnia, sedation, and nightmares, less so with captopril and other angiotensin-converting enzyme inhibitors.
Corticosteroids	Prednisone	Generally disturb sleep, especially if taken late in the day; suppress REM sleep.
Hypnotics	Zopiclone (Imovane)	Effective for sleep-onset insomnia because of rapid absorption.
	Zolpidem (Ambien), zaleplon (Sonata), eszopiclone (Lunesta)	Indicated for treatment of insomnia by U.S. Food and Drug Administration.
	Flurazepam (Dalmane)	Longer half-life, useful for sleep onset and maintenance insomnia.

requiring the skills of a specialist. If the insomnia is related primarily to a mental or physical disorder, management of that condition usually brings relief of associated symptoms. (See the Evidence-Based Practice feature on page 509 for a discussion of intervention strategies for insomnia.) Antidepressants are often effective in reducing sleep pattern disturbance before the antidepressant effect can be noticed. When necessary, prescription sleep aids may be prescribed to treat insomnia. The most common of these are zolpidem (Ambien), zaleplon (Sonata), eszopiclone (Lunesta), and ramelteon (Rozerem). These and other medications that affect sleep are discussed in the What Every Medical–Surgical Nurse Should Know feature above.

The interventions that are discussed in this section may be appropriate with clients in a variety of settings. If the insomnia is relatively recent or mild, information on the basic principles of sleep hygiene may be adequate (refer back to the Partnering with Clients and Families feature on page 494). If the insomnia is chronic and more severe, more rigorous intervention is warranted.

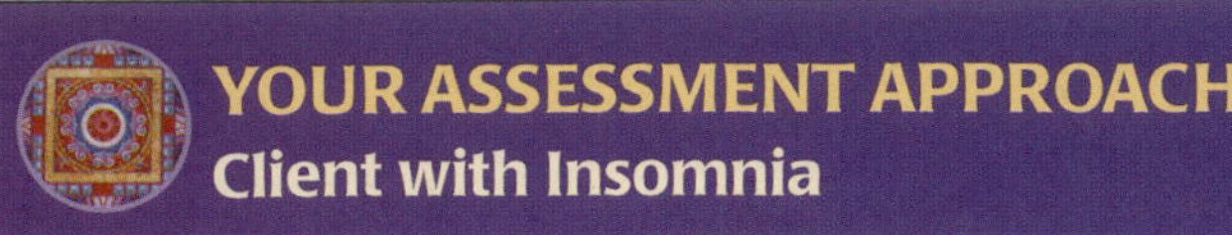

YOUR ASSESSMENT APPROACH
Client with Insomnia

Sample questions to help determine the presence of insomnia are given below.

Nature of the Insomnia

What do you have the most difficulty with:

- Getting to sleep?
- Waking up and then taking a long time to get back to sleep? or
- Waking up earlier than you want to and not being able to get back to sleep?

Possible Contributing Factors

- Does it help if you try to sleep somewhere else in your home?
- Is your sleep better or worse when you are away from home?
- Do you usually sleep with someone? If yes, does it make a difference if they are not with you? (Be alert here for possible disturbance by a partner, or poorer sleep when a habitual partner is not present. Note also that sharing the bed with infants and children varies across and within cultures.)
- How many cups of coffee a day do you drink? (Follow up regarding caffeinated or decaffeinated, timing, other caffeine-containing substances such as tea, chocolate, colas.)
- Do you smoke? How many packs a day?
- What medications and drugs are you using? (Note that many of the psychotropic medications alter sleep patterns, as do most substances of abuse.)

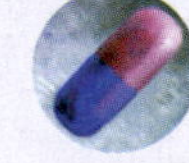

- What do you tend to think about while you are trying to get to sleep?
- What do you associate with sleep?
- What do you think is the single greatest factor affecting your ability to sleep?

Encouraging Hope

Insomnia is such a discouraging and worrisome problem to clients that creating a sense of realistic hope that they will eventually learn to manage the problem is an important part of nursing care. The goal is to change the client's perception of the problem from an event against which they are helpless to an event over which they can gain control.

Providing Information

Clients with severe insomnia are often well acquainted with the self-help literature. However, it is important to review what they have come to understand about managing insomnia. They may have misconceptions or difficulty applying some of the information to themselves. For example, some people are not aware that chocolate is a source of caffeine. Others may not be aware of normal developmental changes in sleep patterns. Normalizing the experience of occasional prolonged sleep latency (more than 30 minutes) or awakening during the night may be helpful as an intervention, as well as facilitating the setting of realistic goals. Clients with insomnia may also need some help in differentiating between myth and research-based evidence, between beliefs and facts. Of particular importance is recognizing that insomnia can be managed and that clients can continue to function adequately even on minimal sleep.

Shortening the Overall Sleep Period with Consistent Rising Time

The time of rising is under voluntary control; the time of actually getting to sleep is not. With shorter total time in bed, sleep usually becomes more consolidated. These two principles are the basis for one of the most effective means of gaining control over insomnia:

1. Clients must not go to bed until they feel sleepy.
2. They must get up at the same time each morning.

Initially, this prescription may seem threatening to clients who have usually gotten into a pattern of getting sleep whenever and wherever they can. They will need support during this initial phase, possibly through a contracting process in which they go one week at a time. Reinforce that they will be able to get by, that the body will eventually begin to respond to the regularity of schedule, and that you believe in their ability to accomplish this goal. Clients with insomnia should not be permitted to nap. (For the very old or very ill, naps should be restricted to a brief, set time period.)

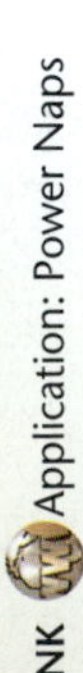

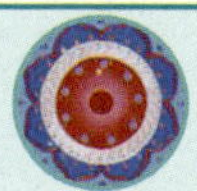

RX COMMUNICATION

CLIENT WITH PRIMARY INSOMNIA

CLIENT: "I'm having a lot of trouble falling asleep."

NURSE RESPONSE 1: "Tell me about your night's sleep and what it means to you."

RATIONALE: This response helps you detect aspects of the sleep pattern that indicate possible insomnia. There may be cultural differences between expectations and actual patterns of sleep.

NURSE RESPONSE 2: "Walk me through what a typical day is like for you."

RATIONALE: This response evaluates the extent to which the client's daily distribution of activities may result in an agitated or nonrelaxed state at bedtime.

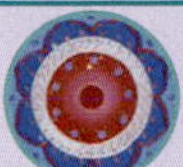

EVIDENCE-BASED PRACTICE

CHRONIC INSOMNIA

Rick Littlejohns is a 42-year-old businessman who has had recurrent episodes of depression and a history of chronic insomnia. He lives alone, except for two cats, having broken up with his wife 7 years ago. He describes himself as always being a light sleeper, but things got worse during his second year of college, when he started drinking heavily and sinking into his first major depression. Rick recently started a new job and since that time has been having increased difficulty getting to sleep and then with wakening again after a few hours. Recently, he missed work a couple of times because he finally managed to get into a sound sleep just as the alarm went off.

As a mental health counselor to whom he has come for help, you formulate a nursing care plan that addresses the following considerations:

1. Rick may have been predisposed to insomnia given his history of always being a light sleeper and history of depression. The current precipitating factor may be occupational stress associated with a new job.
2. Perpetuating factors may include conditioned arousal to his own bedroom and an irregular sleep schedule. Cognitive–behavioral therapy (CBT) is a first-line intervention for chronic insomnia. CBT techniques specific to chronic insomnia such as stimulus control therapy (by which the client is helped to reassociate his bedroom with sleep) and sleep restriction therapy (in which the time the client can spend in bed is temporarily restricted to the usual amount of actual sleep he gets) are among the nonpharmacologic interventions that have been shown to be effective for insomnia. Thus, you arrange referrals for Rick to the appropriate therapists.
3. Studies have shown that residual insomnia is common after remission from depression and can confer greater risk for subsequent depression. Rick's history of recurrent depression and current sleep problems may be related, and thus you will monitor his progress closely. You also consider asking him to keep a sleep diary.

Your plan of care is based on the research evidence summarized in the following journal articles:

Carney, C. E., Segal, Z. V., Edinger, J. D., & Krystal, A. D. (2007). A comparison of rates of residual insomnia symptoms following pharmacotherapy or cognitive–behavioral therapy for major depressive disorder. *Journal of Clinical Psychiatry, 68*(2), 254–260.

Edinger, J. D., Wohlgemuth, W. K., Radtke, R. A., Coffman, C. J., & Carney, C. E. (2007). Dose-response effects of cognitive–behavioral insomnia therapy: A randomized clinical trial. *Sleep, 30*(2), 203–212.

CRITICAL THINKING APPLICATION

1. In what ways would it be useful to determine the current precipitating factor influencing the client's insomnia?
2. In what ways would it be useful to determine the current precipitating factor in the client's depression?
3. How would cognitive therapy help someone with chronic insomnia?
4. Why is sleeping medication not a first-line intervention for chronic insomnia?
5. Why would you want to encourage a client to keep a sleep diary?

Reducing Known Stimulants and Other Sources of Arousal

Help clients with insomnia realize that they are susceptible to any stimulation, even though such stimulating factors may not have been contributory initially. Encourage them to avoid all sources of caffeine, nicotine, and other stimulants. However, in working with psychiatric clients, as with any client population, this intervention and all others must be considered in the context of the overall health problems, goals, and treatment plan as negotiated with the client, family, and other members of the health care team.

You may wish to collaborate with the client in making a list of possible contributing factors to the sleep pattern disturbance. For example, the client may identify interaction with a particular family member as generating a lot of emotion that is tough to deal with before going to bed. If fear or a perceived need for vigilance is a factor, it may be possible to modify the environment. The following clinical example discusses the effect that fear can have on sleep.

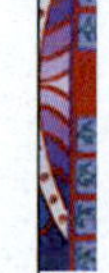

CLINICAL EXAMPLE

An elderly widow, initially referred to a sleep clinic with possible obstructive sleep apnea, had become increasingly depressed. On a recent visit she confided that she had been sexually abused a few years prior and was extremely afraid to venture out of her apartment building. She felt especially vulnerable because of living in a basement suite, which could be readily broken into. Through the efforts of one of the nurse clinicians, the social welfare agency that was involved agreed to pay the slight additional cost involved in moving her to a second-story apartment, where she felt much safer. Through ongoing counseling with the nurse clinician, she began a modest exercise program in her own small apartment, and medical treatment for her sleep disturbance and depression resulted in clinically significant improvement over the next few months.

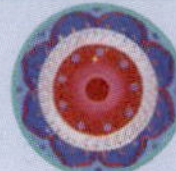

PARTNERING WITH CLIENTS AND FAMILIES

TEACHING ABOUT IMPROVING SLEEP QUALITY

1. Think about the kind of sleep schedule that seems to fit you best.
2. Make a list of things that help you get to sleep (how dark you like it to be, what temperature, how you get ready for bed).
3. Jot down all the "rules" and "suggestions" you have heard about how to get better sleep. Cross out the ones that don't seem to fit. (Some people sleep better by not having a bedtime snack; other people sleep better after having a snack. Do what feels best for you. If you aren't sure, try an experiment doing it one way for a week and then the other way for the next week.) Put a question mark by the rules and suggestions you have never really tried, and underline the ones you think are important for you.
4. Consider what you could change to get an extra half-hour of sleep each night.
5. Keep a sleep diary for 2 weeks. For the first week just keep track of your usual pattern (time you went to bed and got up, number of hours of actual sleep, how you felt in the morning, etc.). At the end of the first week, review the diary and your responses to items 1 through 4 above. In the second week, experiment with one change you think would be helpful to you.
6. Carry on the process a bit longer if you like, but remember:
   - You can manage on very little sleep if you have to.
   - You know better than anyone else what works for you.
   - Your needs and preferences regarding sleep may change as you get older or take on different roles and activities.

As discussed earlier, the state of arousal may be conditioned by objects in the bedroom environment or certain activities. Ways to alter these associations can be explored with the client. An assessment of the bedroom environment and its uses may call for relocating certain activities, such as paying bills or studying, to another part of the home. Rearranging furniture or even changing the color of pillowcases may help to reestablish associating the bedroom with sleep.

Relaxation Training

Relaxation exercises are discussed in Chapter 33∞. The important point in using them as an aid to sleep is that developing the skills should occur apart from the sleep period, so that they, too, do not become associated with the inability to sleep. The Partnering with Clients and Families feature above lists specific interventions that promote overall sleep improvement.

Evaluation

Early collaboration with the client in establishing realistic goals will help result in a satisfactory outcome. Regardless of behavioral or polysomnography-defined changes, it is important that the client can express some sense of mastery over his or her sleep problem. Whether that sense of control is achieved through reframing of essentially the same sleep patterns, a modest improvement in one or more parameters of sleep latency or number and length of awakenings, or an improved sense of energy for the day's activities is not important clinically. However, a better understanding of which interventions are most effective through carefully designed research studies would be a definite asset in helping nurses and others to choose among intervention alternatives.

CASE MANAGEMENT

Case management of the client with primary insomnia involves developing and organizing a program to address the problem. In this regard, you would help the client, to the extent necessary, with the following:

1. Making arrangements for a physical examination with a primary care provider
2. Maintaining a log of sleep activities
3. Keeping track of intake of stimulating substances such as caffeine

It is important to rule out physical factors causing the difficulty and to make the client aware of activities that affect the quality and duration of sleep.

COMMUNITY-BASED CARE

A large segment of clients with insomnia will be treated in the community. Community-based care focuses on management of the problem area within the context of the client's life and activities. Stress, diet and nutrition, exercise, and environment all shape and influence sleep patterns, especially once those patterns become problematic. With this in mind, you would arrange for the client to attend nutrition and stress classes at the local community center.

HOME CARE

When you go into a client's home to provide care, you have the opportunity to directly observe the factors impacting on sleep. Direct observation is a powerful tool in addressing a sleep disorder. Evaluate the environment and the conditions in the client's bedroom or sleep area. Are the lighting and noise level factors of concern? Making observations of the exterior of the residence during a home visit at the usual sleep time can provide additional information. Gradual alterations can be made to resolve whatever issues are detected that cause or contribute to the insomnia.

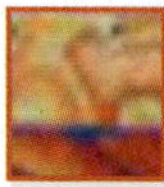

NURSING PROCESS Clients with Primary Hypersomnia

The focus in this section will be on clients with excessive sleepiness as part of their mental disorder. Basic assessments to identify clients who might benefit from referral to a sleep specialist are included. However, principles of treatment for most of the primary sleep disorders characterized by hypersomnia (obstructive sleep apnea, narcolepsy) were discussed earlier.

Assessment

Building from the basic sleep pattern assessment, explore potential contributing factors. With respect to the possibility of sleep apnea or periodic limb movement disorder:

- Try to interview the client's bed partner, or, if the client is institutionalized, to arrange for observation during sleep. If the bed partner describes recurrent periods of erratic breathing, including pauses of 20 seconds or longer interspersed between snoring, gasping, or snorting sounds, the client may have sleep apnea.
- Determine whether the problem disappears when the client is in a side-lying position, is worse after ingesting alcohol (even one or two drinks), or is accompanied by morning headaches or awakening with a feeling of still being tired.
- Ask the bed partner about the client's restlessness, repetitive jerking of one or more limbs, and/or gasping or choking noises.

An occasional apnea or myoclonic (muscular) jerk about the time of sleep onset is not unusual. These are common occurrences as part of the normal wake–sleep transition. It is the recurrent episodes accompanied by some daytime somnolence that are of particular concern.

In the psychiatric context, you will encounter clients whose excessive sleepiness is associated with a coping mechanism, hopelessness, or an underlying mental disorder. Eliciting information about onset, patterns, and perceived causes may be difficult with these clients (see the Rx Communication feature below). Regular observation and recording of states of waking–sleeping in relation to clock time, activities, and environment may provide some clues about the pattern. For example, if the client is sleeping quite soundly whenever left undisturbed, chronic sleep deprivation or posttraumatic hypersomnia could be a factor (AASM, 2005). Clients with secondary depression following a physical illness may also sleep more. In contrast, the lethargy that may accompany a major depressive episode or schizophrenia may be associated with lying with the eyes closed but not actually sleeping. (Such assessment will not be elaborated here, as it is best considered part of the overall assessment for these clients and is discussed in Chapters 16 and 17∞.)

Nursing Diagnosis: NANDA

The list of NANDA nursing diagnoses no longer includes the general diagnosis of sleep pattern disturbance (NANDA International, 2007). Instead, the most appropriate nursing diagnosis for primary hypersomnia is Fatigue, which is defined by the inability to restore energy even after sleep. Further specify and describe the contributing factors, such as depression, if known. Frequently, contributing factors will be unknown or hypothetical at best. It is better to say "Unknown" than to label a client in the absence of adequate evidence. See the Nursing Care Plan for a Depressed Client with Hypersomnia at the end of this chapter.

Outcome Identification: NOC

Sleep efficiency (ratio of total sleep time to total time in bed) will be increased to at least 85%.

Planning and Implementation: NIC

The commonly observed interaction of aging, depression, and concurrent physical disease as contributors to excessive sleepiness illustrates the difficulty of planning and implementing specific interventions. Focus the interventions as follows:

1. Treat the underlying mental and physical disorders.
2. Ensure client safety, because of the frequently associated problems with loss of concentration and memory.

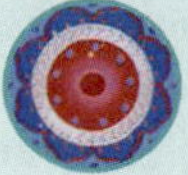

RX COMMUNICATION

CLIENT WITH PRIMARY HYPERSOMNIA

CLIENT: "I seem to fall asleep at unusual times."

NURSE RESPONSE 1: "Tell me about what times you fall asleep." ***RATIONALE:*** This response determines if the pattern of symptoms is indeed unusual.	**NURSE RESPONSE 2:** "Tell me about your overall sleep pattern, both your usual sleeping at night and what happens during these unusual times." ***RATIONALE:*** This response determines whether the client's sleep disturbance can be attributed to fatigue.

3. Regularize the client's schedule, alternating periods of activity and rest, to help the client gain a sense of control over the excessive sleepiness.
4. Expose the client to natural sunlight or light therapy in the morning; encourage walking outdoors.
5. Plan favorite events, such as a television program or visitor.
6. Maximize the use of environmental time cues, such as regular mealtimes and the visibility of a clock and windows.

Evaluation

The setting of short-term, achievable, and meaningful goals is important for clients with this condition. For them, time otherwise seems to become a blur of sleeping and eating.

CASE MANAGEMENT

The case management services needed by the client with hypersomnia focus on training for a healthier sleep pattern (refer back to the Partnering with Clients and Family feature on page 494) and safety. Participation in activities needs to be monitored to ensure that the client is not putting him- or herself in danger due to fatigue and hypersomnia. Times when the client feels most alert could be mapped and activities requiring attentiveness could be scheduled for those times. Arrange for appointments with health care providers specializing in sleep disorders to prioritize which factors play a role in generating fatigue for the client.

COMMUNITY-BASED CARE

Community-based care has similar features and direction to case management services. The client's safety needs must be addressed. Does the hypersomnia interfere with transportation, relationships, nutrition, or the client's abilities to be aware of and respond to environmental conditions? Do physical factors such as obesity or a sedentary lifestyle contribute to the hypersomnia? If so, and after obtaining medical clearance for the activity level, help the client arrange to attend an exercise class.

HOME CARE

Home care with a hypersomnic client will likely involve exploring the client's sleep environment firsthand. Numerous factors contribute to the sleep environment beyond the client's physiologic environment, or internal environment. You will be able to examine and incorporate the following external factors into your plan for maximizing home care:

1. Who the client sleeps with—human and pets.
2. The room size, position within the traffic pattern in the home, and lighting.
3. Bed or sleeping surface.
4. Air circulation and ventilation.
5. Daily schedule—both the client's and that of others in the environment.

Once these features of the external sleep environment have been examined, meet with the client and the entire family. A discussion about how the household functions in relation to sleep is helpful. Cultural features and expectations play a large role in determining sleep pattern expression in a home. A goal could be established with the help of all household members to help regulate the client's times of going to bed, going to sleep, and getting up.

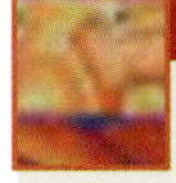

NURSING PROCESS
Clients with Circadian Rhythm Sleep Disorder

This section will focus on clients with circadian rhythm sleep disorders expressed through disorganized sleep–wake patterns. The driving force behind the disorganization could be external events such as shift work or moving among different time zones (jet lag) or internal phenomena such as a mental disorder. Circadian rhythm sleep disorders are common difficulties among depressed and psychotic clients.

Assessment

Much of the information that you need will come from the basic sleep pattern assessment (discussed in the Your Assessment feature on page 495) if clients can participate and recall accurately. The next step is a combined assessment–intervention: a sleep diary. By keeping a diary, clients may confront their own irregularities and be more amenable to developing a regular schedule. Other psychiatric clients may be unable or unwilling to maintain a diary and may require help. See the accompanying Rx Communication feature for examples of assessing this problem.

It is also useful to obtain information about previous patterns, tendencies toward being a morning or evening person, and the type of schedule to which the client will most likely return as his or her condition improves. In that way, the client will not have to cope with further schedule changes upon discharge or resuming family and work roles.

Nursing Diagnosis: NANDA

The nursing diagnosis is Insomnia or Sleep Deprivation as related to impairment of normal sleep pattern, but for this problem it is usually easier to identify contributing factors, such as travel, shift work, or parental responsibilities, at least to the immediate situation. For example, a client may live alone and be on an indefinite leave from work because of a major depressive episode. The mental disorder is an underlying cause, but the immediate and more rectifiable contributing factor is that there are few markers of time in the client's daily life, other than therapy appointments. Some clients, such as those with dementia, may have lost their ability to estimate time or even interpret cues. Other clients who live in a chaotic environment may find it very difficult to achieve any regularity of schedule.

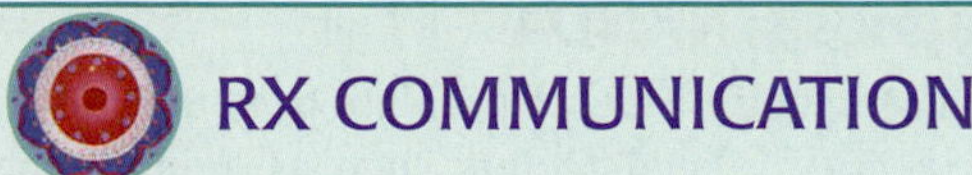

RX COMMUNICATION

CLIENT WITH CIRCADIAN RHYTHM SLEEP DISORDER

CLIENT: "For the last few weeks I wake up too soon and I can't get enough sleep."

NURSE RESPONSE 1: "How many hours of sleep a night are you getting?"

RATIONALE: This response explores the client's perceptions and definitions of symptoms to map out the exact nature of the difficulty.

NURSE RESPONSE 2: "Has anything changed in your schedule over that period of time?"

RATIONALE: This response explores whether any activities could be interfering with usual sleep patterns, including birth of a child, intrusion of a chaotic element in the environment, or a change in work schedules of the client or sleep partner.

Outcome Identification: NOC

Wakeful at appropriate times is the NOC term that best describes the desired outcome for circadian rhythm disorders.

Planning and Implementation: NIC

Interventions will be highly individualized for each client. Establishing sleep regularity is a critical intervention.

For the client who lives alone, external cues may be introduced through the help of family, friends, or social agencies. For example, a family member may agree to phone the client at the same time each day. A volunteer may agree to invite the client and two or three others to dinner every Wednesday evening. A service such as Meals on Wheels may be warranted, providing the combined benefit of better nutrition and another regular daily event. Scheduling morning appointments for these clients gives them a reason to get up early. As their condition gradually improves, they can take increasing responsibility for structuring their own schedule. Markers of the days of the week and even the season may help them to once again participate in the life around them.

Clients who live in a chaotic environment and/or experience multiple role demands present a very different challenge. For example, a young single mother with a colicky baby and a toddler may find her days and nights have become a blur of child care. Sleep deprivation because of caregiving responsibilities may reduce her coping skills. Reliance on alcohol or drugs may further fragment sleep, as may memories of abuse or trauma. A long-term plan of helping her reestablish control in her life will also be an important part of her overall therapy. The Talk About Sleep site at www.talkaboutsleep.com/ has topical research and information for health care providers and clients.

Evaluation

A sleep diary, as suggested for assessment, is an excellent resource for evaluation. Reviewing the diary with the client suffering from sleep–wake disturbance can provide further opportunity for positive reinforcement on accomplishments and for revised goal setting.

CASE MANAGEMENT

The case management of a client with circadian rhythm sleep disorder would depend on the nature of the cause of the disorder. If shift work was the cause, case management could include contacting the client's employee assistance program at work to determine if the work schedule can be made more flexible or different in any manner. With a client who has depressive symptomatology, interventions would focus on structuring the day and nighttime activities in such a way as to maximize sleep hygiene.

COMMUNITY-BASED CARE

The structure of an outpatient's life may depend on community-based care appointments at first. Getting up for an appointment, a group activity, or a day program can shape the sleep schedule. Attention to a variety of activities can be increased once symptomatology decreases and is more comfortably tolerated. If tension has been detected around sleep activities, you may arrange for the client to receive relaxation training in a local adult education program.

HOME CARE

Frequently these disorders occur with clients who experience psychotic symptoms or depression. Home care needs around sleep issues include interventions around these very real and disturbing sleep disruptions. Resolution of active symptoms of the psychiatric–mental health disorder contributes to resolution of many of the sleep difficulties. However, clients may live in circumstances that are chaotic. Make a series of visits to the client's residence at random times over several days during the part of the day the client is having trouble sleeping to determine if there are environmental factors interfering with the client's sleep that can be modified.

MEDIALINK Talk About Sleep

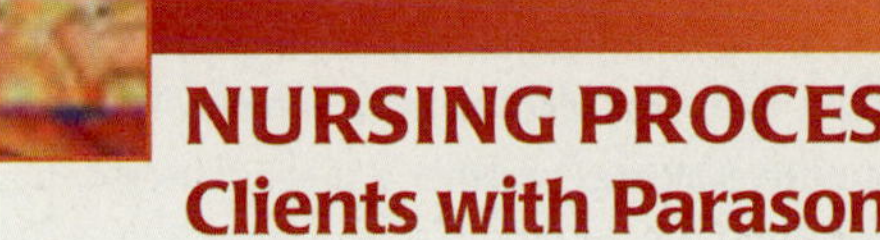

NURSING PROCESS
Clients with Parasomnias

Clients with parasomnias are often encountered in psychiatric settings because of the frequency of associated psychopathologic problems. The exception is young children, in whom parasomnias are considered a normal phenomenon or, at most, a transient sleep disorder (Mason & Pack, 2007). In adults, parasomnias are often associated with major stressful events.

Assessment

Besides the basic sleep pattern assessment, focus on the circumstances at the time of onset of the current and previous episodes and on family history.

- Clients with a single parasomnia may have a history of one or more other parasomnias, so ask about wakening with a sense of terror, vivid nightmares, and the like.
- Clients may be only partially aware of their parasomnias (they are usually amnesic about sleepwalking episodes), so question family members and sleep partners.
- The occurrence of subjective experiences like sleep terrors or sleep paralysis may never have been disclosed out of embarrassment or lack of adequate descriptive language; therefore, use normalizing statements followed by a question, such as, "Many people who have trouble with sleepwalking have also experienced times when they wake up feeling terribly frightened but aren't sure why. Has anything like that ever happened to you?"
- Inquiry about family history should not be limited to the same parasomnia, as there is some mixing of types among family members. The prevalence is higher among first-degree relatives than in the general population.
- Help clients explore stressors that might be associated with initial or recurrent episodes. "What else was happening in your life about then?"
- Ask about current and prior medications. Medication changes may also be a precipitator, particularly of the REM-related parasomnias such as nightmares. Remember that what was prescribed and what the client has actually taken may be different, so be sure to ask.

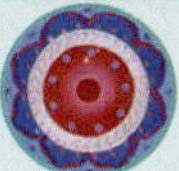

An assessment example for a client with nightmares is in the following Rx Communication feature.

Nursing Diagnosis: NANDA

With parasomnias, specify Sleep Deprivation as the nursing diagnosis and identify related factors such as aging-related sleep change, dementia, narcolepsy, nightmares, periodic limb movement disorder, sleep terror, sleepwalking, and so on. As with the other sleep pattern disturbances, specify the type(s), but the contributing factors may be unknown or hypothesized.

Outcome Identification: NOC

Reduction in frequency of parasomnias would be the desired outcome.

Planning and Implementation: NIC

Promoting client safety and administering medications are the two major nursing interventions.

Promoting Client Safety

Physical and emotional safety is the major goal in planning and implementing interventions for clients with sleep pattern disturbance related to parasomnias. Physically active parasomnias, such as sleepwalking disorder and REM sleep behavior disorder, pose the risk of injury to the client and/or others. At a children's camp, safety may be a matter of seeing that the affected child is assigned a lower bunk and that the cabin counselor is aware of the potential problem. Among older children or adults, the behaviors may be elaborate. Clients have been known to remove barricades, silence alarms, open exterior doors, and cross streets while sleepwalking. Protective intervention must be highly individualized and must involve close collaboration with the family. Caution family members to avoid wakening or arguing with the client.

Subjective parasomnias, such as sleep terror disorder and nightmare disorder, can be extremely frightening to clients, particularly those who are already compromised by a mental disorder. The dreams of clients with post-traumatic stress disorder may likewise be one of the most frightening factors for them.

Clients who are aware that they have sleepwalking disorder or REM sleep behavior disorder also tend to carry some burden of fear as to what might happen during this phenome-

RX COMMUNICATION

CLIENT WITH NIGHTMARES

CLIENT: "For the last couple of months I've been having nightmares."

NURSE RESPONSE 1: "Is there any pattern to the nightmares? For example, are they about one particular theme or subject?" ***RATIONALE:*** This response evaluates whether a specific stressor has played a role in precipitating the parasomnia.	**NURSE RESPONSE 2:** "How often do you get these nightmares, and has anything else changed about the way in which you sleep?" ***RATIONALE:*** This response explores the extent and topography of this sleep difficulty.

non that seems beyond their control. Offer assistance by helping them explore these feelings and understand the physiologic basis. Clients can be guided in the decisions they make about taking their medication and other substances by understanding the possibility of REM rebound.

Administering Medications

Clients with REM sleep behavior disorder respond to the regular administration of clonazepam (Kryger et al., 2005). However, there have been reports of breakthrough behavior even a year after beginning drug therapy. Somnambulism usually responds to clonazepam, diazepam (Valium), or imipramine (Tofranil) (Kryger et al., 2005). As noted earlier, many of the antidepressants suppress REM sleep and therefore offer some protection against nightmares. Caution clients against abruptly discontinuing the medication; REM rebound is less of a problem with gradual reduction of dosage.

Evaluation

Reducing the risk factors is the most important evaluation criterion. It is unrealistic to say you will prevent injury, because that is usually not within your realm of responsibility, nor is it realistic for any other care provider to guarantee injury prevention. In an environment of increasing litigation, the choice of words used in documentation is important.

CASE MANAGEMENT

Case management can work to minimize some of the stressors associated with parasomnias. Initially, you may arrange for the client to spend a series of nights at a sleep laboratory to evaluate the sleep disturbance. Once those data have been analyzed, the case management focus will be to assist the client in moving through the system, getting the help he or she needs for the disorder, and ensuring adherence to overall schedules.

COMMUNITY-BASED CARE

Community-based care is central in the long-term management of a parasomnia. An aspect of this care could concentrate on client access to an evaluation session with a psychiatric–mental health advanced practice nurse to determine whether there are any emotional issues contributing to the parasomnia. Following evaluations, careful examination of the client's particular parasomnia and the sleep environment would direct the plan of care. Cooperation with the family and/or sleep partners is necessary to determine the effectiveness of treatment.

HOME CARE

Parasomnias such as sleepwalking have associated dangers that home care can evaluate and work to decrease. You will be in a unique position to answer the following questions:

1. What is the sleep environment like?
2. Are there stairs, outside doors, or obstacles in the immediate vicinity?
3. What are the distances involved in the sleepwalking?

Meet with the client and family to discuss these factors and to stress the importance of careful monitoring of the situation. It is useful to have a conversation with the client and family or sleep partner to determine whether the response to the client's parasomnia may be positively reinforcing the parasomnia, making change more difficult to accomplish.

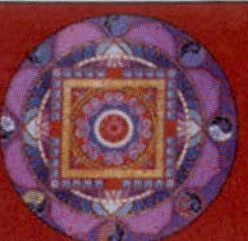

NURSING CARE PLAN
Depressed Client with Hypersomnia

Assessment

Identifying Information

Maha is a 42-year-old woman presently living in a small apartment with her unmarried 22-year-old son. Maha states she has been having trouble with periodic wakening and daytime sleepiness since before her divorce 2 years ago. She has been steadily gaining weight, feels that she has no energy, and says that the only thing she feels like doing is "watching my soaps on TV."

History

Never an energetic person, Maha feels that her present problems started years ago when she had to spend long hours with the children while her husband traveled. His homecomings usually included verbal abuse about her "slovenly" housekeeping and lack of discipline with the children. Having immigrated as a young wife, she misses her family deeply and has made few friends here. Food has always been a source of comfort to her, particularly the traditional dishes of her homeland.

Maha was heavy even as an adolescent and has snored for as long as she can remember. When she was still married, her husband usually slept in another bedroom because of her snoring. Her son describes her snoring as disruptive, with periods of escalating noise culminating in a half minute or more of silence that ends abruptly with a gasp and gradual resumption of quiet breathing until the next episode. She goes to bed about 9:00 PM and stays there until 11:00 or later the next morning, sleeping most of the time. She often wakens with a headache, feeling as tired as she did the night before.

Maha's current depressive episode was diagnosed 6 months ago when her son insisted she see their family doctor. Treatment was initiated with fluoxetine (Prozac) 20 mg, which has now been increased to 40 mg daily in the morning.

Current Mental Status

Maha appears somewhat drowsy, with a paucity of movement. Her speech is slow but coherent. She acknowledges some problems with short-term memory and concentration.

Nursing Diagnosis: Fatigue: Excessive somnolence related to inactivity secondary to depression, obstructive sleep apnea, and obesity

Expected Outcome: Sleep efficiency (ratio of total sleep time to total time in bed will improve to 85%)

Short-Term Goals	Interventions	Rationale
Client sees sleep specialist.	▪ Help client arrange for referral to sleep specialist.	Symptoms (snoring with apneas, daytime sleepiness, obesity) are suggestive of obstructive sleep apnea.
Establish regular sleep.	▪ Negotiate with client to get up every morning at the same time. ▪ Negotiate with client to obtain 8–9 hours of sleep per night.	Shorten time in bed to improve sleep efficiency.
Establish activity schedule.	▪ Encourage her to spend 30 minutes in outdoor activity every morning.	Exposure to natural sunlight early in the day improves sleep consolidation and reduces depression.
Increase activity and exercise.	▪ Explore previously enjoyed activities, involvement in exercise and sports. ▪ Establish a contract based on what client believes she can manage.	Previously enjoyed activities make a good starting point. Contracting can be effective in behavior change.

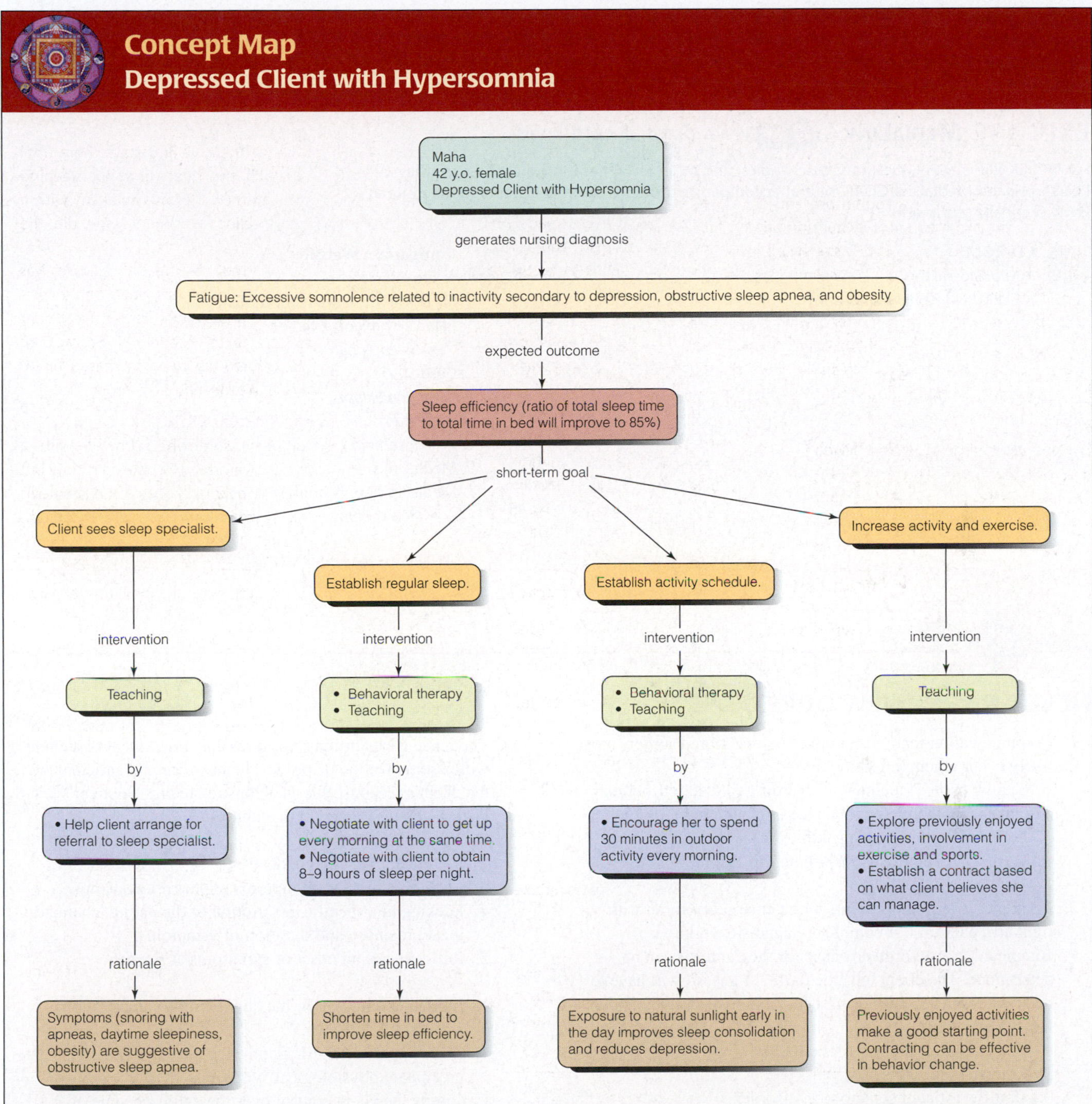
Concept Map
Depressed Client with Hypersomnia
Maha
42 y.o. female
Depressed Client with Hypersomnia
generates nursing diagnosis
Fatigue: Excessive somnolence related to inactivity secondary to depression, obstructive sleep apnea, and obesity
expected outcome
Sleep efficiency (ratio of total sleep time to total time in bed will improve to 85%)
short-term goal
Client sees sleep specialist.
Establish regular sleep.
Establish activity schedule.
Increase activity and exercise.
intervention
Teaching
• Behavioral therapy
• Teaching
• Behavioral therapy
• Teaching
Teaching
by
• Help client arrange for referral to sleep specialist.
• Negotiate with client to get up every morning at the same time.
• Negotiate with client to obtain 8–9 hours of sleep per night.
• Encourage her to spend 30 minutes in outdoor activity every morning.
• Explore previously enjoyed activities, involvement in exercise and sports.
• Establish a contract based on what client believes she can manage.
rationale
Symptoms (snoring with apneas, daytime sleepiness, obesity) are suggestive of obstructive sleep apnea.
Shorten time in bed to improve sleep efficiency.
Exposure to natural sunlight early in the day improves sleep consolidation and reduces depression.
Previously enjoyed activities make a good starting point. Contracting can be effective in behavior change.

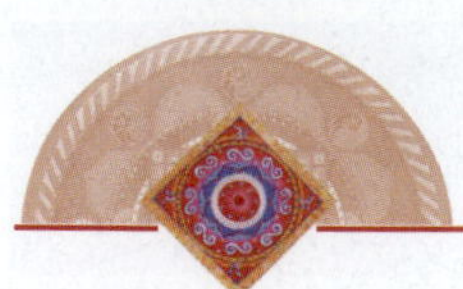

EXPLORE MEDIALINK

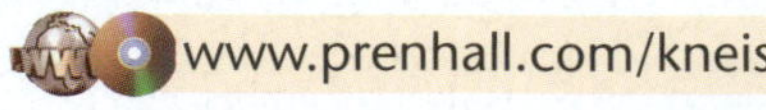

For NCLEX-RN® review questions, case studies, and other resources for this chapter see the Pearson Health MediaLink CD-ROM that accompanies this book and the Companion Website at www.prenhall.com/kneisl.

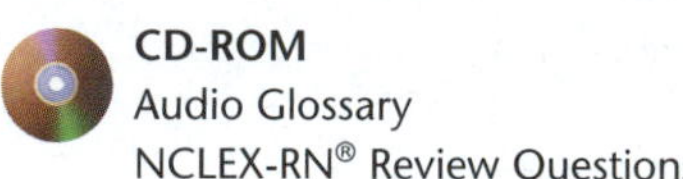

CD-ROM
Audio Glossary
NCLEX-RN® Review Questions

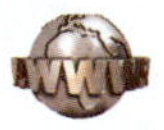

Companion Website
Audio Glossary
NCLEX-RN® Review Questions
Critical Thinking Exercise
- *Sleep Apnea*

Case Study
- *Narcolepsy*

Care Plan
- *Insomnia*

MediaLinks
MediaLink Application
- *Power Naps*

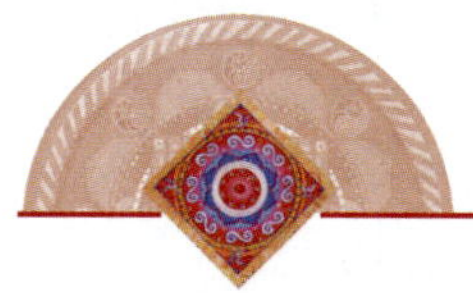

NCLEX-RN® REVIEW QUESTIONS

1. Communication theorists believe somatization disorders most likely occur among clients who:
1. Cannot express feelings for fear of guilt and retribution.
2. Have a biochemical imbalance in the brain.
3. Lack appropriate coping skills.
4. Have a genetic predisposition to this disorder.

2. An adolescent client presents in the emergency room with right arm paralysis. A complete diagnostic workup is completed, but no organic cause for the paralysis can be determined. The client tells the nurse, "I guess I will have to miss my piano recital today." The nurse suspects the client may be experiencing:
1. Body dysmorphic disorder (BDD).
2. Conversion disorder.
3. Undifferentiated somatoform disorder.
4. Malingering.

3. A client with a diagnosis of hypochondriasis tells the nurse in excessive detail about his current physical complaint. The most appropriate response from the nurse would be:
1. "Tell me more about your physical symptoms."
2. "Do you really expect me to believe what you just said? That's absurd."
3. "I will make a note of what you said."
4. "Don't worry. The doctors here know what they are doing."

4. The nurse is performing an admission assessment of a client with a somatization disorder. The nurse should anticipate that the client's responses to questions related to the client's health history will be (select all that apply):
1. Accurate.
2. Presented in excessive detail.
3. Related to how the symptoms impact relationships.
4. Lacking in a specific description of the nature, character, location, onset, and duration of symptoms.
5. Reflective of an onset of symptoms at age 50.

5. Nursing interventions for the client with a somatization disorder include:
1. Assisting the client in identifying stressful situations that precipitate physiological symptoms.
2. Giving the client control over the daily schedule of activities.
3. Setting aside 1 hour per shift for the client to talk about physical concerns.
4. Encouraging the client to verbalize concerns in group therapy.

6. Which of the following factors does not influence the development of primary insomnia?
1. Family history of light sleepers
2. A high need to have control over situations
3. Decreased metabolic rate
4. Environmental conditioning

7. Which of the following would not be included in a basic sleep pattern assessment?
1. Sleep–wake schedule
2. Daytime functioning
3. Satisfaction with sleep
4. 24-hour food diary

8. The belief that clients cope with anxiety by converting the anxiety into physical symptoms but generally do not exhibit psychological symptoms is a concept of which theory?
1. Psychoanalytic
2. Communication
3. Genetic
4. Humanistic

9. A client with acute alcohol intoxication may experience which of the following sleep changes?
1. Significantly reduced sleep time with no complaints of insomnia
2. Extreme anxiety related to falling asleep
3. Fragmented, restless sleep with bizarre dreams
4. Difficulty staying asleep with hyperarousal

10. Nursing interventions to promote sleep in the client experiencing insomnia include:
1. Watching television in bed until the client is ready to fall asleep.
2. Increasing physical exercise during the day.
3. Going to bed 1 hour earlier than usual to encourage falling asleep.
4. Staying up later than usual to ensure the client is tired when going to bed.

See Appendix C for answers.

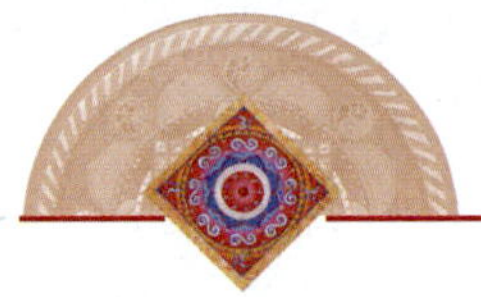

REFERENCES

American Academy of Sleep Medicine. (2005). *The international classification of sleep disorders: Diagnostic and coding manual* (2nd ed.). Rochester, MN: Author.

American Psychiatric Association. (2000). *Diagnostic and statistical manual of mental disorders* (4th ed., Text Revision). Washington, DC: Author.

Arnold, I. A., de Waal, M. W., Eekhof, J. A., & van Hemert, A. M. (2006). Somatoform disorder in primary care: Course and the need for cognitive–behavioral treatment. *Psychomatics, 47*(6), 498–503.

Becker, P. M. (2006). Treatment of sleep dysfunction and psychiatric disorders. *Current Treatment Options in Neurology, 8*(5), 367–375.

Bourne, E. J. (2005). *The anxiety and relaxation workbook* (4th ed.). Oakland, CA: New Harbinger Publications.

Carney, C. E., Segal, Z. V., Edinger, J. D., & Krystal, A. D. (2007). A comparison of rates of residual insomnia symptoms following pharmacotherapy or cognitive–behavioral therapy for major depressive disorder. *Journal of Clinical Psychiatry, 68*(2), 254–260.

Ebisawa, T. (2007). Circadian rhythms in the CNS and peripheral clock disorders: Human sleep disorders and clock genes. *Journal of Pharmacologic Science, 103*(2), 150–154.

Edinger, J. D., Wohlgemuth, W. K., Radtke, R. A., Coffman, C. J., & Carney, C. E. (2007). Dose-response effects of cognitive–behavioral insomnia therapy: A randomized clinical trial. *Sleep, 30*(2), 203–212.

Fink, P., Toft, T., Hansen, M. S., Ornbol, E., & Olesen, F. (2007). Symptoms and syndromes of bodily distress: An exploratory study of 978 internal medical, neurological, and primary care patients. *Psychosomatic Medicine, 69*(1), 30–39.

Griffiths, R. F., & Ellis, P. M. (2007). Visual conversion disorder in a harbor pilot leading to sudden loss of control of a large vessel. *Aviation, Space, & Environmental Medicine, 78*(1), 59–62.

Hening, W. A. (2007). Current guidelines and standards of practice for restless legs syndrome. *American Journal of Medicine, 120*(1 Suppl 1), S22–S27.

Ikawa, M., Yamada, K., & Ikeuchi, S. (2006). Efficacy of amitriptyline for treatment of somatoform pain disorder in the orofacial region: A case series. *Journal of Orofacial Pain, 20*(3), 234–240.

Jackson, J. L., O'Malley, P. G., & Kroenke, K. (2006). Antidepressants and cognitive–behavioral therapy for symptom syndromes. *CNS Spectrum, 11*(3), 212–222.

Karanti, A., & Landen, M. (2007). Treatment refractory psychosis remitted upon treatment with continuous positive airway pressure: A case report. *Psychopharmacology Bulletin, 40*(1), 113–117.

Karst, M., Rahe-Meyer, N., Gueduek, A., Hoy, L., Borsutzky, M., & Passie, T. (2005). Abnormality in the self-monitoring mechanism in patients with fibromyalgia and somatoform pain disorder. *Psychosomatic Medicine, 67*, 111–115.

Kryger, M. H. (2004). *A woman's guide to sleep disorders*. New York: McGraw-Hill.

Kryger, M. H., Roth, T., & Dement, W. C. (2005). *Principles and practice of sleep medicine* (4th ed.). Philadelphia: Saunders.

Kushida, C. A. (2007). Clinical presentation, diagnosis, and quality of life issues in restless legs syndrome. *American Journal of Medicine, 120*(1 Suppl 1), S4–S12.

Lack, L. C., & Wright, H. B. (2007). Clinical management of delayed sleep phase disorder. *Behavioral Sleep Medicine, 5*(1), 57–76.

Longstreth, W. T., Jr., Koepsell, T. D., Ton, T. G., Hendrickson, A. F., & van Belle, G. (2007). The epidemiology of narcolepsy. *Sleep, 30*(1), 13–26.

Malatack, J. J., Consolini, D., Mann, K., & Raab, C. (2006). Taking on the parent to save a child: Munchausen syndrome by proxy. *Contemporary Pediatrics, 23*, 50–63.

Marazzita, D., Giannotti, D., Catena, M. C., Carlini, M., Dell'Osso, B., Presta, S., et al. (2006). Insight in body dysmorphic disorder with and without comorbid obsessive–compulsive disorder. *CNS Spectrums, 11*(7), 494–498.

Mason, T. B., & Pack, A. I. (2007). Pediatric parasomnias. *Sleep, 30*(2), 141–151.

Morin, C. M., Bootzin, R. R., Buysse, D. J., Edinger, J. D., Espie, C. A., & Lichstein, K. L. (2006). Psychological and behavioral treatment of insomnia: Update of the recent evidence (1998–2004). *Sleep, 29*(11), 398–414.

NANDA International. (2007). *Nursing Diagnosis: Definitions & Classifications 2000–2008.* Philadelphia: Author.

National Institutes of Health. (2005). NIH state-of-the-science conference statement on manifestations and management of chronic insomnia in adults. *NIH Consensus State of the Science Statements, 22*(2), 1–30.

Peebles, R., Sabella, C., Franco, K., & Goldfarb, J. (2005). Factitious disorder and malingering in adolescent girls: Case series and literature review. *Clinical Pediatrics, 44*(3), 237–243.

Pressman, M. R. (2007). Factors that predispose, prime, and precipitate NREM parasomnias in adults: Clinical and forensic implications. *Sleep Medicine Review, 11*(1), 5–30.

Ritvo, E. C., Melnick, I., Marcus, G. R., & Glick, I. D. (2006). Psychiatric conditions in cosmetic surgery patients. *Facial Plastic Surgery, 22*(3), 194–197.

Robinson, D. M., & Keating, G. M. (2007). Sodium oxybate. A review of its use in the management of narcolepsy. *CNS Drugs, 21*(4), 337–354.

Roelofs, K., Spinhoven, P., Sandijck, P., Moene, F. C., & Hoogduin, K. A. L. (2005). The impact of early trauma and recent life-events in symptom severity in patients with conversion disorder. *Journal of Nervous & Mental Disease, 193*(8), 508–514.

Sadock, B. J., & Sadock, V. A. (2007). *Kaplan and Sadock's synopsis of psychiatry: Behavioral Sciences/Clinical Psychiatry* (10th ed.). Philadelphia: Lippincott Williams & Wilkins.

Savino, A. C., & Fordtran, J. S. (2006). Factitious diseases: Clinical lessons from case studies at Baylor University Medical Center. *Baylor University Medical Center Proceedings, 19*(3), 195–208.

Schwartz, J. R., & Roth, T. (2006). Shift work sleep disorder: Burden of illness and approaches to management. *Drugs, 66*(18), 2357–2370.

Sivertsen, B., Omvik, S., Pallesen, S., Bjorvatn, B., Havik, O. E., Kvale, G., et al. (2006). Cognitive–behavioral therapy vs. zopiclone for treatment of chronic primary insomnia in older adults: A randomized controlled trial. *Journal of the American Medical Association, 295*(24), 2851–2858.

Smaldone, A., Honig, J. C., & Byrne, M. W. (2007). Sleepless in America: Inadequate sleep and relationships to health and well-being of our nation's children. *Pediatrics, 119*(Suppl 1), S29–S37.

Suresh Kumar, P. N., Andrade, C., Bhakta, S. G., & Singh, N. M. (2007). Melatonin in schizophrenic outpatients with insomnia: A double-blind, placebo-controlled study. *Journal of Clinical Psychiatry, 68*(2), 237–241.

Taylor, D. J., Mallory, L. J., Lichstein, K. L., Durrence, H. H., Riedel, B. W., & Bush, A. J. (2007). Comorbidity of chronic insomnia with medical problems. *Sleep, 30*(2), 213–218.

Thorpy, M. J., & Yager, J. (2006). *Sleeping well: The sourcebook for sleep and sleep disorders.* New York: Checkmark Books.

Valentino, R. M., & Foldvary-Schaefer, N. (2007). Madafinil in the treatment of excessive daytime sleepiness. *Cleveland Clinic Journal of Medicine, 74*(8), 561–566, 568–571.

Waterhouse, J., Reilly, T., Atkinson, G., & Edwards, B. (2007). Jet lag: Trends and coping strategies. *Lancet, 369*(9567), 1117–1129.

Wolkove, N., Elkholy, O., Baltzan, M., & Palayew, M. (2007). Sleep and aging: 1. Sleep disorders commonly found in older people. *Canadian Medical Association Journal, 176*(9), 1299–1304.

Gender Identity and Sexual Disorders

CHAPTER

20

KAREN LEE FONTAINE

LEARNING OUTCOMES

After completing this chapter, you will be able to:

1. Explore the values you hold regarding sexuality.
2. Describe the ranges of transgendered identities and behaviors.
3. Differentiate between adaptive and maladaptive sexual responses.
4. Explain the distinction between noncoercive and coercive paraphilias.
5. Discuss the biopsychosocial theories that help to explain various sexual disorders and gender dysphoria.
6. Elicit a sexual history that includes affective, behavioral, cognitive, and sensation components.
7. Describe the three levels of nursing intervention appropriate to the psychiatric–mental health nurse generalist, and one level appropriate to the psychiatric–mental health advanced practice nurse.
8. Identify the principles common to implementing nursing care for persons with gender dysphoria or sexual disorders.
9. Develop a more comfortable style discussing clients' sexuality and sexual problems.
10. Describe how the psychiatric–mental health nurse can demonstrate sensitivity to the diversity of sexual values in the population.

CRITICAL THINKING CHALLENGE

Charles is a 54-year-old male being treated on the inpatient unit for depression. This is his first hospital stay for a psychiatric problem, although he has had difficulties with depression for months. He has been married for 25 years, has no children, and his relationship with his wife Claudia has been strained for some time.

One of the major problems Charles and Claudia are having is a sexual one. His arousal was based on certain activities in which Claudia no longer wanted to participate. As a couple they decided it would be beneficial to attend therapy focused on this problem. Couples sex therapy provided the opportunity to make some progress on this relationship problem with a specific plan designed for them by a sex therapist. Then Charles's symptoms of depression began affecting their sex life again, and once he began treatment with an antidepressant he experienced significant sexual side effects. The

(continued)

KEY TERMS

androgyny *524*
autoerotic asphyxia *527*
coercive paraphilias *527*
cross-dressers *524*
dyspareunia *531*
erectile dysfunction *530*
exhibitionism *528*
female orgasmic disorder *530*
female sexual arousal disorder *530*
fetishism *525*
frotteurism *528*
gender identity *523*
gender identity disorder *524*
gender roles *523*
hypoactive sexual desire disorder *528*
intersex *524*
male erectile disorder *530*
male orgasmic disorder *531*
noncoercive paraphilias *525*
paraphilias *525*
pedophilia *528*
premature ejaculation *531*
sexual addiction *532*
sexual aversion disorder *530*

(continued)

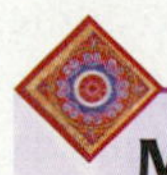

MEDIALINK 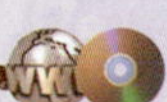 www.prenhall.com/kneisl

Go to the Pearson Health MediaLink CD-ROM and the Companion Website at www.prenhall.com/kneisl for interactive resources for this chapter.

KEY TERMS *(continued)*

sexual dysfunctions *528*
sexual pain disorder *531*
transgender *523*
transsexuals *524*
transvestic fetishism *526*
vaginismus *532*
voyeurism *528*

CRITICAL THINKING CHALLENGE *(continued)*

sexual challenge in this relationship was heightened by the problems caused by Charles's antidepressant medication.

When clients are admitted to inpatient settings for treatment of mental disorders, their sexual needs are rarely addressed. Clients and their partners/spouses are expected to remain celibate throughout the hospital stay. Privacy is often not provided for clients and their loved ones. Visiting is limited and usually restricted to public areas.

1. Do you agree that clients on an inpatient unit should be expected to be celibate?
2. Are professionals imposing their sexual practice values on clients in this situation?
3. When clients are admitted, do they lose their right to consensual sexual activity with their partner?

All humans are sexual beings. Regardless of gender, age, race, socioeconomic status, religious beliefs, physical and mental health, or other demographic factors, we express our sexuality in a variety of ways throughout our lives.

Human sexuality is difficult to define. Sexuality is an individually expressed and highly personal phenomenon whose meaning evolves from objective and subjective experiences. Physiologic, psychosocial, and cultural factors influence a person's sexuality and lead to the wide range of attitudes and behaviors seen in humans. There are no normal, universal sexual behaviors. Satisfying or "normal" sexual expression can generally be described as whatever behaviors give pleasure and satisfaction to the adults involved, without threat of coercion or injury to others. The United States is a multicultural society that has a sexually diverse population. As nurses, we should work toward the goal of acknowledging and appreciating the rich sexual diversity of our clients.

Sexual health is an individual and constantly changing phenomenon falling within the wide range of human sexual thoughts, feelings, needs, and desires. A person's degree of sexual health is best determined by that individual, sometimes with the assistance of a qualified professional.

Sexual health includes both *freedoms* and *responsibilities.* Sexually healthy people engage in activities that are freely chosen, including both self-pleasuring and consensually shared-pleasuring activities. Individuals also have freedom of sexual thought, feeling, and fantasy. Sexually healthy people are ethically motivated to exercise behavioral, emotional, economic, and social responsibility for themselves (Vision of Sexual Health, 2004).

Sexual health care is a relatively new area of involvement for psychiatric–mental health nurses. Until recently, sexuality has not been viewed as falling within their scope of practice. Currently, sexuality is increasingly recognized as an important component of a holistic approach to overall health status. Sexual health care is a legitimate and appropriate nursing concern. The close and often extended relationships that psychiatric–mental health nurses have with clients and families foster the rapport necessary to discuss this private area of clients' health status.

Nursing roles in the area of human sexuality are evolving gradually. Psychiatric–mental health nurses involved in nursing activities related to human sexual functioning need the following:

- Acceptance of, and comfort with, their own sexual values and expressions
- Concrete and comprehensive knowledge about sexual function and dysfunction
- Skill in communication techniques
- A willingness to explore and separate personal values and attitudes from those of clients
- The nurse generalist should be proficient in using the nursing process to assess the client's sexual health and sexual concerns, promote optimal sexual health, play a supportive role, and refer the client to an advanced practice nurse or other health care professional with expertise in this area
- The advanced practice clinical nurse specialist or nurse practitioner with special training and interest in gender identity and sexual disorders can diagnose, intervene, and evaluate care to promote optimal sexual health

Historically, human sexuality has been shrouded in myth and controversy. This history has hindered both the delivery and the receipt of services that promote sexual health and well-being. Although scientific knowledge has expanded immensely during the past several decades, modern North Americans continue to view sex and sexuality with discomfort. Our confusion is complicated by our traditional religious and social values. Basic to nursing is the notion that the nurse's personal beliefs should not influence the quality of care given a client. If nurses hold negative, inappropriate, or stereotyped opinions and ideas, they must confront them before they can meet professional standards of care in helping clients attain optimal sexual health. It is easier for nurses to live up to this standard if they engage in value clarification before providing sexual health care. Giving nonjudgmental nursing care does not mean that the nurse has to agree with others' beliefs and values about sexuality. However, self-awareness can help

YOUR SELF-AWARENESS
Check Your Knowledge and Attitudes About Sex

Use this checklist periodically to assess changes in your knowledge and attitudes.

Knowledge

Circle True or False for each statement.

Women can and do have orgasms while sleeping.	T	F
It is dangerous to engage in intercourse during menstruation.	T	F
Sex drive usually diminishes after a vasectomy.	T	F
The older male may actually have some advantages over the younger male in sexual activity.	T	F
Masturbation is a relatively common practice of both women and men.	T	F
Females have two kinds of orgasm: clitoral and vaginal.	T	F
Children raised by homosexual couples are very likely to become homosexual.	T	F
An adult male who has been castrated immediately loses his sex drive.	T	F
Intercourse should always be avoided during the last trimester of pregnancy.	T	F
Oral–genital stimulation is unhygienic.	T	F

Attitudes

Circle the letter corresponding to your level of agreement with each statement.

A: Strongly agree; **B:** Agree; **C:** Uncertain; **D:** Disagree; **E:** Strongly disagree

Sex education has caused a rise in premarital intercourse.	A	B	C	D	E
Extramarital relations are almost always harmful to a marriage.	A	B	C	D	E
Relieving tension by masturbation is a healthy practice.	A	B	C	D	E
Premarital intercourse is morally undesirable.	A	B	C	D	E
Parents should stop their children from masturbating.	A	B	C	D	E
Women should have sexual experience before marriage.	A	B	C	D	E
Homosexual and bisexual behavior should be against the law.	A	B	C	D	E
Seeing family members nude arouses undue curiosity in children.	A	B	C	D	E
Promiscuity is widespread on college campuses today.	A	B	C	D	E
Men should have sexual experience before marriage.	A	B	C	D	E

psychiatric–mental health nurses respect their clients' sexual rights and needs. Use the Your Self-Awareness feature above to assess your sexual knowledge and attitudes.

GENDER AND TRANSGENDER

Western culture is deeply committed to the idea that there are only two sexes. Biologically speaking, however, there are many gradations running from female to male; these gradations are known collectively as **transgender**. In some cases gender is clear, in some it is unclear, and in other cases there is a blending of both genders within the same individual. This diversity of gender represents normal variations in the human population.

Gender Identity

Gender identity is an individual's personal or private sense of identity as female or male. Gender identity develops from an interaction of biology, identity imposed by others, and self-identity. A newborn is assigned a gender (identity imposed by others) according to the appearance of the external genitals (biology); by 3 years of age, the child says, "I am a girl" or "I am a boy" (self-identity).

Gender identity can be viewed as a continuum. At one end of the continuum are those whose gender identity is congruent with their anatomic sex. In the middle are people who have both male and female gender identities. At the other end of the continuum are those whose gender identity conflicts with their anatomic sex. In addition, sexual identity is fixed for some people, while for others it is more variable and changing.

Gender Roles

Gender roles are the roles a person is expected to perform as a result of being male or female in a particular culture. The expectation that people will exhibit certain behaviors because they are female or male is referred to as *gender role stereotyping*. Stereotypical images of people do not take into account individual differences. The danger of such stereotypes is that people take them seriously and act on them, turning a blind eye to the qualities and interests of individuals. In North American culture, gender roles are more strictly enforced for males than for females, and males are socially punished for female behavior.

MEDIALINK Gender Identity Disorder Video

MEDIALINK Application: Born with the Wrong Body

WHY I BECAME A PSYCHIATRIC–MENTAL HEALTH NURSE

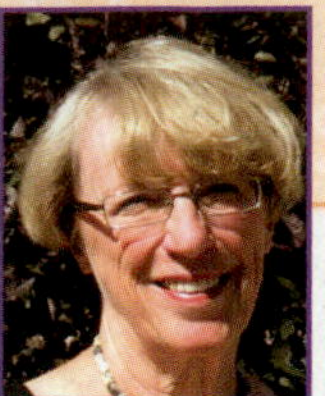

Karen Lee Fontaine
Contributor, Chapters 20, 21, and 24

I was a young nurse in the 1960s when Masters and Johnson published the first scientific studies of human sexuality. Growing up, my family never discussed sex, and in nursing school we studied all body processes *except* sexual behavior. It was a conspiracy of silence. I was fascinated by this new information and was determined to become a sex therapist. Achieving a master's degree in psychiatric nursing was my route to becoming a sex therapist. One has to be proficient in individual and relationship therapy before specializing in sex therapy.

After earning my MSN in psychiatric nursing, I spent a year interning in sex therapy in one of the few early programs. With the proper preparation, I became certified by the American Association of Sexuality Educators, Counselors, and Therapists. I believe that, as a nurse, I bring a unique perspective to the field with my background in physiology, psychology, and spirituality.

I have always been fascinated by human behavior, thoughts, and feelings—in other words, "what makes people tick." Understanding and empowering people is basic to the practice of psychiatric nursing. Being a part of people's growth is a very satisfying professional experience.

Androgyny

Androgyny, or flexibility in gender roles, reflects the belief that most characteristics and behaviors are human qualities that should not be limited to one specific gender or the other. Being androgynous does not mean being sexually neuter, nor does it imply anything about one's sexual orientation. Rather, it describes the degree of flexibility a person has regarding gender-stereotypic behaviors. Adults who can behave flexibly regarding their sexual roles may be able to adapt better than those who adopt rigid, stereotyped gender roles.

Intersex

About 1 in every 2,000 babies is born with an **intersex** condition, in which there are contradictions among chromosomal gender, gonadal gender, internal organs, and external genital appearance. The gender of such an infant is ambiguous; he or she has some parts usually associated with males and some parts usually associated with females (Melby, 2002).

Transsexuals

The medical profession considers **transsexuals** to have a condition called *gender dysphoria* (strong and persistent feelings of discomfort with one's assigned sex) or **gender identity disorder**. For the transsexual person, sexual anatomy is not consistent with gender identity. Those who are born physically male but are emotionally and psychologically female are called Male to Female or MtFs. Those who are born female but are emotionally and psychologically male are called Female to Male or FtMs. Many consider transsexualism a normal variation and by no means a disorder.

The practical realities of providing health care to this population have been addressed in a number of treatment centers in the United States. Such centers are designated LGBT, that is, they provide services for the lesbian, gay, bisexual, and transgender (LGBT) individual. Access to treatment is available without stigmatization or discrimination.

Most transsexuals report that they have felt gender dysphoria since earliest childhood. They often suffer for many years and try to hide the situation from family and friends for fear of being considered "crazy." Being transgendered puts women and men at extreme risk of being:

- Ridiculed and humiliated
- In constant jeopardy about getting and keeping a job
- Evicted without cause from restaurants and stores
- Denied housing
- Refused medical treatment, even to save a life (Lips, 2004)

As self-understanding and acceptance increase, many transsexuals live part time or full time as members of the other sex. Cross-dressing (dressing in the clothing of the other sex) not only makes their outward appearance consistent with their inner identity and gender role but also increases their comfort with themselves. A number of individuals elect sex reassignment surgery so that their bodies match their gender identity. The vast majority report a high level of satisfaction with their surgery. Their sexual orientation pre- and postoperatively may be heterosexual, homosexual, or bisexual (Lawrence, 2005). The DSM-IV-TR diagnostic criteria for gender identity disorder are on page 525.

Cross-Dressers

Cross-dressers are typically males who cross-dress to express the feminine side of their personality. In most instances cross-dressers are not interested in permanently altering their bodies through surgical means, especially since the majority of them are comfortable with their original birth gender. Most cross-dressers exhibit stereotypic masculine identity and behavior in their public and professional lives.

Cross-dressing is a conscious choice and may occur at home or in public settings. The frequency of the activity ranges from rarely to often. It is not unusual for cross-dressers to adopt a female name to go with the female personality and wardrobe. Cross-dressing occurs more frequently in cultures in which males are expected to be strong, independent, and unemotional protectors. If the social climate is perceived as one with rigid gender roles, some men may need to express gentleness and dependence by creating a separate world and female persona within that social climate (Barnett & Rivers, 2004).

Often, cross-dressers do not tell their spouses about the cross-dressing before the marriage. Some are embarrassed and do not know how to bring up the subject. Others view the need to cross-dress as a problem and hope it will disappear after the marriage. Most wives eventually find out. For some women

DSM-IV-TR Diagnostic Criteria for Gender Identity Disorder

A. A strong and persistent cross-gender identification (not merely a desire for any perceived cultural advantages of being the other sex).

In children, the disturbance is manifested by four (or more) of the following:

1. repeatedly stated desire to be, or insistence that he or she is, the other sex
2. in boys, preference for cross-dressing or simulating female attire; in girls, insistence on wearing only stereotypical masculine clothing
3. strong and persistent preferences for cross-sex roles in make-believe play or persistent fantasies of being the other sex
4. intense desire to participate in the stereotypical games and pastimes of the other sex
5. strong preference for playmates of the other sex

In adolescents and adults, the disturbance is manifested by symptoms such as a stated desire to be the other sex, frequent passing as the other sex, or the convinction that he or she has the typical feelings and reactions of the other sex.

B. Persistent discomfort with his or her sex or sense of inappropriateness in the gender role of that sex.

In children, the disturbance is manifested by any of the following: in boys, assertion that his penis or testes are disgusting or will disappear or assertion that it would be better not to have a penis, or aversion toward rough-and-tumble play and rejection of male stereotypical toys, games, and activities; in girls, rejection of urinating in a sitting position, assertion that she has or will grow a penis, or assertion that she does not want to grow breasts or menstruate, or marked aversion toward normative feminine clothing.

In adolescents and adults, the disturbance is manifested by symptoms such as preoccupation with getting rid of primary and secondary sex characteristics (e.g., request for hormones, surgery, or other procedures to physically alter sexual characteristics to simulate the other sex) or belief that he or she was born the wrong sex.

C. The disturbance is not concurrent with a physical intersex condition.

D. The disturbance causes clinically significant distress or impairment in social, occupational, or other important areas of functioning.

Source: Reprinted with permission from the *Diagnostic and Statistical Manual of Mental Disorders,* Fourth Edition, Text Revision. (Copyright 2000). American Psychiatric Association.

USING DSM-IV-TR

Health care providers often use language unfamiliar to clients and their families. Explain the statement "The disturbance is not concurrent with a physical intersex condition" in such a way that clients and family members can understand.

the discovery raises doubts about their own sexuality and self-worth, and they may decide to terminate the relationship. Some women are not threatened by the cross-dressing but fear it will become public knowledge. Other women move on to full acceptance and understanding of their partner's cross-dressing.

PARAPHILIAS

The DSM-IV-TR classifies **paraphilias** as a group of psychosexual disorders characterized by unconventional sexual behaviors. The person, usually a male, has learned to associate sexual arousal with some environmental stimulus, which triggers the unusual behavior.

Paraphilias have a strong obsessive–compulsive component. Affected individuals are often preoccupied with, and feel compelled to engage in, their particular sexual behaviors. One of the distinguishing characteristics of paraphilias is the person's inability to control or stop the behavior.

Noncoercive Paraphilias

Noncoercive paraphilias are unconventional sexual behaviors engaged in by oneself or with a consenting adult. Many people engage in mild forms of the noncoercive behaviors and consider them simply love play. According to the DSM-IV-TR the behavior becomes pathologic when it is severe, insistent, coercive, and harmful to self or others. There is a movement to remove the category of noncoercive paraphilias from the DSM-IV-TR by those who believe these behaviors are normal activities that have been labeled inaccurately as pathological by conservative health care providers. See the DSM-IV-TR Diagnostic Criteria for Noncoercive Paraphilias on page 526.

Fetishism

Humans respond to a wealth of sexual stimuli. Some people are aroused by the strident beat of rock music, while others are aroused by romantic music. Some people prefer making love in a brightly lit room; others, by candlelight; still others, in the dark. Everyone associates sexual arousal with an individual set of stimuli.

An association or stimulus that is not typical for the culture is called a fetish. A fetish is the sexualization of a body part, such as feet or hair, or an inanimate object, such as shoes, leather, or rubber. In **fetishism**, early associations of a particular object or body part with sexual arousal condition the person to respond sexually to that stimulus. Once the initial association is made, repeated viewing or use (fantasized or actual) of the part or object during sexual activity (usually masturbation) reinforces its arousing nature. For instance, a boy may get an erection after trying on his mother's panties. The erection is pleasurable. The next time the boy masturbates he puts the panties on or fantasizes about them. With repeated experiences, seeing the panties or putting them on becomes a sexual stimulus.

The following clinical example illustrates how a fetish can become an obsessive–compulsive behavior.

DSM-IV-TR Diagnostic Criteria for Noncoercive Paraphilias

Exhibitionism

A. Over a period of at least 6 months, recurrent, intense sexually arousing fantasies, sexual urges, or behaviors involving the exposure of one's genitals to an unsuspecting stranger.

B. The person has acted on these sexual urges, or the sexual urges or fantasies cause marked distress or interpersonal difficulty.

Fetishism

A. Over a period of at least 6 months, recurrent, intense sexually arousing fantasies, sexual urges, or behaviors involving the use of nonliving objects (e.g., female undergarments).

B. The fantasies, sexual urges, or behaviors cause clinically significant distress or impairment in social, occupational, or other important areas of functioning.

C. The fetish objects are not limited to articles of female clothing used in cross-dressing (as in Transvestic Fetishism) or devices designed for the purpose of tactile genital stimulation (e.g., a vibrator).

Transvestic Fetishism

A. Over a period of at least 6 months, in a heterosexual male, recurrent, intense sexually arousing fantasies, sexual urges, or behaviors involving cross-dressing.

B. The fantasies, sexual urges, or behaviors cause clinically significant distress of impairment in social, occupational, or other important areas of functioning.

Source: Reprinted with permission from the *Diagnostic and Statistical Manual of Mental Disorders,* Fourth Edition, Text Revision. (Copyright 2000). American Psychiatric Association.

USING DSM-IV-TR

Health care providers often use language unfamiliar to clients and their families. To help clients and families understand noncoercive paraphilias, reword the DSM statement that exhibitionism may be characterized by the sexual urges or fantasies that cause marked distress or interpersonal difficulty.

CLINICAL EXAMPLE

LaDarius, a 24-year-old college graduate with a major in accounting, was unable to hold a job because of his foot fetish. LaDarius spent a considerable amount of time fantasizing about women's feet—bare feet, pretty feet, long, narrow feet—and how they looked, felt, tasted, and smelled. He fantasized at work, at the grocery store, and at the library (where he even went under tables to look at women's feet). LaDarius's fantasies made it impossible for him to work effectively or to maintain satisfactory interpersonal relationships with others. LaDarius refused therapy, preferring instead to pray that he would "get over it."

As with all people, fetishists' responses are highly individual. Fetishism is not considered a problem as long as it is not harmful and occurs in the context of consenting adult partners.

Transvestic Fetishism

In contrast with cross-dressers, men who become sexually aroused by dressing in women's clothing are considered **transvestic fetishists**. Almost 3% of men report at least one episode of cross-dressing to obtain sexual excitement. They may wear female underclothes or may cross-dress completely. Like other fetishists, they have often undergone conditioning, and female clothing is an intense sexual stimulus. Many report great emotional stress if they try to resist the urge to cross-dress. Like other fetishes, cross-dressing is not considered a problem among consenting adult partners (Langstrom & Zucker, 2005).

Autoerotic Asphyxia

A noncoercive but often fatal sexual behavior is **autoerotic asphyxia**, sometimes referred to as hypoxyphilia. At present it is not categorized as a paraphilia in the DSM-IV-TR, but, like paraphilias, it is a compulsive and unconventional sexual behavior. Called head-rushing or scarfing, this behavior typically begins in adolescence and is primarily a male affliction. The person fashions a tourniquet-like device that constricts the neck, decreasing the blood and oxygen supply to the brain, masturbates, and, at the point of orgasm, releases the bonds to enhance the sensation or sexual high. Emergency Departments may see people who have had an acute event following autoerotic asphyxiation. See the following What Every Emergency Department Nurse Should Know feature.

Tragically, this practice causes many deaths. The vagal nerve complex in the carotid artery is stimulated by pressure around the neck, slowing the heart rate and decreasing oxygen flow to the brain even further. The person becomes un-

WHAT EVERY EMERGENCY DEPARTMENT NURSE SHOULD KNOW

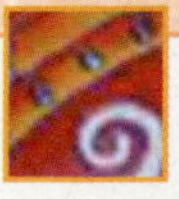

Autoerotic Asphyxia

Some adolescents accidentally kill themselves through autoerotic asphyxia. Professionals may mistake the death for a purposeful hanging suicide. Parents are left confused and guilty because they never saw signs of self-harm. The circumstances of the death, such as nudity and the presence of erotic literature or art, often point to autoerotic asphyxia. Helping the parents understand that this was a tragic accident rather than a suicide helps them cope and grieve the loss of their child.

conscious, slumps forward, and accidentally hangs himself. Many believe the cause of death is suicide, but family and friends cannot understand the reason for the suicide because these young men are not mentally ill or even troubled. Distinguishing features include evidence of sexual activity or a wide range of sexual paraphernalia such as bondage, hoods, and blindfolds.

Coercive Paraphilias

The sexual behaviors known as **coercive paraphilias** are considered criminal acts and are described in the legal code. Coercive paraphiliacs become sexually aroused by including nonconsenting persons in their sexual acts. See the DSM-IV-TR diagnostic criteria for coercive paraphilias below.

Sexual Sadism and Sexual Masochism

Sexual sadism and sexual masochism (S/M) are highly stigmatized in North American culture, and few people admit to being sexually aroused by receiving or inflicting emotional or physical pain. As much as 10% of the population may participate in some form of S/M activity, and all groups—heterosexual, bisexual, homosexual—are represented. Physical behaviors include:

- Intense stimulation (scratching, biting, applying ice)
- Discipline (slapping, spanking, whipping)
- Bondage (holding down, tying down)
- Sensory deprivation (using blindfolds, hoods, ear plugs)

Psychological behaviors include humiliation or degradation, such as verbally berating others or requiring them to perform menial acts. S/M behavior varies in intensity and in its significance in the lives of couples. Some couples engage in the behavior only during sex. Some integrate the roles throughout the relationship, but not at all times. Other couples attempt to live out the dominant/submissive roles continuously.

Thus, S/M may be only a part of foreplay, or it may be a significant component of lifestyle. Most sadomasochists do not engage in S/M behavior unless the partner is willing. Typically, both participants agree to safety "rules," and seldom is the behavior dangerous. Sadomasochists do not see the behavior as a problem and therefore do not wish to change.

A fairly new description, BDSM, has come out of the sexual and gender minority subculture. It combines the behaviors B/D (bondage and discipline), D/S (dominance and submission), and S/M. Thus BDSM refers to any or all of these behaviors. Participants find these activities highly erotic and emotionally charged. Often the activities are subtle and sensual and have little resemblance to pornographic material.

DSM-IV-TR Diagnostic Criteria for Coercive Paraphilias

Pedophilia

A. Over a period of at least 6 months, recurrent, intense sexually arousing fantasies, sexual urges, or behaviors involving sexual activity with a prepubescent child or children (generally age 13 years or younger).

B. The person has acted on these sexual urges, or the sexual urges or fantasies cause marked distress or interpersonal difficulty.

C. The person is at least 16 years and at least 5 years older than the child or children in Criterion A.

Sexual Masochism

A. Over a period of at least 6 months, recurrent intense sexually arousing fantasies, sexual urges, or behaviors involving the act (real, not simulated) of being humiliated, beaten, bound, or otherwise made to suffer.

B. The fantasies, sexual urges, or behaviors cause clinically significant distress or impairment in social, occupational, or other important areas of functioning.

Sexual Sadism

A. Over a period of at least 6 months, recurrent, intense sexually arousing fantasies, sexual urges, or behaviors involving the act (real, not simulated) in which the psychological or physical suffering (including humiliation) of the victim is sexually exciting to the person.

B. The person has acted on these sexual urges with a nonconsenting person, or the sexual urges or fantasies cause marked distress of interpersonal difficulty.

Voyeurism

A. Over a period of at least 6 months, recurrent, intense sexually arousing fantasies, sexual urges, or behaviors involving the act of observing an unsuspecting person who is naked, in the process of disrobing, or engaging in sexual activity.

B. The person has acted on these sexual urges, or the sexual urges or fantasies cause marked distress or interpersonal difficulty.

Frotteurism

A. Over a period of at least 6 months, recurrent, intense sexually arousing fantasies, sexual urges, or behaviors involving touching and rubbing against a nonconsenting person.

B. The person has acted on these sexual urges, or the sexual urges or fantasies cause marked distress or interpersonal difficulty.

Source: Reprinted with permission from the *Diagnostic and Statistical Manual of Mental Disorders,* Fourth Edition, Text Revision. (Copyright 2000). American Psychiatric Association.

USING DSM-IV-TR

Health care providers often use language unfamiliar to clients and their families. To help clients and families understand coercive paraphilias, reword the DSM statement that sexual activity may be characterized by "recurrent, intense sexually arousing fantasies, sexual urges, or behaviors involving the act (real, not simulated) in which the psychological or physical suffering (including humiliation) of the victim is sexually exciting to the person."

Exhibitionism, Voyeurism, and Frotteurism

Exhibitionists and voyeurs, who are almost exclusively men, have powerful urges to display their genitals to strangers (**exhibitionism**) or peep at unsuspecting women involved in intimate behaviors (**voyeurism**). Frotteurs rub up against others, often in a crowded train or elevator, to achieve sexual arousal (**frotteurism**). The frotteur does not attempt to engage in sex with the victim and has no desire to form a relationship. Many describe the urge to peep, expose, or rub themselves against others as something that just "happens" to them and thus have difficulty assuming responsibility for their behavior (King, 2002).

Obscene Phone Calling

A coercive sexual behavior, not categorized as a paraphilia in DSM-IV-TR, is obscene phone calling. Most women and many men have been victims of an obscene phone caller. The caller typically does not know the victim and becomes aroused when the victim reacts with disgust or shock or becomes upset. Some obscene callers breathe heavily, some make sexual noises, and some utter profanities. The caller may tell the victim that he is masturbating or may suggest they get together for sexual activity. Some pretend to have a legitimate reason for talking about sex (posing as researchers conducting a survey, for example) and continue until the victim is offended. The caller is sexually aroused by the combination of proximity (intimate conversation) and anonymity.

Pedophilia

A pedophile is an adult who is sexually aroused by and engages in sexual activity with children. All sexual relationships between adults and children are criminal in North America. The courts consider these acts nonconsensual because minors are presumed to have insufficient knowledge of the consequences of their acts to give meaningful consent. **Pedophilia** activities can include exposure, voyeurism, explicit sex talk, touching, oral sex, intercourse, and anal sex. The child usually knows the pedophile, who may be a family member, neighbor, or friend. For a thorough discussion of the dynamics and consequences of the sexual abuse of children, see Chapters 24 and 26∞.

ALTERED SEXUAL FUNCTION

The ability to engage in sexual behavior is of great importance to most people. Many individuals experience transient problems with their ability to respond to sexual stimulation or to maintain the response. A smaller percentage of people experience problems that are life-long in duration. The problems may be generalized to all sexual interactions and settings, or they may be situational, occurring in a specific setting or with specific types of sexual activity. It is often difficult to sort out the multiple factors contributing to an individual's or couple's sexual problems. Both past factors and situations (lack of sex education, internalizing the belief that sex is dirty) and present (feelings of guilt, anger, or anxiety, fear of failure, spectatoring) contribute to an individual's or couple's sexual problems. For example, spectatoring is the detached appraisal of sexual performance of the body during a sexual act: "Am I going to lose my erection?" "Am I going to have an orgasm this time?" "My stomach is too flabby." "When did his thighs get that fat?" For an overview of past and current factors that may contribute to sexual dysfunction, see Table 20-1 ■.

The DSM-IV-TR classifies problems or difficulties with sexual expression as **sexual dysfunctions**. Male and female prevalence rates for sexual problems are illustrated in Figure 20-1 ■.

Sexual Desire Disorders

Sexual desire disorders are those that include a deficiency or absence of sexual fantasies and a deficiency or absence of desire for sexual behavior, or an aversion to and avoidance of genital sexual contact with a sex partner.

Hypoactive Sexual Desire Disorder

For most people, sexual desire varies from day to day as well as over the years. Some people, however, report a deficiency in or absence of sexual fantasies and persistently low interest or total lack of interest in sexual activity. These clients suffer from **hypoactive sexual desire disorder**. Low desire may be related to relationship problems, other sexual problems, dissatisfaction or boredom with sexual activities, negative messages in childhood, fears, performance anxiety, negative expectations, inaccurate beliefs about sexuality, negative body image, exhaustion, or discordance with sexual orientation.

Table 20-1 ■ Factors Contributing to Sexual Dysfunctions

Type	Past Factors	Current Factors
Physical	■ Trauma: abuse, rape	■ Illness/injuries ■ Organic disorders ■ Medications ■ Substance abuse ■ Failure to engage in effective sexual behavior
Psychological	■ Taught that sex is dirty ■ Childhood sexual abuse	■ Performance anxiety ■ Spectatoring ■ Fear of failure ■ Guilt, anxiety, or anger ■ Negative thoughts
Sociologic	■ Punished as child for normal sex play ■ Lack of sex education	■ Failure to communicate ■ Relationship conflict
Spiritual	■ Taught that sex is sinful ■ Childhood sexual abuse	■ Not feeling connected to partner ■ Lack of intimacy ■ Fear of intimacy

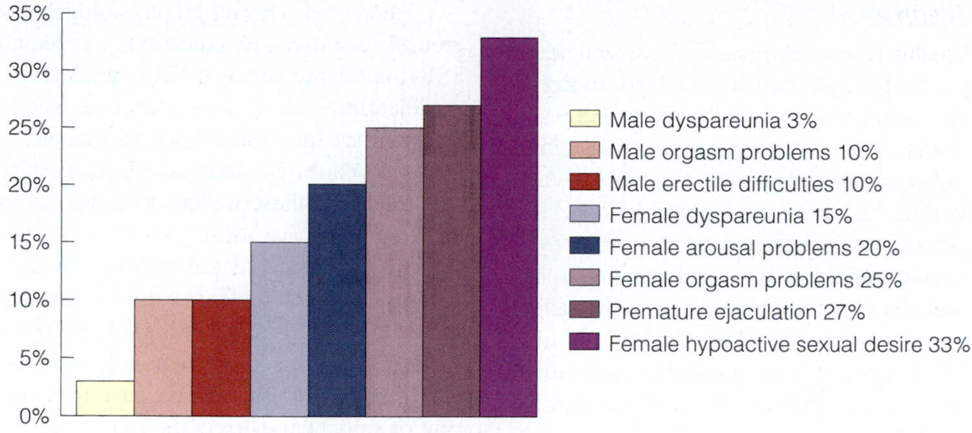

FIGURE 20-1 Male and female prevalence rates of sexual dysfunctions/problems.

The etiology is most often multifactoral, and treatment focuses on all related factors.

If both individuals in a relationship are similarly uninterested in sex, there really is no problem. More typically, there is a disparity of sexual needs, and the person with the greater desire becomes dissatisfied with the sexual relationship and often initiates seeking help. The key issue in the relationship is not frequency but rather neatly fitting together or combining smoothly and efficiently the different partners' needs.

Physiologic factors associated with lack of desire are fatigue, illness, pain, the use of medications, and substance abuse. Maturational factors such as menopause and the effects of surgical procedures that cause menopause can also contribute to decreases in desire. The incidence of hypoactive sexual desire disorder in naturally menopausal women is 9%, and in younger surgically menopausal women the incidence is 26% (Leiblum et al., 2006). The Evidence-Based Practice feature discusses this topic.

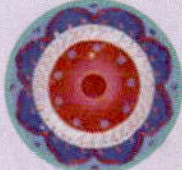

EVIDENCE-BASED PRACTICE

POSTMENOPAUSAL SEXUAL DIFFICULTIES

Peggy is a 57-year-old female who is finding the postmenopausal stage of life a difficult one. Her desire for sexual activity is particularly low, which is affecting her sex life and her relationship with her partner. All physical and psychologic sources for the problem have been ruled out. You work in the gynecology clinic where Peggy is being treated. Peggy asked the nurse practitioner about treatment with testosterone.

Following Peggy's appointment, you and the nurse practitioner discussed testosterone's use in postmenopausal hormone replacement therapy. Available data on its use is conflicting and confusing, but the practice is becoming more widespread. One of the problems with this choice of treatment is that women of Peggy's age group are routinely excluded from research examining effectiveness of treatment; therefore, specific information regarding benefits and risks are lacking.

Currently, there is extensive off-label use by women of a variety of testosterone preparations, including implants, creams, and gels. Some men, especially those with muscle-building as well as sexuality concerns, use testosterone regularly. Because the use of this hormone carries risks, there is reason for some concern.

Further research is needed to determine the role of androgen insufficiency as a cause of low desire in premenopausal as well as postmenopausal women. The role androgens can play in female sexuality will become clearer once practitioners attend to the diurnal variation of testosterone in women and examine these impacts on sexual expression. Research that includes women as participants in testosterone treatment studies and androgen correlation studies, such as the following studies, can shed some light on risk before primary health care providers routinely prescribe testosterone to women experiencing low desire or to postmenopausal women.

El-Hage, G., Eden, J. A., & Manga, R. Z. (2007). A double-blind randomized, placebo-controlled trial of the effect of testosterone cream on the sexual motivation of menopausal hysterectomized women with hypoactive sexual desire disorder. *Climacteric, 10*(4), 335–343.

Turna, B., Apaydin, E., Semerci, B., Altay, B., Cikili, N., & Nazli, O. (2005). Women with low libido: Correlation of decreased androgen levels with female sexual function index. *International Journal of Impotence Research, 17*(2), 148–153.

CRITICAL THINKING APPLICATION

1. If medications are approved for use in specific conditions or illnesses, should off-label use be allowed?
2. Is off-label use an ethical and professionally responsible act?
3. Since menopause is an anticipated maturational transition for women, why not just let the symptoms take their course?
4. If women are not included as research subjects, should study results and recommendations apply to them?

Sexual Aversion Disorder

Sexual aversion disorder is a severe distaste for sexual activity or the thought of sexual activity, which then leads to a phobic avoidance of sex. It occurs in both women and men. Intense emotional dread of an impending sexual interaction also can trigger the physiologic symptoms of anxiety: sweating, increased heart rate, and extreme muscle tension. The client then stops the sexual interaction or prevents it from even beginning. The most common cause of sexual aversion disorder is childhood sexual abuse or adult rape. This severe trauma can lead to a phobic response to sexual activity (McCammon, Knox, & Schacht, 2004). The following clinical example illustrates how sexual trauma can contribute to sexual aversion.

CLINICAL EXAMPLE

Linda and Mike, both 32 years of age, dated all through high school and have been married for 12 years. Linda has a strong aversion to body secretions. She spends hours in the bathtub before she and Mike have sex. Although Mike wears a condom, Linda jumps out of bed before he has finished ejaculating and runs to the bathtub.

Linda can't identify any reasons for her feelings of disgust about body secretions and denies a history of sexual abuse. She does, however, talk about feeling violated by Mike when he "talked me into sex" at age 18. Sometimes she refers to this first sexual experience as date rape.

Despite this problem, Linda and Mike refer to themselves as best friends. Linda has suggested that their marriage be conducted as a platonic relationship. Mike's not sure he wants to live that way the rest of his life. They are in counseling and want to learn how to enjoy one another sexually. Currently, they are learning how to be less genitally focused and to spend more time cuddling, stroking, and touching.

Sexual Arousal Disorders

Sexual arousal refers to the physiologic responses and subjective sense of excitement experienced during sexual activity. Lack of lubrication and failure to attain or maintain an erection are the major disorders of the arousal phase. In **female sexual arousal disorder**, the lack of vaginal lubrication causes discomfort or pain during sexual intercourse. The diagnosis of **male erectile disorder** is usually made when the man has erection problems during 25% or more of his sexual interactions.

Some men cannot attain a full erection, and others lose their erection prior to orgasm. The pejorative term commonly applied to this condition, *impotence*, implies that the man is feeble, inadequate, and incompetent. The accurate term is **erectile dysfunction** (ED), which is objectively descriptive and not judgmental. By the age of 50, slightly more than half of men complain of at least mild ED. Arousal disorder may also be diagnosed even when lubrication and erection are adequate if individuals report a persistent or recurring lack of subjective sexual excitement or pleasure (McCarthy & Fucito, 2005).

There may be other physiological sources for sexual arousal disorders. Medications—especially beta blockers, SSRI antidepressants, SNRI antidepressants, and ADHD medications—can have sexual side effects. In addition, disease processes such as diabetes, hypertension, and cardiovascular disease can cause ED. The side effects of these medications are discussed in Chapters 7 and 32.

Psychological factors may also be a cause of arousal disorders. They include fear of failure, anxiety, anger, poor communication, and relationship conflict. Insufficient vaginal lubrication is less likely than erectile inhibition to create severe distress for couples, because using a water-based lubricant or saliva can correct the immediate problem. An erectile problem may be threatening to a man who feels that his whole sense of masculinity is at stake. Men tend to be dominated by a genital focus more than women are. Therefore, difficulty in getting the penis to "perform" results in humiliation and despair. The following clinical example illustrates how thoughts and expectations can become self-fulfilling prophecies.

CLINICAL EXAMPLE

Paweena and Morufat, both 45 years of age, sought counseling when Morufat found it impossible to achieve an erection. The first time he was unable to achieve an erection was 6 years ago. This was an emotionally traumatic experience for Morufat, who spent a considerable amount of time worrying that it would happen again. Eventually it did, and Morufat found that he could not attain an erection more and more often. About 6 months ago he consulted an urologist. Nighttime penile tumescence studies showed normal functioning.

The couple was referred to a nurse sex therapist, who discovered that Morufat had believed, from an early age, that sexual functioning stopped once the man reached age 49. In working with the couple, the nurse focused on providing sex education and experiential/sensory awareness training. Once it didn't matter whether Morufat achieved an erection, his performance anxiety was decreased and he was able to do so.

Orgasmic Disorders

Orgasmic disorders are those that occur at, or just before, the peaking of sexual pleasure. There are three types of orgasmic disorders: female orgasmic disorder, male orgasmic disorder, and premature ejaculation.

Female Orgasmic Disorder

The pejorative term commonly applied in the past to women who did not experience orgasm, *frigid*, implies that the woman is totally incapable of responding sexually. The more accurate and objective term is **female orgasmic disorder**, which simply means that the sexual response stops before orgasm occurs. Preorgasmic women have never experienced an orgasm; secondarily nonorgasmic women have had orgasms in the past but do not currently experience them; and situationally nonorgasmic women have orgasms in some situations but not in others. Studies indicate that 10% to 15% of women are preorgasmic, and another 20% to 22% report irregular orgasms. Compounding the orgasmic difficulty is the associated anxiety. In the preoccupation with orgasm, the real goal of being sexual—mutual pleasuring and intimacy—is lost, and the interchange becomes one of anxiety, frustration, and anger (Heiman, 2007; McCammon et al., 2004).

Physiologic factors related to inhibited female orgasm include fatigue, illness, neurologic or vascular damage, and medications and drugs that interfere with sexual response. In the physically healthy woman, lack of information or negative attitudes about female sexual response often contribute to orgasmic disorder. Women who were taught that masturbation is wrong or sinful may not have explored their own bodies. If so, they cannot teach a partner where, how, and when to touch.

Male Orgasmic Disorder

Some men suffer from **male orgasmic disorder**. Men with this disorder can maintain an erection for long periods (an hour or more) but have extreme difficulty ejaculating, referred to as *retarded ejaculation*. In heterosexual intercourse, the difficulty may be limited to ejaculation in the vagina. Some men ejaculate after self-stimulation or manual or oral stimulation by the partner, whereas others have great difficulty ejaculating with any type of stimulation. This disorder is much less common than rapid ejaculation.

Organic causes inhibiting orgasm include spinal cord injuries, multiple sclerosis, Parkinson's disease, and use of certain medications. Psychogenic factors include fear of pregnancy, performance pressure, fear of losing control, and anxiety and guilt about engaging in sexual activity. As with other dysfunctions, the difficulty can adversely affect the sexual relationship.

Premature Ejaculation

Rapid ejaculation, or **premature ejaculation**, is one of the most common sexual problems among men. There are many definitions, ranging from ejaculating before being touched, ejaculating before penetration, ejaculating with one internal thrust, to ejaculating within a minute or two of penetration. A more helpful description is the absence of voluntary control of ejaculation. The problem is best self-defined: A man is concerned about his ejaculatory control, or the couple agrees that ejaculation is too rapid for mutual satisfaction.

There is very little information about the mechanisms causing rapid ejaculation. Possible influences include the man's:

- Inability to perceive his arousal level accurately
- Lowered sensory threshold due to infrequent sexual activity
- Early conditioning resulting from hurried masturbation or hurried sexual intercourse

Educating about sexual dysfunction can be enhanced with the information in the Partnering with Clients and Families feature below.

Sexual Pain Disorder

A **sexual pain disorder** is genital pain that occurs during sexual intercourse. The two types of sexual pain disorders are dyspareunia and vaginismus.

Dyspareunia

Both women and men can experience **dyspareunia**, pain during or immediately after intercourse. It is associated with many physiologic causes, especially those that inhibit lubrication. Thus, skin irritations, vaginal infections, estrogen deficiencies, and medications that dry vaginal secretions can cause women to experience discomfort with intercourse.

Pelvic disorders, such as infections, small lesions, endometriosis, scar tissue, or tumors, can result in painful intercourse. Engaging in painful intercourse can lead to vaginismus because the body reflexively becomes guarded and tense. Similarly, in males, infection or inflammation of the glans penis or other genitourinary organs can cause pain with coitus (sexual intercourse). Also, some contraceptive foams, creams, or sponges can irritate either the vagina or the penis, causing pain. For both women and men, fear and anxiety in anticipation of pain can undermine the ability to feel pleasurable sexual responses and may lead to an avoidance of sexual activity.

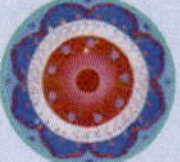

PARTNERING WITH CLIENTS AND FAMILIES

TEACHING ABOUT SEXUAL DESIRE

- Sexual desire varies from day to day as well as over the years.
- Physical factors include low testosterone levels, chronic diseases, and side effects of medications and medical treatments.
- Intrapersonal factors include sexual guilt and anxiety, lack of knowledge, a negative self-concept, and a negative body image.
- Interpersonal factors include conflict, negative communication, fatigue, lack of time, and dislike or fear of the partner.
- Encourage open communication about the situation and each person's feelings about what is or is not happening in their sexual relationship.
- Refer for sex therapy if the issue is not resolved through communication.

Vaginismus

An involuntary spasm of the outer one-third of the vaginal muscles, making penetration of the vagina painful and sometimes impossible, is called **vaginismus**. The woman often experiences desire, excitement, and orgasm with stimulation of the external sexual structures. Attempts at intercourse, however, elicit the involuntary spasm. She may have similar difficulty undergoing pelvic exams and inserting tampons or a diaphragm.

Vulvodynia is constant, unremitting burning that is localized to the vulva with an acute onset. The girl or woman has problems sitting, standing, and sleeping related to the intensity of pain. In contrast, *vestibulitis* causes severe pain only on touch or attempted vaginal entry. Half of women with vestibulitis report lifelong dyspareunia. Women with either of these disorders report a negative impact on their sexual functioning and partner relationship, as well as on their self-esteem and mental health (Metzger, 2005). The DSM-IV-TR diagnostic criteria for sexual dysfunctions are listed in the feature on page 533.

The vaginismic response may develop initially as a protection against real or anticipated pain. It is often associated with sexual trauma, such as childhood sexual abuse or adult rape. Emotional conflicts, such as extreme fear of pregnancy or intense guilt about engaging in sexual activity, may be additional contributing factors.

The partner of a woman with vaginismus often becomes fearful and anxious about hurting her, or may become resentful, believing that she has spasms on purpose. Partners may develop secondary dysfunctions as a result of these negative feelings and interpretations of rejection.

Problems with Satisfaction

Some people experience sexual desire, arousal, and orgasm and yet feel dissatisfied with their sexual relationships. These sexual problems are more commonly related to the emotional tone of the relationship than to the physiologic response. Since giving and receiving pleasure in a mutually intimate relationship are the primary goals of sex for most people, *dissatisfaction problems* may be more disturbing than other types of sexual dysfunctions.

At times, satisfaction problems may be situational. For example, one partner may choose an inconvenient time, or a partner may feel anxious and therefore cannot experience much pleasure or joy. Some people describe their problems as related to lack of extragenital satisfaction. These people describe how much they miss and continue to need all the touching and caressing of their earlier lovemaking experiences. Unfortunately, people who have been relating sexually for a long time often become genitally focused and neglect the rest of the body. One or both partners may feel touch starved, long for more total body touching, and become dissatisfied with sex.

Satisfaction problems are often related to relationship difficulties. The inability to communicate effectively in other relationship areas frequently results in sexual frustration. Partners who are angry at each other and make love without resolving the conflict may feel unhappy about the relationship despite having experienced arousal and orgasm. Couples who define their relationship in terms of rigid, unequal power and gender roles may have difficulty negotiating and compromising about sexual issues. Not infrequently, the person with the least amount of power feels helpless and dissatisfied with the sexual interchanges.

Lack of intimacy or a feeling of connectedness is understandably related to satisfaction problems. If one has sex with a stranger, the body may function well, but there is often a sense of something missing after the sexual experience. Making love to one person while feeling more attracted to or in love with another person can result in feelings of emptiness or disconnection. Even couples in a committed relationship may complain of lack of intimacy. Dissatisfaction issues include lack of romance, love, tenderness, and nurturance. Fulfillment of sexuality, then, depends on the ability to relate to a partner in an intimate and mutually pleasing manner that is compatible with values and chosen lifestyle.

Increased Sexual Interest

An increased interest in sex and sexual activity is symptomatic of the manic phase of bipolar disorder. Elevated mood is accompanied by a corresponding rise in sexual activity, variety of activity, and, often, number of partners. This behavior occurs despite contrary values, is out of the client's control, and puts the client at risk for HIV (see Chapter 25) and other sexually transmitted diseases. The end of the manic episode signals a return to the person's usual level of sexual interest and activity. Since memory is not impaired, the person may feel embarrassed and ashamed about uncontrolled sexual behavior during the manic episode.

Some adult survivors of childhood sexual abuse may go through periods of high sexual activity. This is often a desperate attempt to obtain the nurturance, love, care, and power they were denied in childhood. Having been sexualized at an inappropriately early age, some have learned to survive in a hostile environment by using their sexual availability to make contact with or control others. More information on the impacts of childhood sexual abuse is discussed in Chapter 24.

Sexual Addiction

Frequency of sexual activity can be viewed on a continuum, with most people falling in the middle range. Some people have sex frequently in a way that enhances their lives; others have sex infrequently and report contentment and satisfaction. A sexual pattern that falls at either extreme of the continuum, however, can signal problems. At the low extreme are individuals who have great difficulty in choosing to be sexual; such people may have a sexual dysfunction. At the high extreme are people who have lost their ability to choose or control their sexual behavior; these people are sexual addicts.

Sexual addiction is a disorder in which the central focus of life is sex. People with this addiction spend 50% or more of all waking hours dealing with sex, from fantasy to

DSM-IV-TR Diagnostic Criteria for Sexual Dysfunctions

Sexual Desire Disorders

Hypoactive Sexual Desire Disorder

A. Persistently or recurrently deficient (or absent) sexual fantasies and desire for sexual activity. The judgment of deficiency or absence is made by the clinician, taking into account factors that affect sexual functioning, such as age and the context of the person's life.

B. The disturbance causes marked distress or interpersonal difficulty.

C. The sexual dysfunction is not better accounted for by another Axis I disorder (except another Sexual Dysfunction) and is not due exclusively to the direct physiological effects of a substance (e.g., a drug of abuse, a medication) or a general medical condition.

Sexual Aversion Disorder

A. Persistent or recurrent extreme aversion to, and avoidance of, all (or almost all) genital sexual contact with a sexual partner.

B. The disturbance causes marked distress or interpersonal difficulty.

C. The sexual dysfunction is not better accounted for by another Axis I disorder (except another Sexual Dysfunction).

Sexual Arousal Disorders

Female Sexual Arousal Disorder

A. Persistent or recurrent inability to attain, or to maintain until completion of the sexual activity, an adequate lubrication-swelling response of sexual excitement.

B. The disturbance causes marked distress or interpersonal difficulty.

C. The sexual dysfunction is not better accounted for by another Axis I disorder (except another Sexual Dysfunction) and is not due exclusively to the direct physiological effects of a substance (e.g., a drug of abuse, a medication) or a general medical condition.

Male Erectile Disorder

A. Persistent or recurrent inability to attain, or to maintain until completion of the sexual activity, an adequate erection.

B. The disturbance causes marked distress or interpersonal difficulty.

C. The erectile dysfunction is not better accounted for by another Axis I disorder (other than a Sexual Dysfunction) and is not due exclusively to the direct physiological effects of a substance (e.g., a drug of abuse, a medication) or a general medical condition.

Orgasmic Disorders

Female Orgasmic Disorder

A. Persistent or recurrent delay in, or absence of, orgasm following a normal sexual excitement phase. Women exhibit wide variability in the type or intensity of stimulation that triggers orgasm. The diagnosis of Female Orgasmic Disorder should be based on the clinician's judgment that the woman's orgasmic capacity is less than would be reasonable for her age, sexual experience, and the adequacy of sexual stimulation she receives.

B. The disturbance causes marked distress or interpersonal difficulty.

C. The orgasmic dysfunction is not better accounted for by another Axis I disorder (except another Sexual Dysfunction) and is not due exclusively to the direct physiological effects of a substance (e.g., a drug of abuse, a medication) or a general medical condition.

Male Orgasmic Disorder

A. Persistent or recurrent delay in, or absence of, orgasm following a normal sexual excitement phase during sexual activity that the clinician, taking into account the person's age, judges to be adequate in focus, intensity, and duration.

B. The disturbance causes marked distress or interpersonal difficulty.

C. The orgasmic dysfunction is not better accounted for by another Axis I disorder (except another Sexual Dysfunction) and is not due exclusively to the direct physiological effects of a substance (e.g., a drug of abuse, a medication) or a general medical condition.

Premature Ejaculation

A. Persistent or recurrent ejaculation with minimal sexual stimulation before, on, or shortly after penetration and before the person wishes it. The clinician must take into account factors that affect duration of the excitement phase, such as age, novelty of the sexual partner or situation, and recent frequency of sexual activity.

B. The disturbance causes marked distress or interpersonal difficulty.

C. The premature ejaculation is not due exclusively to the direct effects of a substance (e.g., withdrawal from opioids).

Sexual Pain Disorders

Dyspareunia

A. Recurrent or persistent genital pain associated with sexual intercourse in either a male or a female.

B. The disturbance causes marked distress or interpersonal difficulty.

C. The disturbance is not caused exclusively by Vaginismus or lack of lubrication, is not better accounted for by another Axis I disorder (except another Sexual Dysfunction), and is not due exclusively to the direct physiological effects of a substance (e.g., a drug of abuse, a medication) or a general medical condition.

Vaginismus

A. Recurrent or persistent involuntary spasm of the musculature of the outer third of the vagina that interferes with sexual intercourse.

B. The disturbance causes marked distress or interpersonal difficulty.

C. The disturbance is not better accounted for by another Axis I disorder (e.g., Somatization Disorder) and is not due exclusively to the direct physiological effects of a general medical condition.

USING DSM-IV-TR

Health care providers often use language unfamiliar to clients and their families. Explain *erectile dysfunction* in such a way that clients and family members can understand this sexual dysfunction.

acting-out behavior. Acting-out behaviors are often victimless (the partner is consenting), such as having affairs; overindulging in masturbation, fetishism, pornography use, or commercial telephone sex; or visiting prostitutes. Victimizing behaviors (those with a nonconsenting partner) are less frequent. The incidence of sexual addiction is difficult to determine because of secrecy and shame, but it is estimated that 3% to 6% of the population may be affected. It is predominantly a male disorder, with a gender ratio of 3:1 (Carnes & Wilson, 2002).

It is unethical to label people who do not conform to conventional moral codes as sexual addicts. Sexual addiction is not simply the frequent enjoyment of sexual behaviors. Many people engage in those behaviors without becoming sexual addicts. Rather, sexual addiction is a progressive disorder in which sex is used to numb pain. The payoff is the same as in any other addiction: an intensely pleasurable high, a short-lived release from pain, and an escape from the problems of daily life. The consequences are also the same in that the addict's life eventually becomes unmanageable. The components of sexual addiction are discussed in Box 20-1.

Sexual Problems in Gay Men and Lesbians

Gay men and lesbians may have the same sexual dysfunctions that occur in the heterosexual population. Living in a homophobic culture with fairly strict gender role expectations can cause additional pressures.

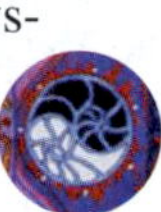

Box 20-1 Components of Sexual Addiction

The components of sexual addiction have the hallmarks of obsessive–compulsive behavior.

1. *Preoccupation.* The person spends hours thinking or obsessing about sex. Preoccupation, in itself, gives a sexual high and is so time consuming that the person cannot fulfill work, school, or family responsibilities.
2. *Ritualization.* The individual engages in specific behaviors done just the "right" way and in the same sequence each time. Ritual behaviors include wearing certain clothing, taking certain steps to get ready, driving certain routes, or looking for partners only in a certain area. The ritual seems to control anxiety; once addicts begin a ritual, they cannot stop until the cycle is completed.
3. *Compulsivity.* The person cannot control sexual behavior, and this behavior becomes the most important aspect of life. Some demonstrate sexually compulsive behavior in a regular pattern; others resist for a time and then have a binge cycle.
4. *Shame and despair.* At the end of the cycle, the person experiences guilt and shame at the loss of control. The pain of despair creates the need to begin the cycle all over again, because the addict seeks to relieve pain by getting high. Like other addicts, these individuals want to stop their behavior, promise to stop, try to stop, and are unable to stop without treatment.

Men, whether gay or straight, may accept stereotyped male gender roles that can lead to ambivalence about intimacy and dependence. Because social norms require that men be unemotional, competitive, and in control, two men in an intimate relationship may experience conflict if both try to be "macho men." The success of the relationship often depends on the partners' ability to negotiate and compromise on issues of power, control, dependence, tenderness, and nurturance. It is not uncommon for gay men to interpret sexual problems in a relationship as a sign that the relationship is over, as opposed to seeing the dysfunction as a problem to be solved.

The most common sexual problem for lesbians, as for heterosexual women, is a lack of interest in sex. There are several differences between lesbian couples and heterosexual couples experiencing low sexual desire. Unlike heterosexual couples, lesbian couples do not typically withdraw from sex because of a lack of intimacy, a power imbalance, or rigid gender roles in the relationship. A lesbian couple is more likely to report that the nonsexual areas of their relationship are pleasing and agreeable and that there is minimal conflict about sex.

It is highly unlikely for lesbian couples to have difficulty with arousal, orgasm, or satisfaction. The explanation for this may be that lesbian couples spend more time making love and include more varied activities than do heterosexual couples (Nichols & Shernoff, 2007).

BIOPSYCHOSOCIAL THEORIES

Human sexual behavior has been studied from various theoretic perspectives. The most significant are biologic, intrapersonal, behavioral, interpersonal, and sociocultural theories.

A review of the various theoretic perspectives shows that human sexuality has been historically characterized by judgments and controversy that have inhibited sexual health care services. It is important for health care professionals to remember that all people to some extent deviate from some physical, social, behavioral, or emotional norm. Some are left-handed, some stutter, some are disabled, some are loners, and some are filled with fears. To achieve the highest level of professional practice, nurses must look beyond the characteristics and respond to the whole person.

Only in the past 40 years has human sexuality been scientifically studied from a multidisciplinary approach. With this knowledge came the beginnings of planned interventions for individuals suffering from a variety of sexual problems and disorders. Nursing has been an active participant in the evolution of treatment approaches and programs to provide sexual health care. The current state of nursing involvement—the nursing diagnoses and therapeutic interventions discussed throughout this chapter—indicates nursing's continued dedication to furthering this area of study.

Biologic Theory

Those individuals who take a biologic approach are concerned with the physiologic aspects of gender identity and sexual behavior. Some believe there is a neurologic basis for gender differences and look to fetal exposure to sex hormones and adult levels of sex hormones as an explanation of gender dysphoria. They explore sexual dysfunctions to discover factors (e.g., organic disease, injury, medications, pain, and/or depression) that interfere with the physiologic reflexes during the sexual response cycle.

It is clear from research over the past several years that the majority of sexual problems are initially physiologic in nature. In middle age, for example, normal physiologic changes (such as decreased hormone production) may interfere with sexual pleasure and interest. Side effects of many medications or medical treatment may contribute to sexual problems. Arteriosclerosis, diabetes, and other medical problems can interfere with the ability to have an erection. Not understanding the physical basis of the problem, people experience anxiety, shame, or guilt, and the stage is set for the emotional component—distress—related to sexual problems.

At this time there is no clear understanding of the etiology of transsexualism. Biologic theory is based on animal studies because experimental research cannot be conducted with humans. When exposed prenatally to increased male hormones, experimental animals exhibit increased male behavior. Decreasing the levels of male hormones prenatally increases female behavior in animals. In humans, the male gonads develop and begin secreting androgen during weeks 8 to 12 of gestation. Differentiation of the hypothalamus to a male pattern, which occurs in months 4 to 5 of gestation, requires high androgen levels. Thus, one explanation of transsexualism is that prenatal androgen levels were sufficient for the development of male anatomy but insufficient for differentiation in the brain. In transsexuals who are anatomically female, the androgenic influences may have been high at the critical time of hypothalamic development, although not at the time of genital formation (Lips, 2004).

Intrapersonal Theory

Intrapersonal theorists view gender dysphoria, paraphilias, and sexual dysfunctions as problems occurring within the individual. Some view them as expressions of arrested psychosexual development, some seek an explanation in sexual guilt, some see the issue as being one of self-punishment, and others see these as normal variations. People who grew up with rigid family and religious taboos about sex often experience guilt and anxiety about their adult sexual roles and behaviors. Inadequate sex education can lead to ignorance and anxiety about sexuality. Performance anxiety, negative self-concept, and negative body image are all seen as contributing to sexual problems. Problems to be solved during the treatment process include fears of:

- Intimacy
- Losing control
- Pain
- Pregnancy
- Sexually transmitted infections

Clients who have difficulties communicating about sexual issues need guidance. You can help clients communicate about sex more clearly and effectively by incorporating the suggestions in the Your Intervention Strategies feature on page 543.

Behavioral Theory

Behaviorists believe that gender dysphoria arises from social learning; that is, that the child was rewarded in some way for adopting behaviors of the other sex. They believe paraphilias are learned responses; the person is conditioned to respond erotically to nonsexual objects or particular sexual acts. In the area of sexual dysfunctions, contributing factors include poor communication skills, lack of sexual experience with oneself or a partner, concern with sexual performance, and ineffective stimulation. The dysfunctions, too, are seen as learned responses.

Interpersonal Factors

Relationship difficulties may cause sexual problems. Negative patterns of communication or dislike or fear of one's partner inhibit sexual expression. Conflict over commonplace issues such as money, schedules, or relatives may lead to a loss of sexual interest. An inability to talk about preferences in initiating sex or determining sexual activities creates problems for some people. Fatigue and lack of time due to family and work obligations are other common causes. Likewise, sexual problems can contribute to relationship difficulties, especially when couples do not openly communicate about the situation. Misunderstanding leads to inappropriate guilt or anger and withdrawal from the relationship. Working with clients who have sexual difficulties requires sensitivity and knowledge about how to communicate effectively. See the Nursing Care Plan at the end of this chapter for a full review of a plan of care for a client with sexual difficulties.

Sociocultural Factors

Ideas about sexuality and sexual behavior are based on cultural values and understanding. What is considered normal or abnormal depends on each group's specific viewpoint. The same behavior may be seen as positive in one culture and pathologic in another. Each culture tends to incorporate ethnocentrism in its beliefs; that is, its members believe their particular sexual values and behaviors are superior and preferable to those of any other culture. Ethnocentrism encourages people to view the sexual behavior of other people as eccentric, exotic, and bizarre. See the Your Assessment Approach feature on page 537 for an example of eliciting a sexuality history that includes cultural factors.

Consider the diversity of sexual values throughout the world. The Mangaia of Polynesia believe that young adolescents of both genders have high sexual drives. However, as they leave young adulthood, they expect their desire to rapidly decline. In contrast, the Dani of New Guinea believe that neither women nor men have high sexual drives and that the primary purpose of sex is reproduction. Following the birth of a child, the husband and wife remain celibate for the next 5 years. Among the Sambrans of New Guinea, young boys around age 7 or 8 have sex with older boys. It is believed that the ingestion of semen is required for physical growth. This pattern of behavior changes to heterosexual interaction as the young men become adults.

Cultures in some parts of Africa and the Middle East practice ritual mutilation of the clitoris, called *female genital mutilation*, as a rite of initiation into womanhood. Because of serious medical complications and psychological trauma, the practice has been outlawed in many countries, although the laws are rarely enforced. Among many cultures throughout the world, there is a third gender. Among the Zuni of New Mexico, this person is called a *berdache*, a male who assumes female dress, gender role, and status. Individuals with this third gender are often considered to have great spiritual power (King, 2002).

The sexual ethics of a culture reflect the culture's assumptions about the purpose of sex. In North American culture, sexual practices have been strongly influenced by the Judeo-Christian tradition, which historically considered procreation to be the primary purpose of sex. As a result, even modern North American culture is fairly sexually intolerant and harshly critical of those whose gender identity or sexual behavior is not in the mainstream. People with little tolerance for cross-gender behavior view transsexuals and cross-dressers as deviants. The sexual acts of noncoercive paraphiliacs conflict with the traditional value of sex for procreation, and they, too, are made to feel like outcasts.

How people communicate about sexuality is culturally determined. In general, North American culture reflects Euro-American values, which include a negative view of public sexual communication, as evidenced by censorship and the attitude that sex is a taboo topic for general discussion. However, there are ethnic differences in communication patterns. African-Americans tend to be very expressive and communicate directly about sexual topics. Latinos from the Caribbean and Central American cultures tend to be restrained in expressing their feelings, while those from Argentina and some other Latin American countries are emotionally expressive. Asian-Americans are often less verbally expressive, so nonverbal communication assumes even more importance. The gay and lesbian subculture has developed private words and expressions in reaction to the homophobia of the dominant culture (Hecht, Collier, & Ribeau, 2002; King, 2002; Ting-Toomey & Chung, 2002).

Sociocultural theories regarding sexual dysfunctions focus on disturbed relationships between partners, negative early learning, and past or present traumatic events. Women who have had sexual problems related to abuse and pregnancy are seen in a variety of settings. See the What Every Obstetric Nurse Should Know feature for a perspective on working with survivors of sexual trauma.

MULTIDISCIPLINARY INTERVENTIONS

Vulvodynia and vestibulitis are systemic problems that take some time and a lot of effort to overcome. A low-glycemic diet—no sugar or white foods—is most helpful. It is also important to test for food allergies, as these seem to contribute to the inflammation. When the pain and inflammation are reduced, pelvic floor therapy by specially trained physical therapists is begun. Hands-on techniques include massage therapy and myofascia and pudendal nerve release. Vaginal dilators may be introduced for home use. An individual exercise program is designed to strengthen weak muscles and stretch tight muscles. Pelvic floor biofeedback measures the tension of the pelvic floor muscles and helps clients learn to relax and strengthen them. Other techniques include pelvic floor electrical stimulation and perineal ultrasound.

Clients who have a true sexual addiction are usually referred to a 12-step-based recovery program. As with other 12-step programs, the initial standard is 90 meetings in 90 days. These programs are generally available in urban settings and have no associated financial cost. There is usually a sense of a "healing community" that includes others with similar hypersexual problems.

Oral medications have been the biggest breakthrough for ED. These medications work by relaxing smooth muscles in the penis, thus allowing arteries to expand and increase blood flow into the penis, causing an erection. These medications are sildenafil (Viagra), vardenafil (Levitra), and tadalafil (Cialis). Although research has been conducted using these medications for female sexual problems, the results have been inconclusive.

Selective serotonin reuptake inhibitors (SSRIs) may be given for rapid ejaculation, as a common side effect is a slowdown in orgasmic response. The doses are usually lower than those given for depression.

WHAT EVERY OBSTETRIC NURSE SHOULD KNOW

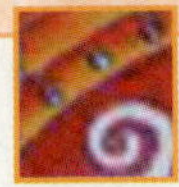

Survivors of Sexual Trauma

Women who are survivors of sexual trauma may experience difficulty during labor and delivery. There is little sense of privacy during this time, as a variety of people check the progress of labor and are present for the delivery. This may trigger flashbacks to the abusive situation. Some survivors may feel they have little or no control over what is happening to their bodies, similar to what they felt when they were victimized. It is important for the staff to know when they are working with survivors so they can anticipate what might occur and intervene in a timely fashion.

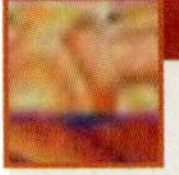

NURSING PROCESS
Clients with Sexual Problems

The specialized nursing care of clients with gender identity and sexual disorders requires extensive background and experience. While nurses at all levels of practice should aim to develop a trusting relationship and assess clients for sexual concerns, they should refer clients to a health care provider with special expertise in dealing with these complex issues. The actual diagnoses and interventions of these clients are best left to the providers with special expertise.

Assessment

Information about a client's sexual health status should always be an integral part of a nursing assessment. The amount and kind of data collected depend on the context of the assessment, that is, the client's reason for seeking health care and how the client's sexuality interacts with other problems.

Including a sexual history as part of the general nursing history is important for some clients and not important for others. It is critical, however, at least to introduce the topic of sexuality to give permission for clients to bring up any concerns or problems.

Subjective Data

The sexual history provides subjective assessment data needed to formulate nursing diagnoses. Elicit sexual information in the same way you elicit a general nursing history. Pay special attention, however, to planning a setting in which privacy and uninterrupted time are available. Such a setting helps clients feel comfortable discussing these private aspects of their lives. It is helpful to begin the interview by explaining why you are asking about sexuality; for example: "Sexuality is a part of people's lives. People often have questions about sexual activity when they have changes in their health. I'd like to take this time to talk with you about your sex life."

Move from general to specific questions. This gradual focus on specific sexual behavior promotes trust and rapport. Initially, questions can relate sexuality to health status. Open-ended questions encourage clients to expand on their sexual experiences and concerns. Reassure clients that it is normal to have sexual concerns and questions, for instance: "It is common for many people to feel concerned about ________. Do you have any questions?" Restate clients' responses to encourage them to expand on their feelings.

All nursing histories should at least include a question such as, "Have there been any changes in your sexual functioning that might be related to your illness or the medications you take?" Nurses might also facilitate communication by saying, "As a nurse, I'm concerned about all aspects of your health. People often have questions about sexual matters, both when they are well and when they are ill. When I take your history, sexual concerns are included to help plan a comprehensive treatment approach." Suggestions for eliciting a sexual history are in the Your Assessment Approach feature.

If clients do identify a sexual problem or if they take medications that affect sexual desire or sexual behavior, you can use the information in Table 20-2 ■ on page 538 to formulate additional questions.

Objective Data

Objective data include observed nonverbal behaviors, laboratory data, test results, medical diagnoses, physical examination results, and other documented sources, such as the chart. Objective data may also include results of physiologic assessment of sexual function.

Erectile Capacity The nocturnal penile tumescence (NPT) procedure provides a direct measure of erectile capacity. The device measures penile engorgement that occurs during sleep. NPT measurement is considered the best available method to determine if a man's erectile difficulties are physiologic. If so, there is minimal penile engorgement during sleep. Men whose erection difficulties appear to be psychological in origin have normal engorgement during sleep.

Female Sexual Function Physiologic assessment of female sexual function is accomplished by the use of vaginal plethysmographs or probes. These devices are inserted into the vagina and measure vasocongestion of the vaginal wall tissue.

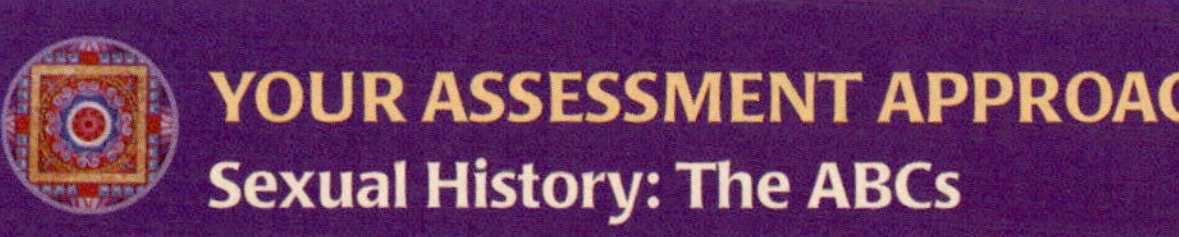

YOUR ASSESSMENT APPROACH
Sexual History: The ABCs

Affective Assessment

- With whom do you feel most intimate and connected?
- Describe the type of love and affection in this relationship.
- In what way do you experience anxiety about sex?
- In what way do you experience guilt about sex?
- How depressed do you feel?
- In what way does anger interfere with your sexual functioning?
- Do you dislike or feel an aversion toward any parts of your body?

Behavioral Assessment

- Describe your level of satisfaction with the frequency of your sexual activity.
- Describe the positive aspects of your own sexual functioning.
- Describe the negative aspects of your own sexual functioning.
- What concerns do you have about your future sexual functioning?
- What are your partner's concerns about current or future sexual functioning?

Cognitive Assessment

- When you were growing up, how did you learn about sex?
- How has your religion influenced your sexual values and behaviors?
- What "shoulds/should nots," "musts/must nots" do you believe about your sexual behavior/relationships?
- How rigidly were gender roles enforced in your family of origin?
- How are gender roles enacted in your present relationship/family?
- Describe the negative thoughts you have about sex.
- Does the use of fantasy increase or decrease your sexual desire?

Sensation Assessment

- Describe any physical discomfort you feel during sexual activity.
- To what degree do you experience pleasure during sexual activity?

TABLE 20-2 ■ **Drugs/Medications and Related Sexual Side Effects**

	Sexual Side Effects						
Drug/Medication	**Increased Sex Drive**	**Decreased Sex Drive**	**Decreased Arousal**	**Retrograde Ejaculation**	**Inhibited Ejaculation**	**Painful Ejaculation**	**Orgasm Problems**
Alcohol	small amts	large amts	yes		yes		
Amphetamines	yes		possible		yes		yes
Antihypertensives		yes	yes		yes		
Antipsychotics (atypical)		yes	yes		yes		yes
Antipsychotics (conventional)		yes	yes	possible	possible		yes
Anxiolytics (very few side effects)							
Beta blockers		yes	yes				
Cocaine	yes				yes		yes
Diuretics		yes	yes				
Hallucinogens (unpredictable side effects)		possible	possible				possible
Heroin		yes	yes		yes		yes
Lithium		yes	yes				
MAO inhibitors		may	may				possible
Marijuana	small amts	large amts	chronic use				
Mood stabilizers		yes	yes				yes
SSRIs			yes				yes
Steroids		yes	yes				
Tricyclic antidepressants		yes	yes		yes	possible	yes

Laboratory Tests Several sophisticated and expensive laboratory tests are designed to assess sexual function. For instance, testosterone (androgen) and estrogen blood levels may be measured. However, laboratory data must be interpreted with caution because test results are not always reliable indicators of actual sexual behavior. Thus, clients' self-reports of sexual performance, feelings, and values (the subjective data) are of primary importance in assessment.

Androgen levels in women peak in early adulthood and decrease slowly with aging. Women in their 40s have approximately one-half the level of women in their 20s. Testosterone has been linked to sexual desire and sexual frequency in menopausal women. At present, it appears that testosterone therapy improves sexual function in women with low levels.

Health factors can interfere with people's expression of sexuality. Physical changes brought on by illness, injury, or surgery may inhibit full sexual expression. Many prescription medications have side effects that affect sexual functioning. The impact is generally negative, but sometimes there is a positive impact. For example, antidepressants may slow ejaculation. This may be a problem for the man who finds himself suddenly feeling unable to ejaculate. If a man is suffering from rapid ejaculation, however, the antidepressant may "cure" this problem. The two antidepressants with the fewest sexual side effects are bupropion (Wellbutrin) and escitalopram (Lexapro). Some street drugs such as marijuana, amphetamine, and cocaine increase sexual drive and activity. Others, such as opioids and anabolic steroids, interfere with sexual functioning.

The following clinical example illustrates how a negative experience with a psychiatric medication can influence the treatment plan.

CLINICAL EXAMPLE

Jared is seeing an advanced practice psychiatric nurse for clinical depression. After several weeks with no improvement, the nurse suggested he consider taking an antidepressant to lift his mood and facilitate the psychotherapy. Jared refused outright, saying, "I took Prozac a couple of years ago and it caused me to lose my orgasms. I'm never taking that stuff again. I would rather be depressed than give up my sex life."

Nursing Diagnosis: NANDA

A number of nursing diagnoses are applicable for clients experiencing gender identity disorders and sexual problems. They are discussed in this section. See Box 20-2 for examples of how you can apply NANDA diagnoses to specific problems.

Anxiety and Fear

Anxiety and fear inhibit the physiologic sexual response as well as the ability to experience pleasure and joy. People who grow up learning that sex is dirty and sinful often experience anxiety in an adult relationship or are so fearful that they develop a phobic avoidance of sex. Adults who have been emotionally, physically, or sexually abused as children often fear intimacy and find they cannot have a trusting relationship with another person. Even individuals with a positive sexual history may at some time feel anxious about their sexual performance and develop a secondary fear of failure as a sex partner.

Spiritual Distress

Lack of fulfillment in a sexual relationship may be related to a temporary feeling of distance from one's partner or an ongoing lack of intimacy in the relationship. Factors relating to lack of intimacy are relationship conflict, multiple fears, adult sexual abuse, or childhood sexual abuse.

Box 20-2 Nursing Diagnoses

Remember to be specific when formulating nursing diagnoses. The list below includes examples relevant to clients with specific problems of sexuality and sexual expression.

- Risk for Self-Directed Violence related to accidental injury or death when experimenting with autoerotic asphyxia
- Risk for Other-Directed Violence related to engaging in coercive sexual paraphilias
- Disturbed Personal Identity related to transgender issues such as cross-dressing or transsexualism
- Pain related to extreme discomfort when vaginal intercourse is attempted
- Ineffective Sexuality Pattern related to the need to engage in noncoercive paraphilias when having a sexual encounter
- Ineffective Sexuality Pattern related to increased sexual interest during the manic phase of bipolar disorder
- Ineffective Sexuality Pattern related to lack of control over compulsive sexual behavior
- Sexual Dysfunction related to the presence of one or more sexual problems affecting a couple's intimate relationship
- Spiritual Distress related to lack of intimacy with partner; multiple fears; history of sexual abuse
- Deficient Knowledge related to a lack of comprehensive sex education when growing up; not knowing how to communicate about sexual needs and desires
- Ineffective Role Performance related to rigidity in gender role expectations and behavior

Compromised Family Coping

It is difficult to experience sexual fulfillment when the relationship is in trouble in nonsexual spheres. The difficulty may be as straightforward as poor communication or as complex as conflict, anger, and unequal power. Other socioeconomic stressors include underemployment, unemployment, and lack of social network support. When one of the partners cross-dresses, the other partner must come to terms with the behavior if a healthy relationship is to be maintained. Being part of a family with a transsexual involves finding ways to reintegrate the person as a member of the other sex, or else reject the transsexual person and distance the family from this particular member.

Disturbed Personal Identity

In cultures with rigid gender roles, transsexuals and cross-dressers suffer a great deal of pain as they struggle with their gender identity. Transsexuals completely reject their anatomic sex, and cross-dressers alternate between their male and their female personas.

Ineffective Role Performance

Sexual addicts often cannot maintain work, family, and social roles. The addiction is so time consuming that the addict cannot devote time or energy to work or relationships.

Ineffective Sexuality Pattern

Some people cannot achieve sexual arousal and orgasm without the stimulation of an unusual object or situation. These individuals are considered to have one of the paraphilias, which may be coercive or noncoercive. Most often they are preoccupied with, and feel compelled to engage in, their particular sexual behaviors.

MEDIALINK Case Study: Sexual Sadism and Masochism

Risk for Violence: Self-Directed or Other-Directed

Autoerotic asphyxia is noncoercive but often fatal. People with this sexual behavior are not suicidal and have no intention of harming themselves but may accidentally kill themselves during sexual activity. Coercive paraphiliacs are considered to be violent against others because the victim is nonconsenting and is offended or hurt by the paraphiliac's sexual behavior.

Pain

A nursing diagnosis of pain applies to women who experience vaginismus. The origin may be past sexual trauma or current emotional conflict. The pain of dyspareunia may occur in both women and men and is typically related to organic factors.

Deficient Knowledge

People who grow up with no or very limited sex education may have difficulties in their adult sexual functioning. For people who don't know what to expect or how to touch themselves or their partners, sexual interactions can be frustrating rather than pleasurable. Lack of knowledge can contribute to ineffective sexual techniques and sexual dysfunctions.

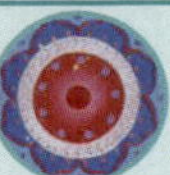

RX COMMUNICATION

CLIENT WITH SEXUAL DYSFUNCTION

CLIENT: "My husband always wants to have sex, and the more he wants, the less I'm interested."

NURSE RESPONSE 1: "Has there ever been a time in your relationship that you enjoyed sexual relations more?"

RATIONALE: This response explores the history of this problem's development in order to clarify whether the difficulty is interactional, intrapersonal, or perhaps medical in origin.

NURSE RESPONSE 2: "Have you spoken with your medical care provider about this problem?"

RATIONALE: This response assesses any contributory medical factors.

Sexual Dysfunction

Many of the previously discussed nursing diagnoses may be contributing factors to the development of sexual dysfunctions. In addition, illness, injury, surgery, medications, or substance abuse may contribute to sexual dysfunction. Problems with satisfaction may be described under either of these diagnoses: Sexual Dysfunction or Spiritual Distress. Communication about sexual dysfunction can be maximized by using the Rx Communication feature above. The impact of aging on sexual expression and satisfaction is explored in Chapter 28.

Outcome Identification

The outcomes expected with this group of clients focuses on the specific problem interfering with normal functioning. If the client has been sexually abused or traumatized and sexual functioning has been affected, then the expected outcome is that the client will have sexual abuse recovery. Other issues, such as menopause and aging impacts, are addressed with physical aging status outcomes.

Risk control is important as an outcome for those with sexual addictions or an increase in sexual interest. Actions need to be taken to reduce or eliminate the behaviors associated with risky sexual behavior so that sexually transmitted diseases are avoided. Outcomes in this overall area of nursing are related to the likelihood of the disorder.

Planning and Implementation: NOC

Developing the nursing plan of care and putting that plan into action can be structured using a format sensitive to clients with sexuality issues.

PLISSIT Model

You can use the PLISSIT model developed by Annon (1974) to help clients with gender identity issues or sexual problems. The model involves four progressive levels represented by the acronym PLISSIT:

P	Permission giving
LI	Limited information
SS	Specific suggestions
IT	Intensive therapy

At each level, nurses provide additional guidance and information to clients and therefore require more specialized and specific knowledge and skill. All professional nurses should be able to function at the first two levels.

Permission Giving Clients may feel that they need permission to be sexual beings, to discuss their gender identity, to ask questions, to show affection, and to express themselves sexually. Giving permission means that you, by attitude or word, let clients know that sexual thoughts, fantasies, and behaviors between informed, consenting adults are allowed. Giving permission begins when you acknowledge clients' spoken and unspoken sexual concerns and convey the attitude that these are important to health and healing.

For example, you might ask a client who is diagnosed with major depressive disorder the following question: "Many people who are depressed experienced a loss of sexual interest. Has this been a problem for you?"

Limited Information Clients need accurate but concise information. You might explain what is usual sexual behavior; how mental disorders and medications affect sexuality; or the impact of cultural expectations on gender role behavior. Continuing with the preceding example, you might say the following: "I notice that you have been on antidepressant medication for two months. Although this medication improves mood and general functioning, there are often some sexual side effects, especially related to orgasms."

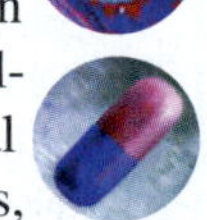

Specific Suggestions At this level, you will need specialized knowledge and skill about specific interventions. You offer suggestions to help clients adapt sexual activity to promote optimal functioning. If you are working on a cardiac unit, you need specialized knowledge about sexual readjustment during cardiac rehabilitation. If you are working with clients with spinal cord injuries, you need information about the sexual consequences of spinal injuries that occur at various levels. If you are working with a client who has gender identity issues you might say the following: "I'm not sure if you are aware of support groups in the area for people who are transgendered. I can give you a list of these groups, if you would like that information."

Intensive Therapy At this level of intervention, nurses must have specialized preparation and knowledge of sexual and

MEDIALINK Critical Thinking Exercise: Gender Identity Disorder

gender identity disorders. Nurses who function in the sex therapist role should meet the qualifications for practice as identified by the American Association of Sex Educators, Counselors, and Therapists (AASECT), which differentiate sex counseling from sex therapy. *Sex counseling* helps clients incorporate their sexual knowledge into satisfying lifestyles and socially responsible behavior. *Sex therapy* is a highly specialized, in-depth treatment to help clients resolve serious sexual problems. AASECT publishes a national directory of professionals certified to provide sex education, counseling, or therapy. This directory is an excellent resource for nurses and clients. A resource link to AASECT can be accessed through the Companion Website for this book.

MediaLink American Association of Sex Educators, Counselors, and Therapists

Some specific sexual counseling strategies are listed in the following Your Intervention Strategies feature.

Reducing Violence Against the Self

The most important nursing intervention regarding autoerotic asphyxia is community education. Warnings about autoerotic asphyxia should be routinely included in adolescent sex-education programs. Teenagers who practice it must be encouraged to seek immediate professional help. Parents should be taught to look for physical signs of trauma to the neck such as bruising, abrasions, pressure marks, or rope burns. Ropes, knotted sheets, knotted T-shirts, or the like hidden in the bedroom may be warning signs.

Reducing Violence Against Others

Individuals who practice coercive paraphilias typically do not stop their behavior and usually end up in the criminal justice system. The court may or may not mandate therapy. Therapy for sex offenders is a specialized area that should not be undertaken lightly. Although behavior modification techniques, group therapy, and hypnosis are used, they are generally unsuccessful. In severe cases, male sex offenders are treated with the antiandrogen medication medroxyprogesterone acetate (Provera or Depo-Provera), which induces a reversible chemical castration. The medication reduces the male sex drive, erections, and ejaculation, and decreases the obsessional focus on sex.

Promoting Comfort with Gender Identity

People who experience gender dysphoria have many options for managing the transgendered part of themselves. Physically they may undergo hormonal treatment, genital reassignment surgery, electrolysis, breast surgery, or other cosmetic surgery. They may decide to live in the other gender role part time or full time, prefer to have sex as a woman or as a man

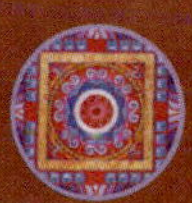

YOUR INTERVENTION STRATEGIES
Guidelines for Working with Clients with Sexual Difficulties

Some of the intensive therapy interventions listed below require more specialized and specific knowledge and skills. Refer back to the PLISSIT model on page 540 to identify which are within your area of expertise and which are level 4 interventions.

Male Orgasmic Disorder
Reestablish a climate of comfort and acceptance for sexual interaction. Encourage the client to masturbate and enjoy touch and body stimulation in general.

Premature Ejaculation
Instruct the client to stimulate the erect penis until the premonitory sensations of impending orgasm are felt. Then the client stops penile stimulation abruptly. This process is repeated to lower the threshold of excitability and make the client more tolerant of the stimuli. Sometimes the client uses the squeeze technique: At the point of orgasm, she squeezes the head of the penis with thumb and first two fingers for 3 to 4 seconds. This stops the urge to ejaculate.

Female Orgasmic Disorder
Instruct the client to avoid genital sex. Nongenital caressing exercises begin with the partners alternating as the initiator of a session of caressing, thus sharing responsibility for sexual interaction.

Next, genital stimulation is added to provide positive sexual experiences without intercourse. When intercourse is attempted, the woman is instructed to assume the superior position and insert the man's penis into her vagina. When setbacks occur, the couple is advised to rely on sexual techniques that do not involve intercourse. The woman is to place her hand lightly on her partner's to indicate her preference for contact. The emphasis is not on achieving orgasm but on learning erotic preferences.

The couple is instructed to use the side-by-side position, which enables both partners to move freely with emphasis on slow, exploratory thrusting. The goal is to develop an ability to enjoy pelvic play with the penis inside the vagina.

Vaginismus
Begin with a physical demonstration to the woman of her involuntary vaginal spasm by inserting an examining finger into her vagina. Then insert Hegar dilators in graduated sizes into the vagina, beginning with the smallest ones. After larger dilators are successfully inserted, instruct the client to retain the dilator for several hours each night. Most involuntary spasms can be relieved in 3 to 5 days with the daily use of dilators.

In addition to physical relief from spastic constriction, therapy is directed toward alleviating the fear that led to the onset of symptoms.

Vulvodynia and Vestibulitis
Clients with these disorders need a great deal of empathy and support as they have been living with acute pain for a significant period of time. Instruct them to use nonirritating substances on the vulva such as Lipocream, Aquaphor, or even olive oil or Crisco. Test for food allergies and environmental allergies, as these may be contributing causes. Specially trained physical therapists provide pelvic floor therapy which includes myofascial release, pudendal nerve release, and biofeedback. Yoga and acupuncture may also be helpful.

with a female, male, both, or neither. They may view themselves as female, male, both, a third gender, or transgendered. Interventions focus on promoting comfort with the chosen gender role.

Transsexuals are usually referred to therapists who specialize in this area or to gender identity disorder clinics. Because gender identity is stable, the goal of treatment with transsexuals is to help them live and function in society in the cross-gender role. Helping people find comfort in their sexual self-esteem is explored in the Caring for the Spirit box below.

If cross-dressing is a newly divulged secret to the partner, offer education and support. If the relationship is to continue, both partners need to agree on where and how cross-dressing will take place. Some couples compromise; for instance, a husband may agree never to cross-dress in front of his wife, and she may agree to give him privacy. Some agree to limit cross-dressing to the home; others are comfortable going out in public with the partner cross-dressed. The long-term success of the relationship depends on the couple's ability to negotiate these issues.

Reducing Pain

Whenever pain is associated with intercourse, a thorough physical examination is necessary to find and treat the organic cause of the pain. During vaginal examinations, careful attention must be paid to tiny tears in the vaginal wall, which are often overlooked. Even very small tears can cause great pain during intercourse. Vaginismus is treated with education, dilators, and supportive psychotherapy. The initial treatment for vulvodynia and vestibulitis involves decreasing the inflammation, followed by pelvic floor therapy by specially trained physical therapists.

Educating about Noncoercive Sex Patterns

Once paraphilias are a programmed part of arousal, they are very difficult to deprogram. The response to certain sexual or erotic stimuli tends to persist throughout life. A noncoercive, nonharmful paraphilia practiced with a consenting adult partner requires no nursing intervention other than client and partner education and possible couple negotiation about the behavior.

Reinforcing Sexual Health

Clients in a manic episode often exhibit impulsive increases in their sexual activity. Explain to family members that such behavior is a symptom of the manic state, is not within the client's control, and is not an indication of a change in ethics and values. As much as possible, clients should be protected from sexual acting out until they are able to assume control over this behavior. Set firm limits on inappropriate verbal and physical sexual behaviors. Chapter 17∞ discusses details on hypersexuality during mania.

Managing Compulsive Sexual Behavior

Sex addicts, like other people with addictions, respond well to community-based programs. Specific programs are discussed in the section on Community-Based Care.

Addressing Sexual Dysfunctions

Accurate identification of feelings is the first step in the problem-solving process, and clients may need help labeling the feelings they are experiencing. Following this step, help clients identify one anxiety-producing situation within their sexual interactions. At this stage, it is productive to focus diffuse anxiety on a manageable single situation or event. With the client, analyze the situation or event to discover negative anticipatory thoughts that may be the source of the anxiety. Together, review how the client has handled anxiety in the past and evaluate the range and effectiveness of this past coping behavior. It may be appropriate to help the client redefine the sensations of anxiety as sensations of sexual excitement, which is more likely to result in positive expectations. Together, explore alternative coping behaviors, and have the client evaluate their effectiveness after implementing them.

Many adult survivors of childhood sexual abuse are periodically overwhelmed by anxiety, fear, and panic (see Chapter 23∞). Refer adult survivors to support groups

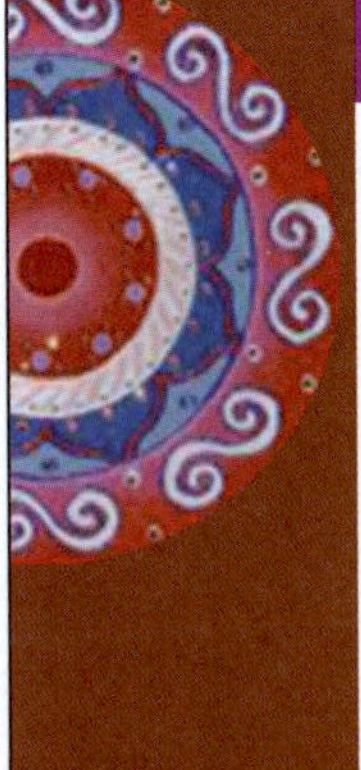

CARING FOR THE SPIRIT

Experiencing Pleasure and Fulfillment in Relationships

Sexual problems can create feelings such as guilt, anxiety, or fear that interfere with the ability to experience pleasure and joy. Some people experience guilt when they simply enjoy sex or participate in what they label "unusual" sexual activities, or guilt regarding the choice of partner. Some people internalize negative expectations and beliefs. Those with low self-esteem may not understand how another person could value and love them and also find them sexually attractive. For those who have not yet accepted their sexual orientation or gender identity, this conflict may interfere with sexual relationships.

Help clients identify and label the feelings they are experiencing. Then help them identify one anxiety- or guilt-producing situation within their sexual interactions. Together, review how feelings have been handled in the past and evaluate the range and effectiveness of this past coping behavior. Explore alternative coping behaviors and have clients evaluate their effectiveness after trying them.

Help clients identify the significance of culture, religion, race, gender, and age on their sexual self-esteem. Assist them in setting realistic goals to achieve higher self-esteem. Ask them to formulate positive self-statements and to repeat these aloud several times a day. Help them develop confidence in their ability to experience pleasure and fulfillment in relationships that are best suited for them.

Box 20-3 Common Components of Sex Therapy Programs

- **Information and education about sexual functions.** The therapist gives clients specific information about their particular needs. The therapist may discuss the information or assign books to read.
- **Experiential/sensory awareness.** The therapist helps clients recognize feelings of anxiety, anger, and pleasure by tuning into bodily cues. Clients focus on and describe feelings both in therapy sessions and at home. If they believe their genitals are ugly and unclean, the therapist assigns desensitization exercises at home that allow clients to become familiar with their own bodies. Some clients need fantasy training if nonsexual thoughts interfere with sexual arousal.
- **Insight.** The therapist attempts to understand what is causing and perpetuating the sexual problem. The goal is for clients to assume responsibility for their own behavior and recognize that change is possible.
- **Cognitive restructuring.** Clients identify and evaluate their fears about sexual interaction. The therapist encourages them to identify and eliminate negative self-statements and irrational expectations.
- **Behavioral interventions.** Since the focus is on changing nonsexual behavior that contributes to sexual problems, the therapist may assign assertiveness training, communication training, stress-reduction exercises, and problem-solving techniques. Behavioral interventions include assigned pleasuring sessions to discover what is arousing and pleasing to the self and partner.

such as Incest Anonymous or VOICES, as well as individual therapy with a therapist who specializes in this field.

Sexual disorders are explained in comfortable lay terms on the Sexual Disorders website that can be accessed through the Companion Website for this book. Since most psychotherapists are not sex therapists, make a referral through AASECT, mentioned earlier in this chapter. The common components of sex therapy programs are listed in Box 20-3.

Enhancing Communication

Good communication is an important part of a sexually fulfilling relationship. Apart from setting specific times to share feelings and beliefs, some couples need training in more effective communication skills. If they give ambiguous signals to indicate sexual interest, they need to learn how to state their interest clearly. Some people expect their partners to "read their minds" about sexual needs and desires; these people need encouragement to assert their needs tactfully. Teach couples to avoid "you" language, which evokes a defensive response and results in arguments, and to use "I" language, which expresses personal thoughts, feelings, and needs. Some examples of accusatory "you" statements and answerable "I" statements are in the Your Intervention Strategies feature at right.

If couples are able to reduce anxiety and improve communication but still have sexual problems, a referral is appropriate.

Reducing Spiritual Distress

Because the origin of spiritual distress is often a lack of intimacy or connection, the goal of nursing intervention is to help clients achieve and maintain a level of intimacy each partner finds comfortable. In the context of therapy, couples discuss their individual needs for closeness and identify barriers to intimacy. They are instructed to make three or four half-hour "dates" each week, during which they share warmth and intimacy. They spend some of the time discussing specific sexual issues; during other "dates," the couple explores intimate, nonsexual topics, such as hopes and expectations for the future. Couples should give these dates top priority, because a common way of avoiding intimacy is by not setting time aside for each other.

Increasing Knowledge

Providing education for sexual health is an important component of nursing implementation. Many sexual problems exist because of sexual ignorance; many others can be prevented with effective sexual health teaching.

You can assist clients to understand their anatomies and how their bodies function. For example, understanding the anatomy of the clitoris may help women learn how their bodies respond to sexual stimulation. Both women and men need to learn the kind of stimulation that is pleasing and causes arousal. Open communication between partners should also be encouraged. Details about physiologic changes that occur throughout the life span should be provided as part of general health care. For example, you discuss the effects of puberty, pregnancy, menopause, and the male climacteric on sexual function at the appropriate times.

Although there is an increasing awareness today of sexuality and sexual functioning, some people still hold certain

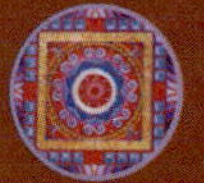

YOUR INTERVENTION STRATEGIES
Asserting Sexual Needs Tactfully

Couples who communicate about emotionally difficult subjects such as sex convey messages more competently through "I" language than through accusatory "you" language.

"You" Language

- "You only have sex on your mind. You're a pervert."
- "You keep grabbing at me like I'm always ready to go to bed with you."
- "You never pay attention to what turns me on. Are you dumb or hard of hearing?"

"I" Language

- "I'm concerned because we seem to have different expectations of how often we would like to make love."
- "I miss all the hugging and caressing we used to do even when we couldn't make love afterward."
- "I feel frustrated and hurt when it seems like I'm repeating myself. Maybe I'm not communicating my needs very clearly."

MediaLink Support Groups

MediaLink AtHealth.com

MediaLink Care Plan: Sexual Disorders and Communication

myths and misconceptions about sexuality. Many of these are handed down in families and are part of beliefs in a particular culture. It is highly important that you learn about the beliefs clients hold and provide up-to-date information. You are encouraged to visit the website of the Sexuality Information and Education Council of the United States, which has a wealth of information on various aspects of sexuality. The website can be accessed through the Companion Website for this book.

Evaluation

Examining your care for effectiveness is especially important where discomfort and bias could interfere with treatment for a client's sexual dysfunction.

Violence

Community and family education programs addressing the danger of autoerotic asphyxia will be established. Victims of this disorder will be identified and referred for immediate treatment. Clients with this disorder will remain safe. Clients with coercive paraphilias will curb their behavior, or society will set strict limits to protect potential victims.

Gender Identity

Clients will report increasing comfort and satisfaction in their new gender role, which will be congruent with their gender identity. Each will be able to function socially and economically as a person of that gender.

Pain

Individuals will report less pain or no pain during intercourse. Clients suffering from vaginismus will report success in using conscious control to relax vaginal muscles, allowing for pain-free intercourse.

Noncoercive Sexuality Patterns

Clients and partners will verbalize an understanding that noncoercive paraphilias are lifelong patterns. Couples will be able to negotiate the behavior in a way that is mutually satisfying.

Compulsive Sexual Behavior

Clients will attend a 12-step program for sexual addicts. Partners will attend appropriate self-help groups.

Sexual Dysfunction

Clients will report a satisfying and fulfilling sex life. They will experience minimal difficulty with desire, arousal, or orgasm. They will be able to identify and label feelings and acknowledge responsibility for their own behavior. They will implement a chosen variety of sexual techniques.

Spiritual Distress

Couples will report an acceptable and meaningful level of intimacy in their relationships. They will continue to set aside time for each other and engage in meaningful intimate time.

CASE MANAGEMENT

Case management services tend to revolve around the coercive paraphilias and autoerotic asphyxia. The criminal justice system is involved in the former, and may or may not be involved in the latter case. Case management consists mainly of making arrangements for services for the client, but the majority of effort is focused on protecting others. Treatment for coercive paraphilias has not been successful to any significant extent and recidivism is all too common.

COMMUNITY-BASED CARE

Transsexuals need a great deal of support and assistance as they establish themselves in their new role. If the present job is not gender-role stereotyped, they may be able to remain in the same or similar position. Others may need retraining programs to find acceptable employment. A multidisciplinary approach is most effective in helping transsexuals adjust to their situation. Family and friends need support and counseling to reintegrate this person into their lives as a person of the other sex.

For sex addicts, the cornerstone of recovery is a 12-step program modeled on the Alcoholics Anonymous program. Partners and codependents are also referred to appropriate self-help groups. A variety of groups, such as Sexaholics Anonymous, Sex Addicts Anonymous, Sex and Love Addicts Anonymous, S-Anon, and Co-Dependents of Sexual Addicts, have been formed throughout the country.

For cross-dressers, a community-based plan of care may include joining a club, such as Tri-Ess, where they can express their female personality in a safe social situation. Counseling for the individual or the couple at a community mental health clinic frequently focuses on the development of compromise within the relationship around cross-dressing issues.

HOME CARE

Sex therapy typically involves one hour a week with a sex therapist. The therapist gives clients specific information about their particular needs. The therapist may assign books to read or discuss the information. The therapist attempts to learn and understand what is causing and perpetuating the sexual problem. Clients identify and reevaluate their fears about sexual interaction. The therapist encourages them to identify and eliminate negative self-statements and irrational expectations.

Clients focus on and describe feelings both in therapy sessions and at home. If they believe their genitals are ugly and unclean, the therapist assigns desensitization exercises at home for clients to explore and become familiar with their own bodies. Some clients need fantasy training if nonsexual thoughts interfere with sexual arousal. Since the focus is on changing nonsexual behavior that contributes to sexual problems, the therapist may assign assertiveness training, communication training, stress-reduction exercises, and problem-solving techniques. Behavioral interventions include assigned pleasuring sessions to discover what is arousing and pleasing to both partners.

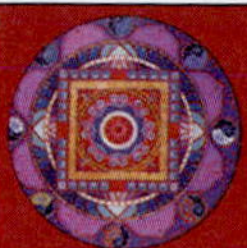

NURSING CARE PLAN
Client with Low Sexual Desire and Orgasmic Disorder

Assessment

Identifying Information

Susan is a 46-year-old married woman who has come with her 48-year-old husband, Brad, to the local mental health outpatient clinic. Neither of them has received mental health services prior to this time.

Client's Description of the Problem

Both Susan and Brad agree that there is a disparity of sexual needs. Susan is satisfied to have sex once a month, and Brad wants to have sex several times a week. Susan has never been orgasmic with Brad but does admit to achieving orgasms during masturbation, a fact she has never been able to tell Brad. Susan states that she would probably like to have sex more often if she would enjoy it. Her fear is that she will not become orgasmic. Brad thinks that entering therapy is the first big step, and he is hopeful that their sexual relationship will improve.

They both describe their sex life at the beginning of their marriage as fine for the first several years, although Susan states that she was never orgasmic during that time. They never talked about their sex life. Some years ago, after reading a "sex book," Susan experimented with masturbation for the first time and began to experience orgasms. She was never able to share this information with Brad because she felt guilty about touching herself when she was alone. They are verbally and physically affectionate with one another, but, they say, not as much as they used to be. They seldom express their anger to one another, and they manage most relationship conflicts by avoiding the issue.

History

No prior psychiatric history with either party. Both Susan and Brad are second-generation Americans of Eastern European descent with a common culture. Both describe their parents as very modest and noncommunicative about any sexual issues. No sex education was given in the family. Susan and Brad have been married 25 years and have two children: a daughter, 19, and a son, 14. They are both pleased with their occupations—Brad in sales, and Susan as a bookkeeper.

The couple describe their routine as Brad initiating sexual activity, primarily nonverbally. Sex typically occurs in the bedroom, after midnight, when they are both tired. Susan determines the length of foreplay, which usually lasts 5 to 10 minutes. The only position they use is man-on-top, but both agree they would like to try other positions. Brad has minimal verbal communication during sex, and Susan says she is too shy to say anything while they are making love. They both have difficulty talking about their sex life with one another. Susan states she is somewhat uncomfortable when Brad touches her body, except for her genitals and breasts. She is comfortable touching Brad's genitals but not touching her own genitals in front of him. She likes to receive oral sex but is uncomfortable giving it because she is afraid Brad will ejaculate in her mouth. Their mutual goals in therapy are to have sex more often, to feel freer to experiment, to discuss sex openly, and to have Susan experience pleasure and orgasms.

Brad has no current or past medical problems. Susan had a hysterectomy 5 years ago for endometriosis and is on hormone replacement therapy.

Current Mental Status

They are both quiet-spoken but articulate individuals. Eye contact is appropriate, mood is stable and appropriate, thought processes are logical, and there are no obvious symptoms of stress. Although they were both uncomfortable discussing sex, it became easier during a 2-hour history-taking time.

Nursing Diagnosis: Ineffective Sexuality Pattern related to disparity of needs.

Expected Outcome: Client will demonstrate an understanding of sexual anatomy and physiology, and openly communicate about sex.

Short-Term Goals	Interventions	Rationale
Susan will be able to discuss the frequency of sexual activity with Brad.	▪ Explore unspoken expectations and the potential for hurt feelings. ▪ Discuss and train on the meaning of, and process of, compromising. ▪ Discuss alternative ways to meet sexual needs besides intercourse.	Sexual expectations are seldom similar, and coming to a compromise regarding sex contributes to a healthy relationship. Masturbation and fantasy may not be readily accessible intercourse alternatives.
The couple will be able to discuss personal preferences for sexual activities.	▪ Encourage communication during sex such as what they like and how they like things between them.	Practice establishes behavior. Information describes Susan's ability to achieve orgasm.
Susan will be able to achieve orgasm during sexual activity with Brad.	▪ Give homework assignments designed to address sexual communication. ▪ Discuss physiology of Susan's sexuality related to orgasmic functioning. ▪ Encourage activities in which Susan has achieved orgasm.	

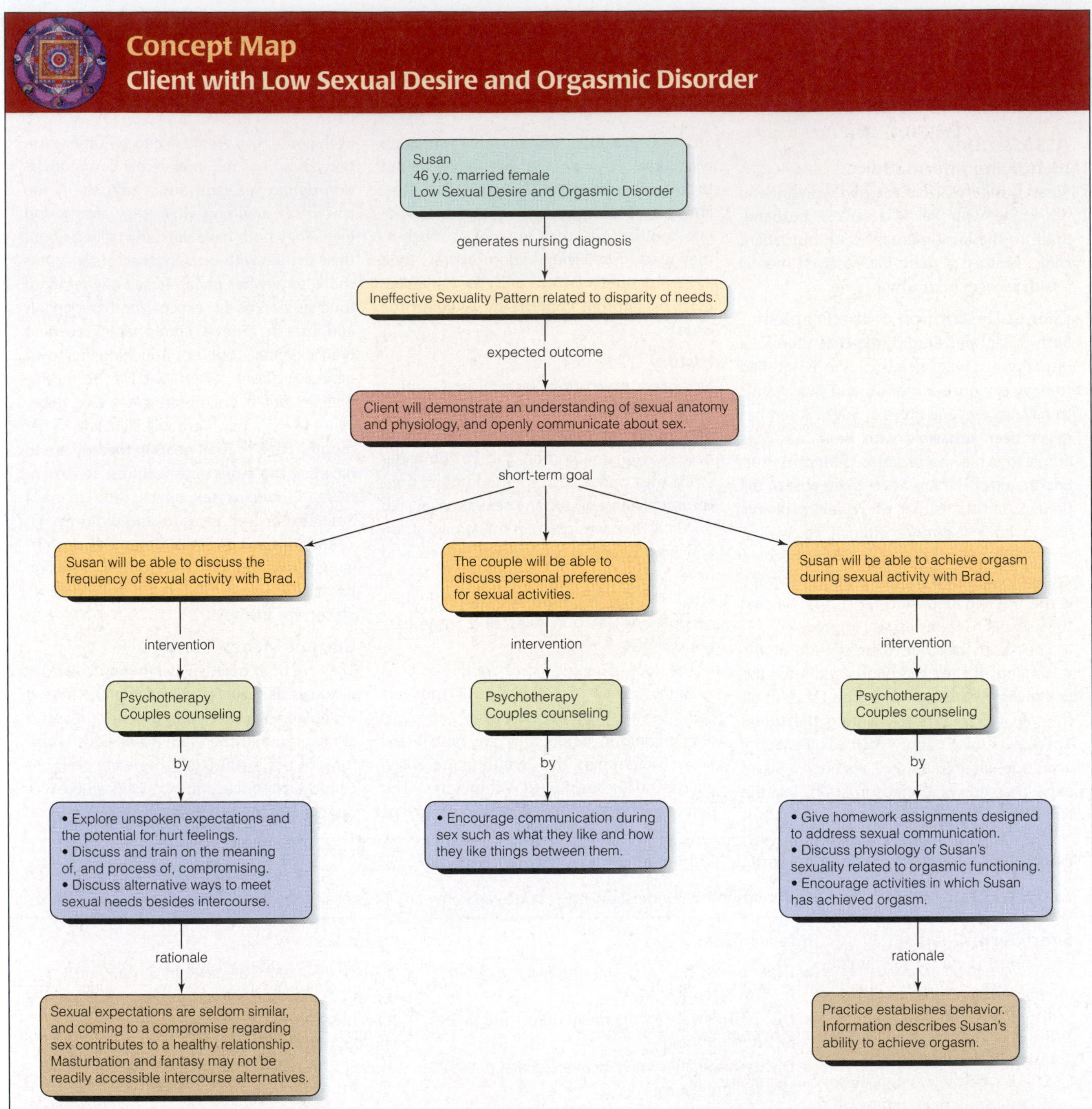
Concept Map
Client with Low Sexual Desire and Orgasmic Disorder
Susan
46 y.o. married female
Low Sexual Desire and Orgasmic Disorder
generates nursing diagnosis
Ineffective Sexuality Pattern related to disparity of needs.
expected outcome
Client will demonstrate an understanding of sexual anatomy and physiology, and openly communicate about sex.
short-term goal
Susan will be able to discuss the frequency of sexual activity with Brad.
The couple will be able to discuss personal preferences for sexual activities.
Susan will be able to achieve orgasm during sexual activity with Brad.
intervention
Psychotherapy
Couples counseling
by
• Explore unspoken expectations and the potential for hurt feelings.
• Discuss and train on the meaning of, and process of, compromising.
• Discuss alternative ways to meet sexual needs besides intercourse.
• Encourage communication during sex such as what they like and how they like things between them.
• Give homework assignments designed to address sexual communication.
• Discuss physiology of Susan's sexuality related to orgasmic functioning.
• Encourage activities in which Susan has achieved orgasm.
rationale
Sexual expectations are seldom similar, and coming to a compromise regarding sex contributes to a healthy relationship. Masturbation and fantasy may not be readily accessible intercourse alternatives.
Practice establishes behavior. Information describes Susan's ability to achieve orgasm.

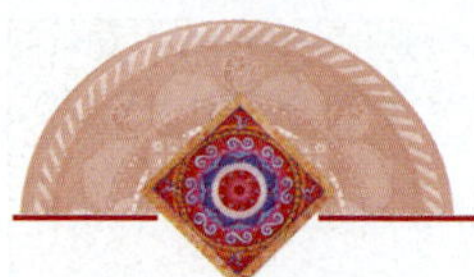

EXPLORE MEDIALINK 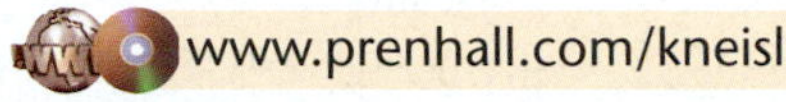

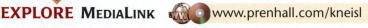

For NCLEX-RN® review questions, case studies, and other resources for this chapter see the Pearson Health MediaLink CD-ROM that accompanies this book and the Companion Website at www.prenhall.com/kneisl.

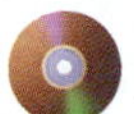

CD-ROM
Audio Glossary
NCLEX-RN® Review Questions
Video
- *Gender Identity Disorder*

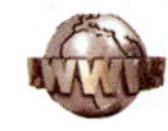

Companion Website
Audio Glossary
NCLEX-RN® Review Questions
Critical Thinking Exercise
- *Gender Identity Disorder*

Case Study
- *Sexual Sadism and Masochism*

Care Plan
- *Sexual Disorders and Communication*

MediaLinks
MediaLink Application
- *Born with the Wrong Body*

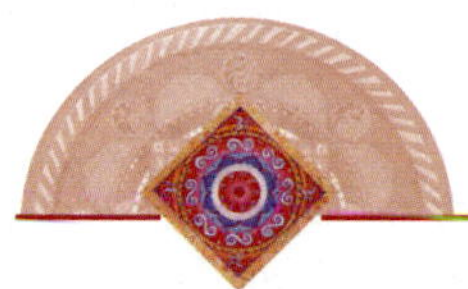

NCLEX-RN® REVIEW QUESTIONS

1. Gender identity can best be described as:
1. The role a person is expected to perform as a result of being male or female.
2. The degree of flexibility a person has regarding gender-stereotypic behaviors.
3. A contradiction between chromosomal gender and external genital appearance.
4. An individual's personal or private sense of identity as male or female.

2. A holistic approach to nursing care of the client with sexual disorders requires the nurse generalist to have which of the following?
1. Extensive experience in caring for clients with sexual disorders
2. The ability to diagnose sexual disorders
3. A basic understanding of the nursing process
4. Proficiency in the use of the nursing process and ability to assess the client's sexual health

3. The client reports a history of rubbing up against others to achieve sexual arousal. This behavior is known as:
1. Exhibitionism.
2. Frotteurism.
3. Pedophilia.
4. Voyeurism.

4. An example of a coercive paraphilia is:
1. Fetishism.
2. Cross-dressing.
3. Obscene phone calling.
4. Gender dysphoria.

5. According to behavior theory, gender dysphoria can result from:
1. The child being rewarded for adopting behaviors of the other sex.
2. Fetal exposure to adult levels of sex hormones.
3. Arrested psychosexual development.
4. Past or present traumatic events.

6. Which of the following questions would be asked as part of the cognitive assessment of a sexual history?
1. "In what way do you experience guilt about sex?"
2. "What is your level of satisfaction with the frequency of your sexual activity?"
3. "How has your religion influenced your sexual values and behaviors?"
4. "To what degree do you experience pleasure during sexual activity?"

7. The components of a sexual addiction include which of the following behaviors? (Select all that apply.)
1. Preoccupation
2. Ritualization
3. Compulsivity
4. Indifference
5. Despair

8. The nurse is utilizing the PLISSIT model of treatment in working with a couple who are experiencing sexual problems within their relationship. What is the purpose of permission-giving (P) in this model?

1. The clients give each other permission to experiment with their sexual fantasies.
2. The nurse conveys the attitude to the clients that sexual thoughts and fantasies between consenting adults are allowed.
3. The nurse provides specific interventions to promote optimal sexual functioning.
4. The nurse gives the couple concise information about treatment options.

9. The priority nursing intervention to prevent autoerotic asphyxia is:

1. Reducing violence against others.
2. Community education and awareness.
3. Exploring alternative coping skills.
4. Reducing spiritual distress.

10. Which of the following is needed for the psychiatric–mental health nurse generalist to work effectively with clients who are experiencing sexual problems?

1. Specialized training related to sexual disorders and gender identity
2. The ability to explore personal values and attitudes related to sexual health
3. Knowledge of the theoretical bases of human sexuality
4. Personal experience with sexual disorders or dysfunction

See Appendix C for answers.

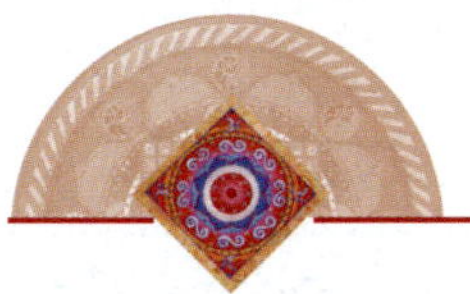

REFERENCES

Annon, J. (1974). *The behavioral treatment of sexual problems: Vol. 1, Brief therapy.* New York: Harper & Row.

Barnett, R., & Rivers, C. (2004). *Same difference.* New York: Basic Books.

Carnes, P. J., & Wilson, M. (2002). The sexual addiction assessment process. In: P. J. Carnes & K. M. Adams (Eds.), *Clinical management of sex addiction* (pp. 3–19). New York: Brunner-Routledge.

El-Hage, G., Eden, J. A., & Manga, R. Z. (2007). A double-blind, randomized, placebo-controlled trial of the effect of testosterone cream on the sexual motivation of menopausal hysterectomized women with hypoactive sexual desire disorder. *Climacteric, 10*(4), 335–343.

Hecht, M., Collier, M. J., & Ribeau, S. (2002). *African American communication* (2nd ed.). Mahwah, NJ: Lawrence Erlbaum Associates.

Heiman, J. R. (2007). Orgasmic disorders in women. In S. R. Leiblum (Ed.), *Principles and practice of sex therapy* (4th ed.) (pp. 84–123). New York: Guilford Press.

King, B. M. (2002). *Human sexuality today* (4th ed.). Upper Saddle River, NJ: Prentice Hall.

Langstrom, N., & Zucker, K. J. (2005). Transvestic fetishism in the general population. *Journal of Sex & Marital Therapy, 31*(1), 87–95.

Lawrence, A. A. (2005). Sexuality before and after male-to-female sex reassignment surgery. *Archives of Sexual Behavior, 34*(2), 147–166.

Leiblum, S. R., Koochaki, P. E., Rodenburg, C. A., Barton, I, P., & Rosen, R. C. (2006). Hypoactive sexual desire disorder in postmenopausal women: U.S. results from the Women's International Study of Health and Sexuality. *Menopause, 13*(1), 46–56.

Lips, H. M. (2004). *Sex and gender* (5th ed.). Mountain View, CA: Mayfield Publishing.

McCammon, S. L., Knox, D., & Schacht, C. (2004). *Choices in sexuality* (2nd ed.). Cincinnati, OH: Atomic Dog Publishing.

McCarthy, B. W., & Fucito, L. M. (2005). Integrating medication, realistic expectations, and therapeutic interventions in the treatment of male sexual dysfunction. *Journal of Sex & Marital Therapy, 31*(4), 319–328.

Melby, T. (2002). Intersex interrupted. *Contemporary Sexuality, 36*(12), 1–6.

Metzger, D. A. (2005). When pleasure becomes a pain. Conference proceedings: *Women's Sexual Health.* The Berman Center and Northwestern University, Feinberg School of Medicine, Department of Obstetrics and Gynecology.

Nichols, M., & Shernoff, M. (2007). Therapy with sexual minorities. In S. R. Leiblum (Ed.), *Principles and practice of sex therapy* (4th ed.) (pp. 379–415). New York: Guilford Press.

Ting-Toomey, S., & Chung, L. (2002). *Understanding intercultural communication.* Los Angeles: Roxbury.

Turna, B., Apaydin, E., Semerci, B., Altay, B., Cikili, N., & Nazli, O. (2005). Women with low libido: Correlation of decreased androgen levels with female sexual function index. *International Journal of Impotence Research, 17*(2), 148–153.

Vision of Sexual Health. (2004). *Contemporary Sexuality, 38*(7), 1–5.

ADDITIONAL REFERENCES

Kafka, M. P. (2000). The paraphilia-related disorders. In S. R. Leiblum & R. C. Rosen (Eds.), *Principles and practice of sex therapy* (3rd ed.) (pp. 471–503). New York: Guilford Press.

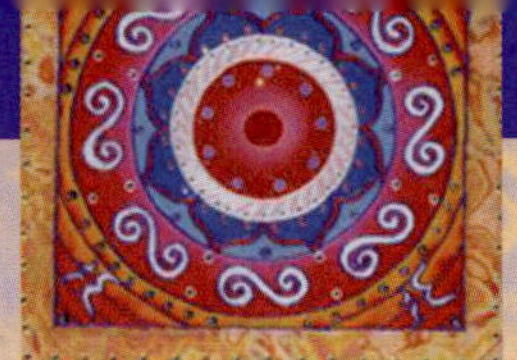

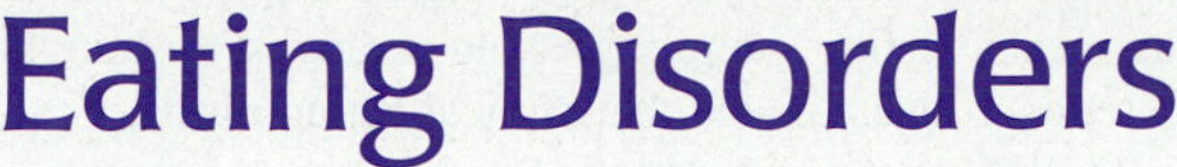

Eating Disorders

CHAPTER

21

KAREN LEE FONTAINE AND KAY K. CHITTY

LEARNING OUTCOMES

After completing this chapter, you will be able to:

1. Describe the roles of culture and biology in the development of eating disorders.
2. Distinguish among the various eating disorders.
3. Compare and contrast the various theories for the causes of eating disorders.
4. Explain how psychological and social pressures can influence the course of eating disorders.
5. Assess individual and family problems of clients with eating disorders.
6. Partner with clients and their families in both the prevention and treatment of eating disorders.
7. Identify the intermediate goals in the treatment of clients with eating disorders.
8. Implement appropriate nursing interventions for clients with eating disorders and their families.
9. Describe methods to prevent or minimize eating disorders.

CRITICAL THINKING CHALLENGE

A school health nurse in a large public high school is aware that a number of girls diet constantly and throw up in the bathroom following lunch period. She also learns that boys on the wrestling team use vomiting as a means of "making weight." When the nurse takes her concerns to the principal to ask his support for an eating disorders educational program, he replies: "This is a health problem, not an educational problem. We just don't have time for this kind of thing. It's really up to the parents."

1. In your opinion, what is the responsibility of nurses in educating the public about prevention of eating disorders?
2. What kinds of information do people—particularly parents, teachers, and coaches—need to communicate about eating and health?
3. What messages have you received that have helped or hindered you in developing healthy eating attitudes and behaviors?

KEY TERMS

anorexia nervosa *551*
binge eating *552*
binge-eating disorder *553*
bulimia nervosa *552*
obesity *554*
purging *552*

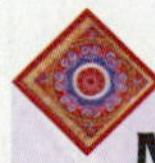

MEDIALINK 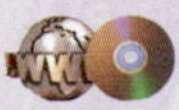 www.prenhall.com/kneisl

Go to the Pearson Health MediaLink CD-ROM and the Companion Website at www.prenhall.com/kneisl for interactive resources for this chapter.

For many, eating symbolizes parental nurturing—the love and care that are the prototype of, and basis for, all future intimate relationships. For some, however, eating creates anxiety because of its association with unsatisfactory and unpleasant parent–child interactions. Clearly, food and eating have greater individual and cultural meaning and importance than merely sustaining life. Disturbed eating patterns may develop as a means of coping with stress.

The three major eating disorders discussed in this chapter—anorexia nervosa, bulimia nervosa, and binge-eating disorder—create biologic, psychologic, and social imbalances that interfere with the individual's normal functioning. Changes in biochemistry, metabolic rate, emotional state, family relationships, and social status brought about by eating disorders can create depression, isolation, and sometimes self-destructive behavior.

Cultural stereotypes contribute to women's preoccupation with their bodies. Attractiveness is determined by how closely a woman's appearance matches the cultural ideal of thinness. Thus, identity and self-esteem are dependent on physical appearance. Being disgusted with one's flesh is the same as having an adversarial relationship with the body—a relationship that often results in eating disorders. The Evidence-Based Practice feature discusses the impact of anorexia on life roles and functioning.

Determining the incidence of anorexia and bulimia is difficult because of the variety of definitions that exist. Certainly the frequency of these disorders has been increasing, but the increase may be due partly to increased reporting. Ninety percent of women and 25% of men diet at some time in their lives. Over half of teenage girls and one-third of teenage boys use unhealthy weight control behaviors such as skipping meals, fasting, vomiting, using laxatives, and smoking cigarettes. It is estimated that clinical eating disorders affect 8% to 20% of the population. They are more commonly seen among females, with estimates of the male–female ratio ranging from 1:6 to 1:10, although 19% to 30% of younger people with anorexia are male. The estimate may be low, as primary health care providers are less likely to diagnose an eating disorder in a male than in a female (Tozzi et al., 2005).

For those with anorexia or bulimia, the most frequently observed disorder is depression. In some cases, this may be the result of abnormal eating and weight loss. In other cases the depression is the primary disorder to which the eating disorder is a response. And for yet another group of people, the depression and abnormal eating both are primary disorders.

There is a high prevalence of several anxiety disorders associated with eating disorders. Social phobias may occur in people with eating disorders, possibly in response to others' awareness of their abnormal eating behaviors. Obsessive–compulsive symptoms are common, especially among people with anorexia. Obsessive–compulsive symptoms often continue even after weight is restored in anorexia. Panic attacks are likely when people with anorexia are prohibited from exercising their usual behavior patterns. It is unclear whether these are primary disorders or are secondary to the eating disorders (Godart et al., 2006).

Anorexia nervosa and bulimia nervosa are not single diseases but syndromes with multiple predisposing factors and a variety of characteristics. Although the most obvious symptom is the eating problem, these disorders are not simply a matter of eating too much or too little. It is because of

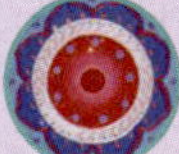

EVIDENCE-BASED PRACTICE

LIFE ROLES AND ANOREXIA NERVOSA

Suzy is a 45-year-old woman who is extremely thin and jogs several miles every day to maintain her (under)weight. She is 5'7" and weighs 112 pounds. You work with her in an outpatient clinic where she is receiving counseling for marital problems.

Suzy has maintained the same weight since she was 17 years old. Her eating habits have always been tied to her weight. Since she was a teenager, Suzy has added extra miles to her running route, decreased her calorie count, or fasted whenever she was one or two pounds over what she considered her ideal weight. The literature reports that adolescence is the peak time for developing eating disorders; however, longitudinal studies would be most helpful to you in understanding and working with Suzy.

As indicated in the following research, many people grow out of eating disorders as they mature. Events such as committing to a relationship, forming a family, and settling into an identity and occupation all serve to provide a stable platform for overall functioning. Women's drive to be thin tends to decline as they age (conversely, men's drive to be thin tends to increase as they age), but Suzy does not follow that trend. You will explore her life roles with her (is she a wife, a mother, a daughter, a business executive, a socialite, a student, an athlete, etc.) to determine if her perception of herself in these roles contributes to perpetuating the eating disorder.

Action should be based on more than one study, but the following research would be helpful in this situation.

Keel, P. K., Baxter, M. G., Heatherton, T. F., & Joiner, T. E. Jr. (2007). A 20-year longitudinal study of body weight, dieting, and eating disorder symptoms. *Journal of Abnormal Psychology, 116*(2), 422–432.

CRITICAL THINKING APPLICATION

1. If Suzy has been maintaining an underweight condition since the age of 17, what are her chances for improvement?
2. What conditions would be necessary for improvement to take place?

the complex interaction of biological, psychological, developmental, familial, and sociocultural factors that certain people develop eating disorders.

There is no clear-cut distinction between the two disorders, and they have many features in common. The traditional division of anorexia and bulimia is still appropriate until more is known about eating disorders. Body weight may be a significant distinguishing characteristic; people with anorexia are severely underweight and people with bulimia are at normal or near-normal weight. About 30% of people with bulimia have a history of anorexia. As many as 62% of people with anorexia exhibit bulimic behaviors. Conversion from anorexia to bulimia may be a way of moving from a "visible" to an "invisible" eating disorder to deceive family, friends, and health care providers. Thus, the two disorders can occur in the same person, or the person can go from one disorder to the other. There are far more similarities than differences between anorexia and bulimia (Tozzi et al., 2005). However, to help you understand the differences, the disorders have been separated in this chapter.

ANOREXIA NERVOSA

Anorexia nervosa is a potentially life-threatening disorder characterized by extreme perfectionism, weight fear, significant weight loss, body image disturbances, strenuous exercising, peculiar food-handling patterns, and reductions in heart rate, blood pressure, metabolic rate, and the production of estrogen or testosterone. The DSM-IV-TR diagnostic criteria for anorexia nervosa follow. A well-known pioneer in the treatment of eating-disordered clients, Hilde Bruch (1978), called anorexia nervosa "the relentless pursuit of thinness."

Rigidity and overcontrol are the hallmarks of anorexia. To control themselves and their environment, these individuals develop rigid rules. Such rigidity often develops into *obsessive rituals*, particularly concerning eating and exercise. Cutting all food into a predetermined size or number of pieces, chewing all food a certain number of times, allowing only certain combinations of foods in a meal, accomplishing a fixed number of exercise routines, and having an inflexible pattern of exercises are rituals common to anorexic people. These rules and rituals help keep anxiety beyond conscious awareness. If the rituals are disrupted, the anxiety becomes intolerable. Paradoxically, all these efforts to stay in control lead to out-of-control behaviors (Tozzi et al., 2005).

Many people with anorexia are hyperactive and discover that overexercise is a way to increase their weight loss. Solitary running tends to be the exercise of choice, and there are often obsessional qualities to it. For example, they believe that before they can eat, they have to earn calories by exercising. Conversely, if they overeat, they believe they must punish themselves with excessive exercise. Excessive exercise signifies the triumph of will over the body and is a possible indication of poor prognosis in recovery (Neumark-Sztainer, 2005).

Anorexic young women have a desperate need to please others. Their self-worth depends on responses from others rather than on their own self-approval. Thus, their behavior is often overcompliant; they always try to meet the expectations of others in order to be accepted. They may overachieve in academic and extracurricular activities, but these accomplishments are usually an attempt to please parents rather than a source of self-satisfaction.

People with anorexia often feel hopeless, helpless, and ineffective. Because of being overcompliant with their parents, they believe they have always been controlled by others. Their refusal to eat may be an attempt to assert themselves and gain some control within the family. As weight is lost, they are rewarded with praise, admiration, and envy from their peers, which reinforces the restricted eating pattern.

MEDIALINK Anorexia Nervosa Video

DSM-IV-TR Diagnostic Criteria for Anorexia Nervosa

A. Refusal to maintain body weight at or above a minimally normal weight for age and height (e.g., weight loss leading to maintenance of body weight less than 85% of that expected; or failure to make expected weight gain during period of growth, leading to body weight less than 85% of that expected).

B. Intense fear of gaining weight or becoming fat, even though underweight.

C. Disturbance in the way in which one's body image or shape is experienced, undue influence of body weight or shape on self-evaluation, or denial of the seriousness of the current low body weight.

D. In postmenarcheal females, amenorrhea, i.e., the absence of at least three consecutive menstrual cycles. (A woman is considered to have amenorrhea if her periods occur only following hormone—e.g., estrogen—administration.)

Restricting Type

During the current episode of Anorexia Nervosa, the person has not regularly engaged in binge eating or purging behavior (i.e., self-induced vomiting or the misuse of laxatives, diuretics, or enemas).

Binge-Eating/Purging Type

During the current episode of Anorexia Nervosa, the person has regularly engaged in binge eating or purging behavior (i.e., self-induced vomiting or the misuse of laxatives, diuretics, or enemas).

Source: Reprinted with permission from the *Diagnostic and Statistical Manual of Mental Disorders,* Fourth Edition, Text Revision. (Copyright 2000). American Psychiatric Association.

USING DSM-IV-TR

Health care providers often use language unfamiliar to clients and their families. Explain *amenorrhea in postmenarcheal females* in a way that would help a family understand the characteristics of anorexia nervosa.

The following clinical example illustrates overcompliant behavior and phobia related to weight gain.

CLINICAL EXAMPLE

Simone is a tall, quiet girl who was considered polite, well-liked, and a good student. She was given responsibility beyond her years at both school and home because of her quiet competence and maturity. When she was 15, she entered a beauty contest at a local amusement park as a lark but did not win. She became convinced that she lost because her legs were too large and her abdomen protruded. She decided to diet. To radically control her own intake without arousing the family's suspicions, she began preparing all the family's meals. She herself did not eat, but played with her food during mealtimes.

Simone spent long hours alone in her room studying, dancing, and exercising vigorously. She weighed herself several times daily, and if the scales showed an unacceptable number, she exercised even more frenziedly. As she lost weight, Simone disguised her gauntness with loose, layered clothes. One day, when she and her mother were shopping, her mother saw her disrobed and was dismayed. She insisted that Simone see the family physician, who encouraged her to eat more and prescribed nutritional supplements.

When Simone collapsed at a shopping mall a few weeks later, her parents prevailed on the family doctor to admit her to the psychiatric unit of the community hospital. As an IV was started in the emergency room, Simone asked the nurse, "How many calories are in that bag?"

BULIMIA NERVOSA

There is a cyclic behavioral pattern in **bulimia nervosa**. It begins with skipping meals sporadically and overstrict dieting or fasting. In an effort to refrain from eating, the person may use amphetamines, which can lead to extreme hunger, fatigue, and low blood glucose levels. The next part of the cycle is a period of **binge eating**, in which the person ingests huge amounts of food (about 3,500 kcal) within a short time (about 1 hour). Binges can last up to 8 hours, with consumption of 12,000 kcal. Binge eating usually occurs when the person is alone and at home, and most frequently during the evening. The cycle may occur once or twice a month for some and as often as five or ten times a day for others. The binge part of the cycle may be triggered by the ingestion of certain foods, but this is not consistent for everyone. Although eating binges may involve any kind of food, they usually consist of junk foods, fast foods, and high-calorie foods.

The final part of the cycle is **purging** the body of the ingested food. After excessive eating, people with bulimia force themselves to vomit. They often abuse laxatives and diuretics to further purge their bodies of the food. Some use as many as 50 to 100 laxatives per day. In rare cases, they may resort to Syrup of Ipecac to induce vomiting. Purging becomes a purification rite and a means of regaining self-control. Some describe it as feeling "completely fresh and clean again." The DSM-IV-TR diagnostic criteria for bulimia nervosa follow.

After the purging, the cycle begins all over again, with a return to strict dieting or fasting. Some people with bulimia

DSM-IV-TR Diagnostic Criteria for Bulimia Nervosa

A. Recurrent episodes of binge eating. An episode of binge eating is characterized by both of the following:
   1. eating, in a discrete period of time (e.g., within any 2-hour period), an amount of food that is definitely larger than most people would eat during a similar period of time and under similar circumstances
   2. a sense of lack of control over eating during the episode (e.g., a feeling that one cannot stop eating or control what or how much one is eating)

B. Recurrent inappropriate compensatory behavior in order to prevent weight gain, such as self-induced vomiting; misuse of laxatives, diuretics, enemas, or other medications; fasting; or excessive exercise.

C. The binge eating and inappropriate compensatory behaviors both occur, on average, at least twice a week for 3 months.

D. Self-evaluation is unduly influenced by body shape and weight.

E. The disturbance does not occur exclusively during episodes of Anorexia Nervosa.

Purging Type

During the current episode of Bulimia Nervosa, the person has regularly engaged in self-induced vomiting or the misuse of laxatives, diuretics, or enemas.

Nonpurging Type

During the current episode of Bulimia Nervosa, the person has used other inappropriate compensatory behaviors, such as fasting or excessive exercise, but has not regularly engaged in self-induced vomiting or the misuse of laxatives, diuretics, or enemas.

Source: Reprinted with permission from the *Diagnostic and Statistical Manual of Mental Disorders,* Fourth Edition, Text Revision. (Copyright 2000). American Psychiatric Association.

USING DSM-IV-TR

Health care providers often use language unfamiliar to clients and their families. Explain purging behaviors in such a way that a family might better understand the characteristics of bulimia nervosa.

eat highly nutritious meals when not binge eating/purging to repair harm done to the body.

Binge eating and purging begin as a way to eat and stay slim. Before long, the behavior becomes a response to stress and a way to cope with negative feelings such as anger, anxiety, and depression. For some it is poor impulse control, and for others it is an expression of rebellion against family members.

People with bulimia may engage in sporadic excessive exercise, but they usually do not develop compulsive exercise routines. They are more likely to abuse street drugs to decrease their appetite and alcohol to reduce their anxiety. Since their binges are often expensive, costing as much as $100 per day, they may resort to stealing food or money to buy the food. The binge–purge cycle can become so consuming that activities and relationships are disrupted. To keep the behavior secret, the person often resorts to excuses and lies. The following clinical example illustrates the progression of bulimia.

CLINICAL EXAMPLE

Beth is a 17-year-old high school student who had been binge eating and purging with vomiting and over-the-counter diuretics and laxatives for about 2 years. She was referred to the mental health center by her school nurse. Beth stated that her school friends became concerned about her increasing preoccupation with purging, even after eating very small amounts of food. She was spending a lot of time in the girls' restroom; after lengthy bouts of self-induced vomiting following lunch period, she was sometimes too exhausted to attend class. Her friends had been "covering" for her but had become frightened and went to the school nurse with their concerns.

Beth is of average weight for her height but admitted that she would be quite heavy if she didn't purge herself of the large amounts of food she consumes in her room at night after her parents have gone to bed. "I'm so embarrassed. My whole life is totally out of control," she told the intake worker.

BINGE-EATING DISORDER

The bulimic pattern is different from **binge-eating disorder**, which is often associated with obesity. This disorder is a proposed new category that needs further study before inclusion in the *Diagnostic and Statistical Manual of Mental Disorders* (4th ed., text revision) (DSM-IV-TR) (APA, 2000). The research criteria for binge-eating disorder are in the following DSM-IV-TR feature. The prevalence in the general population is 1–3% and as high as 25% among people seeking help for weight loss (Pull, 2004).

Obese individuals who overeat tend to follow one of two patterns, neither of which includes purging the body after excessive food intake. The first pattern is overeating and feeling out of control in response to a number of feelings such as anxiety or depression. The diagnosis of binge-eating disorder is given when bingeing occurs at least twice a week for 6 months. Some individuals binge in response to losing control over a weight-loss diet. Although these people lose weight in weight-control programs, they regain it after going

DSM-IV-TR Research Criteria for Binge-Eating Disorder

A. Recurrent episodes of binge eating. An episode of binge eating is characterized by both of the following:
   1. eating, in a discrete period of time (e.g., within any 2-hour period), an amount of food that is definitely larger than most people would eat in a similar period of time under similar circumstances
   2. a sense of lack of control over eating during the episode (e.g., a feeling that one cannot stop eating or control what or how much one is eating)

B. The binge-eating episodes are associated with three (or more) of the following:
   1. eating much more rapidly than normal
   2. eating until feeling uncomfortably full
   3. eating large amounts of food when not feeling physically hungry
   4. eating alone because of being embarrassed by how much one is eating
   5. feeling disgusted with oneself, depressed, or very guilty after overeating

C. Marked distress regarding binge eating is present.

D. The binge eating occurs, on average, at least 2 days a week for 6 months.

   Note: The method of determining frequency differs from that used for Bulimia Nervosa; future research should address whether the preferred method of setting a frequency threshold is counting the number of days on which binges occur or counting the number of episodes of binge eating.

E. The binge eating is not associated with the regular use of inappropriate compensatory behaviors (e.g., purging, fasting, excessive exercise) and does not occur exclusively during the course of Anorexia Nervosa or Bulimia Nervosa.

Source: Reprinted with permission from the *Diagnostic and Statistical Manual of Mental Disorders,* Fourth Edition, Text Revision. (Copyright 2000). American Psychiatric Association.

USING DSM-IV-TR

Health care providers often use language unfamiliar to clients and their families. Explain *inappropriate compensatory behavior* in a way that would help a family better understand the characteristics of binge-eating disorder.

off the diet. People with this eating pattern say that their eating or weight interferes with their relationships and their self-esteem. Women are more likely to have this eating pattern than are men. There is evidence that several medications are effective for this disorder including sibutramine (Meridia), an appetite suppressant; citalopram (Celexa), a selective serotonin reuptake inhibitor (SSRI) antidepressant; and topiramate (Topamax), an anticonvulsant and mood stabilizer (Appolinario et al., 2003; Pull, 2004). The following clinical example discusses overeating in response to emotional distress.

CLINICAL EXAMPLE

Joan is a 45-year-old secretary who is 5′3″ tall and weighs 167 pounds. She came to the outpatient department of a private psychiatric hospital because of depression over her weight. She reported that she had always struggled with her weight but that it became a real problem after her husband left her 10 years ago. She experienced severe financial and emotional stress as a result of her divorce and had become dependent on her aging parents for companionship, financial help, and assistance in raising her son, now 18 years old.

Joan described herself as "tense and angry all the time." She had tried many diets but the problems remained, and eating seemed to be the only way to dull the pain. "When I look at myself in the mirror, I am so discouraged that I eat a whole bag of cookies just to feel better. Then I hate myself even more. I am trapped in a body and a life that I don't want."

The second pattern is overeating because of the enjoyment of food. Seldom attempting to diet, these people have no sense of loss of control. They are more accepting of their body size and understand it to be the result of their enjoyment of eating.

OBESITY

Obesity is the most common form of malnourishment in the United States. Using the body mass index (a calculation based on height and weight), it is estimated that 59 million adults in the United States are obese and 9 million youth are overweight. The prevalence of obesity has increased in all age, gender, and ethnic/racial groups during the past three decades. Since the mental health of obese people is comparable to that of the general population, obesity is not considered a mental disorder. The only similarity between obesity and anorexia and bulimia is dissatisfaction with body size and shape. Therefore, a brief overview is presented here, and you are encouraged to consult other resources, books, and journals for a more comprehensive description.

Obesity is thought to result from a variety of combinations of psychosocial and physiological factors. There is no universal cause and therefore no single treatment approach. There are many ways of becoming and staying obese.

A variety of psychosocial factors may contribute to the development and maintenance of obesity. Eating habits are primarily learned patterns of behavior in response to hunger (a physiological sensation) and appetite (social and psychological cues). Some people manage negative feelings—such as anxiety, anger, and loneliness—by overeating. Others may view eating as a reward. These patterns may have been learned in childhood if parents used food as a way to decrease stress or reward good behavior. Because social events are frequently associated with food, some people make a connection between pleasure and eating—a connection that may predispose them to overeating. Increased caloric and fat intake and decreased physical activity also contribute to the rise in obesity.

Many researchers believe physiological factors are more significant than psychosocial factors. More than 200 genes have been identified that contribute to appetite, hunger, satiety, metabolism, fat storage, and activity tendencies. Recently, a gene for obesity, *ob*, and its protein product *leptin* were discovered. Leptin is produced in fat cells and travels to the brain, where it decreases appetite and increases metabolic rate. A hormone produced in the stomach called *ghrelin* boosts appetite. A competing hormone, *obestatin*, suppresses the appetite. Adoption, twin, and family studies note that obesity has a strong heritable component: 30% to 80% of variability in body weight or fat mass is genetically determined (Devlin et al., 2000).

In obese and nonobese people, the amount of *body fat* seems to be precisely regulated and maintained. This explains the difficulty most people have in changing the amount of their body fat. There is frequently no clear difference between the amount of food eaten by obese people and nonobese people. The belief that all obese people overeat is inaccurate and underlies many of our culture's negative stereotypes about obesity.

Weight gain is among the most problematic side effects of psychotropic medications and is one of the most frequent reasons individuals discontinue their medications. Weight gain is a side effect for all the antipsychotic agents, lithium and other mood stabilizers, and many of the antidepressants.

People who are 35% or more above ideal body weight are at high risk for developing a number of medical conditions. These include diabetes mellitus, hypertension, cardiovascular disease, hyperlipidemia, gallbladder disease, arthritis, polycystic ovary syndrome, sleep apnea, and complications of pregnancy. The risk of death is higher for women than men and higher for the young than the old (Eissa & Gunner, 2004).

Obesity is among the easiest of medical conditions to recognize and the most difficult to treat. A wide variety of treatment approaches have been tried. In all the approaches there is a general tendency to regain lost weight. At this point, preventing obesity is more effective than treating it.

BIOPSYCHOSOCIAL THEORIES

Although many clinical studies have been published, the literature on eating disorders shows no theoretic consensus on etiology and treatment. Psychoanalytic theory, family systems theory, cognitive/behavioral theories, sociocultural theories, and biologic theories all contribute to an understanding of the development and dynamics of eating disorders. Only by understanding the interrelatedness of the factors in eating disor-

MEDIALINK Application: Eating Disorders Can Be Prevented

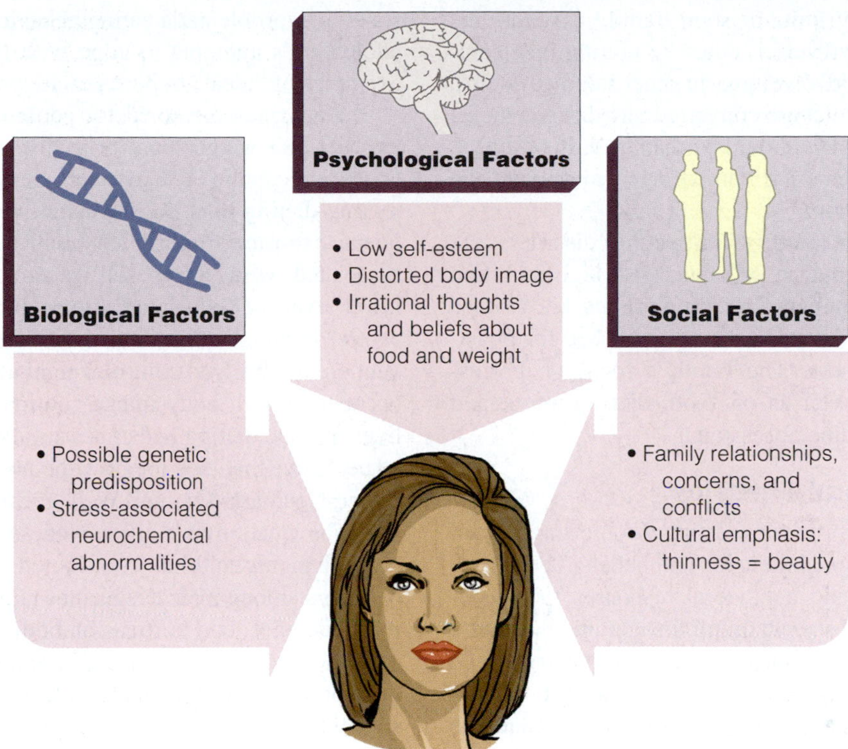

FIGURE 21-1 ■ Biopsychosocial factors in eating disorders. Nurses who understand the interplay among biopsychosocial factors involved in eating disorders are able to take a holistic approach to client care.

ders can psychiatric nurses take a holistic approach to the care of affected individuals and their families. The interrelationship among these biopsychosocial theories is illustrated in FIGURE 21-1 ■.

Psychoanalytic Theory

Since Freud first identified it as such, eating has been regarded as a critical aspect of psychological growth and development. An infant at the breast is already beginning to internalize a rudimentary understanding about life through the quality of the feeding experience.

Psychoanalytic theory considers eating disorders to be symptomatic of unconscious conflicts. Little attention is paid to biologic or cultural factors. Psychoanalytic theory relates eating disorders to regression to prepuberty and repudiation of developing sexuality. Anorexics are thought to fear sexual maturity; the anorexia is seen as a rejection of the feminine form and a desperate attempt to regain the contours and dimensions of a prepubertal child.

In psychoanalytic thinking, compulsive overeating represents overcompensation for unmet oral needs during infancy. In other words, people eat to compensate for emptiness in their lives. Obesity is also thought to represent a defense against intimacy with the opposite sex.

The basic treatment modality in the psychoanalytic model is long-term individual psychotherapy, sometimes accompanied by group therapy. The goal of therapy is the development of insight and subsequent "working through" of underlying issues to resolve the unconscious conflicts manifested by the eating disorder. There is little empirical evidence of the effectiveness of psychotherapy in the treatment of eating disorders (Kaplan, 2002). Promising new approaches include motivational enhancement therapy and psychotherapies aimed at relapse prevention.

Family Systems Theory

Most family theorists believe family issues are not specific to eating disorders. The family is viewed more as an enabler of the disorder than as a primary causative factor. Some people with eating disorders are survivors of childhood or adolescent sexual abuse, which may or may not have occurred within the family or extended family system.

As the result of anorexia, some families become enmeshed; that is, the boundaries between the members are weak, interactions are intense, dependency on one another is high, and autonomy is minimal. Everybody is involved in each member's concerns, and there is minimal privacy. The enmeshed family system becomes overprotective of the child, and the entire family system becomes preoccupied with food, eating, and rituals involving meals. In contrast, current research indicates that families of people with bulimia are less enmeshed than those of anorexic people. Family members tend to be isolated from one another, and eating behavior may be an attempt to decrease feelings of loneliness and boredom.

Many families of individuals with eating disorders have difficulty with conflict resolution. An ethical or religious value against disagreements within the family supports the avoidance of conflict. When problems are denied for the sake of family harmony, they cannot be resolved, and growth of the family system is inhibited. The anorexic child may protect and maintain the family unit. In some family systems, the parents avoid conflict with each other by uniting in a common concern for the child's welfare. In other family systems, the issues of marital conflict are converted into disagreements over how the anorexic child should be managed. In both systems, the marital problems are camouflaged to prevent the disruption of the family unit.

Many families of clients with eating disorders are achievement and performance oriented, with high ambition for the success of all members. In these families, body shape is related to success, and priorities are established for physical appearance and fitness. The family's focus on professional achievement as well as on food, diet, exercise, and weight control may become obsessional.

Cognitive Behavioral Theories

Cognitive behavioral theories view eating disorders as learned behaviors based on irrational thoughts and beliefs. They focus on changing cognitive and behavioral responses to physiologic, psychological, and social stimuli. Insight into the nature of the maladaptive behavior (the eating disorder) is integrated with new and healthier responses to emotional stimuli. Education about the psychology of compulsive behavior and the physiologic effects of starvation and purging behaviors is usually incorporated into the therapy. Other cognitive approaches include correction of perceptual disturbances of body size and elimination of irrational thoughts and beliefs linking weight to self-esteem, such as, "I've gained a pound; I must run 5 miles today and eat nothing," or "I'd rather be dead than fat."

Cognitive behavioral therapy has been found to be a successful treatment method for reducing the symptomatology associated with bulimia nervosa (Martin & Pear, 2007) and to result in more rapid treatment than with interpersonal psychotherapy (Ball & Bindler, 2006). These approaches are also useful in the treatment of binge-eating disorder (Ford, 2007).

Sociocultural Theory

In American society, female attractiveness is strongly equated with thinness. Models, actresses, and the media glamorize extreme thinness, which is then equated with success and happiness. The cultural obsession with an extremely thin female body has led to widespread prejudice against overweight people. This prejudice has a significant impact on overall self-esteem and self-acceptance. Self-worth is enhanced for those who are judged attractive and diminished for those deemed unattractive (Stein & Corte, 2003).

The status of American adolescent boys and girls among their peers is established through weight-related behaviors and cognitions (Wang, Houshyar, & Prinstein, 2006). Body size and dieting behaviors can determine popularity with peers. Having a heavier body shape was associated with lower popularity for females in this research. Adolescent males were less popular if they did not fit the male ideal in either direction—that is, if they were heavier and if they were not muscular or fit. When you consider how important peer relationships are at this stage of development, you can understand how problematic eating behaviors could result from the adolescent's attempts to cope with these pressures. Current examples of "ideal" body types are presented in FIGURE 21-2 ■.

Magazines marketed for adolescent women often present diet and weight control as the solutions for adolescent crises and contain 90% more articles and advertisements promoting dieting than do magazines read by young men. Frequent exposure to articles about dieting is significantly associated with lower self-esteem, depressed mood, and lower levels of body satisfaction. Thus, the body becomes the central focus of existence, and self-esteem becomes dependent on the ability to control weight and food intake. This preoccupation with body image continues throughout women's lives. In fact, dieting and concerns about weight have become so pervasive that they are now the norm for American women (Utter, Neumark-Sztainer, Wall, & Story, 2003).

The ideal of male attractiveness in American society has been changing and has contributed to an increase in eating disorders among men. Magazines targeted to a predominantly male audience tend to focus on body building, weight lifting, or muscle toning. The "ideal" male body is one with well-developed muscles on the chest, arms, and shoulders and a slim waist and hips. This ideal is becoming more and more difficult for the average boy or man to attain. Little boys are

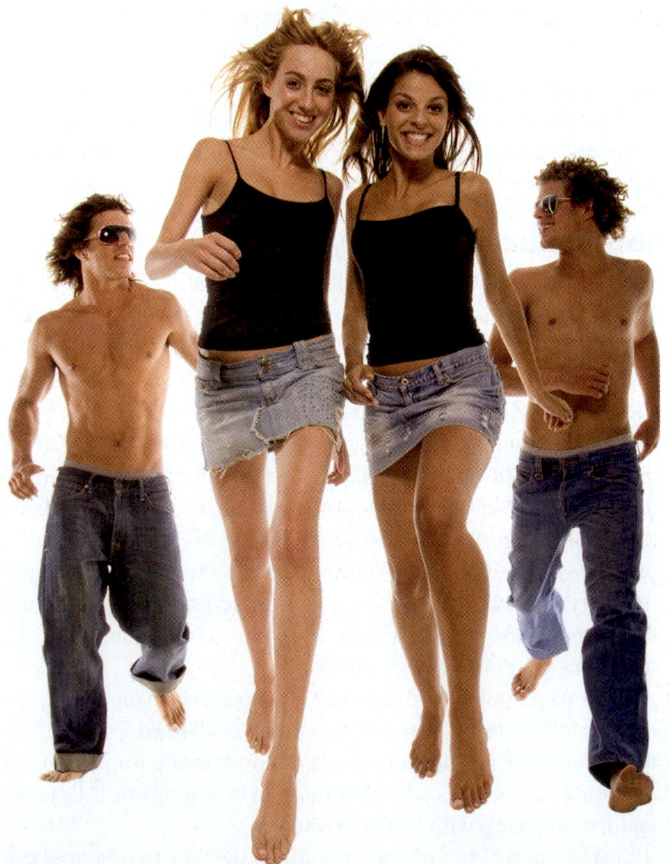

FIGURE 21-2 ■ Advertisements influence our views of attractiveness. The "ideal" female body is excessively thin. The "ideal" male body is well-toned with a slim waist and hips.

Source: Getty Images/Digital Vision, Win Initiative.

being taught to base their self-esteem on strength and athleticism. Their action toys have washboard abdominal muscles, and their heroes are members of World Wrestling Entertainment (WWE). Men with eating disorders have an overwhelming fear of fatness and a desire to maintain a masculine appearance or shape. It is not uncommon to see males with eating disorders use anabolic steroids to improve muscle tone and build strength (Keel, 2005).

Research has shown that a disproportionately high number of men with eating disorders are gay or bisexual. Much like expectations for women, within the gay male culture there are strong pressures on men to be physically attractive, thin, and youthful looking, especially among gay men whose social life is centered on the "gay scene"—clubbing, drinking, and similar activities. Less likely to be satisfied with their body weight and shape, gay men have an increased risk for developing anorexia or bulimia (Keel, 2005).

There is considerable evidence that eating disorders occur predominantly in industrialized, developed countries and less often in traditional societies. For example, Native Canadians (Ojibway-Cree) tend to show a preference for heavier body types than the Euro-Canadian population does. The incidence is changing, however, as cultures around the world become more Westernized. In a sense, anorexia and bulimia could be considered culture-reactive syndromes in the Western world (Keel, Baxter, Heatherton, & Joiner, 2007).

Eating disorders are not solely a problem of specific cultural groups, however. South Asian women were studied to determine the relationship between teasing about body size and subsequent maladaptive eating behavior (Reddy & Crowther, 2007). Study results indicated that negative body image and body dissatisfaction lead to problematic eating behaviors. It seems that, culture notwithstanding, negative interactions about body size can create stress and challenges that affect eating behaviors.

A surprising influence in a girl's vulnerability may be her ethnic background. Recent studies have found, for instance, that African-American women's perceptions of beauty are less media driven than those of Euro-American women. Dieting is less rampant, as are unhealthy weight management practices, and African-American teens may be more accepting of the way they look. African-American women and men are more positive about higher weights in women than are Euro-American women and men. African-American women who are obese have a more positive body image than their Euro-American counterparts. In the Caribbean island of Curacao, the incidence of anorexia among the majority Black population is zero, whereas the incidence among the minority mixed and White population is similar to that in the United States (Hoek et al., 2005; Striegel-Moore et al., 2003).

Typically, Asian-American and Latino women were less likely to describe themselves as fat, were less dissatisfied with their body size, and were less likely to diet. Recent research, however, indicates that a cultural shift is occurring. Asian-American and Latino women are becoming less satisfied with their bodies, and cultural media are presenting thin ideal body sizes for women, similar to those presented in the Anglo media.

Biologic Theory

Family risk studies show that relatives of clients with eating disorders are 5 to 10 times more likely to develop an eating disorder. It appears that in anorexia, the more severe the disorder, the more likely a strong genetic predisposition. Twin studies for anorexia show that the concordance rate for monozygotic twins is 55% to 71% and for dizygotic twins is 0% to 32%. These data suggest that there may be a genetic predisposition to anorexia. Concordance rates for bulimia range from 23% to 83% for monozygotic twins and 0% to 27% for dizygotic twins (Slof-Op't Landt et al., 2005).

Genetic research focuses on behavioral, neurobiological, and temperamental variables that may represent core features of these disorders. These features include perfectionism, orderliness, low tolerance for new situations, low self-esteem, and overall high anxiety. Even if an individual has a high genetic risk, however, he or she might develop an eating disorder even if he or she did not live in a culture that stresses dieting and thinness (Bulik, 2005).

Recent studies indicate that neurotransmitter dysregulation may be involved in eating disorders, particularly serotonin (5-HT). Being full of food to the point of satisfaction is referred to as *satiety*. Normally, a low level of 5-HT decreases a person's satiety and thereby increases food intake. In contrast, a high level of 5-HT increases satiety and thereby decreases food intake. Carbohydrates (CHOs) are involved in the synthesis of 5-HT by increasing tryptophan, the precursor of 5-HT. The neurotransmitter hypothesis of bulimia is that recurrent binge episodes may result from a deficiency in 5-HT and low satiety levels. The tendency of people with bulimia to binge on high-CHO foods may be a reflection of the body's adaptive attempt to increase 5-HT levels. The neurotransmitter hypothesis of anorexia is that decreased food intake is related to excess 5-HT and increased satiety (Romano, Halmi, Sarkar, Koke, & Lee, 2002).

The level of spontaneous physical activity appears to be related to energy expenditure and thus to body weight. Orexin neurons in the lateral hypothalamus appear to integrate this activity with feeding behavior (Kotz, 2006).

Other neurotransmitters affect eating behavior. Norepinephrine (NE) and neuropeptide Y (NPY) increase eating behavior, while dopamine (DA) suppresses food intake. DA agonists such as amphetamines and cocaine are appetite suppressants.

Endogenous opioids, such as endorphins, are associated with food intake and mood. Opioids increase food intake and enhance positive mood states; therefore, insufficient levels of endogenous opioids cause decreased food intake and depressed mood. It has been found that underweight people have significantly lower levels of endorphins compared to healthy volunteers. When the person's weight is returned to normal levels, the endorphin level is also within normal limits.

Neuroimaging studies have shown a low level of functioning in the frontal lobes, parietal lobes, and the anterior cingulate of individuals with anorexia and bulimia. When these individuals viewed high-calorie foods, they experienced abnormally increased activity in those same brain regions (Uher et al., 2004). In the future, research will undoubtedly lead to greater knowledge about the biology of eating disorders. But biologic factors, sociocultural factors, and intrapersonal or interpersonal conflicts cannot—and should not—be dealt with separately. The interaction of these factors is extremely important. For example, clients suffering from severe obesity may experience shame and helplessness as they attempt to cope with fears of rejection and loss of love. These feelings can lead to compensatory overeating, which in turn can create interpersonal conflict with family members. The client may withdraw from others, thus reinforcing the feelings of rejection and increasing social isolation.

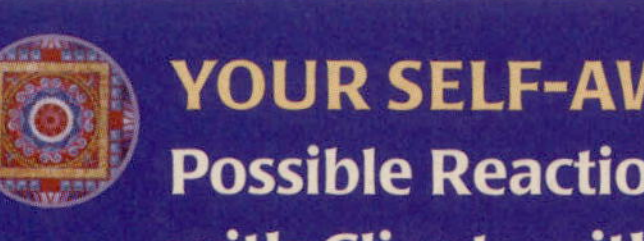

YOUR SELF-AWARENESS
Possible Reactions to Working with Clients with Eating Disorders

In order to explore your reactions to clients with eating disorders, determine which, if any, of the following apply to you.

- You feel exhausted and defeated by the structured demands of the client's care plan.
- You feel resentment at the client's efforts to manipulate and attempts at "staff splitting."
- You identify with the client because of your own personal body image concerns.
- You feel overprotective of the client and allow a coalition between yourself and the client to form.
- You feel annoyance and anger toward the client and are unnecessarily rough during physical care.
- You have difficulty recognizing that the client's symptoms are as serious as those of a hallucinating or delusional client.
- You fail to monitor the client's mealtime and after-meal behaviors, allowing the client to continue maladaptive patterns of coping.
- You allow the client to reenact power struggles from home, such as those about food, weight, and exercising.
- You believe that the client is deliberately engaging in maladaptive coping behaviors to upset the staff and family.
- You feel repelled by the client's eating habits or the appearance of the client's body.
- You feel hopeless and are affected by the client's despondency.

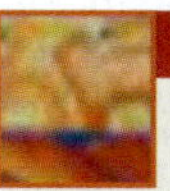

NURSING PROCESS
The Client with Anorexia Nervosa

The following section discusses the specific steps of the nursing process for clients with anorexia nervosa. Be aware of your own potential reactions to clients with eating disorders. Self-aware nurses recognize their own emotional reactions to clients and view clients' self-absorption and manipulativeness as symptoms of the disorder. The Your Self-Awareness feature will help you assess your reactions.

MEDIALINK Case Study: A Teen with Anorexia Nervosa

Assessment

When assessing clients with dramatic weight loss or gain, you must not lose sight of the fact that both can be caused by physical conditions. Certain illnesses must be ruled out before an eating disorder diagnosis can be made. Wasting conditions such as advanced cancer, tuberculosis, AIDS, hyperthyroidism, pyloric obstruction, and drug abuse must be considered when weight loss is a feature. Rapid weight gain can result from a brain tumor, an endocrine disorder, or as a side effect of medications. A good history and physical examination are often needed to provide information to eliminate the possibility of a physical basis for sudden weight loss or gain. After the presence of an eating disorder is established, you will assess the client using the following subjective and objective data.

Subjective Data

Clients with anorexia nervosa perceive themselves as overweight, no matter how thin they may be. However emaciated their bodies, they can always find some body part they believe is fat. They are preoccupied with thoughts of food and simultaneously obsessed with rigidly controlling their own intake. They often collect cookbooks, cook prodigious amounts of food, and insist that others eat while not taking a morsel for themselves. They are fearful of even the slightest weight gain and view with suspicion anyone who encourages them to eat.

Another preoccupation is with exercise. It is not uncommon for anorexics to engage in extremely lengthy sessions of aerobics or calisthenics, or to run, bike, or walk to excess, even when in an emaciated condition. They push themselves to greater and greater levels of endurance and deprive themselves of sleep as a measure of self-control.

Anorexics frequently deny that they have a weight problem. They insist they have never felt better and simply wish to be left alone about food. They report feeling strong, powerful, and good as a result of self-denial. They report feeling guilty, self-indulgent, and weak when they eat. They therefore resist treatment, although they may admit to feeling isolated and lonely and may even describe themselves as exhausted with the effort it takes to achieve the perfection they seek. They tend to have difficulty accepting nurturing behavior from others and therefore have difficulty forming therapeutic alliances. They report a loss of interest in sex but do not perceive this as a problem.

Objective Data

People with anorexia usually experience a weight loss of 25% but a loss as high as 50% is possible. Amenorrhea is extremely common and is thought to be related to the degree of stress the woman is experiencing, the percentage of body fat lost, and altered hypothalamic function. With low estrogen levels, these young women are at higher risk for osteopenia leading to osteoporosis. This is a serious medical complication with no known effective treatment.

The anorexic client is emaciated, with sunken eyes and a skeletal appearence. In very young clients, growth failure may be present. Lanugo growth (babylike, fine hair) on the face, extremities, and trunk may occur. Other physical symptoms include bradycardia, hypotension, arrhythmias, delayed gastric motility, and a hypothyroid-like state manifested by dry skin, listlessness, and dry hair that falls out at a higher-than-normal rate. Peripheral edema may be a feature in advanced starvation. Laboratory tests may reveal leukopenia, anemia, low serum potassium, and elevated blood urea nitrogen (BUN). There may also be low thyroid levels and elevated serum cortisol.

Nursing Diagnosis: NANDA

Once the assessment process is completed, determine appropriate nursing diagnoses.

Imbalanced Nutrition: Less than Body Requirements

By the time anorexic clients are seen in treatment, their physical condition is often so deteriorated from self-imposed starvation that it becomes the priority for nursing care. Life-threatening malnourishment is seen in 5% to 20% of these clients. Death may occur from malnutrition, infection, or cardiac abnormalities related to electrolyte imbalances. Intravenous therapy, tube feedings, and total parenteral hyperalimentation (TPH) are required in cases of medical emergency.

The client's preoccupation with food, evidenced by reading recipes, discussing food, and preparing food for others, is due to suppression and sublimation of the client's own hunger. Overexercising creates even more extreme nutritional deficits. In those anorexic clients who also purge by vomiting or using laxatives, nutritional status is further endangered.

Clients in a state of starvation experience hormonal, metabolic, and emotional changes. Some of those changes are manifested in amenorrhea or delay of onset of menses, ketosis, severe vitamin deficiencies, depressed immune response, lethargy, weakness, and irritability—conditions that also vitally affect nurse–client relationships.

Ineffective Individual Coping

Clients experiencing anorexia nervosa demonstrate impairment of adaptive behaviors, such as self-care in activities of daily living. They have difficulty meeting daily demands, and role performance may be affected. Their preoccupation with the pursuit of thinness deprives them of the energy necessary for adaptive behavior and distracts them from interest in role fulfillment. The quest for thinness is the entire focus of their lives.

In addition, developmental issues such as the desire for independence and the longing for dependence combine with traditionally adolescent resentment of authority to influence the quality and character of the nurse–client relationship. Family enmeshment and unwillingness to allow the client to separate contribute to self-doubt and the inability to accept responsibility for self.

Disturbed Body Image

Clients with anorexia nervosa are unable to make realistic appraisals of their own body size, although they can accurately evaluate the size of others. They drastically underestimate their own bodily needs, even in the face of overwhelming evidence of malnutrition. Profound disturbances in accurate perception of size and intense client denial indicate a poor prognosis. The client's body image disturbance is often the source of conflict in family and therapeutic relationships.

Chronic Low Self-Esteem

Anorexic clients' lack of confidence in themselves and feelings of inferiority are main factors in the disorder. Their self-deprivation and self-denial make them feel powerful and superior to others who cannot muster such profound self-control. The quest for perfection is never-ending, but they can never achieve a level of thinness that is satisfying; there are always a few more pounds to shed. They often present the picture of "model clients," in contrast to seemingly more disturbed clients. As a result, novice nurses may have difficulty assessing the severity of the illness accurately.

The low self-esteem of anorexic clients stems from unrealistic expectations by self and others, complicated by unmet dependency needs. The clinical picture is further complicated because cultural norms of thinness reinforce maladaptive behavior. The nurse–client relationship is affected by the extreme difficulty these clients have in accepting positive feedback and by their nonparticipation in self-care and therapeutic activities. Their preoccupation with their appearance and with others' perceptions of them may be irritating to other clients. The nurse–client relationship is also affected by the client's need to control, which often leads to manipulative behaviors.

Outcome Identification: NOC

Suggested outcomes for each NANDA diagnosis in the previous section follow.

Imbalanced Nutrition: Less than Body Requirements

This diagnosis inevitably leads to the desired outcome of improvement of Nutritional Status: Adequate nutrients taken into the body for height, frame, gender, and activity level.

Ineffective Individual Coping

Several NOC outcomes are relevant to anorexic clients with this nursing diagnosis. They include Coping: Actions to manage stressors that tax an individual's resources; Impulse Control: Ability to self-restrain compulsive or impulsive behavior; and Information Processing: Ability to acquire, organize, and use information.

Disturbed Body Image

For the anorexic client, who invariably has a distorted body image, NOC outcomes include Body Image: Positive perception of own appearance; and Distorted Thought Control: Ability to self-restrain altered perceptions.

Chronic Low Self-Esteem

As in many psychiatric disorders, low self-esteem plays a major role in anorexia nervosa, leading to the NOC outcome of Self-Esteem: Personal judgment of self-worth.

Planning and Implementation: NIC

When a client's behavior meets the criteria for a diagnosis of anorexia nervosa, effective nursing intervention is directed toward ensuring that the client will not die and helping the client learn more effective ways of coping with the demands of life. A variety of approaches, including behavioral, insight-oriented, and cognitive therapies, may be useful; pharmacologic therapy may be used also. As a feature of behavioral therapy, a behavioral contract can be very effective. An explanation of how to develop and use behavioral contracts is in Chapter 31 ∞.

Symptoms can be extreme and dangerous with this disorder. Protection and improvement may require more intensive and constant treatment. In severely debilitated clients, inpatient treatment is indicated. Box 21-1 lists behavioral characteristics that indicate the need for hospitalization. Recovery from eating disorders is a long process. Individuals with anorexia are ambivalent about treatment and often terminate treatment early. Symptoms correlated with early termination include higher levels of weight concerns, greater maturity fears, and impulsivity. For those who continue treatment, about 40% recover and the rest experience a chronic course, some with fewer symptoms and some with the same symptoms (Finfgeld, 2002; Woodside, Carter, & Blackmore, 2004).

Managing Nutrition

To establish adequate eating patterns and fluid and electrolyte balance, assume a calm, matter-of-fact attitude and a positive expectation of the client. Meeting minimal nutritional goals, with the overall goal of gradual weight restoration, is nonnegotiable. A caloric intake of 1,200 to 1,500 cal/day is the usual range. Changing the eating pattern to a healthier one (called refeeding) involves timing, education, and reinforcement. The Your Intervention Strategies feature lists guidelines for refeeding.

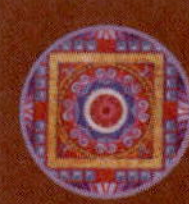

YOUR INTERVENTION STRATEGIES
Guidelines for Refeeding

Strategy	Rationale
■ Validate the client's fears of weight gain.	■ Reassures the client that fears are expected and not unique.
■ Collaborate with the client and dietitian to plan a flexible refeeding program for gradual weight gain.	■ Enlists the client as an active participant in treatment.
■ Adopt a matter-of-fact, consistent, and nonjudgmental attitude.	■ Conveys your confidence and acceptance of the client.
■ Contract with the client for food and fluid intake adequate to meet the weight-restoration goal.	■ Meets the client's need for structure and control.
■ Support the client during refeeding sensations of fullness and bloating; teach that these are normal and transient feelings.	■ The client's gastrointestinal tract must readjust to unaccustomed intake.
■ Encourage the expression of feelings of loss of control.	■ Upon resuming adequate intake, clients fear "losing control" and "becoming fat."
■ Monitor fluid and electrolyte intake and output, vital signs, body temperature, and mood.	■ Refeeding may precipitate both psychologic and metabolic emergencies. Monitor both physiologic and psychologic effects.

Source: Love, C. C., & Seaton, H. (1991). Eating Disorders: Highlights of nursing assessment and therapeutics. *Nursing Clinics of North America, 26*(3), 687. With permission from Elsevier Science.

Box 21-1 Criteria for Inpatient Admission

Inpatient admission is recommended for eating disordered clients who have:

- Suicidal or severely out of control behavior (self-mutilating; abusing large amounts of laxatives, emetics, and diuretics; abusing street drugs)
- Loss of 25–30% of body weight, resulting in severe emaciation
- Cardiac arrhythmias
- Fluid and electrolyte imbalances
- The need for more intensive inpatient contacts and therapy if outpatient treatment has proved insufficient
- The need for extensive diagnostic evaluation to rule out comorbidities

Nursing interventions may include tube feedings or intravenous therapy, which are administered in a nonjudgmental manner. Weighing the client daily, recording intake and output, observing the client during meals, and observing bathroom behavior may be necessary if you suspect the client is discarding food or inducing vomiting. Avoid discussing food, recipes, restaurants, and eating with the client because these conversations reinforce maladaptive behaviors. Providing a pleasant mealtime environment and adopting realistic expectations of how much the client will eat are critically important aspects of nursing care. Clients find frequent small meals more acceptable than three large meals. Setting a time limit of about a half hour is a good way to forestall mealtime "marathons"—protracted meals during which the client eats little.

Mandatory tube feedings, a controversial intervention, may be the therapeutic regimen in some treatment centers. Although tube feedings will manage a dangerously low weight with perilously disordered electrolytes, tube feedings have a conditioned effect that must be taken into account. (See Chapter 31 on the therapeutic resonance of conditioned responses.) Tube feedings do give a message—that is, taking in calories through food is beneficial to overall health. On the other hand, tube feedings can also deliver the message that the problem is too severe for the client to overcome with voluntary action. This message can be demoralizing to the client and may be further amplified by negative associations with treatment providers because of the unpleasant aspects of the experience.

Acknowledge and recognize the efforts of clients who meet weight gain goals, but avoid praise or flattery. Education about adequate eating patterns is a necessary part of discharge planning.

Consistency and coordination among staff members are essential to avoid manipulation by clients. Interdisciplinary planning conferences and adherence to written care plans promote effective care. Behavior modification programs, which base privileges on weight gain, may be useful for focusing on emotional issues, not just eating behaviors. You and the client may engage in a contract for weight gain, such as the one in FIGURE 21-3 ■.

A target weight is usually chosen by the treatment team in collaboration with a dietitian. Target weight for discharge from treatment is usually 90% of average for age and height.

Date: ____________________

Client's Name: ______________________________ Age: ____________

Height: ____________ Weight: ____________ Goal Weight (range): ____________

1. You will be weighed: ____ daily ____twice a week ____weekly

upon arising and after voiding while wearing nightclothes. You should not eat or drink prior to weighing.

Frequency of weighing will change as you progress.

2. No exercising, jogging, or calisthenics are to be done without approval by your treatment team. As you progress, this privilege may be gradually reinstated.

3. Nutritional supplements will be required until made optional by your treatment team.

You will drink ____ cans of supplement per day if your weight gain is less than 1/4 pound over your last highest weight.

You will drink ____ cans of supplement per day if your weight gain is more than 1/4 pound over your last highest weight.

You will drink the nutritional supplement under nursing supervision at regular medication times of:

__________________________. You will consume each can within 15 minutes.

4. Your privilege status will depend upon your progress in weight gain. Your treatment team has determined weights to be attained for privilege status:

1:1 monitoring status:	________ pounds		
Independent status:	________ pounds for	________	consecutive days
Buddy status:	________ pounds		
Pass status:	________ pounds for	________	consectuive days

5. Other issues:

I agree to abide by the provisions of this contract:

Signature of Client ______________________________

Signature of Treatment Team Leader ______________________________

FIGURE 21-3 ■ Sample contract for weight gain. A client contract for weight gain fosters client self-responsibility and nurse–client collaboration.

MEDIALINK Critical Thinking Exercise: The Client with a Feeding Tube

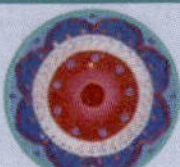

PARTNERING WITH CLIENTS AND FAMILIES

TEACHING ABOUT EATING DISORDERS

Friends and family members of people with eating disorders are often at a loss as to how to help. Heather L. Howard, former administrator for the National Association of Anorexia Nervosa and Associated Disorders (ANAD), recommends the following guidelines:

- Accept that there are no quick and easy solutions. Attitudes and behaviors must change.
- Change takes time and requires the cooperation of the person with the disorder.
- Family and friends must also change to accommodate the person's growth.
- Cooperate fully with the person's therapist.
- Avoid arguments about weight and food.
- Express love and affection both verbally and physically.
- Admit your anger, frustration, helplessness, and powerlessness and help the person see that these feelings do not mean you don't love him/her.
- Do things with the person that do not involve food.
- Don't diet yourself or talk about food, calories, fat grams, and the like.
- Avoid power struggles.
- Recognize that the person will make progress, then retreat into rituals for a time.
- Learn all you can about the disorder (see resource list).
- If the person will not seek help, CONFRONT in the following way:

  Concern—The reason you are confronting is that you care about the person.

  Organize—Decide who will be involved, when and where the confrontation will occur, and what to say.

  Needs—What resources will be needed after the confrontation? Therapist or support group; other resources.

  Face—Face the actual confrontation. Be direct; do not back down if the person angrily denies having a problem.

  Respond—Respond after listening carefully.

  Offer—Offer help and suggestions; offer yourself as a sounding-board.

  Negotiate—Negotiate another time to talk and set a time frame for the person to seek professional help.

  Time—Time to begin work. Remember to stress that recovery takes time and patience but that it is time to begin the process. There is much to be gained by seeking help and much to lose if the behaviors continue.

Resources*

Anorexia Nervosa and Related Eating Disorders
P.O. Box 5102
Eugene, OR 97405
503–344–1144
www.anred.com

National Association of Anorexia Nervosa and Associated Disorders
P.O. Box 7
Highland Park, IL 60035
847–831–3438
www.anad.org

National Eating Disorders Association
603 Steward St., Suite 803
Seattle, WA 98101
206–382–3587
www.nationaleatingdisorders.org

Office on Women's Health
200 Independence Avenue SW, Room 730B
Washington, DC 20201
202–690–7650
www.4woman.gov/bodyimage

Weight-Control Information Network (WIN)
1 Win Way
Bethesda, MD 20892–3665
877–946–4627
http://win.niddk.nih.gov/index.htm

Source: Heather L. Howard, former administrator, National Association of Anorexia Nervosa and Associated Disorders (ANAD). Retrieved September 11, 2007, from www.anad.org.

*These resources can be found on the Companion Website for this book.

MEDIALINK Self-Help Groups

Discharge planning can include referral to self-help groups such as the American Anorexia/Bulimia Association, Anorexia Nervosa and Related Eating Disorders, and National Association of Anorexia Nervosa and Associated Disorders. The websites for these self-help groups are included in the Partnering with Clients and Families feature. These resources can be accessed through links on the Companion Website for this book.

Facilitating Coping

The best way to promote individual coping is by involving clients in their own treatment planning. Self-determination fosters adaptive coping mechanisms in clients' day-to-day hospital experiences; this process carries over to daily life outside the hospital setting and helps clients meet its demands.

Although trust is difficult to establish with anorexic clients, it is the basis for all therapeutic relationships. Being honest, available, and matter-of-fact helps establish trust and encourages clients to express their feelings. If necessary, allow clients to assume a dependent role at first, but as trust is developed and physical condition improves, encourage them to take more responsibility for themselves. Participating in the planning of care gives clients opportunities to practice making decisions. Letting clients have input into their treatment plans also fosters adherence. Provide flexibility in activities of daily living, type and timing of exercise, and choice of occupational and recreational therapy activities. This autonomy increases clients' sense of responsibility for themselves.

Giving clients the opportunity to practice problem solving may lead to power struggles if you disagree with clients' choices. Demonstrate positive belief in their ability to regain healthy functioning and a willingness to tolerate "mistakes." The treatment team must set firm and clear limits, however, to provide the secure environment clients need to learn more effective coping behaviors. Also help clients identify ways to feel in control by other than anorexic and manipulative behaviors.

Clients need to explore their extreme fears of gaining weight before they can relinquish maladaptive behaviors. It is helpful to explore with clients their feelings about their family, their role in the family, and their autonomy within the family system.

Enhancing Body Image

To help clients regain an accurate perception of their body size and nutritional needs, first encourage them to express feelings about body size. An example is shown in the Rx Communication feature below. Reframe clients' misperceptions by using language that emphasizes health, strength, and evaluation. For example, if the client says "My thighs are huge," reply "Your thighs are becoming stronger now that you're gaining weight. Healthy muscles are rounded and firm, like yours." With practice, clients can replace negative thinking with positive self-talk. Teach and reinforce this skill, and help them practice it. For example, ask clients to make three positive statements (positive affirmations) about their bodies each day.

If clients are unable or unwilling to discuss their feelings about body size, ask them to draw themselves as they are now and as they desire to be. These drawings not only focus the discussion of body size and nutritional needs but also help you understand how clients view their bodies. Because clients with bulimia nervosa and compulsive overeating also have distorted body images, this activity can be incorporated into their plans of care as well. You could also use a more structured tool such as the one illustrated in FIGURE 21-4 ■ on page 564. In addition, BodyImage, a software program for the assessment of body image disturbance, can be accessed through a link on the Companion Website for this book.

MEDIALINK BodyImage

When clients share feelings honestly, show improvement in accurate perception of body image, or demonstrate healthier eating behaviors, reinforce their efforts through verbal recognition. It is also useful to examine with clients the ways in which the fashion and advertising industries support unrealistic cultural norms of excessive thinness incompatible with healthy functioning.

Improving Self-Esteem

Help clients reexamine negative feelings about themselves and identify their positive attributes. Encourage clients to record in a diary those thoughts that are difficult to share directly. Be nonjudgmental in your acceptance of negative feelings and positively reinforce the honest expression of all feelings. Encouragement is particularly important when clients experiment with independently made decisions, even when outcomes are not entirely positive. The client needs to interpret each experience as worthwhile. Emphasize the feeling of control gained through independent decision making.

Together, you and the client explore the client's attempt to achieve perfection by controlling weight. The idea is for the client to realize that perfection is an unrealistic goal. You are a role model for the person who accepts imperfection yet retains self-esteem. One way to model strong self-esteem is to admit errors willingly. Also model appropriate expressions of anger and teach clients the destructive effects of unexpressed anger.

Evaluation

Evaluation of the effectiveness of nursing interventions with these disorders is an ongoing part of the nursing process.

Nutritional Status

Clients will regain and maintain at least 90% of normal weight for their height and age. Clients will follow eating patterns that demonstrate they recognize the importance of adequate nutrition. They will regain and maintain normal elimination patterns, vital signs, fluid and electrolyte balance, and muscle tone. Female clients will have normal menstrual cycles.

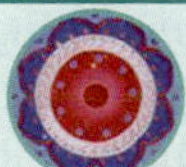

RX COMMUNICATION

CLIENT WITH ANOREXIA NERVOSA

CLIENT: [Tearfully] "My doctor says I have to eat and gain weight but I still have this little fat tummy."

NURSE RESPONSE 1: "Tell me what you are feeling right now."

RATIONALE: Asking the client to focus on her feelings assists her in becoming more self-aware. Obtaining additional subjective data from the client enables you to better understand her.

NURSE RESPONSE 2: "It sounds as though you feel caught in the middle of the doctor's expectations and your own."

RATIONALE: Nonjudgmental acknowledgement of the client's conflict shows empathy and encourages her to clarify the dilemma from her doctor's point of view as well as her own. Avoids directly challenging the client's distorted perception of her body image.°

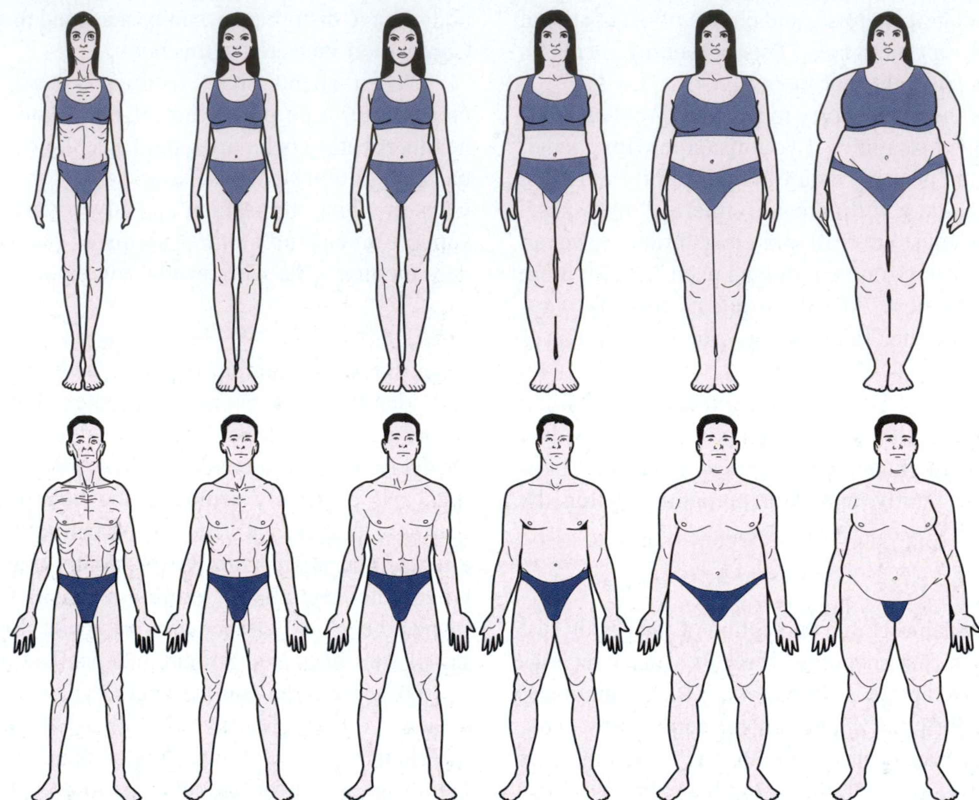

FIGURE 21-4 ■ Assessing body image. A drawing such as this can be used in several ways: (1) Clients can be asked which image best represents them. This assesses the accuracy of the client's body image. Anorexic clients often believe themselves to be larger than they really are. (2) Clients can be asked which image best represents the ideal for them. This assesses whether a client has a positive (image is similar to the client's own body) or a negative (dissimilar image) body image.

Coping

Clients will demonstrate effective coping when they participate actively in treatment planning and discharge planning using problem-solving skills. They will demonstrate interest and competence in self-care activities such as hygiene, sleep, activity, rest, diversional activities, and nutrition. They will accurately identify both maladaptive coping behaviors and adaptive coping behaviors that can be integrated into daily routines. Clients will express less anxiety about weight gain and will verbalize other means of feeling in control of their lives.

Body Image

Body image disturbance will have been alleviated when clients accurately assess their own body size and nutritional needs. They will use criteria such as strength and health, rather than appearance alone, to evaluate body size. They will verbalize less preoccupation with body size. Clients will verbalize positive statements about their own bodies.

Self-Esteem

Clients will demonstrate self-esteem when they verbalize their own positive attributes. They will demonstrate less preoccupation with their own appearance and will focus increasingly on others. They will accept compliments and positive feedback and show greater interest in activities around them. They will verbalize that perfection is an unrealistic life goal. Clients will express anger appropriately without experiencing incapacitating guilt. They will demonstrate interpersonal relationships substantially free of manipulation. Clients will work toward success experiences in work, school, and/or social groups.

CASE MANAGEMENT

Case managers working with clients who have eating disorders must understand the risk factors and possible complications of these disorders. This awareness enables the case manager to recognize symptoms early, mobilize the treatment team and family resources, ensure a smooth transition to inpatient therapy if needed, and ensure adequate follow-up. Failure to respond to treatment occurs in about 50% of cases.

Desired case management outcomes include weight gain/loss, normalization of exercise periods, cessation of binge eating and purging behaviors, and decreased preoccupation with food and body size. Avoidance of hospitalization or the briefest possible hospital stay is a case management priority.

The ultimate case management goal is early detection of symptoms, effective symptom reduction, and rapid return to maximal premorbid function. Despite the best efforts, about half of clients with eating disorders progress from acute to chronic illness, which presents them, their families, and case managers with lifelong challenges.

COMMUNITY-BASED CARE

Although many, if not most, clients with bulimia nervosa and binge-eating disorder can be safely treated in community-based settings, severely anorexic clients usually are admitted to an inpatient program. There are residential treatment facilities for longer-term care of approximately 3 months. Day hospitals are another option. Criteria for hospitalization are found in Box 21-1 on page 560. Nurses in community-based settings, such as school nurses, occupational health nurses, and nurses in doctors' offices, play a major role in recognizing symptoms of eating disorders; providing screening, information, and support to clients and families; and referring clients for specialized treatment. Eating disorders are not self-limiting and specialized care is required.

Prevention of eating disorders is receiving increased attention as an appropriate and much-needed focus for community-based nurses, particularly those in schools. Due to the early onset of anorexic thinking, education programs as early as grade school should be developed. Eating disorders have become more commonly recognized and, to some extent, normalized. The media have contributed to the idea that the ideal body shape is slimness to the point of extreme thinness. Most recently, the media have called the public's attention to eating-disordered public figures (especially in the entertainment field), thus influencing the public's perception of the illness and the community reaction to treatment and relapse.

Nurses in community-based settings can play a valuable role in the education, support, and referral of clients and their families, often enabling clients to remain in the community while in treatment.

HOME CARE

Historically, clients with eating disorders were isolated from their families during treatment. It was thought that ongoing family conflict would jeopardize their recovery. This approach has been challenged, and attitudes toward home-based care are gradually changing. Having a therapeutic alliance with clients and parents is an important aspect of recovery. Some studies have found that increasing family involvement and integration into the treatment program contributes to improved outcomes (Hillege, Beale, & McMaster, 2006).

Just as it is important that families are aware of the helpful websites discussed earlier, it is vital for the family to be aware of Internet websites that are pro-anorexia and promote treatment sabotage. These websites contain information that promote and support anorexia. Content includes lifestyle descriptions, inspirational photos that serve as motivators for weight loss, and "tips and tricks" on being anorexic. Using the information on these websites disrupts the healing process.

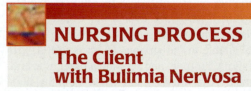

NURSING PROCESS
The Client with Bulimia Nervosa

The following section discusses the nursing process for clients with bulimia nervosa. Since some clients with bulimia may also be anorexic, refer also to the earlier nursing process section on pages 558–564.

Assessment

Although the two disorders are described separately, the boundary between anorexia and bulimia is blurred. Many bulimics were formerly anorexic, while others may become people with anorexia in the future. It is estimated that as many as half of all people with anorexia binge and purge at some time during their illness. During the assessment phase of the nursing process, keep in mind that these two conditions, although distinctly different, often coexist.

Subjective Data

Clients with bulimia nervosa have feelings of low self-esteem, worthlessness, inadequacy, and guilt. They experience shame and embarrassment over their secret binges (eating several quarts of ice cream, buckets of popcorn, or eight or more candy bars is not unusual) and subsequent purging activities. This shame may be manifested in self-deprecating remarks. Clients report feeling out of control, but at the same time they feel an excessive need to control. Unlike anorexics, clients with bulimia nervosa recognize that their eating behaviors are abnormal and bizarre.

Anxiety and unsatisfactory interpersonal relationships are features of this disorder. Anxiety is intensified when others see the bulimic as successful and in control, and they often appear so to others. They are impulsive and cannot delay gratification. Preoccupation with food, weight, and dieting is a prominent feature. Bulimic clients may report feeling weak and lethargic.

Objective Data

Like anorexic clients, bulimic clients tend to be young females. Bulimia first manifests itself later than anorexia, typically during late adolescence or young adulthood. Clients with bulimia are usually of normal or slightly above-average weight. Appearance does not provide diagnostic clues; hence the term *normal-weight bulimic*. Weight tends to fluctuate but does not become dangerously low unless anorexia occurs concurrently.

Clients with bulimia nervosa are more outgoing than those with anorexia and tend to be more comfortable with sexual relationships. They sometimes manifest impulsive behaviors such as substance abuse, shoplifting, and self-inflicted injury. In inpatient settings, they may steal others' food and hoard food in their rooms.

Physical signs of bulimia nervosa include hoarseness and esophagitis, dental enamel erosion, enlarged parotid glands, abrasions or calluses on knuckles from inducing vomiting, and amenorrhea in about 40% of cases. The client may also have symptoms of fluid volume deficit: concentrated urine, decreased urine output, hypotension, elevated temperature, poor skin turgor, and weakness.

Laboratory tests may reveal electrolyte abnormalities, particularly low serum potassium. Potentially fatal cardiac arrythmias may result. The overuse of Syrup of Ipecac, an emetic agent, can create cumulative systemic toxicity affecting the gastrointestinal, neuromuscular, and cardiovascular systems, potentially leading to death from cardiotoxicity.

Another concern is the fact that the frequency of bulimia in diabetics is increasing, particularly among young women. This is a potentially deadly combination because binge eating and purging increase the risk for both hypoglycemic episodes and diabetic ketoacidosis (DKA). Closely monitoring blood glucose levels is indicated for these clients.

Nursing Diagnosis: NANDA

Four major nursing diagnoses for clients with bulimia are discussed next.

Anxiety

Clients with bulimia nervosa experience anxiety: vague, uneasy feelings of moderate to intense severity related to preoccupation with body image. A rise in the client's anxiety level is usually a forerunner of binge/purge behaviors and may lead to purchasing or hoarding food in preparation for a binge.

Deficient Fluid Volume

Depletion of body fluids in clients with bulimia nervosa is usually related to self-induced vomiting and the excessive use of laxatives and diuretics, combined with decreased fluid intake. Extreme dehydration may lead to changes in electrolyte balance, causing altered mental status. Lethargy and confusion are symptoms of advanced dehydration. Edema may also be present.

Ineffective Individual Coping

Binge and purge behaviors are ineffective ways to cope with the stresses of life. Other impulse control problems, such as alcohol abuse, drug abuse, and shoplifting, are equally ineffective ways to reduce stress. The bulimic client's ineffective coping is related to issues such as independence/dependence, identity, and self-determination. Ineffective coping is manifested in the bulimic client's preoccupation with body size, poor self-esteem, distorted body image, and excessive overeating followed by purging.

Compromised Family Coping

The families of clients with bulimia nervosa perceive themselves as unable to deal effectively with the client's eating disorder related to the family's distorted perceptions of the problem. Parents may have difficulty allowing the client to grow up and may be overprotective; at the same time, they may have overly high expectations of the client. The bulimic client's behavior may become the family's focus, preventing the fulfillment of essential family roles. If disruption is extreme, the family may not be able to interact effectively with the larger community. Usual problem-solving methods are only partially adequate to deal with the stress of having a bulimic family member.

Outcome Identification: NOC

Suggested outcomes for each NANDA diagnosis in the previous section follow.

Anxiety

Desired outcomes related to anxiety in bulimic clients may involve Coping: Actions to manage stressors that tax an individual's resources; and Impulse Control: Ability to self-restrain compulsive or impulsive behavior.

Deficient Fluid Volume

Two nursing outcomes that are useful with this nursing diagnosis are Electrolyte and Acid–Base Balance: Balance of electrolytes and nonelectrolytes in the intracellular and extracellular compartments of the body; and Hydration: Amount of water in the intracellular and extracellular compartments of the body.

Ineffective Individual Coping

Similar to the anorexic client, several NOC outcomes are relevant to bulimic clients with this nursing diagnosis. They include Coping: Actions to manage stressors that tax an individual's resources; Impulse Control: Ability to self-restrain compulsive or impulsive behavior; and Information Processing: Ability to acquire, organize, and use information.

Compromised Family Coping

NOC outcome statements relevant to the NANDA diagnosis of Compromised Family Coping have not yet been developed. Appropriate outcomes might include those related to improving family communication, reducing family stress, learning developmental needs of family members, and seeking community resources.

Planning and Implementation: NIC

Several nursing interventions have been somewhat useful in treating bulimia nervosa.

Managing Medication

Medications, primarily antidepressants, are used to reduce the frequency of disturbed eating behaviors such as binge eating and vomiting. In addition, medications are used to ease symptoms that may accompany eating disorders such as depression, anxiety, obsessions, or impulse control problems.

Fluoxetine (Prozac), an SSRI, is effective for clients with bulimia when given at the higher dose of 50 to 60 mg per day. Typically, the medication is continued until 6 months following the disappearance of symptoms. In the past, tricyclic antidepressants have been used, but the dropout rate is higher than with the SSRIs (Bacaltchuk & Hay, 2003).

Reducing Anxiety

The goal of nursing interventions with anxious bulimic clients is to help them recognize events that create anxiety and to avoid binge eating and purging in response to anxiety. Initially, being available to the anxious client is useful. Project a calm, reassuring attitude, and provide a quiet, nonstimulating environment. After trust is established, help the client identify anxiety-producing situations. Clients experience anxiety as occurring "out of the blue" and are often unaware that

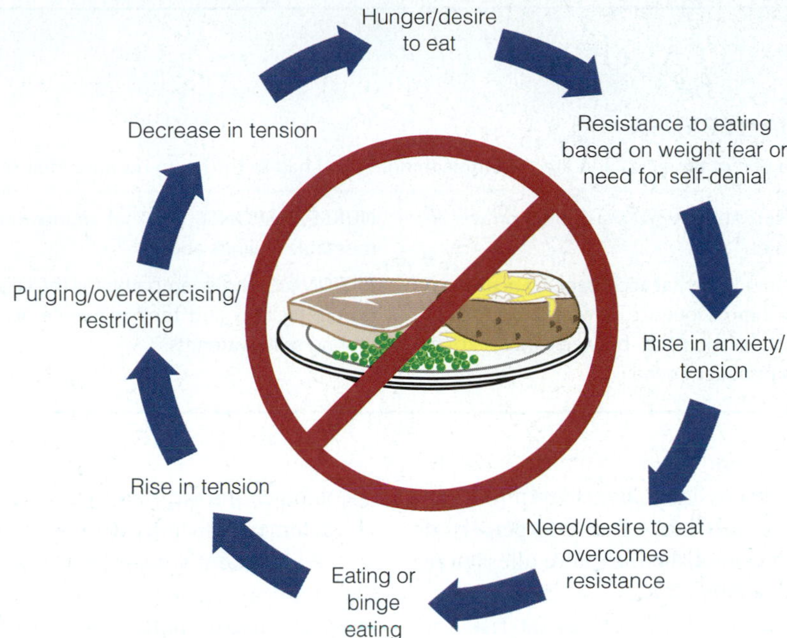

FIGURE 21-5 ■ A disordered eating cycle in bulimia nervosa. A nursing intervention to improve client self-awareness and anxiety reduction involves assisting clients to identify their personal eating cycle, which varies with the individual.

it is related to emotional issues and situations. Help clients identify previously used coping behaviors to determine whether they might be useful in current situations. How did the client handle anxiety before starting to binge and purge? Help bulimic clients identify feelings that precede binge/purge episodes such as those illustrated in FIGURE 21-5 ■, and explore healthier ways of dealing with those feelings.

Teach clients to recognize anxiety early, before it is severe, and to manage increasing anxiety. Energy-consuming activities, such as walking, running, and exercising, are useful but must be used very judiciously if the client's behavior includes overexercising. Clients can benefit from being taught progressive relaxation techniques and meditation (see Chapter 33). Administer antianxiety medications as ordered, but use caution because of the tendency to habituation. Also review the anxiety sections of Chapters 8 and 18.

Client contracts are useful with bulimic clients. The contract is jointly developed with the client and renegotiated at periodic intervals, depending on the client's goals, severity of symptoms, and compliance with the contract. Such a contract might include agreements about binge eating, vomiting, or hoarding food, such as those in the Your Intervention Strategies feature at right. Agreeing to a contract encourages clients to assume self-responsibility.

Managing Fluids and Electrolytes

The importance of accurate intake and output records cannot be overstated. Daily consumption of 2,000 to 3,000 mL of liquid promotes rehydration. Accurate daily weights are needed. Always weigh the client at the same time of day (immediately upon arising is preferred) and on the same scale. Assess and document the condition of the skin and oral mucous membranes as well as pulses and blood pressure daily, and monitor laboratory values, particularly urine specific gravity, reporting significant alterations to the physician. Observe clients for at least an hour after meals to prevent purging. To promote comfort in the dehydrated client, give frequent mouth care.

Facilitating Coping

Clients with bulimia nervosa can learn adaptive coping mechanisms to replace the out-of-control, binge/purge cycle. Once trust is developed, help the client plan and practice strategies for dealing effectively with intense feelings and the demands of daily living. It is important for clients to identify situations and patterns of events that precede binge/purge episodes. The following Rx Communication feature provides an example of

YOUR INTERVENTION STRATEGIES
Sample Contract for a Client with Bulimia

- I will sit at the nurses' station for a half hour following my meals.
- I will not vomit after my meals.
- I will not take laxatives or diuretics.
- I will not bring any such substances onto the unit.
- I will tell the nursing staff if I feel like binge eating.
- I will stay away from the kitchen if I feel like going on a binge.

Client ____________________
Nurse ____________________
Date ____________________

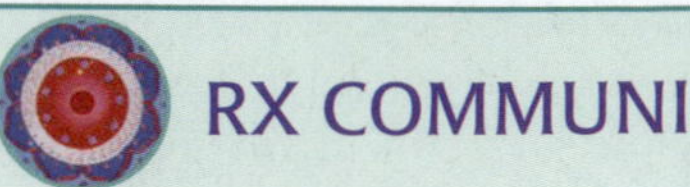

CLIENT WITH BULIMIA NERVOSA

CLIENT: "Last night I made a pan of brownies and ate the whole thing. Then I had to throw up because I felt so miserable."

NURSE RESPONSE 1: "Let's talk about what was going on yesterday before you ate the brownies." *RATIONALE:* Demonstrates nonjudgmental acceptance. Encourages the client to place events in time sequence. This enables her to connect the cause-and-effect relationship between her experiences, her feelings, and her subsequent behavior.	**NURSE RESPONSE 2:** "That sounds uncomfortable. What are the miserable feelings about?" *RATIONALE:* Shows empathy for the client. Encourages her to focus on her feelings and their influence on her behavior, thereby promoting self-awareness.

how you might open up the discussion. Clients learn to identify, name, and express feelings that they formerly perceived only as "bad." Once this is accomplished, explore alternative ways for clients to express those feelings.

Help clients identify times when they are at risk for binge eating and lack impulse control, such as when they are bored, frustrated, angry, lonely, or feeling unloved. Teach clients ways to nurture themselves during these times other than eating and purging. Suggest taking a warm bath, calling or visiting an old friend, or a hobby not involving food.

Clients with bulimia nervosa often perceive feelings of guilt and underlying resentment as overwhelming. They need to learn effective ways of expressing these feelings and assertiveness techniques to diminish guilty interactions in the future. Role-playing with the client helps the client practice assertiveness.

The worsening of both mood and bulimic symptoms during the winter has been reported in eating disorder literature with increasing frequency. Bright white light treatment has proven effective in treating bulimics with seasonal mood and symptom patterns. See Chapter 17 ∞ for a discussion of light treatment.

Involve the client in discharge planning. Topics covered in discharge planning include the productive use of time, identification of diversional activities not related to food, and participation in support groups.

Mobilizing the Family

Certain family dynamics reinforce maladaptive eating behaviors; therefore, families must also develop effective coping mechanisms to support the client's healthier coping behaviors. Assess the family's feelings and perceptions of the client's bulimia, listening carefully for what is most stressful and threatening to family members. Correct misperceptions about the disorder. Encourage family members to explore together their usual coping strategies, and determine if any previously used strategies can be useful in the present situation.

Help the family identify their strengths and weaknesses. Encourage family members to share their thoughts and feelings, including feelings of guilt, blame, and resentment, with one another and with the client. Teach family members to use "I" statements, thereby acknowledging their feelings.

If the client's disorder impairs family functioning, help the family reorganize roles to reduce stress and ensure that members' needs continue to be met during the client's recovery. Help the family understand that two normal developmental needs of adolescents and young adults are to develop autonomy and to establish identities outside the family. Make appropriate referrals to community resources, such as the American Anorexia/Bulimia Association, Anorexia Nervosa and Related Eating Disorders, and Anorexia Nervosa and Associated Disorders groups. (See Resources in the Partnering with Clients and Family feature on page 562.)

Home visits for an evening or weekend can help both the client and the family learn to use their new coping behaviors. Planning before visits and evaluating the success of visits afterward are essential parts of nurse–client and nurse–family interventions.

Evaluation

The evaluation process determines the effectiveness of the nursing interventions.

Anxiety

Clients will demonstrate anxiety control when they verbally identify situations and events that evoke anxiety. They will communicate needs and negative feelings appropriately. Clients will identify symptoms that indicate their own anxiety. They will identify ways of structuring the environment to prevent stressful situations that result in feeling out of control. Clients will eliminate binge/purge behaviors and demonstrate the use of anxiety-reduction strategies unrelated to eating. They will verbalize their acceptance of normal body weight without intense anxiety or will continue healthy eating patterns even though anxiety persists.

Fluid Volume

Dryness of oral mucosa and skin will not be evident. Skin turgor will be normal. Clients' vital signs and results of laboratory studies will be within normal limits. Input and output are balanced over 24-hour periods. Clients will verbalize their understanding of the relationship between dehydration and self-induced vomiting, laxative abuse, and diuretic abuse. Clients will verbalize understanding the physiologic and psychologic consequences of dehydration.

Individual Coping

Clients will demonstrate effective coping when they accurately assess maladaptive coping behaviors. They will demonstrate healthier ways to deal with stress and intense feelings. They will identify times of risk and verbalize alternative self-nurturing behaviors. They will demonstrate assertive communication techniques. Clients will demonstrate self-control in eating behaviors, gradually maintaining without supervision. They will verbalize increased self-confidence in the ability to handle the demands of daily life. They will follow through with recommended self-help or support groups and therapy following discharge.

Family Coping

Families will verbalize accurate perceptions of their situation. They will verbalize their feelings about having a family member with an eating disorder. They will acknowledge the needs of both the client and the family unit. They will identify useful strategies for coping with the impact of bulimia nervosa on the family. They will use "I" statements during communication with one another, the client, and the nurse. They will verbalize an understanding of the developmental needs of family members. They will use more flexible problem-solving strategies. The family will reorganize family roles as necessary. They will identify community resources available to them and will follow through on referrals.

For additional information about the nursing process with clients with bulimia nervosa, see the Nursing Care Plan at the end of the chapter.

CASE MANAGEMENT, COMMUNITY-BASED CARE, AND HOME CARE

Community-based care, case management, and home care for clients with eating disorders have been discussed earlier in this chapter. Refer to pages 564–565.

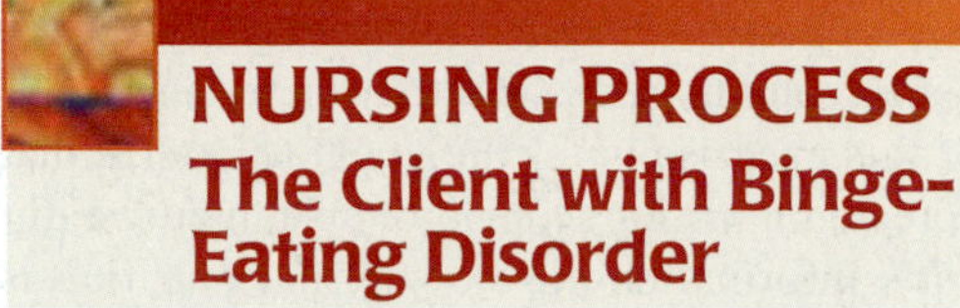

NURSING PROCESS The Client with Binge-Eating Disorder

The nursing process for clients with binge-eating disorder is discussed in the following section. See the Nursing Care Plan at the end of this chapter for a detailed view of this approach.

Assessment

The assessment of binge-eating disorder is not as straightforward as it might seem. Many obese individuals are apparently content and well adjusted. Do not assume that all obese people are emotionally distressed. The following discussion pertains to those clients who suffer psychologically from their excessive weight and who seek treatment for the resulting emotional pain.

Subjective Data

Clients with binge-eating disorder report that a rise in tension usually leads to impaired control over eating and precipitates binges. Types and sources of tension vary among individuals, but all report being significantly distressed by their binge eating. They describe eating large amounts of food rapidly, usually alone, due to embarrassment over their behavior (APA, 2000). They report feeling disgust, guilt, anger, depression, low self-esteem, and feelings of isolation during and after the binge. These feelings in turn create the desire to eat, and the pathologic cycle begins again. Most clients with binge-eating disorder report using food as a substitute for other forms of gratification such as companionship, attention from others, and emotional nurturing. They may also binge when happy or to reward themselves. These clients often report impaired social functioning, leading to withdrawal. Social isolation, however, only intensifies the obsessive preoccupation with food. Numerous attempts to lose weight are reported. Clients may describe a family history of marital conflict. Having one or more depressed parents is often reported.

Objective Data

Unlike anorexia and bulimia, which are found predominantly in women, binge-eating disorder is about equally prevalent in men and women. These clients are also older, averaging 40 years when seeking treatment, although they describe having started binge eating in their late teens or early twenties. Binge-eating disorder clients are almost universally obese, which is defined as having body weight that exceeds by 20% the recommended weight on standard height and weight tables. The binge eating occurs, on average, at least 2 days a week for at least 6 months (APA, 2000). Clients tend to be sedentary and have one or more obesity-related disorders including hypertension, shortness of breath, and palpitations upon exertion.

Be sure to obtain a medication history during assessment. A number of medications, including birth control pills, some antipsychotics, steroids, antidepressants, and antacids, may contribute to weight gain.

Nursing Diagnosis: NANDA

Several nursing diagnoses are appropriate for clients with binge-eating disorder.

Deficient Knowledge: Diet

Despite their preoccupation with food and eating, clients with binge-eating disorder often lack sufficient information about nutrition to make healthy decisions about diet. This knowledge deficit may be related to lack of interest, anxiety, denial of the need for information, confusion, misinformation, or other factors.

Evidence of deficient nutritional knowledge includes a history of nonadherence to dietary regimens, questions and statements indicating a lack of knowledge, misconceptions about the diet plan, and requests for information.

Imbalanced Nutrition: More than Body Requirements

The obese client's nutritional alteration is related to consuming more calories than required while expending few calories in exercise and activity. A sedentary lifestyle and occupation are common. Unhealthy eating patterns, such as night eating and binge eating, complicate the picture.

Recognize that the client's negative self-concept reinforces the desire for nurturance—that is, food—and that all negative feelings may be identified as hunger. These clients often ignore internal cues to hunger and eat in response to external cues, such as the time of day or stressful situations.

Obese clients with binge-eating disorder are vulnerable to a variety of weight-loss fads such as appetite suppressants, fad diets, and expensive "get-thin-quick" programs at diet centers. Some 95% of dieters are unsuccessful, and in general only 5% of obese individuals maintain a weight loss of at least 20 pounds for 2 years or more. The failure of these efforts leads to guilt and a sense of hopelessness about ever losing weight. Depression and loss of faith in self are common in obese clients.

Hopelessness

Clients who compulsively overeat frequently feel hopelessness related to their repeated failure to lose weight or to control their eating behavior. The inability to feel positive about their present life situation is manifested in a despondent and passive approach to living. Any effort seems too extreme; every task is too great. "What's the use?" is a question characteristically posed by hopeless clients.

Hopelessness is debilitating because clients cannot mobilize energy on their own behalf; nor do they believe that anyone else can help. Hopelessness is demonstrated by apathy and a lack of involvement in activities. Clients may lose interest in self-care activities. Oversleeping, decreased affect, and decreased response to stimuli are associated features. The speech of hopeless clients is filled with despondency. They may verbalize a loss of faith in God or another higher power.

MediaLink Care Plan: Binge-Eating Disorder

Social Isolation

The social isolation reported by clients is related to rejection by others or self-imposed withdrawal from social interaction because of self-consciousness and fear of rejection. Regardless of the cause of social isolation, the resulting alienation and loneliness increase the client's depression and preoccupation with food. Obese clients want to participate in social situations, but their negative past experiences have conditioned them to expect ridicule and rejection.

Outcome Identification: NOC

Suggested outcomes for each NANDA diagnosis in the previous section follow.

Deficient Knowledge: Diet

The desired outcome related to this diagnosis involves improvement of the extent of the client's understanding about diet.

Imbalanced Nutrition: More than Body Requirements

Clients with binge-eating disorder are nearly universally obese and often binge on easily consumed, high-calorie foods such as cookies, chips, and doughnuts. Outcomes relevant to this nursing diagnosis therefore include modifications in Nutritional Status: Food and Fluid Intake: Amount of food and fluids taken in a 24-hour period; and Nutritional Status: Nutrient Intake: Adequacy of nutrients taken into the body.

Hopelessness

Several outcomes are relevant to binge-eating disorder clients with the nursing diagnosis of Hopelessness. They include Hope: Presence of internal state of optimism that is personally satisfying and life supporting; Mood Equilibrium: Appropriate adjustment of prevailing emotional tone in response to circumstances; and Quality of Life: An individual's expressed satisfaction with current life circumstances.

Social Isolation

Isolation increases the preoccupation with food and the opportunities for binge eating. Therefore, NOC outcomes helpful to binge-eating disorder clients include Social Involvement: Frequency of an individual's social interactions with persons, groups, or organizations; and Social Support: Perceived availability and actual provision of reliable assistance from other persons.

Planning and Implementation: NIC

Several important nursing interventions for clients with binge-eating disorder are discussed next.

Providing Nutrition Education

Providing basic nutritional education is the goal of interventions with clients who have deficient knowledge in this area. First determine what knowledge or misconceptions the client has, and begin teaching at that level. Asking clients to write down and share with you the history of their numerous attempts to lose weight may be helpful. This provides an opportunity to establish rapport by demonstrating empathy for the anguish, helplessness, and hopelessness they experience.

The goal of this exercise is for the client to realize that dieting has not created a lasting change or sustained weight loss. If the client's information base of normal nutrition is minimal, begin by showing pictures of the basic food groups. Provide lists of foods in each group, and encourage the client to select favorite foods in each group. Discuss the body's need for proteins, carbohydrates, fats, vitamins, and minerals. Help the client plan a day's menus, keeping the client's food preferences in mind. This is also a good time to discuss cultural influences on food choices. Teach the client to analyze labels on prepared foods to determine foods with high nutrient value and reasonable caloric content. Supplement educational sessions with written materials the client can keep for later reference. Opportunities for teaching clients about nutrition can be used as a trust-building strategy.

Assisting with Nutrition Management and Weight Reduction

In planning interventions to help binge-eating disorder clients improve their nutritional status, collaborative goal setting is essential. The client must set a personal goal of controlling eating behaviors and establish a realistic weight loss goal. Help the client explore measures for changing eating habits. For instance, clients can keep a food diary to monitor the types and amounts of foods they eat. Slowing the rate of eating by chewing more thoroughly, placing implements on the plate between bites, conversing with table companions, and avoiding eating alone are helpful. Establishing a program of gradually increasing physical activity helps narrow the gap between caloric intake and energy expenditure.

Encourage clients to voice feelings, maintaining a calm and accepting attitude as they do. Help clients develop new, nonfood-related coping strategies for dealing with troublesome feelings.

Cognitive restructuring techniques, such as correcting clients' irrational beliefs, are helpful. Help the client practice replacing negative self-talk with positive self-talk. Affirming thoughts for compulsive overeaters are in Box 21-2. Cognitive restructuring techniques are discussed in greater detail in Chapter 31∞.

Give positive reinforcement and recognition when clients achieve any small weight loss. Do not allow small "slips" to assume major importance or impede steady progress. Teach the client how to select balanced, nutritionally sound meals when dining outside the home.

Provide information about community resources for exercise, such as the YMCA and YWCA. Make referrals to support groups and self-help groups, such as Overeaters Anonymous, Weight Watchers, and the National Association to Advance Fat Acceptance. Some support groups, such as Overeaters Anonymous, make use of sponsors for new members. Sponsors are individuals who are successfully coping with eating disorders and who can provide encouragement and support at difficult points in the recovery process. These individuals are a particularly valuable resource to people struggling to overcome reliance on compulsive overeating behaviors. Weight Watchers, an organization recommended by many health care professionals, provides healthful basic nutritional information, group support, and written educational materials that clients can use for reference. Resource links for these organizations can be accessed through the Companion Website of this book.

Box 21-2 Affirmations for Compulsive Overeaters

1. I cherish my mind, body, and spirit every day in every way.
2. My actions show that I care for myself and for my loved ones.
3. I encourage myself to grow as a kind and loving person.
4. I am honest with other people and true to myself.
5. My body is nourished and satisfied by moderate meals every day.
6. I know that my feelings guide me to my true self—therefore I tolerate them, welcome them, and think about them.
7. I am reliable and trustworthy, to myself and to others.
8. I am lovable as I am and deserve love and respect.
9. A mild level of anxiety stimulates my creativity.
10. I am honorable to myself by keeping my word to myself.

MEDIALINK Self-Help and Support Groups

Instilling Hope

Personal hygiene and good grooming promote a sense of well-being. Spending time conversing with clients at mealtimes can slow the eating process and demonstrate that change is possible. Assume an unhurried and caring attitude.

Unresponsive, apathetic clients become more responsive when exercise becomes part of their daily routine. Encourage daily exercise or activity.

Also encourage clients to express both positive and negative feelings as an important step toward accepting their feelings as valid. The following Rx Communication feature demonstrates how to encourage expression of feelings. Adopt

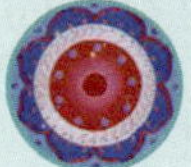

RX COMMUNICATION

CLIENT WITH BINGE-EATING DISORDER

CLIENT: "I hate the way I look now! I was a size 6 when I got married and now I wear a size 14!"

NURSE RESPONSE 1: "You sound upset. How are you feeling?"

RATIONALE: Shows empathy and nonjudgmental acceptance. Assists the client to become aware of her feelings and how feelings influence her behavior.

NURSE RESPONSE 2: "Give me an example of a time when you felt this way and what you did to feel better."

RATIONALE: Gathering more data from the client helps you understand her better. By asking her to describe a concrete incident you assist her to make connections between her feelings and her coping patterns. Fosters a nurse–client partnership to engage in problem solving.

an empathic, nonjudgmental attitude, and over time, help clients move from expressing feelings to exploring ways of coping other than by eating.

Attaining an intellectual understanding of one's condition promotes hope and a sense of control. Helping compulsive overeaters learn to feel and respond to their internal body cues, particularly cues to hunger and satisfaction, is essential. This is a lengthy process that requires external support and inward self-examination. The purpose of the extra weight also must be explored. What protective function does being fat provide? The advantages and disadvantages of being both overweight and having normal weight should be examined. Keeping a diary or journal may be helpful to clients as they struggle to experience and express their feelings without the numbing effect of overeating.

Visualization and guided imagery are useful with clients who feel hopeless (see Chapter 33∞). Encourage them to focus on happy experiences from the past and to envision themselves as they wish to be—healthy, energetic, and filled with vitality. Reinforce any expression of hopefulness, no matter how tentative.

Enhancing Socialization

For the socially isolated client, the goal of nursing interventions is to increase time voluntarily spent in group settings. The first step is to offer companionship; just sitting quietly with the client while making no demands for interaction signifies your acceptance. Frequent, brief contacts indicate interest and foster the development of a therapeutic nurse–client relationship. Next, engage the socially isolated client in a noncompetitive one-to-one activity, such as working on a jigsaw puzzle. After the client feels comfortable during one-to-one activities, offer to accompany the client to a group activity. Help the client plan ahead, making sure the client realizes that leaving is okay if anxiety becomes too high. Positively reinforce any amount of time in groups, however brief.

As the client becomes more comfortable in groups, withdraw gradually, but remain available. Role-playing social skills helps clients increase their repertoire of socially acceptable behaviors. Teach assertiveness techniques (see Chapter 3∞), because both passivity and aggressiveness invite rejection by others.

Evaluation

Evaluating the effectiveness of nursing interventions is an essential ongoing component of the nursing process.

Nutrition Knowledge

Clients will demonstrate knowledge of nutrition by identifying the correct food group for each food in a sample daily menu, recognizing missing food groups, and identifying overrepresented groups. Clients will accurately assess the nutritional value of prepared foods, using label information. They will demonstrate the ability to select a nutritious, low-calorie, balanced daily diet for themselves. They will perform self-monitoring activities.

Nutritional Status

Clients will demonstrate improved nutritional status when they acknowledge their weight problems, verbalize the desire to lose weight, identify and verbalize feelings that trigger overeating, refrain from binge eating, and actively participate in a structured weight loss plan. They will verbalize feelings of increased self-control and greater self-esteem. Clients will progress steadily toward their personal weight loss goals. They will demonstrate slower eating behaviors and avoid eating alone. They will describe how to order food in a restaurant yet adhere to their meal plans. They will participate in regular, structured exercise programs as well as self-help and/or support groups.

Hopefulness

Clients will demonstrate hopefulness when they voluntarily assume responsibility for hygiene and grooming. They will demonstrate commitment to a program of daily exercise. Clients will verbalize both positive and negative feelings and recognize life events over which they have no control. Clients will verbalize an intellectual understanding of the meaning of their compulsive overeating and techniques for its management.

Social Involvement

Clients will demonstrate social involvement when they willingly socialize with others. They will voluntarily attend and participate in client group activities. Clients will approach other people appropriately for one-to-one interactions and will report minimal anxiety during social interactions. They will participate in clubs or volunteer groups and will verbalize fewer feelings or experiences of being excluded.

CASE MANAGEMENT, COMMUNITY-BASED CARE, AND HOME CARE

Community-based care, case management, and home care for clients with eating disorders have been discussed earlier in this chapter. See pages 564–565.

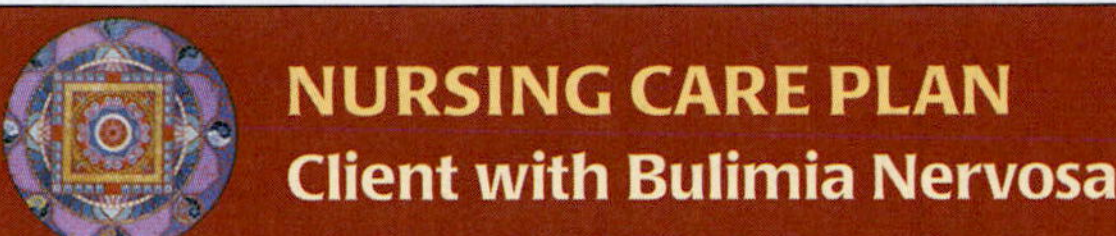

NURSING CARE PLAN
Client with Bulimia Nervosa

Assessment

Identifying Information

Lauren, a 28-year-old married woman, was admitted to the psychiatric unit from the emergency department where she was taken after collapsing during a marathon. She is a master's-prepared social worker who works in a drug abuse prevention program.

Lauren reports that she has been training for the marathon for about a year, running at least 35 miles a week. She believes that she had to be hospitalized because she did not ingest sufficient carbohydrates and fluids before the race.

Lauren states that she has been binge eating and purging for about 3 years, ever since she read about ballet dancers' and gymnasts' use of purging for weight control. On a typical day she arises at 5:00 a.m., runs at least 5 miles, then gets ready for work. On the way to work she buys and consumes a dozen doughnuts. She arrives at work before anyone else and vomits in the employees' bathroom. She eats no lunch unless she can be sure of access to a "good" bathroom, which she describes as one with a single toilet and an outside door that locks. In the evening while preparing dinner she consumes a can of salted peanuts and four or five glasses of wine. She denies ever getting "high." After a large dinner she showers, vomiting while the shower is running. Her husband of 4 years is unaware of her "problem" but worries about her drinking and wonders how she can eat so much and never gain weight.

History

No prior psychiatric history. Lauren is the oldest of three children and the only female. Her parents, both retired schoolteachers, live in a nearby town. She sees them infrequently because "they still treat me like I'm a little girl." She rarely sees her younger brothers and feels closer to her husband's family. There is no family history of eating disorders or substance abuse.

As the daughter of two schoolteachers, Lauren was expected to be the top student in her school. She had few friends because she was "the class geek." In college she excelled academically but was a "social failure." She states that she can drink an entire bottle of wine, vomit, and "sober up instantly." She has few friends or interests except running. She describes her job as "not fulfilling."

Lauren has no significant health problems. Vital signs: T, 98.2; P, 68; R, 14; Ht, 5′ 7″; Wt, 110 lb; BP, 108/68.

Current Mental Status

Lauren is slim, neatly groomed, and cooperative, but reluctant. She is alert and oriented to time, place, and person. Her judgment is good and her ability to think abstractly is unimpaired. She is articulate; affect is appropriate to verbal content; no delusions, illusions, hallucinations, or other signs of thought disorder. She fidgets in her seat but makes good eye contact. She expresses embarrassment about hospitalization and shame about her behavior. She emphatically does not want her husband or office informed of the extent and details of her "problem." She maintains that she does not need to be hospitalized and can handle this herself.

Other Subjective or Objective Clinical Data

Lauren reports that she has not had a menstrual period in over 1 year. She takes no medications.

Nursing Diagnosis: Anxiety related to low self-esteem.

Expected Outcome: Coping: Actions to manage stressors that tax an individual's resources.
Impulse Control: Ability to self-restrain compulsive or impulsive behavior.

Short-Term Goals	Interventions	Rationales
Client will identify at least three sources of anxiety.	■ Adopt a calm, reassuring attitude.	A calm approach conveys safety and confidence.
	■ Provide a quiet, nonstimulating environment.	Reducing stimuli minimizes client's anxiety.
	■ Help client recognize situations and events that create anxiety.	Client's self-awareness is enhanced.
	■ Encourage client to identify previously used, successful coping behaviors.	Recognizing successful behaviors promotes self-esteem.
	■ Encourage client to identify alternatives to alcohol abuse, binge eating, and purging in response to anxiety.	Client's coping skills are expanded.
	■ Limit overexercising.	Limits counteract unhealthy preoccupations.
	■ Negotiate a client contract to limit hoarding, vomiting, and other compulsive behaviors.	Contracts promote self-responsibility and self-control
Client will demonstrate the use of relaxation techniques to manage anxiety.	■ Teach progressive relaxation techniques and meditation.	Relaxation techniques improve coping skills.
	■ Assist client to use techniques when feeling tension that would formerly lead to binge eating and purging.	Techniques reinforce and support effective coping.

(continued)

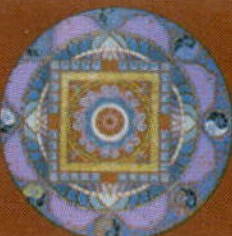

NURSING CARE PLAN
Client with Bulimia Nervosa *(continued)*

Nursing Diagnosis: Deficient Fluid Volume related to self-induced vomiting and excessive exercising.

Expected Outcome: Electrolyte and Acid–Base Balance: Balance of electrolytes and nonelectrolytes in the intracellular and extracellular compartments of the body.
Hydration: Amount of water in the intracellular and extracellular compartments of the body.

Short-Term Goals	Interventions	Rationales
Client will drink a minimum of 2 oz of fluids per hour.	▪ Teach client the importance of adequate fluid intake.	This is information every client should know.
	▪ Offer client her favorite beverages frequently during the day.	Adequate fluid intake maintains hydration.
	▪ Weigh client daily to evaluate rehydration.	Hydration status is monitored.
	▪ Keep accurate intake and output records.	
	▪ Assess skin turgor and condition of mucous membranes daily and record.	
	▪ Encourage frequent mouth care to promote comfort.	Comfort measures promote adherence.
	▪ Monitor laboratory values, reporting significant alterations to the physician.	Lab values provide information on electrolyte status.
Client will not vomit following meals.	▪ Establish a no-purging contract with client.	Contracts promote self-responsibility and self-control.
	▪ Observe client for at least 1 hour after meals to prevent purging.	Monitoring provides support and reinforcement.
	▪ Give positive recognition when progress is shown.	Recognizing progress reinforces healthy behaviors.

Nursing Diagnosis: Ineffective Individual Coping related to feelings of helplessness and lack of control in life situation.

Expected Outcome: Coping: Actions to manage stressors that tax an individual's resources.
Impulse Control: Ability to self-restrain compulsive or impulsive behavior.

Short-Term Goals	Interventions	Rationales
Client will eat regularly within 1 week.	▪ Help client establish a trust relationship with you.	Trust is the basis for a positive nurse–client relationship.
	▪ Assist client to plan for and practice dealing with daily demands.	Practice decreases helplessness, promotes self-responsibility and self-control.
	▪ Assist client to identify events preceding binge/purge episodes.	Self-awareness is an important step toward self-control.
	▪ Encourage client to identify ways of nurturing herself without using food or alcohol.	Concepts of choice, self-determination, and self-control are validated for the client.
Client will refrain from discussing body image dissatisfactions within 1 week.	▪ Engage client in a process of identifying, naming, and expressing negative feelings.	Expressing negative feelings in a responsible manner promotes self-control.
	▪ Assist client to identify and practice alternative ways of expressing negative feelings.	Exploring alternative means of expression increases coping skill, improves impulse control, and decreases helplessness.

Concept Map
Client with Bulimia Nervosa

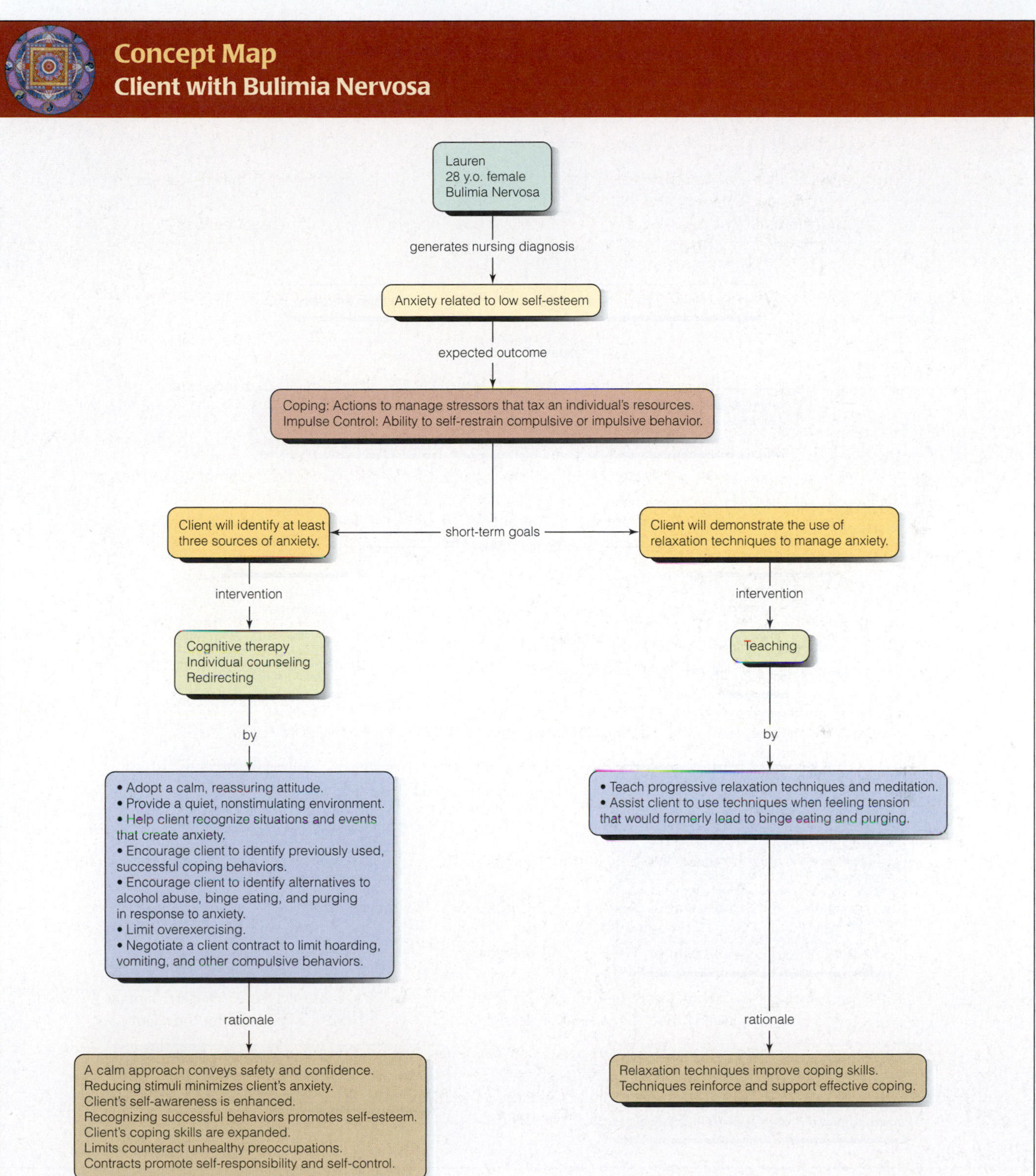
Lauren
28 y.o. female
Bulimia Nervosa
generates nursing diagnosis
Anxiety related to low self-esteem
expected outcome
Coping: Actions to manage stressors that tax an individual's resources.
Impulse Control: Ability to self-restrain compulsive or impulsive behavior.
short-term goals
Client will identify at least three sources of anxiety.
Client will demonstrate the use of relaxation techniques to manage anxiety.
intervention
Cognitive therapy
Individual counseling
Redirecting
intervention
Teaching
by
• Adopt a calm, reassuring attitude.
• Provide a quiet, nonstimulating environment.
• Help client recognize situations and events that create anxiety.
• Encourage client to identify previously used, successful coping behaviors.
• Encourage client to identify alternatives to alcohol abuse, binge eating, and purging in response to anxiety.
• Limit overexercising.
• Negotiate a client contract to limit hoarding, vomiting, and other compulsive behaviors.
by
• Teach progressive relaxation techniques and meditation.
• Assist client to use techniques when feeling tension that would formerly lead to binge eating and purging.
rationale
A calm approach conveys safety and confidence.
Reducing stimuli minimizes client's anxiety.
Client's self-awareness is enhanced.
Recognizing successful behaviors promotes self-esteem.
Client's coping skills are expanded.
Limits counteract unhealthy preoccupations.
Contracts promote self-responsibility and self-control.
rationale
Relaxation techniques improve coping skills.
Techniques reinforce and support effective coping.

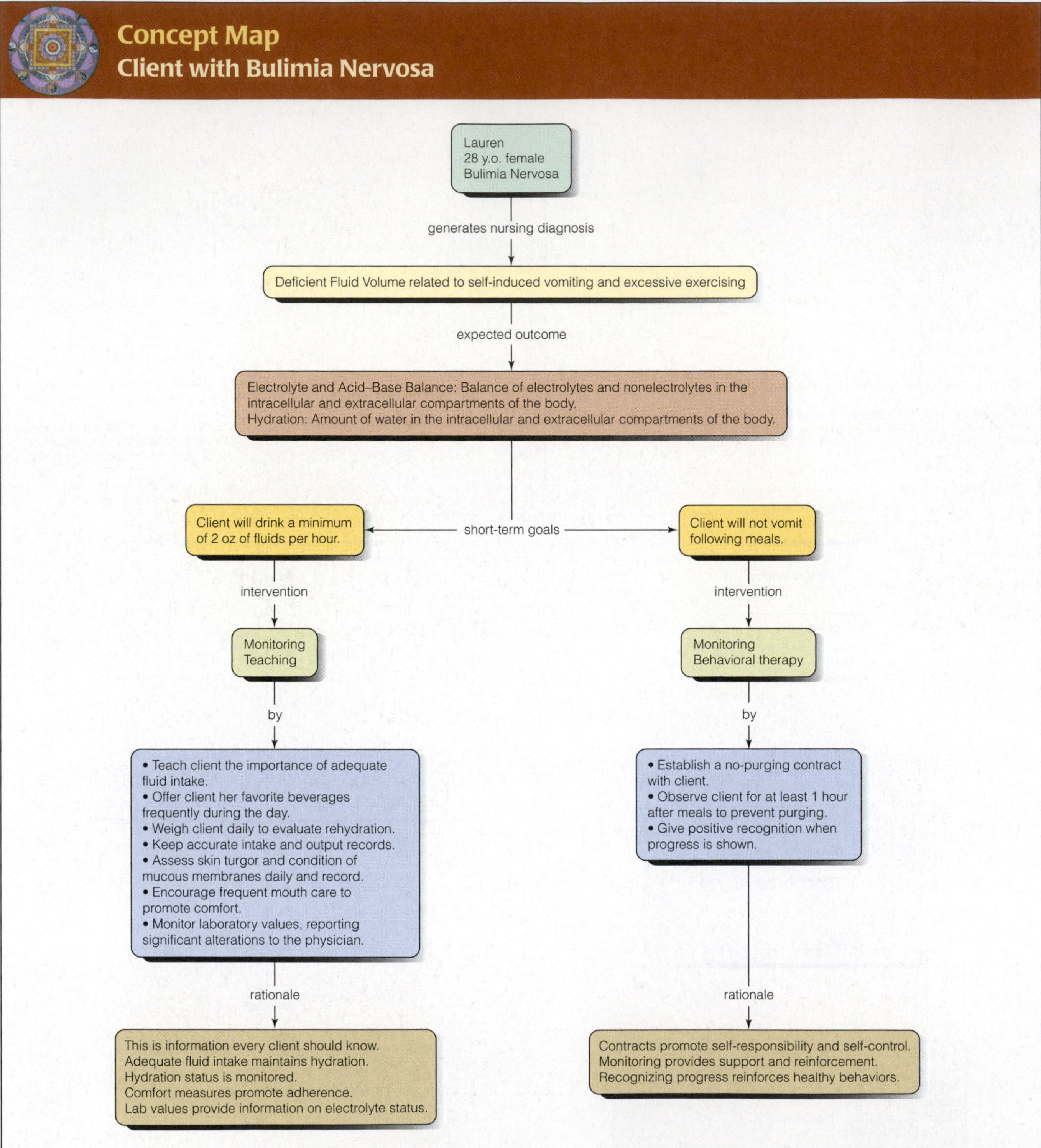
Concept Map
Client with Bulimia Nervosa
Lauren
28 y.o. female
Bulimia Nervosa
generates nursing diagnosis
Deficient Fluid Volume related to self-induced vomiting and excessive exercising
expected outcome
Electrolyte and Acid–Base Balance: Balance of electrolytes and nonelectrolytes in the intracellular and extracellular compartments of the body.
Hydration: Amount of water in the intracellular and extracellular compartments of the body.
short-term goals
Client will drink a minimum of 2 oz of fluids per hour.
Client will not vomit following meals.
intervention
Monitoring
Teaching
intervention
Monitoring
Behavioral therapy
by
• Teach client the importance of adequate fluid intake.
• Offer client her favorite beverages frequently during the day.
• Weigh client daily to evaluate rehydration.
• Keep accurate intake and output records.
• Assess skin turgor and condition of mucous membranes daily and record.
• Encourage frequent mouth care to promote comfort.
• Monitor laboratory values, reporting significant alterations to the physician.
by
• Establish a no-purging contract with client.
• Observe client for at least 1 hour after meals to prevent purging.
• Give positive recognition when progress is shown.
rationale
This is information every client should know.
Adequate fluid intake maintains hydration.
Hydration status is monitored.
Comfort measures promote adherence.
Lab values provide information on electrolyte status.
rationale
Contracts promote self-responsibility and self-control.
Monitoring provides support and reinforcement.
Recognizing progress reinforces healthy behaviors.

Concept Map
Client with Bulimia Nervosa

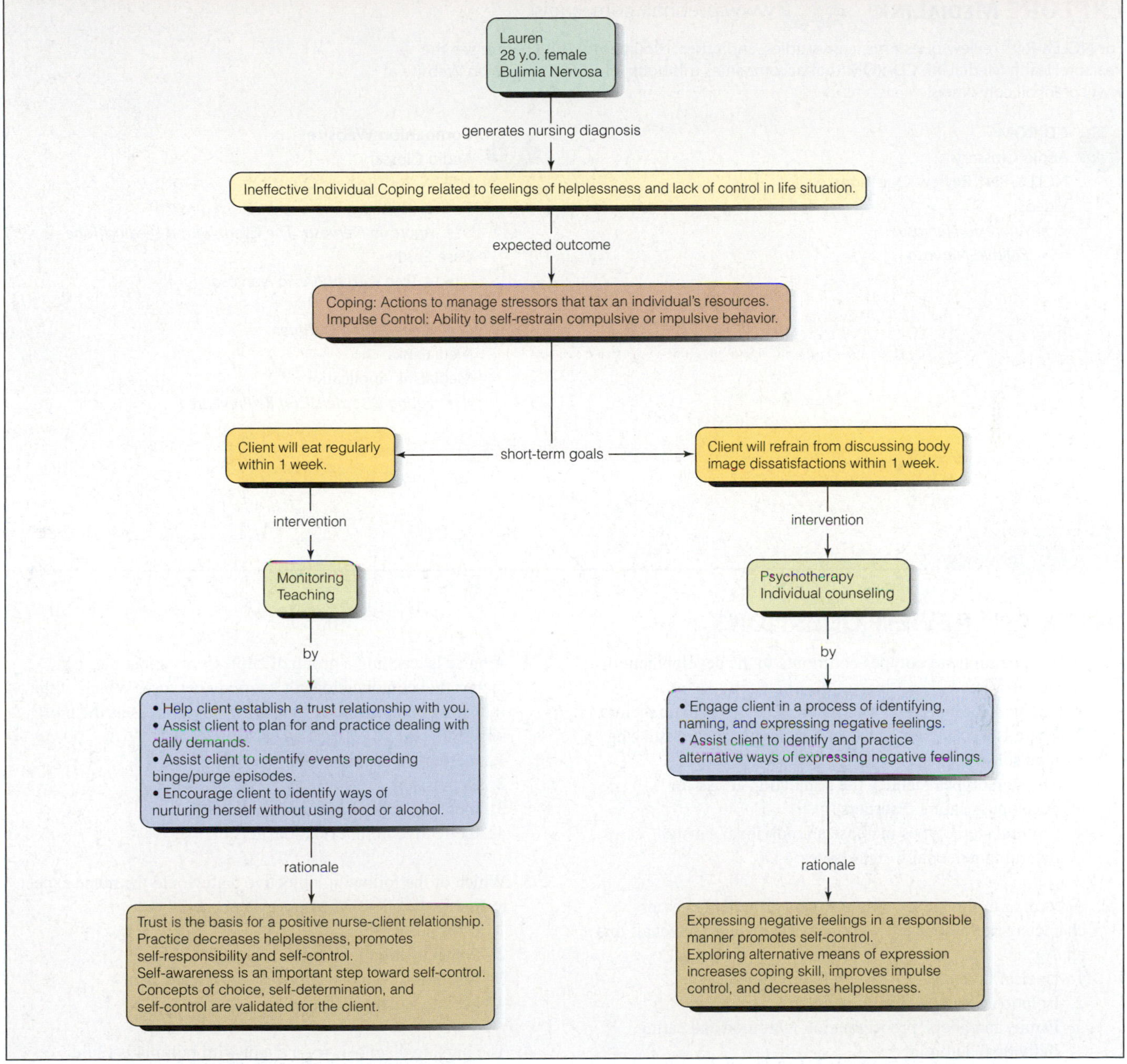

Lauren
28 y.o. female
Bulimia Nervosa

generates nursing diagnosis

Ineffective Individual Coping related to feelings of helplessness and lack of control in life situation.

expected outcome

Coping: Actions to manage stressors that tax an individual's resources.
Impulse Control: Ability to self-restrain compulsive or impulsive behavior.

short-term goals

Client will eat regularly within 1 week.

intervention

Monitoring
Teaching

by

- Help client establish a trust relationship with you.
- Assist client to plan for and practice dealing with daily demands.
- Assist client to identify events preceding binge/purge episodes.
- Encourage client to identify ways of nurturing herself without using food or alcohol.

rationale

Trust is the basis for a positive nurse-client relationship.
Practice decreases helplessness, promotes self-responsibility and self-control.
Self-awareness is an important step toward self-control.
Concepts of choice, self-determination, and self-control are validated for the client.

Client will refrain from discussing body image dissatisfactions within 1 week.

intervention

Psychotherapy
Individual counseling

by

- Engage client in a process of identifying, naming, and expressing negative feelings.
- Assist client to identify and practice alternative ways of expressing negative feelings.

rationale

Expressing negative feelings in a responsible manner promotes self-control.
Exploring alternative means of expression increases coping skill, improves impulse control, and decreases helplessness.

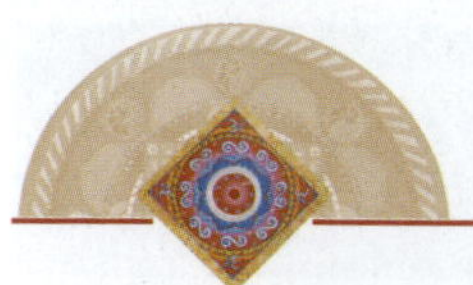

EXPLORE MEDIALINK

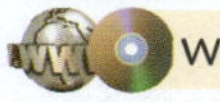 www.prenhall.com/kneisl

For NCLEX-RN® review questions, case studies, and other resources for this chapter see the Pearson Health MediaLink CD-ROM that accompanies this book and the Companion Website at www.prenhall.com/kneisl.

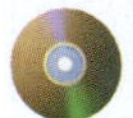

CD-ROM
Audio Glossary
NCLEX-RN® Review Questions
Videos
- *Anorexia Nervosa*
- *Bulimia Nervosa*

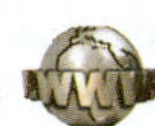

Companion Website
Audio Glossary
NCLEX-RN® Review Questions
Critical Thinking Exercise
- *Anorexia Nervosa: The Client with a Feeding Tube*

Case Study
- *A Teen with Anorexia Nervosa*

Care Plan
- *Binge-Eating Disorder*

MediaLinks
MediaLink Application
- *Eating Disorders Can Be Prevented*

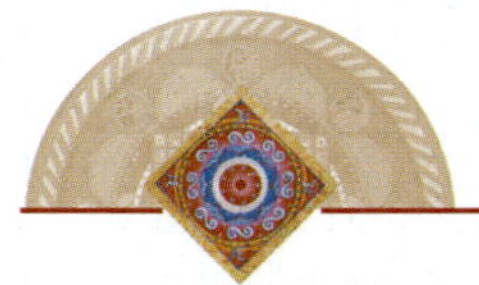

NCLEX-RN® REVIEW QUESTIONS

1. How do cultural stereotypes contribute to the development of eating disorders?
1. Eating disorders result from biological and genetic factors.
2. There is a strong emphasis on low body weight justifying high self-esteem.
3. The stereotypes identify the population at risk for developing eating disorders.
4. Cultural stereotypes increase an individual's insight regarding personal weight issues.

2. According to the family systems theory, family behavior characteristics associated with anorexia include (select all that apply):
1. Unclear boundaries between family members.
2. Isolation between family members.
3. Family members' preoccupation with food and eating.
4. Individual autonomy.
5. Successful conflict resolution.

3. The most common coexisting mental health issue associated with anorexia and bulimia is:
1. Anxiety.
2. Panic attacks.
3. Agoraphobia.
4. Depression.

4. A nurse is teaching a group of adolescents about the risk factors and complications of anorexia nervosa. Which of the following complications should the nurse stress as the most serious?
1. Ineffective coping skills
2. Depression
3. Increased risk of mortality
4. Ineffective family relationships

5. Which of the following objective data would the nurse expect to find in the client with anorexia nervosa?
1. Osteoporosis
2. Preoccupation with food
3. A score of 13 on the Mini-Mental Sate Exam
4. Feeling isolated and lonely

6. The nursing diagnosis for a client with bulimia is Fluid Volume Deficit. Nursing interventions specific to the fluid volume deficit include:
1. Ensuring daily consumption of 1,000 to 2,000 mL of liquid.
2. Weighing the client after each meal.
3. Monitoring the client for at least 1 hour after meals.
4. Monitoring body temperature every 4 hours.

7. Educational guidelines for family members of clients with eating disorders include:
   1. Scheduling family activities that include food.
   2. Expecting a full recovery within 6 months of starting treatment.
   3. Recognizing the client's need to have his or her behaviors controlled by family members.
   4. Expressing love and affection both verbally and physically.

8. The nurse observes a client admitted with anorexia nervosa doing repeated, vigorous sit-ups. The most appropriate action from the nurse is to:
   1. Tell the client she cannot do exercises.
   2. Allow the client to complete the exercise routine.
   3. Interrupt the behavior and offer to walk with the client.
   4. Take away the client's visitor privileges.

9. The nurse is assessing a client with severe anorexia nervosa. Which of the following physical findings should be immediately reported to the physician?
   1. Amenorrhea
   2. Blood pressure of 80/40 mm Hg
   3. Urine output of 50 cc/hour
   4. Pulse rate of 102

10. An effective intervention to facilitate individual coping for clients with eating disorders is to:
   1. Provide flexibility in activities of daily living.
   2. Have the treatment team determine the client's plan of care.
   3. Prohibit the client from making decisions regarding care.
   4. Provide the client with limited information on a need-to-know basis.

See Appendix C for answers.

REFERENCES

American Psychiatric Association. (2000). *Diagnostic and statistical manual of mental disorders* (4th ed., Text Revision). Washington, DC: Author.

Appolinario, J. C., Bacaltchuk, J., Sichieri, R., Claudino, A. M., Godoy-Matos, A., Morgan, C., et al. (2003). A randomized, double-blind, placebo-controlled study of sibutramine in the treatment of binge-eating disorder. *Archives of General Psychiatry, 60*(11), 1109–1116.

Bacaltchuk, J., & Hay, P. (2003). Antidepressants versus placebo for people with bulimia nervosa. *Cochrane Database of Systematic Reviews*, 4, CD003391.

Ball, J. W., & Bindler, R. C. (2006). *Child health nursing: Partnering with children and families.* Upper Saddle River, NJ: Pearson Education.

Bruch, H. (1978). *The golden cage: The enigma of anorexia nervosa.* Cambridge, MA: Harvard University Press.

Bulik, C. M. (2005). Exploring the gene-environment nexus in eating disorders. *Journal of Psychiatry & Neuroscience, 30*(5), 335–339.

Devlin, M. J., Yanovski, S. Z., & Wilson, G. T. (2000). Obesity: What mental health professionals need to know. *American Journal of Psychiatry, 157*(6), 854–866.

Eissa, M. A. H., & Gunner, K. B. (2004). Evaluation and management of obesity in children and adolescents. *Journal of Pediatric Health Care, 18*(1), 35–38.

Finfgeld, D. L. (2002). Anorexia nervosa: Analysis of long-term outcomes and clinical implications. *Archives of Psychiatric Nursing, 16*(4), 176–186.

Ford, L. (2007). *Human relations: A game plan for improving personal adjustment* (4th ed.). Upper Saddle River, NJ: Pearson Education.

Godart, N., Berthoz, S., Rein, Z., Perdereau, F., Lang, F., Venisse, J. L., et al. (2006). Does the frequency of anxiety and depressive disorders differ between diagnostic subtypes of anorexia nervosa and bulimia? *International Journal of Eating Disorders, 39*(8), 772–780.

Hillege, S., Beale, B., & McMaster, R. (2006). Impact of eating disorders on family life. *Journal of Clinical Nursing, 15*(8), 1016–1022.

Hoek, H. W., van Harten, P. N., Hermans, K. M. E., Katzman, M. A., Matroos, G. E., & Susser, E. S. (2005). The incidence of anorexia nervosa on Curacao. *American Journal of Psychiatry, 162*(4), 748–752.

Kaplan, A. S. (2002). Psychological treatments for anorexia nervosa: A review of published studies and promising new directions. *Canadian Journal of Psychiatry, 47*(3), 235–242.

Keel, P. K. (2005). *Eating disorders.* Upper Saddle River, NJ: Prentice Hall.

Keel, P. K., Baxter, M. G., Heatherton, T. F., & Joiner, T. E., Jr. (2007). A 20-year longitudinal study of body weight, dieting, and eating disorder symptoms. *Journal of Abnormal Psychology, 116*(2), 422–432.

Kotz, C. M. (2006). Integration of feeding and spontaneous physical activity. *Physiology & Behavior, 88*(3), 294–301.

Martin, G., & Pear, J. (2007). *Behavioral modification: What it is and how to do it* (8th ed.). Upper Saddle River, NJ: Pearson Education.

Neumark-Sztainer, D. (2005). *"I'm, like, SO fat!"* New York: Guilford Press.

Pull, C. B. (2004). Binge eating disorder. *Current Opinions in Psychiatry, 17*(1), 43–48.

Reddy, S. D., & Crowther, J. H. (2007). Teasing, acculturation, and cultural conflict: Psychosocial correlates of body image and eating behavior among South Asian women. *Cultural Diversity & Ethnic Minority Psychology, 13*(1), 45–53.

Romano, S. J., Halmi, K. A., Sarkar, N. P., Koke, S. C., & Lee, J. S. (2002). A placebo-controlled study of fluoxetine in continued treatment of bulimia nervosa after successful acute fluoxetine treatment. *American Journal of Psychiatry, 159*(1), 96–102.

Slof-Op't Landt, M. C., van Furth, E. F., Meulenbelt, I., Slagboom, P. E., Bartels, M., Boomsma, D. I., et al. (2005). Eating disorders: From twin studies to candidate genes and beyond. *Twin Research and Human Genetics, 8*(5), 467–482.

Stein, K. F., & Corte, C. (2003). Reconceptualizing causative factors and intervention strategies in the eating disorders: A shift from body image to self-concept impairments. *Archives of Psychiatric Nursing, 17(2)*, 57–66.

Striegel-Moore, R. H., Dohm, F. A., Kraemer, H. C., Taylor, C. B., Daniels, S., Crawford. P. B., et al. (2003). Eating disorders in White and Black women. *American Journal of Psychiatry, 160*(7), 1326–1331.

Tozzi, F., Thornton, L. M., Klump, K. L., Fichter, M. M., Halmi, K. A., Kaplan, A. S., et al. (2005). Symptom fluctuation in eating disorders. *American Journal of Psychiatry, 162*(4), 732–740.

Uher, R., Murphy, T., Brammer, M. J., Dalgleish, T., Phillips, M. L., Ng, V. W., et al. (2004). Medial prefrontal cortex activity associated with symptom provocation in eating disorders. *American Journal of Psychiatry, 161*(7), 1238–1246.

Utter, J., Neumark-Sztainer, D., Wall, M., & Story, M. (2003). Reading magazine articles about dieting and associated weight control behaviors among adolescents. *Journal of Adolescent Health, 32*(1), 78–82.

Wang, S. S., Houshyar, S., & Prinstein, M. J. (2006). Adolescent girls' and boys' weight-related health behaviors and cognitions: Associations with reputation- and preference-based peer status. *Health Psychology, 25*(5), 658–663.

Woodside, D. B., Carter, J. C., & Blackmore, E. (2004). Predictors of premature termination of inpatient treatment for anorexia nervosa. *American Journal of Psychiatry, 161*(12), 2277–2281.

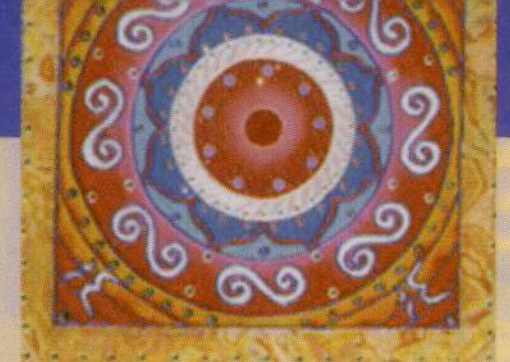

CHAPTER

22

Personality Disorders

SUE C. DELAUNE

KEY TERMS

abandonment 595
antisocial personality disorder 590
avoidant personality disorder 591
borderline personality disorder 585
countertransference 595
dependent personality disorder 591
depersonalization 584
derealization 584
enmeshment 595
histrionic personality disorder 588
hypervigilance 583
identity diffusion 595
impulsiveness 581
manipulation 581
narcissism 581
narcissistic personality disorder 589
obsessive–compulsive personality disorder 593
paranoid personality disorder 582
personality 581
personality disorder (PD) 581
personality traits 581
schizoid personality disorder 583
schizotypal personality disorder 584
splitting 587

LEARNING OUTCOMES

After completing this chapter, you will be able to:

1. Differentiate personality traits and styles from personality disorders.
2. Identify the characteristics common to all three clusters or major categories of personality disorders.
3. Compare the biopsychosocial characteristics of various personality disorders.
4. Identify the developmental and psychobiologic characteristics that distinguish Odd–Eccentric (Cluster A), Dramatic–Emotional (Cluster B), and Anxious–Fearful (Cluster C) personality disorders from one another.
5. Explain the concepts that would help the psychiatric–mental health nurse apply the nursing process to the care of clients with personality disorders.
6. Manage the triad of manipulation, narcissism, and impulsiveness when demonstrated by clients with personality disorders.
7. Focus nursing intervention on a client's specific and unique response to the disorder.
8. Modify the possible effects of the nurse's positive and negative emotional responses to clients who have personality disorders.

CRITICAL THINKING CHALLENGE

A client requests that you, a newly employed nurse on a crisis inpatient unit, bend the rules for her by extending her therapeutic leave for 2 hours so that she may meet her boyfriend for dinner. When you question the legitimacy of this request and suggest that she needs to have approval from the treatment team, the client becomes angry and accuses you of "not being the caring nurse I thought you were." The client states that she will remember this incident and warn her friends about the uncaring nurses at this facility.

1. What would be wrong with bending the rules a little?
2. Shouldn't nurses be flexible and autonomous enough not to require approval from the treatment team?
3. What purpose could the client's accusations serve?
4. How would you handle this situation with the client? What is your rationale?

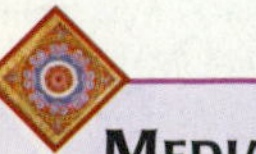

MEDIALINK 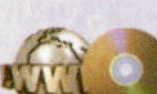 www.prenhall.com/kneisl

Go to the Pearson Health MediaLink CD-ROM and the Companion Website at www.prenhall.com/kneisl for interactive resources for this chapter.

At times, every individual demonstrates behavior that challenges others. However, working with clients who consistently demonstrate impatient, manipulative, self-centered, or overly suspicious behaviors can be especially challenging. This chapter is designed specifically to help you deal with these difficult behaviors and also asks you to evaluate your responses to interpersonally difficult clients. If you did not familiarize yourself with Chapter 3 before you began your clinical work in psychiatric–mental health nursing, make sure you do so before you begin this chapter. Chapter 3 emphasizes the need for the nurse's self-awareness and personal integration.

What distinguishes an individual is referred to as **personality**, which is defined as the individual qualities, including habitual behavior patterns, that make a person unique. **Personality traits** are persistent behavioral patterns. Even though the behaviors may be annoying or frustrating to others, they do not significantly interfere with the person's life. Both personality and personality traits tend to be stable over time. On the other hand, a **personality disorder (PD)** is a rigid, stereotyped behavioral pattern that deviates markedly from the norm of an individual's culture and persists throughout the person's life. A PD is a lifelong maladaptive pattern of perceiving, thinking, and relating that impairs social or occupational functioning and can be traced back to at least adolescence or early adulthood.

Individuals who have a PD have unique ways of perceiving themselves, other people, and the events in their lives. The range, intensity, and appropriateness of their emotional responses are often out of order. They lack insight; that is, they have no understanding of the impact of their behavior on the environment. They fail to accept the consequences of their own behavior and, when feeling threatened, attempt to ease the stress by changing the environment rather than changing their own behavior. Personality-disordered individuals' relationships are usually characterized by superficiality.

This chapter discusses the various types of PDs and the major characteristics of each. Note that the goal of therapeutic approaches is not to restructure the client's basic personality, which is likely to be an impossible task. It is a well-known psychiatric axiom that one's basic personality is fixed by the age of 6. Instead, interventions are implemented to help those with PDs learn to deal with others in more productive, less stressful ways.

PERSONALITY DISORDERS

There are three major categories of PDs, referred to as *clusters* by the American Psychiatric Association (APA). Each cluster is discussed separately in this section. Even though there are some differences among the three clusters, three traits are common to people with all types of PDs:

- Lack of insight—individuals lack understanding of the impact of their behavior on others.
- External response to stress—when feeling threatened, individuals try to change the environment instead of changing themselves.
- Failure to accept the consequences of their own behavior.

The essential characteristics of personality disorders are chronicity, pervasiveness, and maladaptation. The individual with a PD often goes through life repeating the same dysfunctional pattern. The PD affects every dimension of life and seriously impairs interpersonal and functional abilities.

Other problematic behaviors that are characteristic of people with PDs include manipulation, narcissism, and impulsiveness. **Manipulation** is control behavior; the manipulative individual uses and exploits others for personal gain. **Narcissism** is self-centered behavior in which the individual feels entitled to special favors due to a mistaken perception of oneself as the "center of the universe." **Impulsiveness** describes the actions of those who act without considering the consequences of their behavior.

The DSM-IV-TR delineates diagnostic criteria for PDs on Axis II. Essential features of these disorders include significant distress or impairment in at least two of the following areas of functioning:

- Cognition
- Affect
- Interpersonal relationships
- Impulse control

These behavior patterns must be evident by early adulthood and not be a result of other mental disorders or substance abuse (APA, 2000). It is important to distinguish the behaviors that define personality disorders from responses that may emerge as a result of specific situational stressors or transient mental states. Therefore, it is often necessary and important to conduct more than one interview with the client over a period of time. While personality-disordered people display enduring, inflexible, and pervasive maladaptive behaviors in a broad variety of personal, occupational, and social situations, they may not view their lifestyles as abnormal. Typically, they do not seek professional help unless they are very stressed.

Personality disorders may coexist with extreme psychopathology, such as the disorders included in DSM-IV-TR Axis I groupings. In addition, under stress, the individual with a personality disorder may progressively deteriorate even to the point of psychosis.

Cluster A Personality Disorders: Odd–Eccentric

Cluster A consists of the paranoid, schizoid, and schizotypal personality disorders. The major features of these disorders are pervasive distrust, social detachment, and subsequent impairment in social and occupational functioning. People with odd–eccentric personality disorders have the most cognitive impairments as well as the most peculiar behaviors and maladaptive defensive styles of people with PDs. A description of the characteristics of persons with odd–eccentric

DSM-IV-TR Diagnostic Criteria for Personality Disorders: Cluster A (Odd–Eccentric)

Paranoid Personality Disorder

A pervasive distrust and suspiciousness of others such that their motives are interpreted as malevolent, beginning by early adulthood and present in a variety of contexts, as indicated by four (or more) of the following:

1. suspects, without sufficient basis, that others are exploiting, harming, or deceiving him or her
2. is preoccupied with unjustified doubts about the loyalty or trustworthiness of friends or associates
3. is reluctant to confide in others because of unwarranted fear that the information will be used maliciously against him or her
4. reads hidden demeaning or threatening meanings into benign remarks or events
5. persistently bears grudges (i.e., is unforgiving of insults, injuries, or slights)
6. perceives attacks on his or her character or reputation that are not apparent to others and is quick to react angrily or to counter-attack
7. has recurrent suspicions, without justification, regarding fidelity of spouse or sexual partner

Schizoid Personality Disorder

A pervasive pattern of detachment from social relationships and a restricted range of expression of emotions in interpersonal settings, beginning by early adulthood and present in a variety of contexts, as indicated by four (or more) of the following:

1. neither desires nor enjoys close relationships, including being part of a family
2. almost always chooses solitary activities
3. has little, if any, interest in having sexual experiences with another person
4. takes pleasure in few, if any, activities
5. lacks close friends or confidants other than first-degree relatives
6. appears indifferent to the praise or criticism of others
7. shows emotional coldness, detachment, or flattened affect
8. considers relationships to be more intimate than they actually are

Schizotypal Personality Disorder

A pervasive pattern of social and interpersonal deficits marked by acute discomfort with, and reduced capacity for, close relationships as well as by cognitive or perceptual distortions and eccentricities of behavior, beginning by early adulthood and present in a variety of contexts, as indicated by five (or more) of the following:

1. ideas of reference (excluding delusions of reference)
2. odd beliefs or magical thinking that influences behavior and is inconsistent with subcultural norms (e.g., superstitiousness, belief in clairvoyance, telepathy, or "sixth sense"; in children and adolescents, bizarre fantasies or preoccupations)
3. unusual perceptual experiences, including bodily illusions
4. odd thinking and speech (e.g., vague, circumstantial, metaphorical, overelaborate, or stereotyped)
5. suspiciousness or paranoid ideation
6. inappropriate or constricted affect
7. behavior or appearance that is odd, eccentric, or peculiar
8. lack of close friends or confidants other than first-degree relatives
9. excessive social anxiety that does not diminish with familiarity and tends to be associated with paranoid fears rather than negative judgments about self

Source: Reprinted with permission from the *Diagnostic and Statistical Manual of Mental Disorders,* Fourth Edition, Text Revision. (Copyright 2000). American Psychiatric Association.

USING DSM-IV-TR

Health care providers often use language unfamiliar to clients and their families. Explain *ideas of reference* in such a way that clients and family members can understand its meaning in relationship to schizotypal personality disorder.

personality disorders is in the DSM-IV-TR Diagnostic Criteria feature above.

Paranoid Personality Disorder

Clients with **paranoid personality disorder** engage in a pattern of pervasive mistrust of others, interpreting as malevolent the motives of others. They often report that others plot against them or attempt to use or deceive them. They talk about disloyal friends and coworkers and the irreversible harm others' actions have caused. They may be surprised but mistrustful of loyalty shown to them and often refuse to answer questions, saying, "That is no one's business." A frequent theme of clients with a paranoid personality disorder is pathologic suspicion of spousal or partner infidelity. Unrealistic grandiose fantasies often emerge; clients may discuss activities with others who share their beliefs, such as special interest groups or cults. Client affect may be labile, with hostile, stubborn sarcasm being predominant.

Suspiciousness and Mistrust Suspiciousness and mistrust reflect an attitude of doubt toward the trustworthiness of objects or people. Suspiciousness is also a way of thinking and includes such manifestations as expectations of trickery or harm, guardedness, secretiveness, pathologic jealousy, and overconcern with hidden motives and special meanings. For example, the suspicious person may perceive a birthday gift as a trick to create an obligation. Legal disputes may arise from the client's response to perceived threats. In the following clinical example, Jim's situation exemplifies the outcome of paranoid feelings and behaviors.

CLINICAL EXAMPLE

Jim, a 39-year-old engineer, suspects that his employer is withholding significant data from him pertaining to an important job assignment. Jim began to question others about the reliability and integrity of his boss. He went to the plant one

Sunday morning without authorization. A security guard found him going through the filing cabinets of his employer, who confronted him the following day and sent him to the employee assistance program nurse. During the interview, Jim states, "I knew my boss was dishonest from the start. He never could give me a straight answer. As soon as I was almost on him, he sets me up to lose face and maybe my job."

Rigidity People with paranoid personality disorder are inflexible in their perception of the world. They are preoccupied with their expectations of others and relentlessly try to confirm these expectations, often through argumentation. They closely examine arguments and information, with prejudice. The person with paranoid personality disorder justifies a position by excessive rationalization, rejecting any evidence that refutes the distorted thought, and goes to great lengths to prove a point. It is not unusual for a paranoid person to be suspicious of people with opposing ideas. The need to be in control is another characteristic, as is a preoccupation with rank and status. The need to be self-sufficient often results in difficulty working with others. The rigidity in thinking patterns reinforces the individual's need to always be "right."

Hypervigilance **Hypervigilance** is an increased state of watchfulness in which the person is always on guard and unable to relax. There is constant sensitivity to nuances, interpretation of both open and hidden attitudes of others, and scrutiny of others and the environment. As a result, interpersonal relationships are greatly impaired and the person becomes socially isolated.

Distortions of Reality Although paranoid people perceive facts accurately, they may attribute a special significance to events. In this way, they create a private reality. These individuals have a special interest in hidden motives, underlying purposes, and special meanings. They do not necessarily disagree with the average observer about the existence of any given fact, only about its significance. Therefore, even severely paranoid people can recognize various essential facts well enough to achieve a limited adjustment to the normal social world. But they often have difficulty distinguishing real from imagined offenses. Their distorted attitudes antagonize others and may lead to real discrimination, as demonstrated in the following clinical example.

CLINICAL EXAMPLE

Ellen is quick to detect signs of anger, jealousy, and rejection in the actions of her coworkers. She magnifies these negative aspects and overlooks such positive behaviors as humor, support, and empathy. Eventually, Ellen's coworkers begin to snicker when she makes public statements, and they gossip about her.

Projection People who are paranoid attribute their own ego-alien (intolerable) motivations, drives, or feelings to others. Projection is used to attribute to others the harmful intentions that they themselves feel. In this way, the idea that one may be harmed really reflects one's own wish to harm others. Projection and other mental mechanisms (defense mechanisms) are discussed in Chapter 8 ∞.

Restricted Affect Labile emotional expressiveness and a lack of spontaneity characterize people with paranoid personality disorder. They often appear cold, humorless, and devoid of tender, sensitive feelings. Although they may demonstrate temper outbursts, they pride themselves on remaining objective and reasonable and frequently use intellectualization and rationalization to avoid affective experiences. Some paranoid people may appear friendly, but in fact this friendliness is a "script" that helps them adapt to social situations or achieve their goals.

Exclusion Because of the paranoid person's antagonism and suspiciousness, tension develops between the person and significant others. The persistent strain on relationships causes others to define the paranoid person as more than simply "different." Instead, they see the individual as unreliable or untrustworthy, and others begin to interact according to their perceptions. These behaviors reinforce the suspicions and beliefs of the paranoid person. The effects of this process include:

- Blocked communication, which increases the process of exclusion
- Emergence of a crisis, which formally excludes the paranoid person
- Reinforcement of the paranoid person's beliefs, interpretations, or ideas of reference

Because paranoid people are generally intelligent, persuasive, and creative in justifying their beliefs, they often try to adapt by one of two ways. They may join quasi-political groups, esoteric religions, cults, or quasi-scientific organizations that reinforce their interpretations of reality. Or they may join organizations that challenge societal norms and trends in an effort to direct and thus control hostile feelings.

You may encounter clients with paranoid personality disorder in any health care setting. Important information for nurses in emergency departments, where clients are under great stress and their usual coping abilities are taxed, is discussed in the feature What Every Emergency Department Nurse Should Know on page 584.

Schizoid Personality Disorder

People with **schizoid personality disorder** generally have a detached and aloof social style and display a range of adjustment. Some are fairly well-adjusted individuals who are loners; others live out their lives in protective environments, such as group homes, mental hospitals, and prisons.

Schizoid personality disorder is found in about 3% of the population (APA, 2000). Individuals who are diagnosed with schizoid personality disorder are rarely seen in clinical settings, but when they are it is usually for treatment of symptoms associated with anxiety, depression, or dysphoric affect. They may experience transient psychotic episodes which may last a few minutes to several hours.

WHAT EVERY EMERGENCY DEPARTMENT NURSE SHOULD KNOW

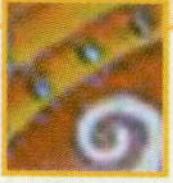

The Client with Paranoid Personality Disorder

- Carefully observe the client for signs of paranoia (e.g., hypersensitivity, guarding).
- Avoid personalizing the client's remarks.
- Approach the client with a calm, quiet demeanor in order to increase the client's sense of security.
- Avoid laughing or whispering within the client's line of vision.
- Explain the parameters of confidentiality to the client.
- Maintain reasonable safety precautions at all times when dealing with this client, depending on the extent of the client's paranoia (e.g., if the client is highly paranoid, face the client at all times rather than turning your back on the client; avoid being cornered by ensuring that you have an available exit).
- Call for security immediately if the client's behavior shows signs of escalation.

Individuals with schizoid personality disorder show a preference for solitary interests—they claim to enjoy being alone—and occupations that require minimal social interaction. They tend to choose solitary hobbies such as solitaire and computer games, and jobs such as night security guard or bridge tender. They may decline job promotions because social demands (meetings, supervisory responsibilities) accompany the promotion. When questioned about sexual activity, clients with schizoid PD usually deny interest or involvement in intimate relationships. They may appear cool, aloof, or bored, and may seem to be cognitively impaired. When asked if they think their loner-type behavior is unusual, a typical response is, "I never thought about it much . . . it doesn't much matter to me." Schizoid clients acknowledge that they rarely become excited, angry, upset, or joyful. Indifference and humorlessness are hallmarks of the individual with schizoid personality disorder.

Schizotypal Personality Disorder

Suspicion, including paranoid ideation, is usually noted in the schizotypal client. Maintaining eye contact may be difficult, and communication strategies such as humor to defuse anxiety may be met with a stare and questions about the meaning or purpose of the joking. Be careful about using humor with mentally disordered people. Their interpretation of humor or joking will not always match yours.

Clients with **schizotypal personality disorder** report a great deal of subjective anxiety in social situations, have cognitive or perceptual distortions, and display eccentric behavior. They often report bizarre fantasies, especially of paranormal events. During an interview, they may remark, "I know what you're going to ask me before you say it," believing they are endowed with special powers or have the ability to control others' behavior by simply "willing it to happen." Often, these clients have speech patterns that are so loose, digressive, or vague that an interview is difficult to conduct. The client may acknowledge this behavior by stating, "I was never talkative" (APA, 2000). Clients with schizotypal PD appear absentminded; they daydream, are vague about goals, are indecisive, and lack social skills. Often, they act as if they are "in a fog." They fail to respond in a usual manner to social cues and seem like social misfits.

The schizotypal personality-disordered client demonstrates eccentricities in communication and behavior not seen in a person with schizoid personality. Examples include such oddities of thought as magical thinking and ideas of reference; altered perceptions, such as illusions, **depersonalization** (a feeling of strangeness or unreality about the self), and **derealization** (a feeling of disconnection from the environment); speech alterations, including circumstantiality (giving detailed, factual but nonessential information), digression, metaphoric speech patterns, and overly concrete or abstract responses; and an odd or unkempt manner of dress, which includes ill-fitting, stained, and mismatched clothing.

They have a history of being loners and neither desire nor enjoy close relationships. They are indifferent to feedback and insensitive to others. The detachment from social relationships is also noted in the client's lack of interest in having intimate or sexual relationships.

Onset of schizotypal PD is believed to be in childhood or early adolescence. Clients report poor academic achievement and poor peer relationships as well as social anxiety, even as children. Clients with schizotypal personality disorders may experience psychotic episodes of very short duration, lasting from a few minutes to several hours (APA, 2000).

Cluster B Personality Disorders: Dramatic–Emotional

The DSM-IV-TR identifies the borderline, histrionic, narcissistic, and antisocial personality disorders as dramatic, emotional, and erratic dysfunctions. Individuals with these disorders are often in conflict with society because of their impulsive behavior. Impulsive people view the world as a discontinuous, fragmented collection of opportunities, frustrations, and affective experiences. They live only in the present moment and, therefore, lack the ability to formulate long-range plans. They act decisively without critical evaluation of consequences. The focus of their intellectual and emotional goals is to achieve immediate satisfaction. This lack of impulse control and inability to delay gratification often result in both verbal and nonverbal outbursts of anger, which may be self-directed or other-directed. Indeed, clients with dramatic–emotional personality disorders may experience rapid escalation of anxiety when their own angry impulses are not controlled by others. A description of the Cluster B personality disorders is in the following DSM-IV-TR Diagnostic Criteria feature.

DSM-IV-TR Diagnostic Criteria for Personality Disorders: Cluster B (Dramatic–Emotional)

Borderline Personality Disorder

A pervasive pattern of instability of interpersonal relationships, self-image, and affects, and marked impulsivity beginning by early adulthood and present in a variety of contexts, as indicated by five (or more) of the following:

1. frantic efforts to avoid real or imagined abandonment. **Note:** Do not include suicidal or self-mutilating behavior covered in Criterion 5.
2. a pattern of unstable and intense interpersonal relationships characterized by alternating between extremes of idealization and devaluation
3. identity disturbance: markedly and persistently unstable self-image or sense of self
4. impulsivity in at least two areas that are potentially self-damaging (e.g., spending, sex, substance abuse, reckless driving, binge eating)
5. recurrent suicidal behavior, gestures, or threats, or self-mutilating behavior
6. affective instability due to a marked reactivity of mood (e.g., intense episodic dysphoria, irritability, or anxiety usually lasting a few hours and only rarely more than a few days)
7. chronic feelings of emptiness
8. inappropriate, intense anger or difficulty controlling anger (e.g., frequent displays of temper, constant anger, recurrent physical fights)
9. transient, stress-related paranoid ideation or severe dissociative symptoms

Histrionic Personality Disorder

A pervasive pattern of excessive emotionality and attention seeking, beginning by early adulthood and present in a variety of contexts, as indicated by five (or more) of the following:

1. is uncomfortable in situations in which he or she is not the center of attention
2. interaction with others is often characterized by inappropriate sexually seductive or provocative behavior
3. displays rapidly shifting and shallow expression of emotions
4. consistently uses physical appearance to draw attention to self
5. has a style of speech that is excessively impressionistic and lacking in detail
6. shows self-dramatization, theatricality, and exaggerated expression of emotion
7. is suggestible (i.e., easily influenced by others or circumstances)

Narcissistic Personality Disorder

A pervasive pattern of grandiosity (in fantasy or behavior), need for admiration, and lack of empathy, beginning by early adulthood and present in a variety of contexts, as indicated by five (or more) of the following:

1. has a grandiose sense of self-importance (e.g., exaggerates achievements and talents, expects to be recognized as superior without commensurate achievements)
2. is preoccupied with fantasies of unlimited success, power, brilliance, beauty, or ideal love
3. believes that he or she is "special" and unique and can only be understood by, or should associate with, other special or high-status people (or institutions)
4. requires excessive admiration
5. has a sense of entitlement (i.e., unreasonable expectations of especially favorable treatment or automatic compliance with his or her expectations)
6. is interpersonally exploitative (i.e., takes advantage of others to achieve his or her own ends)
7. lacks empathy: is unwilling to recognize or identify with the feelings and needs of others
8. is often envious of others or believes that others are envious of him or her
9. shows arrogant, haughty behaviors or attitudes

Antisocial Personality Disorder

There is a pervasive pattern of disregard for and violation of the rights of others occurring since age 15 years, as indicated by three (or more) of the following:

1. failure to conform to social norms with respect to lawful behaviors as indicated by repeatedly performing acts that are grounds for arrest
2. deceitfulness, as indicated by repeated lying, use of aliases, or conning others for personal profit or pleasure
3. impulsivity or failure to plan ahead
4. irritability and aggressiveness, as indicated by repeated physical fights or assaults
5. reckless disregard for safety of self or others
6. consistent irresponsibility, as indicated by repeated failure to sustain consistent work behavior or honor financial obligations
7. lack of remorse, as indicated by being indifferent to or rationalizing having hurt, mistreated, or stolen from another

Source: Reprinted with permission from the *Diagnostic and Statistical Manual of Mental Disorders,* Fourth Edition, Text Revision. (Copyright 2000). American Psychiatric Association.

USING DSM-IV-TR

Health care providers often use language unfamiliar to clients and their families. Explain *idealization and devaluation* in such a way that clients and family members can understand its meaning in relationship to borderline personality disorder.

Borderline Personality Disorder

Individuals with **borderline personality disorder** (BPD) have unstable interpersonal relationships, self-image, and affect, and are impulsive. It is common for such clients to experience psychotic breaks from reality whenever they experience severe stress. Prevalence of this disorder is about 2% (APA, 2000).

Approximately 50% of individuals with BPD also have other coexisting mental disorders, such as major depression, bipolar disorder, eating disorders, and substance abuse

MEDIALINK Application: Borderline Personality Disorder

WHAT EVERY MEDICAL–SURGICAL NURSE SHOULD KNOW

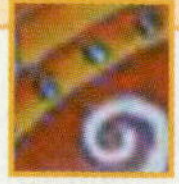

The Client with Borderline Personality Disorder

- When a client constantly makes demands, look for the underlying meaning (e.g., does the client really want more water or is it a bid for your attention?).
- Assess the client's anxiety level; expect that the demands will increase as anxiety escalates.
- Teach the client relaxation techniques and encourage their utilization as soon as you notice an increase in anxiety level.
- Provide attention to the client when appropriate behaviors are exhibited in order to avoid reinforcing the unacceptable behaviors.
- Be sure to communicate often with coworkers about the client in order to reduce the possibility of manipulation.

(National Alliance on Mental Illness, 2007). Individuals with BPD may also have coexisting physical problems. Medical–surgical nurses may meet them as clients in general hospital settings. Helpful guidelines are given in the feature above, What Every Medical–Surgical Nurse Should Know.

Impulsivity Impulsiveness may be expressed in self-damaging ways, demonstrating a lack of responsibility and disregard for the consequences of one's behavior. The responses of individuals with BPD fluctuate in situations that are subjectively interpreted and often distorted. These individuals do not learn from their mistakes and, therefore, do not change their behavior, which reinforces their impulsive responses (de Bruijn et al., 2006). Impulsiveness is manifested in spending habits, sexual promiscuity, substance use, abnormal eating habits, shoplifting, and frequent job changes. "I just told my boss to take this job and shove it" may be the response to a work situation that is perceived as intolerable. "I just got another credit card with a $5,000 limit, so I don't have to worry about going over the limit on my other three cards." "I only drink wine when I'm driving, so I don't worry about DUIs." "I don't worry about AIDS; all my partners come from high-rent districts, so they are clean and safe." Responses such as "I don't know why I did it, I just did" are common when clients are questioned about the reasons for particular actions.

Intense Anger Clients with BPD tend to instigate problems as they become involved in therapeutic relationships. The anger may manifest itself in accusations, frequent displays of temper, inability to control anger (acting out), irritability, sarcasm, argumentativeness, devaluing others, and overreaction to minor irritants. Such behaviors usually sabotage their treatment.

These clients are unable to tolerate their own "bad" image and therefore project it onto others, often raging at the perceived attributes of the other. Anger tends to be greatest toward those people who remind them of a nurturing/frustrating parent, as shown in the following clinical example.

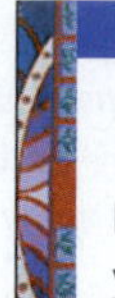

CLINICAL EXAMPLE

During a community meeting on an inpatient unit, Raul, a 34-year-old client, states, "I can't stand that fat slob of a nurse. She acts like God went on vacation and appointed her to substitute for Him." When confronted by the group leader, Raul responds, "So what if I yell when I get angry? I'm paying a lot of money to be here. If you don't like it, leave."

Identity Diffusion Clients with BPD display behaviors that show confusion about values and goals in life. These clients are described as chameleon-like because they are constantly changing their behavior to match the behavior of those around them. An intense fear of rejection causes borderline individuals to say what they think others want to hear and to behave in a manner that they believe will win them popularity or special favors. It is difficult to determine what borderline individuals really think or feel. They cannot genuinely experience feelings and emotions; their core personality is hollow. They do not assume responsibility for their actions but project blame and credit onto others.

Unstable Interpersonal Relationships Clients relate stories of "one-night stands" in search of the perfect partner. Any real or perceived threat of abandonment results in the client's "switching" to another partner. "He's never there when I need him" may be used in conjunction with "I always see to it that his shirts are ironed and his dinner is ready when he gets home from work." These clients need a payback in return for any giving they do. The failure to resolve the separation–individuation process described by Mahler, Pine, and Bergman (1975) in their classic work is reflected in the person's attitudes toward self and others.

Interpersonal relationships may include such behaviors as:

- Manipulation of others
- Pitting individuals against one another
- Intense attachment
- Explosive separations
- Sudden shifts in attitude toward others perceived as good or bad
- Clinging, demanding
- Controlling, exploiting
- Sadism or masochism in close relationships
- Relationships motivated by a need to avoid being alone rather than a need to be with others
- Lack of empathy
- Diminished capacity to evaluate others realistically
- Transient, superficial relationships

Problems of identity diffusion are also apparent in the areas of sexual intimacy and gender identity. Sexual intimacy is disturbed as a result of the person's fears of being either

WHY I BECAME A PSYCHIATRIC–MENTAL HEALTH NURSE

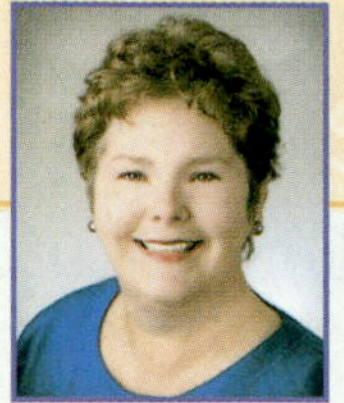

Sue C. DeLaune
Contributor, Chapters 18, 19, 22, and 35

I am so glad that I became a "psych nurse." The reasons for my selecting psychiatric–mental health nursing as a specialty are numerous. I have always been fascinated by trying to determine what motivates behavior. The ability to be comfortable with ambiguity is a real asset for a nurse who is considering mental health as a specialty area. My basic belief is that people do the best they can with what they have at the moment. This belief has been invaluable in dealing with clients experiencing depression, suicidal ideation, and other problems.

The concepts of psychiatric–mental health are applicable to every area of nursing. In fact, a nurse must utilize communication skills, empathy, and self-esteem-boosting approaches with every client. Throughout my 36 years as a nurse I have used psychiatric–mental health nursing skills in every area (emergency department, surgery, psychiatry, and primary-care clinic) and every role (staff nurse, administrator, educator, and business owner).

engulfed and destroyed or else abandoned by another. An approach–avoidance conflict emerges as a consequence of the parent or caretaker having thwarted independence and rewarded dependent behavior. As a result, the borderline client develops two major fears: the fear of abandonment, which leads to clinging behavior, and fear of engulfment, which leads to distancing from others. The client desperately wants intimate relationships but is terrified of losing the self. These fears are reminiscent of the early choice between parent's love and autonomy, which is the core of the borderline conflict.

This conflict is managed by using the primitive dissociation defense, also called **splitting**, which can best be described as the inability to integrate contradictory experiences. Splitting is based on dichotomous thinking, a cognitive distortion in which the person has an "all-or-none" mentality about others; people are viewed as either all "good" or all "bad."

Gender identity disturbance may be manifested by the selection of rejecting or abusive partners, the preference for homosexual relationships while maintaining a heterosexual lifestyle, and bizarre fantasies.

Another area of identity diffusion is temporal discontinuity, which is manifested by a searching for one's origins or keeping detailed chronologic journals. Borderline individuals seem unable to integrate past, present, and future into a continuum. They may frantically plan for the future while reminiscing about past events. These behaviors often lead to difficulty in choosing long-term goals, making career choices, and reassessing personal values. "I can't make up my mind if I should stay in nursing or try interior design" (after completing 1 year in a 2-year nursing program).

Affective Instability The failure to resolve the issues described previously is also related to the inability of the person with BPD to maintain a consistent, satisfying, affective state. Characteristics of this disorder include intense fluctuations of mood, normally of short duration (a few hours or a few days); intense, discrete episodes of depression with accompanying suicidal ideation and gestures; and hypomanic or elated episodes. "Of course I knew I wouldn't kill myself when I took those pills—do you think I'm stupid or something?" "I only told him [partner] I was HIV positive to see if he really cared for me as much as he said."

Feelings of Emptiness and Aloneness Individuals with borderline personality disorder report hollow, empty feelings, lack of peaceful solitude, a sense of being disconnected, and anhedonia (absence of pleasure in performing ordinarily pleasurable acts). The person may attempt to combat these feelings by compulsive eating, drinking, drug abuse, sexual encounters, and self-mutilation. "I get depressed and I think about taking some pills, but then my boyfriend calls and we'll go out and I won't be depressed anymore," or, "I feel so totally empty inside. I burned my wrist with the cigarette just to see if I could still feel."

Self-Damaging Acts Impulsiveness, together with identity disturbances, often leads to self-destructive behaviors. People with BPD are often depressed, but they may make self-destructive gestures in an attempt to affirm their reality and relieve tension rather than to express a wish to die. Self-damaging behaviors such as those illustrated in FIGURE 22-1 ■ include self-mutilation (cigarette burns, cutting, taking drug overdoses), recurrent accidents, and physical fights. Individuals who engage in self-mutilating behaviors often experience boundary disturbances and lack insight. "I don't see what's the big deal, so I tried to cut my wrists a couple of times—doesn't everybody?" "Yeah, I vomit after I eat; it keeps my weight down and I still get to have all the desserts I want."

Distortions of Reality When identity diffusion reaches panic proportions, the borderline individual may experience both

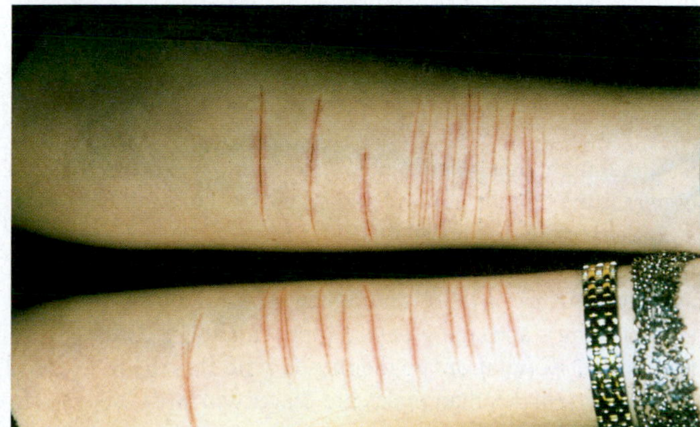

FIGURE 22-1 ■ An example of self-mutilation. The arms of this young woman, who was diagnosed with borderline personality disorder, have numerous recent and healed cuts. Self-mutilating acts should alert you to the need for suicide risk assessment.

Source: Photo Researchers, Inc., Dr. P. Marazzi/Science Photo Library.

depersonalization (feeling of strangeness or unreality about one's self) and derealization (feeling of disconnectedness from the environment). The following clinical example illustrates derealization as experienced by one individual.

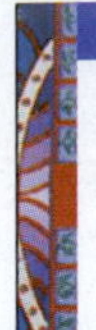

CLINICAL EXAMPLE

Steve has multiple cigarette burns but reports no pain or discomfort and smiles when the nurse is cleaning and dressing his lesions. He tells the nurse, "It doesn't even hurt much. At least I can tell where my arm begins and ends."

Histrionic Personality Disorder

People with **histrionic personality disorder** (HPD) show a lifelong tendency for dramatic, egocentric, attention-seeking response patterns. Their seeming lack of sincerity and emotional commitment contributes to disturbances in interpersonal relationships. These people appear to be continually "on stage" and acting a role. Their coping patterns are based on repression, denial, and dissociation. In the following clinical example, Linda exhibits many of the characteristic behaviors of histrionic personality disorder.

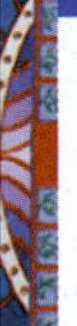

CLINICAL EXAMPLE

Linda, a 33-year-old woman who is twice divorced, was observed at the outpatient clinic responding flirtatiously to male staff members. She was neatly groomed and seductively dressed in a low-cut peasant blouse, a tight miniskirt, and bright red knee-high boots. When called by the female therapist for her appointment, Linda screamed that the wait was too long and complained loudly about patients' rights to rapid treatment. She quickly captured the attention of others in the waiting room. Then Linda feigned dizziness and "fell" as she arose from her chair. During the ensuing session, Linda complained that several men had made passes at her on the bus. When the therapist failed to share her outrage, Linda accused her of being jealous. Linda terminated the interview at that point and left the office, slamming the door behind her and stating, "My problems are physical, and no one cares whether I live or die. You'll be sorry for treating me this way!"

As with other personality disorders, it is important to consider the client's cultural and ethnic background before assuming that the diagnosis of HPD is correct because norms for interpersonal behavior, dress and appearance, and emotional expression vary widely among cultures, genders (sex role stereotyping), and age groups. Approximately 3% of the general population are diagnosed with this disorder. More females than males are diagnosed with this condition (APA, 2000).

Dramatic, Exhibitionistic, and Egocentric Responses The behaviors of individuals with HPD are characterized by exaggerated emotional expression. They demonstrate an excessive craving for attention, activity, and excitement. Often, these individuals behave frivolously, acting silly and making nuisances of themselves.

When confronted with minor stressors, the individual with HPD overreacts with irrational emotional outbursts and temper tantrums. Such a response is illustrated in the following clinical example.

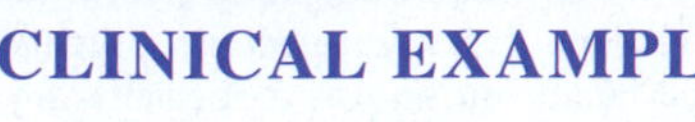

CLINICAL EXAMPLE

Josephine has been waiting 15 minutes for her appointment in the mental health clinic. She grabs the attention of the other clients in the waiting room when she leaps to her feet, rushes to the receptionist's desk, dramatically points to herself, and says in a loud voice, "I need someone to see me right now. What kind of people staff this place—sadists?"

Dysfunctional Interpersonal Relationships People with HPD constantly need love, reassurance, and validation of their existence because of their feelings of dependence and helplessness. For this reason, they have problems with significant relationships. They are likely to manipulate others in order to hold on to them while at the same time being highly inconsiderate and lacking empathy, as described in the following clinical example.

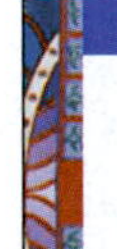

CLINICAL EXAMPLE

Calling her current boyfriend at 3:00 in the morning, Mary says, "Oh, Jim, I couldn't sleep and I knew you would want to be with me, at least in spirit."

Impaired Sexual Expression People with HPD are generally provocative and seductive and use sexual expression to manipulate and control others in relationships. Clients are often unaware of this flamboyance and how others perceive it. They are often competitive with those of the same sex and seductive with members of the opposite sex. A potential problem is promiscuous sexual activity and the risk of developing and spreading sexually transmitted diseases (Chapter 25 discusses the relationship between mental disorder and STDs, specifically the spread of the HIV virus). Disregard for the welfare and safety of others may be noted in sexual acting-out, including intimate relationships with others on the unit. When confronted, the client may say, "I've been talking to the social worker about the need for conjugal visits; maybe now you'll understand how important it is for us to get sex as well as therapy."

Dysphoric Mood Clients may express dysphoria as a sense of disquiet or restlessness. Histrionic clients may experience dysphoria when their demands for attention and affection are not met. They may act out in a suicidal fashion to manipulate or coerce others.

Cognitive Alterations Clients with HPD are much more interested in creative or imaginative pursuits than in analytic or academic achievements. They tend to be impressionable and highly suggestible and tend to look to authority figures for magical solutions to problems.

Impaired Health Patterns Regression and the development of somatic and/or dissociative symptoms are frequent among histrionic people. These disabling symptoms may serve the purpose of calling attention to themselves. Generally, the symptoms occur when an audience is present or when an unpleasant situation is anticipated. Substance use, depression, seizure-like activity, blackouts, falling, dizziness, or reactive psychoses may lead to hospitalization.

Narcissistic Personality Disorder

People with **narcissistic personality disorder** (NPD) engage in a pattern of grandiosity, have difficulty regulating self-esteem, and need admiration and attention from others. Their self-evaluation is dependent on admiration and devotion from others. The constant desire to be the center of attention is based on a strong sense of entitlement; narcissistic people feel they deserve to be treated in a special manner. When their need for constant attention is not met, the narcissistic person feels rejected and may retaliate through acting-out behavior. Characteristics most frequently observed include a sense of entitlement, lack of empathy, indifference toward others, and interpersonal manipulation, as described in the following clinical example.

CLINICAL EXAMPLE

Michael and his spouse have frequent arguments about his sense of entitlement and his need to be at the center of the family's universe. Michael does not believe that his wife treats him the way he should be treated. He expects her to put his needs above her own as well as the needs of their children. When Michael feels rejected, he shouts at them, refuses to talk to them, or leaves the house after banging shut the door. After Michael refused to entertain the notion of family or couples counseling, his wife said she couldn't take it any more and threatened to leave him. Michael's response was "If you won't stay with me, there's no point in living. You'll be very sorry if you do this."

About 1% of the general population has NPD, and the incidence is increasing steadily. Of those diagnosed, 50% to 75% are male (APA, 2000). There may be a higher than usual risk in children of narcissistic parents who impart to them an unrealistic sense of omnipotence, grandiosity, beauty, and talent (Sadock & Sadock, 2005). While narcissistic traits are quite common (and developmentally appropriate) in adolescents, the majority of teens who exhibit narcissism do not necessarily develop NPD as adults (APA, 2000).

Grandiosity Grandiosity is evidenced by expressions of exaggerated self-importance, self-absorption, and egocentricity. This inflated self-concept may be a compensation for feelings of diminished self-worth. Isolating a child from the feedback of others and the parents' failing to mirror the child's behavior may contribute to the development of grandiosity. Mirroring, or mirror images, reflect what the parents think of and how they treat the child. When coming in contact with people outside the home, the child may discover a discrepancy between treatment from others and the mirror images developed at home. Excessive boasting may result from the inconsistency in self-concept. Humility is not a characteristic of people with NPD, as shown in the following clinical example.

CLINICAL EXAMPLE

Alicia is a 40-year-old teacher who seeks professional counseling after dropping out of a graduate program. When questioned about dropping out of graduate school, Alicia rationalizes her failure by blaming it on a "hostile major professor" and further proclaiming, "I know more than he does." She describes herself as the "leader" in her group of six graduate students and interprets this to mean that they have great respect for her.

Exhibitionism Exhibitionistic behavior is demonstrated by the constant seeking of support and admiration from others. Because of their limited interests, these clients boast about themselves to the point of boring others. Concern over declining physical attractiveness and occupational limitations may lead them to seek cosmetic surgery.

MEDIALINK 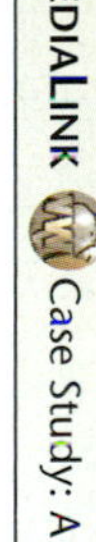 Case Study: A Narcissistic Client

Labile Affective Response Despite the narcissistic individual's extensive use of rationalization for failures, there is an underlying sense of rage, shame, and diminished self-esteem. The perceptive nurse may observe cool indifference, emptiness, humiliation, uncontrolled anger, or desire for revenge. The following clinical example illustrates this lack of empathy.

CLINICAL EXAMPLE

Alicia tells the therapist that she attempted to call two friends following her withdrawal from school. She dramatically and self-righteously expresses anger and disappointment that they were not available to her. (One was vacationing out of state and the other was hospitalized for major surgery.) When the therapist inquired how her friend was doing following surgery, Alicia responded, "How in the world should I know? That's not my problem. She never even bothered to call me back."

Dysfunctional Interpersonal Relationships Clients with NPD feel entitled to special favors and attention. Further, they refuse to assume mutual responsibilities in relationships and tend to exploit and disregard the rights of others. They lack empathy, especially toward those whom they perceive to be of lower status. The following clinical example describes these characteristics of entitlement and exploitation.

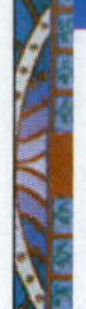

CLINICAL EXAMPLE

Alicia requests that the therapist set up Saturday morning appointments (no office hours are normally scheduled on this day) because she becomes very tired in the afternoons and always takes a nap. When the therapist refuses to meet this request, Alicia becomes angry and shouts, "You're just like all the rest of them. No one considers my needs! I'll see to it that your supervisor hears about this, and I'll let all my friends know how incompetent you are as a therapist."

In his classic work on narcissism that remains the standard for understanding this disorder, Kernberg (1975) emphasizes that chronic, intense envy and defenses against envy lead to idealization or devaluation of others. Responses to others may include lack of concern, mistrust, lack of intimacy, accusations of incompetence, and demand for unattainable perfection. Clients with NPD see interpersonal relationships as a means of enhancing their own self-esteem. A narcissistic person often selects a spouse or partner who will be dutiful and subservient in return for assurances of security and faithfulness. More recently, Kernberg has identified what he calls the "almost untreatable" narcissistic client (Kernberg, 2007). These are clients who combine the characteristics of NPD and BPD, and possibly antisocial personality disorder as well, representing the most severe cases of pathological narcissism.

Impaired Sexual Expression Perverse sexual fantasies and promiscuity may be associated with NPD. There may be confusion regarding sex-role behavior. Sexual favors may be used as bartering tools with partners.

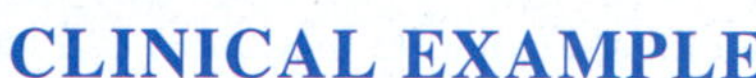

CLINICAL EXAMPLE

Alicia makes it clear on initial contact that she has a wide circle of friends. Indeed, she devotes the first 30 minutes of the session to recounting sexual encounters and venting anger that concern about AIDS is limiting her sex partners. She states she had a live-in relationship with one partner for 15 years but that recently this partner became discontented with her need to "party." Consequently, the two are "not communicating." Alicia defends her desire to seek out a variety of partners by focusing on her personal needs and the "lack of consideration" of her significant other.

MEDIALINK Antisocial Personality Disorder Video

Antisocial Personality Disorder

Antisocial personality disorder (ASPD), a pattern of disregard for and violation of the rights of others, was one of the earliest personality disorders to be identified. It has been labeled *psychopathy*, *sociopathy*, *dyssocial disorder*, and *moral insanity*. Most people with ASPD do not seek medical help but often come to the attention of authorities because of criminal activity that leads to judicial commitment to psychiatric facilities or incarceration in correctional facilities. In clinical settings, 3% to 30% of the population may have this disorder. Higher prevalence rates are found in substance abuse treatment centers and forensic settings (APA, 2000).

Manipulation, which is a hallmark of the antisocial client's behavior, can be a normal, nondestructive mode of meeting one's needs. However, when used to control others, manipulation interferes with interpersonal relationships. In antisocial clients, the drive to manipulate others is paramount, because these clients feel a need to be "number one" at all times. Manipulation may be evident in the client's attempt to form alliances with the staff. Once alliances are formed, splitting occurs and the client is in control, as shown in the following clinical example.

CLINICAL EXAMPLE

"You know, you are the only nurse on this unit who knows anything about the meds that we get. I always feel so safe when you are at the med station. You know when I really need my tranquilizers. The other nurses look at me suspiciously like I'm some kind of criminal. Thank God you're on duty tonight." This same client may tell the nurse on the following shift, "That night nurse does nothing but pass pills all night long; she never spends time with the patients or even tries to talk to them before she drugs them up. I think something should be done about her."

In your contacts with antisocial people, you may find them initially charming. They are often intellectually bright, conversationally glib, and they tell you what you want to hear. Because they are so astute in identifying others' vulnerabilities, nurses are frequently amazed at the "empathy" they show for others. These behaviors are manipulative and are used to create a situation that the person with ASPD can control.

During the initial assessment interview, it is common for the person diagnosed with ASPD to refuse responsibility for admission to the mental health or forensic facility. In fact, this individual will probably claim that the victim of his or her actions is at fault; in addition, no remorse will be shown, as in the following clinical example.

CLINICAL EXAMPLE

Jason says to his arresting officers, "Well, you know, the only reason I'm here is because those cops made a mistake and thought I was the one who was assaulting that woman. Actually I stopped to help her and she told them I was trying to rape her. You know, if she hadn't parked her car in the mall garage, then she wouldn't have been at risk for an assault in the first place."

Impulsiveness is manifested in the client's making quick decisions without regard for the consequences. "I'm going on pass right now; it doesn't matter if you discharge me AMA [against medical advice]." Aggression may be exhibited by instigating fights with other clients, often when the client feels a need for excitement or has not received sufficient attention from the staff. The client's explanation might be: "Hey, if you guys would get more sports going for us here, we wouldn't be getting on each other's nerves so much."

Lack of anxiety is notable with antisocial individuals, unless there is extreme external stress, in which case they may act out in ways that put them at high risk for accidents, physical injury, or suicidal acts. History of violence toward others is very common, including sex offenses (i.e., rape, child pornography, child molestation) and murder. These clients often have histories of drug dealing and substance abuse, prostitution, homelessness, erratic job histories, and exploitive sexual relationships. While these individuals can identify what is correct and appropriate behavior, they do not believe the rules apply to them.

People with ASPD need immediate gratification in most situations but can delay rewards to the extent that they need planning time to achieve what they want. They are often admitted to mental health facilities for depressive symptoms, suicidal attempts, substance abuse, somatic disorders, and/or anxiety disorders.

Cluster C Personality Disorders: Anxious–Fearful

According to the DSM-IV-TR, personality-disordered individuals who are primarily anxious or fearful may be diagnosed with avoidant, dependent, or obsessive–compulsive personality disorder. Anxious–fearful people generally experience both social and occupational impairments as a result of their restricted affect, nonassertiveness, problems expressing feelings, unrealistic expectations of others, and impaired decision making and problem solving. The lifestyle of the anxious–fearful person is characterized by intense emotional repression and behaviors that are socially isolating and self-defeating. The behaviors of anxious–fearful personalities tend to overlap, and common diagnostic features are described in the DSM-IV-TR Diagnostic Criteria feature on page 592.

Avoidant Personality Disorder

The essential feature of people with **avoidant personality disorder** (APD) is a pattern of social withdrawal along with a sense of inadequacy, fear, and hypersensitivity to potential rejection or shame. These people withdraw socially even though they deeply desire affection and acceptance. Their avoidant behavior results in visiting public places (movies, museums, and ballparks) simply to experience the presence of other people because they do not enjoy being alone. When in public places, however, they maintain a safe distance from others. For example, in a movie theater, one can be physically close to people without feeling that one's personal space is being invaded.

Avoidant people devalue their own achievements. They appear overly serious, humorless, and painfully shy. Speech is often slow, and they do not readily express their feelings. Thought content is generally serious. In the following clinical example, Mary Jane exhibits the characteristics of APD.

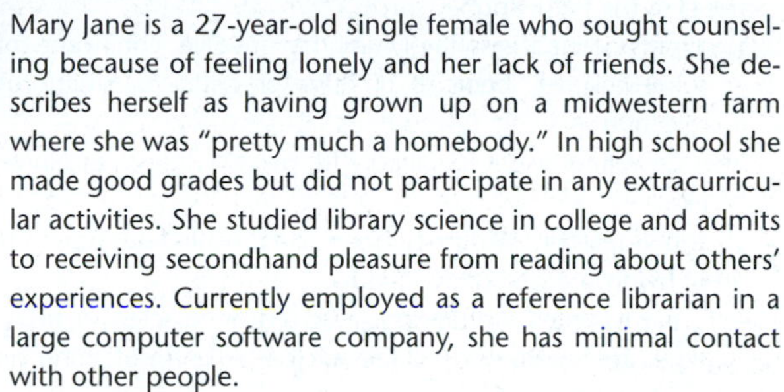

CLINICAL EXAMPLE

Mary Jane is a 27-year-old single female who sought counseling because of feeling lonely and her lack of friends. She describes herself as having grown up on a midwestern farm where she was "pretty much a homebody." In high school she made good grades but did not participate in any extracurricular activities. She studied library science in college and admits to receiving secondhand pleasure from reading about others' experiences. Currently employed as a reference librarian in a large computer software company, she has minimal contact with other people.

She says she wants to establish both male and female friendships but feels afraid that people will laugh at her. Mary Jane joined the company bowling team at the suggestion of a coworker but quit after the first evening because she felt she would "hold them back." Mary Jane rationalized her decision by stating, "I think I would be more comfortable pursuing an intellectual hobby."

Dependent Personality Disorder

The essential features of **dependent personality disorder** (DPD) include a pervasive, excessive, and unrealistic need to be cared for; fear of separation; lack of self-confidence; an inability to make decisions; and an inability to function independently. In sharp contrast to the avoidant person, dependent people cling to others and passively accept their dictates and leadership. Dependent people view themselves as "helpless" or "stupid" and seek out dominant others to rely on for guidance, control, and support as well as for "permission" to behave. These individuals have difficulty initiating projects and function adequately only when assured of approval and supervision.

In dependent people, the normal symbiotic parent–child relationship has been excessively prolonged, impairing their capacity for thinking, feeling, and responding on their own. They believe they must be taken care of and consequently rely on others to mirror their feelings to them.

Dependent people subordinate their desires and needs to the wishes of others in order to maintain relationships. They often appear friendly, helpful, and indispensable. Indeed, they will volunteer for unpleasant tasks if they think they will be reciprocated with nurturing. When the dominant other is unavailable, or perceived as unavailable, dependent people experience intense anxiety. This may lead to feelings of unhappiness, anger, resentment, or depression. It is also noteworthy that significant others may eventually respond to dependent people with anger and resentment because of their continuous clinging and ingratiating behaviors. The following clinical example illustrates how a dependent client might behave.

MediaLink Critical Thinking Exercise: Antisocial Behavior

DSM-IV-TR Diagnostic Criteria for Personality Disorders: Cluster C (Fearful–Anxious)

Avoidant Personality Disorder

A pervasive pattern of social inhibition, feelings of inadequacy, and hypersensitivity to negative evaluation, beginning by early adulthood and present in a variety of contexts, as indicated by four (or more) of the following:

1. avoids occupational activities that involve significant interpersonal contact, because of fears of criticism, disapproval, or rejection
2. is unwilling to get involved with people unless certain of being liked
3. shows restraint within intimate relationships because of the fear of being shamed or ridiculed
4. is preoccupied with being criticized or rejected in social situations. **Note:** Do not include suicidal or self-mutilating behavior covered in Criterion 5.
5. is inhibited in new interpersonal situations because of feelings of inadequacy
6. views self as socially inept, personally unappealing, or inferior to others
7. is unusually reluctant to take personal risks or to engage in any new activities because they may prove embarrassing

Dependent Personality Disorder

A pervasive and excessive need to be taken care of that leads to submissive and clinging behavior and fears of separation, beginning by early adulthood and present in a variety of contexts, as indicated by five (or more) of the following:

1. has difficulty making everyday decisions without an excessive amount of advice and reassurance from others
2. needs others to assume responsibility for most major areas of his or her life
3. has difficulty expressing disagreement with others because of fear of loss of support or approval. **Note:** Do not include realistic fears of retribution.
4. has difficulty initiating projects or doing things on his or her own (because of a lack of self-confidence in judgment or abilities rather than a lack of motivation or energy)
5. goes to excessive lengths to obtain nurturance and support from others, to the point of volunteering to do things that are unpleasant
6. feels uncomfortable or helpless when alone because of exaggerated fears of being unable to care for himself or herself
7. urgently seeks another relationship as a source of care and support when a close relationship ends
8. is unrealistically preoccupied with fears of being left to take care of himself or herself

Obsessive–Compulsive Personality Disorder

A pervasive pattern of preoccupation with orderliness, perfectionism, and mental and interpersonal control—at the expense of flexibility, openness, and efficiency—beginning by early adulthood and present in a variety of contexts, as indicated by four (or more) of the following:

1. is preoccupied with details, rules, lists, order, organization, or schedules to the extent that the major point of the activity is lost
2. shows perfectionism that interferes with task completion (e.g., is unable to complete a project because his or her own overly strict standards are not met)
3. is excessively devoted to work and productivity to the exclusion of leisure activities and friendships (not accounted for by obvious economic necessity)
4. is overconscientious, scrupulous, and inflexible about matters of morality, ethics, or values (not accounted for by cultural or religious identification)
5. is unable to discard worn-out or worthless objects even when they have no sentimental value
6. is reluctant to delegate tasks or to work with others unless they submit to exactly his or her way of doing things
7. adopts a miserly spending style toward both self and others; money is viewed as something to be hoarded for future catastrophes
8. shows rigidity and stubbornness

Source: Reprinted with permission from the *Diagnostic and Statistical Manual of Mental Disorders,* Fourth Edition, Text Revision. (Copyright 2000). American Psychiatric Association.

USING DSM-IV-TR

Health care providers often use language unfamiliar to clients and their families. Explain *a pervasive pattern of social inhibition* in such a way that clients and family members can understand its meaning in relationship to avoidant personality disorder.

CLINICAL EXAMPLE

Marie is a 40-year-old single parent of two teenage daughters. She has gained 70 pounds since her divorce 2 years ago. Currently, Marie is sporadically attending a group for displaced homemakers, where she has shared a great deal of information about herself. She states that she is essentially a "homebody" and feels most satisfied when baking, cooking, and sewing for her daughters. Marie describes her secondhand pleasure in their activities, including ballet, gymnastics, and modeling. In fact, Marie becomes visibly saddened when she discusses her daughters' eventual departure for college. When her daughters expressed concern about Marie's weight gain and general health, Marie giggled and said, "Better to be fat and jolly than skinny and mean."

Marie has made no attempt to develop new friendships or social outlets since her divorce. She is poorly groomed and haphazardly dressed, in contrast to her impeccably groomed daughters. When confronted by group members about setting priorities and the need to direct some energy toward herself, Marie responded, "My life is devoted to my daughters. Their needs are more important than mine, and that's why I agreed to make 30 costumes for their dance recital next week."

WHAT EVERY MATERNAL–CHILD NURSE SHOULD KNOW

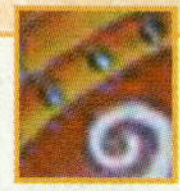

The Client with Dependent Personality Disorder

- Be alert for signs of depression in the new mother.
- Assess the woman's history for indicators of domestic abuse.
- Women who are excessively dependent may have difficulty in assuming care for a newborn.
- Be attuned to your own feelings of helplessness to ensure that apathy does not interfere with your ability to deliver quality care.
- Avoid the tendency to rescue the dependent client; this will only reinforce the woman's sense of helplessness.
- Encourage the client to do as much for herself and her infant as possible.
- Praise the client's assumption of personal responsibility.

Like people with other personality disorders, the dependent person may have multiple DSM Axis II diagnoses. Because DPD is among the most frequently reported of the personality disorders (APA, 2000), you may encounter dependent persons in other health care settings. For example, maternal–child nurses should be aware of the key factors outlined in the feature What Every Maternal–Child Nurse Should Know.

Obsessive–Compulsive Personality Disorder

People with **obsessive–compulsive personality disorder** (OCPD) demonstrate fear and anxiety concerning loss of control over situations, objects, or people. They demonstrate perfectionism, preoccupation with details, and hoarding behavior. The person with OCPD strives at all times to keep the world predictable and organized. The major features of this disorder are an excessive need for order, extreme dedication to work and productivity, and perfectionism to the exclusion of feelings and pleasure. A person with OCPD may be likened to a drill sergeant in the military who is rigid, serious, detail-oriented, and stingy with emotions.

People with OCPD tend to focus on trivial details. Although they may be highly praised for their organizational skills and work ethic, eventually their rigidity causes them to fear making mistakes. Because they repeatedly check their work, they are not good time managers; thus, projects may not get completed. They are self-critical and adhere strictly and concretely to rules. Consequently, they postpone making decisions. They tend to resent authority but rarely express this resentment openly. Instead, they may engage in passive–aggressive behavior, such as procrastination and stubbornness.

People who are excessively conscientious and rigid often exhibit a contradictory pattern of slovenliness, which is also compulsive. Thus, a compulsive housewife may scrub her kitchen floor daily but allow bags of garbage to accumulate and become infested. When clients with OCPD describe their lifestyle, you will quickly become aware of their rigidity, concreteness, and need for order and perfection. In the following clinical example, John demonstrates extreme orderliness.

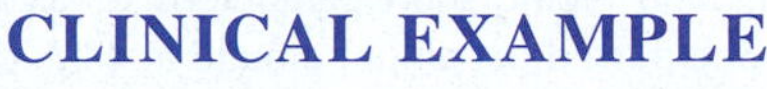

CLINICAL EXAMPLE

John explained, "I have all my clothes hanging in the closet according to the day of the week, including my shoes, socks and underwear, so I know if it's a Tuesday after a long weekend with a Monday holiday that I need to wear the clothing on the hanger marked Tuesday."

Jerlinda has her linen closet and her silverware drawer scrupulously organized. The towels and washcloths are all folded and stacked in the same direction. The forks are lined up in a row in the silverware drawer. However, Jerlinda's kitchen and bathroom floors are a mess.

To manage their procrastination, obsessive–compulsive people often initiate work on a project far in advance of the due date. In the following clinical example, Peter appears to be concerned with his family and interpersonal relationships, but he is really more concerned with meeting the Christmas deadline and checking off his list than in his relatives' enjoyment of their gifts.

CLINICAL EXAMPLE

Peter set himself an early-fall deadline every year for ordering his family's Christmas gifts. His family found this deadline something of an annoyance. Yet Peter persisted in his attempts to get commitments from everyone about what they wanted. Often he was unable to make his early purchases before Christmas and would rush out to do last-minute shopping anyway.

Although Peter suffers under the pressure of his deadlines, he sets them for himself. He functions as his own overseer, issuing commands, directives, reminders, warnings, and admonitions about what should be done.

People with OCPD are also keenly aware of other people's expectations, of the threat of possible criticism, of the weight and direction of authority, of rules, regulations, and conventions, and of a great collection of moral principles. They feel required to fulfill unending duties, responsibilities, and tasks. Obsessive–compulsive people do not view taking work home and working long hours as an imposition, since work organizes their lives and binds their anxiety. Indeed, they will manage to make work out of pleasurable activities, as demonstrated in the following clinical example.

CLINICAL EXAMPLE

Jennifer planned her European vacation in meticulous detail. She scheduled exhausting daily tours and activities from 6:30 a.m. until midnight. Jennifer planned to visit every attraction available as quickly as possible. So as not to waste time, she wrote postcards to her family while she rode tour buses. The cards were crammed with information about weather, prices of goods and services, menus, and daily timetables. She wrote nothing about how she felt or what she was experiencing.

Upon returning home, she spent two weeks cataloging all her photographs and typing short paragraphs to accompany each photo. She passed her album around at work during lunch hour, expecting that her coworkers would read all the captions. She was insulted and irate when several coworkers flipped through the album quickly. Jennifer found it difficult to forgive them for "slighting" her in this way.

OCPD appears in males more often than females and in about 1% of the general population (APA, 2000). Because many cultures emphasize and positively reinforce adherence to a strong work ethic, it is important that you consider cultural factors when assessing clients with OCPD.

BIOPSYCHOSOCIAL THEORIES

As the individual experiences life, adaptive mechanisms solidify, ultimately resulting in an automatic response style. When the response style is based on misperceptions or distortions, a personality disorder may develop. Therefore, the psychiatric–mental health nurse using a biopsychosocial model views clients with personality disorders as people whose communication and behavior are greatly influenced by past experiences, a need to maintain self-direction and control, and a unique style of interpreting their world.

Biologic Factors

Biologic factors associated with personality-disordered individuals as reported by Sadock and Sadock (2005) include alterations in hormone levels and platelet monoamine oxidase (MAO) levels, smooth-pursuit eye movements, levels of endorphin and 5-HIAA (a metabolite of serotonin), and electroencephalographic (EEG) changes.

Recent research addresses the role of biologic factors in the genesis of BPD. Hormones are being implicated to the extent that increased levels of testosterone, 17-estradiol, and estrone have been observed in people with impulse control problems. Dexamethasone suppression test (see Chapters 6 and 17) findings have also been abnormal in some people with depressive symptoms who are diagnosed with BPD. The serotonin metabolite 5-HIAA has been shown to be low in people who attempt suicide and in those with aggression and impulse control problems (Sadock & Sadock, 2005). The following are some examples of brain research findings that support neurobiology as a major contributing factor to PDs:

- Poor cognitive performance and symptoms of schizotypal PD are associated with smaller caudate volume (Koo, Levitt, et al., 2006).
- Functioning of the anterior cortical regions that affects memory recall is impaired in people with schizotypal personality disorder (Harvey, Romero, Richenberg, Granholm, & Siever, 2006; Koenisberg et al., 2005).
- Structural brain abnormalilties have been observed in males who have schizotypal personality disorder. This study states that the smaller neocortical gray matter volume and larger cerebrospinal fluid volumes are evidence of the brain's role in the origin of SPD (Koo, Dickey, et al., 2006).
- People with borderline personality disorder have higher pain thresholds than individuals not affected by BPD. This is theorized to be a result of the interaction between the pain response center in the prefrontal cortex and changes in the cingulate and amygdala (Schmahl, Bohus, et al., 2006).
- Structural and functional imaging studies of the brain indicate that frontolimbic dysfunction contributes to a majority of symptoms associated with borderline personality disorder (Schmahl & Bremner, 2006).
- The fact that many people with borderline personality disorder respond effectively to antispychotic medications supports the conclusion that neurotransmitters are altered in BPD. Quetiapine therapy is especially effective in reducing impulsive and aggressive symptoms in those with BPD (Bellino, Paradiso, & Bogetto, 2006).
- Diminished cerebral blood flow in the orbitofrontal cortex is related to antisocial symptoms in some individuals (Nakano et al., 2006).
- Chronic inflammation, as evidenced by the presence of elevated levels of C-reactive protein (pCRP), are associated with higher levels of aggression and hostility in personality-disorderd individuals (Coccaro, 2005).

Genetic Theories

Following are some current research studies that support a genetic cause of personality disorders:

- Using studies from 15,000 pairs of monozygotic and dizygotic twins in the United States, Sadock and Sadock (2005) identified significant familial correlations of schizotypal personality disorders among people with family members who are schizophrenic.
- Cluster B illnesses (borderline, histrionic, narcissistic, and antisocial) are often correlated with histories of mood disorders, alcoholism, and somatization disorders among family members (Sadock & Sadock, 2005).
- Research indicates strong familial tendencies toward antisocial PD. It is more common among first-degree relatives; having a female biologic relative with the disorder tends to increase the risk. Adoption studies show that both genetic and environmental factors contribute to the risk (APA, 2000).
- Schizoid and schizotypal PDs are significantly more common among first-degree relatives of schizophrenic clients. At this time, however, there is no substantial evidence that these PDs are early

indicators of a future schizophrenic process (Sadock & Sadock, 2005).

- People affected by schizotypal personality disorder demonstrate several deficits in tasks dependent on functioning of the prefrontal and temporal lobes (Minzenberg et al., 2006).
- A preliminary study (Light et al., 2006) indicates an association between a dopamine D_3 receptor gene variant and OCPD. People with this genetic variation are approximately 2.5 times more likely to be diganosed with obsessive–compulsive personality disorder.
- Another recent study suggests that the gene responsible for serotonin transmission may contribute to the development of borderline personality disorder (Ni et al., 2006).

Psychosocial Theories

The sense of self originates with the earliest parent–child interactions. If parents are not sensitive and attuned to the child's needs, they fail to confirm the child's emerging sense of reality. Consequently, the child distorts reality and develops an unreal "as-if" personality that shifts to meet the demands of cues in the outer world. According to Figueiredo (2006), children who have difficulty establishing a sense of reality are those who develop borderline defense mechanisms.

Parental deprivation; inadequate, excessive, or inconsistent discipline; and failure of the child to develop integrated cognitive, affective, and behavioral modes in early life may lead to Cluster B disorders. Clients have generalized feelings of low self-esteem, need to control people and situations, and are unable to delay gratification. In response, dramatic–emotional clients tend to interact by negatively manipulating others. Although manipulation is a standard response in the repertoire of people with these PDs, its occurrence escalates with increased stress.

According to intrapsychic theory, psychological fixations in the genital stage of development may account for many of the behaviors noted in some PDs. For example, it is developmentally appropriate for a toddler to expect immediate gratification of needs. However, many adults with PDs display developmental immaturity through an inability to postpone immediate gratification of needs and wants. Impulsive and self-centered behaviors are examples of this type of developmental fixation.

Individuals with PDs have serious impairments related to establishing and maintaining healthy interpersonal boundaries. Intimacy is characterized by the ability to be close to another while maintaining a sense of separateness. Those with PDs generally have issues related to enmeshment and/or abandonment, which interfere with intimacy. **Enmeshment** refers to a feeling of being engulfed by others or of being overpowered by dominant others. Common signs of enmeshment include speaking for another person, answering for someone else, or responding to an event as another person would. Enmeshment in families is discussed in Chapter 30∞. **Abandonment** refers to feelings of being left alone; many people with PDs are vulnerable to feelings of abandonment as their sometimes bizarre, demanding behaviors push others away, resulting in alienation and isolation. Due to a fear of intimacy, some individuals sabotage relationships by provoking rejection while simultaneously fearing it.

Erikson (1964) coined the term **identity diffusion** to describe the failure to integrate various childhood identifications into a harmonious adult psychosocial identity. Kernberg (1975) suggests that when, as children, borderline clients perceive the parenting figure as both nurturing and punishing, they learn to reduce anxiety and resolve resulting conflicts by such primitive defensive strategies as splitting, projective identification, primitive idealization, omnipotence, devaluation, and denial. It is theorized that children of women with BPD are at greater risk for emotional, behavioral, and somatic problems because they are exposed to a combination of risk factors (Barnow, Spitzer, Grabe, Kessler, & Freyberger, 2006).

Humanistic Theories

Individuals need to feel that they are a part of something greater than themselves. In their search for meaning, some individuals with personality disorder often engage in self-damaging acts. For example, after slitting her wrists with a razor, a client may state, "When I hurt, I feel real." While attempting to negate existential emptiness, the client actually threatens his or her own well-being. The fear of abandonment and alienation that is experienced by many people with personality disorders leads to existential dilemmas, such as "Am I real?" and fear of discovering emptiness within if left alone.

When considering the cause of personality disorders, it is wise to think of a culmination of factors. There is no one definitive cause of personality disorders. However, the humanistic holistic perspective considers that a variety of factors contribute to the problem. For example, according to Bornovalova, Gratz, Delany-Brumsey, Paulson, and Lejuez (2006), BPD is widely considered the result of biological vulnerability and environmental adversity.

SELF-AWARENESS

Self-awareness is the first step in developing therapeutic approaches to clients with any personality disorder. By examining your responses and feelings toward the client, you will be better able to prevent **countertransference** from occurring (see Chapter 29∞). The behaviors demonstrated by personality-disordered clients often evoke strong negative feelings and responses in nurses, which puts clients at risk for stigmatization. Clients may be labeled or stereotyped, which leads to depersonalization and inadequate treatment.

Your responses to clients who have Cluster B personality disorders may be similar to the behaviors displayed by the clients themselves. You must be attuned to your own feelings and reactions when working with clients with NPD. Do not criticize their haughty, uncaring attitude, but demonstrate by actions that they are accepted regardless of wealth, position, or status.

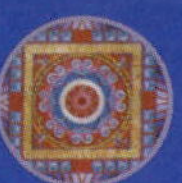

YOUR SELF-AWARENESS
Exploring Your Thoughts and Feelings Toward Clients with Personality Disorders

Pay attention to your feelings when interacting with clients with PDs. The following questions will help you assess your reactions:

- How do you respond when you become angry with a client?
- What do you do when you feel helpless to effect change?
- What do you do when you feel guilty about being unable to help a client?
- Can you detect your early physiologic and emotional responses to stress?
- How great is your need to rescue or "save" clients from unhealthy situations?
- How do you know when you are becoming defensive?
- What is your behavioral response when you feel that you have been "used"?

The arousal of feelings of anger, powerlessness, a sense of having been "conned," disappointment, and even guilt and shame is common among nurses who work with PD clients. Nurses are often unaware of their own beliefs, which may be countertherapeutic. The Your Self-Awareness feature above will direct you toward introspection. By using introspection and clinical supervision, you can become more aware of the impact of your feelings and behaviors on others. Only then will you be able to respond more appropriately to all clients.

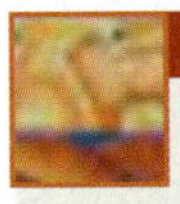

NURSING PROCESS
Clients with Cluster A (Odd–Eccentric) Personality Disorders

This section focuses on information specific to the nursing care of individuals with Cluster A personality disorders: schizoid, schizotypal, and paranoid types.

Assessment

Of the disorders in this group, the one most commonly seen in inpatient psychiatric settings is paranoid personality disorder (APA, 2000). You will also see clients with paranoid personality disorders in outpatient settings, emergency departments (refer back to What Every Emergency Department Nurse Should Know on page 584), and prisons. When conducting assessment interviews with clients with paranoid personality disorder, it is very important to remember that behavior is culturally defined. Many individuals, particularly those from minority and/or immigrant groups, are erroneously labeled mentally ill because their behaviors are not congruent with the expected standards of the health care team. Indeed, the clinical evaluation may reinforce suspiciousness, hostility, and acting-out behavior because the client is unfamiliar with and frightened by the assessment process. Remember that paranoid traits may be adaptive in threatening situations.

When assessing both schizoid and schizotypal clients, it is imperative to consider the person's ethnicity, cultural milieu, and spiritual belief system. Within many cultures, speaking in tongues and psychic phenomena are natural experiences and should not be deemed pathologic. People who are making a transition from one environment to another—from a rural to an urban setting, for instance—may seem different because of their constricted affect and solitary activities. Immigrants must be assessed from a multicultural viewpoint in order to differentiate between lack of understanding and indifference. What may seem odd in Parker, Georgia, may be commonplace in New York City.

Nursing Diagnosis: NANDA

Effective nursing diagnosis depends on collecting accurate data in a thorough, organized assessment. There is much overlap among the problematic behaviors in the various types of personality disorders, and in addition, a person can have more than one personality disorder at the same time. Therefore, nursing diagnoses are focused on the client's response to a disorder rather than on a specific diagnostic category. Since nursing is client-centered rather than disease-oriented, this section will describe the primary nursing diagnoses for each type of PD.

The major nursing diagnoses for clients with Cluster A (odd–eccentric) PDs are:

- Ineffective coping
- Impaired social interaction

Outcome Identification: NOC

Expected outcomes must be individualized for each client, considering the unique situation and cultural context. The major goal is that clients with Cluster A (odd–eccentric) PDs will interact with others in a socially appropriate manner. Specific outcomes that indicate progress toward achievement of this goal include:

- Participates in activity groups
- Copes effectively with stressful situations
- Approaches staff and other clients without encouragement
- Verbalizes thoughts and feelings that interfere with socialization
- Identifies behaviors that maximize social interaction
- Verbalizes trust in other clients, staff, and family

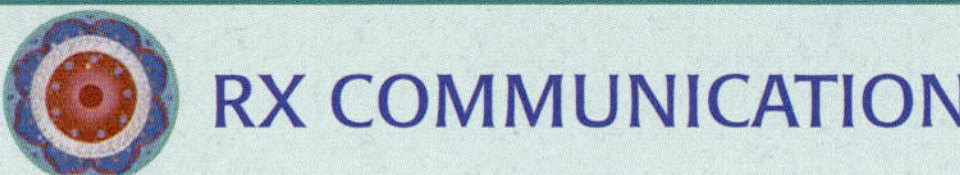

RX COMMUNICATION

THE CLIENT WITH PARANOID PERSONALITY DISORDER

CLIENT: "What did you mean by that remark? People are always making fun of me."

NURSE RESPONSE 1: "That remark was not meant for you, Jerry. It was directed at everyone in the group."

RATIONALE: This response provides a simple explanation without being argumentative or overly detailed in explanation. It also reinforces reality for the client.

NURSE RESPONSE 2: "You feel others are picking on you."

RATIONALE: This statement encourages the client to verbalize feelings of mistrust. It is stated in a nonjudgmental manner while maintaining appropriate eye contact, which is a behavior that promotes trust.

Planning and Implementation: NIC

When interviewing a client who has paranoid personality disorder, maintain an open, nonthreatening style of questioning. The example in the Rx Communication feature above gives some suggestions.

Do not argue with or interpret the client's responses. Because these clients may hold grudges and are quick to attack, consider safety provisions for yourself and other staff as well as the clients. For other intervention guidelines, see the following feature, Your Intervention Strategies: Guidelines for the Client with Paranoid Personality Disorder.

Aggressive Behavior

Clients with paranoid personality disorder, antisocial personality disorder, and borderline personality disorder are those most likely to demonstrate aggressive behavior. You need to help clients learn to differentiate anger and aggression. Anger is an emotion, and aggression is a behavior. Everyone is entitled to feel the way they feel; however, the way in which those feelings are expressed must be modified to avoid causing harm to others. Limit setting and assertiveness training (discussed in Chapter 3) are important interventions for helping clients learn to change aggressive acts to behavior

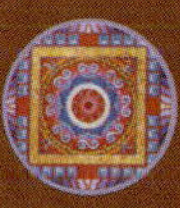

YOUR INTERVENTION STRATEGIES
Guidelines for the Client with Paranoid Personality Disorder

Nursing Intervention	Rationale
Respect personal space.	Promotes a sense of security.
Respect client's preferences as much as is reasonable.	Increases self-esteem.
Give feedback to client based on observed nonverbal cues of responsiveness, such as eye movement, posturing, voice tones.	Improves interpersonal effectiveness.
Provide client with a daily schedule of activities and inform client of changes.	Activity schedules will diminish anxiety about social interactions and may help ensure participation.
Help client identify adaptive diversionary activities (leisure, recreation) in one–to–one sessions and groups.	Participation in groups may increase client's support system.
Use role-playing to help client identify feelings, thoughts, and responses brought on by stressful situations.	Rehearsing social behaviors in a safe environment provides immediate feedback and time for altering responses.
Encourage client to evaluate how client behaviors led to the current crisis.	Points out cause-and-effect aspects of interaction.
Use an objective, matter-of-fact approach with client.	Client will identify the nurse as a reliable person who gives respect without argument.
Use concrete, specific words rather than global abstractions.	Keeps intended message clear by decreasing ambiguity.
Respond to suspicious ideas by focusing on feelings: "It must be distressing." "You see him as vindictive."	Communicates empathy.
Conduct brief one–to–one sessions daily (avoid lengthy sessions).	Shortened sessions decrease fear and anxiety.
Gradually introduce client to group situations.	Trust-building is a slow process.

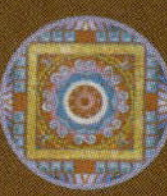

YOUR INTERVENTION STRATEGIES
Guidelines for the Angry Client

Nursing Intervention	Rationale
Use a calm, unhurried approach.	Calmness promotes security.
Do not touch client indiscriminately.	Touch may be misinterpreted as aggressive or sexual.
Respect personal space.	Space provides insulation/protection.
Use active listening skills.	Attention and direct eye contact promote trust.
Remain aware of your feelings.	Helps to avoid counter-transference reactions.
Use statements to provide feedback and identify sources of anger: "I notice your fists are clenched—what's happening?"	Feedback on feelings increases client awareness.
Assure client that staff will not allow the client to hurt self or others.	Conveys the presence of external controls.
Observe for escalation of anger (increased activity, verbal and nonverbal acting-out).	Early awareness prevents crisis.
Institute precautions against suicide, homicide, assault, or escape, as indicated.	Ensures safety of client and others.
Discuss alternate means of releasing tension and physical energy.	Increases self-esteem through adaptive outlets.
Provide physical outlets to reduce tension, such as exercise, gardening, clay work, music, art (avoid competitive or contact sports).	Exercise releases anxiety/tension.
Protect other clients from verbal/physical abuse.	Ensures safety of all clients.
Clearly communicate and enforce agency regulations concerning acting-out behavior.	People behave according to expectations.
Postpone discussion of consequences of acting-out until client is in control.	Avoids triggering aggressive behavior.
Role-model appropriate assertions of angry feelings: "I dislike it when—"	New behaviors can be learned by watching others.
Communicate desire to help client maintain/regain control.	Offering self helps to establish trust.
Hold client responsible for behavior; remind client of the ability to make choices.	Promotes internal control.
Use contracts for behavioral control, including seeking out staff people when feelings emerge.	Reinforces personal responsibility.
Teach assertiveness skills, relaxation, imagery, thought stopping, thought control.	Defuses anxiety and reinforces ability for self-control.

that is appropriate. Another important facet of nursing intervention and psychiatric treatment is helping clients understand and appreciate the rights and needs of others; these concepts can be effectively taught in group settings.

It is important to avoid personalizing the client's aggression. "Taking it personally" will increase your defensiveness, which in turn increases the client's perception of threat and can result in escalation of inappropriate behavior. Nurses who personalize clients' behavior lose their professional credibility. When you look at clients' inappropriate behavior as a clinical manifestation of a disorder instead of an act deliberately intended to harm, you are less likely to personalize the behavior.

When working with aggressive clients, safety is of utmost importance. Many clients with PDs, especially borderline, antisocial, and paranoid types, are at high risk of hurting themselves or others. See the feature above, Your Intervention Strategies: Guidelines for the Angry Client, as well as Chapters 23, 24, and 35.

Evaluation

Remember to use all your observation and interviewing skills when evaluating the progress of clients with Cluster A PDs. Such clients tend to share little of their feelings and will go to great lengths to avoid interacting with staff members. For more information on evaluating care provided to clients with PDs, see the other evaluation sections on pages 602 and 604–605.

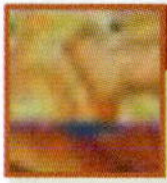

NURSING PROCESS
Clients with Cluster B (Dramatic–Emotional) Personality Disorders

You may often experience feelings of frustration and helplessness when caring for clients with Cluster B personality disorders (borderline, narcissistic, histrionic, and antisocial). Following the structure the nursing process provides will help you remain objective, focused, and organized when providing care.

Assessment

When assessing clients with dramatic–emotional PDs, be sure that your words and actions are congruent—that is, your nonverbal behaviors match what you say. To avoid being drawn in by a client's manipulative behaviors, you must maintain professional distance by using empathy. Specific questions you can ask clients and their families are outlined in the Your Assessment Approach feature below.

Nursing Diagnosis: NANDA

Individuals with Cluster B (dramatic–emotional) personality disorders are likely to experience:

- Chronic low self-esteem
- Risk for self-directed violence
- Risk for other-directed violence

Note that these nursing diagnoses may apply to a client with any type of PD. Clients may also have several other diagnoses, based on their unique situations.

Outcome Identification: NOC

Clients with Cluster B (dramatic–emotional) personality disorders have several issues that need to be resolved, such as learning to act in a less impulsive manner, controlling aggressive behavior, and improving self-esteem. Decreased impulsivity can be measured by the following expected outcomes:

- Identifies consequences of impulsive behavior
- Verbalizes the need to act less impulsively
- Uses techniques to control impulsive behavior (e.g., deep breathing, counting to ten before acting, taking a "time out" for decision making)
- Demonstrates a decreased incidence of impulsive acts (e.g., criminal acts, substance abuse, sexual promiscuity)

The following expected outcomes help measure the client's potential for violence directed at self and others.

- Identifies feelings of anger and/or frustration
- Verbalizes feelings appropriately
- Copes effectively with feelings
- Remains injury-free

Expected outcomes that are relevant to self-esteem include the following:

- Identifies own positive characteristics
- Gives and receives compliments
- Demonstrates assertive behavior
- Demonstrates appropriate eye contact

Planning and Implementation: NIC

Manipulation, impulsivity, and self-destructive behaviors are characteristic of individuals with Cluster B personality disorders. Providing care to individuals with BPD is especially difficult for some nurses and one of the greatest challenges facing mental health professionals today (Osborne & McComish, 2006). This section provides guidelines for responding to clients who exhibit such behaviors.

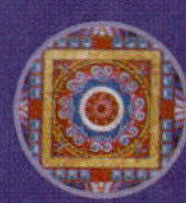

YOUR ASSESSMENT APPROACH
Guidelines for the Client with Dramatic–Emotional Personality Disorders

Ask the client the following questions:	Ask the client's significant others the following questions:
How often do you notice rapid mood changes?	Do you often feel that the client takes advantage of you?
When was the last time you lost your temper?	How does the client express feelings of concern for others?
How do you get along with others?	What does the client do when he/she becomes angry?
What happens when things do not go as you wish they would?	Is the client able to postpone getting what he/she wants?
How do you describe your ability to make decisions?	How would you describe the client's judgment?
What do you do when you feel bored?	Is the client able to share attention with others, or does he/she need to be the center of attention?
What important lessons did you learn from your last mistake?	
Do you ever feel depressed? If so, tell me about that.	

Manipulation

Manipulation is pervasive in the life of someone with a personality disorder, and it is extremely difficult for most clients to change behaviors that are so ingrained. Learning to meet one's needs directly is the major challenge for those who demonstrate manipulative behavior. By establishing an interpersonal relationship with the personality-disordered client, you will be better able to role-model appropriate behavior.

Because of their charm, air of superiority, and persuasiveness, people with ASPD sometimes manipulate nurses to assume the roles of nurturers and rescuers. These clients have lifelong patterns of victimizing and exploiting others. Never give out your telephone number, assign special privileges, or make yourself available to these clients outside the therapeutic relationship. Specific guidelines and their rationales are discussed in the Your Intervention Strategies feature at right.

Incorporate clear, concise, and consistent limit setting and directions into all intervention strategies. Develop these strategies using a team approach, and contract with the client. When infractions of the rules or manipulative behavior occur, apply consequences immediately.

Splitting or playing one staff member against another is a common manipulative ploy used by clients with PDs. A team approach is the only way to successfully counter this behavior. You must communicate continuously with colleagues, both individually and in team meetings, in order to know what the client is telling each staff member. Responding consistently to the manipulative behavior will help gradually lessen its intensity. Examples of appropriate responses to manipulative behavior are listed below in the Rx Communication: The Client with Borderline Personality Disorder feature.

A major intervention in dealing with manipulative behavior is limit setting. It is important to set limits only on the behavior that is most dysfunctional and problematic. If limits are imposed globally, the client is more likely to rebel and the dysfunctional behavior will escalate. Limit setting is done for three fundamental reasons:

1. To prevent escalation of negative behavior
2. To establish boundaries
3. To counteract resistance

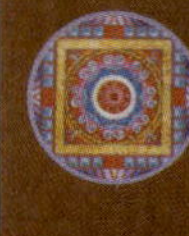

YOUR INTERVENTION STRATEGIES
Guidelines for the Client with Antisocial Personality Disorder

Nursing Intervention	Rationale
Use a concerned, matter-of-fact approach.	A nonargumentative response decreases manipulative attempts.
Set, communicate, and maintain consistent rules and regulations for all clients.	Provides a sense of security.
Do not argue, bargain, or rationalize.	Decreases power struggles.
Confront inappropriate behaviors without anger, punitiveness, or personalization.	The behavior, not the person, should be addressed.
Do not seek approval, or coax; use choices and consequences.	A professional relationship increases client self-control.
Be alert for flattery or verbal attacks.	Being prepared decreases the chance of being manipulated.
Use contracts to help client delay immediate gratification and impulsiveness.	Increases client's personal responsibility for behavior.
Use peer pressure (groups, buddy systems) to modify manipulative behaviors.	Peer feedback is a better reinforcer than staff input.
Role-model self-discipline.	New behaviors can be patterned after those of others.

Boundaries are established by providing consistent expectations and guidelines for self-control. Nursing interventions that provide structure encourage a sense of security in the client; thus, the need to manipulate is decreased. Trying to coerce a client to change is nontherapeutic and counterproductive. The use of confrontation and appropriate self-disclosure

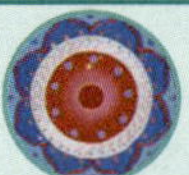

RX COMMUNICATION

THE CLIENT WITH BORDERLINE PERSONALITY DISORDER

CLIENT: "You're the sweetest nurse on the unit. I know you can help me get a pass for next Friday."

NURSE RESPONSE 1: "Darlene, whenever you compliment me, you usually want something from me."

RATIONALE: Confronting the client about her manipulative behavior will help her identify maladaptive approaches. If the nurse fails to confront the behavior consistently, the client will assume the behavior is tolerated and acceptable.

NURSE RESPONSE 2: "Darlene, when you compliment people because you want something from them, they are not likely to trust anything you say."

RATIONALE: This response points out the negative consequences of the manipulative behavior. It encourages the client to consider other ways of interacting

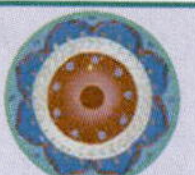

EVIDENCE-BASED PRACTICE

INTERVENTION OPTIONS IN BORDERLINE PERSONALITY DISORDER

Darlene is a 28-year-old woman admitted to an inpatient psychiatric unit from the emergency department, where she was treated for a fractured arm, black eye, and multiple bruises as a reported result of being beaten by her boyfriend. She also had several superficial slashes on her wrists that she stated she inflicted herself in order to "feel real." On this admission, Darlene is screaming hysterically, "Leave me alone. Just let me die because no one loves me." Darlene has been married three times and is currently in an abusive relationship with a man who sells drugs. You know from current literature (Kantojarvi et al., 2006) that substance abuse occurs often in clients with borderline personality disorder. "I hope you go to prison this time!" Darlene yelled at her male partner; however, she refuses to file criminal charges against him.

This is Darlene's fourth admission to the unit, where staff members are very familiar with her history and diagnosis of borderline personality disorder (BPD). On the last admission, Darlene manipulated the staff through splitting. She told three nurses that they were "special" and said, "You are the only one who ever really cared about me" to each nurse.

Your plan for intervention options is based on current research results. For example, in your review of cognitive behavioral therapy (CBT) and BPD, you understand that Darlene will likely experience positive long-lasting effects by participating in Dialectical Behavior Therapy (DBT) groups. After observing Darlene in the group sessions, you determine to spend one-to-one time with her in order to establish a trusting relationship, which you know is a foundation for therapeutic intervention with clients experiencing BPD.

The multidisciplinary treatment team working with Darlene understands that current research shows the efficacy of antipsychotic medications in the treatment of BPD. Therefore, Darlene is prescribed quetiapine as an adjunct to the DBT sessions and other cognitive treatment approaches.

This set of multiple intervention strategies is based on the following research:

Bellino, S., Paradiso, E., & Bogetto, F. (2006). Efficacy and tolerability of quetiapine in the treatment of borderline personality disorder: A pilot study. *The Journal of Clinical Psychiatry, 67*, 1042–1046.

Langley, G. C., & Klopper, H. (2005). Trust as a foundation for the therapeutic intervention for patients with borderline personality disorder. *Journal of Psychiatric & Mental Health Nursing, 12*, 23–32.

Poole, J., & Grant, A. (2005). Stepping out of the box: Broadening the dialogue around the organizational implementation of cognitive behavioral psychotherapy. *Journal of Psychiatric & Mental Health Nursing, 12*, 456–463.

CRITICAL THINKING APPLICATION

1. What are the positives and negatives in having Darlene on a unit where she has been hospitalized before?
2. Is it helpful to know ahead of time that a client has attempted to split the staff?
3. On what basis is quetiapine helpful for clients with BPD?

are techniques that may help reduce the client's resistance. A set of multiple intervention strategies is suggested in the Evidence-Based Practice feature above.

In addition to consistency and limit-setting, other strategies for dealing with manipulative behavior are teaching the client relaxation skills (Chapter 33 provides specific guidelines) and encouraging the client to ask directly for what is needed instead of demonstrating the need through acting-out behavior. All of these approaches require your commitment and patience, whether you are working on inpatient psychiatric or forensic units or in outpatient settings. A variety of intervention strategies and their rationales are suggested in the feature Your Intervention Strategies: Guidelines for the Client with Manipulative Behavior on page 602.

Impulsiveness

Clients with PDs often act before thinking about the potential consequences of their actions. As a result, many clients find themselves in dangerous situations that could have been prevented with forethought and planning. Safety maintenance is a primary concern when working with impulsive clients. Helping clients learn to face the consequences of their own actions is difficult for nurses who want to always protect clients. Implementation of consequences must be done consistently by all staff to be effective. Behavioral contracts can be useful for some clients in curbing their impulsive urges. The group setting is often a safe place for impulsive clients to learn to increase their capacity to tolerate frustration.

Self-Destructive Behavior

As a result of impulsiveness and low self-esteem, many clients with PDs inflict harm on themselves. Such behavior is upsetting to many nurses. Never dismiss or negate a suicidal gesture or self-mutilation as "just" attention-seeking behavior. All acts of self-mutilation or verbalizations of intent to harm oneself must be thoroughly assessed (assessment of clients at risk for suicide and self-destructive behavior is thoroughly discussed in Chapter 23).

Milieu maintenance is one of the most effective nursing interventions in preventing clients' self-destructive behaviors. Physical precautions (e.g., locking doors, removing sharp objects) are some basic measures to ensure client safety. Establishing an environment that is psychologically safe is equally important. Nurses who demonstrate trustworthiness help clients feel more secure. Clearly explaining expectations and consequences for inappropriate behavior also adds to a sense

MEDIALINK Care Plan: The Client Who Self-Mutilates

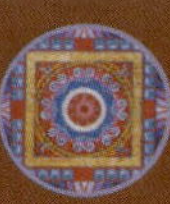

YOUR INTERVENTION STRATEGIES
Guidelines for the Client with Manipulative Behavior

Nursing Intervention	Rationale
Assign one staff member as primary resource person.	Consistency prevents opportunities for splitting staff.
Make limits realistic, with enforceable consequences.	Unpleasant consequences may help decrease negative behavior.
Give reasons for limits and consequences.	Helps client make appropriate choices.
Model respect, honesty, openness, and assertiveness.	Demonstrates expected behavior.
Interact with client when client is not acting out.	Reinforces positive behavior.
Confront client each time manipulation occurs.	Consequences must follow behavior closely.
Discuss with the client alternative ways of dealing with people or situations.	Promotes personal responsibility.
Help client identify assets.	Promotes self-esteem.
Remove limits from treatment plan when client adheres to objectives consistently.	Rewards appropriate behavior.
Evaluate effectiveness of limit setting.	Clarifies discharge planning goals.
Jointly develop contracts for behavioral change.	Establishes client responsibility.
Offer support to other clients who may be targets of manipulation.	Ensures safety of all clients.
Teach stress-reduction techniques (guided imagery, relaxation, thought stopping).	Defuses anxiety and reinforces ability for self-control.
Involve client in assertiveness training and problem solving.	Teaches assertion as opposed to aggression.

of stability. Letting clients know that they are in a safe environment and will not be allowed to harm themselves is especially crucial for people with BPD. The use of no-harm contracts is often therapeutic. A no-harm contract is an agreement between you and the client that the client will contact you or another staff member whenever the feeling to hurt him- or herself is experienced. A sample no-harm contract is illustrated in the Your Intervention Strategies feature on page 629 in Chapter 23.

Dialectical behavior therapy (DBT) is an effective treatment approach for clients with BPD, especially those who are suicidal (Linehan et al., 2006). DBT combines broadly based behavioral strategies—skill training, exposure, and problem solving—with the more general principles of supportive psychotherapy. The goal is to help the client improve interpersonal relationships, tolerate distress, and regulate emotional responses. See Chapter 31 for more detailed information on DBT. Also, the Nursing Care Plan at the end of the chapter is developed for a client experiencing borderline personality disorder.

Evaluation

When evaluating any client with a PD, consider the potential existence of major psychiatric conditions such as depression and anxiety-related disturbances. For example, people with obsessive–compulsive personalities often seek treatment for subjective distress, and the course of treatment may be ineffective as a result of the rigidity of the client's defensive operations. If the behavior is confronted directly, the client might develop acute psychiatric conditions because of intense anxiety. For more information about evaluating care provided to clients with PDs, see also the evaluation section under Cluster C Personality Disorders.

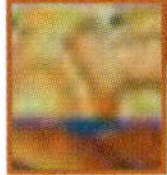

NURSING PROCESS
Clients with Cluster C (Anxious–Fearful) Personality Disorders

The clinging, demanding, excessively helpless, perfectionist, and rigid behaviors typically demonstrated by clients with anxious–fearful personality disorders (avoidant, dependent, and obsessive–compulsive PDs) may create distance between you and the client. However, establishing a therapeutic relationship is your key to helping clients cope more effectively.

Assessment

Because anxious–fearful people tend to be nonassertive and have problems expressing feelings, an accurate assessment will require enough structure and direction to help clients explain themselves and their situations. Rely on the communication techniques discussed in Chapter 10 to encourage clients to provide the information you need. The sense of inadequacy and fear of rejection or shame that many clients feel may interfere with their responses. Remember also that speech is often slow, especially for clients with avoidant PD.

Dependent clients, because of their cloying, clinging, and demanding behaviors, have experienced dislike and avoidance in social, as well as health care, settings. This avoidance response tends to reinforce the clients' perceptions that other people are unwilling to help and that they are unable to help themselves. As a result, clients increase their clinging responses because they know no other way to behave. This increased clinging only leads to further avoidance by others. Therefore, self-awareness is your key to being effective in working with clients who demonstrate dependent behavior.

Nursing Diagnosis: NANDA

Several nursing diagnoses apply to those with anxious–fearful personality disorders. However, the two primary diagnoses are:

- Social isolation
- Defensive coping

Outcome Identification: NOC

Clients with Cluster C (anxious–fearful) personality disorders primarily need to develop more appropriate interpersonal relationships and learn to cope with stressors in a functional manner. Suggested expected outcomes include:

- Identifies feelings about threatening events and situations
- Identifies the consequences of perfectionist tendencies on relationships
- Identifies feelings and beliefs that interfere with asking for help in an appropriate manner
- Makes decisions independently
- Demonstrates ability for self-care

Planning and Implementation: NIC

When you interact with clients experiencing anxious–fearful PDs, you need to consider the impact of your communication on them. Your patience will often be challenged by clients with these disorders. Examples of therapeutic communication techniques are shown in the following Rx Communication: The Client with Dependent Personality Disorder feature.

Impaired Social Interaction

Whether it is the paranoid individual who mistrusts others, the borderline person who makes numerous demands, the antisocial person who exploits others, the obsessive–compulsive person who orders others about, or the dependent person with an excessive and unrealistic need to be cared for, dysfunctional interpersonal relationships are typical of persons with personality disorders. Intervention strategies and their rationales for the client with DPD are in the feature Your Intervention Strategies: Guidelines for the Client with Dependent Personality Disorder on page 604.

Nurses often experience a range of responses to obsessive–compulsive clients, including pity, disgust, anger, frustration, anxiety, and intense discomfort. Always consider how clients with OCPD will react to the realization that years of denying themselves satisfaction, working hard, saving, and restricting their quality of life have not produced the expected rewards (e.g., career advancement, status, promotions). This realization often leads to the potential for depression, especially during middle life. Because anxiety may be contagious, it is wise to limit the duration of one–to–one sessions and make contracts with clients to avoid spending an entire session on obsessional material.

Confront the client's illogical perceptions of others as the first step in helping the client increase his or her capacity for intimacy. Establishing a therapeutic relationship with personality-disordered individuals is challenging because it goes against the basic nature of most personality-disordered clients to trust others and express their true feelings. It is helpful to start with a one–to–one interaction (see Chapter 29∞), then encourage the client to interact in a group setting (see Chapter 30∞). Assertiveness training, which is appropriate for helping clients differentiate aggressive, dependent, and healthy functional behaviors, involves learning how to say no and how to get one's needs met without violating others' rights. (Assertiveness is discussed in Chapter 3∞.)

Remember to use a matter-of-fact approach when responding to the client. It is also important to provide feedback to the client about emotional cues sent to others (e.g., suspiciousness, contempt, intimidation). Role-play and group process are tools that are often useful in helping clients understand the impact of their behavior on others.

Chronic Low Self-Esteem

A common thread in all personality disorders is a pervasive sense of inferiority. Nursing interventions aimed at helping

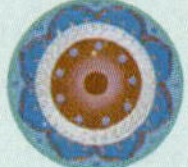

RX COMMUNICATION

THE CLIENT WITH DEPENDENT PERSONALITY DISORDER

CLIENT: "You must help me right now! It's too hard for me to do by myself."

NURSE RESPONSE 1: "Nancy, in the past you have made your appointments very well on your own." ***RATIONALE:*** This response reinforces the clients' sense of mastery by pointing out previous success.	**NURSE RESPONSE 2:** "Nancy, demanding help with tasks you can do for yourself will cause others to leave you alone. It's more effective to ask for help only with tasks that are really difficult for you." ***RATIONALE:*** This response confronts the client with the clinging, demanding behavior and points out the results of such behavior.

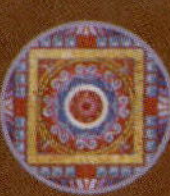

YOUR INTERVENTION STRATEGIES
Guidelines for the Client with Dependent Personality Disorder

Nursing Intervention	Rationale
Evaluate client's ability to perform self-care activities; encourage grooming and personal hygiene.	Fosters independent living skills.
Avoid doing for the client those things the client is capable of doing without help.	Promotes independence.
Schedule regular sessions as a way to anticipate client needs *before* the client demands attention through inappropriate responses.	Anticipatory guidance minimizes anxiety and acting-out.
Help client identify assets and liabilities, including plans for change; emphasize strengths and potential.	Self-assessment can enhance a positive self-concept.
Encourage client to take responsibility for own opinions; point out when client negates own feelings or opinions.	Fosters independence.
Share with client your observations of client's manipulative behavior.	Feedback from staff and peers fosters self-awareness.
Set realistic limits on what will and will not be done for the client.	Minimizes client dependence on others.
Explore with client the consequences of behavior (e.g., clinging tends to result in avoidance by others).	Increases client's self-awareness.
Discuss personal responsibilities and the fact that client has choices.	Choices optimize independent functioning.
Give positive reinforcement for successful achievements.	Reinforces client's ability to succeed.

clients develop higher levels of self-esteem is appropriate for all those with PDs. It is important to confront clients' negative beliefs about themselves and help clients learn to replace the thoughts with more realistic ones. Cognitive behavioral techniques (such as thought stopping) are useful in countering the irrational thoughts; these are discussed in detail in Chapter 31 ∞.

Another way to help clients develop greater self-esteem is to encourage them to identify their strengths. Once identified, these assets are the tools for building a better view of themselves. Applying the concept of unconditional positive regard (Rogers, 1957) with every client helps them feel more valued as individuals. Other techniques that can help clients improve self-esteem include journaling, exercise, and relaxation skills (see Chapter 33 ∞).

Evaluation

Whenever possible, include family members or significant others in some aspects of therapy. Families and significant others can be taught in every setting, both inpatient and outpatient. Inclusion of families helps increase the support necessary for clients to function more independently. Psychoeducation guidelines for clients and their families are given in the Partnering with Clients and Families feature on page 605.

Clients should be able to identify and verbalize their fears and some specific areas in which change is indicated. The following are among the factors that influence the likelihood of successful change:

- The severity of the client's emotional deprivation
- The rigidity of the client's personality structure
- The client's ego strengths
- The client's motivation to change
- The nurse's skill and commitment
- Social support systems in the client's family or milieu that favor the desired change

Evaluation focuses on both the client's expected outcomes and the process of nursing care delivery. When assessing personality-disordered clients for progress, it is essential that the outcome criteria focus on resolution of short-term crises rather than global changes in the client's lifestyle. Keep in mind that PDs are lifelong traits and behaviors, so it is unrealistic to expect a client to change easily or in a short period of time. Using specific outcome criteria for measurement is necessary for evaluation to be meaningful. It is also important to include the client and significant others in evaluating the response to treatment.

When evaluating the delivery of nursing care, do not judge your effectiveness only by the client's progress or lack thereof. Instead, evaluation of nursing interventions should consider how you responded to the client, what milieu was maintained for the client, and whether you consis-

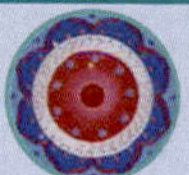

PARTNERING WITH CLIENTS AND FAMILIES

TEACHING ABOUT PERSONALITY DISORDERS

- Provide information about the specific disorder.
- Help client learn to verbally express needs instead of acting out.
- Provide social skills training (cooking, money management) as needed.
- Teach problem-solving techniques, including goal setting, identifying alternative responses, and evaluating consequences.
- Teach stress-reduction techniques (e.g., guided imagery, relaxation).
- Provide instruction in cognitive–behavioral techniques (e.g., thought stopping).
- Teach client and family members about the proper use of medications, including: target symptoms, side effects and adverse medication reactions, contraindications, and when to call for help.
- Practice and/or role-play newly acquired skills (e.g., assertiveness).
- Teach client and family members about signs of relapse or indicators for emergency treatment.
- Emphasize the importance of follow-up care as indicated.

tently set appropriate limits in an attempt to teach the client the skills necessary for living as an independent adult. A determination of whether stability and safety were maintained is just as important as considering the client's response to the treatment plan.

CASE MANAGEMENT

The case manager plays an essential role by collaborating with clients and families/significant others by providing information on when and where to seek help. The case manager also monitors clients for adherence to the aftercare plan, including the client's medication usage. Clients usually need help in identifying community support services and in developing a support system. These tasks can be facilitated by asking the client to identify one family member or friend he or she would trust to help with personal needs.

COMMUNITY-BASED CARE

Individuals with personality disorders lack insight about their behavior; that is, they are generally unaware that their behaviors are problematic to themselves and others. As a result, few people with PDs voluntarily seek inpatient treatment unless they are experiencing a crisis. Many people with PDs are, therefore, treated in the community—in mental health clinics, crisis centers, and through routine visits to therapists' offices. Early intervention and long-term follow-up care are essential for clients with personality disorders. It is essential to identify severe personality disorders early in order to improve community services. Anticipating and adjusting to the effects of personality disorders is likely to improve treatment plans and prognosis (Tyrer & Mulder, 2006).

When working with personality-disordered clients on an outpatient basis, it is especially important to help them identify their personal strengths to use as building blocks for therapy. Referral to outpatient classes on dialectical behavior therapy is especially appropriate. Also, you need to help clients develop a realistic time frame in which to achieve expected outcomes.

HOME CARE

Nurses who provide psychiatric–mental health care in the home setting are significant in helping clients with personality disorders improve their social interactions and in helping to shape behavior. Role-play can be an effective tool for helping clients learn to detect social cues given by others. Predictable environments (schedules, consistent caregivers, etc.) decrease anxiety and foster trust. The following interventions are especially helpful for homebound clients experiencing PD:

- Meet with the client and a family member or significant other to discuss realistic expectations for the client.
- Teach the client home management skills necessary for independent living.
- Ask if the client desires testing, placement services, or job skill retraining.
- Refer to community agencies as needed.

A list of resources for people who care for someone with BPD is available at www.bpdcentral.com and can be accessed through the Companion Website for this book.

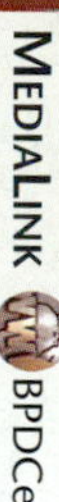

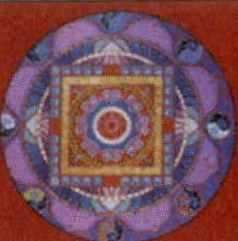

NURSING CARE PLAN
Client with Borderline Personality Disorder

Assessment

Identifying Information

Wendy is a 27-year-old divorced woman who was admitted to the hospital after threatening to commit suicide. She is a dental hygienist who has been employed for 6 months. Her employer confronted her 1 week ago about her rapid mood swings, irritability, and absenteeism related to chemical dependence.

Wendy states that she does not need to be on a psychiatric unit because she really was not going to kill herself; she was merely looking for some attention. She states that her employer, a female dentist, is jealous that the male patients are attracted to her. She thinks it is unfair that her employer asked her not to see patients socially after hours. She also states that her employer is jealous of Wendy's physical appearance and decided that she needs to be treated for an alcohol problem that Wendy denies having. Wendy states that she only drinks to unwind.

History

Wendy reports a history of being unable to relate well with previous female employers. She prefers the company of men, even though she states she was abused physically and sexually by males as a child. Wendy does state that she began drinking more often after her second abortion.

Current Mental Status

The mental status assessment shows Wendy to be hyperactive. She is oriented to time, place, and person. Her judgment is impaired, and her affect is labile. Mood swings alternate between crying and excessive smiling. She denies delusions or hallucinations. Her speech is clear and coherent, though pressured at times. Wendy states she is being treated unjustly and blames others for her hospitalization.

Nursing Diagnosis: Ineffective Coping related to inadequate level of confidence in ability to cope.

Expected Outcome: Client will demonstrate the ability to self-control impulsive behaviors.

Short-Term Goals	Interventions	Rationales
Client will verbalize decreased need to act impulsively.	▪ Point out incidences of impulsive behavior to client.	Confrontation makes the client more aware of problematic behaviors.
	▪ Use active listening during all interactions with client.	Active listening promotes expression of feelings.
	▪ Assign nonjudgmental staff to work with client.	A nonjudgmental approach helps client feel accepted and more willing to express feelings.
Client will use relaxation techniques to control impulsive behaviors.	▪ Teach relaxation techniques (e.g., deep breathing, visualization).	Anxiety interferes with the ability to plan ahead.
	▪ Have client demonstrate newly learned techniques.	Demonstration and repetition reinforce learning.
Client will demonstrate a decreased incidence of impulsive acts.	▪ Encourage client to state negative outcomes of impulsive behavior.	Considering negative consequences of behavior is an incentive to change.
	▪ Allow time for the client to modify old patterns of behavior.	Changing ingrained behaviors is a gradual process.
	▪ Set limits on client behavior to maintain safety.	Setting external limits establishes boundaries for behavior that are appropriate and safe.

Nursing Diagnosis: Ineffective Coping related to manipulative attempts to control others.

Expected Outcome: Client will state needs directly and engage in active problem solving independently.

Short-Term Goals	Interventions	Rationales
Client will demonstrate a decreased incidence of manipulative behaviors.	▪ Inform client of acceptable behaviors.	Knowledge of expectations increases likelihood of adherence.
	▪ Consistently enforce limits when client attempts to manipulate.	Consistency reduces effectiveness of manipulative attempts.
	▪ Avoid seeking client's approval.	People-pleasing behavior provides opportunity for manipulation to occur.

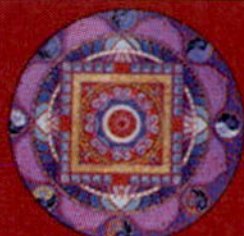

NURSING CARE PLAN
Client with Borderline Personality Disorder *(continued)*

Short-Term Goals	Interventions	Rationales
	▪ Remain neutral to client's comments, being neither flattered nor offended.	Flattery is a form of manipulation; using a matter-of-fact approach removes the effect of manipulative attempts.
	▪ Use group techniques to teach self-responsibility.	Peer feedback is often effective in shaping behavior.
	▪ Avoid rescuing or rejecting client.	Rescuing behaviors reinforce client's sense of powerlessness and inadequacy; rejecting behaviors increase client's perception of threat. Both behaviors lead to escalation of manipulation.
	▪ Provide feedback to client about the effects of behavior on others.	Awareness of consequences of behavior may serve as catalyst to change.
Client will demonstrate independence in daily activities.	▪ Encourage client to be independent while being available to help only when necessary.	Providing assistance only when absolutely necessary encourages client's self-reliance.
	▪ Give positive reinforcement for achievement of goals.	Encourages development of a sense of mastery and boosts self-esteem.
	▪ Help client evaluate personal progress (e.g., through one-to-one, group, journaling).	Seeing progress encourages independence and success.

Nursing Diagnosis: Risk for Self-Directed Violence related to intense rage.

Expected Outcome: Client will remain free from self-inflicted injury.

Short-Term Goals	Interventions	Rationales
Client will verbalize feelings of anger and self-destructive ideation.	▪ Establish a trusting relationship with client.	Trust encourages the expression of feelings.
	▪ Use a nonjudgmental attitude when client discusses suicidal/self-destructive thoughts.	A nonjudgmental attitude promotes continued dialogue.
	▪ Assess history of previous suicidal/self-mutilating thoughts.	Previous self-damaging acts increase the potential for such behavior to be repeated.
Client will remain safe from harm.	▪ Inform clients that they are in a safe place and will be protected from self-harm.	Reassurance decreases anxiety.
	▪ Set limits on destructive behavior.	External limits maintain safety until client learns inner control of impulses.
	▪ Implement safety precautions (e.g., close observation of behavior, searching client belongings for contraband, suicide precautions).	Precautions maintain client safety at all times.

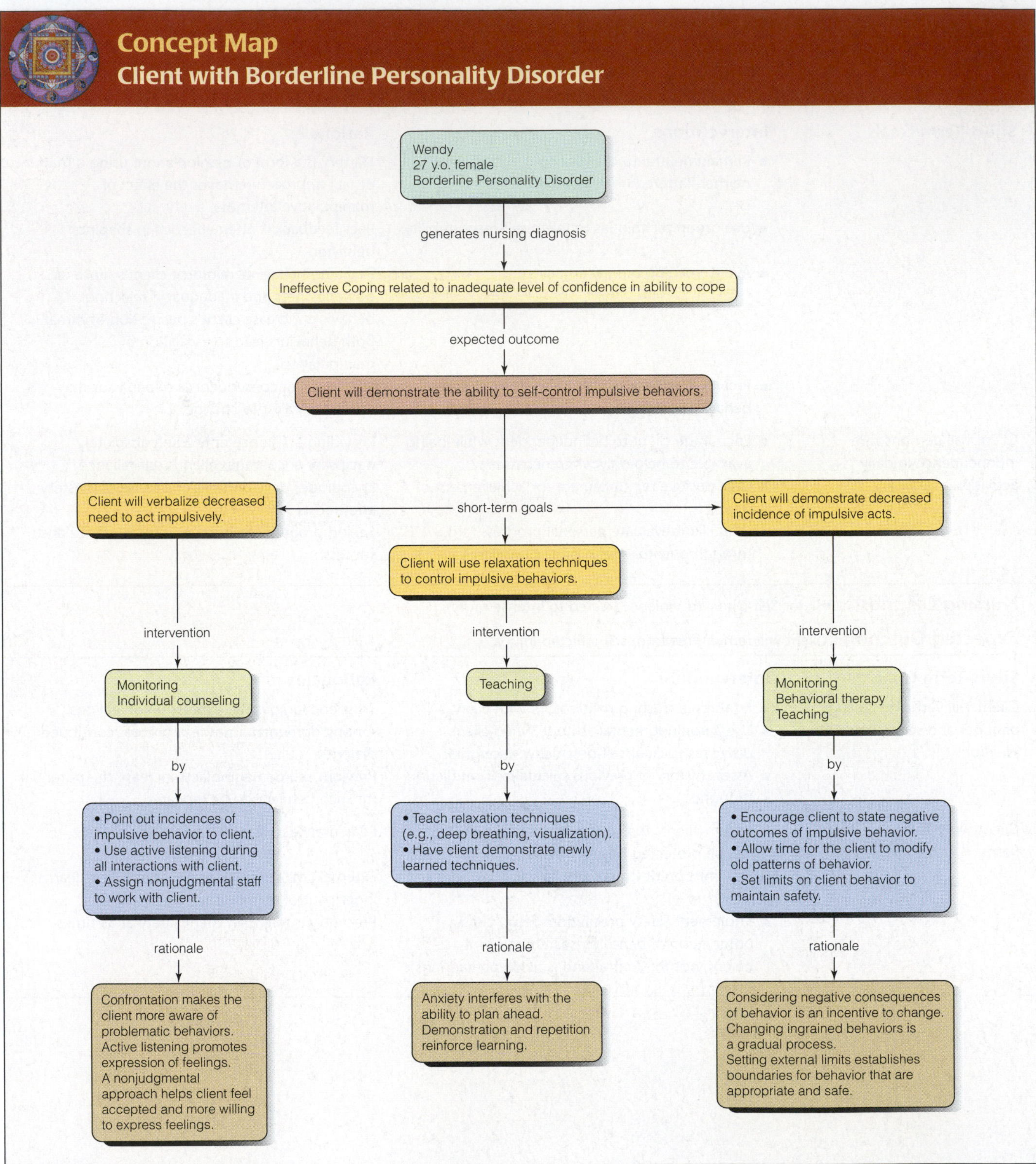
Concept Map
Client with Borderline Personality Disorder
Wendy
27 y.o. female
Borderline Personality Disorder
generates nursing diagnosis
Ineffective Coping related to inadequate level of confidence in ability to cope
expected outcome
Client will demonstrate the ability to self-control impulsive behaviors.
short-term goals
Client will verbalize decreased need to act impulsively.
Client will use relaxation techniques to control impulsive behaviors.
Client will demonstrate decreased incidence of impulsive acts.
intervention
Monitoring
Individual counseling
by
• Point out incidences of impulsive behavior to client.
• Use active listening during all interactions with client.
• Assign nonjudgmental staff to work with client.
rationale
Confrontation makes the client more aware of problematic behaviors.
Active listening promotes expression of feelings.
A nonjudgmental approach helps client feel accepted and more willing to express feelings.
intervention
Teaching
by
• Teach relaxation techniques (e.g., deep breathing, visualization).
• Have client demonstrate newly learned techniques.
rationale
Anxiety interferes with the ability to plan ahead.
Demonstration and repetition reinforce learning.
intervention
Monitoring
Behavioral therapy
Teaching
by
• Encourage client to state negative outcomes of impulsive behavior.
• Allow time for the client to modify old patterns of behavior.
• Set limits on client behavior to maintain safety.
rationale
Considering negative consequences of behavior is an incentive to change.
Changing ingrained behaviors is a gradual process.
Setting external limits establishes boundaries for behavior that are appropriate and safe.

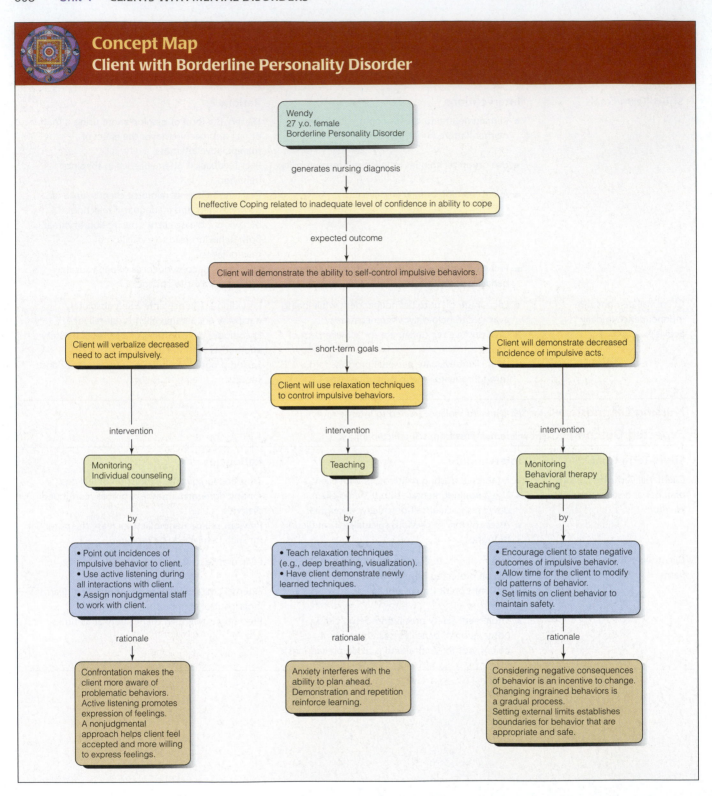

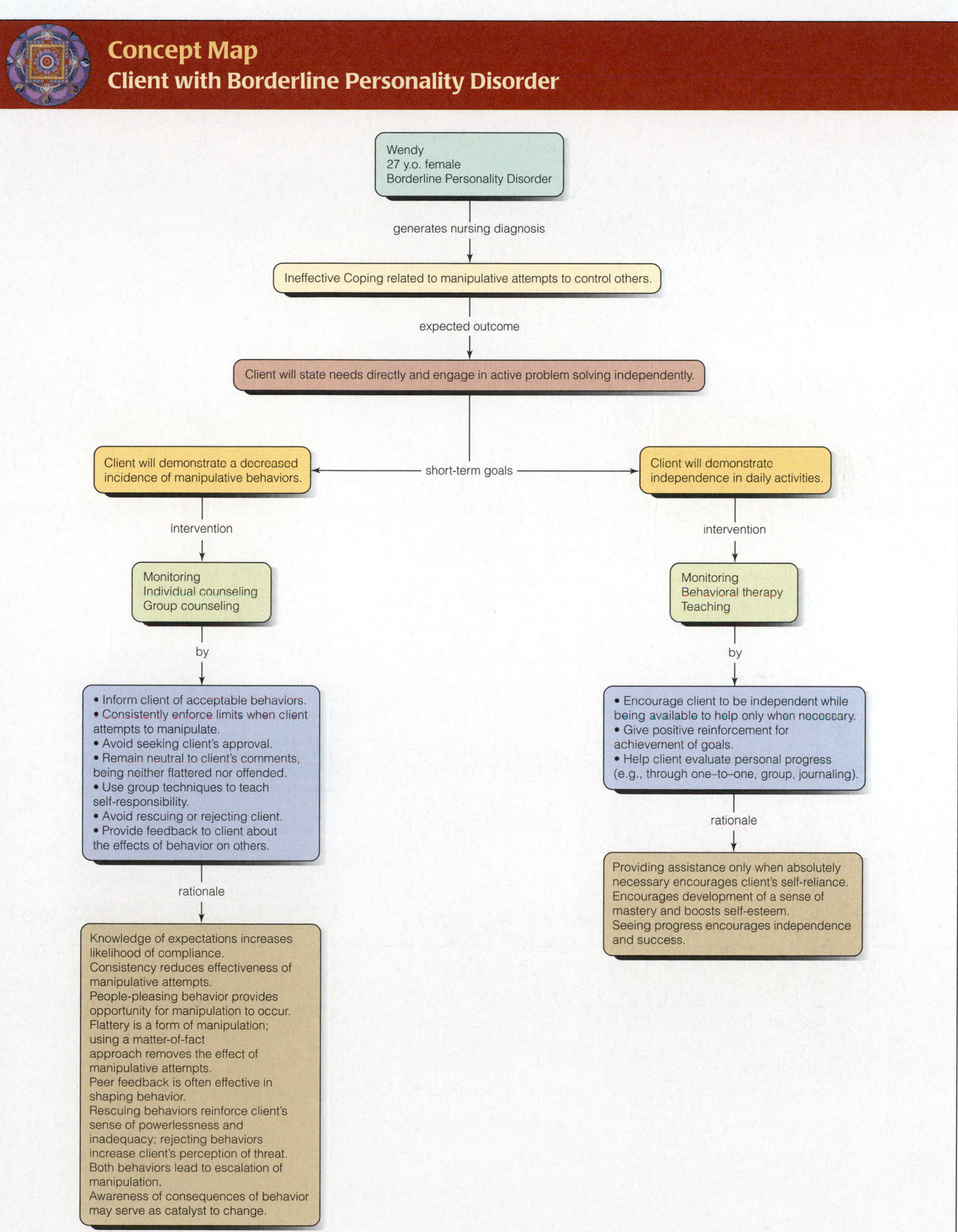
Concept Map
Client with Borderline Personality Disorder
Wendy
27 y.o. female
Borderline Personality Disorder
generates nursing diagnosis
Ineffective Coping related to manipulative attempts to control others.
expected outcome
Client will state needs directly and engage in active problem solving independently.
short-term goals
Client will demonstrate a decreased incidence of manipulative behaviors.
Client will demonstrate independence in daily activities.
intervention
Monitoring
Individual counseling
Group counseling
intervention
Monitoring
Behavioral therapy
Teaching
by
• Inform client of acceptable behaviors.
• Consistently enforce limits when client attempts to manipulate.
• Avoid seeking client's approval.
• Remain neutral to client's comments, being neither flattered nor offended.
• Use group techniques to teach self-responsibility.
• Avoid rescuing or rejecting client.
• Provide feedback to client about the effects of behavior on others.
by
• Encourage client to be independent while being available to help only when necessary.
• Give positive reinforcement for achievement of goals.
• Help client evaluate personal progress (e.g., through one–to–one, group, journaling).
rationale
Knowledge of expectations increases likelihood of compliance.
Consistency reduces effectiveness of manipulative attempts.
People-pleasing behavior provides opportunity for manipulation to occur.
Flattery is a form of manipulation; using a matter-of-fact approach removes the effect of manipulative attempts.
Peer feedback is often effective in shaping behavior.
Rescuing behaviors reinforce client's sense of powerlessness and inadequacy; rejecting behaviors increase client's perception of threat. Both behaviors lead to escalation of manipulation.
Awareness of consequences of behavior may serve as catalyst to change.
rationale
Providing assistance only when absolutely necessary encourages client's self-reliance.
Encourages development of a sense of mastery and boosts self-esteem.
Seeing progress encourages independence and success.

Concept Map
Client with Borderline Personality Disorder

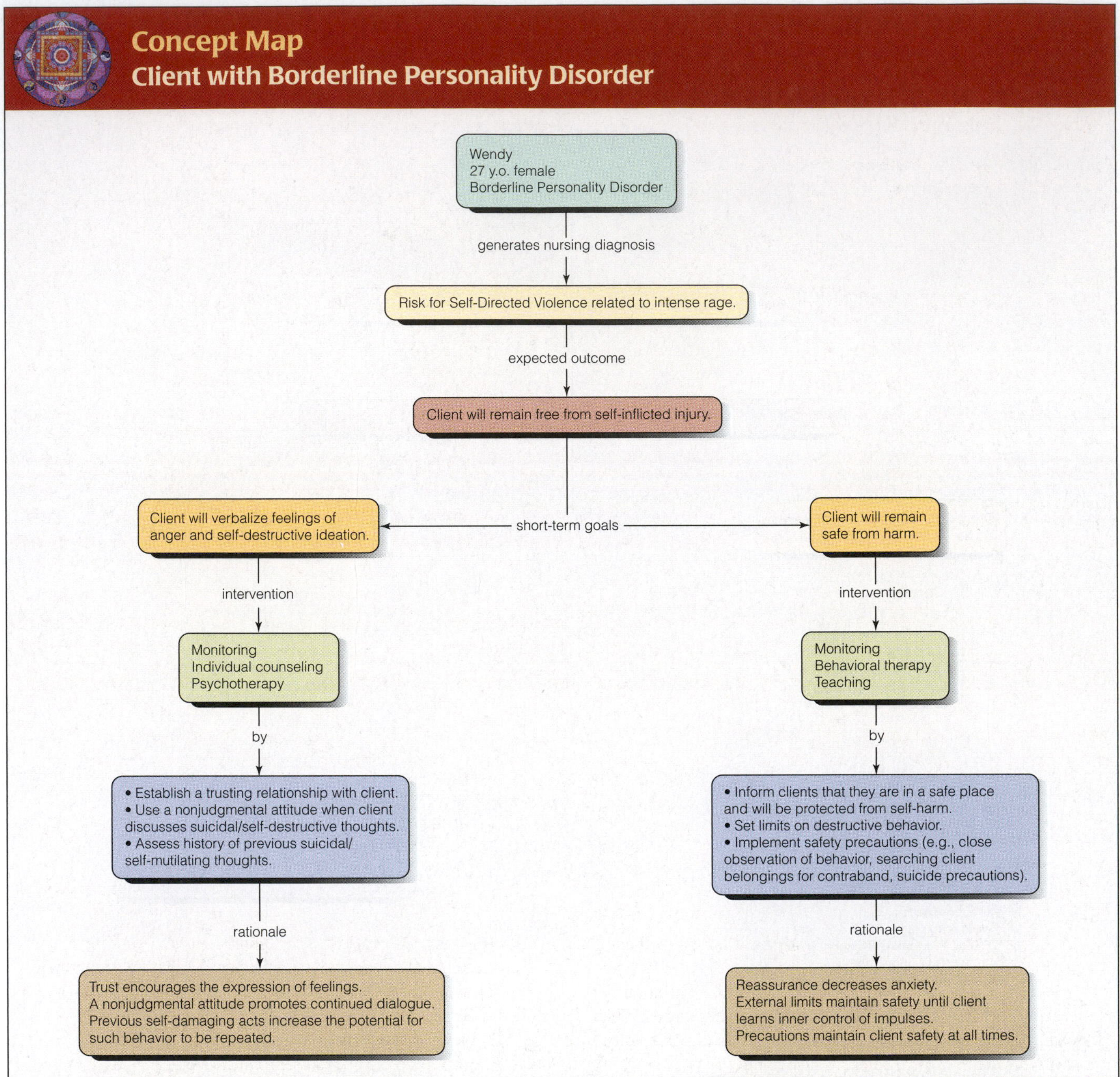

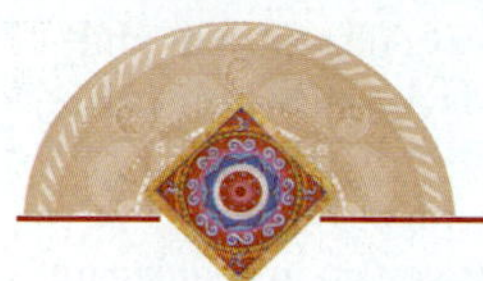

EXPLORE MEDIALINK

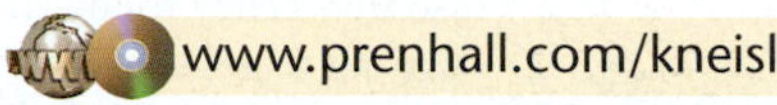

For NCLEX-RN® review questions, case studies, and other resources for this chapter see the Pearson Health MediaLink CD-ROM that accompanies this book and the Companion Website at www.prenhall.com/kneisl.

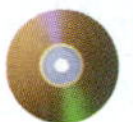

CD-ROM
Audio Glossary
NCLEX-RN® Review Questions
Video
- *Antisocial Personality Disorder*

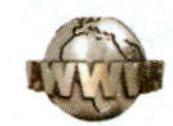

Companion Website
Audio Glossary
NCLEX-RN® Review Questions
Critical Thinking Exercise
- *Antisocial Behavior*

Case Study
- *A Narcissistic Client*

Care Plan
- *The Client Who Self-Mutilates*

MediaLinks
MediaLink Application
- *Borderline Personality Disorder*

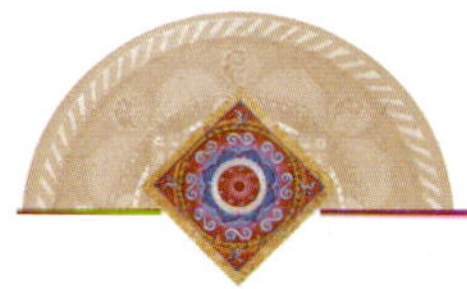

NCLEX-RN® REVIEW QUESTIONS

1. Personality disorders differ from personality traits in that personality disorders:
1. Interfere with role functioning.
2. Remain stable over time.
3. Assist clinicians in predicting behavior.
4. May cause distress in other people.

2. In a final exam in a comparative literature course, a student compares James Joyce to a bowl of soggy corn flakes. She grieves her low grade with the department chair, flirtatiously arguing that her professor did not appreciate her thesis. Which characteristics common to all three categories of personality disorders are evident? (Select all that apply.)
1. Suspiciousness
2. Lack of insight
3. External response to stress
4. Impulsivity
5. Failure to accept consequences

3. Increased levels of testosterone and estrogens and decreased levels of 5-HIAA are associated primarily with which of the following?
1. Cluster A personality disorders
2. Cluster B personality disorders
3. Cluster C personality disorders
4. Cluster A–C personality disorders

4. A dopamine D_3 receptor gene variant is associated with which of the following disorders?
1. Antisocial personality disorder
2. Obsessive–compulsive personality disorder
3. Cluster A personality disorders
4. Cluster B personality disorders

5. The nurse states, "In the past you have made your appointments very well on your own." What is the rationale for the nurse's action?
1. Show consistency in nursing actions
2. Reward appropriate behavior
3. Reinforce the client's sense of mastery by pointing out previous success
4. Clarify discharge goals

6. Your client with a personality disorder has a nursing care plan which includes the nursing diagnosis "Impaired Social Interaction." Applying the principles for caring with this client, which of the following interventions is essential to the care plan?
1. Demonstrate honesty and sincerity in all interactions with the client.
2. Assist the client in identifying personal strengths.
3. Demonstrate unconditional positive regard when confronting inappropriate behavior.
4. Role-model assertive communication.

7. Your client with a personality disorder informs you, "A novice like you couldn't possibly help me. What I need right now is to leave this hospital." What is your best initial response?
1. "What makes you think I cannot help you?"
2. "What are you experiencing right now?"
3. "I will notify your physician."
4. "Where will you go?"

8. Your client has been diagnosed with a personality disorder. The care plan includes the intervention: "Encourage client to direct all requests to assigned staff." Which of the following statements provides a rationale? (Select all that apply.)
1. Consistency minimizes the opportunity for the client to split staff.
2. This is the most efficient way to deliver care.
3. This approach meets the narcissistic needs of the client.
4. Staff members are more likely to detect subtle changes in the client's behavior.
5. Predictability may increase the client's sense of trust and security.

9. Your peer informs you, "This client always disrupts our unit and leaves against medical advice. She is a typical borderline." What is your best initial response?
1. "You cannot get away from people with personality disorders. They follow you wherever you go in health care."
2. "Try not to get angry. It is a waste of your energy, and she will never change."
3. "Be sure to take care of yourself, because working with these clients is not gratifying."
4. "I wish we could identify what she needs and provide it before she acts out on the unit."

10. After being discharged from the hospital less than 24 hours ago, your client with a personality disorder attempts suicide and is readmitted. You overhear a staff member saying, "Why doesn't she just kill herself and put herself out of our misery?" Which of the following is your best response?
1. "She would rather not see you, either."
2. "It is frustrating to care for people with persistent behaviors."
3. "That's a hostile thing to say."
4. "She probably knows you feel that way about her."

See Appendix C for answers.

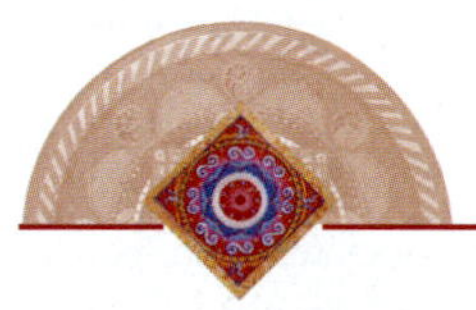

REFERENCES

American Psychiatric Association. (2000). *Diagnostic and statistical manual of mental disorders* (4th ed., Text Revision). Washington, DC: Author.

Barnow, S., Spitzer, C., Grabe, H. J., Kessler, C., & Freyberger, H. J. (2006). Individual characteristics, familial experience, and psychopathology in child mothers with borderline personality disorder. *Journal of the American Academy of Child and Adolescent Psychiatry, 45,* 965–972.

Bellino, S., Paradiso, E., & Bogetto, F. (2006). Efficacy and tolerability of quetiapine in the treatment of borderline personality disorder: A pilot study. *The Journal of Clinical Psychiatry, 67,* 1042–1046.

Bornovalova, M. A., Gratz, K. L., Delany-Brumsey, A., Paulson, A., & Lejuez, C. W. (2006). Temperamental and environmental risk factors for borderline personality disorder among inner-city substance users in residential treatment. *Journal of Personality Disorders, 20,* 218–231.

Coccaro, E. F. (2005). Association of C-reactive protein elevation with trait aggression and hostility in personality disordered subjects: A pilot study. *Journal of Psychiatric Research, 40,* 460–465.

de Bruijn, E. R., Grooten, K. P., Verkes, R. J., Buchholz, V., Hummelen, J. W., & Hulstijn, W. (2006). Neural correlates of impulsive responding in borderline personality disorder: EFP evidence for reduced action monitoring. *Journal of Psychiatric Research, 40,* 428–437.

Erikson, E. H. (1964). *Childhood and society*. New York: Norton.

Figueiredo, L. C. (2006). Sense of reality, reality testing and reality processing in borderline patients. *The International Journal of Psycho-Analysis, 18,* 769–787.

Harvey, P. D., Romero, M., Richenberg, A., Granholm, E., & Siever, L. J. (2006). Dual-task information processing in schizotypal personality disorder: Evidence of impaired processing capacity. *Neuropsychology, 20*(4), 453–460.

Kantojarvi, L., Veijola, J., Laksy, K., Jokelainen, J., Herva, A., Karvonen, J. T., et al. (2006). Co-occurrence of personality disorders with mood, anxiety, and substance use disorders in a young adult population. *Journal of Personality Disorders, 20,* 102–112.

Kernberg, O. (1975). *Borderline conditions and pathological narcissism*. New York: Aronson.

Kernberg, O. F. (2007). The almost untreatable narcissistic patient. *Journal of the American Psychoanalytic Association, 55*(2), 503–539.

Koenisberg, H. W., Buchsbaum, M. S., Buchsbaum, B. R., Schneiderman, J. S, Tang, C. Y., & News, A. (2005). Functional MRI of visuospatial memory in schizotypal personality disorder: A region of interest analysis. *Psychological Medicine, 35,* 1019–1030.

Koo, M. S., Dickey, C. C., Park, H. J., Kubicki, M., Ji, N. Y., Bouix, S., et al. (2006). Smaller neocortical gray matter and larger sulcal cerebrospinal fluid volumes in neuroleptic-naïve women with schizotypal personality disorder. *Archives of General Psychiatry, 63,* 1090–1100.

Koo, M. S., Levitt, J. J., McCarley, R. W., Seidman, L. J., Dickey, C. C., Niznikiewicz, M. A., et al. (2006). Reduction of caudate nucleus volumes in neuroleptic-naïve female subjects with schizotypal personality disorder. *Biological Psychiatry, 60*(1), 40–48.

Langley, G. C., & Klopper, H. (2005). Trust as a foundation for the therapeutic intervention for patients with borderline personality disorder. *Journal of Psychiatric & Mental Health Nursing, 12,* 23–32.

Light, K. J., Joyce, P. R., Luty, S. E., Mulder, R. T., Frampton, C. M., Joyce, L. R., et al. (2006). Preliminary evidence for an association between a dopamine D_3 receptor gene variant and obsessive–compulsive personality disorder in patients with major depression. *American Journal of Medical Genetics. Part B, Neuropsychiatric Genetics, 141,* 409–413.

Linehan, M. M., Comtois, K. A., Murray, A. M., Brown, M. Z., Gallop, R. J., Heard, H. L., et al. (2006). Two-year randomized controlled trial and follow-up of dialectical behavior therapy vs. therapy by experts for suicidal behaviors and borderline personality disorder. *Archives of General Psychiatry, 63,* 757–766.

Mahler, M. S., Pine, F., & Bergman, A. (1975). *The psychological birth of the human infant: Symbiosis and individuation.* New York: Basic Books.

Minzenberg, M. J., Xu, K., Mitropoulou, V., Harvey, P. D., Finch, T., Flory, J. D., et al. (2006). Catechol-O-methyltransferase Val158Met genotype variation is associated with prefrontal-dependent task performance in schizotypal personality disorder patients and comparison groups. *Psychiatric Genetics, 16,* 117–124.

Nakano, S., Asada, T., Yamashita, F., Kitamura, N., Hatsuda, H., Hiral, S. et al. (2006). Relationship between antisocial behavior and regional cerebral blood flow in frontotemporal dementia. *Neuroimage, 32,* 301–306.

National Alliance on Mental Illness. (2007). *Borderline personality disorder.* Retrieved January 2007 from www.nami.org/PrinterTemplate.cfm?Section=By_Illness&Template=TaggedPage

Ni, X., Chan, K., Bulgin, N., Sicard, T., Bismil, R., McMain, S. et al. (2006). Association between serotonin transporter gene and borderline personality disorder. *Journal of Psychiatric Research, 40,* 448–453.

Osborne, U. L., & McComish, J. F. (2006). Borderline personality disorder: Nursing interventions using dialectical behavioral therapy. *Journal of Psychosocial Nursing and Mental Health Services, 44,* 40–47.

Poole, J., & Grant, A. (2005). Stepping out of the box: Broadening the dialogue around the organizational implementation of cognitive behavioral psychotherapy. *Journal of Psychiatric & Mental Health Nursing, 12,* 456–463.

Rogers, C. (1957). The necessary and sufficient conditions for therapeutic personality change. *Journal of Consulting Psychology, 21,* 95–103.

Sadock, B. J., & Sadock, V. A. (2005). *Kaplan & Sadock's pocket handbook of clinical psychiatry* (4th ed.). Philadelphia: Lippincott Williams & Wilkins.

Schmahl, C., Bohus, M., Esposito, F., Treede, R. D., Di Salle, F., Greffrath, W., et al. (2006). Neural correlates of antinociception in borderline personality disorder. *Archives of General Psychiatry, 63,* 659–667.

Schmahl, C., & Bremner, J. D. (2006). Neuroimaging in borderline personality disorder. *Journal of Psychiatric Research, 40,* 419–427.

Tyrer, P., & Mulder, R. (2006). Management of complex and severe personality disorders in community mental health services. *Current Opinion in Psychiatry, 19,* 400–404.

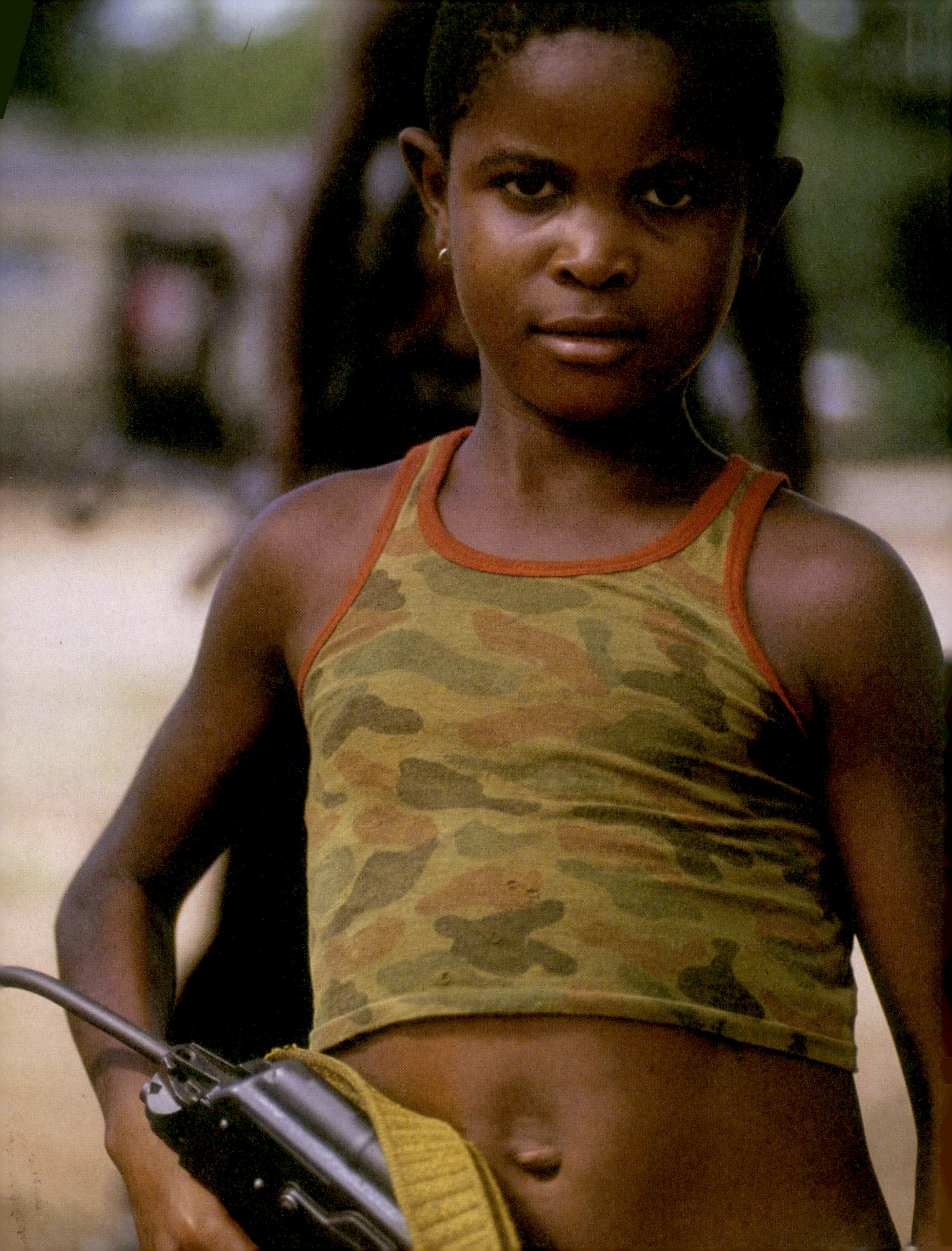

Unit 5

VULNERABLE POPULATIONS

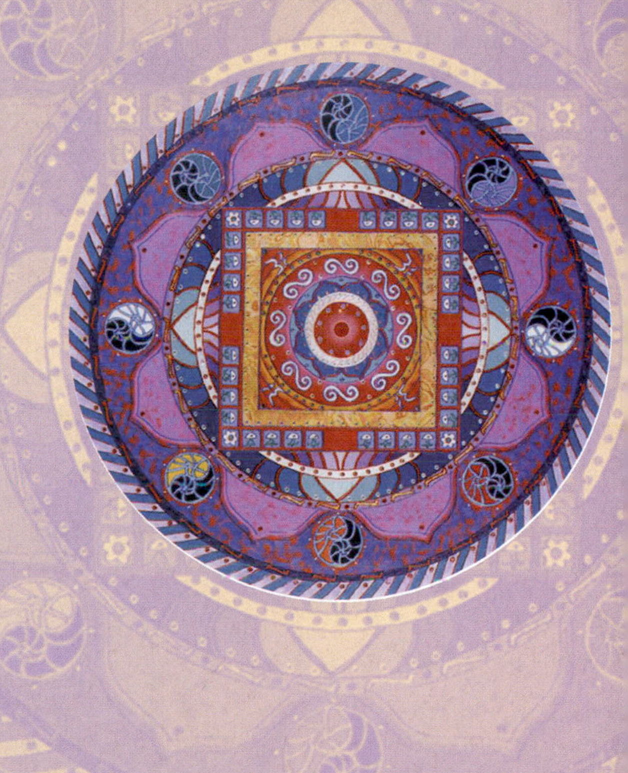

FLORIBÉRT, 11 years old, is a *kadogo,* a child soldier. He is one of an estimated 250,000 child victims who have been systematically exploited as combatants in Africa. A militant warring faction in opposition to the government kidnapped Floribért while he was on his way home from school in Goma in the Democratic Republic of the Congo. "To this very day," says Floribért, "I don't know if my parents are alive or what will become of me." During several weeks of military training, he has been tortured, raped, beaten, and deprived of food or sleep. In active combat, he has been forced to act as a human shield and to kill acquaintances in a nearby village. His friend, Séraphine, was beaten and raped by the other soldiers and forced to sexually service the unit's commander. Floribért lives in mutual fear and hatred in a land divided along ethnic lines. Many *kadogos* have nightmares and panic attacks. Some are emotionally bland to repress memories of the crimes they have witnessed or committed. It will take years, if ever, for Floribért to come to terms with what he has done. As nurses, we must develop a *common fire,* a shared vision of core values respectful of the common good in the shifting complexities and circumstances of vulnerable populations and in the face of the unknowns of contemporary times.

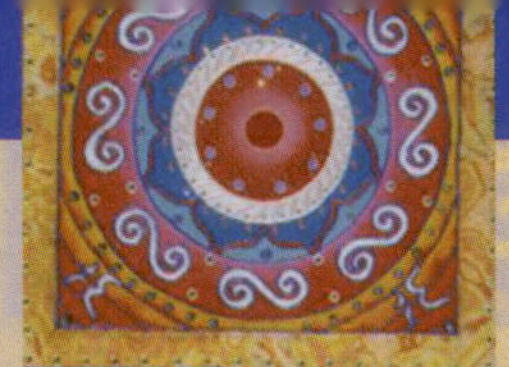

CHAPTER

23

Clients at Risk for Suicide and Self-Destructive Behavior

CAROL REN KNEISL

KEY TERMS

ambivalence *623*
chronic self-destructive behavior *618*
cluster suicide *634*
lethality assessment *627*
psychological autopsy *619*
self-destructive behaviors *617*
self-mutilation *618*
suicidal ideation *618*
suicide *617*
suicide attempt *618*
suicide precautions *630*
suicide threat *618*

LEARNING OUTCOMES

After completing this chapter, you will be able to:

1. Identify the social, demographic, and clinical variables that influence suicidal or self-destructive behavior.
2. Explain the most common reasons for suicide.
3. Describe the characteristics of people who successfully commit suicide.
4. Compare and contrast the similarities and differences in suicide rates among various racial and demographic groups.
5. Discuss the sociocultural, interpersonal, and biologic theories that enhance our understanding of self-destructive behavior.
6. Carry out a lethality assessment.
7. Distinguish between the crucial components of basic suicide precautions and maximum suicide precautions.
8. Describe the nursing interventions to prevent suicide that can and should be implemented in any health care setting.
9. Describe how you would include family members in the plan of care for the suicidal client.
10. Explain why you might feel anxious when working with suicidal or other self-destructive clients.
11. Identify the strategies for intervention that are helpful to survivors of suicide.

CRITICAL THINKING CHALLENGE

Despite your attempts to convince Maureen that her family would not be better off without her, Maureen insists that she is determined to commit suicide. She plans to run from the inpatient unit and jump in front of a moving car. In considering how best to help her, a staff member suggests that taking her shoes away would prevent Maureen from running away.

1. How do you feel about taking belongings away from someone who is suicidal?
2. Do you agree with this practice?
3. How can you best help to maintain Maureen's safety?

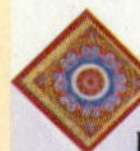

MEDIALINK 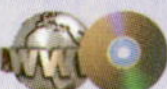 www.prenhall.com/kneisl

Go to the Pearson Health MediaLink CD-ROM and the Companion Website at www.prenhall.com/kneisl for interactive resources for this chapter.

Self-destructive behavior has been a part of the human experience since time began. **Self-destructive behaviors** are maladaptive measures a person uses to restore inner equilibrium when overwhelmed or unable to cope with stressful life events. Distressed and unable to see that they have other options, people attempt to harm themselves or commit suicide thinking that they can take away unbearable emotional pain.

Did you know that **suicide**, the willful act of ending one's own life, is the 11th leading cause of death among Americans, that over 31,000 people kill themselves each year (Centers for Disease Control and Prevention [CDC], 2007a), and that approximately 325,000 to 425,000 people with self-inflicted injuries are treated in emergency departments each year (Corso, Mercy, Simon, Finkelstein, & Miller, 2007)? Did you also know that many people who commit suicide have seen a nurse, physician, or other health care professional the same month they commit suicide? Over 90% of people who commit suicide have a psychiatric illness, and over 50% are under active psychiatric or mental health care.

Stigma and ignorance about mental illness, depression, and suicide may embarrass, shame, and silence individuals who want to speak with others about their pain. Clients may believe that others, including nurses and other health care providers, will label them "crazy" if they speak of suicide. In fact, discussions of suicide do arouse intense and complicated emotions in others.

Suicide is a major public health problem in North America and in many countries around the globe. FIGURE 23-1 ■ depicts U.S. suicide rates by age, gender, and race. The information in Box 23-1 demonstrates that suicide affects all age groups, both genders, and all cultures, religions, and socioeconomic classes. Be aware that any client in a health care, occupational, or community setting may, given the right circumstances, contemplate suicide.

Box 23-1 Suicide Facts

- Every **18 minutes**, a life is lost to suicide.
- Suicide is now the **11th leading cause of death** in the United States across all age groups.
- There are **more than 30,000 deaths** from suicide in the United States each year.
- More people kill themselves each year than are murdered; for every **two people who are murdered**, there are **three persons who take their own lives**.
- In the past 50 years, the number of deaths from **suicide in young adults has tripled**.
- There are **twice** as many suicides as deaths due to HIV/AIDS.
- In the month prior to their suicide, 75% of older suicide victims **had visited a primary care provider**; many had a depressive illness that was not detected.
- **More men than women** die by suicide; the gender ratio is four males to every one female.
- Over half the deaths from suicide are in **adult men ages 25–65**.
- Many suicidal people **never** seek professional care.

Source: National Institute of Mental Health, *Suicide Facts*, 2007.

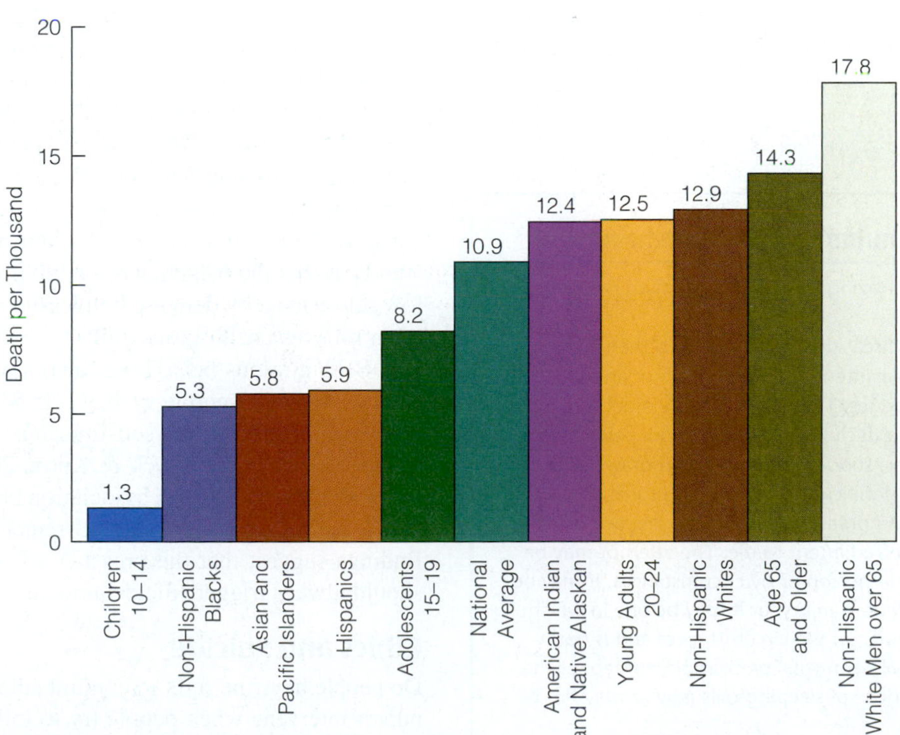

FIGURE 23-1 ■ Death by suicide according to age, ethnicity, and gender—2004 (latest available figures). Almost four times as many men as women die by suicide.

Source: Centers for Disease Control and Prevention, National Center for Injury Prevention and Control. Web-based Injury Statistics Query and Reporting System (WISQARS): www.cdc.gov/ncipc/wisqars.

As psychiatric–mental health nurses, we frequently find ourselves face to face with suicidal or self-destructive people. Few clients elicit such intense feelings of anxiety and helplessness. Suicidal individuals will cause you to question your abilities to help others and preserve life. Thus, it is critically important to be prepared for all the emotional reactions—fear, anxiety, anger, and so on—that a suicidal client may evoke in you. Unless you understand them, these reactions may interfere with your ability to establish rapport. This chapter will help you to understand self-destructive people more clearly so that you can be more comfortable in assessing and intervening with suicidal clients.

SELF-DESTRUCTIVE BEHAVIOR

In addition to suicide, other typical self-destructive behaviors and self-damaging acts include, but are not limited to, nail biting, hair pulling, self-mutilating behaviors such as scratching or cutting one's wrist or another part of the body, smoking cigarettes, driving recklessly, gambling, drinking alcohol, and using drugs. **Chronic self-destructive behavior** is behavior that harms the self, is habitual, and generally poses a low level of lethality. In general, these behaviors range from relatively innocuous acts at one end of the continuum, such as overeating and gambling, to more lethal ones at the other, such as driving recklessly in a blinding snowstorm. Such self-destructive behaviors can injure one's health and sometimes hasten one's death.

A completed suicide is the most violent self-destructive behavior. It is important to understand that not all self-destructive individuals (in fact, only about 10% of those who purposefully injure themselves) go on to kill themselves. People who are suicidal may manifest several of the behaviors listed in Box 23-2.

Box 23-2 Continuum of Suicidal Behavior

- **Suicidal ideation:** Having thoughts of harming or killing oneself.
- **Suicide threat:** A threat that is more serious than a casual statement of suicidal intent and that is accompanied by other behavior changes. These may include mood swings, temper outbursts, a decline in school or work performance, personality changes, sudden or gradual withdrawal from friends, and other significant changes in attitude.
- **Suicide attempt:** A nonfatal, self-inflicted destructive act with explicit or inferred intent to die. The attempt may be thwarted by another person or by circumstances, it may be planned to avoid serious injury, or it may be one in which the outcome depends on the circumstances and is not under the individual's control. For example, someone who takes a heavy overdose of sleeping pills may or may not be discovered in time.
- **Suicide:** A fatal, self-inflicted destructive act with explicit or inferred intent to die.

Self-Mutilation

People who have experienced early childhood neglect, abuse, or trauma frequently have difficulty understanding how to process feelings verbally and how to manage situations in a productive fashion—that is, to avoid problems. Many of these individuals use **self-mutilation**—such as cutting themselves, burning themselves with cigarettes, burning themselves on a stove, pulling out their hair, biting their fingernails into the cuticles—to deal with anxiety and distress. Clients with borderline personality disorder (see Chapter 22∞), such as Katy in the following clinical example, fit this picture.

CLINICAL EXAMPLE

Katy, 29 years old, has had trouble adjusting and being a part of things since "as far back as she remembers." She has no idea how to effectively manage her life problems and her increasing stress. She often cuts her abdomen or her arms. Katy is quick to point out that this is in no way a plan to kill herself. Rather, she finds that it helps relieve tension and changes her perspective.

Individuals who mutilate themselves do not see the behaviors as particularly problematic until the behaviors are out of control. These clients feel that experiencing pain helps change or improve their mood and their level of awareness, thereby enabling them to reconnect with themselves. Individuals such as those described in the previous clinical example perceive their painful behavior as adaptive and helpful to them in dealing with their anxiety and distress.

The exact reason for self-mutilating behavior is unknown, although there is much speculation about it. Several interpretations are possible. For example, it may help people cope with a crisis, or deny mental pain or cope with it, thus avoiding depression. Self-mutilating behavior may also result from impulsivity in people who are unable or unwilling to consider the long-term effects of their behavior. Another possibility is that the behavior is a coping mechanism that raises low self-esteem by denying helplessness. A self-punishing act often relieves unconscious guilt.

Self-injurious behavior is also associated with suicidality. In a random sample of 8,300 U.S. college-age students, 40.3% of those reporting self-injurious behavior also reported suicidal ideation (Whitlock & Knox, 2007). A study in Germany also found a strong association between deliberate self-harm and suicidal behavior (Brunner et al., 2007). These findings suggest that the presence of self-injurious behavior should always trigger suicide assessment.

Ethics and Suicide

Do people have the right to commit suicide, and can or should nurses intervene when people try to kill themselves? The traditional belief is that mental health care professionals should do everything possible to prevent suicide. You should know that, ethical concerns aside, you may be prosecuted under state laws that make it a crime to aid or abet a suicide under any circumstance, even when a terminally ill person decides to end his or her life. Questions about a client's right to suicide and society's right to control suicide are still being debated. Engaging in the process of ethical reasoning presented in Chapter 13 will help you in your search for a personal position.

Meaning and Motivation in Suicide

Suicide is never a random act. Whether committed impulsively or after painstaking consideration, the act has both a message and a purpose. In general, the purpose or reason for suicide is to escape or end an intolerable situation, crisis, or relationship, such as:

- A terminal (especially painful) illness (see What Every Primary Care Nurse Should Know)
- Being a burden to others
- An untenable family situation
- An untenable personal situation
- Punishment or exposure of socially or personally unacceptable behavior

These situations are illustrated in the clinical examples that follow.

CLINICAL EXAMPLE

Antwon's lung cancer has metastasized to his bones; any exertion causes spontaneous fractures and he is in constant pain. He has asked friends, family, and health care workers to help him escape his illness by ending his life.

Joan, a widow, fell three times last year and is now in a nursing home. She decided on suicide so that she would no longer be a burden to her family. Joan has not eaten in 7 days.

Jeremy, age 7, attempted to run into the path of a car. He had heard his mother say many times, "If it weren't for you, your Daddy and I would never have broken up." Jeremy believed that if he were dead, his parents would reunite, thus solving what he believes to be an untenable family situation.

Serena, age 33, had been admitted for the third time to a psychiatric unit because of thoughts of suicide. Jorge, her husband, has broken the last two family therapy appointments and went on vacation when she came into the hospital this time. Serena believes that she is unlovable and will attempt to leave the hospital tonight to finally stop the pain.

Fletcher, 34, was a successful businessman. Last night, he was charged with drunken driving and vehicular homicide. Horrified that his unacceptable behavior would be exposed, he committed suicide after learning that his picture and the story would be in the morning newspaper.

Many people who are self-destructive have lifelong difficulties communicating their needs to others. Some people cannot express their needs or feelings; or, when they do, they do not obtain the results they hoped for. For them, self-mutilation or suicide becomes a clear and direct, if violent, form of communication. See the Rx Communication feature on page 620 for an example of communicating with a client who self-mutilates.

WHAT EVERY PRIMARY CARE NURSE SHOULD KNOW

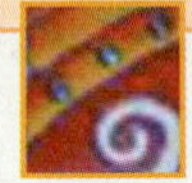

Suicidal Ideation in Primary Care

It is not unusual in primary care settings to see clients with suicidal ideation or at high risk for suicide. It is also not unusual for primary care providers to fail to recognize those at high risk for suicide. Suicidal risk is increased in both physical and psychiatric illness, especially when both are present. Remember that there is also a strong association between depression, risk for suicide, and chronic medical illness (Gaynes et al., 2007). Consider the possibility of suicide risk in all chronically ill clients, including those with solely physical symptoms.

Although there are more effective medications available to primary care practitioners to treat depression, the suicide rate has not declined, and neither has the incidence of unexplained deaths. In instances where mystery surrounds a person's death, a psychological autopsy may be performed (Scott, Swartz, & Warburton, 2006). A **psychological autopsy** is an assessment tool that reviews the circumstances and events that preceded an individual's completed suicide. A review of psychological autopsies revealed that more than 90% of suicide victims have a comorbid mental disorder (most of them mood disorders and/or substance use disorders) and, furthermore, that they were undertreated, despite contact with psychiatric or other health care services (Isometsa, 2001). Recognizing this association, screening for it, and providing treatment is a primary care imperative and may prevent unnecessary tragedies.

The message inherent in suicide is often aimed at a specific person, usually the significant other. Interrupting a suicide plan or suicidal thoughts requires hearing, understanding, and responding appropriately to messages of pain, loneliness, and hopelessness.

BIOPSYCHOSOCIAL THEORIES

Suicide and self-destructive behavior are still not well understood by the public or by the scientific community. In fact, many people's understanding of suicide has been influenced by misconceptions. These myths, and the corresponding explanatory facts that negate them, are discussed in Box 23-3 on page 620.

Suicide is a complex phenomenon, and there is no single explanation for its complicated process; however, sociocultural, interpersonal and intrapsychic, cognitive, and biologic theories seem to contribute the most to our understanding of suicide. In addition to the section that follows, careful study of Chapters 17 and 22 will help you to understand the behaviors discussed in this chapter.

Sociocultural Theory

Sociocultural theories about suicide propose that the social and cultural contexts in which the individual lives influence

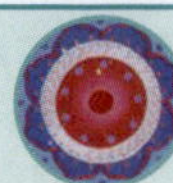

RX COMMUNICATION

THE CLIENT WHO SELF-MUTILATES

CLIENT: "I just had to cut myself. There's no other way I can feel anything."

NURSE RESPONSE 1: "I'm wondering how you felt when you cut yourself."

RATIONALE: Gathering more data will help you to understand the client better. You can help the client consider triggers and behaviors if you first encourage the client to identify and describe feelings and emotions around the event.

NURSE RESPONSE 2: "Let's talk about what led up to your cutting yourself."

RATIONALE: While this response validates the behavior as real, it also asks the client to begin examining cause and effect.

the expression of suicidality. The following clinical examples describe two possible social and cultural contexts for suicide:

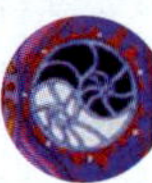

- Experiencing a precipitous deterioration in one's relationship with society (such as the loss of a job or a close friend)
- Considering self-inflicted death as honorable

CLINICAL EXAMPLE

Emma, who is without family or friends, had decided that life was not worth living after retiring from her job with the federal government. She realized that no one would even know or care if she succeeded in killing himself.

In the Gaza Strip, a suicide bomber detonated explosives strapped to his body as he rode his bicycle into an Israeli checkpoint, killing himself and three soldiers and wounding several bystanders. Those who claimed responsibility for the attack indicated their belief that the suicide bomber's death was an honorable one.

Age and Gender

Similarities and differences exist in suicide rates among various ethnic and racial groups and among people of different ages. Adolescent suicide is the third leading cause of death in the United States (Groves, Stanley, & Sher, 2007). A nationwide survey of youth in grades 9 through 12 in public and private schools in the United States found that 17% of students reported seriously considering suicide, 13% reported creating a plan, and 8% reported trying to take their own life in the 12 months preceding the survey (Eaton et al., 2006). Suicide is also a significant public health problem for older adults.

Box 23-3 Suicide Myths versus Suicide Facts

Myth: A suicide threat is just a bid for attention and should not be taken seriously.
Fact: All suicidal behavior should be taken seriously; a bid for attention may be a cry for help.

Myth: It is harmful for a person to talk about suicidal thoughts. The person's attention should be diverted when this occurs.
Fact: Of prime importance in helping a suicidal person is talking with that person in order to assess the lethality of the person's suicide plan.

Myth: Only psychotic people commit suicide.
Fact: The majority of completed suicides are committed by people who are not psychotic.

Myth: People who talk about suicide won't do it.
Fact: Most people do talk about their suicide intention before making a suicide attempt.

Myth: A nice home, good job, or an intact family prevents suicide.
Fact: People of all social and economic backgrounds commit suicide.

Myth: A failed suicide attempt should be treated as manipulative behavior.
Fact: Failed attempts are more likely evidence of a person's ambivalence toward suicide.

Myth: People who commit suicide are always depressed.
Fact: People who commit suicide are not always depressed, although depression is common. People can also be psychotic, agitated, organically impaired, or have personality disorders.

Myth: Suicide is more common in the winter months.
Fact: Contrary to popular belief, suicides peak during spring and early summer months in the Northern hemisphere.

Myth: There is no connection between alcohol or drug use and suicide.
Fact: Alcohol, drugs, and suicide are often closely connected. A person who commits suicide may have become depressed, impulsive, and suicidal after using alcohol or other drugs.

Myth: Once suicidal, always suicidal.
Fact: Suicide attempts are often made during particularly stressful times in people's lives. If the suicide attempt is managed properly, people can and do go on with their lives without recurrent thoughts of suicide.

Myth: Suicidal people rarely seek medical help.
Fact: According to studies, 50% to 60% of suicidal people sought help within the 6 months that preceded the suicide.

For white males, suicide rates jump precipitously after age 60. Refer back to Figure 23-1 and Box 23-1 on page 617.

When gender is considered, males who are Native Americans, white non-Hispanics, African-Americans, Hispanics, and Asian/Pacific Islanders have higher suicide rates than females. When age is considered, Native Americans and African-Americans have the highest suicide rates during the adolescent and young adult years, while the highest suicide rates in those over 65 years of age occur in European-American non-Hispanics, Hispanics, and Asian/Pacific Islanders (Center for Mental Health Services, 2002). The percentage of suicide attempts was significantly higher among Hispanic Latina girls (19.3%) than in African-American or Caucasian groups (Rew, Thomas, Horner, Resnick, & Beuhring, 2001).

Alcohol Use and Adolescents

Alcohol consumption is estimated to cause adolescent males to be up to 17 times more likely to attempt suicide, and females 3 times more likely to attempt suicide (Groves et al., 2007). In this same study, Caucasian adolescents were twice as likely as African-American adolescents to have used alcohol before committing suicide. Among all ethnic groups, alcohol use among adolescents was associated with increased suicidal behavior.

One study indicated a statistically significant correlation between alcohol use and subsequent suicidal ideation and attempts among preteens as compared to boys and girls who did not drink (Swahn & Bossarte, 2007). This suggests that efforts to delay and reduce early alcohol use may reduce suicide attempts.

Ethnicity

Another study compared the relationship between suicide and major depression among whites, Puerto Ricans, Mexican-Americans, and Cuban-Americans. According to Oquendo et al. (2001), the rate of depression was significantly higher for Puerto Ricans (6.9%) and significantly lower in Mexican-Americans (2.8%) and Cuban-Americans (2.6%) compared to the 1-year prevalence rate for major depression for whites (3.6%). This study also found that annual suicide rates were higher for males than for females, and Mexican-American and Puerto Rican males had lower suicide rates than white males. The researchers raised the possibilities that depression differs in form or severity in these groups or that unidentified factors protect against suicide in different subgroups.

A more recent study also found that suicide and suicide attempt rates vary across different ethnicities. An exhaustive review of the literature by Groves et al. (2007) found that depressed Asian-American youth were 4 times more likely to display suicidal behavior when compared to other Asian youths with other diagnoses, and depressed African-American females were more likely to report suicidal ideation than male adolescents. This same study found that conflict with parents is a significant factor. Asian-Americans who experience high parental conflict are 30 times more likely to engage in suicidal behavior than are Asian-American adolescents with low parental conflict. African-American adolescents are almost 7 times more likely to attempt suicide as a result of parental conflict.

Interpersonal and Intrapsychic Theory

The notion that suicide is an expression of interpersonal and intrapsychic as well as societal conflict is perhaps the most significant contribution that psychiatry and psychology have made to our understanding of suicide. The following clinical examples describe some possible interpersonal and intrapsychic contexts for suicide:

- Having no close relationships with others
- Having no personal freedoms and no hope of getting them

CLINICAL EXAMPLE

Daniel thought that suicide was the best way to solve his problems after he lost his job at a local factory and his girlfriend of 10 years precipitously broke off their engagement, left the area, and married someone else.

Jamie, who is a battered woman, believes that it doesn't make any sense to go on living. She has no close friends or relatives. Her husband will not allow her to drive, go shopping, or go to work. She is unable to see an alternative and decides that a life regulated to this extent is not worth living.

According to the classic work of Edwin Schneidman (1996), a clinical psychologist and leading authority on suicide, suicide is more accurately described as a dyadic event between two unhappy people, motivated by real or perceived rejection, abandonment, guilt, revenge, or pity. Suicide can be better understood if viewed in the context of the relationship between two people: the suicidal person and the significant other. Broadly defined, the significant other can be a spouse, child, boss, landlord, friend, nurse, or other health care worker.

Suicidal people almost always communicate their intent to significant others before the fact or attempt, although the meaning of the message may not be clear until after the attempt or death. Schneidman found a clear communication of intent in 80% of cases studied. A suicide threat or suicide attempt can arouse feelings of sympathy, anger, hostility, anxiety, or desire for connectedness on the part of a significant other, thus altering the current relationship to meet the need of the suicidal person. Although there is no one cause associated with suicide, there are several interpersonal and intrapsychic elements that are commonly associated with it. The list in Box 23-4 on page 622 summarizes common characteristics based on Schneidman's work (1996).

Biologic Theory

Several biologic and medical markers have been studied in relation to the biologic foundation of suicidal behavior. The most promising biologic markers to date appear to be decreased central serotonergic function, reduced serum cholesterol levels, decreased platelet 5-HT, low cerebrospinal fluid 5-HIAA,

Box 23-4 Characteristics Most Closely Associated with Suicide

1. The common purpose of suicide is to seek a solution to what appears to be an otherwise insoluble problem.
2. The common goal of suicide is cessation of consciousness or oblivion.
3. The common stimulus in suicide is unbearable psychological pain that may arise from any number of sources.
4. The common stressor in suicide is frustrated psychological needs that often result from family turmoil and occupational and interpersonal difficulties.
5. The common emotion in suicide is a pervasive sense of hopelessness coupled with helplessness.
6. The common cognitive state in suicide is ambivalence—desiring to die, but wishing there were another way out of the dilemma.
7. The common perceptual state in suicide is constriction of thought (tunnel vision) that prevents effective problem solving.
8. The common action in suicide is escape from intolerable circumstances.
9. The common interpersonal act in suicide is communication of intention (estimated to be 80% in completed suicides).
10. The common pattern in suicide is consistency of lifelong styles; suicidal people generally employ the same coping styles they have used throughout their lives.

and hypothalamic–pituitary–adrenocortical axis (HPA axis) dysfunction. These biologic markers are discussed next.

Neurotransmitter Receptor Hypothesis

The neurotransmitter receptor hypothesis of depression (see Chapters 7 and 17∞) holds that errors in the receptors for the specific neurotransmitter, serotonin, are critical in the development of depression and suicide. The research indicates that serotogenic hypofunction is associated with suicide and serious suicide attempts (Gibbons, Brown, Hur, Marcus, Bhaumik, & Mann, 2007). There is considerable evidence that the serotonergic system is partly under genetic control and that as yet unknown genetic factors influence the risk for suicidal behavior. These genetic factors are thought to be independent of the factors responsible for the heritability of major psychiatric conditions associated with suicide.

Normally, serotonin is released from one nerve cell, received by the next nerve cell, and then reabsorbed back into the first nerve cell. Many factors influence how much serotonin is passed from the first cell to the second cell, and how much is reabsorbed back into the first cell. Transmission can be influenced by:

1. The number of receptors
2. The ability of the receptors to function properly
3. Whether the body produces monoamine oxidase, which catabolizes serotonin (as well as norepinephrine and dopamine)

Positron emission tomography (PET) has helped researchers examine how serotonin affects the brain after the person has ingested the serotonin-releasing compound fenfluramine. Mann (2000) found that serotonin-induced brain metabolic activity was reduced throughout the frontal cortex. When the same study was repeated on persons who had attempted suicide (Mann, Brent, & Arango, 2001), serotonin activity was reduced in a small, specific area of the frontal cortex, immediately above the eyes. This area of the brain has been thought to be associated with the control of impulsive behaviors; thus, this may be an underlying cause of a person's reduced ability to resist impulses to act on suicidal thoughts. Whatever the exact mechanism may be when serotonin and serotonin metabolic activity are reduced, more violent lethal suicides and attempted suicides occur in these circumstances. Therefore, enhancing serotonin function may reduce suicide risk.

FDA Advisory on Antidepressants Of special interest has been the recently announced dramatic spike in youth suicide (NIMH, 2007). In the fall of 2004, following months of public hearings and preliminary warnings linking antidepressants with increased risk of suicidal thinking, the U.S. Food and Drug Administration (FDA) decided to require a black box warning on antidepressants for youth, and in 2007 recommended that the warnings be extended to young adults up to age 24. However, an analysis of 19 published studies offered no evidence that suicide risks increase with antidepressant treatment (Baldessarini et al., 2007). In fact, the incidence of youth suicide spiked dramatically when fewer SSRI prescriptions were written for adolescents following warnings from regulatory agencies (Gibbons, Brown, Hur, Marcus, Bhaumik, Erkens, et al., 2007). FIGURE 23-2 ■ presents the latest available figures of youth suicide. This is an important area in which intense research is ongoing.

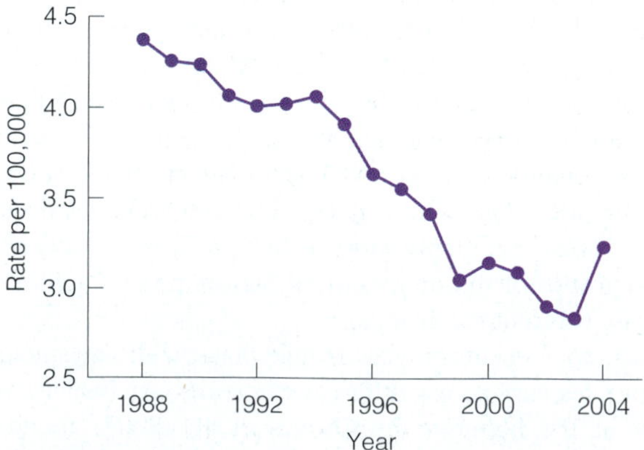

FIGURE 23-2 ■ The youth suicide rate (ages 5–19) in the United States increased conspicuously in 2004, according to statistics released in 2007 by the National Institute of Mental Health. At the same time that suicide rates for youth increased, SSRI prescription rates in the United States declined. Adolescents showed the steepest increase in suicide rates.

Source: National Institute of Mental Health. *Drops in SSRI prescription rates may coincide with increases in youth suicides.* Retrieved on September 19, 2007, from http://www.nimh.nih.gov/science-news/2007.

Genetics

A family history of suicide is a recognized marker for the increased risk of suicide, suggesting that there may be a genetic trait that predisposes some people to suicidal behavior. Various studies provide consistent evidence for a genetic component in suicidal behavior (Rujescu, Thalmeier, Moller, Bronisch, & Giegling, 2007). Genetic studies at the molecular level have concentrated on the genes of the serotonergic system since there is evidence, discussed earlier in this chapter, that serotonergic neurotransmission is implicated in suicidal behavior. Genes of the dopaminergic and noradrenergic neurotransmitter systems have also been investigated. Some epidemiological and clinical studies showed that low serum cholesterol levels and decreased platelet 5-HT levels are associated with suicidal behavior (Marcinko et al., 2007), as is hypothalamic–pituitary–adrenocortical axis (HPA axis) dysfunction (Mann & Currier, 2007). The genes involved in these pathways are also being investigated.

Cognitive Theory

Suicidologists have speculated about the cognitive style (method of thought processing) of clients who commit or attempt suicide. Although there is no single suicidal logic, some cognitive styles predispose to suicidal behavior (Bateman, Hansen, Turkington, & Kingdon, 2007).

Dichotomous thinking (the belief that there is only an either/or choice) is commonly seen in the suicidal person. The person falls into an imminently suicidal state when death seems the only escape. The thought processing of suicidal clients is generally constricted; that is, people who are suicidal have great difficulty (if they can do it at all) considering alternatives to their current dilemma. *Constriction in thought* generally results in the belief that there are only two choices: a magical solution or death. Clients whose prior suicide attempts were highly lethal performed significantly worse than other groups on tests of executive functioning (logical reasoning, verbal learning, integrating old and new information). These differences could not be explained by prior education, occupation, or intellectual capacity (Keilp et al., 2001).

People who are considering suicide are divided within themselves. They have two conflicting desires at the same time (**ambivalence**): to live and to die. Understanding the thinking of someone who is acutely suicidal requires an understanding of the concept of ambivalence. Ambivalence accounts for the fact that a suicidal person often takes lethal or near-lethal action but leaves open the possibility for rescue, allowing for the possibility of intervention. Failing to intervene and provide life choices increases the person's desperation, and death becomes the more focused choice.

The effectiveness of cognitive behavior therapy (CBT) in moderating suicidal risk in people with multiple suicide attempts and significant mental disorders (schizophrenia and borderline personality disorder, for example) is a subject of current study. One such study (Bateman et al., 2007) revealed that CBT provided signficant reductions in suicidal ideation in people with schizophrenia. The results were not accounted for by the administration of medication since the subjects were resistant to conventional antipsychotic medication. The decrease in suicidal ideation at the end of therapy was sustained at follow-up. Further research is indicated to substantiate these findings and determine how and why CBT works. Continued study in this area is important—there is a 10% lifetime risk of suicide in persons with schizophrenia (Schultz, North, & Shields, 2007).

SUICIDE PREVENTION

Suicide is a serious public health problem. However, many suicides are preventable.

In the 1960s, the federal government established the first special suicide unit at the National Institute of Mental Health in Bethesda, Maryland. Since that time, we have seen the growth of prevention efforts. Suicide prevention programs have developed at both the micro- and macro-levels in mental health agencies, with the development of suicide crisis centers and hotlines at local levels; in schools, colleges, and universities; at work sites; in correctional institutions; in aging programs; and in family, youth, and community serivce programs.

Risk Factors and Protective Factors

A combination of individual, interpersonal, community, and societal factors contribute to the risk of suicide as well as the protective factors for suicide. Risk factors are the characteristics that are associated with suicide. They may or may not be direct causes. Protective factors serve as buffers from suicidial thoughts and behavior. Both are equally important, and both need more extensive and rigorous research.

Identifying people at risk allows us to engage them in effective treatments, support the presence of protective factors, and improve clinical practices. Risk factors and protective factors for suicide are discussed in Box 23-5 on page 623.

National Suicide Prevention Initiative

The National Strategy for Suicide Prevention is the first coordinated effort of resources and culturally appropriate services between all levels of government and the private sector. It is a collaborative, multiproject initiative designed to incorporate best practices and research toward reducing the incidence of suicide nationwide (Substance Abuse and Mental Health Services Administration, 2007). The goals and objectives for action are:

- Changing procedures and policies in hospital emergency departments, substance abuse treatment centers, and mental health treatment centers designed to assess suicide risk
- Incorporating suicide-risk screening in primary care
- Ensuring that those who provide services to suicide survivors (emergency medical technicians, firefighters, police, funeral directors) have been trained to respond appropriately to their unique needs
- Increasing the numbers of people with mood disorders who receive and maintain treatment
- Ensuring that persons treated for trauma, sexual assault, or physical abuse in emergency departments receive mental health services

MEDIALINK Application: "If you are thinking about suicide, read this first."

Box 23-5 Risk Factors and Protective Factors for Suicide

Risk Factors

- Family history of suicide
- Family history of child maltreatment
- Previous suicide attempt(s)
- History of mental disorders, particularly depression
- History of alcohol and substance abuse
- Feelings of hopelessness
- Impulsive or aggressive tendencies
- Cultural and religious beliefs (e.g., suicide is a noble resolution of a personal dilemma)
- Local epidemics of suicide (cluster suicides)
- Isolation (feeling cut off from other people)
- Barriers to accessing mental health treatment
- Loss (relational, social, work, or financial)
- Physical illness
- Easy access to lethal methods
- Unwillingness to seek help because of the stigma attached to mental health and substance abuse disorders or to suicidal thoughts

Protective Factors

- Effective clinical care for mental, physical, and substance abuse disorders
- Easy access to a variety of clinical interventions and support for help seeking
- Family and community support
- Support from ongoing medical and mental health care relationships
- Skills in problem solving, conflict resolution, and the nonviolent management of disputes
- Cultural and religious beliefs that discourage suicide and support the instinct for self-preservation

Sources: Centers for Disease Control. (2007c). *Suicide prevention scientific information: Risk and protective factors.* Retrieved on September 10, 2007, from www.cdc.gov/ncipc/dvp/Suicide-risk-p-factors.htm; DeLeo, D., Bertolote, J., & Lester, D. (2002). "Self-directed violence." In E. Krug, L. L. Dahlberg, J. A. Mercy, A. Zwi, & R. Lozano, (Eds.), *World report on violence and health*, pp. 184–212. Geneva: World Health Organization; Goldsmith, S. K., Pellmar, T. C., Kleinman, A. M., & Bunney, W. E. (Eds.). (2007). *Reducing suicide: A national imperative. Washington*, DC: National Academy Press; U.S. Public Health Service. (1999). *The surgeon general's call to action to prevent suicide.* Washington, DC: U.S. Department of Health and Human Services.

- Fostering the education of family members and significant others of those receiving care for the treatment of mental health and substance abuse disorders with risk of suicide
- Eliminating barriers to health care (financial, structural, personal, and cultural)

Reducing barriers to health care is an important advocacy strategy for all nurses. Large numbers of people have inadequate health insurance and do not have the financial capacity to pay for services outside their health plan or insurance program. Others have no health insurance at all. Structural barriers are the lack of primary care providers or other health care professionals and a lack of health care facilities to meet needs. Cultural and spiritual differences, language, and concerns about confidentiality or discrimination are personal barriers.

MEDIALINK Suicide Prevention Resources

Suicide Hotlines and Crisis Centers

For people contemplating suicide or families concerned about loved ones, the **National Suicide Prevention Lifeline 1–800–213–TALK** circumvents the barriers described earlier and provides immediate assistance around the clock. This lifeline consists of a network of more than 120 crisis centers in communities around the country that are committed to suicide prevention. Standards for the assessment of suicide risk to effectively guide crisis hotline workers in assessing callers have been developed and are in the process of being implemented (Joiner et al., 2007). A study of 1,085 suicide callers showed significant decreases in suicidality during the course of the telephone session, with continuing decreases in hopelessness and psychological pain in a 3-week follow-up (Gould, Kalafat, Harrismunfakh, & Kleinman, 2007). Having empathy, respect, a supportive approach, good contact, and collaborative problem solving are helper behaviors and intervention styles that are significantly related to positive outcomes in telephone suicide intervention (Mishara et al., 2007).

Individual states also have suicide hotlines and suicide prevention web pages with information about suicide prevention efforts, including statistical data, suicide prevention plans, and suicide prevention coalitions. Links to individual state websites can be found at the website of the Suicide Prevention Resource Center (SPRC) at www.sprc.org.

As a collaborative effort, SPRC and the American Foundation for Suicide Prevention maintain a best-practices registry for suicide prevention (www.sprc.org.) to disseminate information about the best practices that address the National Strategy for Suicide Prevention.

NURSE'S SELF-ASSESSMENT

When working with a suicidal client, it is imperative that you are aware of and monitor your own reactions to this potentially life-threatening situation, because your reactions may interfere with your ability to accurately assess the situation and intervene. The suicidal client presents a unique challenge and will call on all your resources. You must be able to ask the right questions and make the right decisions as well as manage your own fears and anxieties. Helping a person who not only may not want your assistance but wants deliberately to harm or kill himself is a very complicated process.

You must be compassionate enough to be able to form an effective link with a suicidal client. The goal is to encourage the client to see you as an ally, yet maintain enough de-

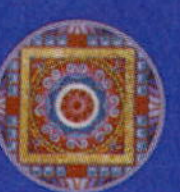

YOUR SELF-AWARENESS
An Attitude Inventory for Working with Suicidal Clients

To increase self-awareness about managing your own anxiety when working with clients who are suicidal, ask yourself the following questions:

- What kinds of things frighten me?
- How do I feel about asking for someone else's help with a client if I'm unsure of myself or uncomfortable?
- Are suicidal clients asking me to take responsibility for their behavior?
- Are suicidal clients able to assume responsibility for their own behavior?

To increase self-awareness of your own feelings about self-destructive people, ask yourself the following questions:

- How do I feel about people who deliberately harm themselves?
- How do I understand self-destructive behavior?
- Do I believe that clients are capable of change?
- Do I believe that people ultimately have the responsibility for their own lives?
- Can a person who is mentally ill choose suicide as a reasonable course?

To increase self-awareness about your own anger, ask yourself the following questions:

- What kinds of things make me angry?
- How do I deal with my own anger? Do I tend to ignore it or hide it?
- How do I react to others when they are angry?
- How do I feel about people who don't change immediately?
- How do I deal with people who appear to do illogical things?
- How do I feel when people don't change their behavior when I've asked them to or when I talk to them about it?

To increase self-awareness about your own feeling of control, ask yourself the following questions:

- In what areas of my life and my work do I feel the need to take control?
- How do I feel when interventions do not go the way I would like them to?
- How do I handle control issues with clients?
- How do I feel about control issues with clients?
- How do I feel about my lack of control over others?

tachment to avoid being overwhelmed by the client's pain. The client will also bring many feelings into the interaction. Whether the feeling is anger, fear, anxiety, irritability, or hostility, remember that all emotions need to be tolerated, worked through, and evaluated.

Our attitudes toward suicidal clients have many sources. In addition to direct experience with suicidal clients, societal, familial, and ethical issues, as well as historical antecedents, influence what we think and how we feel about suicide and self-destructive behavior, euthanasia, abortion rights, the right to commit suicide, and the responsibility to prevent suicide. We can get caught up in the dilemma of how much responsibility to take for the self-destructive person and for how long. (Ethical issues are discussed in Chapter 13.)

All nurses must be competent not only to assess but also to intervene effectively with a suicidal client. This is not easy. Suicidal and self-destructive people seemingly defeat our best efforts by choosing death over life, or by being self-destructive. Although it is our responsibility to promote and maintain life, we cannot force the client to stay alive. Instead, we encourage clients to examine and understand how it is that they have reached this point and to expand their repertoire of coping methods.

Nurses working with self-destructive, self-injurious, or suicidal clients may have a variety of feelings—frustration and anger among them. Before working with someone who is suicidal or self-destructive, it is critically important to assess personal feelings, experiences, conflicts, and memories that may either impede or facilitate your effectiveness. The inventory in the Your Self-Awareness feature will help you to explore your own attitudes.

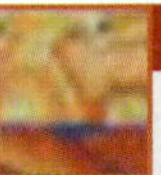

NURSING PROCESS
The Suicidal or Self-Destructive Client

Working effectively with a self-destructive client requires understanding the meaning the self-destructive behavior has for the client, performing a lethality assessment, keeping the client safe, and helping enlarge the client's repertoire of adaptive coping behaviors. An example of how this can be done in clinical practice is in the Evidence-Based Practice feature.

Review these other chapters for information on suicide in specific populations: children, Chapter 26; adolescents, Chapter 27; elders, Chapter 28; substance abusers, Chapter 15; people with HIV disease, Chapter 25.

Assessment

A thorough assessment always includes a self-assessment by the nurse, the identification of clues or cries for help, and an accurate lethality assessment. Because assessment of suicide risk involves a degree of clinical judgment, you should seek sound mentorship if you are a novice practitioner.

Clues or Cries for Help

People intent on suicide almost always give either verbal or nonverbal clues of their plans or ideas. Up to 80% of all individuals who commit suicide may signal their need for help by making contact with the health care system 1 to 2 months before the suicide because of various physical complaints (Mann, 2000). Unfortunately, the cry for help is not always

MEDIALINK Case Study: The Suicidal Client

MEDIALINK Care Plan: Assessing Suicide Attempts

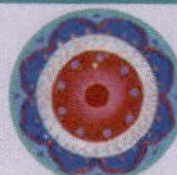

EVIDENCE-BASED PRACTICE

FINDING ALTERNATIVES TO SUICIDE

Carolyn D., a 19-year-old college student majoring in theater arts, has been admitted to the inpatient unit after a heavy night of drinking alcohol that culminated in a suicide attempt. Carolyn's boyfriend has just dropped out of the college they attend—well-known as a "party school"—and returned to his hometown, 1,375 miles away. Within the 3 months prior to this admission, she experienced a major injury to her knee. The injury was severe enough to prevent her from achieving her life plan—being a dancer. Her family reports that she became increasingly despondent, saying she had nothing left to live for. They also worry that Carolyn will revert to the drinking problem she had in high school.

While on the unit, she has been unwilling to attend group therapy, saying that she "can't talk right," that her "head isn't working," and that she "can't talk in front of others." Her DSM-IV-TR diagnosis is Major Depression, and she has begun taking appropriate antidepressant medications. As her psychiatric–mental health nurse, you formulate a nursing care plan that addresses the following considerations:

1. Carolyn is depressed and is working through multiple losses. In order to be able to find alternatives to suicide, she will need to think and process her feelings in a less rigid fashion.
2. Providing a less demanding but secure environment will allow time to demonstrate to her that she has the flexibility to develop new coping skills and behaviors in response to her losses.
3. Cognitive behavioral therapy can help Carolyn learn to identify and respond more appropriately to circumstances that elicit maladaptive responses (alcohol abuse, depression).
4. Helping her to express feelings and perceptions will increase her self-awareness and her ability to plan methods for meeting her needs in the future. Validating Carolyn's perceptions provides reassurance and can decrease her anxiety.
5. Carolyn's hospitalization is likely to be short-term. The likelihood of suicide attempts is elevated in the month after starting treatment when Carolyn will be back at school. Referrals in her college and in the community for suicide prevention and alcohol abuse prevention services for both Carolyn and her family will be important.

The interventions for Carolyn are based on the following research:

Bateman, K., Hansen, L., Turkington, D., & Kingdon, D. (2007). Cognitive behavioral therapy reduces suicidal ideation in schizophrenia: Results from a randomized controlled trial. *Suicide and Life-Threatening Behavior, 37*(3), 284–290.

Simon, G. E., & Savarino, J. (2007). Suicide attempts among patients starting depression treatment with medications or psychotherapy. *American Journal of Psychiatry, 164*(7), 1029–1034.

Swahn, M. H., & Bossarte, R. M. (2007). Gender, early alcohol use, and suicide ideation and attempts: Findings from the 2005 youth risk behavior survey. *Journal of Adolescent Health, 41*(2), 175–181.

CRITICAL THINKING APPLICATION

1. If Carolyn needs to become less rigid in her thinking and more flexible in her coping skills, how can a structured program such as cognitive behavioral therapy help her?
2. Is a short-term hospitalization such as Carolyn's appropriate for someone at increased risk for suicide? Should Carolyn remain hospitalized until the threat of suicide is over?
3. What is the likelihood that Carolyn will abuse alcohol once she is back in her college environment?

clear until after the event. Because people do want help, it is important that you ask questions about depression and suicide. Always be alert to patterns that may at first seem coincidental, as in the following clinical example.

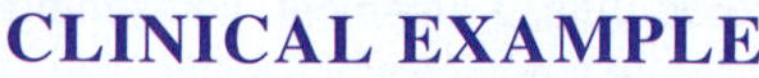

CLINICAL EXAMPLE

Yusef, a 21-year-old man, was referred to a therapist by his physician. Although he described chronic "aches and pains" and "not feeling well," a physical exam revealed no physical problems. He did talk about how life was just not worth living, and he had a recent history of driving recklessly. After further discussion, he said that he had recently broken up with his girlfriend and admitted that his reckless driving had a suicidal intent.

The cry for help may be indirect or subtle. Examples of what a person might say are: "I just can't take it anymore," "There's no reason to go on," "Sometimes I think I'd be better off dead," "I won't be seeing you anymore," "Take care of my dog and cat," "Too bad I won't get to see my little brother grow up," and "Will you be sorry when I'm gone?" Sometimes the behavior of people intent on suicide provides the clue. They may:

- Give away prized possessions
- Make out or change a will
- Take out, or add to, an insurance policy
- Cancel all social engagements
- Be despondent or behave in unusual ways
- Be unable to sleep
- Feel hopeless
- Have trouble concentrating at school or on the job

- Suddenly lose interest in friends, organizations, and activities
- Have a sudden, unexplained recovery from a depression
- Plan their funeral
- Cry for no apparent reason

Be alert to both clear and veiled communications about suicide. Once clues have been identified, the next step is to perform an accurate lethality assessment. An assessment for suicide should *always* be done whenever you suspect suicidal thought or intent.

Lethality Assessment

A **lethality assessment** is an attempt to predict the likelihood of suicide. An accurate lethality assessment is essential in formulating a plan for helping a suicidal person. Assessment of risk factors is essential in order to determine the client's need for hospitalization (Brooker, Ricketts, Bennett, & Lemme, 2007) or the extent of watchful precautions to take when clients are hospitalized. Carrying out a lethality assessment requires direct communication with the client about the client's intent. The Your Assessment Approach feature presents a lethality assessment scale.

Another component of assessing lethality is a consideration of the lethality of the proposed suicide method. Box 23-6 compares the lethality of various suicide methods. There are some gender differences in suicide methods. Women tend to use less violent methods—drugs and carbon monoxide poisoning—while men tend to use more violent methods—firearms and hanging (Denning, Conwell, King, & Cox, 2000). The top three methods used in suicides of young people are hanging/suffocation, poisoning, and firearms (CDC, 2007b).

It is critical that you evaluate the client's ability and intent to act on an idea or plan. Beyond inquiring into the existence of a plan for suicidal action, ask questions and pay particular attention to whether or not steps have already been

Box 23-6 Lethality of Suicide Methods

Less Lethal Methods

- Wrist cutting
- House gas
- Nonprescription medications (excluding aspirin and acetaminophen [Tylenol])
- Tranquilizers

Highly Lethal Methods

- Gun
- Jumping
- Hanging
- Drowning
- Carbon monoxide poisoning
- Barbiturates and prescribed sleeping pills
- High doses of aspirin and acetaminophen (Tylenol)
- Car crash
- Exposure to extreme cold
- Antidepressants

YOUR ASSESSMENT APPROACH
Lethality Assessment Scale

Key to Scale	Danger to Self	Typical Indicators
1	No predictable risk of immediate suicide	No notion of suicide or history of attempts; satisfactory social support network; in close contact with significant others.
2	Low risk of immediate suicide	Has considered suicide with less lethal method; no history of attempts or recent serious loss; satisfactory support network; no alcohol problems; basically wants to live.
3	Moderate risk of immediate suicide	Has considered suicide with highly lethal method but has no specific plan or threats; or has plan with less lethal method, history of less lethal attempts, tumultuous family history, reliance on drugs or medications for stress relief; weighing the odds between life and death.
4	High risk of imminent suicide	Current highly lethal plan with obtainable means; history of previous attempts; unable to communicate with close friends; drinking problem; feels depressed and wants to die.
5	Very high risk of imminent suicide	Current highly lethal plan with obtainable means; history of highly lethal attempts; cut off from resources; depressed and uses alcohol to excess; threatened with a serious loss (unemployment, divorce, failure in school).

Source: Adapted from Hoff, L. A. (1995). *People in crisis: Understanding and helping* (4th ed.). Menlo Park, CA: Addison-Wesley. This material is used by permission of John Wiley & Sons, Inc.

MEDIALINK Critical Thinking Exercise: Assessing the Client for Suicide Potential

taken to implement such a plan. For example, has the person already stockpiled medication, written a suicide note, obtained (or have access to) knives or guns, spoken to others about purchasing a gun, written a will, given away valued objects, or recently purchased insurance? Also obtain information about prior suicide attempts as well as the client's history of violence and impulsiveness, alcohol and drug use, and family history of suicide or violence.

Assessment of suicide risk is not easily accomplished. One barrier is the fear inexperienced nurses have of asking inappropriate or possibly harmful questions. It is important that you understand that *it is not possible to "cause" a person's suicide by assessing feelings and thoughts.* Inquiring about suicidal thoughts may alleviate a person's anxiety about considering suicide, not "give them the idea."

These are some suggestions for questions that you might ask:

- "How bad are things for you?"
- "How down do you get?"
- "Are you worried about yourself?"
- "Do you ever think of harming yourself when you're down?"

Then proceed with questioning the client gently, but directly asking:

- "Have you ever thought of taking your own life?"
- "Have you ever been so sad that you wanted to end it all, maybe by dying?"
- "How long have you been feeling that way?"
- "How are you thinking of hurting/harming yourself?"

Do not use euphemisms—be direct and clear in your communication.

The client who asks you to promise not to tell anyone about a suicide plan poses a serious assessment problem. Never promise to keep clinical information of any kind a secret, and explain to the client that information is shared with the treatment team. You will probably need to discuss the issue of confidentiality further and explore the dynamics of the nurse–client relationship.

A comprehensive assessment, including a lethality assessment, will help you decide which interventions are indicated for the client. For example, a complete assessment of level of lethality can prevent unnecessary hospitalizations. Hospitalizations in and of themselves can create a crisis. However, when the suicide plan is lethal and there are inadequate supports to maintain the client in the community, hospitalization is the optimal option.

Nursing Diagnosis: NANDA

Core nursing diagnoses apply to most self-destructive clients:

- Risk for Self-Directed Violence
- Risk for Suicide
- Risk for Self-Mutilation
- Powerlessness
- Hopelessness
- Spiritual Distress
- Ineffective Individual Coping
- Low Self-Esteem

Several other nursing diagnoses (Anxiety, Impaired Verbal Communication, Dysfunctional Grieving, Impaired Thought Processes, and Dysfunctional Family Processes, among others) may be appropriate, depending on the situation.

Outcome Identification: NOC

Outcome criteria for the self-destructive client are:

- Acknowledge self-harm thoughts.
- Admit to use of self-harm behavior if it occurs.
- Be able to identify personal triggers.
- Learn to properly identify and tolerate uncomfortable feelings.
- Choose alternatives that are not harmful.
- Admit to the use of self-harm behavior if it occurs.
- Attempt to identify stressors.
- Cooperate with interventions designed to reduce suicidal thoughts and control behavior.

Planning and Implementation: NIC

The nursing interventions in the following section are based on the traditional belief that mental health care professionals should do everything possible to prevent suicide.

General Guidelines for Any Setting

The priority task is to work with the client to stop the constricted processing of suicidal thinking, long enough to enable the client and family members to consider alternatives to suicide.

The nature of the nursing interventions is in large part determined by the setting in which you encounter the suicidal client. The following list of interventions and suggestions offers general guidelines that are applicable in most settings.

- Take any threat seriously. Evaluate the threat before dismissing it.
- Talk about suicide openly and directly. Remember, asking about it will not put the notion into the client's head.
- Implement suicide precautions/restrictive status (discussed in greater detail later in this chapter).
- Search the client's room, especially if suicidal thoughts or a suicide attempt occur after admission.
- Decide (along with other members of the team) if a no self-harm/no-suicide contract will be used (a sample contract is in the Your Intervention Strategies feature).
- House the client in an area that is accessible for easy observation. Select a room that is near the nurses' station. A two-person room is best.
- Be careful not to encourage staff behaviors that give clients or staff members a false sense of security.
- Organize a plan of care with the client. Discuss all important problems, prioritize them, and list several

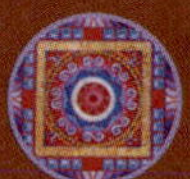

YOUR INTERVENTION STRATEGIES
How to Develop No Self-Harm/No Suicide Contracts

No self-harm/no suicide contracts are effective in many situations, and they work well with certain clients. They can be used in hospital or outpatient settings as a means of providing additional support to people who are likely to harm themselves.

Do

- Do fully assess the client to determine if a contract will be helpful.
- Do establish a relationship with the client prior to initiating the contract.
- Do use the contract as a way of connecting with and staying connected to the client.
- Do specify in the contract the intervals for reevaluation. In outpatient settings, the interval may be 1 week; the inpatient interval may range from every shift to every 1 to 3 days.
- Do have both nurse and client sign the contract and date it.
- Do have the client write out the contract if at all possible. Be creative if a client is unable or unwilling to write it out (the contract could be audiotaped, or the client and the nurse might each write half).

Don't

- Don't use a no suicide contract before performing a thorough assessment.
- Don't place more trust in or more emphasis on a contract than you would on clinical judgment. A contract is a helpful therapeutic tool, but it does not replace good clinical judgment and is not a guarantee against legal liability.

Clients who are acutely suicidal may agree to the contract even though they have no intention of adhering to it.

Sample No Self-Harm/No Suicide Contract

I, Cathy Smith, will not harm myself in any way. If I feel as if I am going to lose control, I will tell the staff (inform my nurse, call the crisis unit, call my therapist, etc.).

I will not bring, nor will I ask others to bring, harmful articles or substances onto the unit.

This contract lasts until __________(date) and is renewable at that time.

Signed (and dated)

___________________________, Client

___________________________, Nurse

approaches to each problem. Write down this plan, noting who is responsible for which actions.

- Do not make unrealistic promises such as, "Don't worry, I won't let you kill yourself." Remain honest but hopeful. Making unrealistic promises diminishes your credibility with the client.
- Encourage the client to continue daily activities and self-care as much as possible. Assign tasks for the client that are distracting but not taxing.
- Decide with the client which family members and friends are to be contacted and by whom.
- Be prepared to deal with family members who may be confused, angry, or uninterested. Strive to remain neutral, and do not make assumptions about the family's behavior.
- Expect that the client will be experiencing shame, and work to help the client toward self-acceptance.
- Remove the client from immediate danger by confiscating pills or other harmful objects in the client's possession, or by moving the client to a physically safe environment.
- Relieve the client's obvious immediate distress. Does the client need a bath, clean clothing, food, sleep?
- Find out what, in the client's view, is the most pressing need. This may be seeing a friend or family member, or arranging for someone to pick up the children after school.
- Assume a nonjudgmental, caring attitude that does not engender self-pity in the client.
- Ask why the client chose to attempt suicide at this particular moment. The client's answer will shed light on the meaning suicide has for the client and may provide information that can lead to other helpful interventions.
- Provide for the client's safety through close observation and careful monitoring (see the section on client safety).
- Review the safety of the environment (see the section on safety in the therapeutic environment).
- Evaluate the client's need for medication.
- Evaluate the plan developed in collaboration with the client, and arrange for appropriate follow-up.
- Monitor your personal feelings about the client, and decide how they may be influencing your clinical work.
- Work with other team members to evaluate the issues fully. You don't always have all the pieces of the puzzle.
- Perform a physical examination. One woman had cut herself severely prior to coming to the hospital, but this injury was not discovered until the physical examination was performed.
- Recognize that people can and do hang or strangle themselves with shoelaces, brassiere straps, pantyhose, robe belts, craft materials, and so on. Remain alert: Razor blades may be found in pages of books; matches are relatively easy to hide; pills may be hidden in plastic wrap in a cake box or stuffed

animals; light bulbs can be broken and used to cut oneself, as can wire from spiral notebooks. Clients are also able to drown in a bathtub, throw themselves through a plate-glass window, set themselves on fire, or drink bleach from the cleaning person's cart.

General Guidelines for the Emergency Department

Suicidal behavior is prevalent in the psychiatric emergency department. As many as 38% of psychiatric emergency department clients are thought to be at increased risk for suicide (Dhossche, 2000).

In the emergency department, whether in a psychiatric hospital or a general hospital medical center, the main goal of treatment is to save the person's life. Although the emergency staff may be excellent at technical interventions, they may voice or feel contempt for the client who is a "repeater," especially if the attempt is not a serious one. The client needs a professional, nonpunitive approach and a smooth transition to other caregivers or agencies. Leaving the person alone or with access to harmful objects is obviously a hazard to be avoided in a busy emergency department.

Suicide Precautions/Restrictive Status

Maintain the client's safety in the least restrictive manner possible (client right of treatment in the least restrictive setting is discussed in Chapter 13). The length of time on restrictive status is of concern to the client as well as the staff. Remember that restrictions meet the safety needs of the client, but they do not constitute treatment. On an inpatient unit, times of highest risk for suicide are evenings, nights, and weekends. Two factors account for this. During these periods, clients' time is less structured, and fewer staff members are available.

Suicide Protocols Most psychiatric inpatient units have developed a set of protocols or guidelines for observing and monitoring client behavior, often referred to as **suicide precautions**. Systems of observation may have three to six levels. Restrictions may require a physician's order but can and should be implemented on an emergency basis by nurses or other clinical staff. These protocols are often labeled to reflect the rationale for their use. In addition to suicide precautions, they may be known by such names as *special awareness*, *observation*, *constant observation*, and *constant visual observation*. For sample protocols, see the Your Intervention Strategies feature on page 631.

It is of critical importance that all staff members be familiar with the system being used and understand the rationale for its use. Maintaining and observing clients on these protocols is an important nursing responsibility.

Restrictive status should be reserved for the safety management of suicidal clients. Restrictions can confound therapeutic management, and their use simply to restrict the free movement of clients diminishes their effectiveness. In general, privileges and other components of unit restriction are better dealt with by other measures such as privilege systems. If there is doubt about the appropriate safety status, the client should remain on a more restrictive status until the team decides what measures are appropriate. If there is doubt or concern about moving a client to a different status, it is best to retain the more restrictive status until the clinical direction of treatment is clarified.

Signs of Clinical Improvement Once a client has been recognized as a suicide risk and a safety plan has been implemented, the therapeutic work of addressing depression, psychosis, and precipitating factors must begin. The treatment focus shifts as the client begins to show signs of clinical improvement.

The following signs usually indicate clinical improvement and signal the need to review or change treatment plans, grant privileges, or plan discharges:

- Verbalizing a range of options other than suicide
- Making long-term plans or discussing future events
- Verbalizing hope
- Responding to antidepressant and/or antipsychotic medications

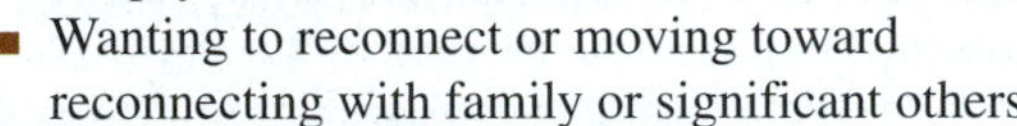

- Wanting to reconnect or moving toward reconnecting with family or significant others
- Showing more energy
- Sleeping better
- Feeling less hopeless
- Demonstrating a wider range of affective responses to situations that occur on the unit

Removing Suicide Precautions/Restrictive Status Restrictions should be changed gradually, rather than all at once. A realistic plan is to change one or, at the most, two variables at a time while observing, monitoring, and documenting client responses.

As the team begins to move the client off special status, it is important for all team members to keep communicating openly about the client. As the client begins to improve, the risk of suicide increases temporarily (especially if the client has increased energy and ability finally to act on the suicidal ideation). The following times are critical and call for careful evaluation:

- *When the decision is made to move the client off suicide precaution status.* Clients, especially those who have come to depend on the around-the-clock safety, comfort, and nurturance provided by a staff member, may experience the discontinuing of suicide precaution status as a loss. Gradual removal from suicide precaution status and careful monitoring of its impact on clients is indicated in these cases.
- *When the decision is made to increase access to "sharps" (dangerous objects).* This increased access may make it possible for a client to act on a suicidal impulse. Assess the client carefully before granting this access.
- *During the second or third week of antidepressant medication therapy.* At this time, clients have increased energy but their depression has not been resolved.

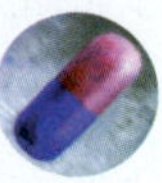

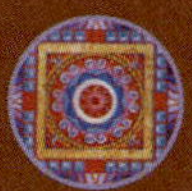

YOUR INTERVENTION STRATEGIES
Sample Protocols for Suicide Precautions

Note that these are sample protocols. Check with the policies and procedures of the specific mental health facility.

Basic Suicide Precautions

Basic suicide precautions may be started without a physician's order, but a psychiatric consultation must be obtained as soon as possible.

- The client is to remain in the room with the door open unless accompanied by a staff or family member. The client may use the bathroom alone.
- Check the client's whereabouts and safety every 15 minutes. Place a check-off sheet on the client's door to document safety checks.
- Stay with the client while all medications are taken.
- Look through the client's belongings for potentially harmful objects. Make the search in the client's presence, and ask for the client's assistance while doing so.
- Check all articles brought in by visitors.
- Allow the client to have a regular food tray, but be sure to check whether the glass or any utensils are missing when collecting the tray.
- Allow visitors and telephone calls unless the client wishes otherwise.
- Check that visitors do not leave potentially dangerous objects in the client's room.
- Maintain the protocol until it is canceled by a psychiatrist.
- Inform the client of the reasons for and details of precautionary measures. This explanation must be made by the nurse and by the psychiatrist and documented in the chart.

Maximum Suicide Precautions

Maximum suicide precautions can be instituted without a physician's order under emergency conditions, but a psychiatric consultation must be obtained as soon as possible.

- Provide one–to–one nursing supervision. The nurse must be in the room within arm's reach of the client at *all* times. When the client uses the bathroom, the bathroom door must remain open. A staff member should sit next to the client's bed at night.
- Do not allow the client to leave the unit for tests or procedures.
- Allow visitors and telephone calls unless the client wishes otherwise. Maintain one–to–one supervision during visits.
- Look through the client's belongings in the client's presence, and remove any potentially harmful objects, such as pills, matches, belts, shoelaces, pantyhose, brassieres, razors, tweezers, mirrors or other glass objects (such as light bulbs), wire, and craft materials.
- If suicide precautions are initiated after the client has been on the unit for any length of time, make a complete search of the room.
- Check that visitors do not leave potentially harmful objects in the client's room.
- Serve the client's meals in an isolation meal tray that contains no glass or metal silverware.
- Prior to instituting these measures, explain to the client what you will be doing and why. A physician must also explain this to the client. Document the explanation in the chart.
- Do not discontinue these measures without an order from a psychiatrist.

- *When the decision is made to grant a pass.* Decisions to grant pass privileges should be evaluated carefully. Where is the client going, and with whom? What time frame is being considered, and why? Perform a careful assessment both before and after the client goes on a pass. Additional searches may be needed at these times.
- *Prior to discharge and while formulating the discharge plan.* Remember that while clients are inpatients, they have staff available to them at a moment's notice. This is not the case once the client is discharged. It is crucial to evaluate the "holding environment" in the community. Refer the client to resources in the community, and schedule a follow-up appointment at the time of discharge. Family and significant others should participate in discharge planning. It is generally not a good idea to discharge a client (especially one who lacks immediate family support and must rely on agencies or clinics) on a Friday, over a long weekend, or when the mental health care provider will be on vacation or otherwise unavailable.

Monitoring Safety of the Therapeutic Environment

The safety of the therapeutic environment should be evaluated periodically. Does it meet the needs of the current client population, and is the level of restrictions consistent with the milieu philosophy? Here are specific questions to consider:

- Are areas free of glass or sharps?
- Are hazardous objects and areas kept locked?
- Are closet or shower rods of the breakaway type?
- Are craft items safe?
- How many clients are there? What is the client population like now? Do they have character disorders? Serious depression?
- If the therapeutic environment is temporarily deemed to be unsafe—that is, if there are objects (such as liquor, razors, drugs) on the unit that can harm others—is there also a need to conduct a thorough "health-and-welfare search," in order to completely examine all areas of the unit for further contraband or other potential hazards?

It is also very important to educate the client's family and visitors about safety measures and their rationale. Taking

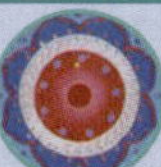

PARTNERING WITH CLIENTS AND FAMILIES

HELPING AN INDIVIDUAL DEVELOP A FAMILY SUICIDE CRISIS PLAN

For most people, thinking about committing suicide is temporary. It is important that when suicidal ideas occur to you that you have a crisis plan in place. This plan will help you avoid acting on suicidal thoughts when those thoughts occur. Your plan should contain the following elements:

- **Tell those you trust about your condition.** It is important for the people close to you to be totally familiar with your condition before it becomes a crisis. Discuss your plan with family and friends so that they can respond quickly and effectively if you need their help.
- **Recognize the earliest warning signs of a suicidal episode.** Learn to be sensitive to subtle warnings of illness. This is a time to take care of yourself with the utmost care. *Do not become angry or disgusted with yourself.*
- **Avoid drugs and alcohol.** Most deaths by suicide are the result of sudden, uncontrolled impulses. Since drugs and alcohol contribute to such impulses, it is essential to avoid them. Drugs and alcohol also interfere with the effectiveness of medications prescribed for depression.
- **Don't despair if your suicidal thinking recurs.** Suicidal thinking is the signal of a neurochemical imbalance. Call for help.
- **Contact your mental health provider, primary care provider, or clinic.** Have these phone numbers with you along with a back-up number such as a psychiatric emergency room or a suicide crisis line.
- **Predial your telephone with emergency numbers.** Having these numbers available will get you help sooner if you are feeling desperate.

MEDIALINK Family Resources

this step helps ensure that family members and other visitors do not bring unsafe objects on the unit. Visitors must understand visit limits and unit policies in relation to passes. It is also necessary to explain the need for searches. Families and friends who repeatedly violate safety measures of the unit may require additional attention, and their visiting privileges may have to be restricted.

Documenting Client Behavior and Treatment

Documentation is essential for those working with suicidal clients on an inpatient unit. Documentation helps all staff members understand the rationale for changes and comply with ethical and legal requirements. In general, follow agency rules about documentation. Also be sure to document:

- All team reviews of client status and the names of the team members involved
- Any decision to remove the client from a more restrictive status to a less restrictive one
- The rationale for any changes in the treatment approach, especially changes in the level of restriction
- Statements from clients about self-harm or denial of self-harm
- Client responses to changes, passes, family, visitors
- All telephone calls or interactions with family members
- All searches carried out and the reason for them

Working with Families

Including family members in the plan of care for the client is extremely important. Hospitalizations for suicidal ideation or a suicide attempt may be brief and may be terminated before antidepressant medication has had a chance to work. There are two important strategies that families need to know:

1. How to prevent suicide
2. How to help their loved one avoid acting on suicidal thoughts when those thoughts occur

Guidelines for families in preventing suicide are given in the Partnering with Clients and Families feature. You can also suggest some helpful websites to family members, such as American Association of Suicidology, American Foundation for Suicide Prevention, and Suicide Prevention Action Network USA. Direct links to these resources can be found on the Companion Website for this book. The websites in the section on Suicide Prevention on page 624 will also be useful to family and friends.

Evaluation

Suicide, like all crisis situations, calls for ongoing evaluation of the plan made by the nurse and client. Because events often occur rapidly, initial care plans may need to be changed almost daily. In addition to evaluating individual care plans, staff members who work with suicidal clients need to evaluate their overall approach and philosophy periodically.

CASE MANAGEMENT

Case managers can ensure that planned therapeutic linkages occur once the client has been discharged. Linkages might be established with public health or home health nurses, community mental health nurses, or psychiatric–mental health nurse practitioners. Discharged suicidal clients should also be linked with a mobile crisis unit.

Make sure that discharged clients and their families have all the telephone numbers they need—suicide/crisis hotline, mobile crisis unit, therapists, community resources. Case managers can also find other appropriate resources in the community to meet an individual client's needs. Clients should also have the time and date of their follow-up appointment.

COMMUNITY-BASED CARE

The treatment team needs to have a realistic approach when planning the care of a suicidal client. It is usually not possible to meet all therapeutic goals in an inpatient setting. Even clients who are suicidal are often discharged well before antidepressant medication is at full therapeutic response (see Chapters 7 and 32∞ for a discussion of antidepressant medications). These clients will need intensive monitoring in the community and should be encouraged to maintain contact with a mental health professional in a mental health facility, private office, or suicide and crisis center. A good case manager will have armed the client with hotline and mobile crisis unit telephone numbers.

HOME CARE

In addition to helping family members learn how to be gatekeepers to prevent suicide (see Partnering with Clients and Families: Helping Families Prevent Suicide), the suicidal client and the family should have a suicide crisis plan in place that will help the client avoid acting on suicidal impulses. The Partnering with Clients and Families feature that follows recommends specific elements for a family suicide crisis plan.

Parents and friends can be instrumental in preventing suicide. A study of youth suicide in Utah identified which contacts in the decedent's life recognized risk factors for suicidal behavior, symptoms of mental illness, and barriers to mental health treatment for the decedent (Moskos, Olson, Halbern, Keller, & Gray, 2005). Most symptoms were universally recognized by parents and friends, although friends were better able to recognize symptoms of substance abuse. This study suggested that parents and friends are the most appropriate individuals for gatekeeper training.

SURVIVORS OF SUICIDE

The act of suicide has long-lasting ramifications for the survivors. Nurses who are working with the families or staff who have worked with the deceased must be alert to the potential aftereffects of the death. (Staff reactions are described later in the chapter.)

Farberow (1992), a suicidologist who studied the effects of suicide on survivors, identified these emotional experiences of survivors of suicide:

- Strong feelings of loss accompanied by sorrow and mourning
- Anger at being made to feel responsible for the behavior of the suicidal person
- Feelings of separation because their help was refused
- Anxiety, guilt, shame, or embarrassment because the person committed suicide
- Relief that the nagging, insistent demands of the suicidal person have ceased
- Feelings of desertion
- The arousal of impulses toward suicide
- Anger caused by the belief that the suicide represents a rejection of social and moral responsibilities

Survivors rarely seek assistance from mental health care professionals. They may be angry and believe mental health care professionals "should have prevented this." Those who work with survivors, including nurses, must be prepared for this reaction. The American Association of Suicidology maintains a website for professionals and suicide survivors at www.suicidology.org.

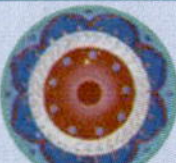

PARTNERING WITH CLIENTS AND FAMILIES

HELPING FAMILIES PREVENT SUICIDE

If you strongly believe that someone is close to a suicidal act, or the person has indicated that he or she is close to acting on a suicidal impulse, taking these steps can help you to prevent suicide.

- **Take the person seriously.** Stay calm, listen, but don't underreact. Express concern.
- **Listen attentively.** Maintain eye contact. Use body language to show concern, such as moving close to the person or holding his or her hand, if appropriate.
- **Do not promise secrecy.** You may need to speak to the person's health care professional in order to protect the person from him- or herself. Don't make promises that would endanger your loved one's life.
- **Ask direct questions.** Find out whether the person has a specific plan for suicide. If you can, determine what method of suicide is being considered.
- **Offer reassurance.** Stress that suicide is a permanent solution to a temporary problem. Remind the person that help is available and that things will get better.
- **Involve other people.** Don't try to handle the crisis alone or jeopardize your own health or safety. Call 911 if necessary. Contact the suicidal person's mental health professional, a crisis intervention team, a suicide hotline, a hospital emergency room, or others who are trained to help.
- **If possible, do not leave the person alone.** Make sure that arrangements are made for your loved one to be in professional hands.

Family and Friends Survivors

Families and friends may not receive the same degree of support as bereaved people whose loved ones died because of illness or accident. People in the support network (including other family members or friends) may be uncomfortable and embarrassed and may stay away rather than help. If there is shame associated with suicide, that shame may be directed toward the survivors of suicide. When comparing subjects' feelings about survivors whose loved ones died by suicide with their feelings about survivors whose loved ones died by accident or natural causes, Jordan (2001) found that survivors of suicide were viewed as more psychologically disturbed and ashamed. The respondents also believed that the suicide survivor could have done more to prevent the death.

Very often, suicide is denied or concealed by family members who wish to avoid feelings of shame or avoid being blamed for the death. This secrecy further impedes grief work, because survivors cannot resolve the loss unless they discuss it openly. Suicide exacerbates dysfunctional family dynamics, such as scapegoating or blaming other family members.

Besides making the usual preparations after death, which are stressful enough in themselves, families must deal with police investigations, the media, and insurance companies. This can precipitate extreme stress, especially if only limited support is available.

Families and all significant others who survive a suicide need nursing intervention, but it is especially warranted for the following:

- Families who lack support from usual sources
- Dysfunctional families who react by blaming, scapegoating, or covering up the death as an accident
- Children whose parent has committed suicide
- Adolescents exposed to the suicide of a friend

Plan outreach services for these groups. A typical plan might include telephoning the family immediately after the suicide and periodically until the first anniversary of the death, and arranging for staff or a staff representative to attend services, if appropriate. Consider involving the family in a bereavement support group. Families (first-degree relatives and spouses of someone who had committed suicide) were found to experience a significant reduction in maladaptive grief reactions and perceptions of blame in a nurse-led cognitive behavior counseling program (de Groot et al., 2007). Psychoeducational services and family network intervention have also been found to be helpful (Jordan, 2001). Support from family and friends has been found to be the strongest protective factor (Callahan, 2000).

MediaLink Resources for Survivors

Families who need assistance toward the positive resolution of grief can contact Compassionate Friends at www.compassionatefriends.com. Peer support services for people affected by a death by suicide of a child of any age may wish to access www.friendsforsurvival.org.

Child and Adolescent Survivors

Children who experience a loss as the result of a parental suicide require urgent intervention to deal with the trauma. Be particularly sensitive with these children, as they often have problems with grieving. A child who loses a parent is also at greater risk for suicide and depression.

Adolescents who are exposed to the suicide of a friend are at high risk for development of major depression and should be carefully screened, observed, and treated for depressive symptoms. A close relationship with the victim, visual exposure to the victim at the scene of death, having a conversation with the victim the day of the suicide, and both a personal and a family history of depression are all predictive of the development of depression subsequent to the suicide.

Cluster Suicide

Cluster suicide—an excessive number of suicides occurring in close temporal or geographic proximity to each other—is a phenomenon of great concern to those who work with adolescents. Clustering is most prevalent in the age group of 14 to 24, where it is two to four times more frequent than in older age groups.

Because of the influence of and close connections with their peer group, adolescents are at risk for cluster suicide. At highest risk are hospitalized or institutionalized adolescents. Clustering has been estimated to account for about 5% of teenage suicides in the United States. While that may seem at first glance to be a small number, it is an important one and a particular public health concern.

Staff Survivors of Client Suicide

Staff members are also survivors of a client's suicide. Client suicide during a course of treatment has sometimes been referred to as an "occupational hazard."

The reactions of staff members can be as varied as the roles they perform with clients. For example, the exact memories and reactions will vary with a nurse who finds a client hanging and administers first aid, a therapist who saw a client for his or her last session, and a psychiatrist who was the last person to evaluate the client. All are likely to experience the suicide as a traumatic event.

Support for staff members is critical after client suicide. Typical reactions to the suicide of a client may include sadness, anger, denial, and shame. Some may have the erroneous belief that if you are "a good enough" nurse or therapist, you will be able to effectively prevent all suicides. Staff members may lack confidence and be unable to function. This would be a good time for nurses to review their reasons for becoming nurses in the first place. Thoughts of reconsidering what they do or where they work are common. The range of other common reactions among nurses, therapists, and physicians range from refusing to admit suicidal clients to their caseloads or units to recognizing what the particular problems were and how they might manage them better in the future. Clinicians who have lost a client to suicide can access the

American Association of Suicidology's website created by its Clinician Survivor Task Force via the Companion Website for this book.

Outside therapists or crisis workers can be helpful for counseling and implementing critical incident stress debriefing (CISD). CISD is a seven-stage structured group in which those who have been affected by a traumatic event are given the opportunity to discuss their thoughts and feelings. See Chapter 30 for a complete discussion of CISD.

Staff members with little medical training or experience suffer more than those who have previously encountered illness and death. These workers need extra attention.

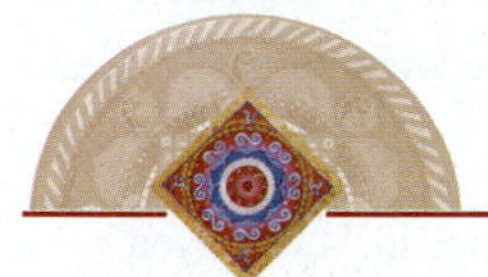

EXPLORE MediaLink

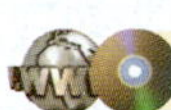 www.prenhall.com/kneisl

For NCLEX-RN® review questions, case studies, and other resources for this chapter see the Pearson Health MediaLink CD-ROM that accompanies this book and the Companion Website at www.prenhall.com/kneisl.

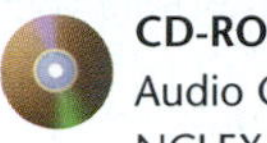

CD-ROM
Audio Glossary
NCLEX-RN® Review Questions

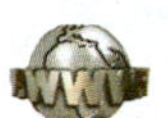

Companion Website
Audio Glossary
NCLEX-RN® Review Questions
Critical Thinking Exercise
- *Assessing the Client for Suicide Potential*

Case Study
- *The Suicidal Client*

Care Plan
- *Assessing Suicide Attempts*

MediaLinks
MediaLink Application
- *"If you are thinking about suicide, read this first."*

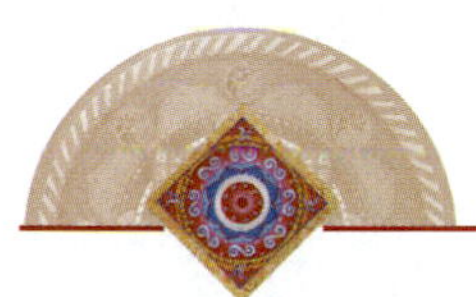

NCLEX-RN® REVIEW QUESTIONS

1. Which variables influence suicide? (Select all that apply.)
1. Presence of psychiatric illness
2. Receiving psychiatric–mental health care
3. History of self-injurious behavior
4. Ability to openly communicate needs to others
5. Use of alcohol

2. According to Schneidman's research, which client statement addresses the most common reason for suicide?
1. "I just had to succeed in school. When I failed, I could think of no other answer to my situation."
2. "My husband had just left me, and I thought if I showed him how much I loved him, he would come back."
3. "I was overwhelmed with flashbacks and terror and wanted relief from my pain."
4. "I was cutting myself so that I could feel real again. It was an accident."

3. You volunteer in your community as a telephone crisis hotline worker. You know that during the course of a telephone session, the caller's decrease in suicidality will be most accurately evaluated by which of the following?
1. Ability to communicate with a significant other
2. Changes in ambivalence
3. Decreased constriction in thought
4. Stated intent to abstain from alcohol consumption

4. Increased suicidal behavior is associated with which of the following? (Select all that apply.)
1. Reduced serotonin activity in the frontal cortex
2. Dichotomous thinking
3. Increased availability of serotonin
4. Use of SSRIs
5. Dysfunction of the hypothalamic–pituitary–adrenocorticoid axis

5. Your client is a 55-year-old white, non-Hispanic male who was just forced to retire. Within the past month, his social drinking has increased from one drink per week to one six-pack of beer per day. Ten years ago, he attempted suicide with opiates and alcohol after his wife died from cancer and the associated debt resulted in bankruptcy. He is unable to share suicidal ideation in his church community because "we worship the sanctity of life" and "the people there would not understand; they would shun me." He admits to having opiates in his possession. Based on the Lethality Assessment Scale, your client is best described as:
1. Low risk of immediate suicide.
2. Moderate risk of immediate suicide.
3. High risk of imminent suicide.
4. Very high risk of imminent suicide.

6. On your inpatient unit, a client reports increased suicidal thoughts with voices in his head screaming, "Do it! Do it! Do it!" Which action should you take to provide for the client's safety?
1. Remain with the client.
2. Provide the client with a private room, furnished with only a mattress, blanket, and sheet.
3. Request the client to remain in the day area with other clients until you have obtained physician's orders for suicide precautions and a room search.
4. Direct the client to a quiet, secluded area of the unit to decrease stimulation.

7. A client informs the nurse, "I am thinking more about death, but I'm not going to hurt myself." Which statements by the nurse would be appropriate and therapeutic within any hospital setting? (Select all that apply.)
1. "It is hard not to think about death in the hospital, is it not?"
2. "We're going to check on you at least every 15 minutes and we'll help keep you safe."
3. "Tell me more about your thoughts."
4. "Sometimes clients who feel hopeless think about killing themselves. Have you had any thoughts about killing yourself?"
5. "You have told me that you have not had thoughts about hurting yourself. If you start having these thoughts, can you tell me or another staff member before you act on them?"

8. After a chronically suicidal client is admitted through the emergency room, a family member informs you, "I am so tired of this. Sometimes I wish this person would succeed at suicide." What is your best response?
1. "It is important for you to get what you need. What do you need for yourself at this time?"
2. "This must be a stressful time for you and your family."
3. "Hopefully, things will be better by the time your family member is discharged."
4. "You may feel that way now, but you would probably feel worse if that actually happened."

9. Halfway through your assessment of a suicidal client, you identify your own feelings of discomfort, anger, and apathy. When you conclude your assessment, which of the following actions should you take? (Select all that apply.)
1. Consider whether you need an opinion from another clinician.
2. Allow time for yourself to explore the thoughts behind your emotional response to this situation.
3. Examine the ethical conflict of autonomy versus beneficence/nonmaleficence.
4. Consider relocating to another health care setting where there are fewer people who require suicide assessment.
5. Consider the issues of control and responsibility in the interaction with this client.

10. Which factors interfere with health care providers offering assistance to family survivors of suicide? (Select all that apply.)
1. Feelings that family members did everything possible to help the client
2. The belief that health care providers should wait for family members to approach them
3. Fear of being blamed for the client's suicide
4. The belief that family members will receive adequate support from their own support network
5. Concerns about litigation, with management directives not to interact with family members

See Appendix C for answers.

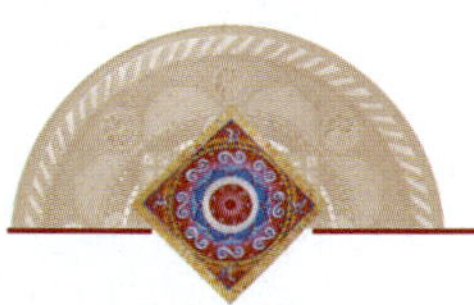

REFERENCES

Baldessarini, R. J., Tondo, L., Strombom, I. M., Dominguez, S., Fawcett, J., Licinio, J., et al. (2007). Ecological studies of antidepressant treatment and suicidal risks. *Harvard Review of Psychiatry, 15*(4), 133–145.

Bateman, K., Hansen, L., Turkington, D., & Kingdon, D. (2007). Cognitive behavioral therapy reduces suicidal ideation in schizophrenia: Results from a randomized controlled trial. *Suicide and Life-Threatening Behavior, 37*(3), 284–290.

Brooker, C., Ricketts, T., Bennett, S., & Lemme, F. (2007). Admission decisions following contact with an emergency mental health assessment and intervention service. *Journal of Clinical Nursing, 16*(7), 1313–1322.

Brunner, R., Parzer, P., Haffner, J., Steen, R., Roos, J., Klett, M., et al. (2007). Prevalence and psychological correlates of occasional and repetitive deliberate self-harm in adolescents. *Archives of Pediatric and Adolescent Medicine, 161*(7), 641–649.

Callahan, J. (2000). Predictors and correlates of bereavement in suicide support group participants. *Suicide and Life-Threatening Behavior, 30*(2), 104–124.

Center for Mental Health Services. (2002). *At a glance—Suicide among diverse populations*. Retrieved June 30, 2002, from www.mentalhealth.org/suicideprevention/diverse.asp.

Centers for Disease Control and Prevention. (2007a) Web-based Injury Statistics Query and Reporting System (WISQARS). Retrieved on September 10, 2007, from www.cdc.gov/ncipc/wisqars.

Centers for Disease Control and Prevention. (2007b). Suicide rate trends among youth ages 10–24 years, United States, 1990–2004. *Morbidity & Mortality Weekly Report, 56*(SS–35).

Centers for Disease Control and Prevention. (2007c). *Suicide prevention scientific information: Risk and protective factors*. Retrieved on September 10, 2007, from www.cdc.gov/ncipc/dvp/Suicide-risk-p-factors.htm.

Corso, P. S., Mercy, J. A., Simon, T. R., Finkelstein, E. A., & Miller, T. R. (2007). Medical costs and productivity losses due to interpersonal violence and self-directed violence. *American Journal of Preventive Medicine, 32*(6), 474–478.

de Groot, M., de Keijser, J., Neeleman, J., Kerkhof, A., Nolen, W., & Burger, H. (2007). Cognitive behaviour therapy to prevent complicated grief among relatives and spouses bereaved by suicide: Cluster randomized controlled trial. *British Medical Journal, 334*(7601), 994–999.

DeLeo, D., Bertolote, J., & Lester, D. (2002). Self-directed violence. In E. Krug, L. L. Dahlberg, J. A. Mercy, A. Zwi, & R. Lozano (Eds.), *World report on violence and health* (pp. 184–212). Geneva: World Health Organization.

Denning, S. G., Conwell, Y., King, D., & Cox, C. (2000). Method choice, intent, and gender in completed suicide. *Suicide and Life-Threatening Behavior, 30*(3), 282–288.

Dhossche, D. M. (2000). Suicidal behavior in psychiatric emergency room patients. *Southern Medical Journal, 93*(3), 310–314.

Eaton, D. K., Kann, L., Kinchen, S. A., Ross, J. D., Hawkins, J., Harris, W. A., et al. (2006). Youth risk behavior surveillance—United States, 2005. *Morbidity & Mortality Weekly Report, 55*(No. SS–5), 1–108.

Farberow, N. L. (1992). The Los Angeles survivors—after suicide program: An evaluation. *Crisis, 13*, 23–24.

Gaynes, B. N., Rush, A. J., Trivedi, M. H., Wisniewski, S. R., Balasubramani, G. K., Spencer, D. C., et al. (2007). Major depression symptoms in primary care and psychiatric care settings: A cross-sectional analysis. *Annals of Family Medicine, 5*(2), 126–134.

Gibbons, R. D., Brown, C. H., Hur, K., Marcus, S. M., Bhaumik, D. K., & Mann, J. J. (2007). Relationship between antidepressants and suicide attempts: An analysis of the Veterans Health Administration Data Sets. *American Journal of Psychiatry, 164*(7), 1044–1049.

Gibbons, R. D., Brown, C. H., Hur, K., Marcus, S. M., Bhaumik, D. K., Erkens, J. A., et al. (2007). Early evidence on the effects of regulators' suicidality warnings on SSRI prescriptions and suicide in children and adolescents. *American Journal of Psychiatry, 164*(9), 1356–1363.

Goldsmith, S. K., Pellmar, T. C., Kleinman, A. M., & Bunney, W. E. (Eds.). (2007). *Reducing suicide: A national imperative*. Washington, DC: National Academy Press.

Gould, M. S., Kalafat, J., Harrismunfakh, J. L., & Kleinman, M. (2007). An evaluation of crisis hotline outcomes. Part 2: Suicidal callers. *Suicide and Life-Threatening Behavior, 37*(3), 338–352.

Groves, S. A., Stanley, B. H., & Sher, L. (2007). Ethnicity and the relationship between adolescent alcohol use and suicidal behavior. *International Journal of Adolescent Medicine and Health, 19*(1), 19–25.

Isometsa, E. T. (2001). Psychological autopsy studies—A review. *European Psychiatry, 16*(7), 379–385.

Joiner, T., Kalafat, J., Draper, J., Stokes, H., Knudson, M., Berman, A., et al. (2007). Establishing standards for the assessment of suicide risk among callers to the national suicide prevention lifeline. *Suicide and Life Threatening Behavior, 37*(3), 353–365.

Jordan, J. R. (2001). Is suicide bereavement different? A reassessment of the literature. *Suicide and Life-Threatening Behavior, 31*(1), 91–102.

Keilp, J. G., Sackheim, H. A., Brodsky, B. S., Oquendo, M. A., Malone, K. M., & Mann, J. J. (2001). Neuropsychological dysfunction in depressed suicide attempters. *American Journal of Psychiatry, 158*(5), 735–741.

Mann, J. J. (2000). Serotonin activity in suicidal patients different from depressed patients. *Psychiatric News*. Retrieved from www.psych.org/pnews/00-04-07/serotonin.html.

Mann, J. J., Brent, D. A., & Arango, V. (2001). The neurobiology and genetics of suicide and attempted suicide: A focus on the serotonergic system. *Neuropsychopharmacology, 24*(5), 467–477.

Mann, J. J., & Currier, D. (2007). A review of prospective studies of biologic predictors of suicidal behavior in mood disorders. *Archives of Suicide Research, 11(1)*, 3–16.

Marcinko, D., Pivac, N., Martinac, M., Jakovljevic, M., Mihaljevic-Peles, A., & Muck-Seler, D. (2007). Platelet serotonin and serum cholesterol concentrations in suicidal and non-suicidal patients with a first episode of psychosis. *Psychiatric Research, 150*(1), 105–108.

Mishara, B. L., Chagnon, F., Daigle, M., Balan, B., Raymond, S., Marcoux, I., et al. (2007). Which helper behaviors and intervention styles are related to better short-term outcomes in telephone crisis intervention? Results from a silent monitoring study of calls to the U.S. 1-800-SUICIDE Network. *Suicide and Life-Threatening Behavior, 37*(3), 308–321.

Moskos, M., Olson, L., Halbern, S., Keller, T., & Gray, D. (2005). Utah youth suicide study: Psychological autopsy. *Suicide and Life-Threatening Behavior, 35*(5), 536–546.

National Institute of Mental Health. *Drops in SSRI prescription rates may coincide with increases in youth suicides*. Retrieved on September 19, 2007, from www.nimh.nih.gov/science-news/2007.

Oquendo, M. A., Ellis, S. P., Greenwald, S., Malone, K. M., Weissman, M. M., & Mann, J. J. (2001). Ethnic and sex differences in suicide rates relative to major depression in the United States. *American Journal of Psychiatry, 158*(10), 1652–1658.

Rew, L., Thomas, N., Horner, S. D., Resnick, M. D., & Beuhring, T. (2001). Correlates of recent suicide attempts in a triethnic group of adolescents. *Journal of Nursing Scholarship, 33*(4), 361–367.

Rujescu, D., Thalmeier, A., Moller, H. J., Bronisch, T., & Giegling, I. (2007). Molecular genetic findings in suicidal behavior: What is beyond the serotonergic system? *Archives of Suicide Research, 11*(1), 17–40.

Schneidman, E. S. (1996). *The suicidal mind*. New York: Oxford University Press.

Schultz, S. H., North, S. W., & Shields, C. G. (2007). Schizophrenia: A review. *American Family Physician, 75*(12), 1821–1829.

Scott, C. L., Swartz, E., & Warburton, K. (2006). The psychological autopsy: Solving the mysteries of death. *Psychiatric Clinics of North America, 29*(3), 805–822.

Simon, G. E., & Savarino, J. (2007). Suicide attempts among patients starting depression treatment with medications or psychotherapy. *American Journal of Psychiatry, 164*(7), 1029–1034.

Substance Abuse and Mental Health Services Administration. (2007). *National suicide prevention initiative*. Retrieved on September 10, 2007, from www.mentalhealth.samhsa.gov.

Swahn, M. H., & Bossarte, R. M. (2007). Gender, early alcohol use, and suicide ideation and attempts: Findings from the 2005 youth risk behavior survey. *Journal of Adolescent Health, 41*(2), 175–181.

U.S. Public Health Service. (1999). *The surgeon general's call to action to prevent suicide*. Washington, DC: U.S. Department of Health and Human Services.

Whitlock, J., & Knox, K. L. (2007). The relationship between self-injurious behavior and suicide in a young adult population. *Archives of Pediatric and Adolescent Medicine, 161*(7), 634–640.

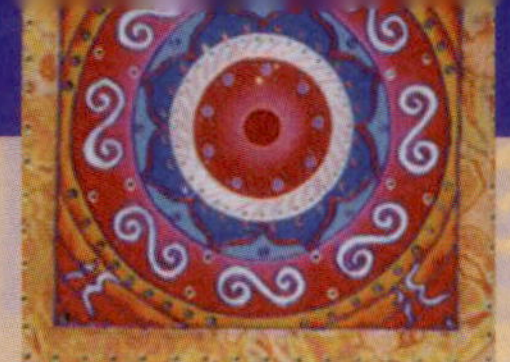

CHAPTER

24

Persons at Risk for Abuse or Violence

KAREN LEE FONTAINE

KEY TERMS

battering *645*
neglect *646*
physical abuse *648*
psychological abuse *648*
rape *639*
rape-trauma syndrome *639*
sexual abuse *655*
shaken baby syndrome *646*
stalking *648*

LEARNING OUTCOMES

After completing this chapter, you will be able to:

1. Describe the biopsychosocial causes of rape, intrafamily physical abuse, and intrafamily sexual abuse.
2. Discuss the short-term and long-term effects on victims of rape and intrafamily violence.
3. Identify those at greatest risk for intrafamily physical and sexual abuse.
4. Identify the principles common to most treatment plans for victims of violence.
5. Explain why spiritual recovery is important for persons who have been victims of violence.
6. Identify specific actions you could take to advocate for the reduction of family violence.
7. Discuss personal feelings and attitudes that may affect professional practice when caring for victims of rape or violence.

CRITICAL THINKING CHALLENGE

Beth is a 40-year-old professional woman in a long-term abusive relationship with Pat. Each time Pat beats Beth, he screams at her that she made him so angry that he had no choice but to hit her. Even though she is a competent professional, Beth has difficulty seeing that she is not responsible for Pat's loss of control.

Much of the current sociocultural climate encourages beliefs and practices about abuse that can subtly, or overtly, support abuse.

1. Is Pat abusive because Beth has made him angry?
2. If a person yells at or nags another incessantly, does that individual have a right to strike out?
3. Does violence in families continue to exist because the legal and criminal justice systems tolerate it?

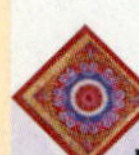

MEDIALINK 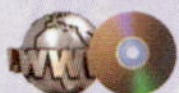 www.prenhall.com/kneisl

Go to the Pearson Health MediaLink CD-ROM and the Companion Website at www.prenhall.com/kneisl for interactive resources for this chapter.

Violence that is demonstrated as rape, or that occurs as physical or sexual abuse within the family, is a national health problem that confronts nurses in many different clinical settings. Victims are seen in the community, in pediatric units, in intensive care units, in medical–surgical units, in maternal care settings, in ambulatory care facilities, in geriatric units, and in psychiatric–mental health settings.

As nurses, we assess and provide appropriate intervention for the emotional and physical consequences of violence and abuse—including rape. We may be called on to give legal evidence in the prosecution of a rapist. Within the community, we can establish, or refer victims to, support groups. We can also become active in increasing public awareness of rape through formal and informal teaching activities. Because of our unique position, we can be active in the prevention of rape and the treatment of rape survivors.

Nurses also are key persons in the prevention, detection, and treatment of intrafamily violence. It is important to develop a knowledge base and be able to identify factors that contribute to domestic violence in order to assume a preventive role. Part of this role is providing public education and advocating for changes in public policy. This knowledge, along with increased awareness of the extent of the problem, helps us arrive at earlier, more accurate detection of intrafamily violence. When intrafamily violence is detected, nurses must comply with state laws on the reporting of violence and referral for treatment. Nurses with advanced education in family therapy are part of the therapy teams that intervene with violent families.

RAPE

Rape is a crime of violence. It is second only to homicide in its violation of a person. The issue is not one of sex but one of force, domination, and humiliation. If you think rape is about sex, you have confused the weapon with the motivation. **Rape** refers to any forced sexual activity; the key factor is the absence of consent. For discussion purposes, a rape victim will be referred to as a female throughout this chapter. However, as Box 24-1 illustrates, there is no typical rape victim.

Exposure of men to videos and other media sources is believed to be a factor in why rape appears to be more acceptable to them (Kaestle, Halpern, & Brown, 2007). Women very rarely report rapes when they know their attackers, especially if they were involved with their attacker in a dating relationship. The victim is often blamed, by herself and others, for being naïve or provocative. A cultural value, slow to die, is: If a woman accepts a date and allows the man to pay all the expenses, she somehow "owes" him sexual access and has no right to refuse. The Office on Violence against Women, in the U.S. Department of Justice, has a website of interest (http://www.usdoj.gov/ovw) that can also be accessed through the Companion Website for this book.

Traditionally, husbands have not been charged when they raped their wives. It was not until 1974 in the United States and 1991 in Great Britain that the first cases of marital rape were prosecuted. Marital rape is often accompanied by extreme violence and is the most underreported type of rape (Rauch & Foa, 2004). The attacks range from assaults that are relatively quick to those that involve sadistic, torturous episodes that last for hours. In some instances, women are forced to have sex with other people while their husbands/lovers watch.

Box 24-1 **There Is No Typical Rape Victim**

- 90% to 95% of rape victims are female.
- 90% of the perpetrators are male.
- One can be a victim of rape at any age, from childhood through old age.
- A woman is raped every 6 minutes in the United States.
- 80% of rapes are unreported.
- One out of every three or four American women will be raped or sexually assaulted at least once in her lifetime.
- 50% of victims are raped by a spouse, partner, relative, or friend.
- 50% of rapes on college campuses are date rapes.
- Alcohol is involved in 81% of sexual assault cases.
- Teens now account for 18% to 20% of rapes. Forcible rape by juveniles in both the United States and the United Kingdom is on the increase.

Source: French, K., Beynon, C., & Delaforce, J. (2007). Alcohol is the true "rape drug." *Nursing Standard, 21*(29), 26–27; Rauch, S.A.M., & Foa, E. B. (2004). Sexual trauma. In B. T. Litz (Ed.), *Early interventions for trauma and traumatic loss* (pp. 216–240). New York: Guilford Press; Thoreson, E. J. (2006). In times of crises: Care of adolescent rape patients. *Journal for Undergraduate Nursing Scholarship, 8*(1), 4.

The myth of male rape has been that it occurs only in situations where heterosexual contact is not possible, such as in prisons or in isolated living conditions. As more male rape victims report the crime, however, this myth is being shattered. Male rape is not a homosexual attack. Just as in female rape, the issue is one of violence and domination rather than one of sex. Some perpetrators are gay males who coerce partners or dates into sexual activity by use of threats or intimidation, as in date rape. Other perpetrators are heterosexual males who rape other males as a way of punishing and degrading them; this can occur among prison inmates or as part of gay bashing. Inmates who are sexually assaulted are often viewed by the public as deserving of their fate because of the crimes they have committed against society (Yeager & Fogel, 2006). Similarly, many people believe that gay men deserve to be raped as punishment for their "perverse" lifestyle (Lips, 2004).

MediaLink Office on Violence Against Women

Rape-Trauma Syndrome

Rape is a violent act against an innocent person. It changes lives forever because once people become victims, they never again feel completely safe. The victim's response to this act of violence is referred to as **rape-trauma syndrome**. Some rape survivors do not develop major symptoms in response to the trauma, while as many as 25% continue to have signs of impairment a year after the assault.

Responses to Rape

A variety of factors contribute to the response, including age or developmental state, a history of prior victimization, the relationship to the offender, precrisis coping abilities, and the ability to use support resources. Response factors related to the rape itself include the severity of the rape, the duration, the frequency, the number of offenders, and the degree of violence. Environmental factors contributing to a rape victim's response are the quality and continuity of social supports and community attitudes and values. In a sample of 1,253 university women, 216 of whom were raped, feelings of self-blame for the assault and the negative reactions of others were important predictors of avoidance coping, a psychologically unhealthy behavior (Littleton & Breitkopf, 2006).

During the actual rape, some victims use the defense mechanism of depersonalization or dissociation to cope with the attack (defense mechanisms are discussed in Chapter 8 ∞). By perceiving the attack as "not really happening to me," a victim protects her sense of integrity. Other victims rely on denial to block out the traumatic experience. The use of these defense mechanisms may continue through initial treatment and should be supported until the person is able to face the reality of the attack. The following clinical example illustrates a client's reaction to rape.

CLINICAL EXAMPLE

Doreen, a graduate student at the local university, was brought to the hospital by the police, who had found her running down the street half-clothed. In the hospital she was able to tell the staff that she had been raped by her date, Mike, another graduate student. She exhibited outward calmness but kept repeating, "This cannot have happened to me. My friends introduced us and he seemed so nice." She was unable to decide whom to call to take her back to the dorm or what to tell her friends.

Some rape victims respond immediately with agitated and nonpurposeful behavior. They appear in the emergency department emotionally distraught and unable to respond to questions about the rape. Their level of anxiety may be so high that they may not be able to follow simple directions. After a period of shock and disbelief, many experience episodes of fear.

Fears may arise in response to any stimulus that brings back the rape memories. There are also fears of rape consequences such as pregnancy, sexually transmitted diseases (especially HIV), talking to the police, and testifying in court. In addition, there are fears related to the potential for future attacks, which underlie fears of establishing close relationships with men, being alone, and being in a strange place.

Physical Injuries

Rape usually results in a number of physical injuries as the result of being beaten, stabbed, or shot. Profuse bleeding and trauma to vital organs may be critical problems. Most likely, the vagina or rectum will be painful or swollen. There may be tearing of the vaginal or rectal wall from forceful insertion of the penis or a foreign object. The throat may be traumatized from forced oral sex or pressure on the throat during the attack.

Long-Term Consequences

Rape trauma syndrome may have long-term consequences. Depression frequently develops within a few weeks of the assault. This posttrauma depression usually lasts about 3 months, and it is not unusual for the survivor to experience suicidal ideation during that time. For some, the depression will develop into a major depressive disorder requiring medical intervention (Symes, 2000). Some survivors develop obsessional thoughts about the rape, which may be severe enough to interfere with daily functioning. Some experience flashbacks, some have violent dreams, and others may be preoccupied with thoughts of future danger.

Rape profoundly affects beliefs about the environment. If the assault occurred in the home, the normal feeling of safety within the home will most likely be destroyed. Belief in an inability to protect oneself in the future may lead to social withdrawal or phobic avoidance. A woman who is a survivor of marital rape suffers additional problems. Often, she must continue to interact with her rapist because she is dependent on him. She may be forced to pretend, to herself and to family members and friends, that the rape never occurred.

Sexual problems are one of the longest-lasting effects of rape. Nearly all adult rape survivors feel the need to withdraw from sexual activity for a period of time. For some, a period of celibacy is necessary to reestablish control and autonomy. Others may choose abstinence because they feel unclean or contaminated. Both the survivor and the sex partner must understand that the need for closeness and nondemanding physical contact continues. Expressing caring and affection through nonsexual touching minimizes the partner's feelings of rejection and reduces the rape survivor's feelings of self-blame and uncleanliness. Box 24-2 describes the phases of response to rape.

BIOPSYCHOSOCIAL THEORIES

Theorists in many disciplines have studied the crime of rape in an effort to understand the causes and develop preventive measures. Most agree that rape is a crime of violence generated by issues of power and anger rather than by sex drive.

Intrapersonal Theory

The intrapersonal perspective views rapists as emotionally immature individuals who feel powerless and unsure of themselves. They are incapable of managing the normal stresses of everyday life. The causes of rape are many, but the dynamics of the act are that perpetrators abuse their own and others' sexuality as a method of discharging anger and frustration. From this perspective, there are five types of rape (McCabe & Wauchope, 2005):

1. Anger rape
2. Power rape
3. Sadistic rape
4. Gang rape
5. Date or acquaintance rape

Box 24-2 Phases of Response to Rape

Anticipatory Phase

- This phase begins when the victim realizes the situation is potentially dangerous.
- The victim may think about how to get away, may reason or argue with the offender, and recall advice others have given about rape.
- The victim may dissociate, suppress, or rationalize to preserve the illusion of invulnerability.
- The victim may take physical action.

Impact Phase

- This phase includes the period of actual assault and its immediate aftermath.
- The victim may have an intense fear of death or serious injury.
- The victim may display any of the following expressive styles:
  - Open expression of feelings—crying, sobbing, pacing
  - Controlled style—numbness, shock, disbelief
  - Compound reaction—reactivated symptoms of previous conditions, such as psychotic behavior, depression, suicidal behavior, substance abuse
- The victim may have somatic reactions—tension headache, fatigue, increased startle reaction, nausea, gagging.

Reconstitution Phase

- This phase has the outward appearance of adjustment with an attempt to restore equilibrium.
- The victim reengages in life activities, but superficially and mechanically.
- At the same time, the victim may experience periods of anxiety, fear, nightmares, depression, guilt, shame, vulnerability, helplessness, isolation, or sexual dysfunction.

Resolution Phase

- In this phase, the survivor comes to terms with the event.
- The survivor may be angry with the assailant, society, and the judicial system.
- The survivor has the need to talk to resolve feelings.
- The survivor seeks family and professional support.

Anger Rape

An *anger rape* is characterized by physical violence and cruelty to the victim. Believing that he is the victim of an unjust society, the rapist takes revenge on others by raping. He uses extreme force and viciousness to demean and humiliate the victim. The ability to injure, traumatize, and shame the victim provides an outlet for his rage and temporary relief from his turmoil. Rapes occur episodically as the rage builds up and he strikes out at others to relieve his pain.

Power Rape

In a *power rape*, the intent of the rapist is not to injure someone but to command and master another person sexually. The rapist has an insecure self-image, with feelings of incompetence and inadequacy. The rape becomes the vehicle for expressing power and strength. Seeing his victim as a conquest, the rapist temporarily has the feeling of omnipotence.

Sadistic Rape

A *sadistic rape* involves brutality, bondage, and torture as stimulants for the rapist's own sexual excitement. For the rapist, the assault is an erotic experience. He plans very carefully, and the process of rape may be ritualized. Victims are often murdered after being raped.

Gang Rape

A *gang rape* involves a number of perpetrators and may be part of a group ritual that confirms masculinity, power, and authority. The perpetrators may range in age from 10 to 30, but they are most typically adolescents. Victims are usually the same age as the gang members.

Date or Acquaintance Rape

A *date rape*, or *acquaintance rape*, is forced sexual activity by a perpetrator who is known to the victim. Typically, there is less physical violence and more coercion and deception involved. Even during the high school years, it is estimated that 30% of female students are sexually or physically abused in their dating relationships (McCabe & Wauchope, 2005).

Interpersonal Theory

Most rapists do not have normal interpersonal involvements. Preoccupied with their own fantasies, they want to control and dominate others rather than engage in mutually satisfying relationships. With this model in mind, a rapist sees no need for consent to sexual activity, particularly from his wife. The husband may view the rape as merely a disagreement over sexual behavior. If the wife has said she does not want to engage in sex and the husband uses force, her control and autonomy have been violated. When sex occurs without consent, it is, in fact, rape.

Social Learning Theory

The acceptance of interpersonal violence in a culture contributes to a higher incidence of rape. Society's approval of the use of intimidation, coercion, and force to achieve a goal promotes an excessive level of violence. Violent behavior is an expression of power and strength, and individual rights are disregarded.

Aggression is learned from three primary sources: family and peers, culture/subculture, and the mass media. The modeling effect occurs when potential offenders see rape scenes and other acts of violence against women in real life—in their families or their peers. The media, through slasher and horror films and in violent pornography, also model violence. The media contribute to the process of desensitization; with repeated exposure, viewers become numb to the pain, fear, and humiliation of sexual aggression.

Gender Bias Theory

From the gender bias perspective, rape is the result of long and deeply rooted socioeconomic traditions. In this perspective, men dominate most political and economic activities, and women are viewed as subservient and relatively powerless. At the farthest extreme, women are viewed as property. Sexual gratification is not the prime motive in rape; rather, it is used to establish or maintain control of one person by another. When women are considered inferior to men, tacit approval is given for coercion and force. These stereotypes support the false beliefs that at times women deserve to be raped, that they may want or need to be raped, and that rape does not cause them much physical or emotional damage.

One study (Yamawaki, 2007) explored the roles of gender bias in minimizing rape, blaming the victim, and excusing the rapist. As predicted, hostile sexists minimize the seriousness of the rape in both stranger and date-rape scenarios. These results show that external observers make different assumptions about a rape incident based on whether they have traditional views of gender roles and whether they have hostile gender bias attitudes.

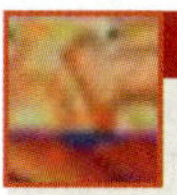

NURSING PROCESS
The Client Who Has Been Raped

Rape victims must be physically assessed thoroughly for any serious or critical injuries that may have resulted from the assault. Critical injuries have the highest priority of care. Before any further medical intervention occurs, clients must be informed of their rights, which include the following:

- A rape crisis advocate is present in the emergency department.
- The client's personal physician is notified.
- The client has privacy during the assessment and treatment process.
- Family, friends, or an advocate can be present during the questioning and examination.
- Confidentiality is maintained by all members of the staff.
- The client receives gentle and sensitive treatment.
- The client receives detailed explanations of, and gives consent for, all tests and procedures, including photographs.
- The client is given referrals for follow-up treatment and counseling.

Remember to respect the victim's autonomy and give the victim as much control as possible through every step of the assessment and treatment process. If this is not done, the client is susceptible to revictimization by members of the health care team.

MEDIALINK Critical Thinking Exercise: Assessing the Rape Victim

Assessment

With the victim's permission, a vaginal or rectal examination is performed to determine necessary treatment and to provide evidence for legal action. With permission, photographs of the injuries may be taken for legal documentation. The physiologic assessment process must be carefully documented in writing to assist with possible prosecution of the perpetrator. Guidelines for physical assessment are given in Your Assessment Approach: Physical Assessment of the Rape Victim below.

Victims who respond to rape in a controlled manner may be able to answer assessment questions, but those in a state of emotional shock and disbelief may find it difficult to engage actively in the assessment process. The method by which you complete the assessment depends on the person's response to the trauma. Documentation of assessment should be in subjective terms and objective quotes. Clear and concise depicting of the client is necessary for possible court proceedings. Guidelines for assessing the victim's mental status are given in Your Assessment Approach: Nursing History Tool for Assessment of the Rape Victim on page 643.

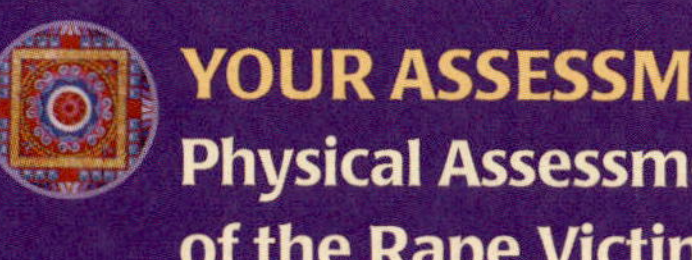

YOUR ASSESSMENT APPROACH
Physical Assessment of the Rape Victim

Complete a head-to-toe physical assessment with particular attention to the following:

Head and Neck
- Evidence of trauma
- Facial bruises
- Facial fractures
- Eyes: swollen, bruised, hemorrhages

Skin
- Bruises
- Genital trauma
- Rectal trauma

Musculoskeletal
- Fractures of the ribs
- Fractures of arms/legs
- Dislocated joints
- Impaired mobility

Abdomen
- Bruises or wounds
- Evidence of internal injuries

Other
- Have physical injuries such as scratches, bruises, and cuts been recorded and photographed?
- Have fingernail scrapings been taken and preserved?
- Has blood typing been done?
- Have smears for sexually transmitted infections been taken of the mouth, throat, vagina, and rectum?
- Have combings of the pubic hair been made and preserved?
- Has genital trauma been recorded and photographed?
- Has rectal trauma been recorded and photographed?
- Have semen specimens been preserved?
- When was the client's last menstrual period?
- Has the clothing been inspected for rips, blood, and stains?
- Has the clothing been preserved?

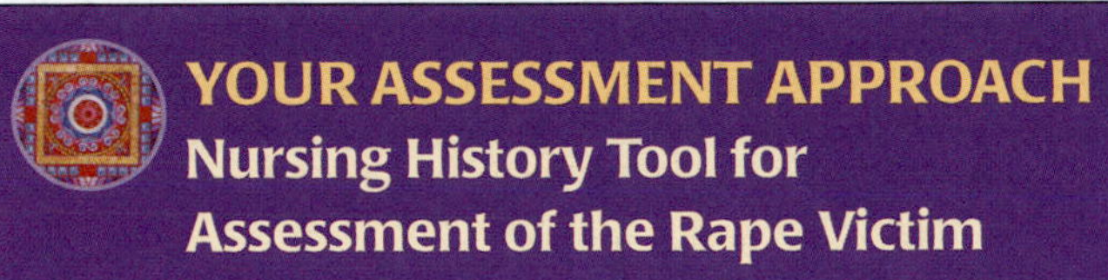

YOUR ASSESSMENT APPROACH
Nursing History Tool for Assessment of the Rape Victim

Behavioral Assessment

- Is the client able to respond verbally to questions?
- Is the client able to follow simple directions?
- Has the client bathed, douched, changed clothes, or done any self-treatment before coming to the hospital?

Affective Assessment

Which of the following emotions is the client experiencing? Describe with objective and subjective data.

- Disbelief
- Shame
- Embarrassment
- Humiliation
- Hopelessness
- Vulnerability
- Anxiety
- Fear
- Guilt
- Anger
- Depression
- Alienation from others

Cognitive Assessment

- Is there evidence of defense mechanisms?
- Is the client confused?
- Has the client been informed of her rights?
- What is the client's attention span like?
- Is the client able to describe what occurred?
- Is the client able to make decisions?
- Whom has the client informed about the rape? Family? Friends? Police?
- Does the client need assistance in telling others?
- Is the client blaming herself for the attack?
- Is the client experiencing flashbacks to the attack?
- What does this event represent to the client?

Sociocultural Assessment

- Who and where are the available support systems for the client? Family? Friends? Advocate? Clergy?
- Is the client in need of temporary shelter?
- Does the client know about available counseling?

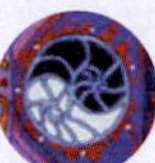

Nursing Diagnosis: NANDA

The health care team must quickly establish physical and mental status priorities. Attention must then be given to long-range physical, emotional, social, and legal concerns of the survivor.

The nursing diagnosis for clients who have been raped is Rape-Trauma Syndrome. If clients suffer from reactivated symptoms of a previous physical illness or mental disorder, or if they rely on alcohol or drugs to manage their trauma, they are given the more specific nursing diagnosis of Rape-Trauma Syndrome: Compound Reaction. The nursing diagnosis of Rape-Trauma Syndrome: Silent Reaction is applied when the client experiences high levels of anxiety, an inability to discuss the trauma, abrupt changes in relationships with men and/or changes in sexual behavior, and the onset of phobic reactions.

There is no corresponding DSM-IV-TR diagnosis for Rape-Trauma Syndrome. Rape is, however, mentioned specifically as the type of trauma that may result in posttraumatic stress disorder. Rape victims may also experience one of the anxiety disorders, mood disorders, or sexual dysfunctions discussed in the DSM-IV-TR.

Outcome Identification: NOC

The long-term goal of intervention is to help survivors of rape return to their precrisis level, or achieve a higher level of functioning. The following outcome behaviors demonstrate that the crisis has been resolved in an adaptive fashion:

- Control over remembering—the client can elect to recall or not recall the rape; flashbacks and nightmares decrease.
- Affect tolerance—feelings can be felt, named, and endured without overwhelming arousal or numbing.
- Symptom mastery—anxiety, fear, depression, and sexual problems have decreased and are more manageable.
- Reconnection—ability to trust and attach to others increases.
- Meaning—the client has discovered some tolerable meaning for the trauma and for the self as a trauma survivor; feels empowered.

Planning and Implementation: NIC

It is important to support defense mechanisms until the client is able to cope with the reality of the assault. Give her ample time to respond to simple questions; anxiety will decrease her ability to perceive input, thereby slowing her response time. If the client is unable to express her feelings, acknowledge the difficulty by saying, "I understand that it's difficult for you to describe your feelings right now. That's okay. You may be able to talk about them later." Communicate your knowledge and understanding of the usual emotional responses to rape. Statements such as "People usually experience a number of feelings, like anxiety, fear, embarrassment, guilt, and anger" will reassure her that her feelings are a normal reaction to rape. Use the Your Self-Awareness feature on page 644 to help you understand your own feelings and attitudes.

Encouraging Coping

Encourage the client to talk about the rape. Many clients will have a compulsive need to recount the assault. The emotional arousal of the trauma contributes to this intense pressure to talk. Listen patiently and supportively, understanding that compulsive retelling is a natural way the victim uses to gradually desensitize herself to the trauma.

Identify specific coping behaviors clients used during the rape such as screaming, fighting, talking, blacking out, and/or remaining passive. Initially, clients may experience distortions related to self-blame or guilt. Recognizing that their behavior was an adaptive mechanism for survival will raise their self-esteem and decrease their feelings of guilt. Repeatedly tell clients it was not their fault. Emphasize that survival is the most important outcome. Reassure them that they did the best they could under the degree of fear that rape

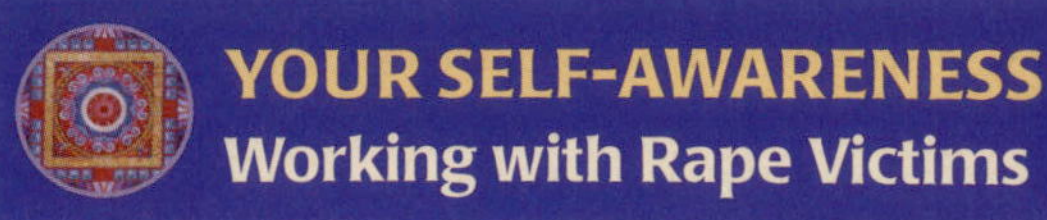

YOUR SELF-AWARENESS
Working with Rape Victims

Take some time to think about and consider your reactions to the following questions:

- Are people being conditioned by their families, movies, and television into accepting rape as something allowable?
- Have you ever been in a situation in which genital or oral sex occurred without your complete consent or your partner's complete consent? How did you feel after it was over?
- Is acquaintance rape more emotionally destructive than stranger rape?
- Is it rape if the victim is under the influence of alcohol or drugs?
- Can a person who is mentally retarded or suffering from a mental disorder give consent to sexual activity?
- Is our society too tolerant of rapists?

induces. A helpful statement might be, "I know you handled the situation right because you are alive."

Identifying and Prioritizing Concerns

Help clients identify and prioritize immediate concerns. Focusing on immediate problems lessens the client's confusion and the feeling of being overwhelmed. Next, help the client use the problem-solving process. Clients need to be empowered to make their own decisions and act on their own behalf. Restoring personal choice is a primary antidote to rape trauma. Informed choices help clients regain control and autonomy, both of which were violated during the rape.

Providing Anticipatory Guidance

Help clients identify who should be told about the rape. Rape is both a personal and a family crisis. Victims often fear how family and friends will respond to the situation. Anticipatory guidance on your part will help them take advantage of available support systems. When significant others are involved, prepare them before they join the victim because they may not know how to best support their loved one. Common myths about rape are discussed in the Partnering with Clients and Families feature below.

Discuss beliefs about postcoital contraception and abortion if appropriate. Pregnancy may result from the rape, and clients must have information about available options. The most common medical intervention is a course of hormonal treatment. Elevated doses of an oral contraceptive or DES (diethylstilbestrol) may be administered if the woman chooses to prevent conception. Mifepristone (RU-486), also known as the "morning-after pill," is a chemical that greatly diminishes the chances that a fertilized ovum will be implanted or that a placenta will develop. Inform clients about the need for follow-up medical evaluation and treatment for sexually transmitted infections, including HIV/AIDS.

Connecting Clients with Helpful Resources

Provide a written list of referrals of community resources before clients are discharged from the emergency department. Crisis intervention counseling can help minimize the long-term emotional impact of rape. Every effort should be made to connect clients with aftercare services while they are still in the emergency department. Links to these resources can be found on the Companion Website for this book.

Group therapy provides an opportunity for victims to meet with other survivors of rape in a safe, supportive, and egalitarian setting. In this therapeutic environment, clients have their feelings validated as normal reactions to the assault and receive confirmation of their survival behaviors. The long-term goal of group therapy is to help survivors understand their distress and take charge of their own recovery. Recovery is accomplished by counteracting self-blame, sharing grief, and affirming the self and life.

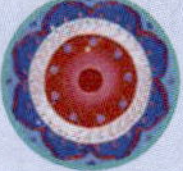

PARTNERING WITH CLIENTS AND FAMILIES

TEACHING ABOUT RAPE

Myths and Facts

Myth: Sexual assault is caused by uncontrollable sex drives.
Fact: Sexual assault is an act of physical and emotional violence, not of sexual gratification. Men assault to dominate, humiliate, control, degrade, terrify, and violate. Studies show that power and anger are the primary motivating factors.

Myth: Women provoke sexual assault, and sex appeal is of prime importance in selecting targets.
Fact: Women who have been sexually assaulted range in age from infants to elders. Appearance and attractiveness are not relevant; accessibility and vulnerability are.

Myth: Women are usually sexually assaulted by strangers.
Fact: Studies show that the majority of sexually assaulted women are acquainted with their assailants.

Myth: Sexual assault is unplanned and spontaneous.
Fact: Studies show that a majority of sexual assaults are planned in advance.

Myth: Women make false reports of sexual assault.
Fact: Statistics show that unfounded reports of alleged rape are the same proportion as for all other crimes.

Myth: Men do not have to be concerned about sexual assault because it affects women.
Fact: Men, both straight and gay, are sexually assaulted. In addition, men have wives, friends, mothers, and daughters who may someday need help coping with the aftereffects of sexual assault.

Evaluation

When assessing the rape client for progress, it is best to use specific outcome criteria. There are a number of areas to be measured for the evaluation to be meaningful. Expressing feelings in an appropriate way, reducing personal responsibility or guilt in the rape, feeling empowered, making her own decisions, and being actively involved in self-care decisions and behaviors are all appropriate outcomes. You can evaluate the effectiveness of nursing interventions by observing the client's progress throughout the various stages of her crisis. The client and her significant others should participate in evaluating the response to treatment.

COMMUNITY-BASED CARE AND HOME CARE

In the 1990s Sexual Assault Nurse Examiner (SANE) programs were established to improve community response to sexual assault victims. In the past, the retraumatization of victims in the medical setting included long waits in busy public areas; not being allowed to eat, drink, or urinate to avoid destroying evidence; and encounters with health care professionals untrained in forensic evidence collection procedures.

A SANE is a registered nurse who has advanced education and clinical preparation in forensic examination of sexual assault victims. SANEs provide respectful and prompt emergency medical–legal treatment. They offer victims compassionate care for both physical and psychological traumas. In some instances, this humane contact may be the first appropriate, adult interaction child victims have (Rawson, 2007). SANEs know what forensic and other legal evidence to collect and how to document injuries. SANE programs provide improved medical and legal response to sexual assault victims (Stermac, Dunlap, & Bainbridge, 2005).

As a nurse, regardless of the clinical setting in which you practice, it is important that you challenge cultural values and beliefs that promote and condone sexual violence. Confront myths that support rape in any way so that a new understanding of rape and rape victims can be developed. Changing the stereotypes of gender roles and the inequality of power inherent in heterosexual relationships can decrease the prevalence of sexual violence. It is only through this process that long-term changes will occur.

INTRAFAMILY VIOLENCE: PHYSICAL ABUSE

Domestic violence—violence within the family—occurs at all levels of society. The myth is that violence occurs only among the poor and undereducated; the reality is that violence also occurs among the middle and upper classes as well as the professional elite. In the past, these problems among wealthy or prominent people were kept hidden from the general public. With an increase in national concern, however, more publicity is being given to cases of domestic violence at all socioeconomic levels.

In this text, the word *family* refers to any one of these three categories of people who are:

- Related by birth, adoption, or marriage
- In an intimate relationship
- In a domestic relationship; that is, sharing the same household

Although the image of the American family is one of happiness and harmony, this ideal is often in conflict with the underlying reality of domestic violence. The home is the most frequent place for violence of all types. Women and children are more likely to be assaulted, raped, and killed by people who claim to love them than they are by strangers. Perpetrators of violence do to intimates in their homes what they would not dare do anyplace else. Our culture does not condone violence in schools, at work, or on the streets, but continues to "allow" it within the privacy of the family. Family members often appear to believe they have a license to strike other family members. **Battering**, a pattern of repeated physical assault, can be considered an epidemic in North America.

The incidence of domestic violence can only be estimated. Studies often include only those people who are willing to respond to surveys. Typically underrepresented in such studies are those who do not speak English or are illiterate, the very poor, the homeless, and those who are hospitalized or incarcerated at the time of the survey. The actual rates of domestic violence are probably much higher than reported. A good source of information on domestic violence is the NIH website, www.nlm.nih.gov/medlineplus/domesticviolence.html.

Domestic violence is a violent crime against which the victim has the right to be protected and for which the perpetrator can be arrested and prosecuted. In all 50 states of the United States, nurses are required by law to report suspected incidents of child abuse, and in every state there is a penalty—civil, criminal, or both—for failure to report child abuse. In addition, not reporting child abuse is considered to be nursing malpractice. Laws on reporting the abuse of adults and elders vary by state. Be sure to know the laws in the state in which you practice. The far-reaching impacts of violence on a child's life are explored in the Evidence-Based Practice feature on page 646.

Sibling Abuse

A form of domestic violence that is very common but not necessarily acknowledged occurs between siblings. Many people assume it is natural and even appropriate for children to use physical force with one another. Parents may say, "It's a good chance for him to learn how to defend himself," "She had a right to hit him; he was teasing her," and "Kids will be kids." With these attitudes, children learn that physical force is an appropriate method of resolving conflict among themselves. Children who are hit by their parents exhibit more than double the rate of violence against siblings than children whose parents do not hit them. Hitting children increases the probability that they will be violent. Parents should not be complacent about sibling aggression; siblings cause 3% of all child homicides in the United States. Even though violence

MediaLink Application: Parenting in the Context of Domestic Violence

MediaLink National Library of Medicine

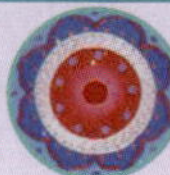

EVIDENCE-BASED PRACTICE

IMPACT OF VIOLENCE ON CHILDREN'S LIVES

In your role as a community health nurse, you have been conducting health classes for children at a local school. You have noted the prevalence of violence in young children's lives and the negative effects of exposure to violence on development. During your class discussions, several children spoke about their fears regarding abuse and violence. It is not hard to imagine how violence can become "normalized" in the lives of children. It becomes apparent to you that those in direct contact with young children need further education about childhood violence.

In your review of the literature you become aware of one antiviolence program, the ACT (Adults and Children Together) Against Violence Training Program. It is aimed specifically at the role models in young children's lives (their parents or caregivers, teachers, and others who work directly with them). As a nurse, you are in an ideal position to disseminate information to the role models in children's lives.

The ACT program is reportedly effective in terms of participants' increased awareness of the prevalence and impacts of childhood violence. Other professionals involved in health care for abused children consider this program an effective intervention.

Action should be based on more than one study, but in this situation the following study was helpful in developing appropriate interventions:

Guttman, M., Mowder, B. A., & Yasik, A. E. (2006). The ACT against violence training program: A preliminary investigation of knowledge gained by early childhood professionals. *Professional Psychology: Research and Practice, 37*(6), 717–723.

CRITICAL THINKING APPLICATION

1. Whom would you identify as important to contact in order to initiate an effort to reduce violence toward children?
2. Why would it be useful to identify the major role models in a child's life?
3. How would an increased awareness of childhood violence make a difference?
4. Why would involving adults in reducing childhood violence likely be helpful?
5. What would be the purpose of talking about violence as if it were not normal?

decreases with age, studies indicate that 63% to 68% of adolescent siblings use physical violence to resolve conflict (Marleau, 2005).

Child Abuse

Each year, approximately 2.8 million American children experience at least one act of physical violence, and 1.4 million are otherwise abused or neglected. Children who live in a home in which a parent is being abused are 1,500 times more likely to be abused than the national average. Younger parents are more likely to engage in physical abuse against children than older parents, and the abuse is often disguised as discipline. For many, hitting begins when they are infants and does not end until they leave home. Younger children are spanked, punched, grabbed, slapped, kicked, bitten, and hit with fists or objects. Adolescents are more likely to be beaten up and have a knife or gun used against them. Men and women are equally likely to abuse young children. During adolescence, however, the abuser is more likely to be male (Edwards, Holden, Felitti, & Anda, 2003).

Acts of violence against children range from a light slap to a severe beating to homicide. In some families or cultures, hitting or spanking children is condoned and even approved as being necessary and good for the child. Many parents, however, do not realize the underlying messages they are giving the child by hitting:

- If you are small and weak, you deserve to be hit.
- People who love you hit you.
- It is appropriate to hit people you love.
- Violence is appropriate if the end result is good.
- Violence is an appropriate method of resolving conflict.

Generally, violence against children can compromise the child's physical and mental health (Terra & dos Santos, 2006).

Shaken Baby Syndrome

Shaken baby syndrome is one of the most serious, yet frequently overlooked, forms of child abuse. It involves the vigorous shaking of a baby held by the extremities or shoulders that causes whiplash-induced intracranial and intraocular bleeding. It is estimated that one-third of victims have significant and permanent brain damage, and one-third die. Not recognizing the danger, many parents shake rather than hit the child, mistakenly believing it is less violent.

Child Neglect

Neglect is the most frequently reported type of child maltreatment. It differs from abuse in that it is an act of omission that results in harm. Neglect includes lack of adequate physical care (including not medicating as prescribed), nutrition, and shelter. It also includes unsanitary conditions that often contribute to health and developmental problems. Lack of human contact and nurturance is considered emotional neglect.

Homicide of Child

In the United States, homicide is one of the five leading causes of death before the age of 18. Sixty-one percent of children who are killed by their parents or caretakers are under the age of four, and 40% are less than one year old. Most of these deaths are the result of battering in response to colic in the infant and toilet training difficulties in the toddler. A small percentage of children are killed because they are unwanted, as the result of mercy killings, at the hands of a mentally ill parent, or in retaliation when one parent kills the child to inflict hurt on the other parent. Compared to other developed countries, the United States has the highest rate of child homicide at all ages (Friedman, Horwitz, & Resnick, 2005; Patton, 2003).

The children of parents who have psychiatric disabilities are at relatively high risk for homicide. A 5- to 10-fold increase in risk for being murdered was seen in young and older children of affected mothers or fathers (Webb, Pickles, Appleby, Mortensen, & Abel, 2007).

In judicial documentation, mothers who killed their children were frequently mentally disordered. Postpartum depression has been documented as the primary cause of infanticide. A disproportionately large number of biologic mothers who killed their offspring, especially older children, had a mental illness and received relatively short sentences, if convicted. Murder of a son or daughter by biologic fathers were disproportionately accompanied by marital discord, suicide, and murder of a wife by her husband. Murders of children by stepparents were disproportionately common and likely to involve ongoing abuse and death by beating. Moreover, if parents also had biologic offspring, their stepchildren were at increased risk of ongoing abuse and neglect prior to death (Harris, Hilton, Rice, & Eke, 2007).

Homicide of Parent

Although it is a rare event, each year more than 300 parents are killed by their children in the United States. This number accounts for 1.5% to 2.5% of all homicides. Both victims and perpetrators tend to be European-Americans, and 30% of the perpetrators are under age 18. The most frequent situation—90% of the cases—is one in which the teen has been severely abused and/or the mother is a victim of abuse. The adolescent's attempts to get help have failed, and the family situation becomes increasingly intolerable prior to the murder. A critical factor is the easy availability of guns in the home. The other 10% of cases involve either severely mentally ill children who experience hallucinations and delusions or dangerously antisocial children who have extreme conduct problems (Ewing, 1997).

Partner Abuse—Heterosexual

Although no socioeconomic class, ethnic group, religion, or age group is immune to domestic violence, most victims are women. If the abused are mothers of dependent children, their children are also likely to be victims. Female partner abuse in heterosexual relationships is the most widespread form of family violence in the United States. It is thought that 1 woman in 5 is physically abused by her partner, and that 3 to 4 million women are severely assaulted every year (Daniels, 2005). Half the women who are abused suffer beatings several times a year. The other half may be beaten as often as once a week. The intensity and frequency of attacks tend to escalate over time. If verbal and emotional assaults were included, the numbers would be much higher. Violence is the single largest cause of injury to women in the United States, with 20% of women's emergency department visits resulting from physical abuse. Three to four battered women are killed every day in the United States (Zlotnick, Johnson, & Kohn, 2006).

Overwhelmingly, the first acts of partner violence occur in dating relationships. Physical abuse occurs among as many as 30% to 50% of adolescent and college students who are dating. Sadly, many victims and offenders interpret violence as a sign of love. Common reasons teens and young adults give for the violence is betrayal and jealousy (Amar & Gennaro, 2005; Close, 2005).

It is important to be aware of female abuse of heterosexual males. It is estimated that 100,000 to 150,000 heterosexual male partners are abused by women who initiate the violence. They are generally not recognized as "real" victims, and when they do tell others, they are criticized for not standing up for themselves or for not fighting back. This may account for underreporting by male victims; admitting the occurrence would be a sign of weakness or a cause for embarrassment.

Partner Abuse—Homosexual

Until very recently, the existence of physical abuse in lesbian and gay relationships has been downplayed or even denied. This denial has been supported by the myths that women are not violent people and that men can defend themselves. In reality, violence does occur in some gay and lesbian families, for the same reasons as in heterosexual families: to demonstrate, achieve, and maintain power and control over one's partner. In addition to physical or emotional abuse, the violent partner may use homophobic control—the threat of telling ("outing") family, friends, neighbors, or employers about the victim's sexual orientation.

In the United States, domestic violence is the third largest health problem for gay men, following substance abuse and AIDS. It is estimated that 20% to 25% of coupled gay men are victims. Men rarely talk about being victims for fear of being considered feminine if they admit that their partners are hurting them. Looking at violence in same-sex relationships demonstrates clearly that violence is not a gender issue but rather a power issue (Heintz & Melendez, 2006).

Homophobia and hatred of homosexuals in the United States contribute to the difficulties of battered lesbians and gays. They are cut off from the usual support systems available to heterosexual victims such as specialized counseling services and shelters. Most state laws regarding domestic violence exclude gays and lesbians by using limiting terms such as *spouse* and *battered wife*. Gays and lesbians of color and those who live in rural areas are even more isolated than their counterparts. Since same-sex partnerships are not recognized as "legitimate," victims have no access to the legal system. Being victimized by one's lover can be less frightening than being victimized by the legal system. Fear of being identified as gay or losing custody of children adds to the silence about the violence. Members of lesbian and gay communities are currently making an attempt to intervene with and support victims.

Elder Abuse

Two million older adults are mistreated each year nationwide (Pearsall, 2005). Elder abuse is any deliberate action or negligence that harms an older adult. **Physical abuse** is the nonaccidental use of physical force that results in bodily injury, pain, or impairment. Some older adults may have their basic physical needs neglected and suffer from dehydration, malnutrition, and oversedation. They may be deprived of necessities such as glasses, hearing aids, and walkers. Emotional neglect can mean leaving a person alone for long periods of time or failing to provide social contact. Some older people are subjected to **psychological abuse** in the form of verbal assaults, threats, humiliation, and/or harassment. Remarks such as "One of these days I am going to poison your food and you won't know when" and "I am the only thing standing between you and a nursing home" are considered psychological abuse.

Families may violate an older person's rights by refusing appropriate medical treatment, forcing isolation or unreasonable confinement, denying privacy, providing an unsafe environment, or demanding involuntary servitude. Some elders are financially exploited through theft or misuse of property or funds. Others are beaten and even sexually abused or raped.

The perpetrator of elder abuse may be a spouse, child, grandchild, niece, nephew, some other relative, or a nonrelated caretaker. The abuse is most likely to be inflicted by a person with whom the victim lives. A number of factors contribute to the abuse of older adults. Perpetrators may have personal problems such as lack of support in caring for the older family member, alcohol or drug addiction, or a family history of violence. Family factors include unresolved previous conflicts and power struggles. The perpetrator may be retaliating for previous abuse suffered at the hands of the older person. Elders are often resistant to intervention because they fear that losing a caregiver will mean having to be put in an institution.

Emotional Abuse

Although the focus of violence in this chapter is on physical abuse, it must be remembered that emotional abuse is often equally damaging. Words can hit as hard as a fist, and the damage to self-esteem can last a lifetime. Emotional abuse involves one person's shaming, embarrassing, ridiculing, or insulting another either in private or in public. It may include destruction of personal property or the killing of pets in an effort to frighten or control the victim. Such statements as "You can't do anything right," "You're ugly and stupid—no one else would want you," and "I wish you had never been born" are devastating to one's self-esteem.

Abuse of Pregnant Women

Pregnancy is a time of increased risk for abuse. There are more incidents of violence during pregnancy than of hypertension, gestational diabetes, or placenta previa, all of which are screened for regularly. Indeed, 21% to 43% of women report abuse during pregnancy (Levendosky, Leahy, Bogat, Davidson, & von Eye, 2006). A past history of abuse is one of the strongest predictors of abuse during pregnancy. Nonpregnant women are usually beaten in the face and chest. But pregnant women tend to be beaten in the abdomen, which can lead to miscarriage, placenta abruptio, fetal loss, premature labor, fetal fractures, pelvic fractures, rupture of the uterus, and hemorrhage. Battering during pregnancy is associated with severity of abuse. The man who beats his pregnant partner is an extremely violent and dangerous man. Battering during pregnancy is also a risk factor for eventual homicide of the female partner (Kearney, Haggerty, Munro, & Hawkins, 2003).

The timing of the first prenatal visit is often related to abuse status. Abused women are twice as likely to delay prenatal care until the third trimester. Many abused women report that the abuser forced them to avoid prenatal care by denying them access to transportation. The feature What Every Obstetric Nurse Should Know gives you specific questions to ask and cues to incorporate into your assessment of the pregnant woman.

Physical abuse during pregnancy may be related to ambivalent feelings about the pregnancy, competition for attention with the developing fetus, increased vulnerability of the woman, increased economic pressures, and decreased sexual availability. Unfortunately, the abuse of pregnant women is often overlooked by health care professionals even when the victim appears in the emergency department with bruises, cuts, broken bones, and abdominal injuries.

Stalking

The term *stalking* has become not only a part of the American vocabulary but also a new classification of crime, and all

WHAT EVERY OBSTETRIC NURSE SHOULD KNOW

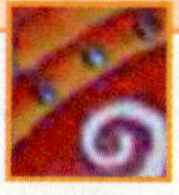

Assessing for Abuse

At the first prenatal visit, you should explain to the client that you will be asking her questions related to emotional and physical abuse throughout her pregnancy since pregnancy is a time of increased risk for abuse. Determine if there is a prior history of physical or emotional abuse in the current relationship. Avoid making assumptions based on cultural myths (upper-class women are not abused, lesbian women do not abuse their partners, women could leave abusive situations if they chose to, and so on). In addition to assessing for physical injuries, at each prenatal visit, ask the following questions:

- Do you feel valued as a person by your partner?
- Do you feel safe in your home?
- Are you isolated from others for long periods of time?
- Have you been hurt in any way since your last visit here?

50 states have passed stalking laws. **Stalking** is the act of following, viewing, communicating with, or moving threateningly toward another person. Property damage and assault may accompany stalking. Victims often feel trapped in an environment filled with anxiety, stress, and fear that often results in their having to make drastic changes in how they live their lives.

Domestic stalking occurs when a former partner, spouse, or family member threatens or harasses a person. The stalker often makes it clear that the victim is his "property." The stalker is usually motivated by a desire to continue the relationship, which can evolve into an attitude of "If I can't have her/him, no one can." In some cases the stalker is angry and retaliating against the victim, whom he perceives as rejecting him. Frequently, there is a history of domestic violence, and the stalking often ends in a violent attack on or killing of the victim (Muscari, 2005).

Cycle of Violence

Domestic violence is the deliberate and systematic pattern of abuse used to gain control over the victim. The behavior is always intentional. Perpetrators choose to be violent and give themselves permission to be violent. Perpetrators are not out of control, as is commonly assumed. They may be enraged or cool and calculating, but in either case they have made a choice. The victim cannot "make them do it." Generally, perpetrators of domestic violence are law-abiding citizens who are dangerous only to their loved ones.

To the victim, domestic violence often happens without warning and without a buildup of tension. A pattern of violence usually develops. The first incident may be precipitated by frustration or stress. If the victim immediately refuses to accept the violence and seeks outside help, there are often no further episodes. If the victim submits to the violence, then physical force, without the stimulus of frustration or stress, becomes a way of relating, and the pattern becomes resistant to change. A typical cycle occurs when conflict escalates into a violent episode, after which the perpetrator begs for the victim's forgiveness. The victim stays in the system because of promises to reform. With the next episode of conflict, the cycle of violence begins again and becomes part of the family dynamics.

Violent people are often extremely jealous and possessive. They view other family members in terms of property and ownership. Abusers use violence in an attempt to prove to themselves and others that they are superior and in control. Their use of physical force temporarily obliterates their sense of inadequacy and compensates for a lack of internal resources.

The abuser is the most powerful person in the life of the abused. The abuser's purpose is to enslave the victim, while simultaneously demanding respect, gratitude, and love. Control over the victim is established by repetitive emotional abuse that instills terror and helplessness. Threats of serious harm or threats against other family members keep the victim in a constant state of fear.

In order to have complete domination, the abuser isolates the victim. She often is forced to give up work, friends, and family. He may stalk her, eavesdrop, and intercept letters and phone calls. Control and scrutiny of the victim's body and bodily functions, finances, and transportation further destroy her sense of autonomy. She is shamed and demoralized when told what to eat, when to sleep, what to wear, when to go to the bathroom, and so on. For a victim who has been deprived long enough, the hope of a meal, a bath, or a kind word can be a powerful reward. This ongoing abusive behavior is punctuated by unpredictable outbursts of physical violence. Such domestic captivity of women, along with traumatic bonding to the abuser, often goes unrecognized. Recognize also that some abusers may adopt only one or two of these behaviors.

Victims can be further immobilized by feelings of anxiety and depression. Feelings of self-blame may be expressed in such statements as "If I hadn't talked back to my mother, she wouldn't have hit me," and "If I were a better wife, he wouldn't beat me." Guilt can contribute to depression, which further immobilizes victims and keeps them from leaving or seeking help for the family system.

Fear contributes to women's inability to leave abusive relationships. Often threatened with death at the idea of leaving, they live in fear of physical reprisal. Fearing loneliness, some women may believe that being in a bad relationship is better than being alone, and leaving the relationship would not necessarily ensure the end of the abuse. They may become dependent and believe they are incapable of "making it on my own." The abuser is often most dangerous when threatened or faced with separation. The following clinical example illustrates the tragic outcome in one situation.

CLINICAL EXAMPLE

Sandy, age 20, met Jack at work. In the beginning of their dating relationship, Jack bought her small gifts and said sweet things to her. He told Sandy he'd never loved anyone else as much. Sandy believed him, quickly fell in love, and moved in with Jack. Several months later she called her parents from work and begged them to come and get her. Sandy told them that she didn't like the relationship with Jack but she didn't know how to get out of it. Jack had taken over Sandy's life, even controlling the use of the car her parents had helped her buy. He followed her everywhere and rarely let her out of his sight.

Sandy insisted on returning to the apartment that night to get her car, telling her parents that Jack was not a violent person. However, Jack brutally beat her for having called her parents. Sandy moved back home and began trying to put her life back together. Even so, Jack continued to make harassing phone calls to Sandy. Because she had moved out so quickly, there were still financial matters she and Jack needed to clear up, so Sandy agreed to meet with him one evening. But instead of allowing her to end their 16-month relationship, Jack pulled out a gun and shot Sandy once in the back of the head.

For a partial list of reasons people remain in abusive relationships, see Box 24-3 on page 650.

Box 24-3 Why Do They Stay? Why Do They Go Back?

Fear: Victims are afraid of physical reprisal if they resist, of being found and beaten again, and of their children being hurt. Those who attempt to leave risk suffering worse violence and even death.

Learned helplessness: Victims believe they have no choices and no control; they have come to believe that violence is an acceptable way of life.

Traumatic bonding: Victims stay loyal in the relationship, hoping and searching for meaning in the indifference and abuse. Traumatic bonding results from alternating good and bad treatment; the victim has no sense of autonomy and puts energy into keeping the relationship intact.

Emotional dependence: Victims are convinced they are weak, inferior, and do not deserve better treatment; they are insecure about their potential autonomy.

Financial dependence: Victims may not have a source of income; if the abuser is arrested, he may lose his job and the family will have no income. Victims have been taught that they must be submissive in exchange for financial support.

Guilt and/or shame: Victims have been convinced that they provoked the abuse. They feel guilt over the failure of the relationship or shame for remaining in the relationship despite the abuse. They may feel pressured by family, religious, or cultural values against divorce or separation.

Isolation: Victims have few, if any, friends; little support from family; and/or no car, phone, or mail.

Children: Victims may believe two parents are better than one. They may be threatened with loss of custody; the abuser may threaten to harm or kidnap the children.

Hope: Victims hope that if they change in the way the abuser wants them to, the abuse will stop. They hope the abuser will keep his promise to stop the assaults.

Fear also contributes to the inability to leave a partner in an abusive gay or lesbian relationship. Because many couples share close friends within the same community, victims may fear shaming their partners. They may also fear that friends will either deny the problem or take the abuser's side. Homophobia contributes to the victim's reluctance to seek help. Calling the police may result in ridicule or hostile responses from the officers. Victims may not seek help from family members to avoid reinforcing negative stereotypes about homosexuality, which might exacerbate the family's homophobia.

MEDIALINK Care Plan: Abuse in a Cultural Context

BIOPSYCHOSOCIAL THEORIES

Domestic violence is easy to describe but difficult to explain. There is no single cause of this type of violence. It results from an interaction of neurobiologic, personality, situational, and societal factors that have an impact on families.

Neurobiologic Theory

Neurobiologic theorists propose that genes and neurotransmitters may contribute to causing violent behavior. Although a genetic predisposition may make certain behaviors more likely, it does not make them inevitable. Serotonin (5-HT) plays an important role in mood and aggressive behavior. 5-HT calms us through inhibitory control over aggression. Abnormally low levels of 5-HT result in a lack of control, loss of temper, and explosive rage.

Childhood abuse and neglect lead to permanent alterations in the parts of the central nervous system that are known to be stress-responsive. Corticotropin-releasing factor (CRF) is a major regulator of the endocrine, autonomic, immune, and behavioral stress responses. It is thought that stress early in life results in sensitization of the brain to even mild stressors in adulthood, thus contributing to mood and anxiety disorders long after the abuse or neglect has stopped (Griffin, Resick, & Yehuda, 2005). As a result, changes in the way CRF performs its function make it more difficult for the adult to cope with stress.

Intrapersonal Theory

Intrapersonal theory suggests that the cause of violence lies in the personality of the abuser. It is thought that people who are violent are unable to control their impulsive expressions of anger and hostility. As many as 80% of male abusers grew up in homes in which they were abused or observed their mothers being abused. With these family dynamics, the child sees the father as frightening and intimidating and sees the mother as helpless and nonprotective. This early emotional deprivation contributes to the formation of an adult who has an excessive need for nurturing and support. He comes to adult relationships with unrealistic demands for time and attention. As the relationship develops, he discourages his partner's relationships with other people because of his low self-esteem and fear of abandonment.

Social Learning Theory

Social learning theory proposes that violence is a learned behavior and people are conditioned to respond aggressively and violently. Children learn about violence from observing it, from being victims, and/or from behaving violently themselves. If the use of violence is rewarded by a gain in power, the behavior is reinforced. If there is immediate negative reinforcement within the family, a decrease in violent behavior will result. Learning to abuse is the first step in the battering process, but it does not necessarily lead vulnerable individuals to abuse. The social environment affects how the potentially abusive person behaves: the person must have the *opportunity to abuse* without suffering negative consequences. He has the perception that he can "get away with it." Although learning may have occurred and opportunity is present, the potentially abusive person makes a *conscious choice* to abuse. The batterer is solely responsible for the violence.

In addition to family models, the media provide many models of violence to which children are exposed. Some movies and television shows demonstrate that "good" people use force to achieve "good" ends. Many of the stories make no attempt to justify the use of force for "good" ends; they simply present endless, senseless acts of cruelty by one human being upon another—violence without consequences.

With these types of family and media examples, children develop values that tolerate, and even accept as normal, everyday violence between people.

Gender Bias Theory

The sexist structure of the family and society is an important factor in domestic violence. It is a common belief that men have the right to keep women subordinate through power and privilege. If there is nothing to contradict this ethos within the family system, then reaching the goal of maintaining female subordinance will be accomplished using any means possible. Domestic violence is a way to promote that goal, as it uses the power automatically granted a male in that family system. Victims are sometimes labeled as codependent in the abusive relationship, but such labeling is just another way of blaming the victim for the abuse.

The economic system helps entrap women, who are often forced to choose between poverty and abuse. It is often difficult for women to find advocates and solutions within the male-dominated legal, religious, mental health, and medical systems. Society sanctions male violence by neglecting female victims. The ultimate outcome of the cycle of abuse from which women cannot extricate themselves is that they become a built-in, ready target. Statistics validate this outcome by documenting that women are being murdered on a regular basis, not by strangers, but by husbands and lovers.

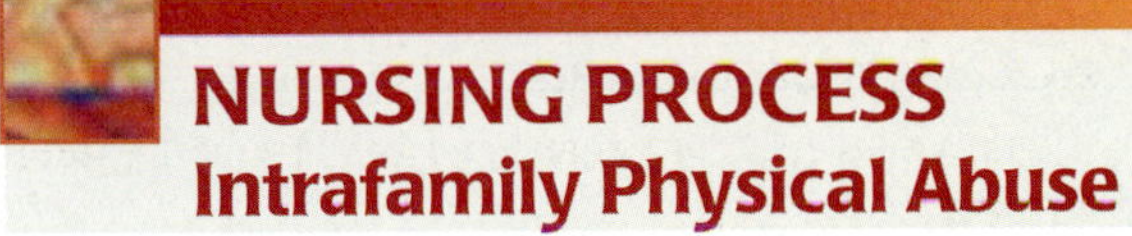

NURSING PROCESS Intrafamily Physical Abuse

Addressing abuse that occurs within the family system requires an approach that is sensitive and effective.

Assessment

Nurses in all clinical settings must routinely assess clients for evidence of intrafamily violence. Considering how extensive this problem is, ask one or two introductory questions of every client. In assessing a child, say, for example, "Moms and dads try to help their children learn how to behave well. What happens to you when you do something wrong?" Or ask, "What is the worst punishment you ever received?" In assessing adults, you may begin with this approach: "One of the sources of stress in our lives is family disagreement. Could you describe how disagreements affect you? What happens when you disagree?" If the responses to these questions are indicative of violence, conduct a more in-depth nursing assessment. Guidelines for assessment are given in the Your Assessment Approach nursing history tool on page 652.

Nursing Diagnosis: NANDA

The most important outcome of nursing assessment is identifying the existence of domestic violence. Priority must be given to critical and serious physical injuries. The severity and potential fatality of the situation must be considered, as well as the needs of dependent children and legal issues surrounding the case. Consider the following nursing diagnoses when analyzing your assessment data:

- Disabled Family Coping related to an inability to manage conflict without violence
- Ineffective Coping related to being a victim of violence
- Impaired Parenting related to the physical abuse of children
- Powerlessness related to feelings of being dependent on the abuser
- Low Self-Esteem, Situational, related to feeling guilty and responsible for being a victim
- Social Isolation related to shame about family violence
- Risk for Other-Directed Violence related to a history of the use of physical force within the family

Outcome Identification: NOC

Achievement of the following outcome criteria is evidence that the intervention plan was successful. The victims have:

- Recognized that they are not to blame for the violence of others
- Ended the denial and minimization of domestic violence
- Demonstrated an awareness of their own strengths, skills, and competence
- Reestablished a sense of power over their own lives
- Verbalized their right to express their own needs and to satisfy them
- Established social networks to decrease isolation and secrecy

Planning and Implementation: NIC

Most victims of domestic violence would like it to end, but they may not know how to seek the help they need. It is extremely important that you be nonjudgmental in your interactions with all family members. Initially, clients may be unwilling to trust you because of family shame and fear of being judged for remaining in the violent relationship. It is vital that you not impose your own values by offering quick and easy solutions to the very complicated problem of domestic violence. The features on pages 652 and 653, Your Self-Awareness and Partnering with Clients and Families, will help you to debunk myths about family violence and understand your own feelings and attitudes.

The treatment of families experiencing violence requires a multidisciplinary approach, with a broad range of interventions. Nurses, social workers, physicians, family therapists, vocational trainers, police, protective services personnel, and lawyers must coordinate to intervene effectively in a situation of intrafamily violence.

In the initial contact with family members, ensure their physical safety as much as possible. It is critical to assess the level of danger for the victim; homicide may be a real possibility if previous threats have been made. Also assess the level of danger for the abuser. The severity and duration of

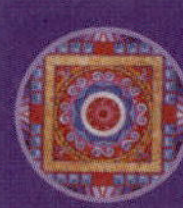

YOUR ASSESSMENT APPROACH
Nursing History Tool for Assessing Victims of Family Violence

Behavioral Assessment

- Tell me about how people communicate within your family.
- What types of things cause conflict within your family?
- How is conflict managed or resolved?
- Who in your family loses control of themselves when angry?
- Have you received verbal threats of harm?
- Have you ever been threatened with a knife or gun?
- What happens to you when a family member has violent outbursts? Are you slapped? Hit? Punched? Thrown? Shoved? Kicked? Burned? Beaten up?
- Who in your family has needed emergency medical treatment?
- In what ways have you attempted to stop the violence?
- Have you attempted to leave the situation in the past?
- What happened when you attempted to leave?
- Describe the use of alcohol in your family.
- Describe the use of drugs in your family.

Affective Assessment

- Who do you think is responsible for the use of physical force within your family?
- In what way is this person(s) responsible?
- How much guilt are you experiencing at this time?
- Tell me about your fears. Lack of security? Financial problems? Child care problems? Living apart from spouse? Further physical injury?
- What factors contribute to your feeling of helplessness to leave or stop the abuse?
- How hopeless do you feel about your situation?
- How would you describe your level of depression?

Cognitive Assessment

- Describe your strengths and abilities as a person.
- If you were describing yourself to a stranger, what would you say?
- What are your beliefs about keeping your family together?
- Tell me about your reasons for remaining in this situation. Promises of reform? Material rewards?
- Do you believe or hope the violence will not recur?
- What are your expectations of how children should behave?
- What rights do parents have with their children?
- What rights do spouses have with each other?
- What are the rules about physical force within your family?

Sociocultural Assessment

- How did your parents relate to each other?
- Who enforced discipline when you were a child?
- What type of discipline was used when you were a child?
- What was/is your relationship like with your mother?
- What was/is your relationship like with your father?
- How did you get along with your siblings?
- In your present family, who is the head of the household?
- How are decisions made in your family?
- How are household jobs assigned in your family?
- Describe recent and current stresses on your family. Unemployment? Financial problems? Illness? New family members? Deaths or separations? Child-rearing problems? Change in job status? Increase in conflict? Change in residence?
- To whom can you turn for support in times of stress?
- Describe your social life.
- What types of contact have you had with the legal system? Phoned police? Obtained an order of protection? Obtained a lawyer? Court cases? Protective services?

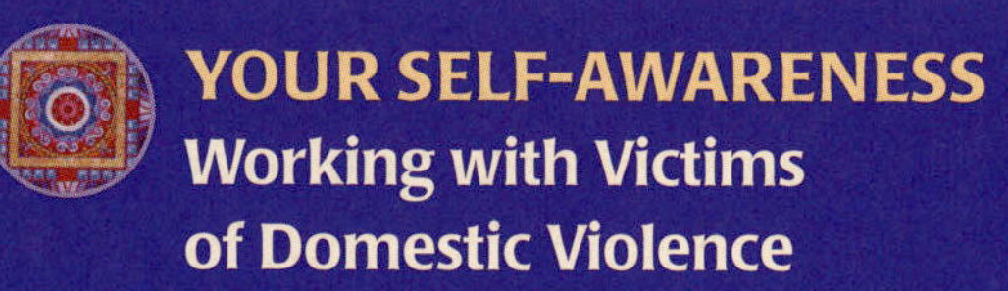

YOUR SELF-AWARENESS
Working with Victims of Domestic Violence

Take some time to think about and consider your reactions to the following questions:

- Is American culture violent compared to other cultures?
- The United States was founded by violence. How has this influenced the values and behavior of present-day Americans?
- What is the difference between spanking a child and beating a child?
- Do you think the stalking laws are decreasing the level of violence in the United States?
- Are you for or against gun control?
- Would it be more difficult for a person to stab a family member than to shoot that person?

the violence are the factors that contribute most directly to victims killing their abusers in self-defense. If the level of danger is high, contact protective services or the police for emergency custody placement or removal to a shelter.

Providing Psychoeducation

Provide interventions to improve communication. Families experiencing violence often have poor communication skills. Teach active listening with feedback (see Chapter 10), clear and direct communication, and communication that does not attack the personhood of others.

Identify the normality of conflict within all families by discussing how disagreements are inevitable. From there, discuss the use of the democratic process in conflict resolution and decision making. It is best to practice with simple, unemotional family problems at first.

Help family members identify methods to manage anger appropriately. All family members must assume responsibility for their own behavior. They can practice talking about

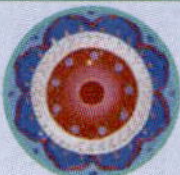

PARTNERING WITH CLIENTS AND FAMILIES

TEACHING ABOUT DOMESTIC VIOLENCE

Myths and Facts

Myth: Family violence is rare.

Fact: Every year, 10 million Americans are abused by a family member.

Myth: Family violence is confined to mentally disturbed or sick people.

Fact: Fewer than 10% of all cases involve an abuser who is mentally ill. The vast majority seem totally normal and are often charming, persuasive, and rational.

Myth: Violence is trivial—a joking matter.

Fact: A woman is beaten every 15 seconds in the United States, and 2,000 to 4,000 women are murdered by their husbands or boyfriends every year. Every year, 2.5 million children are abused, and 1,200 die from the abuse. There are 1 million cases of elder abuse annually.

Myth: Family violence is confined to the lower classes.

Fact: Social factors are not relevant. There are doctors, ministers, psychologists, and nurses who beat their family members. Violence occurs at least once in two-thirds of all marriages.

Myth: All members of the family participate in the family dynamics; therefore, all must change in order for the violence to stop.

Fact: Only the perpetrator has the ability to stop the violence. A change in the victim's behavior will not cause the abuser to become nonviolent.

Myth: Family violence is usually a one-time event, an isolated incident.

Fact: Violence is a pattern, a reign of force and terror. It becomes more frequent and severe over time.

Myth: Abused women like being hit; otherwise, they would leave.

Fact: Abused women are forced to stay in the relationship for many reasons. The perpetrator dramatically escalates the violence when a woman tries to leave.

angry feelings as they occur. Make suggestions for appropriate expression, such as relaxation, physical exercise, and striking safe, inanimate objects (a pillow, a couch, or a punching bag). Guide the family in establishing limits and defining consequences if violence recurs. Emphasize that violence within the family will not be tolerated.

Help parents who are physically abusive develop and improve their parenting skills. Begin by recognizing their current positive parenting skills to increase their self-worth and help them engage in the learning process. Share your understanding that the use of violence is often a desperate attempt by parents to cope with their children. Confirming that they care about their children will increase the likelihood of their active participation in the treatment process.

Because domestic violence is often transgenerational, discuss with the parents how they were punished as children. Teach them about the normal growth and development of children. Unrealistic demands for children to comply beyond their developmental ability often result in violence. The first step in the problem-solving process is helping parents identify specific problems they experience with raising children. They can then go on to identify solutions, other than physical force, that are age-appropriate for their children. They need support in implementing, practicing, and evaluating these new skills.

Empowering Victims

One of the primary goals of therapy is the empowerment of victims. The process of violence removes all power and control from the victim, resulting in low self-esteem, anxiety, depression, and somatic problems. The following principles are basic to the empowerment of victims:

- A commitment to the belief that women and men are inherently equal
- An egalitarian approach to the nurse–client relationship. The client is viewed as an equal partner rather than a helpless recipient of nursing interventions
- An emphasis on the victim's strengths and abilities
- Respect for the victim's ability to understand his or her own experiences
- An emphasis on altering destructive roles and expectations within the family system
- A willingness to state clear value positions about domestic violence

Through this approach, clients can become aware that they have choices in, and control over, their lives. Avoid trying to convince adult victims to leave their abuser. As difficult as it may be, you must be willing to support clients in their pain, rather than telling them what to do about their problems. For the most positive adaptive outcome, adult victims must be their own rescuers and take charge of their own safety and protection plan. If they need help with this process, teach them to ask for that help directly. This is not meant to imply in any way that you would abandon clients; rather, you stand by, support, and affirm the positive choices and decisions they make.

Help adult clients begin identifying ways in which they are dependent on their abusers. High levels of dependence make it difficult for victims to leave abusers without intense support. You can help them identify intrapersonal and interpersonal strengths to decrease their feelings of powerlessness. From there, clients can move on to identifying aspects of life that are under their control. Offer assertiveness training to help them develop new skills for relating to others in the future (see Chapter 3). If they are still in the abusive relationship, however, caution them that assertive behavior may escalate the violence.

Treating the Abuser

Most abusers do not seek treatment unless it is court ordered or there are custody issues involved. It is frustrating to intervene with abusers who deny the reality of or responsibility for the violence. Group therapy for abusers is sometimes helpful. The group setting is more effective than individual therapy because interactions with a number of people more successfully address the anger and control problems. The responsibility for aggression is always placed on the aggressor. Issues regarding the patriarchal and power views of relationships are discussed in great depth. Participants are asked to specify their abusive behaviors, identify the intentions behind those behaviors, and examine the effects of the abuse on their victims. Abusers learn that anger can be controlled and that violence is always a *choice*.

Evaluation

Nurses in acute care settings may not have the opportunity for long-term evaluation of the family system. Short-term evaluation focuses on:

1. The identification of domestic violence
2. The family's ability to recognize that a problem exists
3. The willingness of the family to accept assistance by following through with referrals
4. The removal of the victim from a volatile situation

Nurses in long-term settings or within the community have an opportunity to evaluate the effectiveness of the multidisciplinary treatment plan over an extended period of time. When violence no longer exists within the family system, the plan has succeeded. Sharing in the process of family growth and adaptation can be a tremendous source of professional satisfaction.

All nurses should evaluate their professional obligations and practice in counteracting those aspects of society that foster domestic violence. Domestic violence is a mental health problem of national and international importance, and we can be leaders in helping prevent it in future generations. Primary prevention includes the nursing interventions of parent education, family life education in schools, referral for appropriate child or elder care, establishment of support groups, and education of fellow nurses about the problem of domestic violence. It also includes community education about the pervasive effects of media violence on individuals and society. An example of a cultural perspective on domestic violence can be found at the website of the Institute on Domestic Violence in the African American Community (www.dvinstitute.org/).

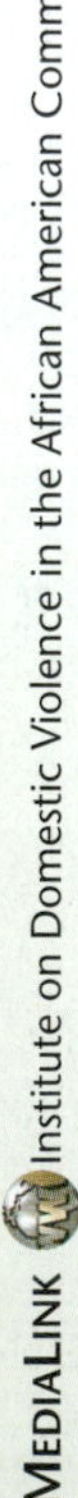

Secondary prevention of domestic violence includes working with children who are victims or who have seen their mothers beaten, and making referrals for multidisciplinary intervention. Nurses must be community advocates in supporting hotlines, crisis centers, and shelters for victims of domestic violence. On the political level, nurses must make their voices heard in regard to policies and laws affecting children, women, and older people. Questions to guide the evaluation of nursing practice and the extent of your advocacy activities include:

- Have I, as a nurse, assessed each client for possible abuse?
- What actions have I taken to decrease violence in the media?
- Have I considered the issue of gun control?
- Have I confronted the use of physical punishment within families?
- Have I volunteered to teach parenting classes at grade schools and high schools?
- Have I written to legislators to protest funding cuts in programs designed to help children, women, and older people?
- Have I spoken out on the need to increase the number of bilingual/bicultural counselors, lawyers, nurses, and physicians to attend to the needs of ethnic families?

CASE MANAGEMENT

Case managers coordinate care for victims of domestic violence. The goal is to focus on the immediate problems. Intervention is directed toward developing rapport with the victim, clarifying the presenting problems, and enhancing the victim's existing problem-solving ability. Safety of the victim(s) is of primary importance. Once safety is ensured, case management interventions include:

- Identification of effective and ineffective coping skills
- Emphasis on victim's strengths and abilities
- Development of problem-solving skills and new coping behaviors
- Identification of available support systems
- Group therapy with other victims and survivors of domestic violence
- Evaluation of the effectiveness of new coping strategies (McCloskey & Bulechek, 1996)

Although necessary, case management services present certain issues. Unless attention is paid to the contexts of the problems, these marginalized women's complex needs will be ill-served. A more holistic approach to case management can ease overall struggling (Smyth, Goodman, & Glenn, 2006).

COMMUNITY-BASED CARE

Prevention of child abuse is a community function that involves the identification of risk factors and crisis intervention. Risk factors include:

- Parents who were abused as children
- Adult relationship dysfunction
- Poor self-esteem
- Social isolation
- Unrealistic expectations of children's abilities
- Having a child with special needs

Interventions are geared toward improving adult–adult relationships as well as adult–child relationships. Helping families connect with other families decreases their sense of isolation. Parenting classes help families develop realistic expectations of their children according to developmental levels. It is very important that families of special-needs children be referred to appropriate support groups.

Prevention of elder abuse involves supporting older individuals and caretakers in identifying and expanding social support networks. These community resources may be able to help with activities of daily living (ADLs), transportation, financial advice, and assistance with personal problems. Assist the caretakers in exploring their feelings about the older people in their care. Help them identify factors that are disturbing to them and that may contribute to neglect or abuse. Determine the caretakers' ability to meet their loved one's needs, and provide appropriate teaching. Provide community resource information, including addresses and phone numbers of agencies that offer senior service assistance.

The federal Gun Control Act of 1968 prohibits anyone who has been convicted of a felony from owning or possessing a firearm or ammunition. The 1996 amendment to the Act prohibits anyone who has been convicted of a misdemeanor involving domestic violence from owning or possessing a firearm or ammunition. There are no exceptions to this law, including police or military personnel. Violation of this Act results in 10 years in prison and a fine of $250,000. Victims of domestic violence should be able to turn to the police and have their perpetrator arrested. This law, however, has been difficult to enforce.

HOME CARE

Nurses involved in home care help women develop a "safe plan" or an "escape plan" to use when their safety is threatened. They should plan a quick, safe exit from their home and have a safe place to go once they do leave. The plan should be easy and complete, and it must be taught to their children. As part of the plan, you may suggest that they have all important documents (such as birth certificates and orders of protection), some money, a list of important phone numbers, and a couple of days' clothing gathered in one secure location. They should have a second set of car keys so they can leave quickly if the need arises.

INTRAFAMILY VIOLENCE: SEXUAL ABUSE

Childhood sexual abuse is a major health problem in the United States. The majority of cases are probably unreported. **Sexual abuse** is defined as inappropriate sexual behavior, instigated by a perpetrator, for the purpose of the perpetrator's sexual pleasure or economic gain through child prostitution or pornography. Behavior ranges from exhibitionism, peeping, explicit sexual talk, touching, caressing, masturbation, oral sex, vaginal sex, and anal sex to forcing children to engage in sex with one another or with animals.

Health care professionals, as well as families, have used denial to cope with ambiguous evidence of the cultural taboos of incest and sex with children.

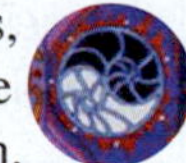

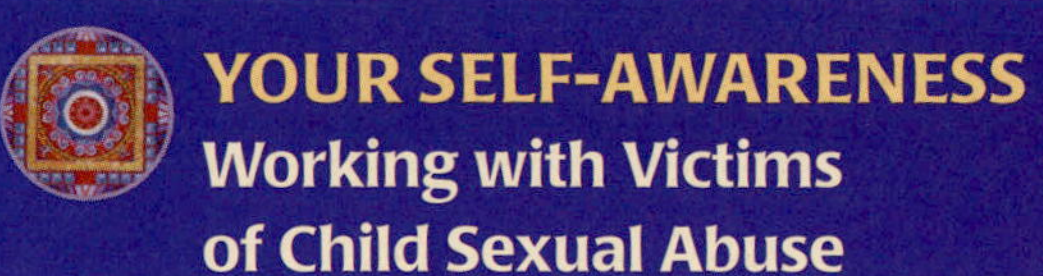

YOUR SELF-AWARENESS
Working with Victims of Child Sexual Abuse

Take some time to think about and consider your reactions to the following questions:

- Do you think the rate of child sexual abuse is increasing, or is there just better reporting?
- Do you think sex education can decrease the rate of sexual abuse?
- Which situation do you think is more devastating in child sexual abuse—when force is used or when no force is used?
- Does the fact that most perpetrators were sexually abused as children excuse their behavior? What if the perpetrator is only 11 years old?
- Far fewer women than men are accused of sexually abusing their children. How do you explain this?
- What needs to be done to decrease the incidence of child sexual abuse?

(Use the Your Self-Awareness feature above to help you understand your own feelings and attitudes.) In order to respond appropriately to cues that signal sexual abuse, you need to understand the characteristics and dynamics of families involved. A note of caution, however: With the recent increased publicity about the prevalence of child sexual abuse, there is a real danger of jumping to conclusions; any hint or accusation of sexual abuse may be interpreted as absolute proof of guilt. Rumors and false accusations have destroyed individuals and families. You must assess carefully and maintain a balance between the extremes of denial and automatic belief of guilt.

Sexually abused children and adult survivors of childhood sexual abuse (hereafter referred to as adult survivors) are crying out for help. A few cry out loudly in protest, but most cry inwardly in silence. It is thought that as many as 1 in 3 girls and 1 in 7 boys are sexually abused before the age of 18. Many of these are single, isolated incidents. Boys are more frequently molested outside the family system than are girls. The period of abuse tends to begin and end at a younger age in boys and is less likely to be disclosed (Valente, 2005).

MediaLink Sexual Abuse Interview Video

Sexual abuse occurs in all ethnic, religious, economic, and cultural subgroups. Affinity systems—immediate family, relatives, friends, neighbors, clergy, scout leaders—account for 75% to 80% of the abusers. Male perpetrators are involved in 90% of reported cases. Although father–daughter incest is most reported, it is believed that sibling incest is the most widespread. Some siblings turn to each other for emotional nurturance and acceptance. In other instances a sibling uses coercion or violence to perpetrate the abuse (National Center for Victims of Crime, 2004; Valente, 2005).

Types of Offenders

Some offenders prefer girls, others prefer boys, and some abuse both, as long as the victim is a child. Some are interested in adolescents or preteens, some in toddlers, and some in infants. Some offenders do not abuse until they are adults, but more than half start in their teens.

Juvenile Offenders

Many, if not most, cases involving juvenile offenders are unreported. Family members often want to protect and shield the young offender. Sometimes the behavior is rationalized as adolescent male experimentation. Between 50% and 60% of juvenile offenders were sexually abused as children; they gradually develop offending behaviors as they reach adolescence. The other 40% to 50% show fairly high rates of other delinquent behaviors, and most are diagnosed with conduct disorder. Those offenders who were child victims tend to begin abusing at a younger age, to have more victims, and to have male victims when compared with nonabused teen sex offenders. Juvenile offenders may seek victims within or outside the family system. The type of sexual offense often parallels their own experiences of abuse. The most frequent offense is sexual touching, which often escalates to rape and other sex crimes.

Male Offenders

One research study focusing on fathers who abused their daughters established five types of incestuous fathers (Schetky, 1999):

1. *Sexually preoccupied abusers* (26% of the fathers) have a conscious and often obsessive sexual interest in their daughters. Many of them regard their daughters as sex objects, in some cases as early as birth.
2. *Adolescent regressors* (33% of the fathers) become sexually interested in their pubescent daughters. These men sound and act like adolescents around their daughters.
3. *Self-gratifiers* (20% of the fathers) are not sexually attracted to their daughters per se, and during the abuse, they fantasize about someone else. In effect, they are simply using their daughters' bodies.
4. *Emotional dependents* (10% of the fathers) see themselves as failures and feel lonely and depressed. They see their daughters as romantic figures in their lives.
5. *Angry retaliators* (10% of the fathers) abuse out of anger, either at the daughter or at the mother. This type of offender is most likely to have a criminal history of assault and rape.

Female Offenders

Female perpetrators have been largely overlooked but commit between 3% and 13% of sexual abuse cases. The most common types of sexual abuse by women are fondling, oral sex, and group sex.

Female offenders fall into four major types:

1. Teacher-lovers are older women who teach children about lovemaking.
2. Experimenter-exploiters are often girls who have had no sex education growing up. Babysitting is often an opportunity to explore younger children. Many of the girls in this group do not even realize what they are doing or that it is inappropriate.
3. Predisposers usually come from a family with a long history of physical and sexual abuse. These families have been dysfunctional over many generations.
4. Women coerced by males abuse children because men have forced them to abuse. Usually, they have been victims as children and are easily manipulated and intimidated (McCloskey & Raphael, 2005).

Abusive Behavior Patterns

Typically, adult perpetrators initiate sexual behavior in a manipulative or coercive manner. Often, the adult misrepresents the abuse as a game or "fun" activity. The behavior usually follows a progression of sexual activity, from exposure and fondling to oral, vaginal, and/or anal sex. Secrecy is imposed on the child by persuasion or threat. The abuser may make threatening statements such as those in Box 24-4. Secrecy and silence are used by abusers to escape accountability. When secrecy fails and the child victims or adult survivors begin to talk to others about the abuse, perpetrators usually attack the credibility of the victims and try to make sure no one will listen. Other perpetrators acknowledge the abuse but minimize the impact, while some use the defense mechanism of projection and blame the child for the abuse.

Box 24-4 Typical Threatening Statements by Sexual Abusers

To Obtain Secrecy and Silence

- "If you tell, you'll be sent away."
- "If you tell, I won't love you anymore."
- "If you tell, I will kill you."
- "If you tell, I'll do the same thing to your baby brother."

To Attack the Victim's Credibility

- "It never happened, she's lying."
- "He's exaggerating some innocent touching."

To Acknowledge the Abuse While Minimizing the Impact

- "Better for her to learn about sex from her father than from some horny teenager."
- "She didn't really mind; in fact, we have a very close relationship."
- "Even if it did happen, it's time to forget the past and move on."

To Use the Defense Mechanism of Projection and Blame the Child

- "She's a very provocative child, and she seduced me."
- "If he hadn't enjoyed it so much, I wouldn't have kept doing it."

Child Victims

Children know that adults have absolute power over them, so they obey. When they have been threatened with abandonment or harm, they frequently choose to protect others. When asked, "Why didn't you tell sooner?" the answers are, "I didn't know who to tell," "I was scared," and/or "I did tell and no one believed me."

Children often feel responsible for the adult's behavior and ashamed that they have not been able to stop the abuse. Secrecy and guilt keep these children isolated, causing them to feel alienated from their peers. They may act out sexually by initiating oral or genital sex with other children or adults. The feeling of powerlessness is extremely potent because what the victim says and does makes no difference. When the repressed rage comes to the surface, it may be directed against the self in self-defeating and self-destructive ways, such as self-mutilation and suicide (Salter et al., 2003).

Adolescent victims may run away from home to escape an intolerable situation. Because they have learned, at home, that sexual behavior is rewarded by affection, love, and attention, some turn to prostitution. Others are forced into prostitution as a way to support themselves while living on the streets.

Some child victims use denial to cope with the trauma. Acknowledging the abuse would mean acknowledging that the world is dangerous and that those who are supposed to protect and nurture failed instead and caused harm. Other victims minimize the impact, saying things like "It's not so bad; it only happens once a month" or "It's all right because it stopped when I was 11 years old." The following clinical example illustrates the impact on one child victim.

CLINICAL EXAMPLE

Sonja describes her current sexual life as one of promiscuity and relates this to being sexually molested from age 4 through age 7 by her grandfather.

This is her description of the abuse: "Whenever I was alone with him in the car, he would fondle me and expose his penis to me. He would tell me I could touch it, it would be all right.

So much of the time I tried to block everything out—it's hard for me to recall exactly what happened. Some of the things I remember clearly. I remember Grandpa's easy chair. When we were alone he would make me sit on his lap in that chair, and he would stick his fingers in me. This happened many times. One time he parked in an isolated area and played with me and made me touch him and kiss his penis. He tried to coax me to have intercourse. He told me it wouldn't hurt. But I cried and he masturbated into his handkerchief instead. He made me promise never to tell anyone.

He always bought me things or gave me money. I remember the day he died. I came home from school and when my mom told me, I cried. But deep down I was glad. I was really safe from him now. And I hated him for hurting me and making me tell lies all the time."

Frequently, dissociation is the victim's major defense. The mind is "separated" from the body so the victim is not emotionally present during the sexual attack. Dissociation is evidenced by such statements as "I put myself in the wall, where he couldn't reach all of me" and "When he would come into my room, I would close my eyes and go to my favorite place. Only my body stayed on the bed; the rest of me wasn't there." When sexual abuse is severe and sadistic, the victim may develop dissociative identity disorder (DID). DID is discussed in Chapter 22.

Adult Survivors

Many adult survivors continue to believe that they were to blame for the abuse and should have been able to resist the adult. This self-blame often contributes to depression, anxiety, panic attacks, and low self-esteem. They feel worthless and different from other people. For some, anger is the only emotion experienced and expressed; all other feelings are repressed. Many adult survivors continue to hate their perpetrators, as well as the nonabusing significant adults who did not protect them.

Sexual Difficulties

Adult survivors may believe they are only sex objects, to be used and abused by others. Some have a very strong aversion to sex and are filled with terror in sexual situations. Some are sexually inhibited and experience discomfort with sexual thoughts, feelings, and behaviors. Some engage in compulsive sexual behavior, perhaps as an unconscious way to validate their shame and guilt, or as a way to feel powerful. Many adult survivors go through a period of celibacy as they try to manage fear, anger, and distrust.

Confusion about sexuality is very common among male survivors. Sexual victimization of a male by a male carries a hidden implication that the victim is less than a man. Heterosexual survivors fear that the abuse has made, or will make, them homosexual. Intense homophobia and/or hypermasculine behavior may be an effort to disprove their fears. Gay survivors worry that their sexual preference may have caused the abuse. It must be remembered that childhood sexual abuse is not related to adult sexual orientation.

Self-Mutilation

Some adult survivors engage in *self-mutilation*, as in cutting, slashing, or burning themselves. It is important to understand the meaning of such behavior. For some, the pain of self-mutilation proves their existence and reassures them that they are alive and real. Self-mutilation may be a plea for nurturance, as they come to the emergency department seeking care. Others nurture themselves by cleaning up the wounds after self-mutilation. For those who dissociate, self-mutilation may be a way to stop the dissociation, to focus on the here-and-now with physical pain. Others self-mutilate as a form of self-punishment and a way to decrease guilt feelings. And finally, some self-mutilate as a way to reduce emotional pain through the feeling of physical pain. It is important to understand the function of the behavior in order to replace it with healthier behaviors that satisfy the same need.

Memory of Sexual Abuse

Research shows that many memories of past events are not reports but reconstructions. It is the difference between remembering facts and remembering events. What is remembered is the overall impression rather than the specific details. The details we add when we reconstruct our experience depend on our personality traits and cognitive styles. We may also create pseudomemories of events that never actually occurred, especially after being told of such "events" by trusted individuals. Reports of remembered child abuse in adults, therefore, should ideally be corroborated by other people. See the Caring for the Spirit feature on page 151 in Chapter 8.

BIOPSYCHOSOCIAL THEORIES

There is no single cause of childhood sexual abuse. Rather, the abuse results from a combination of personality, family, and cultural factors.

Intrapersonal Theory

There are many types of perpetrators of sexual abuse of children. Some traits are contradictory, and there is no agreement on a composite personality. Certain characteristics apply to many people, not just abusers. The descriptions that follow are guidelines for assessment, not proof that the person actually committed sexual abuse:

1. Perpetrators usually have low self-esteem and feel more secure in interactions with children than with adults.
2. Some were emotionally deprived as children and thus have a great need for constant, unconditional love, which is more easily obtained from children than from adults.
3. Some perpetrators are described as lacking impulse control and the ability to experience feelings of guilt.
4. Some are described as rigid and overcontrolled, while others are dominant and aggressive.

If perpetrators were sexually abused themselves as children, they may have learned to associate all feelings of love with sexual behavior. Most people who were sexually abused as children do not go on to sexually abuse others. Some victimized children, however, develop offending behavior in late childhood, adolescence, or adulthood. Most likely, there are a number of factors involved in why some abuse and others do not. The world of abuse is comprised only of victims (powerless) and perpetrators (powerful). Victims become perpetrators in an unconscious attempt to master the trauma of their own experiences and retrieve power. The move from victim to offender may also result when anger and hostility concerning the past are externalized and projected onto new victims.

Family Systems Theory

Intrafamily sexual abuse most typically occurs in families that have difficulty with structure, cohesion, adaptability, and communication.

Family structure is usually hierarchical according to age, roles, and distribution of power. Typically, the adults, who are older, assume the parental roles and are the most influential. The structure of incestuous families, however, is often quite different as the result of dysfunctional boundary patterns. An adult may move "down" in the structure or a child may move "up" in terms of roles and influence (boundaries). If the father moves downward, he assumes a childlike role and is cared for and nurtured like a child in the family. In this position, the father assumes little parental responsibility. He may then turn to the daughter as a "peer" for sexual and emotional gratification.

As another example, the daughter may move upward and replace the mother in the hierarchy. The mother does not usually move downward but rather moves out of the structure by distancing herself emotionally or physically from the family. As the daughter assumes the parental role and responsibilities, the father may turn to her for fulfillment of his emotional and sexual needs.

Families that are enmeshed—that is, the members are immersed in and absorbed by one another—may be at risk for sexual abuse. In addition, incestuous families tend to be either rigid or chaotic in their adaptability. Rigid family systems have strict rules and stereotyped gender-role expectations, with minimal emotional interaction. Children have no power or authority, even over their own bodies. They are not allowed to question or protest inappropriate sexual behavior. In contrast, chaotic family systems have either no rules or constantly changing rules. Within the chaotic system, there may be no assigned roles or no rules regarding appropriate sexual behavior, which may contribute to the incidence of sexual abuse.

Communication patterns within the family system may contribute to the occurrence of sexual abuse. Incest depends on keeping the secret within the family. In family systems that avoid conflict, accusations of sexual abuse are not tolerated. Peace, and therefore silence, must be kept at all costs. (See Chapter 30 for a complete discussion of family dynamics.)

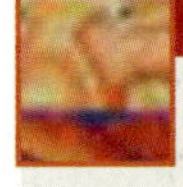

NURSING PROCESS
Intrafamily Sexual Abuse

A nursing care plan for an adult survivor of childhood sexual abuse is at the end of the chapter.

Assessment

It is vitally important that you acknowledge the reality of childhood sexual abuse. Nurses who deny the existence of the problem will miss the cues and fail to complete a detailed assessment. If you are knowledgeable about the incidence and characteristics of the problem, you will be alert for cues that demand nursing assessment. Guidelines for assessment are given in the Your Assessment Approach features on pages 659 and 660.

When assessing children, remember that some will exhibit most of the symptoms presented in this chapter, others will exhibit only some, and still others will exhibit none. Also

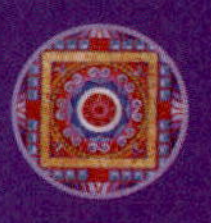

YOUR ASSESSMENT APPROACH
Nursing History Tool for Assessment of Individuals and Families for Intrafamily Sexual Abuse

Behavioral Assessment

Individual Child

- Have there been any signs of regressive behavior in the child?
- Is the child having sleeping problems?
- Is the child exhibiting clinging behavior to the parents or others?
- Does the child have friendships with other children?
- Has there been any sexual acting-out on the part of the child?
- Has the child ever run away or threatened to run away?
- Has the child ever attempted suicide?

Perpetrator

- Describe how discipline is handled in the family.
- Do you see yourself as the dominant person in the family?
- At what age do you believe parents should give up control of their children?
- How many adult friends do you have?
- Describe your relationships with these friends.
- Describe your relationship with your spouse.
- What kinds of sexual difficulties are you and your spouse experiencing?
- When you were young, who was the closest family member with whom you had any sexual activity?

Family System

- Describe who has responsibility (mother, father, both parents, or children) in the following areas of home management:
  - Caring for the younger children
  - Cooking
  - Cleaning
  - Paying bills
  - Shopping
  - Outside home maintenance
  - Budget planning
  - Decisions about leisure time
  - Supervising children's homework
  - Taking children to activities
  - Putting children to bed
- Who are the best communicators in the family?
- Who talks to whom the most?
- Who is unable to talk to whom very much?
- How are secrets kept from one another within the family?
- How are secrets prevented from leaking outside the family?

Affective Assessment

Individual Child

- How helpless does the child feel about changing any of the family's problems?
- Does the child feel responsible for family problems?
- Does the child get enough love within the family?
- Is the child more loved than the other children in the family?
- Ask about the fears the child may have if any family secrets are told:
  - Fear of not being believed
  - Fear of being blamed for the problems
  - Fear that your parents will not love you
  - Fear that you will be moved to a foster home
  - Fear that your parents will be taken away
  - Fear of physical abuse

Perpetrator

- Who loves you most within the family?
- Who is able to give you unconditional support and affection?
- Do you see yourself as responsible for family problems?
- How does fear of failure affect your life?

Family System

- Describe the emotional relationships among family members.
- Does everybody know each family member's business?
- How is privacy protected within the family?
- Do you have any fears of the family unit disintegrating?
- What will happen if the family is separated?

Cognitive Assessment

Individual Child

- Tell me about your nightmares.
- How would you describe the family's problems?
- What effect do these problems have on you?
- What effect do these problems have on the rest of the family?
- Who do you believe is responsible for these problems?

Perpetrator

- Describe what kind of a person you are.
- What are your personal strengths?
- What are your personal limitations?
- Describe how you handle new situations.
- Do you enjoy changing situations?

Family System

- Who sets the family rules?
- Tell me about the most important family rules.
- How do rules get changed within the family?
- What are the expectations of the males in the family?
- What are the expectations of the females in the family?

Sociocultural Assessment

- What significant events have occurred for your family in the past year?
- What support systems do you have outside the family?
- How often do you visit with friends?
- Who are the problem drinkers in the family?
- How is the issue of drugs managed within the family?

MEDIALINK Case Study: Assessing the Needs of a Victim of Sexual Abuse

remember that these same behavioral, affective, and cognitive characteristics may be symptoms of other emotional problems. Once it has been discovered that one child in a family is a victim of sexual abuse, suspect the abuse of siblings, both boys and girls, as well. Sometimes entire families are sexually abused before someone "tells."

You must appreciate the power of secrecy and how difficult it is for adult survivors to disclose such information,

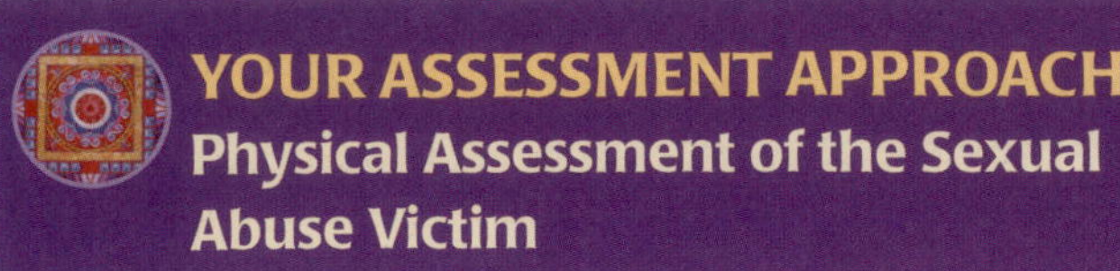

YOUR ASSESSMENT APPROACH Physical Assessment of the Sexual Abuse Victim

Complete a head-to-toe physical assessment with emphasis on the following:

- Weight and nutritional status
- Throat irritation
- Gag reflex
- Episodes of vomiting
- Abdominal pain near diaphragm
- Smears of the mouth, throat, vagina, and rectum for sexually transmitted infections
- Genital irritation or trauma
- Rectal irritation or trauma
- Chronic vaginal infections
- Chronic urinary tract infections
- Pregnancy

especially for men, who, in our society, are expected to be anything other than victimized. Routine questions on nursing histories may provide an opportunity for survivors to share their pain and obtain treatment as adults.

Be responsible for initiating the topic. Shame and confusion may keep the adult survivor from doing so. If you avoid the topic, you will be contributing to pathology by supporting the client's denial of reality. Failure to initiate a discussion of sexual abuse sends a message to clients that such abuse does not occur or does not matter. Now that childhood sexual abuse has been identified as a major health problem, nurses in every clinical setting must be alert for cues from both individuals and families.

When working with adult survivors, you must continuously assess the client's comfort level with the physical setting. Closed doors increase anxiety in some clients, while other clients request that doors never remain open. Some are uncomfortable in a room with a couch or a bed rather than chairs. How close you sit can be an issue for some clients. Even normally appropriate physical contact, such as a handshake, may increase anxiety. Always ask permission before touching a client.

Nursing Diagnosis: NANDA

Based on assessment data, nursing diagnoses are formulated for the individual child victim, the family members, and/or the adult survivor. Possible diagnoses for the child victim include:

- Ineffective Individual Coping related to being a victim of sexual abuse
- Powerlessness related to being helpless to stop the abuse
- Post-Trauma Syndrome related to being a victim of sexual abuse
- Social Isolation related to keeping the family secret of sexual abuse

For families experiencing sexual abuse, some possible diagnoses are:

- Ineffective Family Coping, Compromised, related to a child being sexually abused
- Ineffective Family Coping, Disabled, related to an enmeshed family system that is either rigid or chaotic
- Impaired Parenting related to being a perpetrator of sexual abuse
- Dysfunctional Family Process related to disruption of the family unit when abuse is discovered

For adult survivors of childhood sexual abuse, some possible diagnoses are:

- Post-Trauma Syndrome related to being an adult survivor
- Spiritual Distress related to issues about fairness and justice in life or not being protected by a supreme being
- Chronic Low Self-Esteem related to self-blame for the abuse
- Ineffective Denial related to amnesia for childhood events
- Social Isolation related to difficulty in forming intimate relationships, mistrust of others
- Sexual Dysfunction related to the trauma of abuse

Outcome Identification: NOC

Once you have established outcomes, you, the client, and the family mutually identify goals for change. Goals are specific behavioral measures by which you, clients, and significant others determine progress toward healing. The following are examples of some of the goals appropriate to people who have experienced childhood sexual abuse:

- Remains safe and free from harm
- Utilizes a variety of therapies to express feelings about the sexual abuse
- Verbalizes improved self-esteem
- Manages negative emotions in an appropriate manner
- Verbalizes a feeling of connectedness to significant others
- Verbalizes improvement in sexual functioning
- Utilizes community resources

Planning and Implementation: NIC

The first priority of care with child victims is to ensure the safety of the child. Nurses are mandated by law to report any suspected child sexual abuse. See the Case Management section for details on a plan.

When families are enmeshed and either rigid or chaotic, help family members move to a moderate position between the extremes. Teach the family the problem-solving process. With a rigid family, problem-solve ways in which the members can increase their flexibility of roles and rules. With a chaotic family, problem-solve ways to organize appropriate roles and formulate consistent rules.

Working with Children

Facilitate the child's ability to talk and to think about the abuse with decreasing anxiety. Create a safe and predictable environment in which the child feels supported. Make it clear to the child that you understand that talking about the abuse is difficult.

Plan interventions that will encourage affective release in a supportive environment. Child victims must be able to experience a range of emotions. Play therapy helps these children play out traumatic themes, fears, and distorted beliefs. It is a nonthreatening way to process thoughts and feelings associated with the abuse, both symbolically and directly. Art therapy provides an opportunity to express feelings for which there are no words. Therapeutic stories present the traumatic issues of abuse, link victims' feelings and behavior, and describe new coping methods. Journal writing can help children over age 10 cope with intrusive thoughts and feelings. They often choose to bring their journal into the one–to–one sessions with their therapist.

Empowering Survivors

Because the process of sexual abuse is disempowering, it is important to empower survivors. The focus on traumatic stress therapy treats the trauma while acknowledging the process and result of victimization. Developmental therapy focuses on the "gaps" in the personality that occurred during the abusive process such as trust issues, identity issues, and relationship issues. Loss therapy focuses on helping the survivors identify and grieve over the things they have lost during their childhood sexual abuse such as innocence, trust, nurturing, and memories.

In working with adult survivors, remember that they have been robbed of a sense of power and feel detached from others. Recovery includes restoring power and control. Be sure to avoid becoming a "rescuer," as that might send the message that clients are not capable of acting for themselves. Also be careful not to set yourself up as a powerful authority because that might recreate the type of relationship in which the abuse occurred. The most helpful approach is being an ally, collaborator, and supporter as clients struggle through the healing process. Point out instances in which they have taken control of their lives, and help them identify situations in which they are able to make self-respecting choices.

Supporting Spiritual Recovery

To recover from sexual abuse, survivors must place responsibility for the abuse where it belongs—100% with the offender. If they fail to do this, they will continue to be paralyzed by self-blame and guilt. For this reason, it is essential that you support the client's need for spiritual healing. Strategies for doing so are in the Caring for the Spirit feature.

Increasing Self-Esteem

Design interventions to increase self-esteem. Adult survivors have a continuous internal monologue of negative statements such as "You're weak, stupid, incompetent, unlovable, and unattractive." Negative statements become self-administered abuse and keep the survivor weak and powerless. Help clients become aware of the frequency and intensity of these negative thoughts. Teach them to consciously replace negative thoughts with positive ones. While this is often difficult at first, it becomes easier with practice.

Reducing Anxiety

Because adult survivors are often anxious, interventions to reduce anxiety are also necessary. Clients who learn progressive relaxation and controlled breathing are often able to avoid full-blown panic attacks. Teach the process, and talk clients through the stages of relaxation until they are able to reduce anxiety by themselves. When they are relaxed, instruct them to imagine a scene in which they feel safe and comfortable. Anytime they need to, they can return to this safe scene where they are in total control. Daily practice increases the effectiveness of these techniques (see Chapter 33∞).

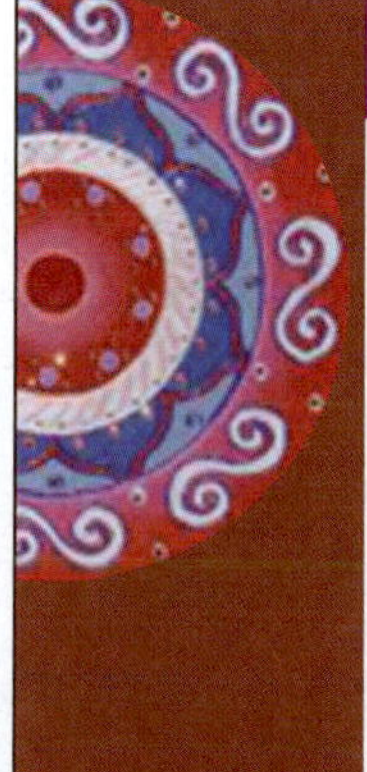

CARING FOR THE SPIRIT

Supporting Spiritual Recovery from Sexual Abuse

Betrayal by abusing adults is a spiritual issue. Therefore be sure to acknowledge a client's need for spiritual healing. Victims and survivors are consumed with spiritual questions such as "Why did it happen to me?", "What's wrong with me?", and "Am I an evil person?" When people are sexually abused, they must struggle with questions of a God who either overlooked their pain and did not respond or did not even see their pain at all. Questions arise, such as "What's wrong with God?" and "Why didn't God stop it?" It is not unusual for survivors to be angry with God and hold God responsible for the abuse. This anger may in turn trigger fear and guilt for hating someone so powerful.

Spirituality includes a sense of connectedness to others. Survivors must begin the long journey of developing trusting relationships. The adult self needs to reach out and care for the hurt inner child by breaking down the walls that have isolated that child. Fully experiencing the rage and grief enables the survivor to move on to self-forgiveness and more complete healing. Survivors need to experience human contact and the warmth of the nurse–client relationship. When requested, refer clients to religious counselors who understand the emotional issues surrounding sexual abuse and who are sensitive to the need of survivors to work slowly through their spiritual struggles.

Facilitating Healing

Art therapy helps adults in the healing process. Making group murals to express both individual progress and a sense of unity among clients can be very effective. Music therapy, combined with movement or dance, may be a way for clients to experience very early memories. Journal writing is used more than any other expressive therapy and can be expanded to include poetry, songs, and plays.

Group therapy allows survivors to share their feelings and experiences with others who believe their stories. The group setting fosters mutual understanding and decreases the sense of isolation. Many adult survivors find self-help groups to be very supportive in the process of healing (see Chapter 30).

Evaluation

Nurses in acute care settings may not have the opportunity for long-term evaluation. Short-term evaluation focuses mainly on identifying child victims and adult survivors and referring them to appropriate community resources.

Nurses in long-term or community settings can evaluate the effectiveness of the treatment plan over an extended period. Questions to guide the evaluation of the child victim and family include the following:

- Has the child remained safe from further harm?
- Has the child returned to functioning at an appropriate developmental level?
- Is the child able to express feelings either verbally or through play or art therapy?
- Is the child verbalizing decreasing feelings of guilt and/or responsibility?
- Is the child developing peer friendships?
- Has the family structure become more flexible?
- Is communication more open within the family?

As a nurse, you have the opportunity to influence the care of adult survivors of childhood sexual abuse. Explain to others that the survivors' behavior is a posttrauma response that makes sense as an adaptation to trauma and to a possibly dysfunctional family. Intervene if staff members recreate the dynamics of the abusive relationship by assuming a position of power and control.

Questions to guide the evaluation of adult survivors include:

- Has the client remained safe from further harm in adult relationships?
- Is the client able to talk about the childhood trauma? If not, is art therapy, music therapy, movement therapy, or journal writing effective in facilitating expression?
- Is the client able to identify situations in which he or she has been able, or hopes to be able, to make self-respecting choices?
- Is the client verbalizing increased spiritual comfort regarding the trauma?
- Is the client verbalizing less self-blame?
- Is the client verbalizing improved self-image?
- Is there evidence that the client is able to develop trusting and respectful relationships with adults?

Although, as a culture, we say that we protect our children, we do not in reality live out this value. We do not invest many of our energies—time, caring, and money—in the prevention of childhood sexual abuse. Our present approaches to treatment and to the social control of sexual abuse are not yet effective enough so we are assured of the long-term safety of children. Be encouraged to become active in the battle to stop childhood sexual abuse.

CASE MANAGEMENT

The first priority of care with child victims is to ensure the safety of the child. Nurses are mandated by law to report any suspected child sexual abuse. Protective services will implement one of four plans if the abuse is occurring within the family system:

1. The most frequent option is removing the abuser from the family. The nonabusing parent must protect the child from any contact with the abuser.
2. When the nonabusing parent is unable to protect the child, both the child and the abuser are removed from the home. This option maximizes the child's safety and decreases the child's feelings of responsibility.
3. In a few cases in which families have not used physical violence, there is no substance abuse, and there is someone who can ensure the child's safety, the family may be allowed to remain intact while participating in intensive therapy.
4. In a few instances, the child may be removed from the family when that is the safest option. Unfortunately, this decision may place additional guilt on the child.

COMMUNITY-BASED CARE AND HOME CARE

A community issue that touches the lives of women, in particular, is how women are treated by men in the workplace. If the environment is one that tacitly supports keeping women subordinate, then those women are being discriminated against. Sexual harassment of women in the workplace and in schools has always existed as a hidden crime. Only recently has it been recognized for what it is—discrimination against and violation of the victim. It is on one end of the continuum of sexual violence, the other end being childhood sexual abuse and rape. Girls and boys and women and men must be taught that they do not have to tolerate harassing behaviors. These behaviors include:

- Engaging in sexual teasing, jokes, remarks, or demeaning comments
- Making sexually stereotypical comments
- Showing offensive pictures

- Asking invasive questions regarding personal life
- Pressuring persistently for dates
- Communicating through letters, telephone calls, or e-mails of a sexual nature
- Making sexual gestures
- Deliberately touching, cornering, or pinching
- Watching invasively (such as leering, staring, following all actions)
- Pressuring for sexual favors
- Attempting or committing rape

Sexual harassment can lead to severe stress in the victims. Many experience depression, isolation, feelings of powerlessness, helplessness, fear, restlessness, inability to concentrate, somatic complaints, sexual problems, and loss of self-esteem. At its most severe, harassment resembles the other sexual traumas of rape and child sexual abuse and may result in post-traumatic stress disorder. The U.S. Equal Employment Opportunity Commission (EEOC) is the government agency that interprets and enforces employment laws. In 1980, the EEOC issued a position statement clearly stating that sexual harassment is a form of sexual discrimination and, therefore, an unlawful employment act. The intent of the law is to ensure a work environment that is free from sex-based discrimination and harassment.

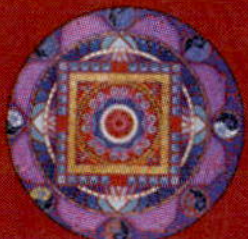

NURSING CARE PLAN
An Adult Survivor of Childhood Sexual Abuse

Identifying Information

Jill is a 35-year-old woman who is a full-time homemaker. Her husband, John, is president of an advertising firm. Jill and John have been married for 15 years and have three children, ages 14, 12, and 7.

Jill was sexually abused by her grandfather from a very young age until she was about 11 or 12. Sometimes the grandfather would involve Jill's brother, who is 3 years older, by forcing Jill and her brother to have sex for the grandfather's enjoyment. She states that she told her mother about the abuse when she was 9 or 10 but that her mother just ignored it. Her mother now denies that Jill told her about the abuse when it was occurring. Jill has tried to ignore her abuse history until several months ago when she saw a television program about incest. She has periods when she is filled with rage at her parents and grandfather.

History

No prior psychiatric history.

Jill was born and raised in Ohio and is the third child of five in an intact family. Jill describes her mother as "strict . . . she would threaten by saying 'wait until your dad comes home.'" When asked about her father, Jill states, "He wasn't around . . . he was working . . . he was always distant." She describes the family communication as "dysfunctional; only certain people talked to certain other people. For example, none of us kids could talk directly to our father. We always had to go through our mother."

Jill describes herself as a "homebody." In the past, she attended social functions with her husband as required by his professional position. These functions were not a great source of pleasure for her, however. Lately she has had no desire to participate in any activities outside the home. She states that she has never had close friends. Her only friend is her husband, and she feels somewhat intimidated by him. She has a very close relationship with her children.

Jill has no current or past medical problems. She states she is in good health except for feeling "terrible at times."

Current Mental Status

Jill is oriented to person, place, and time. Her affect appears dysphoric, irritable, and constricted in range. At times she is filled with rage, saying, "I am mad . . . mad at the world in general and at having to deal with all of this." She states that during her entire life she has spent much of her energy in "not thinking," "not imagining," and "not remembering" the abuse. She has attempted to keep a sense of distance from her inner emotional life. After viewing the television program on incest, she now experiences "painful, bitter, brooding thoughts about the abuse." Jill is an anxious and angry woman with extremely low self-esteem and intense feelings of inadequacy. She views herself as unable to function in an autonomous, self-directed, and self-reliant fashion and sees the world as untrustworthy, betraying, and often cruel. Unable to rely on her own resources or depend on the support of others, Jill feels a sense of bitter futility and resignation. She identifies herself as a victim who is inevitably betrayed and disappointed. Many of her dynamics are consistent with those of adult survivors of sexual abuse. She feels intense rage at her parents for being unsupportive, unprotective, and unable to provide her with a sense of safety and security in herself and in the world around her. This contributes to Jill's fear of autonomy and the conflict between her need to depend on others and her intense mistrust of the sincerity and commitment that others can offer. There is no evidence of psychotic illness or of a manifest thought disturbance.

Other Subjective or Objective Clinical Data

Jill states that she needs more emotional support from her husband. Her husband states that he has been unable to give it to her lately because he is often irritated at the mess and dirt in the house. She thinks he is being perfectionistic. He has offered to hire someone to help, but Jill sees that as another failure on her part.

(continued)

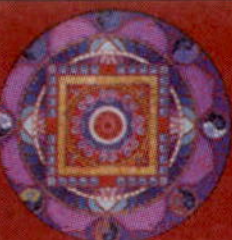

NURSING CARE PLAN
An Adult Survivor of Childhood Sexual Abuse *(continued)*

Nursing Diagnosis: Post-Trauma Syndrome related to being an adult survivor of incest.

Expected Outcome: Client will resolve associated anger and anxiety.

Short-Term Goals	Interventions	Rationales
Jill discharges the energy of her anger appropriately.	■ Discuss feelings of guilt. Repeat often that children are never responsible for the incest but rather that her grandfather is totally responsible.	Jill needs to place the responsibility for this abuse where it belongs.
	■ Discuss her feelings of anger toward the grandfather and her parents for not protecting her as a child.	Survivors of abuse frequently take blame for the incest.
	■ Connect feelings of low self-esteem to feelings of guilt and anger.	Jill's current interactions with others are based on what she learned from these experiences as a child.
	■ Assign journal keeping for recording feelings, thoughts, and memories.	
	■ Help Jill identify and grieve over things lost in childhood, such as innocence and trust.	
Jill uses relaxation exercises.	■ Teach anxiety-reducing techniques such as muscle relaxation, deep breathing, and physical exercise.	Handling stress and taking care of herself were not taught to her as a child by the adults who

Nursing Diagnosis: Social Isolation related to withdrawal and decreased desire to interact with others.

Expected Outcome: Client will increase interactions with people outside her family.

Short-Term Goals	Interventions	Rationales
Jill will be able to initiate relationships outside the family.	■ Help Jill identify the benefits of social interactions. ■ Help Jill identify a variety of available supportive people.	Jill may not know that she could feel better when she is in regular contact with other people.
	■ Give Jill positive feedback when she expresses an interest in or engages in interactions with others.	Jill will respond to positive feedback and be likely to continue to discover others by answering where, how, and when questions on social interactions.
	■ Provide assertiveness training.	Jill's ability to say "No" comfortably through assertiveness training will increase her comfort in relationships with others.
Jill will receive support and help from a self-help group.	■ Provide information on self-help groups for adult survivors where Jill can share with others and establish trusting relationships.	Self-help groups provide the opportunity to realize that one is not alone.

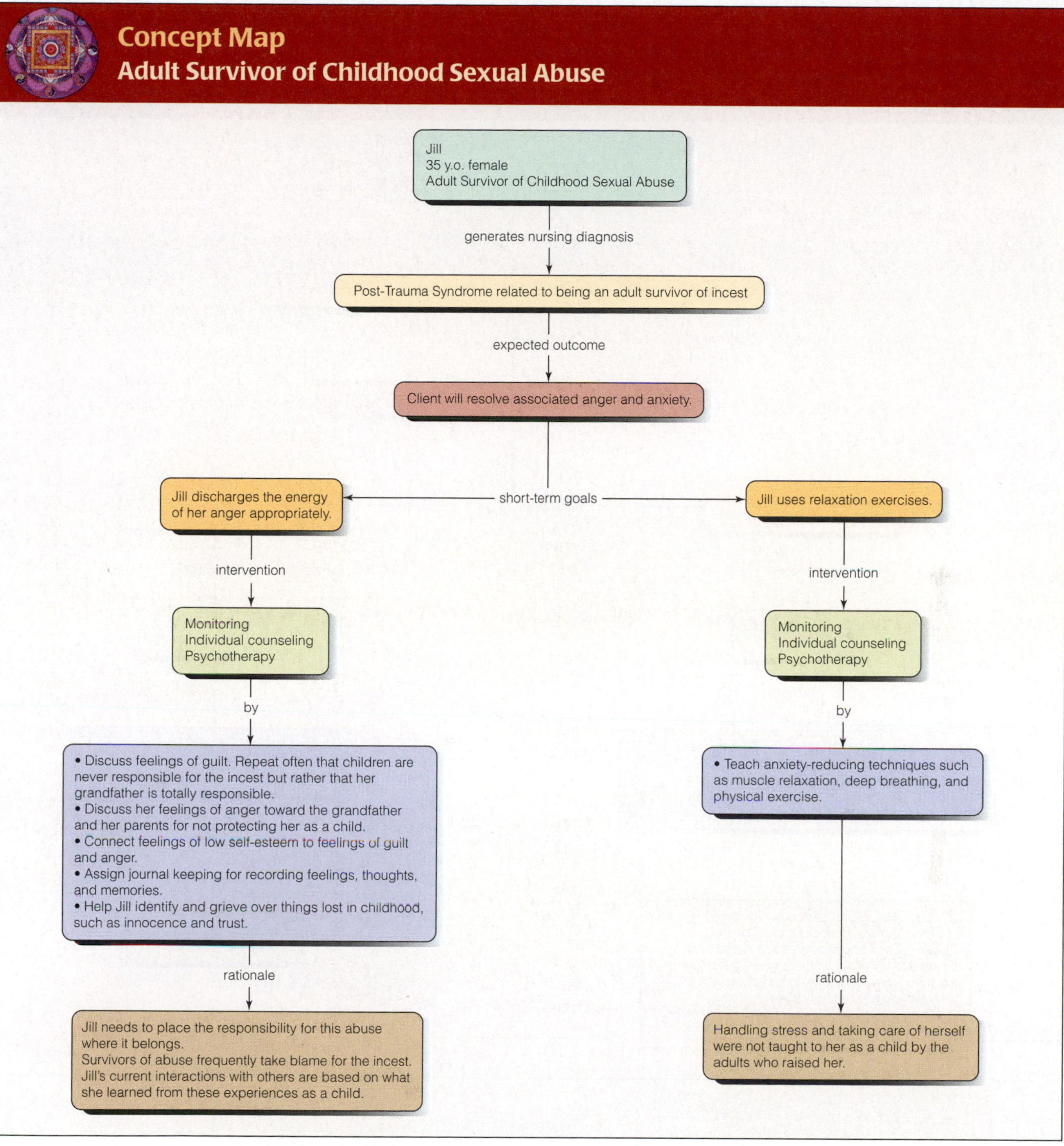
Concept Map
Adult Survivor of Childhood Sexual Abuse
Jill
35 y.o. female
Adult Survivor of Childhood Sexual Abuse
generates nursing diagnosis
Post-Trauma Syndrome related to being an adult survivor of incest
expected outcome
Client will resolve associated anger and anxiety.
short-term goals
Jill discharges the energy of her anger appropriately.
Jill uses relaxation exercises.
intervention
Monitoring
Individual counseling
Psychotherapy
by
• Discuss feelings of guilt. Repeat often that children are never responsible for the incest but rather that her grandfather is totally responsible.
• Discuss her feelings of anger toward the grandfather and her parents for not protecting her as a child.
• Connect feelings of low self-esteem to feelings of guilt and anger.
• Assign journal keeping for recording feelings, thoughts, and memories.
• Help Jill identify and grieve over things lost in childhood, such as innocence and trust.
rationale
Jill needs to place the responsibility for this abuse where it belongs.
Survivors of abuse frequently take blame for the incest.
Jill's current interactions with others are based on what she learned from these experiences as a child.
intervention
Monitoring
Individual counseling
Psychotherapy
by
• Teach anxiety-reducing techniques such as muscle relaxation, deep breathing, and physical exercise.
rationale
Handling stress and taking care of herself were not taught to her as a child by the adults who raised her.

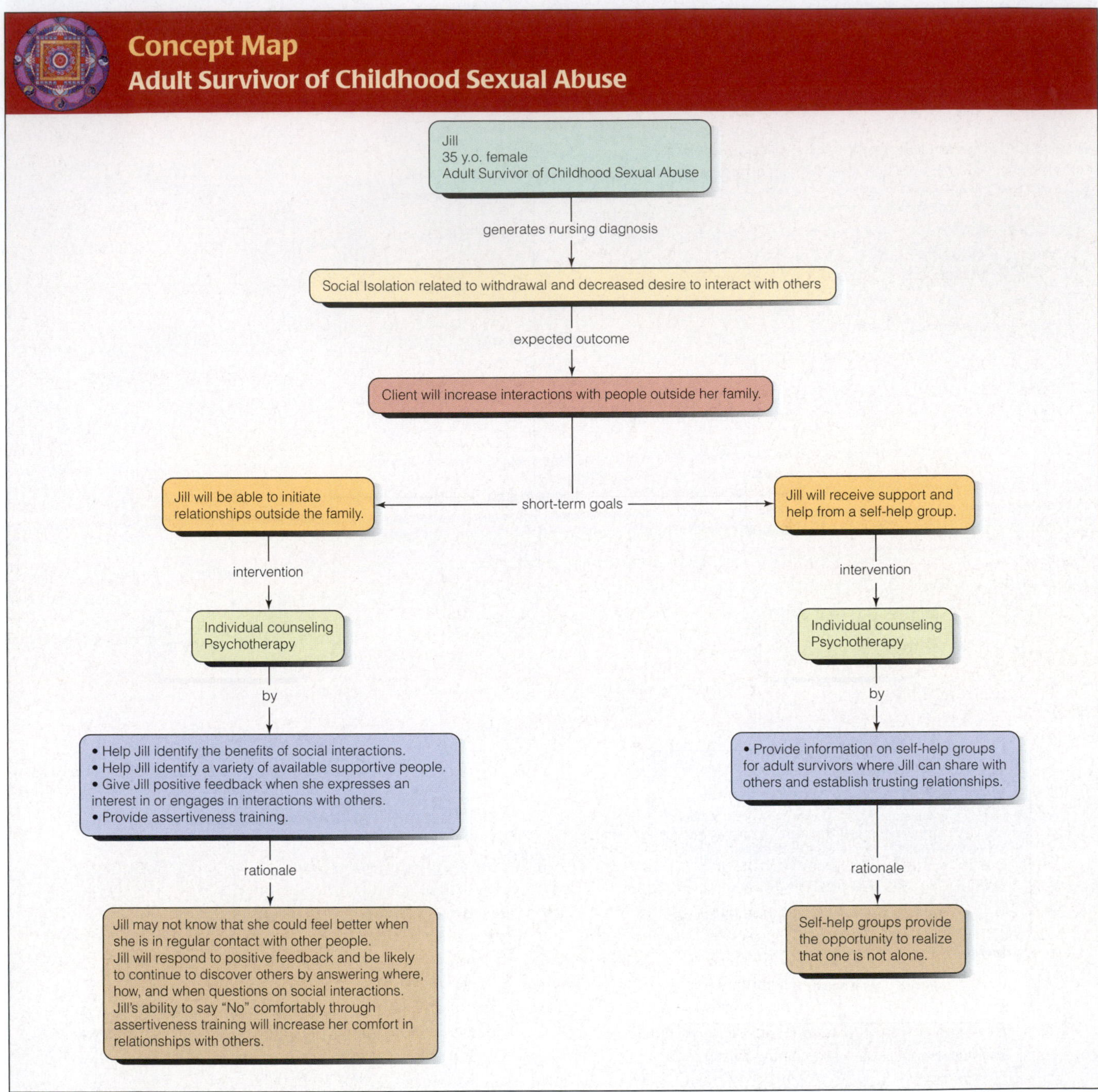
Concept Map
Adult Survivor of Childhood Sexual Abuse
Jill
35 y.o. female
Adult Survivor of Childhood Sexual Abuse
generates nursing diagnosis
Social Isolation related to withdrawal and decreased desire to interact with others
expected outcome
Client will increase interactions with people outside her family.
short-term goals
Jill will be able to initiate relationships outside the family.
intervention
Individual counseling
Psychotherapy
by
• Help Jill identify the benefits of social interactions.
• Help Jill identify a variety of available supportive people.
• Give Jill positive feedback when she expresses an interest in or engages in interactions with others.
• Provide assertiveness training.
rationale
Jill may not know that she could feel better when she is in regular contact with other people.
Jill will respond to positive feedback and be likely to continue to discover others by answering where, how, and when questions on social interactions.
Jill's ability to say "No" comfortably through assertiveness training will increase her comfort in relationships with others.
Jill will receive support and help from a self-help group.
intervention
Individual counseling
Psychotherapy
by
• Provide information on self-help groups for adult survivors where Jill can share with others and establish trusting relationships.
rationale
Self-help groups provide the opportunity to realize that one is not alone.

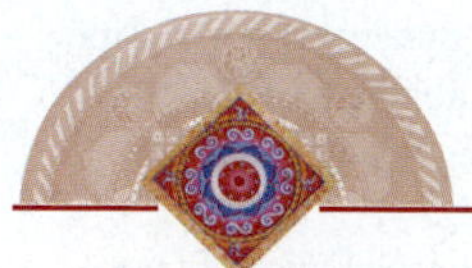

EXPLORE MEDIALINK

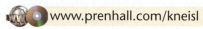

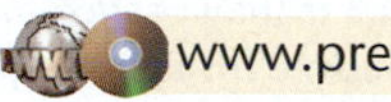 www.prenhall.com/kneisl

For NCLEX-RN® review questions, case studies, and other resources for this chapter see the Pearson Health MediaLink CD-ROM that accompanies this book and the Companion Website at www.prenhall.com/kneisl.

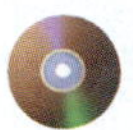

CD-ROM
Audio Glossary
NCLEX-RN® Review Questions
Video
- *Sexual Abuse Interview*

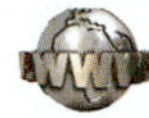

Companion Website
Audio Glossary
NCLEX-RN® Review Questions
Critical Thinking Exercise
- *Assessing the Rape Victim*

Case Study
- *Assessing the Needs of a Victim of Violence and Sexual Abuse*

Care Plan
- *Abuse in a Cultural Context*

MediaLinks
MediaLink Application
- *Understanding Women's Experiences Parenting in the Context of Domestic Violence*

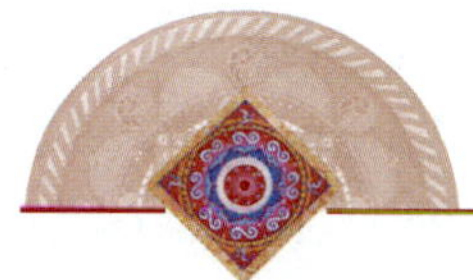

NCLEX-RN® REVIEW QUESTIONS

1. There are several biopsychosocial theories associated with causation of rape and intrafamily abuse. However, the nurse knows that:
1. Inability to control impulses is a consistent finding.
2. None of the contributing factors consistently results in or is predictive of rape or intrafamily abuse.
3. Stranger rape has a sexual connotation, while dynamics associated with family abuse relate to power and control.
4. The greatest predictor for intrafamily abuse is the perpetrator's history of abuse as a child.

2. According to systems theory, families in which sexual abuse occurs are characterized by which of the following?
1. Fluid boundaries
2. Openness with nonfamily members
3. Consistent equality within their structure and roles
4. High expressed emotion

3. The care plan formulated with your client includes the following goals: "Client reports fear, depression, and stranger anxiety as 'tolerable.' Client reports increased control over remembering. Client describes self as a rape 'survivor.' " For which client are these goals not appropriate?
1. Client in emergency room with a panic attack that the client associates with rape 6 months ago
2. Client in individual therapy 1 month after the rape
3. Client in primary care setting 3 months after the rape
4. Client in the emergency room immediately after the rape

4. Risk factors for intrafamily physical and sexual abuse include which of the following? (Select all that apply.)
1. Residence in low-income housing
2. Family's immigrant or refugee status
3. Family's primary language other than community's dominant language
4. Breadwinner's active military status
5. Continuous socioeconomic functioning below the poverty level

5. The interventions common to treatment plans for survivors include which of the following? (Select all that apply.)
1. Identify areas of control.
2. Remove the client from the home.
3. Support the client in the decisions he/she makes.
4. Encourage the client to pursue legal action.
5. Establish trust and rapport.

6. During an assessment in the emergency room, in the family's presence, you develop concerns about caregiver abuse. Your state requires you to report cases of suspected abuse. The family members repeat their explanation of the client's injuries. What do you say to them?
1. "I am required by law to report suspected abuse."
2. "I believe what you are telling me. Another health care provider may report this as suspected abuse, but I will not report this."

3. "Some state officials will be calling you in the next few days. Tell them what you told me."
4. You do not discuss your obligation to report with the family.

7. Spiritual distress is an important issue for survivors of violence because survivors often report a sense of:
1. Shame.
2. Responsibility for the violence.
3. Isolation.
4. Loss of control.

8. Your peer in the emergency department expresses frustration at the incidence of domestic violence in modern society and her inability to have an impact upon it. You respond, "I address my frustration by acting to decrease the incidence of domestic violence with activities every day." Your activities include which of the following? (Select all that apply.)
1. You role-model self-respect in the workplace.
2. You confront sexual harassment among pre-adolescents and adolescents.
3. During your assessment, you consider only certain clients at risk for experiencing violence.
4. During your assessment, you inquire about parenting challenges and interventions.
5. Your community association assists new residents to develop social support networks.

9. Self-awareness is essential in caring for the survivors of rape or violence. Possible outcomes from an absence of self-awareness include which of the following? (Select all that apply.)
1. The nurse may convey to the client that the client is not responsible for the violence.
2. The nurse may assume the perpetrator was a stranger.
3. The perpetrator's safety may be jeopardized.
4. The nurse may "normalize" behavior the client perceives as violent.
5. The client may feel obligated to defend the perpetrator.

10. Your peer, who works in the emergency department, asks you to identify characteristics of the typical perpetrator of child abuse. Which of the following statements should you include in your response?
1. "Abusers often have a long history of violent, criminal behavior."
2. "Perpetrators often present as pleasant, concerned individuals."
3. "Be alert to family members who appear agitated or almost out of control."
4. "As you interact with the perpetrators, it will become obvious they are mentally ill."

See Appendix C for answers.

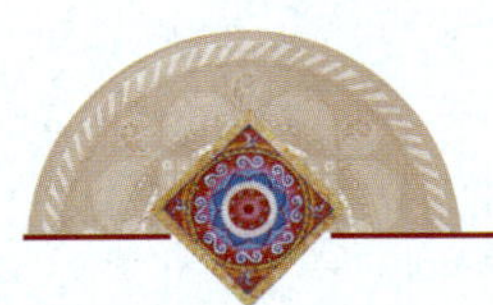

REFERENCES

Amar, A. F., & Gennaro, S. (2005). Dating violence in college women. *Nursing Research, 54*(4), 235–242.

Close, S. M. (2005). Dating violence prevention in middle school and high school youth. *Journal of Child and Adolescent Psychiatric Nursing, 18*(1), 2–9.

Daniels, K. (2005). Violence and depression. *Journal of Psychosocial Nursing, 43*(1), 45–51.

Edwards, V. J., Holden, G. W., Felitti, V. J., & Anda, R. F. (2003). Relationship between multiple forms of childhood maltreatment and adult mental health in community respondents. *American Journal of Psychiatry, 160*(8), 1453–1460.

Ewing, C. P. (1997). *Fatal families*. Thousand Oaks, CA: Sage.

French, K., Beynon, C., & Delaforce, J. (2007). Alcohol is the true "rape drug." *Nursing Standard, 21*(29), 26–27.

Friedman, S. H., Horwitz, S. M., & Resnick, P .J. (2005). Child murder by mothers. *American Journal of Psychiatry, 162*(9), 1578–1587.

Griffin, M. G., Resick. P. J., & Yehuda, R. (2005). Enhanced cortisol suppression following dexamethasone administration in domestic violence survivors. *American Journal of Psychiatry, 162*(6), 1192–1199.

Guttman, M., Mowder, B. A., & Yasik, A. E. (2006). The ACT against violence training program: A preliminary investigation of knowledge gained by early childhood professionals. *Professional Psychology: Research and Practice, 37*(6), 717–723.

Harris, G. T., Hilton, N. Z., Rice, M. E., & Eke, A. W. (2007). Children killed by genetic parents versus stepparents. *Evolution and Human Behavior, 28*(2), 8–95.

Heintz, A. J., & Melendez, R. M. (2006). Intimate partner violence and HIV/STD risk among lesbian, gay, bisexual, and transgender individuals. *Journal of Interpersonal Violence, 21*(2), 193–208.

Kaestle, C. E., Halpern, C. T., & Brown, J. D. (2007). Music videos, pro wrestling, and acceptance of date rape among middle school males and females: An exploratory analysis. *Journal of Adolescent Health, 40*(2), 185–187.

Kearney, M. H., Haggerty, L. A., Munro, B. H., & Hawkins, J. W. (2003). Birth outcomes and maternal morbidity in abused pregnant women with public versus private health insurance. *Journal of Nursing Scholarship, 35*(4), 345–349.

Levendosky, A. A., Leahy, K. L., Bogat, G. A., Davidson, W. S., & von Eye, A. (2006). Domestic violence, maternal parenting, maternal mental health, and infant externalizing behavior. *Journal of Family Psychology, 20*(4), 544–552.

Lips, H. M. (2004). *Sex and gender* (5th ed.). New York: McGraw-Hill.

Littleton, H., & Breitkopf, C. R. (2006). Coping with the experience of rape. *Psychology of Women Quarterly, 30*(1), 106–116.

Marleau, J. D. (2005). Birth order and fratricide. *Medicine, Science, and the Law, 45*(1), 52–56.

McCabe, M. P., & Wauchope, M. (2005). Behavioral characteristics of men accused of rape. *Archives of Sexual Behavior, 34*(2), 24–253.

McCloskey, J., & Bulechek, G. M. (1996). *Nursing interventions classification (NIC)* (2nd ed.). St. Louis, MO: Mosby.

McCloskey, K. A., & Raphael, D. N. (2005). Adult perpetrator gender asymmetries in child sexual assault victim selection. *Journal of Child Sexual Abuse, 14*(4), 1–24.

Muscari, M. E. (2005). What should I do when a client is being stalked? *Medscape Ask the Experts Advance Practice Nurse*. Retrieved February 4, 2005, from http://www.medscape.com/viewarticle/502450.

National Center for Victims of Crime. (2004). Domestic Violence Statistics. Retrieved March 1, 2006, from http://www.ncvc.org.

Patton, S. B. (2003). Understanding the murder of children and intervening to reduce the risk. *Topics in Advanced Practice Nursing eJournal, 3*(3), 1–8.

Pearsall, C. (2005). Forensic biomarkers of elder abuse. *Journal of Forensic Nursing, 19*(4), 182–186.

Rauch, S. A. M., & Foa, E. B. (2004). Sexual trauma. In B. T. Litz (Ed.), *Early interventions for trauma and traumatic loss* (pp. 216–240). New York: Guilford Press.

Rawson, C. (2007). Touch of kindness. *American Nurse Today, 2*(5), 64.

Salter, D., McMillan, D., Richards, M., Talbot, T., Hodges, J., Bentovim, A., et al. (2003). Development of sexually abusive behaviour in sexually victimised males: A longitudinal study. *Lancet, 361*(9356), 471–476.

Schetky, K. H. (1999). Sexual victimization of children. In J. A. Shaw (Ed.), *Sexual aggression* (pp. 107–128). Washington, DC: American Psychiatric Press.

Smyth, K. F., Goodman, L., & Glenn, C. (2006). The full-frame approach: A new response to marginalized women left behind by specialized services. *American Journal of Orthopsychiatry, 76*(4), 489–502.

Stermac, L., Dunlap, H., & Bainbridge, D. (2005). Sexual assault services delivered by SANES. *Journal of Forensic Nursing, 1*(3), 124–128.

Symes, L. (2000). Arriving at readiness to recover emotionally after sexual assault. *Archives of Psychiatric Nursing, 14*(1), 30–38.

Terra, F. S., & dos Santos, L. E. S. (2006). Domestic violence and children. *Revista Mineira de Enfermagem, 10*(3), 271–276.

Thoreson, E. J. (2006). In times of crises: Care of adolescent rape patients. *Journal for Undergraduate Nursing Scholarship, 8*(1), 4.

Valente, S. M. (2005). Sexual abuse of boys. *Journal of Child and Adolescent Psychiatric Nursing, 18*(1), 10–16.

Webb, R. T., Pickles, A. R., Appleby, L., Mortensen, P. B., & Abel, K. M. (2007). Death by unnatural causes during childhood and early adulthood in offspring of psychiatric inpatients. *Archives of General Psychiatry, 64*(3), 345–352.

Yamawaki, N. (2007). Rape perception and the function of ambivalent sexism and gender-role traditionality. *Journal of Interpersonal Violence, 22*(4), 406–423.

Yeager, J. C., & Fogel, J. (2006). Male disclosure of sexual abuse and rape. *Topics in Advanced Practice Nursing eJournal, 6*(1), 1–10.

Zlotnick, C., Johnson, D. M., & Kohn, R. (2006). Intimate partner violence and long-term psychosocial function in a national sample of American women. *Journal of Interpersonal Violence, 21*(2), 262–275.

ADDITIONAL REFERENCES

Bishop, S. E., Ellison, P. J., Ellisor, D. M., & Harper, C. J. (2007). Is your patient being abused? *Men in Nursing, 2*(3), 41–51.

Straus, M. A. (1994). *Beating the devil out of them: Corporal punishment in American families*. Lexington, MA: Lexington Books.

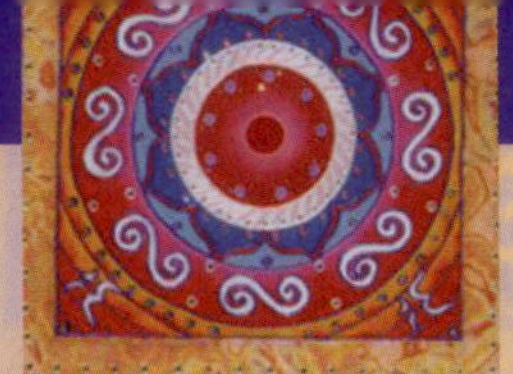

CHAPTER

25

Psychiatric–Mental Health Clients with HIV/AIDS

CAROL REN KNEISL

KEY TERMS

acquired immune deficiency syndrome (AIDS) *671*
harm reduction *683*
HIV-related dementia *677*
safer sex practices *682*

LEARNING OUTCOMES

After completing this chapter, you will be able to:

1. Explain why certain psychiatric populations are at risk for acquired immune deficiency syndrome (AIDS).
2. Describe the biopsychosocial impact of human immunodeficiency virus (HIV) infection.
3. Synthesize knowledge about neuropsychiatric manifestations into the care of psychiatric–mental health clients with HIV.
4. Modify the provision of direct nursing care to people with HIV disease in psychiatric settings.
5. Educate psychiatric–mental health clients, their families and friends, and people in the community about HIV risk-reduction education strategies related to sexual behavior and substance abuse.
6. Partner with and support caregivers of mental health clients with HIV and AIDS.
7. Provide comfort and mental health services to individuals experiencing AIDS-related bereavements.
8. Analyze personal feelings that may affect professional practice when caring for mentally disordered persons with HIV or AIDS.

CRITICAL THINKING CHALLENGE

The community in which you live is against a needle and syringe prescription program for injection drug users (IDUs), but is considering establishing a needle and syringe exchange program as an HIV/AIDS prevention strategy. At the town meeting, several people voice their concern that a needle and syringe exchange program would not only facilitate but also encourage illicit drug injection. Because you are a psychiatric–mental health nurse, you are asked to comment.

1. Does having access to clean needles and syringes make life easier for injection drug users?
2. Would having clean needles and syringes actually encourage people in the community to become illicit drug users?
3. Does a community have a responsibility to educate its members to prevent the transmission of HIV?
4. When you get up to speak, what would you say?

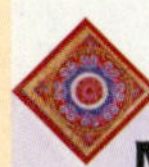

MEDIALINK 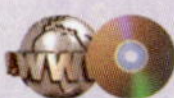 www.prenhall.com/kneisl

Go to the Pearson Health MediaLink CD-ROM and the Companion Website at www.prenhall.com/kneisl for interactive resources for this chapter.

A chronic, potentially life-threatening illness, **acquired immune deficiency syndrome (AIDS)** is of clinical concern to all nurses, but especially to psychiatric–mental health nurses, who, by nature of their commitment and responsibility, become involved in human experiences. Clients with the human immunodeficiency virus (HIV), the virus that causes AIDS, require care that promotes quality of life and personal growth now that HIV is a chronic disease with long-term survival.

Mood and anxiety disorders, particularly depression, and substance abuse commonly co-occur with HIV infection. It is not uncommon in HIV treatment settings to see clients with a mood or anxiety diagnosis (76% of whom had clinically relevant depression), a substance use diagnosis (21%), or both (8%) (Pence, Miller, Whetten, Eron, & Gaynes, 2006). Posttraumatic stress disorder was also frequent (11%). The burden of psychiatric disorders in this mixed urban and rural clinic population in the southeastern United States is comparable to that reported from other HIV-positive populations. These numbers exceed general population estimates of the comorbidity of mood and anxiety disorders with substance use disorders (Conway, Compton, Stinson, & Grant, 2006).

Promoting quality of life and personal growth can be achieved only when psychiatric–mental health nurses are knowledgeable about the disease itself and its comorbidity with mental disorders, and are sensitive to the issues common to the communities hardest hit by this chronic illness:

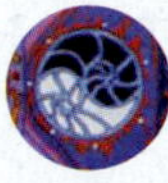

- Men who have sex with men, their partners, friends, children, and families of origin
- Male and female injection drug users (IDUs), their partners, friends, children, and families of origin, disproportionately represented in the African-American and Latino communities
- The fastest growing group of persons newly infected with HIV—heterosexual women

FIGURE 25-1 ■ illustrates the problem of AIDS in the United States by gender and transmission category among adults and adolescents. As you can see, high-risk heterosexual contact constitutes the largest transmission category. Second is injection drug use.

The focus of this chapter is on the understanding and skills essential to providing HIV/AIDS care to vulnerable psychiatric populations. This chapter is written with the assumption that, from earlier courses, you have basic knowledge of HIV disease, its cause, incidence and distribution, and modes of transmission; that you understand the basics of instituting universal precautions to protect yourself and others; and that you know how to provide physical care to people with HIV disease.

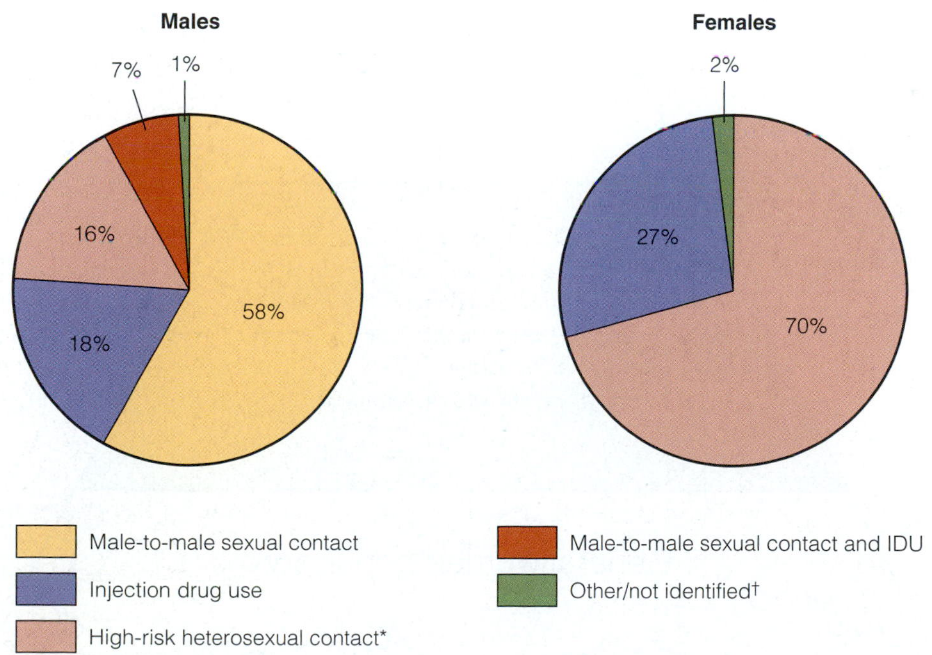

FIGURE 25-1 ■ Proportion of AIDS cases among adults and adolescents by sex and transmission category.

Source: Centers for Disease Control and Prevention. (2007). *HIV/AIDS surveillance report, 17*(6).

THE HIV MENTAL HEALTH SPECTRUM

Knox, Davis, and Friedrich (1994) identified a broad spectrum of people in the population with growing mental health care needs that are related to HIV. Their model of the HIV mental health spectrum remains relevant today and is illustrated in FIGURE 25-2 ■.

The General Worried Population

The general worried population makes up the majority of people in this country. Although worried about transmission of HIV, they perceive themselves to be personally unaffected—that is, they are not infected, are not close to someone who is infected, and believe, perhaps naively, that they do not practice behaviors that put them at high risk. Identifying and reducing fears, promoting knowledge and reducing social naivete, and encouraging behavioral change are crucial roles of mental health care providers with this population.

Health Care Providers

Irrational fears, prejudice, and stress can lead to burnout and reduce the quality of health care. Although it is crucial that mental health care workers help set the tone and example for others in the community for appropriate attitudes and practices regarding HIV infection, some are reluctant to work with HIV-infected individuals. They cite fear of contagion (as the result of an accidental needlestick or being cut with a sharp instrument) as a primary concern. However, studies of health care workers that documented parenteral or mucous membrane exposure to the blood or body fluids of HIV-infected people indicate that the incidence is extremely low. Additional concerns are discomfort in working with the terminally ill and discomfort with IDUs and men who have sex with men.

Worries about how best to protect themselves and their families are also common concerns. Providing empathic, supportive care requires confronting your own and your family's

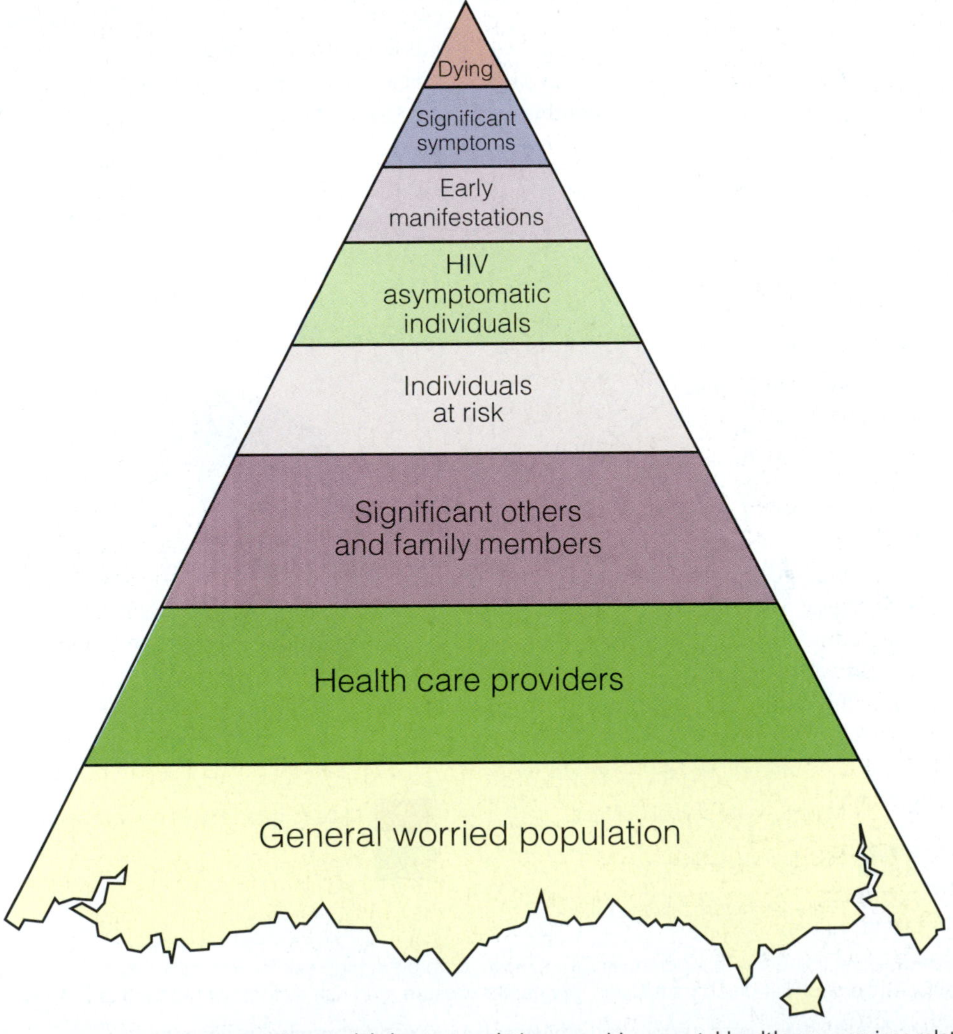

FIGURE 25-2 ■ The HIV–mental health spectrum. This model shows populations requiring mental health care services related to HIV. Cross-sectional size represents population size and diversity. Distance from the base represents increasingly direct emotional effects of HIV infection and the increasing need for mental health intervention.

Source: Adapted from Knox, M. D., Davis, M., & Friedrich, M. A. (1994). The HIV mental health spectrum. *Community Mental Health Journal, 30*(1), 77. Kluwer Academic/Plenum Publishers. Reprinted with kind permission from Springer Science and Business Media.

fear of infection as well as your own values and prejudices. (See also the section on ethical concerns and the Your Self-Awareness feature on page 679.)

Significant Others and Family Members

Significant others and family members face many emotional challenges. Many families are facing the emotional challenge of multiple HIV diagnoses and injection drug use within the family. Family secrets about sexual or drug use behavior may be publicly disclosed along with an HIV diagnosis. At the same time they cope with these problems, significant others and family members are often the mainstay of emotional support for the person with HIV. They assume the burden of providing emotional support while coping with their own fears, providing physical care, and anticipating, then grieving, their loss. The issue of bereavement associated with HIV and AIDS is addressed later in the chapter. Family burden is discussed in Chapter 30∞.

Individuals at Risk

Individuals at risk are those who are most likely to have or to contract HIV, due to past or current participation in high-risk activities. This specific group includes people who have not been tested for HIV and those who have received negative HIV antibody test results but are still considered at risk. Maladaptive human responses in individuals at risk could result in self-destructive and irresponsible behaviors such as unsafe sexual practices.

HIV-Seropositive (Asymptomatic) Individuals

One category of individuals affected by HIV is referred to in the Centers for Disease Control and Prevention (CDC) classification system as HIV-seropositive (asymptomatic). This group consists of people whose HIV antibody tests confirm the presence of the virus but as yet exhibit no symptoms associated with immune system suppression.

People who are HIV-seropositive (asymptomatic) may experience many of the same responses as individuals at risk, in addition to problems of impaired adjustment and the development of a sense of powerlessness. This may be manifested in a variety of ways, including chronic depression and decreasing motivation. As asymptomatic people begin to deal with the reality of their condition, you may be able to help them engage in health-seeking behaviors. Wellness activities not only promote physical health but also empower the individual, thus promoting mental health.

Individuals with HIV-Related Conditions

This category on the HIV mental health spectrum includes individuals with HIV-related conditions (HRCs). These people are referred to in the CDC classification system as HIV-seropositive (symptomatic).

Individuals with HRC have begun to experience the physical effects of immune system deterioration. In addition to having physical manifestations, they may experience complex psychosocial responses as well as the other human responses previously discussed. These may include altered role performance and self-concept disturbance related to losses, and changes in their perceptions and abilities secondary to the development of physical symptoms and limitations.

Individuals with AIDS

People with significant symptoms are those with a formal diagnosis of AIDS, as defined by CDC guidelines. They have potentially life-threatening complications because of extensive immune system suppression.

People with AIDS (PWAs) may experience any of the human responses of individuals throughout the HIV mental health spectrum. In addition, PWAs may experience a sense of hopelessness, social isolation, impaired social interactions, or spiritual distress associated with the effects of a chronic life-threatening illness.

Long-Term Survivors

Although not listed in the HIV mental health spectrum, there is one other group of people of clinical concern to psychiatric–mental health nurses. People who have outlived the generally expected life span for people with HIV and AIDS are called long-term survivors. As more individuals with HIV infection are identified and new treatments are discovered to slow or halt HIV progression in a predictable fashion, the number of long-term survivors will continue to increase. This has obvious implications for mental health care professionals working with people affected by HIV infection. As the number of long-term survivors who have benefited from highly active antiretroviral therapy (HAART) increases, psychiatric–mental health nurses should expect to see increasing numbers of people struggling with issues related to HIV infection.

HIV TRANSMISSION RISKS IN PSYCHIATRIC POPULATIONS

The research overwhelmingly indicates that the major modes of transmission of the virus are:

- Intimate unprotected sexual contact with an HIV-infected person (oral sex, vaginally insertive heterosexual intercourse, anally receptive sex)
- Parenteral injection of blood or blood products infected with HIV
- Transfer of the virus from an HIV-infected mother to a fetus or newborn infant in utero, during labor or delivery, or in the early newborn period during breastfeeding

Because of the nature of these major modes of transmission and the epidemiology of the epidemic in the United States, the following psychiatric–mental health populations are at high risk for contracting HIV:

- Intravenous drug users (because intravenous transmission is a major mode of transmission of the virus)
- The seriously mentally ill (because their judgment and problem-solving ability are compromised and they are likely to engage in unprotected sex)

MediaLink Application: Case Studies: HIV/AIDS

MediaLink Critical Thinking Exercise: Psychiatric Populations at Risk for HIV/AIDS

- The homeless mentally ill (because they often trade sex for drugs or money)
- Clients whose mental disorder causes them to act recklessly (because they are likely to engage in unprotected sex or inject drugs)

Substance Users

The literature evaluating the relationship between substance abuse and HIV has primarily focused on injection drug users (IDUs). The second largest transmission category for HIV in North America, Europe, and parts of Asia is injection drug use through the transfer of small amounts of blood in shared needles or syringes. Active IDUs who are also hazardous alcohol users are thought to be at particularly high risk. Injection drug users also constitute a bridge to others—their fetuses, newborns, and sex partners—putting them at increased risk. Unfortunately, 60.4% of IDUs minimize their HIV risk, appraising their risk of infection as nil or small (Brown, Outlaw, & Simpson, 2000).

More than 60% of people with AIDS in the United States are IDUs or the sexual partners of IDUs (Centers for Disease Control and Prevention [CDC], 2007). Of heterosexuals whose only known exposure was through sex with a person at risk, approximately two-thirds are female partners of male IDUs. Figure 25-3 ■ illustrates the distribution of IDU-associated AIDS cases by exposure category.

Research on the relationship between HIV and alcohol and cocaine use is of increased interest since substantially elevated rates of HIV infection are also present among crack cocaine users and individuals with at-risk drinking. Studies have found that drug use, both injection and noninjection, substantially increases the risk for HIV infection (Chander, Himelhoch, & Moore, 2006; Klinkenberg & Sacks, 2004). A population of concern because of persistent drug and sex risk behaviors is adolescents, especially those who have been brought to the attention of the juvenile justice system. Two studies that randomly sampled 800 juvenile detainees, aged 10 to 18 years, found that more than 60% of youths with a substance use disorder, either alone or with a comorbid major mental disorder, engaged in five or more sexual risk behaviors such as having multiple partners or unprotected vaginal sex (Romero et al., 2007; Teplin et al., 2005). Additionally, across all types and patterns of drug use, drug users were less likely to take antiretroviral medications and more likely to:

- Have suboptimal ambulatory care
- Miss scheduled appointments
- Use the emergency department
- Have unmet support services needs (Sohler et al., 2007)

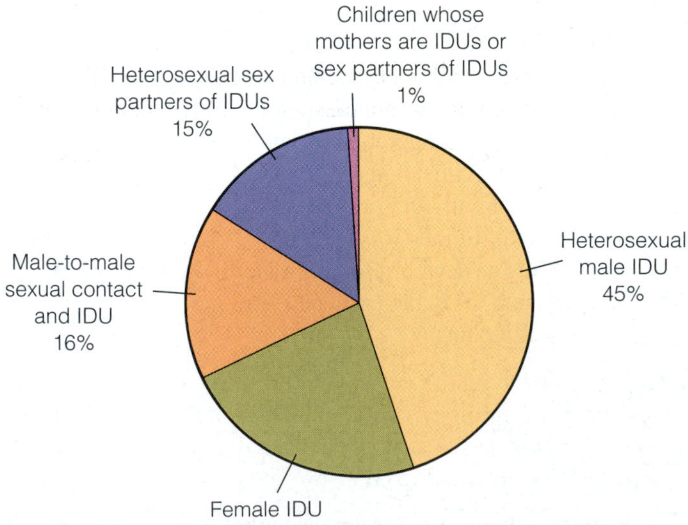

Figure 25-3 ■ IDU-associated AIDS cases by exposure category, United States.

Source: Centers for Disease Control and Prevention. (2007). *HIV/AIDS surveillance report, 17*(6).

Studies that look at age and gender differences in comorbid HIV and substance use report that older-aged adults (especially those with illicit drug use and at-risk drinking) were less likely to be receiving behavioral health care when there was evidence of need (Zanjani, Saboe, & Oslin, 2007), and women have unique vulnerabilities, especially those related to violence, physical abuse, and other traumatic events (Klinkenberg & Sacks, 2004).

The Seriously Mentally Ill

People with severe and persistent mental disorder are disproportionately affected by HIV/AIDS. Fully 50% of severely mentally ill adults in the United States are dually diagnosed with co-occurring substance use disorders and are at risk for HIV and hepatitis C infection (Rosenberg, Drake, Brunette, Wolford, & Marsh, 2005). It is for this reason that the Office on AIDS Research of the National Institutes of Health has identified the prevention and treatment of HIV in persons with serious mental illness as one of its highest priority research initiatives.

People with serious mental illness often engage in sexually risky behaviors that put them at elevated risk for HIV and other sexually transmitted infections (Meade, 2006). For example, a survey of adults with severe mental illness receiving outpatient psychiatric treatment found that the majority were sexually active (73%), had multiple sexual partners (45%), and had traded sex for drugs (21%) in the previous year (Meade & Sikkema, 2007). They were also eight times more likely to have injected illicit drugs and shared needles 7.4% of the time. In most studies of HIV among the seriously mentally ill, there are several consistent findings:

- Multiple sex partners
- Sex partners who are IDUs
- Absence of, or inconsistency in, condom use
- Frequent use of alcohol and drugs in conjunction with sex
- A history of sexually transmitted infections

According to Brown and Jemmott (2000), seriously and mentally ill persons are thought to be especially susceptible to HIV risk-related behaviors for the following reasons:

1. Poor judgment
2. Limited impulse control
3. Deficits in problem-solving skills
4. Suicidal intent
5. Self-destructive tendencies

Several of these risk-related behaviors are evident in the clinical example that follows.

CLINICAL EXAMPLE

On her last admission to the inpatient unit for treatment of a manic episode, Sadie had a persistent vaginal fungal infection that resisted treatment. HIV testing came back positive for the presence of HIV. Prior to this last admission, Sadie had not taken her lithium for 2 months. As Sadie's mania increased, so did her risk behavior. When elated, Sadie was game to try anything, from alcohol to crack cocaine to unprotected sex with men she met at several bars she frequented. Sadie felt invulnerable.

It is not unusual for mentally ill clients to meet sex partners in bars or mental health clinics or, as you have learned previously in this chapter, for their sexual activities to involve the exchange of money or drugs for sex.

In addition, mentally disordered clients are often ambivalent about abstinence and the need to reduce the risk of infection with a sex partner. They may see themselves as more helpless than others in the general population when it comes to reducing risk, or, on the contrary, they may view themselves as invincible.

Whether clients with HIV and severe mental illness receive adequate care is uncertain, and current research is attempting to answer this question. Generally, it seems that HIV clients with severe mental illness were more likely than those without severe mental illness to have difficulty obtaining care, according to interviews and chart reviews carried out in Los Angeles and New York City (Fremont et al., 2007). It is believed that case management and specialized programs that provide assistance to this specific population with HIV may be helping to narrow HIV health care disparities as a result of having serious mental illness (Bogart et al., 2006).

The Homeless Mentally Ill

The homeless mentally ill who live in urban areas, particularly those who live in municipal shelters, are at particular risk for HIV and other communicable diseases. The high incidence of injection drug use in this population, along with exchanging sex for drugs or money, makes them extremely vulnerable. The homeless mentally ill are likely to experience several barriers to beginning, maintaining, and completing treatment. Several practical matters—establishing a medication routine, having access to health care providers, having an actual address or telephone, and being supported by friends and family—are the usual barriers faced by homeless people. The specific cognitive barriers that result from mental illness and HIV infection add to the difficulty of obtaining prophylactic or early treatment.

THE BIOPSYCHOSOCIAL IMPACT OF HIV/AIDS

HIV affects the neurologic, neurocognitive, psychologic, developmental, sociocultural, economic, and ethical spheres of human life. One particularly exciting field of research that has contributed toward answering these questions is *psychoneuroimmunology* (discussed in Chapter 6∞), the study of the communication between the mind, the brain, the endocrine system, and the immune system. In particular, a growing body of evidence has demonstrated the interrelatedness of the body–mind–spirit connection and the immune system.

Belief in the interconnectedness of mind, body, and spirit has long been a tradition of nursing. Recent scientific advances in psychoneuroimmunology are important to nurses because they support the mind–body–spirit connection. There is widespread support for the use of holistic nursing practices and treatment approaches to boost the immune system. The Caring for the Spirit feature on page 676 discusses long-term survival from a psychoneuroimmunology perspective.

Neuropsychiatric

Studies suggest that physiologically based clinical neuropsychiatric manifestations or disorders are common among adult PWAs, although abnormal neurological signs have been found in children diagnosed with HIV before 3 years of age (Foster et al., 2006). A neurologic syndrome or neurocognitive impairment may be the first clinical manifestation of HIV disease. Neurocognitive changes associated with HIV consist of cognitive, behavior, and motor dysfunction (Ances & Ellis, 2007). Significant numbers of people with HIV experience neuropsychiatric manifestations for two major reasons:

1. Because the virus is capable of invading central nervous system (CNS) tissue, several of the opportunistic infections and neoplasms associated with AIDS also affect the CNS (see FIGURE 25-4 ■ on page 676).
2. Prescribed pharmacologic treatment may have neuropsychiatric side effects.

In addition to neurocognitive changes, more ominous changes—delirium, dementia, and coma—can occur.

Focal Brain Processes

The most common focal brain processes are toxoplasmosis (a parasitic opportunistic infection), cryptococcal meningitis (a fungal opportunistic infection), cytomegalovirus (CMV) encephalitis (a viral opportunistic infection), progressive multifocal leukoencephalopathy (PML, a viral opportunistic

MEDIALINK Case Study: The Biopsychosocial Impact of AIDS

MEDIALINK T-Cell Destruction by HIV Animation

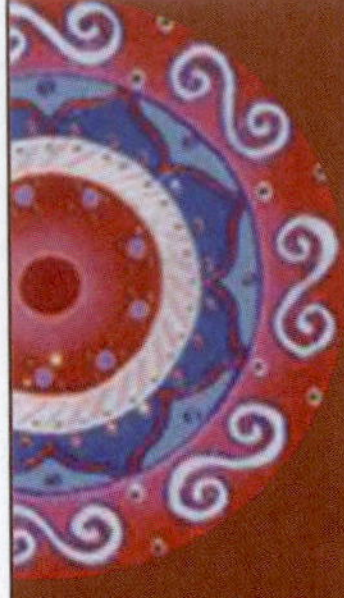

CARING FOR THE SPIRIT

Long-Term Survivors of HIV

Wars wage within our bodies every minute of every day. Most of the time we are unaware of the battles that go on within us. We have evolved legions of defenders—specialized cells that silently rout the unseen enemy. Their victories go unheralded. When our defenses are penetrated, our defenders are caught unprepared, or our defenders are routed and we've lost the battle. Then we develop a cold, the flu, or something worse. Why did I catch a cold from the sick toddler on the airplane when the woman next to me did not? Why didn't you come down with the flu when your roommate was sick? Why do only some of the people exposed to HIV develop the disease? Why do some people with HIV die within a year or two while others have survived, or even thrived, for 10, 20, or more years? We don't, as yet, have all the answers to these questions.

Perhaps the most common characteristics of people with AIDS who live long past the time predicted for them is their refusal to accept the diagnosis of HIV disease as a death sentence. They do not deny the diagnosis, but *they do defy the fatal outcome* that is supposed to be connected to it. Long-term survivors are extremely goal oriented and social. They treat their symptoms as if they were minor impediments in their lives; they are determined to prevail. Their immune systems seem to function better. They have higher T-cell counts and, in many cases, other immune system cells compensate for the ravaged T cells. Emotional distress, on the other hand, has been found to accompany negative immune function factors in HIV-infected individuals.

The highest incidence of illness and death occurs in people who experience stress after infection with HIV. This suggests that HIV-seropositive people should reduce their exposure to stressful events. Assertive coping, less stress, more self-nurturing, regular exercise, and a spiritual outlook have been associated with better immune status, suggesting that stress-reduction behaviors may be helpful in slowing the progression of HIV disease.

While we cannot promote the idea that clients are in total control of the disease process and the state of their health, or that the mind or the spirit can cure AIDS, we can and should teach clients the self-care and self-nurturing behaviors that long-term survivors are using to maintain their health. Assess the level of stress, quality of social support, and mood factors that influence the quality of life of people with HIV disease. Nursing interventions to help clients enhance neurologic, immunologic, and cognitive functioning should focus on improved nutrition, adequate sleep–wake patterns, hygiene, stress reduction, and social and spiritual support.

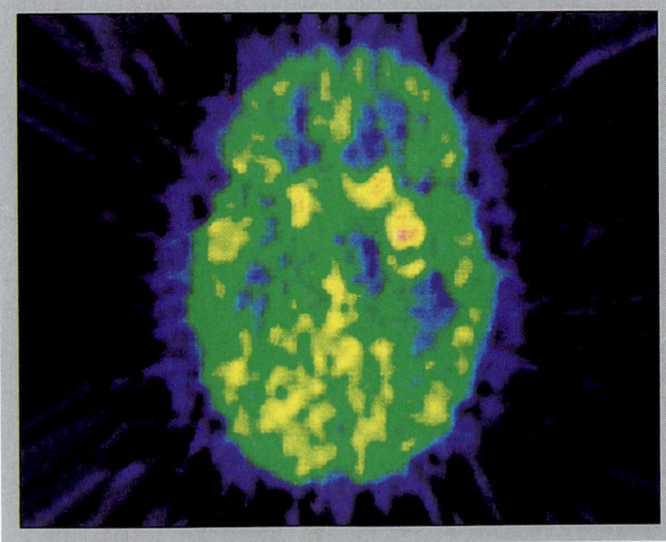

A

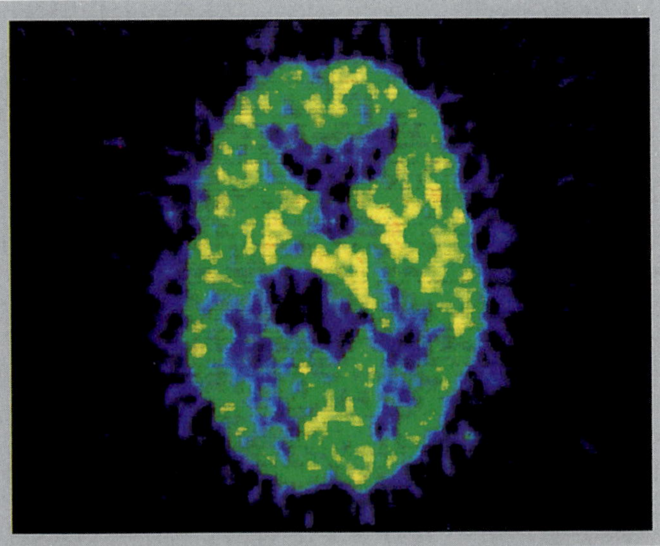

B

FIGURE 25-4 ■ Opportunistic HIV Diseases of the Brain. PET scans facilitate a neurologic diagnosis by distinguishing between hot lymphomas and metabolically cold toxoplasmosis. (A) PET scan of an HIV-related lymphoma, the metabolically hot tumor on the right side of the scan. (B) In contrast, this scan shows HIV-related toxoplasmosis, indicated by the dramatic "hole" of a metabolically cold area.

Source: Courtesy of Dr. Giovanni DiChiro and Dr. Ramesh Raman of the Neuroimaging Branch, National Institute of Neurological Disorders and Stroke, National Institute of Health.

infection), and CNS lymphoma (a neoplastic process). Signs and symptoms associated with these processes include focal deficits, altered level of consciousness, confusion, memory disturbances, headaches, and seizures.

Medication Side Effects

Several antiretroviral medications and medications used to treat associated symptoms and opportunistic infections cause significant neuropsychiatric side effects. For example, acyclovir, isoniazid, pentamidine, thiabendazole, vincristine, and zidovudine may cause hallucinations. Sleep disturbances—including insomnia, vivid dreams, and nightmares—can be a side effect of most of the medications listed earlier, as well as amphotericin B, cotrimoxazole, didanosine (ddI), interferon, procarbazine, stavudine (d4T), and steroids. Isoniazid can cause memory impairment. Several cause one or more of the following: agitation, anxiety, confusion, delirium, depression, headache, and irritability. Be sure to know which medications your clients receive in order to assess accurately the presence of neurological and emotional signs and symptoms.

HIV-Related Dementia

A syndrome caused by direct HIV infection of the CNS, **HIV-related dementia** (HIV-D) is characterized as a progressive dementia that involves a progressive slowing and loss of precision in both cognitive and motor functions, with accompanying behavioral disturbances. Its cause is not yet fully known. HIV infection is the most common preventable and treatable cause of dementia in persons under 50 years of age (Ances & Ellis, 2007).

The signs and symptoms of HIV-D include the following:

- Cognitive dysfunction: forgetfulness, loss of concentration, confusion, and slowness of thought
- Declining motor performance: loss of balance, muscle weakness, and deterioration in fine motor skills such as handwriting
- Behavioral changes: apathy, withdrawal, dysphoric mood, and regressed behavior
- Other symptoms such as headaches or seizures

HIV-D is often initially confused with psychiatric depression but may progress in a period of months to the point at which the affected individual is bedridden. Individuals with HIV-D also may quickly succumb to opportunistic infections because they are unable to take care of themselves.

The incidence of HIV-D has declined by 40% to 50% (McArthur, 2004) since the introduction of HAART in the 1990s. In addition, the progression of HIV-D appears to have been slowed by HAART, with most individuals now showing an attenuated form of dementia. Therefore, it is important to encourage clients to follow their medication regimen precisely.

Psychological

HIV disease threatens psychological integrity as well as physiologic integrity. Psychological syndromes associated with HIV infection are generally related to the initial diagnosis of HIV, crisis points along the HIV mental health spectrum, or adjustment to the experience of chronic illness or chronic loss. Increased suicide risk is relatively common among HIV-positive individuals and can result from illness-related burdens, alcohol and substance abuse, anxiety, and depression (Carrico et al., 2007), although people who identified themselves as Hispanic/Latino, were in a primary romantic relationship, and had greater self-efficacy for coping were less likely to report suicidal ideation.

The inherent lack of predictability and control, the fear of rejection and abandonment, hopelessness, and problems such as memory deficit and confusion also play a role. These factors, especially anxiety and depression, not only affect the client's quality of life but may also determine how closely the client adheres to the treatment plan (Holzemer, 2002).

Loss

The concept of loss is central to an understanding of the psychological impact of HIV and the depression, anxiety, and suicidal ideation that often accompany it. HIV disease is frequently linked with several different loss experiences for people with HIV and their families, friends, and caregivers. These include loss of the following:

- Energy, appetite, strength, and physical stamina
- Control of body functions such as elimination, mobility, speech, sight, hearing, and tactile sensations
- Control of body appearance due to dramatic weight loss, oozing wounds, skin breakdown, hair loss, skin lesions, or side effects of antiviral medications (e.g., persistent lipodystrophy syndrome)
- Self-worth and personal competence
- Mental clarity and cognitive ability
- Privacy
- Self-sufficiency and self-determination
- Employment, health insurance, salary
- Physical intimacy, including sexual expression
- Friends and lovers to earlier deaths from AIDS
- Social support
- Hope
- Peace of mind and spirit
- Life itself

Developmental

Most people with HIV disease are young adults or adults in their middle years. The period known as young adulthood is normally the healthiest and is characterized by peaks in muscular strength. Cognitive development should be completed and cognitive abilities should be refined at this stage. Recall that the psychosocial task of identity consolidation is the major developmental task of young adulthood. HIV disease may disrupt the person's ability to negotiate this challenge successfully.

Typically, the middle years are very productive in the arenas of work and family. During this period, adults consolidate relationships and occupational status and goals. HIV disease may interfere with the individual's ability to accept the responsibilities inherent in such roles as parent, worker, mate or partner, and so on. Questions of dependence and independence, thought to have been resolved previously, are reawakened as illness forces a return to earlier developmental phases.

Children and adolescents with HIV infection face delays or changes in skills on all developmental fronts—physical, cognitive, and psychosocial—as they confront acute life-threatening illness and chronic disability. In addition to the neurological difficulties discussed earlier in this chapter, children with severe HIV infection have more significant developmental delays on standardized developmental assessments than children with milder symptomatology (Foster et al., 2006). Increasing numbers of developmentally delayed children with HIV in industrialized countries are surviving into adult life.

Sociocultural and Economic

Although HIV/AIDS continues to be a leading public health issue in the United States, public focus on the epidemic as a significant social and political issue has waned in the new millennium. Webber (2000) believes that this waning of interest is taking place because HIV increasingly affects low-income people of color in urban areas, as well as women. Stigma and economic factors, including homelessness, combine to cause inequality in access to HIV care. In general, the poor have limited access to health services (Burnam et al., 2001).

Stigma

The sociocultural environment of people affected by HIV can be hostile to them. Most people with HIV are in one of two risk categories—men who have sex with men and injection drug users—that engender fear, anger, and prejudice. Persons in both risk categories experience stigma during hospitalization. There is some evidence to suggest that stigmatization by nurses of clients with HIV is based on the means by which HIV had been contracted. People who are IDUs express the greatest feeling of having been stigmatized (Surlis & Hyde, 2001). On the other hand, children with HIV disease or individuals who have contracted HIV from the transfusion of blood or a blood product are usually perceived as "innocents." However, they too may be feared and subject to discrimination.

Economic Factors

Days lost from work because of illness may cost people with HIV infection or AIDS their jobs and insurance benefits. Some insurers are avoiding or reducing claims by isolating high-risk applicants with HIV antibody tests, denying new policies to those at risk, and aggressively fighting existing policyholders' claims in court. Family and friends may be unable or unwilling to assist financially. Young adults find themselves having to seek public assistance such as Medicaid or rely on pharmaceutical companies for help in meeting the costs associated with HIV disease.

Adults who have a triple diagnosis—a combination of HIV, mental illness, and substance abuse problems—face significant income and employment problems. A study of the labor market found that for these clients the average income was below the poverty level, with more than two-thirds of their money coming from public income sources (Conover, Arno, Weaver, Ang, & Ettner, 2006). Although most private income comes from employment, less than 15% of this population had either full-time or part-time employment. Further, the likelihood of receiving disability or retirement income was lower among persons with the worst mental health.

AIDS services organizations (ASOs) provide a social and economic lifeline for people with AIDS. They provide emotional support counselors and pastoral counselors to the dying and their families; send out workers to clean, cook, shop, and provide transportation; run low-cost residences; and shuttle PWAs back and forth to hospital and clinic appointments. Programs such as these have helped lessen the financial impact of the disease. Unquestionably, HIV/AIDS presents an economic problem of severe proportions.

Homelessness

An increasingly critical problem is the lack of decent, appropriate housing for the growing number of people with HIV disease. HIV disease is disproportionately prevalent among individuals already at the economic edge and those who are targets of discrimination in housing and medical care: people of color, homosexuals, injection drug users, and homeless and runaway youths. In many communities around the country, available housing and services fall short of the need for appropriate residential care for thousands of people who have been made homeless by HIV-related illnesses, or whose struggle to survive on the streets has been worsened by the disease. Fatigue, repeated hospitalizations, and recurring illnesses all require time off from work, resulting first in the loss of employment, then in the loss of housing. The lack of effective risk-reduction education programs among the homeless has led to predictable and dramatic increases in HIV-seropositivity among them. Studies estimate the predicted number of homeless with HIV to be between 3% and 20% (National Coalition for the Homeless, 2002).

Although most people with an impaired immune system can live independently, they require a safe environment that helps them avoid exposure to infectious diseases, get adequate rest, meet their special nutritional needs, and have access to support services and home help when necessary.

ROLES FOR PSYCHIATRIC–MENTAL HEALTH NURSES

Psychiatric–mental health nurses work with clients all along the continuum of HIV infection and disability. You may be involved in working with people with HIV disease in inpatient settings in psychiatric hospitals, psychiatric units in general hospitals, mental health clinics, community health agencies, HIV day treatment programs, hospices or homes, private practice, industry, schools, or even as a citizen and neighbor. In addition, you will have an active role with healthy people, the family and friends of people with HIV, and bereaved survivors.

Delivering Ethical Care

Be aware that HIV-infected people are doubly stigmatized. They have an HIV diagnosis, and many are already members of other stigmatized groups. The ethical issues surrounding HIV/AIDS prompt many emotional responses. Review the ethical questions in the Your Self-Awareness feature while being conscious of your own emotional responses.

Several state nurses associations and national nursing organizations have published statements relative to nursing practice that clarify the professional nurse's responsibility in relation to the care of HIV-infected people. These statements and the Code of Ethics for Nurses of the American Nurses Association (ANA) (2001) address the need to provide appropriate care (both direct and indirect), health teaching, and advocacy regardless of the nature of the client's illness because of moral obligation. Be sure to familiarize yourself with your state nurses association's statement on the care of HIV-infected people. The advocacy role of nursing organizations in the United States, Canada, Australia, and New Zealand is discussed later in this chapter.

Providing a Therapeutic Milieu

Proactive preparation and programming are critical in allaying the anxiety of staff members and clients when incorporating people with HIV disease into a psychiatric–mental health setting. Both staff members and clients may have concerns about disease transmission, inadequate knowledge regarding HIV and AIDS, and lack of understanding of the needs and behavior of people with HIV disease.

Protecting Privacy

Be concerned with protecting clients' privacy. Clients experience breaches in confidentiality because of institutional policies that make their disease conspicuous and from nurses' nonchalance in handling information about their disease (Surlis & Hyde, 2001). Clients also consider the sharing of stigmatizing medical information among nurses and other medical personnel, without their prior consent, a breach of confidentiality and make decisions on where to seek care based on the staff's degree of professionalism. Obviously, clients who do not trust that you will respect their privacy are likely not to be forthcoming.

Modifying Agency Policies and Procedures

Special arrangements may need to be made for the scheduling of activities, visiting policies in an inpatient setting, and the provision of physical treatments, depending on the physical and neuropsychiatric manifestations of the disease and the extent of HIV disease progression. Staff will need to make individual decisions on a case-by-case basis. Clear communication with staff members and other clients is necessary for promoting consistency and preventing disruption of the milieu as a result of perceived inequities.

Clients with neurologic manifestations may present a special challenge to the staff and to the therapeutic environment. Their behavior may be erratic, frightening, and unlike that of the usual psychiatric client. This may require modification of usual unit procedure or activities. It may become necessary to exclude some clients, such as those with HIV dementia, from certain activities that risk their safety or to bend the rules to keep clients involved.

Not all clients react favorably to the presence of PWAs. Clients with paranoid disorders tend to have the greatest difficulty in accepting clients with HIV. They may become hostile, incorporate AIDS into paranoid delusions, insist on being transferred to another mental health facility, or insist that PWAs be transferred elsewhere.

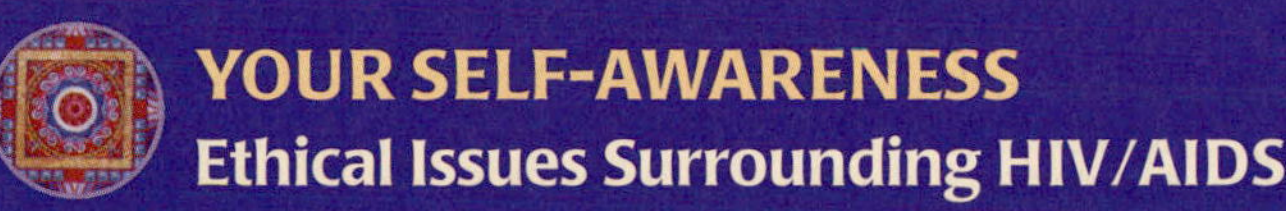

YOUR SELF-AWARENESS
Ethical Issues Surrounding HIV/AIDS

Engage in the process of ethical reflection discussed in Chapter 13 to analyze these and other issues to avoid further stigmatizing people with HIV disease.

- Should HIV antibody testing be made mandatory? If so, who should be tested: gay men, IDUs, pregnant women, people admitted to hospitals, prisoners, couples applying for marriage licenses, food handlers, health care workers, child care workers, people applying for health and life insurance—everyone?
- Is it in the public interest to identify, report, and make public the names of HIV-infected individuals or those at risk for HIV?
- Should people with HIV/AIDS be placed in quarantine for the public good?
- Can or should employers suspend, terminate, or refuse to hire people with HIV/AIDS? If they are teachers? Food handlers? Health care workers?
- Can or should insurance companies deny HIV-related medical insurance claims and life insurance policy claims?
- Should people who have had sexual contact with people with HIV or have received infected blood products be traced and informed by public health authorities?
- Should people infected with HIV be tattooed to protect potential sex partners from infection?
- Do health care workers have a duty to inform those at risk when a person with HIV does not modify high-risk behavior?
- Can, or should, nurses or other health care professionals refuse to provide care to people with HIV disease?

You can help other clients by providing education, offering support, allowing them to vent their fears and express their concerns, and emphasizing that the care of HIV clients is an important and normal part of the facility's routine.

Implementing Infection Control Precautions

The use of standard infection control precautions in a psychiatric–mental health setting can also help minimize staff and client anxiety. Not all people with HIV (both staff and clients) are aware of their status or feel comfortable disclosing the information even if they are aware. Standard precautions, as prescribed by the CDC, will protect all staff members and clients against the transmission of HIV. This approach promotes confidentiality because appropriate precautions are taken in the care of all clients.

Giving Direct Care

Psychiatric hospitalization may be needed because the client is depressed, suicidal, or psychotic or has an AIDS-related behavior disturbance, probably because of a focal brain disorder or HIV-related dementia. Nursing care for clients with depression, suicidal ideation, psychosis, dementia, and delirium has been discussed in earlier chapters in this text (see Chapters 17, 23, 16, and 14). Incorporate these principles into your care of clients with HIV as appropriate.

Psychiatric–mental health nurses caring for clients with HIV or AIDS on inpatient units encounter a number of issues that are uncommon in psychiatric settings:

- The client may have a multitude of physical problems.
- The client has a condition that calls for infection control precautions.
- The quality of the nurse–client relationship is intensified through the additional contact required in giving physical care.
- The common problems of adherence to prescribed psychotropic medication become more complex because clients need also to be faithful to antiretroviral and other AIDS-related pharmacologic regimens (see Chapter 32 and Your Intervention Strategies: Adherence Enhancers on page 392 in Chapter 16 for guidelines to enhance adherence) and must contend with unwelcome side effects from antiretrovirals and antipsychotics.
- Physical problems can be mistaken as psychiatric problems, and vice versa. For example, it is important not to mistake delirium for depression (see Table 14-1 on page 300).
- Psychiatric–mental health nurses, who very seldom work with dying clients, find it necessary to confront the issue of caring for clients with life-threatening illnesses.

Using Touch

A necessary modification in the care of clients with HIV/AIDS has to do with the use of touch. The physical care needs of AIDS clients require modifying the usual psychiatric injunction of limiting physical contact with clients. Because AIDS is such an isolating and stigmatizing condition, giving a massage or holding the client's hand has therapeutic value.

A variety of complementary and alternative therapies may be appropriate. For example, you might incorporate some of the complementary and alternative therapies, such as relaxation techniques, visualization, imagery, or massage, that are discussed in Chapter 33. Caring for clients with a dual diagnosis that includes HIV disease requires creative modification.

Providing Support Group Services

It may be beneficial to set up a separate support group for people with HIV disease, where they can discuss issues specific to HIV/AIDS in a supportive setting. If there aren't enough HIV clients for a group, then an AIDS service organization, such as the one described in the clinical example that follows, may provide support group services.

CLINICAL EXAMPLE

Jorge, an outpatient client at a mental health clinic based in a medium-size northeastern city, has both bipolar disorder and HIV disease. Jorge and Bill, his life partner, had recently returned to the city of their birth after an absence of 15 years. Although Jorge comes from a large family, he has very limited contact with his family. Most of his family members are having trouble accepting Jorge's homosexuality. Bill and his family have taken on the caregiving responsibility for Jorge; however, Bill is becoming concerned about the extent of the emotional and physical care he needs to provide for Jorge since Bill is trying to manage his own alcohol abuse.

The psychiatric–mental health nurse at the mental health clinic made a phone call to a local ASO, AIDS Family Services, and referred Jorge and Bill. The ASO offers several services—a support group for family members, friends, and partners; and a 12-step spirituality group—from which both Jorge and Bill could benefit.

An ASO can also be an important resource for HIV clients after discharge. The range of services available depends on the structure of the ASO but frequently includes counseling, support groups, buddy programs, educational programs, pastoral care, spirituality programs, financial assistance, housing referral, legal aid, and client advocacy.

Clients with neuropsychiatric disorders such as HIV dementia may offer the greatest challenge to staff members. Three important but frequently ignored nursing diagnoses that apply to clients with neuropsychiatric disorders are:

1. Impaired Verbal Communication
2. Spiritual Distress
3. Impaired Home Maintenance

Clients with neuropsychiatric manifestations of HIV disease often have special discharge planning needs or experience

MEDIALINK Care Plan: The Care of Clients with Mental Illness Who Have AIDS

placement problems. Intervention strategies appropriate to these three selected nursing diagnoses are discussed in the following sections.

Intervening in Impaired Communication

Evidence exists that clients with both HIV infection and psychiatric disorders may not receive optimal care because their psychiatric disorders are a barrier to communication with health care workers. Incorporate the facilitative communication principles discussed in Chapter 10 in your work with these clients.

Dementia and other cognitive problems are also barriers to communication. Because a client's symptoms are generally progressive, interventions do not reverse the dementia but may enhance the quality of life for both the client and the primary caregiver. Here are several strategies:

- Convey unconditional positive regard, maintain a relationship, and maintain a sense of normality in interactions.
- Make verbal communication clear, concise, and unhurried; be sure to have the person's attention before starting; encourage the person to communicate; be comfortable with periods of silence; be aware of tone and volume of voice (this may prevent misperceptions).
- Use brief, direct statements: "Bob, eat this pudding" rather than "Why don't you and I have some pudding for dessert?"
- Ask questions that require only simple yes or no answers, and make only one request at a time.
- Be sensitive to the need to restate statements or questions at intervals.
- Reintroduce yourself as often as necessary; the client may have memory loss.
- Remember that nonverbal communication and touch are important; nonverbal communication may eventually become the primary communication mode between the client and the nurse or the client and the primary caregiver.
- Remember who the person was in the past, because reminiscence and validation are important; provide familiar stimuli.
- Use empathy and carefully analyze behaviors and statements to understand what is happening (for example, when a person who is at home says, "I want to go home"); support the person's feelings.
- Provide an environment of sheltered freedom, that is, the least restrictive level that is safe (unhurried, consistent, structured, with decreased external stimulation).
- Avoid mechanical or chemical restraints as much as possible.
- Avoid infantilizing the person, but remember that you may need to set firm limits.
- Be flexible, try different approaches, and share information.

Intervening in Spiritual Distress

Spiritual distress is usually evidenced by guilt, recriminations and self-blame, hyperreligiosity, rejection of significant others, and expressions of despair. Guidelines for working with clients experiencing spiritual distress include:

- Give the person permission to experience personal feelings, no matter what they are, and encourage appropriate expression of these feelings.
- Accept the fact that primary caregivers may not be able to listen to the client's feelings. If the primary caregiver delegates this job, recognize the distress it may cause both the client and the primary caregiver.
- Recognize the stages of grieving, and allow people to progress at their own rate; don't push the client into a stage that you think is necessary.
- Share spiritual resources as appropriate; encourage the person to find comforting spiritual outlets (poetry or other literature may be used to encourage reflection).

Be sure to familiarize yourself with the nursing strategies recommended earlier in the Caring for the Spirit feature on page 676.

Prayer as a complementary health strategy to cope with HIV-related anxiety, depression, fatigue, and nausea is an interest of nurse researchers. When data were analyzed from an ethnically diverse convenience sample of 1,071 adults, the researchers found that older African-Americans, Hispanics, and females were more like to use prayer (Coleman, Eller, et al., 2006). A study of African-American men and women and their use of prayer found the following: More women than men were likely to use prayer as a means of coping with fatigue, while men were more likely to use prayer to cope with nausea and depression. There was no gender difference in the use of prayer to manage anxiety (Coleman, Holzemer, et al., 2006). Prayer was reported as a self-care strategy by over 50% of those who participated in the study for three of the four symptoms (fatigue, nausea, anxiety, depression). The respondents rated prayer as highly effective as a self-care strategy for symptom management.

Having a spiritual connection was found to be a positive factor for long-term survivors. In a study designed to measure both spirituality and religiousness, Ironson et al. (2002) found that long-term survivors scored higher than an HIV-positive comparison group on four factors—sense of peace, faith in God, religious behavior, and compassionate view of others. Long-term survival was also correlated positively to frequency of prayer and negatively to judgmental attitude.

Enhancing Home Maintenance Management

The following list gives guidelines for enhancing care in the home and community:

- If the client is in an inpatient setting, begin planning for discharge as soon as the client is admitted to the facility.

MEDIALINK Centers for Disease Control and Prevention

- Assess the client's abilities to function in the home as well as the family's or primary caregiver's abilities to function in the home and the housing or home environment itself.
- Make referrals to home care professionals and other community agencies.
- Help the primary caregiver determine the appropriate level of care and realistically assess his or her own ability to provide home care; explore all role responsibilities and related factors; assist in redefining and prioritizing roles and functions.
- Determine the primary caregiver's learning needs, and facilitate the development of skills by identifying specific symptoms (such as memory loss) and developing strategies to address those symptoms.
- Arrange for respite care for primary caregivers.
- Provide emotional support to clients and primary caregivers, and refer them to additional support systems.

You can also refer clients and their families to a guide for home care of persons with HIV/AIDS from the Centers for Disease Control and Prevention. The CDC site can be accessed through a resource link on the Companion Website for this book.

Providing Risk Reduction Education and Counseling

Taking a leading role in risk reduction education and counseling is a crucial responsibility of all nurses. Teaching risk reduction can best be accomplished by listening, informing, and supporting clients in making choices that reduce their risk. Risk reduction education is directed toward three broad goals:

1. Educating clients, the public, other professionals, colleagues, friends, and neighbors in strategies to reduce the risk of contracting or spreading HIV
2. Counteracting the myths, stereotypes, and hysteria that surround HIV and AIDS
3. Correcting misinformation

Before implementing risk reduction and prevention programs for people at risk for contracting HIV, consult current CDC guidelines at http://www.cdc.gov, which is available through a resource link on the Companion Website for this book.

Sexual Behavior

Some experts fear that educating people about **safer sex practices** (avoiding the risk of HIV infection by preventing the transmission of body fluids during sexual activity) generates a false sense of security. These experts say the only safe sex is no sex. Realistically, however, abstinence is not a lifelong change that will be maintained by many. Counseling about high-risk sexual behaviors, low-risk sexual behaviors, and risk-free sexual behaviors makes more sense, especially in terms of the goals outlined in the previous list.

High-risk sexual behaviors are those in which there is an exchange of blood or body fluids. Receptive anal intercourse is thought to be of highest risk because of the trauma caused to the mucous membranes of the rectum. Any sexual activities that involve tissue trauma or exchange of blood or body fluids that may transmit HIV are high risk. This includes wet kissing (French kissing), fellatio (oral–penile contact), and cunnilingus (oral–vaginal contact) when there are breaks in the mucous membrane of the mouth, as well as the sharing of sex toys.

The use of condoms (a barrier protection placed on the penis to prevent the transmission of body fluids during sexual activity) is important in minimizing risk, but in order to be effective they must be used, and they must be used correctly. The Partnering with Clients and Families feature will provide you with information about effective condom use to share with clients and their significant others. As you will note, effective use requires more than simply rolling a condom onto a penis.

Since HIV is most commonly transmitted through sex, being sexually active without taking proper precautions is definitely high-risk behavior. It is crucial to understand that a person does not simply go to bed with one other person. When one calculates the possible length of the HIV latency period, a person goes to bed with everyone in the other person's entire sex history for approximately the past 10 years. FIGURE 25-5 ■ is a sobering illustration of one couple's hypothetical sex history.

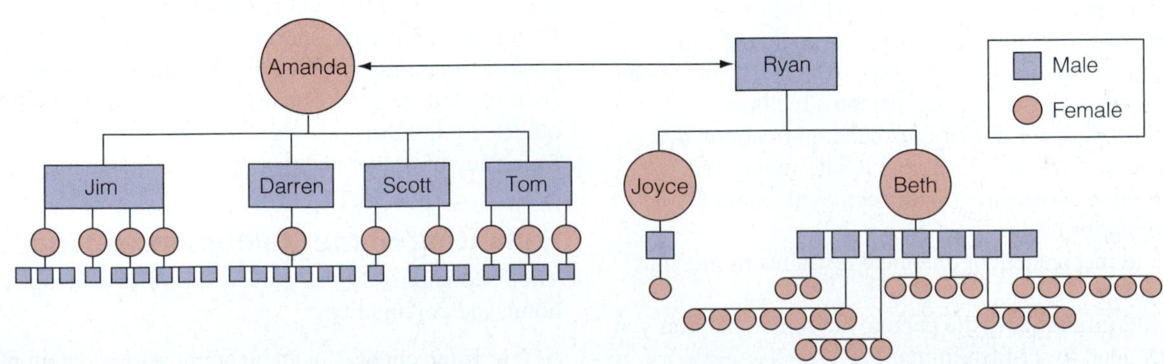

FIGURE 25-5 ■ A Hypothetical Sex History. Amanda and Ryan think that they are only having sex with one another. However, they are hypothetically having sex with each other's sex partners for approximately the past 10 years (the HIV latency period). Imagine tracing the sex history of the last row of sex partners. The explosive geometric progression could not be contained on one page.

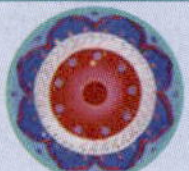

PARTNERING WITH CLIENTS AND FAMILIES

TEACHING ABOUT EFFECTIVE CONDOM USE

Remember to include the following information about condoms in any risk-reduction program. Remind clients to use a new condom for each act of vaginal, anal, or oral sex.

- Latex condoms are safer to use than natural or lambskin condoms. *HIV may be small enough to pass through the pores in natural condoms.*
- Condoms with reservoir tips are safer than those without. *A reservoir tip provides space for the semen and helps prevent breakage.*
- Do not open condom packages until use. Open packages carefully. *This helps to prevent damage from rough handling or jagged fingernails.*
- Store condoms in a dark, cool, dry place. *Excessive heat or cold, sunlight, and moisture can damage the latex. Therefore, a wallet is not a good place to store a condom.*
- Apply the condom before any genital contact. Use the condom throughout sex from start to finish. *Semen and seminal fluid may be discharged in advance of ejaculation.*
- Place the condom at the tip of the erect penis and gently press the air out of the condom tip. *Air bubbles can cause condoms to break.*
- Hold the condom at the tip, roll it down, and smooth it over the entire erect penis. Uncircumcised men should pull back the foreskin before applying the condom. *This provides a more effective seal.*
- Use a water-based product for lubrication. *Insufficient lubrication can cause condoms to tear or pull off. Oil-based lubricants such as petroleum jelly, baby oil, vegetable oil, mineral oil, cold cream, or hand lotion may cause the latex to disintegrate.*
- After ejaculating, but before losing the erection, the man should hold the base of the condom firmly while gently withdrawing the penis. *This prevents the escape of semen from the condom.*
- Safely discard, and never reuse, a condom.

Substance Use

Prevention of risk to sex partners is important because IDUs who use heroin, cocaine, or amphetamine serve as a bridge for transmitting HIV to their sex partners or to fetuses and newborns. However, there are other less well-known links to noninjection substance use and HIV. The use of poppers (volatile amyl and butyl nitrates in breakable glass capsules inhaled to enhance sexual pleasure) may be a cofactor in the susceptibility to HIV and in the development of AIDS because they are thought to lead to a generalized suppression of the immune system. Alcohol, as well as drugs such as amphetamines, cocaine, and marijuana, are also thought to damage the immune system. Another factor is lessened inhibition; that is, with loss of inhibition, a person under the influence of alcohol or drugs is more likely to engage in high-risk activities.

A general counseling plan for clients with a dual diagnosis of HIV disease and substance use is given in the Your Intervention Strategies feature.

Harm Reduction Realistic approaches to HIV risk-reduction education for IDUs consist of more than information about, and encouragement to obtain treatment for, substance abuse. According to the **harm reduction** approach, those who are not ready for treatment must be counseled on how to reduce the risk to themselves and to others. As a concept, harm reduction respects work on any positive change as a person defines it for himself or herself (Bigg, 2001) and focuses on minimizing the personal and social harms and costs associated with the spread of HIV through drug use. The major goal is to see to it that IDUs protect themselves against HIV and other life-threatening diseases such as hepatitis C. Because harm reduction does not seek to eliminate drug use, it is considered controversial in several quarters. You can learn more about harm reduction by accessing the website of the Harm Reduction Coalition, a national advocacy organization for individuals and communities affected by drug use, through a link on this text's Companion Website.

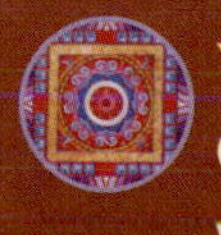

YOUR INTERVENTION STRATEGIES
Counseling Plan for Clients with a Dual Diagnosis of HIV and Substance Use

In addition to the general counseling and risk-prevention teaching for anyone with HIV, incorporate the following steps into an intervention plan for a substance-using client with HIV.

- Confront denial or lack of commitment to minimize risk behavior.
- Check the need for, and the depth of, motivation for referral to chemical dependence or alcohol treatment programs.
- Encourage joining or continuing a commitment to the recovery process in treatment for chemical dependence or alcoholism.
- Help the client verbalize feelings of anger, grief, and loss generated by the diagnosis; the need for change in sexual and drug use behavior; possible delay in childbearing; or the fear of having exposed others to HIV or doing so through continued risk behavior.
- Stress the need to use tools learned in recovery from chemical dependence and alcoholism in coping with this life crisis.
- Continue to confront the drug abuse as you would with clients not diagnosed with HIV.
- Involve the client in a harm reduction program.

MEDIALINK Harm Reduction Coalition

The best way to prevent transmission is, of course, to stop injecting drugs. IDUs' risks to themselves derive from the practice of sharing drug use equipment with others. In a realistic world, many people will be unable or unwilling to discontinue injecting drugs. Teach these clients to never share injectable drugs, needles, syringes, cookers (for heating solutions) or cottons (for filtering solutions) or other drug paraphernalia with others. The next best way to prevent transmission is for clients to use new, sterile needles and syringes, from a reliable source, each time they inject drugs. As an HIV prevention strategy, increasing numbers of states (approximately 40) are providing needle and syringe exchange programs or writing laws to allow health care providers to prescribe needles and syringes, and pharmacists to dispense them. The ANA has supported needle and syringe exchange programs since 1993 (ANA, 1997).

If the user cannot stop injecting; does not have a new, sterile syringe; and is about to inject with a syringe that has been used before, then a backup prevention strategy is for the client to clean his or her "works" (syringe and needle) (Abdala, Crowe, Tolstov, & Heimer, 2004). Remind clients to clean needles immediately after use to reduce sterilization problems caused by clotted blood. First, fill the syringe with water and shake—this dislodges particles and thoroughly mixes the water with material in the syringe—as often as necessary to remove blood or other debris. Then, flush with fresh, full-strength bleach (held for 30 seconds) and then with water, three separate times. You should, however, inform clients that *cleaning used "works" with bleach does not guarantee that all viruses have been killed and should be done only when there is no safer alternative*. Plastic syringes are usually designed for one-time use and can be damaged by bleach. External conditions may also affect the reliability of cleaning one's "works." For example, withdrawal symptoms or the threat of being seen by others (police, family) may drive an IDU to inject without disinfecting.

Studies report that needle and syringe exchange programs have played a significant role in lowering the rates of needle sharing in the Netherlands, Australia, the United Kingdom, and the United States. Studies also report that needle and syringe exchange programs have served as sources of referrals into drug treatment programs. Additionally, these programs recapture used and potentially infectious syringes for safe disposal. The Evidence-Based Practice feature provides an example of the nursing role in risk prevention and harm reduction.

Supporting Caregivers

You can be a vital support link for the wide spectrum of people who are caregivers of persons with HIV disease. This spectrum includes nurses and other health care professionals; the family members, friends, and same-sex partners of people with HIV; firefighters, police officers, and correction officers; and community volunteers. Nurses are now and will continue to be the health care professionals who are the front-line workers in providing health care to increasing numbers of people with HIV/AIDS.

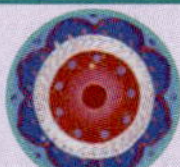

EVIDENCE-BASED PRACTICE

HIV RISK PREVENTION AND HARM REDUCTION

Donald is a 35-year-old client on the inpatient unit in which you work. He is ready for discharge after his second admission for schizophrenia. Donald is also an IDU. He has injected drugs for 8 years and been in several substance abuse programs over this period of time. Each time, Donald has returned to using heroin.

During this admission, Donald consented to testing for the presence of HIV. The test came back positive. Donald is being treated with several medications to control the symptoms of his schizophrenia and to treat the HIV. In a conversation with Donald, you discover that he has been sharing needles with others. When you express concern, Donald tells you not to worry; he rinses his syringes and needles with water when he uses them, and sometimes with bleach.

You immediately institute risk prevention and harm reduction teaching. You tell Donald that HIV is often transmitted through shared injection equipment, that cleansing with water will not wash away HIV, and that bleach is not a safe alternative. Using sterile, never-used needles and syringes is the best answer. You plan to meet with Donald later in the afternoon after you've had an opportunity to investigate needle and syringe exchange programs in your community and the availability of physician prescription and/or pharmacist dispensing programs for IDUs. You will also contact the mental health outreach team that services Donald's neighborhood and the buddy program of AIDS Family Services to link Donald with a support group and a medication maintenance program.

These suggestions stem from the following research:

Abdala, N., Crowe, M., Tolstov, Y., & Heimer, R. (2004). Survival of human immunodeficiency virus type 1 after rinsing injection syringes with different cleaning solutions. *Substance Use and Misuse, 39*(4), 581–600.

Hilton, B. A., Thompson, R., Moore-Dempsey, L., & Janzen, R. G. (2001). Harm reduction theories and strategies for control of human immunodeficiency virus: A review of the literature. *Journal of Advanced Nursing, 33*(3), 357–370.

CRITICAL THINKING APPLICATION

1. Donald keeps injecting drugs despite having participated in several substance abuse programs. What circumstances probably interfere with Donald's ability to be successful at kicking his habit?
2. What can the buddy program of AIDS Family Services provide that you cannot?
3. What problems of adherence to antiretroviral medications would you anticipate with Donald?

Caring for people with HIV requires participation as a client advocate, effective multidisciplinary collaboration, and the ability to make appropriate referrals. To address the needs of this group adequately, one needs the ability to empathize with the individual with HIV and with primary caregivers and to act on the basis of that empathy. A primary caregiver is a person who is generally responsible for providing or coordinating daily care for a PWA who cannot perform self-care activities. Usually, a primary caregiver is a nonprofessional who is a significant other (life partner, spouse, family member, or close friend) of the person with AIDS.

Special emotional stamina is needed to care for PWAs. Not only must nurses and other caregivers care for and comfort those who face great suffering and death, they also care for and comfort those infected with the virus who have not developed the disease. At the same time they provide help, nurses must cope with their fears for their own and their family's health (especially if the nurses themselves are members of a risk group) and their own pain in caring for people who do not get well or whose future is uncertain.

Specifically, our skills and knowledge make us able to:

- Facilitate caregivers' expression of fears and concerns
- Help caregivers acknowledge their susceptibility to increased stress and burnout in AIDS work
- Instruct caregivers in complementary and alternative therapies (see Chapter 33∞)
- Identify what needs to be reorganized and renegotiated in the work environment to maintain the health of caregivers and clients, such as: staff support groups, networking with AIDS providers in other agencies and communities, respite time for staff, time off to attend funerals or memorial services, rearranging staff assignments to avoid overloading or overburdening particular staff members, or creating getaway space for staff in the work setting
- Provide help to caregivers unaccustomed to dealing with delirium and dementia, who may have unrealistic expectations about the client's ability to adhere to procedures and treatment as mental capacities diminish (see Chapter 14∞)

Providing Bereavement Support

Millions of people will experience AIDS-related bereavements. There are several groups of people to whom the psychiatric–mental health nurse can provide bereavement support. The most obvious is the person with AIDS who grieves over a potentially fatal diagnosis, the loss of other friends or family to the disease, or any of the several other losses discussed in the section on the biopsychosocial impact of HIV/AIDS. In particular, clients who have sustained multiple and repetitive losses are at risk for depression. The bereavement coping challenges they face can be especially difficult and pronounced.

Bereavement support to family, friends, same-sex partners, and caregivers should continue after death has occurred. Home visits to friends, lovers, and family members demonstrate your continuing interest and concern for the survivors' well-being, as illustrated in the following clinical example.

CLINICAL EXAMPLE

When Antoine died of complications of AIDS, Jim, his nurse, made a home visit to Antoine's family. Jim helped Antoine's wife, children, mother, and three brothers plan remembrance rituals for a memorial service for Antoine. They asked Jim to participate in the memorial service by sharing his memories of Antoine's personal resilience and love of his family and friends.

Bereavement support groups and individual and family counseling can all be helpful, depending on individual situations and the availability of volunteers and professionals.

To provide adequate bereavement support to the survivors of people with AIDS (SOPWAs), it is important to consider a number of factors. SOPWAs represent a diverse segment of society:

1. Sex partners of PWAs
2. Children of PWAs
3. Parents and siblings of PWAs
4. Friends of PWAs
5. Health care providers of PWAs

Some SOPWAs may be in high-risk groups or may have HIV disease themselves, while some may have been unaware of the significant other's sexuality or lifestyle until diagnosis or death. Some survivors may have been responsible for the transmission of HIV, and many are members of minority groups and have few resources.

SOPWAs are often characterized by several factors that place them at high risk for complicated grief reaction. These factors are identified in the Your Assessment Approach feature on page 686. It is important to assess survivors for the presence of these factors, which can interfere with adaptive grieving. Be aware that many SOPWAs have been on a hope roller-coaster ride as hope waxes and wanes with the arrival or perceived failure of treatment (Kelly, 2007). For many survivors, caregiving became a part of the self and the death of the loved one results in the loss of a relationship that contributed significance and meaning to life (Cadell & Marshall, 2007). Individual or group bereavement interventions can help survivors engage in the grief process in an adaptive fashion.

Promoting Self-Help and Social Support

Self-help is one way in which persons with HIV disease can move to reestablish a sense of self-control and reduce feelings of helplessness and powerlessness. Self-help can occur on several levels, depending on the client's physical and mental abilities and motivation. Clients should participate as much as possible in their own care and in decision making that affects them. Encourage clients to join peer support groups and engage in HIV/AIDS advocacy activities in their communities.

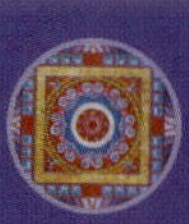

YOUR ASSESSMENT APPROACH
High-Risk Bereavement Factors for SOPWAs

Stigma

Sources

- Discomfort with illness, death, and grief
- Sexuality and drug use often associated with HIV/AIDS
- Confusion and hysteria associated with HIV/AIDS

Results for SOPWAs

- May need to mask the cause of death to self and others
- Community may not recognize the significance of the loss
- Support from others in mourning the loss or expressing feelings associated with bereavement may be absent

Ambivalence

Sources

- Strained relationship with PWA

Results for SOPWAs

- May feel guilt
- Progress in the grief process may be blocked

Untimely Nature of Death

Sources

- Facing issues of mortality
- Generally young age of PWAs

Results for SOPWAs

- Anxiety, despair
- Unprepared to accept the death

Concurrent Life Crises

Sources

- Fear of the possibility of having been exposed to a fatal illness
- Guilt if the survivor feels he or she may have transmitted HIV
- Experiencing the deaths of many other PWAs

Results for SOPWAs

- Anger associated with being a SOPWA
- Helplessness associated with being a SOPWA
- Recurring need to grieve for many other PWAs

MediaLink Self-Help and Social Support Resources

Peer support may be associated with higher adherence to treatment regimens and lower depressive symptomatology (Simoni, Pantalone, Plummer, & Huang, 2007). Negative mood and lower social support are related to avoidance-oriented coping strategies. Use of these coping strategies by clients on HAART is related to poorer medication adherence and, subsequently, higher viral load (Weaver et al., 2005). Some of the many resources available to you and your clients are as follows:

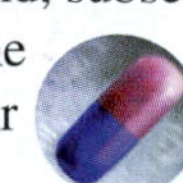

- For general information on prevention, see www.cdcnpin.org (CDC National Prevention Information Network)
- For general information and lists of AIDS organizations and support groups, see www.aegis.com (AIDS Education Global Information System)
- For general information on treatment and clinical trials, see www.amfar.org (American Foundation for AIDS Research)
- For information on research on AIDS and mental health, see www.nih.gov/oa/ (NIH Center for Mental Health Research on AIDS)

Direct links to all of these resources can be found on the Companion Website for this book.

Clients may benefit from such activities as nutritional counseling and psychological counseling. Boosting the immune system also helps keep people healthy. Stress-management techniques and visualization and imagery for self-healing and pain and symptom control (such as those discussed in Chapter 33) are believed to boost the immune system by reducing stress.

Incorporating Research

Psychiatric–mental health nurses have a direct role in research and an indirect role in supporting ongoing research and encouraging the undertaking and funding of new research. Being knowledgeable about the current research and incorporating it into clinical practice enables the psychiatric–mental health nurse to act on the basis of what is currently known or supposed (see Chapter 4). For example, there is a growing body of knowledge about quality of life and how it affects the physical, psychological, and social well-being of people affected by HIV.

Participating in Advocacy and Political Activism

Persons with HIV disease and their loved ones need advocates. Psychiatric–mental health nurses can be effective advocates, as shown in the clinical example that follows, by speaking out against dehumanizing measures that threaten well-being.

CLINICAL EXAMPLE

A proposition was introduced in California that could have forced public health officials to establish camps to quarantine people with AIDS, as well as anyone infected by HIV, whether healthy or unhealthy. This measure would also have flatly banned HIV-seropositive people from attending or teaching in public schools or holding jobs that involve food handling. The California Nurses Association was among the groups that actively spoke against the proposition and contributed to its failure.

As a citizen and an advocate, you need to be politically aware of pending legislation and move to influence it in a positive direction.

Earlier in this chapter, brief mention was made of nurses associations with published statements about the care of people with AIDS and the role of nurses. National specialty groups such as the Association of Nurses in AIDS Care (ANAC) are also active in mobilizing the professional and political resources of the nursing community in the United States. In association with the ANA, ANAC has published a set of standards of practice for nurses who work with clients with HIV infection (2006). You can access the website of ANAC via the Companion Website for this book. Canadian nurses can contact the Canadian Association of Nurses in AIDS Care (CANAC). AIDS nursing organizations in Australia and New Zealand are affiliated with ANAC, as are several AIDS nursing organizations around the globe.

It is every nurse's responsibility to find out what nursing groups are accomplishing or not accomplishing at local, state, and national levels. A good place to start is at the local level, by becoming involved in community AIDS councils, self-help groups, and nursing organizations. Local involvement is a bridge to state and national involvement. You can also be part of a nationwide effort to lobby for adequate public and private funding for research, education, prevention, treatment, and a cure for HIV/AIDS.

MEDIALINK AIDS Nursing Organizations

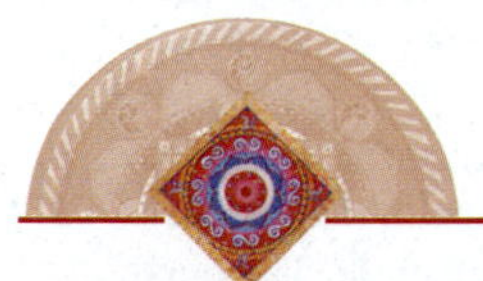

EXPLORE MEDIALINK

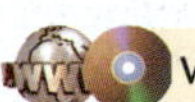

www.prenhall.com/kneisl

For NCLEX-RN® review questions, case studies, and other resources for this chapter see the Pearson Health MediaLink CD-ROM that accompanies this book and the Companion Website at www.prenhall.com/kneisl.

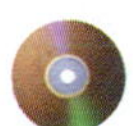

CD-ROM
Audio Glossary
NCLEX-RN® Review Questions
Animation
- *T-Cell Destruction by HIV*

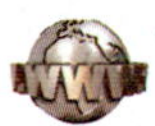

Companion Website
Audio Glossary
NCLEX-RN® Review Questions
Critical Thinking Exercise
- *Psychiatric Populations at Risk for HIV/AIDS*

Case Study
- *The Biopsychosocial Impact of HIV/AIDS*

Care Plan
- *The Care of Clients with Mental Illness Who Have AIDS*

MediaLinks
MediaLink Application
- *Case Studies: HIV/AIDS*

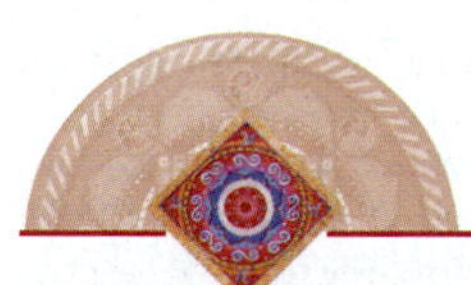

NCLEX-RN® REVIEW QUESTIONS

1. Risk factors that increase the risk of the individual with serious mental illness being affected by human immunodeficiency virus (HIV)/acquired immune deficiency syndrome (AIDS) include (select all that apply):
1. Controlled psychiatric symptoms due to adherence with medications.
2. Deficits in problem-solving skills.
3. Limited impulse control.
4. Limited use of drugs or alcohol in conjunction with sex.
5. Impaired judgment.

2. The neuropsychiatric changes observed in HIV are a result of (select all that apply):
1. The client's previous drug use.
2. The side effects of the pharmacological treatment.
3. An underlying psychiatric disorder.
4. A viral invasion of the renal system.
5. A viral invasion of the central nervous system (CNS).

3. A priority nursing diagnosis for the client with HIV-related dementia is:
1. Risk for Injury.
2. Ineffective Protection.
3. Impaired Mobility.
4. Powerlessness.

4. The cognitive changes associated with HIV-related dementia include:
1. Regressed behavior.
2. Dysphoric mood.

3. Muscle weakness.
4. Slowness of thought.

5. The nurse is interacting with a client with HIV-related dementia. Appropriate communication techniques include:
1. Asking open-ended questions.
2. Asking abstract questions that encourage the client to elaborate on the answer.
3. Using brief, direct statements.
4. Asking multiple questions at a time.

6. A nurse is instructing a group of teenagers about high-risk sexual behaviors. The nurse recognizes that a student did not understand the concepts when the student states:
1. "I can French-kiss my girlfriend and will not contract HIV."
2. "High-risk behaviors include the exchange of body fluids."
3. "If I use a condom I have to make sure I put it on correctly."
4. "Having unprotected sex increases the risk of contracting HIV."

7. The purpose of a harm reduction approach to HIV risk reduction education is to:
1. Educate the public about safe sex behaviors.
2. Convince the client with a current history of intravenous drug use (IDU) to enter a detoxification program.
3. Offer sterile needles to intravenous drug users (IDU).
4. Protect the intravenous drug user (IDU) from contracting HIV and other life-threatening diseases.

8. Which of the following is not a high-risk factor for dysfunctional bereavement for survivors of people with AIDS (SOPWAs)?
1. Lack of community recognition of the significance of the loss
2. Untimely nature of death
3. Fear of exposure to HIV
4. Support of others who have experienced a similar death

9. Which of the following statements by the nursing student indicates a need for additional education on how to care for the client who has both HIV/AIDS and a psychiatric disorder?
1. "I can't touch the client or I will get HIV/AIDS."
2. "Relaxation techniques can be used to help the client relax."
3. "I can give the client a backrub."
4. "The client's psychiatric symptomatology may be related to HIV/AIDS."

10. A client with depression and AIDS is prescribed acyclovir, zidovudine, and isoniazid. The client reports that he has insomnia and disturbing nightmares each night. The nurse observes that the client is agitated, confused, and anxious. The nurse suspects the client's symptoms are related to:
1. Depression.
2. Central nervous system (CNS) lymphoma.
3. Side effect of the antiretroviral medication.
4. HIV-related dementia.

See Appendix C for answers.

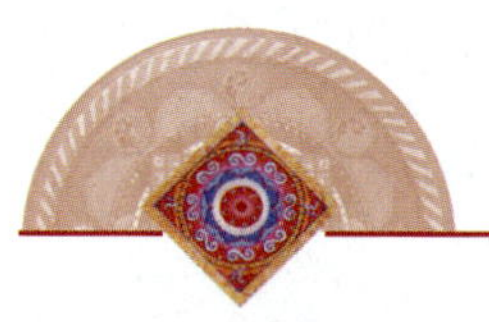

REFERENCES

Abdala, N., Crowe, M., Tolstov, Y., & Heimer, R. (2004). Survival of human immunodeficiency virus type 1 after rinsing injection syringes with different cleaning solutions. *Substance Use and Misuse, 39*(4), 581–600.

American Nurses Association. (1997). *Position statement: Needle exchange and HIV*. Washington, DC: Author.

American Nurses Association. (2001). *Code of ethics for nurses*. Washington, DC: Author.

American Nurses Association and Association of Nurses in AIDS Care. (2006). *HIV/AIDS nursing: Scope and standards of practice*. Silver Spring, MD: nursebooks.org.

Ances, B. M., & Ellis, R. J. (2007). Dementia and neurocognitive disorders due to HIV-1 infection. *Seminars in Neurology, 27*(1), 86–92.

Bigg, D. (2001). Substance use management: A harm reduction-principled approach to assisting the relief of drug-related problems. *Journal of Psychoactive Drugs, 33*(1), 33–38.

Bogart, L. M., Fremont, A. M., Young, A. S., Pantoja, P., Chinman, M., Morton, S., et al. (2006). Patterns of HIV care for patients with serious mental illness. *AIDS Patient Care STDS, 20*(3), 175–182.

Brown, E. J., & Jemmott, L. S. (2000). HIV among people with mental illness: Contributing factors, prevention needs, barriers, and strategies. *Journal of Psychosocial Nursing, 38*(4), 14–19.

Brown, E. J., Outlaw, F. H., & Simpson, E. M. (2000). Theoretical antecedents to HIV risk perception. *Journal of American Psychiatric Nurses Association, 6*(6), 177–182.

Burnam, M. A., Bing, E. G., Morton, S. C., Sherbourne, C., Fleishman, J. A., London, A. S., et al. (2001). Use of mental health and substance abuse treatment services among adults with HIV in the United States. *Archives of General Psychiatry, 58*(8), 729–736.

Cadell, S., & Marshall, S. (2007). The (re)construction of self after the death of a partner to HIV/AIDS. *Death Studies, 31*(6), 537–548.

Carrico, A. W., Johnson, M. O., Morin, S. F., Remien, R. H., Charlebois, E. D., Steward, W. T., et al. (NIMH Healthy Living Project Team). (2007). Correlates of suicidal ideation among HIV-positive persons. *AIDS, 21*(9), 1199–1203.

Centers for Disease Control and Prevention. (2007). *HIV/AIDS surveillance report, 17*(6).

Chander, G., Himelhoch, S., & Moore, R. D. (2006). Substance abuse and psychiatric disorders in HIV-positive patients: Epidemiology and impact on antiretroviral therapy. *Drugs, 66*(6), 769–789.

Coleman, C. L., Eller, L. S., Nokes, K. M., Bunch, E., Reynolds, N. R., Corless, I. B., et al. (2006). Prayer as a complementary health strategy for managing HIV-related symptoms among ethnically diverse patients. *Holistic Nursing Practice, 20*(2), 65–72.

Coleman, C. L., Holzemer, W. L., Eller, L. S., Corless, I., Reynolds, N., Nokes, K. M., et al. (2006). Gender differences in use of prayer as a self-care strategy for managing symptoms in African Americans living with HIV/AIDS. *Journal of the Association of Nurses in AIDS Care, 17*(4), 16–23.

Conover, C. J., Arno, P., Weaver, M., Ang, A., & Ettner, S. L. (2006). Income and employment of people living with combined HIV/AIDS, chronic mental illness, and substance abuse disorders. *Journal of Mental Health Policy and Economics, 9*(2), 71–86.

Conway, K. P., Compton, W., Stinson, F. S., & Grant, B. F. (2006). Lifetime cormorbidity of DSM-IV mood and anxiety disorders and specific drug use disorders: Results from the National Epidemiologic Survey on Alcohol and Related Conditions. *Journal of Clinical Psychiatry, 67*(2), 247–257.

Foster, C. J., Biggs, R. L., Melvin, D., Walters, M. D., Tudor-Williams, G., & Lyall, E. G. (2006). Neurodevelopmental outcomes in children with HIV infection under 3 years of age. *Developments in Medicine and Child Neurology. 48*(8), 677–682.

Fremont, A. M., Young, A. S., Chinman, M., Pantoja, P., Morton, S., Koegel, P., et al. (2007). Differences in HIV care between patients with and without severe mental illness. *Psychiatric Services, 58*(5), 681–688.

Hilton, B. A., Thompson, R., Moore-Dempsey, L., & Janzen, R. G. (2001). Harm reduction theories and strategies for control of human immunodeficiency virus: A review of the literature. *Journal of Advanced Nursing, 33*(3), 357–370.

Holzemer, W. L. (2002). HIV and AIDS: The symptom experience. *American Journal of Nursing, 102*(4), 48–52.

Ironson, G., Solomon, G. F., Balbin, E. G., O'Cleirigh, C., George, A., Kumar, M., et al. (2002). The Ironson-Woods spirituality/religiousness index is associated with long survival, health behaviors, less distress, and low cortisol in people with HIV/AIDS. *Annals of Behavioral Medicine, 24*(1), 34–48.

Kelly, A. (2007). Hope is forked: Hope, loss, treatments, and AIDS dementia. *Qualitative Health Research, 17*(7), 866–872.

Klinkenberg, W. D., & Sacks, S. (HIV/AIDS Treatment Adherence, Health Outcomes and Cost Study Group). (2004). Mental disorders and drug abuse in persons living with HIV/AIDS. *AIDS Care, 16 Suppl 1*, 522–542.

Knox, M. D., Davis, M., & Friedrich, M. A. (1994). The HIV mental health spectrum. *Community Mental Health Journal, 30*(1), 75–89.

McArthur, J. C. (2004). HIV dementia: An evolving disease. *Journal of Neuroimmunology, 157*(1–2), 3–10.

Meade, C. S. (2006). Sexual risk behavior among persons dually diagnosed with severe mental illness and substance use disorder. *Journal of Substance Abuse Treatment, 30*(2), 147–157.

Meade, C. S., & Sikkema, K. J. (2007). Psychiatric and psychosocial correlates of sexual risk behavior among adults with severe mental illness. *Community Mental Health Journal, 43*(2), 153–169.

National Coalition for the Homeless. (2002). *HIV/AIDS and homelessness*. Washington, DC: Author.

Pence, B. W., Miller, W. C., Whetten, K., Eron, J. J., & Gaynes, B. N. (2006). Prevalence of DSM-IV-defined mood, anxiety, and substance use disorders in an HIV clinic in the southeastern United States. *Journal of Acquired Immune Deficiency Syndromes, 42*(3), 298–306.

Romero, E. G., Teplin, L. A., McClelland, G. M., Abram, K. M., Welty, L. J., & Washburn, J. J. (2007). A longitudinal study of the prevalence, development, and persistence of HIV/sexually transmitted infection risk behaviors in delinquent youth: Implications for health care in the community. *Pediatrics, 119*(5), 1126–1141.

Rosenberg, S. D., Drake, R. E., Brunette, M. F., Wolford, G. L., & Marsh, B. J. (2005). Hepatitis C virus and HIV co-infection in people with severe mental illness and substance use disorders. *AIDS, 19 Suppl 3*, S26–S33.

Simoni, J. M., Pantalone, D. W., Plummer, M. D., & Huang, B. (2007). A randomized controlled trial of a peer support intervention targeting antiretroviral medication adherence and depressive symptomatology in HIV-positive men and women. *Health Psychology, 26*(4), 488–495.

Sohler, N. L., Wong, M. D., Cunningham, W. E., Cabral, H., Drainoni, M. L., & Cunningham, C. O. (2007). Type and pattern of illicit drug use and access to health care services for HIV-infected people. *AIDS Patient Care STDS, 21 Suppl 1*, 568–576.

Surlis, S., & Hyde, A. (2001). HIV-positive patients' experiences of stigma during hospitalization. *Journal of the Association of Nurses in AIDS Care, 12*(6), 68–77.

Teplin, L. A., Elkington, K. S., McClelland, G. M., Abram, K. M., Mericle, A. A., & Washburn, J. J. (2005). Major mental disorders, substance use disorders, comorbidity, and HIV-AIDS risk behaviors in juvenile detainees. *Psychiatric Services, 56*(7), 823–828.

Weaver, K. E., Liabre, M. M., Duran, R. E., Antoni, M. H., Ironson, G., Penedo, F. J., et al. (2005). A stress and coping model of medication adherence and viral load in HIV-positive men and women on highly active antiretroviral therapy (HAART). *Health Psychology, 24*(4), 385–392.

Webber, D. W. (2000). HIV/AIDS legal issues in the United States. *Canadian HIV AIDS Policy Law Review, 5*(4), 38–41.

Zanjani, F., Saboe, K., & Oslin, D. (2007). Age difference in rates of mental health/substance abuse and behavioral care in HIV-positive adults. *AIDS Patient Care STDS, 21*(5), 347–355.

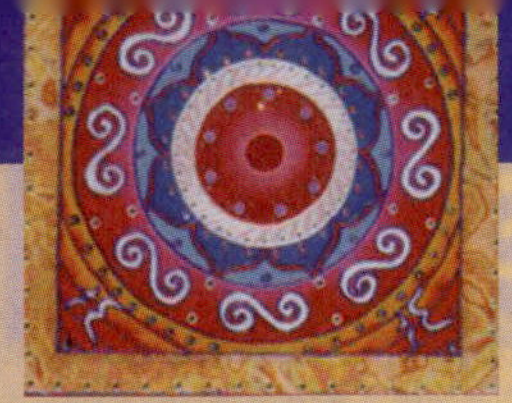

CHAPTER

26 Children

SANDRA J. WEISS AND SANDRA NIEMANN

KEY TERMS

Asperger's disorder *694*
attention deficit hyperactivity disorder (ADHD) *695*
autism spectrum disorders (ASD) *692*
autistic disorder *693*
conduct disorder (CD) *696*
developmental disorders *691*
disruptive behavior disorders *694*
elimination disorders *700*
encopresis *700*
enuresis *700*
feeding and eating disorders *697*
feeding disorder *697*
mental retardation *691*
oppositional defiant disorder (ODD) *697*
pica *697*
reactive attachment disorder (RAD) *698*
Rett's disorder *694*
rumination disorder *697*
selective mutism *701*
separation anxiety disorder *700*
tic disorders *702*
Tourette's disorder *702*

LEARNING OUTCOMES

After completing this chapter, you will be able to:

1. Compare the similarities and differences between generalist and specialist roles in child psychiatric nursing.
2. Discuss the key ideas in the biopsychosocial theories that aid in understanding the development of childhood psychiatric disorders.
3. Explain the multicausal or interactive model of child mental illness.
4. List the potential risk factors for childhood mental illness.
5. Describe the signs and symptoms associated with each of the common psychiatric disorders of children.
6. Conduct an assessment of a child with a mental health problem.
7. Discuss various therapeutic approaches that child psychiatric–mental health nurses might use in working with child clients.
8. Discuss various therapeutic approaches that child psychiatric–mental health nurses might use in working with the parents of child clients.
9. Monitor the impact of psychopharmacologic agents on children at various developmental levels.
10. Become aware of your own attitudes and behavior toward child psychiatric clients and their parents and how they affect the therapeutic outcomes of your work with them.

CRITICAL THINKING CHALLENGE

You are checking the charts of the children who will be your clients on the shift you have just begun. A nurse who is finishing her shift says to you as she is leaving, "So you'll be working with Kevin tonight, the little red-haired guy with autism. I warn you . . . his mother is a real pain. She is constantly asking questions and telling the staff what to do. I don't think they should even let her visit. If you ask me, she is the reason for all the kid's problems."

1. How might the nurse's attitude influence the care that Kevin and his family receive?
2. What are the possible effects of autistic disorder on family relationships?

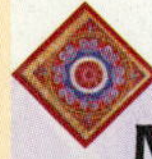

MEDIALINK 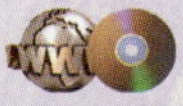 www.prenhall.com/kneisl

Go to the Pearson Health MediaLink CD-ROM and the Companion Website at www.prenhall.com/kneisl for interactive resources for this chapter.

There are more children in need of psychiatric care than ever before. About 1 in 10 children in the United States suffers from mental illness (National Institute of Mental Health [NIMH], 2006) but fewer than one in five of these children receive treatment. Available resources for prevention and treatment of mental illness are minimal and the number of mental health professionals prepared to work with children has dwindled.

The Office of the U.S. Surgeon General produced a report indicating that the unmet mental health needs of children and their families is a public health crisis (Department of Health and Human Services [DHHS], 2001). The report calls for a national action agenda to promote mental health in children and treat more effectively their mental disorders. Among the many important goals in this national agenda are plans to:

- Improve assessment and recognition of children's mental health needs.
- Eliminate racial/ethnic and socioeconomic disparities in access to care.
- Educate mental health providers as well as front-line, primary care providers to better recognize and manage children's mental health issues.

A number of mental health problems typically appear in childhood, although they may continue into adulthood or lead to other psychiatric disorders in later life. Each type of disorder has a particular constellation of symptoms or descriptive features that sets it apart from others. Keep in mind that the disorders described in this chapter are not the only ones found in childhood.

CHILD PSYCHIATRIC–MENTAL HEALTH NURSING AS A SPECIALTY

Nurses are in a key position to advance the Surgeon General's goals. Growing recognition of the psychobiologic underpinnings of mental illness has resulted in a greater interest in using nurses for a variety of roles that demand knowledge of both mental and physical health. For example, nurses in child psychiatry must assess psychologic and physical symptoms, explain laboratory tests to children, administer medications that require strict and systematic monitoring, and work with children having a dual medical and psychiatric diagnosis (such as diabetes and conduct disorder). They educate children about their illness; promote wellness, self-esteem, and more effective interpersonal relationships; and help children to identify and label their feelings, deal with stress, and manage anxiety. Child psychiatric–mental health nurses have the knowledge to perform these diverse clinical functions at a reasonable cost to society.

As a specialty, child psychiatric–mental health nursing had its inception in the early 1950s, when graduate programs opened and training funds became available through the National Institute of Mental Health (NIMH). The early child mental health teams did not include the nurse. In some residential programs, the majority of milieu staff were from other disciplines, and only one nurse was included for each shift, primarily to attend to the physical needs of the children and administer medications. As the community mental health movement developed, programs specifically for children began to offer appropriate roles for the child psychiatric–mental health nurse, including treatment, consultation, education, and medication supervision.

Today, advanced practice nurses are often the primary caregivers for children with mental health problems, providing direct counseling, working with the family, and managing the child's medications. This comprehensive role is especially common in rural or inner city areas. Child psychiatric–mental health nurses also are the mainstay of hospital treatment programs, where they are responsible for daily treatment plans, ongoing one-on-one or group counseling, and management of the child's medication regimen.

A growing role for child psychiatric–mental health nurses involves promotion of infant mental health in high-risk families in which the infants have medical complications or the parents have a history of mental illness or substance abuse. They also function as liaisons to pediatric inpatient and outpatient settings, providing psychiatric consultation to the pediatric staff. In most cases, the nurse functions as part of an interdisciplinary team, along with child psychiatrists, social workers, psychologists, occupational therapists, recreational therapists, special educators, pediatricians, and child care workers. (For more information, refer to Chapter 2 and visit the website of the Association of Child and Adolescent Psychiatric Nurses via the Companion Website for this book.) Other specialists are used for consultations as indicated, particularly child neurologists, speech and language specialists, child protective services, clergy, and physical therapists.

DEVELOPMENTAL DISORDERS

All **developmental disorders** involve a lack of expected development or a regression after normal development. These impairments are sometimes in single areas or can involve a spectrum of deficits.

Mental Retardation

The major feature of **mental retardation** is significantly subaverage intellectual functioning (an IQ below 70 in children, or, in infants, clinical judgment based on cognitive tests). The degree of severity of intellectual impairment is described as mild (IQ 50/55–70), moderate (IQ 35/40–50/55), severe (IQ 20/25–35/40), or profound (IQ below 20/25). The child must also show deficits or impairments in adaptive functioning in at least two areas of life—for example, communication, social/interpersonal skills, or safety. The onset of this disorder occurs before the age of 18.

Mental retardation is found in approximately 1% of the population (American Psychiatric Association [APA], 2000). The major risk factor for retardation is the early alteration of embryonic development as a result of exposure to toxins in utero (maternal drug use, for example) or chromosomal changes (such as Down syndrome). Other predisposing factors include inherited errors of metabolism (such as fragile X syndrome), pregnancy and perinatal problems such as prematurity or trauma, medical conditions acquired in infancy or childhood, and early environmental influences such as deprivation of nurturance or other stimulation.

Specific Developmental Disorders

Three categories of developmental disorders involve specific cognitive impairments that are presumed to result from dysfunctions in the cortex of the brain: learning disorders, motor skills disorder, and communication disorders. These dysfunctions have been associated with genetic vulnerabilities, organic damage, and delayed maturation. Children from disadvantaged socioeconomic circumstances tend to receive these diagnoses more frequently, particularly boys.

Learning Disorders

A learning disorder may be diagnosed when a child's achievement on standardized tests in reading, mathematics, or written expression is substantially below what is expected for his or her age, schooling, or intelligence level. The problems are so major as to significantly interfere with the child's activities of daily living or academic progress.

Learning disorders affect 2% to 10% of the population and about 5% of all public school students (APA, 2000). Reading is the major learning problem.

Motor Skills Disorder

A motor skills disorder, marked impairment in the development of motor coordination, occurs in approximately 6% of all children (APA, 2000). You may first notice this problem in a child's delay in achieving motor milestones such as walking or crawling, in "clumsiness," and in poor handwriting or sports performance. To be considered a psychiatric disorder, the impairment must significantly interfere with the child's academic achievement or activities of daily living and not be the result of a physical health problem such as cerebral palsy.

Communication Disorders

Communication disorders can be one of four different problems: impairments in language expression, in the understanding of language, in phonology, or stuttering:

1. Problems in language expression may include a markedly limited vocabulary, errors in tense, or difficulty recalling words or producing sentences of developmentally appropriate length or complexity.
2. Problems in understanding language include difficulty understanding words, sentences, or specific types of words.
3. The symptom of a phonological disorder is the failure to use developmentally expected speech sounds appropriate for a child's age and dialect. For example, the child may substitute one sound for another ("t" for "k") or omit sounds in words.
4. Stuttering is a disturbance in the normal timing and fluency of speech; for instance, frequent repetitions, prolonged sounds, or pauses in the middle of a word.

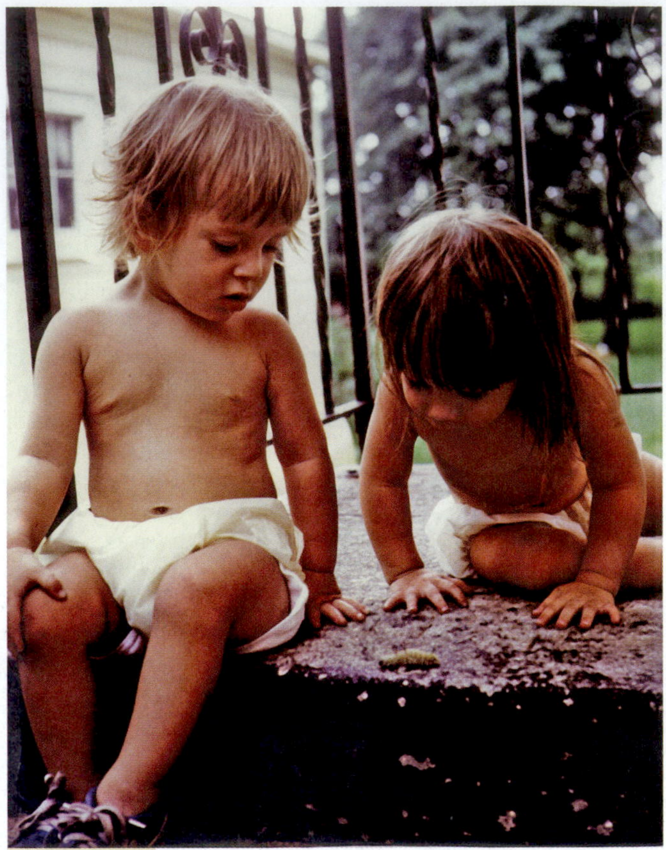

FIGURE 26-1 ■ Toddlers looking at a "calipitter" (caterpillar), a classic language flip.

Word substitution is often used by a child to avoid problematic words (see FIGURE 26-1 ■). These impairments must be severe enough to interfere with academic achievement or social communication.

While stuttering occurs in about 1% of prepubertal children, the prevalence of the other communication disorders is somewhat greater: about 3% to 5% of all children. However, under the age of 3, language delays occur in up to 25% of all children (Tanner, 2006). Remember to evaluate any communication problems within the child's cultural and language context, especially if the child is bilingual. The only known predisposing factor for the development of a communication disorder is a family history of the disorder. For stuttering, especially, family and twin studies provide strong evidence of a genetic factor in its etiology.

AUTISM SPECTRUM DISORDERS

The **autism spectrum disorders (ASD)**, called pervasive developmental disorders (PDD) in the DSM-IV-TR (2000), include autistic disorder, Rett's disorder, childhood disintegrative disorder, and Asperger's disorder. Each of these psychiatric conditions usually arises in the first years of life and is characterized by severe developmental impairment in several areas.

Autistic, disintegrative, and Asperger's disorders are much more common in boys, with rates of autism four to five times higher than for girls. Rett's disorder has been found to

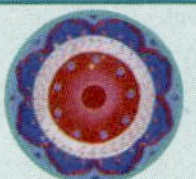

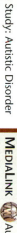

RX COMMUNICATION

COMMUNICATING WITH THE PARENT OF A CHILD WITH AUTISM

PARENT: "I've had it. I just can't take this anymore. Kaetlin screams and flaps her arms every time I touch her. I can't even give her a bath without a huge scene. It's exhausting."

NURSE RESPONSE 1: "I hear how frustrated and exhausted you are. Let's talk about your needs for a bit and figure out ways to get you some support and relief."

RATIONALE: This response shows the parent that the nurse empathizes with the parent's situation. It also provides an opportunity (a) for the parent to discuss her feelings in more detail, and (b) for the nurse to make concrete suggestions for decreasing the burden the parent is experiencing.

NURSE RESPONSE 2: "Yes, it can be very exhausting. Other families I work with have these same experiences. Let's talk about some approaches that you might use to help Kaetlin handle her bath without getting so upset."

RATIONALE: First, this response provides comfort to the parent that the problem is not unique to her family but is shared by others. The nurse then offers her the opportunity to learn some specific strategies to better manage the child's behavior.

occur only in girls. The reasons for these gender differences are not yet understood for autistic, distintegrative, and Asperger's disorders. A probable explanation for the occurrence of Rett's disorder in girls is explained later in this section.

All of these disorders are rare, with autistic disorder having the highest incidence. It occurs in 5 children per 10,000 (APA, 2000). Regardless of the small percentage of children affected by pervasive developmental disorders, their impact on children and families is enormous. They also represent a substantial segment of the families to whom child psychiatric–mental health nurses provide care, because the problems these families encounter are severe and require significant professional support (see the Rx Communication feature above).

Autistic Disorder

Sometimes referred to as autism, **autistic disorder** is a lifelong condition that involves difficulties in the quality of both the social interaction and the communication of the child. In social interaction, the child may have problems making eye contact, fail to develop appropriate peer relationships, fail to spontaneously seek out shared enjoyment with other people, or show no social or emotional reciprocity. In communication, the child may have a delay in developing language or a total absence of speech; use language in a stereotyped, repetitive, or idiosyncratic fashion; show deficits in spontaneous, imaginative play; or have a restricted, repetitive repertoire of interests or behaviors (as in folding a facial tissue repeatedly or flapping the hands up and down). The DSM-IV-TR feature on page 694 describes the specific features of this disorder.

About 75% of children with autism also have a diagnosis of mental retardation, usually in the moderate range (Tanner, 2006). Autism appears prior to age 3. Parents may tell you that their baby does not want to cuddle, shows indifference to touch and affection, does not make eye contact, or is not facially responsive. Children may also have many associated behavioral problems such as hyperactivity, aggressiveness, self-injurious behaviors such as head banging, temper tantrums, and unusual sensitivity to sensory stimuli (such as an oversensitivity to touch or a high threshold for pain). You may notice abnormal mood or affect as well; for example, a child may overreact or not react at all to the environment.

Autism is growing at the startling rate of 10–17% per year. It is the fastest-growing serious developmental disability in the United States. Based on statistics from the U.S. Department of Education, the Centers for Disease Control and Prevention, and other government agencies, we can expect the following:

- A new case of autism will be diagnosed approximately every 20 minutes (or, 67 children per day).
- More children will be diagnosed with autism this year than with cancer, diabetes, and AIDS combined.
- One in every 150 children will have some form of autism.
- Approximately 1.5 million Americans will have some form of autism.
- The prevalence of autism may reach 4 million Americans in the next decade (Autism Society of America, 2008).

These and other facts about autism are available at the website of the Autism Society of America, which can be accessed through a link on the Companion Website for this text. It is possible also that the increase, or a least part of it, is due to a broader definition of autism (Freitag, 2007).

Several current clinical trials for ASD are listed in the National Institute of Mental Health (NIMH) clinical trials registry (NIMH, 2008). They include studies of the effectiveness of medications such as atomoxetine (Strattera), olanzapine (Zyprexa), aripiprazole (Abilify), D-cycloserine (Seromycin, a drug more commonly used for the treatment of tuberculosis), methylphenidate (Ritalin), fluoxetine (Prozac), and risperidone (Risperdal). Autism clinical trials of school- and home-based early intervention for toddlers, relationship training for children and their peers, factors that distinguish autism from delayed development and normal development, and the interaction of diet and behavior are also in the NIMH pipeline (NIMH, 2008). You can counsel parents to obtain information on current clinical trials through the NIMH website via a link on the Companion Website for this book.

MEDIALINK Autism: What Is It? Video

MEDIALINK Case Study: Autistic Disorder

MEDIALINK Autism Society of America

MEDIALINK National Institute of Mental Health

DSM-IV-TR Diagnostic Criteria for Autistic Disorder

A. A total of six (or more) items from (1), (2), and (3), with at least two from (1), and one each from (2) and (3):
   1. qualitative impairment in social interaction, as manifested by at least two of the following:
      a. marked impairment in the use of multiple nonverbal behaviors such as eye–to–eye gaze, facial expression, body postures, and gestures to regulate social interaction
      b. failure to develop peer relationships at appropriate developmental level
      c. a lack of spontaneous seeking to share enjoyment, interests, or achievements with other people (e.g., by a lack of showing, bringing, or pointing out objects of interest)
      d. lack of social or emotional reciprocity
   2. qualitative impairments in communication as manifested by at least one of the following:
      a. delay in, or total lack of, the development of spoken language (not accompanied by an attempt to compensate through alternate modes of communication such as gesture or mime)
      b. in individuals with adequate speech, marked impairment in the ability to initiate or sustain a conversation with others
      c. stereotyped and repetitive use of language or idiosyncratic language
      d. lack of varied, spontaneous make-believe play or social imitative play appropriate to developmental level
   3. restricted repetitive and stereotyped patterns of behavior, interests, and activities, as manifested by at least one of the following:
      a. encompassing preoccupation with one or more stereotyped and restricted patterns of interest that is abnormal either in intensity or focus
      b. apparently inflexible adherence to specific, nonfunctional routines or rituals
      c. stereotyped and repetitive motor mannerisms (e.g., hand or finger flapping or twisting, or complex whole-body movements)
      d. persistent preoccupation with parts of objects

B. Delays or abnormal functioning in at least one of the following areas, with onset prior to age 3 years: (1) social interaction, (2) languages as used in social communication, or (3) symbolic or imaginative play.

C. The disturbance is not better accounted for by Rett's Disorder or Childhood Disintegrative Disorder.

Source: Reprinted with permission from the *Diagnostic and Statistical Manual of Mental Disorders*, Fourth Edition, Text Revision. (Copyright 2000). American Psychiatric Association.

USING DSM-IV-TR

Health care providers often use language unfamiliar to clients and their families. Define *emotional reciprocity* in terms that a client and family members can easily understand.

Rett's Disorder

Rett's disorder is the accumulation of multiple developmental deficits by a child following normal development during the first 5 months of life. Within the first or second year of life, the baby begins to show deceleration in head growth, loss of previously acquired hand skills and eventual stereotypic hand movements (repetitive movements that serve no purpose), loss of social engagement, poorly coordinated gait or trunk movements, and severely impaired language development with psychomotor retardation. Rett's disorder primarily affects females due to the lethality of the disorder in male children, according to the City of Hope National Medical Center in Duarte, California (2008). The disorder is lifelong, with persistent and progressive loss of skills. Only modest developmental gains have been noted in a few children later in their childhood or adolescence.

Childhood Disintegrative Disorder

Childhood disintegrative disorder (CDD) is quite similar to Rett's disorder except that its period of normal development is much longer, with symptoms not appearing until ages 2 through 10. In addition, there is no head growth deceleration or loss of hand skills. Instead, the losses involve skills in expressive or receptive language, social skills, play, and bowel or bladder control. Some of the abnormalities of functioning that develop are similar to those in autistic disorder, such as impairments in social interaction, communication, and repetitive, restricted, stereotypic behavior. However, in autistic disorder, the abnormalities are usually noticed within the first year of life and do not reflect the pattern of developmental regression found in CDD.

Asperger's Disorder

Asperger's disorder has some but not all of the features of autism. Children with this disorder show the same problems with social interaction and restricted, repetitive behavior as in autism. However, there is no delay in language, in cognitive development, in age-appropriate self-help and adaptive skills, or in curiosity about the environment. The onset of the disorder is also later than in autism, most commonly in the preschool period. In contrast to CDD, there is no loss of previously acquired skills in Asperger's disorder.

ATTENTION DEFICIT AND DISRUPTIVE BEHAVIOR DISORDERS

This category of child psychiatric problems includes attention deficit hyperactivity disorder and two **disruptive behavior disorders**: conduct disorder and oppositional defiant disorder. Disruptive behavior disorders are a group of mental disorders in which behavior problems cause significant impairment in social, academic, or occupational functioning. The symptoms common to all of these disorders involve behavior that is externally manifested or directed, often called *externalizing disorders*.

Attention Deficit Hyperactivity Disorder

The most distinctive features of **attention deficit hyperactivity disorder (ADHD)** are the child's inattention to the surrounding environment, and hyperactivity and/or impulsiveness. Both of these symptoms must persist for at least 6 months, be apparent in two or more settings, be inconsistent with the child's developmental level, and cause clinically significant impairment in functioning. In addition, some of these symptoms must have been present prior to age 7.

To determine whether inattention exists, look for behaviors such as making careless mistakes in schoolwork, not listening when spoken to, disliking tasks that require sustained mental effort, and being easily distracted. You will be able to observe hyperactivity in fidgeting or squirming, running around when the child is asked to stay seated, or talking excessively. Signs of impulsiveness are a child's difficulty waiting for his or her turn in activities, or interrupting others.

Most children with this disorder have a combination of symptoms indicating both inattention and hyperactivity–impulsiveness, but some children have predominantly one or the other. Girls are more likely to have symptoms only of inattention. The details of the diagnostic criteria are included in the DSM-IV-TR feature on ADHD.

ADHD is most commonly diagnosed in early school years, when demands for sustained attention increase. (See the feature What Every School Nurse Should Know on page 696.) By late childhood and adolescence, excesses in gross motor activity become less apparent, and symptoms may reflect primarily fidgetiness or even inner feelings of restlessness without any observable signs. A clinical example that includes ADHD is in the next section on conduct disorder.

DSM-IV-TR Diagnostic Criteria for Attention Deficit Hyperactivity Disorder

A. Either (1) or (2):
1. six (or more) of the following symptoms of inattention have persisted for least 6 months to a degree that is maladaptive and inconsistent with developmental level:
   Inattention
   a. often fails to give close attention to details or makes careless mistakes in schoolwork, work, or other activities
   b. often has difficulty sustaining attention in tasks or play activities
   c. often does not seem to listen when spoken to directly
   d. often does not follow through on instructions and fails to finish schoolwork, chores, or duties in the workplace (not due to oppositional behavior or failure to understand instructions)
   e. often has difficulty organizing tasks and activities
   f. often avoids, dislikes, or is reluctant to engage in tasks that require sustained mental effort (such as schoolwork or homework)
   g. often loses things necessary for tasks or activities (e.g., toys, school assignments, pencils, books, or tools)
   h. is often easily distracted by extraneous stimuli
   i. is often forgetful in daily activities
2. six (or more) of the following symptoms of hyperactivity–impulsivity have persisted for at least 6 months to a degree that it is maladaptive and inconsistent with developmental level:
   Hyperactivity
   a. often fidgets with hands or feet or squirms in seat
   b. often leaves seat in classroom or in other situations in which remaining seated is expected
   c. often runs about or climbs excessively in situations in which it is inappropriate (in adolescents or adults, may be limited to subjective feelings of restlessness)
   d. often has difficulty playing or engaging in leisure activities quietly
   e. is often "on the go" or often acts as if "driven by a motor"
   f. often talks excessively
   Impulsivity
   g. often blurts out answers before questions have been completed
   h. often has difficulty awaiting turn
   i. often interrupts or intrudes on others (e.g., butts into conversations or games)

B. Some hyperactive–impulsive or inattentive symptoms that caused impairment were present before age 7 years.

C. Some impairment from the symptoms is present in two or more settings (e.g., at school [or work] and at home).

D. There must be clear evidence of clinically significant impairment in social, academic, or occupational functioning.

E. The symptoms do not occur exclusively during the course of a Pervasive Developmental Disorder, Schizophrenia, or other Psychotic Disorder and are not better accounted for by another mental disorder (e.g., Mood Disorder, Anxiety Disorder, Dissociative Disorder, or a Personality Disorder).

Source: Reprinted with permission from the *Diagnostic and Statistical Manual of Mental Disorders*, Fourth Edition, Text Revision. (Copyright 2000). American Psychiatric Association.

USING DSM-IV-TR

Health care providers often use language unfamiliar to clients and their families. Explain *inattention* in a way that helps a client and family members better understand ADHD.

WHAT EVERY SCHOOL NURSE SHOULD KNOW

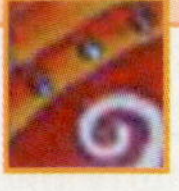

ADHD Assistance

Children with ADHD may be eligible for assistance under the Individuals with Disabilities Education Act (IDEA) of 2004 or section 504 of the Rehabilitation Act. To help children receive accommodations, families often need:

- Education about the school district's protocol for identifying, assessing, and intervening with children with ADHD
- Help finding a provider who is knowledgeable about ADHD
- A nursing liaison between their child's teacher and the child's psychiatric or primary care provider, especially when children are on medication and need monitoring to determine the optimal dose and schedule

Controversy has grown about the number of children being diagnosed with ADHD. National statistics indicate that approximately 7% of all children have ADHD, but this figure can increase to 17% for elementary-school-aged boys in specific communities and from 40% to 70% of child psychiatric inpatients (Bloom & Dey, 2006). In light of these numbers, concerns have developed regarding possible overdiagnosis and overtreatment of ADHD. Some mental health professionals question whether the growing trend toward assessment and management of the disorder by pediatricians and family physicians is a problem because they may not be as skilled in the differential diagnosis or treatment of psychiatric disorders. Another concern relates to the pressures by school personnel to control children's behavior, pressures that may influence parents and/or primary care practitioners to prescribe medication for ADHD when psychosocial management of the behavioral problems would be better.

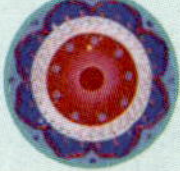

In response to these public and professional concerns, a number of studies have assessed the effectiveness of stimulants. Outcomes of these studies suggest that psychostimulants are highly effective at reducing symptoms, improve the child's quality of life, and typically have mild and short-lived side effects (King et al., 2006). However, there is limited information on the long-term effects of stimulants or the impact of treatment when the child is on medication for 10 years or more.

Conduct Disorder

Conduct disorder (CD) is also one of the most frequently diagnosed problems for children. Boys show an incidence 3 to 5 times greater than girls. The prevalence of CD is up to 10% in inner-city areas (DHHS, 2001). The central feature of CD is repetitive and persistent behavior in which the basic rights of others or major age-appropriate societal norms or rules are violated. Look for behaviors that show aggression toward people and animals, destruction of property, deceitfulness or theft, or serious violation of parental or school rules. These symptoms may appear as early as 5–6 years of age, but occur more typically in later childhood or early adolescence. The diagnosis of CD is made only when the behavior is symptomatic of a problem within the child and not a reaction to a social context of war, poverty, high crime, or fear for one's well-being.

There are two subtypes of conduct disorder: childhood onset and adolescent onset. Childhood onset must show at least one symptom prior to 10 years of age. In the majority of cases, the disorder remits by adulthood, but individuals with childhood onset are more likely to develop adult antisocial personality disorder (APD; see Chapter 22) than are those with onset in adolescence.

Children with conduct disorder may have little empathy toward others, and in ambiguous situations, they often misinterpret the intentions of others as hostile and threatening, responding with aggressive behavior that they view as reasonable and justified (see the accompanying Rx Communication feature). Self-esteem is commonly low but covered up by a facade of toughness.

Boys with the disorder are more likely to fight, steal, vandalize, or have school problems, whereas girls are more likely to run away, be truant, use drugs, or become involved in prostitution. Girls usually do not show confrontational behavior, although in recent years this has become more com-

RX COMMUNICATION

COMMUNICATING WITH A CHILD WITH CONDUCT DISORDER

CHILD: "I'm going to beat the crap out of that kid!"

NURSE RESPONSE 1: "You sound very angry at him. What is it that has made you feel so angry?"

RATIONALE: This response reflects back to the child the feelings underlying the aggressive behavior and helps to facilitate the child's awareness of his anger. The follow-up question encourages the child to develop some insight regarding his anger and is general enough to allow issues to surface that may actually be unrelated to the other child.

NURSE RESPONSE 2: "You know, Rob, that you will not be allowed to hurt anyone on the unit. If you're angry about something, I'll help you find ways to deal with your anger."

RATIONALE: This response clearly establishes limits on the child's behavior, reinforcing what is appropriate versus inappropriate behavior. The nurse also makes it clear that there are constructive ways to handle anger and that she will be there to help the child learn how to manage his feelings more effectively.

mon. While almost all cases of CD in childhood involve boys, there is a more even gender balance in adolescent onset. The following clinical example illustrates the constellation of symptoms often found in boys.

CLINICAL EXAMPLE

Rob, a 9-year-old boy, was recently diagnosed with CD in addition to an earlier diagnosis of ADHD. Rob has been in numerous fights at school for the past 2 months. His grades have dropped substantially, and he was caught vandalizing school property. At home, he refuses to talk to his parents and hit his mother when she was yelling at him for stealing money from her purse.

Rob's long history of behavioral problems began with temper tantrums at 6 months of age. At the age of 3, he cut up the family sofa. His parents took him out of preschool because the teachers couldn't handle his behavior, especially the shoving of other children and running around. During his early school years he had difficulty concentrating and focusing on an activity for a sustained period of time and interrupted ongoing class activities. He has almost no friends in school.

Rob views his problems as the result of others' hostility and threats toward him. He expresses much anger toward the "school bullies" and all authority figures in his life.

Oppositional Defiant Disorder

All the features of **oppositional defiant disorder (ODD)** are usually present in conduct disorder, so it is not diagnosed if it meets the criteria for CD. ODD is a recurrent and hostile pattern of behavior toward authority figures. However, it does not involve the physical aggression, destructive behavior, deceitfulness, theft, or serious violation of rules shown in CD.

ODD has a prevalence rate of 2% to 16% (APA, 2000). It is more common in children from families in which the child experiences many different caregivers; in which harsh, inconsistent, or neglectful child-rearing practices are used; in which mothers are depressed; or in which serious marital discord exists. The disorder is associated with problematic temperament in the preschool years and a high degree of motor activity. ODD usually becomes apparent before age 8, with symptoms first appearing in the home and then later within other settings. The child may show low self-esteem, minimal frustration tolerance, swearing, mood lability, and precocious use of tobacco, alcohol, or illegal drugs.

FEEDING AND EATING DISORDERS

Three **feeding and eating disorders**—pica, rumination disorder, and feeding disorder of infancy or early childhood—are persistent feeding and eating disturbances that include problems with what is being eaten, how much is being eaten, and the activities and behaviors around eating. Anorexia nervosa and bulimia nervosa may also occur during later childhood. These disorders are discussed in Chapter 21 because they are not unique to childhood, nor do they necessarily first appear in childhood.

Pica

Pica is a disorder in which the child persistently eats nonnutritive substances (such as paint, plaster, string, hair, cloth, animal droppings, insects, or leaves). To be considered a disorder, the behavior must be inappropriate for the developmental level of the child and not part of a culturally sanctioned practice. This disorder is most frequently seen in preschool children and in individuals who have mental retardation. Lack of adequate supervision, neglect, and poverty increase the possibility of the problem. Usually, the disorder lasts only for a few months, but it can continue into adolescence or adulthood.

Rumination Disorder

Rumination disorder is the repeated regurgitation and rechewing of food. It appears after a period of normal eating behavior in an infant or child. The child brings up partially digested food into the mouth, with no evidence of nausea or retching, and then chews and reswallows it. Sometimes the food is spit out. These symptoms are not associated with any medical condition or with any other eating disorder. Rumination disorder is most common in male infants between 3 and 12 months of age. You will observe a characteristic straining and arching of the back in these babies, and they make sucking movements with the tongue, appearing to enjoy the process very much. However, between regurgitations, babies are often irritable and hungry, and they eat a lot when fed. Because they regurgitate immediately after eating, either weight loss or failure to gain expected weight is common.

Certain factors place an infant at risk for the disorder, including lack of stimulation, neglect, and problems in the parent–child relationship. In turn, the unsuccessful nature of the feeding experience and the aversive nature of the regurgitation may result in a parent's difficulty in providing responsive or loving care.

Feeding Disorder of Infancy or Early Childhood

In a **feeding disorder**, there is a persistent failure to eat adequately, accompanied by either a failure to gain weight or significant weight loss. This state is described sometimes as "failure to thrive." Resulting malnutrition can threaten the child's life. As with other disorders in this category, there is no medical condition causing the behavior.

Children with this problem are particularly irritable and difficult to console during feeding. At other times, they may appear apathetic or withdrawn. Infants who have preexisting developmental impairments or problems with regulation of the nervous system (for example, sleep–wake irregularities) may be less responsive to the parent, creating difficulties in the feeding process. See the DSM-IV-TR feature on Feeding Disorder on page 698 for a description of the necessary elements for diagnosis.

In addition, parent behavior can make the feeding problem worse. For example, a parent may force the food into a baby's mouth too roughly or at too rapid a pace. There is a high incidence of parental psychopathology as well as child

MediaLink: Care Plan: Oppositional Defiant Disorder

DSM-IV-TR Diagnostic Criteria for Feeding Disorder of Infancy or Early Childhood

A. Feeding disturbance is manifested by persistent failure to eat adequately with significant failure to gain weight or significant loss of weight over at least 1 month.
B. The disturbance is not due to an associated gastrointestinal or other general medical condition (e.g., esophageal reflux).
C. The disturbance is not better accounted for by another mental disorder (e.g., Rumination Disorder) or by lack of available food.
D. The onset is before age 6 years.

Source: Reprinted with permission from the *Diagnostic and Statistical Manual of Mental Disorders*, Fourth Edition, Text Revision. (Copyright 2000). American Psychiatric Association.

USING DSM-IV-TR
Health care providers often use language unfamiliar to clients and their families. Explain *associated gastrointestinal or other general medical condition* in terms that family members can easily understand.

abuse or neglect associated with the condition. Although the disorder is most common in infancy (about 1% to 5% of all pediatric hospital admissions are for failure to thrive), it may have its onset as late as age 2 to 3 (APA, 2000). Most children eventually achieve improved growth patterns. This clinical example illustrates how both child and parental factors can contribute to a feeding disorder.

CLINICAL EXAMPLE

Chang, an 8-month-old Asian-American boy, was referred to the child psychiatric clinic by pediatrics for an assessment. Chang's mother was dependent on alcohol and had several bouts of drinking during her pregnancy with Chang. As a result, he had low birth weight and many neurobehavioral problems at birth. Chang continued to have tremors and an increased startle response throughout his first 6 months of life. He was also highly irritable and difficult for his mother to console, especially during feeding. His health care was being conducted by a nurse practitioner, Dawn, since the time he was 3 months of age.

Dawn reported that he had not eaten well from the time he was born, was quite undernourished, and failed to gain weight. Chang's failure to thrive became such a concern that Dawn hospitalized him for treatment of a number of resulting medical problems. During his hospitalizations, an extensive diagnostic workup produced no clear reasons for his failure to eat and develop normally. The pediatric nurses, however, had noted his mother's frustration with Chang's lack of interest in eating. Her frustration was often accompanied by impatience and she would simply stop trying to get Chang to eat. They also charted some concern about her current alcohol use. They could smell alcohol on her breath when she came to the unit and sometimes she was verbally abusive to the staff.

The child psychiatric–mental health nurse noted that, most of the time, Chang's mother related to him with very little emotion. His mother commented to the nurse, "Chang has always been a difficult and stubborn baby, never happy with anything. I've given up trying to please him. He has a personality just like his father." The nurse also noticed that Chang's facial expression was solemn and he rarely made eye contact with anyone. He seemed listless and lethargic much of the time. When attempts were made to feed him, Chang would become very distressed, crying, and trying to bang his head against the wall or floor. His mother commented that, because of such behavior, she rarely tried to pick him up anymore and would prop the bottle during his feeding.

When parents are interacting with a child who has these responses, it is not uncommon for the parents to become less involved.

REACTIVE ATTACHMENT DISORDER OF INFANCY OR EARLY CHILDHOOD

Reactive attachment disorder (RAD) of infancy or early childhood is a markedly disturbed and developmentally inappropriate way of relating that is presumed to be the result of extremely inadequate or negligent caregiving. Inadequate or negligent care may involve any of the following:

- Persistent disregard of the child's basic emotional needs for comfort, stimulation, or affection
- Persistent disregard of the child's basic physical needs
- Repeated changes of caregivers that prevent the formation of stable attachments

However, not all children who experience extremely inadequate care develop the disorder. The DSM-IV-TR feature on page 699 lists the diagnostic criteria for reactive attachment disorder.

The two types of this disorder are distinctly opposite in their symptoms:

- The *inhibited type* involves a failure to initiate and respond to most social interactions in a developmentally appropriate way. Children show excessively inhibited, hypervigilant, or ambivalent responses. Examples are a look of frozen watchfulness, resistance to comfort, and a mixture of approach and avoidance.
- In contrast, the *disinhibited type* involves an indiscriminate sociability or lack of selectivity in the choice of attachment figures. The child may be excessively familiar with strangers—hugging and

DSM-IV-TR Diagnostic Criteria for Reactive Attachment Disorder of Infancy or Early Childhood

A. Markedly disturbed and developmentally inappropriate social relatedness in most contexts, beginning before age 5 years, as evidenced by either (1) or (2):
   1. Persistent failure to initiate or respond in a developmentally appropriate fashion to most social interactions, as manifest by excessively inhibited, hypervigilant, or highly ambivalent and contradictory responses (e.g., the child may respond to caregivers with a mixture of approach, avoidance, and resistance to comforting, or may exhibit frozen watchfulness)
   2. Diffuse attachments as manifest by indiscriminate sociability with marked inability to exhibit appropriate selective attachments (e.g., excessive familiarity with relative strangers or lack of selectivity in choice of attachment figures)

B. The disturbance in Criterion A is not accounted for solely by developmental delay (as in Mental Retardation) and does not meet criteria for a Pervasive Developmental Disorder.

C. Pathogenic care as evidenced by at least one of the following:
   1. Persistent disregard of the child's basic emotional needs for comfort, stimulation, and affection
   2. Persistent disregard of the child's basic physical needs
   3. Repeated changes of primary caregiver that prevent formation of stable attachments (e.g., frequent changes in foster care)

D. There is a presumption that the care in Criteron C is responsible for the disturbed behavior in Criterion A (e.g., the disturbances in Criterion A began following the pathogenic care in Criterion C).

Source: Reprinted with permission from the *Diagnostic and Statistical Manual of Mental Disorders*, Fourth Edition, Text Revision. (Copyright 2000). American Psychiatric Association.

USING DSM-IV-TR

Health care providers often use language unfamiliar to clients and their families. Explain *indiscriminate sociability* in such a way that family members can more easily understand reactive attachment disorder.

cuddling an adult stranger in a store, for example—or may seek comfort and affection from a variety of adults who are not well known to the child.

The severity and duration of the disorder depend on the degree of psychosocial deprivation and the nature of any intervention. If a supportive environment is provided, improvement does occur. Children with this disorder commonly have a feeding and eating disorder as well. See how parental trauma affects a child's mental health in the Evidence-Based Practice feature.

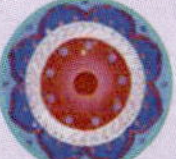

EVIDENCE-BASED PRACTICE

THE EFFECT OF PARENTAL TRAUMA ON CHILDREN'S MENTAL HEALTH

Elena Vasquez is being seen at your family mental health clinic for PTSD and depression. She is a recent refugee who experienced many traumatic events, most notably seeing her parents shot and killed. She was also the victim of domestic violence, being frequently beaten by her partner. You notice that Ms. Vasquez regularly brings her 2-year-old son Mario with her to her treatment sessions. He sits in the hallway while his mother meets with her therapist. You are concerned that Mario shows very little facial expression, seems uninterested in his toys, and is distant toward his mother. You are concerned about Mario's affect. You also recently read a research report that identified disengagement between mother and child as a sign of potential attachment problems. Concerned about Mario, you approach the mother's therapist and propose that Mario have a clinical assessment.

With the mother's agreement, you perform a mental status exam with Mario and interview the mother about his behavior. The assessment indicates that Mario has symptoms of major depression as well as indications of reactive attachment disorder. You then develop a care plan that includes both play therapy and child–parent psychotherapy. Your interventions are based upon the following evidence:

Chaffin, M., Hanson, R., Saunders, B. E., Nichols, T., Barnett, D., Zeanah, C., et al. (2006). Report of the APSAC task force on attachment therapy, reactive attachment disorder, and attachment problems. *Child Maltreatment, 11*, 76–89.

Bratton, S., Ray, D., Rhine, T., & Jones, L. (2005). The efficacy of play therapy with children: A meta-analytic review of treatment outcomes. *Professional Psychology: Research and Practice, 36*, 376–390.

CRITICAL THINKING APPLICATION

1. Is routine assessment of children of traumatized adults appropriate clinical practice?
2. Is it reasonable to do play therapy with a 2-year-old child?
3. Will the symptoms of depression and attachment disorder resolve on their own in due course?
4. Generally, few children are used as research subjects. What are some possible reasons?

SEPARATION ANXIETY DISORDER

Separation anxiety disorder involves a developmentally inappropriate and excessive anxiety over separation from home or from attachment figures. Symptoms may include fear and worry about possible harm befalling attachment figures or about being separated from them. There is usually a reluctance or refusal to go to school, be without attachment figures, or go to sleep without them nearby. It is also common for the child to have somatic complaints when separation occurs or is anticipated.

Children with this disorder frequently come from close-knit families and are often described as demanding, intrusive, or in need of constant attention. They may also be unusually compliant, conscientious, or eager to please. You may also see a depressed mood that increases over time.

The disorder occurs in about 4% of children and may appear after a stressful life event such as the death of a pet, a family illness, or immigration (APA, 2000). There are periods of exacerbation and remission over the course of the disorder that persist for many years, including into adulthood. The diagnostic criteria for separation anxiety disorder are described in the following DSM-IV-TR feature.

ELIMINATION DISORDERS

The **elimination disorders**, in which passing urine and stool involve problematic behaviors, are encopresis and enuresis. In order to be classified as a mental disorder, these problems must not be due to any medical condition or to the physiologic effects of a laxative, diuretic, or other substance.

Encopresis

Encopresis is the repeated passing of feces by the child into inappropriate places such as clothing or a corner of the room. This is usually involuntary behavior, but it may be intentional in some situations.

There are two subtypes of the disorder. The first involves constipation and continuous leakage of feces during the day and during sleep. Incontinence stops once the constipation is treated. The constipation may develop for psychological reasons, often related to a general pattern of anxious or oppositional behavior that leads the child to avoid defecation. Health problems causing dehydration, or the side effects of medication, may also initially create the constipation, but once it has developed, a child may retain stool because of painful defecation or anal fissure.

The second subtype does not involve constipation or incontinence. Feces are normal and soiling is intermittent, with feces usually found in an obvious place. Children with this subtype often have a dual diagnosis of ODD or CD.

With either subtype, smearing the feces may result from attempts to clean or hide the feces, or it may be a deliberate effort to make a mess.

Enuresis

Enuresis is the repeated voiding of urine into the bed or clothes, either during the day or at night:

- The *nocturnal type* is most common and typically occurs during the first part of the night.
- The *diurnal type* (during waking hours) happens most typically in the early afternoon of school days. This

DSM-IV-TR Diagnostic Criteria for Separation Anxiety Disorder

A. Developmentally inappropriate and excessive anxiety concerning separation from home or from those to whom the individual is attached, as evidenced by three (or more) of the following:
   1. recurrent excessive distress when separation from home or major attachment figures occurs or is anticipated
   2. persistent and excessive worry about losing, or about possible harm befalling, major attachment figures
   3. persistent and excessive worry that an untoward event will lead to separation from a major attachment figure (e.g., getting lost or being kidnapped)
   4. persistent reluctance or refusal to go to school or elsewhere because of fear of separation
   5. persistently and excessively fearful or reluctant to be alone or without major attachment figures at home or without significant adults in other settings
   6. persistent reluctance or refusal to go to sleep without being near a major attachment figure or to sleep away from home
   7. repeated nightmares involving the theme of separation
   8. repeated complaints of physical symptoms (such as headaches, stomachaches, nausea, or vomiting) when separation from major attachment figures occurs or is anticipated

B. The duration of the disturbance is at least 4 weeks.

C. The onset is before age 18 years.

D. The disturbance causes clinically significant distress or impairment in social, academic (occupational), or other important areas of functioning.

E. The disturbance does not occur exclusively during the course of a Pervasive Developmental Disorder, Schizophrenia, or other Psychotic Disorder and, in adolescents and adults, is not better accounted for by Panic Disorder with Agoraphobia.

Source: Reprinted with permission from the *Diagnostic and Statistical Manual of Mental Disorders*, Fourth Edition, Text Revision. (Copyright 2000). American Psychiatric Association.

USING DSM-IV-TR

Health care providers often use language unfamiliar to clients and their families. Define *major attachment figure* in terms that family members can easily understand.

type may be related to social anxiety and a resulting reluctance to use the toilet, or it may be because the child becomes preoccupied with play or other activities.

Some children show a combination of both day and night enuresis.

For both encopresis and enuresis, there is a primary and secondary type:

- With the *primary type*, the child has never been toilet trained.
- In the *secondary type*, the disturbance develops after a period of using the toilet appropriately.

Of course, the problem is not diagnosed as a mental disorder unless the child has reached a chronological age at which elimination problems should not be apparent (at least age 4 for encopresis and age 5 for enuresis).

Predisposing factors for both disorders include inconsistent or lax toilet training, or psychosocial stressors such as entry to school or a sibling birth. In contrast to encopresis, about 75% of all children with enuresis have a parent or sibling who had the disorder (APA, 2000).

Both disorders are more common in boys, with prevalence rates for enuresis being higher (5% to 10% of 5-year-olds) than for encopresis (1% of all 5-year-olds) (APA, 2000). Neither disorder is typically chronic. Most children become continent by adolescence. The degree of immediate and long-term impairment depends to a great extent on the amount of resulting peer rejection, punishment and rejection by the caregiver, and a child's overall self-esteem.

OTHER IMPORTANT DISORDERS OF INFANCY OR CHILDHOOD

Two other disorders are typically diagnosed in childhood and rarely continue past childhood. Features or components of these disorders may have relevance for adult behaviors.

Selective Mutism

Selective mutism is the persistent failure to speak in specific social situations, even though the child can speak in other situations. Of course, the failure to speak must not be the result of a lack of normal language skills or knowledge of a certain language. The child can be excessively shy, fearful of embarrassment, withdrawn, clinging, and negative; or you may observe temper tantrums or oppositional behavior, especially at home. Mutism is rare, but slightly more common in girls. Usually, the disturbance lasts for only a few months, but it can continue for several years.

Stereotypic Movement Disorder

Stereotypic movement disorder is a pattern of motor behavior that is repetitive and nonfunctional and one that the child appears driven to do. Examples of such movements are rocking, twirling objects, head banging, self-biting, picking at skin or body orifices, or hitting parts of one's own body. The specific behaviors may change over time from one type to another. The disorder can result in self-injurious behavior (see Chapter 23 ∞) that causes tissue damage or is life threatening. The behavior is frequently associated with mental retardation; however, it may also occur in children with severe sensory deficits—blindness or deafness, for example—or in institutional environments in which there is insufficient stimulation.

Sometimes children try to restrain themselves from the behavior—for example, by putting their hands in their pockets—but if the restraint is interfered with, the behaviors resume. Onset of the disorder may follow a stressful event. See the DSM-IV-TR feature for diagnostic criteria related to this condition.

TIC DISORDERS

There are three disorders classified as tics:

1. Tourette's disorder
2. Chronic motor or vocal tics disorder
3. Transient tic disorder

DSM-IV-TR Diagnostic Criteria for Stereotypic Movement Disorder

A. Repetitive, seemingly driven, and nonfunctional motor behavior (e.g., hands shaking or waving, body rocking, head banging, mouthing of objects, self-biting, picking at skin or bodily orifices, hitting own body).

B. The behavior markedly interferes with normal activities or results in self-inflicted bodily injury that requires medical treatment (or would result in injury if preventive measures were not used).

C. If Mental Retardation is present, the stereotypic or self-injurious behavior is of sufficient severity to become a focus of treatment.

D. The behavior is not better accounted for by a compulsion (as in Obsessive–Compulsive Disorder), a tic (as in Tic Disorder), a stereotypy that is part of a Pervasive Developmental Disorder, or hair pulling (as in Trichotillomania).

E. The behavior is not due to the direct physiological effects of a substance or general medical condition.

F. The behavior persists for four weeks or longer.

Source: Reprinted with permission from the *Diagnostic and Statistical Manual of Mental Disorders*, Fourth Edition, Text Revision. (Copyright 2000). American Psychiatric Association.

USING DSM-IV-TR

Health care providers often use language unfamiliar to clients and their families. Explain *nonfunctional motor behavior* in terms that a client and family members can easily understand.

DSM-IV-TR Diagnostic Criteria for Tourette's Disorder

A. Both multiple motor and one or more vocal tics have been present at some time during the illness, although not necessarily concurrently. (A tic is a sudden, rapid, recurrent, nonrhythmic, stereotyped motor movement or vocalization.)

B. The tics occur many times a day (usually in bouts) nearly every day or intermittently throughout a period of more than 1 year, and during this period there was never a tic-free period of more than three consecutive months.

C. The onset is before age 18 years.

D. The disturbance is not due to the direct physiological effects of a substance (e.g., stimulants) or general medical condition (e.g., Huntington's disease or postviral encephalitis).

Source: Reprinted with permission from the *Diagnostic and Statistical Manual of Mental Disorders*, Fourth Edition, Text Revision. (Copyright 2000). American Psychiatric Association.

USING DSM-IV-TR

Health care providers often use language unfamiliar to clients and their families. Define *vocal tics* in such a way that a client and family members can more fully understand Tourette's disorder.

Tic disorders are characterized by rapid, recurring, nonrhythmic, stereotypic movements or vocalizations that occur suddenly and involuntarily. Tic disorders are worse during stress but occur less frequently when the child is focused intently on an activity such as reading.

Most tic disorders appear to be transmitted through a genetic or constitutional factor, which gives the child a vulnerability to developing the disorder. However, about 10% of children with the disorder have a "nongenetic" form; these children frequently have a dual diagnosis with another mental disorder or a medical condition such as epilepsy (APA, 2000). Regardless of type, boys are more likely to develop tic disorders than girls.

The symptoms of children who have tic disorders (or other disorders such as obsessive–compulsive disorder) may worsen following streptococcal infections (e.g., strep throat). The mental health problems resulting from such an exacerbation of symptoms are referred to as PANDAS (pediatric autoimmune neuropsychiatric disorders associated with streptococci). (See Chapter 18 ∞ for a more detailed discussion.)

Tourette's Disorder

Tourette's disorder involves multiple motor tics and one or more vocal tics, which can occur simultaneously or at different periods during the illness. The diagnosis requires that there is never a tic-free period longer than 3 months. Vocal tics are words or sounds such as yelps, barks, snorts, or coughs. *Coprolalia* is a specific type of vocal tic in which obscenities are uttered. *Motor tics* include such behavior as eye blinking, protruding the tongue, sniffing, retracing steps, or twirling when walking.

The disorder may begin as early as age 2, but more often it starts during childhood or early adolescence. Tourette's disorder normally lasts for a lifetime with periods of remission, but in most cases the symptoms decrease during adolescence and adulthood. The diagnostic criteria for Tourette's disorder are in the DSM-IV-TR feature above.

Chronic versus Transient Tic Disorders

Chronic motor or vocal tic disorder differs from Tourette's disorder in that it involves *either* motor tics or vocal tics, but not both, as is required for a diagnosis of Tourette's disorder. Transient tic disorder differs from chronic motor or vocal tic disorder and Tourette's disorder in its duration. While the others require that the problems have occurred for at least a year, transient tic disorder does not last longer than 12 months.

ADULT DISORDERS THAT MAY BEGIN IN CHILDHOOD

A few disorders that are diagnosed more frequently in adulthood may begin in childhood. These include anxiety disorders, mood disorders, and schizophrenia.

Anxiety Disorders

In addition to separation anxiety, which was described earlier, children can have many other anxiety disorders (anxiety disorders are thoroughly discussed in Chapter 18 ∞). Panic disorder and agoraphobia are rare in children. Specific phobias, however, may be seen in children even before age 5 and are common childhood anxiety disorders. Children develop fears, especially of animals and blood-related events. Severe social phobia is also found in children and may lead to school avoidance.

The onset of obsessive–compulsive disorder (OCD) is common for children aged 9 to 11. Because children may not have developed "insight" yet, the requirement for OCD that they recognize the excessive nature of their behavior is waived for children. Generalized anxiety disorder (GAD) and post-traumatic stress disorder (PTSD) are also found in children. Children with GAD are often shy and may act more mature and serious than expected for their age. They often are perfectionistic and highly compliant to demands of authority figures.

PTSD in children is often associated with child abuse. In contrast to the adult experience of "flashbacks" of the traumatic event, children typically reexperience traumatic events as nightmares or through repetitive reenactment during play. Remember that children can have strong memories of events even though they cannot describe them verbally. These memories can be brought forth in play or dreams by children who are as young as 2 or 3 years of age.

Early treatment of all types of anxiety disorders in children is very important because they can lead to many social problems, including rejection or neglect by peers, academic failure, and inadequate development into an autonomous, secure adult. In general, the symptoms of anxiety disorders are similar in children and adults.

Mood Disorders

Mood disorders are discussed fully in Chapter 17, so they will not be covered in detail here. However, a few issues related to mood disorders in children are important to note. Diagnoses of mood disorders are usually not made during infancy, because developmentally, children often do not have the ability to reflect on their feelings even if the feelings are strongly affecting them. Remember also that children may not be able to accurately report symptoms even if they are experiencing them.

Bipolar disorder was considered very rare in childhood but this disorder is now being better recognized and diagnosed. Hyperactivity can easily be confused with symptoms of mania in children. Children with bipolar disorder often have a chronic mixed state of depression and mania or rapid cycling. In addition to hyperactivity, observe for aggressive, long-lasting temper outbursts, excessive risk taking, and highly energized affect as signs of mania in children.

Depressive disorders are quite common in children, with depressive symptoms occurring even in the first year of life. Although there is a greater incidence of depressive disorders among women in adulthood, the prepubertal incidence is about 2% for both boys and girls (APA, 2000). The two types of depressive disorders are major depression and dysthymia.

Major depression involves a definite change in behavior from the child's normal functioning. The child begins to show a depressed or sad mood or a lack of pleasure (anhedonia) in almost all activities at least 50% of the time. There are some important differences in how children and adults may manifest these symptoms. Children may describe things as bad, gloomy, blue, or empty when they are depressed. You may see a bland, frozen look on their faces or only fleeting smiles, as if they are smiling because it is socially expected rather than because they feel like smiling. On the other hand, you may see no evidence of sadness in children but rather a persistent irritability around even small matters. Pervasive boredom is a common sign of anhedonia in children. Another sign is social withdrawal, especially when a child avoids or rejects opportunities to play.

Other symptoms of depression in children include unexplained somatic complaints, poor school performance, sleep and appetite changes, and/or psychomotor agitation and increased risk taking. The most common type of depression in children is called reactive depression, which occurs in response to a particular situation, such as the trauma of hospitalization or an extended separation from a parent.

Dysthymia is a chronic disorder in which periods of depressed affect are interspersed with normal mood. Symptoms of later adult dysthymia often begin in childhood, even if not diagnosed until later. Because of this early and chronic quality, the person is often described as a "depressive personality." Although the symptoms of dysthymia are the same for children and adults, children are likely to show greater evidence of irritability, not simply depressed affect, and may react negatively or shyly to praise. They may respond to positive relationships with testing, anger, or avoidance.

Other symptoms of dysthymia are similar to those described for major depression, except that the child may show more evidence of low energy and low self-esteem. A key predisposing factor for childhood dysthymia is the presence of an inadequate, rejecting, or chaotic home environment.

Schizophrenia

Occuring as early as age 5 or 6, childhood-onset schizophrenia is rare. Its incidence is about 1 in every 1,000 children, mostly boys (APA, 2000). The features of schizophrenia (delusions, hallucinations, disorganized speech and behavior, and negative symptoms) are the same in children as adults. Be aware, however, that failure to reach expected levels of speech and behavior may be seen in children rather than a deterioration into disorganization. (Schizophrenia is discussed fully in Chapter 16.) The following clinical example illustrates one girl's symptoms that led to the diagnosis of schizophrenia.

CLINICAL EXAMPLE

Shauna, an 11-year-old, described hearing the voice of her mother calling her name and yelling at her, although her mother was not present. At times, she heard her own voice telling her to do things such as chores for her mother. She experienced her mother's voice as coming from outside her head and her own voice as coming from inside her head. She reported seeing a woman who looked like her mother and she thought was her mother. She also believed that her mother was watching her.

Shauna described going to the bathroom in the morning and "daydreaming" that objects were weapons (e.g., cotton swabs were sticks to stab people, and washcloths were used to smother people). All these experiences seemed real to Shauna as they happened. Shauna also believed that the world was coming to an end. She described hearing on the news that a hole was breaking apart pieces of the earth, and she thought this was going to happen. She also expressed concern that a heat wave might result in there not being enough air to breathe.

It is difficult to make the diagnosis in children, however, because delusions and hallucinations are less detailed and more accepted developmentally as normal fantasy or imaginary playmates. Visual hallucinations are more common in children than in adults but are almost always accompanied by auditory hallucinations. Disorganized speech (such as in communication disorders) or disorganized behavior (as in ADHD or autistic disorder) may result in other diagnoses when they are actually symptoms of schizophrenia.

BIOPSYCHOSOCIAL THEORIES

Five major theories guide existing views of the etiology of childhood psychopathology and the therapeutic approaches underlying its prevention and treatment. These are psychodynamic theory, object-relations theory, attachment theory, cognitive behavioral theory, and biological theory. Although many specific schools of thought fall within these perspectives, only the central features of these overarching theories will be discussed here.

Psychodynamic Theory

Psychodynamic theory originated with Sigmund Freud in his conceptualization of psychoanalysis but has evolved substantially since its original formulation (Gabbard, 2004). Much of Freud's speculation regarding psychosexual stages of development has been rejected, but many components of his personality theory continue to serve as a foundation for assessment and treatment in child psychiatry (Muratori et al., 2002).

A central component of this theory is the concept of *psychic determinism*, which proposes that the child's initial perceptions of the world are defined substantially during the first 5 to 6 years of life and will influence the child's later views and behavior in a causal way. While this stance seems almost a given in today's world, the concept was unheard of when Freud first proposed it.

Psychodynamic theory also holds that the child is born with instincts or drives for the gratification of needs to ensure survival. *Libido* is described as the psychic energy that makes the child try to meet these needs. If the needs are not satisfied during development, the child may become so fixated on meeting the needs that they influence much of his or her behavior.

Because the ego and superego prevent the id from getting all needs met, Freud proposed that children attempt to cope with the anxiety associated with need deprivation through the unconscious mental processes known as defense mechanisms (see Chapter 8 ∞). Defense mechanisms commonly employed by children are repression, reaction formation, and projection. The child comes to deal with the world through these distorted views in an attempt to defend against painful unconscious issues. However, the unconscious content continues to influence the behavior and conscious thoughts of the child, often in ways that severely impair his or her ability to function in life. Defense mechanisms are, therefore, considered to be symptoms of mental health problems.

The focus of treatment is attempting to bring repressed conflicts and issues into awareness so that they can be addressed and resolved. A primary way in which this occurs is through *transference*, a process whereby the child unconsciously directs feelings and desires from other relationships in life onto the therapist. So the relationship between therapist and child is used as a focus for interpretation and change. Transference is more fully discussed in Chapter 29 ∞.

Object-Relations Theory

Object-relations theory is built on the foundation of psychodynamic theory and is based on the work of Fairbairn, Winnicott, Klein, Mahler, Stern, and others (Kaslow & Magnavita, 2002). In this theory, an object is defined as a person or thing in the child's environment that has psychological significance to the child. A major assumption of the theory is that rather than being driven simply by physical needs or instincts that enhance survival, infants have an innate biologic need for relationships. These relationships increase in quality and complexity as a child develops.

Initially infants are undifferentiated from the object they seek (the primary caregiver) and are in a state of diffuse, unorganized experiences. The child is totally dependent on the mother to organize the child's different experiences into an understandable whole. As the young child begins to differentiate—that is, separate and develop a sense of his or her own self as an individual—the relationships with interpersonal "objects" in the world of the child are internalized and become the internal mental representations that form the self.

The differentiated self forms the basis for the child's future views of his or her own worth and the availability and responsiveness of others. Ultimately, it determines whether or not the child becomes healthy, strong, and creative. Development of the self is considered to depend primarily on the relationship between parent and child, and how effectively a parent responds to the baby's needs and assists in organizing experience. Object-relations theorists maintain that an individual will repeat in relationships throughout life what is learned about self and others from initial experiences with the primary caregiver.

Attachment Theory

Attachment theory builds on the psychodynamic concepts of psychic determinism and the impact of unconscious processes. As in object-relations theory, relationships are viewed as the organizing principle for the development of psychologic well-being in the child. However, the concept of *security* within the relationship is the main focus of attachment theory. Attachment theory was originally described by Bowlby and later extended by Ainsworth and others (Hankin & Abela, 2005).

Attachment refers to the socioemotional bond of the child to another person (the attachment figure) who is perceived as strong or powerful and who can be turned to for protection and support in situations of perceived danger or adversity. Infants are viewed as coming into the world with an innate neurobiologic structure called the attachment behavioral system. This evolutionary-based adaptive system monitors and processes information regarding uncertainty, stress, or potential danger as well as the accessibility of the attachment figure during these situations. The infant appraises both the environmental conditions and his or her emotional state to determine how much proximity or contact is needed in order to feel secure. The child then uses attachment behaviors (proximity or contact-promoting behaviors such as calling, approaching, or clinging) to acquire a sense of security.

The ways the attachment figure responds to the child's attachment behaviors are considered critical to the foundation of the child's internal working models (Belsky, 2006). These models are ways of viewing relationships that will come to guide the child's evaluation of his or her own capacity to han-

TABLE 26-1 ■ Patterns of Attachment

Attachment Pattern	Characteristics of the Child	Characteristics of the Caregiver
Secure	■ Readily seeks out caregivers in times of stress and is reassured by the caregiver's presence.	■ Is available and responsive to the child's attachment needs. ■ Encourages the child to seek security through proximity and contact.
Insecure–avoidant	■ Appears indifferent to stress and uncertainty, although physiologic responses suggest otherwise. ■ Actively avoids the attachment figure during stressful times and focuses on other things, such as play.	■ Is insensitive to the child's needs. ■ Actively rebuffs the child's attempts to be comforted during distress.
Insecure–resistant	■ Resists interaction and contact with caregivers when it is available. ■ Shows proximity-seeking behavior when contact is unavailable. ■ Shifts between seeking comfort excessively and being difficult to settle or soothe when contact is acquired.	■ Tends to be unpredictable in accessibility to child. ■ Is less able to adapt than typical children, is hesitant, and is occupied with caregiving routines.
Disorganized	■ Shows unexplainable or disoriented behavior toward the attachment figure during distress (e.g., frightened expressions and freezing while greeting the parent with raised arms, smiling while forcefully striking the parent's face, or extended rocking or ear pulling).	■ May behave in frightening or threatening ways toward the child. ■ May reverse roles, acting timid or deferential toward the child.

dle stress, as well as the responses he or she expects of others in times of need. Four major patterns of attachment have been identified as resulting from the initial experiences with the primary attachment figure (see TABLE 26-1 ■). While the first three patterns reflect different internal working models, the last pattern is viewed as a lack of any integrated or consolidated model to guide attachment behavior during situations where comfort or felt security is needed. Felt security is the emotional security a child feels when either physical or emotional caretaking indicates a bond between child and caretaker.

These various patterns can be seen in children by 12 months of age and eventually stabilize into cognitive frameworks that influence all of their intimate relationships in adulthood. While the primary attachment relationship is seen as central to the development of these life patterns, other significant relationships and the child's own degree of resilience or temperamental vulnerability are recognized as important mediators in developing secure or insecure attachment patterns.

Cognitive Behavioral Theory

The origins of cognitive behavioral theory stem from Skinner's behavioral learning school of thought. However, current views integrate more recent cognitive theory and social learning theory traditions (Friedberg & McClure, 2002). The basis of this theory is the importance of the environment in the child's psychologic development. The environment encompasses everything to which the child is exposed, including the immediate caregiving environment (the family, school, and neighborhood), as well as the larger sociocultural milieu within which values and expectations are developed. Infants are viewed as coming into the world with a relatively "blank slate," and they develop personality by being conditioned to respond in certain ways by others in the environment. Modeling is important as well, whereby children learn by watching others and what happens to those people as a result of their behavior.

The original views of behavioral theory were that positive and negative reinforcement alone could condition a child's behavior. These views expanded to recognize the child's ability to deliberate consciously on what occurs and make certain choices about which behaviors are used. This process is called reciprocal determinism. The environment provides information that influences the child in choosing how to behave, but *interpretation* of the environment is the determinant of the child's behavior, not the environment itself. However, without the environment, the child has no stimulus toward growth or development.

Cognitive theorists emphasize that psychopathology results from particular mental sets or cognitive schemata that involve distortions of reality. Children's experiences with the environment create these schemata, or ways of viewing the world, which then influence what is perceived and how it is processed and understood in all future interactions. Biased or inaccurate ways of thinking or processing information can take a number of forms; for instance:

- Interpreting things as worse than they are
- Overgeneralizing
- Selective perception
- Disqualifying the positive
- Jumping to conclusions
- Personalizing events that are not actually related to the child

These distortions are brought about by the irrational beliefs stemming from the child's schemata. External events and relationships set off particular schemata that have been established early in life and that can create major problems in the child's ability to function appropriately, or that are adaptive for the child. Treatment is thus focused on a reeducation or relearning process aimed at the child's irrational beliefs and their related behaviors (Stallard, 2005). This process can occur individually or in a group situation.

Biologic Theory

There are many hypotheses regarding the particular biologic characteristics that may make children vulnerable to developing certain psychiatric disorders (Hankin & Abela, 2005). While the exact relationship between various biological factors and mental illness is not yet understood, several hypotheses are discussed next.

Neurobiologic Factors

There is considerable evidence for the role of neurobiologic factors in the development of disorders such as autistic disorder and childhood-onset schizophrenia. Children with these disorders have more physical anomalies, neurologic soft signs, and brain abnormalities on electroencephalograms (EEGs) and in computed tomography (CT) and magnetic resonance imaging (MRI) scans. Similarly, lead poisoning, central nervous system (CNS) trauma, and infections in childhood have all been implicated as possible causative factors. These problems are considered potential causes of the mental disorder.

There has been great concern among parents, consumer advocacy groups, and health care professionals that vaccines given to infants may be linked to the increase in autism. Because of this concern, some parents have been reluctant to have their children protected from childhood diseases through vaccination. Two reasons are generally given for this concern. The first is the use of thimerosol (a preservative in vaccines that contains trace amounts of ethylmercury). The second is related to the measles–mumps–rubella immunization schedule for infants. The data do not support the hypothesis that exposure to thimerosol causes autism. The rate of autism has increased even with the exclusion of thimerosol from childhood vaccines (Schecter & Getcher, 2008). Studies in Canada yield similar results. In fact, one study (Fombonne, Zakarian, Bennett, Mung, & McLean-Heywood, 2006) found that the increase was higher for thimerosol-free children than for thimerosol-exposed children. This same study also determined that autism was not related to the one- or two-dose measles–mumps–rubella immunization schedule.

MEDIALINK City of Hope

Neurotransmitter Secretion

There is growing support for the existence of certain abnormalities in neurotransmitter secretion (Hankin & Abela, 2005). Dopamine and serotonin (5-HT) have been of major interest in a number of disorders. For instance, studies suggest that 5-HT levels may be elevated in autism but depleted in childhood depression. However, it is often unclear whether the dysfunction in neurotransmitter levels causes the disorder, or whether the disorder may create nervous system changes that cause the neurotransmitter abnormality.

Nervous System Responsiveness

Studies also indicate that problems with nervous system responsiveness may be related to certain psychiatric disorders. For example, children with schizophrenia have unusually high autonomic system reactivity when in baseline or resting states, and children with ADHD appear to have a lowered excitability in the reticular activating system of the brain, requiring more stimulation in order to feel optimally aroused.

Neuroendocrine Reactivity

A related biological vulnerability is the child's neuroendocrine reactivity. The hypothalamic–pituitary–adrenal axis regulates the nervous system's release of stress hormones such as cortisol. The feedback mechanism controlling these hormones appears dysfunctional in certain psychiatric disorders. For instance, children with PTSD show excessive secretion of stress hormones, with neurotoxic effects on brain development and function (van der Kolk, 2003).

Genetic Predisposition

Twin and adoption studies continue to provide evidence in support of genetic etiology for many disorders, including pervasive developmental disorders, schizophrenia, and depression. Adopted children and their biologic parents show a much stronger likelihood of both having these disorders than adoptive parents and children. In addition, when one twin has a disorder, the other is much more likely to have the disorder than is another sibling, parent, or other relative. There is also strong evidence of a familial pattern for both major depression and dysthymia, with clear support for a genetic, biochemical etiology (Hankin & Abela, 2005).

Rett's disorder has been found to be an X-linked dominant inheritance disorder associated with mutations in the MECP2 gene (City of Hope, 2008). In addition, there is evidence that other milder mutations in the MECP2 gene may predispose to autism and mental retardation. Information on DNA testing for the MECP2 gene is available at the website of the City of Hope's Clinical Molecular Diagnostic Laboratory, accessible via the Companion Website for this text.

New research that has emerged from the Autism Genome Project Consortium at NIMH has implicated the brain's glutamate chemical messenger system and a previously overlooked site on chromosome 11. Based on studies of 1,168 families with at least two affected members, the research adds to evidence that tiny, rare variations in genes may heighten the risk for ASD (NIMH, 2008). Another Consortium study has identified a defect—a missing segment—on chromosome 16 (Weiss et al., 2008). None of the parents in this study had the chromosomal defect, leading researchers to conclude that some cases of genetically caused autism are due to a random accident while the egg or sperm is being formed and not to heritability.

WHAT EVERY NEONATAL NURSE SHOULD KNOW

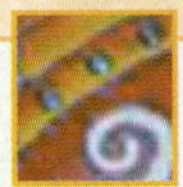

Prematurity and Mental Health Problems

Infants born prematurely are at greater risk of developing mental health problems. Neonatal nurses who help parents learn parenting skills in caring for their infant can improve the child's mental health outcomes. Important parenting skills include attending to the infant's behavioral cues, understanding the potential meaning of various infant behaviors, and reducing the infant's distress through soothing, consoling, and other stress reduction techniques.

Box 26-1 Risk Factors for Developing Mental Health Problems in Childhood

- Inherited metabolic deficiencies or nervous system abnormalities
- Injury, toxic exposure, or physical complications in utero or during the perinatal period
- Medical conditions of infancy or childhood (such as epilepsy, low birth weight)
- Early deprivation of nurturance or stimulation (parental absence or loss, neglect or rejection, large family size, foster placement)
- Traumatic experience (such as abuse or life-threatening event)
- Family history of a psychiatric disorder
- A chaotic home environment (family violence or severe marital discord)
- Disadvantaged socioeconomic status (poverty, violence, hopelessness)

Perinatal Complications

Perinatal complications, including perinatal asphyxia, congenital anomalies, and intrauterine exposure to drugs and alcohol, have also been associated with psychiatric disorders (Delobel-Ayoub et al., 2006; Linares et al., 2006). Refer to the feature What Every Neonatal Nurse Should Know regarding potential effects of premature birth.

Brain Structure and Function

Finally, there is a growing body of research that suggests that early psychological trauma from severe neglect or abuse may create deficits or abnormalities in brain structure and function. It was previously thought that a child's biologic makeup could influence his or her psychosocial outcomes but not the reverse. Evidence now indicates that psychological trauma in the first few years of life can create changes in the size of the brain, the number of neuronal pathways affecting certain brain functions (such as emotion), and the amount and function of neurotransmitters in the brain (van der Kolk, 2003).

Multicausal Model

While each of the perspectives just described is often considered in isolation, there is growing acceptance of a multicausal, multidimensional nature in any etiology of mental illness. Box 26-1 lists potential risk factors that have been identified for childhood mental illness.

Although various schools of thought may emphasize specific risk factors, as nurses, we need to view mental health in an integrative, interactive way. In this view, the child's genetically determined attributes or vulnerabilities are seen to interact with life experience to influence mental health outcomes (see FIGURE 26-2 ■).

Many children show tremendous hardiness and resilience in the face of horrible life experiences, while other, more vulnerable children may be severely affected by even a minimally stressful or adverse experience. Not only do the child's characteristics affect how the child will respond to and internalize what is experienced, but he or she can influence what the environment provides as a result of a genetically given temperament or biomedical status.

It is important to remember that children both:

- Actively elicit and seek out certain responses and experiences
- Perceive what is given by the environment through the looking glass of their unique genotype

These factors interact with what is actually available in the environment to determine the degree to which a child achieves mental health or develops a mental illness. In a multicausal model, there is no certain etiology, no predictable set of risk factors, and no specific therapeutic approach having a standard effectiveness. The unique fit between a particular child and a particular set of life experiences must be considered to understand the child's mental health problems and develop an appropriate intervention (Fonagy, Target, Cottrell, Phillips, & Kurtz, 2005).

Genetic Predisposition
• Metabolic Deficiencies
• Nervous System Abnormalities
Interaction Between Genotype and Experience
Life Experience
• Injury/Illness
• Toxic Exposure
• Deprivation/Neglect
• Abuse/Rejection
• Other Major Stressors (e.g., death of a parent)

FIGURE 26-2 ■ Interactive model of child mental illness.

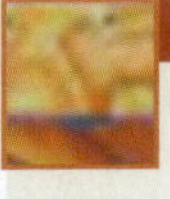

NURSING PROCESS Children

The assessment, diagnosis, planning, implementation, and evaluation activities undertaken by the child psychiatric–mental health nurse are always in collaboration with the child, the family, and professional colleagues who are part of the child's care. The degree to which these individuals are active partners in the nursing process will influence the resulting quality and efficacy of your nursing care.

Assessment

The basics of an effective assessment include gathering cultural and developmental information, eliciting a history from the parents, and undertaking a clinical assessment of the child.

Cultural and Developmental Context

MEDIALINK Autism Case Study Video

Your ability to perform a valid assessment depends on your knowledge of developmental norms and your cultural sensitivity, including gathering pertinent cultural information within which to consider a particular child's behavior. Your nursing assessment must occur within the context of a child's cultural background and developmental stage. What can be defined as "normal or functional" versus "abnormal or dysfunctional" is relative to the meaning certain behaviors have within a culture and the child's developmental capabilities.

For instance, temper tantrums can be viewed very differently within different cultures. In one culture, tantrums may be viewed as the result of a nervous temperament or a fragile personality. Families of another culture may think that tantrums are the disobedient acts of a stubborn child. These different perceptions bring about different responses by the parent, which may, in turn, affect the child's behavior over time.

Asking families what they believe about the cause of their child's problems is a good way to assess their culture-specific beliefs. You can also find out what their parents and grandparents have said about the problems as well as traditional resource people within their communities (such as spiritual advisors or healers). Also be sure to ask whether they have used any traditional remedies or cultural practices to deal with the child's problems. It is important to show respect for a family's unique views of mental illness and to build a mutually acceptable approach to your assessment. As the following clinical example illustrates, you may also need to help family members reconcile different cultural beliefs within the family.

CLINICAL EXAMPLE

The maternal grandmother of a suicidal child who was scheduled for admission to an inpatient unit tried to block the admission. She insisted that the child was possessed by a demon and wanted the child to stay with her so she could pray over her and give her healing herbs.

The child psychiatrist and the child psychiatric nurse spent time with the parents discussing the pressure they experienced from the child's grandmother. They mentioned to the parents that psychiatric services were unfamiliar to the grandmother's generation and cultural beliefs. They also reviewed the basis for the recommendation of hospitalization. The parents were encouraged to make their own decision based on their experience with their child and their concerns for her safety. Ways to involve the grandmother and her traditional medicines were suggested, and the professionals offered to be available to discuss the grandmother's questions and concerns.

Regarding developmental norms, you must determine whether a behavior (such as temper tantrums or separation anxiety) is understandable or appropriate based on the child's age. Stage of development affects the symptoms you will see, a child's expected responses to life stress, and the child's ability to understand and communicate with you about certain problems. Be sure to allow adequate time for full responses to open-ended questions, active listening, and careful observation of patterns of behavior. Assessment should be an ongoing process rather than a one-time session. Do not assume that observations can be generalized to other times and settings.

The History-Taking Interview

When taking a history, include the child as well as the parents in the discussion. Although parents are a better source of facts such as onset, developmental milestones, or context surrounding the symptoms, including the child is helpful because it:

- Decreases the child's feelings of being left out, talked about, or powerless in the situation
- Helps you learn the child's perspective. Children are the best informants regarding their feelings and thoughts. You will also find it very useful to hear an older child's response to the parents on certain issues or how the child's view may differ.
- Allows you to observe the nonverbal communication among family members. The way in which they interact will give important clues regarding the family's functioning in areas such as closeness, conflict, decision making, and flexibility.

Since parents may not be comfortable discussing certain information in front of their child, be sure to give them some time with you alone in addition to this total family approach. Specific areas to cover in the history-taking interview are outlined in the Your Assessment Approach feature. You may also wish to refer to Chapter 30 for specific suggestions on assessing family process.

Clinical Assessment of the Child

The clinical assessment of the child involves a mental status exam by the nurse and referral of the child for a complete physical and neuropsychologic evaluation. These latter evaluations are important in order to rule out any medical condi-

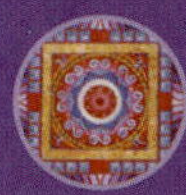

YOUR ASSESSMENT APPROACH
Areas to Cover in the History-Taking Interview

1. ***The child's current problems.*** Discuss the history of the problems, including major concerns or complaints, how long it has been since the problem(s) first began, the specific symptoms, and the parents' previous and current efforts to address the problem(s).
2. ***Family history and process.*** Talk with the family about their own history and family process. This aspect of the assessment can include a genogram or family time line (see the description in Chapter 30), discussion of child-rearing beliefs and behaviors, supports and stressors for the family, the history of any separations between parents and child, and any psychiatric or other illness in the family.
3. ***The child's medical history.*** Find out about any childhood illnesses, allergies, medications, and physical health problems.
4. ***The child's developmental history.*** Starting with pregnancy or birth complications, progress through the child's development to identify any lags or events in achieving developmental milestones.
5. ***The child's characteristics and psychosocial environment.*** Find out both the parents' and the child's view of the child's temperament, interests, and skills. During this aspect of the interview, also identify the nature of the child's sociocultural environment (home, neighborhood, school) and how it may support or inhibit the achievement of developmental tasks. Be sure to find out about the number and type of friends the child has.

tions and identify any neurologic or cognitive problems that may be associated with the child's psychiatric symptoms.

A mental status exam consists of both a semistructured interview and an unstructured play session with the child. Areas for assessment during the mental status exam are shown in Your Assessment Approach: Guidelines for Children. If the child is nearing adolescence or is ambivalent about unstructured play, try games instead as a medium through which you can observe the child's way of relating and approaching various situations.

For both aspects of the exam, a relaxed, conversational approach is the most effective, where the child has the opportunity to tell you his story about problems he may be having and his relationships with family, peers, and teachers. Research has shown that children are a better source than their parents regarding the nature and extent of their symptoms. Frame questions in ways that are developmentally appropriate for the child. Even 3- to 6-year-olds can give excellent feedback about their symptoms if questions are developmentally appropriate. Asking simple, informal questions such as what

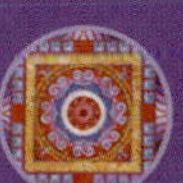

YOUR ASSESSMENT APPROACH
Guidelines for Children

Areas to Assess During the Mental Status Exam

General Appearance and Demeanor
- Grooming, alertness, eye contact, and overall attitude toward clinician

Motor Behavior and Coordination
- Activity level, gross motor and fine motor control, nature of movements, posture

Mood and Affect
- Overall mood state, manner of expressing feelings, range and intensity of emotions, evidence of dysphoric state (anger, anxiety, sadness)

Speech and Language
- Clarity and articulation, rhythm and organization, appropriateness of word choice

Thought Process
- Ability to understand and express meaning in an age-appropriate way, evidence of any loss of connectedness between ideas (loose associations), repeated behaviors or mannerisms (perseveration), or tangentiality of child's response to your questions

Thought Content
- Themes in play and talk, fears, evidence of beliefs that have no basis in reality

Perceptual Disturbances
- Threshold and tolerance for sensory input, evidence of hallucinations or illusions

Cognitive Function
- Orientation to person, time, and place; ability to follow through on requests; attention and concentration; distractability

Impulse Control
- Ability to manage behavior appropriately in response to needs and desires

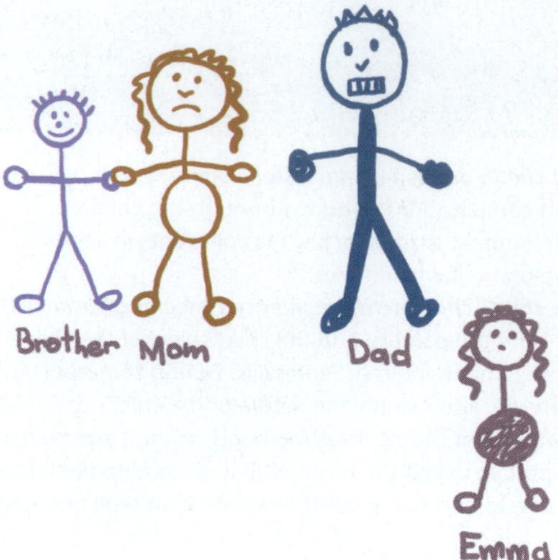

FIGURE 26-3 ■ Family drawing by Emma, a 6-year-old girl. Emma's drawing has a number of distinctive features. She has placed herself at a distance from the rest of the family, suggesting feelings of isolation, rejection, or perhaps fear. The heavy lines around her father's body may indicate that he is seen as aggressive or angry. This interpretation is supported by the father's mouth, which appears to be open as if shouting or showing his teeth. Her brother looks happy, and her mother's downturned mouth looks a bit sad. Emma's drawing of herself is quite small, in contrast to others in the family (especially her brother, who is actually younger and smaller than Emma). Her smallness could indicate some insecurity, low self-esteem, or perhaps a desire to withdraw from the world and not be noticed. The center of Emma's body is shaded, suggesting some anxiety about that part of her body. She is also missing her mouth and hands. This could imply a sense of inadequacy or powerlessness to act or speak.

kind of animal they would like to be, what they would want if they could have three wishes, or what was the saddest thing that ever happened to them can provide a great deal of information regarding speech, modes of thinking and perception, and feeling states. Having children draw and discuss pictures of themselves and their family can be very useful for understanding their view of the world. The drawing in FIGURE 26-3 ■ by a 6-year-old girl named Emma is an excellent example.

Observing a child at play with puppets, clay, or a sand tray can also provide invaluable information about motor behavior, thought content, affect, and impulse control. In addition, there are many children's books using stories about abuse, depression, divorce, or hospitalization as themes. These stories portray children and animals with problems that relate to a variety of mental health challenges faced by children. They can serve as a stimulus for questions such as "How do you think that puppy might feel?" or "What would you do if you were that little girl?" These stories offer children opportunities to project their own thoughts and feelings onto the characters in the stories and share them with you.

Assessing Possible Maltreatment

You should always be alert for possible signs of maltreatment during your psychiatric assessment. Maltreatment is frequently identified in emergency departments as well (see the What Every Emergency Department Nurse Should Know feature). Some of the most important signs of maltreatment in a child are detailed in Your Assessment Approach: Signs of Maltreatment of a Child.

Maltreatment can involve child neglect or outright abuse. In neglect, parents fail to recognize when a problem exists or to meet their child's normal emotional and physical needs. Abuse can take many forms. It may be physical, involving severe disciplinary practices (e.g., beatings) or unexplained injury to the child (e.g., burns or bruises). Before age 12, boys are at greater risk of physical abuse but girls are more at risk as teenagers. Abuse can also be emotional, such as a child being verbally demeaned or rejected. And, of course, sexual abuse is possible. Sexual abuse can include exposure to exhibitionism, molestation or fondling, nonassaultive intercourse, or rape. Girls are more likely than boys to be victims of sexual abuse by a 10-to-1 ratio. Chapter 24∞ has more information on physical and sexual child abuse.

WHAT EVERY EMERGENCY DEPARTMENT NURSE SHOULD KNOW

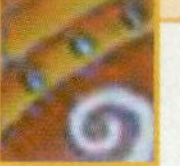

Assessing Physical Abuse in Children

Physical abuse of children can be addressed through careful observation in the emergency department (ED). Take special notice if:

- A child seems hypervigilant or hyperreactive to your touch
- A parent seems evasive, unconcerned, or resistant to your questions or any follow-up procedures

Collect further information if the following risk indicators are present:

- The child has been admitted to the ED for previous injuries.
- There are inconsistencies between your clinical exam and the parent's or child's description of what occurred.
- There was a delay in bringing the child for medical attention.

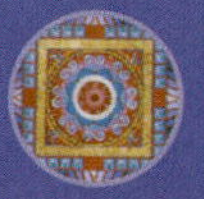

YOUR ASSESSMENT APPROACH
Signs of Maltreatment of a Child

When performing a clinical assessment of a child, be alert for any of the following:

- Unexplained or unusual history of physical injuries
- Fearful and withdrawn or hyperalert and placating behavior
- Unexplained developmental delays in language or motor behavior
- Malnutrition and dehydration
- Medical problems such as vaginal bleeding or recurrent urinary tract infections

Assessing Suicide Risk

Suicide by children, while always a difficult and devastating situation, has become more of a problem as we are not entirely sure what causes the rate to rise or fall. There is a continuing discussion over the role of antidepressants in youth suicide (see Chapters 23 and 32). NIMH notes that rate changes in youth suicide can be linked to the competent use of appropriate antidepressant treatment (NIMH, 2006). Studies report a decline in suicide attempts and completed suicides among adults and adolescents who are prescribed antidepressant medications (Gibbons, Hur, Bhaumik, & Mann, 2006). All child suicide statistics are confounded by the ages included in the report and by the tendency of professionals and families to label suicidal acts as accidents. Depending on age, children may not conceptualize death as an irreversible state, and to that degree, suicide may be accidental.

Some people cannot believe that children can be depressed or would want to end their lives. Suicide attempts by children belie the myth of the "happy child" in our culture. The following clinical example illustrates denial and lack of information on the part of the parents of a suicidal child.

CLINICAL EXAMPLE

A 7-year-old boy set up a rope over a door to hang himself. His attempt was stopped by his parents. The door, a second entrance to the room, was nailed shut and painted, but the subject of suicide was not discussed. His parents failed to recognize the same symptoms in the child 2 years later. At this time, however, severe behavioral problems in school, and pressure by school personnel, forced the parents to seek a psychiatric evaluation.

Although suicide in children under 12 occurs infrequently, suicidal ideation or suicide threats by a child always deserve attention and merit careful study. Even the most obvious gesture can prove fatal, especially in a child whose assessment of physical danger is immature and unrealistic. Children commit suicide by simple but lethal methods such as poisoning, shooting themselves with firearms, hanging, or darting into the path of moving cars.

It is unclear what drives a child to suicide. However, there are characteristic presuicidal symptoms and life circumstances of the suicidal child. The symptoms are known as depressive equivalents; that is, the symptoms may indicate a masked depression (see the feature What Every Pediatric Nurse Should Know). Life circumstances that put the child at higher risk for suicide are experiences of significant loss, family discord, abuse, neglect, or the presence of other psychiatric problems, such as depression and related disorders.

A careful assessment of suicide risk should be done whenever a child expresses ideas about suicide or makes an attempt. The assessment interview should consider the degree of risk while exploring the family situation and the external events that preceded the thoughts or the attempt. The meaning behind the attempt must be explored. Young children are less able to verbalize, and thus require more structure and planned activities before an appropriate assessment can be made. You may, for example, want to use books that help children talk about suicide.

Also see Chapter 23 for a discussion of youth suicide and child survivors of the death by suicide of a parent.

WHAT EVERY PEDIATRIC NURSE SHOULD KNOW

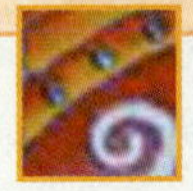

Childhood Depression

Parents are often unaware of their child's sadness or depression and do not recognize suicide risk. A confidential discussion with the child is essential in assessing suicidal thoughts or actions. Signs of depression can be masked, so take note if a parent or child reports the following symptoms:

- Boredom or lethargy
- Irritability or restlessness
- Difficulty concentrating
- Purposeful misbehavior
- Somatic preoccupation
- Isolation from others or excessive dependence on others

Nursing Diagnosis: NANDA

Your nursing assessment will provide information for both a psychiatric diagnosis using DSM-IV-TR criteria and nursing diagnoses.

Nursing diagnoses are the critical foundation underlying all planning, implementation, and evaluation activities with a child. Once you identify a child's problems, determine which of the NANDA diagnoses best match the problems. Then, prioritize the diagnoses based on their urgency or their need for attention before other problems can be addressed. There are some diagnoses specific to children in the NANDA classification system, such as:

- Disorganized Infant Behavior
- Risk for Delayed Development
- Risk for Impaired Parent/Child Attachment

Many other general diagnoses are relevant to children, such as Impaired Verbal Communication, Anxiety, Disturbed Sensory Perception, Ineffective Coping, Impaired Social Interactions, Risk for Violence, Post-Trauma Syndrome, and Chronic or Situational Low Self-Esteem. Many family and parent-related diagnoses are also quite relevant.

Outcome Identification: NOC

After determining your nursing diagnoses, identify outcomes that are important for the child and/or family to achieve specific to each diagnosis. These outcomes are behaviors or skills that are necessary to bring about positive mental health changes. For instance, you may have identified a diagnosis of disturbed sensory perception in a young child with autism who is highly sensitive to being touched. You could then work with the child's parents to identify specific outcomes they would like to achieve, such as the child being able to receive an affectionate stroke from the parent or have her hair cut without becoming agitated and emotionally distressed.

Planning and Implementation: NIC

Planning and implementation of nursing care depend on the nursing diagnoses for the child and family. The treatment approaches most commonly used by child psychiatric–mental health professionals are shown in the following Your Intervention Strategies feature, along with a rationale for when each is likely to be useful. There are, however, many other approaches that can be used.

Child–Parent Psychotherapy

Child–parent psychotherapy should be considered by the advanced-practice child psychiatric nurse when a parent or caregiver has beliefs or a caregiving style that may be contributing to the child's mental health problems (Timmer, Urquiza, Zebell, & McGrath, 2005). It can also be very effective when the child has temperament or behavioral characteristics that are creating special challenges for a parent. There are many approaches to child–parent psychotherapy, depending on the clinician's theoretical perspective. It is used with a wide variety of problems, including pervasive developmental disorders, feeding disorders, disruptive behavior disorders, maltreatment, and reactive attachment disorder (Landreth & Bratton, 2006). In child–parent psychotherapy, the nurse works closely with both the primary caregiver (usually the mother) and the child, focusing on three components: the child's behavior, the parent's attitudes and feelings about the child, and the interaction between parent and child. Depending on the particular problems being addressed, greater focus may be placed on one of these components.

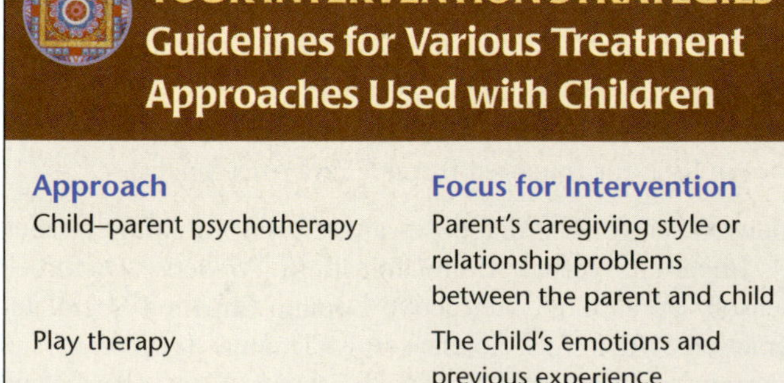

YOUR INTERVENTION STRATEGIES
Guidelines for Various Treatment Approaches Used with Children

Approach	Focus for Intervention
Child–parent psychotherapy	Parent's caregiving style or relationship problems between the parent and child
Play therapy	The child's emotions and previous experience
Cognitive behavioral therapy	The child's attitudes, beliefs, and behaviors
Family therapy	The dynamics of family interaction
Medication	A neurobiologic deficit or abnormality

WHY I BECAME A PSYCHIATRIC–MENTAL HEALTH NURSE

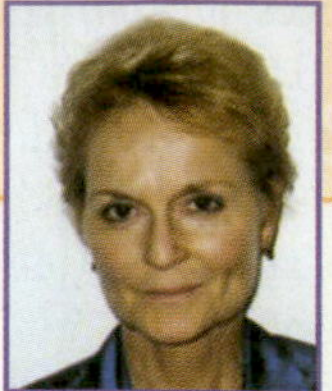

Sandra Weiss
Contributor, Chapter 26

When I began my nursing career, I worked in critical care nursing, where much of the emphasis was on assessment and management of the individual's biological processes. While I found that focus stimulating and important, I was drawn to the psychological issues being faced by my patients and their families. I became the resident "expert" on the unit to whom "psychologically difficult" patients and families were assigned. Because of my growing interest in the psychological components of care, I returned to graduate school to increase my knowledge and skills in mental health nursing. Never had I been so excited about a field of study.

To this day, I continue to feel the same excitement when I read a new article about some aspect of the field or design and conduct some new research project that I believe can ultimately improve mental health care. I have felt privileged, throughout my career, to be trusted with the deep psychological struggles and emotional pain that children and their families have shared with me and to help them address these struggles or find ways to resolve and manage their pain. The field has provided me with the tools to enhance my own personal growth and address my own psychological struggles in a meaningful way. This self-growth has improved my mental health care of others and my own quality of life. I feel very fortunate to have chosen this field as the medium for my life's work. There is simply nothing that interests me more!

Child Behavior The focus on the child aims to identify specific difficulties in the child's temperament or behavior and to help manage these difficulties more effectively. *Temperament* is the constitutional makeup of the child at birth, specifically the child's behavioral and psychophysiologic attributes. For instance, infants who have been exposed to drugs in utero may be very sensitive to stimulation from lights, sounds, or touch; may cry frequently and be difficult to console; and have trouble developing regular patterns of sleep. An infant with such a temperament will need help to develop better regulation of sleep patterns and responses to distress through a variety of activities that reduce stimulation and help calm and soothe the infant. In this way, the child may feel less distressed and begin to feel more secure with people.

You may also work to improve a child's interpersonal skills or capacity to respond through interventions that help the child learn how to be a more active social partner. These skills are important to the child's ability to engage the parents and respond in ways that reward their caregiving. Parents watch the nurse work with the child to develop a better understanding of the child's unique temperament and needs.

Parental Attitudes and Feelings Focusing on the parent's attitudes and feelings toward the child is essential, especially for caregivers whose feelings about the child or attitudes about parenting are distorted in some way. For example, distortions can occur as a result of a parent's own maltreatment as a child or current mental illness. Interventions with the parent may include exploration of feelings about the parent's own history and family relations and how they are affecting the care of the child. Parents who receive your empathy and support may experience less psychological distress and be able to rework the model they hold in their mind of their relationship with their child. The goal of these interventions is to increase the capacity of the parent to nurture the child and find satisfaction in the role of caregiver.

Interaction Between Parent and Child. Child–parent psychotherapy provides interaction guidance in order to sensitize the parents to appropriate caregiving practices. You can do this by modeling specific ways of interacting with the child, suggesting approaches for the parents to try, supporting and praising the use of positive interactions, and speaking for the child so the parents become more aware of the child's potential experience during caregiving (e.g., "Oh, I feel so safe and loved when you snuggle me close like this . . ."). You can also teach the parent certain approaches that will help reduce a child's symptoms or encourage growth in an area where the child is having difficulties.

Each of the components of child–parent psychotherapy attempts to enhance the *goodness-of-fit* between parent and child in order to increase their enjoyment in one another and provide the child with a more supportive foundation for optimal mental health. This therapeutic approach can change the way the child behaves toward the parent, the way the parent interprets the child's behavior and defines the parent role, and the way the parent behaves toward the child. The theoretical orientation of clinicians who use child–parent psychotherapy may vary, but it typically reflects an interactive model of mental illness and integrates the theories described earlier.

Play Therapy

Play therapy is child-centered (Landreth, 2002) and typically builds on the foundation of the psychodynamic, object-relations, and attachment theories described earlier. Although play therapy is used as part of most assessment protocols and to treat a variety of mental health problems, you may find it quite helpful for nursing diagnoses associated with posttraumatic stress disorder, disruptive behavior disorders, mood disorders, and reactive attachment disorder. Play therapy can be used by advanced-practice child psychiatric nurses with children who are around 3 years of age or older. The generalist nurse does therapeutic play with children, but not play therapy. The generalist nurse uses reflection, but not interpretation (discussed later in this section).

Nondirective play is normally viewed as the best way to begin play therapy. The symbols and themes that emerge in play provide a core of information for assessment and subsequent treatment. They give us the same type of information that we gather through verbal communication with adults. Remember that symbols (such as aggressive behavior toward a father doll) can have several meanings and should never be interpreted in a standardized fashion. Always consider the way a symbol is used in the play as it may relate to the particular context of the child's life before you interpret a symbol's subjective meaning to a child. Your impressions must be verified or refuted based on a variety of different types of information collected over time. The following clinical example illustrates the multiple subjective meanings in a symbol.

CLINICAL EXAMPLE

When she was a preschooler, 12-year-old Laura had been sexually molested by her father. Her father was sent to prison for the sexual molestation of another preschooler. During Laura's therapy session, she built a fortress of large multicolored blocks. She put a chair inside the structure and sat down, stating, "This is a dungeon. A rainbow dungeon." As the nurse used gentle questions to help Laura talk about what the dungeon meant to her, she began to speak hesitantly of her father and the ambivalence she had about his sexual abuse. Although the dungeon symbolized how trapped and tormented she felt during the times she was molested, they also were the only times she felt loved and cared for by her father. This was the feeling symbolized by the rainbow dungeon.

There is a general belief that toys with ambiguous meaning and diverse uses foster symbolic play more effectively because they allow the child to project his or her own identity and function onto the toys. However, there may be times when you want to move the child more directly into specific play themes through structured play. In these situations, toys with an obvious identity or function may be selected for a play session (as in addressing themes of parental separation or abuse). Structured play is rarely used until nondirective play has enabled a full assessment of relevant themes and issues, and the child's trust around anxiety-laden issues has been developed.

Purposes of Play Therapy Play therapy can serve many purposes. A major use is for *catharsis*, the release of strong emotions in order to provide relief from the inner tension they may be causing the child. It is also believed that expressing emotions, interactions, and relationships, even though they may not be conscious for the child, provides some kind of cognitive relief. Catharsis can be facilitated through many forms of play, including drawings, doll play, clay modeling, or the acting-out of certain feelings through pounding toys or punching dolls or bags.

Another purpose of play therapy is *abreaction*, the reliving through play of past events and their related feelings. Through abreaction, the child gradually can assimilate previous experiences that have been traumatic or painful. Assimilation occurs through the release of related emotions, as well as through integrating what happened into the child's ongoing view of himself and the world. The basis of this integration is the opportunity, through play, to gain mastery over an experience in which the child most likely had no control. Mastery comes from reenacting the event in the child's own way, working through the feelings that were part of the experience,

MediaLink Critical Thinking Exercise: Working with Child Psychiatric Clients and modifying, over time, how it happened and what the outcome may have been.

Another frequent use of play therapy is to help the child try out other ways of relating to the world or responding to situations. At about 3 years of age, children have the capacity for role-play (Russ, 2004). In taking on certain roles, they can learn how others may feel or think (by putting themselves in somebody else's shoes). Role-play can occur through the child taking on a character himself or projecting that character onto a puppet or doll.

Therapeutic Interventions Regardless of the specific purpose of play therapy, your interventions should involve a combination of reflection and interpretation to help the child gain greater awareness of the unconscious issues that are becoming apparent (see the following Your Intervention Strategies feature).

Reflection involves simple commenting on what is happening in the child's play—for example, "The boy doll is hitting the father doll again." Such a statement includes no interpretation but has the potential to help the child become more aware of what is happening in the play. Reflection is the major intervention used by more inexperienced clinicians, including the generalist nurse. It is also the mainstay for clinical specialists during their initial work with the child. However, there should be a few sessions of play observation without any reflective comment, to allow the child to gain comfort in the play, before eliciting any anxiety that may arise as a result of reflection.

The use of *interpretation* begins after rapport and trust have been established, and it can range from subtle to very direct. Subtle interpretations are more removed from the child and speak to the potential meaning behind the toy's behavior—for instance, "The boy doll is hitting the father doll because he's very angry at him." More direct interpretations are used over time as the advanced-practice nurse develops greater confidence in the validity of the interpretations for the child—for example, "I wonder if you feel like the boy doll. You seem angry at your dad for leaving." Obviously, these more direct interpretations must integrate anything observed in the play with your total assessment of the child's issues and problems in the real world.

YOUR INTERVENTION STRATEGIES
Play Therapy

In either nondirective or more structured play therapy, you can use these two key strategies:

Strategy	Rationale
Reflection (describing what the child is doing or saying during play)	■ Helps establish rapport and trust because the child feels seen and heard ■ Increases the child's awareness of his/her behavior during play
Interpretation (commenting on the potential meaning of the child's play)	■ Helps the child become more aware of the issues that may be causing distress ■ Creates opportunities for the child to release pent-up emotions (catharsis) ■ Helps the child to assimilate painful experiences (abreaction)

Cognitive Behavioral Therapy

The approaches used in cognitive behavioral therapy stem from cognitive behavioral theory, described earlier. Two major differences exist between this modality and traditional play therapy:

1. First, cognitive behavioral approaches focus on the child's conscious rather than unconscious issues.
2. Second, emphasis is placed on more effective coping in the present rather than on mastery over unresolved feelings associated with the child's past experiences.

Cognitive behavioral approaches have been particularly successful in treating problems associated with depression, conduct disorder, ADHD, and anxiety in children 7 and older (Martin & Pear, 2007). Behavioral techniques, without the cognitive component, are also widely used to address therapeutic goals for 3- to 6-year-old children and those with mental retardation, learning and communication disorders, pervasive developmental disorders, tic disorders, and elimination disorders.

Cognitive Restructuring Cognitive behavioral treatment is a reeducation and relearning process involving the development of new ways of thinking about life and new behaviors that are more adaptive and more functional for the child. The cognitive aspects of therapy attempt to modify inaccurate or biased ways of processing information that result in distortions of what is actually occurring in the child's world (Martin & Pear, 2007; Stallard, 2005).

The process of cognitive restructuring involves strategies such as finding out what the child means by statements he makes, teaching him to question the "evidence" he's using to maintain any irrational beliefs, helping him identify other options for what a situation might mean, listing advantages and disadvantages of a particular belief, and teaching him to use self-talk or directives to himself to help change or reframe a situation—for example, "Stop and wait; don't get angry until you find out more." You can coach the child to think differently about problems, thereby helping him more effectively make sense of the world. In this way, the child begins to modify his perceptions of interactions with others and his expectations for the future.

Behavioral Approaches The behavioral aspects of therapy are based to a great extent on classical and operant conditioning techniques. The major classical conditioning technique is systematic desensitization, which involves the pairing of a nega-

WHY I BECAME A PSYCHIATRIC–MENTAL HEALTH NURSE

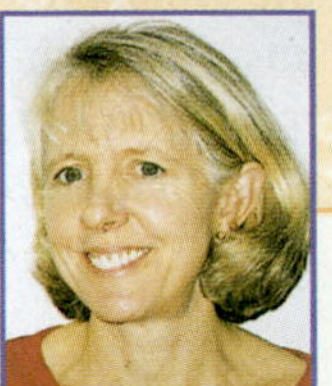

Sandra Niemann
Contributor, Chapter 26

Although I didn't plan to become a psychiatric nurse when I entered nursing school, a clinical rotation at a state mental hospital during my last semester changed all that. That semester I cared for a client with chronic schizophrenia. Although in retrospect I realize I understood very little about her world, her aloneness and daily struggle touched me. And her obvious pleasure in my visits solidified something I'd recently learned but didn't yet believe—that a relationship is often the most powerful treatment of all.

This same realization brought me back to a doctoral program in nursing many years later, this time to do research in infant mental health. I had recently adopted my daughter from Taiwan, where she spent her first seven months in an orphanage. I could see the imprint of these early months on her development, but there was very little research to tell me what lay ahead or the best practices for mitigating early deprivation. I would like to contribute to this field by conducting research that helps clarify what those best practices are.

tive stimulus (such as a feared situation or animal) with a positive stimulus (such as candy or relaxation exercises).

The pairing is done in a progressive way, so the child begins to handle situations that are increasingly fearful or aversive. For example, a child may initially look at pictures of a dog that scares him while having a favorite snack, and progress through a series of more frightening situations. Eventually, the child is asked to touch a dog and receives more positive rewards, such as a favorite snack, which counteract the negative impact.

Examples of operant conditioning techniques are contingency contracting, the use of tokens, modeling, and behavioral role-play groups. *Contracting* involves setting goals with a child, with specific consequences (positive and negative) clearly identified for achieving or not achieving the goals. *Tokens* can also be used in contracting, whereby points are accumulated or lost depending on the child's following through with agreed-upon behavior. These tokens can then be exchanged for various rewards that are important to the child. When a *modeling* intervention is used, children with specific problems are exposed to real or filmed examples of other children who model effective responses to difficult situations. *Behavioral role-play* takes modeling a step further to help the child try out new behaviors before applying them in the real world.

Milieu Therapy Based on Behavioral Approaches Cognitive behavioral approaches, such as the ones just described, serve as the basis for most milieu therapy in child psychiatric inpatient settings. These settings are for children with more severe mental health problems, who may require around-the-clock assessment to determine an exact diagnosis or intensive, consistent care for life-threatening or violent conditions.

The use of behavioral interventions on inpatient units allows nursing staff to give continuous feedback to the children about the appropriateness of their behavior. The children receive rewards such as verbal praise, a sticker, or points for appropriate behavior. For example, children who have a problem hitting others all the time may receive a sticker and verbal praise for no hits hourly, until they associate their behavior with the reward. At that time, the need for feedback may decrease to a less-frequent schedule, and later to only verbal reminders of the desired behavior.

At the same time staff members are trying to reward children for positive behavior, the children also need to know that certain hostile or aggressive behaviors cannot be tolerated. When children cannot behave in acceptable ways, they can take a time-out from the activity by sitting in chairs until they are able to pull themselves together. If that does not work, the time-out may be taken in a quiet room free of objects and stimulation. If isolation from others is also too difficult, you may need to help a child calm down by firmly holding him in place.

As the child calms down, help him see why he needed a time-out and what he can do differently next time. The goals are to have children learn what precedes episodes during which they lose control and learn ways to avoid the negative consequences of out-of-control behavior such as fights with other children. It is through effective limit-setting that you can help children separate their feelings from their behavior and learn more adaptive ways of expressing themselves.

The following clinical example illustrates how a program of rewards and sanctions helped one boy learn to control his anger at his peers.

MediaLink Application: Talking to Children About Community Violence

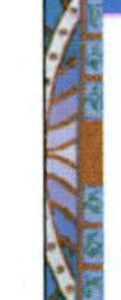

CLINICAL EXAMPLE

Jervis was a strong, very large 8-year-old boy with mild retardation. He was on a child psychiatric unit for evaluation after he severely injured another child during a fight. When the other children on the unit made fun of him or made faces at him, Jervis would strike out at them, often punching and knocking them to the floor.

The child psychiatric clinical nurse specialist, Rita, brought the unit staff together to develop a behavioral program for Jervis. Rita also met with Jervis to discuss a behavioral contract with him. Part of this discussion was to identify the things Jervis liked most and least on the unit because these would be used as part of his rewards or sanctions for fulfilling his part of the contract. For instance, he loved his television time, making cookies with the staff, and playing ball outside in the courtyard. But he disliked helping with cleanup after meals and sitting in the corner for a time-out from games or other activities. The purpose of the contract was to help Jervis learn to better control his anger when other children teased him. If he ignored the children or came to one of the staff to express his frustration or get their help in resolving the problem, he got a red star. If he struck out at the children, he got a blue dot. These were kept on a bulletin board in his room. For each red star, he could negotiate with staff for an extra something on his list of "likes." For each blue dot, he would either lose a chance to participate in one of his favorite activities or he would have to do something on his list of "dislikes."

Family Therapy

Family therapy goes beyond family involvement in the child's treatment to focus on treatment of the entire family (Nichols & Schwartz, 2005). This method is selected when interactions among family members need attention in order to address specific problems exhibited by the child. The goal is to increase the likelihood that improvements in the child's mental health will occur and will be supported in the home with consistent and sustained family patterns (Diamond & Josephson, 2005). The following clinical example illustrates how parents may need to be involved in order for treatment to progress.

CLINICAL EXAMPLE

The staff on an inpatient unit found they needed to help the parents of Nathan, a 12-year-old boy with conduct disorder, plan his weekend day passes. Nathan reported that he barely saw his parents while home on pass. Both parents worked most of the time, and when they were home, they argued a lot. So Nathan hung out at the local mall with his friends and got into trouble. This situation was interfering with Nathan's recovery and his transition back into the home.

The family therapist and primary nurse brought the family together to talk about the issues related to Nathan's use of time on his weekend passes. The overt goal of the first meeting was to help the family better structure Nathan's time and their availability to him. But it became clear that there was a great deal of conflict between the parents as well as much hostility directed at Nathan during the family discussions. Because the family conflict had implications for the success of Nathan's treatment, the entire family was scheduled for a number of therapy sessions.

Family therapy is described fully in Chapter 30, but there are a few issues specific to family therapy when children are included (Karver, Handelsman, Fields, & Bickman, 2005).

If children under age 7 are involved in family therapy, the nurse may choose to alternate between having the child present and seeing the parents or other family members only. The child's presence provides information for clinical assessment, allows for direct comment on and discussion of the dynamics that occur among parents and children, and provides opportunities for the nurse to model effective interaction with the child, as well as teach the family about normal development and positive parenting. However, there may be issues for discussion that are beyond the child's capacity to understand and/or inappropriate for discussion in front of the child. Meeting with the parents alone enables these issues to be more openly addressed in a setting with fewer distractions.

Family play therapy is another option with young children that enables their full participation. Usually, the first half of the family session involves either directive or nondirective play. In the second half, the parents talk with the therapist about family issues that arose during the play, while the child continues to play or engages in discussion as desired or when invited.

Older children can be involved with more typical family therapy approaches. The developmental status of the child's capabilities and the nature of the child's problems should guide the nurse's decisions with the family regarding the specific strategies to use.

Psychopharmacology

The nature of medication therapy is detailed in Chapters 7 and 32. However, there are important considerations in using medications with children. First, never assume that the actions and side effects of any medication will be the same for children as for adults. The size of a child's liver relative to the child's overall body size is different proportionately than in adults. This means that dosing for children could be lower than for adults of the same size.

Only recently have studies been undertaken to carefully examine the impact of medications on children at various developmental stages (Luby, 2006). Not only do children at various stages have different medication needs in terms of rates of absorption, excretion, sites of action, and toxicity, but these may change for the same child as he or she develops. You will need to monitor children carefully, with ongoing titration, if they are kept on a medication over extended periods of time.

Second, the developmental impact of a medication on a child must be weighed alongside its potential benefits for a specific mental health problem. Some research has shown that the developing neurotransmitter systems of young children can be very sensitive to medications and it is unclear how this sensitivity may affect their brain development (NIMH, 2006). Medications are often used to address a behavioral problem that may be disturbing to the child's family or teachers, yet their use may interfere with the child's developmental capacity. For instance, antipsychotic medications such as chlorpromazine (Thorazine) cause cognitive dulling and may interfere with learning. They also cause tardive dyskinesia, movement disorders that occur after chronic use. Stimulants may increase learning potential for children with ADHD, but they can also affect their physical growth potential. Such risks have significant implications for children who are developing and who may experience cumulative effects of medications over many years. All the benefits and risks must be balanced against one another in a full and open discussion with the child's family.

Three classes of medications are most commonly used with children: stimulants, antidepressants, and low-dose antipsychotics. Mood stabilizers and antianxiety agents are also prescribed. TABLE 26-2 ■ outlines these major classes of medications, their uses, and common side effects. Refer to Chapters 7 and 32 for a detailed discussion of psychopharmacology. You can refer families to the American Academy of Child and Adolescent Psychiatry website (http://www.aacap.org) for information on children and psychiatric medications.

MEDIALINK American Academy of Child and Adolescent Psychiatry

TABLE 26-2 Classes of Medications Used with Children

Medication Class	Disorders Treated	Side Effects
Stimulants	ADHD PDD Mental retardation	Anorexia and weight loss Abdominal pain Headache Sadness or mood lability, irritability Insomnia
Antidepressants	Major depression OCD Enuresis Separation anxiety ADHD Tourette's disorder PTSD Panic disorder Phobias	Fatigue, drowsiness, insomnia Nausea, upset stomach, diarrhea Cognitive dulling Tachycardia and hypotension Weight gain Restlessness, agitation Headaches, dizziness Dry mouth
Antipsychotics	Schizophrenia Tourette's disorder Severe aggression in PDD and CD	Sedation, lethargy Cognitive dulling Tremor, rigidity, drooling Nausea, diarrhea or constipation, abdominal discomfort Weight gain
Mood stabilizers	Bipolar disorder Mental retardation PDD	Tremor Weight gain Polyuria Nausea, abdominal discomfort, diarrhea Hypothyroidism Fatigue, lethargy, cognitive dulling
Antianxiety agents	Anxiety disorders Sleep disorders	Fatigue, drowsiness Addiction Disinhibition

Stimulants The stimulants most frequently used with children are methylphenidate (Ritalin, Concerta), dextroamphetamine sulfate (Dexedrine), and mixed amphetamine salts (Adderall), primarily for the treatment of ADHD. Some stimulants have been approved only for children over 6 years of age, while others may be used for ages 3 and up. Methylphenidate appears to have fewer side effects, although dextroamphetamine sulfate has a longer duration of action and is less expensive. A nonstimulant medication, atomoxetine (Strattera), is effective for some children and adults with ADHD.

It is very important to monitor for vital sign changes or signs of depression. An increase in symptoms (rebound effect) may occur as each dose wears off every 3 to 4 hours, so maintaining a consistent schedule for taking the medication is important for the parent or for you as the nurse who manages a child's medication.

There has been a fair amount of controversy regarding the long-term effects of stimulants on the growth of children (Martin, 2006). Some studies have found deficits in weight and height for children treated with these medications. But other research suggests that growth catches up once the stimulant is discontinued. Little is known about the effects of stimulants on children treated continually from childhood through adolescence. As a result, we cannot be sure about the persistence of growth deficits and whether they are the result of stimulant use versus maturational delays related to ADHD itself.

Antidepressants Antidepressants are used primarily to treat major depressive disorder and many anxiety disorders in children. They may also be used for enuresis, bulimia, and ADHD. Until recently, tricyclic antidepressants (TCAs) have been the most widely used with children, especially imipramine (Tofranil). But they can create cardiac rate and rhythm changes (a greater risk for children than adults) and can be highly toxic if overdosed accidentally by a child. So adults must closely supervise their administration and keep the medication in a safe place.

Because they have fewer side effects, selective serotonin reuptake inhibitors (SSRIs) have become the first-line medications of choice for treating depression, anxiety, and obsessive–compulsive behavior in children (Rihmer, 2007)). The SSRIs used with children include fluoxetine (Prozac), paroxetine (Paxil), citalopram (Celexa), sertraline (Zoloft), and fluvoxamine (Luvox). Because of the disinhibition that can occur when using antidepressants, some children may become more impulsive and uninhibited about harming themselves. Therefore, you will need to assess regularly the child's suicidal ideation and risk-taking behavior and teach the parents to monitor these as well.

Monoamine oxidase inhibitors (MAOIs) are rarely used for children because they require careful dietary control to prevent untoward interactions. Such control is very difficult for children.

Antipsychotics Antipsychotics (also called neuroleptics) may be used to treat psychosis, bipolar disorder, severe aggression, Tourette's disorder, or schizophrenia in children. However, antipsychotics are less effective in reducing psychotic symptoms in children than in adults. In addition, children don't respond as well to the medication used to control the acute extrapyramidal side effects (e.g., tremor or drooling) of the more traditional antipsychotic medications. Last, tardive dyskinesia and cognitive blunting can have major implications for a child's academic potential and ability to function effectively later in life. The newer atypical antipsychotics have fewer of these side effects than the typical antipsychotics such as haloperidol (Haldol) or thioridazine (Mellaril) and also appear to be more effective in reducing psychotic symptoms in children. Risperidone (Risperdal), olanzapine (Zyprexa), and quetiapine (Seroquel) have the most support for use with children (McKim, 2007).

You should be aware of the sometimes inappropriate use of antipsychotics to reduce agitated behavior or sedate children with mental retardation or pervasive developmental disorders (PDD). Although medications like haloperidol may be appropriate for some children who could injure themselves or others, medications should not be used as a substitute for careful supervision or behavioral interventions that could modify and control problem behaviors.

Mood Stabilizers Lithium carbonate (Lithobid) is the mood stabilizer used with children. Its primary use, however, is for severe aggression and agitation across a variety of disorders (e.g., mental retardation or PDD) rather than for managing mania. In general, children have a poorer response to lithium than do adults. In addition, children under 7 are more prone to toxic side effects of lithium than are older youth or adults, so its use must be cautiously considered. Seizures and coma may occur; it can be lethal in overdose. In addition, potential hypothyroidism from the use of lithium has especially negative consequences for a child because of the impact of thyroid disease on so many facets of development. Selected anticonvulsants such as carbamazepine (Tegretol) and valproic acid (Depakote) are also effective mood stabilizers for children.

Anxiolytics Benzodiazepines such as clonazepam (Klonopin) and lorazapam (Ativan) are only infrequently used with children. Most clinicians believe that symptoms of anxiety or sleep disturbances should be treated first with psychosocial interventions or perhaps SSRIs unless these methods have proved unsuccessful and the symptoms are causing severe impairment or distress for the child. Remember that benzodiazepines can become addictive if used over a period of time, so they are normally discontinued after a few weeks.

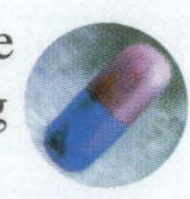

Nursing Interventions Nurses play an important role in monitoring the child on medication and educating the child and parents about the medication.

- Monitor side effects daily in inpatient settings and weekly in outpatient settings.
- If the child is being treated in an outpatient setting, work closely with parents and teachers to record the child's behavior.
- Assess the child's concerns about side effects and stigmatization by peers related to the medication.
- Take time to assess the parents' beliefs and fears about the medication. Parents are often concerned about side effects and the potential for dependency. Give them an opportunity to discuss their worries and questions as you educate them about the medication.
- Prepare the child and the parents for the possibility that symptoms will worsen when a medication is removed or decreased. Plan other interventions to help the child and family at this time.
- Discuss any risk that the medication may increase suicidal tendencies in the child, and review signs of masked depression with the parents (see the section "Assessing Suicide Risk" on page 711).

Responding to Suicide Risk

If your assessment of a child indicates that the child is at risk of attempting self-harm, you need to take immediate action.

1. Determine the seriousness of the attempt by talking to the child confidentially and asking questions such as the following:
   - Do you have a plan to hurt yourself? If so, tell me about it.
   - What would you do if you were thinking about hurting yourself? Would you let someone know before you did anything?
   - Do you want to be dead?

   Well-thought-out plans that avoid discovery and plans to use lethal methods indicate a greater risk for suicide completion.
2. If you are concerned by the child's responses, be sure that the child is seen by a psychiatrist or an advanced-practice psychiatric nurse for a comprehensive evaluation. The need for hospitalization must be considered.
3. If there is agreement by the psychiatric team that the child does not require hospitalization, you can do the following:
   - Obtain a promise from the child, in the form of a contract, not to cause self-harm for a specified period of time (see the discussion of no suicide/no self-harm contracts on page 629 in Chapter 23∞).
   - Obtain the support of the family in creating a safe environment for their child by making sure that all potentially lethal objects and medications are secured and out of sight.

If the child and family are unable or unwilling to agree to the contract or to create a safe home environment, it may be necessary to hospitalize the child.

Evaluation

The purpose of evaluation is to determine whether interventions are effective and how you should modify your care if necessary. The focus of evaluation should be on the nursing outcomes you have identified in your work with a particular child. But it is important to choose concrete and observable aspects of the child's behavior. Tangible changes or improvements are more readily assessed than vague statements that cannot be measured or observed in some way. For example, assessing an increase in the child's self-esteem is very difficult, but evaluating specific behaviors indicating esteem (such as positive statements about self or improved grooming) will make your evaluation easier and more useful.

Acquiring input from as many sources as possible is also essential to effective evaluation of the child. Have you obtained information from the child, parents, other nursing staff, or school personnel? Depending on the situation, it may or may not be possible to conduct a comprehensive evaluation, but it should be your goal whenever possible.

Remember that outcome criteria for evaluation must be congruent with appropriate developmental and sociocultural expectations. Frustration tolerance, for example, is much lower in the 4-year-old than the 14-year-old. For this reason, an accurate evaluation must consider the norms for age-appropriateness. Similarly, expectations should take into consideration the child's sociocultural norms. For instance, a child who exhibits aggressiveness or informality with adults may have had such behaviors encouraged at home but is viewed by the larger society as disrespectful toward authority. Children need to fit in with their own communities and social context as well as society as a whole, so these factors must be weighed as various outcomes are identified for interventions.

NURSE'S SELF-AWARENESS

In addition to the outcome criteria you establish to assess the effectiveness of your interventions, another critical feature of evaluation is the ongoing review and evaluation of your own process as a child psychiatric nurse. The following clinical example illustrates one instance in which staff feelings must be addressed in order for the staff to work effectively with a child and her family.

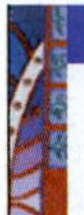

CLINICAL EXAMPLE

Eleven-year-old Luisa had a history of living with extended family and several hospitalizations. Luisa's mother was ambivalent toward her, often openly rejecting her (by visiting rarely, missing family sessions, and so on). Luisa's predicament stimulated a lot of feeling among the staff about bad mothers and good mothers, and staff members were protective of the child and angry at the mother. They were encouraged to examine the mother's own deprivation by an abusive mother and her difficulties in raising this very troubled child.

Are you aware of your attitudes and behaviors in working with specific children? How are these affecting your interventions with each child? For some key areas to consider in evaluating your potential impact, see the Your Self-Awareness feature below.

Working with children, particularly children with emotional problems, may activate feelings about your own unresolved issues with your family of origin or current family. You may then react as if the child is feeling or acting in ways that you might have felt or acted, and project your own issues onto the child, rather than responding to the child's actual therapeutic needs. Nurses may also respond to children or parents with certain stereotyped attitudes or beliefs, rather than being open to each child and parent as individuals. Self-awareness and ongoing self-monitoring and self-evaluation are essential skills for child psychiatric nurses. Without this capacity, you have little assurance that you can provide truly therapeutic nursing care.

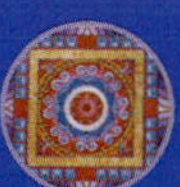

YOUR SELF-AWARENESS
Attitudes and Behavior Toward Child Psychiatric Clients

Honestly examining your attitudes and behavior toward child psychiatric clients can enhance your personal and professional growth. Consider the following:

Attitudes

- What do I like about this child?
- What don't I like about this child?
- Is there anything about this child's personality or problems that reminds me of myself or my own childhood?
- What feelings arise in me when I work with this child? What is it about the child or me that might cause these feelings?

Behavior

- How are my views/feelings about this child affecting the way I relate to the child? How are they helping my therapeutic work? How are they hindering my therapeutic work?
- How is the child responding to my interventions?

Personal Growth

- What am I learning about myself as I work with this child?
- Am I fully exploring these issues with my supervisor so that I can improve both my working relationship with this child and my insight as a child psychiatric nurse?

CASE MANAGEMENT

Community-based care and home care are dependent on effective case management. Case management by a child psychiatric–mental health nurse includes multiple responsibilities. In a full-service model, the nurse may work with a multidisciplinary team to provide most, if not all, of the major clinical and support services needed by a child. In another type of case management, the nurse serves as a broker for the child and family, identifying and arranging services that are then provided by other agencies or professionals. While this latter approach is frequently used when the case manager is not a nurse, it is less common for psychiatric nurses because of their multiple skills. Advanced-practice child psychiatric nurses can provide psychiatric assessment, medication prescribing and monitoring, symptom management, direct psychotherapy, supportive counseling, teaching, and coordination of overall care. Case management is especially useful for children with serious mental illness or those who do not respond well to standard treatment programs. As part of community-based care, a major feature of case management is collaboration with other agencies to improve care across the continuum of services. Effective collaboration requires nursing skills in communication, relationship building, and conflict resolution.

See the Partnering with Clients and Families feature for examples of useful information to share with families at various stages in the child's treatment.

COMMUNITY-BASED CARE

The focus of this chapter is on the care of children in both inpatient and outpatient settings. It is important to note, however, that advanced-practice nurses who are specialists in child psychiatry are now assuming growing responsibilities as primary care providers, case managers, counselors, and crisis team members in community mental health agencies and public health departments. Because mental health work with children entails close relationships with parents and school systems, the nurse's role in the community typically involves visits to the home and school as well as contacts with the juvenile justice system, family shelters, foster care placements, and social services. Child psychiatric nurses work in clinics, daycare programs, residential treatment programs, and school-based mental health programs. These sites may provide general mental health services or specialized care such as treatment for children who have been sexually abused, children in correctional facilities, or children with life-threatening illnesses.

HOME CARE

Resources for inpatient care have been reduced in recent years. As a result, children with serious mental health problems are often living at home. Home care presents numerous challenges that family members must face. You will need to engage parents as active members of their child's treatment. Develop a strong relationship with the family and work closely with the parents to help them learn strategies for managing their child's symptoms while promoting his or her mental health. Develop a care plan with parents for the daily management of the child's illness. Adherence to the plan will be enhanced if you do the following:

- Discuss the purpose and goals of each aspect of the child's treatment with the family. Be sure they understand what you have said by asking questions to assess their understanding.
- Educate the family about the child's symptoms and ways to manage them. Give the information in simply written handouts that will reinforce what you tell them.
- Give the family written reminders of days and times for therapy sessions, medications, and other treatments the child may have.
- Give the family information about whom to call if the child's mental health deteriorates or emergency management is needed.
- Schedule regular visits with the family to reinforce, support, and monitor their care of the child.

Involving parents as active members of their child's treatment team has a profound impact on the degree to which the treatment is effective.

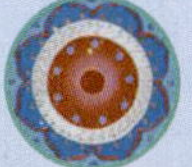

PARTNERING WITH CLIENTS AND FAMILIES

IMPORTANT TYPES OF INFORMATION TO DISCUSS WITH FAMILIES

- These are the symptoms your child may have as a result of his mental health problems. . .
- Some theories about the causes of your child's problems are. . .
- These are the options for treating your child's symptoms. . .
- This is the rationale for the recommended treatment. . .
- You can do these things to help reduce your child's symptoms. . .
- These are the potential side effects of the medications your child is receiving. . .
- This is what you can do to reduce the likelihood of side effects. . .
- Here are some specific suggestions for how to manage various side effects if they do occur. . .
- Here is the number of the person to contact if you have concerns about your child's symptoms or medications. . .
- Here are some strategies for coping with your own stress related to your child's problems. . .
- Here is some information and the number of a support group that may help you. . .

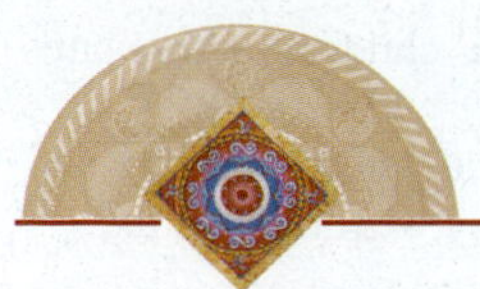

EXPLORE MEDIALINK 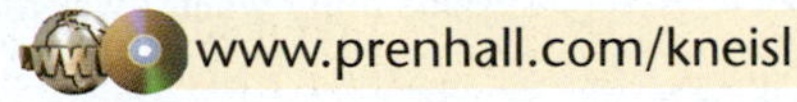

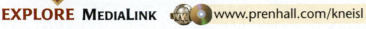

For NCLEX-RN® review questions, case studies, and other resources for this chapter see the Pearson Health MediaLink CD-ROM that accompanies this book and the Companion Website at www.prenhall.com/kneisl.

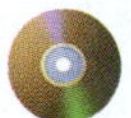

CD-ROM
Audio Glossary
NCLEX-RN® Review Questions
Videos
- *Autism Case Study*
- *Autism: What Is It?*

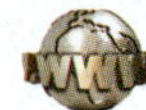

Companion Website
Audio Glossary
NCLEX-RN® Review Questions
Critical Thinking Exercise
- *Working with Child Psychiatric Clients*

Case Study
- *Autistic Disorder*

Care Plan
- *Oppositional Defiant Disorder*

MediaLinks
MediaLink Application
- *Talking to Children About Community Violence*

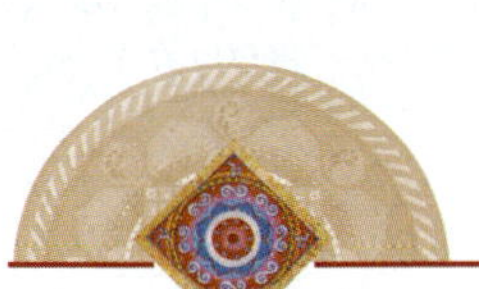

NCLEX-RN® REVIEW QUESTIONS

1. Of the following roles, which one is not within the scope of practice for the child psychiatric–mental health nurse?
1. Member of an interdisciplinary team
2. Assessing high-risk families
3. Identifying psychiatric diagnoses
4. Providing one–to–one counseling

2. The idea that a child's behavior is determined by how the child interprets his/her environment is consistent with which biopsychosocial theory?
1. Psychodynamic theory
2. Object-relations theory
3. Attachment theory
4. Cognitive behavioral theory

3. According to the multicausal or interactive model of childhood mental illness, which of the following statements is true?
1. The etiology of mental illness is known.
2. There is no predictable set of risk factors.
3. Therapeutic interventions are specific to the mental disorder.
4. The child's genetic predisposition does not influence mental health outcomes.

4. Which of the following is not considered a risk factor for developing mental health problems in childhood?
1. Physical complications in utero
2. Low birth weight
3. Family history of mental health well-being
4. Large family size

5. The difference between autism and Asperger's disorder is that children with Asperger's disorder:
1. Experience no loss of previously acquired skills.
2. Demonstrate delays in language development.
3. Exhibit delays in cognitive development.
4. Exhibit a lack of interest in the environment.

6. The nurse is assessing a child with a mental health problem. Which of the following questions would assist the nurse in gathering data regarding the family's cultural beliefs related to the child's problem?
1. Is there anyone else in your family who has a mental health problem?
2. Why do you think your child has a problem?
3. What do you believe to be the cause of your child's problem?
4. Tell me about your child's developmental milestones.

7. The purpose of abreaction in play therapy is to allow the child to:
1. Relive past events and feelings through play.
2. Establish a rapport with the therapist.
3. Identify more appropriate behaviors to deal with stress.
4. Systematically desensitize to fearful situations.

8. The nurse is working with the child and primary caregiver on issues related to the child's disruptive behaviors in school and at home. The nurse will focus on:
1. Interactions between the child's parents.
2. The child's behavior.
3. The primary caregiver's attitudes and feelings toward the nurse.
4. Interactions between the child and the teacher.

9. A 7-year-old child who had been prescribed lithium as a mood stabilizer is found to have lithium toxicity. The priority nursing diagnosis for this child is:
1. Activity Intolerance.
2. Risk for Aspiration.

3. Ineffective Therapeutic Regimen Management.
4. Disturbed Thought Process.

10. Which of the following statements by the nurse who works with children with psychiatric disorders is reason for concern?
1. "When the child becomes violent I need to protect the other clients on the unit."
2. "Since I have been working with this child, his acting-out behavior has lessened."
3. "I cannot get personally involved with the children."
4. "I know exactly how the child feels. I went through the same thing when I was that age."

See Appendix C for answers.

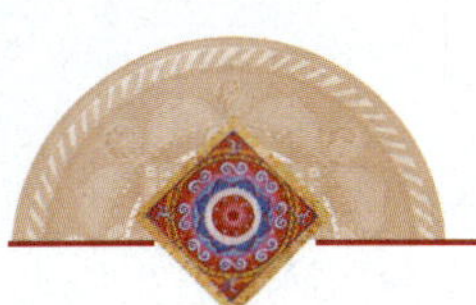

REFERENCES

American Psychiatric Association. (2000). *Diagnostic and statistical manual of mental disorders* (4th ed., Text Revision) (DSM-IV-TR). Washington, DC: Author.

Autism Society of America. (2008). Defining autism. Retrieved January 3, 2008, from www.autism-society.org

Belsky, J. (2006). Determinants and consequences of infant-parent attachment. In L. Balter & C. S. Tamis-LeMonda (Eds.), *Child psychology: A handbook of contemporary issues* (2nd ed.) (pp. 53–77). New York: Psychology Press.

Bloom, B., & Dey, A. (2006). Summary health statistics for U.S. children: National health interview survey, 2004. *Vital Health Statistics, 10*, 1–85.

Bratton, S., Ray, D., Rhine, T., & Jones, L. (2005). The efficacy of play therapy with children: A meta-analytic review of treatment outcomes. *Professional Psychology: Research and Practice, 36*, 376–390.

Chaffin, M., Hanson, R., Saunders, B. E., Nichols, T., Barnett, D., Zeanah, C., et al. (2006). Report of the APSAC task force on attachment therapy, reactive attachment disorder, and attachment problems. *Child Maltreatment, 11*, 76–89.

City of Hope. (2008). MECP2 (Methyl-Cp-G-Binding Protein 2) gene DNA testing. Retrieved January 3, 2008, from www.cityofhope.org/cmdl/MECP2.

Delobel-Ayoub, M., Kaminski, M., Marret, S., Burguet, A., Marchand, L., N'Guyen, S., et al. (2006). Behavioral outcome at 3 years of age in very preterm infants: The EPIPAGE study. *Pediatrics, 117*, 1996–2005.

Department of Health and Human Services. (2001). *Surgeon General's report on child mental health*. Rockville, MD: Public Health Service.

Diamond, G., & Josephson, A. (2005). Family-based treatment research: A 10 year update. *Journal of the American Academy of Child and Adolescent Psychiatry, 44*, 872–887.

Fombonne, E., Zakarian, R., Bennett, A., Mung, L., & McLean-Heywood, D. (2006). Pervasive developmental disorders in Montreal, Quebec, Canada: Prevalence and links with immunizations. *Pediatrics, 118*(1), 139–150.

Fonagy, P., Target, M., Cottrell, D., Phillips, J., & Kurtz, Z. (2005). *What works for whom? A critical review of treatments for children and adolescents*. New York: Guilford.

Freitag, C. M. (2007). The genetics of autistic disorders and its clinical relevance: A review of the literature. *Molecular Psychiatry, 12*(1), 2–22.

Friedberg, R., & McClure, J. (2002). Review of clinical practice of cognitive therapy with children and adolescents. *Journal of Developmental & Behavioral Pediatrics, 23*(6), 457–458.

Gabbard, G. (2004). *Long-term psychodynamic psychotherapy*. New York: American Psychiatric Association.

Gibbons, R. D., Hur, K., Bhaumik, D. K., & Mann, J. J. (2006). The relationships between antidepressant prescription rates and rate of early adolescent suicide. *American Journal of Psychiatry*, *163*(11), 1898–1904.

Hankin, B., & Abela, J. (2005). *Development of psychopathology: A vulnerability-stress perspective*. Thousand Oaks, CA: Sage Publications.

Karver, M., Handelsman, J., Fields, S., & Bickman, L. (2005). A theoretical model of common process factors in youth and family therapy. *Mental Health Services Research, 7*, 35–51.

Kaslow, F., & Magnavita, J. (2002). *Comprehensive handbook of psychotherapy*. Hoboken, NJ: John Wiley & Sons.

King, S., Griffin, S., Hodges, Z., Weatherly, H., Asseburg, C., Richardson, G., et al. (2006). A systematic review and economic model of the effectiveness and cost-effectivenes of methylphenidate, dexamfetamine and atomoxetine for the treatment of attention deficit hyperactivity disorder in children and adolescents. *Health Technology and Assessment, 10*, 1–162.

Landreth, G. (2002). *Play therapy: The art of the relationship*. New York: Brunner-Routledge.

Landreth, G., & Bratton, S. (2006). *Child-parent relationship therapy*. New York: Routledge.

Linares, T., Singer, L., Kirchner, H., Short, E., Min, M., Hussey, P., et al. (2006). Mental health outcomes of cocaine-exposed children at 6 years of age. *Journal of Pediatric Psychology, 31*, 85–97.

Luby, J. L. (2006). Psychopharmacology. In J. L. Luby (Ed.), *Handbook of Preschool Mental Health: Development, Disorders, and Treatment* (pp. 311–330). New York: Guilford Press.

Martin, A. (2006). Stimulating: Prescribing amidst controversy. *American Journal of Psychiatry, 163*, 574–577.

Martin, G., & Pear, J. (2007). *Behavioral modification: What it is and how to do it* (8th ed.). Upper Saddle River, NJ: Pearson Education.

McKim, W. A. (2007). *Drugs and behavior: An introduction to behavioral pharmacology* (6th ed.). Upper Saddle River, NJ: Pearson Education.

Muratori, F., Picchi, L., Casella, C., Tancredi, R., Milone, A., & Patarnello, M. (2002). Efficacy of brief dynamic psychotherapy for children with emotional disorders. *Psychotherapy and Psychosomatics, 71*, 28–38.

National Institute of Mental Health. (2006). *Treatment of children with mental disorders*. Rockville, MD: Department of Health and Human Services, Public Health Service. NIH Publication # 00–4702.

National Institute of Mental Health. (2008). *Clinical trials: Autism spectrum disorders (pervasive developmental disorders)*. Retrieved January 3, 2008, from http://www.nimh.nih.gov/health/trials/autism-spectrum-disorders-pervasive-developmental-disorders.shtml.

National Institute of Mental Health. (2008). *Largest-ever search for autism genes reveals new clues*. Retrieved January 3, 2008, from www.nimh.nih.gov/science-news/2007.

Nichols, M., & Schwartz, R. (2005). *Family therapy: Concepts and methods*. London: Allyn & Bacon.

Rihmer, Z. (2007). Suicide risk in mood disorders. *Current Opinion in Psychiatry, 20*(1), 17–22.

Russ, S. (2004). *Play in child development and psychotherapy*. Mahwah, NJ: Lawrence Erlbaum.

Schecter, R., & Getcher, J. K. (2008). Continuing increases in autism reported to California's developmental services system: Mercury in retrograde. *Archive of General Psychiatry, 65*(1), 19–24.

Stallard, P. (2005). *A clinician's guide to think good-feel good: Using CBT with children and young people*. New York: Guilford Press.

Tanner, D. C. (2006). *Case studies in communication sciences and disorders*. Upper Saddle River, NJ: Prentice Hall.

Timmer, S., Urquiza, A., Zebell, N., & McGrath, J. (2005). Parent–child interaction therapy: Application to maltreating parent–child dyads. *Child Abuse and Neglect, 29*, 825–842.

van der Kolk, B. (2003). The neurobiology of childhood trauma and abuse. *Child and Adolescent Psychiatric Clinics of North America, 12*, 293–317.

Weiss, L. A., Shen, Y., Korn, J. M., Arking, D. E., Miller, D. T., Ragnheider, F., et al. (2008). Association between microdeletion and microduplication at 16p11.2 and autism. *New England Journal of Medicine* (10.1056/NEJMoa075974). Retrieved January 9, 2008, from www.nejm.org.

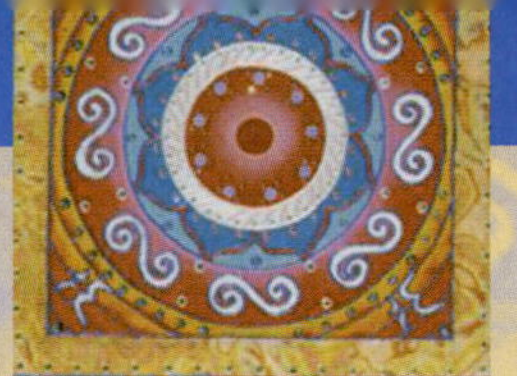

Adolescents

CHAPTER

27

CAROL BRADLEY-CORPUEL

LEARNING OUTCOMES

After completing this chapter, you will be able to:

1. Discuss the biopsychosocial theories important to an understanding of adolescents.
2. Incorporate relevant biologic and developmental data in the assessment of adolescents.
3. Explain the importance of a humanistic interactionist perspective in a comprehensive assessment of adolescent problems.
4. Describe the roles and functions of psychiatric–mental health nurses who work with adolescents in outpatient and inpatient settings.
5. Determine intervention strategies for adolescent clients who act out a "life script" in their behavior and their interpersonal relationships.
6. Determine intervention strategies for adolescent clients who are angry or hostile, test the staff, scapegoat others, engage in problematic sexual behaviors, or abuse substances.
7. Construct a client contract for use with an adolescent in treatment.
8. Analyze personal feelings and attitudes or unresolved issues about adolescence that may affect professional practice when caring for adolescent clients.

KEY TERMS

acting out *731*
Ecstasy (MDMA) *739*
life script *731*
scapegoating *743*
seduction *736*

CRITICAL THINKING CHALLENGE

Your 15-year-old client, Angela Cook, informs you that her mother has sent her to your community clinic for contraception and information on "safe sex." Your own personal beliefs advocate sexual abstinence before marriage for religious as well as preventive health reasons. Moreover, you feel compelled to be a "better parent" to this young girl than her mother has been and feel inclined to dissuade her from sexual intercourse at this early age.

1. Why do you suppose Angela's mother sent her to the community clinic rather than educating Angela at home?
2. How might your own personal convictions interfere with or influence the preventive health care and education you provide?
3. Can you be a "better parent" to Angela? Should you?

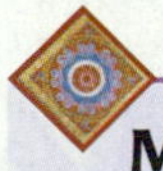

MEDIALINK 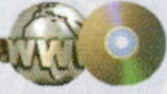 www.prenhall.com/kneisl

Go to the Pearson Health MediaLink CD-ROM and the Companion Website at www.prenhall.com/kneisl for interactive resources for this chapter.

What is adolescence? Some sources define it simply as the time of physical and psychosocial development between the ages of 12 and 20. Others describe it as a period of "normal psychosis." Still others see it as an attempt by a tyrannical subculture to overtake adult America. It is not necessary to accept the latter two definitions verbatim to understand their implications. Most people recognize the immense stress that occurs during adolescence and the importance to an adolescent's future of managing that stress.

Whether a generalist, clinical specialist, or nurse practitioner, the nurse in today's health care setting integrates professional capabilities, skills, and roles to intervene with adolescents to achieve optimal social, emotional, cognitive, and physical development. Using expertise to identify relevant deviations in the developmental process, the nurse works closely with the systems (family, school, community, and institution) on which adolescents are emotionally and economically dependent.

Trying to understand adolescents is a challenge to anyone. For the nurse who chooses to work with adolescents, the challenge offers considerable rewards. Nurses who can recollect their own experiences and reactions during this tumultuous time will better appreciate the dilemmas that adolescent clients face.

BIOPSYCHOSOCIAL THEORIES

A sound theoretic knowledge base helps you differentiate between the "normal" and "abnormal," or the usual and unusual, behaviors of adolescents. In particular, you can do a comprehensive assessment by focusing on the psychologic development of the individual and the evolution of the adolescent as a biopsychosocial being. You can accomplish the first task with an understanding of developmental theory and the second with an appreciation of biologic and humanistic interactionist theories.

Biologic Theory

Psychiatric–mental health nursing in the 21st century requires that you integrate a biologic focus into your practice, to accommodate both changing client needs and an expanding biologic knowledge base. An appreciation of hormonal changes, growth spurts, stress and immune function, chronic illness, depression, and other mental disorders can help you evaluate adolescents from a more effective and comprehensive perspective.

Neurobiology and Biochemistry

In recent years, clinician researchers have carried out studies using neuroimaging, magnetic resonance imaging (MRI), and spectroscopy in children and adolescents in order to better delineate the anatomic, functional, and biochemical imbalances of mood disorders in children and adolescents. As a result, for example, we have learned that bipolar disorder in children and adolescents is similar to that in adults. Equally important, neuroscientists have established a correlation between aggressiveness and brain levels of corresponding neurochemical changes.

With advancements in molecular biology and biochemistry, scientists are now investigating gene expressions in specific neuronal systems of the brain. Such studies reveal that metabolic functions, neurobiological systems, and specific neuropeptides and hormones are as important as behavioral and familial habits in abnormal body weight regulation. Specifically, researchers are able to examine different neurochemical and humoral substances related to traits of overeating, weight gain, and eating disorders that could directly affect preventive treatment and abnormal body weight regulation in conditions such as obesity, type 2 diabetes, and eating disorders (Leibowitz, 2006). These discoveries are important in themselves for clinical treatment. Moreover, knowledge regarding the biochemical and physiological etiology for these physical conditions could help positively influence society's tendency to discriminate against people who have these conditions. Realizing that biochemical and neuronal systems are contributing to these medical conditions could alleviate some of the bias and prejudice that, for example, the obese adolescent receives from his peers who believe "All he has to do is push himself away from the table" or that the adolescent with an eating disorder endures from her peers who may say, "Doesn't she know that's disgusting?"

Chronic Illness

Of equal importance is the effect of chronic illness on the adolescent's mental health. Asthma, head injury, diabetes, epilepsy, and many of the less common chronic physical diseases can result in depression. Equally at risk for depression are adolescents with various learning disabilities or specific neuropsychiatric illnesses, such as attention deficit/hyperactivity disorders (ADD/ADHD); disruptive behavior disorders; tic disorders; eating disorders; anxiety disorders, including obsessive–compulsive disorder (OCD) and post-traumatic stress disorder (PTSD); and schizophrenia and related conditions (American Psychiatric Association [APA], 2000).

Moreover, the proportion of obese and overweight children and adolescents in the United States nearly doubled in the last two decades, and the numbers continue to rise. Currently more than 25% of youth between the ages of 2 and 19 years are overweight or obese (Owens, 2006). In addition to the more publicized comorbid medical conditions (such as diabetes, cardiac abnormalities, and hypertension) associated with excessive weight, there is the psychological impact of depression and suicidal tendencies that burden the obese teen (Boggs, 2006; Latner, Stunkard, & Wilson, 2005).

Health care professionals who treat adolescents, including pediatric practitioners, need to be aware of the stressors inherent in having a chronic illness. The feature What Every Pediatric Nurse Should Know discusses some of this information.

Psychopharmacology

There is increasing impetus to study the clinically significant effects that various psychotropic medications may have on the brain when administered during the developing phase that spans from birth through adolescence. The National Institute of Mental Health (NIMH), the

WHAT EVERY PEDIATRIC NURSE SHOULD KNOW

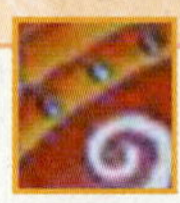

Allaying the Stress of Parents and Family Members

In the pediatrics acute care or critical care arenas where adolescents are treated, emotions and fears can run high. Parents and family members frequently feel guilt, anger, and helplessness as they watch their adolescent undergoing invasive procedures. You can help allay their fears as well as obtain much-needed assessment data by talking with them about their stress. Consider comments such as, "This must be very stressful for you. The diagnosis of diabetes was such a shock. This is beyond the usual day-to-day stressors. How do you usually cope?" Such questions can yield adaptive measures they can draw on or reveal maladaptive measures, such as physical abuse.

National Institute of Child Health and Human Development (NICHD), and the National Institute on Drug Abuse (NIDA) continue to study the clinical use of psychotherapeutic medications in children and adolescents. This program incentive, entitled "Developmental Psychopharmacology," is related to Mental Health and Mental Disorders and Biology of Brain Disorders, one of the priority areas of the *Healthy People 2010* initiative. The U.S. Public Health Service is committed to achieving the health promotion and disease prevention objectives of this comprehensive, nationwide agenda. *Healthy People 2010* contains 467 objectives organized into 28 focus areas, reflecting the identified major health concerns in the United States at the beginning of the 21st century. A limited set of the objectives, known as the Leading Health Indicators, are:

1. Physical Activity
2. Overweight and Obesity
3. Tobacco Use
4. Substance Abuse
5. Responsible Sexual Behavior
6. Mental Health
7. Injury and Violence
8. Environmental Quality
9. Immunization
10. Access to Health Care (U.S. Department of Health and Human Services [DHHS], 2005)

Developmental Theory

An understanding of developmental theory helps you identify deviations in adolescent growth and development processes and intervene appropriately. The theories of Freud, Erikson, and Sullivan provide considerable insight into the adolescent's struggle to attain adulthood. These developmental theories are discussed in Chapter 5.

The development of an adolescent's sense of identity entails a preoccupation with self-image. It also entails a connection between future role and past experiences. In the search for a new sense of sameness and continuity, many adolescents must repeat the crisis resolutions of earlier years to integrate these past elements and establish the lasting ideals of a final identity. According to Erikson, these crisis periods or stages are reviews of the adolescent's sense of trust, autonomy, initiative, and industry, in that order.

Equally important for an adolescent's development is cognition. Piaget's research revealed three stages of cognitive development. The third stage, called formal operations, develops between ages 12 and 14 and results in the adolescent's ability to conceptualize on an adult level. The adolescent has the capacity to think abstractly, to be self-reflective, and to adopt a multidimensional perspective on problems. (For a discussion of developmental theories in general, see Chapter 5.)

Humanistic–Interactionist Theory

As a psychiatric–mental health nurse, you not only need knowledge about developmental theories and psychobiology, you must also integrate humanistic–interactionist principles into assessment and interventions to develop a trusting, caring interpersonal relationship with adolescent clients. The adolescent developmental period is a time when identity, values, and goals are in a state of flux. You should take into account not only the immediate situation but also the impact of the developmental stage; the social, ethnic, and cultural factors; family influences; and psychodynamic conflicts on the adolescent's behavior. To accomplish this, explore the meaning of the identified problem or behavior. The list of questions in the Your Assessment Approach feature can help guide this exploration.

It is insufficient to base the nursing response to the adolescent's needs and dilemmas solely on behaviors without a

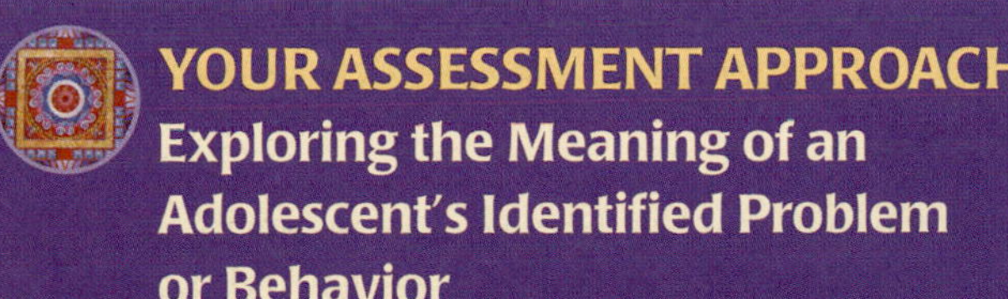

YOUR ASSESSMENT APPROACH

Exploring the Meaning of an Adolescent's Identified Problem or Behavior

- What meaning does this behavior or problem hold for the adolescent?
- What message is he or she conveying through this behavior?
- What impact does this problem have on the client in this developmental stage? Is this a usual or unusual problem or behavior for the adolescent's peer group?
- How have resulting changes, if any, affected the adolescent and his or her relationships with others?
- What goals does the client have for the immediate and distant future?
- What personal strengths does the adolescent have to help deal with this problem?
- What considerations have you and the client given to other developmental, familial, biologic, or sociocultural factors involved?

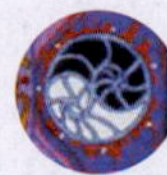

more comprehensive evaluation of these other factors. This approach can lead to ineffective treatment, a temporary ceasing of the initial behaviors with an upheaval of symptoms in another area, and possibly a sterile treatment environment with no meaningful therapeutic alliance. Only by considering all aspects of the adolescent client as a biopsychosocial being can you truly understand the meanings of such behaviors to the client and intervene effectively.

THE ROLE OF THE NURSE

Psychiatric–mental health nurses can assume numerous roles within a variety of treatment modalities to help maintain the health and well-being of adolescent clients and identify abnormal or problem-causing behavior during this difficult period of development. In the past decade studies have determined that as many as 7 million youth have had a mental health problem, with higher rates of medication use, primary care visits, and specialty care visits than youth without such problems (Schapiro, 2005).

WHAT EVERY SCHOOL NURSE SHOULD KNOW

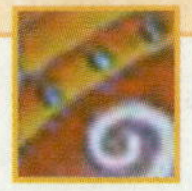

Teen Pregnancy

The prospect of more than a million pregnancies in females under the age of 20, with fewer choices for alternatives to continuing the pregnancy, is of utmost concern. Recent challenges in the court system to the adolescent's right to access abortion and contraception are eroding the *Roe v. Wade* decision. New regulation enforcement under HIPAA (Health Insurance Portability and Accountability Act) in 2007 is further complicating adolescent care. Nurses need to familiarize themselves with legal issues pertaining to their specialty areas in order to fully address the health and psychological needs of adolescents.

In the Outpatient Setting

In the changing world of health care, the outpatient arena for services to adolescents yields numerous diverse roles for the psychiatric–mental health nurse.

Community Health Nurse

In the school, clinic, or community health agency, the community health nurse has excellent opportunities to observe adolescents engaging in the normal activities of daily living. There are frequent occasions to counsel adolescents in the problems that confront them daily such as teen pregnancy and substance abuse and to advise school or clinic staff members in their encounters with adolescents. The feature What Every School Nurse Should Know discusses teen pregnancy. The nurse who knows how to deal with normal adolescent problems will also be adept at identifying obstacles to effective resolution of emotional problems and suggesting further treatment.

Within the School School is the most influential experience in an adolescent's life outside the home. Adolescents spend more waking time in school activities than in any other activity, and most of their successes, problems, and conflicts are demonstrated in the school setting. Even adolescents who are supposedly truant from school are often on the school grounds, perhaps meeting their friends at lunchtime, playing cards in the library, or "hanging out" on the school steps. Such an "absent" student may suddenly appear at the school nurse's door because of "boredom" or a physical complaint.

Unfortunately, the school nurse's role in the early recognition and treatment of predelinquent individuals has been minimized or has gone unrecognized. There are several reasons for this. One reason is that school administrators and teachers tend to view the school nurse as a person who deals only with physical sickness and medical emergencies. They may not be aware that because of the intimate quality of a nurse–client relationship or the comprehensive and holistic nature of nursing assessments, the nurse may be helpful in exploring an area of conflict in an adolescent's life or intervening with a disruptive student. Such early intervention could prevent more serious problems in later years. Box 27-1 outlines problems in the school setting that should warrant early intervention.

Another reason is that administrators tend to limit the nurse's activities to the school itself. They may see no need for the nurse to make home visits to meet with a sick student's family or view problems firsthand. Many school districts lack the time and money to provide for counseling families or individuals in a formal setting. As the role of the independent nursing practitioner expands, and as legislation for third-party reimbursement for independent practice becomes a reality in more states, nurses will be better able to assume more autonomy and responsibility in meeting student needs more comprehensively and effectively.

Box 27-1 Adolescent Behaviors in the School Setting That Call for Early Intervention

- Antisocial behaviors such as stealing, setting fires, bullying others
- Avoidance behavior
- Chronic illness
- Depression
- Disruptive classroom behavior
- Substance abuse
- Excessive daydreaming
- Hypochondriasis
- Learning difficulties
- Poor school performance or a dramatic shift in school performance
- Temper tantrums

Within Community-Based Care The nurse who is employed in a community agency can seize every opportunity to provide an active school health program and educate school administrators and faculty members about the importance of preventive care. For example, the nurse in a viable school health program can provide preventive counseling not only to troubled adolescents in school but also to their preschool siblings during routine home visits. Nurses can establish productive relationships with teachers, help other faculty members, encourage parent–teacher conferences, take an active part in developing the curriculum, and help adolescents on probation or parole return to school.

Within Social Programs The many problems encountered by today's youth—substance abuse, teenage pregnancy, family and school violence, street crime, and school failure—are increasingly being recognized in professional, community, and social arenas. The American Academy of Child and Adolescent Psychiatry (AACAP) has developed various tools to disseminate information. The AACAP Facts for Families and the Children and Firearms Fact Sheet are two such options to inform lay persons and professionals of the incidence of violent behavior among our youth. See Box 27-2 for a summary of the Children and Firearms Fact Sheet (AACAP, 2004).

Moreover, among its six categories of priority health-risk behaviors among youth and young adults, the Youth Risk Behavior Surveillance (YRBS) system monitors sexual behaviors, including dating violence, that contribute to unintended pregnancy and sexually transmitted diseases (STDs) including human immunodeficiency virus (HIV) infections. During the 12 months preceding a study based on this data (Eaton et al., 2006), 9.2% of students nationwide had reported being hit, slapped, or physically hurt on purpose by their boyfriend or girlfriend. Overall, the prevalence of dating violence was higher among black males (11.8%) and Hispanic males (10.9%) than among white males (8%). Nationwide 7.5% of students had even been physically forced to have sexual intercourse when they did not want to. Overall, the prevalence of forced sexual intercourse was higher among female (10.8%) than male (4.2%) students and higher among white female (10.8%), black female (11.5%), and Hispanic female (9.4%) than white male (3.1%), black male (7.1%), and Hispanic male (6.4%) students. Overall, the prevalence of forced sexual intercourse was higher among black (9.3%) than white (6.9%) students and higher among black male (7.1%) and Hispanic male (6.4%) than white male (3.1%) students.

The National Library of Medicine has compiled the Current Bibliography on Youth Violence Prevention Resources. This extensive listing can be found through a resource link provided on the Companion Website for this book.

MEDIALINK NLM Youth Violence Prevention Resources

Box 27-2 AACAP Children and Firearms Fact Sheet

The following is a summary of the information collected on children and firearms.

- In 1998 more than 10 children and teenagers, ages 19 and under, were killed with guns every day. Many more were wounded.
- In 1998 77% of murdered juveniles ages 13–19 were killed with a firearm.
- Currently an estimated 39% of households have a gun, and 24% of all households have a handgun.
- Guns kept in the home for self-protection are 22 times more likely to kill a family member or friend than they are to be used to kill a stranger in self-defense.
- Youth victims of suicide who used firearms were 5 times more likely to have been drinking alcohol than those who used other means to harm themselves.

Source: Reprinted with the permission of the American Academy of Child and Adolescent Psychiatry, Copyright 2004.

Nurse Counselor/Therapist

Whether in the clinic, home, school, or community health setting, the psychiatric–mental health nurse has many opportunities to organize individual, group, or family counseling sessions. Nurses can function within a variety of treatment roles, according to their experience and capabilities.

Individual Therapist The nurse's qualifications and role in the clinic, school, or community setting may allow for counseling adolescents on an individual basis. Sometimes the nurse can establish a trusting alliance and facilitate communication with the client. (See Chapter 29 regarding counseling the individual.) Sometimes, however, the adolescent is too threatened to talk openly with the nurse in this intimate setting. Some adolescents view the nurse as an authority figure and resist all efforts to communicate. You may make more headway with this mode of treatment when you use it in conjunction with group therapy. Unless educated at the graduate level and certified to provide this service, you should counsel the adolescent only for the purposes of identifying the problem area and referring the client to a qualified professional for individual psychotherapy.

MEDIALINK Application: Psychological Trauma in the Juvenile Justice Population

Group Therapist It is usually more effective to work with adolescents in a group. Because the values, acceptance, and recognition of peers are so important during adolescence, the group can provide support for dealing with problems and effecting change. In addition, involving the adolescent's peers helps dilute the conflict with adults that may exist in one–to–one work. In the school setting, health education groups can provide an acceptable forum for peer interaction and discussion of difficult topics. Otherwise, the nurse should practice as a group therapist only with graduate preparation as an advanced-practice nurse, with certification, or with adequate supervision by a certified individual. Knowledge of group dynamics is crucial to being an effective group leader. Chapter 30 discusses the group leader role for generalist nurses and the group therapist role for advanced-practice nurses.

WHY I BECAME A PSYCHIATRIC–MENTAL HEALTH NURSE

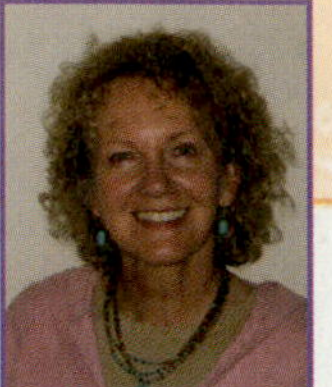

Carol Bradley-Corpuel
Contributor, Chapter 27

Like so many new graduates, I wanted "to make a difference" in people's lives and believed that the only way to do that was in the medical–surgical acute care arena. Starting out in the ICU soon after graduation, I was thrust into the thick of things in an ICU multispecialty trauma unit where clients and their families grappled with bleak prognoses and the need to cope with a loved one's new disability. Despite the diverse technical and clinical challenges, collegial relationships, and great on-the-job education, I still felt dissatisfied. Something was missing. I wanted my nursing care to have a greater interpersonal impact than what my meds, IVs, or physical procedures were doing.

I feel truly blessed as a psychiatric–mental health nurse to be able to get to know my clients intimately and to help them to more fully know themselves. I have been afforded opportunities for satisfaction and diverse roles in varied employment settings. Having expertise as a psychiatric–mental health nurse can open doors for you that didn't exist before—in hospitals, private offices, the corporate world, schools, and the community. I encourage you to talk to psychiatric nurses. Conduct an information interview with them to explore their daily challenges and rewards and discover how you can be the best you can be in your professional life.

Family Therapist Being a parent of a "normal" adolescent is difficult, at best. As the child grows into adulthood, with all its perplexing questions and problems, parents normally worry about the child's safety and well-being. They may feel rejected because they are no longer needed in the same way. Because many parents of relatively normal adolescents share this plight, they can usually find receptive listeners who will give them comfort and support.

The problems of the parents of emotionally disturbed adolescents are more complicated. Many such parents have a strong sense of failure because their children did not turn out "right." Their feelings of guilt, frustration, and helplessness are likely to increase if their child is institutionalized. They probably felt confused and resentful when experts offered them smug and guilt-provoking advice. Unlike the parents of other adolescents, these parents may have no one in whom to confide, either because they lack the support and understanding of others or because their own self-reproach prevents them from seeking out confidantes.

Meetings with family members may be indicated if the adolescent's role in the family seems to compound the problems presented in the school or agency setting. An important part of the problem-solving process is organizing initial interviews with parents and family members. Use the information gathered during these meetings to determine whether the problems stem from difficulties posed by the larger system (the family), and, if so, whether family therapy is indicated (refer to Chapter 30 ∞).

Show compassion and understanding for the parents' dilemma without blaming them or their offspring. Parents will be more receptive to family therapy and to exploring their part in the adolescent's problems if they sense that you will support them, too. Stress and psychologic symptoms evidenced by parents can serve as markers for emotional or behavioral problems in adolescents.

Any tendency to feel self-righteous or superior to the disturbed adolescent's parents is an obstacle to effective treatment. These feelings are readily communicated to parents and can only validate their fear of blame and increase their reluctance to participate in therapy with their child. By the same token, resist any temptation to overidentify with the parents, thereby inadvertently perpetuating the family system's problems. The adolescent and the family need a neutral party who can play an objective, knowledgeable, and supportive role in helping them change. The adolescent's chances for resolving the underlying conflicts and maintaining a healthy life are virtually nonexistent if the family system remains unchanged.

Parents, school, and agency staff must understand the objectives and goals of treatment to appreciate the progress the client has made and avoid reinforcing the client's previously maladaptive behavior. The following clinical example illustrates the problems that arise when parents and school authorities, particularly those who must deal directly with behavior problems in the classroom, lack psychological sophistication.

CLINICAL EXAMPLE

Jeremy, a 13-year-old boy, was referred to the school nurse because he was introverted and isolated. He made no contact with either his peers or his teachers and rarely spoke unless addressed directly. After he had spent 3 months in group and individual counseling sessions with the nurse, Jeremy started going to the grade counselor's office of his own accord to talk about his depression and the problems he had been having in his family. Both the grade counselor and the boy's family believed this to be an indication that his difficulties had worsened, and they began to complain to the nurse about his illness! Not only were Jeremy's parents and counselor ignorant of the goals of treatment and the behaviors expected to come with change, but apparently they were also uncomfortable with the changes in Jeremy's behavior and with the implications of these changes for their relationships with him.

The client's siblings may experience many different feelings. Sometimes they share in the parents' guilt and shame. Sometimes, however, they are pleased and relieved when the "troublemaker" is out of the family and hospitalized. You should extend the same understanding to the siblings as to the parents, helping them see how each member of the family contributes to the problem. If the troubled adolescent is hospitalized, another member of the family, usually a sibling, may assume the role of the "bad" or "sick" person in the family because the identified "bad" person is no longer at home. Be aware of this tendency. If you are not skilled in assessing the need for family therapy or in providing this service, refer the family to a competent family therapist (see Chapter 30).

You may identify a need for all of these therapies in dealing with a client's problems. In some cases, an informal discussion with you is all that is warranted. In other cases, you may identify problems that require considerable attention. Sometimes a period of unsuccessful treatment is necessary to determine that outpatient therapy is ineffective and that hospitalization is indicated. Before making such a recommendation, you need to establish a trusting relationship with the client and the client's parents. An excellent resource, Facts for Families, has been developed by the AACAP that will help you provide concise and current information on issues that affect children, adolescents, and their families. The AACAP has produced these materials in English and Spanish. They are accessible via their website, www.aacap.org, and through a resource link on the Companion Website of this book.

In the Inpatient Setting

Admission into a hospital or other residential treatment facility may be indicated under the following circumstances:

- If the adolescent is unable to control impulsivity
- If the degree of destructive or antisocial behavior escalates beyond normal limits
- If the adolescent cannot form meaningful, stable relationships within the everyday environment (as in the case of family dysfunction)

The existence of any of these conditions warrants counseling or professional treatment. A combination of two or more is likely to make treatment on an outpatient basis virtually ineffective, indicating the need for hospital or residential treatment.

Hospitalization of the disturbed adolescent has these possible advantages:

- It provides additional structure within which to handle the physically and psychologically destructive elements of the adolescent's behavior.
- It removes the individual from the stresses of a disturbed family environment.
- It offers opportunities for supporting existing ego strengths and promoting whatever ability the client has for forming relationships.

Adolescents are sometimes institutionalized because their ideas are strange or threatening to their families, or because the responsible authorities seek to punish the adolescent's unacceptable behavior. The results can be disastrous. Therefore, it is important to make accurate assessments and to implement early treatment when indicated. You can play a crucial role in making assessments, undertaking appropriate interventions, and educating parents, teachers, and school officials to recognize these needs.

Staff Nurse in a General Hospital Setting

Adolescents with emotional problems may have symptoms of physical illness and as a result may be admitted to a general hospital setting for evaluation and treatment. Clients with anorexia nervosa, in particular, may be referred for inpatient treatment on general adolescent medical units. As a medical unit staff nurse, you can take the opportunity to reach out to adolescents who have emotional problems.

Consultant in a General Hospital Setting

Staff nurses from a psychiatric inpatient unit of a general hospital may be consulted by other nursing staff about emotionally disturbed adolescents who have been admitted to their general medical or surgical units. Some general hospital settings have advanced practice registered nurses (APRNs) who are clinical nurse specialists or nurse practitioners in psychiatric liaison positions as consultants.

Staff Nurse or Advanced Practice Nurse in a Psychiatric Setting

In inpatient psychiatric settings, the staff nurse or APRN may assume any of the previously mentioned roles. Nurses in inpatient settings also have numerous opportunities to observe and assess the family dynamics among the adolescent's family members and possibly to intervene. Nurses involved in family therapy sessions can perceive maladaptive ways of relating and take direct steps to work toward change. However, you need not work within the structured format of a therapy hour to have an impact on the family system. The Your Intervention Strategies feature on page 730 delineates specific parent behaviors and corresponding interventions by the nurse in the therapeutic environment.

Because inpatient nursing entails around-the-clock care, the nurse has the responsibility to maintain the therapeutic environment. The role of the inpatient staff nurse includes the following:

- Maintaining physical and psychologic safety of the unit
- Setting verbal and physical limits on client behavior
- Establishing meaningful one–to–one relationships with clients
- Identifying client strengths and promoting more adaptive coping skills
- Role-modeling socially acceptable behaviors
- Participating in group therapies and other structured activities

Milieu Therapist

Many authors have described the importance of the therapeutic environment, indicating the strong influence of the treatment environment on the treatment outcome. (For a complete discussion, see Chapter 12.)

Because of adolescents' needs for peer acceptance, their overwhelming uncertainties and fears, and their ever-changing behaviors and attitudes about identity, their chances for success in inpatient treatment are increased by a peer group setting. Much has been written about the value of the therapeutic environment in dealing with adolescent problems, including the problems of substance abuse and similar destructive activities. Without the social interaction and living–learning situations provided by the peer group, psychotherapy may be sterile and ineffective.

MediaLink American Academy of Child & Adolescent Psychiatry

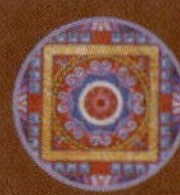

YOUR INTERVENTION STRATEGIES
Encouraging More Effective Parenting Behaviors

Parent Behavior

- Initiates loud verbal arguments during visits with adolescent

Nursing Interventions

- Stop the immediate behavior, pointing out the disruptiveness to the unit.
- Refer adolescent and family to family therapist to resolve differences and learn more adaptive ways of relating in supportive atmosphere of family therapy.
- Suggest that family therapist contract with family for one or more of the following:
  - Staff will monitor visits.
  - Family will bring up potentially volatile topics only within the structure of family meetings and not on the unit during visits.
  - Staff will intervene if arguments ensue on unit.
  - Staff may limit visiting time on unit.

Parent Behavior

- Has history of physical violence against adolescent

Nursing Interventions

- Upon admission, contract with adolescent and family for no acts of violence against people or property.
- Monitor parent visits with adolescent on unit.
- Limit or deny passes with parents until progress is demonstrated.
- Depending on parent's level of self-control, refuse visiting privileges with adolescent until progress is seen in family therapy.

Parent Behavior

- Is unable to set limits with adolescent during unit visits (is adversely influenced by manipulative attempts, tolerates verbal abuse, etc.)

Nursing Interventions

- Intervene if demands or behavior could lead to physical harm, unit rule breaking, or other negative results.
- Point out problem and refer adolescent and parents to family therapy.
- Role-model appropriate and effective limit setting with adolescent, if necessary.
- Offer to discuss situation with parents and adolescent if desirable in immediate situation.
- Offer emotional support to parent who needs to talk.

Parent Behavior

- Has limited interaction with adolescent during unit visits

Nursing Interventions

- Initiate discussion among adolescent and family members related to visit and treatment goals.
- Communicate observations to family therapist.
- Initiate discussion with parents to allow exploration of difficulty, if desired.
- Suggest that family members and adolescent discuss problem in family therapy.
- Plan outings or special-occasion celebrations to include family, if appropriate.

The therapeutic environment provides valuable experiences for adolescents for the following reasons:

- Adolescents more readily hear and accept limits from peers than from adults.
- Adolescents more readily respond to feedback, both negative and positive, from peers than from adults.
- Shared goals and objectives facilitate group processes and the development of cohesion among adolescent group members.
- Group interaction allows for the expression of appropriate feelings and identification with peers with similar feelings.
- Group interaction provides opportunities for learning how to develop relationships with others.
- Group structure allows for the testing of new, more adaptive behaviors.
- Adolescents receive feedback from the peer group and have the opportunity to give feedback in a supportive environment.
- The group format provides an opportunity to work out specific issues of conflict with adult group leaders while receiving the support and understanding of peers.

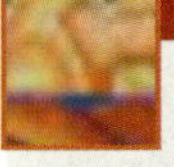

NURSING PROCESS
Adolescents

Adolescents present behaviors and problems unique to their developmental stage. Without knowledge and understanding about potentially difficult areas, you may respond with confusion, anger, and even hostility, which will cause feelings of frustration and failure for both yourself and your adolescent clients. The following pages contain numerous examples of either typical behaviors expected of the "normal" adolescent or problem behaviors that may provide the impetus for referral to a treatment setting, or both. In many situations, you may simply need to focus on the difficult issues encountered in working with adolescents. That information is given in the Assessment section. Situations that represent an identified problem necessitating treatment are discussed under Planning and Implementation.

Assessment

It will be important for you to keep in mind that over the course of normal development, children and adolescents experience symptoms of anxiety, dysphoria, oppositionality, or conduct disorder. On the other hand, there are factors that can contribute to missed or inaccurate diagnoses in the assessment of an adolescent:

- Symptom overlap, which can blur diagnostic boundaries
- Effects of normal development on symptom presentation
- High rates of comorbidity in youth with mental illness
- Perception of informants (i.e., parents/guardians, teachers, or other family members)

Moreover, two other factors that can minimize the effectiveness and comprehensive nature of an adequate assessment in the adolescent are:

- The impact of managed care, with its emphasis on brevity of client contact in inpatient and outpatient settings
- The emphasis in some clinical training on the rigid adherence to DSM-IV-TR criteria without the exploration of developmental stages, risk and protective factors, current stressors, temperament, cultural issues, and/or family dynamics

Accurate and comprehensive assessments can be obtained only by viewing the adolescent as a biopsychosocial being. Only by integrating knowledge from biology, psychology, and humanistic interactionist theory can you understand what a particular behavior means to an adolescent. If you can remember your own adolescent experiences—the conflicts and uncertainty as well as the elation and the triumphs—you will better appreciate the adolescent's turmoil. It is equally important that you discover who the individual adolescent is.

Meanings of behavior, values, and actions can vary from client to client and may not reflect meanings or values that you hold. For example, the client who has trouble with competitive feelings may be reluctant to accept an invitation to play a game of Trivial Pursuit. And because adolescents are developmentally between childhood and adulthood, they frequently have the feelings and choices of adulthood without an adult's abilities in verbal discourse and impulse control. As a result, adolescents may "act out" feelings and decisions nonverbally, in a childlike way. This is particularly true of the emotionally disturbed adolescent. In settings where tension and anxiety are typically high, such as the Emergency Department of a hospital, the high emotionality of an adolescent can be potentiated. See the feature What Every Emergency Department Nurse Should Know for assessment and intervention information.

Acting Out

The concept of **acting out** is complex. The term has been used to describe a variety of behaviors, ranging from antisocial, destructive acts to unconscious impulses expressed in action rather than in symbolic words or symptoms. Acting out may, and often does, include destructive actions and seemingly undefinable behaviors. The term describes a re-creation of the client's life experiences, relationships with significant others, and resulting unresolved conflicts.

These are all components of what is commonly called the client's **life script**, which unfolds as the client relates, reacts, and behaves in accustomed ways. Through observation of and interaction with the client, you can uncover the meanings that various behaviors and actions hold for the individual. For example, the child who has assumed the "black sheep" role in the family seeks to re-create that familiar role with others outside the home, particularly in the inpatient setting. This clinical example illustrates one girl's relationship with her parents as replayed with the staff on an inpatient unit.

WHAT EVERY EMERGENCY DEPARTMENT NURSE SHOULD KNOW

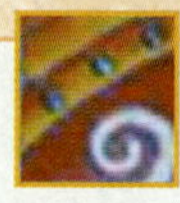

Helping Upset Adolescents

If the hospital is often a frightening place for adults, you can imagine what the emergency department (ED) is like for an adolescent. Adolescents come to the ED as clients, as family members of a client, or as friends of a client. In fact, if there is an injury or accident at the local school, an onslaught of teens may show up to support their injured or sick schoolmate. Whether as clients or supporters of a client, adolescents can be histrionic and exaggerate the nature of a problem. You may find it helpful to deal with the upset adolescent by suggesting deep-breathing or de-escalation techniques. Having the teens focus on their breathing can provide a focus for their anxiety, allow them to concentrate, and increase their oxygen level. When they are able to "hear" what you have to say, ask questions with simple answers while also encouraging positive expectations. An example might be, "Have you felt this way before?" If the answer is yes, ask, "What did you do to help yourself at that time?"

CLINICAL EXAMPLE

Liza is 14 years old. She has been on the unit for 6 days. She is an attractive, engaging young person who has been friendly with both staff and clients. Liza has been on the periphery of several rule-breaking incidents but has not been directly involved. She has begun to establish close ties with Jim, a nurse, and engages in frequent lengthy discussions with him about her innermost feelings and fears. One evening she candidly talks to him about the callous way in which she was treated by one of the other nurses, a woman, in regard to a gynecologic problem. Liza says with undisguised fear and embarrassment that she is afraid the situation will repeat itself. She expresses great respect for Jim's knowledge and style and asks him to attend to any subsequent problems himself rather than interact herself with Jane, the other nurse.

The implications for treatment are many. The most important factors for Jim to consider are what meaning Liza's behavior has for her and what would be the most therapeutically effective way to deal with the situation. The client's presenting problems and the expectation that the client will act out previous conflicts and life scripts have provided Jim adequate information on which to base an appropriate intervention. The client's attempt to manipulate (seduce) the nurse, and the need for nurses to examine their own behavior and motivations, are discussed in detail later in this chapter.

CLINICAL EXAMPLE

In the previous clinical example Jim recognizes how Liza is unconsciously acting out her life script by re-creating her relationships with her parents with Jim and Jane, a female nurse on the unit. Jim remembers that Liza's home situation is chaotic. Liza's mother and father frequently fight over who is the better parent. Jim surmises that Liza also plays a part in these fights. Jim recognizes the "pull" from Liza to feel that only he can adequately handle the situation. The present situation seems to indicate that he is about to be pitted against Jane, just as Liza perhaps plays one parent against the other. Jim responds by reiterating his concern for her dilemma and suggesting that Liza speak with Jane about the situation that is causing her concern.

In this example, it is clear that the client is attempting to re-create her home situation, using two of the nurses to reenact the roles of her parents. Had Jim been seduced into playing the father's role in the script, he would have re-created the family's conflict on the unit. The ideal solution is for staff to interrupt this pathologic process by substituting a healthier way of resolving the problem. Thus, Jim does not react with compliance or with anger to Liza's attempts. Instead, he recognizes the significance of her behavior and deals with the situation in a concerned yet healthy way, suggesting a resolution to the immediate problem that demonstrates respect for both Liza's and Jane's abilities to resolve the conflict.

Such situations are commonplace with adolescents. They require nursing staff to evaluate the client's psychodynamics and psychopathology as well as their own inner feelings and behavior. For these reasons, it is imperative to identify transference and countertransference issues and to discuss them with your clinical supervisor. Transference and countertransference are discussed in Chapter 29∞. But these situations are not limited to the inpatient setting. This fact alone obliges you to be alert in observing and assessing verbal and nonverbal communication and to understand your own feelings and behavior in order to make accurate assessments and appropriate interventions. In this way, you will be most effective when working with adolescents.

The Evidence-Based Practice feature provides an illustration of how research can help shape interventions to maximize resilience in an adolescent who is acting out a self-destructive life script.

Communication

Communication with adolescents is an art in itself. To become proficient in this area, you must accept and understand the following:

- Adolescents tend to act out feelings and conflicts rather than verbalize them.
- Adolescents have an unconventional language of their own.
- Adolescents, especially disturbed ones, may use profanity frequently.
- Many clues can be obtained simply by observing an adolescent's behavior, dress, or environment.

If you learn the verbal and nonverbal communication skills discussed in Chapter 10∞, you can use them comfortably and naturally in communicating with adolescents.

Nonverbal Cues Adolescents give many nonverbal cues to their specific emotional struggles, underlying confusion, or transitory moods. A glance around their rooms or a brief study of their dress can tell you more than several direct questions would elicit.

Sometimes adolescents give obvious cues. A client who wears a coat around the unit may be planning to run away. Other less obvious behaviors, which are often outside the client's conscious awareness or control, can also yield vital information. A sudden escalation of horseplay among the boys around bedtime is an example. You would probably be correct in identifying this behavior as an expression of anxiety related to sexual identity and fears of homosexual feelings. Interactionist theory holds that the adolescent boy's newfound sexual feelings and changing body image provide unfamiliar ways of relating to members of his own sex. As a result, he regresses to preadolescent behavior, which served him well in handling close feelings then, but now proves inappropriate. In this instance, firm limit setting is in order. Avoid interpreting the behavior or paying undue attention to the specifics. (Testing and limit setting are discussed later in the chapter.)

Slang and Obscenities Adolescents create a language all their own. This takes some understanding and acceptance. In seeking their identity, adolescents establish a form of communication unique to the group. To gain acceptance into the adolescent world, the adult must accept this need to use ambiguous (to the adult) yet specific (to the adolescent) terms to express themselves. In many cases, you must communicate with adolescents by using their slang.

This slang often includes obscene and profane words. This is particularly true of disturbed adolescents, who have an especially difficult time expressing anger and fear appropriately. The words they use often reveal the nature of the emotional conflict. For example, a young male adolescent grappling with his sexual identity and aggressive feelings may resort to sexually graphic words when he feels anxious or afraid. You may sometimes find it productive to use similar words to give explanations or to clarify communication. Understandably, some nurses have difficulty tolerating profane or

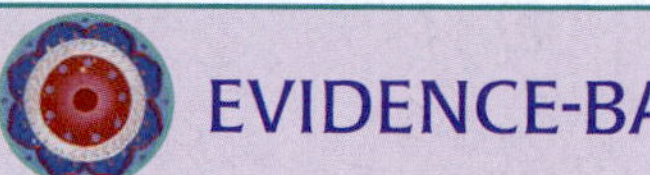

EVIDENCE-BASED PRACTICE

MAXIMIZING RESILIENCE

Danny is a slightly underweight 15-year-old who was admitted to the crisis unit in your community after treatment in the ED for an "accidental" overdose of his insulin. After admitting to his parents that he had intentionally drawn up too much insulin in a suicide attempt "to get what's coming anyway," he was admitted to the unit for observation and treatment.

Your initial nursing assessment revealed that Danny's depression and guilt seem to have evolved over time as he endured the loss of several relatives close to him, who died following complications from diabetes. He fears for himself and also feels guilty for "surviving" the illness that has taken his loved ones. Talking to him and his family about his diabetes condition reveals a similarly fatalistic attitude among his family members.

Your plan for intervention options is based on current research results. For example, in your review of studies of building resilience in adolescents, you know that optimism is a trait that contributes to resilience and has been identified as the most influential adolescent cognitive factor to moderate the effects of life stressors. Danny's parents commented that they had always regarded him as the "most positive" of their three children. Prior to puberty (his female cousin with diabetes died at age 12) he had been active in all sports and was "upbeat in every way." You recall that the design and delivery of an intervention to maximize resilience in adolescents require gender-specific strategies that are attractive, engaging, and easily accessible. You ask his parents to bring in pictures of him when he was active in sports. You encourage him to talk about his exploits and remind him about his physical abilities and competitive nature. You encourage him to be conscientious about managing his diabetes while inviting him to envision his goals for the future after high school. You incorporate these values and resiliency-building interventions in the nursing care plan and in all staff treatment meetings.

Furthermore, your readings and experiences have yielded information regarding the financial and staffing limits of community and school resources. As a result, you understand that local resources may tend to be problem-focused and disease-oriented because they do not have the funds or time to provide preventive or creative activities. You expect to put a plan in motion that will use preexisting resources as well as connect Danny with new supports, perhaps even identifying a program or resource to enhance Danny's school and social environments. With the help of Danny's school nurse, you set up a "surprise" visit from a local sports celebrity, an adult who has managed his diabetes since childhood. Danny is thrilled to meet him but, more importantly, is surprised to learn of his lifelong diabetes self-management and to see firsthand the positive results of his efforts. Over the next few weeks of his treatment Danny demonstrates a renewal of his optimism and displays a newfound autonomy and self-assurance in his diabetes self-management skills. Moreover, he agrees to explore serving as a counselor to younger kids in a local diabetes camp who might feel the way he "used to."

This set of multiple intervention strategies is based on the following research:

Davis, T. K. (2005). Beyond the physical examination: The nurse practitioner's role in adolescent risk reduction and resiliency building in a school-based health center. *Nursing Clinics of North America, 40*(4), 649–660, viii.

Tusaie, K. R., & Patterson, K. (2006). Relationships among trait, situational, and comparative optimism: Clarifying concepts for a theoretically consistent and evidence-based intervention to maximize resilience. *Archives of Psychiatric Nursing, 20*(3), 144–150.

CRITICAL THINKING APPLICATION

1. How would knowing how the adolescent has coped with earlier problems in life help you to design strategies for intervention?
2. Would an increased awareness of ways to be resilient make a difference in an adolescent client's life? How?
3. Why would involving others in Danny's goal of increased resilience be helpful?
4. Of what value are reminders of earlier active times in Danny's life? Would they be discouraging rather than encouraging?

sexually graphic language. However, you must evaluate your clients' underlying reasons for using such language, to help them understand their feelings. Only then can you encourage clients to use more appropriate means of expression. If clients sense that the reason you want them to speak more appropriately is only to make you, the nurse, feel more comfortable, the end result will not be satisfactory. The Rx Communication feature on page 734 further demonstrates two examples of this.

The adolescent psychiatric client often has symptoms of disturbed communication, which can affect all realms of daily living, particularly in relationships with peers, family members, and nonparental authority figures. Giving information is one way you can help decrease communication deficits and facilitate relationships with others. Other nursing behaviors are outlined in the Planning and Implementation section. (For the general principles of therapeutic communication, see Chapter 10∞.)

Confidentiality An emerging body of research underscores the importance of discussing confidentiality with the adolescent. There will be health concerns, thoughts, and feelings that the adolescent client will want to keep private. Assurances of confidentiality will increase the likelihood that the adolescent will disclose sensitive personal information to you. Confidentiality, however, cannot be unconditional in that some information, such as sexual abuse, must be disclosed by law, and other information, such as a suicide plan, must be discussed with the parents and the rest of the treatment team.

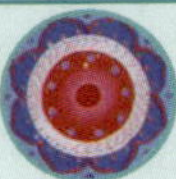

RX COMMUNICATION

CLIENT USING PROFANITY OR OBSCENITIES

CLIENT: "Hey, bee-atch! [Slang word for "bitch."] When is dinner served around this hell-hole? [Other clients are snickering in the background.]"

NURSE RESPONSE 1: [with an exaggerated look of surprise] "Rocky, you're new to the unit. I will give you information about the unit and about mealtimes but you need to understand something first. Profanity is not an acceptable way to get to know anyone here. I expect you to treat me with respect, as I will you. Now I'll show you your room and you can put your things away." [She then proceeds with him to a less public space where she talks with him without the other clients for an audience.]

RATIONALE: The client was newly admitted to the unit and may be attempting to overcompensate for his anxiety and fears as "the new kid" with bravado and intimidation. He needs an adequate orientation to the unit and unit expectations. The nurse believes she can give information to allay his anxiety while verbally setting limits on his provocative behavior. In this way she expects to avoid an escalation of such bravado, which might lead to the need for physical controls.

NURSE RESPONSE 2: [with an obvious look of surprise] "Rocky, you need to learn about the unit. That includes information about acceptable behaviors as well as mealtimes. Let that be the last time you address me or anyone else here that way. If you have trouble controlling your behavior we can assist you in taking a time-out until you're able to control yourself and are ready to be with the rest of the group. Steve and I will show you to your room, and you can ask us any other questions there." She and a male staff member escort him to his room, soliciting information as they evaluate his reactions and degree of control.]

RATIONALE: The client was newly admitted to the unit. Knowing his history of violent outbursts at home and at school, the nurse assesses his behavior as an attempt to assert his domination over the staff and intimidate the other clients. She sets limits immediately, with consequences spelled out to deter any continuation of his provocative behavior.

In discussing confidentiality with the adolescent, one way of clarifying this dilemma might be to simply state, "What you and I discuss is confidential. However, you need to know that *if it means harm to you or to someone else* [emphasize these words], it will be important for me to talk it over with your parents/other members of the team [whoever is most appropriate to the situation]. In that case, I will first discuss it with you to determine the best way in which to present our concerns to others."

Anger and Hostility

Expressions of anger and hostility are common on an adolescent unit. Anger expressed verbally usually takes the form of profanity. How effectively you deal with expressions of anger and hostility depends on how effectively you handle your own angry or hostile feelings. You will compromise your effectiveness as a nurse if you are uncomfortable with expressions of anger or hostility, or view anger and hostility as negative or to be avoided at all costs.

Nurse's Self-Assessment A subject that is rarely considered is anger felt and expressed by the nurse toward the client. The general focus on the client's need for understanding and good care seem to make it unacceptable to display negative feelings toward the client. In the nursing care of adolescents, however, a constant all-giving and all-accepting attitude by the nurse, particularly during times of testing, would be not only nontherapeutic but also illogical and dishonest, and adolescents need honest feedback. The adolescent sometimes escalates the provocative behavior to test your response or to evoke an angry reaction. For you to pretend that you are not angry in such a situation is as undesirable for treatment as it would be to pretend that you are fond of the client.

Being honest about your feelings is a prime prerequisite in establishing and maintaining meaningful and productive relationships with adolescent clients. This does not mean that you should vent all your thoughts or impulses. Be aware of your reactions, and use good judgment in handling them. This is also an opportunity to model adult modes of anger expression. The questions in the Your Self-Awareness feature will help you assess your own ways of dealing with anger.

Anxiety and Resistance

Normal adolescents frequently feel anxious as they experience change and inner turmoil in adapting to a new identity. The anxiety evidenced by disturbed adolescents in treatment can indicate many other things. The changes required are much more threatening to disturbed adolescents than to normal adolescents. If treatment is to be successful, clients must look at the meaning of their behavior and must change many of their earlier interactional patterns. This can be frightening. For example, it is more comfortable to play the role of the "bad seed" or "bad kid," with its known pitfalls and expectations, than to attempt a change that entails many uncertainties and unknowns.

Clients feel threatened and anxious when the nurse does not act according to their expectations, because they must then find other ways of handling the situation. They must also deal with the anxiety. Frequently this anxiety is channeled into a game of "cops and robbers," as the client once again assumes a familiar role and maintains the negative or unhealthy image. The anxiety caused by unfamiliar roles is dissipated by further testing and acting out. Do not take this as

MEDIALINK Case Study: Assessing the Resistant Client

YOUR SELF-AWARENESS
A Self-Awareness Inventory for Working with Adolescents

To increase self-awareness about your own way of dealing with anger, ask yourself these questions:

- What kinds of things make me angry?
- How do I deal with my anger? Do I tend to ignore or hide it, or do I show that I am angry?
- Do I sometimes use profanity or act out my feelings in a physical way? How do I feel about others who do this?
- What do I think about how I handle anger? Am I proud of the way I handle anger?
- How do I react to others when they are angry?

To increase self-awareness about your tendency to be seduced or manipulated, ask yourself these questions:

- Is this client's friendliness compromising the professional role boundaries between us and "personalizing" our relationship?
- Do I feel compelled to respond in a personal rather than therapeutic way, possibly revealing information about my own life and lifestyle?
- Do I feel uncomfortable with the client's flattering comments or probing questions?
- Do I tend to forget that this person is a client?
- Is the client encouraging me to keep secrets from other staff or to "side" with the client against other staff?

To increase self-awareness about your own sexual attitudes and feelings, ask yourself these questions:

- How would I describe my adolescence as it related to my developing sexuality?
- What do I remember about the development and changes in my body?
- How did I feel about these changes?
- How would I describe my adolescent relationships with members of my own sex?
- How would I describe my adolescent relationships with members of the opposite sex?
- What events stand out in my mind when I recall my sexual experiences during adolescence?
- How have these past relationships, events, and feelings influenced me today?

an indication that therapy is not working. It may simply indicate that the client needs to move ahead more slowly with insightful discoveries and needs your support in doing so.

Keep in mind that to these adolescents, "opening up" in a trusting way does not hold the same positive promise that it might for you. Adolescents who have been rejected or have experienced loss following close relationships in the past will be wary of your expressions of interest or concern and will be cautious about repeating such experiences. They may respond to you with testing behaviors, anger and mistrust, or outright rejection. Adolescents who expect rejection gain some control over the relationship if they reject others before being rejected themselves.

Nurse's Self-Assessment Sometimes nurses find it difficult to allow adolescents to grapple with their anxieties and fears. At other times, you may not recognize the client's behavior as a symptom of anxiety or depression. The following clinical example demonstrates the value of a comprehensive assessment, of exploring all possible reasons for a client's resistance to your efforts, before implementing action.

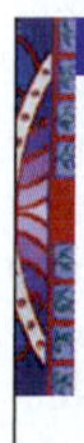

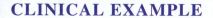

CLINICAL EXAMPLE

Kathy was the quietest and most aloof client on the unit. She had isolated herself from the other clients during the week that followed admission and avoided conversing with staff members outside meetings. One evening she seemed unusually receptive to the new nurse, Ellie, who was able to interest her in a sewing project. Ellie, who was a new graduate, felt pleased that Kathy had responded warmly to her during their time together. The next day, Kathy did not speak to Ellie and seemed to avoid her at all costs. Later, Ellie noticed that the dress Kathy had been sewing had been torn into shreds and stuffed into the wastepaper basket. Ellie interpreted this quite personally. She felt deeply hurt and rejected.

In her discussion with her supervisor, Ellie showed her disappointment and anger. Her supervisor observed that, although the good time and feelings that Ellie and Kathy had shared the evening before were genuine, Kathy had not experienced many such times before with her parents or other adults. She suggested that Kathy was probably angry with Ellie for pointing out what she, Kathy, had missed. The supervisor suggested that Ellie be patient with Kathy. Perhaps later Ellie could reestablish the bond, and they would be able to talk about what had happened.

Fortunately, Ellie did not act on her angry feelings. Had she done so, she might have impulsively assessed Kathy's behavior as "hopeless," interpreting Kathy's anxiety and resistance as an inability to trust, or she may have begun to relate to the client in a vindictive way, withdrawing from Kathy in turn. Instead, she sought advice. Ellie's supervisor recognized that Ellie wanted to do well and needed positive feedback. She also realized that Ellie did not understand the nature of giving to emotionally disturbed adolescents. Had Ellie not sought advice, she might have acted on her angry feelings, further alienating Kathy and causing herself more anger and frustration. Without an understanding of Kathy's actions,

Ellie would have continued to expect kindness in return for kindness and would have been keenly disappointed.

Seduction and Manipulation of the Nurse

In working with adolescents, there is always the risk of **seduction** of the nurse—that is, manipulation of the nurse by the client into relating in a nontherapeutic way. (Thus, the word *seduction* is not necessarily linked to *sexual* in psychiatric settings.) These factors contribute to the problem:

- The intimate nature of the nurse's involvement with the adolescent client
- The narcissism inherent in this age group
- The nurse's all-accepting attitude in working with the adolescent client

Narcissism in this age group is caused by the child's withdrawal from the parents and their value system. This withdrawal leads to a general self-centeredness, overevaluation of the self, heightened self-perception, decreased ability for reality testing, and extreme self-absorption. The result is that the people to whom adolescents turn become all-important and perfect in their eyes. Nurses may be strongly tempted to respond accordingly.

Nurse's Self-Assessment The dangers inherent in this situation are not simply the two possible extremes: total submission to temptation, resulting in a sexual relationship with the client; or strong denial of temptation by maintaining a rigid, unapproachable stance that makes it impossible to establish a meaningful, trusting relationship. Neither of these extremes is unknown.

It is tempting to respond to the adolescent's idealized view, to be the "savior" who succeeds with this difficult person where everyone else has failed, to feel superior to the imperfect parents, the harassed school teacher, the skeptical juvenile judge, or other members of the staff on the unit. However, you should not give in to such temptations. Complications will most certainly develop that at best will temporarily compromise your effectiveness and at worst will render the treatment program completely ineffective. Liza's example of acting out demonstrates this. Jim, the evening nurse, could have been seduced by Liza to collude with her against the day nurse, Jane, had he not been keenly aware of that possibility.

Nurses who work intensively with adolescents often face situations in which their own unresolved feelings are aroused. You must choose whether to act on these impulses or to explore their origin. Of course, one is not always conscious of these unresolved feelings. It would be unrealistic to expect you to be totally aware of the meaning of your behavior at any given moment. Nonetheless, the skilled clinician is usually acquainted with the issues or conflicts that have caused problems in the past. In doubtful cases, the knowledgeable nurse will seek consultation from a clinician. The clinician can help you assess the situation and understand what part you may have played in initiating it. Nurses who wish to explore their personal conflicts further may then seek counseling or therapy. The questions in the Your Self-Awareness feature on page 735 can help you assess the nature of your interactions with clients.

In addition, nursing staff would benefit from establishing one or more of the following to provide a consistent format for assessing and evaluating ongoing situations with adolescent clients:

- Each nurse's own ongoing supervision with a preceptor or nurse supervisor
- A regularly scheduled meeting (perhaps monthly) for all nursing staff to discuss difficult situations and conflicting feelings
- Staff meetings (perhaps weekly) in which all disciplines identify interpersonal obstacles and plan interventions toward more optimal treatment

Sexual Behavior of the Adolescent

The biologic changes that occur in late childhood and early adolescence are rapid and pervasive. Do not underestimate the importance of the adolescent's experimentation and attitude in sexual matters.

Likewise, evaluate your own attitudes and feelings about sexual issues as they relate to past experiences and current activities. Conflicts in such matters or resentments left over from the past will certainly affect your decisions or interactions with clients regarding sexual matters. Again, while it is not necessary for you to resolve all these issues, it is highly desirable to be aware of areas of conflict that might make it difficult to view a situation objectively or to set rational limits. Refer again to the Your Self-Awareness feature to increase your self-awareness about sexual attitudes and feelings. The feature What Every Community Health Nurse Should Know discusses the sexual behavior of adolescents and is a useful component in understanding this age group.

Until adolescents master their anxieties and fears about their sexual identity and gain control over sexual urges, they will exhibit a variety of behaviors and attitudes that may confuse or trouble you. In the past decade, rates of sexual activity,

WHAT EVERY COMMUNITY HEALTH NURSE SHOULD KNOW

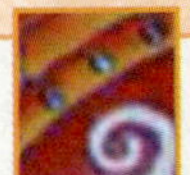

Discussing Sexuality with Adolescents

Discussing sexual matters with adolescents may be easier and more practical if you use a structured, user-friendly tool to "break the ice" and acquire the information you need. Nurses in a community clinic used an Event History Calendar (EHC) for sexual risk assessment with Latina females aged 15 to 19 years. The EHC is a way to track the elevation of risk factors and the effect on young women of their environment. It uses familiar language to discuss these topics. The EHC proved to be a time-efficient and adolescent-friendly risk assessment tool that helped identify and encourage discussion of sexual risk and comorbid risk behaviors (Martyn, 2006).

pregnancy, and live births among adolescents have stabilized and perhaps even begun to decline as there appears to have been a decrease in sexual activity among youth and a reported increase in the use of more effective contraceptive methods. Although these trends are encouraging, it is estimated that 25% of sexually active teenagers have an STD (sexually transmitted disease), with equivalent health risk of pelvic inflammatory disease, genital herpes, and gonorrhea (Herrman, 2006).

Heterosexual Behavior Heterosexual activity is normal and desirable during adolescence. However, nurses working with either normal or disturbed adolescents will sometimes see them engage in sexual activities that do not seem healthy or growth producing. For example, the adolescent girl who seeks punishment rather than true pleasure in her sexual exploits will display them in an overt, exhibitionistic way in a place where a particularly moralistic person will discover her and give her the reprimands she desires. She may be testing a parent's values in an attempt to resolve her own inner conflicts.

Adolescents in an inpatient treatment setting where sexual intercourse is forbidden may engage in sexual intercourse where you or another staff member will be sure to discover them. The experience may reinforce their image of sexual behavior as "bad" behavior. Or it may simply provide a means of acting out their defiance of the rules, thereby earning the familiar "bad kid" label. The incident involving the clients Laurie and Bill in the following Rx Communication feature is an excellent example of this situation.

Homosexual Behavior Homosexuality is the persistent sexual and emotional attraction to someone of the same sex. It is part of the range of sexual expression and has existed throughout history and across cultures. Preadolescents usually choose a member of the same sex with whom to experience intimate or loving feelings. This does not necessarily mean that a sexual relationship will ensue, although it often does. Homosexual activity may continue into the adolescent years. Many gay, lesbian, and bisexual individuals first become aware of their sexual thoughts and feelings and may have their first experiences during adolescence. Recent changes in society's attitude toward sexuality, including homosexual issues, have helped gay, lesbian, and bisexual youth feel more comfortable with their sexual orientation. Moreover, AACAP has designed a Fact Sheet to assist parents and professionals alike in meeting the developmental needs of the homosexual or bisexual adolescent (AACAP, 2005).

Although the causes of homosexuality or bisexuality are not fully understood, the AACAP position makes it clear that sexual orientation is not a mental disorder. Nor is it a matter of choice. Individuals are no more able to "choose" whether or not to be homosexual than to be heterosexual.

Like their heterosexual counterparts, gay, lesbian, and bisexual teens have many concerns, including: feeling different from their peers; fearing ridicule, rejection, or harassment by others; worrying about a negative response from their families or loved ones; and worrying about sexually transmitted diseases, including HIV infection. Moreover, they have an additional fear of discrimination due to their sexual orientation when seeking employment, applying to college, or joining clubs or sports activities. They can become socially isolated, withdraw from friends and activities, have trouble concentrating, develop low self-esteem, become depressed, and feel suicidal. Counseling may be helpful for teens who are uncomfortable with their homosexuality or who are unable to express it. Regardless of setting or sexual orientation, adolescents do have a choice about how and where to express their sexual feelings, just as they do their other emotions.

Generally speaking, however, adolescents view homosexual feelings as a threat to the development of their identity. As a result, they may ward off such feelings by engaging in frantic sexual activity with a member of the opposite sex. This is particularly true for boys. It is normal for an adolescent boy to be afraid of his own passive wishes and to label

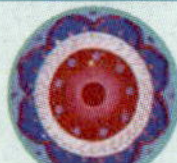

RX COMMUNICATION

CLIENT WITH SEXUAL ACTING-OUT BEHAVIOR

CLIENT: [A male and female client are discovered making out in a closet on the unit.] "Hey, a little privacy, if you don't mind!"

NURSE RESPONSE 1: "Laurie, Bill, not cool, guys. What's going on? You knew I was coming in here to get more towels. Laurie, does this have to do with your pass home tomorrow? Let's talk about this in the office. C'mon." [She escorts the two clients to the office to talk.]

RATIONALE: Both adolescents are "veterans" on the unit and know full well the rules and expectations. The nurse believes that the behavior is a display of Laurie's anxiety about her pass home tomorrow and may be an attempt to sabotage the privilege. Rather than addressing the rules as the focus for their discussion, she talks with them about the underlying meaning of their behavior.

NURSE RESPONSE 2: "What are you guys doing in here? What am I supposed to do with this? You know sex is not allowed. Come out of there and go into the dining room with everyone else. We'll have a community meeting right after dinner and talk about this."

RATIONALE: The nurse is new to the unit and inexperienced in dealing with such acting-out behaviors. She expects to use the format and support of the group meeting to both deal with the inappropriate behavior and observe the interventions of the veteran staff.

them homosexual. He had probably been brought up to identify with physical displays of strength or aggressive displays of power. Thus, an incident in which he feels threatened or powerless would produce feelings of sexual impotence, a feeling of dependence or weakness, and a greater fear of homosexuality. The adolescent boy in treatment may act out these feelings, or he may attempt to reaffirm his masculinity with inappropriate displays of aggression or destructive behavior. Likewise, the adolescent girl who feels a need to ward off intense feelings for female peers may engage in frantic sexual activity with numerous male partners for similar reasons. Clients who use homosexuality to express hostility toward their parents will undoubtedly act out with the staff as well.

Nurses who work with adolescents may encounter any of these situations and they must attempt to understand the meaning that homosexual behavior has for the client. The clients may need to explore their feelings and anxieties openly. Open discussion with an understanding yet knowledgeable professional may help resolve many of the concerns and conflicts inherent in adolescent sexual behavior. Remain objective and nonjudgmental with these clients, allowing them to deal with the feelings of anger or depression that may result from addressing the conflict.

Although homosexual behavior during adolescence does not predict adult sexual preference, some adolescents make a lasting identification as homosexuals during these years. These adolescents will not experience conflicts about homosexual relationships or need to flaunt them or act out with the staff in an angry or hostile way. In these cases, however, you may have to deal with your own negative feelings about homosexuality, if any exist. It is important for you to consider what clients' relationships mean to them and to respect them.

Pregnancy Adolescent pregnancy may reflect social and family expectations and unconscious motivations. Some teenage girls are quite pleased to be pregnant and suffer no emotional consequences from motherhood. In general, however, a conscious, deliberate decision to become pregnant at this age is manipulative. The goal may be to escape a difficult family situation, to express hostility toward parents, or to act out a life script in which the daughter is seen as "bad." The adolescent girl who did not receive adequate nurturing as a child could be acting out dependency needs by giving her baby the love and caring she herself did not receive. In so doing, she feels loved and cared for in turn.

Be sensitive to motivational factors in dealing with emotionally deprived adolescents. Use existing educational tools and interpersonal relationships to help adolescent girls understand their needs and motivations to become pregnant. It is also important to educate adolescents of both sexes about sex and birth control. Many high schools are now recognizing this need and providing information in birth control clinics or through health education classes. Too often parents and professionals alike deny the adolescent's sexual activity until an unwanted pregnancy occurs.

MEDIALINK Care Plan: Violence and Self-Mutilation

Dietary Problems and Eating Disorders

The eating habits and food preferences of disturbed adolescents can reveal a great deal about the nature of their inner turmoil. A comparison between the client's diet and that of a normal, healthy adolescent may show little difference in variety but probably a great difference in quantity.

Adolescents who have been deprived of early nurturing tend to eat more than others and probably place a higher value on mealtimes and on receiving their "share" of the food. You may notice that adolescents consume more milk than usual during periods of stress or anxiety. In general, girls want to follow food fads or unreasonable dietary regimens to become slim and attractive. This usually gives you an opportunity to engage in health teaching about nutrition and exercise, and to express a cooperative interest in their developing feminine identity. (Eating disorders are discussed in Chapter 21.)

Depression and Suicide

Both depression and suicide are thought to be underreported among adolescents. Suicide rates among adolescents remain unacceptably high, and recently rates have spiked significantly (see Figure 23-2 on page 622 and the discussion of youth suicide in Chapter 23).

The National Center for Injury Prevention and Control (NCIPC) has designed a Suicide Fact Sheet including Prevention Strategies and Links for further study and resources. The Center reports that few schools and communities have suicide prevention plans that include screening, referral, and crisis intervention programs for youth (NCIPC, 2006).

The Youth Risk Behavior Surveillance system (YRBS) monitors six categories of priority health-risk behaviors among youth and young adults, including behaviors that contribute to unintentional injuries and violence (Eaton et al., 2006). In the United States 71% of all deaths among youth and young adults aged 10–24 resulted from four causes: motor vehicle crashes (31%), other unintentional injuries (14%), homicide (15%), and suicide (11%) (Centers for Disease Control and Prevention [CDC], 2006). During the 30 days preceding the survey, many high school students engaged in behaviors that increased their likelihood of death from four causes: 9.9% had driven a vehicle when they had been drinking alcohol; 18.5% had carried a weapon; 43.3% had consumed alcohol; and 20.2% had used marijuana. During the 12 months preceding the survey, 35.9% had been in a physical fight and 8.4% had attempted suicide. In addition to these dramatic statistics there were equally important data regarding implications for sexuality and ethnicity. These facts concerning suicide among the young are in Box 27-3. (See Chapter 23 for a complete discussion of suicide, including assessment and nursing intervention.)

Repetitive deliberate self-injury and self-mutilation (cutting one's arms or abdomen, burning oneself) are also underreported and associated with both depression and suicidality. As many as 4% of 9th-grade students reported repetitive self-harm, and an even larger number, 10.9%, reported occasional deliberate self-harm (Brunner et al., 2007). In another study,

Box 27-3 **At a Glance: Suicide Among the Young**

- For young people 15 to 24 years old, suicide is the third leading cause of death, behind unintentional injury and homicide. In 2001, 3,971 suicides were reported in this age group.
- In 2001, of the total number of suicides among young people ages 15 to 24, 86% were male and 14% were female.
- American Indian and Alaskan Natives have the highest rate of suicide in the 15-to-24 age group.
- In 2001, firearms were used in 54% of youth suicides.
- In 2005, 8.4% of high school students had actually attempted suicide one or more times during the 12 months preceding the survey with the prevalence of having actually attempted suicide higher among females (10.8%) than males (6.0%).
- The prevalence of having seriously considered attempting suicide was higher among white (16.9%) and Hispanic (17.9%) than black (12.2%) students.
- It has been widely reported that gay and lesbian youth are 2 to 3 times more likely to commit suicide than other youth and that 30% of all attempted or completed youth suicides are related to issues of sexual identity. There are no empirical data on completed suicides to support such assertions, but there is growing concern about an association between suicide risk and bisexuality or homosexuality for youth, particularly males. Increased attention has been focused on the need for empirically based and culturally competent research on the topic of gay, lesbian, and bisexual suicide.

Source: National Center for Injury Prevention and Control. (2006). *Suicide: Fact sheet*. Retrieved July 18, 2006, from http://www.cdc.gov/ncipc/factsheets/suifacts.htm; Eaton, D. K., Kann, L., Kinchen, S., Ross, J., Hawkins, J., Harris, W. A., et al. (2006). *Youth risk behavior surveillance—United States, 2005*. Retrieved July 18, 2006, from http://www.cdc.gov/mmwr/preview/mmwrhtml/ss5505a1.htm; American Academy of Child & Adolescent Psychiatry. (2004). *Facts for families: Teen suicide*. Retrieved September 18, 2007, from http://www.aacap.org/cs/root/facts_for_families/teen_suicide.

40.3% of students reporting self-injurious behavior were suicidal as well (Whitlock & Knox, 2007). The presence of self-injurious behavior should always trigger a suicide assessment.

Substance Use and Abuse

According to the 2005 Monitoring the Future survey of approximately 50,000 students in 8th, 10th, and 12th grades, there was a decline of almost 19% in the previous month's usage of any illicit drug by these groups between 2001 and 2005. In addition, use of the drug **Ecstasy (MDMA)**, a synthetic compound with both stimulant and mildly hallucinogenic properties, also declined. On the other hand, nonmedical use of prescription medications, in particular Vicodin and OxyContin, continue to be high, with long-term trends showing a significant increase in the abuse of OxyContin from 2002 to 2005 among 12th graders (NIDA, 2005).

Adolescents give many reasons for using drugs: to experiment, to get high, to "get inside my head," to have fun, to understand more about life. Adolescents may also use drugs to cope with feelings of worthlessness or loneliness or to avoid uncomfortable feelings, as in the following clinical example.

CLINICAL EXAMPLE

Cindy is a 15-year-old high school sophomore who has been abusing drugs since age 12. According to Cindy, her 3-year history of substance abuse has involved regular marijuana use one to two times a week, occasional use of Valium (which she sneaks from her mother's 5-mg tablet prescription bottle), Seconal ("street reds") on two occasions, and LSD on two occasions.

Cindy describes herself as a "loner" who has few friends and keeps to herself at home and at school. She leaves the house each morning for school before the others are awake "to avoid the hassles with my mother and sisters." She describes one female classmate to whom she feels close but states that their time together is usually brief and usually involves smoking marijuana in the morning just before school. Cindy has recently been suspended from school as a result of the school principal's discovery of Cindy and her friend smoking marijuana outside the cafeteria.

Cindy is lonely and depressed, and has extreme feelings of worthlessness. She characterizes herself as "bored," "bad," and "hopeless." Cindy says that when she uses drugs, her situation doesn't seem as bad.

Although the general public may disagree about whether drugs are harmful, the fact remains that using drugs—or at least experimenting with them—is acceptable to many adolescents.

Assessing Drug Abuse How can you determine when drug *use* becomes drug *abuse*? Generally, the adolescent who abuses drugs or alcohol exhibits at least one of these following characteristics:

- The adolescent's performance at school or work increasingly deteriorates.
- The adolescent is frequently caught high or in the act of getting high by parents or other authority figures.
- The adolescent increasingly resorts to alcohol or drugs in times of stress or boredom.
- The adolescent has seriously deficient interpersonal relationships and can relate only when under the influence of drugs or alcohol.
- The adolescent may lose interest in interpersonal relationships altogether, preferring to be high alone rather than to be with others.

Nurses are most effective when they can determine what the particular drug or high does for the client. A boy with a poor self-image and low-esteem may say that it makes him "feel like a man." A particularly shy or introverted girl may say that it makes her "outgoing and friendly." You may discover that being high helps rid disturbed adolescents of angry or depressed feelings. Indeed, in the treatment setting, the client frequently resorts to smoking marijuana or "popping"

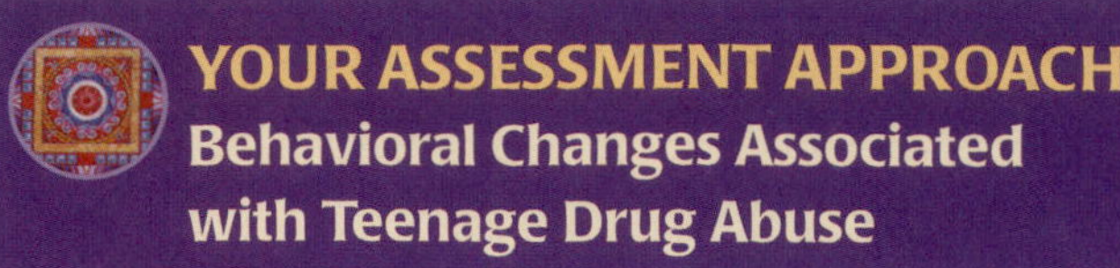

YOUR ASSESSMENT APPROACH
Behavioral Changes Associated with Teenage Drug Abuse

- Unexplained periods or reactions of moodiness, depression, anxiety, irritability, oversensitivity, or hostility
- Strongly inappropriate overreaction to mild criticism or simple requests
- Lessening in warmth toward family; avoids interaction and communication with parents, withdraws from family activities
- Preoccupation with self, less concern for the feelings of others
- Loss of interest in previously important hobbies, sports, activities
- Loss of motivation and enthusiasm (amotivational syndrome)
- Lethargy, lack of energy and vitality
- Loss of ability to self-discipline and assume responsibility
- Need for instant gratification
- Change in values, ideals, beliefs
- Changes in friends, unwillingness to introduce friends
- Secretive phone calls; callers refuse to identify themselves or hang up when someone other than the adolescent answers
- Unexplained absences from home
- Disappearance of money or items of value from home; handling of money becomes secretive
- Desire for increased sensory stimuli

uppers or downers to escape uncomfortable feelings. The Your Assessment Approach feature highlights some of the behavioral changes that may be observed in adolescents using drugs.

Nursing Diagnosis: NANDA

The use of nursing diagnoses with adolescent clients can lend meaning and substance to the clients' behavior that might be overlooked with a DSM-IV-TR diagnosis alone. For example, look back at Cindy, the 15-year-old with a 3-year history of substance abuse. Limiting your assessment to a DSM-IV-TR diagnosis alone might yield a substance use disorder, a marijuana cannabis use disorder, or a substance-induced mood disorder. While this tells you something about her drug history, it does not reveal any specifics such as current stressors; temperament; or cultural, social, or family dynamics that might contribute to or even underlie her drug abuse.

Specifically, your assessments (and interventions) become more comprehensive and universally informative with an exploration of any or all of the following: Ineffective Coping, Compromised Family Coping, Chronic Low Self-Esteem, and/or Hopelessness. By using the various subsystems provided by nursing diagnoses, you can establish a more comprehensive picture of the client's difficulty and immediately become more goal-oriented in assessing and planning care.

Moreover, in many treatment settings, mental health care professionals are reluctant to give adolescents a DSM-IV-TR diagnosis during these formative years to avoid labeling them (possibly erroneously). Such labeling may result in inadequate treatment, self-fulfilling prophecy, or both, in subsequent mental health care contacts (see also the Your Self-Awareness feature on standardized terminology interfering with individualized client care on page 265 in Chapter 13). For a more thorough discussion of DSM-IV-TR diagnoses with psychiatric clients, see Chapter 11.

For nurses, the dilemmas described here make the language of nursing diagnosis even more beneficial and user-friendly. We can use nursing diagnoses as tools to adequately describe the client's behavior without rigidly adhering to a medically diagnostic label. We can then communicate the adolescent's experience to family, lay personnel, and non–mental health professionals without having to resort to specialized terminology.

Outcome Identification: NOC

Your choice of NOC expected outcomes and NIC interventions will depend primarily on your individualized assessment and the adolescent's stated goals. As a result, your goals and your interventions for the client have depth and are more likely to be effective.

With 15-year-old Cindy, for example, an expected outcome that she will no longer use drugs after discharge might be unrealistic. Expected outcomes that would yield more success, yet demonstrate client improvement, might be one or all of the following:

- Client approaches a nurse to discuss temptation to use drugs.
- Client attends and participates in family meetings.
- Client verbalizes negative feelings.
- Client correlates negative feelings with temptation to use drugs.
- Client demonstrates alternative ways of dealing with stressful situations, such as talking to others, becoming involved in peer group activities, or using "quiet time" in anticipation of family meetings.

Successful treatment with adolescents may translate into their use of new skills the vast majority of the time, but not 100% of the time. Adolescents will take some time to "try out" new behaviors and coping mechanisms. It is important to acknowledge that clients may need to take two steps forward and one backward as progress is made. Moreover, as stressful situations arise, adolescents will be inclined to resort to previous and maladaptive patterns of behavior. In Cindy's situation, she may resist attending a difficult family meeting or may even bolt from the room when confronted with her behaviors or feelings. Either behavior alone does not mean that she is not showing progress or improvement.

Likewise, correlating interventions to support the above expected outcomes might include one or all of the following:

- Establish a no-drug contract with the client.
- Adopt a neutral, matter-of-fact attitude when discussing drug usage.
- Encourage the client to seek out a nurse when feeling tempted to use drugs.

- Draw a parallel for the client between drug usage and sad or angry feelings.
- Encourage the client to talk about feelings in individual therapy, group meetings, and family meetings.

Planning and Implementation: NIC

Nurses in numerous roles and diverse settings are in prime positions to recognize and intervene early with pathologic symptoms and behaviors.

Planning for Prevention

By preventing certain circumstances in the early stages of life, such as smoking or drug use as coping mechanisms, health improvements are more probable at later stages. The progression from primary prevention (education/self-care) to secondary prevention (early problem recognition and treatment) to tertiary prevention (more complicated and serious forms of illness and risky behaviors) includes services that become increasingly more technological, expensive, and exclusive.

Establishing a Contract with the Adolescent

Contracts can be particularly useful with adolescents. Adolescents can feel powerless in a treatment setting, especially when referred to treatment by parents or the legal system. Moreover, with this increased sense of control over their own behavior, adolescents become your collaborators in their treatment rather than objects of your treatment plan.

With most adolescents, a written contract is best, for these reasons:

- The goals and expectations are less easily forgotten.
- The process seems more formal and "serious."
- The adolescent has more responsibility as a signee, indicating increased awareness of responsibility and choice of behavior.
- There is less room for misinterpretation and manipulation.

Contracts seem especially helpful in situations of substance abuse, eating disorders, suicidal behavior, and impulsive or manipulative behaviors. Whether verbal or written, the contract can be simply stated to promote clarity, consistency, and cooperation. Here is an example:

- I will not take drugs or bring drugs onto the unit.
- I will not call or accept calls from my drug friends while in the treatment program.
- I will go directly to my outpatient therapy appointment and return immediately to the unit.
- I will not harm myself or others. If I feel like hurting myself, others, or property, I will tell the staff.

If written, the contract is signed by the client, dated, and cosigned by you. The contract is renegotiated at regular intervals (hourly, daily, or weekly), depending on the goals, the severity of the symptoms, and the degree of adherence with the agreement. The form of the contract is less important than the way you and the client jointly set the goals and expectations, carry out the contract, set limits and renegotiate changes, and evaluate the final outcome. Chapter 23 discusses and illustrates no-suicide contracts.

Intervening into Anger and Hostility

Depending on the degree to which the client is experiencing and expressing anger and hostility, you may choose any of a variety of interventions. These range from observing and assessing the client's behavior to physically restraining someone who is attempting destructive action (see Chapter 35).

Choosing an Appropriate Intervention In some situations, a disturbed adolescent's ability to express anger directly to another person can be a sign of success in treatment. The choice of interventions also depends on your own experiences with these feelings, your knowledge and understanding of this client's life experiences with anger, and the external limits imposed by the mental health agency.

Attempt to discover what meaning anger and hostility have for the client by asking the following questions:

- How has this client handled anger in the past?
- Does the client have a history of aggression toward objects or people?
- If so, what were the consequences of this behavior?
- What does this adolescent describe feeling after such a reaction?
- What kinds of things make this client angry? Which of these would be most likely to occur on the unit or in this setting?

The clinical example that follows illustrates a situation in which you might choose to observe and assess rather than intervene in response to a client's anger and hostility.

CLINICAL EXAMPLE

Steve had expressed great interest in building a model airplane. He saved up his money and took a long time to choose "just the right one" at the hobby shop. After spending most of the afternoon constructing and painting it, he was interrupted by a phone call from his mother. She told him that she would not be able to attend the family meeting that week, giving a number of reasons. This was the third consecutive week that she had missed a family meeting. Each time, she gave questionable reasons for being unable to attend.

Steve was disappointed and angry. He slammed down the receiver, yelling obscenities in response to the nurse's questions, and ran into his room. There he destroyed the plane by throwing it repeatedly against the floor.

In this example, Steve was not hurting himself or another. Although he did destroy property, the plane belonged to him, and he was free to do with it as he chose. The nurse resisted any impulse to stop Steve from damaging his plane. Because it was of significant value to him, he later regretted having taken out his anger on it. However, the situation provided Steve with an opportunity to explore his actions, and he later asked the nurse why he would destroy something that he valued so much after his mother had disappointed and angered him. The parallel between this situation and hurting himself with drugs right after he had argued with his mother was only too apparent.

Anger Directed Toward the Nurse Incidents in which the nurse bears the brunt of a client's anger or hostility do not offer obvious solutions. Disturbed adolescents may not think twice about addressing a female nurse as "bitch" and coupling such a greeting with a request for a favor. Adolescents direct insults and hostile remarks at nurses for many reasons, most of which have little to do with the nurses as people but a lot to do with nurses as adults or authority figures.

In choosing interventions, consider the meaning behind the client's behavior, your own relationship with this client, your immediate feelings, and the desired result. For example, if the client calls you "bitch" the first time you meet, you may interpret this as a form of testing and may choose to respond immediately with a bewildered look at this unwarranted display of hostility. Later, you may approach the client, expressing a naïve curiosity as to the origin of the hostile feelings: "Hey, I don't understand what happened between us a few minutes ago. We just met, and you're calling me a bitch. What's that all about?" This simple question conveys two messages. First, it indicates to the client that you are not accustomed to this kind of salutation. Second, it indicates that you are more interested in the motivation for the remark than in curtailing its use.

If the client resorts to name calling only when angry or under stress, you may decide to ignore the words and deal only with the feelings involved. For example, if a client has angrily left an ongoing family meeting and then calls you a bitch, you can probably assume that the anger is displaced. It is probably a result of overwhelming feelings experienced during the meeting. You may elect simply to say, "I know you're not angry at me right now. It seems like the meeting was pretty heavy, though. Do you want to talk about why you don't want to be in there now?" In neither situation is the name calling intended as a personal affront. However, the way you handle it determines both the outcome of the immediate situation and your chances of furthering your relationship with the client.

Client Reactions The adolescent's reaction to your intervention largely determines its effectiveness. For example, with Steve, the boy who destroyed his plane, the nurse's goal was to help Steve understand the impulsive reaction that destroyed something he loved and to encourage a more appropriate and direct expression of anger at his mother. He was able to do this as well as draw a parallel between anger at his mother and his drug abuse, which hurt himself. If the nurse's goal had been simply to stop the destruction of his property, Steve could have felt even greater anger and frustration, and he might have turned his aggression toward himself, the nurse, or the environment. Certainly if Steve had escalated his destructive behavior, turning his aggression toward himself or others, then direct limit setting, including physical restraints, would have been indicated.

In first-time encounters with any client new to the setting, do not be surprised or dismayed about less-than-optimal success with interventions. It may take some time and trial and error to assess the client's behaviors and choose the most effective interventions.

Intervening into Testing and Limit Setting

As young adolescents attempt to adjust to the upheaval in their emotional lives and begin to emancipate themselves from parental figures, a good deal of testing is to be expected. This is normal. However, the meaning that testing holds for the disturbed adolescent is a more complicated matter.

Adolescents who lack early nurturing have difficulty with interpersonal relationships. In many cases, parents were emotionally unable to provide adequate parenting. In other cases, they chose not to impose their values on their children. In either case, the children never developed the internalized values that reduce conflict and avert crisis during adolescence. This causes identity diffusion (the failure to maintain a cohesive self-concept), which in turn results in emptiness, a lack of basic trust, and difficulties with intimacy on any level.

In the treatment setting, these clients test by making limitless and absolute demands. Although these clients often react to imposed limits with cries of injustice, they often really seem to be asking for limits as an indication of caring, as Julie did in the clinical example that follows.

CLINICAL EXAMPLE

Julie had been on the unit only 2 days. During that time she had seen several of the older clients run away from the unit, commonly known as "going AWOL," and had witnessed the staff members' attempts to encourage those remaining on the ward to deal with whatever feelings they were experiencing. Toward the end of her second evening, Julie abruptly jumped up from a conversation with a nurse and ran toward the open door. The surprised nurse immediately followed, running down the stairs after her. A smiling Julie was waiting at the bottom step when the nurse arrived, breathless and confused, asking why Julie ran away. Julie quickly answered, "I just wanted to see if you cared enough to come after me."

In this situation, no further action was necessary.

Sometimes the client may use annoying or destructive behavior to test you. At these times, setting firm limits without further interpretation or exploration may be indicated. In other instances, the client may be reacting to some real threat, as in the clinical example that follows, or to an uncomfortable situation.

CLINICAL EXAMPLE

Joanne was quietly playing pool by herself when she noticed her therapist talking to a new female client. Joanne's volatile nature gave rise to jealousy and rage, and she began to hit the billiard balls off the table, making a lot of noise and startling everyone around her.

The nurse who had been observing her witnessed the change in her behavior and understood it as a reaction to sharing her therapist's attention with the new client. Without questioning Joanne's apparent anger, she stepped up to the table and challenged her to a game, which Joanne immediately accepted. Because Joanne prided herself on her pool-playing ability, she quickly channeled her energy and competitive feelings into the game and won. She then sought out her therapist and happily announced her victory.

Had the nurse not understood what had triggered Joanne's outburst, she might have become angry with her for making noise and set limits on her privilege to play pool. This would certainly have produced a helpless and even angrier Joanne, whose destructive behavior probably would have escalated. Because of the nurse's perceptive action, Joanne was able to save face by winning at pool and was not forced into a situation that would have made her feel more helpless.

Think about what other interventions might have been equally effective with Joanne. In your relationships with adolescent clients, you might find yourself inclined to respond with myriad, seemingly unrelated, interventions. With a combination of increased clinical experience, a personalized assessment of the adolescent and the immediate situation, and knowledge of current practice studies, you will be most effective in your interventions.

Intervening into Scapegoating

Scapegoating—a process by which an individual or group of individuals is identified as different from others and becomes the object of the group's fears, frustrations, or anger—is common in many groups, but particularly in adolescent groups. It occurs in three stages:

1. Frustration generates aggression.
2. The aggression is then displaced onto other people.
3. A process of blaming, projecting, and stereotyping follows. This displaced aggression is rationalized and finally justified, because the identified scapegoat is "different" in some real way.

The members of a group tend to attack the scapegoat because they are afraid to attack the person, group, or institution on whom their feelings are actually focused. Adolescents readily identify peers who are "different" and project on them their own fears and insecurities about their changing images. The client identified as the scapegoat is the object of much teasing and many hostile remarks.

Refrain from attempting merely to rescue the scapegoat, as this may augment the other clients' anger and frustration and encourage an escalation of the hostility. Set limits on the behavior and then ask the group to focus on what is going on, to acknowledge the anxiety or other uncomfortable feeling that preceded the scapegoating incident. If possible, anticipate the occurrence of scapegoating in times of stress and try to circumvent the process before it gets out of control.

Also be aware that identified scapegoats share some responsibility for their predicament by presenting themselves to the other clients in a different or provocative stance. In some instances the scapegoat is accustomed to this role or has an inner need to be punished and meets the group's urgent need to punish as well. You can be valuable to these clients by helping them explore whatever function this role serves for them.

Intervening into Sexual Behaviors

With self-awareness and an understanding of your feelings and attitudes about sexual issues, you can more readily plan interventions to deal with the sexual behaviors of the adolescent client.

Masturbation Masturbation is a normal sexual activity for people of all ages, from the beginning of sexual awareness to senescence. If you have a relatively healthy attitude toward masturbation, you are not likely to run into problems unless the client masturbates in inappropriate places or uses masturbation to express hostility.

You may be confronted with an adolescent boy who fondles his genitals when he is anxious or feels threatened. Understanding his behavior as an indication of anxiety, you may elect to ignore the gesture and explore the nature of his anxiety with him. At other times, the boy may make a masturbatory gesture to convey contempt or hostility. In this case it would be ludicrous to feign indifference in response.

Your reaction depends on all the previously mentioned factors, such as the nurse–client relationship and the behavior that preceded the gesture. Generally, however, it is wise to comment on the client's gesture—for example, by mentioning it as an attempt to "make me uncomfortable"—and then to allow the client the opportunity to express his feelings verbally. It is unlikely that this intervention will produce a tumultuous outpouring of feeling resulting in immediate resolution. However, it does allow you to acknowledge both the client's and your own feelings, perhaps paving the way for a more appropriate exchange in the future.

Heterosexual Behavior The adolescent often uses sexual behavior as a means of acting out other conflicts and as a testing ground for the nursing staff's feelings and attitudes. The clinical example of Barbara and Laurie illustrates both issues.

CLINICAL EXAMPLE

This was the third time Barbara, a nurse, had gone into Laurie's room to check on two clients, Laurie and Bill, who were an identified couple on the unit. Although there was a rule against clients having sexual intercourse with each other, Laurie and Bill had been discovered in the act each evening Barbara was on duty. Barbara found these discoveries disconcerting. She wondered if she was the only staff member who checked on clients, as no one else had reported any sexual activity. She decided to bring up the subject at the next treatment planning meeting to find a more effective way to deal with the situation.

Imagine Barbara's surprise when her peers agreed that Barbara was actually partly responsible for Laurie and Bill's acting-out. It seemed that her frequent checking on clients conveyed her expectation that they were "up to something." Barbara acknowledged that she expected that sort of behavior and was quite afraid of discovering Laurie and Bill in the act of intercourse.

The team helped Barbara see that her own expectations were being met. Laurie and Bill were doing exactly what she expected them to do—maybe even wanted them to do. Laurie and Bill were following their scripts of being "bad" and expressing their hostility toward Barbara. When Barbara heard how other staff members spent time with the couple to encourage them in indirect ways to join the larger group activities, she realized how obvious her anxiety and unconscious messages actually were. She then began to question her own attitudes about sexual matters and to explore why she feared discovering the couple engaged in sexual intercourse.

In this example, the client couple used sexual behaviors to act out their own underlying feelings. Had Barbara's assessment been limited to each immediate situation, she would have focused only on the couple's unacceptable behavior and would not have been open to the implications their behavior had for her. By seeking out information and feedback from her peers, she made a discovery about herself and realized it was more effective to anticipate and possibly circumvent such client behaviors than to intervene after the fact. Had Barbara not asked for feedback, the problem would have continued with an increase in the sexual behaviors and in Barbara's frustration. The situation would then have required intervention by an astute supervisor or an empathic colleague.

Homosexual Behavior In situations in which homosexual behavior is an expected developmental step or a lifestyle without expressions of anger or hostility toward parents or staff, little or no intervention may be indicated. As mentioned in the Assessment section, it is as important for the nurse to understand and provide emotional support for the homosexual or bisexual teen as for the heterosexual teen dealing with sexual identity and other developmental issues. Moreover, adolescents should be allowed to decide when and to whom to disclose their sexual orientation.

Counseling directed specifically at insisting that one's sexual orientation be the norm, when it is not, may be traumatic and cause lasting harm for an unwilling adolescent. Professionals and laypersons alike can obtain understanding and support from organizations such as Parents, Families, and Friends of Lesbians and Gays (PFLAG, http://www.pflag.org).

On the other hand, when homosexual behavior is used to act out feelings of impotence, or aggressive behavior is used to counteract feelings of intimacy, limits must be imposed. Try to anticipate this behavior and provide other ways for the adolescent client to work with the anxiety. As one example, with a male needing to demonstrate his masculinity, perhaps you could organize a game of football or tennis, if he is fairly proficient at these skills, or engage him in some other activity in which he excels. With a female fearing intimate feelings, anticipate and circumvent a similar display of acting-out, perhaps with a group activity where intimate or competitive feelings can be channeled in a more socially appropriate way. The point is to reestablish the adolescent's feeling of competence and control. Without these interventions, feelings of impotence will escalate to the point where the client will act them out in a negative way. The client who uses homosexuality to express defiance against authority figures will flaunt homosexual activities and consistently incur the anger, embarrassment, or both, of staff and clients alike.

MediaLink Parents, Families, and Friends of Lesbians and Gays

Intervening into Substance Abuse

While the 2005 Monitoring the Future Survey shows a continuing general decline in illicit drug use (due to the decreasing rates of marijuana use among 8th, 10th, and 12th graders between 2001 and 2005), there are continued high rates of nonmedical use of prescription medications, especially opioids. Also of concern has been the significant increase in the use of sedatives, including barbiturates, among 12th graders since 2001 (NIDA, 2005).

You will benefit from self-awareness and an understanding of the feelings that working with substance abusers can evoke. For example, the nurse who feels angry and punitive with the client who abuses drugs, or who overidentifies with the client and finds adventure in the client's drug stories, cannot establish a therapeutic relationship with the client. Feelings of disdain or envy can compromise nursing care and, indeed, may make the client's treatment ineffective. Only by viewing substance abuse as a symptom of a broader illness can you be effective in dealing with adolescents. Nurses who have contact with adolescents, especially in school or community settings, should familiarize themselves with the general effects of various drugs and the first aid treatment for each (see Chapter 15∞).

Interventions are determined to be effective or ineffective by the use of subjective and objective behavioral criteria, as described in the outcome identification section on pages 740–741. These criteria should reflect your individualized plan of care and the goals you and the client agreed on. Only then can you expect to see the merits of your professional interventions and reap the rewards that can come from working with this special population.

Evaluation

Evaluating nursing interventions with adolescent clients can be tricky for numerous reasons:

- The adolescent client may need to test the limit one more time following a nursing intervention to avoid appearing "too compliant" or to "save face" with the group.
- Although it is important to set limits, it is equally important to be flexible. To set a limit and immediately "draw the line" with the next infraction is to invite the client to step over that line to test its seriousness.
- This is a slow process. Quick judgments should not be made if immediate results are not obtained.
- The behaviors that brought the adolescent to psychiatric treatment will continue long after treatment and nursing interventions have begun. Despite a well-designed nursing care plan and client

contract, the adolescent will resort to previous maladaptive ways, immature and impulsive acts, or destructive behaviors in the face of change, particularly if this change represents improvement or growth (such as an increase in privileges or an impending discharge). The nurse who thinks this means that the nursing interventions are not effective may feel hopeless about progress and convey that hopelessness to the client and the rest of the treatment team.

- Using a behavioral contract without understanding the underlying reasons or factors contributing to the adolescent's problems will result in a superficial approach with an equally superficial evaluation.

If the adolescent had the desire or the impulse control simply to "act right" after being given the rules and consequences, then the client would be doing so already, and psychiatric treatment would not have been necessary. The adolescent needs the structure and consistency of a nursing care plan and a client contract without the rigidity that can be imposed by a "now or never" behavioral plan with absolute consequences.

You can make a more adequate evaluation if you are aware of the social context and the meaning of the behavior to the adolescent. For example, you may be wrong in determining that an indicator of increased self-esteem for a female client would be to stop dyeing her hair purple. Dyeing one's hair an unusual color may have been an indication of low self-esteem during your adolescent years, but for the client in question, that may or may not be the case. For that adolescent client and her peer group, purple hair may be a well-defined status symbol.

CASE MANAGEMENT, COMMUNITY-BASED CARE, AND HOME CARE

Psychiatric–mental health nurses who work with adolescents need to be able to function as case managers and to work in community-based and home care settings. The skills required in these roles include:

- Assessing conflicted adolescents and problematic families wherever you encounter them
- Educating faculty, school administrators, and parents about the importance of preventive attention and the resources available to help teens and their families
- Preventing youth violence and drug abuse if possible
- Advocating for home-based therapy models
- Refining skills as an individual, group, and family therapist with adolescents and their families
- Teaching about sensitive health topics such as drug use, STDs, unwanted pregnancy, and the consequences of violence
- Advocating for social policies and programs that help keep families out of poverty, a major risk factor for adolescents

Psychiatric–mental health nurses are most likely to encounter troubled adolescents in community-based settings such as schools, emergency rooms, jails and detention centers, detoxification programs, sexually transmitted disease (STD) clinics, and other outpatient settings that provide programs for angry, abused, neglected, or otherwise troubled teenagers. Psychiatric–mental health nurses may also encounter adolescents who are experiencing a temporary crisis and are in need of support and counseling while in abortion clinics, group homes, homes for young mothers, and drunk-driver programs. The section earlier in this chapter on psychiatric–mental health nursing roles in outpatient settings (pages 726–729) addresses in detail the skills you will need to address these client problems.

The *Healthy People 2010* initiative presents a special opportunity to promote the health, safety, and well-being of adolescents and young adults. Of the 467 objectives, 107 are important to adolescents and young adults (DHHS, 2005). Because of the large number of objectives relevant to this population, 21 Critical Health Objectives were identified. Table 27-1 ■ on page 746 outlines 12 of the most serious health and safety issues for adolescents and young adults, including mortality, unintentional injury, violence, substance use and mental health, reproductive health, and prevention of adult chronic diseases. Nurses in school and community settings are vital to establishing more effective health programs and other policy and programmatic interventions to reduce risk, highlight protective factors, and improve health outcomes among adolescents. The feature What Every Pediatric, Oncology, and Hospice Nurse Should Know addresses the health risks of adolescents.

In response to the *Healthy People 2010* initiative, numerous agencies, professional and research organizations, foundations, and advocacy groups have developed various programs and activities. The National Adolescent Health Information Center (NAHIC), based within the University of

WHAT EVERY PEDIATRIC, ONCOLOGY, AND HOSPICE NURSE SHOULD KNOW

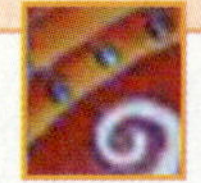

Cancer-Related Deaths Among Adolescents

Approximately 2,300 children and adolescents in the United States die from cancer-related causes each year (Stutzer et al., 2005). Although the numbers are relatively small, each death is "one too many." You will want to familiarize yourself with evidence-based standards for end-of-life care for young clients in order to provide the physical, cognitive, emotional, spiritual, and social strategies to prepare both the client and the family for the process of dying. Tending to the physical symptoms of distress (such as dyspnea, fatigue, and nutritional concerns) will provide you with the opportunity to deal with the psychological and spiritual distress as well.

MediaLink Critical Thinking Exercise: Promoting Mental Health Among Adolescents

TABLE 27-1 ■ **Top 12 of the 21 Critical Health Objectives for Adolescents and Young Adults**

Critical Health Issues	1998–1999 Data	2010 Objective
Reduce deaths of adolescents and young adults (per 100,000)		
10- to 14-year-olds	21.5	16.8
15- to 19-year-olds	69.5	39.8
Reduce deaths caused by motor vehicle crashes (per 100,000)	25.6	*
Reduce deaths and injuries caused by alcohol- and drug-related motor vehicle crashes (per 100,000)	13.5	*
Increase use of safety belts, 9th–12th graders	84%	92%
Reduce the proportion of adolescents who report that they rode, during the previous 30 days, with a driver who had been drinking alcohol	33%	30%
Reduce homicides (per 100,000)		
10- to 14-year-olds	1.2	*
15- to 19-year-olds	10.4	*
Reduce physical fighting among adolescents	36%	32%
Reduce weapon carrying by adolescents on school property, 9th–12th graders	6.9%	4.9%
Reduce the proportion of 12–17-year-olds engaging in binge drinking of alcoholic beverages	7.7%	2%
Reduce past-month use of illicit substances (marijuana) in 12–17-year-olds	8.3%	0.7%
Reduce the suicide rate (per 100,000)		
10- to 14-year-olds	1.2	*
15- to 19-year-olds	8.0	*
Reduce the rate of suicide attempts by adolescents that require medical attention	2.6%	1%

*2010 target not provided for age group.

Source: U.S. Department of Health and Human Services. (2005). *Healthy people 2010*. Retrieved July 18, 2006, from www.health.gov/healthypeople/LHI/lhiwhat.htm.

California, San Francisco, was established with the overall goal of serving as a national resource for adolescent health information. Information can be obtained on topics as diverse as "components of managed care for adolescents" and "the impact of Hurricanes Katrina and Rita on youth" (NAHIC, 2006). Numerous resources and publications are available at the center's website, which can be accessed through the Companion Website for this book.

Of particular interest to psychiatric–mental health nurses who are committed to advocating for troubled and troublesome teens are opportunities to effect change at the state and national level. AACAP has been particularly effective in advocating for youth through postings on its website, also accessible via the Companion Website. During the first annual Society of Professors of Child and Adolescent Psychiatry (SPCAP) Advocacy Day in Washington, DC (April 29, 2006), several important bills were addressed. Specifically, the Child Health Care Crisis Relief Act, H.R. 1106, addressed the critical national shortage of child and adolescent psychiatrists and other mental health professionals, including psychiatric–mental health nurses, by creating education incentives to encourage recruitment (AACAP, 2006). You can peruse details of any bill, including whether your Representative is a cosponsor of the bill, at http://thomas.loc.gov and via the Companion Website. Simply enter the bill number and click on "Bill summary and status." AACAP posts talking points on various bills on its website as well.

With the promise for change that these innovations bring, community health nurses are in a prime position to play a key role in the movement toward proactive partnerships among schools, families, and the community in enhancing the health and ensuring the future of our nation's youth.

MEDIALINK Library of Congress

MEDIALINK NAHIC

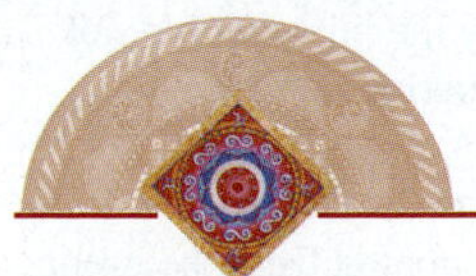

EXPLORE MEDIALINK

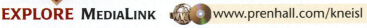

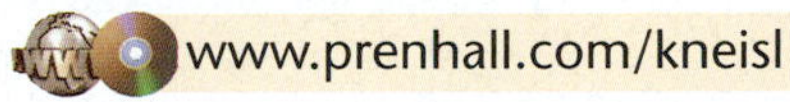

For NCLEX-RN® review questions, case studies, and other resources for this chapter see the Pearson Health MediaLink CD-ROM that accompanies this book and the Companion Website at www.prenhall.com/kneisl.

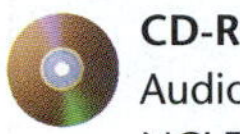

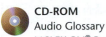

CD-ROM
Audio Glossary
NCLEX-RN® Review Questions

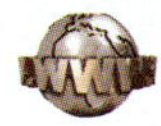

Companion Website
Audio Glossary
NCLEX-RN® Review Questions
Critical Thinking Exercise
- *Promoting Mental Health Among Adolescents*

Case Study
- *Assessing the Resistant Client*

Care Plan
- *Risk for Violence and Self-Mutilation*

MediaLinks
MediaLink Application
- *Assessing Exposure to Psychological Trauma and Post-traumatic Stress in the Juvenile Justice Population*

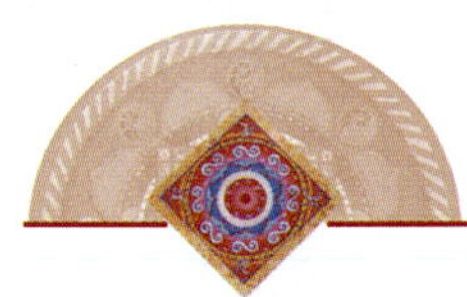

NCLEX-RN® REVIEW QUESTIONS

1. The relationship between adolescent obesity and biochemical and neuronal systems is important because it:
1. Identifies the underlying psychological causes of obesity.
2. Provides guidelines for treatment providers in developing behavior modification programs for obese adolescents.
3. Explains the biochemical and physiological causes of obesity.
4. Reinforces the need for the obese adolescent to consume fewer calories.

2. Which of the following should be included in the assessment of an adolescent's mental health and related behaviors? (Select all that apply.)
1. Hormonal changes
2. Chronic illnesses
3. Immune function
4. Growth spurts
5. Health insurance coverage

3. In planning care for the adolescent with behavioral problems, which of the following would not be incorporated into the treatment planning process?
1. The client's strengths and weaknesses
2. The client's goals for retirement
3. The client's developmental stage
4. The underlying meaning of the behavior or problem

4. Which of the following actions by the community health nurse would increase the nurse's visibility within the school environment?
1. Establish a separate and distinct clinic to provide treatment to school-age children with mental health problems.
2. Request a meeting with the school administrators to develop strategies to improve faculty awareness of mental health problems in children.
3. Actively participate in curriculum development within the school.
4. Work with those faculty members who have mental health issues.

5. An adolescent is acting out on the inpatient unit. An appropriate intervention by the staff nurse would include:
1. Ignoring the behavior.
2. Confronting the behavior
3. Restricting the adolescent's privileges on the unit.
4. Identifying an effective way to resolve the problem.

6. An appropriate nursing intervention for a client who is verbally aggressive toward staff and other clients would include:
1. Ignoring the behavior.
2. Role-modeling socially acceptable behaviors.
3. Letting your anger show when you inform the client that the verbal aggression will not be tolerated under any circumstances.
4. Requesting a PRN order for a sedative for the client.

7. Which of the following statements would not be included in a written contract with an adolescent client on an inpatient mental health unit?
   1. "I will not accept phone calls from my family while in the treatment program."
   2. "I will not accept phone calls from my drug friends while in the treatment program."
   3. "If I feel like hurting myself, I will notify the staff immediately."
   4. "I will abide by the unit's behavior conduct code or I will have my free time privileges revoked."

8. A client says to the nurse, "Hey, you dumb blonde, what are you looking at?" Which of the following responses would be inappropriate for the nurse to make?
   1. "Don't you ever speak to me like that again."
   2. "What's this all about?"
   3. Initially ignore the behavior and speak with the client after the client calms down.
   4. "I don't understand where that comment came from."

9. Which of the following interventions by the nurse would not be appropriate when addressing scapegoating behaviors on a mental health unit?
   1. Set limits on the behaviors.
   2. Rescue the client who is being scapegoated from the group.
   3. Ask the group to focus on their behaviors and feelings prior to the scapegoating.
   4. Anticipate the behavior and try to circumvent the process.

10. Which of the following behaviors by the nurse would be nontherapeutic when working with adolescent clients?
    1. Provide honest feedback to the adolescent.
    2. Accept and support all behaviors exhibited by clients without question.
    3. Acknowledge feelings of anger precipitated by a client's behaviors.
    4. Set limits on unacceptable client behaviors.

See Appendix C for answers.

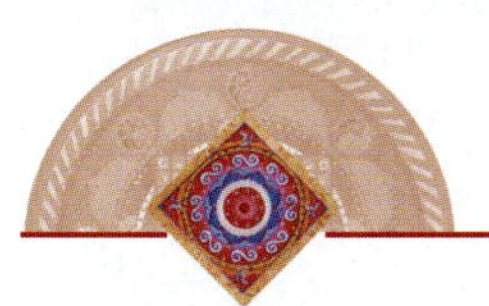

REFERENCES

American Academy of Child and Adolescent Psychiatry. (2004). *Facts for families: Children and firearms*. Retrieved July 18, 2006, from http://www.aacap.org/cs/root/facts_for_families/facts_for_families.

American Academy of Child and Adolescent Psychiatry. (2005). *Gay, lesbian and bisexual adolescents*. Retrieved July 12, 2006, from http://www.aacap.org/.

American Academy of Child and Adolescent Psychiatry. (2006). Legislative Action 109th Congress. Retrieved July 18, 2006, from http://aacap.browsermedia.com/.

American Psychiatric Association. (2000). *Diagnostic and statistical manual of mental disorders* (4th ed., Text Revision) (DSM-IV-TR). Washington, DC: Author.

Boggs, W. (2006). *Obesity linked to cardiac abnormalities in adolescents*. Retrieved July 17, 2006, from http://www.nursingconsult.com.

Brunner, R., Parzer, P., Haffner, J., Steen, R., Roos, J., Klett, M., et al. (2007). Prevalence and psychological correlates of occasional and repetitive deliberate self-harm in adolescents. *Archives of Pediatric and Adolescent Medicine, 161*(7), 641–649.

Centers for Disease Control and Prevention. (2006). *Public use data file and documentation: Multiple causes of death for ICD-10 2003 data*. Retrieved July 18, 2006, from http://www.cdc.gov/nchs/about/major/dvs/icd10des.htm.

Davis, T. K. (2005). Beyond the physical examination: The nurse practitioner's role in adolescent risk reduction and resiliency building in a school-based health center. *Nursing Clinics of North America, 40*(4), 649–660, viii.

Eaton, D. K., Kann, L., Kinchen, S., Ross, J., Hawkins, J., Harris, W. A., et al. (2006). *Youth risk behavior surveillance—United States, 2005*. Retrieved July 18, 2006, from http://www.cdc.gov/mmwr/preview/mmwrhtml/ss5505a1.htm.

Herrman, J. W. (2006). Position statement on the role of the pediatric nurse working with sexually active teens, pregnant adolescents, and young parents. *Journal of Pediatric Nursing, 21*(3), 250–252.

Leibowitz, S. F. (2006). *Laboratory of behavioral neuroscience*. Retrieved July 20, 2006, from http://www.rockefeller.edu/labheads/leibowitz/.

Latner, J. D., Stunkard, A. J., & Wilson, G. T. (2005). Stigmatized students: Age, sex, and ethnicity effects in the stigmatization of obesity. *Obesity Research, 13*, 1226–1231.

Martyn, K. K. (2006). Improving adolescent sexual risk assessment with event history calendars: A feasibility study. *Journal of Pediatric Health Care, 20*(2), 19–26.

National Adolescent Health Information Center. (2006). *National initiative to improve adolescent health*. Retrieved July 18, 2006, from http://nahic.ucsf.edu/index.php/partner_resources/publications.

National Center for Injury Prevention and Control. (2006). *Suicide: Fact sheet*. Retrieved July 18, 2006, from http://www.cdc.gov/ncipc/factsheets/suifacts.htm.

National Institute on Drug Abuse. (2005). *2005 Monitoring the Future Study shows continued decline in drug use by students*. NIDA News Release. Retrieved July 18, 2006, from http://www.drugabuse.gov/newsroom/.

Owens, T. M. (2006). Bariatric surgery risks, benefits, and care of the morbidly obese. *Nursing Clinics of North America, 41*(2). Retrieved July 10, 2006, from http://www.nursingconsult.com.

Schapiro, N. A. (2005). Bipolar disorders in children and adolescents. *Journal of Pediatric Health Care, 19*(3), 131–141.

Stutzer, C. A., Drew, D., Himelsein, B. P., Hinds, P. S., LaFond, D. A., Nuss, S. L., et al. (2005). Consensus statement: Collaborative clinical research on end-of-life care in pediatric oncology. *Seminars in Oncology Nursing, 21*(2). Retrieved July 10, 2006, from http://www.nursingconsult.com.

Tusaie, K. R., & Patterson, K. (2006). Relationships among trait, situational, and comparative optimism: Clarifying concepts for a theoretically consistent and evidence-based intervention to maximize resilience. *Archives of Psychiatric Nursing, 20*(3), 144–150.

U.S. Department of Health and Human Services. (2005). *Healthy people 2010*. Retrieved July 18, 2006, from http://www.health.gov/healthypeople/LHI/lhiwhat.htm.

Whitlock, J., & Knox, K. L. (2007). The relationship between self-injurious behavior and suicide in a young adult population. *Archives of Pediatric and Adolescent Medicine, 161*(7), 634–640.

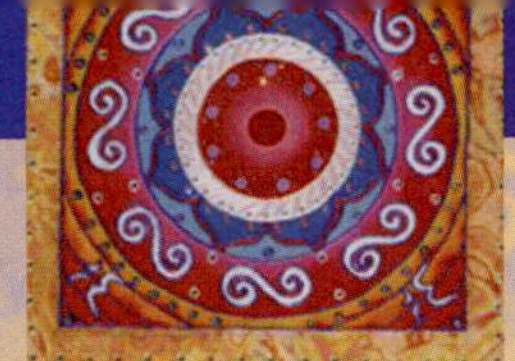

Elders

CHAPTER

28

EILEEN TRIGOBOFF

LEARNING OUTCOMES

After completing this chapter, you will be able to:

1. Identify the age-related demographic projections that have implications for planning future mental health services for elders.
2. Discuss the major theories of aging and the ideas associated with each one.
3. Differentiate the normal physical and psychosocial changes that accompany aging from mental disorders affecting elders.
4. Synthesize the key components of a biopsychosocial assessment into the plan of care for an older client.
5. Provide reminiscence therapy, life review, reality orientation, and socialization enhancement for elders.
6. Incorporate available community support programs such as adult day care, restorative programs, and assisted living for elders and their families into your plan of care.
7. Analyze personal biases, feelings, and attitudes that may be experienced in professional practice when caring for elders who suffer from mental disorders.

KEY TERMS

geropsychiatry *750*
life review *765*
palliative care *758*
psychogerontology *750*
reality orientation *765*
reminiscence therapy *765*
remotivation therapy *766*
resocialization groups *766*
respite *768*
restorative care *768*

CRITICAL THINKING CHALLENGE

A recently retired 65-year-old man is brought to your clinic by his wife, who states he "just sits around all day watching TV and won't do anything." She tells you that he had a very active career and loved it. He also played golf or spent time in his garden on the weekends. She reveals that he has changed considerably now in that he seems unable to concentrate and has become bitter and difficult. Upon interviewing the client, you find that he had been a successful owner of a small hardware store with his younger brother, who recently died of a heart attack while working at the store. Your client retired from the business soon thereafter at his family's insistence. He goes on to tell you that his memory is impaired, he has difficulty sleeping, and he has lost his robust appetite. You would like to gather further data, including assessing his grieving skills (for his younger brother, for his career, for confidence in his own longevity), and assessing for depression and dementia.

1. What areas of his functioning and interactions with others would be important to assess?
2. How would you determine whether physical problems contribute to his symptoms?

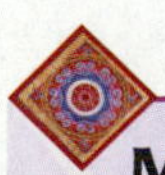

MEDIALINK 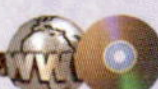 www.prenhall.com/kneisl

Go to the Pearson Health MediaLink CD-ROM and the Companion Website at www.prenhall.com/kneisl for interactive resources for this chapter.

The population of American elders is growing faster than the nation as a whole. In 2000, the U.S. Census Bureau reported that by the year 2050, 21% of the population will be age 65 and older. The over-65 population exceeded 35 million (or more than 12% of the U.S. population) in 2000. The U.S. Census Bureau predicts that by the year 2030, the number will be 71 million. The rest of the world experienced a similar population explosion in the over-65 age group. According to the Census Bureau's (2000) estimate for the world population, by the year 2050 the numbers of those over 85 years of age will continue to increase dramatically, especially in the United States, China, and India.

With this booming section of the population, the term "elderly" or even "geriatric"—meaning those over the age of 65—is insufficient to discuss a group of people whose ages may span four decades. The descriptive terms used to specifically group elders into relevant age categories include *young-old* (65 to 74), *middle-old* (75 to 84), and *old-old* (85 and older).

As a consequence of improved pharmacologic and other treatments, individuals affected by dementia and mood disorders (once associated with decreased longevity) will experience a relatively normal life span. An unprecedented growth in the number of elders with chronic mental illness will have a significant impact on the need for quality geropsychiatric care. **Geropsychiatry** is the treatment of psychiatric problems in older adults. At the same time, family caregivers, who themselves are aging, will also strain geropsychiatric care resources.

It is important to examine the age distribution of the over-65 population carefully. Grouping elders into an aggregate of all persons over the age of 65 tends to blur important distinctions. The old-old group tends to have the greatest incidences of depression, delirium, dementia, and other chronic disabling conditions. Of this group, 49% have some limitation in their ability to perform activities of daily living (Kondo et al., 2007; Miller & Reynolds, 2007). The frail older adults who consume many health care resources and maintenance services constitute only 5% of the over-65 population. A large proportion of healthy older people, particularly single older women (who outnumber single older men by 2.5 to 1), will benefit most from supportive psychosocial services often provided by psychiatric–mental health nurses.

Anticipating the varied mental health needs of a growing population of aging "baby boomers" is important for program planning and funding allocation. The data clearly underscore a need for an increased number of health professionals who recognize that older adults have multiple needs. Nursing's role in psychogerontology and in geriatrics is expanding as the needs and real numbers of elders increase (Crewe, 2007; Dyck, Culp, & Cacchione, 2007; Gum, Arean, & Bostrom, 2007). **Psychogerontology** is a subspecialty within gerontology that studies the psychosocial needs of elders.

The aim of this chapter is to provide a comprehensive discussion of health promotion and advocacy for elders with mental health needs. Contemporary issues including end-of-life care, restorative programs, and community-based support are also addressed. We do not discuss the nursing care of elders with cognitive disorders in this chapter. Refer to Chapter 14 ∞ for nursing care strategies for cognitively impaired elders.

ROADBLOCKS TO MENTAL HEALTH SERVICES FOR ELDERS

Elders are the most underserved population in need of supportive and tertiary mental health care. This discussion highlights four roadblocks to mental health care services—ageism, myths, stigma, and health care financing—and examines the demographic realities that compel us to break through these disabling roadblocks through self-awareness, health promotion, and client advocacy (see Figure 28-1 ■).

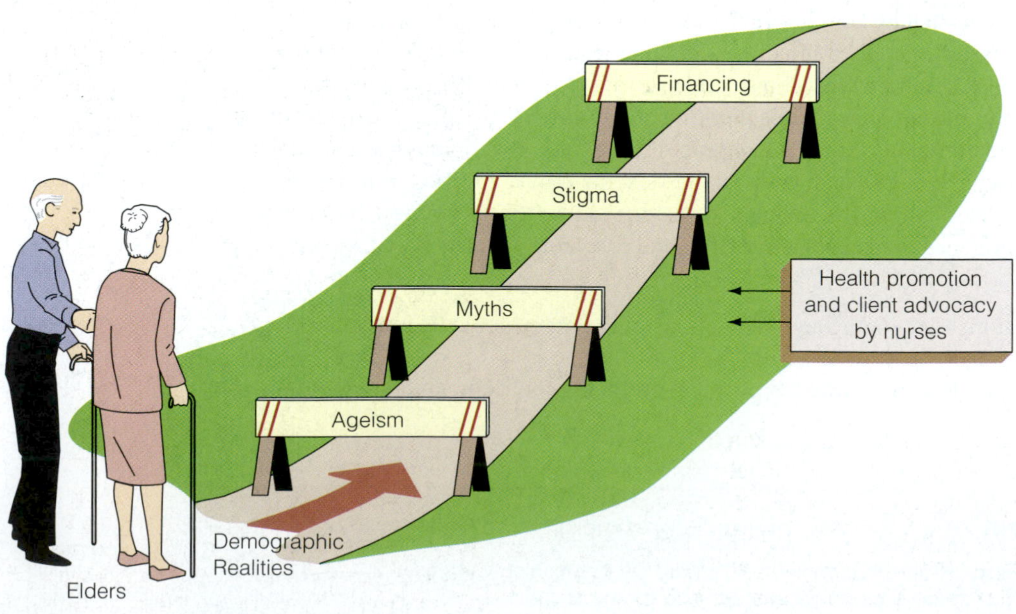

Figure 28-1 ■ Roadblocks to mental health services for elders.

YOUR SELF-AWARENESS
Attitudes Toward Aging

A bias against elders because of their age can result in discrimination against them even by mental health professionals. Ask yourself the following questions and discuss your responses with other students, faculty, or colleagues.

1. Am I uncomfortable around people who are old, infirm, or confused?
2. Do I have positive role models for aging with grace?
3. Do I dread growing old myself?
4. Should elders be encouraged to do as much as possible for themselves or be cared for by others?
5. How do I feel about old people who are sexually active and insist on trying to look and act young?
6. Do most elders become rigid and set in their ways once they age?
7. Am I well informed about the differences between mental disorder in elders and the normal aging process?
8. Do I equate advanced age with unattractiveness, incompetence, and senility?
9. Am I well informed about community resources and support systems available for elders and their family caregivers?
10. How do I feel when caring for an elderly person who is demanding and dependent?

Reflection on such questions can promote your beginning awareness of any attitudes that might interfere with quality care for elders.

Ageism

A primary roadblock to adequate mental health services for elders is ageism—prejudice against people because they are old. In many contemporary Western cultures, aging is often viewed with disdain, dislike, and trepidation. Elders are criticized for being unattractive, incompetent, socially irrelevant, and unhealthy. Thompson (2007) states that ageism, by marginalizing and dehumanizing older people, has the potential to undermine selfhood and self-worth. Ageism stems from the belief that elders present a financial and emotional drain on the family and society. Ageism results from our fears of facing our own aging process and mortality. Ageist attitudes can be internalized by elders, causing decreased self-worth and self-esteem, whatever the source.

When caring for older clients, be aware of their feelings and your own. Your personal biases can influence your clinical assessment and your decisions about interventions. You can provide invaluable support, insight, and feedback to colleagues who are working with older adults. Consider using the Your Self-Awareness feature as a discussion point. We know that elders are as responsive to mental health services as are members of any other age group. By modeling positive attitudes toward aging and by advocating quality of life and health care for elders in all settings and at all levels of function, you can help dispel ageist influences. See Figure 28-2 ■ for a photograph of an elder and the supportive, candid, and loving comments her family made about her.

Myths

Mental health care professionals and elders themselves often equate growing old with growing sad, lonely, disengaged, inactive, socially isolated, and dependent. Such myths all too often inhibit people from seeking treatment for feelings and behaviors that they believe are a normal part of aging. Misled by these myths, health professionals can be less inclined to refer elders for mental health services. We know that advancing age does not condemn an individual to senility, social isolation, loneliness, or dependence. Most elders live independently and contentedly—well into late life—unless they can no longer drive and live alone, live in rural areas without transportation, or live in urban areas with limited access to health care resources.

Psychiatric–mental health nurses can serve as elder advocates by educating the public, other health care professionals, and elders and their families about the differences between

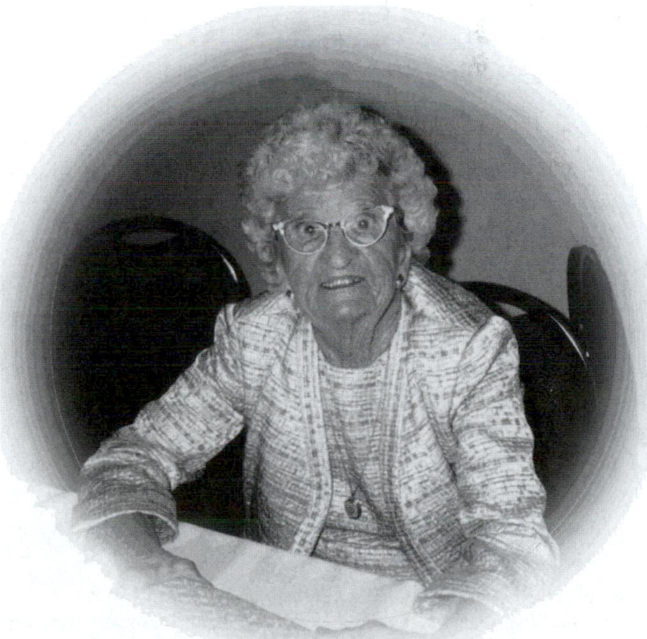

Figure 28-2 ■ In the eyes of her family and friends, this was a woman worthy of respect and admiration. She was "strong-willed" and "the epitome of aging with style and grace." "She had a sense of humor, kept moving, spent 80 years living a full life rather than 50 years preparing to die, and enjoyed it to the last." "She was her own person, no matter what."

normal aging and changes associated with pathologic conditions (Ito, Takahashi, & Liehr, 2007; Roriz-Cruz et al., 2007). Recognizing that aging itself is not a problem increases the likelihood that problems that do arise will be assessed and appropriately treated.

Stigma

MediaLink National Alliance on Mental Illness

Despite recent advances in mental health care, the stigma associated with mental illness remains very real to elderly people. Elders may not seek mental health services as readily as they should and may hide their psychic pain for fear of being labeled "crazy" or losing control and being institutionalized.

Nurses have the opportunity to educate the public about mental disorders and state-of-the-art treatments that are available to all age groups. In so doing, we can help to decrease the stigma associated with psychiatric illness and treatment. The National Alliance on Mental Illness (NAMI) has made important advances in this direction by circulating information about the biological basis for many psychiatric disorders. You can refer elders who feel reluctant about acknowledging a psychiatric problem to the NAMI website at http://www.nami.org, which can be accessed through a resource link on the Companion Website for this text.

As people learn more about research that confirms brain mechanisms associated with psychiatric disorders, traditional stigma associated with seeking mental health services is likely to decrease. At the present time, however, the primary care provider for many mentally ill elders is their family physician or adult nurse practitioner.

Elders are seen by their general health care providers, surgeons, specialists for chronic illnesses such as arthritis or diabetes, and in clinics where they receive medications and have laboratory tests evaluated on a regular basis. Because of the likelihood that they will need specialized care, nurses specializing in a variety of settings need specific information about elders. The feature What Every Rehabilitation Nurse Should Know has information that is useful for nurses in rehabilitation services.

Health Care Financing

Financial barriers, physical disability, and transportation problems are some factors that limit access to services, especially elders diagnosed with mental disorders. The financial barriers are particularly serious. Medicare, the major form of health care financing for elders, covers only a portion of the costs for its beneficiaries. Long-term care coverage and coverage for chronic conditions are sorely lacking.

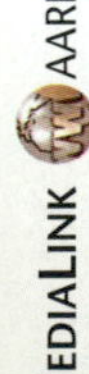

Medicare initiated its Part D program to address the costs of pharmaceutical management of health care problems. Expensive prescription medication plans and large copayments for services reimbursed through Medicare add to an older person's psychosocial stressors. Although Medicare Part D provides options for elders in an effort to minimize costs and maximize treatment adherence, the program is difficult to understand. Working through the many options can be daunting, and high costs are still very likely.

WHAT EVERY REHABILITATION NURSE SHOULD KNOW

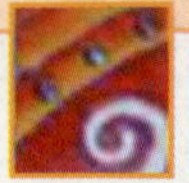

Psychological Symptoms an Elder May Exhibit

A rehabilitation nurse needs to be familiar with the likely symptoms that people over the age of 65 years may exhibit when placed in rehabilitation centers. The reason for the placement—post-stroke care, joint replacement, respite for family members, recovery from a fall—can direct you to anticipate what is likely to occur emotionally with the individual. Each of these events carries meaning for an elder that would not apply to someone younger. Stress, staying in an unfamiliar environment, and struggling to adapt to body and emotional changes take a larger toll on older adults. There are three reasons why rehabilitation nurses should be familiar with these symptoms:

1. These symptoms could be part of an emotional response requiring treatment.
2. The presence of symptoms can distort or mask the presentation of symptoms of physical illnesses.
3. Severe psychiatric distress can impair healing from medical and surgical procedures and injuries.

When a rehabilitation client has symptoms that appear to be behavioral or psychiatric, be prepared and able to document, classify, and report these symptoms correctly so that the client receives necessary treatment. Knowing the proper interventions, pharmacologic and nonpharmacologic, can speed stabilization and improve the quality of life your clients experience.

Community and home-based care for elders is limited at best, and Medicare does not cover many mental health services at all. Few practitioners across the nation specialize in ongoing psychotherapy for the elderly. As baby boomers reach old age and require long-term care services, these gaps and lack of coverage will reach crisis levels unless service needs are addressed and resolved. For the mentally ill elders, the crisis is even more acute as long-term care facilities selectively admit identified geropsychiatric clients. It is important for us to become active voices in lobbying for policy changes to improve financing for elder care that covers the broad range of acute and chronic illnesses. The American Association of Retired Persons (AARP) is an excellent source of information related to these topics. The AARP website, http://www.aarp.org, can be found through a resource link on the Companion Website for this text.

BIOPSYCHOSOCIAL THEORIES OF AGING

Distinguishing between changes associated with aging and mental disorder in later life is a challenge. Many variables affect mental health as a person ages. Not all theories identified here have been fully confirmed through systematic research, and some, such as the disengagement theory, remain controversial.

Biologic Theories

Biologic theories of aging include genetic, wear-and-tear, immunology, nutritional, and environmental theories.

Genetic Theory

Throughout the Human Genome Project (initiated in 1990) of the Department of Energy and the National Institutes of Health, which aimed to map and sequence the human genome in its entirety, definitions of health, illness, and healthy aging have been transformed by knowledge of genetics (Blazer, 2007). According to genetic theories, aging is a process that operates over time to alter cellular structures. Harmful genes activate in late life to stop cell growth and division. This theory supports the idea that the life span is predetermined and people's aging experience is programmed by their genetic makeup. The website of the National Coalition for Health Professional Education in Genetics (http://www.nchpeg.org), initiated by the American Nurses Association, the American Medical Association, and the National Human Genome Research Institute, can be accessed through this text's Companion Website.

MEDIALINK National Coalition for Health Professional Education in Genetics

Wear-and-Tear Theory

The wear-and-tear theory proposes that the accumulation of waste products from metabolism damages DNA synthesis, leading eventually to organ malfunction (Muravchick, 2003). In short, cells wear out. Even though the theory allows for individual rates of cell decline that can be accelerated from abuse and slowed by care, the emphasis is one of loss and decline in later life.

Immunology Theory

The immunology theory explains age-related decline in the immune system. As a person ages, his or her ability to defend against foreign organisms declines, with a corresponding increase in susceptibility to diseases, including cancer and serious infections. Theorists suggest that the changes that take place with aging allow the body to misidentify old, irregular cells as foreign bodies and the body then attacks these cells (Crighton & Puppione, 2006). Multiple neurochemical and viral theories are being developed as cellular research advances. For example, free radical theory posits that free radicals cause the damage to cell membranes as one ages.

Nutritional Theory

Nutritional theory focuses on the idea that diet affects how one ages (Cappellano, 2007; Glowacki, 2007). The quality of one's diet (amounts of Vitamin D, fresh fruits and vegetables especially) is as important as the quantity because vitamin and nutrient deficiencies or excesses have an influence on disease processes. How an older body metabolizes nutrients is also a theoretical issue. For example, there may be more than enough Vitamin D in a meal, but if an elder cannot fully metabolize it, calculations of the actual amount of Vitamin D that are bioavailable to that individual would need to be revised.

Environmental Theory

A number of environmental factors are known to threaten health and may be associated with aging. The ingestion of lead, arsenic, pesticides, and other substances can seriously harm the body, as can smoking, exposure to secondhand smoke, and air pollution. Environmental factors such as crowded living conditions and high levels of noise are known to be stressful and to drain a person's coping capacity. An elder's primary activities can also be an indication of health status or a threat to health; for example, sedentary TV watching contributes to metabolic syndrome in elders (Gao, Nelson, & Tucker, 2007). All these factors can affect one's vulnerability or vigor while aging.

Psychosocial Theories

Psychosocial theories of aging include the activity and disengagement theories, which contrast sharply with each other.

Activity Theory

The activity theory proposes that the way to age successfully is to stay active and involved. Exercise and social interaction are believed to contribute to mental health and satisfaction in late life. Consequently, elders are encouraged to remain as active as possible for as long as possible (Signorile et al., 2007). A number of consumer products, including computer and card-based activities, have been developed to encourage motor activity and mental activity contributing to successful aging. The Evidence-Based Practice feature on page 754 includes culturally competent activities. Elders in assisted living facilities benefit from the newer video games—especially bowling, tennis, and interactive World War II games. They are often inspired by video documentaries of elders surfing in Hawaii, ballroom dancing, and traveling in elder hostel groups.

Disengagement Theory

Disengagement theory is quite the opposite of activity theory. First proposed in the 1960s, the disengagement theory described what was considered an inevitable process in which elders willingly withdrew from social contact and responsibilities, relieved to turn matters over to the younger generation (Bergstom & Holmes, 2000). This theory has become controversial because many older adults continue to be engaged and responsible well into later life unless limited by immobility, which can lead to involuntary social isolation. Recent research discusses the negative impact of apathy on elder health and wellness (Onyike et al., 2007) and emphasizes the need for continued mental activity in order to sustain health throughout the life span. See the section on restorative care later in this chapter.

PSYCHIATRIC DISORDERS IN ELDERS

Ageist attitudes in our culture account for some of the misconceptions about the prevalence of mental disorders among elders. Older people are believed to be more prone to mental illness than are young people. For several reasons, however, it is difficult to obtain exact incidence and prevalence rates for mental disorders in later life. Elders are often difficult to reach

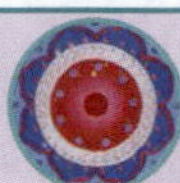

EVIDENCE-BASED PRACTICE

CULTURALLY COMPETENT AND FAMILY-FOCUSED ELDER CARE

Doris is 72 years old and attends a geriatric care program during the day. Her family is very close to her and is concerned that Doris, a member of an ethnic minority, may not receive culturally competent care.

The program Doris is involved in is a family-centered program in which family members and clients are recognized as active members of the health care team. In order to practice these ideals thoroughly, the geriatric day program is culturally sensitive and sophisticated. The client's cultural background, beliefs, and values are incorporated into the treatment plan. Nursing staff are trained to be more culturally competent. The training focuses on multiethnic values, Eastern and Western medicine and activities, culturally sensitive geriatric assessment, and health care interventions that are relevant for this population. Action should be based on more than one study, but for this training program the following research evidence was helpful.

Salman, A., McCabe, D., Easter, T., Callahan, B., Goldstein, D., Smith, T. D., et al. (2007). Cultural competence among staff nurses who participated in a family-centered geriatric care program. *Journal for Nurses in Staff Development, 23*(3), 103–111.

CRITICAL THINKING APPLICATION

1. Describe what other evidence you would need to review before designing an intervention for Doris.
2. Why is specific training needed to help nurses become culturally aware?
3. Are the family's concerns valid?

with community-wide surveys, they are reluctant to respond to personal questions that deal with emotional problems, and most either do not seek treatment for emotional problems or consult primary care providers rather than psychiatric professionals.

The need for psychiatric–mental health nursing among this population has been supported by research and by clinical observation (Moyle & Evans, 2007). When physical deterioration becomes a significant feature of an elder's life, the risk of comorbid psychiatric illness rises. Social isolation and financial burdens are additional common difficulties elders experience. The sequelae of these social and physical pressures can evolve into symptoms of a psychiatric nature, to the extent that psychiatric diagnoses are not unusual. Results of lifetime prevalence and longitudinal studies (Blow, Serras, & Barry, 2007; Hudson, Hiripi, Pope, & Kessler, 2007; Moyle & Evans, 2007) indicate that psychiatric disorders including eating disorders, depressive symptoms, and psychosocial stress are public health concerns.

Symptoms of mental illness in the older population often differ from those in other age groups. While the DSM-IV-TR (American Psychiatric Association [APA], 2000) has enhanced our ability to make valid and reliable diagnoses of mental disorders, there are few age-specific categories. Thus, despite the DSM-IV-TR's extensive, detailed descriptions of each problem category, clinicians and researchers continue to have difficulty applying the written descriptions of symptoms to older adults.

MEDIALINK Application: Depression in the Elderly

Mood Disorders

Mood disorders are primarily characterized by disturbed affect or emotional experience. When they occur in elders they may present as:

- Sustained elation and hyperactivity, such as in a manic episode
- Changes from elation to depression, such as in bipolar disorder
- Pervasive depressed mood not accompanied by mania, such as in major depression

Depression is the most preventable and most treatable mental disorder in later life (Gum et al., 2007; Miller & Reynolds, 2007).

Depression in Elders

Depression among elders is widespread in general practice and even higher in hospitals and nursing homes. Depression robs the person of later-life satisfaction, inhibits ego integrity, and may substantially decrease life expectancy. Elders have the highest rate of suicide of any age group and a range of physical disturbances intensified by depression (Chan, Lyness, & Conwell, 2007; Chiriboga, Jang, Banks, & Kim, 2007).

Although the signs and symptoms of depression are relatively consistent throughout the life span, certain characteristics of depression are particular to elders. It is crucial for clinicians to remember that depression in older adults that responds well to treatment may appear with cognitive changes similar to those that accompany other organically based, irreversible disorders. Loss of executive function (often a diagnostic clue to dementia) includes disturbances in planning, sequencing, organizing, and abstracting. Such cognitive impairment can also be a sign of depression.

In addition to cognitive changes, another sign of depression in older adults is an excessive preoccupation with physical symptoms known as *somatization*. Expressing discomfort through the body may be more familiar and comfortable than recognizing and describing psychic pain. Such is the case in the following example.

CLINICAL EXAMPLE

Mr. Gambino, a 79-year-old widower, came to his physician's office complaining of "not feeling well." After a physical examination, the doctor told Mr. Gambino that he had a weight loss of 10 pounds, mild chronic obstructive pulmonary disease (COPD), and slight hypertension, but was otherwise in good health for his age. Mr. Gambino responded angrily, "I know I'm dying but it doesn't matter because I have nothing to live for now that my wife is dead. She's been gone for 6 months and everyone says I should be feeling better, but I feel worse! I can't eat, can't sleep, and I don't have enough energy to even wash my car!" Mr. Gambino says he is tired all day but cannot sleep at night. "I'm up at 3:00 A.M. and can't go back to sleep." He says he tries to eat but does not cook well and "the food just doesn't taste right."

Clearly, Mr. Gambino has a number of physical complaints that may shift the focus away from distressing emotions to more acceptable medical conditions that are less stigmatizing. Other possible somatic signs of depression to watch for include:

- Chronic constipation
- Muscular pain
- Chest tightness
- Headaches
- Difficulty breathing
- Chronic gastrointestinal upset

It is important to be persistent and perceptive in looking for signs of depression. Depressed, apathetic elders may believe they are supposed to feel blue and "down in the dumps" as they age. We need to educate them and their families about depression as a pathologic condition often caused by biochemical imbalances that can be corrected. Interventions for depression in older adults should be instituted as aggressively and comprehensively as they are with any other age group.

Depressive symptoms may also result from social and economic circumstances such as social isolation and neglect. They may be the result of an acute or chronic medical condition such as a stroke, Parkinson's disease, or even a hip fracture. Consequently, it is imperative to include a comprehensive geriatric assessment of elders before beginning a treatment regimen. An older person's response to traumatic events may be tied to functional disability and requires multiple areas of intervention.

Suicide Among Elders

Data from nearly all industrialized countries report that suicide rates rise progressively with age. The highest rates occur in men age 75 and older (Baker, 2007). Compared with the general population, suicide attempts are more lethal and approached with a greater degree of premeditation and planning when made by elders. Older adults who are at greater suicide risk include:

- Men
- Widowed or divorced people
- Caucasians
- Those of lower socioeconomic status
- Those with chronic pain and terminal illness
- Alcoholics
- Those with mental disorders
- Those with neurologic deficits due to stroke and brain injury
- Those who fear becoming a burden

Suicidal elders have been known to seek help in the emergency room, often for a vague nonspecific physical problem, prior to their self-destructive act. Accurate assessment of suicide potential requires active listening and direct questioning (Piechniczekbuczek, 2007). A suicidal older client needs to be assessed when any of the following are present:

- Verbal cues (I'm going to end it all; life is not worth living; I won't be around much longer; I won't be here for the next holiday)
- Behavioral cues (completing a will, making funeral plans, acting out, withdrawing, somatic complaints)
- Situational cues (a recent move, loss of a loved one, the diagnosis of a terminal illness)

For detailed information on suicide and the assessment of suicide potential, including a lethality assessment, see Chapter 23.

Schizophrenia

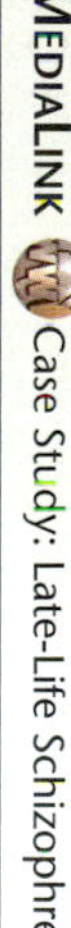

The number and proportion of older adults with schizophrenia will increase considerably with the movement of baby boomers into this population group over the next 30 years. This generation of people with chronic mental illness has not spent years in institutions as the mentally ill elders of past generations did. There is limited research on late-life schizophrenia and less on its treatment. This population of clients poses a particularly critical issue—85% of older individuals with schizophrenia live in the community and are approaching the age when long-term care may become necessary. At the same time, nursing homes are severely restricting admission of psychiatric clients.

An individual with *late-life schizophrenia* may be a psychotic person who has grown old or may be a person who did not experience psychotic symptoms until late in life. People with late-onset schizophrenia are often women with less severe negative symptoms, better premorbid functioning in early adulthood, and less impairment in the areas of learning, abstraction, and cognitive flexibility. They also require smaller doses of neuroleptic medication to manage their psychotic symptoms.

Adjustment Disorders

Elders often experience dramatic life changes because of losses due to death, relocation, dependence, loss of autonomy, retirement, illness, and financial stress. One or a combination of life changes and losses may contribute to the development of an *adjustment disorder*. The essential feature of adjustment disorders is a maladaptive reaction to an identifiable psychosocial stressor or stressors that occurs within 3 months after the onset of the stressor and has persisted for no longer than 6 months (APA, 2000). People experiencing adjustment disorders may have a variety of psychiatric symptoms, including:

- Anxious mood
- Depressed mood
- Mixed emotional features
- Physical complaints
- Withdrawal

Talk therapies can be enormously successful in the treatment of persons with adjustment disorders.

Anxiety Disorders

Anxiety is common across age groups and increases in frequency with advancing age (Ito et al., 2007). Adjustments to physical, emotional, and socioeconomic changes add to the variety of causes for anxiety. Anxiety reactions in the aging individual may manifest themselves as somatic complaints, rigid thinking and behavior, insomnia, fatigue, hostility, restlessness, confusion, and increased dependence. Physiologic indicators of anxiety include increased blood pressure, pulse, respirations, psychomotor restlessness, and frequent voiding. Many of these manifestations are present in the following clinical example.

CLINICAL EXAMPLE

Mrs. Pyun, age 82, was rushed to the emergency room by her bridge group with what they think might be a heart attack. She is short of breath and sweating, her pulse is rapid, her hands are shaking, and she cannot sit still during the assessment. She is tearful and cannot tell the triage nurse what is wrong. Mrs. Pyun says, "I don't know why I feel this way. I just know something bad is going to happen. I have to leave and get home. Why are you asking me all these questions? No, I don't have chest pain. I tried to tell them I was just nervous. I get this way sometimes."

Unfortunately, anxiety disorders and panic attacks are often overlooked in older clients because, as with depression, these clients have a predominance of physical complaints that mask the underlying disorder. In addition, anxiety in older people often co-occurs with depression. The anxiety is treated but the depression persists, leading to a cycle of anxiety–depression and physical illness.

Delusional Disorders

Delusions in elders are considered a cognitive mechanism for maintaining a sense of power and control. The delusions may be comforting ("I know I'm being guarded by an angel from God") or threatening ("The UPS driver has reported me to Homeland Security because he thinks I am a terrorist"), but whatever the content, they customarily form a structure for understanding a situation that otherwise seems unmanageable. Delusions may also result from internalized ageist attitudes, sensory losses (particularly hearing impairment), and social isolation, as in the following clinical example.

CLINICAL EXAMPLE

Ms. Colgán is an 88-year-old woman living alone in a rural suburb of Calgary, Canada. Her cottage is on a country road with few neighbors nearby, and the long winters have kept her indoors and isolated. A sister who has financial power of attorney pays her bills, and she primarily eats canned soups that she heats herself. Ms. Colgán rarely wears her hearing aids and spends most of her time watching TV with the sound turned up to the highest volume. Recently, she called her sister demanding to know "what all these people are doing in my house." She believed people were there to take her money and poison her food. After a careful assessment by the community mental health nurse, it became clear that Ms. Colgán was mistaking the actors on TV for people in her home.

The delusions of elders are often associated with delirium, depression, dementia, or anxiety disorders.

Persecutory delusions involve the belief that one is under investigation, being harassed, or at the mercy of some powerful force. Persecutory delusions may be a response to an older person's diminishing sense of self-mastery. Delusions involving suspiciousness and persecutory ideation are among the most unsettling for elders' caregivers and families. As older adults gradually give up important areas of function, such as financial management, driving, cooking, and shopping, they may begin to develop delusions that people are robbing them or poisoning their food. They respond to these delusions by "dismissing" or rejecting their caregivers in an effort to regain control over these areas of life.

With somatic delusions, the predominant theme is an imagined physical disorder or abnormality of appearance. Somatic delusions in older people are frequently characterized by extremely morbid content ("My blood is leaking into my skin and will poison anyone who touches me").

As a psychiatric–mental health nurse, you will find it crucial to establish trust and consistency with delusional elders. It is important to assess the situation to validate that any persecutory and somatic content is not based in reality. Clients need social interaction with caring people and consistent reality orientation. Relieving social isolation and correcting sensory losses may go far to solve the problem. Delusional processes associated with delirium often abate when the cause of the delirium is treated. Medication in small doses, geared toward relieving underlying anxiety or depressive disorder, may be helpful, although adherence is often a problem because of the client's suspiciousness.

Substance-Related Disorders

A growing body of information suggests that substance use disorders, particularly alcoholism and prescription medication abuse, are more serious problems among elders than had been thought in the past (Blow et al., 2007; Lang, Guralnik, Wallace, & Melzer, 2007). Later-life losses and poor coping skills can lead to increased use of alcohol as a self-medication. Alcohol is both a psychological and physical depressant, thereby raising the risk for both depression and substance dependence. The multiplicity of prescription medications elders are frequently given can create problems with side effects, cognitive impairments, drug-drug interactions, and metabolism. Prescribing practices can also inadvertently mask a substance abuse issue. See the following clinical example about an elder's benzodiazepine misuse.

CLINICAL EXAMPLE

Agnes Szczechowski, a 78-year-old woman, was brought by her family to an assisted living facility. Over the previous couple of years she had had increasing difficulty taking care of herself at home. The family reported the following problems prior to making the decision to place Mrs. Szczechowski: leaving a stove burner turned on long after she had stopped cooking, putting household objects away in unusual places (frying pan in the dryer, for example), and leaving the house dressed inappropriately for the weather. The family also noticed that medication bottles were in a state of disarray, and she could not give them a coherent account of which medications she was taking or on what schedule.

Several days after Mrs. Szczechowski moved to Green Meadow Assisted Living Facility, staff members noticed that she was developing increasing symptoms of anxiety. These included physiological symptoms such as hyperventilation and diaphoresis, behavioral symptoms such as pacing and an inability to relax, and cognitive symptoms such as catastrophic thinking. However, she was not able to specify any cause for the anxiety. It appeared to be an adjustment disorder related to moving to the facility.

A psychiatric–mental health nurse interviewed Mrs. Szczechowski and found, in the course of researching the problem, that the client's primary care physician had been prescribing diazepam (Valium) for her for at least 5 years prior to admission. In gathering collateral information from family members, the nurse discovered that the client had taken larger doses of diazepam than prescribed over several periods. Recently, Mrs. Szczechowski appeared to be consistently taking more diazepam on a daily basis than prescribed, six to eight pills a day rather than the prescribed three. Since admission to the assisted living facility, the diazepam has been administered by the staff exactly as prescribed. Therefore the client's effective dose of diazepam has suddenly been reduced by 50% to 75%.

The upsurge in Mrs. Szczechowski's anxiety appeared to be a consequence of her previously undetected diazepam abuse, as she had difficulty tolerating the reduction in the dose. To address this problem, the psychiatric–mental health nurse worked with the other health care providers to reformulate the diazepam regimen so that the client could be safely and slowly titrated off the diazepam and be prescribed a safer agent for the treatment of her anxiety.

The extent of alcoholism and drug- and alcohol-related problems among older adults, while a definite problem, is not clearly known. In previous generations it was believed that the elderly constituted the age group with the lowest rate of alcohol and illegal drug use because of influences in early life such as Prohibition and a historic disapproval of drinking by women. With the societal changes in subsequent generations, these beliefs are changing as baby boomers age.

It is important to note that elders are more vulnerable than younger people to the effects of alcohol and other substances and that they consume more over-the-counter (OTC) preparations and prescribed medications than other population groups (Lang et al., 2007). Alcohol abuse and drug dependence among elders are now recognized as serious problems. Alcohol abuse can predispose older people to accidents, nutritional deficiencies, and diseases that may lead to loss of autonomy. When older drinkers seek medical help for alcohol-related problems such as malnutrition, injuries from falls, and sleep problems, they rarely report alcoholism as their primary complaint. Unfortunately, the presenting problems may be treated and other symptoms mistakenly attributed to the aging process.

Clinical manifestations of alcohol abuse in elders include:

- Tolerance (requiring more of the substance for the same effect)
- Alcohol-related physical health problems such as gastritis, liver problems, and pancreatitis
- Physiologic dependence on alcohol (the experience of withdrawal symptoms)
- Unexpected reaction to prescription medications
- Poor response to antipsychotic medications
- Multiple social complications (problems with family relationships and social isolation)
- Frequent behavioral problems such as aggression, memory gaps, driving while impaired by alcohol, and traffic accidents
- Self-care neglect such as incontinence, malnutrition, dehydration, and poor hygiene and home maintenance

Many late-onset alcoholics are believed to have turned to drinking in response to stressful life events such as bereavement, illness, divorce, retirement, marital stress, or depression. Assessment for drug and alcohol abuse in elders, especially socially isolated elders who have suffered recent losses, should be respectful; approach elders in a nonjudgmental way when addressing this topic. All clients must be educated about the risks of mixing medications with alcohol. Preventing drinking as a reaction to stress may be accomplished by providing social support and mental health services for elders at risk for social isolation and depression. Referral to resources such as Alcoholics Anonymous (http://www.alcoholics-anonymous.org) is a recommended intervention, especially when combined with other psychiatric supports (see Chapter 15 for information about treating people with the dual diagnosis of mentally ill chemical abuser).

MEDIALINK Alcoholics Anonymous

Disorders of Arousal and Sleep

Elders frequently experience sleep disruptions that may or may not meet the diagnostic criteria for a formal sleep disorder. For example, a lighter sleep phase pattern occurs with less deep sleep, as well as a common circadian rhythm sleep disorder called advanced sleep-phase cycle (*advanced* in terms of direction rather than severity, e.g., sleep and wake times are far earlier than desired). The result in elders is an inability to stay awake past 7:00 p.m. and then awakening—unable to return to sleep—at 3:00 a.m. (Grigg-Damberger, 2007). This pattern can be mistakenly diagnosed as depression. Because older adults do have a disproportionately high incidence of depression, determining the presence of depression is also important.

The quantity and quality of sleep change with the aging process. For example, the amount of REM sleep decreases with aging. Elders experience more frequent awakenings during the night, spend increased total time awake at night, and take longer to fall asleep. Changes in sleep architecture and resulting sleep patterns are believed to be related to changes in internal body rhythm, emotional stress, physical illness, and the effects of medications or drugs. Over one-third of people over 60 years of age complain of sleep disturbances (Grigg-Damberger, 2007; Yaffe, Blackwell, Barnes, Ancoli-Israel, & Stone, 2007). Elders nap more during the day and use a disproportionately high amount of OTC and prescription sleeping aids. Yet the chronic use of sedatives and hypnotics by elders has not been shown to improve their quality of sleep and can lead to many undesirable and dangerous side effects. Elders excrete these medications more slowly than the young and thus are prone to developing toxic effects, including delirium, daytime drowsiness, and loss of equilibrium. Respiration can be significantly disturbed with the use of sleeping medication.

Clinicians and clients alike must be cognizant of the risks associated with medications, especially when combined with alcohol or even herbal and other supplements. Frequently, sleep disturbances are treated with medications that treat the underlying cause of the sleep problem. Examples include mirtazapine (Remeron), an antidepressant that helps with the sleep and appetite problems of depression, and alprazolam (Xanax) if the sleep difficulty is associated with anxiety. The National Council on Patient Information and Education and the Federal Drug Agency launched a campaign called "Be MedWise" to educate consumers on OTC medication use. For information go to http://www.bemedwise.org or use the Companion Website for this textbook.

MediaLink Be Medwise

Clients and health care providers should be more willing to try nonpharmacologic therapies if indicated. Nonpharmacologic guidelines that are recommended for improving sleep for elders include:

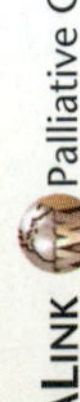

- Consistent daily physical activity
- A cool, well-ventilated room
- A light bedtime snack
- Stress reduction to promote relaxation
- Regular arousal time
- Avoiding long naps during the day
- Clean bed linens
- Avoiding caffeine, tobacco, and alcohol

Sleep disorders are also discussed in Chapter 19.

PALLIATIVE AND END-OF-LIFE ISSUES WITH MENTALLY ILL ELDERS

Death and dying have been characterized in two entirely different directions: as a crisis that is a natural part of life and as a part of life constituting another transition. Death has been referred to as the ultimate loss; a uniquely personal experience that each of us faces alone. While more imminent for older adults, the need for improved care near the end of life is not unique to elders. Each death evokes different needs and behaviors and provides an opportunity for you to address physical, psychological, social, and spiritual needs of clients and their families. The increased use of technology at the end of life, diminished inpatient care resources, and an aging population have all created a demand for palliative care.

Precepts of Palliative Care

The World Health Organization (WHO) defines **palliative care** as the active total care of clients whose disease is not responsive to curative treatment. Not all palliative care occurs at the end of life, and much of it aims to help clients and their families reach personal goals, reconcile conflicts, and derive meaning at the end of life (McGrath & Patton, 2007). Addressing such end-of-life issues is especially complicated when an elder client is exhibiting alteration in mental status due to delirium or dementia or associated with a preexisting psychiatric illness.

Palliative care requires attention to helping clients achieve comfort, the amelioration of pain and distress, and the best possible death. While fears of pain, abandonment, and loss of control are among the most common symptoms for which nurses must provide relief, other end-of-life symptoms of particular concern to psychiatric–mental health nurses include:

- Delirium
- Agitation
- Anxiety
- Depression
- Loneliness
- Hopelessness
- Grief
- Social isolation
- Suffering
- Spiritual distress

The American Association of Colleges of Nursing (AACN) developed guidelines concerning end-of-life care. These guidelines are considered the definitive statement on the knowledge and skills needed by nurses who are committed to improving palliative care. The statement, entitled *Peaceful Death: Recommended Competencies and Curricular Guidelines for End-of-Life Nursing Care*, can be found at http://www.aacn.nche.edu/Publications/deathfin.htm or through the Companion Website for this text. An additional Web-based resource can be found at the City of Hope Pain & Palliative Care Resource Center at http://www.cityofhope.org/prc/.

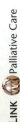

An understanding of family dynamics as well as social, cultural, and religious beliefs may result in the need for the additional supportive services of social workers, hospital chaplains, or other members of the interdisciplinary team. The entire team should be aware of the client's wishes and respond in an appropriate manner to his or her requests.

Spirituality and End-of-Life Care

One of the precepts of palliative care is honoring the preferences, values, and culture of the client and family, especially with respect to suffering, whether physical, psychosocial, or spiritual. Spiritual assessment and care are significant components of end-of-life care. Spiritual integrity gives meaning, purpose, and fulfillment to life and death. The spiritual dimension has been described as a striving for self-transcendence or a search for a higher power and meaning that is greater than the self. Spirituality may or may not include formal religious participation. According to the Joint Commission (2007) standards, the dying client requires a comprehensive spiritual assessment and care that maximizes the client's comfort and dignity and addresses spiritual needs. Staff members must be educated about the needs of: (1) clients receiving care at the end of their life, (2) those who are being treated for emotional or behavioral disorders, and (3) those in recovery from alcohol or drug dependence. Spiritual care according to hospice philosophy is nonjudgmental and all-inclusive and focuses on healing, forgiveness, and acceptance. Spiritual interventions can include any of the practices identified in the Caring for the Spirit feature.

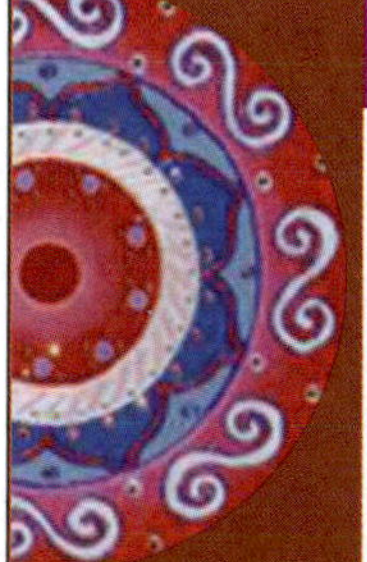

CARING FOR THE SPIRIT

Supporting and Nurturing Spirituality of Elders in End-of-Life Care

The word *spirituality* is rooted in the Greek language as a word for breath, breathing, and inspiration. Spirituality has evolved to mean something more than religiosity in nursing literature due to the influence of holism and humanism (as described in Chapter 5). Spirituality is recognized as a source of inner peace, hope, trust, faith, meaning, and strength and can be said to incorporate our sense of identity and understanding of our place and status in the world.

Attending to a client's spiritual quality of life and spiritual well-being has emerged as an important role for nurses. Spiritual needs, problems, concerns, distress, and pain all have been considered as nursing diagnoses, particularly among those receiving end-of-life care. In addition to conducting and documenting a spiritual assessment and facilitating religious practices if the client wishes, a number of strategies are available to you as you attempt to provide care that supports and nurtures the spirituality of your clients. Consider learning more about each of them and adding them to your repertoire.

Engaging Spirituality Through Nature

Feelings of wonder, awe, and transcendence; a renewed sense of vigor; increased mindfulness; the sense of being present in the moment; an awareness of humility; and a better perspective all have been recognized as benefits of experiencing nature. Bringing elements of the natural environment to clients who are confined in nursing homes, hospice care, or hospitals can help them draw strength and courage from things as simple as the image of a rainbow or the fragrance of pine needles.

Listening to Storytelling, Life Review, and Reminiscence

Encouraging a client to make an audiotape, dictate letters, create a photo album or scrapbook, or create other artistic expressions to depict the wholeness of his or her life can help the client establish a sense of satisfaction from a life well lived. Reminiscence and life review are identified as useful nursing interventions later in this chapter. Experts who teach about listening to clients' stories suggest guidelines for nurses using this approach. A major guideline is the idea of developing a list of questions that encourage awareness of positive aspects of a life story and reflection and enthusiasm on the part of the client telling the story. Questions might include: "How would you like the rest of your story to be?" "How has what has happened to you shaped who you are today?" "What do you think are the major themes in your life story?"

Assisting with Journal or Diary Writing

Keeping a journal offers a client a way to express inner thoughts. A journal can consist of narratives on topics such as "What do I stand for?", "What personal quality do I feel best about?", or "What makes me feel joy?" However, a journal can also take the form of sketches, song lyrics, descriptions of dreams, poetry, or prayers that can be original or collected from various sources.

Making and Appreciating Art as Spiritual Expression

Creating art and sharing it with others allow clients to leave a legacy, build a sense of community, and make sense of experiences. You can encourage clients to participate actively by drawing, painting, or sculpting or passively by collecting healing images such as mandalas, icons, or wilderness landscapes or photographs. Listening to music can help decrease anxiety, depression, agitation, and aggressive behavior as well as improve relaxation and peace of mind.

The strategies for supporting and nurturing spirituality described here represent only a sample of the possibilities. They all require self-disclosure on the part of clients who may feel vulnerable. Extreme sensitivity is required of the nurse who uses them in practice. Some clients prefer to discuss these topics with a member of the clergy or a spiritual advisor. Their wishes must be respected.

Suffering is defined as a highly personal state of severe distress that transcends the physical, psychological, social, and spiritual dimensions and threatens the intactness of the person. Efforts to reduce suffering involve collaborative care at this fragile time in the client's life. Responding to the spiritual needs of clients and families coping with end-of-life issues may ameliorate the depth of suffering. Gerdner, Yang, Cha, and Tripp-Reimer (2007) highlight the bereavement process of the family-oriented Hmong (a Southeast Asian ethnic minority). The interplay of culture, spirituality, and the meaning of life and death is vital to Hmong family decision-making and rituals. In this culture there is a high level of family involvement in a family member's milestones.

Historically, the role of the psychiatric–mental health nurse did not require expertise in palliative and end-of-life care. However, as the current population of psychiatric clients age and geropsychiatric care settings expand, addressing end-of-life care issues will become a major challenge and critical to the management of a client's psychiatric illness. Effective communication with clients and their loved ones is essential. Communication strategies require that you accomplish the following:

- Be clear about the client's goals and expectations of care and treatment.
- Avoid euphemisms for words like *death* and *dying*.
- Be specific when using words such as *hope* and *better*.
- Listen to and honor the preferences, values, and cultural beliefs of clients and their loved ones (Gerdner et al., 2007; Peters, 2007).

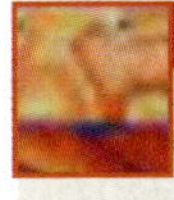

NURSING PROCESS Elders

The following sections provide specific strategies for applying the nursing process when providing care to elders.

Assessment

Assessment of the elder includes the assessment interview, a biologic assessment, consideration of cognitive status, an assessment of psychological/emotional status, an assessment of strengths and coping strategies, an assessment of sexuality, an attempt to determine social and financial status, and a focused effort to be alert for any indicators of elder abuse.

The Assessment Interview

The variety of theories on aging and the complex interrelationship of physical, emotional, and environmental factors affecting the mental health of elders require an individualized, comprehensive, and multidimensional approach. If feasible, a multidisciplinary team approach is most effective in providing validation of assessment impressions, accurate diagnoses, and appropriate intervention strategies.

The interview is the initial step in the assessment process and important in differentiating between psychiatric disorders and the normal aging process. Chapter 11 offers a comprehensive overview of assessment procedures that should be adapted for elders. Specific guidelines for interviewing elders appear in the Your Assessment Approach feature.

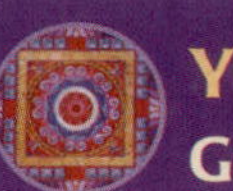

YOUR ASSESSMENT APPROACH
Guidelines for Interviewing Elders

1. Try to make the assessment interview as pleasant as possible by conveying a sense of respect and caring.
2. Be close to the client; use touch when appropriate.
3. Be clear in stating the purpose of the interview and the length of time it will take.
4. Attend to verbal, nonverbal, and environmental cues as well as to the cognitive and behavior status of the client.
5. Repeat the purpose and the time frame of the interview if the client forgets.

Interviewing requires skill and heightened sensitivity and may take more time with older adults than with members of other age groups. Sensory loss, confusion, agitation, wandering, communication disorders, cultural influences, shame, and the fear of stigmatization may inhibit the expression of feelings in elders. They may be unaware of their behavior or expect negative changes as a normal part of aging. It is imperative to solicit interpretations from family and other staff members to help fill in aspects of the clinical picture and validate information provided by the client in the individual interview. See the Rx Communication feature for an illustration of communicating with a confused elder.

A holistic assessment of elders should include objective and subjective data regarding the client's status on a number of levels: biologic, cognitive, psychological, strengths and coping strategies, sexual, social, and financial. A variety of self-report screening tools have been designed for use specifically with older clients. These require minimal special training to administer and can help you obtain subjective assessment information. These tools may also be used as objective measures of the outcomes of interventions. Several of the most commonly used tools and scales are listed in the Your Assessment Approach feature that follows.

Biologic Assessment

Before a definitive psychiatric diagnosis can be made, all medically based illnesses with psychiatric symptoms (depression, confusion, restlessness, and anxiety) must be ruled out. In addition, a complete medical and neurologic examination is necessary to differentiate irreversible conditions from treatable conditions such as pseudodementia (discussed in Chapter 14). There are conditions, both chronic and systemic, that can predispose an elderly individual to confusion. A urinary tract infection (UTI) is a common and debilitating problem for the elderly that has accompanying pain and cognitive symptoms. A client exhibiting confusion must be examined for anemia, infections, organ failure, or cardiovascular disease (Neal-Boylan, 2007). Many emergency room

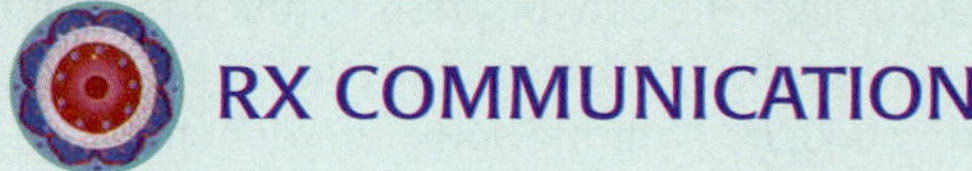

COMMUNICATING WITH A CONFUSED ELDER

CLIENT: "I don't know why I'm here. My brother takes care of my finances. He doesn't think I take proper care of myself, but I am as I am and I want him to leave me ALONE!"

NURSE RESPONSE 1: "Give me an example of something that your brother told you was your 'not taking proper care of yourself.'"

RATIONALE: This response focuses on collecting more information about the genuine safety risks faced by this 84-year-old woman who lives alone in a small New York City apartment. She has been referred to your clinic to have her safety skills assessed.

NURSE RESPONSE 2: "What has your brother told you about why you are here at the clinic?"

RATIONALE: This response requests concrete information from the client rather than any interpretations. It also has the potential to provide a picture of memory impairments she might be experiencing.

YOUR ASSESSMENT APPROACH
Screening Instruments Frequently Used in Assessing Elders

- *Cornell Scale for Depression in Dementia*—Specifically developed to assess signs and symptoms of major depression in clients with dementia
- *Geriatric Depression Scale*—Useful for collecting information about symptoms of depression
- *Iowa Self-Assessment Inventory*—Useful for obtaining a functional assessment of elders in a variety of settings
- *Mini Mental State Examination*—Also used to assess mental status of elders
- *Short Portable Mental Status Questionnaire (SPMSQ)*—Useful for assessing mental status, including orientation, memory, and other cognitive functions
- *Zung Self-Rating Anxiety Scale*—A self-reporting instrument with 20 questions for clients being evaluated for anxiety-associated symptoms

admissions for psychiatric problems in the elderly prove to have an underlying biologic etiology such as an infection or dehydration.

Objective assessment information includes laboratory results, a complete history, and physical examination including weight, vital signs, and a description of the physical appearance of the client. Standard diagnostic laboratory analyses appear in FIGURE 28-3 ■. Your medical–surgical nursing or general nursing texts offer specific biological assessment guides for elders.

Other procedures important for ruling out infections, space-occupying lesions, drug and medication toxicities, and cancers include chest radiography, drug toxicology screening, computed tomography (CT) scanning, positron-emission tomography (PET) scanning, electrocardiogram (ECG), electroencephalogram (EEG), and lumbar puncture. A dementia workup should include serologic tests for syphilis; folate, B_{12}, and trace mineral levels; and a thyroid panel.

Subjective assessment information includes clients' perceptions of their physical health and a description of their chronic illnesses, symptoms, self-care activities, and concerns and fears about their current situation.

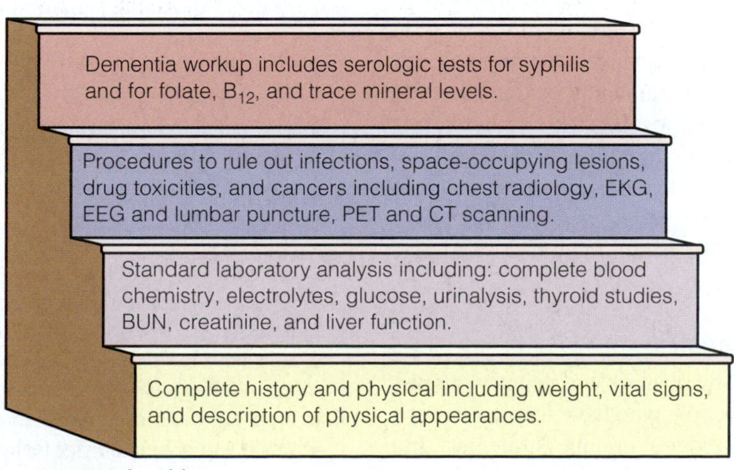

FIGURE 28-3 ■ Levels of biologic assessment for elders.

Cognitive Status

A thorough mental status examination is essential. Objective information includes the presence and extent of cognitive impairment. Include the family and other caregivers to determine the course of any mental changes. Ask: "Did the changes happen gradually (dementia of the Alzheimer's type, drug/medication toxicity, metabolic imbalances), suddenly (depression, cerebrovascular accident, drug/medication toxicity), or in a graduated, stepwise fashion (multi-infarct dementia)?" Family and other caregivers may have noticed changes at certain times of the day that could indicate specific problems. Ask: "Have there been changes in mood, or has there been agitation in the late afternoon or early evening (sundowning)?" "Has the client been observed to have or complained of having trouble making decisions or concentrating (depression)?"

The *Short Portable Mental Status Questionnaire* (SPMSQ) is a simple, reliable, and valid 10-item cognitive performance evaluation tool. It was designed to assess and monitor cognitive changes in an elderly client. Keep in mind, however, three important points when using standardized assessment tools with elders:

1. Older people are sensitive to fatigue, boredom, medications, and environmental influences that can affect results on a mental status measurement tool.
2. Tools like the SPMSQ cannot distinguish delirium from dementia.
3. Assessment instruments designed for use with other age groups may not be accurate or complete for use with elders.

Subjective information regarding cognitive status includes clients' own perceptions of their mental status. Questions to ask include:

- How has your thinking been lately?
- Is your memory as good as it used to be?
- Have you been able to keep track of your medications? The days of the week? Mealtimes?

Psychological/Emotional Status

Objective data about the client's psychological and emotional status require synthesis of impressions from both the content and process of the assessment interview and mental status examination. Avoid the overuse of psychiatric terminology but rather strive for descriptions accompanied by examples of the client's behavior and direct quotations. Be sure to include significant negative findings such as the absence of delusional thoughts, the absence of suicidal ideation, and the absence of hallucinations. Your assessment should include not only pathology and problems but also health, adaptive strengths, and personal assets.

Strengths and Coping Strategies

Aging is a process punctuated by positive and negative stress-producing events. Elders are people who have learned to cope with stress. Data about an elder's coping strategies and strengths are as important as information about psychiatric symptoms. You can shift the conversation in this direction by making a statement such as, "You certainly have lived a long, full life. Would you share with me some of your survival secrets?" The following Your Assessment Approach feature provides sample questions to help you gather data about an elder's strengths and coping strategies, such as spiritual practices, playing a musical instrument, or reaching out to help others. With this information you can develop a cogent plan of care that supports weak areas and activates those areas in which the client excels.

Spirituality can be a psychological support and a coping mechanism. Often, people who are facing novel stressors or significant threats to their security turn to religion or spirituality for the first time in their lives, or after an absence for a significant period of time. Assess clients to determine whether a recent focus on spirituality is a new addition to their support structure. If so, explore the concepts, meanings, and emotions that spiritual expression offers the client.

Sexuality

Sexuality is an important area often overlooked when assessing elders. Remember that sexual activity can and does continue into later life and that sexuality is a broad, multidimensional component of personal identity. Films such as *Harold and Maude* and *Innocence* portray richly, and with humor, sexual expression among elders. Sexual expression includes body image, affection, love, flirtation, social roles, and interaction. Older people who do abstain from sexual expression often do so because they lack the opportunity or perceive negative social pressure about sexuality in people their age.

Approach the topic of sexuality in a tactful, caring, and nonjudgmental manner. An elder who does not wish to discuss sexual issues most likely will make that clear by stating it directly, not answering the question, or changing the sub-

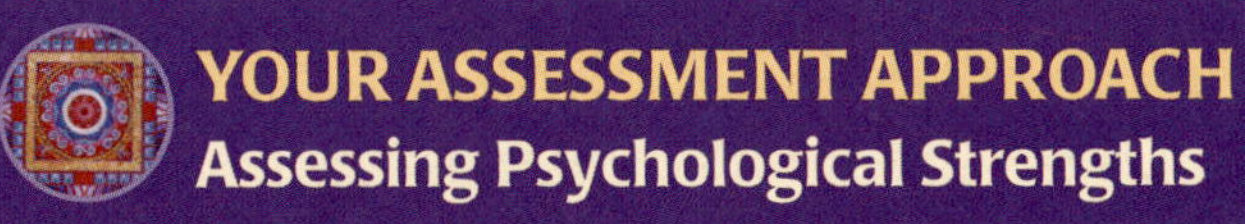

YOUR ASSESSMENT APPROACH
Assessing Psychological Strengths

- What are some of the things you like about yourself?
- What are some of the upsetting, stressful, difficult times you can remember?
- What did you do to comfort yourself when your spouse/partner died?
- How did you make it through the death of your child (or friend)?
- What kinds of things do you do to cheer yourself up?
- What makes you happy or content?
- How do you nurture yourself?
- What do you do to have fun? To relax?
- What things do you think you can do to get through rough times?
- How have the passing years affected your sexuality?
- Are you happily married or partnered?
- What are you most concerned about right now?
- What kind of help do you feel you need?

ject. An elder who was socialized in a different, more conservative era may not be comfortable discussing sex. Older adults who matured in the 1960s, however, may have entirely different attitudes toward their continuing sexuality.

Social and Financial Status

Also assess the quality and quantity of social support (past and present) available to an elder. Social support has been confirmed as important for optimal functioning even with psychiatric disturbances. Maintaining a meaningful social network suggests strong interpersonal skills that can be mobilized to help negotiate stresses and losses in later life. Formation of a new social network when others have dissolved is easier for an elder with social skills and the personal resources of assertiveness, friendliness, and warmth. Consider the following clinical example.

CLINICAL EXAMPLE

Irene is a 75-year-old widow who recently broke her hip while cross-country skiing. At first she felt depressed, embarrassed, and socially isolated by her injury and immobilization. She longed for her usual schedule of hiking, swimming, traveling, and attending plays and concerts. Because Irene had a wide circle of friends, had regularly hosted holiday parties at her home, and was generous with her time and energy with her adult children and grandchildren, her social support network rallied to help her as soon as they learned of her condition.

Friends and family brought in the health food Irene loved and stayed with her to keep her company while she ate. Others sent clever, encouraging cards and notes. One friend telephoned her each day until she was able to be out and about. One of her sons sent her some of his favorite books, and her other son set up Internet and e-mail connections for her computer. Irene made a rapid and full recovery both physically and psychologically. She rose to the challenge of an unexpected injury and recovery period with cheerfulness and resilience. Instead of being derailed by her accident, she emerged even stronger.

Elders who get by on a low, fixed income may be plagued by financial problems that affect their mental and physical health. Some communities offer services to help older people manage their finances. The removal of financial strain can dramatically improve the health of an aging person.

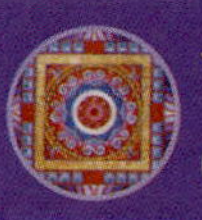

YOUR ASSESSMENT APPROACH
Guidelines for Assessing Social and Financial Status

- How many phone calls and e-mails do you get in a week?
- How frequently do you have visitors?
- How frequently do you visit others?
- Are you happily married/partnered?
- How would you describe your relationship with your family members?
- Do you have someone you can trust and confide in?
- Do you find yourself feeling lonely?
- Do you have transportation to get to doctor/nurse appointments or to the hospital if needed?
- How is your financial situation? Do you worry about spending or running out of money?

Learning about available financial aid and assistance programs will help you be an effective case manager for older clients. Sample questions for obtaining information about a client's social and financial status are listed in the Your Assessment Approach feature.

Elder Abuse

The mistreatment of elders is a serious, underreported, underdetected phenomenon. Elder mistreatment may take many forms, including physical abuse, neglect, exploitation, abandonment, and psychological abuse (see TABLE 28-1 ■).

Elders who are at greatest risk for abuse and neglect are those who are dependent on others for care (Baker, 2007). The degree of dependence may overwhelm the caregiver, who may then harm the elder. Stressors related to caregiving can overwhelm any caregiver, but the caregiver of a frail elder is often an adult child with additional family and work responsibilities or a spouse who is also aging (Gallagher-Thompson & Coon, 2007). (See Chapter 30 for more information on family stress and the burdens of caregiving.)

A growing number of states provide legal alternatives for the removal of an elder to a protective situation. Long-term care centers or respite care placement, discussed later in this chapter, may be necessary. However, most elders react

TABLE 28-1 ■ Forms of Mistreatment of Elders

Physical Abuse	Neglect	Exploitation	Abandonment	Psychological Abuse
■ Direct beatings ■ Infliction of pain ■ Coercion (abrasions, sprains, dislocation)	■ Withholding food ■ Withholding fluids ■ Withholding medical attention	■ Taking Social Security or pension checks ■ Taking possessions against elder's will	■ Dropping elder off at ER ■ Leaving incapacitated elder alone at home ■ Failing to provide for basic services	■ Continuous degrading ■ Threatening ■ Using other scare tactics when the elder cannot provide for his or her own needs

negatively to such placement and want to return to the potentially harmful home situation. In-home assistance is becoming available in most areas, and such home health services can decrease the strain on caregivers. Home visits made by a case manager or community health nurse can provide an opportunity to assess the possibility of elder abuse in any of its forms, or to prevent it by planning for services to meet the needs of elders and their family caregivers.

Nursing Diagnosis: NANDA

Once a comprehensive, multidimensional assessment is accomplished, nursing diagnoses are identified. The NANDA nursing diagnoses likely to be associated with DSM-IV-TR disorders in elders are covered in this section.

Major Depression

NANDA diagnoses associated with the DSM-IV-TR disorder of major depression include the following.

Chronic or Situational Low Self-Esteem Low self-esteem is a hallmark feature of depression. Not only do elders internalize social ageist biases, but they are also often plagued with irrational guilt in the form of intrusive, obsessional, and self-deprecating thoughts.

Risk for Self-Directed Violence Feelings of hopelessness, low self-esteem, obsessive–compulsive symptoms, apathy, and powerlessness often contribute to suicidal ideation and suicide attempts in depressed elders.

Activity Intolerance Psychomotor agitation and/or retardation are both symptoms of depression. Psychomotor agitation affects social interaction, self-care abilities, and the sleep–wake cycle. Psychomotor retardation is a common vegetative sign of depression in elders. People with psychomotor retardation experience compromised self-care abilities and lack of physical exercise, and are at risk for developing complications of decreased mobility.

Feeding Self-Care Deficit, and Imbalanced Nutrition: More or Less than Body Requirements Many depressed elders lose weight dramatically. A weight gain secondary to overeating and decreased activity occurs less frequently.

Ineffective Health Maintenance Depressed elders are at risk for developing physical health complications secondary to poor self-care and poor health maintenance habits.

Sleep Deprivation or Insomnia Often, older clients with depression experience sleep pattern disturbances, particularly early morning awakening. Occasionally, depressed elders report excessive sleeping.

Disturbed Thought Processes Elders may have cognitive changes such as short-term memory loss that accompany depression. Concentration may be impaired, and lack of motivation hinders the ability to learn new information and avoid social isolation. Chapter 14 ∞ provides detailed information on memory impairment.

Adjustment Disorder

NANDA diagnoses most likely to be found in elders with adjustment disorder are described next.

Dysfunctional Grieving Elders may become immobilized by stress associated with loss. Often, depression ensues, with an identified stressor as the only factor differentiating an adjustment disorder from major depression.

Self-Care Deficit Individuals may lose interest in self-care activities. Grooming, hygiene, and other activities of daily living are neglected. In some cases, elders are at risk for developing serious physical illnesses as a result of failing to adhere to medication regimens and refusing to eat or engage in other health care practices.

Ineffective Role Performance The experience of losses often leads to changes in social interaction and role performance. Social withdrawal and loneliness as well as changes in mental status can occur due to lack of social stimulation.

Hopelessness The experience of loss coupled with a pervasive dysphoria can place an older person at risk for developing dependence and loss of function as self-concept and motivation wane.

Anxiety Disorders

Elders with anxiety disorders may have the following NANDA diagnoses.

Ineffective Coping Anxiety symptoms often impair a person's ability to concentrate and think clearly. Consequently, judgment is affected and the client decreases activities in order to avoid stressful situations.

Activity Intolerance Anxiety is often associated with psychomotor agitation and restlessness.

Delusional Disorders

NANDA diagnoses most likely to be found in elders with delusional disorder are covered next.

Disturbed Thought Processes Older people with delusional disorders often become paranoid and suspect others of trying to rob them, cheat them, or harm them in some way. They may also have delusions about their body or bodily functions. Delusions may be accompanied by feelings of fear, paranoia, anger, and anxiety. Behavioral manifestations of these feelings include suspiciousness, aggression, lashing out, social isolation, and unusual eating behaviors.

Impaired Social Interaction Delusions that are centered on family members and caregivers strain interpersonal relationships and may make them impossible to maintain.

Outcome Identification: NOC

Outcomes associated with NANDA diagnoses common among elders are described in the following section.

Improvement in Disturbed Thought Processes

Subjective indications of improvement in thought processes include client reports of thinking more clearly, improved concentration, and ability to remember recent and remote events. Individuals with delusions and other signs of psychosis will note that they feel more like themselves and will be able to make more accurate, reality-based interpretations. Other NOC outcomes specific to this nursing diagnosis include:

- Cognitive orientation: Ability to identify person, place, time, and purpose
- Concentration: Ability to focus on a specific stimulus
- Decision making: Ability to choose between two or more alternatives
- Information processing: Ability to acquire, organize, and use information
- Memory: Ability to cognitively retrieve and report previously stored information
- Consciousness: Ability to arouse, orient, and attend to environment

Renewed Hope and Self-Acceptance

Expressions of hope and self-acceptance, renewed involvement, and motivation in activities and planning for the future indicate improvement and replace dependence, apathy, and negative self-talk.

Other NOC outcomes relevant to this diagnosis in elders include:

- Expressions of faith, will to live, reasons to live, meaning in life, optimism, and belief in self and others
- Ability to identify personal strengths
- Ability to recognize behaviors that reduce feelings of hopelessness
- Interest in social and personal relationships
- Interest in and satisfaction with life goals

Resumption of Self-Care and Health Maintenance

Elder clients will resume their prior level of self-care and health maintenance. Other NOC outcomes relevant to this nursing diagnosis with elders include:

- Ability to perform most basic physical tasks and personal care activities
- Ability to dress self
- Ability to maintain neat appearance
- Ability to maintain own hygiene

Appropriately Paced Activity, Rest, and Psychomotor Activity

Vegetative signs will be replaced with more appropriately paced activities, movement, gait, speech, appetite, and sleep–wake cycle. Anxiety and fear will be replaced with subjective feelings of calm, restfulness, and well-being.

Pleasure in Eating and Normal Weight

Clients will report that their appetites are returning to premorbid level with increased pleasure associated with eating. Weight will return to normal range.

Decreased Preoccupation with Death and Dying

Clients will report that suicidal ideation has markedly decreased if not resolved. Morbid preoccupation with death and dying will also decrease.

Planning and Implementation: NIC

The following psychiatric–mental health interventions are frequently effective when working with elders.

Reminiscence Therapy and Life Review

Reminiscence therapy and life review are useful interventions for elders who are experiencing self-esteem disturbance, grief, hopelessness, powerlessness, altered role performance, and social isolation. **Reminiscence therapy** uses the recall of past events, feelings, and thoughts to facilitate pleasure, quality of life, or adaptation to present circumstances. Although it can be used throughout the life span, it is of special significance when working with elders.

Reminiscing can and should be encouraged for elders individually and in groups. Creative use of food, music, pets, and special events can facilitate the process and make it fun. Materials such as photo albums, journals, cameras, and video recorders provide ways for older people to establish a record of their lives, creating a legacy for those who follow.

Life review is a structured process involving the recall of past events in one's life in an effort to find meaning in those events. The process systematically reviews remote memories and addresses the expression of related feelings and the recognition of conflicts. A life review is a chance to reexamine one's life, solve old problems, make amends, and restore harmony. As life review becomes an integral part of clinical care, it provides emotional and spiritual support. Approaching the second half of life with a positive perspective—a journey filled with new possibilities and enriched by wisdom and learning from life experience—provides an opportunity to reflect on personal intentions, values, interpersonal relationships, and a personal legacy (Jenko, Gonzalez, & Seymour, 2007). Initiating and therapeutically directing the life review process requires your use of effective therapeutic listening skills (refer to Chapter 10∞) in order to enhance the psychological growth that can emerge as a result of this process.

Reality Orientation

Reality orientation is a structured program for elderly clients that emphasizes awareness of time, place, person, and purpose. The approach provides consistency and a constant reminder to clients of where they are, why they are there, and what is expected. The periodic use of reality orientation tests the elder's level of confusion and disorientation. The rationale for reality orientation is the need to use the part of the person's mind that remains intact.

MediaLink Critical Thinking Exercise: Psychosocial Care of Elders

Socialization Enhancement

Socialization enhancement with elders usually takes place in **resocialization groups** conducted in senior centers, adult day care, rehabilitation, and long-term care facilities. The goal of resocialization groups is to facilitate the elder's ability to interact with others and to renew interest in his or her surroundings. One form of resocialization group focuses on **remotivation therapy**, in which the emphasis is on stimulating interest in the environment and relationships with others. Group discussion focuses on topics chosen by members of the group and may include world affairs, current local activities, and happy experiences. In the discussions, group members are encouraged to pool knowledge and develop stimulating discussions related to the topic at hand.

Animal-Assisted Therapy

Animal-assisted therapy or pet therapy involves the purposeful use of animals to provide affection, attention, diversion, and relaxation to clients. The animals may be certified therapy animals, may be obtained from a variety of sources such as community-based SPCA/Humane Society volunteer programs or the local zoo, or may live on the grounds of the facility. Animals that have physical contact with elders are trained to respond in a calm, nonthreatening manner. Small animals can be held in an older person's lap, larger animals are trained to stand next to a chair and allow the client to stroke or pet them without having to hold them, and aviaries of birds provide sound, movement, and interaction.

Exercise and Movement Therapy

Exercise and movement therapy can help induce relaxation, maintain flexibility, restore balance, and enhance joy in older clients. Such interventions may include stretching and reaching activities, complex exercises such as Tai Chi for those able to mirror the leader, or simple and concrete movements such as handholding for those who are physically or cognitively incapacitated. See the feature What Every Radiology Nurse Should Know for information on specific challenges posed by elders in the Radiology Department.

Support Groups

Social support and group interventions are useful when working with clients who experience dysfunctional or interrupted family processes, knowledge deficits, ineffective coping, dysfunctional grieving, social isolation, and spiritual distress. The group situation or social environment provides emotional support as well as information for its members. Groups are the treatment of choice for many older clients, especially those in long-term care facilities, because several people can benefit and transportation is not a problem.

Medication Administration

Used judiciously, medications can be an effective adjunct to other interventions when working with clients with mental disorders in later life. A key axiom to remember about medication dosing with elders is: "Start low, go slow." The high incidence of adverse medication reactions in older clients underscores the need for careful monitoring and conservative dosages. Table 28-2 ■ summarizes recommended dosages for categories of psychotropic medications used with elders. In general, information about dose adjustments and special considerations with elders are catalogued in medication references such as drug guides and medication manuals. (See also Chapter 32 of this text for in-depth information.)

WHAT EVERY INTERVENTIONAL RADIOLOGY NURSE SHOULD KNOW

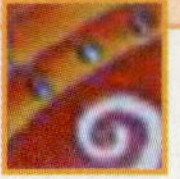

Needs of Elders Differ from Those of Other Age Groups

Treating an elder in radiology differs from treating younger clients. In a number of ways elders are more restricted in their movements and their ability to accommodate change. For example, many elders have a lower tolerance for cool temperatures than others, and radiology departments tend to be very cool. Whatever keeps older clients comfortable should be done to ensure their continued interest in treatment. Other issues include positioning difficulties due to injuries, surgery, arthritis, or scoliosis. Positioning can and should be made more comfortable with a little extra effort and creativity. Attending to the elder's particular needs will enhance treatment and allow for more effective nursing assessment (Barba, Barba, & Rankin, 2007).

It is important that you recognize that elders are more prone to side effects from psychiatric medications and observe for their occurrence. Among these side effects are:

- Extrapyramidal symptoms (dystonias, akathisia, tremor, pseudoparkinsonism)
- Constipation
- Anticholinergic effects (urinary retention, cognitive impairments, blurred vision, dry mouth, hallucinations, sexual dysfunction)
- Cardiovascular effects (postural hypotension, arrhythmias)
- Drug interactions resulting in delirium, confusion, or disorientation
- Sedation
- Paradoxical effects, especially common with diphenhydramine (Benadryl) and meperidine (Demerol)

Medications within each psychotropic class vary widely in intensity of side effects and ideally should be monitored by a specially prepared psychogerontologist who is knowledgeable about the appropriate doses and possible side effects of these medications.

Evaluation

Identified outcomes and their measurement in both subjective and objective terms guide the evaluation step in the nursing

Table 28-2 ■ Dosage Ranges of Psychotropic Medications Used with Elders

Category	Dosage Range
Antipsychotics: Atypical	
Olanzapine (Zyprexa)	5–10 mg/day
Risperidone (Risperdal)	0.25–6 mg/day
Antipsychotics: Conventional	
Chlorpromazine (Thorazine)	10–800 mg/day
Fluphenazine (Prolixin)	PO: 0.25–20 mg/day, IM: 2.5–10 mg/day, Decanoate: 12.5–25 mg/1–4 wk
Haloperidol (Haldol)	PO: 0.25–15 mg/day, IM: 2–5 mg q4h PRN, Decanoate: 50–100 mg/4 wk
Trifluoperazine (Stelazine)	PO: 0.5–40 mg/day, IM: 1–2 mg q4–6h, Max 10 mg/day
Anxiolytic Agents	
Buspirone (BuSpar)	10–60 mg/day
Anxiolytic Agents (Benzodiazepines)	
Clonazepam (Klonopin)	1.5–20 mg/day
Lorazepam (Ativan)	0.5–2.0 mg/day
Oxazepam (Serax)	10–30 mg/day
Mood Stabilizers	
Carbamazepine (Tegretol)	400–1,200 mg/day
Lithium	300 mg tid
Valproate (Depakote)	125 mg bid to max 60 mg/kg/day
Monoamine Oxidase Inhibitors (MAOIs)	
Isocarboxazid (Marplan)	10–30 mg/day
Phenelzine (Nardil)	15–90 mg/day
Tranylcypromine (Parnate)	30–60 mg/day
Sedative/Hypnotic Benzodiazepines	
Flurazepam (Dalmane)	15–30 mg/bedtime
Temazepam (Restoril)	7.5–15 mg/bedtime
Atypical Antidepressants	
Bupropion (Wellbutrin)	50–300 mg/day
Nefazodone (Serzone)	50–600 mg/day
Trazodone (Desyrel)	25–150 mg/day
Selective Serotonin Reuptake Inhibitors (SSRIs)	
Citalopram (Celexa)	20 mg/day
Fluoxetine (Prozac)	10–80 mg/day
Paroxetine (Paxil)	10–80 mg/day
Sertraline (Zoloft)	25–200 mg/day
Tricyclic Antidepressants	
Amitriptyline (Elavil)	10–150 mg/day
Desipramine (Norpramin)	75–150 mg/day
Imipramine (Tofranil)	PO: 75–300 mg/day
Nortriptyline (Pamelor)	10–150 mg/day

Source: Trigoboff, E., Wilson, B. A., Shannon, M. T., & Stang, C. L. (2005). *Psychiatric drug guide*. Upper Saddle River, NJ: Prentice Hall. Adapted by permission of Pearson Education, Inc., Upper Saddle River, NJ.

process. When working with older mentally ill clients, expectations must be realistic. The aging process has normal, nonpathological impacts on behavioral speed, rate of learning new information, and adaptation to degeneration of sensory input. Once these characteristics of aging are taken into account, evaluation of an older client's response to nursing interventions can proceed. As with clients in other age groups, psychiatric symptoms are evaluated for reduction in intensity, intrusiveness, and interference with functioning.

Elder clients have a repertoire of learning, coping, communicating, and adjusting that is useful in evaluating nursing interventions. Ultimately, clients' own values, culture, and preferences, particularly in the late stages of life, should be honored as the gold standard. Families and significant others should, whenever possible, be involved along with the client in the evaluation process.

CASE MANAGEMENT, COMMUNITY-BASED CARE, AND HOME CARE

Care of mentally ill elders takes place in a variety of settings, including at home, in day care programs, in geropsychiatric or dementia units of hospitals, in outpatient clinics, in assisted living programs, and in long-term care facilities. Goals for care provided in the community emphasize:

- Maintaining optimal functional independence
- Supporting clients and families across settings
- Delaying institutionalization
- Enhancing self-esteem and personal integrity
- Educating clients and family caregivers about treatment strategies
- Ensuring coordinated supportive daily activities that enhance the client's ability to cope and compensate for deficits

Restorative Care

Restorative care is a planned, systematic program that focuses on restoration and maintenance of optimal function and assisting adults to compensate for impairments. It also emphasizes prevention of deterioration whenever possible.

In order for it to be successful, everyone working in the environment must adopt the philosophy of restorative care. This approach is particularly relevant in long-term care facilities. Staff from the living units, the social work staff, dietary staff, and activities staff are all involved in promoting and restoring function and ability.

Community-Based Programs

While the philosophy of restorative care is clearly applicable to the care of elders who live in nursing homes or other long-term care facilities, it also guides many other community-based programs. Senior centers, adult day care, respite centers, and community support services such as Meals on Wheels and Whistle Stop Wheels, which respectively bring prepared food and transportation to elders being cared for at home, are all designed to promote the elder's optimal independent functioning and reduce the stress and burden on family caregivers.

Community-based programs offer alternatives to institutionalization. In the case of senior centers, the emphasis is on (1) health and wellness promotion, and (2) social, educational, and recreational activities. Adult day care programs are another alternative to institutionalization. Adult day care programs represent a community resource for elders who need nursing, medical, and rehabilitative services beyond socialization and education. Many adult day care facilities and assisted living centers offer a **respite** option wherein elders can remain overnight in order to relieve family caregivers if they are feeling burdened. Both of these community programs allow elders to continue living at home.

Assisted living communities are a relatively new option for elders who require support and can no longer remain in their own homes. Such communities take several forms but usually offer a range of assistance levels from independent apartment units through nursing home–like complete care. Unfortunately, this option is rarely available to elders who have sparse financial resources.

The next level of care for frail or mentally disordered elders is admission to a nursing home or other long-term care facility. Even when long-term care is an option, the decision to institutionalize a loved one with dementia is usually made only when family caregivers have reached the brink of their own tolerance levels, putting their own health at risk; when the elder no longer recognizes them; or when it becomes physically impossible to manage the elder due to violence or incapacity. As a nurse, especially when serving as case manager, you should be well informed about your community's resources for mentally ill elders and their family caregivers.

Resistance to Care

Descriptions such as *uncooperative*, *stubborn*, *noncompliant*, and *aggressive* have all been used to characterize elders who are resistant to care. These behaviors are commonly noted as the biggest problems when caring for a mentally disordered elder in a community or home setting. The research by Werner, Tabak, Albert, and Bergman (2002) on interventions used by nurses with psychogeriatric clients resisting care identified frequently mentioned reasons for disruptive behavior and resistance to care among elders. These included:

- Cognitive impairment
- Fear
- Excessive demands
- Acute illness and pain
- Environmental stress such as noise

This team of nursing and health care researchers defines *resistance to care* as client behaviors that prevent, oppose, or interfere with the caregiver's efforts to provide help. Resistance to care by mentally disordered elders can take the form of pushing, hitting, screaming, and cursing. Werner and associates' research, as well as research by others, suggest the following as potentially useful nursing interventions:

MediaLink Care Plan: Adjustment to Nursing Home

- Consult with the primary caregiver (family member or nursing staff member) who is in most frequent contact with the client about strategies that worked in the past.
- Talk and reason with the client.
- Allow the client to eat or dress independently.
- Distract the client by initiating social activity.
- Wait and return at a later time to resume the activity.
- Allow the client to refuse care, such as getting dressed, that involves few health consequences.

Try to discover the reason for resistance to care. Is it pain? Fatigue? Fear of caregivers who are strangers to the client? Confusion because of an unfamiliar environment? Not knowing what is wanted or expected by caregivers?

Dealing with mentally ill elders can be challenging, particularly in the home or community. More nursing research is needed to determine strategies that are effective, especially with elders who are resistant to care.

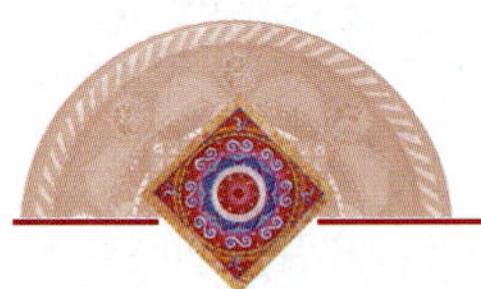

EXPLORE MEDIALINK 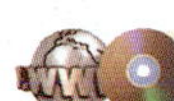 www.prenhall.com/kneisl

For NCLEX-RN® review questions, case studies, and other resources for this chapter see the Pearson Health MediaLink CD-ROM that accompanies this book and the Companion Website at www.prenhall.com/kneisl.

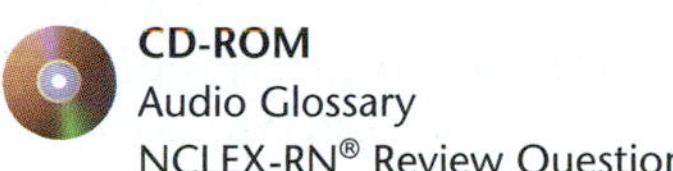

CD-ROM
Audio Glossary
NCLEX-RN® Review Questions

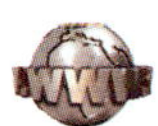

Companion Website
Audio Glossary
NCLEX-RN® Review Questions
Critical Thinking Exercise
- *Psychosocial Care of Elders*

Case Study
- *Late-Life Schizophrenia*

Care Plan
- *Adjustment to Nursing Home*

MediaLinks
MediaLink Application
- *Depression in the Elderly*

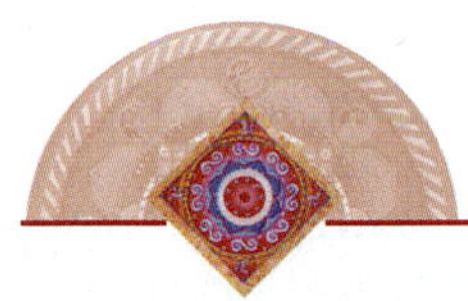

NCLEX-RN® REVIEW QUESTIONS

1. As the population age 85 and older increases dramatically, which of the following consequences are health care implications for both the national and world populations? (Select all that apply.)
1. Decreased incidence of depression, delirium, and dementia
2. Increased incidence of other chronic disabling conditions
3. Increased numbers of chronically disabled individuals requiring assistance with activities of daily living
4. Increased numbers of frail older adults (who consume many health care resources, maintenance services, and residential placements)
5. Increased numbers of underfunctioning older adults due to inadequate intervention associated with stigma and ignorance

2. Which of the major theories of aging suggests that individual older adults have a limited impact on the aging process, as most of the damage to the body has already been done?
1. Disengagement theory
2. Nutritional theory
3. Environmental theory
4. Wear-and-tear theory

3. Which of the major theories of aging suggests that older adults may decelerate the aging process?
1. Disengagement theory
2. Activity theory
3. Genetic theory
4. Immunology theory

4. Which of the following is a guiding principle for the nurse in distinguishing mental disorders from the expected changes associated with aging?
1. The clinical presentation of mental illness in older adults differs from that in other age groups.
2. Older people are believed to be more prone to mental illness than young people.
3. When physical deterioration becomes a significant feature of an elder's life, the risk of comorbid psychiatric illness rises.
4. A competent clinician can readily distinguish mental disorders from the expected changes associated with aging.

5. A tearful elder client presents at a mental health clinic for an initial evaluation accompanied by her daughter. The nurse has reviewed the health care records from the primary health care provider, remarkable for a "history of somatization" and "several episodes of depression." The client's daughter informs the nurse that the client has been sleeping more lately and is "always tearful" when awake, reporting that she "has no energy." The nurse decides to ask several questions before she attempts to complete the lengthy, holistic assessment form. Which of the following questions are essential to address? (Select all that apply.)
1. "How did this current problem start?"
2. "You've never had this before, correct?"
3. "What type of health insurance do you have?"
4. "What other changes have you experienced recently?"
5. "What has it been like for you in the past when you experienced sadness and body complaints?"

6. A 75-year-old client presenting with cognitive changes is prescribed citalopram (Celexa). The client's adult child asks the nurse, "Does this look like depression or dementia to you?" Which of the following is the nurse's best response?
1. "Cognitive changes can be associated with depression, dementia, and other medical, nonpsychiatric conditions. Your parent may respond well to this intervention."
2. "This medication will help, whether it is depression or dementia."
3. "Has your parent had episodes of depression in the past?"
4. "We will not know until your parent tries the medication."

7. An elder nursing home client, a war veteran and career military man, has alcoholic encephalopathy with short-term memory impairment and diabetes. One month ago, he had bilateral below-the-knee amputations. The client initiated a cutoff from his family 20 years ago. He is angry and irritable around most other residents. Which of the following group activities is he initially most likely to find pleasurable? (Select all that apply.)
1. Current Events, during which residents discuss world, state, and local news
2. Animal Afternoon, during which residents interact with certified therapy animals
3. Time Line, during which residents make collages for each decade of life
4. Music Night, during which a stage band plays requests from the residents
5. Here and Now, during which residents assist each other in reality orientation

8. A family member states, "My mother wants to know the benefits of going to adult day care rather than staying home with me. I could not answer, because I know nothing about adult day care." Which of the following should the nurse include in her response? (Select all that apply.)
1. "Some adult day care facilities offer respite services so that your mother could stay overnight once in a while to ease your burden."
2. "Attending an adult day care would give her something to anticipate each day and would provide a schedule with structure."
3. "If you have a particular adult day care in mind, it might be worth scheduling a visit to see what it is like."
4. "It could free you up so that you would have more energy to interact with her when she is home with you."
5. "She would have the opportunity to meet other people and engage in activities that you do not do at home."

9. A psychiatric nursing home resident says to another nurse, "Most of the other residents are a lot older than I am, and a lot sicker than I am. Is that just what happens when you get older?" Which of the following is the nurse's best initial response?
1. "Everybody is here for a different reason."
2. "They are not that much older than you, and they are not sicker than you."
3. "Everyone ages a little differently, but there are very few changes to the mind that are associated with age alone."
4. "Just concentrate on taking good care of yourself."

10. In the shift-to-shift report, a nurse reports a client's recent behavior change. In the emergency room 36 hours ago, the client was described as "oriented x 4, clear, coherent, and organized." Currently, the client is agitated and fearful, repeating incessantly, "My brain is being eaten by worms." A nursing assistant responds, "What do you expect? This client is 95!" Which of the following is the nurse's best initial response?
1. "That change has nothing to do with age. When the client changes that dramatically in a short period of time, there is something really wrong with that client."
2. "If it were just due to age, the client would not have been so clear in the emergency room."
3. "The client probably has too much sensory stimuli in the hospital room."
4. "It's probably an adjustment disorder with depression."

See Appendix C for answers.

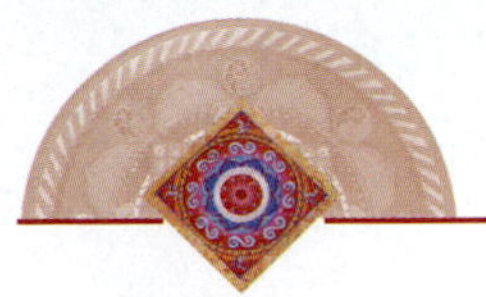

REFERENCES

American Psychiatric Association. (2000). *Diagnostic and statistical manual of mental disorders* (4th ed., Text Revision). Washington, DC: Author.

Baker, M. W. (2007). Elder mistreatment: Risk, vulnerability, and early mortality. *Journal of the American Psychiatric Nurses Association, 12*, 313–321.

Barba, B. E., Barba, J. R., & Rankin, C. (2007). Caring for older adults in the radiology department. Are you prepared? *Journal of Radiology Nursing, 26*(1), 11–14.

Bergstom, M. J., & Holmes, M. E. (2000). Lay theories of successful aging after the death of a spouse—review. *Health Communication, 12*, 377–406.

Blazer, D. G. (2007). Religious beliefs, practices and mental health outcomes: What is the research question? *American Journal of Geriatric Psychiatry, 15*(4), 269–272.

Blow, F. C., Serras, A. M., & Barry, K. L. (2007). Late-life depression and alcoholism. *Current Psychiatry Reports, 9*(1), 14–19.

Cappellano, K. L. (2007). Connecting your senior clients to Web health and nutrition resources. *Nutrition Today, 42*(3), 139–142.

Chan, S. S., Lyness, J. M., & Conwell, Y. (2007). Do cerebrovascular risk factors confer risk for suicide in later life? A case-control study. *American Journal of Geriatric Psychiatry, 15*(6), 541–544.

Chiriboga, D. A., Jang, Y., Banks, S., & Kim, G. (2007). Acculturation and its effect on depressive symptom structure in a sample of Mexican American elders. *Hispanic Journal of Behavioral Sciences, 29*(1), 83–100.

Crewe, S. E. (2007). Joy of living: A community-based mental health promotion program for African American elders. *Journal of Gerontological Social Work, 48*(3–4), 421–438.

Crighton, M. H., & Puppione, A. A. (2006). Geriatric neutrophils: Implications for older adults. *Seminars in Oncology Nursing, 22*(1), 3–9.

Dyck , M. J., Culp, K., & Cacchione, P. Z. (2007). Data quality strategies in cohort studies: Lessons from a study on delirium in nursing home elders. *Applied Nursing Research, 20*(1), 39–43.

Gallagher-Thompson, D., & Coon, D. W. (2007). Evidence-based psychological treatments for distress in family caregivers of older adults. *Psychology & Aging, 22*(1), 37–51.

Gao, X., Nelson, M. E., & Tucker, K. L. (2007). Television viewing is associated with prevalence of metabolic syndrome in Hispanic elders. *Diabetes Care, 30*(3), 694–700.

Gerdner, L. A., Yang, D., Cha, D., & Tripp-Reimer, T. (2007). The circle of life. *Journal of Gerontological Nursing, 33*(5), 20–31.

Glowacki, J. (2007). Vitamin D inadequacy in 2007: What it is and how to manage it. *Current Opinion in Orthopedics, 18*(5), 480–485.

Grigg-Damberger, M. (2007). Normal sleep: Impact of age, circadian rhythms, and sleep debt. *CONTINUUM: Lifelong Learning in Neurology, 13*(3), 31–84.

Gum, A. M., Arean, P. A., & Bostrom, A. (2007). Low-income depressed older adults with psychiatric comorbidity: Secondary analyses of response to psychotherapy and case management. *International Journal of Geriatric Psychiatry, 22*(2), 124–130.

Hudson, J., Hiripi, E., Pope, H., & Kessler, R. (2007). The prevalence and correlates of eating disorders in the National Comorbidity Survey Replication. *Biological Psychiatry, 61*(3), 348–358.

Ito, M., Takahashi, R., & Liehr, P. (2007). Heeding the behavioral message of elders with dementia in day care. *Holistic Nursing Practice, 21*(1), 12–18.

Jenko, M., Gonzalez, L., & Seymour, M. J. (2007). Life review with the terminally ill. *Journal of Hospice & Palliative Nursing, 9*(3), 159–167.

Joint Commission. (2007). *Hospital accreditation standards*. Oakbrook, IL: Author.

Kondo, D. G., Speer, M. C., Krishnan, K., Ranga, M. B., McQuoid, D. R., Slifer, S. H., et al. (2007). Association of AGTR1 with 18-month treatment outcome in late-life depression. *American Journal of Geriatric Psychiatry, 15*(7), 564–572.

Lang, I., Guralnik, J., Wallace, R. B., & Melzer, D. (2007). What level of alcohol consumption is hazardous for older people? Functioning and mortality in U.S. and English national cohorts. *Journal of the American Geriatrics Society, 55*(1), 49–57.

McGrath, P., & Patton, M. A. (2007). Indigenous understanding of hospice and palliative care: Findings from an Australian study. *Journal of Hospice & Palliative Nursing, 9*(4), 189–197.

Miller, M. D., & Reynolds, C. F. III (2007). Expanding the usefulness of interpersonal psychotherapy (IPT) for depressed elders with co-morbid cognitive impairment. *International Journal of Geriatric Psychiatry, 22*(2), 101–105.

Moyle, W., & Evans, K. (2007). Models of mental health care for older adults: A review of the literature. *International Journal of Older People Nursing, 2*(2), 132–140, 149.

Muravchick, S. (2003). Physiological changes of aging. *ASA Refresher Courses in Anesthesiology, 31*(1), 139–149.

Neal-Boylan, L. (2007). Health assessment of the very old person at home. *Home Healthcare Nurse, 25*(6), 388–398.

Onyike, C. U., Sheppard, J. E., Tschanz, J. T., Norton, M. C., Green, R. C., Steinberg, M., et al. (2007). Epidemiology of apathy in older adults: The Cache County study. *American Journal of Geriatric Psychiatry, 15*(5), 365–375.

Peters, A. (2007). A world of difference. *Nursing Older People, 19*(4), 12–14.

Piechniczekbuczek, J. (2007). Psychiatric emergencies in the elderly population. *Emergency Medicine Clinics of North America, 24*(2), 467–490.

Roriz-Cruz, M., Rosset, I., Wada, T., Sakagami, T., Ishine, M., Roriz-Filho, J. S., et al. (2007). Stroke-independent association between metabolic syndrome and functional dependence, depression, and low quality of life in elderly community-dwelling Brazilian people. *Journal of the American Geriatrics Society, 55*(3), 374–382.

Salman, A., McCabe, D., Easter, T., Callahan, B., Goldstein, D., Smith, T. D., et al. (2007). Cultural competence among staff nurses who participated in a family-centered geriatric care program. *Journal for Nurses in Staff Development, 23*(3), 103–111.

Signorile, J. F., Sandler, D., Ma, F., Bamel, S., Stanziano, D., Smith, W., et al. (2007). The Gallon-Jug Shelf-Transfer Test: An instrument to evaluate deteriorating function in older adults. *Journal of Aging and Physical Activity, 15*(1), 56–74.

Thompson, S. (2007). Spirituality and old age. *Illness, Crisis & Loss, 15*(2), 167–178.

Trigoboff, E., Wilson, B. A., Shannon, M. T., & Stang, C. L. (2005). *Psychiatric drug guide*. Upper Saddle River, NJ: Prentice Hall.

U.S. Census Bureau. (2000). *Sixty-five plus in the United States*. Statistical brief. Washington, DC: U.S. Department of Commerce, Economic and Statistics Administration.

Werner, P., Tabak, N., Albert, R., & Bergman, R. (2002). Interventions used by nursing staff members with psychogeriatric patients resisting care. *International Journal of Nursing Studies, 39*(4), 461–467.

Yaffe, K., Blackwell, T., Barnes, D. E., Ancoli-Israel, S., & Stone, K. L. (2007). For the Study of Osteoporotic Fractures Group: Preclinical cognitive decline and subsequent sleep disturbance in older women. *Neurology, 69*(3), 237–242.

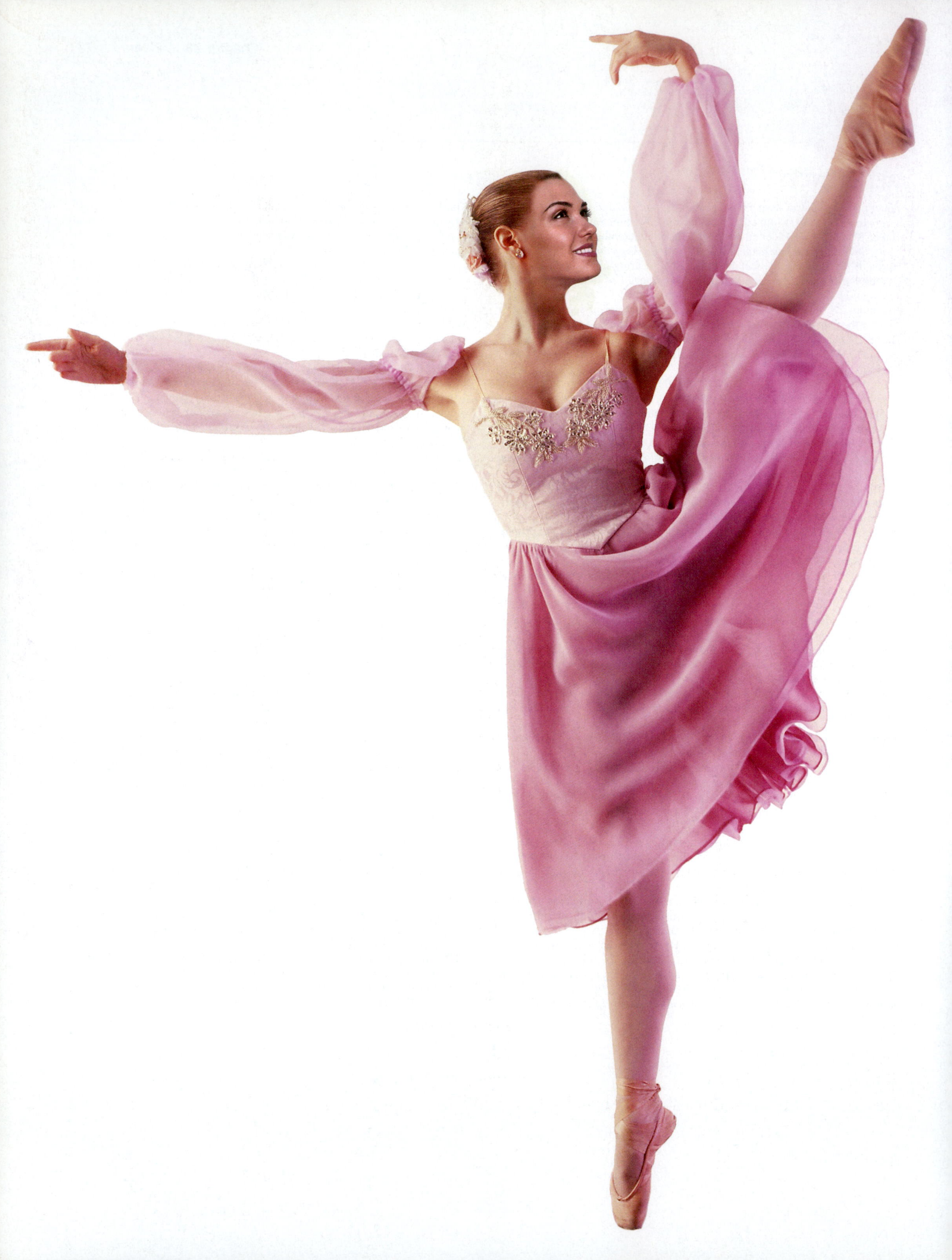

Unit 6

INTERVENTION STRATEGIES AND OUTCOMES

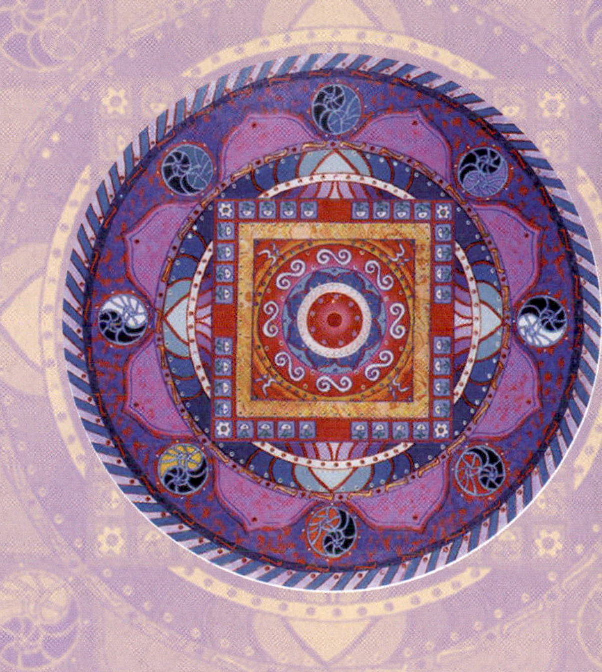

GALINA, a prima ballerina for the Kirov Ballet in St. Petersburg, Russia, is in dress rehearsal for the part of Maria in the ballet *The Nutcracker.* A graduate of the prestigious Vaganova Ballet Academy in St. Petersburg, Galina is known for her matchless precision, elegance, and technical excellence. She has danced major roles in acclaimed productions of *Swan Lake, Giselle,* and *Orpheus and Eurydice.* Galina worries about her brother, Aleksandr. He is being treated for heroin addiction in St. Petersburg, where drug users' names are listed in a government registry, they receive extreme sedation during withdrawal from heroin, psychological support is minimal or nonexistent, prescribing oral medications such as methadone or buprenorphine to reduce dependence is illegal, and 90–100% of addicts return to illicit drugs. Rather than sparking a reexamination of this approach to treatment, the length of internment for heroin addicts like Aleksandr has been increased. Our mental health interventions must reflect the capacity to respond creatively to the challenges, vulnerabilities, and strengths in the global community based on evidence and cultural competence.

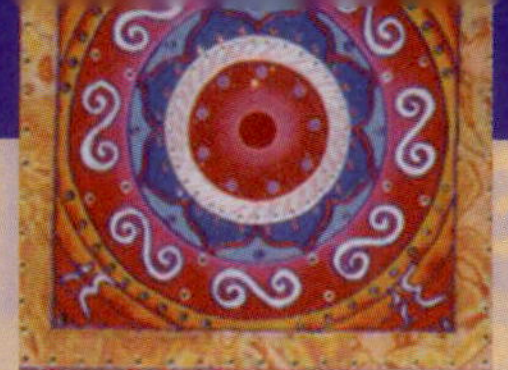

CHAPTER

29

Counseling the Individual

BETH MOSCATO
EILEEN TRIGOBOFF

KEY TERMS

LEARNING OUTCOMES

After completing this chapter, you will be able to:

1. Explain the common shared characteristics of one–to–one relationships.
2. Encourage the client's systematic use of abilities and behaviors most often associated with growth-producing outcomes.
3. Analyze how phenomena such as resistance, transference, countertransference, critical distance, gift giving, the use of touch, and the values held by both client and nurse affect the therapeutic relationship.
4. Incorporate an understanding of the three phases of the therapeutic nurse–client relationship and the main objectives and therapeutic tasks of each phase into one–to–one work with clients.
5. Apply the nursing process to the three phases of the nurse–client relationship.
6. Establish and maintain one–to–one relationships within the context of the client's cultural background.

CRITICAL THINKING CHALLENGE

You have just met with your first psychiatric–mental health client to develop a therapeutic nurse–client relationship. Despite your best efforts, your client, Sammy, gave you "a hard time." There were long periods of silence broken by angry and explosive statements about your abilities. You are uncertain whether Sammy will meet with you again.

1. What are your ideas about why Sammy behaved the way he did?
2. How might your feelings about Sammy's behavior influence your performance as a nursing student?
3. What steps can you take to deal with this first contact and the uncertainty of subsequent contacts with this client?

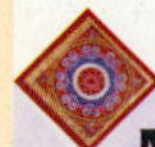

MEDIALINK 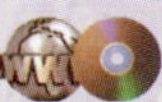 www.prenhall.com/kneisl

Go to the Pearson Health MediaLink CD-ROM and the Companion Website at www.prenhall.com/kneisl for interactive resources for this chapter.

In the 21st century, psychiatric–mental health nursing continues to expand its neuropsychiatric focus. There has been an explosion of knowledge concerning the neurobiologic basis of mental illness, in diagnostic technology, and in the discovery of newer and better psychopharmacologic approaches (see Chapters 7 and 32) that has moved us toward a neuropsychiatric paradigm of care. A neuropsychiatric paradigm is less stigmatizing and allows treatment to reach more people than a psychosocial view alone. At the same time that clients may have their needs for safety, structure, and medication met, they may also express their longing for a deeper connection to mental health staff and more insight-oriented treatment. The real time constraints on our practice in the current health care environment present an additional factor that determines how well we connect with clients: Is there enough time? The challenge for us is to integrate both biologic and psychosocial concepts while maintaining our nursing focus on caring. The therapeutic nurse–client relationship provides the opportunity to meet this challenge.

The **therapeutic nurse–client relationship**, also called the one–to–one relationship, is one in which the nurse uses theoretical understandings, personal attributes, and appropriate clinical techniques such as those in Figure 29-1 ■ to provide the opportunity for a corrective emotional experience for clients. It has evolved as the cornerstone of psychiatric–mental health nursing theory and practice, largely based on nearly five decades of work by Hildegard Peplau. Memorial tributes to Peplau upon her death in 1999 by nurses around the world recognized her as the "mother of psychiatric nursing" (Barker, 1999). Her theory of interpersonal relations in nursing, including the stages of the nurse–client relationship, was the basis for psychotherapeutic nursing (Peplau, 1952, 1997).

We are challenged to creatively adapt the time-honored principles of Peplau's work under changing conditions such as the brevity of inpatient psychiatric treatment and the increase in outpatient and community treatment. The current health care economic climate, with its focus on managed care, has changed the face of the traditional therapeutic nurse–client relationship advocated by Peplau. Nevertheless, we incorporate the principles in our everyday work—brief encounters as well as consistent long-term relationships.

This chapter demystifies the characteristics, processes, phases, and problems of one–to–one relationships so that beginning psychiatric–mental health nurses can approach them with increased awareness of their own interpersonal effectiveness. Practical guidelines on how to facilitate interpersonal effectiveness with clients are included. The principles, processes, and phases discussed in this chapter also apply to family, group, and community interventions or therapies.

THE ONE–TO–ONE RELATIONSHIP

The one–to–one relationship between psychiatric–mental health nurse and client is a mutually defined, collaborative, and goal-oriented professional relationship. It may be viewed as a series of sequential nurse–client interactions with the following additional elements:

- The interactions occur over a designated period of time (daily, weekly, monthly).

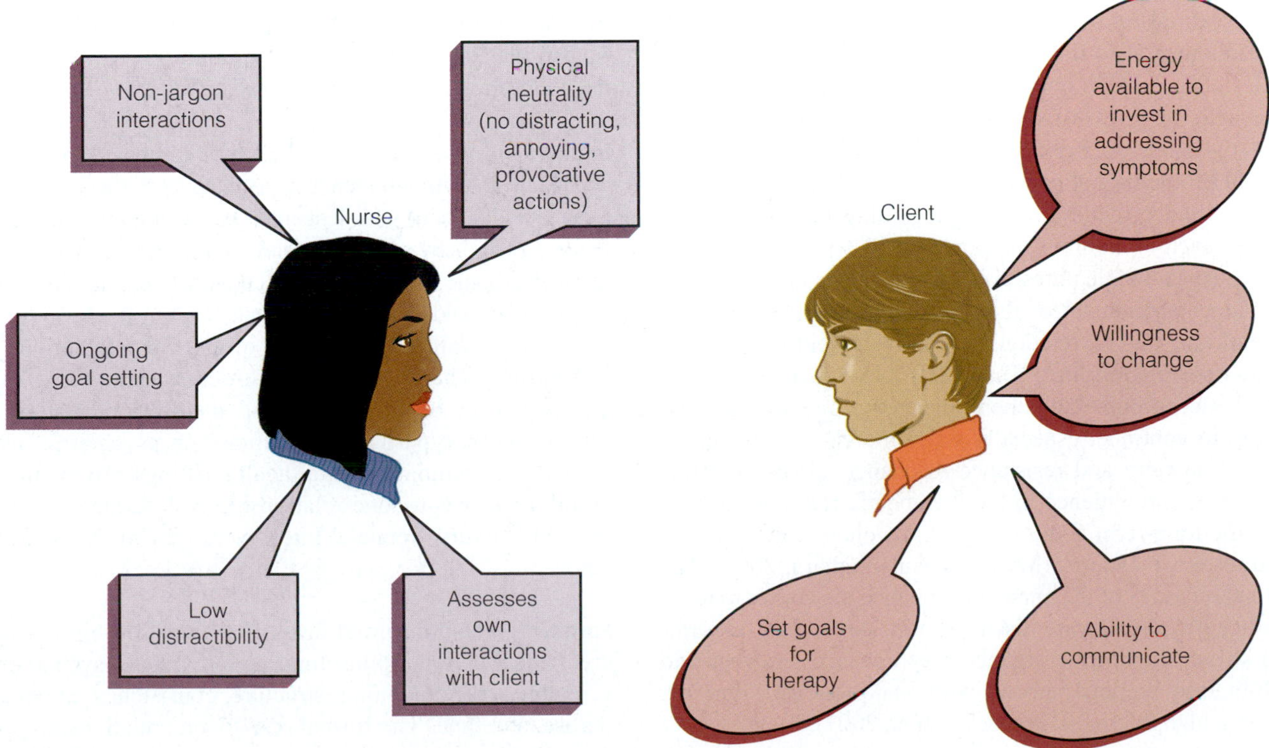

Figure 29-1 ■ Nurse and client characteristics that enhance the one–to–one therapeutic relationship.

- The interactions take place in a unique nurse–client structure, characterized by specific phases, processes, and problems.
- The interactions occur in a designated setting that tends to remain stable over time (home, private practice office, mental health clinic, inpatient psychiatric unit, medical unit).

A one–to–one relationship has three distinct phases:

1. The orientation (beginning) phase, characterized by the establishment of contact with the client
2. The working (middle) phase, characterized by the maintenance and analysis of contact
3. The termination (end) phase, characterized by the termination of contact with the client. Each phase of a one–to–one relationship is distinguished by important goals and therapeutic tasks, discussed in detail in the nursing process section of the chapter.

Shorter hospital stays for inpatient clients change the timing of, and expectations for, the inpatient one–to–one relationship. Although the components themselves do not change, the schedule will. Inform the inpatient client of the brevity of the length of the relationship. Announce the time frame during the beginning phase, and reinforce it throughout the other phases, so it does not come as a surprise when the termination phase arrives.

Therapeutic Alliance

The major task and overriding characteristic of the one–to–one relationship is the creation of a therapeutic alliance between nurse and client. The **therapeutic alliance** is a conscious relationship between a facilitative person and a client. It is fundamental to the process of making adaptive change (Ford, 2007). In this process, the nurse forms a mature alliance with the growth-facilitating aspects of the client. Each implicitly agrees to work together to help the client address personal problems and concerns. More specifically, the nurse identifies and provides feedback regarding the client's patterns of reaction, abilities, and potentials. The client can use these assets to handle unresolved problems constructively.

The establishment of the therapeutic alliance enhances informal one–to–one relationships and is essential in formal one–to–one relationships (Gary, 2007). Such a binding alliance between nurse and client allows the one–to–one relationship to continue, especially when the client experiences increased anxiety and resistance to change. Investing time, persistence, and patience in the therapeutic relationship promotes the long-term goal of helping the client change established response patterns (Mynatt & Cunningham, 2007). The personal qualities of the nurse that enhance the ability to forge a therapeutic alliance are discussed in Chapter 3. Forming a strong therapeutic alliance may enhance recovery and rehabilitation among persons with major mental illnesses such as schizophrenia (Davis & Lysaker, 2007).

MediaLink Application: Therapeutic Alliance

Cultural Context

Because cultural context influences nursing care, a sensitive and systematic consideration of the client's cultural and ethnic background is an essential part of the psychiatric nursing process in one–to–one relationship work. Cultural forces shape the expression of distress and the formation of symptoms (Mackin, Targum, Kalali, Rom, & Young, 2007). Culture also influences the client's expectations of the nurse–client relationship and the client's interpretations of the events that take place within it. The nurse consistently evaluates the influence of culture within the one–to–one relationship as well as the effects of the therapeutic relationship on the client's values and life experiences. General considerations of cultural diversity are interwoven throughout this chapter and are further described in Chapter 9.

Characteristics

In addition to having three distinct phases, discussed later in this chapter, the therapeutic nurse–client relationship has several specific, inherent characteristics.

Professional

One–to–one relationships reflect a professional, rather than a social, relationship. Psychiatric–mental health nurses use their personalities, interpersonal skills and techniques, and theoretic knowledge of psychiatric–mental health nursing practice in a purposeful, goal-directed manner to facilitate a useful change in their client's lives. This professional relationship differs from a social relationship in several significant ways. Table 29-1 ■ summarizes the major differences between professional and social relationships.

A professional one–to–one relationship can be either informal or formal. Spontaneous, informal nurse–client relationships are at one end of the continuum, and formal individual counseling or psychotherapy is at the other end.

Informal Informal nurse–client relationships may be prearranged and planned, but more often they occur spontaneously— between a nurse and a client with leukemia, between a nurse and an offender in jail, between a nurse and a high-risk pregnant woman, between a home care nurse and a client with emphysema, or between a nurse and a psychiatric client.

These relationships consist of a set of interactions limited in time. There is minimum structure and a sense of immediacy. They occur in numerous medical and nonmedical settings and are particularly common in psychiatric institutions and community mental health settings. An example of an informal one–to–one relationship is described in the feature What Every Neonatal Intensive Care Unit Nurse Should Know.

Formal The more formal one–to–one relationship is used in crisis intervention, counseling, or individual psychotherapy. It requires more planning, structure, consistency, nursing expertise, and time. The formal one–to–one relationship occurs

Table 29-1 ■ Differences Between Professional and Social Relationships

Characteristic	Professional Relationship	Social Relationship
Purpose	Systematic working-through of troublesome thoughts, feelings, and behaviors	Companionship, pleasure, sharing of interests
	Planned evaluation (through stages)	Evolves spontaneously
Role delineation	Roles for nurse and client with explicit use of psychiatric nursing skills and interventions	Generally not present, except for broad social norms governing the particular type of relationship (friend versus lover)
Satisfaction of needs	Client is encouraged to identify, develop, and assess ways to meet own needs more effectively	Mutual sharing and satisfaction of personal and interpersonal needs
	Does not address personal needs of the nurse	
Time frame	Usually time-limited interactions with an expected termination	Usually not time limited, in either duration or frequency of contact
		No planned termination

in various psychiatric settings, including psychiatric institutions, community mental health centers, and private practice.

The choice and effectiveness of informal or formal relationships depend on:

- The client's level of functioning
- The psychiatric–mental health nurse's current abilities and skills
- To some degree, the time that is available to both participants

High levels of symptoms can compromise the client's level of functioning, and thus the ability to establish a formal relationship. If a one–to–one relationship already exists when symptoms exacerbate, your therapeutic interactions must be skilled and flexible enough to change your pace and expectations (Stanton, 2007). When the goal of the therapeutic relationship is to promote major changes in emotional states, the client must be able to participate in a focused and abstract effort (Smith & Greenberg, 2007). The nurse must be an expert partner in achieving that goal. The amount of time a client may have available to establish a one–to–one formal relationship can be contingent on a variety of circumstances. If the client has made a commitment to address a main source of discomfort or distress, ancillary issues may need to be tabled. The client's health care insurance resources may restrict access to mental health care services. A reality of health care, particularly mental health care, is the time frame imposed from without, often without a surplus of options.

Table 29-2 ■ on page 778 highlights the similarities and differences of informal and formal relationship work. The differences are discussed throughout this chapter.

Mutually Defined

A one–to–one relationship is mutually defined by the two participants. Both psychiatric–mental health nurse and client voluntarily enter the relationship and specify the conditions under which it is to evolve. For example, the client may seek immediate alleviation of symptoms rather than long-term individual psychotherapy. Nurse and client identify together where and when they will meet and other conditions of their participation. This contractual aspect of the one–to–one relationship is explored further in the discussion of the beginning (orientation) phase of therapy later in the chapter. Once the

WHAT EVERY NEONATAL INTENSIVE CARE UNIT NURSE SHOULD KNOW

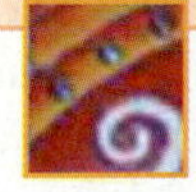

The Therapeutic Relationship with Parents of a Premature Infant

When an infant has been born prematurely or has physical problems upon birth (such as low birth weight) the infant may be placed in a neonatal intensive care nursery (NICU). The infant's parents may develop a relationship with the NICU nurse involved in their infant's care. As a NICU nurse, you will need to know how to respond to the demands of this one–to–one relationship.

Emotions can run high in the NICU as the infant's health fluctuates. Crises and chronicity blend in an unusual manner. Your ability to act as a liaison between the medical system and the parents throughout the infant's tenure in the NICU will likely take place within a one–to–one relationship. You will incorporate a number of one–to–one strategies when you work with parents: recognizing and respecting the boundaries of the therapeutic relationship, acknowledging how the parents' anxiety affects communication with their infant as well as the NICU staff, adjusting the speed and volume of your information sharing so as not to overwhelm the stressed adults, and discussing the emotional tone the parents have while interacting with their infant. You can use the information in this chapter, specifically information about the therapeutic alliance, cultural context, and goal-directed behaviors, to shape how you proceed.

TABLE 29-2 ■ **Similarities and Differences of Informal and Formal One–to–One Relationships**

Characteristic	Informal Relationship	Formal Relationship
Setting	Varied	Generally psychiatric settings
Frequency and duration of contact	Flexible, depending on client need or tolerance; example: short, frequent intervals daily	Structured; example: once weekly, with possible crisis sessions; duration usually set at 30 minutes or 1 hour
Duration of relationship	May or may not involve time commitment Generally a few days to a few weeks	Involves time commitment: weeks to months, for short-term work; months to years, for long-term work
Type of dysfunction	In general, more effective with severe dysfunction	In severe dysfunction, may be useful after client is stabilized on medication
Use of therapeutic contract	May involve simple therapeutic contract	Utilizes therapeutic contract; the more specific, the better
Fees	Usually not relevant	May be relevant; may be part of therapeutic contract
Degree of skill required	Nursing student or psychiatric nurse	Advanced degree beneficial but not essential
Degree of supervision	Some degree and type of supervision always necessary	Consistent supervision or consultation usually necessary
Degree of effectiveness	Depends on client's level of functioning, skills of the psychiatric–mental health nurse, and time allotment	Depends on client's level of functioning, skills of the psychiatric–mental health nurse, and time allotment

one–to–one relationship is established, its maintenance depends on the commitment of both participants.

Collaborative

Both participants enter a relationship in which goals, strategies, and outcomes evolve within the context of the therapeutic work together. Mutual collaboration implies that each participant brings personal abilities, capabilities, and power to the relationship. Thus, the psychiatric–mental health nurse does not assume responsibility for client behaviors but actively works with the client to assess the self-defeating and growth-promoting aspects of specific behaviors.

The client is in charge of change following a joint assessment of problematic behaviors and emotional states (Huss & Baer, 2007). Working in concert with a nursing professional in a therapeutic alliance has the added effect of supporting psychological well-being by crafting healthy interdependence (Steelman, 2007). Mutual collaboration also means that nurses assess and are accountable for their own behavior with clients. Ongoing supervision often helps the nurse meet these particular goals.

Goal-Directed

A therapeutic nurse–client relationship is always goal directed. The client is expected to identify and achieve specific physical, emotional, and social goals within the context of the relationship. Client goals vary widely in type and depth. For example, in informal relationship work a client's goal may be to initiate one peer relationship within an inpatient psychiatric unit. Other examples include resolution of a divorce involving children and shared personal possessions, or coming to terms with the client's impending death. Often the client's initial goal is to solve an immediate problem, and this serves as a basis for establishing more extensive psychosocial goals.

The psychiatric–mental health nurse also formulates therapeutic goals to enhance the growth-producing elements of the relationship. Inpatient clients with serious symptomatology may have difficulty connecting and modifying behaviors in the time allotted. Goals that can be worked on in the future and in various settings are more likely to be achieved.

Open

The one–to–one relationship between nurse and client may be viewed as an experience in *shared dignity*. The psychiatric–mental health nurse adapts to allow clients to reveal their humanness freely and openly. Each aspect of the nurse's verbal and nonverbal behavior either encourages or inhibits clients from being open themselves. The Evidence-Based Practice feature shows how one nurse demonstrated openness using several interventions to encourage a client to discuss a difficult topic.

Negotiated

In the one–to–one relationship, the client is an active decision maker and is personally accountable for the work. The atmosphere of give-and-take within the relationship emphasizes mutuality, reciprocity, and interpersonal fairness. Establishing a clearly defined, mutually agreed-upon therapeutic contract represents a prime example of negotiation in one–to–one work. (The therapeutic contract is covered later in the chapter.)

Committed

Commitment is based on the therapeutic contract between nurse and client. The contract establishes the limits of the relationship as well as the time and energy allotted to it. At some point in the relationship, the nurse is confronted by the reality of the client's dysfunction. Because of personal discomfort, the beginning psychiatric–mental health nurse

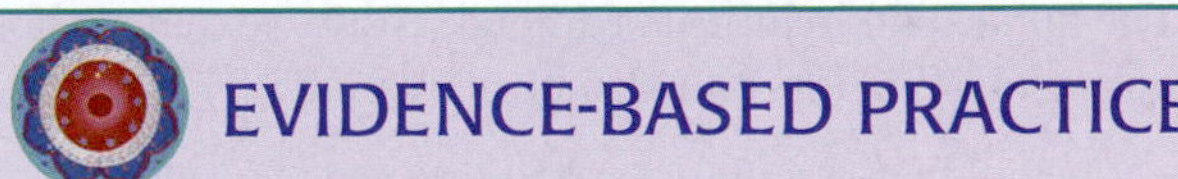

PREGNANCY AND ANTIDEPRESSANTS

Sharon is a 25-year-old with a history of depression. She is currently pregnant and is wondering if she should continue taking antidepressant medications during her pregnancy or stop and risk having her symptoms return. Sharon has been discussing her concerns with you and the rest of the team during her prenatal care appointments. She has not discussed them with anyone besides her health care providers, as she is afraid of what they might say.

During your one–to–one interactions with Sharon, you state your concern for her welfare and assure her that her concerns will be discussed on a regular basis. You tell her that you and she will work on a solution together as you have in the past with other problems.

The one–to–one relationship maintained in this situation has a positive effect on Sharon's ability to discuss a difficult topic. You remain available, without withdrawing, despite Sharon's distress, fears, or silence. You promote trust by stating your concern for Sharon's welfare and offering to discuss the issue together. Your nursing intervention should be based on more than one study, but the research cited below would be helpful in this case.

O'Brien, L., Schachtschneider, A. M., Koren, G., Walker, J. H., & Einarson, A. (2007). Longitudinal study of depression, anxiety, irritability, and stress in pregnancy following evidence-based counseling on the use of antidepressants. *Journal of Psychiatric Practice, 13*(1), 33–39.

CRITICAL THINKING APPLICATION

1. If antidepressants have even an unlikely potential to affect the baby, should Sharon stop taking them?
2. Should women who take psychotropic medications avoid pregnancy?
3. Why is it important that Sharon's depressive symptoms do not return?

may respond by actively colluding with the client to deny or ignore the dysfunction and remain on a superficial, social level of communication. This collusion protects the nurse from having to address the client's helplessness, desperation, hostility, or raw grief. The nurse who does not let the client express these feelings is not sufficiently committed to the client.

The opposite is also nontherapeutic. The overcommitted psychiatric–mental health nurse may assume an omnipotent or rescuer role to "cure" the client. This role robs the client of active decision-making power and accountability.

The client will test the nurse's commitment in some phase of the relationship. Both nurse and client need to deal with this test explicitly on verbal and nonverbal levels. A sense of positive connectedness with the client strengthens the sense of commitment.

PHENOMENA OCCURRING IN ONE–TO–ONE RELATIONSHIPS

Sometimes you may initially feel a sense of unease or confusion about what is happening in the nurse–client therapeutic relationship. This uneasiness may be difficult to identify, describe, and explore. Remember to keep the following phenomena in mind when you are attempting to "make sense" of a one–to–one relationship.

Resistance

Resistance refers to all the phenomena that interfere with and disrupt the smooth flow of feelings, memories, and thoughts. It inevitably surfaces in the course of psychotherapeutic work and most often occurs as the client begins to address self-defeating thoughts, feelings, and behaviors.

Resistance is often mistakenly seen as the client's struggle against the nurse. Instead, the client is struggling against the anxiety associated with change, against self-awareness, and against responsibility for actions (Smith & Greenberg, 2007). Be aware of the tendency to react adversely to client resistance and make the effort to use it to propel the client toward growth. Although the client's behavior patterns may have self-defeating aspects, they have also provided some satisfaction to the client or prevented some discomfort (Epstein et al., 2007). The client may also resist giving up a defense that offered protection from the anxiety associated with unbearable thoughts and impulses. Thus, resistance in therapeutic one–to–one relationships is best understood as the client's struggle against change.

Manifestations

In general, you may suspect resistance when the client's behavior appears to block the progress of the relationship. Resistance is usually expressed in five different forms (Messer, 2002):

1. Resistance to the recognition of feelings, fantasies, and motives
2. Resistance to revealing feelings toward the nurse or therapist
3. Resistance as a way of demonstrating self-sufficiency
4. Resistance as the client's reluctance to change behavior outside of the nurse–client relationship
5. Resistance as a result of the failure of empathy on the part of the nurse or therapist

You must exercise caution in evaluating a client's behavior as resistive. There may be other explanations for the emotional atmosphere in the one–to–one interaction. The client's silence may indicate pensiveness, a pause before emotive expression, or a sense of completion. The client who is habitually late may have real difficulties adjusting a full personal schedule to accommodate the sessions. Resistance to specific topics or concerns may indicate that the client is not ready for investigative work. Likewise, the client may resist giving up a defense because it is desperately needed to keep anxiety about a present situation at manageable levels.

Remember that the client has a right to resist one aspect of, or the entire, therapeutic process as a matter of choice. However, the client's resistive behavior should be openly discussed, rather than ignored.

Acting Out

Acting out is a particularly destructive form of resistance in which the client puts into action (that is, "acts out") emotional conflicts. It is important to recognize that the client is externalizing an inner conflict to people in the immediate environment.

Rather than verbalizing conflicts or feelings, the client displays inappropriate behaviors. Examples of acting out include forcefully slamming a door, dressing provocatively, or slapping someone. In acting out, the client acts toward a mate, friend, relative, or other person those feelings and attitudes that the client does not express toward the nurse. An example of acting out is developing third-person relationships to absorb the emotions and fantasies that belong in the therapeutic relationship. Exaggerated feelings of intense hostility toward the nurse may lead to violence or physical harm to the client, nurse, or the third person. Intense feelings of love for the nurse or therapist may precipitate an affair or marriage with the third person.

Acting out contains a vital seed for change. That is, it can form the basis for the client's understanding of, and eventual giving up of, destructive and inappropriate behaviors. The one–to–one therapeutic relationship can transform a client's acting out (for example, rageful behaviors) into adaptive emotions and behaviors by facilitating change (Smith & Greenberg, 2007). Acting out is difficult to deal with because the client does not talk about the feelings that precipitate the behavior and later tends to conceal or rationalize the behavior. Acting out can abruptly disrupt treatment, unless it is identified and dealt with explicitly.

Specific nursing interventions relating to acting out include the following:

- Bring acting out to the attention of the client.
- Encourage the client to *talk about* impulses rather than to act them out.
- Encourage identification of feelings *before* putting them into action.
- Increase frequency of contact.
- Look for evidence of transference phenomena toward the nurse.
- With repeated dangerous acting out, consider withdrawing from the relationship unless the client sets limits on these behaviors.

The nurse who manifests parental, erotic, sexual, or hostile nonverbal behaviors can also be acting out:

- Placing hands on hips or pointing a finger while setting limits on a client's behavior (parental)
- Patting a client on the shoulder and offering reassurance (parental)
- Dressing suggestively (erotic)
- Blushing and giggling when a client makes a sexual remark (sexual)
- Being sarcastic in response to a client's concern (hostile)

These behaviors by the nurse encourage acting out by the client.

Parental or caretaker behaviors that express the need to nurture the client are the most common among beginning psychiatric–mental health nurses. These behaviors may indicate a countertransference problem (discussed later in this chapter) for the nurse and discount the client's ability to ensure his or her own well-being. Recognition of acting out by the psychiatric–mental health nurse is essential and reinforces the need for formal supervision.

General Intervention Strategies

Several consecutive approaches are used as general nursing intervention strategies for resistance. They begin with the nurse's awareness of the resistance. Helpful intervention strategies include the following:

- Label the resistant behavior with the client. The nurse may allow the resistance to occur several times to demonstrate its presence to the client. It is as if the nurse were holding up a mirror for the client, reflecting and clarifying the specific resistant behavior.
- Explore the accompanying emotion and the history of its development.
- Explore what function the resistance may serve, especially any self-defeating aspects.
- Facilitate working through the resistance by fully understanding and appreciating its implications in the client's life.

This sequence may occur repeatedly before a resistant behavior is resolved.

Transference

Transference is a normal phenomenon that may surface and inhibit effectiveness in any phase of one–to–one relationship work and in any setting, including nonpsychiatric settings. **Transference** is a set of feelings and thoughts about significant others in the client's past and current life that is transferred to the caregiver. Transference can be considered a lens through which the client sees his or her relationships. Transference typically happens quickly, and generally unconsciously, in the therapeutic relationship (Boag, 2007). Therapeutic effectiveness requires working with transference issues within the client's cultural framework and developing options for the client to emote and behave adaptively in interpersonal relationships.

A study of early transference reactions (Beretta et al., 2007) noted that people tend to have a limited number of types of relationship patterns (parents, romantic, family, friendship, colleague, and impersonal). It is likely that clients will repeat their particular patterns with you and reenact the patterns they use outside the therapeutic relationship. The recognition of transference signals that it is time to explore this interaction. Expect that clients will have transference issues. Work collaboratively with clients, using the transference as a therapeutic tool, to foster adaptive and positive changes in their relationships.

Explore the meaning of individual words, gestures, events, and situations in the current one–to–one relationship to determine how these reflect or replay distortions in other past or current relationships. The therapeutic task is to separate feelings, thoughts, and behaviors that belong to the current one–to–one relationship from those that represent unresolved conflicts in other relationships.

Increasing awareness of the transference process often frees the client to work through conflicts and explore the more creative, self-actualizing aspects of personal identity as they evolve. You must not interact as the client's parent or any other transference figure. Rather, help the client bring an unconscious event into consciousness, to examine its cause and meaning. The following clinical example illustrates how transference may surface in a clinical setting.

CLINICAL EXAMPLE

Conrad Weber, hospitalized for depression, was assigned to a primary counselor, a male psychiatric–mental health nurse. Over the course of several meetings with his counselor, Conrad assumed a cowering, ingratiating manner. He seemed to resemble a little boy awaiting punishment from an intimidating, punitive father. This interpersonal orientation was observed by other male staff members who informally initiated interaction with Conrad on the unit.

The counselor chose not to explore Conrad's past relationships. The aim of short-term work was to focus on concrete ways to decrease depressed feelings in Conrad's present life situation. The counselor addressed ingratiating behaviors in the nurse–client relationship only when they had an adverse effect on their short-term work together.

In this example, the primary counselor chose to focus on present rather than past relationships in an effort to stabilize the hospitalized client. Transference may be dealt with in many ways, depending on the client's functioning, the counselor's theoretic orientation, and the type of therapy.

Positive Transference

Transference may be positive or negative. *Positive transference*—that is, positive feelings for the therapist—occurs when the client generally has had satisfying past relationships with significant others during childhood. The therapeutic relationship is usually able to progress in this instance.

Negative Transference

In *negative transference*, the client shows a number of reactions based on forms of hate (hostility, loathing, bitterness, contempt, annoyance). Although there are both positive and negative aspects to every transference, a predominantly negative transference is uncomfortable for client and nurse alike. The client does not like to be aware of and express this hate, and the nurse does not like to be the target of it. When negative transference appears unresolvable, it may be advisable to terminate the relationship work rather than run the risk of further client dysfunction.

Countertransference

While transference involves the client's reactions to the psychiatric nurse, **countertransference** involves the nurse's reactions to the client. The psychiatric–mental health nurse may develop powerful counterproductive fantasies, feelings, and attitudes in response to the client's transference or personality. Countertransference is now thought to be almost inevitable in psychotherapeutic situations (Ellis, 2001).

Countertransference is suspected when the nurse repeatedly assigns meaning to the nurse–client relationship that belongs to the nurse's other relationships. In countertransference, the psychiatric–mental health nurse's ability to assess nurse–client interactions becomes confused or thwarted by unresolved conflicts. Thus, the nurse may unconsciously use behaviors (as parent, sibling, lover, or friend) that attempt to replay in the current situation some conflict with significant others. Countertransference indicates unresolved conflict in the nurse. This conflict may be expressed in acts of omission or commission, and they may be covert or overt. Be alert for actions with clients that are out of line with standard expectations for professional psychiatric–mental health nursing care. The Your Self-Awareness feature includes cues to the presence of countertransference.

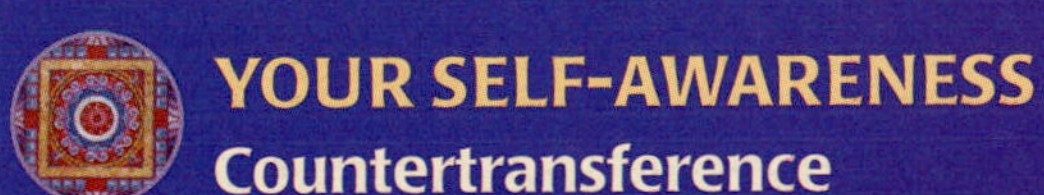

YOUR SELF-AWARENESS
Countertransference

Look for the following cues in your own behavior that signal the presence of countertransference:

- Irrational friendliness toward the client
- Irrational concern about the client
- Reacting with annoyance or irrational hostility toward the client
- Feeling uneasy during or after meeting with the client
- Dreaming about or fantasizing about the client
- Being preoccupied with thoughts of the client during leisure time
- Any actions that are out of line with standard expectations for therapist behaviors

Countertransference is a normal occurrence, requiring clinical supervision or consultation to prevent degeneration of the one–to–one relationship. Clinical supervision may enable the nurse to separate feelings, thoughts, and behaviors that belong to the current relationship from those that represent unfinished conflicts in other relationships.

It is reassuring that most countertransference problems can be resolved by self-assessment with professional supervision. Once the countertransference process is identified, the nurse can consciously develop therapeutic, goal-directed responses. Avoid self-disclosure of countertransference to clients. Sharing these feelings may overwhelm clients and burden them in a destructive way (Beretta et al., 2007). In rare instances, however, referral to another nurse is appropriate when the first nurse cannot control the disturbed attitudes and emotions.

Conflict Between Caretaker and Therapist Roles

Nurses may erect rigid defenses aimed at denying their personal feelings because of the emotional demands of nursing. For example, some procedures actually require the nurse to violate a client's emotional or physical state (injections, dressings). Defending against feelings becomes one way for the nurse to cope with inflicting pain on another person. You can deal effectively with the feelings of clients only to the extent that you explore your own personal feelings.

Continued assumption of the caretaker role also undermines your therapeutic effectiveness. The caretaker role tends to involve sympathy rather than empathy. The difference between these two responses is significant to therapeutic outcomes. How effective you are when you interact with a client in a one–to–one relationship is based on your intentions and emotions. The path of the relationship depends on your self-knowledge of these factors. Interpersonal boundaries such as accountability and sympathy versus empathy are discussed in Chapter 3.

A one–to–one relationship requires that you help the client actively explore the meaning underlying the client's personal pain, distress, or discomfort. Avoid the caretaker role in which you alleviate pain. Rather, encourage clients to develop ways to do so for themselves. Similarly, the caretaker role requires nurses to make decisions for clients. It does not encourage clients to be accountable for their own decisions.

Critical Distance

It is important to observe how the client uses physical space. Individual preferences as well as culture will dictate the specific distance between individuals, depending on the relationship between them. Psychiatric–mental health nurses allow physical distance between themselves and clients, especially early in a relationship. This distance promotes verbal communication and minimizes any existing anxiety and hostility. Moving rapidly toward closeness, especially in establishing the nurse–client relationship, may overwhelm the client and increase anxiety.

The physical distance between the psychiatric–mental health nurse and the client can be indicative of other therapeutic processes. For example, a client may sit in a chair at a great distance from you during initial meetings but move closer and closer as the working relationship is established. Assess the possible interpersonal implications of proximity (nearness) for each client. As the relationship progresses, assess whether physical distance or proximity reduces client anxiety. The client's need for critical distance during the therapeutic process usually increases as the client experiences panic or near-panic levels of anxiety. See Chapter 10 and Figure 10-3.

Gift Giving

The giving of gifts may be a special concern in therapeutic relationships. Gift giving may take various forms: a fleeting social amenity (the purchase of a cup of coffee), a gesture (the loan of a favorite book), or the presentation of a valued object (the giving of an original painting). Like self-disclosure (discussed in Chapter 3), gift giving in any instance must be met with ongoing assessment and evaluation to determine its form, intent, appropriateness, and meaning in the context of the therapeutic relationship (Shapiro & Ginzberg, 2002). Nurses from specialty areas other than psychiatry may have more leeway in this regard (Weeks, Cowell, Scullion, & Tanton, 2007). However, professional ethics and therapeutic integrity bar many but the most token of gifts. No rule covers all instances of gift giving. Several broad guidelines discussed in this section can help you evaluate each particular situation.

During Orientation Phase

During the orientation phase of a therapeutic relationship, the client may overtly offer or ask for a gift. This gesture may be as incidental as offering you (or asking for) a cigarette. Examine this overture, keeping in mind several possible motivations:

- The client may seek to bribe or manipulate you, thereby seeking to control the direction of the therapeutic relationship. (Chapter 22 deals with manipulation.)
- The client may seek to "buy" your time and attention.
- The client may ask for small gifts to reinforce a helpless, "take-care-of-me" interpersonal stance.
- Of course, the client may have no covert intent and may simply need a cigarette.

In the orientation phase, it may be helpful not to accept or give any gift you feel uncomfortable about. Explore the client's intent. Often, this mutual exploration not only clarifies the client's intent but also helps define the parameters of the evolving relationship and models the exploratory process for the client.

During Working Phase

During the working phase, particularly after the client has shown positive growth, the client may offer a gift in the form of a craft or skill. As in the orientation phase, the intent of the gift needs to be made explicit. Some governing bodies—in Great Britain, for example—have suggested regulatory restrictions on receiving work-related gifts (even those that express hospitality), but are being challenged in that country (Duffin, 2007). Most ethics and professional conduct boards set overall limits on the monetary value of gifts and agree that professionals must consider the symbolic meaning of the gift. Encourage this exploration by asking questions such as, "How is it that you're sharing this gift with me?" or "What feelings might you want to share with this gift?"

A client might give a gift during the working phase for several reasons:

- The client may wish to acknowledge the mutual work that has taken place.
- The client may wish to show appreciation for being allowed to share concerns with another person.
- The gift may be a smoke screen to block further exploration of a major dynamic.
- The gift may outwardly cover up anger or frustration felt inwardly.
- Finally, the gift may indicate the client's perception that the therapeutic work is finished.

In every instance, assess the intent of the gift, as well as its timing and appropriateness, in the context of the therapeutic relationship.

During Termination Phase

Gifts are most often given during the termination phase of one–to–one relationships. In this phase, a gift may have several overt and covert meanings:

- The client may wish to give a token of appreciation for positive personal growth that has taken place.
- The client may desire to change the therapeutic relationship into a social one.
- The client may wish to prolong sessions to avoid the final goodbye.

Some nurses accept a small gift from a client at the time of termination if feelings regarding the gift have been explored and clarified. (The gift may be an appropriate remembrance of a mutual and positive growth experience.) Exploring the significance of a termination gift will ensure the maximum therapeutic benefit for the client. A nurse's refusal to accept a gift of any type may prevent the client from learning the important skill of being able to accept gifts from others (Duffin, 2007). The nurse, as role model, has an opportunity to model appropriate gift-giving and gift-receiving. You may find receiving a gift at times awkward and "artificial." Yet such a situation gives you the opportunity to help the client toward further self-expression and self-knowledge.

Use of Touch

Physical contact is used cautiously in therapeutic work. It is best to avoid unplanned physical contact without therapeutic rationale. Clients with poor ego boundaries may become intensely threatened and feel overwhelmed by physical contact. For example, a client may lose the ability to distinguish self from the nurse during simple hand contact. Such contact may be perceived as a hostile or sexual gesture, although you do not intend it that way. In contrast, an acutely grief-stricken client, too distraught to focus on words, might receive needed support from being held. When considering any use of touch, ask yourself:

1. Does touch meet the client's therapeutic goals, or does it meet my needs?
2. Does touch foster a more productive therapeutic relationship?

Evaluate the use of touch, like self-disclosure, in the context of the therapeutic relationship, paying attention to its timing, appropriateness, and type. For example, a client is thrilled to achieve an on-the-job goal that has taken much personal time and effort. You determine that a firm handshake and a statement of congratulations are facilitative in this instance and at this working phase of the relationship. If you are unsure of the effect of such a gesture, a frank inquiry may be in order: "How did you feel when I shook your hand a few moments ago?" Again, the client's reaction and subsequent exploration can be a gauge for measuring how the client perceives and responds to the use of touch.

Culture, Values, and Beliefs

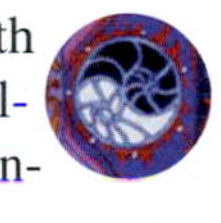

Address client values and beliefs that interfere with adaptive functioning. The following people hold cultural values and beliefs that may interfere with constructive change:

- The abusive spouse who believes the partner should be subservient, and, conversely, the partner who defers personal needs to preserve the relationship
- The abusive parent who believes that to "spare the rod" is to "spoil the child"
- The child raised with the family injunction that family problems should not be discussed outside the home, who may view the nurse's actions as an invasion of privacy

It is also possible that religious beliefs may interfere with change. For example, a client may believe that since God takes care of His people, there is no need to solve personal problems. Or, a client may believe that divorce or homosexuality is a sin, and therefore will never be forgiven (or forgive self).

Initially, you should become aware of the specific values and beliefs that influence the immediate relationship work. It is often useful to label the value or belief with the client, exploring its history, importance, cultural context, and impact. Nonjudgmental, alternative values may be discussed if the client initiates such an exploration. The humanistic nurse respects the client's values and beliefs and the client's ultimate choices regarding personal value systems. Your earnest interest in how the client is coping with emotional stressors provides the encouragement and support that facilitates health-related behavior change (Weiss & Lewis, 2007).

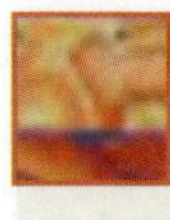

NURSING PROCESS
Orientation (Beginning) Phase

The primary goal of the orientation phase is to establish contact and begin developing a working relationship with the client. Establishing contact includes the initial encounters between nurse and client—how they approach and interact with each other, both verbally and nonverbally. You and the client meet to discuss how you will work together toward a common goal. See the Rx Communication feature for an example of an early dialogue related to goal setting. You are aware of having an impact on the client and acknowledge the client's personal impact on you. A sensitive and systematic consideration of the client's cultural and ethnic background is important at each phase of the one–to–one relationship.

MEDIALINK Case Study: Orientation Phase

The time required for each phase ideally depends on the severity of client dysfunction, the number and types of problems surfacing during treatment, and the type of therapeutic contract. Although these phases are presented here in their entirety to develop a comprehensive theoretic framework, nurses rarely experience them in such detail and sequence. You are more likely to experience the development of several short-term goals and to experiment with several subsequent interventions in any phase of relationship work. Nevertheless, an exploration of each phase will increase your familiarity with the flow—that is, "what comes next"—and may also provide a framework in which you can see client and nurse behaviors as partial expressions of a specific phase.

In informal relationships, contact usually begins when the nurse seeks out the client. Establishing contact may involve developing client awareness of your presence, followed by working to communicate with the client verbally. In formal relationships, contact may begin when the client inquires about services or when the psychiatric–mental health nurse contacts the client following referral. In formal relationships, the sense of working together in a therapeutic alliance enables the client to endure anxiety and deal with resistance to change, which inevitably surface during the course of one–to–one relationships. This phase of the therapeutic relationship concludes with mutual agreement on a therapeutic contract, which may be verbal and quite simple. The contract spells out the client's goals for treatment and the nurse's professional responsibilities.

Assessment

Client assessment begins at the first moment of contact. Assessment continues throughout the therapeutic relationship but is particularly important during the orientation phase. Remember that shortcuts taken in assessment procedures almost always jeopardize the ultimate quality of care. Crucial areas of concern may go unaddressed or be treated superficially.

An important part of client assessment is to determine what the client is likely to accomplish in the time allotted. Consider the extent of the client's responsiveness to you during this early stage of relating, the severity of the client's symptoms, the client's level of resistance, and the priorities for the care of the client. Emphasize the treatment needed to reach the most important and obtainable goals. Together, you and the client take this opportunity to shape the nature of the client's care within the limits of the current health care environment.

Subjective Data

Observation, a process long regarded as essential to clinical nursing practice, is of particular importance in one–to–one relationship work. Note elements in the nurse–client interaction that are missing, distorted, or imbalanced. What the client avoids discussing is often more crucial than what is shared.

An effective one–to–one relationship requires observation of the client's behavior and facial expressions, the content of the client's communication, and other cues about the client's involvement in the process. Keep in mind that you will also be sending the message that you understand, care about, and respect the client. Being aware of and using the cues you observe helps you adjust your interventions as necessary during the session. Your goal is to promote the therapeutic relationship and allow the therapeutic process to continue.

An awareness of changes in the client's nonverbal behavior—such as crossing the arms across the chest, leaning back in the chair, and appearing to withdraw from the interaction with you—is an important component of maintaining a one–to–one relationship. In this instance, an appropriate therapeutic response is, "I'm noticing as we're talking that you've crossed your arms and leaned back in the chair away from me. I wonder how you're feeling right now."

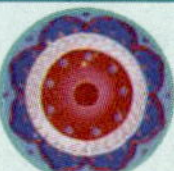

RX COMMUNICATION

THE INITIAL CONTRACT

CLIENT: "What, exactly, are we supposed to be doing together?"

NURSE RESPONSE 1: "I'd like to meet with you every day while you're here. This will give you an opportunity to talk about yourself and the things that are of concern to you."

RATIONALE: In addition to providing structure about the sessions, the nurse lays the groundwork for the focus on the client.

NURSE RESPONSE 2: "That's something that you and I can decide together tomorrow morning when we meet here at 9:30."

RATIONALE: The nurse reminds the client of the time for their meeting and sets the stage for mutual collaboration and negotiation.

Objective Data

Objective data collection ideally includes the following: mental status examination, complete physical examination, nursing history, and psychologic testing, as needed. Which examinations are done and by whom are generally determined by the agency or institution in which the psychiatric–mental health nurse works, and by the psychiatric–mental health nurse's expertise in these specific areas.

Interview

Interviewing is a process that generally occurs in the orientation phase of one–to–one relationships. Although a psychiatric–mental health nurse may use the structured initial interview in formal one–to–one work, it is rarely used in informal relationships.

The initial interview has the following purposes:

- Initiate trust building
- Establish rapport with the client
- Obtain pertinent client data
- Initiate client assessment
- Make practical arrangements for treatment

The initial interview is crucial because it sets the stage for subsequent therapeutic contact. As you begin to work together with the client to identify the issues the client intends to work on, you facilitate establishment of the one–to–one relationship. You are more likely to intervene effectively if you understand how a therapeutic relationship will fit into the client's life and consider the direction the client wishes to take (Gary, 2007).

Amount of Structuring Structure the initial interview to establish rapport, decrease anxiety, and convey willingness to address the client's distress. Begin by introducing yourself, inviting the client to be seated, and making a statement about information thus far known about the client's seeking of services. An open-ended question, such as, "How is it that you are here today?" provides an opportunity for the client to talk about concerns. Inform the client that the purpose of the initial interview is to obtain an overview of the client's current situation and then determine the availability of appropriate services.

Essential Data One primary purpose of structuring the initial interview is to collect essential data (see Chapter 11∞). Address client resistance if it surfaces during the initial interview. This resistance may occur when the client has initiated services at someone else's request or insistence, has fears and misconceptions about therapy, or has had an unsatisfactory therapeutic experience in the past. Nursing intervention calls for explicit exploration of the specific resistance before further data collection.

Anxious clients may be confused about or misinterpret information given during the initial interview. You may need to repeat information several times or in subsequent meetings. Manifestations of anxiety must be differentiated from manifestations of resistance, as in the clinical example that follows.

CLINICAL EXAMPLE

Selena, a 35-year-old woman, has been referred to the outpatient mental health clinic following several visits for minor medical problems. You note from the record a pattern of medication refills for antianxiety medication from her primary care provider. You also note that she was referred for mental health care on two other occasions, but failed to keep those appointments.

In thinking about the information Selena presented in the first session, you review her comments on her failures to follow through on the other two referrals. There are many possible reasons a client may miss appointments, some having to do with insufficient motivation for treatment, some having to do with psychiatric symptoms, and others attributable to unavoidable life circumstances. Selena's explanations indicate no external interfering life stressors or difficulties with transportation.

During that first session Selena was distraught and apologetic for not following through on the referrals, which she attributed to her anxiety symptoms. Specifically, she has been experiencing increasing difficulty leaving her home. The farther she gets from home, the more anxious she becomes. She told you that she cannot leave home, even to run important errands, without taking antianxiety medications. She cannot really specify the reason for her anxiety other than a sense of impending catastrophe.

Because these symptoms are consistent with a known anxiety disorder, you begin to think of agoraphobia as a potential initial working diagnosis. Selena's behavior, self-reports, and history are all consistent with what would be expected in a case of agoraphobia. However, because this is only the first session, you will collect further data in subsequent sessions that may lead to other potential alternative diagnoses. You note the lack of defensiveness in her presentation and you conclude that, at this point, there are no defense mechanisms such as avoidance or resistance that would sabotage the initiation of treatment. Of course, the client may employ other defenses as the treatment for her emotional difficulties proceeds.

Knowing about a client's typical emotions and defenses is valuable because it provides direction for appropriate nursing diagnoses related to both behavior and affect, identifying appropriate outcomes, setting specific client-centered goals, and implementing appropriate interventions.

Nursing Diagnosis: NANDA

Following a comprehensive assessment, you will need to organize all the data collected and formulate preliminary nursing diagnoses. The word *preliminary* is used to imply the ongoing potential for revision as client behaviors unfold during the course of the nurse–client relationship.

The goal in organizing the data is to understand the data as they reflect the client's unique, private world. Look for dominant themes or central issues in the client's responses. The dominant themes and central issues will be unique to each individual client. Select NANDA nursing diagnoses that derive from these themes and issues.

Outcome Identification: NOC

The major outcomes of the orientation phase are establishing contact and beginning to form a working relationship between client and nurse. The working relationship in this initial phase is the framework on which the client constructs behavioral change, a challenging task, in the next phase. The Your Assessment Approach feature highlights common signs of a working relationship. Other individual outcomes will be determined by the specific dominant themes and central issues of the client.

Planning and Implementation: NIC

The following interventions are common elements during the orientation phase. The development of additional interventions is based on assessment and nursing diagnoses for each individual client.

Therapeutic Contract

A plan for action actually forms the *therapeutic contract* negotiated in a one–to–one relationship. The therapeutic contract is a concrete, detailed, and mutually negotiated acknowledgment of the client's personal goals for treatment plus the nurse's professional responsibilities.

The contract may be modified over time but always serves as a tool for evaluating the benefit to the client and the effectiveness of the nurse. In an informal therapeutic relationship, the therapeutic contract may differ from the usual care plan often developed in outpatient and inpatient settings. For example, an initial contract may begin as a very simple agreement concerning the time and place of subsequent meetings together.

The client's personal goals for treatment may be long-term or short-term goals, but they always specify detailed, observable outcomes, as in the following clinical example.

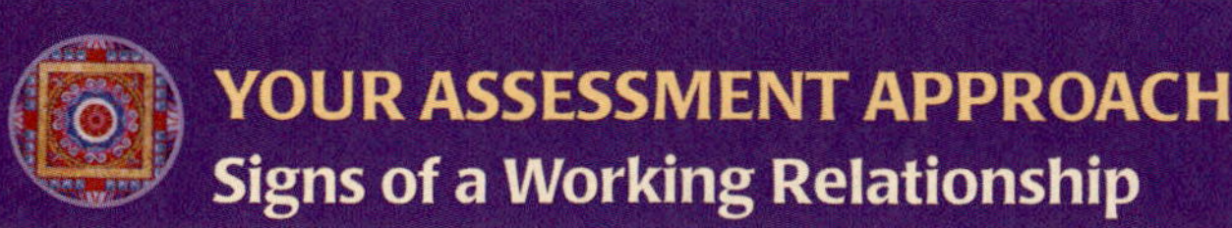

CLINICAL EXAMPLE

Nicole is a 30-year-old woman admitted to an inpatient psychiatric unit following an overdose of risperidone (Risperdal). During past hospitalizations, Nicole has been emotionally labile, has had trouble following her treatment schedule, was easily frustrated by the limits and compromises of living in the hospital, demanded medication, and threatened suicide. Nicole's primary nurse proposed that they work together to identify goals and behaviors for improved personal and interpersonal functioning. Nicole identified problems of feeling empty, having poor relationships with others, and being angry; she chose to focus on the overall goal of improved social skills. Nicole agreed to the following expectations:

- I will participate in a one–to–one relationship with my nurse and express my feelings verbally.
- I will identify uncomfortable situations involving other people and discuss the interactions with my nurse at appointed times.
- I will continue my routine treatment activities until the appropriate time to meet with my nurse.

Strive for the most concise, detailed, and accurate description of client goals in the beginning phase. Clearly stated goals facilitate subsequent mutual evaluation during the middle and end phases of one–to–one work. Goals may focus on:

- Decreasing or eliminating troublesome behaviors
- Increasing socialization
- Increasing living skills

Client goals most often contribute to the establishment of a working relationship when they are specific, address intrapersonal or interpersonal behavior patterns, and specifically delineate the degree of change necessary for client self-satisfaction.

At times, client goals may be long-term or even inappropriate. In this situation, help the client define initial steps toward the long-term goal. For example, a readmitted mentally ill client may pinpoint discharge as an important goal. You may then work with this client to identify the steps needed to achieve this goal. One step may be to maintain self-care in the area of bathing/hygiene. When severe dysfunction limits client input into planning, the nursing staff may supplement goals that are determined to be beneficial to the client.

In a formal therapeutic relationship, as in individual psychotherapy, the therapeutic contract is more detailed and generally includes three practical matters:

1. Determining the place, duration, and time of the meetings

YOUR ASSESSMENT APPROACH
Signs of a Working Relationship

The following criteria may be useful in determining whether a one–to–one relationship is moving into the working, or middle, phase.

For Nurse	For Client
▪ Sense of making contact with the client	▪ Nonverbal and verbal evidence of liking the nurse
▪ Sense that the client is responding well to the relationship	▪ Sense of relaxation with the nurse
▪ Sense that the nurse can facilitate client growth regardless of the severity of client dysfunction	▪ Sense of confidence in the nurse
▪ Sense of commitment to addressing the client's problems	▪ Nonsuperficial (in nature and depth) problems addressed

2. Establishing fees and payment intervals, if any
3. Considering optional referral sources, should the client be unable to negotiate an agreement on the first two matters

In formal therapeutic relationships, the therapeutic contract may not reflect client problems and strengths in their entirety. At that moment, the client may not determine that an area is, in fact, a problem. Thus, the therapeutic contract in formal relationship work reflects the *client's* definition of personal goals at one moment in time. The psychiatric–mental health nurse, in this instance, remains aware of other probable problem areas and assesses these areas with the client in an ongoing manner, as appropriate.

Regardless of the form that goal identification takes, the therapeutic contract serves the following purposes:

- Facilitating humanistic involvement with the client as an individual
- Involving the client as a full partner in the therapeutic process
- Serving as a basis for communication in the therapeutic process
- Providing continuity for the client and everyone involved with the client

The initial goals of the therapeutic contract may be modified or deleted in subsequent phases of the one–to–one relationship as appropriate or necessary.

Trust

Concerns about trust surface in this first phase of the relationship. Trust between nurse and client evolves over time as the client tests the emotional climate of sessions, risks self-disclosure, and observes the nurse's follow-through on responsibilities delineated in the therapeutic contract. You can promote trust by responding to all of the client's feeling states without being judgmental or attempting to control emotive expression. The process recording in Table 29-3 ■ on page 788 demonstrates how one nurse began to promote trust early in the orientation phase. Note that she was self-assured enough to encourage the client to share his concerns about trust. It is important to be consistent and to be self-aware of the part your feelings play in the interactions (Paris, 2007). The nurse's self-awareness of personal feeling states also enhances trust. It allows the client to disclose uncomfortable, even forbidden, feelings in safety.

The following interventions enhance initial trust:

- Listening attentively to client feelings
- Responding to client feelings
- Exhibiting consistency, especially regarding appointment times
- Viewing situations from the client's perspective

These behaviors constitute positive, helpful influences in encouraging trust.

A common failing among those learning relationship skills is focusing on technique. This produces mechanical, unfeeling responses. It is also important to avoid giving premature reassurances about trust, which may inhibit exploration of this vital therapeutic issue and create distance between nurse and client.

Confidentiality

Client concerns about the level of confidentiality also surface in this first phase of the therapeutic relationship. Keeping clients' confidentiality is not only a legal responsibility, but describing the encompassing issues and the limits of the confidence uphold caring behaviors. Circumstances do exist (for example, intent to commit suicide, intent to harm others) in which disclosure of a client's information is necessary. Keeping clients' confidentiality is your legal responsibility (see pages 282–284 in Chapter 13).

In addition, it is crucial to be aware of your responsibilities in relation to confidentiality (Beech, 2007). The issue of confidentiality must be explicitly addressed when the client makes even vague reference to it. Explicitly state which people will have access to client revelations (clinical instructor, case supervisor, consultant, colleague), and explore how the client feels in response to this information.

Tuning into Process

The beginning nurse often attends carefully to the *content* of the client sessions—what the client says—and only after considerable experience becomes actively attuned to *process*. Process here does not mean nursing process but rather a complex communication skill that enables the nurse to focus on several aspects of the nurse–client relationship at the same time. Process involves attending to all nonverbal and verbal client behaviors. It involves responding to client themes, such as anger, hopelessness, and powerlessness. The challenge for the nurse is to become savvy enough to learn what to ignore and sensitive enough to know what to emphasize (Guy & Brady, 2001). The experienced nurse is simultaneously aware of both content and process, interweaving both for maximum therapeutic effectiveness. Processing is discussed in Chapter 30.

Addressing the Client's Suffering

Interventions during the orientation phase are valid and important, even if you do not reach the working phase with a particular client (because of time limitations or because the client is unable to agree on goals). The psychiatric–mental health nurse intervenes by directly addressing the client's suffering within the context of the client's cultural and ethnic background. This intervention allows clients to share how they perceive, experience, and manifest the problem. The following clinical example illustrates how the nurse encourages a depressed client to "move outside himself."

CLINICAL EXAMPLE

Client: "This depression is like a big log weighing on my chest."

Nurse: "How might I, or someone else, know that you are suffering in this way?"

Client: "Well . . . I sigh a lot . . . I don't move a lot, only when I have to . . . I wouldn't look at you, or bother to talk to you. I guess when I feel like this, I close people out. Yeah, I close everyone out, even my wife."

Nurse: "So when you suffer in this way, you close people out. And what is this like for you?"

Client: "I'm alone and lonely. Not a soul on earth cares for me."

Clarifying Purpose, Roles, and Responsibilities

An additional therapeutic task is to intervene directly in clarifying the purpose of the relationship work, the role of the nurse, and the responsibilities of the client. When this preliminary exploration of purpose, roles, and responsibilities is explicit and detailed, each participant better understands how to move within the relationship. It also decreases anxiety and the chance that a client may use the relationship to obtain special privileges. From the first meeting the nurse also intervenes to reinforce effective coping skills and increase client self-esteem. The following Your Intervention Strategies feature summarizes the goals, tasks, and subsequent nursing interventions of the orientation phase of one–to–one relationships.

Evaluation

In the orientation phase, evaluation includes your initial comprehensive evaluation of client behaviors, any initial steps toward the development of client self-evaluation, and your ongoing self-evaluation. The more specific and goal-oriented the therapeutic contract, the easier it is for the client and nurse to evaluate the effectiveness of the therapeutic relationship.

Table 29-3 ■ Process Recording of an Orientation Phase Session

Verbatim Interaction	Nursing Intervention	Rationale
Client: "It's so difficult for me to talk . . . to let you know about me." (30-second pause.)	None	Allows client to proceed at own pace; if silence is uncomfortably long to client in first few contacts, you may use reflection, e.g., "I sense how difficult talking is for you."
Client: "Every time I start to tell anybody about myself, they usually end up laughing at me."		
Nurse: "Give me an example."	Encourage elaboration.	Explores meaning of this statement to the client.
Client: "Well, just last week I started talking to my neighbor. I told him that I was laid off from work again. Next thing you know, he's laughing, slapping my back, and saying, 'Hey, hard times, eh?'" (Shifts in chair, avoids eye contact.)		
Nurse: "What was this like for you?"	Explore client's personal reaction, especially accompanying feelings.	Further explores meaning of this specific incident as perceived by the client.
Client: "Awful . . . lousy . . . that's all." (Pause.)		
Nurse: "I wonder if you're concerned that the same might happen here—that you'll be laughed at?"	Connect the client's concern regarding this emotionally difficult interaction to the here–and–now, i.e., the one–to–one therapeutic relationship.	Issues concerning client's immediate life situations often reflect parallel issues in nurse–client relationship.
Client: "Well, maybe . . . I don't know you, so how do I know what you might do? You don't look like the type, but then again, how do I know?"		
Nurse: "It sounds like you're wondering if it's safe to trust me."	Identify what appears to be the underlying central concern or theme.	Reflection of what appears to be the central concern (theme) encourages client assessment by validation or correction of your statement.
Client: "Yeah . . . no offense, though."		
Nurse: "Let's talk about how safe you feel today and as we continue to work together."	Focus on trust as an issue for further exploration; acknowledge that there is stress in evolving a working relationship.	Avoid premature reassurances so that trust can evolve and be assessed periodically.

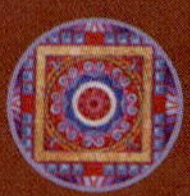

YOUR INTERVENTION STRATEGIES
Goals, Tasks, and Interventions of the Orientation Phase

Goal: Establish contact and begin to form a working relationship with the client.

Therapeutic Tasks	Nursing Interventions
Clarify the purpose of relationship work, the role of the nurse, and responsibilities of the client.	Provide information regarding purpose, roles, and responsibilities in relationship work to alleviate initial client anxiety. Immediately and explicitly address any misconceptions, fantasies, and fears regarding relationship work and/or the nurse.
Address client suffering directly, offering to work with the client toward its alleviation.	Use facilitative characteristics, especially empathic understanding. Avoid premature reassurance (allow trust to evolve). Be explicit about who has access to client's revelations (degree of confidentiality).
Negotiate therapeutic contract (client's definition of personal goals for treatment and the nurse's professional responsibilities).	Whenever possible, encourage delineation of goals that are specific, address intrapersonal and interpersonal behavioral patterns, and designate the degree of change necessary for client self-satisfaction. In informal relationship work, the contract generally includes a determination of time and place for working together to the extent that client ability permits. In formal relationship work, the contract generally includes place, duration, and time of therapy; fees and payment intervals, if any; and optional referral sources.

In addition to evaluating the effectiveness of each therapeutic task, you must evaluate the important goal of the orientation phase: Has a working relationship evolved between the client and nurse, and, if so, to what degree? Review Your Assessment Approach: Signs of a Working Relationship on page 786 to assess the extent of the working relationship.

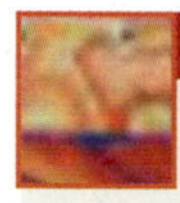

NURSING PROCESS
Working (Middle) Phase

Once contact is established, attention turns to maintenance and analysis of contact in the working phase. *Analysis of contact* refers to an in-depth exploration of how the client relates to others as manifested in the nurse–client relationship. In this working phase, the client may address developmental and situational problems, as well as interpersonal problems. It is called the *working phase* because during this phase, the nurse and client actively and systematically identify, explore, link, modify, and evaluate specific behaviors, especially those determined to be dysfunctional for the client.

The client's clearly stated goals in the therapeutic contract are now explored. The nurse has the following two therapeutic goals:

- *Behavioral analysis*. The nurse and client determine the dynamics of the client's response patterns, especially those considered to be dysfunctional. Such analysis also addresses dysfunctional thought and emotive patterns, because these inevitably alter the client's behavior.
- *Constructive change in behavior*. This applies particularly to dysfunctional response patterns.

Thus, the psychiatric–mental health nurse and client work together to analyze behavior and institute behavioral change.

Assessment

Assessment is continued, detailed, and expanded upon. Your observations of nonverbal, verbal, and environmental responses continue to have vital importance as the client begins to address personal response patterns. In addition, you continue to assess emotive, cognitive, cultural, and behavioral aspects. By filling in gaps of information not obtained in the orientation phase, you may now acquire a detailed assessment about a subject the client was unable to share or ignored earlier. The following clinical example illustrates that what is not said (that is, what is avoided, blocked, rejected) by the client may have more significance than what the client shares.

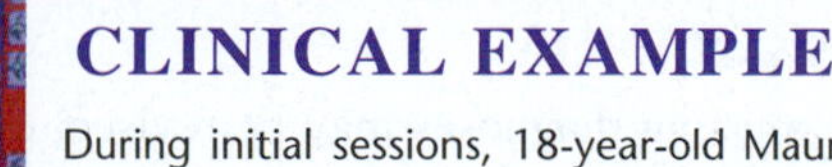

CLINICAL EXAMPLE

During initial sessions, 18-year-old Maureen avoided any inquiries about her parents, other than to say that she lived alone. After several sessions, the nurse again asked about the parents. Maureen replied softly, with tears welling in her eyes,

"They're dead. They died in a car crash 2 years ago." She slowly related how, since their deaths, she had spent so much energy trying to survive that she barely felt much of anything. Subsequent sessions dealt with her apparent delayed grief reaction.

The new data caused the nurse to revise and update the tentative nursing diagnoses and initiate a marked change in the direction of the sessions. Such shifting is not uncommon in one–to–one relationships. When a change in direction occurs, assess if the sudden change indicates either the need to avoid a certain topic or a move toward a deeper level of emotive expression.

In the working phase, you facilitate many aspects of assessment with the client. First, collaborate with the client in identifying important behavioral trends and patterns. Once a pattern is identified, explore it in elaborate detail to determine its origin, causes, operation, and effects on the client and the people in the client's world. Environmental factors (familial, political, economic, or cultural) are separated from intrapersonal factors (depression or anxiety) contributing to the pattern. The client figuratively holds the pattern to the light to examine and make sense of its every aspect. The elements of one pattern will inevitably link with others, so that the major life patterns gradually unfold. The first part of the Your Intervention Strategies feature on page 791 summarizes the therapeutic tasks undertaken to achieve the objective of behavioral analysis and offers specific nursing approaches to helping the client.

There are two noteworthy considerations regarding therapeutic tasks of the first goal, behavioral analysis:

1. As clients begin to describe and re-experience conflict, they consciously or unconsciously use defenses to ward off the anxiety this awakens. The development of a good working relationship enables clients to tolerate increased anxiety in the working phase.
2. As clients become familiar with self-assessment, they may modify original personal goals, or develop additional goals, in keeping with what they have learned.

It is important during the working phase to encourage the client's self-assessment of growth-facilitating and growth-inhibiting behaviors. After assessing one specific response, the client is often able to transfer this skill to begin assessing other aspects of life as well. A realistic self-assessment process is perhaps the most valuable skill that the client can "take home." It is often thrilling to experience the client "taking over" and further applying realistic assessment skills developed in one–to–one work.

Nursing Diagnosis: NANDA

In the working phase, nursing diagnoses may be revised, expanded, or deleted to more accurately reflect a central pattern of concern in the evolving one–to–one relationship. As the working phase proceeds, the priority assigned to a nursing diagnosis may change—for example, when the client is able to implement positive change in some areas. Those nursing diagnoses designated as "risk for" may move up or down on the priority list, depending on what interventions, if any, have been effective. A potential diagnosis may decrease in priority after preventive health education, if both the client and the nurse evaluate this intervention as beneficial.

Outcome Identification: NOC

The initial goal of behavioral analysis of the client's response patterns continues throughout the working phase. The major identified outcomes are:

- The client develops an awareness of current behavioral patterns.
- The client understands how and when those patterns manifest themselves.
- The client may gain insight into the potential causes of those patterns.
- The client assesses which behavioral patterns are ineffective and self-defeating.
- The client attempts to change ineffective behavioral patterns and develop new, more effective behaviors.

Planning and Implementation: NIC

In the working phase, planning is ideally done collaboratively between client and nurse. Such planning involves frequent consideration of the client's initial goals. When planning has been systematic and thorough, there is hardly a moment to worry about "what to do." The short-term and long-term treatment goals in the form of the therapeutic contract are a map indicating the direction, momentum, and the steps that are needed to reach a designated point.

There is, however, a potential danger in the implementation of the planning component: moving too quickly and incompletely through an exploration of the client's feelings and thoughts in an attempt to reach a designated goal. *Slowness* and *thoroughness* are all-important here. Change needs to take place in the client's feelings, thoughts, and behaviors. If change does not occur in all aspects, then it is destined to be short-lived and ineffectual in the long run and may contribute to client discouragement.

When the client is working on an issue that is unresolved at the end of a meeting, it is often helpful to summarize the unfinished work for the next meeting. This technique may help the client anticipate, plan, or prepare to tackle this area of concern again. Personal experiments, such as trying out new behaviors in real situations, may be encouraged between sessions. Some clients may be able to continue working through a problem on their own between meetings.

Active intervention is especially important to achieve the second goal of the working phase, constructive changes in behavior, particularly in self-defeating, growth-inhibiting behavior patterns. Behavioral change flows from the first goal of behavioral analysis. The objectives are interrelated and essential for successful therapeutic work. Understanding and insight need to be complemented by behavioral implementation (Mar-

MediaLink Critical Thinking Exercise: Working Phase

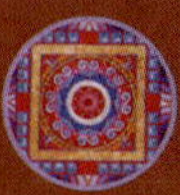

YOUR INTERVENTION STRATEGIES
Goals, Tasks, and Interventions of the Working Phase

Goal: Behavioral analysis (mutual determination of dynamics of response patterns identified by client, especially those considered dysfunctional)

Therapeutic Tasks	Nursing Interventions
Identify and explore important response patterns in detail.	Explore response pattern in depth, including origin, causes, operation, and effect of pattern (intrapersonally and interpersonally). Separate environmental factors (familial, political, economic, cultural) from intrapersonal factors. Link elements of one response pattern to other patterns as appropriate, for a gradual unfolding of central life patterns.
Analyze, with the client, client's mode of conflict resolution.	Encourage a detailed exploration of how the client reacts to reduce anxiety associated with conflict. Increase awareness of defenses employed to ward off anxiety awakened by such exploration.
Facilitate client self-assessment of growth-producing and growth-inhibiting response patterns.	Encourage client to evaluate each response pattern to determine which are self-defeating and/or thwart gratification of basic needs.

Goal: Constructive change in behavior, especially in dysfunctional response patterns identified by the client

Therapeutic Tasks	Nursing Interventions
Address forces that inhibit desired change (troublesome thoughts, feelings, and behaviors).	Help the client challenge personal resistance to change. Use problem-solving strategies, active decision making, and personal accountability. Help the client learn and apply problem-solving strategies. Encourage the client to assert own needs when external environmental conditions (group, agency, institution) are an inhibiting force.
Create an atmosphere offering permission for active experimentation to test and assess the effectiveness of new behaviors.	Allow freedom to make and assess mistakes and blunders. Avoid parental judgment of any behavioral experimentation; encourage client self-assessment instead.
Facilitate the development of coping skills to deal with anxiety associated with constructive changes in behavior.	Address, rather than avoid, anxiety and its manifestations. Strengthen existing growth-promoting coping skills, especially regarding unalterable conditions (terminal illness, physical deformity, loss of significant other by death). Encourage the development of new coping skills and their application to actual life experiences.

tin & Pear, 2007). The client's failure to make adaptive behavioral changes stymies progress and sabotages the therapeutic experience (Martin & Pear, 2007). Chapter 31 highlights behavioral interventions. Clients may consistently generate and thrive on sophisticated insights while continuing to assume a powerless stance about implementing constructive change in their condition. The Your Intervention Strategies feature above highlights therapeutic tasks and specific nursing interventions for the second goal, constructive change in behavior, in the working phase.

You can also use active experimentation to test the effect of new behaviors. The introverted male client who resolved to establish relationships with women may assume various postures (cavalier, paternal, seductive) with a female nurse to determine the appropriateness of these behaviors before displaying them outside of sessions. Permission to "try on" or role-play new behaviors must also include the freedom to make mistakes. Errors and blunders are rich sources of additional learning and occasional fun. Clients who can see humor in errors in a nondefeatist manner have acquired a new skill. Encourage them to apply this skill, and any other coping skills learned in relationship work, to normal maturational and situational crises encountered throughout life.

In inpatient settings, work with other staff members to make the whole team aware of the meaning of the client's behavior as positive actions that may be exaggerated at first. For example, some staff members may encourage a depressed client to verbalize anger and begin by shouting. If there is no staff collaboration, the client may receive negative feedback (room restrictions) for testing out new coping skills.

Dialectical behavioral therapy (DBT), a specialized subset of the cognitive behavioral treatment modalities, is a useful working-phase intervention strategy (Sambrook, Abba, & Chadwick, 2007). DBT promotes the client's attention to an emotional experience, enhanced effectiveness in interpersonal relationships, regulating of emotions in a productive manner, and ability to tolerate distress. Chapter 31 provides details about DBT and its use in therapeutic relationships.

Problem-Solving Strategies

Problem-solving strategies, as a mode of intervention, are particularly important in the working phase. Problem-solving strategies are essential after the client has identified, explored, and assessed important behavioral patterns. Encourage clients to use the sequential problem-solving strategies discussed in the Your Intervention Strategies feature that follows. Reminding clients to be patient is supportive and reassuring. Problem-solving abilities improve with time and experience.

Challenging the Client's Resistance to Change

Challenging the client's resistance to change is an appropriate intervention in the working phase. There are two major categories of forces that inhibit desired change:

1. Intrapersonal forces, which may arise from troublesome thoughts, feelings, or behaviors. Examples include thoughts that hamper the client's sense of worth, the client's inability to control and express emotion appropriately, or the client's inability to relate to others in a meaningful manner.
2. The client's personal resistance to change, which is the greatest inhibiting force. In fact, the client's challenge to this resistance constitutes the major work in one–to–one relationships.

Problems of resistance and general intervention strategies were discussed earlier in the chapter. Of equal significance is the previous discussion of transference and countertransference phenomena, since these may require careful, planned nursing interventions. Sometimes transference and countertransference are so intense that they become a problem for the beginning psychiatric–mental health nurse.

Evaluation

Several levels of evaluation occur simultaneously in the working phase. First, do an ongoing evaluation of the client's various levels of intrapersonal and interpersonal functioning. Feedback from family, community agencies, or the client's employer may enhance any current comprehensive evaluation. For example, does the client seem to be facing an impending crisis? If so, you may choose to switch from intrapersonal exploration to a crisis intervention strategy. Second, encourage client self-evaluation, as explored in previous discussion. Finally, constantly perform self-evaluation as a helping person growing in skill and experience. Nursing self-evaluation is done by informal discussions with staff and other mental health care personnel and by formal clinical supervision.

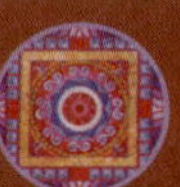

YOUR INTERVENTION STRATEGIES
Problem-Solving Strategies

- **Observation.** Observation as a problem-solving strategy involves gathering and analyzing facts about a potential problem area. It eliminates opinions and impressions and emphasizes facts. (Observation as an aspect of assessment is discussed in the section on subjective assessment)
- **Definition.** Definition is perhaps the most significant and far-reaching problem-solving strategy. It involves an initial specification of a problem, followed by a question. Starting a problem-solving exploration with the word "How" ("How is it?" "How does it manifest itself?" "How has this come about?") puts the focus on the process of a specific problem. It is generally more useful than asking "Why?" which emphasizes rationale. (Questioning as a communication technique is explored in Chapter 10.)
- **Preparation.** Preparation involves collecting additional pertinent data related to the basic problem that may prove useful in later stages of problem-solving strategies. This enables the nurse and client to anticipate which data might be most useful.
- **Analysis.** As a problem-solving strategy, analysis involves breaking down the relevant material into subproblems so that each subproblem may be assessed separately.
- **Ideation.** Ideation involves accumulating alternative ideas on how to resolve the basic problem.
- **Incubation.** Incubation is used when the problem-solving process or one aspect of it is set aside for a period of time to allow for illumination.
- **Synthesis.** As a problem-solving strategy, synthesis involves putting together all elements of the basic problem, subproblems, and possible alternatives.
- **Evaluation.** Evaluation consists of making judgments about the ideas that result.
- **Development.** As a final problem-solving strategy, development involves planning the implementation of these ideas.

On-the-spot evaluations of relevant short-term and long-term goals can occur during any meeting with the client. For example, as the client talks about increasing socialization skills, the nurse may reflect: "Let's look at our contract together. You originally wanted to date a woman of your choice for two hours during an evening without leaving the situation. How do you think this compares with what you're now saying has happened?" Support any effort at evaluation on the part of the client and explore what else needs to happen for the client to achieve the short-term goal. An additional area of evaluation involves the client's "trying on" alternative behaviors to determine whether these new behaviors may work.

The client and nurse should mutually evaluate the appropriateness of goals in any one of the following areas in light of the client's current functioning:

- Degree of the client's success in achieving specific goals

- The client's growth-producing and growth-inhibiting behavior patterns
- Unfinished business that must be resolved to achieve a desired goal

The working phase may also involve ongoing evaluations of the status, characteristics, and depth of the nurse–client relationship. The client may view the nurse in different ways (parent, sibling, friend) at various times. It is only when the client makes these views explicit that the nurse may intervene to clarify roles and responsibilities in a facilitative manner.

The psychiatric–mental health nurse and the client have moved through the first two phases of therapeutic relationships when:

- They have established a working relationship.
- They have analyzed the dynamics of the client's behavioral patterns.
- The client has effectively instituted behavioral changes in keeping with the therapeutic contract.

In informal relationship work, the nurse may touch on only one or two aspects of the working phase. Even the advanced psychiatric–mental health nurse rarely addresses all therapeutic tasks in this phase of relationship work.

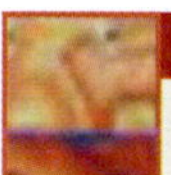

NURSING PROCESS Termination (End) Phase

During the termination or resolution phase of one–to–one relationships, the psychiatric–mental health nurse works toward discontinuing contact. This phase is as important as the previous two phases, although both the nurse and the client frequently avoid it because of past difficulties with separation.

The goal of the end phase is termination of the one–to–one relationship in a mutually planned, satisfying manner. Remind the client that termination was first addressed in the orientation phase, when the duration of the relationship was discussed. Also emphasize the growth and positive aspects of the relationship, rather than focusing exclusively on separation.

A smooth and complete termination sometimes occurs in actual practice. In informal relationship work in inpatient settings, termination more often occurs with the client's abrupt departure or planned medical discharge. Even in formal relationship work in community settings, contact often ceases without explanation after a series of missed appointments, or with a phone call by the client to inform the therapist of the client's decision to terminate, or with the client abruptly leaving a session and failing to resume subsequent contact. In these instances, the nurse can call or write the client and suggest an additional session to deal with either the therapeutic good-bye or a willingness to continue the relationship work. Termination requires careful preparation, adequate time for the client to work through the feelings about ending, and an opportunity for the nurse to explore personal reactions with a clinical instructor, colleague, supervisor, or consultant.

Assessment

Assessment as a component of the nursing process in the resolution phase deals primarily with determining when the client may be ready to terminate, how the client deals with termination, and how the nurse deals with termination. Criteria that indicate a client's readiness for termination are presented in the following Your Assessment Approach feature.

Many factors influence how the client reacts to termination. These factors include:

- *Degree of client involvement.* The greater the degree of client involvement, the more intense the client's reaction to termination.
- *Length of treatment.* In general, the longer the nurse–client relationship lasts, the more time should be spent in exploring all aspects of termination.
- *Client's past history of significant losses.* A client who has lost significant others may reexperience past conflicts and emotional responses.
- *Ability to separate from others.* The reaction to termination is influenced by how well the client has mastered the early separation–individuation phase of development.
- *Degree of success achieved.* Reaction to termination depends on how successful and satisfying the relationship has been for the client.
- *Degree of transference in the relationship.* The greater the transference in the nurse–client relationship, the more intense the client's reaction to termination.

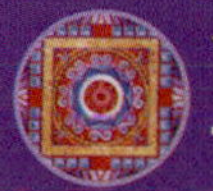

YOUR ASSESSMENT APPROACH Termination Readiness

The following criteria may be useful to determine whether the client is ready to terminate:

- **Relief from the presenting problem.** Symptoms no longer interfere with the client's comfort.
- **Achievement of treatment goals.** These ideally are planned goals included in the therapeutic contract between the nurse and client.
- **Improvement in social functioning.** The client experiences increased satisfaction in interpersonal relationships.
- **Acquisition of adaptive coping strategies.** Ideally, these strategies include the client's use of effective problem-solving strategies on a daily basis.
- **Acquisition of more effective defense mechanisms.** A client who cannot achieve adaptive coping strategies should develop more effective defense mechanisms to ensure stabilization.
- **Attainment of identity.** The client experiences self-satisfaction and no longer needs to depend on the nurse for a sense of well-being.
- **Disruption due to a major impasse in the one–to–one relationship.** Stubborn resistances may surface and persist on the part of the client. Uncontrollable countertransference may develop on the part of the nurse.

MediaLink Care Plan: Termination Phase

Be alert to client responses during termination. Any number of responses—repression, regression, anger, denial, sadness, withdrawal, avoidance, acceptance, joy—may surface, and it is not unusual for several to surface at once. When repressing, the client shows no emotional response. Regression on the part of the client is an extremely common response to termination. Regressive behavior may range from statements of abandonment and hopelessness to an inability to tend to personal hygiene. The central message conveyed is: "See? I can't make it without you!"

Nurse's Self-Awareness

Finally, assessment involves how you personally manage separation in the one–to–one relationship. Like the client, you can have any number of responses. Some common responses are:

- Regret that the client did not achieve more than the client actually did
- Hesitation to give up the dependence elements of the relationship
- Collusion with the client to prolong sessions to avoid the inevitability of separation

Nursing Diagnosis: NANDA

Nursing diagnoses during termination should reflect the termination behaviors manifested by the client. A wide variety of nursing diagnoses may be relevant. Potential nursing diagnoses that stem from regression during the termination phase may be: Self-Care Deficit, Hopelessness, Powerlessness, and Ineffective Coping. Nursing diagnoses should be modified as necessary, as the client moves through the termination experience.

Outcome Identification: NOC

The ideal outcome occurs when the nurse–client relationship terminates after achieving all identified and measurable personal behavioral changes. Such resolution seldom occurs in psychiatric practice, especially since brief hospital stays are now the rule rather than the exception. Often, the client achieves more limited behavioral changes and agrees to return for future work or referral as necessary. At other times, the client achieves symptom relief only.

Outcomes are compromised when the client is unable to make progress due to lack of insight or mental capacity. Chronic catastrophic life circumstances (such as severe medical illness, life-threatening poverty, prison, etc.) may interfere with growth-producing behaviors. On rare occasions, the client's condition deteriorates and the client is unable to benefit from the nurse–client relationship.

Planning and Implementation: NIC

Planning involves preparing for the final good-bye (the subject of this section) and mutual planning about where the client may seek future help if the need arises (the subject of the next section).

Intervention strategies vary according to the client's behaviors. You may respond to the client who is repressing the reality of termination by repeatedly observing that he or she is not addressing the issue of the impending separation. You may then attempt to explore this avoidance with the client. Useful interventions for clients who are regressing in response to termination include:

- Addressing the possible underlying fears of abandonment
- Emphasizing the growth achieved by the client
- Continuing to focus on the realities of separation

The acting-out client may protest termination in numerous ways before the termination date, such as attempting suicide, psychiatric hospitalization, quitting a job, or rejecting the nurse. In general, the underlying feelings, fears, and fantasies need ventilation, exploration, and working through, as do reactions of anger, depression, and grief. An exception to this general guideline is the client who uses distraction maneuvers to prevent termination, such as introducing explosive new material in final sessions. In this situation, you may use limit setting rather than exploration because of time constraints. In other words, there may be "unfinished business" despite planning and effort.

The nurse has the final task of participating in an *explicit and therapeutic good-bye* with the client. Nursing responsibilities in this final phase include anticipating your own personal reaction to separation and, optionally, expressing this reaction in a manner that does not burden the client. In addition, you may share a special wish for the client, based on the client's particular assets within the therapeutic relationship.

A therapeutic good-bye gives the client a sense of freedom to move on to other relationships. The end phase may take from one meeting to several months of meetings, depending on the duration of the one–to–one relationship. In general, the longer the duration of the relationship, the longer the time needed to deal explicitly with the termination of contact. The Your Intervention Strategies feature on page 795 summarizes the goal, therapeutic tasks, and specific nursing interventions of the termination phase.

Ideally, the client can completely work through feelings regarding separation so that there is no unfinished business between nurse and client. The nurse–client relationship has given the client the opportunity to depend on another in a realistic and mature manner. The direct, explicit good-bye is frequently the first such experience for the client. It is usually a moment of unique humanness for both the nurse and the client.

Evaluation

Evaluation is a vital component of the nursing process during the termination phase. You have the task of helping the client evaluate the therapeutic contract. The criteria for evaluation are the goals formulated in the orientation and working phases of the one–to–one relationship. Each goal is evaluated in terms of measurable, observable behavior. Were the goals appropriate, practical, and specific to the client? What are the therapeutic gains? What are the areas for possible further therapeutic work? How does the client evaluate motivation, effort, progress, and outcome? Has the client worked through most feelings about separation from the nurse?

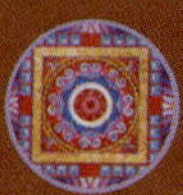

YOUR INTERVENTION STRATEGIES
Goals, Tasks, and Interventions of the Termination Phase

Goal: Terminate contact in a mutually planned, satisfying manner.

Therapeutic Tasks	Nursing Interventions
Help the client evaluate the therapeutic contract and the therapeutic experience in general.	Encourage the client's realistic appraisal of personal therapeutic goals (motivation, effort, progress, outcome) as these evolved in treatment. Provide appropriate feedback regarding the appraisal of goals. Review the client's assets and therapeutic gains. Review areas for further therapeutic work.
Encourage the transference of dependence to other support systems.	Encourage the client to develop reliance on others in client's immediate environment (spouse, relative, employer, neighbor, friend) for empathic, emotional support.
Participate in explicit therapeutic good-bye with the client.	Be alert to the surfacing of any behavior arising on termination (repression, regression, acting out, anger, withdrawal, acceptance). Help the client work through feelings associated with these behaviors. Anticipate own reaction to separation and share in a manner that does not burden the client. Allow time and space for termination; the longer the duration of the one–to–one relationship, the more time is needed for the termination phase.

You will also help the client evaluate the therapeutic experience in general, which may set the stage for future psychotherapeutic work. Would the client seek a similar experience in the future, if deemed necessary? Having the opportunity to discuss the work and the outcome is an empowering exercise for clients.

The nurse's own personal, ongoing self-evaluation also warrants emphasis here. It is essential to continuously evaluate which of your own behaviors consciously or unconsciously promote, inhibit, or actively block growth-producing client abilities.

Clinical Supervision

Clinical supervision is essential if the one–to–one relationship is to be effective. Professional supervision helps you use transference effectively and recognize countertransference phenomena. The supportive function of supervision may be used to monitor your own needs, thereby minimizing the likelihood of severe clinical stress and burnout. There are various methods of evaluation: process recordings, videotapes, client evaluations, audiotapes, didactic instruction, and referral to specific clinical readings. There are several kinds of supervision available, such as intradisciplinary supervision with a psychiatric–mental health clinical nurse specialist, or interdisciplinary supervision by another mental health care professional (psychologist, psychiatrist, psychiatric social worker). An ethnic consultant can help to evaluate the influence of transcultural issues, including specific culture-bound syndromes (see Chapter 9). All of these people can be helpful, depending on their skills and availability. Supervision helps the psychiatric–mental health nurse effectively define, initiate, use, and evaluate client and self in any therapeutic relationship.

CASE MANAGEMENT

The likely possibility that not all client goals would be achieved during typical brief hospitalizations makes case management and community-based care more important than ever. Performing case management functions involves assisting the client on an almost daily basis in managing frequent challenges or problems associated with dysfunction. You will need to work at promoting the client's confidence in your skills during the therapeutic relationship to ensure the client makes the effort to seek help to manage problems. The client's confidence in your knowledge promotes improved health maintenance behaviors so that he or she does not sabotage the treatment or recovery process.

Guiding or accompanying clients through the mental health care system is another facet of the case manager role. Each geographic area differs in the kind of services that are available. In order to obtain treatment, the psychiatric client has to know how to work the system. Case management services assist clients in this process. Working the system may involve the nurse making appointments for clients, accompanying clients to disability interviews, and explaining forms and paperwork required by agencies or providers. Maneuvering around barriers or obstacles is a special skill of the nurse case manager.

COMMUNITY-BASED CARE

Community-based care is a commonly used forum for treating people who have psychiatric problems. It is much more cost-effective to treat clients on an outpatient than an inpatient basis. The nurse working in a community care setting will likely see particular outpatients repeatedly in that setting. Even though considerable time may elapse between sessions, you will want to help the client develop a strong, ongoing relationship with the provider, thus encouraging the client to seek needed help and to disclose important information. Information about symptoms, side effects, and recovery throughout the client's care in the community is essential to determining appropriate and effective interventions.

HOME CARE

Home care involves entering a sensitive space for the client—the home. Home care nurses need to effectively communicate respect for the client's customs and living arrangements while managing to deliver needed care in a setting that may require quick thinking and improvisation. Acceptance of home care and other services by the client and the client's significant others involves a variety of cultural, demographic, and personal preferences. In one study, there was resistance to several types of home care services. However, ethnic and racial minority clients accepted services from psychiatric nurses (Joosten, 2007), demonstrating that the decision to accept counseling at home can be positively influenced by the interaction between nurse and client. Counseling an individual in his or her home requires sensitivity—about both the therapeutic process and the therapeutic content.

A major consideration in psychiatric–mental health nursing is continuity of care. An important feature of effective care is making sure the same nurse who had a one-to-one relationship with the client sees the client afterward, during home care. Organizations could create new positions or expand duties within existing positions to achieve this continuity. Sometimes, to maximize available services and budgets, mental health systems combine the duties of nurses providing care to clients. This leads to multitasking, not an unusual feature of nursing positions. The clinical example that follows illustrates how a primary nurse in an inpatient setting can continue the therapeutic nurse–client relationship after discharge and can also function as a case manager.

CLINICAL EXAMPLE

You have worked with Francisco, a 65-year-old male, during his brief 5-day stay on your unit. The treatment team's goal was to stabilize his mood and begin antidepressant medication. You have spent 45 minutes each day developing a therapeutic nurse–client relationship with Francisco.

Following his discharge, you function as his case manager, connecting him with a job training program, a social club for mental health clients, and a medication psychoeducation group. You also meet with Francisco in the outpatient clinic weekly for 4 weeks, then every 2 weeks for the next 2 months, and finally, monthly for the next 4 months.

When a referral is made to another psychiatric–mental health nurse or therapist, a home care nurse, a self-help group, a community agency, or a job training program, it is often wise to arrange for an initial contact with the referred person or agency before the nurse–client relationship terminates. This is a way to identify and deal with any initial misconceptions about what will take place after discharge and to ensure follow-up. The shift to dependence on other support systems (family, friends, referrals) is a therapeutic task that should be jointly managed, at least initially, by the nurse and the case manager.

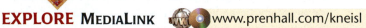

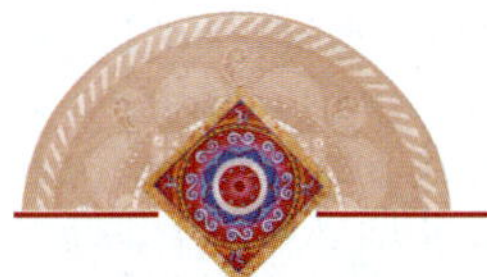

EXPLORE MEDIALINK

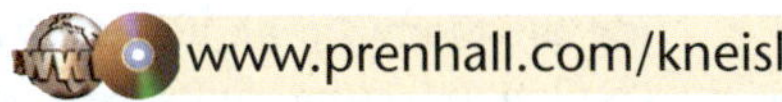

For NCLEX-RN® review questions, case studies, and other resources for this chapter see the Pearson Health MediaLink CD-ROM that accompanies this book and the Companion Website at www.prenhall.com/kneisl.

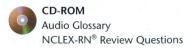

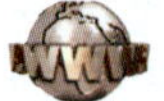

Companion Website
Audio Glossary
NCLEX-RN® Review Questions
Critical Thinking Exercise
- *Working Phase*

Case Study
- *Orientation Phase*

Care Plan
- *Termination Phase*

MediaLinks
MediaLink Application
- *Therapeutic Alliance*

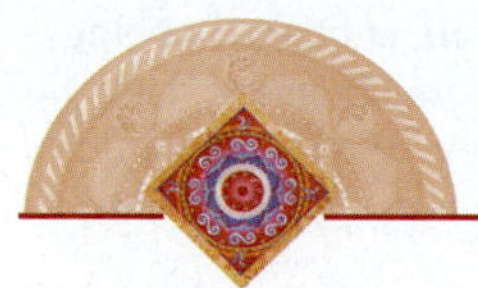

NCLEX-RN® REVIEW QUESTIONS

1. Which of the following client statements does not reflect a characteristic of the functional one–to–one relationship?
1. "We agreed to meet twice monthly for a year in her office at the clinic."
2. "My nurse wants to focus on anger management techniques, and I want to examine my early childhood."
3. "When I move in December, our relationship will end. My nurse plans to refer me to a clinic near my new home. I will miss her, because I will not see her again."
4. "The nurse and I decided to address physical safety issues first, and then focus on sources of social support."

2. The client identifies a behavior that is self-defeating. After 30 seconds of silence, the client states, "I don't want to deal with that right now." Which of the following nurse responses is most therapeutic?
1. "One of the goals you had set was to identify more self-actualizing coping strategies. You just identified a problem."
2. "We can deal with that when you feel more comfortable."
3. "How about telling me about something you did well?"
4. "If you really trust me, we can face anything together."

3. Halfway through a 45-minute session with a nurse, the client is silent for long periods, off and on, for 10 minutes. The nurse hypothesizes that the client is experiencing resistance. Which of the following responses is the most therapeutic?
1. "It's all right if you do not want to talk today. We can end early."
2. "If you do not want to share your thoughts, I do not know how I can help."
3. "You have been silent for long periods during the last 10 minutes."
4. Maintain the silence for the rest of the session.

4. Within the context of a one–to–one relationship, which of the following nurse's statements is inappropriate?
1. "I received your gift in the mail right after you missed your appointment."
2. "I am not comfortable giving hugs to my clients at the end of each session, but I think it would be fine to shake hands."
3. "You sounded very angry the last time we spoke—when I told you I would have to charge you for the late cancellation."
4. "I thought a lot about your situation this week. Last night, you were in my dream."

5. Which client statement reflects attainment of the most important outcome of the orientation phase?
1. "I feel safe enough with my nurse that I could share my thoughts and feelings."
2. "My nurse is the best nurse in the whole clinic."
3. "I have tried to get a reaction from my nurse, but she does not respond to drama."
4. "My nurse reminds me of my mother."

6. Which client statement reflects a realistic outcome attainment associated with the termination phase?
1. "I did not accomplish everything I wanted to, and now you are abandoning me."
2. "I did not accomplish everything I wanted to, but I will come back for more therapy when I am ready."
3. "I met all my goals, and I could not have done it without you."
4. "There is still more work to be done. Don't you think we could resolve more of my issues with a few more sessions?"

7. The nurse's documentation includes the following: "Client mentions long-term relationships, then jokes about their triviality. When confronted about this topic and avoidance of intimacy, client became tearful and shared fears of inadequacy." Which of the following statements best describe this interaction? (Select all that apply.)
1. The client is regressing.
2. During the next session, the nurse should renegotiate the duration of the therapeutic relationship.
3. It is characteristic of the working phase.
4. The client is finalizing therapeutic work and moving toward termination.
5. The nurse and client may reprioritize therapeutic goals.

8. The nurse's note reads, "Client is tearful: reviewing past losses and identifying new problems." Based on this information, the client is:
1. Experiencing the stressors associated with the termination phase.
2. Manipulating to extend the therapeutic relationship.
3. Beginning the working phase.
4. Avoiding behavioral analysis and constructive change in behavior.

9. During the orientation phase, the nurse validates that the client is distrustful of health care providers. The client views the health care system as having values different from those of her culture. Which of the following modifications does the nurse anticipate?
1. Less constructive behavioral change
2. A shorter relationship
3. Less behavioral reflection and analysis
4. A longer orientation phase

10. In the middle of the working phase, the client begins sobbing and screams at the nurse, "You cannot possibly understand! No one has ever discriminated against you based on your cultural heritage!" Which of the following is the nurse's best initial response?
1. "Do you think you would be more comfortable with a therapist who shares your cultural heritage?"
2. "What have I done to offend you?"
3. "Whether or not that's true, I am right here with you. I will stay with you. You are not alone."
4. "Your anger has less to do with me and more to do with figures from your past."

See Appendix C for answers.

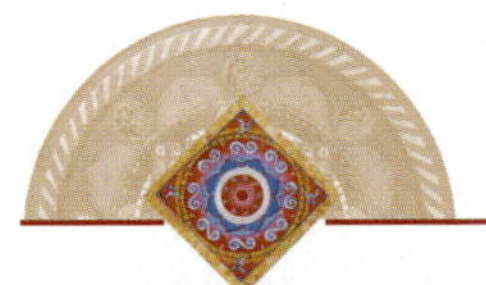

REFERENCES

Barker, P. (1999). Hildegard E. Peplau: The mother of psychiatric nursing. *Journal of Psychiatric and Mental Health Nursing, 6*(3), 175–176.

Beech, M. (2007). Confidentiality in health care: Conflicting legal and ethical issues. *Nursing Standard, 21*(21), 42–46.

Beretta, V., Despland, J. N., Drapeau, M., Michel, L., Kramer, U., Stigler, M., et al. (2007). Are relationship patterns with significant others reenacted with the therapist? A study of early transference reactions. *Journal of Nervous & Mental Disease, 195*(5), 443–450.

Boag, S. (2007). *Decoding the meaning of transference and countertransference: An integrative perspective*. Washington, DC: American Psychological Association.

Davis, L. W., & Lysaker, P. H. (2007). Therapeutic alliance and improvements in work performance over time in patients with schizophrenia. *Journal of Nervous and Mental Disease, 195*(4), 353–357.

Duffin, C. (2007). NMC proposal to ban gifts "could harm staff–patient relationships." *Nursing Standard, 21*(32), 10.

Ellis, A. (2001). Rational and irrational aspects of countertransference. *Journal of Clinical Psychology, 57*(8), 999–1004.

Epstein, E. E., McCrady, B. S., Morgan, T. J., Cook, S. M., Kugler, G., & Ziedonis, D. (2007). The successive cohort design: A model for developing new behavioral therapies for drug use disorders, and application to behavioral couple treatment. *Addictive Disorders & Their Treatment, 6*(1), 1–19.

Ford, L. (2007). *Human relations: A game plan for improving personal adjustment* (4th ed.). Upper Saddle River, NJ: Pearson Education.

Gary, J. M. (2007). Counseling adult learners: Individual interventions, group interventions, and campus resources. In J. A. Lippincott & R. B. Lippincott (Eds.), *Special populations in college counseling: A handbook for mental health professionals* (pp. 99–113). Alexandria, VA: American Counseling Association.

Guy, J. D., & Brady, J. L. (2001). Identifying the faces in the mirror: Untangling transference and countertransference in self psychology. *Journal of Clinical Psychology, 57*(8), 993–997.

Huss, D. B., & Baer, R. A. (2007). Acceptance and change: The integration of mindfulness-based cognitive therapy into ongoing dialectical behavior therapy in a case of borderline personality disorder with depression. *Clinical Case Studies, 6*(1), 17–33.

Joosten, D. (2007). Preferences for accepting prescribed community-based, psychosocial, and in-home services by older adults. *Home Health Care Services Quarterly, 26*(1), 1–18.

Mackin, P., Targum, S. D., Kalali, A., Rom, D., & Young, A. H. (2007). Cultural background may influence the perception of psychiatric symptoms. *British Journal of Psychiatry, 190*(2), 178–179.

Martin, G., & Pear, J. (2007). *Behavioral modification: What it is and how to do it* (8th ed.). Upper Saddle River, NJ: Pearson Education.

Messer, S. B. (2002). A psychodynamic perspective on resistance in psychotherapy: Vive la resistance. *Journal of Clinical Psychology, 58*(2), 157–163.

Mynatt, S., & Cunningham, P. (2007). Unraveling anxiety and depression. *Nurse Practitioner: American Journal of Primary Health Care, 32*(8), 28–37.

O'Brien, L., Schachtschneider, A. M., Koren, G., Walker, J. H., & Einarson, A. (2007). Longitudinal study of depression, anxiety, irritability, and stress in pregnancy following evidence-based counseling on the use of antidepressants. *Journal of Psychiatric Practice, 13*(1), 33–39.

Paris, J. (2007). Intermittent psychotherapy: An alternative to continuous long-term treatment for patients with personality disorders. *Journal of Psychiatric Practice, 13*(3), 153–158.

Peplau, H. E. (1952). *Interpersonal relations in nursing*. New York: Putnam.

Peplau, H. E. (1997). Peplau's theory of interpersonal relations. *Nursing Science Quarterly, 10*(4), 162–167.

Sambrook, S., Abba, N., & Chadwick, P. (2007). Evaluation of DBT emotional coping skills groups for people with parasuicidal behaviours. *Behavioural and Cognitive Psychotherapy, 35*(2), 241–244.

Shapiro, E. L., & Ginzberg, R. (2002). Parting gifts: Termination rituals in group therapy. *International Journal of Group Psychotherapy, 52*(3), 319–336.

Smith, K. W., & Greenberg, L. S. (2007). Internal multiplicity in emotion-focused psychotherapy. *Journal of Clinical Psychology, 63*(2), 175–186.

Stanton, K. (2007). Emergency: Communicating with ED patients who have chronic mental illnesses. *American Journal of Nursing, 107*(2), 61–65.

Steelman, J. R. (2007). Relationship dynamics: Understanding married women's mental health. *Advances in Nursing Science. Women and Aging. 30*(2), 151–158.

Weeks, S., Cowell, R., Scullion, J., & Tanton, E. (2007). Readers panel. Refusing gifts. *Nursing Standard, 21*(39), 26–27.

Weiss, M. A., & Lewis, L. (2007). Respect for the patient. *American Journal of Nursing, 107*(Supp.), 12.

Group and Family Interventions

CHAPTER

30

CAROL REN KNEISL

LEARNING OUTCOMES

After completing this chapter, you will be able to:

1. Create and maintain a therapeutic group.
2. Design a therapeutic group based on the personality characteristics of potential members.
3. Explain the purposes that therapeutic groups fulfill.
4. Apply the process of here-and-now activation to a therapeutic group.
5. Describe families and their dynamics in terms of relationships, associations, and connections.
6. Carry out a family assessment.
7. Partner with clients and their families in recognizing when family interventions or family therapy are appropriate.
8. Incorporate an understanding of group and family processes in promoting and maintaining an individual's mental health.

CRITICAL THINKING CHALLENGE

You are present at a multidisciplinary case conference presentation. Mark James, your 22-year-old client, is being discharged from his first hospital admission for schizophrenia to the home he shares with his father and two sisters. Mark has been alienated from his mother since his parents' divorce when he was 17 years old. Mark's mother has failed to show up for the discharge conference. The mental health team has recommended family therapy to the James family. You perceive what you think is annoyance on Mr. James's face, and one of Mark's sisters appears embarrassed. Although you would not be the James family therapist because you are not a clinical specialist, you recognize how important Mark's family can be to his progress.

1. What might be some of the family's unspoken concerns and needs?
2. What actions can you take to address the family's unspoken needs and concerns?
3. Mark is 22 years old, an adult. Why would family therapy be appropriate, rather than individual therapy?

KEY TERMS

cohesion *803*
family burden *820*
family system *815*
genogram *820*
goblet issues *805*
here-and-now activation *812*
life script *817*
self-fulfilling prophecy *817*
self-reflective loop *811*

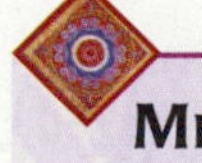

MEDIALINK 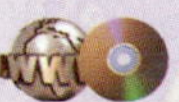 www.prenhall.com/kneisl

Go to the Pearson Health MediaLink CD-ROM and the Companion Website at www.prenhall.com/kneisl for interactive resources for this chapter.

Why are groups and families important? Most people are born into a group—the family—and our survival from the moment of birth depends on relationships formed with other human beings. The sense of self, of being, of personal identity derives from the ways in which other members of the groups to which we belong perceive and respond to us. We interact with others at all stages of our lives in various groups—family groups, peer groups, work groups, play groups, worship groups.

The family is the context in which most people, including nurses, develop their first relationships with other people. Their view of the larger social world outside their own unique family is molded by the events that happen within families and influence the development of the individual. Nurses encounter families in many areas of their practice—in the emergency room, the intensive care unit, the school, the cancer hospital, the community health setting, and the mental health care setting. Preventive approaches to family mental health, assessment of families in trouble, and intervention on their behalf must be based on an understanding of how families grow and interact and how family coping patterns develop.

Many of the goals we set for ourselves cannot be achieved without membership in groups and families. Other people are important to each of us, just as we are important to others. Through cooperation and coordination we can achieve objectives and reach goals that we could not through individual effort alone. In this way, groups and families help us improve the quality of our lives.

Much of our professional life is spent in groups—groups of clients and groups of colleagues with whom we plan and implement the delivery of health care services. Group interventions, relatives' groups, and multiple-family groups will become increasingly more important in this economy as a result of the need to provide treatments that are also cost effective.

To use groups rationally and effectively and to effectively intervene with families, nurses must understand the forces that underlie small group interactional processes and family processes, and recognize their own patterns of participation. Using group and family interventions, psychiatric–mental health nurses can provide psychoeducation for their clients and their families. Group and family interventions also provide the opportunity to seek validation, give and receive interpersonal feedback, and test new and different ways of being that may improve the quality of life. Mental health can be preserved, maintained, and restored through interaction with others in productive groups and families.

Nurses have long been involved in working with clients and their families in small groups brought together for health teaching, psychoeducation, or supportive purposes. All nurses, regardless of level of education, can lead therapeutic groups or psychoeducation groups, and all nurses can assist families, as long as they understand and apply group and family dynamics in their interventions.

Informal groups exist on units in inpatient facilities and in community-based agencies as well. The disciplined application of group and family psychotherapeutic principles is the basis for the nurse's therapeutic use of self in unplanned encounters in these settings. However, the role of the psychiatric–mental health nurse as group psychotherapist or family therapist is reserved for advanced-practice registered nurses prepared at the master's level and above (see Chapter 2, which discusses psychiatric–mental health nursing roles in relationship to education, preparation, and certification).

SMALL GROUP DYNAMICS

Several forces modify and shape groups, influencing their effectiveness. These forces are discussed in the sections that follow.

Trust

Trust develops in relationships when people disclose more and more of their thoughts, perceptions, attitudes, and reactions to one another and find that their disclosures have been made in a safe environment among persons who respect their self-disclosures. The group member who makes a suggestion; discloses an attitude, feeling, experience, or perception; gives feedback; or confronts another member engages in trusting behavior and assumes the risks inherent in trusting. Trusting and being trusted are intimately linked to risk taking. The level of trust among the members of a group determines the extent of risk-taking behavior in the group. When trust exists, individual members will risk sharing more. Since trust takes some time to build, do not expect that trust will necessarily exist in short-term inpatient groups in which membership changes frequently in a brief period of time.

Self-Disclosure and Self-Awareness

There are many ways to think about self-awareness. Some theorists have used the image of multiple masks that people wear under a variety of circumstances. Others have written about the "true self" versus "the false self" or the "good me," the "bad me," and the "real me." Common to all these concepts is the idea that self-awareness is a complex, multidimensional phenomenon, often contradictory and partly undiscovered. The Johari Awareness Model, often called simply the Johari Window, is a theoretical tool used to represent self-awareness and self-disclosure in relation to other people. The notion of self-disclosure has been discussed in general in Chapter 3. This section discusses a theory of self-disclosure that can be applied to the understanding of individuals as well as therapeutic groups.

Luft and Ingham first developed the Johari Awareness Model in 1955. They maintained that interpersonal interaction, in a group setting, for example, is facilitated when people have sufficient knowledge about one another's attitudes, beliefs, actions, and opinions to determine how safe it is to self-disclose to them. The Johari Window is Luft and Ingham's graphic representation of their self-awareness model. It is described here and illustrated in FIGURE 30-1 ■.

- *Johari Window Quadrant 1*—Open Activity. The first quadrant of the window represents aspects of the self that are known about oneself and are readily available and known to others as well. This is the part of the self that engages in daily social conversation.

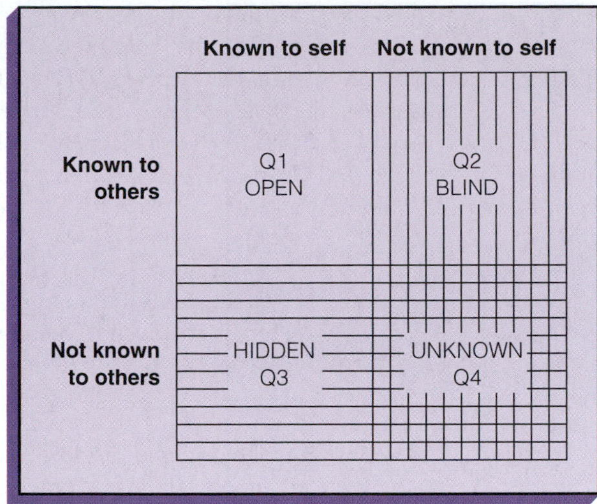

FIGURE 30-1 ■ The Johari Awareness Model.

- *Johari Window Quadrant 2*—Risk. Quadrant 2 contains characteristics that are known to others but not to oneself. In this quadrant is information about how the person affects others intentionally or unintentionally. It is an aspect of self about which a person may get honest, genuine, uncensored feedback from others. It is also an area that influences reactions from others that may surprise and shock the individual.
- *Johari Window Quadrant 3*—Private Life Space. Quadrant 3 represents the knowledge one has about oneself that is not known to others. These are the secrets, the personal and private feelings.
- *Johari Window Quadrant 4*—The Unknown. Quadrant 4 contains knowledge about the self that is unconscious for the individual and unknown to others. This quadrant may be brought into awareness through psychotherapy with special guidance.

Relations Within the Group

Major elements in this awareness model are its assumptions that humans respond to groups and that change or learning can follow opportunities for new interaction. The primary principle of change in relation to the Johari Window is: A change in one quadrant will affect all other quadrants. Certain other general principles of change that derive from the Johari Window are particularly suited to the understanding of small group behavior. These principles are:

- A large open quadrant (Q1) facilitates working with others. Therefore, more of the resources and abilities of group members can be brought to bear on the group task when members have large Q1 areas.
- The open quadrant can be enlarged and awareness can be increased by learning about group processes as they are being experienced.
- The group's value system influences how a group confronts the unknown quadrant.

In a new and immature group, the open quadrant (Q1) is small because free and spontaneous interaction does not occur in new groups. As the group matures, the open quadrant expands and the private quadrant (Q3) shrinks accordingly. This means that members become freer to be themselves and to perceive others as they really are. An atmosphere of increasing trust, risk taking, and self-disclosure begins to form. An enlarged area of free activity means that the group uses more energy to work on the group task than to maintain or defend the hidden or avoided area of Q3. The risk quadrant (Q2) also diminishes as members learn more about themselves. The unknown quadrant (Q4) changes more slowly and to a lesser degree, because it represents an area in which unknown behaviors and motives reside. FIGURE 30-2 ■ compares the degrees of openness in immature and mature groups.

A group can also be understood and diagrammed according to the Johari Windows of the individual members. The Johari Window configurations of the group in the clinical example that follows are illustrated in FIGURE 30-3 ■ on page 802.

CLINICAL EXAMPLE

Sam was a person with limited freedom. Although he was polite, he appeared to be superficial and constricted. He devoted large amounts of energy to walling off the behavior and motivations of the risk, private, and unknown quadrants (Q2, Q3, and Q4) by intellectualizing.

Laura was a group member whose great inner resources allowed her to develop a very large area of free activity.

In contrast, Debbie was what could be termed a "plunger." Debbie's spontaneity and inappropriate openness lacked discretion and created distance in her relationships with other group members.

Van and Maria, the other two members of this group, tended not to take many risks in their interactions with others, although their moderate openness indicated flexibility.

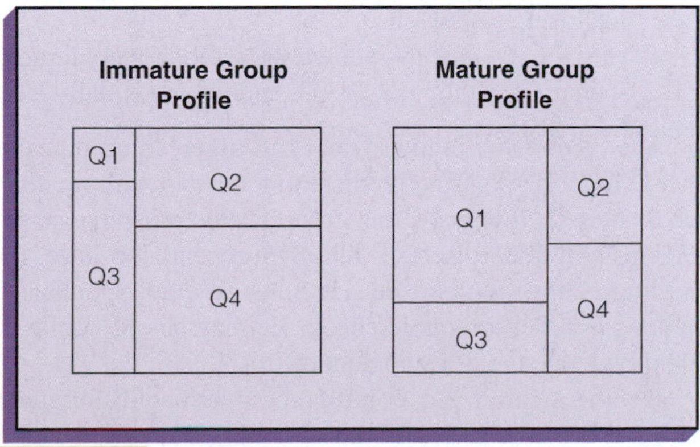

FIGURE 30-2 ■ Johari Window configuration of the immature versus mature group.

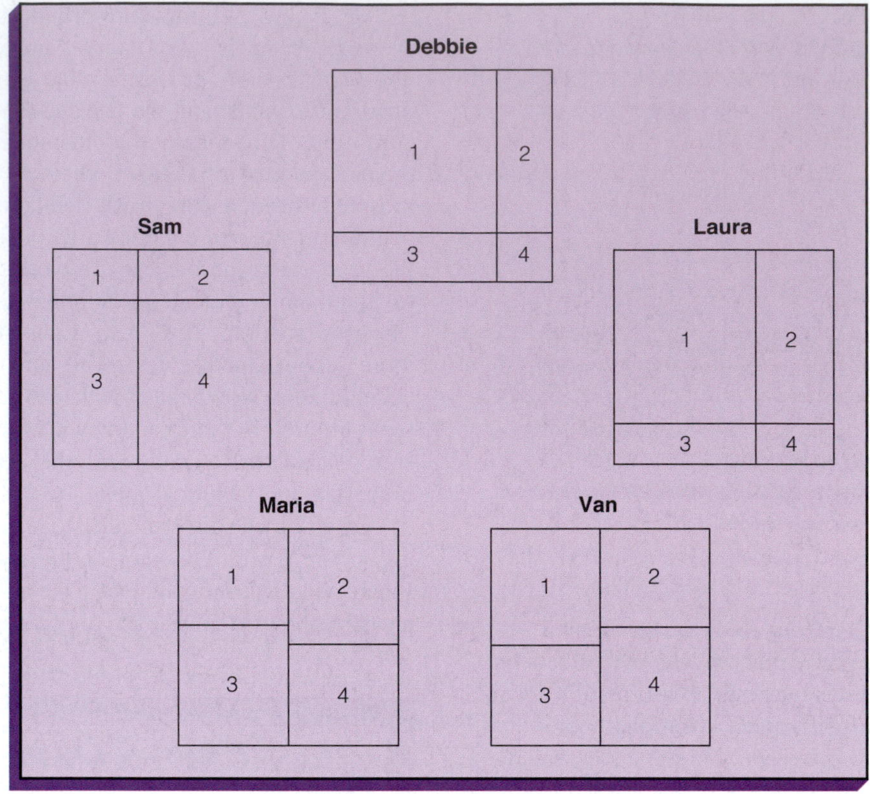

FIGURE 30-3 ■ Awareness configurations of the members of one group.

The Johari Window configurations of this entire group are illustrated in Figure 30-3:

- Sam's window shows a greatly reduced and constricted open quadrant. His behavior and feelings are likely to be limited in range, variety, and scope. His interactions tend to be conventional, and he is likely to be threatened by group behaviors that go beyond the bounds of convention.
- Laura's window represents a person whose interactions are characterized by great openness to the world. Much of her potential has been developed and realized.
- Debbie's window is that of the inappropriately transparent person who deals with others by disclosing too much.
- Maria's and Van's windows show moderately large open areas although Q2, Q3, and Q4 are equally large.

The group's windows raise an interesting question: What behaviors might be predicted in a group with members such as these? Obviously, this group needs to resolve several problems. An underdiscloser like Sam reveals too little, thus reserving control for himself. He tends to quell spontaneous reactions in order to double-check. He may be one of the last to acknowledge the development of trust.

Debbie's failure to control her overdisclosure means that her relationships with others in the group will be either too smothering (because of being too close) or too demanding because she imposes herself on others without considering their intimacy needs. She discloses to everyone because she has not learned to discriminate among relationships. Her behavior forces others to take responsibility for defining the nature of the relationship. Group members are likely to feel threatened by her early, spontaneous disclosures, which they may experience as overwhelming. Problems of trust, intimacy, and risk-taking may arise in her interactions with the other members.

Laura, because of her high degree of self-awareness, will be less preoccupied with defensiveness and differences than other members. She will be able to accept the differences in others and serve as a role model for them.

Van and Maria, whose awareness configurations demonstrate that they have progressed to moderate openness, should continue to move in this direction with minimal discomfort to themselves or the other group members.

Relations with Other Groups

A group can also be viewed as a whole entity in interaction with other groups. Q1 includes the open, available information that is known to the group as well as to others. Q2 is the area that others outside the group see but the group itself does not.

Q3 has to do with the secret, hidden things that the group keeps to itself. Knowledge may be hidden purposefully to enable the group to manipulate other groups. A group of businesspeople who hide the flaws in a company they put up for sale illustrate this. Groups keep things hidden for other reasons as well, such as being ashamed of some activity or attitude or finding an event or belief hard to explain because it refers to idiosyncratic occurrences known only to the members. Hidden things form the *lore* of the group.

Q4 includes behavior and motives that are unknown to the group and to outsiders as well. A covert and unrecognized split among the members with regard to the group goals would be one example. Difficulties in effective group functioning could result from such an unrecognized split.

Cohesion

Cohesion can be defined as a spirit of common purpose. In groups that cohere, the members have a desire for mutual association. Cohesion is the primary factor keeping a group in existence and working effectively.

A group is cohesive when its members are attracted to it. People are attracted to a therapeutic group for a wide variety of reasons. The group may meet their needs for affiliation, interpersonal security, self-knowledge, or therapy. It may have members who not only are available for human interaction but also have important shared attitudes, values, interests, and beliefs. An attractive group has explicit, mutual, and attainable group goals with clear paths to goal attainment.

What indicates that the spirit of cohesion exists in a given group?

- Attendance is high.
- The members arrive on time.
- The members stay with the group.
- The members engage in an interdependence that is cooperative rather than competitive.
- The activities the group undertakes are satisfying and successful.
- There is a high degree of member participation.
- Communication networks are open, central, and flexible in a warm and friendly atmosphere.
- "We" is frequently heard in discussions.
- The members like and trust one another.
- The members enjoy interacting with one another.
- Participation is high.

Cohesive groups are not born—they are developed. Cohesion does not become evident until the group has come together long enough to have shared experiences that provide the basis for attraction. An outpatient group has an existence lengthy enough to provide time for cohesion to develop. Inpatient groups are usually too brief to become cohesive.

How can a group's tendency to cohere be enhanced? Some methods are increasing the trusting and trustworthy behavior of members, the affection expressed among members, the expressions of inclusion and acceptance among members, and the influence that members have on one another. Another method for building cohesion is structuring cooperative relationships among the group members.

Group Roles and Leadership

Group roles center on the influence relationships that exist within the group. The primary influence relationship is leadership. Group dynamics theory tells us that leadership functions within a group can be fulfilled by the person designated as the leader, and by members who engage in leadership behavior. This approach to understanding leadership behavior is called the *distributed functions approach* and stems from the classic research of Benne and Sheats (1948).

The distributed functions approach to group leadership is based on two major beliefs:

1. Any member of a group may become a leader by taking actions that serve group purposes.
2. Different members may perform various roles in a group.

Each member may play more than one role during a meeting of the group and a wide range of roles in successive participations. Any member may play any or all of the roles. The various functional roles may be grouped in two categories:

1. *Task roles* are related to the task of the group. The job of people assuming these roles is to facilitate and coordinate group efforts in the selection, definition, and solution of a group problem.
2. *Maintenance roles* are oriented toward building group-centered attitudes among the members and maintaining and perpetuating group-centered behavior.

Sometimes members of a group satisfy individual needs that are irrelevant to the group task and may also be negatively oriented to group maintenance functions. These are called *self-serving roles*. If a group is to function effectively, it must perform a self-diagnosis to determine what the needs of the group are and how they can be met, so that the self-serving roles no longer present obstacles to effective functioning. Task, maintenance, and self-serving roles are described in Box 30-1 on page 804.

Distributing leadership functions among group members is important because it teaches people the diagnostic skills and behaviors needed to accomplish the group's goals and maintain good interpersonal relationships. Of course, in psychotherapy groups, some functions or activities may be largely, or even solely, the province of the therapist. In psychotherapy groups, the quality of the therapeutic alliance with the group therapist was a consistent predictor of short-term group therapy outcome (Joyce, Piper, & Ogrodniczuk, 2007).

Power and Influence

It is impossible to discuss group dynamics without discussing power because it is impossible to interact without influencing, and being influenced by, others. This process constantly occurs within groups, forcing members to adjust to one another and modify their behavior and, sometimes, their attitudes and beliefs. Power is defined as the ability to do or act, to have possession of command or control over others, to achieve the desired result. The terms *power* and *influence* are used interchangeably in this chapter.

Power and influence are not negative forces. Do not confuse the judicious use of power in building effective groups with the use of power to control, manage, and manipulate

Box 30-1 Group Roles and Functions

Role	Function
Task Roles	
Coordinator	Identifies the relationships among the group suggestions and ideas
Elaborator	Fleshes out ideas and suggestions (arranging seating; distributing handouts)
Information giver	Offers facts, ideas, and own experiences
Information seeker	Asks for information that would clarify issues
Opinion giver	States beliefs about group function and group values
Opinion seeker	Asks for beliefs that would clarify group values
Maintenance Roles	
Compromiser	Minimizes conflict by seeking alternatives
Encourager	Moves the group in a positive direction by encouraging and praising the contributions of others
Follower	Goes along with the group
Group observer	Keeps the group records; interprets data
Harmonizer	Keeps the peace; smoothes over conflict
Standard setter	Reminds group of the standards to be achieved
Self-Serving Roles	
Aggressor	Attacks group members, ideas, or values
Blocker	Disagrees, opposes, and resists
Dominator	Manipulates others, seeks control through excessive talking; interrupts others
Playboy	Fails to become involved in group process
Recognition seeker	Boasts, brags about accomplishments, calls attention to self
Self-confessor	Expresses personal and self-oriented, rather than group-oriented, insights and feelings

Source: Adapted from Benne, K. D., & Sheats, P. (1948). Functional roles of group members. *Journal of Social Issues, 4,* 41–49. Reprinted with permission from Blackwell Publishing.

others. Become aware of how you can employ power and influence in serving your clients and your profession.

A group in which certain members have much power and others have little power is likely to be a group in trouble. The unequal distribution of power affects both the task and the maintenance functions of a group. Members who believe they have little influence within the group are unlikely to feel committed to group goals and to the implementation of group decisions. Their dissatisfaction with the group decreases its attractiveness and reduces its cohesion.

GROUP DEVELOPMENT THEORY

The interpersonal needs approach discussed in this section can be used to understand the development, dynamics, and functioning of small groups, from self-help groups to psychoeducation groups to psychotherapy groups. The interpersonal needs approach helps us to understand how groups develop and the factors that determine how effective they are.

The basic assumption of the interpersonal needs approach known as FIRO (Fundamental Interpersonal Relationship Orientation), a classic group dynamics theory, is that people need people. In addition, people need to establish some equilibrium between themselves and the others in their environment. This equilibrium is determined by the interaction of three basic interpersonal needs, and it appears to be synonymous with interpersonal compatibility (Schutz, 1958b).

Three Basic Interpersonal Needs

An interpersonal need is one that can be satisfied only through relationships with people. Schutz reasoned that every individual has three interpersonal needs: inclusion, control, and affection.

Inclusion

The interpersonal need for *inclusion* is the need to establish and maintain relationships with others that offer interactions and associations satisfying to the individual. To put this another way, the inclusion need consists of the ability to take an interest in others to a satisfactory degree, and the ability to allow other people to take an interest in you to a satisfying degree to yourself. This need determines whether a person is outgoing or prefers privacy. Compare the inclusion needs illustrated in FIGURE 30-4 ■.

Control

The interpersonal need for *control* is the need to establish and maintain a satisfactory relationship between oneself and other people with regard to power and influence. Stated another

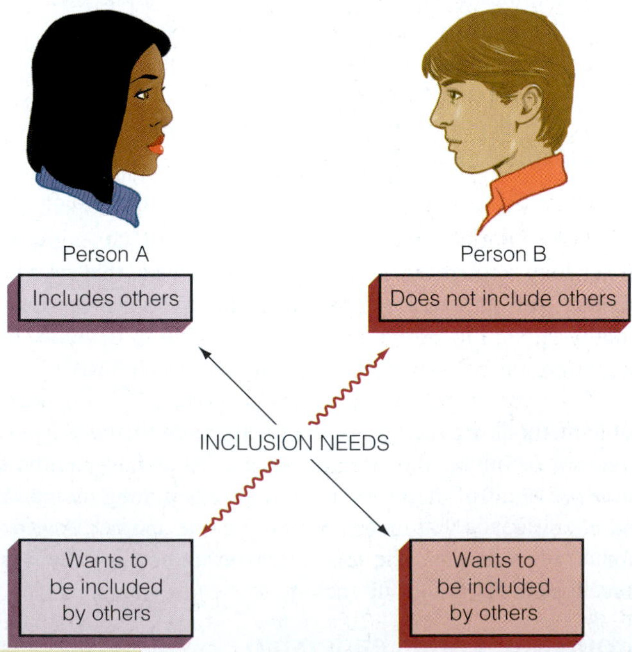

FIGURE 30-4 ■ Inclusion needs. While both people want to be included by others, only one (Person A) includes others. Therefore, Person B's needs for inclusion are met. However, Person A will feel frustrated because her need to be included is not being met.

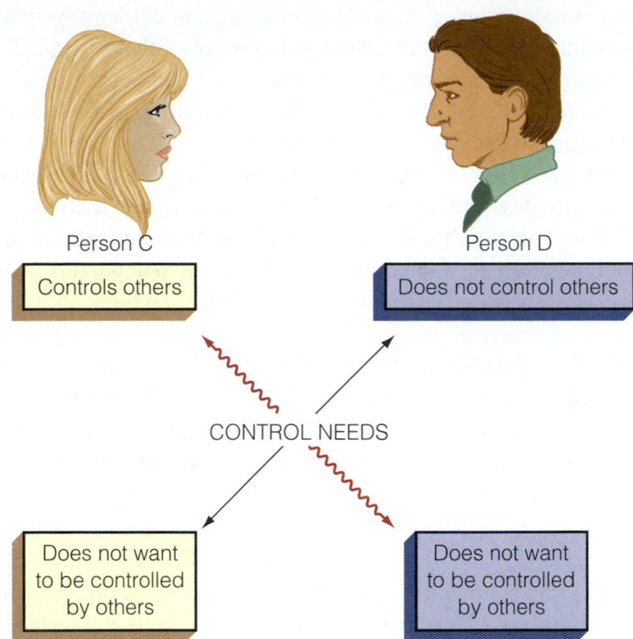

FIGURE 30-5 ■ Control needs. This situation has the potential for great conflict. Person D, who is happiest in a lackadaisical atmosphere, will resent, and perhaps sabotage, Person C's efforts to control. Person C is likely to intensify her control efforts in response.

way, the control need consists of the ability to take charge to a satisfactory degree, and the ability to establish and maintain a feeling of respect for the competence and responsibleness of others to a satisfying degree to yourself. Compare the control needs illustrated in FIGURE 30-5 ■.

Affection

The interpersonal need for *affection* is the need to establish and maintain a satisfactory relationship between the self and other people with regard to love and affection. Put another way, the affection need consists of being able to love other people or to be close and intimate to a satisfactory degree, and having others love you or be close and intimate with you to a satisfactory degree. Compare the affection needs illustrated in FIGURE 30-6 ■.

Group Phases

According to this approach any group, given enough time, moves through three interpersonal phases—inclusion, control, and affection, in that order—that correspond to the three basic interpersonal needs.

Inclusion Phase

The first or inclusion phase is concerned with the problem of *in or out*. People attempt to find their place in the group and are concerned with learning whether they will be acknowledged as individuals or left behind and ignored. Because these concerns give rise to anxiety, this phase is dominated by behavior centered around the self. Overtalking, withdrawal, exhibitionism, and sharing other group experiences and biographies are some examples.

Frequently, what Schutz (1958a) calls **goblet issues** predominate. These are issues of minor importance to the group that help the members get to know one another better and to test each other out. Goblet issues are a vehicle for sizing people up. Goblet issues may revolve around the weather, sports, rules of procedure, and so on. If goblet issues continue to a significant extent beyond this initial phase of the group, they will impede group progress.

Control Phase

The second or control phase is concerned with the problem of *top or bottom*, which becomes central after problems of inclusion have been resolved. Concern about decision-making procedures predominates. The problems that emerge in this phase center around two concerns:

1. How responsibility is shared
2. How power and influence are distributed

There are struggles for leadership and about the structure, rules of procedure, and methods of decision making. Members are attempting to establish comfortable positions for themselves in terms of responsibility and influence.

Affection Phase

The third or affection phase is concerned with the problem of *near or far*, and it follows satisfactory resolution of the preceding two phases. Individual members are now faced with the problem of becoming emotionally involved with one another. Concerns about not being liked by, being too close to, or not being close enough to others become relevant. The behavior in this phase is generally characterized by high emotion—positive feelings, jealousy, hostility, and pairing are some examples. Schutz (1958a) describes this

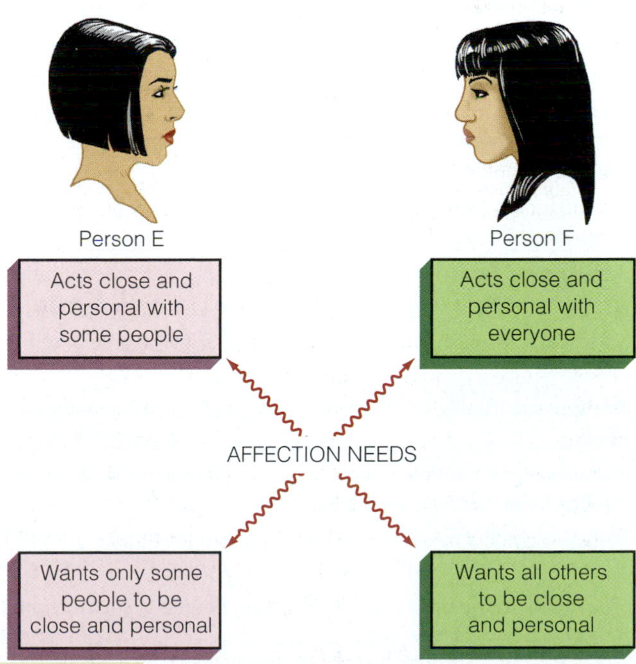

FIGURE 30-6 ■ Affection needs. Both people in this situation are getting some of their affection needs met if Person F is one of the people with whom Person E wishes to be close and personal. If not, Person E could back away emotionally if she views Person F as intrusive. Backing away would likely cause frustration for Person F.

phase as one in which, like porcupines, people attempt to get close enough to receive warmth, yet avoid the pain that sharp quills can inflict.

Interweaving of Phases

None of these phases is distinct, since all three problem areas—in or out, near or far, top or bottom—are present at all times, even though only one predominates. Schutz (1958a) uses a tire-changing analogy, what he calls *tightening the bolts*, to describe the sequence of the phases. Changing a tire is best done by tightening the bolts just enough to hold the wheel in place. Then each bolt is tightened further until it is secured. The leader helps the group work on all three interpersonal need areas in similar fashion, returning to and working over each area to a more satisfactory level than was reached the last time. The interpersonal needs approach of Schutz is based on the belief that the way to attack problems within groups is by investigating what is going on among the individuals in the group and attempting to improve their interpersonal relations. You will discover a parallel between this group development theory and Yalom's group therapy theory, discussed next.

GROUP THERAPY THEORY

There is great diversity and flux in the field of group therapy. Many types of groups are found in mental health care settings or in communities at large. However, certain common principles seem to apply to all therapeutic groups, although specific methods and techniques may vary according to the purpose of the group or the skills and theoretic orientation of the therapist or group leader.

Irvin Yalom (2005) uses the term *interactional group therapy* to describe a process of group therapy in which member interaction plays a crucial role. The common principles that apply to interactional group therapy are discussed next.

The psychiatric–mental health nurse, even if not an advanced-practice nurse qualified as a group psychotherapist, can incorporate many of these principles of group therapy into the leadership role in therapeutic groups as well as in informal groups in the milieu. The principles will have a sense of familiarity—Yalom, like Hildegard Peplau (see Chapter 2∞), was greatly influenced by the interpersonal theory of Harry Stack Sullivan (see Chapter 5∞). The principles will need to be modified for use in short-term groups, such as those in effect on most inpatient units. Modifications for short-term inpatient groups are discussed throughout this section. Essential differences between inpatient and outpatient groups are identified in Table 30-1 ■.

Advantages of Group Therapy

The advantages of group therapy stem from one major factor: the presence of many people, rather than a solitary therapist,

Table 30-1 ■ Differences Between Inpatient and Outpatient Groups

Inpatient Groups	Outpatient Groups
The composition of the group changes depending on who has been admitted and who has been discharged.	The composition of the group is stable, usually over its life.
Members may be selected because they happened to be clients on a particular unit or assigned to a particular therapist.	Selection criteria play a major role in designing the group.
Although clients may be assigned to one or another of available groups depending on appropriateness, selection interviews are not usually conducted.	Selection interviews are standard practice to prepare clients for the group experience and to establish and clarify the group contract.
Attendance is compulsory and clients are often wary of, or ambivalent about, attending the group.	Clients usually choose whether or not to join a group. Those who choose to join are motivated.
Membership length is determined by the length of hospitalization. When the client is discharged, membership in the group ends.	The group continues for a predetermined length of time identified in the group contract—often 1 year or more.
The goal is relief of symptoms and possibly some degree of self-awareness.	The goal is insight-oriented.
Sessions are usually 45–50 minutes long, daily or several times a week.	Most outpatient groups are approximately 1½ hours in length, once a week.
Because of the continually changing membership, inpatient groups rarely become cohesive.	Group cohesion can be expected to develop over time.
Group members have 24-hour exposure to one another.	Members in outpatient groups are discouraged from having relationships with other members outside the meetings.
The inpatient therapist provides a greater degree of structure and takes on a more active role.	The outpatient therapist is less active and waits for the structure and the process to unfold.
Because the therapist has limited ability to select who will be in the group, the group tends to be heterogenous in terms of vulnerability or ego strength as well as personality characteristics.	Outpatient therapists usually design their groups to balance the behavior and characteristics the members bring to the group. The members are more likely to be homogenous in terms of their ego strength.

who participate in the therapeutic experience. Specifically, group therapy provides the following:

- Stimuli from multiple sources, revealing distortions in interpersonal relationships so that they can be examined and resolved
- Multiple sources of feedback
- An interpersonal testing ground that allows members to try out old and new ways of being in an environment specifically structured for that purpose

Qualifications of Group Therapists

Mental health care professionals may believe, in error, that group therapy is less complex and therefore "easier" than one-to-one work—because, for example, the presence of more people makes interactions between therapist and client less intense. Although it is true that the interactions between any one member and the therapist may be less intense because interactions are dispersed among others, it does not follow that anyone can be an effective group therapist. Rather, group processes are very complex because the interactions occur among many different personalities. To be effective, the group therapist should have the following special preparation:

- Education in small group dynamics
- Education in group therapy theory
- Clinical practice with groups
- Expert supervision of the clinical practice (with ongoing supervision and/or consultation, depending on level of expertise)

The scope and standards of practice for psychiatric–mental health nurses (American Nurses Association, American Psychiatric Nurses Association, and International Society of Psychiatric–Mental Health Nurses, 2007) identify the group psychotherapist role as appropriate for advanced-practice registered nurses prepared at the master's level (see Chapter 2∞). Experienced therapists report that it is also valuable to have been a member of a therapy or sensitivity training group before becoming a group leader.

Psychiatric–mental health nurses at the generalist level are qualified, with appropriate preparation, to lead the therapeutic support groups described later in this chapter.

The Curative Factors

Yalom (2005) contends that 11 interdependent curative factors or mechanisms of change in group therapy help people. These factors constitute a rational basis for the therapist's choices of tactics and strategies. They are identified and defined in Table 30-2 ■ on page 808.

Types of Group Leadership

Groups can be led by a therapist working alone or by cotherapists working together in a variety of ways.

Single Therapist Approach

Groups led by a single therapist are common. They have an economic advantage in that only one therapist need be involved. A disadvantage is that the therapist cannot compare analyses of the group process with a cotherapist or get instant feedback or validation from a peer. Therapists working alone, however, do not have to direct their energies toward creating and maintaining a relationship with a colleague.

Cotherapy Approach

Groups led by two therapists, who share responsibility for leadership of the group to varying degrees, are gaining in popularity. The two models seen most often are the junior–senior and the egalitarian styles of cotherapy.

Junior–Senior Cotherapy In the junior–senior approach, the therapists have unequal responsibilities toward the group. The senior member of the team is usually the more experienced or educated. Besides having major responsibility for the success of the group, the senior therapist is responsible for training the junior member of the team.

This approach is commonly used in agency settings, because it provides in-service training of new personnel and nonprofessionals under the guidance and watchful eye of an experienced group leader. However, relationship problems frequently surface when the roles of the leaders are not clear, or when one or both leaders are unable, or unwilling, to remain in the designated roles. The members of the group may also be unclear about the subordinate/superordinate roles and unsure of how to deal with and respond to leaders of unequal abilities and responsibilities.

Egalitarian Cotherapy In the egalitarian approach to cotherapy, two therapists of relatively equal ability and status share equally in responsibility for the group. The method is also used for training, with both cotherapists working under clinical supervision.

Two nurses considering an egalitarian cotherapy relationship with each other need to engage in preliminary work to determine whether such a relationship is feasible for them. Exploration should include:

- Discussing each therapist's theoretic approaches, intervention styles, past experiences with groups, sociocultural background, and personality characteristics
- Considering and resolving such issues as how and when feedback is to be given, how disagreements between them are to be handled in the session, and the general conditions under which they will work together
- Agreeing that decisions on client selection, length and number of sessions, time, and place are made together, and that decisions of an emergency nature made by one therapist in the absence of the other are based on mutually agreed-upon procedures for just such situations

Obviously, egalitarian cotherapists must establish and maintain clear channels of communication. Not only must they expend a great deal of time and energy in preparation for the group experience, they must also plan for presession and postsession meetings, joint analysis of data, and joint supervision or consultation.

TABLE 30-2 ■ Curative Factors of Group Therapy

Factor	Definition
Instilling hope	■ Establishing a sense of optimism for change and the success of the group therapy experience ■ Calling attention to the improvement that group members have made
Universality	■ Confirming that group members experience similar pain and struggles ■ Disconfirming that the client is alone or unique in misery or hurt to provide a powerful sense of relief
Imparting information	■ Sharing didactic information or advice about recovery, strategies, resources, and coping behaviors ■ Providing psychoeducation
Altruism	■ Finding that the members can be of importance to others and have something of value to give ■ Gaining from the act of giving
Corrective recapitulation of the primary family group	■ Reviewing and correctively reliving early familial conflicts and growth-inhibiting relationships in a more supportive environment ■ Challenging and exploring fixed roles ■ Working through unfinished business
Development of socializing techniques	■ Acquiring basic social skills, e.g., preparing for discharge, approaching a prospective employer, asking someone out on a date ■ Acquiring sophisticated social skills, e.g., resolving conflicts, being attuned to process, being facilitative toward others
Imitative behavior	■ Trying out bits and pieces of the behavior of the therapist and the members and experimenting with those that fit well ■ Benefiting by observing the therapy of another member
Interpersonal learning	■ Learning that one authors one's interpersonal world, and therefore, one has the power to change it ■ Comparing one's interpersonal evaluations with those of others and altering distortions (consensual validation) ■ Learning how to adapt and to take on perspectives other than one's own
Group cohesiveness	■ Being attracted to the group and the other members with a sense of "we"-ness rather than "I"-ness ■ Being included, accepted, and involved meaningfully with the other members
Catharsis	■ Being able to express feeling as a way of acquiring skills for the future ■ Feeling a sense of liberation by being able to get relief in a supportive group
Existential factors	■ Being able to "be" with others, to be a part of a group ■ Taking ultimate responsibility ■ Self-realization

Source: Adapted from Yalom, I. D. (2005). *The theory and practice of group psychotherapy* (5th ed.). New York: Basic Books.

Creating the Group

The effectiveness of a group depends greatly on the conditions under which it is created. Much as architects design buildings, therapists design groups with certain functions and characteristics in mind.

Selecting Members

Selecting the members is one of the most important functions of group leaders or group therapists, since the quality of the interpersonal relationships among the members constitutes the core of successful group treatment. This is one of the major differences between group and individual therapy.

Clients may be admitted to an inpatient group on the basis of being hospitalized on a particular unit that mandates group therapy for all clients, being assigned to a particular therapist, or because group therapy has been determined as the most appropriate form of treatment. Group therapists or leaders of therapeutic groups in inpatient units may have little leeway about including specific individuals in the group. Therefore, inpatient groups tend to have a more heterogeneous composition; that is, the members may vary significantly in terms of their personality characteristics, their vulnerabilities, or their ego strengths. They also tend to be more ambivalent about group therapy. You are encouraged to attempt to apply the following principles, regardless of the nature or location of the group.

It is more difficult to identify the characteristics of people who make good candidates for group therapy than those of people who do not make good candidates. We know that a person's motivation for therapy in general, and group therapy in particular, is of primary importance. Personality variables such as extraversion, openness, and conscientiousness have been found to be directly related to favorable treatment outcome (Ogrodniczuk, Piper, Joyce, McCallum, & Rosie, 2003). Inclusion in a therapy group should also be at least partially determined by the effect a prospective member will have on the others, in terms of the prospective member's ability to bring the curative factors into play (Yalom, 1998). The higher the percentage of members in a therapy group with a history of relatively mature relationships, the better the outcome for the group as a whole (Piper, Ogrodniczuk, Joyce, Weideman, & Rosie, 2007).

Selection for a group is also determined by the balance, in terms of behavior or characteristics, a prospective member will bring to the group. Will the person's subdued presentation prevent a member with similar behavior from being marginal and alone in the group? Does the person's age, occupation, cultural background, or sex match another's so that the member will not feel singled out as different or deviant? The factor that appears to be most important, according to Yalom (1998), however, is that members are homogeneous in terms of their vulnerabilities or ego strengths. Highly vulnerable members retard the progress of the less vulnerable, and vice versa. Yalom's research indicates that, if at all possible, avoid including in the group individuals who use denial to a significant extent, differ significantly from others in the group in relation to psychopathology, or have a pervasive dread of self-disclosure (Yalom, 2005).

Selection Interviews

Selection interviews are standard procedure for long-term outpatient groups. They are useful as well for short-term inpatient groups and groups in day hospitals to help determine the most appropriate type of group for each individual client.

The pregroup interview session has two major purposes: selecting the members and establishing the initial contract. Cotherapists should always interview potential members jointly, and both should make all decisions regarding membership. The interview session gives members and therapists the opportunity to be exposed to one another. The therapists should accomplish the following tasks in the selection interview:

- Determine the motivation of the potential member.
- Encourage the client to ask questions about the group.
- Correct erroneous prejudgments or misinformation the client has about group therapy.
- Inquire about any major pending life changes that may prevent the client's full and continued participation in the group.
- Inquire about what hurts—what the client sees as a need to work on.
- Establish and clarify the initial group contract.

During this period, therapists and members have a chance to decide whether they can work together in the specific group under consideration. Outpatient clients as well as therapists can choose whether they will participate or not. Because clients in outpatient groups have the choice of being a member of the group or not, they tend to be motivated to learn and to change.

Group Contract

The group contract identifies the shared rights and responsibilities of therapists and members. It is a negotiated set of rules or arrangements for the structure and functioning of the group. It may be written or verbal, and it should cover the following elements.

Goals and Purposes The purpose of the group must be clear to all involved. In interactive group psychotherapy, the purpose is to bring about enduring behavioral and character change. The interactive group psychotherapy experience takes place largely in the present, in the here-and-now.

Goals may be long term or short term and are both group oriented and individualized. Some goals may be identified as early as the selection interview, and others may be added as they emerge during the life of the group. Goals may be altered as appropriate.

Time, Length, and Frequency of Meetings The time, length, and frequency of meetings should be determined by the therapists after consideration of the clients' needs. Most outpatient clients find one 80- to 90-minute session per week useful. Shorter periods may not allow adequate time for discussion. Longer periods generally tax the endurance and alertness of both members and therapists. Inpatient groups generally meet several times per week, or even daily for about 45 to 50 minutes, although sessions may be longer or shorter depending on the anxiety and tolerance levels of the particular clients.

Place of Meetings The physical environment is important and influences the interaction among members. It is best to choose a pleasant room with comfortable chairs, preferably placed in a circle. The room should be private and free from external distractions.

Starting and Ending Dates If the group has a predetermined life span and the inclusive dates are known, members should be told the dates. Groups without fixed termination dates usually plan termination individually as each member is ready to move away from the group. Starting and ending dates are determined in inpatient groups by the length of the client's hospitalization.

Addition of New Members Open groups accept members after the first session; closed groups begin with a certain number of members and do not add new members. Open groups maintain their size by replacing members who leave the group. They may continue indefinitely or have a predetermined life span. Open groups are more common in short-term inpatient units where there is rapid turnover. Once the client leaves the inpatient setting, membership in the group ends. This means that since most hospitalizations are of 1 to 3 weeks' duration, there is little time for cohesion to develop. Cohesion develops in outpatient groups because of their length—1 or more years in duration, and 52 or more meetings.

Closed groups are more common in settings where the stability of membership is likely. Such settings include private practice settings, residential facilities of various types, and prisons. A major problem with the closed group is that it runs the risk of extinction as members leave the group for various reasons.

Attendance It is important that members make a commitment to attend every session. Absences hinder the establishment of cohesion and have a demoralizing effect, especially when perceived as evidence that a member lacks interest or that the group is not attractive and valuable to its members. Stability of membership and high attendance have been demonstrated to be critical factors in the successful outcome of group therapy (Yalom, 2005).

Confidentiality Some rules regarding confidentiality should be established, and clients' concerns about which people will have access to information concerning them should be explored. Many therapists like to use tape recorders so that their work can be evaluated afterward by supervisors. They must obtain client agreement to use of a tape recorder.

Rules about confidentiality and access may be determined by the therapists' employing agency. In some instances, therapists may be required to make regular notes concerning each member's participation. Therapists may also wish to establish with group members guidelines on confidentiality that allow the therapists to share content with professionals who provide clinical supervision to the therapist, or when clients are dangerous to themselves or others. A good rule of thumb is: *Promise only what you can safely deliver*. Members should also be held accountable for maintaining the confidentiality of the group.

Member Interaction Outside the Group Members in outpatient groups are discouraged from having relationships with other members outside the meetings. Relationships outside of the group are likely to interfere with the group dynamics because of the formation of social coalitions or dyads. Limiting relationships is impossible in inpatient groups because the members may have 24-hour exposure to one another on the hospital unit and may also interact with the group therapist while the therapist is functioning in other roles. In fact, interaction with one another is encouraged in inpatient settings.

Participation of Members and Therapists Therapists and clients should reach an understanding about the responsibilities of participants. Clients should be fully informed participants in the therapeutic process. Participants should share their expectations about the behavior and functions of clients and therapists and should clearly understand the modes of participation. Interaction patterns should form pathways among all members and the therapist, as illustrated in FIGURE 30-7 ■ (left).

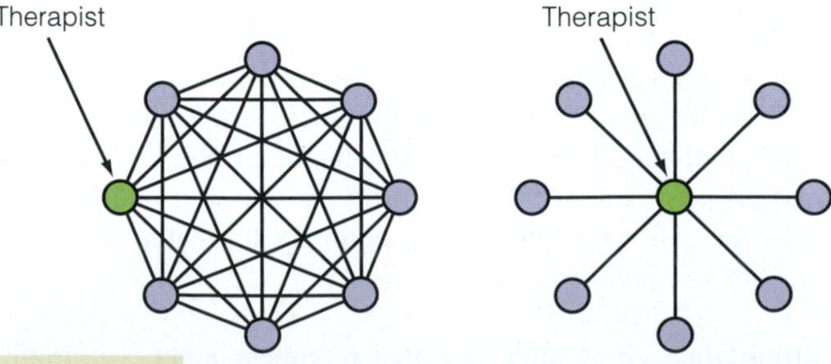

FIGURE 30-7 ■ Comparison of positive and negative interaction patterns in group therapy. The desirable interaction pattern is on the left. The diagram on the right, in which communication is primarily to or through the therapist, is undesirable.

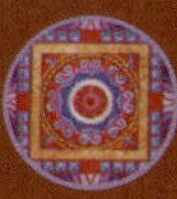

YOUR INTERVENTION STRATEGIES
Structuring an Inpatient Group

1. 3–5 minutes of orientation, warm-up, or preparation
2. 20–30 minutes for an agenda go-around in which each member may share personal concerns or problems
3. 20–30 minutes in which the therapist attempts to fit the members' agendas together by finding commonalities or threads to work on
4. 3–5 minutes to review the work of the group and to identify the issues or concerns that remain unresolved

Source: Adapted from Yalom, I. D. (1998). *The Yalom reader*. New York: Basic Books.

It is important for the inpatient group therapist to provide significantly more structure for the group and to take on a more active role than would be necessary in an outpatient group. Hospitalized inpatients are likely to be in crisis and to be more dysfunctional than outpatients. Passivity on the therapist's part would be destructive to the group and could increase a client's distress. Yalom (1998) suggests a protocol for structuring an inpatient group that is listed in the Your Intervention Strategies feature above.

Fees Fees for outpatients should be determined in advance and arrangements for payment made. Most mental health care agencies have a sliding fee scale that is determined by the client's income and ability to pay. Clients should know whether fees will be charged for missed sessions. Fees for inpatients are included in the cost of hospitalization.

Stages in Therapy Group Development

There is comfort in being able to predict, to some extent, the behavior of members at specific points in the group's life. Therapists organize predictions around stages or phases in the therapeutic experience, hoping to be prepared for expressions of behavior. You must bear in mind, however, that human experiences are dynamic and fluid and do not always progress as neatly as predicted.

The Schutz framework, presented earlier, gives clear indications of how group life develops in terms of meeting inclusion, affection, and control needs. This section focuses on the characteristics of member behavior and therapist interventions in the orientation phase (where inclusion needs are more salient), the working phase (where control needs are more salient), and the termination phase (where affection needs are more salient) of interactional group therapy. As members' problems in living are revealed, group life becomes richer and more complex. Therefore, there is no "cookbook" method that a therapist can follow to respond to every situation. The Your Intervention Strategies feature on page 811 is simply a guide for identifying some common member behaviors and therapist interventions at various points in the life of the group.

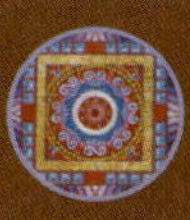

YOUR INTERVENTION STRATEGIES
Characteristic Member Behaviors and Nursing Interventions in Phases of Group Therapy

Member Behavior	Nursing Interventions
Beginning Phase	
Anxiety is high.	Move to reduce anxiety; avoid making demands until group anxiety has abated.
Members are unsure of what to do or say; need to be included.	Be active and provide some structure and direction; suggest members introduce themselves; work to sustain therapeutic rather than social role; include all members and encourage sharing but limit monopolizing.
Members are unclear about contract.	Clarify contract; give information to dispel confusion or misunderstandings.
Members test therapists and other members in terms of trustworthiness, value stances, etc., often through goblet issues.	Capitalize on opportunity to "pass" tests by proving trustworthiness and by being open to and accepting the values of others.
Beginning attempts at self-disclosure and problem identification are made.	Focus on related themes; begin exploration; begin to focus on here-and-now experiences in session.
Members have sense of "I"-ness, little sense of "we"-ness.	Encourage involvement with others through curative factor of *universality*.
Middle Phase	
Sense of "I"-ness is replaced by "we"-ness.	Encourage cohesion; provide opportunity for expression of warm feelings.
Self-disclosure increases.	Encourage exploration and move to problem solving.
Middle Phase (continued)	
Members are more aware of interpersonal interactions in the here-and-now.	Encourage members to participate in observing and commenting on the here-and-now; make process comments.
Additions and losses of members evoke strong reactions.	Prepare members for additions and losses where possible; provide opportunity to talk about addition and loss experience.
Ability to maintain focus on one topic increases.	Encourage exploration of topic area in depth.
Termination Phase	
Feelings about separation may run the gamut (anger, sadness, indifference, joy, etc.).	Provide adequate time in as many sessions as necessary to work through affective responses; be sure members know the termination date in advance; help members leave with positive feelings by identifying positive changes that have occurred in individual members and in the group.
Members may feel lost and rudderless.	Explore support systems available to individual members; bridge the gap where possible (to another agency, another therapist, etc.); keep in focus the task of resolving the loss.

Here-and-Now Emphasis

The core of interactional group therapy is the here-and-now. According to Yalom (2005), the here-and-now work of the interactional group therapist occurs on two levels:

1. Focusing attention on each member's feelings toward other group members, the therapists, and the group
2. Illuminating the process (the relationship implications of interpersonal transactions)

Thus, group members need to become aware of the here-and-now events—what happened—and then reflect back on them—why it happened. Yalom (2005) calls this the **self-reflective loop** (see FIGURE 30-8 ■).

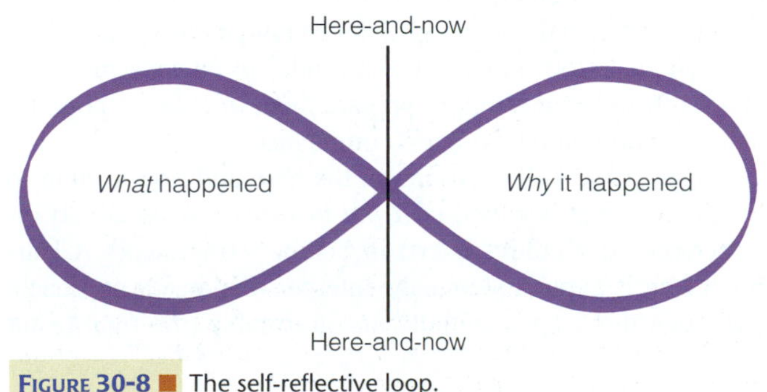

FIGURE 30-8 ■ The self-reflective loop.

Steering the Group into the Here-and-Now

The first task of the therapist is to steer the group into the here-and-now. Yalom calls this process **here-and-now activation**. As the group progresses and becomes comfortable with awareness of the here-and-now, much of the work is taken on by the members. Initially, however, a primary task of the therapist is to actively steer the group discourse toward here-and-now work. In other words, events in the session (the here-and-now) take precedence over those that occur outside or have occurred outside (the there-and-then).

Illuminating the Process

If the group is to engage in interpersonal learning, the therapist must illuminate the process. This is the second task of prime importance. The group must move beyond a focus on content toward a focus on process—the how and the why of an interaction. The process can be considered from any number of perspectives. The perspective chosen should be determined by the mood and needs of the group at that particular time. The group members must recognize, examine, and understand the process and be willing to self-disclose (review the discussion of self-disclosure earlier in this chapter). The task of illuminating the process belongs mainly to the therapist, as in the following clinical example.

CLINICAL EXAMPLE

Every time Jim makes a comment in group, Al either sneers or smirks. As soon as Jim finishes speaking, Al contradicts whatever Jim has said. The group members focus on the content of the disagreements between Jim and Al. Margaret, the clinical nurse specialist who is the group therapist, steers the group in the direction of analyzing the dynamics of the relationship between these members and the possible purposes their disagreements can serve for the group (e.g., controlling the direction of the group's efforts, meeting Al's control needs, or keeping the group anxiety down by keeping the focus away from other, more anxious members).

Process commentary is anxiety-producing for new or inexperienced therapists and group members because there are so many injunctions against it in social situations. For example, commenting on someone's nervousness at a party is generally taboo. It not only makes the nervous person uncomfortable, but also puts the process commentator in a high-risk situation. The comment may well be taken as criticism or viewed as inappropriate to the social context, and the commentator is vulnerable to retaliation from others. It is essential to educate members about this difference and to prepare them to hear, respond to, and eventually initiate process commentary.

The process of focusing on the here-and-now is akin to the process that is called *clearing the air* (making covert interpersonal difficulties overt) in Schutz's framework. Clearing the air is a major step in the interpersonal needs approach. Although this step is initially uncomfortable, the final result is rewarding. The following are common interpersonal difficulties that occur in therapy groups and should be made overt:

- Withdrawal or silence by members
- Inactivity and unintegrated behavior by members
- Overactivity and destructive behavior by members
- Power struggles between members
- Battles for attention among members
- Dissatisfaction with the leader
- Dissatisfaction with the amount of recognition a member receives for contributions
- Dissatisfaction with the amount of affection and warmth demonstrated in the group

In concert with Yalom's principles, Schutz's interpersonal needs approach is based on the belief that the way to attack problems within groups is by investigating what is going on among the individuals in the group, and attempting to improve their interpersonal relations.

Focusing on the here-and-now experience differentiates interactive group psychotherapy from many other group therapies or therapeutic groups such as those discussed later in this chapter.

THERAPEUTIC GROUPS

Nurses at all levels have long been involved in working with clients and their families in small groups brought together for health teaching, psychoeducation, or supportive purposes. This section discusses several different types of therapeutic groups that do not require the nurse to be an advanced-practice registered nurse.

Developing and planning a therapeutic group should be a systematic process. FIGURE 30-9 ■ illustrates a step-by-step investigative process that could be undertaken to determine the clinical need for the group and to develop and implement the group.

Self-Help Groups

The major operating principle in self-help groups is that the help given to members comes from the members themselves. A mental health professional is viewed as unnecessary. In fact, many of these groups developed because of the failure of programs planned and implemented by professionals.

The role of the nurse in self-help groups is that of a resource person. You need to be informed about such groups so that you can refer potential members to groups appropriate to their needs, or to provide consultation when invited to do so. In most self-help groups, leaders are former members. Alcoholics Anonymous is a well-known example of this principle.

There is a wide variety of self-help groups, for example:

- Recovery Incorporated and Schizophrenics Anonymous, concerned with mental disorder
- Alcoholics Anonymous and Narcotics Anonymous, concerned with substance abuse
- Al-Anon and Alateen, concerned with the families of alcoholics
- Rational Recovery, concerned with substance abuse

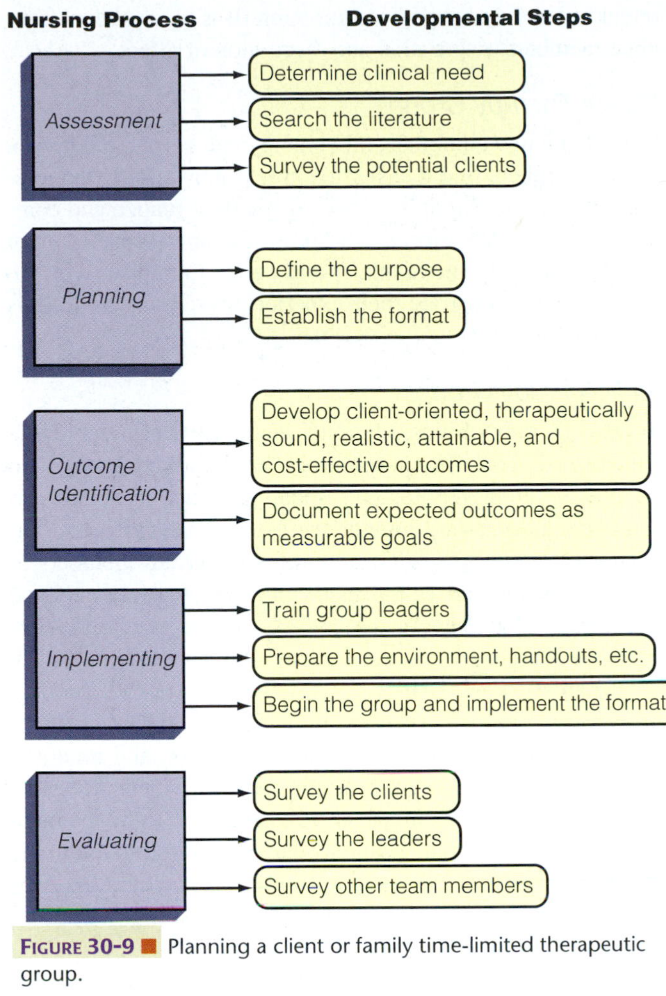

FIGURE 30-9 ■ Planning a client or family time-limited therapeutic group.

- Overeaters Anonymous, concerned with overeating
- Gamblers Anonymous, concerned with compulsive gambling
- Gam-Anon, concerned with the families and friends of compulsive gamblers
- Child Abuse Listening and Mediation (CALM), concerned with child abuse

In Canada, a directory of self-help groups is available through the Canadian Mental Health Association. All of these resources can be accessed through the Companion Website for this book.

Groups for divorced, widowed, or single people, for parents of runaways and troubled adolescents, for parents who abuse their children, and for the recently bereaved are common in most major cities throughout the world. Client clubs for people who have had a colostomy, ileostomy, laryngectomy, mastectomy, or amputation are also popular.

Psychoeducation Groups

Psychoeducation groups led by nurses have the sharing of mental health care information as a primary goal. They also have the secondary benefit of facilitating the discussion of feelings such as isolation, helplessness, sadness, stigmatization, and/or anger and possible strategies for dealing with these feelings. Some examples of nurse-led psychoeducation groups follow.

Medication Teaching Groups

Nonadherence to prescription medication is the leading cause of relapse or recurrence of psychotic illness. Many studies have shown that the causes of medication nonadherence are related to a lack of insight and understanding by clients of their illness and of their medication treatment. In addition, medication side effects such as dry mouth, blurred vision, impotence, sedation, and akathisia can be difficult to tolerate.

Medication teaching groups provide an opportunity for psychiatric–mental health nurses to educate clients about medications, their side effects, the nature and course of their mental disorder, the possibility of relapse without continued medication treatment, and the positive effect medications have on their lives. Research has shown that improved attitudes, adherence to treatment, and insight often result from medication teaching groups (Tay, 2007).

Social Skills Training Groups

Social skills training can be accomplished effectively in groups. Small groups provide structure and support, while clients are coached in simple yet essential social interactions. It is best to form groups of clients who function at similar levels. Provide structure by clearly setting the time for group meetings, beginning and ending each session with a statement of goals, and recapping what the group has accomplished.

Social skills training has been found to decrease anxiety and psychopathology and increase self-control in clients with generalized social phobia (van Dam-Baggen & Kraaimaat, 2000), and to improve community life (recreational, residential, and vocational) for clients with schizophrenia and their family members by enhancing social competence (Magliano, Fiorello, Malangone, De Rosa, & Maj, 2006). Older people with severe and persistent schizophrenia can also learn and maintain new skills and report improved functioning after cognitive behavioral social skills training (Granholm et al., 2007).

Social skills training groups often focus on communication skills. For example, relationship risk factors for couples are reduced by teaching conflict resolution and communication skills (Kirby & Baucom, 2007). Social skills training groups for incarcerated adult offenders focus on role-plays with performance feedback, modeling, and anger reduction (Bourke & Van Hasselt, 2001).

Social skills training is even more effective when combined with cognitive behavior therapy (CBT) or dialectical behavior therapy (DBT), two approaches discussed in detail in Chapter 31∞. CBT, combined with social skills and problem-solving training, improves cognitive insight and functioning in people with schizophrenia (Granholm et al., 2007). DBT has been found to be especially effective with borderline personality clients and suicidal clients and their families (Linehan et al., 2006).

MEDIALINK Self-Help Groups

Groups of Medically Ill Clients and Their Families

Groups composed of medically ill clients are increasingly common, as psychiatric–mental health nurses move into general health care settings offering liaison and consultation services to clients and staff. Group work is useful for chronically ill or disabled clients, preoperative and postoperative clients, clients with regulative medical problems (such as diabetes, cardiac disease, or kidney disease), dying clients, elderly clients, and clients with psychophysiologic disorders, among others.

Such groups generally focus on the stress associated with illness and have as their goal the reduction of stress. While they may not prolong life, as in the case of clients with cancer, they may improve the quality of life, including protection against depression (Kissane et al., 2007). Group therapy has also been helpful for clients with HIV infection, who demonstrated improvements in social, job, and home environments, sexual relationships, and family relationships (Rousaud et al., 2007). Groups may be composed of clients alone, family members alone, or a combination.

Activity Therapy Groups

Activity therapies are manual, recreational, and creative techniques to facilitate personal experiences and increase social responses and self-esteem. Activity therapies are generally the province of health and recreation specialists.

Some activity therapies, such as the creative arts therapies, are organized and conducted in groups. Creative arts therapies provide many people with a comfortable opportunity for social exchange. Although there are specifically educated creative arts therapists, their numbers are small. Nurses may lead such groups or use their principles to reach beyond the ordinary realm of verbal communication with clients.

Poetry Therapy Groups

The goal of poetry therapy groups is to help members get in touch with feelings and emotions through the use of poetry. Poems that are read aloud provide the stimulus for understanding and catharsis. They are selected as the therapeutic medium because they are powerful but not explicit avenues of communication. It is not necessary to be able to write poetry to be a member or leader of a poetry therapy group, although some members or leaders may be stimulated to write poems of their own.

Art Therapy Groups

In art therapy groups, the art produced by each member gives the art therapist or group leader a personal insight into the artist's personality. The art is produced during the session and is used as the basis for discussion and for exploring members' feelings.

Music Therapy Groups

Music therapy consists of singing, rhythm, body movement, and listening. It is designed to increase group members' concentration, memory retention, conceptual development, rhythmic behavior, movement behavior, verbal and nonverbal retention, and auditory discrimination. It is also used to stimulate members' expression and discussion of affect.

Dance Therapy Groups

Dance therapy combines movement and verbal modes. In dance, members find it easier to express nonverbally the feelings and emotions that have been difficult to realize and communicate by other means. The person's inner sense is often reflected in body movements, and dance therapists work to help members integrate their experiences verbally as well as nonverbally.

Bibliotherapy Groups

In bibliotherapy groups, literature is the means for achieving a therapeutic goal. The purpose of a bibliotherapy group is to assimilate the psychological, sociologic, and aesthetic insights books give into human character, personality, and behavior. Literature provides a stimulus for group members to compare events and characters with their own interpersonal and intrapsychic experiences.

Storytelling Groups

Storytelling groups—a process by which group members create a story together—can stimulate interaction and imagination. Wenckus (1994) used an approach in which the group leader or the group members chose one person to be the main character in a story. The group leader can give direction to the story by having an opening question in mind that is likely to determine the direction of the story. Questions a group leader could ask include:

1. Where would you go if you were given a trip?
2. What would you do if you won the lottery?
3. What would you title your autobiography?
4. What would your epitaph say?
5. If your fairy godmother could grant your wish, what would it be?
6. What is your favorite room in the house you grew up in?

Storytelling can be very effective in helping clients talk about feelings they would otherwise have suppressed and to connect with one another. It can assist elders in reminiscence work. In addition, storytelling can be fun, generate laughter, and reduce stress, no matter the client's age.

Community Client Groups

Psychiatric–mental health nurses in community settings are involved in a variety of community groups. These settings include schools, youth centers, industries, neighborhood centers, churches, prisons, summer camps, single-room occupancy boarding houses, transitional facilities such as halfway houses, apartments for the elderly, and residential facilities for delinquent youths and runaways. Clients may also be people who have direct contact with these groups, such as teachers, youth counselors, prison guards, police officers, and camp counselors.

Groups with Nurse Colleagues

Nurses who work together may form discussion and counseling groups to help reduce their job-related stress and to help them deal with problems of interpersonal relationships in more satisfying ways. Nurses in various intensive care and other high-pressure settings identify with increasing frequency the need for group work services that the psychiatric–mental health nurse can provide. The psychiatric–mental health nurse may also identify the need and offer this opportunity to colleagues.

FAMILY DYNAMICS

Over the past 30 years, family interventions have become important components of treatment for a number of psychiatric disorders. It is for this reason that we have integrated discussions of family dynamics, needs, and functioning in the majority of chapters in this text, especially Chapters 14–24.

While there are common factors and mechanisms of change that undergird most forms of successful treatment (Sprenkle & Blow, 2004), there are several unique dynamics that take place in families and influence both family and individual functioning. A selection of relevant theories that help to explain family dynamics and family treatment are discussed next. The section on family therapy will help you to understand and explain family therapy to clients. It does not prepare you as a family therapist. As you will learn later in the chapter, the nurse family therapist role is an advanced–practice role.

Family Structures

The traditional nuclear family is a two-parent, two-generation family consisting of a married couple and their children by birth or adoption. In today's society, fewer than one in five children have grown up in the traditional nuclear family structure. Contemporary families may look like any one of the following:

- A mother, a father, and 2.2 children (traditional nuclear family)
- A couple with eight children—three of hers, three of his, and two of theirs (blended family)
- A 32-year-old single electrical engineer and his three foster children
- A divorced woman and her two teenagers
- A widowed man, his child, and his parents
- A grandmother raising her three grandchildren
- Two lesbian mothers and their child
- Three single women friends sharing an apartment none could afford alone
- Two gay men living together in a committed relationship

North American family forms continue to change. For that reason, sensitive psychiatric–mental health nurses reject a narrow definition of family and adapt their clinical practice to the wide variety of family constellations that exists in contemporary society.

Stages of Family Development

Theories to explain family development were first formulated after World War II. Probably the most important was that originally proposed by Duvall in 1957 and expanded upon by Duvall and Miller in 1985 (Duvall & Miller, 1985). Duvall's formulations focused on the patterns and changes in family development as families move through stages. These family stages are the period of time in which the structure and interactions of role relationships are noticeably distinct from other periods. The stages are inferred from events spurred on by a change in family membership. Family development theory is based on the assumption that families, like individuals, change over a period of time. They progress through a series of similar developmental stages and face similar transition points and developmental tasks.

The notion of universal family stages, however, has attracted criticism over several decades. Critics of family development theory point to it as a limiting way of thinking about ethnically and racially diverse populations, gender, and families without children. They propose that the notion of families moving through rigid, predetermined stages is a less productive method of understanding the dynamics that take place in families. It is also important to recognize that the universality of family developmental tasks have not been empirically validated through research.

However, because the concepts inherent in family development theory can be valuable as general propositions and can help clinicians to understand some families, family developmental tasks throughout the life cycle are discussed in TABLE 30-3 ■ on page 816. Understanding families requires consideration of the challenges they face in each stage, how well they resolve the challenges, and how well they transition to the next stage.

Family Characteristics and Dynamics

Whether they are functional or dysfunctional, families have certain characteristics and dynamics. In a family, each person's behavior is contingent on and affects the behavior of the others. This creates some interesting and complex turns in family relationships.

Family Roles

Members of a family must determine how to accomplish family developmental tasks. They do so by establishing roles, patterns of behavior sanctioned by the culture. Jackson (1968) believes that families set roles by operating as a rule-governed system, an ordered format designed so that members may be aware of their positions in relation to one another. Families decide which roles will exist within the system, socialize members into the roles, and then expend energy maintaining members within their roles.

When members are unable or unwilling to perform assigned roles, the family experiences stress. For the health of the **family system**—which includes not only family members but also their relationships, their communication with one another, and their interactions with the environment—roles often must

TABLE 30-3 ■ Duvall's Stages of Family Development

Stage of the Family Life Cycle	Stage-Sensitive Family Developmental Tasks
Stage 1: Married couples (without children)	■ Establishing a mutually satisfying marital relationship ■ Fitting into the kin network of the partner ■ Adjusting to the promise of parenthood
Stage 2: Childbearing families (oldest child, birth–30 months)	■ Having and adjusting to a child ■ Encouraging the development of the infant ■ Establishing a satisfying home for both parents and child
Stage 3: Families with preschool children (oldest child, 2½–6 years)	■ Coping with energy depletion and lack of privacy as parents ■ Adapting to the needs and interests of preschool children in stimulating, growth-producing ways
Stage 4: Families with schoolchildren (oldest child, 6–13 years)	■ Encouraging children's educational development ■ Fitting into the community of school-age families in constructive ways
Stage 5: Families with teenagers (oldest child, 13–20 years)	■ Establishing postparental interests and careers as growing parents ■ Balancing freedom with responsibility as teenagers mature and emancipate themselves
Stage 6: Families as launching centers (first child gone to last child leaving home)	■ Releasing young adult children into college, work, marriage, military service, and so on with appropriate rituals and assistance ■ Maintaining a supportive home base for young adult children
Stage 7: Middle-age parents ("empty nest" to retirement)	■ Refocusing on the marital relationship ■ Maintaining kinship ties with older and younger generations
Stage 8: Aging family members (retirement to death of both spouses)	■ Coping with bereavement and living alone ■ Adjusting to retirement ■ Closing the family home or adapting it to needs associated with aging

Source: Adapted from Duvall, E. M., & Miller, B. C. (1985). *Marriage and family development.* New York: Harper & Row.

be negotiated in other than stereotyped ways. When the roles are not negotiated satisfactorily, family disequilibrium results.

Family Boundaries

Families have *boundaries* as well. Boundaries define who participates in the family, the amount or intensity of emotional investment in the family, the amount and kind of experiences available outside the family, and particular ways to evaluate experiences in terms of the family.

Boundaries may be clear or conflicting, rigid or diffuse. Rigid boundaries—those in which rules and roles are maintained under all conditions—keep members from having meaningful relationships with and understanding one another. People with rigid boundaries can become isolated or withdrawn. The isolation extends to the outside community as a whole and the family is cut off from others.

A diffuse boundary is the opposite of a rigid boundary. A person with diffuse boundaries has no clear, definable boundaries with others. In families, diffuse boundaries are characterized by family overinvolvement in the lives of its members, leading to loss of independence by one or all family members. Parents and children become increasingly dependent on one another at the expense of relationships outside the family. Diffuse boundaries increase the family's dependence on one another and allow the destructive behavior to continue. Families that struggle with boundaries tend to raise children who struggle with boundaries.

MEDIALINK Critical Thinking Exercise: Family Boundaries

Clear, stable, and healthy boundaries allow for personal and meaningful relationships with others. A person with healthy boundaries has a solid sense of self. There are feelings of belongingness to the family as well as to others outside the family.

Power Structure

Most families have a hierarchical power structure in which the adults wield the power. The power structure is often developed in this way because it creates a safe environment in which young children can grow and develop, and because it is easy to operate. However, stress develops when disagreements exist about who holds the power.

CLINICAL EXAMPLE

Tom, the 17-year-old son in the M family, always used the family car without permission. Although some serious arguments ensued between Tom and his father, no restrictions were placed on Tom's behavior, and the car keys continued to hang on a key rack in the front hall. Tom's paternal grandfather, who lived with the M family, took Tom's side in his arguments with his father. Grandfather M took the stance that "boys will be boys."

One evening when the family car was in a repair shop for some minor work, Tom "borrowed" his grandfather's new car. He was involved in a collision about an hour later. Although no one was injured, Grandfather M's car was extensively damaged and had to be towed away. Later that night, the adults of the M family managed to come together to agree on a stance concerning Tom's use of the family car that they could mutually support.

Once the adults in the M family were able to acknowledge their internal power struggle and come to an agreement on what rules were to be set and by whom, the family system was subject to less stress.

When children mature and become capable of assuming greater responsibility for their own functioning, power is often diffused among all members of a family system in a more democratic fashion. Certain families, however, do not allow power to be redistributed, thus hindering the individual development of the members with less power. In some dysfunctional families, there is chronic discord about power.

Relationship Strains or Conflicts

Relationship strains or conflicts can occur in the family or among various parts of the family, or outside of it. A strain can exist between the individual members of a family—for instance, between two siblings with differing views on an issue. Conflict or strain can also occur between a member of the family and the rest of the family, or between a minority of family members and the other members. This commonly occurs when a previously and unanimously held family view is challenged by one or more members. Strain can also exist between a family and the community when a family view differs from that of the community at large.

Relationship and Communication Intricacies in Families

Some of the relationship complexities described next exist in all families, but dysfunctional families handle them differently than functional families do. Functional families allow for individuation and growth-producing experiences.

Self-Fulfilling Prophecy and Life Scripts

A **self-fulfilling prophecy** is an idea or expectation that is acted out, largely unconsciously, thus "proving" itself. In families, self-fulfilling prophecies are often seen in the guise of family life scripts. A **life script** is a plan decided not by the fates, but by experiences early in life. People with life scripts are following forced, premature, early childhood decisions. Most people live a scripted life, at least to some extent.

There is an endless variety among life scripts. The Miss America script is decided for the 5-year-old girl whose parents enroll her in the Little Miss New York State (or Alabama or Colorado) competition. There are "My Son the Doctor, Delinquent, Alcoholic, Drug Addict" scripts. A person with a script, either "good" or "bad," is terribly disadvantaged in terms of autonomy or life potential. According to self-fulfilling prophecy, unless people recognize what the script is and take steps to change it, they are prevented from living to their potential.

Family Myths and Themes

Family myths and themes help families maintain balance by permitting them to resist change. *Family myths* are well-integrated beliefs, shared by all family members, about each other and their positions in family life. The beliefs are unchallenged, even though family members may have to resort to distortions to maintain the myth. The family myth is related to the family's inner image—how the family appears to its members.

CLINICAL EXAMPLE

A myth in the Lundqvist family was that the father had the ability to make wise decisions. Individual members in this family participated to maintain the myth of the father as a wise man by gearing interactions with him in such a way that he appeared to make high-level family decisions single-handedly.

The *family theme* is the family's perception of its development and history. Family themes are important because they shape the fates of individual members and determine the pressures with which each person must contend.

CLINICAL EXAMPLE

The Weber family had a theme constructed around second-generation grandparents of Austrian descent, who were able to provide their oldest son with a law school education through their hard work. This family conceived of people on welfare as "lazy," thus reaffirming its view of the value of working hard and becoming educated.

Energy in the family is directed toward upholding particular images of the family—as the most hard-working, religious, popular, talented, financially successful, nonconformist, or whatever—in order to maintain the front the family strives to present to others.

Family Coalitions

Of all the forms of communicative exchange, dyadic communication is the most common. In fact, many families begin with a couple, a dyad. The presence of a third person always has an effect on an existing dyad. When the couple gives birth to or adopts a child, or a third person enters the family, the relationship becomes triadic. A triad is not a stable social situation, because it actually consists of a dyad plus one. Shifting alliances characterize triads or triangles in families. For example, adult partners may unite to discipline the child, mother and child may unite to argue for a family vacation, or father and child may join forces to go fishing together. Triangles are dysfunctional when issues are solved by shifting the intimacy among members rather than by working the actual issue through, or when interaction among family members is determined by fixed triangles. Fixed and rigid triangles are an effort to reduce stress and restore balance in a dysfunctional

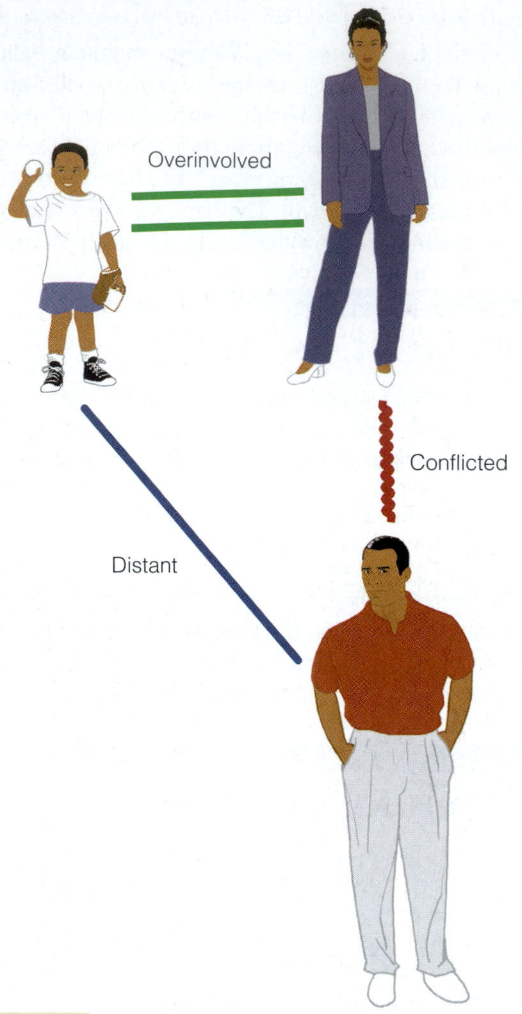

FIGURE 30-10 ■ A family triangle. In this family, the relationship between husband and wife is conflicted. Mother and son are overinvolved. Father and son have a distant relationship.

family. In actuality, fixed and rigid triangles perpetuate problems in families. Such coalitions always result in someone feeling "left out" (Bowen, 1988). A problematic family triangle is illustrated in FIGURE 30-10 ■.

Coalitions arise basically to affect the distribution of power. By joining forces, two people can increase their influence over a third. Parents frequently pair up in order to discipline their child in a consistent manner. However, the child may also attempt to pair up with one parent to avoid discipline. In families with a number of children, typical coalitions involve children closest in age or children of the same sex.

Deviations in the Adult Partners' Coalition

In some families, problems develop from the couple's inability to form a satisfying coalition in terms of intimacy and control. Several common deviations within the family are examined in the sections that follow.

Schism Families in which the children are forced to join one or the other camp of two warring spouses or adult caretakers are called *schismatic families*. The constant fighting in these families is most likely a defense against intimacy or closeness. In schismatic families, the adult partners devalue and undercut each other. This makes it difficult for the children to want to be like either of them.

Skew Families in which one mate is severely dysfunctional are called *skewed families*. The other mate, who is usually aware of the dysfunction of the partner, assumes a passive, peace-making, submissive stance to preserve the relationship. The passive partner is caught between effectively responding to the dysfunctional partner's view of "reality" of the outside world and giving up this view within the home, accepting the dysfunctional mate's view. On the surface, a skewed couple may appear to be complementary. However, their relationship is actually lopsided and unsuited to many basic family tasks.

Enmeshment A fast tempo of interpersonal exchange is characteristic of *enmeshed families*. Interactions within the family are of high intensity and are directed more toward issues of power than toward issues of affection. In enmeshed families, one adult is often overcontrolling and becomes anxious over the possibility of losing control over the children. Enmeshed families have diffuse boundaries.

Disengagement Abandonment—at the other extreme from enmeshment—is characteristic of *disengaged families*. Family members seem oblivious to the effects of their actions on one another. They are unresponsive and unconnected to each other. Structure, order, or authority in the family may be weak or nonexistent. Assuming control and guidance increases the anxiety of the parent, who may feel overwhelmed and depressed. In these families, a child often assumes the parental role.

Pseudomutuality and Pseudohostility

A family in which *pseudomutuality* occurs functions as if it were a close, happy family. This pattern of relating has the following characteristics:

- Persistent sameness in the structuring of roles
- Insistence on the desirability and appropriateness of the role structures within the family, despite evidence to the contrary
- Intense concern over deviations from the role structure or emerging autonomy
- Marked absence of spontaneity, enthusiasm, and humor in participating together

In these families, the members do not form intimate bonds with one another as individuals. Instead, an inordinate amount of energy is expended in maintaining ritualized and stereotyped ways of behaving and relating. Such a family requires its members to give up their sense of personal identity.

Pseudohostility exists in families characterized by chronic conflict, alienation, tension, and inappropriate remoteness. As in pseudomutuality, family members deny the problems in an attempt to negate the hostility. Family members view their differences as only minor ones. Both pseudomutual and pseudohostile family environments are stifling milieus.

FAMILY ASSESSMENT

Assessing and intervening with the families of your clients is an essential role. Unfortunately, some mental health care professionals still have a bias against family involvement. This bias is a remnant of now-discredited theories that poor parenting and dysfunctional family interaction patterns give rise to mental illness. A related bias is the belief by some that if families "cause" schizophrenia, then the family's contact with the client should be limited for the client's sake. Besides violating family rights, this bias prevents social interaction with family members that might serve as a normalizing force by confronting clients with reality (Myin-Germeys, Nicolson, & Delespaul, 2001). Here is a question you can use to check if you have a bias against the family's rights: *Am I responding to this family any differently than I would to the family of a client with a medical condition?*

In addition, your experiences in your own family influence how you perceive and react to your client's family. Truthfully answering the self-assessment questions in the Your Self-Awareness feature will help you to determine how your own family experiences might influence your behavior with your client's family.

The family who has cared for the client with a mental disorder has an in-depth understanding of the client's illness, history, and ability to function in the community. Include the family's insights in the assessment phase, and, if appropriate, use them in the planning of care, particularly care after discharge.

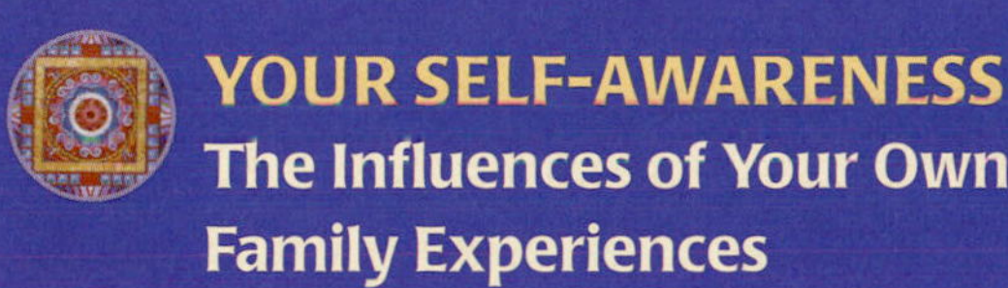

YOUR SELF-AWARENESS
The Influences of Your Own Family Experiences

It is helpful when working with families to first come to an understanding of the experiences you bring with you from your own family. Complete the following statements to facilitate your self-understanding and recognition of the biases you bring to your work with families.

1. When someone in my family talks too much, I usually . . .
2. When one of my family members is silent, I usually . . .
3. When someone in my family cries, I usually . . .
4. When my family members are excessively polite and unwilling to confront each other, I usually . . .
5. When there is conflict in my family, I usually . . .
6. When one individual in my family is verbally attacked, I usually . . .
7. If there is physical violence in my family, I usually . . .
8. My typical intervention "rhythm" (fast/slow) is . . .
9. My style is characteristically more (nurturing/confronting) . . .
10. The things that make me most uncomfortable in my family are . . .

Family assessment involves gathering data in several different areas and can be done both formally and informally. Do not overlook natural opportunities to assess families and their needs. During visits, join the family for a few minutes to learn about their understanding of the treatment program, their concerns, and their questions. More formal assessments using interview guides or strategies such as a family genealogy or time line (discussed later in this chapter) are also available. Whichever methods you use, remember that a trusting relationship with key members of the client's family is essential for establishing a flow of information and planning care. Remember, however, to secure clients' permission before releasing information to their families, and encourage clients to involve their families in their treatment. Clients' rights in relation to sharing of information is discussed in Chapter 13.

Demographic Information

Data pertaining to gender, age, occupation, religion, and ethnicity should be obtained. In addition to gathering discrete bits of information (the father is a 39-year-old Latino, physician's assistant, and a member of St. Ann's Roman Catholic parish), it is important to gather more detailed information that will give insight into family functioning:

- How actively does the family pursue religious/spiritual activities?
- What is the link of religion/spirituality to the family's value system, norms, and practices?
- What is the family's racial, cultural, and ethnic identification in relation to sense of identity and belonging?
- Who in the family is employed? What are their attitudes about employment?

Medical and Mental Health History

Here, substantive information should also be gathered. You want to know about past medical and mental health treatment, past and present illnesses, and pertinent health facts in the family of origin, in the extended family, and in the family history.

Gather information about the developmental stage of the family.

- What were (are) the problems in transition from one developmental level to another?
- How has the family solved problems at earlier stages?
- What shifts in role responsibility have occurred over time?

Family Interactional Data

This is probably the most complex data to obtain. For example, you want to gather information about family rules.

- What family rules foster stability in the family?
- What rules foster maladaptation?
- How are rules modified?
- What happens when all members do not agree about the family rules?

You also need to determine the roles of family members.

- What are the formal roles for each member?
- What are the informal roles (scapegoat [scapegoating is explained in Chapter 27], controller, decision maker, and so on)?
- Do the roles seem to have a good fit in the family?

Most important, gather information on how family members communicate.

- What are the channels of communication—who speaks to whom?
- Are the messages clear?
- What is the extent of unclear or ambiguous messages, mixed messages, or missed messages?
- Do members "hear" one another?

Assess levels of cohesion by noting who accompanies the client and who visits if the client is hospitalized.

- Is it the whole family or just one member?
- Does the client come in alone? (Visits from family are a rich source of information.)
- Who visits, how often, and for how long?
- How do family visitors behave with the client?
- Do the members spend time interacting and sharing activities, do they sit quietly together, or do they maintain physical and emotional distance from one another?

Document these patterns of family interactions, and monitor the effect of family visits on the client.

Family Burden

In a report on the experience of stigma in families with mentally ill members, Muhlbauer (2002) noted that more than 4 million American families live with severely mentally ill members. Most families of mentally disordered individuals report that caring for the ill member is a very important, largely underappreciated, stigmatized, and frequently expensive, all-consuming, and lifelong task (Karp, 2000). **Family burden** is a term that refers to the difficulties and responsibilities of family members who assume a caretaking function for relatives with psychiatric disability.

Family burdens reported most often are financial strain, violence in the household, reductions in the physical and mental health of family caregivers, disruption of family routines, worry about the future, the impact of stigma, the mental health system itself as a stressor, and feeling overwhelmed or unable to cope. Families also report having these needs:

- Information about the disorder itself
- Information about how to manage day-to-day problems due to the client's symptoms
- Information and access to resources about medications and their side effects
- Strategies for helping the seriously mentally ill family member accept treatment
- Support in their role as caregiver

MediaLink Care Plan: Family Dysfunction

Gathering information about the family burden will help you to determine what kind of support would be most helpful to this family: a family support group? Referral to the National Alliance on Mental Illness (NAMI; discussed later in this chapter)? Respite care to give the family a break from their caregiving role? Family therapy?

Family System Data

Determine how the family interacts with the outside world.

- How permeable or rigid are its boundaries?
- What is the extent to which the family fits into the larger culture of which it is a part?
- To what degree could the family be considered deviant from the larger culture?

Within the family, determine the family alliances.

- Who supports whom?
- Which members are in conflict with one another, or with the family as a whole?
- Are there extended family supports?
- What other social supports are available to the family?

Needs, Goals, Values, and Aspirations

Determine whether essential needs are met.

- Are physical needs met?
- At what level does the family meet the social and emotional needs of its members?
- What are the individual needs of family members, and how do they fit with the family needs?
- Is the family willing or able to meet the individual needs of its members?

Determine the extent to which individual family members' goals and values are articulated and understood by the other members.

- Are the goals and values shared by all?
- Do some members compromise?
- Do other members simply give up and give in?
- Does the family as a whole allow individual members to pursue individual goals and values?

Family Genogram

From the study of families in detail, it becomes apparent that patterns are spread over generations. The timeline, or **genogram**, is highly effective as a visual representation of family patterns from one generation to the next. By drawing it on a long, narrow piece of paper and taping it to the wall during the family's sessions, the therapist can use it repeatedly as therapy progresses. Colored lines can differentiate individual family members. Colored flags, pins, or stickers can identify and call attention to significant events in the family history. Births, deaths, marriages, and leave-takings should be noted. Any of several family tree or genealogic tracing formats for the family timeline can be used. One example is illustrated in FIGURE 30-11 ■. Other genograms can be developed to explore specific issues.

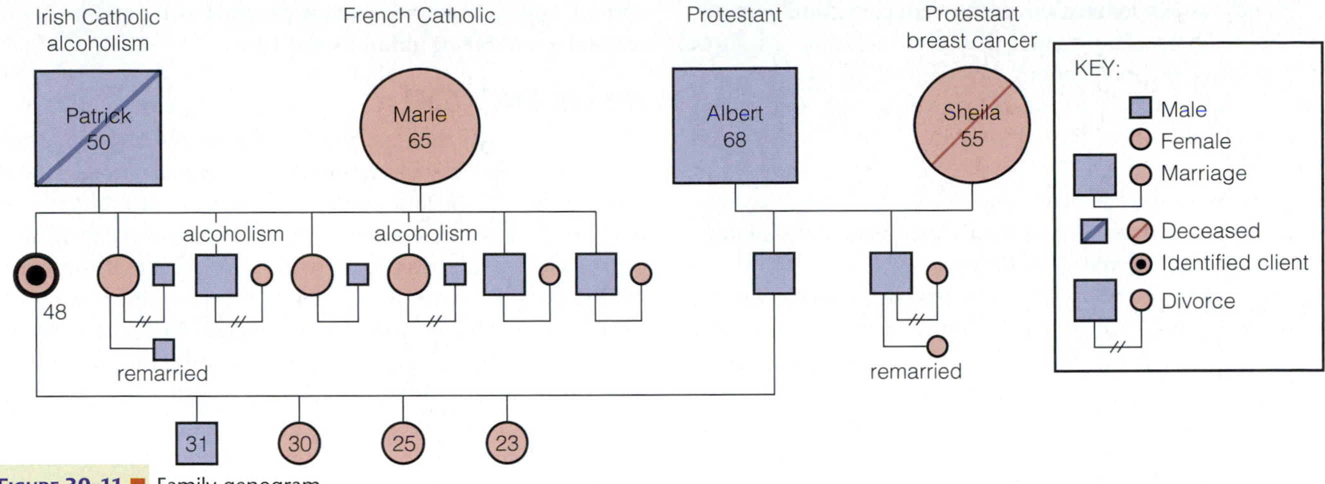

FIGURE 30-11 ■ Family genogram.

Cultural Family Genogram

A cultural family genogram is a useful tool for working with culturally diverse families. You can use a cultural family genogram to become more aware of the cultural differences between yourself and the family and between the family and other families, assess a family's strengths, and point to areas where intervention may be useful. A cultural family genogram might include the following elements:

- What language is spoken at home and in the community?
- What significance does race, skin color, and hair play within the group?
- What role does religion and spirituality play within the everyday lives of the family members?
- What prejudices or stereotypes does this family have about themselves and other members of their cultural group?
- What prejudices or stereotypes does this family have about other cultural groups?
- What are the health beliefs in this family's culture?
- How does this culture view mental health professionals?
- What values does this family have about family, education, and work?
- What are the pride/shame issues of this cultural group? How are they manifested in this family?

Spiritual Family Genogram

A spiritual genogram—a multigenerational map of family members' religious and spiritual affiliations, events, and conflicts—enables clients to make sense of their families' religious/spiritual heritage. It also helps them to explore the ways in which their experiences with spirituality affect couple or family issues. A spiritual family genogram could also be a tool in a spiritual issues discussion group for psychiatric inpatients that helps members explore their spiritual beliefs, past experiences, and spiritual lives in relationship to their mental illness (Popovsky, 2007).

Forensic Family Genogram

A forensic family genogram is a useful tool for forensic nurses for both assessment and intervention purposes. Kent-Wilkinson (1999) suggests a three-generational map to help offenders see the patterns in their lives as a way to begin to understand their personal circumstances. As part of the legal chart, it provides the courts with information about the events and factors in the individual lives of offenders in the form of a graphic database.

FAMILY INTERVENTIONS

Two main goals for involving family members in a client's treatment plan are:

1. Enlisting the family as an ally in promoting and bringing about therapeutic progress (Atwood, 2001)
2. Supporting family caregivers (Doornbos, 2002)

Three main forms of family intervention in current use are: family psychoeducation, referral to the National Alliance on Mental Illness (NAMI), and family therapy.

Services directed toward supporting the family caregivers of persons with serious and persistent mental illnesses may have the potential to improve outcomes for both the caregivers and the clients (Doornbos, 2002). Although there seems to be a consensus about the need for coordinated family-based services, they are not always implemented. This is an area for active advocacy by the psychiatric–mental health nurse.

Family Psychoeducation

Family members can benefit from psychoeducation groups designed specifically to help them cope with their loved one's illness. Family psychoeducation programs have emerged as a strongly supported evidence-based practice in the treatment of schizophrenia, bipolar disorder, depression, obsessive–compulsive disorder, and borderline personality disorder (Murray-Swank & Dixon, 2004). Family psychoeducation has also been found to reduce psychotic relapse and rehospitalization and to improve client recovery and family well-being (McFarlane, Dixon, Lukens, & Lucksted, 2003).

MediaLink Case Study: Family Education and Intervention

MediaLink Application: Services to Families of People with Psychiatric Disabilities

Family psychoeducation groups educate family members about the specific mental disorder, including its signs and symptoms, the medications the client takes, the signs and stages of relapse, the treatment plan, and the fluctuating course of mental illness. They also learn about life events that cause stress for the client, how to prevent relapse, and how to manage behavior that is disturbing to others. Family psychoeducation may also address all family members' emotion regulation and interpersonal skills deficits.

Unfortunately, the use of family psychoeducation in routine clinical practice is limited. Family members are most likely to receive information about diagnosis and medications and least likely to receive information about the treatment plan. However, nurses can be influential in persuading their agencies to develop family psychoeducation programs, as discussed in the Evidence-Based Practice feature.

Dialectical behavior therapy combined with family skills training is being used more often because of its confirmed effectiveness. It is particularly effective in teaching family members (or couples in marital therapy) how to regulate their emotions and helping them to achieve an understanding of how strong feelings affect and are affected by their relationships with one another (Kirby & Baucom, 2007).

Family psychoeducation groups also serve a supportive function in an accepting environment. Family members are informed about local and national groups and organizations that provide educational and counseling services and respite care. A family psychoeducation program is a good bridge to referral to NAMI or to family therapy.

Referral to NAMI

The National Alliance on Mental Illness (NAMI) is a grassroots, self-help, advocacy, and support organization of families, consumers (a term used by NAMI to describe people diagnosed with and receiving treatment for severe mental illness), and friends of people with severe mental disorders. NAMI provides several services to families and consumers, including general information on mental disorders, psychiatric medications, and mental health policy positions; referral to state and local affiliates and support groups throughout the country; and support from trained volunteers—consumers and family members—who know what it's like to have a mental disorder or to have a family member with a mental disorder. One program of special interest to families is the NAMI Family-to-Family Education Program. The special features of this course, prepared by families for families, has both a personal and a social focus and can be found on the NAMI website provided at the end of this section.

NAMI also provides educational services to mental health care providers. The NAMI Provider Education Program for line staff at public agencies who work directly with people with severe and persistent mental illness is a 10-week course to educate providers about how to include families in the care of the client. The program is based on

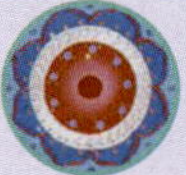

EVIDENCE-BASED PRACTICE

DECREASING FAMILY BURDEN THROUGH PSYCHOEDUCATION

The program development committee at the mental health outreach clinic where you work has challenged you to provide a convincing rationale for your recent proposal. You believe that family psychoeducation helps to reduce family burden. However, in order to commit resources such as staff and funding, the committee has asked you to review the research to determine on what basis the agency can support your proposal.

Your review of the research found significant support for your proposal. Family psychoeducation groups for families with a schizophrenic member show a significant improvement (74%) in clients' social relationships, interest in obtaining a job, and management of social conflicts. Family burden significantly improved, as did relatives' social contacts and perception of professional support. Family distress decreased as the confidence and skills of the members increased. Similar results are found with studies of bipolar disorder, depression, suicide, borderline personality disorder, and dementia of the Alzheimer's type.

Your rationale for implementing family psychoeducation programs is based on the results of the following studies:

Hepburn, K., Lewis, M., Tornatore, J., Sherman, C. W., & Bremer, K. L. (2007). The Savvy Caregiver program: The demonstrated effectiveness of a transportable dementia caregiver psychoeducation program. *Journal of Gerontological Nursing, 33*(3), 30–36.

Magliano, L., Fiorello, A., Malangone, C., De Rosa, C., & Maj, M. (2006). Patient functioning and family burden in a controlled, real-world trial of family psychoeducation for schizophrenia. *Psychiatric Services, 57*(12), 1784–1791.

Morris, C. D., Miklowitz, D. F., & Waxmonsky, J. A. (2007). Family-focused treatment for bipolar disorder in adults and youth. *Journal of Clinical Psychology, 63*(5), 433–445.

Powers, C. E. (2006). The Family Caregiver Program: Design and effectiveness of an education intervention. *Home Healthcare Nurse, 24*(8), 513–516.

CRITICAL THINKING APPLICATION

1. What are the purposes of reviewing the evidence before designing an intervention?
2. What specific areas of research should you review other than studies of family psychoeducation?
3. What might a structured family psychoeducation program look like?

principles of competence (stressing empowerment and collaboration) and adaptation, rather than psychopathology, and shifts the emphasis from the causes to the effects of mental disorders.

You can refer consumers and families in need (as well as other health care providers) to the NAMI HelpLine at 1–800–950–NAMI (6264). You can also suggest the NAMI website at http://www.nami.org, which can be accessed through a direct link on the Companion Website for this book.

Family Therapy

In general, family therapists believe that the emotional symptoms or problems of an individual are an expression of emotional symptoms or problems in a family. Therefore, family therapists view the family system as a unit of treatment. Their concerns are basically with the relationships between the family members, not with the intrapsychic functioning of individual family members.

Traditional family therapy has been criticized for its reliance on outdated theories and ineffective interventions, especially in relationship to the treatment of families with a member with a serious and persistent mental illness (discussed earlier in this chapter in the section on Family Assessment).

Forms of Family Therapy

There are two basic forms of family therapy—insight-oriented family therapy and behavioral-oriented family therapy—into which all schools of family therapy fit. Some examples of insight-oriented family therapy approaches are:

- *Psychodynamic:* Problems are believed to arise because of developmental delays, or current interactions or stresses.
- *Family of origin therapy:* The goal is to foster differentiation among the members and decrease emotional reactivity and triangulation (Bowen, 1988).

Some examples of behavioral-oriented family therapy and the theorists who developed them are:

- *Structural:* The focus is on systems, subsystems, boundaries, and schismatic, skewed, enmeshed, or disengaged families (Minuchin & Fishman, 1981; Navarre, 1998).
- *Strategic:* Problems arise because of inequality of power, flawed communication, and repetitive and maladaptive family interaction patterns (Haley, 1996; Satir, 1983).
- *Cognitive/behavioral:* The focus is on changing thinking and behavior, problem solving, and the development of skills (see Chapter 31 ∞ for a complete discussion of cognitive and behavioral strategies).

These lists are general, not exhaustive. Discussion of these theories and their specific interventions is beyond the scope of this book.

Qualifications of Family Therapists

Being a family therapist requires a firm and clear understanding of all of the dynamics and forces that influence families. Family therapists should be specially educated in the practice of family therapy and strongly committed to a belief in the importance of the family. Nurse family therapists should be clinical specialists or advanced practitioners prepared in graduate programs that provide both theory and supervised clinical practice in this specialized area. Refer families to qualified nurse family therapists or other qualified family therapists. Families can also receive help in finding a therapist on the website of the American Association for Marriage and Family Therapy, which can be accessed through the Companion Website for this book.

MediaLink American Association for Marriage and Family Therapy

The Unit of Treatment

Most family therapists recommend that all people in the family constellation participate in the assessment phase of family therapy. Not all agree on which people comprise the family constellation or the treatment unit. Some include all members of the nuclear family; others include members of the extended family; and still others, large numbers of people in the family's social network. Different coalitions may be seen together at different times to accomplish specific goals. For example, mates are often seen together for the first few sessions.

Children 4 years of age and younger are often not included in ongoing family therapy sessions. They may misinterpret, or be frightened by, the dialogue. In addition, small children tend to be disruptive. Some therapists, however, make it a point to bring all the children into some family therapy sessions to see how the family as a whole operates.

MediaLink National Alliance on Mental Illness

Contract or Goal Negotiation

The negotiation phase of family therapy is begun by identifying what each member would like changed in the family. When each family member and the therapist have identified important goals, they begin negotiating a set of attainable goals that everyone is willing to work on. Compromise is needed to achieve a working goal. At this time, the family therapist, along with the family, may also identify the means—tasks, strategies, and so on—that will be used to reach the negotiated goals.

Intervention

Therapy for a family system involves understanding and use of the here-and-now, and of the basic processes that occur in the system. Guidelines for interventions employed by family therapists are listed in the Your Intervention Strategies feature on page 824.

Terminating Family Therapy

Family therapists use various criteria to determine when termination is appropriate. Family therapy is often terminated when family members can:

- See how they appear to others
- Give feedback to others, telling them how they appear

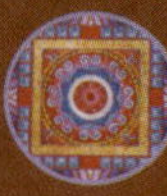

YOUR INTERVENTION STRATEGIES
The Role of the Family Therapist

- Creating a safe setting in which family members can risk looking at themselves and their actions
- Teaching family members how to share their observations with one another
- Asking for and giving information in a matter-of-fact, nonjudgmental, congruent way
- Responding as a role model whose meaning or intent can be checked on without fear
- Setting rules for interaction to ensure that all family members participate; interruptions, acting-out, or making it impossible to converse are not tolerated; no one speaks for anyone else
- Clarifying the content and relationship aspects of messages
- Pointing out significant discrepancies, incongruities, or double-level messages
- Helping everyone speak out clearly so that each can be heard
- Viewing the family as a system and not taking sides
- Showing that anger, pain, and the "forbidden" are safe to examine
- Reeducating family members to be accountable
- Delineating family roles and functions and teaching explicitly about role responses and role choices

- Share their hopes, fears, and expectations with one another
- Openly discuss problems with one another
- Openly disagree with one another when appropriate
- Give clear messages
- Check meaning with one another
- Ask for clarification
- Support one another
- Achieve the family's goals

Termination in family therapy occurs in a flexible way, helping families achieve realistic goals, thus ending therapy with a feeling of accomplishment.

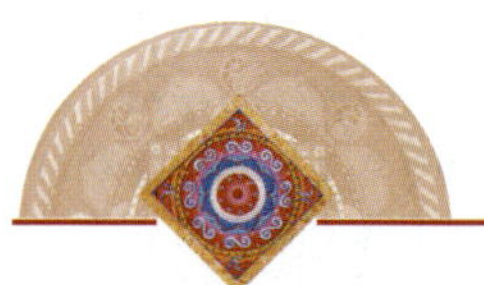

EXPLORE MEDIALINK 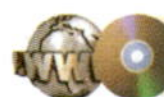 www.prenhall.com/kneisl

For NCLEX-RN® review questions, case studies, and other resources for this chapter see the Pearson Health MediaLink CD-ROM that accompanies this book and the Companion Website at www.prenhall.com/kneisl.

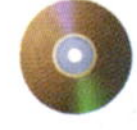

CD-ROM
Audio Glossary
NCLEX-RN® Review Questions

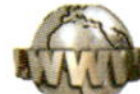

Companion Website
Audio Glossary
NCLEX-RN® Review Questions
Critical Thinking Exercise
- *Family Boundaries*

Case Study
- *Family Education and Intervention*

Care Plan
- *Family Dysfunction*

MediaLinks
MediaLink Application
- *Evidence-Based Practices for Services to Families of People with Psychiatric Disabilities*

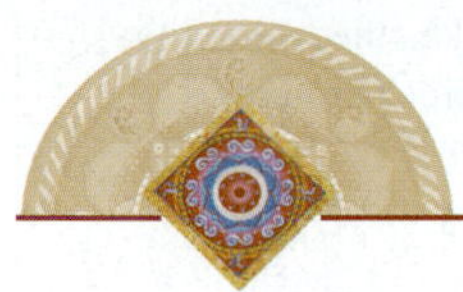

NCLEX-RN® REVIEW QUESTIONS

1. A nurse wants to start an outpatient support group for clients with chronic mental illness. Which of the following statements best describe the nurse's procedure? (Select all that apply.)
   1. Determine how to identify potential members.
   2. Post a sign-up sheet in the outpatient clinic to solicit group members.
   3. At the first meeting, have members identify and vote on the group rules.
   4. At the first meeting, provide a basic list of group rules in writing.
   5. Identify group members, then determine the best time for everyone to meet.

2. A nurse wants to start an outpatient self-help support group for clients with chronic mental illness. Which of the following initial goals is most realistic?
   1. The group will meet weekly to discuss any current concerns of interest to the group members.
   2. The group will help members identify feelings toward other group members, the nurse, and the group.
   3. The nurse will focus on illuminating the group process.
   4. The group members will learn new interpersonal skills from other group members.

3. A client asks the nurse, "How can I benefit from a therapeutic group?" In terms of the Johari Window, which of the following is the nurse's best response?
   1. "Group membership and participation meet the needs for inclusion, control, and affection."
   2. "As you interact with other group members, you will see in them the different aspects of yourself: the 'good me' and the 'bad me,' for example."
   3. "As other members give you feedback about the effect you have on others, you learn to see yourself differently."
   4. "I firmly believe that everyone can benefit from group therapy."

4. Which of the following group member statements is an example of here-and-now activation?
   1. "You became tearful last week. Is there something you can discuss with the group now?"
   2. "You have expressed hurt when people have interrupted you, but for the past 20 minutes you have talked without allowing others to share."
   3. "When the other people were talking, you appeared upset. Did their disruption bring up feelings about something from your past?"
   4. "When you say 'no one listens to me' to an older group member, does it feel like a parent talking to you?"

5. Within a particular adult client's family, the client's mother (the matriarch) makes all decisions. The client's father (patriarch) assists the matriarch in accomplishing her goals and routinely defers to her judgment. In addition, he acts as a liaison between the matriarch and the identified client. The other three married adult children consult the matriarch about decisions regarding their families of procreation. The client reports that the "children-in-law" rebel sometimes but more often accept this arrangement. The client reports a crisis following the matriarch's cerebrovascular accident (CVA), which rendered her unable to speak or perform self-care. The patriarch did not assume leadership or engage in decision making, and none of the four adult siblings assumed the leadership role.

   One month later, the matriarch died before any changes in living arrangements were even discussed. Which of the following descriptors characterizes this family?
   1. Unsatisfactory role negotiation with disequilibrium
   2. Democratic with diffuse boundaries
   3. Traditional nuclear family with satisfactory role negotiation
   4. Sharing of the family burden of mental illness of a family member

6. Which of the following findings supports a nursing diagnosis of Altered Family Processes?
   1. Four family members share a home. Each family member has chronic mental illness.
   2. A stable household, comprised of a married couple with two teenage children, is augmented when a family member with a chronic, debilitating illness moves into a spare room.
   3. A married couple with twins sends the children off to college as the wife enters menopause.
   4. A divorced couple brings their 10-year-old child to a mental health clinic for evaluation. Despite 5 years of pharmacotherapy combined with therapeutic boarding school, the parents are unable to agree on a consistent cognitive–behavioral therapeutic approach.

7. Which of the following assessment findings support a nursing diagnosis of Ineffective Family Coping?
   1. Two adult siblings lived together for 20 years until the mentally ill sibling responded to voices and destroyed the home by fire.
   2. One parent accepted early retirement in order to care for the mentally ill adult child.
   3. Three siblings report sharing the family burden of the mentally ill sibling, while the remaining sibling is uninvolved.
   4. Both parents and two of the four siblings have active chemical dependency problems.

8. The nurse is completing a family mental health assessment. Which of the following data would not be included in this assessment?
1. Employment history of individual family members
2. The informal roles of each family member
3. Decision-making process within the family
4. The food preferences of each family member

9. The nurse is summarizing her assessment findings with the family and tells them she perceives them to be an enmeshed family. What is the best description of enmeshment?
1. Family members are unconnected to each other.
2. Intrafamily boundaries are rigid.
3. The family member perceived to be the weakest is blamed for the family's troubles.
4. Family members do not have a strong sense of self.

10. Following a family meeting, a client makes the following statements. Which client statement requires the nurse's immediate intervention?
1. "Neither my siblings nor my father can deal with the burden I present. I have no options."
2. "I am going to have to rely heavily on resources outside my family."
3. "I wish we could all just turn to my oldest sibling and let her be the leader."
4. "I thought this was how all families function."

See Appendix C for answers.

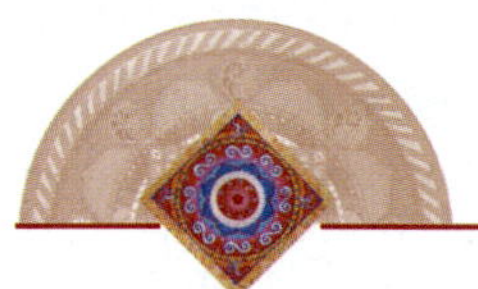

REFERENCES

American Nurses Association, American Psychiatric Nurses Association, & International Society of Psychiatric–Mental Health Nurses. (2007). *Psychiatric–mental health nursing: Scope and standards of practice.* Silver Spring, MD: Nursesbooks.org.

Atwood, N. C. (2001). Combining individual and family treatment: Guidelines for the therapist. *New Direction in Mental Health Services, 91*, 31–46.

Benne, K. D., & Sheats, P. (1948). Functional roles of group members. *Journal of Social Issues, 4*, 41–49.

Bourke, M. L., & Van Hasselt, V. B. (2001). Social problem-solving skills training for incarcerated offenders: A treatment manual. *Behavior Modification, 25*(2), 163–188.

Bowen, M. (1988). *Family therapy in clinical practice* (2nd ed.). Northvale, NJ: Jason Aronson.

Doornbos, M. M. (2002). Family caregivers and the mental health care system: Reality and dreams. *Archives of Psychiatric Nursing, 16*(1), 39–46.

Duvall, E. M., & Miller, B. C. (1985). *Marriage and family development*. New York: Harper & Row.

Granholm, E., McQuaid, J. R., McClure, F. S., Link, P. C., Perivolliotis, D., Gottlieb, J. D., et al. (2007). Randomized controlled trial of cognitive behavioral social skills training for older people with schizophrenia: 12-month follow-up. *Journal of Clinical Psychiatry, 68*(5), 730–737.

Haley, J. (1996). *Learning and teaching therapy*. New York: Guilford Press.

Hepburn, K., Lewis, M., Tornatore, J., Sherman, C. W., & Bremer, K. L. (2007). The Savvy Caregiver program: The demonstrated effectiveness of a transportable dementia caregiver psychoeducation program. *Journal of Gerontological Nursing, 33*(3), 30–36.

Jackson, D. D. (1968). *Communication, family, and marriage*. Palo Alto, CA: Science and Behavior Books.

Joyce, A. S., Piper, W. E., & Ogrodniczuk, J. S. (2007). Therapeutic alliance and cohesion variables as predictors of outcome in short-term group psychotherapy. *International Journal of Group Psychotherapy, 57*(3), 260–296.

Karp, D. A. (2000). *The burden of sympathy: How families cope with mental illness*. London: Oxford University Press.

Kent-Wilkinson, A. (1999). Forensic family genogram: An assessment and intervention tool. *Journal of Psychosocial Nursing and Mental Health Services, 37*(9), 52–56.

Kirby, J. S., & Baucom, D. H. (2007). Treating emotion dysregulation in a couples context: A pilot study of a couples skills group intervention. *Journal of Marital and Family Therapy, 33*(3), 375–391.

Kissane, D. W., Grabsch, B., Clarke, D. M., Smith, G. C., Love, A. W., & Bloch, S., et al. (2007). Supportive-expressive group therapy for women with metastatic breast cancer: Survival and psychosocial outcome from a randomized controlled trial. *Psychooncology, 16*(4), 277–286.

Linehan, M. M., Comtois, K. A., Murray, A. M., Brown, M. Z., Gallop, R. J., Hearde, H. L., et al. (2006). Two-year randomized controlled trial and follow-up of dialectical behavior therapy vs. therapy by experts for suicidal behaviors and borderline personality disorder. *Archives of General Psychiatry, 63*(7), 757–766.

Magliano, L., Fiorello, A., Malangone, C., De Rosa, C., & Maj, M. (2006). Patient functioning and family burden in a controlled, real-world trial of family psychoeducation for schizophrenia. *Psychiatric Services, 57*(12), 1784–1791.

McFarlane, W. R., Dixon, L., Lukens, E., & Lucksted, A. (2003). Family psychoeducation and schizophrenia: A review of the literature. *Journal of Marital and Family Therapy, 29*(2), 223–245.

Minuchin, S., & Fishman, H. (1981). *Family therapy techniques*. Cambridge, MA: Harvard University Press.

Morris, C. D., Miklowitz, D. F., & Waxmonsky, J. A. (2007). Family-focused treatment for bipolar disorder in adults and youth. *Journal of Clinical Psychology, 63*(5), 433–445.

Muhlbauer, S. (2002). Experience of stigma by families with mentally ill members. *Journal of American Psychiatric Nurses Association, 8*(3), 76–83.

Murray-Swank, A. B., & Dixon, L. (2004). Family psychoeducation as an evidence-based practice. *CNS Spectrum, 9*(12), 905–912.

Myin-Germeys, I., Nicolson, N. A., & Delespaul, P. A. (2001). The context of delusional experiences in the daily life of patients with schizophrenia. *Psychological Medicine, 31*(3), 489–498.

Navarre, S. (1998). Salvador Minuchin's structural family therapy and its application to multicultural family systems. *Issues in Mental Health Nursing, 19*, 557–565.

Ogrodniczuk, J. S., Piper, W. E., Joyce, A. S., McCallum, M., & Rosie, J. S. (2003). NEO-five factor personality traits as predictors of response to two forms of group psychotherapy. *International Journal of Group Psychotherapy, 53*(4), 417–442.

Piper, W. E., Ogrodniczuk, J. S., Joyce, A. S., Weideman, R., & Rosie, J. S. (2007). Group composition and group therapy for complicated grief. *Journal of Consulting and Clinical Psychology, 75*(1), 116–125.

Popovsky, M. (2007). A spiritual issues discussion group for psychiatric inpatients. *Pastoral Care and Counseling, 61*(1–2), 119–128.

Powers, C. E. (2006). The Family Caregiver Program: Design and effectiveness of an education intervention. *Home Healthcare Nurse, 24*(8), 513–516.

Rousaud, A., Blanch, J., Hautzinger, M., De Lazzari, E., Peri, J. M., Puig, O., et al. (2007). Improvement of psychosocial adjustment to HIV-1 infection through a cognitive-behavioral oriented group psychotherapy program: A pilot study. *AIDS Patient Care and STDS, 21*(3), 212–222.

Satir, V. (1983). *Conjoint family therapy*. Palo Alto, CA: Science and Behavior Books.

Schutz, W. C. (1958a). Interpersonal underworld. *Harvard Business Review, 36*, 123–135.

Schutz, W. C. (1958b). *The interpersonal underworld: FIRO*. Palo Alto, CA: Science and Behavior Books.

Sprenkle, D. H., & Blow, A. J. (2004). Common factors and our sacred models. *Journal of Marital and Family Therapy, 30*(2), 113–129.

Tay, S. E. (2007). Compliance therapy: An intervention to improve inpatients' attitudes toward treatment. *Journal of Psychosocial Nursing and Mental Health Services, 45*(6), 29–37.

van Dam-Baggen, R., & Kraaimaat, F. (2000). Group social skills training of cognitive group therapy as the clinical treatment of choice for generalized social phobia. *Journal of Anxiety Disorders, 14*(5), 437–451.

Wenckus, E. M. (1994). Storytelling: Using an ancient art to work with groups. *Journal of Psychosocial Nursing and Mental Health Services, 32*, 30–32.

Yalom, I. D. (1998). *The Yalom reader*. New York: Basic Books.

Yalom, I. D. (2005). *The theory and practice of group psychotherapy* (5th ed.). New York: Basic Books.

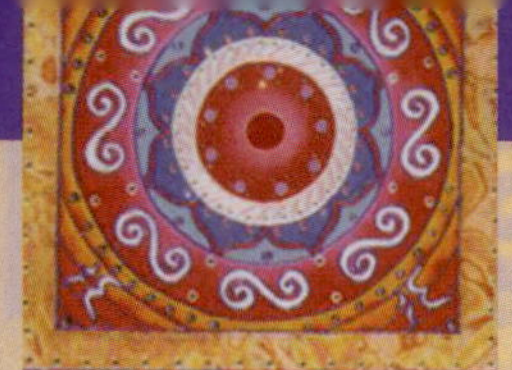

CHAPTER

31 Cognitive and Behavioral Interventions

EILEEN TRIGOBOFF

KEY TERMS

behavior modification *833*
mastery imagery *831*
negative imagery *831*
positive imagery *830*
positive reinforcement *832*
response prevention *833*
systematic desensitization *834*

LEARNING OUTCOMES

After completing this chapter, you will be able to:

1. Describe the central features of cognitive behavioral interventions.
2. Discuss how humans express themselves in cognitive and behavioral ways.
3. Relate conditioning and association to the process of human learning.
4. Design nursing care plans for people with varied diagnoses using cognitive behavioral therapies.
5. Analyze the effectiveness of a behavioral contract to promote a change in health-related behaviors.
6. Modify a nursing care plan to promote and enhance positive outcomes for cognitive behavioral therapies.
7. Describe how your personal characteristics might influence your effectiveness in using cognitive behavioral therapies.

CRITICAL THINKING CHALLENGE

Steven Norah is a full-time college student. He has been depressed for some time and has not made significant progress in long-term psychotherapy specifically focused on his childhood and developmental issues. You discussed his treatment responses with other members of the treatment team during his recent hospitalization for an exacerbation of his depression. Steven has expressed frustration at his inability to "get better and leave the depression behind." His depression and his routine ways of thinking and behaving continue in an unchanged, habitual manner.

The team believes a cognitive behavioral approach would give Steven a better chance at recovery from depression. Changing his thoughts and behaviors could change his feelings and diminish depressive thinking. Once changes occur, Steven would have the opportunity to feel competent and successful, a distinct difference from his current view of himself.

1. How do you explain the notion that a change in thoughts and behaviors results in a change in feelings?
2. What should Steven know about this therapeutic method?
3. What differences would you expect to see in Steven's behavior if the cognitive behavioral approach is effective?

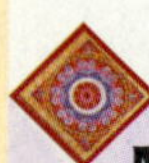

MEDIALINK 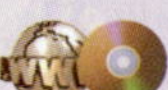 www.prenhall.com/kneisl

Go to the Pearson Health MediaLink CD-ROM and the Companion Website at www.prenhall.com/kneisl for interactive resources for this chapter.

Marcy, a person who is most comfortable with structure and routine in her daily life, has finally decided to seek help to overcome her fear of flying. Her friends have invited Marcy to travel with them to Paris, a place she has always wanted to visit. Marcy always has several reasons why she cannot travel with them. Most of the time she says that she needs to stay home to care for her sister, who has a severe case of arthritis.

How might therapists with a variety of orientations approach Marcy's problem? A biologically oriented therapist would first focus on diagnosing Marcy's problem as a specific phobia—fear of flying—once the presence of other anxiety disorders, specifically panic disorder with agoraphobia, have been ruled out. The biologically oriented therapist would investigate Marcy's family history for the presence of phobias among first-degree biological relatives and prescribe an antianxiety medication to alter her brain chemistry.

In contrast, a psychodynamic therapist would focus on Marcy's defensive style of avoidance. This therapist would identify Marcy's pattern of needing to have structure and control as a way of keeping anxiety in check. Treatment would be a talk therapy in which the therapist provides only minimal direction in the exploration of Marcy's past, her feelings, and her frustrations. The therapeutic goal would be for Marcy to gain insight into her intrapsychic conflicts, interpersonal difficulties, and defenses.

A cognitive behavioral therapist would be aware of the issues in Marcy's life, but would approach therapy quite differently. A believer in the axiom that "actions speak louder than words," the cognitive behavioral therapist looks for treatments that work based on research evidence. The therapist would focus on changing behavior in the present rather than focusing on gaining insight into the past. This change-oriented approach would pair relaxation training (discussed in Chapter 33) and systematic desensitization (discussed later in this chapter) in Marcy's case.

In this chapter you will learn that cognitive (thought) and behavioral (action) interventions have their base in human learning theory and are comprised of diverse treatments based on empirical evidence. While not the only effective treatment—medications and talk therapy can also be effective—cognitive and behavioral strategies lend themselves to integration within a plan of care for clients who may be receiving diverse, but effective, treatments for mental disorders. More recently, the term *cognitive behavioral therapy* has largely replaced the terms *behavior therapy* and *cognitive therapy* as a way of describing these therapeutic techniques. You can access the empirical evidence for cognitive behavioral therapy through the National Science Foundation's website specifically dedicated to behavioral and cognitive sciences, which can be accessed through the Companion Website for this text.

Cognitive and behavioral interventions make use of the principles of cognitive functioning and behavior listed in Box 31-1. They are tailored to individual client needs and may be applied as single therapeutic entities or in combination.

Box 31-1 Principles of Cognitive Functioning and Behavior

Principles of Cognitive Functioning

1. What people think affects how they feel.
2. What people think is often based on thinking habits.
3. If we change our thinking, we can effect a change in our feelings.

Principles of Behavior

People do things:	When they are rewarded in a way that is meaningful for them
	When something they don't like is removed
People don't do things:	When they get punished
	When something they like is taken away from them

COGNITIVE THERAPY

We know that our thoughts (cognitions) affect our feelings. Cognitive therapy is based on making cognitive changes, which, in turn, alters feelings. Consider the routine and habitual thinking of most depressed persons: "I'm no good at anything. I'm a failure in life." With enough repetition, the depressed person comes to accept this particular self-evaluation as accurate. The goal in cognitive therapy is to alter these thoughts to: "There are things that I can do well, and there are things that I need to work on." This type of thinking is more realistic and avoids adhering to an unhealthy perspective. Over time, a change in thinking allows the client to replace disturbing and negative thoughts with neutral and positive thoughts; a cognitive change can influence an emotional change for the better. This process is the basis for cognitive therapy (Skinner, 1974, 1989).

Basic Concepts

Three basic concepts are basic to an understanding of cognitive therapy—attributions, modeling, and self-efficacy.

Attributions

As humans, we constantly ascribe causes to the events in our lives. By labeling or assigning meaning to a circumstance or a set of circumstances we make *attributions* ("I only got a grade of C. I'm no good at anything. Sarah and Francisco got As. They can do anything.") Think of attributions as perceived causes that may or may not be objectively accurate. Depressed people often attribute failure to themselves and success to others. Then we attribute associated features or characteristics to that circumstance or set of circumstances (such as being a good student or knowing the material). Next, we expect a certain outcome from that circumstance and we behave consistently with that expectation. Finally, we have feelings that match, or are congruent with, the experience. The basic idea is that thoughts and behaviors lead to feelings.

MediaLink National Science Foundation

Modeling

Modeling involves imitating another (or others) in the expectation that one will receive rewards such as those other people seem to be receiving. See FIGURE 31-1 ■ for an example of how people learn through modeling the behaviors of others. You have likely experienced modeling throughout your education, especially once you selected nursing as your career. You have doubtless observed nurses who are competent and effective, and you strive for that level of skill in order to receive the same rewards.

Self-Efficacy

Human learning also occurs through self-efficacy. Self-efficacy involves feeling effective through one's own actions. People learn and adapt when they find themselves in circumstances demanding new or different skills. Under those circumstances, people who tend to believe that they can cope successfully with life and problems in living through acquiring skills, practicing them, and observing successful outcomes will gain confidence and a sense of self-efficacy.

Over time, consistently making attributions, modeling behavior, and experiencing self-efficacy set a pattern of thinking in place. The pattern explains events while shaping expectations about interactions and other behaviors. The patterns can be shaped in adaptive or maladaptive ways, depending on the circumstances and the multiple variables that come into play. Unrealistic thought patterns are maladaptive in that they make demands on the individual that cannot be met or cannot be resolved. For example, a 70-year-old woman who was adopted as a child may believe she has no worth because her birth mother gave her away. In her case, it is unrealistic to assume that the reason her mother gave her up for adoption was a malevolent one, and, as her birth mother is not likely to be found or identified in order to explain the circumstances of the adoption, this negative perception taints her life.

Cognitive Therapy Techniques

The purpose of cognitive therapy is first to identify thoughts that are unrealistic, negative, or otherwise problematic. Once these thoughts are identified, they are examined for their impact on the individual. Nurses are instrumental in helping a client see how a particular set of thoughts can create a problem. When this connection is made, substituting neutral or positive thoughts for problematic thinking takes place over time. Correcting automatic problematic thinking is a retraining experience. The individual must unlearn the maladaptive cognitive style, then learn adaptive cognitions. The following clinical example describes why cognitive changes are important to mental health.

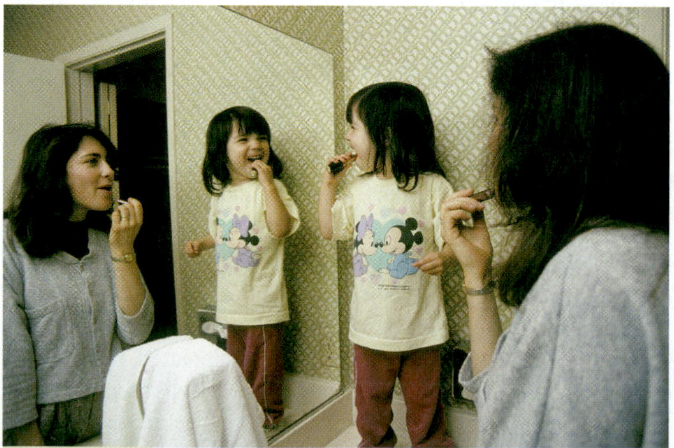

FIGURE 31-1 ■ Modeling. Imitative learning is a form of complex learning.

Source: Elizabeth Crews Photography, Elizabeth Crews.

CLINICAL EXAMPLE

George is a 45-year-old male being treated for schizophrenia. His symptoms are coming under reasonable control with medications and therapy; however, he has been having difficulty lately with his mother. Whenever she cannot visit him at his apartment, he becomes depressed and agitated. The outpatient clinic nurse spoke with him about his current problems, and together they identified an irrational thought George had about his mother. He believed that if she didn't visit him every 7 days, regardless of whether or not she had to work overtime, that meant she did not love him. George thought he would never be able to be "a man" without his mother's love. Once George identified his irrational conclusions about the meaning of her visits, he was able to talk to her about her feelings for him. George had to concentrate and work to replace his automatic and irrational thoughts with more realistic ones; his mother's love does not need to be renewed—it is always there. George recognized that the visiting schedule and their relationship were not connected. He prepared a number of neutral and positive statements that he could repeat to himself whenever the old irrational thoughts appeared. Eventually, George was able to tolerate changes in the frequency of his mother's visits.

Positive Imagery

Positive imagery consists of thinking in a positive way about how an event or experience will unfold rather than anticipating disastrous results. This tends to promote the likelihood of a positive outcome.

Positive imagery can also be applied to past events. It is a reframing of actions taken. For example, a woman is attacked at her parked car and blames herself for being weak, unprepared, and frightened. Positive imagery reframes the woman's actions as perfectly understandable under the circumstances and walks her through the events with this different perspective. It gives her permission to react to frightening events with fear.

When directed toward an upcoming event, positive imagery can be a cognitive rehearsal. Thinking positively in advance about how a set of behaviors or an event will occur helps the individual perform more competently in a variety of situations and with a wider array of skills.

Mastery Imagery

Mastery imagery shapes the individual's thoughts about being in control or having mastery over a particular situation. The point of this technique is to practice imagined successful behavior change. Imagining interacting competently and in an adult manner with someone who abused you in childhood is an example of mastery imagery. In the clinical example that follows, Christine is achieving mastery over her work situation.

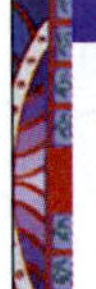

CLINICAL EXAMPLE

Christine imagines and rehearses interacting with her usually demanding, critical, and agitated supervisor. In the past she would typically respond haphazardly and with agitation, which resulted in making errors and feeling ineffective. Christine's mastery imagery establishes a new routine that consists of interacting with her supervisor in a consistently calm and organized manner.

Negative Imagery

Another useful cognitive therapy tool to help change maladaptive behaviors is **negative imagery**, or envisioning negative events and outcomes for maladaptive behavior. Envisioning the negative outcome of maladaptive behavior can serve as a powerful educator. The scenario is played out in the client's thinking and can assist the client in predicting what is likely to happen unless changes are made.

The client is taught to identify the imagery invoked (the thoughts) when beginning a maladaptive behavior, such as substance use. It may be something like: "My favorite drug will be fun" or "I am so much more relaxed and able to interact better when I use this stuff." This is positive imagery. In this case, positive imagery promotes use of the substance even though that behavior will interfere with and damage important relationships with others. The real impact of the behavior is understood only when denial is dispensed with and consequences are recognized. Then substituting with negative imagery can begin.

For example, if a client uses cocaine, the positive imagery may be that the drug will make him feel good. Negatively envisioning cocaine use would consist of the client learning to say and think, "If I use, I will lose control of my thoughts and feelings. It will cost a lot of money, which I don't have, and will put a bigger emotional and physical gap between me and my wife." Replacing positive imagery with negative imagery may reduce the automatic positive associations over time and reduce the urge to use the drug.

Attribution Restructuring

The heart of cognitive therapy lies in recognizing how we think and behave and in identifying problematic learning. People develop patterns of thinking over time, often automatically, without active or conscious effort. Automatic thoughts can develop into specific (and frequently solidly crystallized) sets of automatic thinking. For example, a person who takes the same mental steps over and over comes to the same problematic conclusion. It is important to realize that maladaptive automatic thoughts and attributions require detection prior to intervention.

If a client has had a number of depressive episodes, the resulting cognitive map must be factored into treatment. Each depressive episode generates negative cognitive maps that are likely to be reactivated the next time the client experiences even a mild dysphoric state, so that current experiences are interpreted more negatively (Havermans, Nicolson, & deVries, 2007). Each successive negative experience breeds another.

Attribution restructuring or retraining involves abandoning intuitive strategies in order to change the meanings associated with people, places, and things. Once maladaptive cognitions are detected, evidence-based cognitive interventions are employed to alter and restructure thinking.

BEHAVIOR THERAPY

Behavior has an impact on feelings and thoughts, as the following clinical example demonstrates.

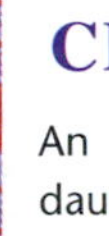

CLINICAL EXAMPLE

An older woman with a hearing deficit is living with her daughter and son-in-law. She wears a hearing aid but, to save on battery power, she removes it and turns it off immediately after dinner every night. When they try to talk to her, she cannot hear. She complains to others that her daughter and son-in-law are not interested in talking or interacting with her in the evening. Her behavior isolates her, but she does not see the connection between her attempts at thriftiness and her feelings of loneliness.

The ways in which particular types of behavioral therapy can affect a variety of conditions are discussed next.

Classical Conditioning

Generally, behavior therapy reduces the occurrence of problematic behaviors. Behavioral therapy is very effective when used with a current problem that is relevant to the client's life (Nsimba, 2007). It focuses on behavioral learning processes, including *classical conditioning*. The principles of classical conditioning are:

- People learn to associate a particular feeling state with a particular circumstance that then becomes a conditioned stimulus for the feeling.
- Over time, the association between the circumstance and the feeling is strengthened through repetition and rehearsal.

The therapist's goal in behavior therapy is to decrease or eliminate the association of a particular circumstance (the conditioned stimulus) with a particular feeling. See FIGURE 31-2 ■ on page 832 for an example of a behavior that responds well to conditioning and intermittent reinforcement.

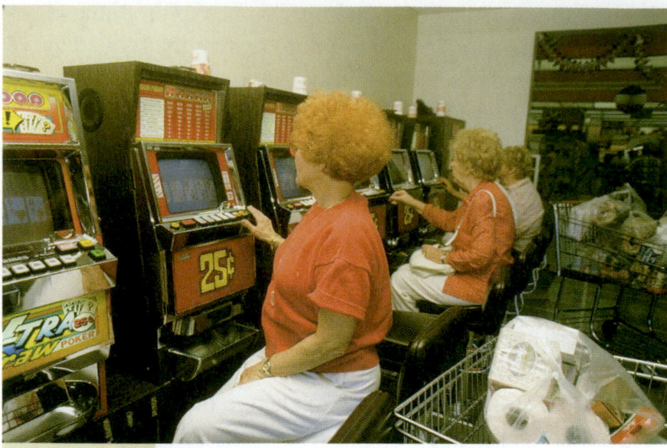

FIGURE 31-2 ■ Intermittent reinforcement. Operant conditioning involves an association between a stimulus and a response. When people are rewarded for pressing the button on a slot machine, they repeat the process.

Source: PhotoEdit Inc., Bonnie Kamin.

Operant Conditioning

Operant conditioning is another behavioral learning process and is based on these concepts:

- People are positively reinforced for certain behaviors.
- People learn to seek further **positive reinforcement** (an environmental event that rewards, and thus increases the probability of, a behavioral response) by increasing that behavior.
- Positive reinforcement results from either getting something desirable or avoiding something unpleasant.

The therapist's goal in operant conditioning is to help the individual increase positive reinforcement through more adaptive and effective behavior. The effort to change health-related behavior can be facilitated with a behavioral contract. An effective behavioral contract must be tailored for the individual, and a comprehensive behavioral assessment is necessary to design such a contract and form practical, measurable, and feasible objectives and goals. Behavioral contracting is covered in the nursing process section of this chapter.

MEDIALINK Rational Emotive Behavioral Therapy

Rational Emotive Behavioral Therapy

Rational emotive therapy (RET) was originated by Albert Ellis (1975) and emphasizes cognitive causes of emotional problems along with the importance of taking personal responsibility for maintaining health-damaging thought habits and irrational beliefs. An irrational belief is a belief that lacks reason and sound judgment. Box 31-2 is a list of some common irrational thoughts that, when incorporated into an individual's belief system, are known to create unhealthy thoughts and feelings. The clinician who is skilled in RET helps identify irrational thought structures with the client and then helps develop a plan to substitute more rational personal life philosophies and attitudes based on accurately perceived realities (Ellis, 1997). Healthy emotional consequences occur when rational thinking drives adequate functional behaviors.

Box 31-2 Irrational Thoughts

- I need someone—often a specific person—to be with and lean on (I can't do everything by myself).
- It is easier for me to overlook or avoid thinking about tense situations than to face the problems and take the responsibility for correcting the situation.
- I should always be able, successful, and "on top of things" (if I'm not, I'm an inadequate, incompetent, hopeless failure).
- Everyone should love and approve of me (if they don't, I feel awful and unlovable).
- When the situation is scary or going badly, I should be—and can't keep from—worrying all the time.
- When things do not go the way I wanted and planned, it is terrible and I am, of course, going to be very disturbed. I can't stand it!
- Things have been this way so long, I can't do anything about these problems now.
- I know there is an answer to every problem. I should find it (if I don't, it will be awful).
- People who are evil and bad should be punished severely (and I have the right to get upset if they aren't stopped and made to pay the price).
- External events, such as other people, a screwed-up society, or bad luck, cause most of my unhappiness. Furthermore, I don't have any control over these external factors, so I can't do anything about my depression or other misery.
- I don't like the way I'm feeling but I can't help it. I just have to accept it and go with my feelings.
- When my close friends and relatives have serious problems, it is only right and natural that I get very upset too.

Source: Ellis, A., & Harper, R. (1975). *A new guide to rational living.* Chatworth, CA: Wilshire Book Co.

Rational emotive behavior therapy (REBT), as it is now known, identifies and corrects irrational beliefs. Rational and irrational beliefs, defined by REBT, form the basis of inferences (conclusions based on reasoning) derived to explain life experiences. Those inferences can be more or less functional depending on the beliefs behind them. People who hold rational beliefs form inferences that are significantly more functional than those formed by people who hold irrational beliefs. The Albert Ellis Institute and the Association for REBT can be accessed through the Companion Website for this text.

The following clinical example illustrates how firmly held irrational beliefs can inhibit functioning.

CLINICAL EXAMPLE

Marvin, a 38-year-old forklift operator, was injured on the job 4 years ago. His back injuries were treated and all tests indicate a complete recovery; however, his ability to function at work is impaired and he continues to complain of back pain. Marvin has been referred to a specialist in psychotherapy for chronic pain.

In an REBT session he describes an early experience of observing his father's lengthy struggle with cancer, during which his father was largely sedentary and his mother reacted hysterically whenever his father tried to be more active. In therapy it emerged that Marvin had acquired an irrational core belief that problems or fears are best handled with rest, withdrawal, and being sedentary. Marvin's past pain symptoms were uncomfortable enough to trigger this response, consistent with his core belief. As he became more sedentary and less functional, his back became increasingly weak and prone to pain. The greater the pain, the less active he became, until he was caught in a vicious cycle of increasing pain and withdrawal.

REBT helped Marvin learn to identify his irrational belief. This was accomplished through a Socratic question-and-answer format whereby Marvin recognized that withdrawal and inactivity led to more rather than fewer problems. The sources for Marvin's irrational belief were clarified as well. The belief was reframed in a more rational direction—that many problems respond best to constructive and productive activity. Specifically, Marvin's chronic pain was likely to improve with exercise, physical therapy, and daily productive activity. Assignments were given between sessions to help Marvin develop his repertoire in these areas. As he successfully proceeded to do so, his pain symptoms diminished and his self-esteem increased.

The Socratic question-and-answer format is an important aspect of REBT. This method, illustrated in Box 31-3, allows the client to explore how a particular line of reasoning was allowed to develop and how it continues to function. It focuses on a logical perspective, which is an appealing and manageable therapeutic style to which many adults can relate. As with all therapeutic styles, however, there must be a fit between the client and the therapeutic intervention. Not all therapies will be useful, or even therapeutic, with all clients in all situations.

Box 31-3 The Socratic Question-and-Answer Format

Marvin:	"I spent the day in bed yesterday because my back hurt."
Therapist:	"What did you hope that would accomplish?"
Marvin:	"That my back would feel better."
Therapist:	"Did it?"
Marvin:	"No."
Therapist:	"Can you ever remember a time when inactivity made your back feel better?"
Marvin:	"No, it just gets worse."
Therapist:	"So where and how did you come to believe that inactivity would make your back feel better?"
Marvin:	"In my family we always rested when we were hurt."
Therapist:	"Did that help your family?"
Marvin:	"Come to think of it, not that I ever saw."
Therapist:	"Maybe too much resting doesn't help?"
Marvin:	"I never thought of it that way."
Therapist:	"If too much resting doesn't help, what else might?"
Marvin:	"Once when my back hurt I went to a chiropractor and did some exercises. I remember that helped."
Therapist:	"What does that tell you about resting too much?"
Marvin:	"Maybe it's not such a good idea."

Behavior Modification

Behavior modification frequently focuses on a target behavior that is problematic for the individual (e.g., overeating) or for the community (e.g., loud verbal outbursts). The behavior is observed and tracked in objective and measurable terms, then addressed with a behavior modification plan. Both nonpharmacologic and pharmacologic interventions may be employed to assist in the modification of behavioral disturbances. We will discuss nonpharmacologic behavioral modification interventions here. Pharmacologic interventions are discussed in Chapters 7 and 32∞.

A behavior modification program begins with the identification of a specific behavior that requires change. It is important to monitor the target behavior and develop a detailed database about it. The problem behavior is carefully observed for:

- Antecedents (what came before)
- Precipitants (what appeared to cause or provoke the behavior)
- How the behavior is expressed
- Timing
- Frequency
- Duration
- Personal strengths to be capitalized on in designing the plan

To enable a client to modify behavior that is undesirable or unhealthy, giving support and involving the client in the plan of action are required. One strategy organizes the client's problem behavior into a hierarchy. In this hierarchy, the least distressing changes are at the lowest level and the most distressing are at the highest. For example, scores are assigned to levels of distress, ranging from zero, or none, to 100, the highest level of difficulty the client can imagine. Someone who overeats may feel only slight distress, or a score of 15, when thinking about not eating at a movie or a sporting event. A much higher distress level, with a score of 85, might occur when the same client considers being in an unfamiliar or uncomfortable social environment and not being able to eat.

Response Prevention

The individual is guided through imagining a situation at the lowest level of distress initially and developing and rehearsing adaptive responses to the distress. This establishes a new pattern that supplants the older, maladaptive response. This is called **response prevention**, meaning the

MEDIALINK Critical Thinking Exercise: Modifying Unhealthy Behavior

MEDIALINK Beck Institute

automatic maladaptive responses are modified and replaced with adaptive behaviors. Gradually, the client advances through his or her hierarchy of distress, learning to develop skills in responding competently at every step.

Systematic Desensitization

Systematic desensitization, another behavioral modification treatment regimen, also uses a hierarchy to arrange treatment. Behaviors are identified and ordered according to level of distress for the client. The client imagines being in certain situations at various levels of distress and learns to cope before moving on to the next level of distress. See the following Your Intervention Strategies feature for a desensitization hierarchy for a phobic fear of heights.

Assignments for graded exposures and response prevention are usually completed as homework, accompanied by self-monitoring (through diaries and/or graphs) and clinical assessment of progress through the behavioral programming. The behavior modification plan requires a realistic appraisal of the difficulties facing the person who wants to make a change and includes a plan for handling those difficulties (Dunbar-Jacob, 2007). A sample plan for someone who wants to quit smoking, for example, must include the following three steps:

1. Understanding the mechanisms that trigger the urge to smoke
2. Substituting other activities for the habit of smoking
3. Recognizing supports that will promote success in unlearning the rituals of smoking behavior

For a client trying to quit smoking, the environment should be smoke free and all smoking materials and accoutrements disposed of in order to minimize relapses. Psychopharmacologic supports are available for the smoking cessation process. See Chapter 32 for more information. Box 31-4 lists behavior modification tips for smoking cessation.

YOUR INTERVENTION STRATEGIES
Desensitization Hierarchy for Phobic Fear of Heights

1. Develop 10 to 12 scenes of increasing levels of fear.
   Example: Tell the client to imagine the scene with the lowest level of fear:
   "You are going up a kitchen stepladder. Step to the third rung, and look around."
   "Now you are going up to the top rung. You are at the top. Look around at the cupboards. Look at the floor."
   "Now you are on the second floor of an office building. Walk toward the window and look out."
2. Continue in this manner, increasing the level of fear attached to the scene each time the client is able to visualize without undue anxiety:
   "Now you go to the top of the Sears Tower. Go over to the guardrail and look straight down."
3. The final steps of the desensitization process include encouraging the client to try some of these behaviors in real life, after the client has successfully coped with the imagined scenes.

Box 31-4 Smoking Cessation Behavior Modification Guidance

Helping a Smoker to Quit

- Set up a timeline of the typical smoking schedule.
- Develop a tracking mechanism for where the individual smoked (couch, corner bar, car).
- Use checklists for situations and interactions with others in which smoking is involved.
- Suggest a set of behaviors to substitute for smoking.
- Provide self-help literature.
- Encourage those in the environment to also quit.
- Provide motivational material related to the client's current health status.
- Problem-solve to enhance coping with stressors.
- Enhance skills for coping with stressors.
- Emphasize positive benefits.
- Provide individual support.
- Reinforce short-term success.
- Provide support through group therapy.

COGNITIVE BEHAVIORAL THERAPY

The goal in cognitive behavioral treatment is to develop healthier labeling and an expectancy strategy that leads to more desirable feelings and a greater feeling of self-efficacy. Beck (1976; Beck, Freeman, & Associates, 1990) indicates that behavioral problems arise in childhood when we learn core beliefs and make associations between what we believe and what we expect to happen. Beck's theories are accessible at the website for the Beck Institute for Cognitive Therapy and Research and through a link on the Companion Website for this text.

Building on what we learn in childhood, our labels and expectations influence the strategies we select to compensate and cope. Webster copes with the following situation according to the particular pattern that he developed over time.

CLINICAL EXAMPLE

Webster is a traveling salesman who must drive long distances to meet with his clients. One day, during a meeting with a client, he experienced a panic attack. His symptoms included shortness of breath, rapid heartbeat, and thoughts of wanting to escape the situation. Afterward he was very tired. He decided to leave work early and drive home. When he got home he felt more relaxed and relieved. He hoped the panic attack was an isolated event that would not happen again.

But Webster had more panic attacks. He longed to be at home when they occurred because he experienced relief and greater comfort there. Soon he began to cut back on face-to-face client meetings and conducted meetings online or by telephone instead. The more he succeeded in staying at home, the more anxious he became when he was required to leave. Eventually he became almost completely unable to leave home, whether for business, social, or any other purposes (such as an emergency with a friend). The mere thought of stepping outside the house precipitated a panic attack. Webster had developed diagnosable panic disorder with agoraphobia at a severe level.

Cognitive and behavioral treatment consists of identifying and recognizing maladaptive thinking styles and working toward the acquisition of new skills for managing stressors. Features of treatment include teaching, interpreting, reframing, and learning and practicing new behaviors (Nsimba, 2007; Reilly-Harrington et al., 2007). Once thoughts and behaviors are realistically and rationally framed and implemented, emotional reactions will be consistent with them. See the Evidence-Based Practice feature for a description of how these treatment strategies are incorporated into a group setting for the treatment of panic disorder.

The cognitive behavioral approach is important in the contemporary treatment of substance dependence. There is sufficient research evidence supporting both drug-free outpatient treatment programs and treatment methods involving medications such as naltrexone and buprenorphine. These programs, combined with psychosocial treatment or behavioral techniques, provide additional promise for outpatient-based drug abuse treatment in the future (Nsimba, 2007).

Thought Stopping

Thought stopping is an example of a cognitive behavioral psychotherapeutic technique that can help a client change thinking processes. This change is important, as cognitive behaviorists maintain that feelings can be strongly influenced by the pattern and process of thoughts (Ford, 2007).

Clients sometimes have difficulty with repetitive, maladaptive thinking. For example, a client worries incessantly about things she cannot control; another client repeatedly has inaccurate, negative thoughts about himself. For these clients the cognitive behavioral therapist may implement the procedure known as thought stopping. The client learns to stop negative or maladaptive thinking by visualizing or imagining a specific image, sensation, or circumstance. Examples of thought stopping include:

- Visualizing a traffic stop sign
- Imagining hearing the word "stop" said loudly
- Imagining the tactile sensation of leaning up against a closed door

Thought stopping is done whenever the identified negative or maladaptive thought occurs. Over time, the client learns to stop such thoughts in an almost reflexive manner. This technique is typically used as part of a larger set of techniques that might also include developing alternative thoughts and mastering behavioral skills to alter outcomes in various problematic circumstances.

Techniques used in cognitive behavioral therapy such as thought stopping are defined and explained on the website of the National Association of Cognitive Behavioral Therapists, accessible through the Companion Website for this text.

MEDIALINK National Association of Cognitive Behavioral Therapists

Dialectical Behavioral Therapy

Linehan specifically developed dialectical behavioral therapy (DBT) for the outpatient treatment of chronically suicidal

MEDIALINK Application: Illness Management and Recovery Program

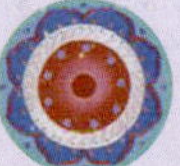

EVIDENCE-BASED PRACTICE

TREATING PANIC ATTACKS

Otis, a 45-year-old man, experienced panic attacks for 6 years. He tried to control the attacks on his own, but after 2 years finally went for treatment. Otis took medications with only moderate success for 4 years and was ready to try something different to address his problem. He agreed to participate in your cognitive behavioral therapy group in an outpatient clinic.

It was noted by Otis's pharmacotherapist and reported to you that Otis had a number of automatic responses to his panic attacks. He would think and feel a particular way whenever he became anxious, was exposed to a stressor, or had a panic attack. His defense mechanisms were frequently immature, although he did not describe them as such.

Over 4 months Otis and several other individuals attended 12 group sessions based on a cognitive behavioral curriculum. Muscle relaxation, diaphragmatic breathing skills, cognitive restructuring, and homework assignments formed the cognitive behavioral aspects of the therapy. At the end of the treatment period, Otis was able to respond to stressors in a more mature, satisfactory manner. His panic attacks and other symptoms were also reduced. Even 1 year after the group concluded, Otis was still benefiting from the cognitive behavioral therapy he received.

Action should be based on more than one study, but these interventions were developed using cognitive behavioral principles in conjunction with the following research:

Heldt, E., Blaya, C., Kipper, L., Salum, G. A., Otto, M. W., & Manfro, G. G. (2007). Defense mechanisms after brief cognitive-behavior group therapy for panic disorder: One-year follow-up. *Journal of Nervous and Mental Disease, 195*(6), 540–543.

CRITICAL THINKING APPLICATION

1. What elements would you take into consideration when planning to introduce behavioral change?
2. How can Otis and his family benefit from psychoeducation?
3. What exercises and rehearsals would be considered priorities for Otis?

people with borderline personality disorder (Linehan et al., 1999). DBT is a specialized subset of the cognitive behavioral treatment modalities. The client with borderline personality disorder tends to be crisis prone, with intense relational episodes (Swales & Heard, 2007). In other words, interactions with others have the potential to disrupt the client powerfully.

DBT is a biosocial behavioral model of treatment that assumes a disorder in how the client regulates emotions and tolerates stress (Lindenboim, Chapman, & Linehan, 2007). The numerous dysfunctional patterns of behavior common in the diagnosis of borderline personality disorder (see Chapter 22), such as self-destructive behavior, the inability to govern impulses, or severe dissociative phenomena, are regarded within the DBT framework as the client's attempts to problem-solve. DBT has also been used successfully in treating the multiproblem adolescent who is at highest risk for suicidal behavior and self-injury (Miller, Rathus, & Linehan, 2007).

DBT is a psychosocial treatment program that focuses on teaching clients four skills:

1. Mindfulness (attention to one's experience)
2. Interpersonal effectiveness
3. Emotional regulation
4. Distress tolerance

This concept of therapy focuses on the continuing balance between the necessity of accepting maladaptive behavior patterns (a cognitive feature) in both an intrapsychic and interactional context while still working to change them (the behavioral feature). Improvements in rates of depression, dissociation, anxiety, and global stress occur with this method (Lindenboim et al., 2007).

DBT is a clearly structured therapy and integrates a wide choice of therapeutic strategies. It is a promising psychosocial intervention for improving interpersonal functioning among severely dysfunctional individuals with borderline personality disorder. For more information, visit the website of the Association for Behavioral and Cognitive Therapies, accessible through the Companion Website for this book.

MEDIALINK Association for Behavioral and Cognitive Therapies

Cultural Aspects of Cognitive and Behavioral Interventions

Cultural considerations involve more than an individual's race or ethnicity. Culture is an envelope that includes, among other characteristics, religion, spirituality, gender, sexual orientation and expression, social status, and age. To be a competent provider of cognitive behavioral interventions, you must, at a minimum, understand these variables, be self-aware, and be comfortable working with those from a culture that differs from your own. The Your Self-Awareness feature will help you sensitize yourself to the forces of a dominant culture. This section will briefly describe how to implement this consciousness within a cognitive behavioral intervention framework. Chapter 9 explores cultural considerations in detail.

The emphasis is on the individual in cognitive behavioral interventions (what the individual thinks, feels, interprets, assigns meanings to, etc.); therefore, it can be the ideal venue to address multiculturalism in treatment. Consider the following clinical example.

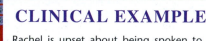

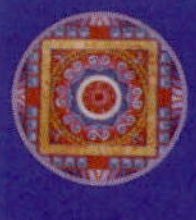

YOUR SELF-AWARENESS
Influence of the Dominant Culture on Cognitive Behavioral Interventions

Can you see differences between a member of a dominant cultural group, yourself, and a client? Listed below are some major cultural characteristics. Think about what behaviors express these characteristics in your culture, and which is the dominant group. Is there a difference? Being a member of the dominant group shapes who you are, just as not being a member of the dominant group has the power to shape your identity. What you think (cognitions) and how you act (behavior) are influenced by your culture. Determine whether there is a difference between you, your client, and the dominant culture on these characteristics in the list. Be alert to the effect these differences will have on your cognitive behavioral interventions.

- Religion
- Spirituality
- Gender
- Ability/disability
- Sexual orientation and expression
- Social status
- Age
- Race
- Ethnicity

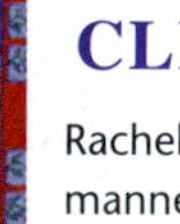

CLINICAL EXAMPLE

Rachel is upset about being spoken to in a harsh and loud manner by her male supervisor at work. She feels demoralized after every interaction with him. She is working with you within a cognitive behavioral framework. Rachel is willing to make several changes in her thinking and behavior in order to feel and function better. She may require cognitive restructuring, mastery imagery, and assertiveness and communication assignments.

You examine each feature of Rachel's situation and Rachel's characteristics to determine if there are any cultural contributions to the overall problem and identify the following factors. Rachel is young, and therefore may not have a lot of experience with supervisors. She has an untreated 20% hearing loss that may prompt people to speak louder to her than normal to ensure she hears all of what is being said. Because Rachel is Egyptian-American, you will want to assess Rachel's comfort level when speaking with males, her expectations when she interacts with males, and whether her heritage could be contributing to the difficulties she is having with her supervisor. When you take cultural considerations into account, you may change the overall structure of her plan (or not), but you would certainly shape your interventions around these issues.

There is a further benefit to blending an understanding of cognitive and behavioral interventions and multiculturalism. Often the emotional reaction to an event is caused more by a client's interpretation of the event than by the event itself (Everly & Lating, 2007). Unlearning maladaptations, learning new skills, practicing them, and ultimately becoming proficient at implementing them is essentially an individual, independent process. It empowers clients to use, rather than deny, their cultural reality. It is also important to know that cognitive behavioral interventions can be easily applied with clients whose primary language is not English because the concepts are concrete (specific thoughts, feelings, events, behaviors), not abstract.

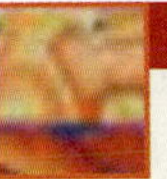

NURSING PROCESS Behavioral Contracting

The effort to change health-related behavior may be facilitated with competent behavioral contracting. A behavioral contract is a behavior modification plan arranged as a specific agreement between the individual and the team of caregivers who identify the behavior and design the plan. To be effective, the behavioral contract must be tailored for the individual client. A comprehensive behavioral assessment is necessary to form such a contract, as is the identification of practical, measurable, and feasible objectives and goals. The components of a behavioral contract for quitting smoking in the form of the nursing process follow.

Assessment

A comprehensive assessment interview is the first step in developing a contract with the goal of behavioral change. The purpose of the interview is to assemble a complete picture of the behavior and what maintains it or keeps it going, so that strategies for changing the behavior have the best chance of success. The interview process identifies problem behavior and divides it into four components, to be explored in turn:

- The *behavioral* component asks what the client is doing.
- The *cognitive* component examines what the client is thinking.
- The *affective* component identifies what the client is feeling.
- The *physiologic* component examines the physical realities of the situation.

What precipitates or precedes this client's problem behavior? Try to identify when it occurs. Does it occur only when the client is anxious, with certain people, or in certain places? What are the consequences of the problem behavior for the client? Assess whether the behavior relaxes or angers the client, or if it endangers the client's life.

Environmental factors (family, economic, and social) may have an effect on the problem behavior and therefore on the success of a behavioral contract. If the client's relatives or friends smoke or if social occasions always take place in smoking areas, the behavioral contract should take this into account.

Assessing the intrapsychic factors influencing the problem behavior can be accomplished during the assessment interview. Determine whether the client:

- Has assertiveness skills
- Experiences stress when asserting needs with other people (such as when stating to friends, "I have trouble staying away from cigarettes when others smoke around me")
- Has fragile, dependent, or abusive relationships

All of these factors would have to be taken into account to develop a viable behavioral contract.

A comprehensive interview also covers any difficulties with depression, irritability, anxiety, psychotic symptomatology (hearing voices, seeing things, or believing in things that are not real), substance or alcohol use/abuse, or addictive/compulsive behavior). Problematic behaviors could also be uncovered during the interview. Such behaviors would include smoking as a type of addictive behavior or refusing to adhere to bed rest instructions as a compulsive and self-destructive behavior.

Current psychosocial variables are essential features to be investigated in a thorough interview and assessment. These variables include present employment, marital and family status, social and romantic functioning, and avocational pursuits. Hobbies are not always constructive. They can be quite destructive, especially if the hobby revolves around a problematic set of behaviors (e.g., drinking beer and smoking while bowling).

If possible, observe the client demonstrating the problem behavior to confirm or disconfirm the client's self-reports. Collateral information on the problem behavior from family, work records, friends, colleagues, and other treatment providers can offer a different perspective. Ultimately, the assessment interview seeks to identify the client's perception of how behavior change might alter his or her life.

Nursing Diagnosis: NANDA

Nursing diagnoses emerge from the comprehensive assessment. The nature and intensity of the problem determines whether it can be addressed immediately or whether other issues are more pressing. Prioritized issues are resolved first. Problems that do not require immediate intervention are monitored and addressed later.

Examples of nursing diagnoses that may derive from a cognitive behavioral assessment in preparation for the development of a behavioral contract include:

- Deficient Knowledge
- Dysfunctional Family Processes
- Interrupted Family Processes
- Impaired Social Interaction
- Hopelessness
- Ineffective Coping
- Ineffective Health Maintenance

MEDIALINK Case Study: Behavior Modification

MediaLink National Association of Cognitive Behavioral Therapists

Outcome Identification: NOC

Knowledge about one's disease process, medication, treatment regimen, or health behaviors would indicate a positive outcome for Deficient Knowledge. Displaying hope would indicate a positive change in Hopelessness. Improved family functioning and coping is evidence of a successful outcome in relation to Dysfunctional Family Processes and Interrupted Family Processes. For a client with the nursing diagnosis of Ineffective Coping, identifying harmful behaviors and what triggers them, then avoiding high-risk situations, constitutes a successful outcome.

In general, outcomes for behavioral change are easily identified. Behaviors are objective criteria by which progress can be tracked. They can be compared to previous behaviors for similarities or differences. If problematic behaviors occur less frequently, they may be considered to have a positive outcome. The following clinical example illustrates positive outcomes with a client experiencing anxiety.

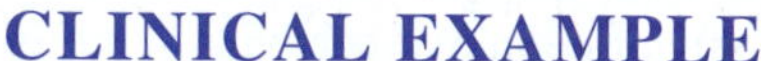

CLINICAL EXAMPLE

Kim, a 29-year-old man with a diagnosis of obsessive–compulsive disorder, obsessively worried that electrical appliances would cause fires. Kim's nurse taught him relaxation exercises and thought-stopping techniques to use when he found himself becoming anxious. The expected outcomes in Kim's situation were: uses coping strategies to reduce anxiety and reports decreased physical manifestations of anxiety. With practice, Kim found that within 1 week he was less anxious when in the kitchen or near other electrical appliances. Although his thoughts about appliance fires and his anxiety had not completely abated, they were definitely more manageable.

Planning and Implementation: NIC

The planning phase of the nursing process with behavioral contracting requires taking into consideration the client's interactions with you during the assessment interview. Consider these components of the mental status exam: appearance; facial expression; motor behavior; cooperativeness; quality of speech, including spontaneity, pace, volume, response time, coherence, and relevance; and goal directedness. Observations of the client's affect (appropriate or inappropriate), mood, lethality, delusions, hallucinations, and orientation to person, place, time, and purpose also contribute information essential to developing a plan of care. The client's immediate, short-term, and long-term memory abilities, along with evidence of executive functioning (such as the ability to carry out multistep activities independently), give direction to how the client thinks. How people think and react and remember is their cognitive style or overall pattern of thought. A cognitive style is the way someone thinks best. For example, some people respond better to audiovisual than to printed material, or they perform tasks more effectively with persistent encouragement versus occasional monitoring. These differences in cognitive style shape several components in your behavioral contract. The website of the National Association of Cognitive Behavioral Therapists has information about cognitive behavioral therapy and its uses in treatment and is accessible through the Companion Website for this text.

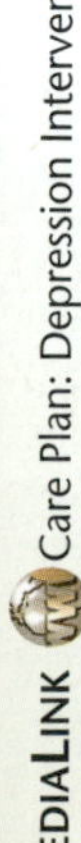

MediaLink Care Plan: Depression Intervention

Forming Practical and Measurable Objectives and Goals

Formulating practical and measurable objectives and goals is the next step in developing a behavioral contract. Objectives are small steps leading to goal attainment; goals represent the overall desired outcomes. Prioritizing the behavioral objectives involves four main features:

1. The goal should contribute directly to the desired result. In other words, how will tracking every cigarette the client smokes, and under what circumstances, help the client stop smoking? (It will sensitize the client and you to factors that contribute to smoking behavior and exactly how much and when the client smokes.)
2. The goal can be objectively monitored. (You know the objective is reached when the client completes the tracking mechanism.)
3. The goal is easily understood by the client and all supportive significant others. (The client knows how to fill out the tracking mechanism and knows why he or she is tracking the behavior.)
4. The goal can be accomplished in the available time. (The client can fill out the form daily for 1 week.)

Behavioral goals should be objectively verifiable as contributing to positive treatment outcome. The change is necessary and relevant, not outlandish (it is relevant to track how often one smokes through daily journaling; it is outlandish to set a goal of never having another craving to smoke). The goal is agreed upon and understood by the client, all significant others, and the treatment team, and is not likely to negatively affect other important aspects of the client's health or psychosocial, interpersonal, or intrapersonal functioning. Remember with whom you are formulating this contract—for example, you will not be asking a lifelong introvert to engage in sensitive self-disclosure in an intense support group.

Negotiating a Behavioral Contract

The basic rules for negotiating a behavioral contract include engaging the client as a colleague, avoiding complex terminology or coercive formats, and making sure the client completely understands, agrees to, and, to the extent possible, feels comfortable with the contract.

Potential problems can have a minimal impact if they are detected early in the process. If you anticipate and address them, the client does not have to experience failure simply because the contract was poorly designed. Possible problems include a lack of understanding, lack of commitment, lack of adequate follow-up monitoring, and lack of a defined format or contingency plan for unforeseen problems. A contract is poorly designed when it is in conflict with important and unchangeable aspects of the client's psychosocial functioning.

YOUR INTERVENTION STRATEGIES
Developing a Behavioral Contract

Step	Purpose	Action	Strategy
1	Comprehensive behavioral assessment	Interview	Interactions
2	Formulating practical and measurable objectives and goals	Prioritizing	Evaluating abilities
3	Negotiating a behavioral contract	Basic rules	Making adjustments
		Potential problems	Evaluating
4	Optimizing the client's ability to adhere to a behavioral contract	Barrier determination ■ Intellectual ■ Emotional ■ Motivational ■ Physiologic	Constructive catalysts ■ Psychotherapy ■ Relaxation Training ■ Biofeedback ■ Family involvement

The Your Intervention Strategies feature above summarizes the behavioral contracting process.

Continuing assessment, regular evaluations, and troubleshooting meetings will determine whether adjustments to the contract are necessary. Designing a contract to which the client can adhere will maximize the chance of success. Contracts can be adjusted in many ways, including formal supports, prioritization of various objectives, and appropriate revisions of goals. Creativity is an essential component in negotiating an effective behavioral contract.

Data on how well the client adheres to the contract can be collected through client self-monitoring, client self-reports at regular meetings, discussions in counseling sessions, and natural or scheduled observations of the client. Further information can be collected from relatives, friends, colleagues, and other treatment providers.

Optimizing the client's ability to adhere to a behavioral contract requires careful determination and assessment of any potential barriers. Check for overall intellectual functioning as well as cognitive style. Emotional perspectives can influence performance and outcome. Does the client manifest depression, irritability, or anxiety that would interfere with contract adherence? It is important to design supports that will address these problems and promote success. Motivation can also play a large part in outcome (Chew, 2007). Was the client poorly motivated to begin with? What was done to address this problem? If design features to address motivation were implemented, check to see how they are working. Is the client demonstrating a decline in motivation? If so, why (psychiatric, social, economic, or medical causation)? Address all underlying causative factors.

Physiology can affect outcome. Is the client experiencing side effects, or is the main effect of a medication (such as mood stabilization for symptoms of mania) bothering the client? If the client perceives this behavioral change as threatening to an established lifestyle and interaction pattern or if the client becomes uncomfortable with the independence or responsibilities expected of him or her following the behavioral change, this could also sabotage adherence.

Provide constructive catalysts, those tools that will enhance the process without interference. Some psychotherapeutic interventions are useful with most clients undergoing stress. These include general stress management, preparing for the likely emotional consequences and adjustment difficulties that changes in health behaviors can cause, the opportunity to ventilate and disclose feelings, and support services. More specialized treatment and techniques include relaxation training and biofeedback (Everly & Lating, 2007). Family involvement is a powerful and useful catalyst for promoting and maintaining behavioral change. Significant others, particularly those with whom the client resides or will reside, are likely to provide important input regarding the level of contract adherence. It is therefore important to involve them as much as appropriate in formulating and implementating the behavioral contract. If the details of the contract do not work for the involved family, they will not work for the client.

FIGURE 31-3 ■ on page 840 is a sample behavioral contract format and gives an overview of how the process of combining medications and behavioral change can be documented. Sections may be expanded or eliminated depending on the targeted behavior and client needs. Imagine a health behavior of your own that could be changed and walk yourself through this contract. If you can develop a plan to change your behavior, you may very well be successful in helping others to change theirs.

Medications

Often, clients feel anxious when faced with making behavioral changes. This anxiety is best handled through supportive and instructive interactions. However, some individuals require physiologic support to prevent their anxiety from reaching panic levels. Anxiolytics, or antianxiety medications, could be administered in sufficient quantities to reduce the problematic affect yet leave the client with enough motivation to learn behavioral techniques for anxiety management where appropriate. Dosing anxiolytics to the extent that anxiety is completely eliminated is considered countertherapeutic. Anxiety at low to moderate levels has been found in many circumstances to enhance learning and motivation.

Sample Behavioral Contract

Client Name ______________________________ Date ______________

Problem Behavior: ______________________________

Problem Behavior Components

Behavioral	Affective
Cognitive	Physiological

Interview Findings

Depression	Anxiety	Substance or Alcohol Use/Abuse
Irritability	Psychotic Symptomatology	Addictive/Compulsive Behavior

Psychosocial Variables

Present Employment	Social/Romantic Functioning	Typical Daily Routines
Marital/Family Status	Avocational Pursuits	Eating/Sleeping/Exercise Habits
The Client's Expectations of How This Behavior Change Might Alter Any of the Above		

Collateral Information ______________________________

____

Cognitive Style ______________________________

____

Which of the following apply for this contract?

- ☐ Psychotherapy for any current psychological problems
- ☐ Relaxation training/biofeedback
- ☐ General stress management
- ☐ Preparation for likely emotional consequences and adjustment difficulties
- ☐ The opportunity to ventilate and disclose feelings
- ☐ Support

Contract Objectives and Goals

This goal is agreed upon and understood by the client, all significant others, and the treatment team.

Signature ______________________________

Signature ______________________________

Signature ______________________________

Signature ______________________________

FIGURE 31-3 ■ Sample behavioral contract.

Evaluation

Evaluating client abilities and strengths, particularly with regard to learning and making changes, will help in the design of the contract. Discover what other situations requiring behavioral change the client has mastered and what specific personal or social strengths the client employed in implementing the change. Evaluate the client's weaknesses with regard to learning and making changes as well. What has the client attempted to change without success? Try to ascertain the specific factors that interfered with the success of that goal.

Formulated objectives and goals should draw on the client's strengths and prior patterns of successful change. What the client is asked to do should mirror as closely as possible what the client has previously done successfully. The best predictor of future behavior is past behavior.

For a contract to lead to a successful outcome, it must be carefully crafted. Frame the components of a behavioral contract in the success (e.g., will maintain abstinence) rather than failure (e.g., will not relapse into use) mode.

CASE MANAGEMENT

It is important to focus on maintaining the routines and schedules of cognitive behavioral interventions once a plan of care has been established. Homework assignments and practicing using more competent responses will ensure that the client retains the skills developed in therapy. The case manager can be helpful in sustaining that structure. The variety of interventions, such as group or individual therapy, behavior modification, and self-study, can all be promoted and supported through case management.

COMMUNITY-BASED CARE AND HOME CARE

Each of the problems addressed with cognitive behavioral interventions benefits from maintaining those interventions in the client's natural setting. Counseling, psychotherapy, and other treatments discussed in this chapter are frequently conducted in the community. The behavioral contract can be designed to address inpatient issues and community living and to enhance the transition from inpatient treatment to an outpatient setting. Additional supports can be built into the contract to ensure the client's success after the transition. These interventions in the community maximize both the quality of life and management of symptoms.

Family psychoeducation can be an integral feature of community-based care and home care. Teaching about symptoms and how to address them with the planned interventions is supportive and reassuring. Involving significant others increases the likelihood that the plan of care is implemented and that frustrations and misunderstandings are minimized.

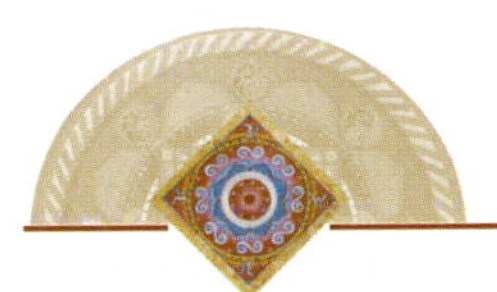

EXPLORE MEDIALINK

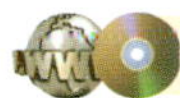

www.prenhall.com/kneisl

For NCLEX-RN® review questions, case studies, and other resources for this chapter see the Pearson Health MediaLink CD-ROM that accompanies this book and the Companion Website at www.prenhall.com/kneisl.

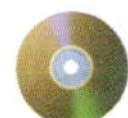

CD-ROM
Audio Glossary
NCLEX-RN® Review Questions

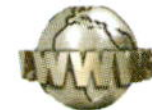

Companion Website
Audio Glossary
NCLEX-RN® Review Questions
Critical Thinking Exercise
- *Modifying Unhealthy Behavior*

Case Study
- *Behavior Modification*

Care Plan
- *Depression Intervention*

MediaLinks
MediaLink Application
- *The Illness and Recovery Management Program*

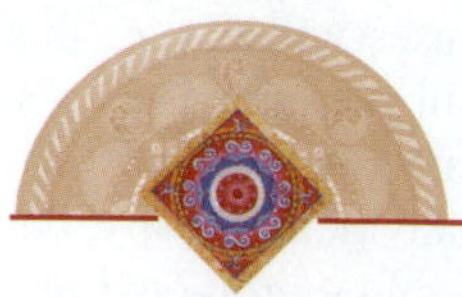

NCLEX-RN® REVIEW QUESTIONS

1. The concepts that are basic to understanding cognitive therapy include (select all that apply):
1. Desensitization.
2. Attribution.
3. Self-efficacy.
4. Modeling.
5. Conditioning.

2. The goal of cognitive therapy is to:
1. Alter a client's feelings.
2. Change maladaptive thoughts.
3. Educate the client about the need for medication to treat maladaptive thoughts.
4. Replace all negative thoughts with positive ones.

3. Which of the following statements is an example of negative cognitions?
1. "If I study for the exam, I think I can be successful."
2. "What's the point of studying? I am never going to graduate."
3. "I've tried to deal with this issue by ignoring it. I think I need to be more direct in my efforts."
4. "Look at me, I'm fat. I think it's time to start exercising."

4. An outcome of operant conditioning is:
1. Learning new and acceptable behaviors through positive thinking.
2. Reinforcing positive behaviors that result in desired learning outcomes.
3. Assigning a meaning to a set of circumstances.
4. Receiving rewards for imitating the behaviors of other individuals.

5. A client with a 30-year history of smoking two packs per day asks the nurse for help with smoking cessation. Which of the following is an appropriate client-related goal?
1. Client will cease all smoking within 7 days.
2. Nurse will educate client on the health risks associated with long-term smoking.
3. Client will identify three feelings associated with smoking.
4. By the end of the shift, nurse will talk with client regarding the desire to quit smoking.

6. A nursing student tells the nursing instructor, "I am such a failure. My parents were right. I will never amount to anything." The best response from the instructor is:
1. To assure the student that this is not true; that every human life has purpose and meaning.
2. To say nothing, but encourage the student to express his or her feelings.
3. To tell the student that parents are often correct in their judgments.
4. To assist the student in identifying recent behaviors or activities that reflect the student's success.

7. Which of the following can result in the negative outcome of a behavioral contract?
1. Have the members of the treatment team develop the contract for the client.
2. Use terminology the client understands.
3. Ensure adequate follow-up monitoring of the client.
4. Monitor the client for any adverse effects of medication.

8. A client with an impulse control disorder is becoming frustrated and angered by an inability to control and stop the impulsive behaviors. Which of the following actions by the nurse will assist the client in controlling impulsive behaviors?
1. Tell the client the behavior is unacceptable and must not happen again.
2. Provide the client with a controlled environment to perform the impulsive behaviors.
3. Assist the client to identify feelings that trigger the impulsive behaviors.
4. Request that the prescriber order an antianxiety medication to control the behaviors.

9. Which of the following statements made by the nurse on a mental health unit is reason for concern?
1. "It is evident that how we were raised directly influences our behaviors and thoughts."
2. "Why are we wasting our time with these people? They are never going to get any better."
3. "If I can help the client identify what triggers the behavior, I can help the client learn how to cope with it."
4. "I can't believe I thought the client was a hopeless case. Her behavioral improvements have opened my eyes."

10. The nurse and the client are developing a care plan that includes mastery imagery. The nurse explains that this technique enables the client to:
1. Behave in a positive manner to enhance self-confidence.
2. Identify the thoughts at the beginning of maladaptive behaviors and recognize the consequences of the actions.
3. Think about being in control throughout a particular situation.
4. Take personal responsibility for maintaining health-damaging thought habits and irrational beliefs.

See Appendix C for answers.

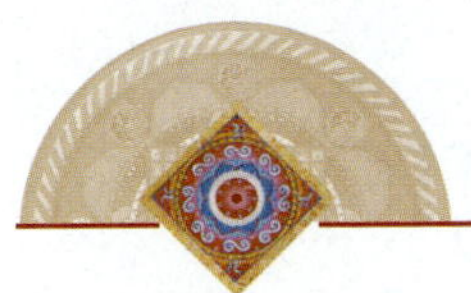

REFERENCES

Beck, A. T. (1976). *Cognitive therapy and the emotional disorders*. New York: International Universities Press.

Beck, A. T., Freeman, A., & Associates. (1990). *Cognitive therapy of personality disorders*. New York: Guilford Press.

Chew, C. E. (2007). The effects of dialectical behavioral therapy on moderately depressed adults. *Dissertation Abstracts International: Section B: The Sciences and Engineering, 67*(8-B), 4701.

Dunbar-Jacob, J. (2007). Models for changing patient behavior. *American Journal of Nursing, 107*(Suppl. 6), 20–25.

Ellis, A. (1997). Albert Ellis on rational emotive behavior therapy. *American Journal of Psychotherapy, 51*, 309–316.

Ellis, A., & Harper, R. (1975). *A new guide to rational living*. Chatworth, CA: Wilshire Book Co.

Everly, G. S., Jr., & Lating, J. M. (2007). Psychotherapy: A cognitive perspective. In A. Monat, R. S. Lazarus, & G. Reevy (Eds.), *The Praeger handbook on stress and coping* (Vol. 2, pp. 497–508). Westport, CT: Praeger Publishers/Greenwood Publishing Group.

Ford, L. (2007). *Human relations: A game plan for improving personal adjustment* (4th ed.). Upper Saddle River, NJ: Pearson Prentice Hall.

Havermans, R., Nicolson, N. A., & deVries, M. W. (2007). Daily hassles, uplifts, and time use in individuals with bipolar disorder in remission. *Journal of Nervous & Mental Disease, 195*(9), 745–751.

Heldt, E., Blaya, C., Kipper, L., Salum, G. A., Otto, M. W., & Manfro, G. G. (2007). Defense mechanisms after brief cognitive-behavior group therapy for panic disorder: One-year follow-up. *Journal of Nervous and Mental Disease, 195*(6), 540–543.

Lindenboim, N., Chapman, A. L., & Linehan, M. M. (2007). Borderline personality disorder. In N. Kazantzis & L. L'Abate (Eds.), *Handbook of homework assignments in psychotherapy: Research, practice, prevention* (pp. 227–245). New York: Springer Science + Business Media.

Linehan, M. M., Schmidt III, H., Dimeff, L. A., Craft, J. C., Kanter, J., & Comtois, K. A. (1999). Dialectical behavior therapy for patients with borderline personality disorder and drug-dependence. *American Journal on Addictions, 8*, 279–292.

Miller, A. L., Rathus, J. H., & Linehan, M. M. (2007). *Dialectical behavior therapy with suicidal adolescents*. New York: Guilford Press.

Nsimba, S. E. D. (2007). Outpatient treatment programs: A review article on substances of abuse outpatients treatment outcomes in the United States. *Addictive Disorders & Their Treatment, 6*(3), 91–99.

Reilly-Harrington, N. A., Deckersbach, T., Knauz, R., Wu, Y., Tran, T., Eidelman, P., et al. (2007). Cognitive behavioral therapy for rapid-cycling bipolar disorder: A pilot study. *Journal of Psychiatric Practice, 13*(5), 291–297.

Skinner, B. F. (1974). *About behaviorism*. New York: Knopf.

Skinner, B. F. (1989). The origins of cognitive thought. *American Psychologist, 44*, 12–18.

Swales, M. A., & Heard, H. L. (2007). The therapy relationship in dialectical behaviour therapy. In P. Gilbert & R. L. Leahy (Eds.), *The therapeutic relationship in the cognitive behavioral psychotherapies* (pp. 185–204). New York: Routledge/Taylor & Francis Group.

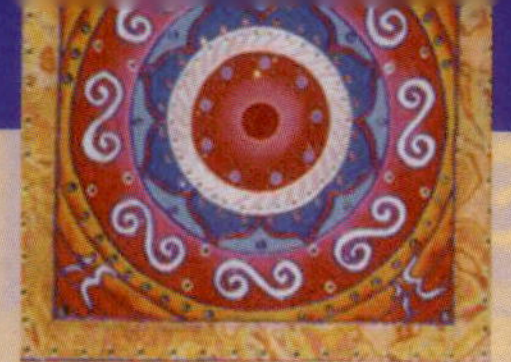

CHAPTER

32

Psychopharmacologic Nursing Interventions

EILEEN TRIGOBOFF

KEY TERMS

akathisia *854*
anticholinergic side effects *851*
extrapyramidal side effects (EPSEs) *853*
neuroleptic malignant syndrome *858*
parkinsonian syndrome *854*
polypharmacy *866*
second-generation antipsychotics (SGAs) *851*
tardive dyskinesia (TD) *855*

LEARNING OUTCOMES

After completing this chapter, you will be able to:

1. Describe how nurses in psychiatric–mental health settings assess the effectiveness of medications.
2. Assess for extrapyramidal side effects and explain them to clients and their families.
3. Recognize the positive and negative effects of psychiatric medications on behavior.
4. Discuss three factors that affect the extent to which clients adhere to prescribed medication treatment regimens.
5. Delineate various aspects of taking these medications for an indefinite period of time.
6. Formulate nursing interventions to address the major side effects associated with psychotropic medications.

CRITICAL THINKING CHALLENGE

Frank is a 42-year-old married man who has had repeated episodes of depression. His symptoms have responded well to SSRI antidepressants in the past. He has been taking fluoxetine (Prozac) as ordered and has experienced a substantial improvement in his symptoms. Frank and his wife are here to talk with you about a sexual problem they are having. After attempting to deal with it on their own, unsuccessfully, they finally decided to speak with you about it. Frank has had a substantial delay in ejaculation and sometimes he is not able to have an orgasm. Both he and his wife are concerned that the problem indicates he is not enjoying sexual activity as he should, one of the symptoms of depression he had in the past. Another possible explanation the couple is concerned about, if he is not depressed, is that Frank may be losing interest in his wife as he recovers from depression. Frank denies losing interest, but they have been through so much with his illness that they feel unsure of many previously held convictions.

1. How would you explain the experiences Frank is having?
2. What key elements should be included in a program designed to address Frank's side effects?

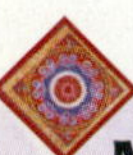

MEDIALINK 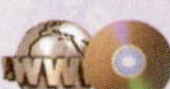 www.prenhall.com/kneisl

Go to the Pearson Health MediaLink CD-ROM and the Companion Website at www.prenhall.com/kneisl for interactive resources for this chapter.

Unlike medications for medical illnesses, psychiatric medications are stigmatizing. Telling a man with diabetes that he must take insulin for the foreseeable future, or possibly suffer unmanageable and life-threatening symptoms, is not equal (yet) in our society to telling a man with bipolar disorder that he must take psychiatric medications for the same purpose. Treating mental illness with psychiatric medications is still relatively new.

It is also more difficult for people to understand the similarities between physical problems and psychological problems. For example, both physical and psychological problems may require medications to help healing, prevent serious problems, and save lives. Because clients can benefit greatly from the neuroprotective effects of psychopharmacologic agents and from the reduced disruption and increased stability that they bring to clients' lives, remember to add advocacy to reduce stigma to your repertoire of nursing interventions related to psychiatric medications.

The safe and effective management of medications by nurses, clients, and family members is the focus of this chapter. We discuss nursing interventions to promote client and family coping with medication side effects or adverse effects, with drug interactions, and with the psychosocial impact of medications. We also focus on specific psychoeducational activities that demonstrate how you can partner with clients and their families in meeting the goal of medication management. An important example of partnering is in the following Evidence-Based Practice feature.

Medication management is a therapeutic challenge that requires you to marshal complex nursing knowledge and resources within a holistic framework. Your goal is to design psychopharmacologic nursing interventions that promote recovery and wellness. Well-designed psychopharmacologic nursing interventions require your understanding of the science of pharmacology, which is discussed in Chapter 7∞. The science of psychopharmacology—medication categories, how they work, safe dosage ranges, and so on—will not be repeated here; therefore, be sure to review Chapter 7∞ before continuing.

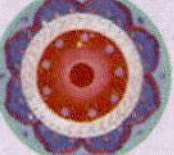

EVIDENCE-BASED PRACTICE

MEDICATION PSYCHOEDUCATION GROUPS

You are conducting an outpatient group consisting of seven people who are all in treatment for depression. This is a psychoeducational group with the goal of educating clients about symptoms of depression, available treatments, and prevention or reduction of relapse.

The group discovers that everyone has a different viewpoint about medications for their depressive symptoms. You are asked about the latest information on these treatments as well as your clinical experience with antidepressants and psychotherapy. You report that research indicates that a combination of talk therapies and antidepressants works well in treating the symptoms of major depression. Other group members wonder about criticisms they've heard about some studies. The popular media occasionally report that antidepressants are no better than placebo treatment and that results indicating otherwise are illusory.

The discussion centers around the most effective treatments and the research that drives competent practice. Overall, the literature shows that antidepressant response rates are approximately 50%, while placebo response rates hover at around 30%. It has been suggested that clinician bias is the cause of the discrepancy, implying that antidepressants are really no more effective than a placebo. The clients who wondered whether their therapists could slant the interpretation of treatment outcomes discuss how the client self-ratings might resolve that problem. Research has shown, however, that the criticism that client self-ratings are more valid than clinician outcome ratings is not supported in any way.

Another aspect of depression care discussed in the popular press is the assertion that psychotherapy could be superior to drugs in treating depression. You have seen journal articles regarding this very issue and share with the group your familiarity with meta-analyses (studies that analyze the analyses of several studies) of studies with severely depressed individuals. It has not been supported that psychotherapy, while necessary in the treatment of depression and very effective as a stand-alone treatment, is superior to psychopharmacology in treatment efficacy.

Psychoeducational groups provide a very important function beyond giving facts about mental illness and treatment. Examining and discussing what the layman hears and reads allows for correction of misconceptions and support for the scientific basis of care. Definitive statements about the role of treatments for depression can be misleading and thereby become a public health concern. If a public figure or a media outlet states that treating depression is wrong for nonscientific reasons (religion, personal opinion, fear, superstition, politics, or economics), clients may assume the public figure is correct and refuse treatment. Keeping current with research and active in critical thinking skills benefits your clients. Findings from antidepressant research, such as the following references, are usually valid, meaning that the treatment of depression is often specifically useful.

Engel, B. (2007). Eagle soaring: The power of the resilient self. *Journal of Psychosocial Nursing and Mental Health Services, 45*(2), 44–48, 49–51.

Ferentz, K. S. (2007). A guide to switching antidepressant therapy. *Patient Care, 41*(1), 16–21.

CRITICAL THINKING APPLICATION

1. Is failing to vehemently deny the possibility of therapist bias a disservice to your group members? Why or why not?
2. Should you refer group members directly to the research articles with which you are familiar? Why or why not?

THE NURSING ROLE IN PSYCHOPHARMACOLOGY

Because psychopharmacology is an integral and important part of a client's life for years, and perhaps a lifetime, psychiatric–mental health nurses must know as much about the many ways that psychiatric medications affect a client as they do about the characteristics of a client's mental disorder. Psychopharmacologic medications affect the client's behavior, body, and thought processes.

Psychopharmacologic treatment is not the only answer. It is combined with various psychologic and social therapies to achieve the goal of promoting hope and recovery from a mental illness. Many clients can manage some symptoms by activating certain thought processes (cognitive therapy), changing beliefs or incorporating different beliefs (which contribute to the effectiveness of cognitive therapy), and changing or activating specific behaviors (behavioral therapy). Certainly, when psychiatric symptoms are severe or hospitalization is required, medication management is a must.

Theorists and clinicians hold a variety of attitudes, beliefs, and philosophies about psychiatric medications. Medications may be used as an adjunct to the psychotherapeutic process to decrease overwhelming arousal (feelings of being overwhelmed by matters raised in psychotherapy), to improve judgment that has been impaired by psychosis, to improve information processing, to reduce anergia (lack of energy), and to improve thinking and motivation. Clients and their family members also hold specific attitudes and beliefs about psychiatric medications. These are discussed in Chapter 7∞.

There are a variety of ways to refer to psychiatric medications. The terms *neuroleptic* and *psychotropic* both describe medications that address psychiatric symptoms. They can be, and often are, used interchangeably and as a general term to describe any medication for a psychiatric diagnosis. For example, an antidepressant could also be called a neuroleptic or a psychotropic. Clients and family members often report having taken "a psychotropic for years." This statement tells you that psychiatric symptoms were being addressed. It does not tell you the category or categories of medication prescribed.

When added to a medication regimen, talk therapies (psychotherapy) are used to treat demoralization and lethality in the interim period before medication has a chance to take effect. Talk therapies can improve medication adherence, decrease irrational thinking, address problems in relationships, modify the triggers that cause a recurrence of symptoms, and treat residual symptoms. With any psychiatric problem, relapse is an issue. Psychotherapy reduces the risk of relapse that persists after pharmacotherapy is discontinued (Knight, Sanchez, Sherritt, Bresnahan, & Fromson, 2007).

The ongoing assessment of a psychiatric client includes assessing how well the medications are helping the client to cope with psychiatric symptoms. An additional observation, one that is inevitable, is whether the psychiatric medication is causing a side effect or an adverse effect. Managing side effects behaviorally and pharmacologically is crucial to our clients' health and to their quality of life. Effective medication management is a critical process that depends upon your understanding of the content in this chapter as well as the content in Chapter 7∞. Remember to review the American Nurses Association's (ANA) Guidelines on Psychopharmacology (given in Box 7-2 on page 113) to evaluate how well you carry out your responsibilities in relationship to psychopharmacology.

The nursing functions described in the next three sections—assessing clients, administering medications, and educating clients and families—are general and can be applied to the care of any client receiving a psychiatric medication. Specific nursing functions are described in the drug category sections later in this chapter.

WHY I BECAME A PSYCHIATRIC–MENTAL HEALTH NURSE

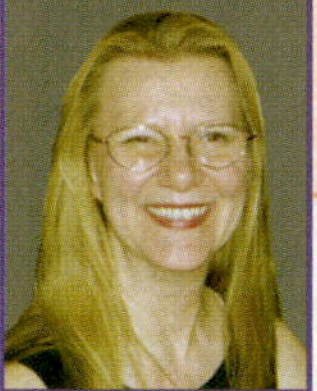

Eileen Trigoboff
Textbook Author

What attracted me to psychiatric–mental health nursing was recognizing the powerful link between the emotional and physiological aspects of my clients. I began my nursing career as a pediatric ICU nurse, talking to parents and siblings about injuries, illnesses, surgery, and recovery. The most demanding interactions were with parents who had abused their children so severely they ended up in the ICU. My coworkers pointed out to me that when I spoke to these parents—not avoiding them, not judging them, and not scolding—I was performing the therapeutic role of a psychiatric nurse.

The idea of psychiatric nursing interested me so much that I enrolled in a graduate program in psychiatric nursing; met some wonderful faculty who shared, taught, mentored (one of them is my coauthor on this book); became a Clinical Nurse Specialist in Psychiatry; then got my doctorate in psychiatric nursing and have never looked back. Working in this field has been wonderfully fulfilling and enriching.

Assessing Clients

Our responsibilities as nurses to clients receiving psychotropic medications are very different from our responsibilities to clients in nonpsychiatric settings. A nurse working with clients having cardiac difficulties, for example, may have clear physiologic indicators for the administration of drugs such as isosorbide dinitrate (Iso-Bid) or nitroglycerin (Nitroglyn), but psychiatric nurses rarely have comparable consistent complexes of symptoms on which to base clinical judgments.

In psychiatric work, nurses must often observe client behaviors closely to be aware of the sometimes subtle nature of the presenting symptom. Pacing, mild diaphoresis, slight increases in blood pressure or pulse, heightened muscle tone, and hypervigilance may indicate escalating anxiety, but they may also point to other problems such as caffeine toxicity, excessive use of tobacco, or side effects of psychopharmacologic agents. Accurate nursing assessment of client behavior is crucial in order to give medications effectively and appropriately. Psychiatric nurses must also be attuned to the circumstances of adjunct pharmacotherapy (taking different medications at the same time). This clinical example demonstrates how symptoms can become unmanageable for a client when adjunctive therapy is discontinued.

CLINICAL EXAMPLE

Evan, a 33-year-old with a diagnosis of bipolar disorder, decided to stop taking his risperidone (Risperdal) and lamotrigine (Lamictal) as mood stabilizers because he did not like the way they made him feel—emotionally stunted and less creative. Evan has difficulty when his manic symptoms are reduced as a result of the main effect of the medication. As he put it, "I miss feeling on top of the world."

Within 2 weeks of stopping the medication, he was unable to sleep and berated his neighbors in the middle of the night for their choice of house siding. Although he liked his job at the local playhouse and knew he would likely earn more money in the near future, he refused to go to work because "they just don't understand my potential as an actor, dancer, and director." He was fired because of poor attendance and belligerence toward other workers. His spiraling symptoms and the loss of a structured schedule exacerbated his deterioration and Evan relapsed, requiring hospitalization.

Assessment is not a static process. It takes shape over time and depends upon activating a wide range of nursing knowledge. A sleepy, isolated client with schizophrenia may be experiencing paranoid ideation, may have negative symptoms of the illness, may be experiencing sedating side effects of the antipsychotic medication, or may be depressed as well as schizophrenic. The behaviors may be similar, but they come from a wide array of vastly different sources. Your assessment of this client and your clinical judgment will direct the nursing care. Whether you decide to administer a PRN (given when needed) antipsychotic, hold the next dose of antipsychotic, develop a treatment plan that includes motivational aspects, or discuss the possibility of depression with the other treatment team members depends on your ongoing assessment of this client.

Administering Medications

Administering psychiatric medications demands more than the six rights: the right medication, the right dose, the right route, the right time, to the right client, with the right technology. These aspects of medication administration are confounded by the psychiatric illness. Knowing the side effects of the medication in addition to the interactive effects with other psychiatric and medical–surgical medications is crucial in psychiatric–mental health nursing.

Administering the right medication in a psychiatric setting depends on your assessment skills. The right medication may be one of a number of choices. A medication may be ordered by mouth (PO) for routine administration, but the client may refuse it. Assessment skills come into play here as well; you must determine whether the client needs a liquid, a pill, a quick-dissolving formulation, or a PRN injection.

Making sure you are administering medications to the right client, a client identification issue, is different than it is in medical–surgical settings. In psychiatric settings, clients usually do not wear wristbands. Clients may be confused or have psychiatric symptoms that encourage them to spontaneously assume the identity of another client for any number of reasons, including an effort to please the staff.

Documenting the effect of medications is an important nursing responsibility. Follow-up documentation on a medication that was given as a PRN will simplify treatment decisions for the client. Did the PRN work? How did you determine the value of the PRN's effect? What behavioral indicators are you using in your evaluation of a medication's effectiveness?

Educating Clients and Families

MEDIALINK Client Education on Medications

Nursing responsibilities include educating clients about their medications as well as educating their family members. The Your Intervention Strategies feature includes guidelines for medication teaching strategies and reminders of general information to include for all clients, no matter the category of psychiatric medication.

Information on client education is also available from a variety of sites. For example, PsychNet-UK and the University of Iowa Virtual Hospital websites offer accessible and relevant information on various psychopharmacologic topics and can be accessed through the Companion Website for this text.

Addressing Individual Differences

Individual differences must be addressed in the course of the teaching–learning process. The Partnering with Clients and Families feature on page 848 helps you to identify which learning strategies have proved successful for the client in the past and suggests new ones to try.

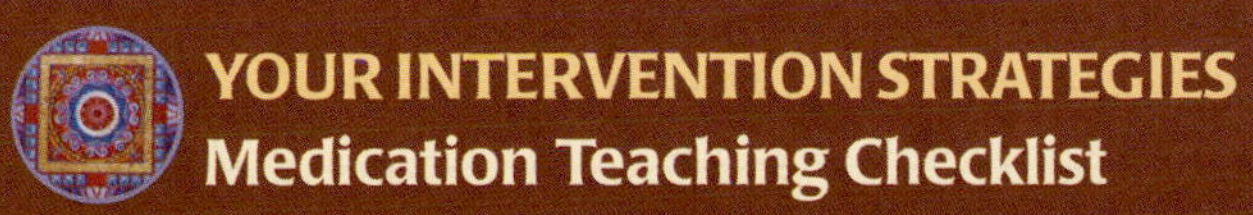

YOUR INTERVENTION STRATEGIES
Medication Teaching Checklist

Be sure to teach clients and families about the following regardless of the category of medication the client is taking. Do not hesitate to repeat instructions. Repetition is a useful tool in psychoeducation.

- Keeping all medications and information about them together in one dry, cool, place (not the bathroom or the kitchen).
- When to report side effects.
- How to report side effects.
- Strategies and tools for managing side effects.
- Strategies and tools for managing residual symptoms.
- The impact of mental illness and psychiatric medications on life goals.
- Reinforce learning by providing an opportunity at some point for the client to teach others about medications.

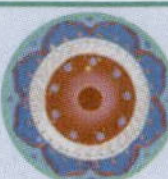

PARTNERING WITH CLIENTS AND FAMILIES

STRATEGIES AND METHODS FOR TEACHING ABOUT MEDICATIONS

Before you begin teaching clients and their family members about medications, identify which learning methods have already proven successful for them:

- **Repetition:** Rehearsing or practicing the skill repeatedly can place it in several areas in the memory, thereby increasing the chances of retrieval.
- **Primacy:** Some learners more easily retrieve the *first* item learned or the first skill performed.
- **Recency:** Some learners more easily retrieve the *last* item learned or the last skill performed.
- **Association:** Learning by hinging one memory to another.
- **Coding:** Shaping a thought in one's memory in a particular way to facilitate retrieval for skill performance.
- **Background information and explanation:** Describing a skill by giving specific details can assist many to learn the skill and perform it reliably. Incorporating the client's value system into this method is most effective.
- **Reminder boxes:** Physical prompts are helpful for clients who need concrete environmental hints.
- **Lists, notebooks:** Making lists and keeping track of tasks and events in a notebook can be a powerful tool for clients with executive functioning deficits.
- **Videos:** Visual learners can make use of a multimedia presentation of materials.
- **Positive transfer:** If the client learned to do task A well, and it is similar enough to task B, then task B can be accomplished through transferring that learned behavior.
- **Positive reinforcement:** Either obtaining something desirable or avoiding something unpleasant

An issue of great concern to many nurses is the planning of teaching–learning experiences for severely and persistently mentally ill clients. Although this population has learning needs concerning care and treatment, teaching is often difficult, depending on the severity and chronicity of the illness. See Box 32-1 for common learning problems associated with specific psychiatric diagnoses.

Recidivism, the tendency to relapse into a previous mode of behavior requiring readmission to a treatment program, can be linked to a psychiatric client's psychoeducation. Helping a client change health-related behavior requires a thoughtful, comprehensive approach. Relevant interventions designed to match the client's learning style can reduce recidivism and promote healthier behavior. Contracting with a client for behavioral change can also help to avoid relapse. See "Designing a Behavioral Contract" in Chapter 31 on page 839.

Another concern for nurses working with psychiatric clients is the need to assess the client's learning capacity at different points in the chronology of the disorder. For example, when clients are first admitted to an inpatient unit, they may be too disorganized and symptomatic to focus on specific learning tasks. Depressed clients may have severe psychomotor retardation because of hormonal shifts and dysfunctional neurotransmission and may be unable to learn. Given appropriate treatment and care, however, a client's psychobiologic disequilibrium may be corrected, making learning possible.

Perceiving that a client is ready to learn—that is, that the client's cognitive abilities are intact—does not necessarily

Box 32-1 Common Interferences to Learning with Specific Psychiatric Diagnoses

Psychoses

- Cognitive difficulties secondary to thought disorder
- Motivational problems secondary to negative symptoms
- Unpleasant side effects from medication
- Persistence of positive symptoms (delusions) mitigating against adherence

Mood Disorders

- Persistent dysphoria leads to amotivation
- Self-destructiveness–lethality
- Manic irresponsibility as a result of impulsivity, thoughtlessness, and cognitive symptoms
- Loss of manic or hypomanic egosyntonic excitement (energy around ideas in harmony with an ideal self-image)
- Unpleasant side effects from medications

Anxiety Disorders

- Addiction to antianxiety medication
- Quick action of many antianxiety agents leads to positive reinforcement of increasing dosages
- Lack of consistent provider knowledge of and expertise in application of effective nonmedication treatment strategies for anxiety problems

Personality Disorders

- Addictive or abusive use of medications
- Sensation seeking
- Manipulation

mean that learning will occur. Many nurses conduct medication groups on an acute psychiatric unit to not only address the importance of assessing cognitive abilities but also to explore affective and social issues that may contribute to effective learning experiences. Once you have considered the client's readiness, knowledge, background, environment, beliefs, preferences, and lifestyle, involving the client and significant others in the design and implementation of the medication treatment plan will help ensure the client's active collaboration in his or her care.

In many ways, psychiatric clients are no different from other learners. When presented with material that has clear benefits for them, they are more likely to be interested in the learning process.

Evaluating the Teaching–Learning Process

An evaluation of teaching efforts and the client's knowledge of the information taught is essential to completing the teaching–learning process. You will not be able to evaluate a client's understanding of information unless, at minimum, the client verbally reiterates information or performs a return demonstration of the skill. A change in behavior over time is a powerful indication that learning has taken place.

If you desire a more extensive evaluation you may consider using a "pretest/posttest" format. You can develop a written test to cover the content of the teaching and have the client complete the test before you begin teaching (a pretest). This provides a written measure of the client's learning needs and level of knowledge. After you implement and complete the teaching plan, the client completes the same examination (a posttest). Comparison of the pretest and posttest results yields a documented measure of how much learning has occurred as a result of your teaching intervention.

Ethical Concerns

Several ethical issues are: Should children and adolescents take psychiatric medications? Do conflicts of interest influence the prescribing of psychiatric medications? Should clients be informed of the risks of taking psychiatric medications and the alternatives to medication? These issues, as well as questions of impaired decision-making, are discussed here. Issues such as limiting individual freedom through chemical controls and an individual's right to refuse treatment are discussed in the ethics and legal sections of Chapter 13∞.

Children and Adolescents

The question of whether children and adolescents are helped or harmed by psychiatric medications continues to arouse concerns, which are often accompanied by intense feelings. Some of the ethical issues are: Should young persons be treated with psychopharmacologic agents because they prevent symptoms from overwhelming and traumatizing the child or adolescent? Or, should children and adolescents not be given psychopharmacologic agents because of their unknown long-term effects? Current clinical practice supports treating symptoms with the minimal effective amount of medication.

Elders

Medication planning for elders is different than for other age groups. Specifically, elders—because of aged organs, injuries, and comorbidities—metabolize medications differently than younger clients. Medications pose several challenges to the physiological functioning of older clients. For example, medications often:

- Are metabolized at a somewhat slower rate
- Take longer to reach therapeutic levels
- May interact with other medications
- May cause side effects or adverse effects at lower doses than for other age groups
- Take longer to clear the system

When older clients begin a regimen of psychotropic medications, the strategy often followed is based on the principle "Start low; go slow." Frequent assessment of the effect of the medication on the targeted symptoms is important. Your vital role is to observe elders to assess and monitor their physiologic functioning along with the effectiveness of the medication.

Pharmaceutical Advertising

The potential impact of advertising in the popular media by the pharmaceutical industry has engendered debate. (This issue is central to the discussion in the Evidence-Based Practice feature presented on page 845.) We are exposed to innumerable print, radio, and television commercials for over-the-counter and prescription agents to address any number of physical and psychological ailments. Two major ethical concerns are:

1. Individuals who are unable to think critically because of psychiatric symptoms could make decisions based on the advertisement.
2. Prescribers, influenced by the media or by those who have a financial interest in the outcome (such as a pharmaceutical representative, for example) may prescribe a medication without considering all the options or accessing the available research evidence.

Both concerns can be minimized with proper action.

When clients approach you with questions about a medication they heard about on the Internet or saw on television, you can give fair and balanced information. In order to do so, your knowledge about available pharmaceuticals must be thorough and complete. Keep up-to-date and absorb relevant information from reliable sources. Employ your critical thinking skills to determine if you have adequate information to satisfactorily address the issue.

Conflicts of Interest

Professionals are required to monitor their relationships for conflict of interest (COI). COI is defined as a situation in which there is an opportunity for bias not in the client's best interests. These are usually situations in which your personal interests, such as a hobby or an investment, can be advanced by what you decide to do professionally. It would be considered a COI if a prescriber who owns stock in a pharmaceutical

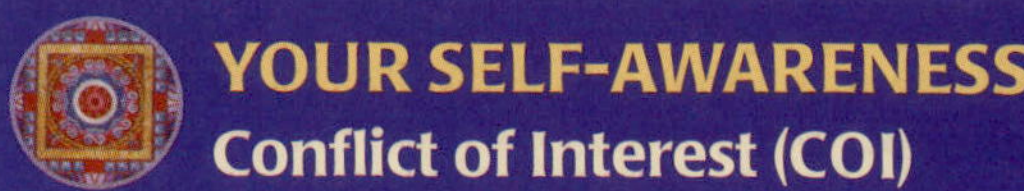

YOUR SELF-AWARENESS
Conflict of Interest (COI)

Does COI affect your objectivity? Review the following and think about what impact each has, if any, on your clinical judgment.

- Your professional and facility policies on ethics
- Your financial interests (monetary or percentage interests in products or sponsors), board memberships, or relationships that may make conflicting demands
- How your financial interest in a product could influence your professional judgment
- Professional, government, and agency or facility policies on the financial amount or percentage of interest you can have in a product, business, or stock
- Whether your loyalties could be divided

Once you have carefully considered these points, expunge the opportunities for bias.

company recommends that company's medication to the exclusion of similar medications manufactured by other pharmaceutical companies. COI is especially worrisome in psychiatry, where clients with interactional and interpersonal difficulties and impaired decision-making abilities may be swayed by subtle influences such as trademarks and branded items. Does COI affect the objectivity of your interactions? See the Your Self-Awareness feature above for information on tracking COI.

Right to Refuse Medications

Another ethical issue involves our duty to inform the client of the risks of, and alternatives to, the proposed treatment, and to accept the client's decision to authorize or refuse that treatment. Clients with psychiatric disorders cannot be assumed to lack capacity. A number of studies have demonstrated that many mentally disordered clients can make unimpaired decisions (Morris, Naimark, & Haroun, 2005). Even a diagnosis of dementia does not inevitably mean that clients do not retain some abilities to decide for themselves. Impairment in decision-making capacity does not equal legal incompetence to make a decision. When the deficit makes it unlikely or impossible to understand the specific information needed to make a decision, then the deficit is relevant. Be sure to work closely with the client's designated decision-maker if the client has a psychiatric advance directive (see Chapter 13∞).

THE CLIENT'S CULTURAL PERSPECTIVE

A vital component of competent care is accounting for the client's cultural perspective. People can have strong feelings about psychopharmacology that arise from their cultural background. Refusing to take medication may indicate more than paranoia or misunderstanding; it may be intrinsically representative of a cultural standard—for example, the perception that any mental strain or mental illness indicates a weakness of spirit or personality. In another culture, its members may believe that illness is caused by a supreme being, and therefore prayer is the only acceptable route to healing.

Learning as much as you can about the culture's ideas about mental health and illness, its perspective on medications, and its belief systems related to caring will help to minimize miscommunication. Summaries of cultural health beliefs and practices for six major cultural groups (Hispanic, African-American, Native American and Alaska Native, Asian-American, Pacific Islander, and Anglo-American/European-American populations) are in the Partnering with Clients and Families feature on pages 172–173. This table also provides helpful suggestions to consider when working toward cultural competence.

Nurses often act as liaisons between the health care system and the client's belief system, translating and reframing so that clients have a better understanding of symptoms and treatment. This can be accomplished by being open and nonjudgmental about a cultural practice while promoting the healthy aspects of its use.

Psychiatric–mental health nurses may be especially challenged by certain cultural differences, however, especially if a client's native language provides a more detailed, or a more restricted, description of events than the English language (Flaskerud, 2007a). Examining interventions and plans for care in light of the client's culture and commonly held views is necessary. For example, individualism is a dominant theme in the Western world; however, this focus may not fit with people of other ethnicities whose values define caretaking as a collective responsibility. How treatment is given and health attained may be decided by the family or a group of significant others rather than by the individual client. Research on the cultural values of individualism versus collectivism shows the strong positive effect of culture on commitments to long-term endeavors such as medications for chronic conditions (Cohen, 2007). The more committed a person is, the more likely that person is to adhere to the medication regimen.

Working with an Interpreter

Flaskerud (2007b) suggests that we use caution when assessing a client from another culture, especially when an interpreter is present. When you work with an interpreter, keep in mind that, in an attempt to make sense of disorganized statements, the interpreter may alter the client's intended meaning. Your assessment of the client's progress may actually be an assessment of the interpreter's progress. The interpreter may edit embarrassing or inappropriate statements, which will interfere with your ability to assess accurately the existence of continued symptoms.

When you must give a client information through an interpreter, avoid using medical euphemisms and Anglocentric health concepts. Be clear and descriptive. When giving feedback, regardless of the cultural orientation, it is best to focus your input on the client's behavior and not on who the client is personally or spiritually. Information about behavior can cut across cultural differences and be useful input. Even when language is not an issue and interpreters are not involved, it has been argued that it is

MEDIALINK Critical Thinking Exercise: Cultural Issues and Medication

difficult to incorporate non-Western sensibilities into our present psychiatric classification system. Your recognition of the validity of cultural backgrounds other than Western will promote client rights and afford clients legitimate entry into health care delivery systems. Remember that the information you share will be shaped by your own culture and beliefs.

Cultural Self-Awareness of Nurses

An awareness of the issues relating to your own as well as the client's culture helps minimize cultural interferences with communication and is necessary for providing quality mental health care. See the Your Self-Awareness feature to determine how your cultural inclinations influence your attitudes toward medications.

The most effective approach to promoting cultural competence is to expose yourself to as many cultures as possible. Becoming involved in culturally diverse communities will provide you with cross-cultural experiences. Implementing your own program of culturally competent education by immersing yourself in an activity that is specific for a particular culture, such as community activities, celebrations, memorials, and festivals, could provide you with an invigorating set of broadening experiences (Chrisman, 2007; Lipson & DeSantis, 2007).

Ethnicity and Metabolism of Psychiatric Medications

Cultural influences can have enormous consequences for the recovery of clients. In addition to assessing for cultural influences on behavior, you must also assess for the biologic effects of medications on ethnically distinct groups. Different races and ethnicities do metabolize psychiatric and other medications in a variety of ways. Dose levels, side effects even at low dose levels, toxicity effects, and physical impacts will be different with diverse groups. Recognizing how ethnicity determines a client's response to medications promotes the provision of culturally competent care. Be sure to discuss the nature of the client's responses to psychopharmacology with the client, and remember that focused and specific documentation of unusual responses to medications communicates the culture-related reality to the interdisciplinary team. The biologic effects of medications on ethnically distinct groups are explored in detail in Chapter 7.

YOUR SELF-AWARENESS
Cultural Competence in Psychopharmacology

Check your cultural competence in psychopharmacology by thinking about your perspective on the following statements.

1. I learn as much as I can about how members of other cultures view mental health symptoms, their perspective on medications, and their belief system on health care.
2. I avoid using medical euphemisms and Anglocentric health concepts when I teach clients and families about psychiatric medications.
3. I am clear and descriptive when I give information on psychiatric medications.
4. I recognize the validity of cultures and values other than Western and their influences on client and family attitudes toward, and beliefs about, psychopharmacology.
5. I promote client rights and advocate for clients of all cultures in issues of psychopharmacology.
6. I maintain awareness of the issues and controversies that involve culture and psychiatric medications.

NURSING RESPONSIBILITIES WITH ANTIPSYCHOTICS

Detailed information on the category of psychiatric medications known as antipsychotics is in Chapter 7. This section discusses the important clinical considerations for psychiatric–mental health nurses.

Medications are frequently referred to in terms of their generation (their discovery, or birth) as a way of characterizing the major features of the medication. Once a newer, more sophisticated and powerful medication is developed, the previous grouping is referred to as the first-generation antipsychotics and the newer group as the **second-generation antipsychotics (SGAs)**. Although the first- and second-generation classifications can apply to other classes of medications, the terms are most often used when discussing antipsychotics. Generational designations can also be determined not just by timing but also by the neurological pathways they use and their effects on neurotransmitters.

Side Effects

Side effects of medications are defined as unintended physical effects. For example, the main effect of an antibiotic prescribed for a sinus infection is to kill the bacteria causing the infection. A side effect, or unintended effect, may be digestive disruption. Of course, not everyone who takes an antibiotic will experience disrupted digestion. However, it occurs often enough to warrant being prepared to cope with this side effect. Side effect issues can and do occur with psychiatric medications. Side effects are sometimes called adverse effects. They are interchangeable terms, although side effects may be a more recognizable phrase for your clients.

Continuous contact with clients in the inpatient psychiatric setting gives nurses an advantage over other mental health professionals who may see a client only every other day or, at best, once a day. Both the dangerous and the more uncomfortable side effects frequently have a rapid onset and require immediate attention. TABLE 32-1 ■ on page 852 lists the side effects of various antipsychotic medications in common use.

Autonomic Nervous System Effects

All antipsychotics possess anticholinergic and antiadrenergic side effects; that is, they interfere with the normal transmission of nerve impulses by acetylcholine and epinephrine, in both central and peripheral nerves. **Anticholinergic side effects** and adverse effects are the most common and are generally drying to the various tissues and systems. They are

TABLE 32-1 ■ **Side Effects of Antipsychotic Medications**

Effect	Chlorpromazine (Thorazine)	Haloperidol (Haldol)	Loxapine (Loxitane)	Molindone (Moban)	Risperidone (Risperdal)	Clozapine (Clozaril)	Thioridazine (Mellaril)
Akathisia	Occasional	Frequent	Occasional	Frequent	Occasional	Occasional	Occasional
Allergic skin reactions	Occasional	Rare	Rare	Rare	Rare	Occasional	Not reported
Anticholinergic effects	Frequent	Not reported	Rare	Occasional	Occasional	Occasional	Frequent
Blood dyscrasia	Occasional	Occasional	Not reported	Rare	Not reported	Occasional	Rare
Cholestatic jaundice	Occasional	Rare	Not reported	Not reported	Not reported	Not reported	Rare
Dystonias	Occasional	Frequent	Rare	Occasional	Rare	Occasional	Occasional
Impotence	Occasional	Not reported	Not reported	Not reported	Rare	Rare	Occasional
Parkinsonism	Occasional	Frequent	Frequent	Occasional	Rare	Rare	Frequent
Photosensitivity	Occasional	Rare	Not reported	Not reported	Not reported	Not reported	Occasional
Postural hypotension	Frequent	Occasional	Rare	Rare	Occasional	Frequent	Frequent
Retinitis pigmentosa	Not reported	Not reported	Not reported	Not reported	Not reported	Not reported	Occasional
Sedation	Frequent	Not reported	Occasional	Rare	Rare	Frequent	Frequent

Effect	Thiothixene (Navane)	Trifluoperazine (Stelazine)	Fluphenazine (Prolixin)	Olanzapine (Zyprexa)	Quetiapine (Seroquel)	Ziprasidone (Geodon)
Akathisia	Occasional	Frequent	Frequent	Frequent	Rare	Occasional
Allergic skin reactions	Rare	Rare	Rare	Rare	Rare	Frequent
Anticholinergic effects	Occasional	Frequent	Frequent	Frequent	Not reported	Common
Blood dyscrasia	Rare	Rare	Rare	Rare	Rare	Rare
Cholestatic jaundice	Rare	Rare	Rare	Not reported	Not reported	Not reported
Dystonias	Occasional	Frequent	Frequent	Not reported	Rare	Occasional
Impotence	Not reported	Occasional	Occasional	Not reported	Not reported	Occasional
Parkinsonism	Occasional	Frequent	Frequent	Not reported	Not reported	Occasional
Photosensitivity	Rare	Occasional	Occasional	Not reported	Not reported	Frequent
Postural hypotension	Occasional	Rare	Rare	Frequent	Occasional	Frequent
Retinitis pigmentosa	Not reported	Not reported	Not reported	Not reported	Not reported	Not reported
Sedation	Frequent	Not reported	Occasional	Frequent	Occasional	Common

usually more pronounced in older adults. See the Your Assessment Approach feature on page 853 for a list of the various anticholinergic side effects that result from interference with acetylcholine transmission.

Constipation Constipation, a burdensome problem for many people, is also a side effect of many psychiatric medications. Medications and supplements that can cause constipation include opioids, anticholinergics, antihistamines, tricyclic antidepressants, antispasmodics, calcium channel blockers, iron supplements, aluminum antacids, and antiemetic, chemotherapeutic, and antiparkinsonian medications (Bisanz, 2007). Strategies for coping with this common and frustrating side effect can be found in the Your Intervention Strategies: Coping with Constipation feature.

Orthostatic Hypotension Orthostatic hypotension, also known as postural hypotension, is a common antiadrenergic effect. The primary danger here is injury from a fall. Clients receiving parenteral medications, such as chlorpromazine in-

YOUR ASSESSMENT APPROACH
Anticholinergic Side Effects

- Nervousness, drowsiness, headache
- Tachycardia
- Blurred vision
- Dry mouth, constipation, nausea, vomiting
- Under rarer circumstances, paralytic ileus
- Urinary hesitancy/retention
- Cognitive functioning impairment and hallucinations (especially with older adults)

tramuscularly, must have their blood pressure monitored both lying down and standing, before and a half hour after each dose. Clients should be advised to rise from a supine position gradually and to sit down if they feel faint. Support stockings and a large intake of fluids may be indicated. Orthostatic hypotension is much less significant with oral administration of the drug. However, nurses working with clients receiving oral antipsychotic medications should take both baseline and routine vital sign readings at regular intervals. This practice establishes the client's tolerance for medications without the untoward side effects of orthostatic hypotension and subsequent falls. The Your Intervention Strategies feature at right includes guidelines for measuring orthostatic blood pressure.

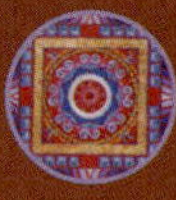

YOUR INTERVENTION STRATEGIES
Guidelines for Measuring Orthostatic Blood Pressure

1. Instruct the client to lie down for approximately 5 minutes. This allows for an equilibration of the blood pressure in the supine position and gives a precise supine reading. *Do not substitute a sitting reading for a supine reading!* Take the client's blood pressure and pulse.
2. Instruct the client to stand. Wait for approximately 30 seconds to 1 minute and retake the blood pressure and pulse. Waiting this brief period allows for a full evaluation of the initial orthostasis.
3. Wait 2 more minutes and retake the vital signs once again. This third set of measurements allows for an evaluation of the client's body mechanisms to compensate for the presence of any orthostasis that may be present.

Extrapyramidal Side Effects

Another common and sometimes frightening group of adverse reactions results from the effects of antipsychotics on the extrapyramidal tracts of the central nervous system, which are involved in the production and control of involuntary movements. This group of reactions is known as **extrapyramidal side effects (EPSEs)**. Animal studies have been useful in examining these problems. One study found that prior administration of buspirone (BuSpar) for 2 weeks may be of help in the improvement of extrapyramidal symptoms induced by antipsychotic drugs (Haleem, Samad, & Haleem, 2007).

The first-generation, conventional, or typical antipsychotics such as haloperidol (Haldol), trifluoperazine (Stelazine), and chlorpromazine (Thorazine) tend to be harsher on the body and cause significant EPSEs. Although many clients are taking second-generation antipsychotics, some respond well to first-generation antipsychotics and must continue taking them. Managing the EPSEs as a long-term treatment option involves careful nursing intervention and client and family education. Four major types of EPSEs are discussed in the following section and in the Your Assessment Approach feature on page 854; each EPSE has distinguishing clinical characteristics and times of onset after the initiation of drug therapy. A fifth category, dopamine-acetylcholine imbalance in the extrapyramidal system, is an uncommon type of EPSE and is also discussed in the Your Assessment Approach feature on page 854.

There are several different types of EPSEs that take unique and distinctive forms. They are discussed next.

Acute Dystonic Reactions The earliest and most dramatic EPSEs are the *acute dystonic reactions*, forms of dystonia. These occur in the first days of medication treatment, sometimes after a single dose of medication. They involve bizarre and severe muscle contractions. These reactions can be physically painful and are almost always frightening to the individual. They are readily reversible. The term *dystonia* describes the experience of the side effect. *Dys* typically means bad, and *tonia* means muscle tone; essentially, these are muscle spasms.

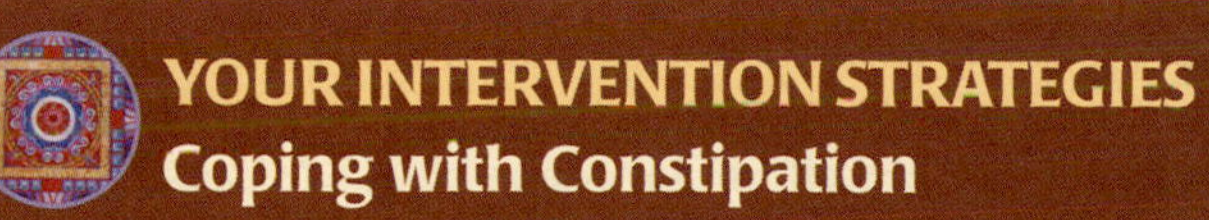

YOUR INTERVENTION STRATEGIES
Coping with Constipation

Several of these strategies may be needed to regularly manage bowel competence:

- Determine the client's usual frequency and type of bowel movement.
- Discuss changes to routine bowel movements and how the client can communicate about constipation.
- Ensure adequate fluid intake to fend off dehydration.
- Ensure soluble and bulk-forming fiber intake daily.
- Assess the number and volume of meals eaten.
- Instruct the client to move around; a sedentary lifestyle is a constipating lifestyle.
- Stool softeners can be very useful.
- Instruct the client to make time in his or her schedule to have a bowel movement.
- If a bowel regimen must be used (refer to a medical–surgical text), find a reliable combination and employ it regularly.
- Keep in mind that some clients may have laxative reactions to alcohol-based sugar substitutes, chocolate, and some grains.

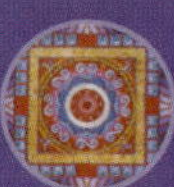

YOUR ASSESSMENT APPROACH
Extrapyramidal Side Effects (EPSEs)

Dystonia

- Usually occurs within 48 hr after beginning treatment but may occur at any time.
- Described by the client as "Sometimes my back tightens up," or "I get tongue-tied when I try to talk."
- Characterized by abnormal tonic contractions of muscle groups.
- Characterized by odd posturing and strange facial expressions such as torticollis (twisting of the neck or pulling the neck down into the shoulders), opisthotonos (spasms of the neck and back, forcing the back to arch and the neck to bend backward), and oculogyric crisis (a fixed gaze that cannot return to lateral once raised vertically).
- Is more common in young males.
- Treated prophylactically by anticholinergics. Some clients may experience a "high" from this treatment.

Drug-Induced Parkinsonism

- Usually occurs after 3 or more weeks of treatment.
- Characterized by rigidity (cogwheeling), tremor, or regular rhythmic oscillations of the extremities, particularly the distal parts, and in the hands (a pill-rolling movement of the fingers).
- Clients are more susceptible to aspiration or to injury by falling.
- Treatment consists of decreasing the medication dosage or administering anticholinergics.

Akathisia

- Usually occurs after 3 or more weeks of treatment.
- Described by the client as "My nerves are jumping," or "I feel like jumping out of my skin."
- A subjective need or desire to move, not a type of pattern or movement.
- Mild akathisia: vague feelings of apprehension and irritability.
- Severe akathisia: an inability to sit (or the feeling one cannot sit) for more than a few seconds, resulting in running, rocking, or agitated dancing.
- Not always responsive to anticholinergics; lowering the medication dosage may be necessary.
- There is an associated dysphoria not treated by anticholinergics or benzodiazepines.

Dopamine–Acetylcholine Imbalance in the Extrapyramidal System

- Characterized by hallucinations, dry mouth, blurred vision, decreased absorption of antipsychotics, decreased gastric motility, tachycardia, and urinary retention.

Tardive Dyskinesia (TD)

- Late onset during the course of treatment with antipsychotics, with frequently irreversible abnormal movements or a neurologic syndrome.
- Characterized by coordinated, arrhythmic, involuntary movements (lip smacking, tongue protrusion, rocking, foot tapping).
- Complications include inability to wear dentures, impaired respirations, weight loss, and impaired gait and posture.
- Treatment is primary prevention through careful initial assessment of the client's needs, as well as continual evaluation of the course of treatment.

MEDIALINK Videos: Extrapyramidal Side Effects

Dystonic movements can occur abruptly and co-occur with other extrapyramidal side effects (Brahm, McElwain, & Brown, 2007). Treatment to resolve the EPSEs is effective in many instances, although the impact on the client is taken into account. Continued experiences that are painful and unpredictable tend to shatter trust in psychophamacology, and discontinuing the medication may be necessary. This clinical example describes one way to address dystonic reactions.

CLINICAL EXAMPLE

Nino has been treated with antipsychotic medications for fixed delusional beliefs that include believing that he must rid the planet of people attempting to "steal" its vibrations and use them as weapons. Years ago Nino had a dystonic reaction during which he could move his eyes from side to side but, when he raised them to look at the ceiling, could not lower them again. The spasms in his eye muscles frightened and angered him. Because Nino requires medication to think more clearly, it is important to prevent dystonic events that might cause pain and damage his trust in both the medication and the prescribers. A prophylactic regimen of the anticholinergic medication trihexyphenidyl (Artane) has proved most effective for Nino.

Parkinsonian Syndrome **Parkinsonian syndrome** (so named because of its striking resemblance to true Parkinson's disease) commonly occurs after a week or two of the medication therapy. It is the result of dopamine blockade caused by psychiatric medications. Treatment with oral medication is usually sufficient, because urgency is seldom a consideration in the management of this syndrome.

Akathisia A third reversible extrapyramidal side effect is known as **akathisia**. The word *akathisia* is derived from the Greek word *kathisia*, meaning "ability to sit" (the prefix *a-* indicates "not" or "without"; hence "inability to sit still"). Akathisia is a motor restlessness perceived subjectively by the client and experienced as an urge to pace, a need to shift weight from one foot to the other, or an inability to sit or stand still. Akathisia can occur weeks to months into the course of therapy.

Your accurate observation of the course of therapy can promote prompt recognition and proper interpretation of EPSEs. If care is not taken, the health care provider may misinterpret the increasing withdrawal, emotional blunting, apathy, and lack of spontaneity as an increase in the severity of schizophrenic symptoms. This error in interpretation may lead to a mistaken increase in the dosage of antipsychotic medication, which will aggravate the condition. Akathisia can also be confused with psychotic agitation, and this error also prompts an increase in medication. Clients with akathisia require a reduction in the dosage of offending agents and/or treatment with an antiparkinsonian drug. You can save the client many uncomfortable and worrisome days. First, be aware of the frequency with which these syndromes complicate treatment. Report any suspicious sign or symptom to the prescriber. Finally, reassure the client of the reversibility of the syndrome in almost all cases.

Tardive Dyskinesia The last EPSE to emerge in the course of treatment, **tardive dyskinesia (TD)**, is also the most severe because it can be irreversible. TD frequently appears after years of antipsychotic drug treatment, although it can occur earlier. It usually appears after a maintenance dose is discontinued or reduced, and it can be masked—but not treated—by reinstituting the medication or increasing the dosage, or by switching to another drug. The term *tardive dyskinesia* is formed from the word *tardive*, meaning "late onset" or "slow" (from the root for tardy and retardation); the prefix *dys-*, and the word *kinesia*, meaning movement. It is essentially a late-arriving bad movement. TD is a neurological syndrome involving the innervation of muscle groups. Typical tardive dyskinesia movements include thrusting the tongue out of the mouth or facial grimacing.

Current estimates put the incidence of TD at 5% per year for young adults and as high as 25% after 1 year in older adults. The limited evidence available clearly indicates that atypical antipsychotics cause less tardive dyskinesia, approximately 1%. Atypical antipsychotics demonstrate antidyskinetic properties in individuals with preexisting tardive dyskinesia. The underlying mechanisms remain unclear, and without such information it is impossible to say under what clinical conditions, if any, these advantages might be diminished or even eliminated (Remington, 2007). Early detection through regular examinations (at least every 6 months) is recommended.

There is no known cure for the adverse event of TD. The recommended intervention is to stop all medication to see if the syndrome resolves spontaneously. This course of action must be weighed against the client's need for medication and the likelihood of relapse into psychosis. Using cholinergic drugs (arecoline, cevimeline, choline, deanol, donepezil, dimethylamino ethanol lecithin, eptastigmine, galantamine, ipidacrine, meclofenoxate, metoxytacrine, metrifonate, physostigmine, rivastigmine, tacrine, xanomeline) to treat neuroleptic-induced TD in people with schizophrenia or other chronic mental illness has had equivocal results (Tammenmaa, Sailas, McGrath, Soares-Weiser, & Wahlbeck, 2004).

With the emergence of the newer antipsychotic medications such as clozapine (Clozaril), aripiprazole (Abilify), and paliperidone (Invega), which have been found to reduce TD, the available choices are expanding. See Chapter 7∞ for detailed discussions of these medications. The seventh and newest antipsychotic, paliperidone, is currently being evaluated in this regard.

TABLE 32-2 ■ Antiparkinsonian Medications

Generic Name	Trade Name	Maximum Daily Dosage	Available in Injectable Form?
Amantadine	Symmetrel	300 mg	No
Benztropine	Cogentin	8 mg	Yes
Biperiden	Akineton	8 mg	Yes
Diphenhydramine	Benadryl	100 mg	Yes
Procyclidine	Kemadrin	15 mg	No
Trihexyphenidyl	Artane	15 mg	No

Prophylactic Treatment of EPSEs In view of the relatively high incidence of EPSEs, the question of whether clients should be treated prophylactically with antiparkinsonian agents is open to debate. Some argue that the use of antiparkinsonian agents eventually leads to relatively higher antipsychotic doses, thereby increasing the probability of serious side effects. Another argument is that antiparkinsonian agents also pose risks and thus should be used only to counteract EPSEs, not to guard against their possible emergence. Moreover, a great many clients never develop the syndromes. If the likelihood of an extrapyramidal reaction is high (if, for example, the client has a history of them) and the possible consequences are significant (the client may discontinue medication or drop out of treatment altogether), antipsychotic and antiparkinsonian agents are frequently initiated simultaneously. TABLE 32-2 ■ lists the commonly used antiparkinsonian medications for addressing EPSEs.

Assessment of EPSEs Nursing assessment of EPSEs is important to the quality care of clients receiving psychotropic medications. One difficulty is consistency of assessment among caregivers. For example, nurses usually assess for the presence of cogwheeling or muscle rigidity in clients receiving psychotropic drugs. However, those assessments are not necessarily reliable or consistent; what one nurse may consider moderate to severe side effects may be assessed as mild to moderate by another nurse. Repeating the assessment after the medication is given helps you assess the amelioration of the side effect. These assessment data chart the course of a client's side effects and the effectiveness of medications to decrease them and are vital to quality nursing care.

Two assessment tools that lend greater objectivity to the assessment of EPSEs are the Simpson Neurological Rating Scale for the assessment of extrapyramidal side effects and the Abnormal Involuntary Movement Scale (AIMS) for the assessment of iatrogenic movements resulting from particular psychotropic drugs. These assessment tools can be found on the Companion Website for this book. They are helpful in quantifying EPSEs prior to administering a medication to counteract the side effect.

An example of the AIMS tool is in the Your Assessment Approach feature on pages 856–857. Directions on the

YOUR ASSESSMENT APPROACH
The Abnormal Involuntary Movement Scale

DEPARTMENT OF HEALTH AND HUMAN SERVICES PUBLIC HEALTH SERVICE Alcohol, Drug Abuse, and Mental Health Administration NIMH Treatment Strategies in Schizophrenia Study	PATIENT NUMBER _ _ _ _	DATA GROUP **aims**	EVALUATION DATE _ _ _ _ _ _ M M D D Y Y
ABNORMAL INVOLUNTARY MOVEMENT SCALE (AIMS)	PATIENT NAME		
	RATER NAME		

RATER NUMBER _ _ _	EVALUATION TYPE (*Circle*)			
	1 Baseline 2 2-Week minor 3 Screening	4 Start double-blind 5 Major evaluation 6 Other	7 Start open meds 8 During open meds 9 Stop open meds	10 Early termination 11 Study completion

INSTRUCTIONS: Complete Examination Procedure before making ratings.
MOVEMENT RATINGS: Rate highest severity observed.

Code: 1 = None; 2 = Minimal, may be extreme normal; 3 = Mild; 4 = Moderate; 5 = Severe

		(Circle One)				
FACIAL AND ORAL MOVEMENTS:	**1. Muscles of Facial Expression** e.g., movements of forehead, eyebrows, periorbital area, cheeks; include frowning, blinking, smiling, grimacing	1	2	3	4	5
	2. Lips and Perioral Area e.g., puckering, pouting, smacking	1	2	3	4	5
	3. Jaw e.g., biting, clenching, chewing, mouth opening, lateral movement	1	2	3	4	5
	4. Tongue Rate only increase in movement both in and out of mouth, NOT inability to sustain movement	1	2	3	4	5
EXTREMITY MOVEMENTS:	**5. Upper** *(arms, wrists, hands, fingers)* Include choreic movements, (i.e., rapid, objectively purposeless, irregular, spontaneous), athetoid movements (i.e., slow, irregular, complex, serpentine). Do NOT include tremor (i.e., repetitive, regular, rhythmic)	1	2	3	4	5
	6. Lower *(legs, knees, ankles, toes)* e.g., lateral knee movement, foot tapping, heel dropping, foot squirming, inversion and eversion of foot	1	2	3	4	5
TRUNK MOVEMENTS:	**7. Neck, shoulders, hips** e.g., rocking, twisting, squirming, pelvic gyrations	1	2	3	4	5

GLOBAL JUDGMENTS:	**8. Severity of abnormal movements**	None, normal Minimal Mild Moderate Severe	1 2 3 4 5
	9. Incapacitation due to abnormal movements	None, normal Minimal Mild Moderate Severe	1 2 3 4 5
	10. Patient's awareness of abnormal movements Rate only patient's report	No awareness Aware, no distress Aware, mild distress Aware, moderate distress Aware, severe distress	1 2 3 4 5
DENTAL STATUS:	**11. Current problems with teeth and/or dentures**	No Yes	1 2
	12. Does patient usually wear dentures?	No Yes	1 2

(continued)

YOUR ASSESSMENT APPROACH
The Abnormal Involuntary Movement Scale *(continued)*

Examination Procedure

Either before or after completing the Examination Procedure observe the patient unobtrusively, at rest (e.g., in waiting room). The chair to be used in this examination should be a hard, firm one without arms.

1. Ask patient to remove shoes and socks.
2. Ask patient whether there is anything in his/her mouth (e.g., gum, candy, etc.) and if there is, to remove it.
3. Ask patient about the current condition of his/her teeth. Ask patient if he/she wears dentures. Do teeth or dentures bother patient *now*?
4. Ask patient whether he/she notices any movements in mouth, face, hands, or feet. If yes, ask to describe and to what extent they *currently* bother patient or interfere with his/her activities.
5. Have patient sit in chair with hands on knees, legs slightly apart, and feet flat on floor. (Look at entire body for movements while in this position.)
6. Ask patient to sit with hands hanging unsupported. If male, between legs, if female and wearing a dress, hanging over knees. (Observe hands and other body areas.)
7. Ask patient to open mouth. (Observe tongue at rest within mouth.) Do this twice.
8. Ask patient to protrude tongue. (Observe abnormalities of tongue movement.) Do this twice.
9. Ask patient to tap thumb, with each finger, as rapidly as possible for 10–15 seconds; separately with right hand, then with left hand. (Observe facial and leg movements.)
10. Flex and extend patient's left and right arms (one at a time). (Note any rigidity.)
11. Ask patient to stand up. (Observe in profile. Observe all body areas again, hips included.)
12. Ask patient to extend both arms outstretched in front with palms down. (Observe trunk, legs, and mouth.)
13. Have patient walk a few paces, turn, and walk back to chair. (Observe hands and gait.) Do this twice.

assessment tool and the accompanying examination procedure guide you through a careful and complete TD screen. It is helpful to use a goose-neck lamp to see minute movements, particularly in the oral/facial areas. Clinical practice dictates an AIMS be completed every 6 months during treatment. Using a video camera allows clinicians to record the client examination and compare results over time.

Other Central Nervous System Effects

Central nervous system (CNS) side effects of antipsychotic medications are sedation and reduction of the seizure threshold. Because antipsychotics vary in their sedative effects, this side effect is troublesome, but it can be managed by changing to a less sedating agent. Seizures are not a contraindication for using these medications. However, their use requires close observation.

Allergic Effects

The principal allergic manifestation of the antipsychotics is cholestatic jaundice. This occurs much less frequently than in the early days of psychopharmacology, and it is usually a benign and self-limiting condition. Chlorpromazine (Thorazine), tricyclic antidepressants, and phenothiazines can all cause cholestatic jaundice, which is not universally thought to always be an allergic reaction. It is suggested that chlorpromazine exerts a direct toxic effect on the bile secretory mechanisms of the liver.

Some clients may have a record of what is thought to be an "allergic" reaction to a psychotropic medication but without documented evidence of cholestatic jaundice or other allergic reactions. When these circumstances are more carefully analyzed, it may turn out that the client either experienced neuroleptic malignant syndrome (NMS; discussed later in this chapter) or a dystonic reaction. The dangers associated with NMS may have prompted an explanation to the client along the lines of the dangers associated with an allergic reaction. This communication may have been misinterpreted and not detected or corrected.

Sometimes clients report dystonia as an allergic reaction to a psychiatric medication. A painful side effect such as dystonia is a negative experience to be avoided and clients may report it as an allergy in an attempt to ensure that the offending medication is not prescribed for them. Careful scrutiny of reports of allergies must be conducted regularly to determine true allergies not only to protect the client from contact, but also to make sure no effective medications are removed from the array of treatments for that client.

Cardiac Effects

Antipsychotics can have an impact on the length of time it takes the heart to go through its electrical and muscular cycle. This cycle is abbreviated as the QT complex, referring to the length of the interval between the first wave identified in an ECG—there are Q, R, S, and T waves—and the last wave. A standardization of the length of this cycle is referred to as the QTc (a corrected QT interval). An interval longer than 450–500 msec can indicate a cardiac problem. An elongated QT interval can lead to arrhythmias and a drug-induced cardiac condition called Torsades de Pointes. Elongated QT intervals can also be traced to a family history of QT prolongation, nonpsychiatric medications that prolong the QT, and lifestyle (Carlo, Bobo, & Meltzer, 2007; Girgis, Huckstep, Oakley, Ferriter, & Nikolaou, 2007; Gupta, Lawrence, Krishnan, Kavinsky, & Trohman, 2007).

High doses of antipsychotics can contribute to the prevalence of QT interval abnormalities. However, in a study

MediaLink Application: Weighty Issues

of clients on high doses of antipsychotics in a psychiatric–forensic setting (Girgis et al., 2007), the incidence of cardiac side effects was lower than expected and the increased risk of QTc abnormalities could be managed.

The highest risk for significant QT prolongation is with thioridazine (Mellaril). This medication was given a black box warning by the FDA to call attention to the risk. Pimozide (Orap), droperidol (Inapsine), and haloperidol (Haldol) also increase cardiac risk. The atypical antipsychotic aripiprazole (Abilify) was first marketed with FDA direction to monitor QTc. Ultimately, as with all other antipsychotics, aripiprazole should be used with caution in clients with known cardiovascular disease (history of myocardial infarction or ischemic heart disease, heart failure, or conduction abnormalities), cerebrovascular disease, and conditions that increase the likelihood of hypotension or hypertension. In clinical trials of aripiprazole, the incidence of QT prolongation was comparable to placebo (Carlo et al., 2007; Girgis et al., 2007).

Blood, Skin, and Eye Effects

Among the other side effects in this category, agranulocytosis is the most serious. It is both potentially fatal and, fortunately, extremely rare. Usually the person acquires an infection and deteriorates rapidly or begins to bleed spontaneously, requiring emergency medical attention. Many medications cause agranulocytosis, including benzodiazepines and antibiotics. (See the discussion on page 117 in Chapter 7∞.)

Skin eruptions, photosensitivity leading to severe sunburn, blue-gray metallic discolorations over the face and hands, and pigmentation changes in the eyes are all potential side effects. Clients are generally advised to avoid prolonged exposure to sunlight or to use a sunscreen agent when outdoors. These conditions usually remit.

One serious and permanent eye change is retinitis pigmentosa. This condition may occur in clients on dosages of thioridazine exceeding 800 mg/day. The condition may lead to blindness. Therefore, doses exceeding 800 mg per day are contraindicated.

Endocrine Effects

Lactation in females and gynecomastia and impotence in males lead a list of endocrine changes that can occur with antipsychotic drug treatments. Hyperprolactinemia is a common side effect that will affect many aspects of the client's sex life. Difficulties with libido, arousal, excitation, orgasm, male ejaculatory volume, and overall performance can occur to a disturbing degree with hyperprolactinemia. You can imagine how these side effects would affect the regular or long-term use of the medication. Hyperprolactinemia is also responsible for oligomenorrhea or amenorrhea in women, galactorrhea in women and rarely in men, and, in cases of prolonged hyperprolactinemia, osteoporosis (Freeman, Levy, & Gorman, 2007). Be alert to these endocrine changes; you are most likely to be the professional told about such problems.

Another endocrine problem is diabetes in people who have schizophrenia. The baseline occurrence of diabetes is elevated with schizophrenia (twice the rate of the general population), and seems to be further escalated by endocrine changes from psychotropics. Although weight gain raises the risk of diabetes, some studies show diabetes occurring in clients who have not gained significant weight. The particular medication used may be a contributing factor. You should be alert to any changes in body functions reported by clients taking these medications.

Weight Gain

Weight gain is a significant side effect that affects self-esteem and poses health risks for the client. Certain antipsychotics, tricyclic antidepressants, lithium, anticonvulsants, and other classes of medications can cause an increase in weight. As mentioned earlier, an increase in weight can put an individual at risk for health problems such as diabetes, hypertension, and coronary artery disease. The impact of weight gain can be more disturbing to clients than EPSEs. Over time, this side effect can be a devastating blow to long-term treatment and quality of life. Paying careful attention to the potential for weight gain from the inception of treatment can help minimize this particular side effect.

Neuroleptic Malignant Syndrome

Although we discuss **neuroleptic malignant syndrome** in this section on antipsychotic medications, be aware that it is a severe and potentially life-threatening side effect of all psychotropic medications. This extreme condition is believed to be the result of either dopamine blockade in the striatum of the brain or dopaminergic antagonism in the CNS. Research is being conducted on the genetic etiology of NMS—its phenotypes and genetic markers (Gurrera, Simpson, & Tsuang, 2007; Kemp, Fitzgerald, & White, 2007).

NMS occurs in 0.2% to 0.5% of clients taking psychiatric medications. Approximately twice as many men are affected as women, and younger clients appear to be more susceptible than older ones (Brunelle, Guigueno, Gouin, Tamion, & Thibaut, 2007). NMS typically occurs within the first 2 weeks of treatment with a new medication or a return to a previously used medication, or when a dosage has been increased. NMS has also been reported months after a new medication regimen has begun. Nurses are in the best position to assess for this condition; symptoms are muscle rigidity, hyperpyrexia, altered consciousness, and diaphoresis. Because NMS often occurs in clients whose presentations are already complex, the nursing assessment can be difficult.

Treatment for NMS includes discontinuing all psychotropic medication immediately and supporting the client medically through the crisis. If cooling and rehydration are not achieved quickly, the client may die. Follow-up care is, of course, important. The pathology of NMS is complex and not completely understood at this time beyond the knowledge that its major symptoms are caused by the blockade of the dopamine receptors.

Client and Family Education

Client and family education about antipsychotics centers upon the individual client's medications, responses to it (or them), side effects exhibited, the client's and family mem-

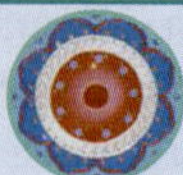

PARTNERING WITH CLIENTS AND FAMILIES

TEACHING ABOUT ANTIPSYCHOTICS

This teaching plan points out the major areas to be addressed when educating clients and their families about antipsychotic medications. Each teaching plan must be individualized for the following issues: the client's specific medication(s), responses to it (or them), side effects, and the client's and family members' abilities and interests in learning. Your documentation of client and family education can be a narrative note or a checklist of the topics discussed.

"What does this medication do?"	"Antipsychotic medications help treat the emotional and thinking problems of schizophrenia or psychosis. It helps organize thinking, keeps you in touch with reality, and reduces the symptoms of your illness. It is not a cure. When you stop taking this medication, the benefits wear off over time and you will have these problems again, possibly at a more disturbing level."
"How should I take this medication?"	"Take it as prescribed on a regular basis. If you feel that you cannot or do not want to continue, notify your therapist or prescriber before you take action."
"What if I miss a dose?"	"Take the dose as soon as you remember if it's only been a few hours. But if it is almost time for your next dose, do not take double or extra doses."
"What other medication does not mix with this antipsychotic?"	Tailor this response to the specific medication prescribed. Mention the major drug interactions with prescribed medications, over-the-counter substances, alternative and complementary supplements, and, of course, alcohol and recreational drug use. There may even be interactions with caffeine, nicotine, and food items that should be discussed in detail.
"What side effects can I expect?"	A discussion of the client's previous side effects with the substance drives this conversation. Although there is no need to overwhelm the client with excess information, the client should know what actions to take when side effects occur. Describe ordinary and extraordinary side effects as well as the actions that should be taken in response to the side effects. Some standard side effects are important to cover: dystonia, akathisia, agitation, confusion, sensitivity to sunlight, and changes in sexual expression.
"Where can I keep my medication?"	"In a safe place at room temperature. Do not keep it in the bathroom where there is a shower or bathtub, in the kitchen where there is a dishwasher, or above or right next to the kitchen sink. Medications should not be kept in a motor vehicle, as temperatures can reach extreme levels within such an enclosed area. Moisture, light, and heat can affect your medication."
"What do I do if I have a problem?"	Give the client and family the names and numbers of health care providers the client can call for questions and in emergencies.

bers' abilities to learn about medications, and their interest in learning. The Partnering with Clients and Families feature above discusses common questions that clients and families ask and suggests responses that you can make.

NURSING RESPONSIBILITIES WITH ANTIDEPRESSANTS

Detailed information on the category of psychiatric medications known as antidepressants is in Chapter 7∞. This section discusses the important clinical considerations for psychiatric–mental health nurses. Atypical antidepressants such as mirtazapine (Remeron) and bupropion (Wellbutrin) are discussed in Chapter 7∞.

It is important to understand that antidepressant medications are not effective in all cases of depressed mood. Evidence from research and clinical practice indicates that only a portion of depressive disorders respond to this category of drugs. For example, tricyclic antidepressants (TCAs), monoamine oxidase inhibitors (MAOIs), and amphetamines are generally contraindicated in depression related to grief reaction or pathologic grief. Other types of depression may be more amenable to psychopharmacologic intervention. Thus, accurate diagnosis is necessary to ensure maximum effectiveness.

Clients for whom antidepressants are indicated usually suffer from characteristic symptoms: a severely depressed mood, loss of interest, an inability to respond to normally pleasurable events or situations, a depression that is worse in the morning and lessens slightly as the day goes on, early morning awakening (and an inability to fall asleep again), marked psychomotor retardation or agitation, appetite and weight changes, and excessive or inappropriate guilt. These symptoms are known as melancholia. In fact, the symptoms of melancholia are the features that most reliably predict a person's response to drug therapy (Clemens, 2007; Parker, 2007). A significant, and commonly overlooked, clinical consideration is that antidepressants have a delayed-reaction onset. A client will not show lessening of depressed mood until 2 to 3 weeks after instituting an adequate dose of TCAs, for example.

The principles guiding the use of MAOI and TCA medications are as follows:

- Drug treatment does not preclude psychotherapy, electroconvulsive therapy, or behavioral treatments if they are also indicated.
- Other antidepressant treatment should be given first unless contraindications are present, there are clinical indications for MAOIs, or there is a past history of unresponsiveness to other antidepressants.
- Dosage may vary and may be limited because of significant side effects.

Clients with recurrent major depressive episodes with melancholia may require long-term maintenance treatment, although doses are usually lower than those needed in acute episodes.

Because clients who do not respond to other classes of antidepressants may respond to MAOIs, clients taking these medications are likely to have had negative experiences with antidepressant medication therapy. This history, in combination with the demands made of clients who take MAOIs, requires careful attention by psychiatric–mental health nurses to the education needs of clients and their family members.

Side Effects of TCAs

Many of the common side effects of tricyclics are autonomic due to the anticholinergic characteristics of the medications (refer to the Your Assessment Approach feature on page 853). These side effects, discussed earlier in the section on antipsychotic medications, include dry mouth, blurred vision, constipation, palpitations, and urinary retention. Clients with glaucoma must be treated with caution. Some allergic skin reactions have been observed.

TCAs also cause changes in the normal electrical conduction of the heart and are cardiotoxic, which is particularly significant in treating clients with a history of cardiovascular disease, especially heart block. Sudden death has occurred during tricyclic treatment. TCAs are contraindicated in clients with mitral valve disease. Clients with known heart disease and most elderly clients require electrocardiograms (ECGs) before, and periodically during, the course of tricyclic therapy. Several CNS effects may occur, including tremor, twitching, paresthesias, ataxia, and convulsions.

Overdose Effects of TCAs

The consequences of overdosing are one aspect of TCA treatment that deserves attention. Significant overdoses may cause delirium, hyperthermia, convulsions, and even coma, shock, and respiratory failure. A lethal dose of an antidepressant such as amitriptyline (Amitril) is estimated at between 10 and 30 times the usual daily therapeutic dose. Drug intake deserves close attention, because many clients treated with these medications are severely suicidal. Serious overdosing is a medical emergency and may require resuscitative measures.

Side Effects of Monoamine Oxidase Inhibitors (MAOIs)

The main adverse effect with MAOIs is hypertensive crisis. Hypertensive crisis is a significant danger when foods, fluids, or medications that contain tyramine are in the digestive tract together with an MAOI. The blood pressure increases precipitously in hypertensive crisis and can cause a cerebral vascular event or a cardiac arrhythmia. Lower levels of side effects are sometimes referred to as "cheese syndrome" because these side effects occur when an MAOI has been combined with any form of cheese. There is no firm formula to determine how much tyramine will cause an adverse event. Clients often test their capacity to tolerate tyramine by ingesting prohibited foods and fluids in small amounts as long as they are unable to detect side effects. (Prohibited foods and fluids are discussed later in this chapter.) The MAOI patch is largely not metabolized through the digestive system and thus is much less likely to require dietary restrictions.

More common side effects of MAOIs include lightheadedness, mild sedation or insomnia, muscle twitching, palpitations, and blurred vision. There are sexual side effects, and typical anticholinergic side effects such as constipation and urinary retention can be a problem. Clients are usually taking MAOIs because no other antidepressant has worked to resolve symptoms or the client only responds to MAOIs. For these clients, side effects need to be managed on a long-term basis. Discuss with the client the side effects the client experiences and develop a plan to address the more durable and annoying ones.

Side Effects of Selective Serotonin Reuptake Inhibitors (SSRIs)

Although the side effects of SSRIs are less severe than those of other antidepressants, some may be intolerable for certain clients. The side effect profile for SSRIs is discussed in Table 32-3 ■. Side effects of SSRIs are thought to be the result of an individual's sensitivity to higher levels of serotonin in the synapse as a consequence of SSRI treatment. Activation, a more energized state that includes decreased sleep and akathisia, is common. Special care must be taken with clients who have histories of hypomania or mania since SSRIs may precipitate a re-emergence or a relapse. The two Your Assessment Approach features on pages 861 and 862 describe the SSRI discontinuation syndrome, and the serotonin syndrome and its management and prevention.

An important consideration with clients taking SSRIs is the proximity of the administration of MAOIs. Fluoxetine (Prozac) and an MAOI together may cause serious and fatal interactions. The half-life of fluoxetine requires a 5-week gap between taking fluoxetine and taking an MAOI, and vice versa. Sertraline (Zoloft), paroxetine (Paxil), citalopram

TABLE 32-3 ■ Side Effects of SSRIs Compared to Those of a Typical Tricyclic (Amitriptyline)

	Fluoxetine (Prozac)	Sertraline (Zoloft)	Paroxetine (Paxil)	Citalopram (Celexa)	Escitalopram (Lexapro)	Amitriptyline (Elavil)
Anticholinergic	0	1	1	1	0–1	4
Sedation	1–2	1–2	0–1	0–1	0–1	3
Activation	1–2	1–2	1–2	1–2	1–2	0
Hypotension	0	0	0	0–1	0	3
GI activation	1–2	1–2	1–2	1–2	1–2	0
Seizures	+	+	0	0	0	+

0 = low; 4 = high; + = present

(Celexa), and escitalopram (Lexapro) have shorter half-lives, and there must be a 1- or 2-week gap (in both directions) between these medications and MAOIs.

Side Effects of Serotonin and Norepinephrine Reuptake Inhibitors (SNRIs)

Venlafaxine (Effexor) was the first in a class of medications called phenethylamine antidepressants. It has two mechanisms of action: inhibiting the reuptake of serotonin and inhibiting the reuptake of norepinephrine. Medications that have this dual action are in a class known as serotonin and norepinephrine reuptake inhibitors (SNRIs). Duloxetine (Cymbalta) has similar neurotransmission action and addresses the pain sensations amplified by depression as well.

Anticholinergic-like side effects may occur with this category of medications. Sustained increases in blood pressure have also been reported with some clients taking venlafaxine. This last side effect seems to be dose-related, so the nursing management of clients taking venlafaxine should include regular blood pressure monitoring. There is also a need for a time buffer with MAOIs: a 14-day gap after discontinuing an MAOI before starting venlafaxine, and at least a 7-day gap after discontinuing venlafaxine before starting an MAOI.

Medications that inhibit the reuptake of serotonin and norepinephrine, as SNRIs do, have an activation component that can cause nervousness. Anorexia may be a difficult side effect for underweight individuals. Other reported side effects include nausea, somnolence, dry mouth, dizziness, constipation, sweating, asthenia, abnormal ejaculation, abnormal orgasm, and anorexia.

The recommended starting dosage for venlafaxine is 75 mg/day, administered in divided doses and taken with food. The dose may be increased to 225 mg/day according to clinical needs, and even further increased to 375 mg/day. It is recommended that clients who have been taking venlafaxine for more than 1 week taper the dose when discontinuing the medication. Clients taking it for 6 weeks or more should time this taper over a 2-week period to minimize the risk of symptoms caused by discontinuing the medication.

Duloxetine dosing focuses on a total dose of 40 mg/day (20 mg twice daily) to 60 mg/day (given either once a day or as 30 mg twice daily). Duloxetine does not have to be taken on an empty or a full stomach; its bioavailability is not dependent on meals. There is no evidence that doses greater than 60 mg/day provide any additional antidepressant benefits. When discontinuing the medication, tapering the dose rather

YOUR ASSESSMENT APPROACH
SSRI Discontinuation Syndrome

- Withdrawal from an SSRI is characterized by symptoms including: dizziness, light-headedness, insomnia, fatigue, anxiety or agitation, nausea, headache, and sensory disturbances. Other possible symptoms include hypomania, worsening of mood, aggressiveness, and suicidality.
- Symptoms have occurred in less than 5% of clients taking long-acting agents, compared to 86% of clients treated with fluvoxamine for panic disorder.
- A possible cause of the syndrome could be a hyposerotonergic state as long-term use of SSRI therapy may downregulate (or desensitize) postsynaptic serotonin receptors. Abrupt discontinuation may restore or even enhance serotonin reuptake, resulting in a depletion of synaptic serotonin. May take 2 to 3 weeks for these systems to readapt.
- Mild, transient symptoms such as jitteriness, sleep disturbance, and heart palpitations have been reported in newborns whose mothers received SSRIs during pregnancy.
- Short-acting SSRIs cause more numerous symptoms that appear earlier after discontinuation and typically last up to 3 weeks.
- Abrupt discontinuation or "drug holidays" should be avoided with short-acting SSRIs.
- These agents should be tapered if discontinued.
- If symptoms appear, the taper needs to be more gradual.

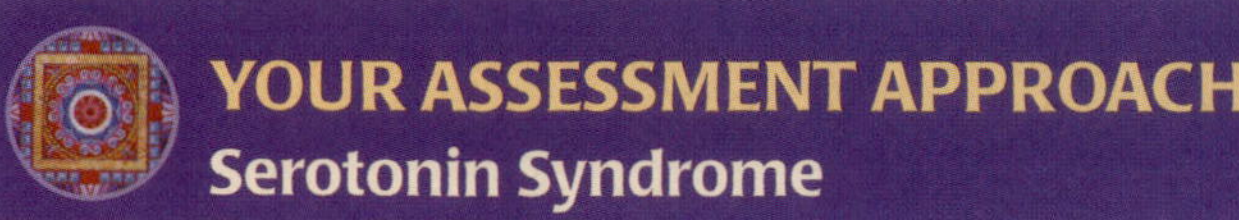

YOUR ASSESSMENT APPROACH
Serotonin Syndrome

Definition

- Mental, autonomic, and neuromuscular changes
- Mild in most people, and with supportive care recovery is complete within 24–72 hours, although it can cause death under certain circumstances (11%)
- Seen in people taking two or more medications that increase the levels of serotonin in the CNS, including SSRIs, TCAs, and MAOIs

Conditions of Diagnosis

- No antipsychotic medication used or increased in dose prior to onset of symptoms
- No other obvious causes of confusion or fever
- Recent addition or increased dose of an agent that raises serotonin levels

Symptoms

Three of the following must be present:

- Mental status changes (confusion, hypomania, anxiety, coma)
- Agitation
- Myoclonus
- Shivering
- Diarrhea
- Hyperreflexia
- Ataxia/incoordination
- Diaphoresis
- Hyperpyrexia

Other Symptoms

Cardiovascular:

- Sinus tachycardia
- Hypertension
- Hypotension

Gastrointestinal:

- Nausea
- Abdominal pain
- Salivation

Motor Abnormalities:

- Muscle rigidity
- Restlessness
- Tremor
- Nystagmus
- Seizures

Other:

- Unreactive pupils
- Tachypnea

Management and Prevention of Serotonin Syndrome

- Supportive measures to reduce hypertension, tachycardia, hyperthermia, and respiratory distress.
- Discontinue suspected agent.
- Discontinue OTCs that increase serotonin levels (dextromethorphan, pseudoephedrine, phenylpropanolamine).
- Benzodiazepines (lorazepam and diazepam) are used commonly to treat myoclonus and resultant hyperthermia.
- Severe cases not responding to benzodiazepines may respond to dantrolene (Dantrium) for relieving muscle rigidity and hyperthermia.
- Severe cases are treated with antiserotonergic agents (cyproheptadine [Periactin], methylsergide [Sansert], propranolol [Inderal]).
- Reconsider using two or more serotonergic medications or consider switching to less serotonergic alternatives.

Note: Clonazepam is ineffective in treating serotonin syndrome.

than abruptly stopping the medication is recommended to minimize discomfort. If intolerable symptoms occur after a decrease in the dose or when the medication is discontinued, then resuming the previously prescribed dose may be considered. Once the client is stabilized, the prescriber may continue decreasing the duloxetine dose but at a more gradual rate.

Age-Related Considerations with Antidepressants

Overall, antidepressants given to any child, adolescent, or young adult must be carefully monitored. The current concern is that antidepressants may contribute to an increased risk of suicidal behavior. Following an FDA Public Health Advisory in 2005, all antidepressants now have labeling that indicates that children, adolescents, and adults treated with antidepressants can experience greater suicidal ideation and behavior during the first few months of treatment. An increase in suicidal ideation following weeks of treatment with antidepressants coincides with the clinical experience of most mental health professionals. Depressed individuals frequently become more activated by their medications and have considerably more energy while they are still actively depressed. Depressed thinking may include lethality. Therefore, closely monitor all clients who have expressed depressed, lethal thoughts and be aware of flight into health (see Chapters 23 and 29∞), changes in behavior, and comments indicating an intention to harm themselves. Unfortunately, along with the decrease in the use of antidepressants with adolescents has come a significant increase in the rate of adolescent suicide. See Chapter 23∞ for a discussion of this phenomenon.

Client and Family Education

Because clients who do not respond to tricyclics may respond to MAOIs, they are likely to have had past negative experiences with antidepressant medication therapy. This, in combination with the demands of taking an MAOI, indicates the need for increased nursing involvement in educating clients and their family members.

MAOI antidepressants require an especially strong, concerted teaching effort from nurses. There are drawbacks to

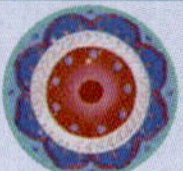

PARTNERING WITH CLIENTS AND FAMILIES

TEACHING ABOUT A LOW-TYRAMINE DIET

MAO inhibitors combine with certain foods and medications to produce a significant increase in blood pressure, which can be a health hazard. In general, foods that can cause this reaction are those that have been pickled, fermented, smoked, or aged. The list below includes the main foods, fluids, and medications that clients should avoid while taking an MAOI and for the 2 weeks after the MAOI is discontinued. Keep in mind that fertilizers and preservatives can be tyramine-based; therefore the dietary restrictions should be updated regularly. This list may not include everything to be avoided (for example, the kind of fertilizer or preservative used may change over time) and may also include items that may be safe to consume at some later point in time.

Note: The monoamine oxidase inhibitor patch Emsam (selegiline) at its lowest strength can be used without the dietary restrictions that apply to all oral MAO inhibitors.

Foods and Beverages to Avoid Completely

Meats and fish	Pickled herring, dried fish, aged/dried/cured meats, unrefrigerated fermented fish, liver, caviar, fermented sausage (bologna, salami, pepperoni, summer sausage), hoisin sauce (fermented oyster sauce used in Asian dishes), any jerky, leftovers that may be partly fermented, meat extracts, commercial gravies, crackers made with cheese, miso (fermented soybean paste), soy sauce, teriyaki sauce, salad dressings with disallowed ingredients
Vegetables	English broad peas, Chinese pea pods, fava beans, banana peels, Italian or broad green beans, kim chee (fermented cabbage), lentils, lima beans, sauerkraut, spoiled or overly ripe fruits, peanuts, spinach
Dairy products	Yogurt, most cheeses (see Allowed Foods for exceptions). Tyramine content of some cheeses, per serving: English Stilton, 17.3 mg; mozzarella, 2.4 mg; grated Parmesan, 0.2 mg; cream cheese, 0
Beverages	Chianti, aged wines, imported beers, aged beers
Combination foods	Breads made with aged cheeses and meats, or yeast extracts, homemade or high-yeast breads, pizza, lasagna, soufflés, macaroni and cheese, quiche, liver pâté, Caesar salad, eggplant parmesan, all yeast products (such as brewer's yeast, bouillon or broth with yeast, and yeast extracts such as Marmite and other yeast spreads)
Medications	Cold medications, nasal decongestants (tablets, drops, sprays, etc.), hay fever and allergy medications, weight reduction preparations, "pep" pills, antiappetite medications, asthma inhalant

Foods and Beverages to Take in Small Amounts

Dairy products	Processed American cheese
Fruits	Raisins, prunes, bananas, avocados, plums, canned figs
Caffeine sources	Coffee, chocolate, colas
Beverages	Domestic jug red wines; domestic beers, ales, and stouts; sherry *(Note: Alcohol is a depressant and should not be ingested by individuals in treatment for depression.)*

Allowed Foods

Beverages	White wines *(Note: Alcohol is a depressant and should not be ingested by individuals in treatment for depression.)*
Any baked goods raised with yeast, but not high yeast	
Dairy products	Cottage cheese, cream cheese, milk, cream, ice cream

Additional Information

St. John's wort	Naturally occurring MAOI, less potent than pharmaceutical grade; is not regulated and may cause inconsistent access to the active ingredient; has the same dietary and medication restrictions as a pharmaceutical-grade MAOI

taking these medications that directly affect nursing intervention. For example, clients on MAOIs must avoid foods that contain even moderate amounts of tyramine; failure to do so will result in hypertensive crisis. The Partnering with Clients and Families feature above outlines the low-tyramine diet for clients taking MAOIs.

NURSING RESPONSIBILITIES WITH MOOD STABILIZERS

Detailed information on the category of psychiatric medications known as mood stabilizers is in Chapter 7∞. This section discusses the important clinical considerations for psychiatric–mental health nurses.

A variety of compounds are used as mood stabilizers. Mood stabilization as well as activating and sedating side effects must be addressed to ensure comfortable and consistent medication adherence. Because of the dangers of unmedicated bipolar disorder, an awareness of side effects and an effective response are important treatment and safety issues.

Lithium has a significant number of side effects that can be troublesome and, in some cases, quite dangerous. Significant side effects are usually correlated with blood levels of lithium above 1.2 mEq/L. Common side effects include tremor, nausea, thirst, and polyuria. Thyroid goiter has also been seen as a side effect.

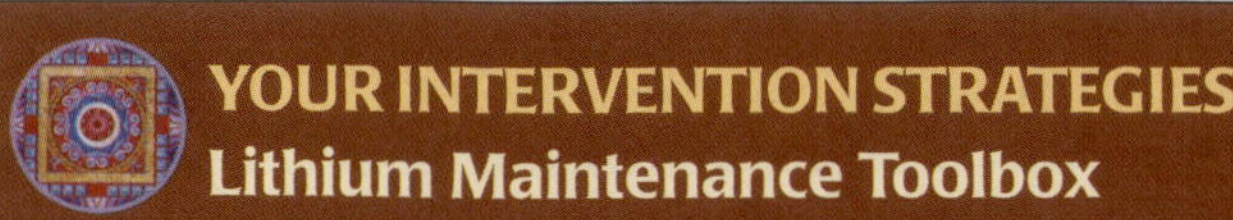

YOUR INTERVENTION STRATEGIES
Lithium Maintenance Toolbox

To keep a stable lithium level, nurses, clients, and family members should know the following:

1. Stabilize dosing schedule (through sustained release formula or divided doses).
2. If a dose is missed, take within 2 hours. If more than 2 hours has elapsed, skip that one dose.
3. Ingest adequate dietary sodium.
4. Maintain hydration.
5. Replace fluids and electrolytes lost during exercise, exertion, GI illness.
6. Monitor for signs of side effects and lithium toxicity.

Watch for these events to cause lithium level increases:

1. Hydration status change
2. Increases in other medications
3. Marijuana use
4. Carbamazepine
5. Lithium overdose
6. Decreased sodium intake
7. Diuretic treatments
8. Medical illness
9. Nonsteroidal antiinflammatory drug therapy
10. Tetracycline use
11. Fluid and electrolyte loss through fever, sweating, diarrhea, vomiting, dehydration

Severe lithium poisoning is a potential medical emergency. Early signs include vomiting and diarrhea, lethargy, and muscle twitching. These may progress to ataxia and slurred speech. The client may become semiconscious or comatose; seizures may occur; and electrolyte imbalances may lead to cardiac arrest. This syndrome of severe toxicity ordinarily occurs only when the client has a blood lithium level of 2 to 3 mEq/L. The client may have overdosed or severely restricted food or salt intake (or taken diuretics) to induce this state.

Occasionally, very violent, agitated, or paranoid individuals with mania require antipsychotic medications as either a mood stabilizer (in the case of atypical antipsychotics) or as an adjunctive medication (for atypical and conventional antipsychotics). Antipsychotic medications used for delusions or agitation can be started simultaneously with the mood stabilizer, increased to whatever level is required to control the disintegrative behavior, then gradually reduced, and finally eliminated after therapeutic mood stabilizer levels have been effective for about 1 week. The Your Intervention Strategies feature above provides practical strategies for the client receiving lithium therapy.

MediaLink Care Plan: The Exercising Client on Lithium

NURSING RESPONSIBILITIES WITH ANXIOLYTICS

Detailed information on the category of psychiatric medications known as anxiolytics, or antianxiety medications, is in Chapter 7. This section discusses the important clinical considerations for psychiatric–mental health nurses.

Anxiolytic medications are used to treat a variety of problems, ranging from high levels of anxiety and panic to insomnia.

Side Effects

Common side effects include problems with daytime functioning, drowsiness, dizziness, and decreased coordination. These side effects can lead to an increase in accidents and falls, especially among older adults. Benzodiazepines induce hypnosis and sedation in addition to their action as muscle relaxant, anxiolytic, and anticonvulsant. Benzodiazepines are also known to induce respiratory depression, and caution should always be used with older adults, those with respiratory diseases, and those taking other medications that depress respiration, such as opiates. Regular use of benzodiazepines can lead to rebound insomnia (see Chapter 19), dependency on the benzodiazepine, and withdrawal symptoms even if tapering is completed after long-term use (Holcomb, 2007).

Client and Family Education

Client teaching is an especially important element in the care of clients taking antianxiety medications. As you know from Chapters 8 and 18, anxiety is a generally uncomfortable experience. Self-medication often becomes the relief-seeking behavior used by many people with severe anxiety. Self-medication can be temporarily helpful in restoring a person's capacities and internal comfort. Many of the anxiolytic drugs (especially benzodiazepines), however, carry a potential for dependence and tolerance. Therefore, nurses have a responsibility to help clients control anxiety in other safer and more effective ways.

Anxious clients often self-medicate when they have trouble sleeping. As with anxiolytics, insomnia preparations are generally intended for either occasional or short-term use. These medications are appropriate for clients newly admitted to a psychiatric inpatient unit or for clients in outpatient therapy who develop sleep disorders. As other medications (antidepressants, lithium, antipsychotics) begin to have a therapeutic effect, however, the need for sedative–hypnotic medication such as alprazolam (Xanax) or diazepam (Valium) should almost, if not completely, abate. Nurses working with clients in these situations need to help them regulate their sleep patterns. Strategies to reinstitute regular sleep patterns are discussed in Chapter 19.

NURSING RESPONSIBILITIES WITH ACETYLCHOLINESTERASE INHIBITORS

Detailed information on the category of psychiatric medications known as acetylcholinesterase inhibitors is in Chapter 7. This section discusses the important clinical considerations for psychiatric–mental health nurses.

Dementia and other cognitive impairments are typically treated with acetylcholinesterase inhibitors (donepezil [Aricept], galantamine [Reminyl], and rivastigmine [Exelon]) and an *N*-methyl-d-aspartate (NMDA) receptor antagonist (memantine or Namenda). These medications perform actions that improve cognitive function.

The first of the acetylcholinesterase inhibitors was tacrine (Cognex). Problems with this medication included liver toxicity, which could be controlled, and several side effects such as GI disturbances and headache. From this beginning, subsequent compounds were developed. Donepezil, galantamine, and rivastigmine are more effective with dementia of the Alzheimer's type and have fewer and less problematic side effects. GI disturbances occur at a much lower level than with the original compound, and headaches are reported at only a slightly higher level than among clients taking a placebo.

Acetylcholinesterase inhibitors are safe, effective, and well tolerated. They promise competent treatment for clients with dementia and other cognitive impairments (Demaerschalk & Wingerchuk, 2007). Chapter 14∞ discusses cognitive disorders.

NURSING RESPONSIBILITIES WITH HERBAL MEDICINES

Detailed information on herbal medicines can also be found in Chapters 7 and 33∞. Table 33-3 on page 887 identifies herbals and dietary supplements commonly used for psychiatric symptoms. This section discusses the important clinical considerations for psychiatric–mental health nurses.

Research involving complementary and alternative (CAM) medications assesses how safe and effective botanicals can be in treating psychiatric symptoms. Herbal side effects and drug–drug interactions should be rigorously assessed as the CAM industry, unlike the pharmaceutical industry, is not regulated and monitored.

One study (Zhang et al., 2007) examined the therapeutic potential of a Chinese herbal CAM called Free and Easy Wanderer Plus (FEWP) for mood disorders as an adjunct to carbamazepine (Tegretol). The adjunctive treatment resulted in significantly better outcomes with depression but failed to produce significantly greater improvement on manic measures and the response rate in manic subjects. There was a lower incidence of dizziness and fatigue in the combination therapy compared to carbamazapine monotherapy. These results suggest that selected adjunctive CAM medications can have additive beneficial effects in clients with bipolar disorders, particularly for those in the depressive phase of the illness (Krishnamurthy & Telles, 2007).

Depression is one of the leading reasons people use CAM products. CAM substances used for depression—St. John's wort, tryptophan/5-hydroxytryptophan, S-adenosyl methionine, folate, and inositol—have been studied. However, no study was conclusively positive. A vital question that concerns the use of CAM substances by people who are depressed is: What happens when a CAM product such as St. John's wort, a naturally occurring MAOI, is used in combination with a prescriptive antidepressant? An earlier discussion in this chapter (see page 861) explores why combining SSRIs and MAOIs is contraindicated. Drug–CAM product interactions can and do occur. Inconclusive results and unequivocally negative results are regularly seen in the literature (Thachil, Mohan, & Bhugra, 2007). If a depression does not respond to St. John's wort or other CAM within a brief and reasonable period of time, it is necessary to address the symptoms with a reliable and regulated medication. Although these results may make clinicians feel uncomfortable with and reluctant to recommend or advocate their use, CAM products may be an alternative for people who are sensitive to pharmaceutical-grade compounds or cannot tolerate the lowest, weakest dosage form available.

Assessing Herbal Consumption

There are a variety of potentially adverse herb–drug interactions based on the pharmacological properties of both herbal and prescription medications. The rate of potential and observed adverse herb–drug interactions seen clinically and in research are reportedly 40% (Bush et al., 2007; Geller & Studee, 2007). This high rate makes it vital that CAM–drug interactions become a topic of discussion for clients and caregivers.

Clients often combine prescription medications with complementary and alternative medications without telling their health care providers, and health care providers often fail to ask clients about CAM use. It is important to introduce a discussion of CAM use when assessing clients in order to avoid CAM–drug interactions. Table 33-4 on page 888 identifies commonly used natural medicines (including herbals) that should not be taken in combination with psychotropics. A nonjudgmental approach and an open dialogue about the use of CAM are more likely to yield relevant information. See the Rx Communication feature on page 132 in Chapter 7 for examples of a conversation about this topic.

INCOMPATIBILITIES AND UNCOMMON MEDICATION COMBINATIONS

Nurses have many responsibilities to clients receiving neuroleptic drugs. To ensure the bioavailability and effectiveness of neuroleptic medications, it is important to understand the relationships between the medication and the liquid (or substance) with which it is administered, as well as the relationships between medications. Some medications are not compatible with all substances. For an overview of the compatibility of medications and typical liquids, see Table 7-5 on page 129.

In addition to liquid and drug compatibilities, you need to be aware of other problematic combinations—for example, the combination of grapefruit juice and several psychiatric medications, such as the anxiolytic medications triazolam (Halcion) and buspirone (BuSpar). When taken with grapefruit juice, triazolam is not metabolized efficiently and therefore remains at higher levels in the body, and buspirone blood levels can be raised to nine times the normal. The explanation for this resides in the furanocoumarins in grapefruit juice and their ability to inhibit a liver enzyme (cytochrome P_{450}3A4 or CYP3A4) from metabolizing the medication out of the system (see Chapter 7∞). This action allows the medication and its metabolites to remain in the system longer than usual, where it accumulates, causing higher blood levels, enhanced effects of the medication, and greater side effects (Laustsen, Gilbert, & Wimett, 2007).

Ultimately, either of these mechanisms, cytochrome P_{450} activation or inhibition, can be accomplished through a variety of interactions among drugs, foods, liquids, or substances (e.g., nicotine). Maintaining a holistic view of your clients and their medications will alert you to drug–drug interactions as well as the dynamism of drug metabolism.

As drug combinations and innovative psychobiologic therapies become more commonplace in the practice of psychiatry, psychiatric–mental health nurses must be observant for idiosyncratic responses among clients. Knowing the interactive effects of medications is an important feature of effective psychopharmacologic nursing. Planning and implementing care for this specialized client subpopulation are likely to be challenging, and you need to be aware of the underlying psychobiology to recognize potential drug-related behaviors among clients who are on multiple-drug regimens (see Chapter 7).

Polypharmacy (using more than one medication to treat a set of symptoms) with second-generation antipsychotics (SGAs) is quite frequent among chronic clients who have severe and persistent mental illness. The practice of adding another medication as an adjunct to address persistent symptoms has become more frequent lately. When one SGA, such as risperidone, is used to treat psychotic symptoms, the client may still experience sleep difficulties. Adding another SGA such as quetiapine (Seroquel) at bedtime could further address the psychosis while providing sedation sufficient to allow quality sleep. Some research does not support the use of polypharmacy with SGAs, but methodological shortcomings have been noted in the research that may have prevented detection of a true, positive effect (Megna et al., 2007).

MediaLink Case Study: Medication Adherence

ADHERENCE ISSUES

The current estimate of treatment adherence by recipients of psychiatric services, including adherence to prescribed medication regimens, is that less than 35% take the medication that they should (Velligan et al., 2007). Responding to this treatment reality—two thirds do not adhere to their medication regimen—involves examining the reasons for nonadherence and generating creative nursing solutions to the problem. The Your Assessment Approach feature lists possible factors that contribute to medication nonadherence.

Many people who take prescribed psychotropic medications find it difficult to continue taking them over the long term. There are many factors that contribute to nonadherence to a medication regimen. Sometimes these medications can have uncomfortable or awkward side effects. Side effects are a major cause of nonadherence. Sometimes clients do not have a proper orientation about what to expect from these medications. The schedule of doses or the route of medication administration may be inconvenient or stressful for the client. Furthermore, the client's friends or relatives may not be entirely supportive of the client's continued adherence to the psychotropic regimen.

Because all these factors can impair medication adherence, it is important that treatment includes interventions designed to help overcome any or all of these difficulties to the extent possible. Efforts to enhance adherence should be a standard feature of psychiatric–mental health nursing care. The Your Intervention Strategies feature on page 867 suggests a number of avenues to explore when partnering with clients in this aspect of care.

These interventions can include supportive individual contacts with clients, family meetings, psychoeducation regarding specific medications and their effects, and communicating a basic interest in how the client is reacting to his or her course of medications. The goal in creating a collaborative environment of care is to incorporate better client-specific interventions than those contributing to nonadherence. Enlisting the cooperation and involvement of families in implementing interventions as appropriate also helps to promote adherence.

YOUR ASSESSMENT APPROACH
Factors That Contribute to Medication Nonadherence

- Experiencing problems with prescribed psychotropic medications
- Severe level of symptomatology
- Cognitive impairments
- Negative effect of the medication on the client's adjustment
- Decreased motivation to collaborate in treatment
- Effect of the medication on the client's interpersonal relationships
- Paternalistic attitudes toward clients that interfere with partnering with clients in medication-based treatment planning decisions
- Substance use or abuse
- Lack of support from significant others
- Cultural attitudes and beliefs
- Insufficient or inadequate care planning

YOUR INTERVENTION STRATEGIES
Adherence Enhancers

The following are ideas you can use to make it easier for clients to maintain their prescribed medication regimen:

- Discuss their health behaviors and perceptions with clients and their families.
- Use atypical antipsychotic medications—they have a lower side effect profile and can increase adherence because they are easier on the body.
- Change to another medication with a different neurotransmitter action that may have a different or more tolerable side effect.
- Employ role playing and assertiveness in practice sessions with clients that teach them how to report the range and severity of side effects, from dry mouth to priapism.
- Teach clients how to manage the side effects (and therefore continue taking the medication) by making side effects more tolerable (e.g., hard candy for dry mouth, rubber pillowcase liner for nighttime drooling [sialorrhea]).
- Arrange for reminders well before discharge from inpatient settings, especially with geriatric clients, to maximize both knowledge and adherence (knowledge can be the number-1 factor that determines whether or not a client adheres to his or her medication regimen).
- Simplify the medication regimen.
- Discuss with clients their expectations of the medication to determine whether those expectations are realistic.
- Use concrete educators that are known to enhance cognition—pamphlets, booklets, handbooks, workbooks, sheets, cards, videos, audiotapes, posters, magnets, logs, journals, computers, MP3 players, etc.
- Enhance the client's control over the treatment regimen by offering real choices.
- Teach the client how to self-administer medications as soon as possible in the inpatient setting.
- Involve the client in planning for and learning to problem solve.
- Provide support from peers who will share how this medication could help with symptoms.
- Give depot medications weekly, biweekly, or monthly so that the client does not have to remember to take pills.
- Repeat relevant information on a number of occasions with patience, especially with clients who have schizophrenia and depression.
- Develop reminders to serve as cues to remembering. Wearing a rubber band on the wrist is a visual cue reminding the client "When I see this I need to take my pills" or "When I eat lunch I need to take my pills." Calendars, to-do lists, and alarm clocks or alarms on wristwatches or cell phones can also be helpful.
- Recommend the use of pillboxes, which come in many shapes, sizes, and organizational styles (marked for multiple daily doses, layers for time of day, timers with small alarm clock feature that opens compartment). If the medication cannot be taken out of its original container without affecting potency, placing a small button or candy in the pillbox will serve as a reminder.
- Keep all medications and information about them in one dry, cool place, not in the bathroom or by the sink or dishwasher in the kitchen.
- Refer the client to social services, where it can be determined whether financial assistance might be available.
- Arrange for the client to teach others (other clients or significant others) about their medications once they have learned sufficiently. Nothing speeds learning as much as teaching others.
- Encourage the client to be hopeful about his or her ability to manage symptoms.

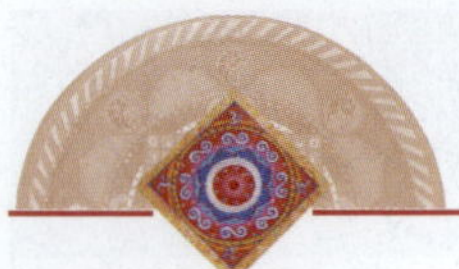

EXPLORE MEDIALINK

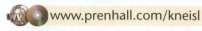

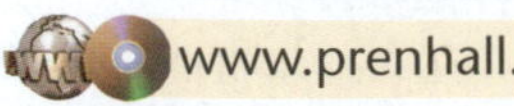

For NCLEX-RN® review questions, case studies, and other resources for this chapter see the Pearson Health MediaLink CD-ROM that accompanies this book and the Companion Website at www.prenhall.com/kneisl.

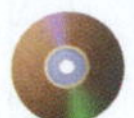

CD-ROM
Audio Glossary
NCLEX-RN® Review Questions
Videos
- *Hands & Arms Tremor*
- *Grasping Tremor*
- *Lateral Tremor*
- *EPSE: Dystonia/Akathisia*
- *EPSE: Akinesia & Pill Rolling*
- *EPSE: Parkinsonism*
- *EPSE: Bradykinesia (Shuffling Gait)*
- *EPSE: Tardive Dyskinesia (Mouth, Trunk, Ambulation)*

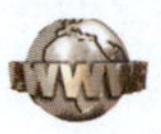

Companion Website
Audio Glossary
NCLEX-RN® Review Questions
Critical Thinking Exercise
- *Cultural Issues and Medication*

Case Study
- *Medication Adherence*

Care Plan
- *The Exercising Client on Lithium*

MediaLinks
MediaLink Application
- *Weighty Issues*

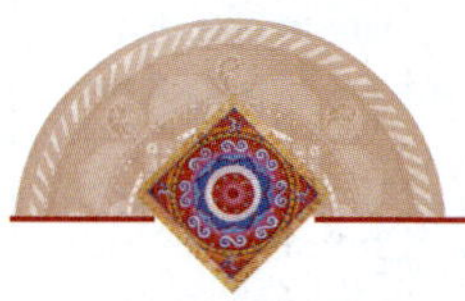

NCLEX-RN® REVIEW QUESTIONS

1. A nurse is assessing a client to determine the effectiveness of the psychotropic medication the client has been taking. Which of the following assessment findings is reason for concern? (Select all that apply.)
1. Elevated blood pressure
2. Increased agitation
3. Bradycardia
4. Increased thirst
5. Restful sleep pattern

2. Within 3 days of beginning a new antipsychotic medication, the client reports severe muscle spasms. This adverse effect is known as:
1. Parkinsonian syndrome.
2. Akathisia.
3. Tardive dyskinesia.
4. Dystonia.

3. The nurse is educating the client and family member on the symptoms associated with drug-induced parkinsonism. What safety factors should the nurse emphasize in the teaching plan?
1. Maintain clear walkways throughout the house.
2. Limit the client's mobility and activity while on the medications.
3. Encourage the client to drink extra fluids to prevent dry mouth.
4. Discontinue the medication if symptoms of drug-induced parkinsonism appear.

4. A client with major depression with suicidal ideations and psychomotor retardation has been taking antidepressants for 2 weeks. What is the priority nursing assessment for this client?
1. Blood pressure
2. Suicidality
3. Sleep patterns
4. Nutrition

5. The nurse plans to provide client education about the side effects of antipsychotic medications to a client with delusions and psychosis. When should the nurse provide the client with the educational material?
1. Prior to administering the first dose of medication
2. Twenty-four hours after the first dose of medication
3. When the client is stabilized and psychotic symptoms are manageable
4. Client education is not required for clients who have psychotic behaviors.

6. A client on antipsychotic medications presents with symptoms of hyperprolactinemia. What symptom should the nurse assess for?
1. Weight gain
2. Dry mouth
3. Constipation
4. Difficulty achieving orgasms

7. A psychotic client with a family history of diabetes and hypertension is started on an antipsychotic. Which of the following symptoms should the nurse monitor the client most closely for?
1. Constipation
2. Decreased libido
3. Insatiable thirst
4. Drowsiness

8. At the 2-month follow-up visit at the mental health clinic, the client tells the nurse he stopped taking the clomipramine (Anafranil) 6 weeks ago because of the side effects. What symptoms should the nurse expect to observe in the client?
1. Increased drowsiness and slurred speech
2. Orthostatic hypotension
3. Repeatedly folding pages in a magazine
4. Increased appetite

9. The nurse is assessing the client with schizophrenia who is taking clozapine (Clozaril). Which of the following findings should the nurse report immediately to the prescriber?
1. Dry mouth
2. Constipation
3. Elevated body temperature
4. Decreased platelet count

10. What is the priority nursing diagnosis for the client experiencing neuroleptic malignant syndrome?
1. Activity Intolerance
2. Risk for Aspiration
3. Risk for Imbalanced Fluid Volume
4. Hyperthermia

See Appendix C for answers.

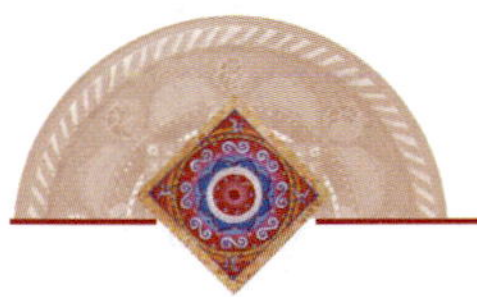

REFERENCES

Bisanz, A. (2007). Chronic constipation. *American Journal of Nursing, 107*(4), 72B–72H.

Brahm, N. C., McElwain, D. L., & Brown, R. C. (2007). Potential aripiprazole-mediated extrapyramidal symptoms in an adult with developmental disabilities. *American Journal of Health-System Pharmacy, 64*(8), 827–829.

Brunelle, J., Guigueno, S., Gouin, P., Tamion, F., & Thibaut, F. (2007). Aripiprazole and neuroleptic malignant syndrome. *Journal of Clinical Psychopharmacology, 27*(2), 212–214.

Bush, T. M., Rayburn, K. S., Holloway, S. W., Sanchez-Yamamoto, D. S., Allen, B. L., Lam, T., et al. (2007). Adverse interactions between herbal and dietary substances and prescription medications: A clinical survey. *Alternative Therapies in Health and Medicine, 13*(2), 30–35.

Carlo, A. A., Bobo, W. V., & Meltzer, H. Y. (2007). Factors affecting outcome in schizophrenia and their relevance for psychopharmacological treatment. *International Clinical Psychopharmacology, 22*(5), 249–267.

Chrisman, N. J. (2007). Extending cultural competence through systems change: Academic, hospital, and community partnerships. *Journal of Transcultural Nursing, 18*(1), Supplement: 68S–76S.

Clemens, N. A. (2007). Deconstructing depression. *Journal of Psychiatric Practice, 13*(2), 106–108.

Cohen, A. (2007). An examination of the relationship between commitments and culture among five cultural groups of Israeli teachers. *Journal of Cross-Cultural Psychology, 38*(1), 34–49.

Demaerschalk, B. M., & Wingerchuk, D. M. (2007). Treatment of vascular dementia and vascular cognitive impairment. *Neurologist, 13*(1), 37–41.

Engel, B. (2007). Eagle soaring: The power of the resilient self. *Journal of Psychosocial Nursing and Mental Health Services, 45*(2), 44–48, 49–51.

Ferentz, K. S. (2007). A guide to switching antidepressant therapy. *Patient Care, 41*(1), 16–21.

Flaskerud, J. H. (2007a). Cultural competence: What is it? *Issues in Mental Health Nursing, 28*(1), 121–123.

Flaskerud, J. H. (2007b). Cultural competence column: What else is necessary? *Issues in Mental Health Nursing, 28*(2), 219–222.

Freeman, B., Levy, W., & Gorman, J. M. (2007). Successful monotherapy treatment with aripiprazole in a patient with schizophrenia and prolactinoma. *Journal of Psychiatric Practice, 13*(2), 120–124.

Geller, S. E., & Studee, L. (2007). Botanical and dietary supplements for mood and anxiety in menopausal women. *Menopause, 14*(3), 541–549.

Girgis, S., Huckstep, B., Oakley, J., Ferriter, M., & Nikolaou, V. (2007). QTc-interval abnormalities in a forensic population. *Criminal Behaviour & Mental Health, 17*(2), 75–88.

Gupta, A., Lawrence, A. T., Krishnan, K., Kavinsky, C. J., & Trohman, R. G. (2007). Current concepts in the mechanisms and management of drug-induced QT prolongation and torsade de pointes. *American Heart Journal, 153*(6), 891–899.

Gurrera, R. J., Simpson, J. C., & Tsuang, M. T. (2007). Meta-analytic evidence of systematic bias in estimates of neuroleptic malignant syndrome incidence. *Comprehensive Psychiatry, 48*(2), 205–211.

Haleem, D. J., Samad, N., & Haleem, M. A. (2007). Reversal of haloperidol-induced extrapyramidal symptoms by buspirone: A time-related study. *Behavioural Pharmacology, 18*(2), 147–153.

Holcomb, S. S. (2007). Putting insomnia to rest. *Nurse Practitioner, 32*(4), 28–34.

Kemp, W. L., Fitzgerald, J., & White, C. L. III. (2007). Undiagnosed progressive supranuclear palsy in a patient with neuroleptic malignant syndrome due to use of neuroleptics: The utility of autopsy in deaths due to known drug reactions. *American Journal of Forensic Medicine & Pathology, 28*(1), 59–62.

Knight, J. R., Sanchez, L. T., Sherritt, L., Bresnahan, L. R., & Fromson, J. A. (2007). Outcomes of a monitoring program for physicians with mental and behavioral health problems. *Journal of Psychiatric Practice, 13*(1), 25–32.

Krishnamurthy, M. N., & Telles, S. (2007). Assessing depression following two ancient Indian interventions. *Journal of Gerontological Nursing, 33*(2), 17–23.

Laustsen, G., Gilbert, M., & Wimett, L. (2007). Drug approvals. *Nurse Practitioner, 32*(2), 43–51.

Lipson, J. G., & DeSantis, L. A. (2007). Current approaches to integrating elements of cultural competence in nursing education. *Journal of Transcultural Nursing, 18*(1), Supplement: 10S–20S.

Megna, J. L., Kunwar, A. R., Mahlotra, K., Sauro, M. D., Devitt, P. J., & Rashid, A. (2007). A study of polypharmacy with second-generation antipsychotics in patients with severe and persistent mental illness. *Journal of Psychiatric Practice, 13*(2), 129–137.

Morris, G. H., Naimark, D., & Haroun, A. M. (2005). Informed consent in psychopharmacology. *Journal of Clinical Psychopharmacology, 25*(5), 403–406.

Parker, G. (2007). Is the diagnosis of melancholia important in shaping clinical management? *Current Opinion in Psychiatry, 20*(3), 197–201.

Remington, G. (2007). Tardive dyskinesia: Eliminated, forgotten, or overshadowed? *Current Opinion in Psychiatry, 20*(2), 131–137.

Tammenmaa, I. A., Sailas, E., McGrath, J. J., Soares-Weiser, K., & Wahlbeck, K. (2004). Systematic review of cholinergic drugs for neuroleptic-induced tardive dyskinesia: A meta-analysis of randomized controlled trials. *Progress in Neuro-Psychopharmacology & Biological Psychiatry, 28*(7), 1099–1107.

Thachil, A. F., Mohan, R., & Bhugra, D. (2007). The evidence base of complementary and alternative therapies in depression. *Journal of Affective Disorders, 97*(1–3), 23–35.

Velligan, D. I., Wang, M., Diamond, P. D., Glahn, D. C., Castillo, D., Bendle, S., et al. (2007). Relationships among subjective and objective measures of adherence to oral antipsychotic medications. *Psychiatric Services, 58,* 1187–1192.

Zhang, Z. J., Kang, W. H., Tan, Q., Li, Q., Gao, C. G., Zhang, F. G., et al. (2007). Adjunctive herbal medicine with carbamazepine for bipolar disorders: A double-blind, randomized, placebo-controlled study. *Journal of Psychiatric Research, 41*(3–4), 360–369.

ADDITIONAL REFERENCES

American Nurses Association Task Force on Psychopharmacology. (1994). *Psychiatric–mental health nursing psychopharmacology project.* Washington, DC: American Nurses Association.

Becker, M. E., Hertzberg, M. A., Moore, S. D., Dennis, M. F., Bukenya, D. S., & Beckham, J. C. (2007). A placebo-controlled trial of bupropion SR in the treatment of chronic posttraumatic stress disorder. *Journal of Clinical Psychopharmacology, 27*(2), 193–197.

Bozikas, V. P., Kosmidis, M. H., Giannakou, M., Anezoulaki, D., Petrikis, P., Fokas, K., et al. (2007). Humor appreciation deficit in schizophrenia: The relevance of basic neurocognitive functioning. *Journal of Nervous & Mental Disease, 195*(4), 325–331.

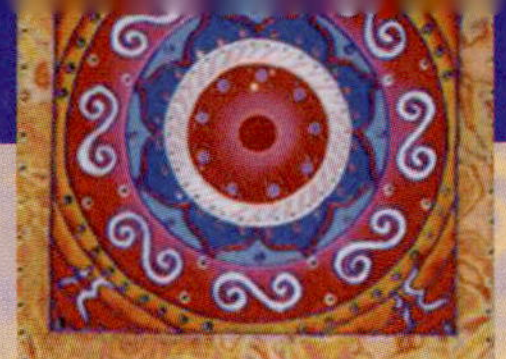

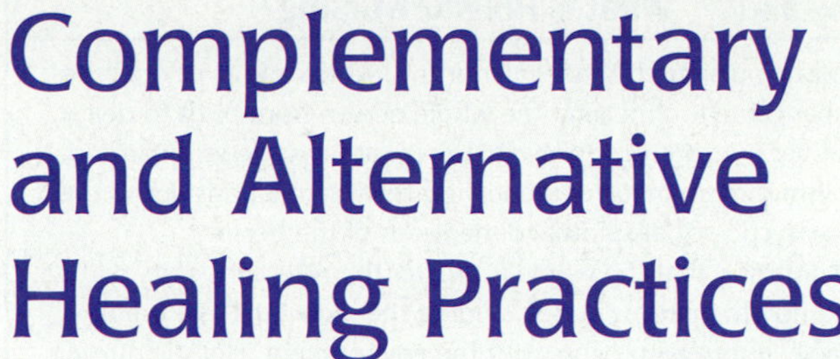

Complementary and Alternative Healing Practices

CHAPTER 33

CAROL REN KNEISL

LEARNING OUTCOMES

After completing this chapter, you will be able to:

1. Identify the therapeutic uses for each of the complementary and alternative medicine (CAM) techniques discussed in this chapter.
2. Compare and contrast various CAM techniques, including their important characteristics and functions.
3. Integrate appropriate CAM techniques into a plan of care to promote, maintain, and restore emotional well-being for clients and their families.
4. Encourage clients and their family members to become educated consumers by educating them about the safety and effectiveness of CAM techniques, quackery and fraud, the qualifications of providers, and quality of service delivery.
5. Educate clients and their families in the effective use of CAM therapies.
6. Identify the natural medicines used for psychiatric symptoms and their effectiveness and safety.
7. Determine when a client should not use natural medicines in combination with prescribed psychopharmacologic medications.
8. Integrate CAM strategies into personal and professional functioning.

CRITICAL THINKING CHALLENGE

You and three of your classmates are discussing your most recent clinical experiences. Jenny tells the story of a toddler she was caring for on the pediatric oncology unit. LaTonya and Shi-An share what it's like to work in the intensive care unit. You discuss the events of your day in the psychiatric emergency room. The four of you agree that stress is, and will continue to be, a part of your nursing life regardless of your area of clinical practice. The four of you also agree that living and working in a high-tech, stressful environment causes you to feel apprehensive and to worry about your ability to live your life to its fullest potential.

1. Should you anticipate that stress will continue to be a part of your nursing life regardless of your area of clinical practice? Why?
2. How can this chapter help you and your classmates cope with the stresses in your nursing life?
3. Why should complementary and alternative healing practices be integrated into the care plan for a client when appropriate?

MEDIALINK 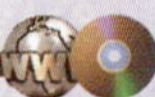 www.prenhall.com/kneisl

Go to the Pearson Health MediaLink CD-ROM and the Companion Website at www.prenhall.com/kneisl for interactive resources for this chapter.

KEY TERMS

acupressure *883*
acupuncture *883*
alternative therapies *872*
biofeedback *886*
chakras *883*
complementary and alternative medicine (CAM) *872*
complementary therapies *872*
deep breathing *878*
eye movement desensitization and reprocessing (EMDR) *886*
guided imagery *879*
imagery *879*
integrative medicine *872*
mantra *882*
massage *885*
medical meditation *882*
meditation *881*
progressive relaxation *878*
reflexology *883*
Reiki *885*
repetitive transcranial magnetic stimulation (rTMS) *886*
Therapeutic Touch (TT) *885*
visualization *879*

In many cultures around the world, health care and medical practices that are not currently an integral part of conventional Western medicine are used to relieve pain and cure illnesses. In Western culture they are referred to as **complementary and alternative medicine (CAM)**. **Complementary therapies** are those used in conjunction with conventional medical practices. **Alternative therapies** are those that are used instead of conventional medicine. **Integrative medicine** or integrative therapies combines conventional medicine and CAM methods for which there is quality evidence of safety and effectiveness. Integrative medicine is being used more often in hospitals, medical centers, and universities in North America as increasing numbers of contemporary Western health care providers incorporate the most appropriate, safe, and effective of ancient traditions and healing approaches into their practice.

Programs in integrative medicine and CAM clinical centers are in existence in several settings such as the University of Arizona in Tucson, Beth Israel Deaconess Medical Center and Harvard University in Boston, University of Maryland, University of Michigan, University of Toronto in Canada, and many other centers in North America. In fact, 95% of U.S. academic centers surveyed in a recent study provide some CAM clinical care (Nedrow, 2006).

Nursing, with its tradition of holistic care—providing care for the whole person (mind, body, and spirit) in all its uniqueness—is especially well suited to deliver integrative therapy. Florence Nightingale herself encouraged holistic care by recognizing the importance of the environment, touch, light, aromatics, music, and quiet reflection to the healing process. Holistic nursing promotes healing in clients, families, social groups, communities, and health care practitioners themselves (Hagedorn & Zahourek, 2007). The tools that holistic nurses use to facilitate healing and help their clients find meaning in their life experiences are presence, intent, unconditional acceptance, love, and compassion (Erickson, 2007). Several schools of nursing—New York University, University of Texas at Austin, and Tennessee State University, among others—offer graduate or certificate programs in holistic nursing. Holistic nursing is described in Box 33-1.

Complementary and alternative approaches such as those described in this chapter provide nurses with yet another way to promote clients' well-being.

Box 33-1 What Is Holistic Nursing?

Holistic nursing embraces all nursing, which has as its goal the enhancement of healing the whole person from birth to death. Holistic nursing recognizes that there are two views regarding holism: holism involves identifying the interrelationships of the bio-psycho-social-spiritual dimensions of the person, recognizing that the whole is greater than the sum of its parts; and holism involves understanding the individual as a unitary whole in mutual process with the environment. Holistic nursing responds to both views, believing that the goals of nursing can be achieved within either framework.

The holistic nurse is an instrument of healing and a facilitator in the healing process. Holistic nurses honor the individual's subjective experience about health, health beliefs, and values. To become therapeutic partners with individuals, families, and communities, holistic nursing practice draws on nursing knowledge, theories, research, expertise, intuition, and creativity. Holistic nursing practice encourages peer review of professional practice in various clinical settings and integrates knowledge of current professional standards, laws, and regulations governing nursing practice.

Practicing holistic nursing requires nurses to integrate self-care, self-responsibility, spirituality, and reflection in their lives. This may lead the nurse to greater awareness of the interconnectedness with self, others, nature, and God/Life Force/Absolute/Transcendent. This awareness may further enhance the nurses' understanding of all individuals and their relationships to the human and global community, and permits nurses to use this awareness to facilitate the healing process.

Source: Reprinted with permission from American Holistic Nurses' Association. (2007). *What is holistic nursing?* Retrieved November 2, 2007, from http://www.ahna.org/about/whatis.html.

DISCOVERING AND REDISCOVERING CAM

Ancient traditions and healing practices such as those discussed in this chapter, as well as prayer and animal-assisted therapy, are being discovered by consumers and rediscovered by providers of health care in Western culture. Increasing numbers of consumers are seeking out CAM on their own, asking questions of their health care providers, and requesting that CAM be added to their plan of care. Health care providers are finding it easier to find articles on CAM in respected non-CAM medical and nursing journals.

National Center for CAM

In 1992, the Office of Alternative Medicine was established at the National Institutes of Health (NIH) in response to increasing interest in CAM among the general population. This office has funded and studied a wide range of CAM therapies. Before this time, most studies of CAM had serious methodologic problems, and their lack of scientific validity was justly criticized. The results of the office's scientifically designed and implemented studies led to greater acceptance by the medical community and increased credibility for CAM. As a result, the office was upgraded in 1998 to a fully recognized national center at the NIH and is now called the National Center for Complementary and Alternative Medicine (NCCAM). Much of the research in CAM today is funded by the NCCAM. You can access the NCCAM database at http://www.nccam.nih.gov through a direct resource link on the Companion Website for this book.

Five major domains of complementary and alternative medicine have been identified by the NCCAM. They are listed, with examples, in Table 33-1 ■.

Consumers of CAM

In national surveys, anywhere from 50% to 80% of respondents report using at least one CAM therapy in their lifetime. Many health care providers are surprised to find that their clients use CAM at the following rates:

MediaLink National Center for Complementary and Alternative Medicine

TABLE 33-1 ■ NCCAM's Major Domains of Complementary and Alternative Therapies

Whole Medical Systems	Mind–Body Medicine	Biologically Based Practices	Manipulative and Body-Based Practices	Energy Therapies
■ Traditional Chinese medicine ■ Ayurveda ■ Homeopathic medicine ■ Naturopathic medicine	■ Meditation ■ Yoga ■ Hypnosis ■ Art, music, and dance therapy ■ Biofeedback ■ Prayer ■ Visual imagery ■ Relaxation	■ Herbal products ■ Special diet therapies and dietary supplements ■ Vitamins or minerals ■ Natural substances such as bee pollen or shark cartilage	■ Chiropractic or osteopathic manipulation ■ Tai chi ■ Rolfing ■ Massage	■ Healing touch ■ Reiki ■ Bioelectromagnetic-based therapies ■ Qi gong

Note: This list represents the major CAM therapies in use. It is not all-inclusive.

Source: Adapted from *Major domains of complementary and alternative medicine*, National Center for Complementary and Alternative Medicine, National Institutes of Health, Bethesda, MD. Retrieved October 12, 2007, from http://nccam.nih.gov/.

- 82% of older adults with anxiety or depression and 65% of older adults without these conditions (Grzywacz et al., 2006)
- 68% of persons treated in emergency departments (Taylor, Walsham, Taylor, & Wong, 2006b)
- Over 1.6 million noninstitutionalized adult U.S. citizens with insomnia or trouble sleeping (Pearson, Johnson, & Nahin, 2006)
- Approximately 66% of people with arthritis (Herman, Dente, Allen, & Hunt, 2006) in one study and more than 80% in another (Katz & Lee, 2007)
- 69% of breast cancer survivors (Matthews, Sellergren, Huo, List, & Fleming, 2007)
- 52% of children with autism spectrum disorders in one study (Wong & Smith, 2006), and 74% in another (Hanson et al., 2007)
- More than half of menopausal women (Gold et al., 2007)
- 20% of people hospitalized with coronary artery disease (Decker et al., 2007)

Similar results are found in studies of persons with stress, allergies, neurologic problems, HIV, gastrointestinal disorders, diabetes, chronic sinusitis, and other physical and emotional problems. There is no question that the move toward CAM reflects a consumer-driven health care environment.

People use CAM methods for several reasons. The most common reasons are listed in Box 33-2.

Sociocultural Aspects

The use of CAM, and the reasons for use, are likely to vary among racial and ethnic groups because its use is related to cultural and health beliefs (Hsiao et al., 2006). A national telephone survey of over 3,000 women found that non-Hispanic white women were most likely to cite personal beliefs for CAM use (Chao, Wade, Kronenberg, Kalmuss, & Cushman, 2006). The cost of conventional medicine was the most prevalent reason among Mexican-American women. Media sources, family and friends, and physician referral were most influential among non-Hispanic white women. Informal networks of family and friends were the most important social influences of CAM use among African-, Mexican-, and Chinese-American women.

A study of Asian Americans found that herbal medicines are used more often by Chinese Americans (32%), and mind/body therapies by Asian Indians (31%) and Filipinos (22%) than by non-Hispanic whites (Mehta, Phillips, Davis, & McCarthy, 2007). This same study reported that Asian Americans are less likely than non-Hispanic whites to disclose the use of CAM methodologies to conventional health care providers. The use of herbal and natural supplements is also prevalent among Hispanics and lowest among African Americans (Kelly, Kaufman, Kelley, Rosenberg, & Mitchell, 2006). Another study found reluctance to disclose CAM use among Hispanics and non-Hispanic blacks (Graham et al., 2005). This suggests that it is particularly important to query these populations about CAM use. In an increasingly diverse society, understanding the rationales, motivations, and differences in and reasons for CAM use will enhance the cultural competence of health care professionals, shed light on cultural and social factors related to health behaviors, and help address the need for health care improvements among minority populations.

Box 33-2 Reasons People Seek CAM Therapies

- Wanting greater control over their lives
- Having a sense of responsibility for their own health care
- Wanting a more holistic orientation in health care so that body, mind, and spirit are addressed
- Concern over the side effects of conventional therapies
- Concern over the financial cost of conventional medicine
- Finding the results of conventional treatments to be inadequate
- Identifying with a particular philosophy or practice because of cultural background

MEDIALINK Application: Older Americans Not Discussing CAM Use with Doctors

MEDIALINK Critical Thinking Exercise: Explaining Allopathy vs. CAM

NURSING ROLE IN CAM

Nurses have several imporant roles in relationship to CAM approaches and integrative therapies. We are often in a position of being able to: identify whether a client is currently using CAM therapies; identify a client's need for CAM; suggest CAM therapies to treatment team members and to clients, their family members, or their friends; encourage clients to consider using a CAM therapy if appropriate; enlist the support of the treatment team, family members, and friends; and help clients to find providers.

Second, we may be CAM practitioners ourselves. Nurses may be practitioners of CAM therapies in a variety of settings—hospital, outpatient clinic, home, community, private practice office, and so on. The most common CAM therapies that nurses provide are relaxation techniques (such as deep breathing, active progressive relaxation, visualization, and meditation), bodywork techniques (such as massage), and energy therapies (such as Therapeutic Touch and Reiki). Some of these therapies, such as the relaxation techniques, visualization, meditation, and therapeutic touch, are discussed in detail in this chapter. CAM therapies that require further training or equipment or are usually provided by others are discussed briefly.

Third, we are teachers of CAM therapies. Nurses play a significant role in making clients and their families aware of these methods and teaching them how to use them effectively. As health care educators, we have an important role in encouraging clients to be informed health consumers. And fourth, we can coordinate the integration of CAM services into a client's plan of care, as illustrated in the Evidence-Based Practice feature.

Helping Clients Become Informed Health Consumers

Integrative CAM approaches are creative and powerful tools under the following circumstances:

1. The approach used has been demonstrated to be safe and effective.
2. The method is appropriate for that particular client.
3. The client learns to use the method properly.

The appropriateness of individual CAM methods and guidelines for proper use are identified later in this chapter in the discussion of techniques. Safety and effectiveness, the expertise of the practitioner, quality of service delivery, inte-

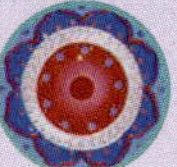

EVIDENCE-BASED PRACTICE

HELPING CLIENTS BECOME INFORMED CAM CONSUMERS

Judy Krasinski is a psychiatric–mental health nurse and a member of the treatment team in the wellness center of a large urban medical center. Jammela, a new client, has recently been referred to the wellness center for evaluation of anxiety and depression, as well as an evaluation of the herbs and other natural medicines she is taking. Jammela has HIV and is on a HAART (highly active antiretroviral therapy) regimen to treat her symptoms. Judy was aware that some HIV clients use CAM as an alternative to their HAART regimen rather than to complement it. Using HAART inconsistently is problematic given its association with drug resistance.

Jammela has been on edge, worries about her future constantly, and has been moody and feeling blue. The results of the Beck Depression Inventory indicated that she is moderately depressed. Her depression has not improved despite treatment with paroxetine (Paxil) and then citalopram (Celexa). When Judy found that Jammela has also been taking garlic supplements, she became even more concerned, knowing that garlic supplements have been found to inhibit the effectiveness of saquinavir, one of the protease inhibitors in Jammela's medication protocol. Judy also learned that Jammela has not informed her prescriber of the herbs and other products she takes because she felt it wasn't important for her doctor to have this information and, that in any case, the doctor might not approve.

In addition to providing Jammela with information about the effects of garlic supplements on protease inhibitors, Judy met with the other members of the team to discuss the possibility of CAM therapies other than herbs or dietary supplements to enhance Jammela's treatment for anxiety and depression. The team has suggested two programs based on the following research to augment her treatment: massage therapy and a mindfulness meditation program.

Carmody, J., & Baer, R. A. (2007, September 25). Relationships between mindfulness practice and levels of mindfulness, medical and psychological symptoms and well-being in a mindfulness-based stress reduction program. *Journal of Behavioral Medicine*, Epub.

Finucane, A., & Mercer, S. W. (2006). An exploratory mixed methods study of the acceptability and effectiveness of Mindfulness-Based Cognitive Therapy for patients with active depression and anxiety in primary care. *BMC Psychiatry, 7*, 6–14.

Owen-Smith, A., Diclemente, R., & Wingood, G. (2007). Complementary and alternative medicine use decreases adherence to HAART in HIV-positive women. *AIDS Care, 19*(5), 589–593.

CRITICAL THINKING APPLICATION

1. Since Jammela is also depressed and anxious, what other herbal or dietary supplements should you assess for?
2. Why did the team recommend massage therapy?
3. How does mindfulness meditation help with anxiety?

grating CAM into a treatment plan, and quackery and fraud are discussed next.

Safety and Effectiveness

Many CAM therapies are not well regulated and researched. Some of the problems in determining the evidence base for CAM have to do with inconsistency across studies, variations in methodology, inadequate sample size, and problematic study design, making it difficult to judge the clinical significance of the results. You can determine the safety and effectiveness of CAM methods and read any consumer advisories and news releases about the most recent research by accessing NCCAM's website at http://www.nccam.nih.gov. Another source is the current literature. The National Library of Medicine (NLM) and NCCAM have jointly developed a means of easy access to the literature on CAM from 1966 to the present. Over 12 million CAM journal citations can be found on NLM's PubMed at http://www.pubmed.gov, which can be accessed through a direct link on this text's Companion Website.

Remember to be an inquiring consumer of research. An investigation of the contents of complementary and alternative medicine journals cautions that fewer articles in 2005 than in the previous 10 years were of clinical trials and the proportion of positive articles was greater, thus suggesting bias and appearing not to adequately reflect the best available effectiveness evidence (Coelho, Pittier, & Ernst, 2007).

Encourage your clients to become informed health consumers. Help them to gather the following information about CAM:

- Advantages and disadvantages
- Risks
- Side effects and adverse effects
- Expected results
- Length of treatment
- Interaction with conventional Western medications

Clients can also gather information in informal ways, such as testimonials by others. However, while testimonials from others who are or have been clients may be helpful, they should not be the sole criterion in selecting a therapy. Informed health care consumers and health care practitioners will seek information on controlled scientific trials such as those summarized on the websites listed earlier.

MediaLink CAM Safety

By helping clients become informed health consumers, you also help them to avoid fraudulently marketed products that:

- Are useless (such as electronic devices that claim to cure serious illnesses by sending electrical energy into the body)
- Have serious medication interaction risks (such as those that may cause a reduction in the therapeutic effect of oral contraceptives and medications used to treat HIV or prevent transplant rejection)

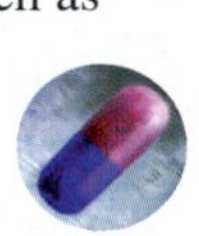

Tips on avoiding fraudulently marketed products are listed in the Partnering with Clients and Families feature. A guide to fraud, quackery, and informed decision making is available on http://www.quackwatch.com, a website maintained by a physician. This data can be accessed through a link on the Companion Website for this text.

Practitioner Expertise

Encourage clients to examine the background, qualifications, and competence of a potential CAM practitioner. If there is licensure or certification for the particular CAM practice, is the practitioner licensed or certified? National organizations of CAM practitioners can provide referrals as well as information on legislation and state registration or licensing. Nurses who practice CAM methods can be credentialed by any one of several specialty bodies and/or the American Holistic Nurses' Association, or licensed to practice specific CAM therapies in states where their use is governmentally regulated. Health regulatory bodies can provide information on state licensure or registration and any complaints lodged against specific practitioners.

Encourage clients to also talk with other health care providers or former clients, who may be able to address the question of competence and the quality of the services the practitioner provides. Clients should actually interview the CAM practitioner, asking about education, licensure, certification, treatment approach, and possible side effects or problems with the specific technique.

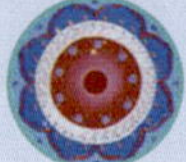

PARTNERING WITH CLIENTS AND FAMILIES

TIPS FOR AVOIDING FRAUDULENT HEALTH CLAIMS

- Be suspicious of claims for a "miracle cure," an "exclusive product," or a "magical discovery."
- Check out claims on the Internet, in advertisements on television and radio, and in newspapers and magazines with reliable sources such as NCCAM.
- Understand that claiming to be "natural" doesn't necessarily mean that the product is safe.
- Be aware that impressive-sounding terminology may be a way to disguise a lack of good science.
- Be skeptical about claims that the government, research scientists, or the medical profession have conspired to suppress a product. Cures for serious disease are widely reported in the media. They are not hidden in obscure magazine ads, paid television advertisements, or website promotions.
- "Quick relief" or "quick cure" claims are unreliable, especially if the disease is serious.
- Beware of products that claim to treat a wide spectrum of unrelated illnesses.

Increasing numbers of hospitals and academic medical centers are integrating CAM therapies, up to 95% in one study (Nedrow, 2006), into conventional medical settings. This study, and another by Cohen and associates (2005), found that hospitals use heterogenous approaches to address licensure, credentialing, hiring, scope of practice, requirements for professional liability insurance, informed consent disclosure, and hiring. The University of Michigan Integrative Medicine Clinical Services division has developed policies for CAM designed to be used as a generalizable template for standard policy development by other institutions that use such modalities as acupuncture (Myklebust et al., 2006) and therapeutic massage (Myklebust & Iler, 2007).

Quality and Costs of Service Delivery

Clients should visit the practitioner's office, clinic, or hospital to personally see the conditions under which treatment will be given. Are conditions safe and clean? Are regulated standards for medical care and safety adhered to?

Cost may also be an important consideration for clients. Although increasing numbers of insurers are covering costs of CAM services, not all do. Clients may have to pay directly for CAM services. Practitioners and health insurers should be able to tell clients which services are reimbursable.

Integrating CAM into a Treatment Plan

Integrating CAM into a treatment plan can take place only when clients discuss all CAM treatments and therapies with their primary physical or mental health care providers. Some CAM treatments affect physical or mental functioning, and certain herbs can interfere with or potentiate treatment with conventional medications.

Selecting Appropriate Clients

Most CAM techniques require that a client is motivated to participate in the interventions, is able to concentrate, and can follow directions, some of which may be quite complex. Assess clients to see if they meet these criteria. Be sure to obtain informed consent before instituting CAM therapies.

Techniques that are lengthy and introspective or meditative should probably not be used with clients who are severely depressed, hallucinating, delusional, or have loss of contact with reality. Introspective techniques may lead to an increased loss of contact with reality, withdrawal, or increased rumination. Brief and externally focused techniques would be better for these clients. Clients who have multiple problems or are in extremely stressful situations may not have the time or energy to focus on or learn complex CAM techniques. Avoid adding another stressor to these clients' lives. Mental health problems that often respond well to CAM therapies are identified in Box 33-3.

Box 33-3 Mental Health Problems and Related CAM Therapies

Alcohol Abuse

- Acupuncture
- Herbal therapy (kudzu)
- Meditation/medical meditation
- Yoga

Alzheimer's Dementia

- Herbal therapy (gingko)
- Dietary supplements (omega-3 fatty acids)
- Massage
- Medical meditation

Anxiety

- Acupressure
- Biofeedback
- Breathing and relaxation techniques
- Guided imagery
- Healing touch/therapeutic touch
- Self-hypnosis
- Massage
- Meditation/medical meditation

Attention Deficit/Hyperactivity Disorder

- Biofeedback

Depression

- Acupuncture
- Healing touch/therapeutic touch
- Herbal therapy (St. John's wort)
- Meditation/medical meditation
- Transcranial magnetic stimulation

Insomnia

- Breathing and relaxation techniques
- Herbal therapy (valerian/melatonin)
- Meditation

Obsessive–Compulsive Disorder

- Acupuncture
- Medical meditation

Stress

- Breathing and relaxation exercises
- Healing touch/therapeutic touch
- Massage
- Meditation/medical meditation

Monitoring the Plan of Care

Clients using CAM therapies should first discuss the program with their health care provider. National population-based surveys and studies in primary care settings have documented inadequate communication about CAM between clients and their conventional health care providers. One study of primary care clinicians—physicians, nurse practitioners, certified nurse midwives, and physician assistants—found that although 94% of clinicians reported CAM use among their clients, few consistently asked their clients about their CAM use (Flannery, Love, Pearce, Luan, &

Elder, 2006). Clients often report they do not inform their primary care practitioner of CAM use, most frequently because they were not asked (Taylor et al., 2006b).

The failure to assess for CAM use is problematic for several reasons. Be aware that some people, because of cultural background, may seek CAM therapies before they even access Western medicine. Because many of these techniques lower blood pressure, decrease heart rate, and reduce pain and anxiety, clients' medications should be closely monitored. Monitoring is particularly important for psychiatric clients receiving psychotropic medications that may cause hypotension. Clients with cardiac problems may be at increased risk for cardiac arrhythmia because of vasovagal stimulation with certain techniques such as active progressive relaxation.

The potential for medication–CAM interaction is considerable. In one study of adults who visited the emergency department, 275 reported using CAM. Of this number, 138 reported that they were also taking a prescription drug. The investigators identified 15 documented potential medication–CAM interactions in 9, and 97 theoretical potential medication–CAM interactions in 51 (Taylor et al., 2006b). Medication–CAM interactions are discussed later in this chapter, especially in the section on herbal therapy on pages 886–887.

Experimenting with What Works

It is not necessary to use every suggestion or technique in this chapter. If one particular CAM technique does not seem to help, encourage the client to move on to another one. What is important is to give each a fair trial and to experiment to find out what works in each person's individual situation. As Mahatma Gandhi once said, "As long as you derive inner help and comfort from anything, keep it."

DEEP BREATHING AND RELAXATION EXERCISES

Unfortunately, many clients do not reduce the stresses in their lives because they do not realize that they are at the mercy of involuntary fight-or-flight responses (such as those discussed in Chapter 8). Many fail to identify environmental, physiologic, or cognitive sources of stress. Like clients in any other health care setting, psychiatric clients must endure time pressures, weather, noise, crowds, interpersonal demands, job performance demands, and various threats to security and self-esteem. And, perhaps more than clients in many of the other settings in which nurses practice, psychiatric clients experience cognitive stress because of how they interpret and label their experiences. For instance, a client might interpret the boss's facial expression as amused rather than pleased or as disgruntled rather than quizzical. This interpretation is likely to provoke anxiety. Dwelling on one's concerns and anxieties causes physical tension in the body, which in turn creates the subjective feeling of uneasiness and leads to more anxious thoughts.

The deep breathing and relaxation exercises that follow are based on the belief that mind and body are interrelated and that the condition of one will eventually affect the condition of the other. A relaxed body is incompatible with anxiety. If the body is relaxed, the mind will feel relaxed as well.

Body Scanning to Assess Body Tension

The importance of body states and their relationship to stress have been emphasized by Eastern philosophies such as yoga and Zen. Because stress and body tension are simultaneous, one of the first steps in recognizing stress and anxiety is recognizing tension in the body. Body scanning helps you to become aware of where tension collects in your body and is an effective way to begin any of the relaxation techniques that follow. Use the step-by-step guide in the Your Self-Awareness feature to help yourself become aware of the tension you carry in your body. You can use the same step-by-step guide to teach body scanning to your clients.

Enhancing Relaxation with Music

Many people find that listening to soothing music is relaxing. Music, on audiotape, compact disc (CD), videotape, or digital video disc (DVD), can help clients reduce anxiety and achieve relaxation (Labbé, Schmidt, Babin, & Pharr, 2007) and can also be a substitute for, or adjunct to, pain medication and tranquilizers. Oncology nurses (Kwekkeboom, Bumpus, Wanta, & Serlin, 2007) and hospice nurses use music as a nondrug pain intervention. Recorded music may be used before or during surgery, dental work, chemotherapy, kidney dialysis, during recovery from spinal injury or burns, and to decrease anxiety in young children during cast room procedures (Liu et al., 2007).

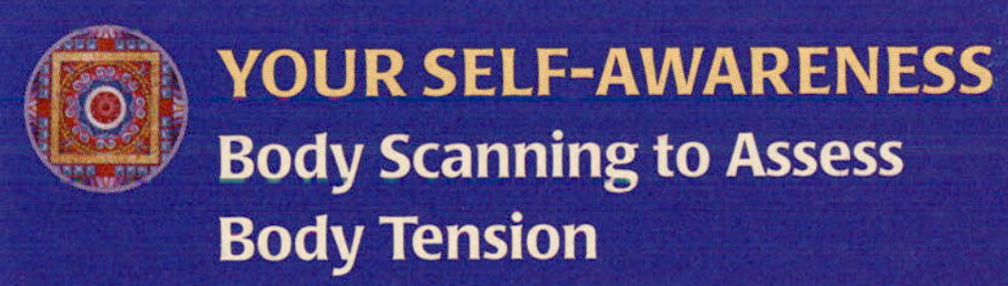

In order to help others become aware of their own body tension, you must first become aware of where you carry tension in your own body. Use the following step-by-step guide to perform a self-assessment. You can follow these same guidelines when teaching clients and their families.

- Make sure that the spine is straight before beginning body scanning or any of the other exercises described in this chapter. Stand, sit, or lie on the floor, whichever is most comfortable, while maintaining good posture.
- Begin by closing your eyes and turning your attention to your own internal world, focusing on your body.
- Focus on your toes and move up slowly.
- As you do this, ask yourself: "Where am I tense?"
- Become aware of all of the muscles in your body and especially the parts of your body that feel tense or tight.
- Notice the location of the tenseness and talk to yourself about it, reminding yourself that muscular tension is self-induced. Perhaps you might say: "The muscles in the back of my neck feel tight. This means that I'm creating tension in my body. Tension causes me problems."

Music can also be effectively used in conjunction with guided imagery (Chou & Lin, 2006). You can teach clients to lower their blood pressure 10 to 20 points by using a combination of visual imagery and music. Music with 60 beats per minute can help those with cardiac arrhythmias achieve a better-regulated heart rate. Guided imagery (visualization) is discussed later in this chapter.

How does music achieve its relaxing effect? Soothing music produces endorphins in the brain, the same "feel-good" chemicals that running and meditation produce. These natural opiates, secreted by the hypothalamus, reduce the intensity with which pain is felt. Because people vary in their response to music, encourage clients to experiment with different kinds of music to discover which has positive effects and then to develop their own personal library. Tapes, CDs, and DVDs specifically for stress reduction are sold in bookstores and through catalogs. They are often available through local public libraries.

Recommend that clients pay attention to their breathing as they listen to music. Slow and deep breathing enhances the relaxing effect of music.

Breathing Exercises

Under most circumstances, people take breathing for granted as an automatic body function. They usually become aware of their pattern of breathing only when it has gone awry, such as when they are out of breath. Breathing properly can, by itself, reduce stress. Breathing calmly and deeply keeps the blood well oxygenated and purified. It helps remove waste materials from the blood and clears thinking. Poorly oxygenated blood may contribute to fatigue, mental confusion, anxiety, muscular tension, and feelings of depression.

As a nursing student, you may find deep breathing especially helpful when preparing for an anxiety-provoking experience such as taking a final examination, embarking upon a new clinical experience, or taking the RN licensure examination. Practicing a stress management technique such as deep breathing on a regular basis helps to decrease test anxiety, nervousness, self-doubt, and concentration loss (Paul, Elam, & Verhulst, 2007). Relaxation techniques may also reduce distraction and increase positive mood states (Jain et al., 2007).

The following exercises are designed to facilitate proper breathing.

Awareness of Breathing

Do you breathe properly, or does your breathing actually deprive you of oxygen? Take time to pay attention to your own breathing. Begin by placing one hand just below your rib cage and taking a deep breath. Notice what happens when you inhale. Does your hand move in? Does your hand move out? Does your hand move at all? If your hand moves out, you are breathing properly. But if your hand moves in or doesn't move at all, it's probably because you learned, as most of us have, to hold your stomach in and push your chest out while breathing. People who breathe this way do not fill the lungs to full capacity; they fill only the top third or top half.

Deep Breathing

During **deep breathing**, you move the diaphragm downward and fill the lower part of the lungs with air. The chest expands as the middle part fills with air, and the shoulders move upward as the upper part fills. To teach yourself or a client how to take deep, healthful breaths, follow the directions in the Partnering with Clients and Families feature on page 879. Remember also to use these same directions when you teach clients to deep-breathe after surgery.

Deep breathing becomes easier with practice. It may become almost automatic. This is an exercise few resist—it is easy to do, it is inconspicuous, and it yields fast results.

Ten-to-One Count

This exercise is also quick and simple. To teach yourself or a client how to perform the ten-to-one exercise, follow the directions in the Partnering with Clients and Families feature on page 879. Some people use an abbreviated version and begin counting at the number 5; others require the full count of 10 to feel calm.

Alternate-Nostril Breathing

Although somewhat more difficult, alternate-nostril breathing, which stems from the practice of yoga, also helps reduce tension and sinus headaches. To teach yourself or a client how to perform alternate-nostril breathing, follow the directions in the Partnering with Clients and Families feature on page 879.

It may be easier to breathe through the right nostril at certain times of the day and through the left nostril at other times. The reason is that people breathe primarily through one nostril for approximately 4 hours and then breathe primarily through the other for the next 4 hours.

Progressive Relaxation

The technique of **progressive relaxation** is based on the premise that muscle tension is the body's physiologic response to anxiety-provoking thoughts. Muscular tension increases the feeling of anxiety and reinforces it. Deep muscle relaxation, by contrast, decreases physiologic tension and blocks anxiety.

Progressive relaxation decreases pulse and respiratory rates, blood pressure, and perspiration. In addition, it helps reduce anxiety. Clients with muscle spasms, lower-back pain, tension headaches, insomnia, anxiety, depression, fatigue, irritable bowel syndrome, hypertension, or mild phobias are among those who can achieve positive results using this technique. Some clients report feeling less alert after either active or passive progressive relaxation. When alertness is important, one of the other deep breathing exercises is probably better.

It may take longer to master progressive relaxation than the deep-breathing techniques discussed earlier. With practice, however, one can learn to relax faster and more easily.

Active Progressive Relaxation

Active progressive relaxation helps people identify which muscles or muscle groups are chronically tense by distinguishing between sensations of tension (purposeful muscle tensing) and deep relaxation (a conscious relaxing of the

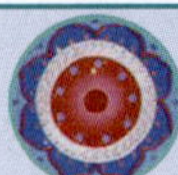

PARTNERING WITH CLIENTS AND FAMILIES

GUIDELINES FOR DEEP-BREATHING EXERCISES

Deep Breathing

- Sit, stand, or lie with your spine straight.
- Scan your body for tension.
- Place one hand on your chest and the other on your abdomen.
- Inhale slowly and deeply so that your abdomen pushes your hand up.
- Visualize your lungs slowly filling with air. Your chest should move only slightly as you inhale, but you should be aware of the movement of your abdomen.
- Exhale through your mouth, making a soft, whooshing sound by blowing gently. Keep your face, mouth, and jaw relaxed.
- Be aware of what it feels like and what you sound like when you breathe properly.
- Continue to take long, slow, deep breaths for at least 10 minutes at a time, once or twice a day.
- Increase the frequency if you wish, once you have mastered the technique.
- Scan your body for tension again, comparing the tension to what it was like before you began the deep-breathing exercise.

Ten-to-One Count

- Sit, stand, or lie with your spine straight.
- Scan your body for tension.
- Incorporate the guidelines in the deep breathing exercise described earlier.
- Inhale, taking a deep breath, while saying the number 10 to yourself.
- Then exhale slowly, letting out all the air in your lungs.
- Inhale again, saying the number 9 to yourself.
- As you exhale, tell yourself: "I feel more relaxed than I did at number 10."
- With your next breath, say the number 8 to yourself.
- As you exhale, remind yourself: "I feel more relaxed than I did at number 9."
- Continue counting down and experience increasing calmness as you approach number 1.
- Scan your body for tension again, comparing the tension to what it was like before you began the deep-breathing exercise.

Alternate-Nostril Breathing

- Sit, stand, or lie with your spine straight.
- Scan your body for tension.
- Close off your right nostril by lightly pressing it with your right thumb.
- Then inhale through your left nostril as slowly and quietly as possible. (Do not exhale yet.)
- Remove your thumb from the right nostril and use your forefinger to close off the left nostril.
- Exhale slowly through your right nostril.
- Inhale through your right nostril as slowly and quietly as possible.
- Follow the procedure outlined earlier, closing your right nostril with your right thumb while exhaling through your left nostril.
- The basic cycle is 10 breaths; this can be increased up to 25 breaths.
- Scan your body for tension again, comparing the tension to what it was like before you began the deep-breathing exercise.

muscles). You can teach yourself or your clients active progressive relaxation by implementing the procedure outlined in the Partnering with Clients and Families feature "Guidelines for Active Progressive Relaxation" on page 880. Be sure to attend to the cautions described in the feature.

Passive Progressive Relaxation

In *passive progressive relaxation*, the muscles are not tensed. The goal is to relax the muscles without first tightening them. The sequence in which body parts are relaxed differs from that of the active progressive method. Begin with muscles easiest to relax (in the toes) and progress to muscles most difficult to relax (in the head). The sequence is as follows: feet, lower legs, knees and upper legs, hips and buttocks, lower back, lower arms and hands, chest and diaphragm, abdomen, pelvis and genitals, neck, forehead and upper face, mouth and jaw.

VISUALIZATION AND IMAGERY

Émile Coué, a French pharmacist, began to use the power of imagination with clients around the turn of the century. Carl Jung used it in his psychiatric practice during the early part of the 20th century. Nurses use it because it is time- and cost-effective and creates a healing partnerhsip between nurse and client (Reed, 2007). Most recently, contemporary clinicians and individual clients have had remarkable success in the use of visualization to achieve control over serious physical illness and emotional discomfort and to improve quality of life (Baird & Sands, 2006).

Positive **visualization**, or **imagery**, uses the healing power of a person's own imagination and positive thinking to create powerful mental pictures or images to reduce stress or promote healing. Because of the vivid mental images that can be created, imagery has been considered by some to be a form of hypnosis (see the following section on hypnotherapy and self-hypnosis). Visualization should be used in conjunction with the body-scanning and deep-breathing exercises discussed earlier.

Not everyone finds using the imagination in this way easy, and the technique may not work for everyone. Constructing a detailed, effective visualization requires time, patience, and practice. Some people find that **guided imagery**—using an outside resource such as an actual person who guides the imagery process or a voice on an audiotape or CD—helps to create a series of images. You can also implement the guidelines in the Partnering with Clients and Families feature "Guidelines for Constructing a Visualization" on page 880 with soft background music to record your own guided imagery experience for relaxation, guidance, or symptom control or pain relief or to record a guided imagery for a client.

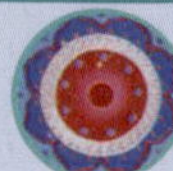

PARTNERING WITH CLIENTS AND FAMILIES

GUIDELINES FOR ACTIVE PROGRESSIVE RELAXATION

In active progressive relaxation, each muscle or muscle grouping is tensed for 5 to 7 seconds and then relaxed for 15 to 20 seconds. Repeat the cycle.

Four major muscle groups are covered in this order: (1) hands, forearms, and biceps; (2) head, face, throat, and shoulders; (3) chest, abdomen, and lower back; (4) thighs, buttocks, calves, and feet using this procedure:

- Practice progressive relaxation while lying down or seated in a chair with feet firmly on the floor.
- Begin active progressive relaxation by tightening the right fist (5 to 7 seconds) and paying attention to the tension. Allow the muscles of the right fist to relax (15 to 20 seconds), while noticing the pleasant difference.
- Do the same with the left fist—tensing, relaxing, and noticing the difference.
- Follow the same procedure for the forearms (tensing and relaxing as explained earlier), and then for the biceps, remembering to compare the difference in sensation between tensed and relaxed muscles.
- Progress through the next major muscle group—head, face, throat, and shoulders.
- Move to the third major muscle group—chest, abdomen, and lower back.
- End with the fourth major muscle group—thighs, buttocks, calves, and feet.
- Remember to return to muscle groups that are only partially relaxed to bring about deeper relaxation.

Caution: Counsel clients to observe some cautions while carrying out this technique. To avoid soft tissue and spinal injury, the muscles of the neck and back should not be excessively tightened. Tightening the muscles of the toes and feet too vigorously could also result in uncomfortable muscle cramps. Clients with cardiac arrhythmias should be cautioned against vasovagal stimulation by tensing muscles too tightly. Postoperative clients should probably avoid active progressive relaxation, a practice that could increase pain in the postoperative period. Teach these clients passive progressive relaxation instead.

MEDIALINK Guided Imagery Certification

Nurses interested in gaining expertise in incorporating guided imagery into their practice might consider a certification program. Both the American Holistic Nurses Association and the Academy for Guided Imagery provide continuing education and certification programs. Such data can be accessed through a direct resource link on the Companion Website for this book. The website of the American Holistic Nurses Association also provides information on programs of study, standards of practice, and student memberships.

Visualization for Relaxation

Relaxing through visualization is enhanced by constructing in one's own mind a relaxing environment. Some people find the soothing sounds of the seashore calming; others prefer to imagine themselves floating above the world on a soft cloud or a magic carpet. Still others relax as they imagine themselves descending on a slow-moving escalator into a calmer and more relaxed state. If visualization seems difficult (and if a warm bath, hot tub, or swimming pool is relaxing), try constructing a

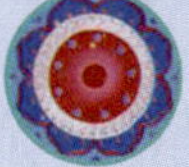

PARTNERING WITH CLIENTS AND FAMILIES

GUIDELINES FOR CONSTRUCTING A VISUALIZATION

- Assume a position of comfort—either lying down or sitting up.
- Take five cleansing deep breaths. With each inhalation, imagine that you are taking in calmness and peacefulness. With each exhalation imagine that you are releasing tension, discomfort, and worry.
- Allow your body to become increasingly relaxed with each deep breath.
- Use all your senses—seeing, hearing, touching, smelling, tasting—as you imagine yourself to be in an especially beautiful and wonderful place for you. What are the colors, shapes, and living things in your special place? What do you hear and smell? What objects and shapes do you feel? What do you usually taste in this place?
- If constructing a *visualization for guidance,* put your wise person into your special place. Use all your senses to imagine this person. What color hair, eyes, and skin does your wise person have? What are the textures of that person's clothes? What smells do you associate with that person? What does it feel like to grasp that person's hand?
- If constructing a *visualization for pain or symptom relief,* the goal is to associate orange or red lights with the pain or symptom, and then to change the orange or red lights to blue lights that signify a change to pain-free or calm or symptom-free areas. Another visualization involves attaching a symbolic visual image to the pain (a lump in the throat, a hammer pounding the head, a dog gnawing on a bone) and then imagining the symbol becoming weakened as the pain or symptom lessens.
- When you're ready, allow the images to fade. Take whatever time you need to bring yourself back to your outer world by slowly opening your eyes and stretching.

visualization while in warm water, combining the physiologic effects of the warm water with the products of the imagination.

Visualization for Guidance

Visualization can also be useful when seeking guidance, direction, or help with decision making. Upon reaching a special soothing place, visualize an "inner advisor" or "wise person." You can ask for an image to appear or use someone you know—a valued teacher, a historical figure (Florence Nightingale, Martin Luther King, Jr., Mother Theresa), a beloved grandparent (see the Partnering with Clients and Families feature "Guidelines for Constructing a Visualization").

Visualization for Symptom Control or Healing

Visualization techniques for symptom control or healing can be part of a well-rounded health program. For example, visualization can be used in conjunction with conventional medical treatment for people with cancer and with preoperative clients to control postoperative pain and enhance tissue healing. Clients with vascular problems—migraine headache, hypertension, or Raynaud's disease—benefit from visualization. Allergies, asthma, rheumatoid arthritis, osteoarthritis (Reed, 2007), gastritis, colitis, peptic ulcer, insomnia, anxiety, depression, and chronic pain all respond to visualization. Guided imagery before and after open heart surgery appeared to reduce pain and tension during early recovery (Kshettry, Carole, Henly, Sendelbach, & Kummer, 2006).

Two suggestions for visualizations are given in the Partnering with Clients and Families feature "Guidelines for Constructing a Visualization."

HYPNOTHERAPY AND SELF-HYPNOSIS

Hypnotherapy is the therapeutic use of suggestion during an altered state of consciousness to effect positive changes in a person's behavior and to treat a wide range of health conditions. It has been used as an adjunct to anesthesia or in place of anesthesia, to decrease pain, to treat tension and migraine headaches, to decrease dependence on tobacco, for weight control, in dentistry, and in trancelike states to access the deepest levels of the mind.

Although hypnotherapy has been practiced in many cultures for thousands of years, its use in health care became more common in the mid-20th century when the American Medical Association approved its use as a valid medical intervention. Self-hypnosis has the potential to provide anxiety relief without undue cost and to reduce pain. When compared with women receiving standard care or structured empathic attention during large core breast biopsy, the anxiety of women in the self-hypnosis group decreased significantly (Lang et al., 2006). In hospitals today, it is not uncommon to find anesthesiologists, nurses, surgeons, psychologists, and social workers who use hypnosis in their therapeutic work.

Nurses who wish to use hypnosis in their clinical practice must recognize that it is an advanced intervention that requires specialized training in hypnotherapy. It is also important to be aware of whether your state board of nursing identifies hypnosis as within the scope of practice of nurses.

People practice self-hypnosis—hypnosis accomplished by oneself without the help of a second party as hypnotist—to achieve significant relaxation, to make positive suggestions for change (to lose weight, to stop smoking, to overcome fear of the dark or insomnia), and to increase learning and remembering. TABLE 33-2 ■ on page 882 gives examples of some life problems and the hypnotic suggestions that can be used to overcome them.

Most people can achieve significant relaxation within 2 days with self-hypnosis. Self-hypnosis can be self-taught through books on the subject. Community adult education programs and holistic health centers often offer courses on self-hypnosis. Self-hypnosis is clinically effective in relieving insomnia, low to moderate levels of chronic pain, tics and tremors, and low to moderate levels of anxiety. It is a well-established treatment for chronic fatigue.

MEDITATION

The increased use of meditation in North America owes much to Herbert Benson, a Harvard physician who identified and promoted the scientific benefits of meditation as a relaxation response almost 40 years ago (Benson & Klipper, 2000). **Meditation** helps one achieve inner peace and harmony by focusing uncritically on one thing at a time. Meditation has been associated with various religious and cultural practices and philosophies for thousands of years. It is seen as a way of becoming one with a higher power or the universe, finding enlightenment, and achieving such virtues as selflessness. However, the person who practices meditation need not associate it with religion or philosophy. It can be practiced as a means of reducing inner discord and increasing self-knowledge.

Effects of Meditation

The state of meditation is equivalent to a state of deep rest. The heart rate slows, the body uses less oxygen, and blood lactate—a waste product of metabolism—decreases sharply. Alpha brain waves, present during states of calm alertness, increase, as does the secretion of dopamine. There appear to be beneficial effects on cardiovascular functioning at rest and during acute stress situations. Meditation was also found to be effective in decreasing mood disturbance and stress symptoms in both males and females of various ages with a wide variety of cancer diagnoses, stages of illness, and educational backgrounds (Carlson, Ursuliak, Goodey, Angen, & Speca, 2001). The regular practice of meditation may even have neuroprotective effects and reduce the cognitive decline associated with aging (Pagnoni & Cekic, 2007).

Meditation, combined with cognitive therapy (discussed in Chapter 31 ∞), has been found to result in statistically significant reductions in mean depression and anxiety scores—72% of clients showed improvements in symptoms of depression and 63% in symptoms of anxiety (Finucane & Mercer, 2006). Mindfulness-based (meditation) cognitive therapy involves an educational protocol (as an 8-session course) delivered to participants in groups. It has been deemed promising as a cost-effective addition to methods of

TABLE 33-2 ■ Life Problems and Related Hypnotic Suggestions

Life Problem	Hypnotic Suggestion
Fear of coming into a dark house at night	I can come in tonight feeling relaxed and glad to be home.
Anxiety that prevents working or studying to meet deadlines	I can work steadily and calmly. My concentration is improving as I become more relaxed.
Insomnia	I will gradually become more and more drowsy. In just a few minutes, I will be able to fall asleep and will sleep peacefully all night.
Chronic fatigue	I can wake up feeling refreshed and relaxed.
Minor chronic headache or backache	As I become more relaxed, my headache (backache) lessens. In just a few minutes, it will go away. Soon, my head will be cool and relaxed. Gradually I will feel the muscles in my back loosen, and in an hour, they will be completely relaxed. Whenever these symptoms come back, I will simply turn my ring a quarter of a turn to the right and the pain will relax away.
Feelings of inferiority	The next time I see ________, I can feel secure in myself. I can feel relaxed and at ease because I am perfectly all right.
Anxiety about an upcoming evaluation or test	Whenever I feel nervous, I can say to myself . . . (insert your special key word or phrase here) . . . and relax.
Chronic anger or chronic guilt	I can turn off anger (guilt) because I am the one who turns it on. I will relax my body and breathe deeply.
Worry about interpersonal rejection	Whenever I lace my fingers together, I will feel confidence flowing through me.
Chronic tension or discomfort in a particular part of the body	I will think about my ________ every hour and let it relax.

addressing depression in old age (Smith, Graham, & Senthinathan, 2007) and improving psychological functioning for persons dealing with stress-related problems, illness, anxiety, and chronic pain (Carmody & Baer, 2007).

Steps in Meditating

Meditation exercises can be relatively easy to learn. Some people experience immediate relief and pleasure in only one session. To experience deeper effects, the person needs to practice meditation regularly for at least a month. There are four major requirements for successful meditation. They are discussed in the Your Intervention Strategies feature.

Many people who meditate prefer to use a **mantra**, a syllable, word, or name that is repeatedly chanted aloud. Some teachers of meditation insist that each person have a special mantra with a specific meaning and vibration to achieve individual effects. Others recommend the use of any word or phrase the individual is drawn to, such as *love* or *calm*. Some popular mantras are *om* (I am), *so-ham* (I am he), *sa-ham* (I am she), *Shalom* (peace), and *The Lord is my shepherd*.

Avoid chanting too loudly or too vigorously. After about 5 minutes, shift to whispering the mantra as you relax more deeply. When it is not possible to chant aloud, you can chant silently.

Medical Meditation

More recently, scientific research has demonstrated that one of the newest and most cutting-edge advances in CAM is medical meditation. **Medical meditation**—meditation combined with adaptations of kundalini yoga (one of several forms of yoga)—as developed by a physician, Darma Singh Khalsa, has specific physiologic effects that can target such disorders as arthritis, anxiety disorder, Alzheimer's, diabetes, depression, hypertension, and many other physical

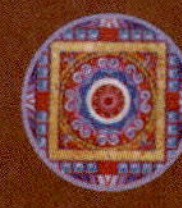

YOUR INTERVENTION STRATEGIES
The Four Major Requirements for Successful Meditation

1. *A quiet place.* The environment for meditation should be one that minimizes distractions—a quiet place set aside as a haven from the urgencies of everyday life.
2. *A comfortable position.* A comfortable position that can be held for 20 minutes without stress facilitates meditation.
3. *An object or thought to focus on.* A repeated word, an object or symbol to look at or think about, or a specific thought or feeling helps keep distracting thoughts from entering the mind.
4. *A passive attitude.* A passive attitude requires understanding that thoughts and distractions will occur and can be cleared from the mind. If they occur, they should be noted and released without concern about their interference. It is counterproductive to worry about how well you are doing at meditating.

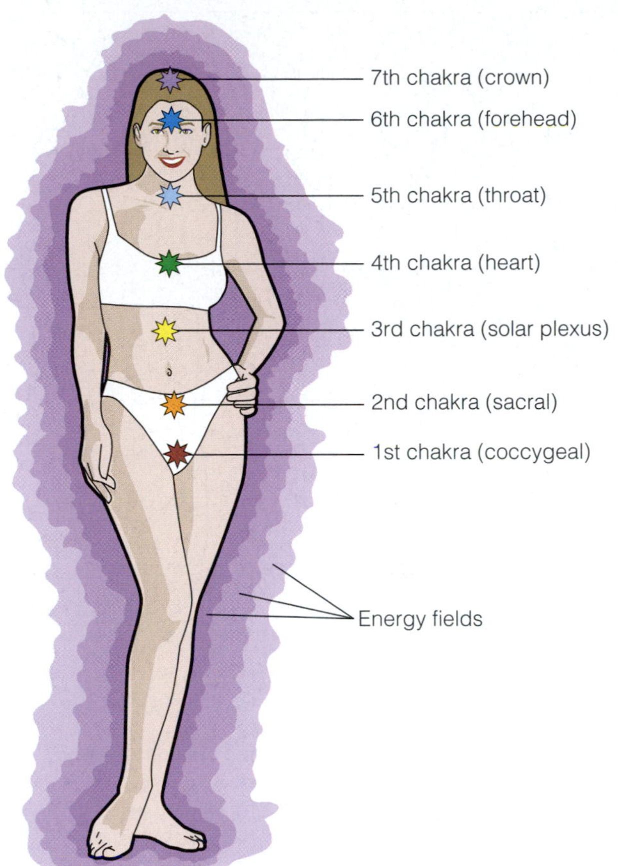

FIGURE 33-1 ■ The seven major chakras, according to Hindu tradition, are concentrated areas of energy.

and mental conditions (Khalsa & Stauth, 2001). Yoga is "a journey of the body, mind, and spirit on a path toward unity" (Fontaine, 2004). Thus, it is much more than simply a fitness-oriented practice.

Medical meditations unite the body, mind, and spirit by amplifying the energy system of the body that is, according to Hindu tradition, located in the seven major **chakras**. Chakras are concentrated areas of energy vertically aligned through the center of the body from the crown of the head to the pelvis (see FIGURE 33-1 ■). The chakras influence the physical body, the emotions, and the spirit. Each chakra corresponds to specific body structures and organs and has specific functions. The three lower chakras are primarily involved with basic elements of life such as survival, power, financial security, and procreation. The four higher chakras are involved with the higher, more advanced elements of life such as intellect, intuition, compassion, and spirituality.

Medical meditations are very specific. They involve special postures and movements, exact positioning of the hands and fingers, specific mantras, and specific breathing patterns in order to activate specific chakras.

PRESSURE POINT THERAPIES

Several approaches use the application of pressure or stimulation to specific points on the body to promote healing, relieve pain, or promote wellness.

Acupuncture

Acupuncture originated in China more than 2,000 years ago and has grown in popularity in the United States over the past 20 years as more anesthesiologists, neurologists, nurses, specialists in physical medicine, and specialists in addictions are becoming trained and certified as practitioners by the National Certification Commission for Acupuncture and Oriental Medicine (http://www.nccaom.org). A national health interview survey of U.S. citizens found that 4.1% of the respondents reported lifetime use of acupuncture, and 1.1% (representing 2.13 million Americans) reported recent use (Burke, Upchurch, Dye, & Chyu, 2006). Musculoskeletal complaints were the most frequently reported condition, led by back pain (34%).

MEDIALINK NCCAOM

Acupuncture is based on the belief that the vital life energy of the body (*qi*, pronounced chee) circulates along 12 major and 8 secondary pathways, called meridians. These pathways are linked to specific organs and organ systems. Hair-thin needles placed at acupuncture sites are used to stimulate the meridians and influence the flow of energy that affects internal organs.

According to the NIH consensus development statement on acupuncture (1997), stimulating acupuncture points causes biochemical changes in the central nervous system that either change the experience of pain or release other chemicals, such as hormones and neurotransmitters, that influence the body's self-regulating systems. The biochemical changes may stimulate the body's natural healing abilities and promote physical and emotional well-being. Promising results have emerged in treating posttraumatic stress disorder (PTSD) (Hollifield, Sinclair-Lian, Warner, & Hammerschlag, 2007), postoperative nausea and vomiting, nausea and vomiting associated with pregnancy and chemotherapy, and for relieving dental pain. The data are equivocal or contradictory for conditions such as irritable bowel syndrome, headache, circulatory problems, mood-related mental disorders, and schizophrenia.

Acupuncture, specifically auricular acupuncture (see FIGURE 33-2 ■ on page 884), is widely used to ease withdrawal and treat addiction in alcoholics, drug addicts, and smokers in North America and in Europe (substance-related disorders are discussed in Chapter 15∞). However, evidence from controlled studies regarding its effectiveness as a treatment for substance addiction has been inconclusive. For example, the use of acupuncture as a stand-alone treatment for cocaine addiction or in situations in which clients receive only minimal concurrent psychosocial treatment has not been supported (Margolin et al., 2002). Further research into the effectiveness of acupuncture as an ancillary therapy in addiction treatment is needed.

Acupressure

Acupressure is based on the same principles as acupuncture, but does not involve needles; finger pressure or implements are used to stimulate the meridians. Shiatsu massage, Jin Shin Jyutsu, and Jin Shin Do are forms of acupressure that stem from the Japanese tradition. **Reflexology** is the practice of acupressure on particular points of

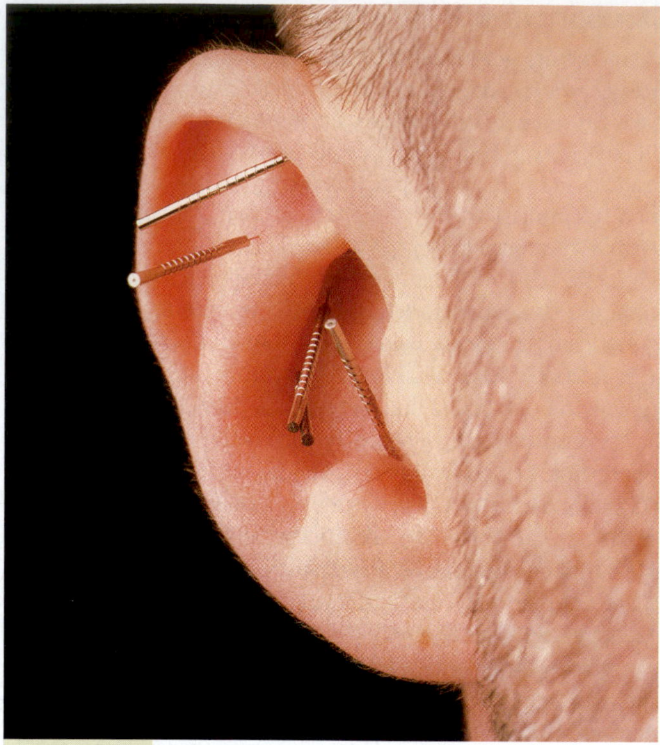

FIGURE 33-2 ■ Auricular acupuncture.

Source: Photo Researchers, Inc., Cordelia Molloy.

the feet, hands, and ears. Foot reflexology points are illustrated in FIGURE 33-3 ■.

While these practices involve advanced training, you can incorporate noninvasive hand, foot, or ear massages into your clinical practice (Fontaine, 2004). The Partnering with Clients and Families feature "Self-Help Pressure Point and Finger Holding Techniques" discusses pressure points and finger holds that you can teach others as a self-help process.

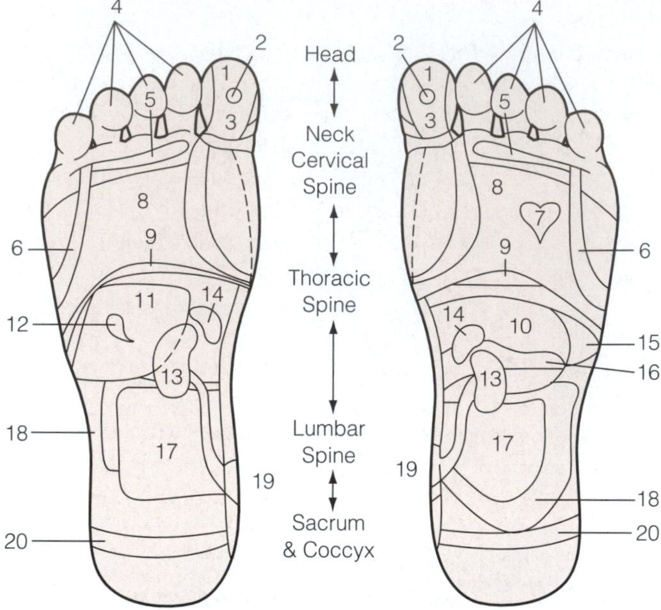

1. Head and brain
2. Pituitary and pineal glands
3. Throat and thyroid gland
4. Sinus
5. Eyes and ears
6. Shoulder
7. Heart
8. Lungs and thymus gland
9. Diaphragm and solar plexus
10. Stomach
11. Liver
12. Gallbladder
13. Kidney
14. Adrenal gland
15. Spleen
16. Pancreas
17. Small intestine
18. Large intestine
19. Bladder
20. Sacrum and sciatic nerve

FIGURE 33-3 ■ Foot reflexology points.

Source: Fontaine, K. L. (2004). *Complementary and alternative healing therapies for nursing practice* (2nd ed.). Upper Saddle River, NJ: Prentice Hall.

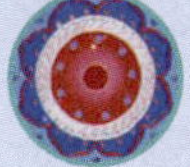

PARTNERING WITH CLIENTS AND FAMILIES

SELF-HELP PRESSURE POINT AND FINGER HOLDING TECHNIQUES

Pressure Point Therapy to Ease Tension and Restore Energy

- Hold your left palm in front of you, fingers together.
- Using your right thumb, massage the fleshy spot between your thumb and index finger for a slow count of 15 (this spot is a key pressure point).
- Then switch hands, and repeat the process.

Finger Holds to Improve General Well-Being

Gently hold the appropriate finger on either hand while imagining negative emotions melting away and physical symptoms easing.

- **Thumb.** Corresponds to worrying, depression, and anxiety. Physical symptoms may be stomachaches, headaches, skin problems, and nervousness.
- **Index finger.** Corresponds to fear, mental confusion, and frustration. Physical symptoms are digestive problems and muscular problems such as backaches.
- **Middle finger.** Corresponds to anger, irritability, and indecisiveness. Physical symptoms are eye or vision problems, fatigue, and circulation problems.
- **Ring finger.** Corresponds to sadness, fear of rejection, grief, and negativity. Physical symptoms are digestive, breathing, or serious skin problems.
- **Little finger.** Corresponds to insecurity, effort, overdoing it, and nervousness. Physical symptoms are sore throat and bone or nerve problems.

Source: Fontaine, K. L. (2004). *Healing practices: Alternative therapies for nursing* (2nd ed.) (p. 214). Upper Saddle River, NJ: Prentice Hall.

TOUCH THERAPIES FOR HEALING

Touch therapies for healing, or the "laying on of hands" to help heal, are as old as history. However, the research on touch therapies is still in the early stages of development. Although the data are promising, to date they can only suggest that touch therapies may reduce anxiety, improve muscle relaxation, aid in promoting wound healing, and reduce pain (Engebretson & Wardell, 2007). There are several CAM modalities that involve the use of touch for healing.

Massage

Massage, probably because it releases endorphins, has been helpful for persons with cancer (Gecsedi, 2002), autistic children (Escalona, Field, Singer-Strunck, Cullen, & Hartshorn, 2001), people who are depressed or addicted (Field, 2002), and, in combination with aromatherapy, for persons with dementia (Smallwood, Brown, Coulter, Irvine, & Copland, 2001). In a review of clinical trials for massage, 26 out of 27 demonstrated significant improvements in comfort and symptoms such as anxiety, emotional distress, nausea, and pain in seriously ill clients needing end-of-life care (Lafferty, Downey, McCarty, Standish, & Patrick, 2006).

Nurses have traditionally used massage to ease a client's discomfort and to develop a connection with the client. Increasing numbers of nurses focus on this CAM modality as licensed massage therapists in private practice and are affiliated with the American Massage Therapy Association (AMTA) (http://www.amtamassage.org, accessible through the Companion Website for this book). Another modality is **Reiki**, a gentle laying on of hands corresponding to the seven main chakras, discussed earlier on page 883.

Most laying-on-of-hands modalities involve the transfer of energy (see the earlier discussion of chakras). Nurses around the globe are using touch therapies to assist in easing pain and anxiety, promoting relaxation, accelerating wound healing, diminishing depression, and increasing the sense of well-being.

Therapeutic Touch (TT)

Therapeutic Touch (TT) was developed by Dolores Krieger (1979, 1993), a nursing professor, as a nursing activity. TT is defined as an intentionally directed process of energy exchange during which the TT practitioner uses the hands as a focus to facilitate the healing process. During this process, the therapist may direct energy from a universal source, or energy is transferred from one place to another within the body of the client. Despite flaws in early research, TT has one of the strongest research bases of the CAM modalities, probably due to the large number of nursing studies devoted to it. For this reason, *disturbed energy field* has become a NANDA diagnosis. Increasingly more sophisticated studies are providing evidence-based support for TT (Stephen, Mackenzie, Sample, & Macdonald, 2007).

Nurse practitioners of TT can be found across North America. In the United States, you can contact nurse practitioners of TT at www.therapeutic-touch.org. In Canada, there are TT groups in Ontario (http://www.therapeutictouchnetwk.com), British Columbia, Alberta, and the Canadian Atlantic Coast. These resources can be found on the Companion Website for this text.

MEDIALINK Therapeutic Touch

Phases in Therapeutic Touch

TT is a conscious, deliberate act composed of four phases: Centering, Assessing/Scanning, Intervention, and Evaluation/Closure. Although the phases are described sequentially in the following section, they are dynamic and often performed concurrently and repeated as often as necessary by experienced practitioners.

MEDIALINK American Massage Therapy Association

1. *Centering:* Centering is a process of bringing the body, mind, and emotions to a quiet, focused state of consciousness in order to find an inner sense of equilibrium and connect with the inner core of wholeness and stillness. This phase serves to gather and focus the healer's energies on the client and exclude extraneous thoughts from the mind, a process akin to meditation. This state of centeredness is maintained throughout the TT process.
2. *Assessing/Scanning:* Holding the hands 2 to 6 inches away from the client's body, the TT practitioner moves the hands from the head to the feet in a rhythmic and symmetric manner to determine the nature of the dynamic energy field. Sensory cues such as warmth, coolness, static, blockage, pulling, and tingling are described by some practitioners. These areas indicate a static condition, an imbalance, or congestion in the client's energy field that extends beyond the person's physical body.
3. *Intervention: Clearing*, also called *unruffling*, is an intentional intervention process of facilitating the flow of energy through the field. Clearing is achieved by using sweeping hand movements, with the palms facing toward the client, from the midline to the outer edge of the body while continuing to move in a rhythmic and symmetric manner from the head to the feet. The intent of this process is *balancing* and *rebalancing* the bioenergetic field. It involves the transfer of energy through the TT practitioner to the client with the intent of bringing balance to areas of imbalance. The TT practitioner projects, directs, and modulates energy to reestablish order in the system.
4. *Evaluation/Closure:* Reassessment of the bioenergy field completes the session. The TT practitioner uses professional, informed, and intuitive judgment to determine when to end the session and elicits feedback from the client. Evaluation is an ongoing process that guides the responses, intention, and knowledgeable interaction of the practitioner.

Effectiveness of Therapeutic Touch

Clients report a sense of relaxation and relief from pain. Krieger's early research (1979) demonstrated experimentally that TT produced a significant change in the hemoglobin component of red blood cells. Advocates of TT have found that, although the freeing of bound energy varies with each recipient, it does seem to facilitate the repatterning of energy necessary for healing. Many small studies of TT have suggested it is effective in a wide variety of conditions such as pain, wound healing, osteoarthritis, migraine headache, and anxiety. Practitioners indicate that TT can also result in a person's emotional and spiritual growth.

HERBALS AND BOTANICALS

Natural herbs have been used as medicines across the ages and across all cultures. Their use has grown tremendously within the past 10 years and has become a billion dollar market (Kaplan et al., 2007). Thousands of natural herbal products are used for symptom relief in a variety of conditions.

However, be aware that there may be insufficient reliable information available to judge the effectiveness or safety of many herbs. Consumers who rely on portrayals in the media for information on herbal and botanicals are not being provided with information sufficient to make informed choices. A study of the media found significant errors of omission in descriptions of clinical trial quality and a serious underreporting of the risks of herbal remedies (Bubela, Koper, Boon, & Caulfield, 2007). Testing in clinical trials is relatively recent, and little long-term random testing has been conducted.

Misconceptions also abound. For example, one common misconception is that the herb goldenseal can be used to mask the results of laboratory tests for illicit drug use. Goldenseal has been found to be ineffective for this purpose. Other misconceptions are that herbals and botanicals are always safe because they are "natural" and that they are more effective than prescription medications (Taylor, Walsham, Taylor, & Wong, 2006a). People who use these products are often unaware of their potential toxicities. Always encourage clients to discuss with their health care provider all natural remedies that they ingest. The safety and effectiveness of herbs can be validated at the following websites:

1. U.S. Food and Drug Administration (FDA): http://www.fda.gov
2. National Center for Complementary and Alternative Medicine: http://www.nccam.nih.gov
3. University of Washington Medicinal Herb Garden: http://www.nnlm.gov/pnr/uwmhg/
4. NIH Office of Dietary Supplements: http://ods.od.nih.gov

MEDIALINK Herbal Safety and Effectiveness

Adverse effects from dietary supplements can be reported to the FDA's MedWatch program at www.fda.gov/medwatch. These data can also be found as resource links on the Companion Website for this book.

Fewer herbs are used for treatment of emotional symptoms or mental disorder. TABLE 33-3 ■ lists the natural medicines that are likely to be effective and safe for clients with psychiatric-related symptoms. Psychotropic medications and the herbs that affect them are listed in TABLE 33-4 ■ on page 888. Some herbals and botanicals may potentiate the effects of psychotropic medications; others may block the effects. Others may increase the extent of adverse side effects.

BIOFEEDBACK

Visceral learning, known as **biofeedback**, is a technique for gaining conscious control over involuntary body functions such as blood pressure and heart rate, which are mediated by the autonomic nervous system. It has been shown, for example, that biofeedback is a promising alternative treatment for attention deficit/hyperactivity disorder (Friel, 2007), which is discussed in Chapter 26, and for migraine headaches, which can be relieved by increasing blood flow to the hands (Scharff, Marcus, & Masek, 2002). Biofeedback has also been found to be useful in treating tension headaches, insomnia (discussed in Chapter 19), muscle or colon spasm, pain, hypertension, asthma, stuttering, bruxism (grinding of the teeth), and epilepsy. The psychological states achieved through biofeedback can be beneficial in decreasing anxiety and phobic reactions.

The technique is based on giving continuous feedback through the use of machines about the results of each attempt at control until the person is able to achieve control without the aid of a machine. In a typical session, a person might be given this feedback by equipment that amplifies body signals and translates them into a flashing light or a steady tone. Once people can "see" a heartbeat, for instance, and observe when it slows down or speeds up, they have the information they need to control their heart rate by slowing a flashing light or altering a tone. Inexpensive equipment for home use is available.

REPETITIVE TRANSCRANIAL MAGNETIC STIMULATION (rTMS)

In **repetitive transcranial magnetic stimulation**, an insulated coil of wire is placed on the client's head. A powerful electrical current, sent through the insulated coil, generates a magnetic field that causes neurochemical changes in specifically targeted structures of the brain. As a therapy, rTMS is still experimental. The most promising beneficial effects of this experimental treatment are in clients with depression and hallucinating clients who are medication-resistant (Rossini & Rossi, 2007). A longitudinal study at 3- and 6-month intervals suggests that rTMS could replace electroconvulsive therapy (ECT) as a treatment for major depression (Dannon, Dolberg, Schreiber, & Grunhaus, 2002). There is no pain involved with rTMS, and no anesthesia is required. More detailed information on rTMS is in Chapter 6.

EYE MOVEMENT DESENSITIZATION AND REPROCESSING (EMDR)

Eye movement desensitization reprocessing is a controversial intervention suggested for PTSD and dissociative identity

TABLE 33-3 Herbals, Botanicals, and Dietary Supplements Used for Psychiatric Symptoms

Psychiatric Symptom	Natural Medicine	Effectiveness and Safety[a]
Anxiety/restlessness	Kava[b]	■ Comparable to low-dose benzodiazepines for short-term treatment of anxiety ■ Possibly unsafe over the long term or in high doses (associated with liver failure)
Dementia	Ginkgo leaf extract	■ Likely effective; effect is similar to that of donezepil (Aricept) ■ Likely safe when used orally ■ Likely unsafe when used intravenously (IV) ■ Warrants large-scale trials
	SAMe (S-Adenosylmethionine)[c]	■ Likely safe orally, IV, and intramuscularly (IM)
Depression	St. John's wort	■ Evidence is contradictory—possibly as effective as fluoxetine (Prozac) and sertraline (Zoloft), or perhaps no more effective than placebo ■ Likely safe when used orally and short term ■ Possibly unsafe in large doses (1,800 mg or more per day) ■ Interferes with prescription medications by metabolizing them and transporting them out of the body
	SAMe	■ Possibly as effective as oral tricyclic antidepressants
Encephalopathy (alcoholic) or peripheral neuropathy	Thiamine (Vitamin B_1)	■ Likely safe when taken orally ■ Rare hypersensitivity when taken IM or IV
Sleep disturbance/ insomnia	Melatonin/Valerian	■ Possibly effective for jet lag and insomnia ■ Likely ineffective for work shift change adjustment ■ Possibly safe when used orally or parenterally
Dementia of the Alzheimer's type	Omega-3 fatty acids[d]	■ May possibly slow the cognitive and functional decline in Alzheimer's

[a]According to the sources listed, these natural medicines are thought likely to be effective and safe when used appropriately. It is important to validate safety and effectiveness with the most up-to-date sources.

[b]NCCAM has placed studies of kava on hold, pending further guidance from the Federal Food and Drug Administration (FDA). To view the FDA advisory, go to www.cfsan.fda.gov/.

[c]Available studies are limited by small numbers of subjects, inconsistent diagnostic criteria, and short treatment periods.

[d]In May 2007, NIH announced the launching of a nationwide trial to test whether omega-3 fatty acids can affect the progression of, and lower the risk of, Alzheimer's disease.

Sources: Brenner, R., Azbel, V., Madhusoodanan, S., & Pawlowska, M. (2000). Comparison of an extract of hypericum (LI 160) and sertraline in the treatment of depression: A double-blind, randomized pilot study. *Clinical Therapies, 22*, 411–419; Freeman, M. P., Hibbeln, J. R., Wisner, K. L., Davis, J. M., Mischoulon, D., Peet, M., et al. (2006). Omega-3 fatty acids: Evidence basis for treatment and future research in psychiatry. *Journal of Clinical Psychiatry, 67*(12), 1954–1967; Jellin, J. M., Gregory, P. J., Batz, F., & Bonakdar, K. (2002). *Pharmacist's letter/prescriber's letter natural medicines comprehensive database* (4th ed.). Stockton, CA: Therapeutic Research Faculty; and Wettstein, A. (2000). Cholinesterase inhibitors and ginkgo extracts—are they comparable in the treatment of dementia? Comparison of published placebo-controlled efficacy studies of at least six months' duration. *PhytoMedicine, 6*, 393–401.

MEDIALINK FDA Center for Food Safety and Applied Nutrition

disorder. Clients are asked to recall traumatic memories or a feared stimulus while making a series of rapid lateral eye movements. There is no definitive theoretical explanation of how EMDR might work other than the suggestion by Stickgold (2002) that it is the repetitive redirection of attention in EMDR that induces a neurobiologic state, similar to that of rapid eye movement (REM) sleep, which assists in the integration of traumatic memories into the cortex of the brain.

There is confusion in the literature about EMDR. For example, there is no empirically validated model that provides a convincing explanation of exactly how EMDR works, and there have been inaccurate and selective reporting of research, inadequately designed studies, and biased or inaccurate reviews. EMDR has been described as having a significant healing outcome for an adult with a childhood memory of medical trauma resulting from a tonsillectomy. However, this study is based on a single case (Broad & Wheeler, 2006). On the other hand, a randomized clinical trial that compared the short- and long-term benefits of medication (fluoxetine) with those of EMDR in subjects diagnosed with PTSD found that 75% of adult-onset subjects at 6-month follow-up were asymptomatic compared with none in the fluoxetine group (van der Kolk et al., 2007). For most childhood-onset trauma victims, neither medication nor EMDR produced complete symptom remission. This is clearly an area in which well-designed empirical studies are needed.

Table 33-4 ■ Commonly Used Natural Medicines That Should Not Be Taken in Combination with Psychotropic Medication[a]

Psychotropic Medication	Natural Medicine
Anticonvulsants	Sage
Carbamazepine (Tegretol)	Grapefruit juice, psyllium
Antidepressants	European mistletoe, SAMe, St. John's wort
Clomipramine (Anafranil)	Grapefruit juice
Monoamine oxidase inhibitors (MAOIs)	American ginseng, black tea, brewer's yeast, caffeine, cocoa, coffee, cola nut, ephedra, fenugreek, ginkgo leaf extract, green tea, guarana, panax ginseng, passionflower, phenylalanine, wine, yohimbe
Serotonin agonists	5-HTP
Serotonin antagonists	5-HTP
SSRIs	St. John's wort, SAMe
Fluoxetine (Prozac)	Melatonin
Fluvoxamine (Luvox)	Melatonin
Tricyclics	Belladonna, St. John's wort, SAMe, yohimbe
Antipsychotics	American ginseng, coffee, panax ginseng, Siberian ginseng (*Eleutherococcus*)
Central nervous system depressants	German chamomile, hawthorn, kava, melatonin, stinging nettle (above-ground parts), wine
Alcohol	Gamma hydroxybutyrate (GHB), kava, Siberian ginseng, valerian
Central nervous system stimulants	American ginseng, panax ginseng
Caffeine	Cocoa, black tea, ephedra, green tea, guarana, panax ginseng
Fenfluramine	St. John's wort
Clozapine (Clozaril)	Black tea, caffeine, cocoa, coffee, cola nut, green tea, guarana
Lithium	Black tea, caffeine, cocoa, coffee, green tea, guarana, psyllium
Phenothiazines	Evening primrose oil, yohimbe
Sedatives	Goldenseal, gotu kola, kava, passionflower, Siberian ginseng, valerian
Barbiturates	Ginger, goldenseal, kava, passionflower, Siberian ginseng, St. John's wort, valerian
Benzodiazepines	Kava, melatonin, valerian
Alprazolam (Xanax)	Kava
Buspirone (BuSpar)	Grapefruit juice
Midazolam (Versed)	
Triazolam (Halcion)	

[a]These combinations result in canceling out the therapeutic effect of the psychotropic medication, potentiating the effects above and beyond what is therapeutically intended, or causing untoward side effects. This table contains only those combinations that are likely to be clinically significant. It does not include all possible problematic combinations, nor does it include all incidents of case reports.

Source: Blumenthal, M., Goldberg, A., & Brinkman, J. (2000). *Expanded commission E monographs*. Newton, MA: Integrative Medicine Communications; and Jellin, J. M., Gregory, P. J., Batz, F., & Bonakdar, K. (2002). *Pharmacist's letter/prescriber's letter natural medicines comprehensive database* (4th ed.). Stockton, CA: Therapeutic Research Faculty.

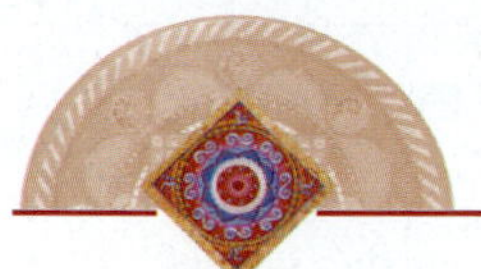

EXPLORE MEDIALINK 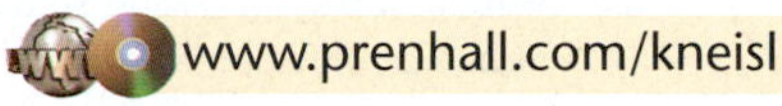

For NCLEX-RN® review questions, case studies, and other resources for this chapter see the Pearson Health MediaLink CD-ROM that accompanies this book and the Companion Website at www.prenhall.com/kneisl.

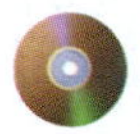

CD-ROM
Audio Glossary
NCLEX-RN® Review Questions

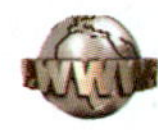

Companion Website
Audio Glossary
NCLEX-RN® Review Questions
Critical Thinking Exercise
- *Explaining Allopathy vs. CAM*

Case Study
- *Serotonin Syndrome*

Care Plan
- *Alcohol Abuse and CAM Care*

MediaLinks
MediaLink Application
- *Older Americans Not Discussing Complementary and Alternative Medicine Use with Doctors*

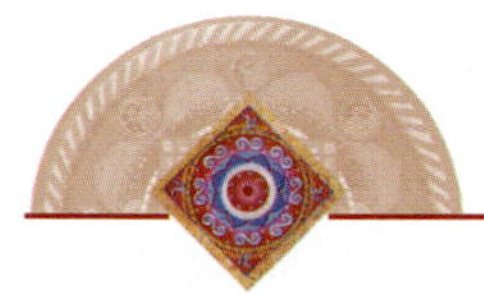

NCLEX-RN® REVIEW QUESTIONS

1. Complementary and alternative healing practices are inappropriate for which of the following clients?
1. A client who has a history of delusional thinking
2. A client who is motivated to try alternative methods of treatment
3. A client who is severely depressed and cannot focus on simple tasks
4. A math teacher with a history of mild depression

2. Which of the following complementary and alternative medicine (CAM) techniques would be appropriate for the client with moderate to severe dementia of the Alzheimer's type?
1. Biofeedback
2. Guided imagery
3. Massage
4. Breathing and relaxation techniques

3. Active progressive relaxation techniques are based on which of the following principles?
1. Muscle tension is the body's physiologic response to anxiety-provoking thoughts.
2. An individual's own imagination creates mental images to reduce stress.
3. Muscles are not purposefully tensed.
4. Relaxation begins at the feet and progresses upward.

4. The nurse is assessing a client to determine if complementary and alternative medicine (CAM) would be appropriate as part of the treatment plan. Which of the following factors should be assessed when making this determination? (Select all that apply.)
1. Client's employment history
2. Client's level of education
3. Client's interest in utilizing alternative medicine techniques
4. History of cardiac disease
5. Medications, herbs, or other nutraceuticals the client is currently taking

5. The nurse is educating a group of health care consumers on how to select complementary alternative medicine techniques and practitioners. The nurse knows a consumer needs additional instructions when the consumer states:
1. "It is important to identify the risks and benefits of the techniques."
2. "I will ask my friends for the name of a practitioner who is good."
3. "I will talk with my health care provider about this."
4. "I think I will meet with the practitioner first to learn more about his or her experience and treatment approaches."

6. The nurse is teaching a client relaxation exercises using music. Music achieves a relaxing effect by:
1. Producing endorphins in the brain.
2. Reducing the amount of endorphins released by the brain.
3. Guiding the client to use positive thinking to reduce stress.
4. Allowing the client to identify a relaxing environment and focusing on it.

7. A client with chronic alcohol abuse asks the nurse if kava would help alleviate some of the anxiety the client is experiencing. The nurse should answer based on knowledge of which of the following?
1. Kava is used to treat depression and is not indicated for anxiety.
2. There is an increased risk of liver failure with long-term use.

3. Kava is indicated for the treatment of sleep disorders and insomnia.
4. Kava may slow the cognitive and functional decline associated with alcohol abuse.

8. Which of the following is contraindicated for the client taking clozapine (Clozaril)?
1. Grapefruit juice
2. Brewer's yeast
3. Caffeine
4. Evening primrose oil

9. Which of the following is not a likely drug interaction between psychotropic medications and natural medicines?
1. Potentiates the effects of the medication to exceed the desired therapeutic effect
2. Untoward side effects
3. Nonadherence with the medications
4. Negates the therapeutic effect of the psychotropic medication

10. Which of the following statements by a nursing student indicates the need for further training on the use of complementary and alternative medicine (CAM) techniques?
1. "It is important to assess the client's motivation to participate in treatment before beginning."
2. "Massage therapy can help alleviate pain for patients with cancer."
3. "These techniques are appropriate for all clients."
4. "I should practice deep breathing exercises before trying to teach a client how to use them."

See Appendix C for answers.

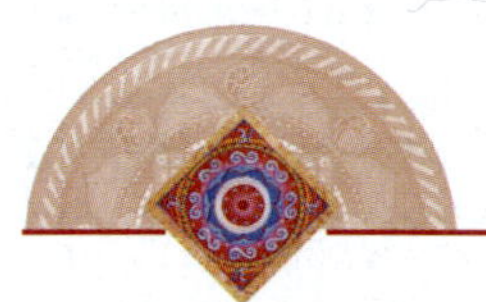

REFERENCES

Baird, C. L., & Sands, L. P. (2006). Effect of guided imagery with relaxation on health-related quality of life in older women with osteoarthritis. *Research in Nursing and Health, 29*(5), 442–451.

Benson, H., & Klipper, M. Z. (2000). *The relaxation response*. New York: William Morrow.

Blumenthal, M., Goldberg, A., & Brinkman, J. (2000). *Expanded commission E monographs*. Newton, MA: Integrative Medicine Communications.

Brenner, R., Azbel, V., Madhusoodanan, S., & Pawlowka, M. (2000). Comparison of an extract of hypericum (LI 160) and sertraline in the treatment of depression: A double-blind, randomized pilot study. *Clinical Therapies, 22*, 411–419.

Broad, R. D., & Wheeler, K. (2006). An adult with childhood medical trauma treated with psychoanalytic psychotherapy and EMDR: A case study. *Perspectives in Psychiatric Care, 42*(2), 95–105.

Bubela, T., Koper, M., Boon, H., & Caulfield, T. (2007). Media portrayal of herbal remedies versus pharmaceutical clinical trials: Impacts on decisions. *Medical Law, 26*(2), 363–373.

Burke, A., Upchurch, D. M., Dye, C., & Chyu, L. (2006). Acupuncture use in the United States: Findings from the National Health Interview Survey. *Journal of Alternative and Complementary Medicine, 12*(7), 639–648.

Carlson, L. E., Ursuliak, Z., Goodey, E., Angen, M., & Speca, M. (2001). The effects of a mindfulness meditation-based stress reduction program on mood and symptoms in cancer outpatients: 6-month follow-up. *Support Care Cancer, 9*(2), 112–123.

Carmody, J., & Baer, R. A. (2007, September 25). Relationships between mindfulness practice and levels of mindfulness, medical and psychological symptoms and well-being in a mindfulness-based stress reduction program. *Journal of Behavioral Medicine*, Epub.

Chao, M. T., Wade, C., Kronenberg, F., Kalmuss, D., & Cushman, L. F. (2006). Women's reasons for complementary and alternative medicine use: Racial/ethnic differences. *Journal of Alternative and Complementary Medicine, 12*(8), 719–720.

Chou, M. H., & Lin, M. F. (2006). Exploring the listening experiences during guided imagery and music therapy of outpatients with depression. *Journal of Nursing Research, 14*(2), 93–102.

Coelho, H. F., Pittier, M. H., & Ernst, E. (2007). An investigation of the contents of complementary and alternative medicine journals. *Alternative Therapies in Health and Medicine, 13*(4), 40–44.

Cohen, M. H., Hrbek, A., Davis, R. B., Schachter, S. C., Kemper, K. J., Boyer, E. W., et al. (2005). Emerging credentialing practices, malpractice liability policies, and guidelines governing complementary and alternative medical practices and dietary supplement recommendations: A descriptive study of 19 integrative health care centers in the United States. *Archives of Internal Medicine, 165*(3), 289–295.

Dannon, P. N., Dolberg, O. T., Schreiber, S., & Grunhaus, L. (2002). Three- and six-month outcome following courses of either ECT or rTMS in a population of severely depressed individuals—preliminary report. *Biological Psychiatry, 51*(8), 687–690.

Decker, C., Huddleston, J., Kosoborod, M., Buchanan, D. M., Stoner, C., Jones, A., et al. (2007). Self-reported use of complementary and alternative medicine in patients with previous acute coronary syndrome. *American Journal of Cardiology, 99*(7), 930–933.

Engebretson, J., & Wardell, D. W. (2007). Energy-based modalities. *Nursing Clinics of North America, 42*(2), 243–259.

Erickson, H. L. (2007). Philosophy and theory of holism. *Nursing Clinics of North America, 42*(2), 139–163.

Escalona, A., Field, T., Singer-Strunck, R., Cullen, C., & Hartshorn, K. (2001). Improvements in the behavior of children with autism following massage therapy. *Journal of Autism and Developmental Disorders, 31*(5), 513–516.

Field, T. (2002). Massage therapy. *Medical Clinics of North America, 86*(1), 163–171.

Finucane, A., & Mercer, S. W. (2006). An exploratory mixed methods study of the acceptability and effectiveness of Mindfulness-Based Cognitive Therapy for patients with active depression and anxiety in primary care. *BMC Psychiatry, 7*, 6–14.

Flannery, M. A., Love, M. M., Pearce, K. A., Luan, J. J., & Elder, W. G. (2006). Communication about complementary and alternative medicine: Perspectives of primary care clinicians. *Alternative Therapies in Health and Medicine, 12*(1), 56–63.

Fontaine, K. L. (2004). *Complementary and alternative therapies for nursing practice* (2nd ed.). Upper Saddle River, NJ: Prentice Hall.

Freeman, M. P., Hibbeln, J. R., Wisner, K. L., Davis, J. M., Mischoulon, D., Peet, M., et al. (2006). Omega-3 fatty acids: Evidence basis for treatment and future research in psychiatry. *Journal of Clinical Psychiatry, 67*(12), 1954–1967.

Friel, P. N. (2007). EEG biofeedback in the treatment of attention deficit hyperactivity disorder. *Alternative Medicine Review, 12*(2), 146–151.

Gecsedi, R. A. (2002). Massage therapy for patients with cancer. *Clinical Journal of Oncological Nursing, 6*(1), 52–54.

Gold, E. B., Bair, Y., Zhang, G., Utts, J., Greendale, G. A., Upchurch, D., et al. (2007). Cross-sectional analysis of specific complementary and alternative medicine (CAM) use by racial-ethnic group and menopausal status: The Study of Women's Health Across the Nation (SWAN). *Menopause, 14*(4), 612–623.

Graham, R. E., Ahn, A. C., Davis, R. B., O'Connor, B. B., Eisenberg, D. M., & Phillips, R. S. (2005). Use of complementary and alternative medical therapies among racial and ethnic minority adults: Results from the 2002

National Health Interview Survey. *Journal of the National Medical Association, 97*(4), 535–545.

Grzywacz, J. G., Suerken, C. K., Quandt, S. A., Bell, R. A., Lang, W., & Arcury, T. A. (2006). Older adults' use of complementary and alternative medicine for mental health: Findings from the 2002 National Health Interview Survey. *Journal of Alternative and Complementary Medicine, 12*(5), 467–473.

Hagedorn, M. E., & Zahourek, R. P. (2007). Research paradigms and methods for investigating holistic nursing concerns. *Nursing Clinics of North America, 42*(2), 335–353.

Hanson, E., Kalish, L. A., Bunce, E., Curtis, C., McDaniel, S., Ware, J., et al. (2007). Use of complementary and alternative medicine among children diagnosed with autism spectrum disorder. *Journal of Autism and Developmental Disorders, 37*(4), 628–636.

Herman, C. J., Dente, J. M., Allen, P., & Hunt, W. C. (2006). Ethnic differences in the use of complementary and alternative therapies among adults with osteoarthritis. *Prevention of Chronic Disease, 3*(3), A80.

Hollifield, M., Sinclair-Lian, N., Warner, T. D., & Hammerschlag, R. (2007). Acupuncture for posttraumatic stress disorder: A randomized controlled pilot study. *Journal of Nervous and Mental Diseases, 195*(6), 504–513.

Hsiao, A. F., Wong, M. D., Goldstein, M. S., Yu, H. J., Andersen, R. M., Brown, E. R., et al. (2006). Variation in complementary and alternative medicine (CAM) use across racial/ethnic groups and the development of ethnic-specific measures of CAM use. *Journal of Alternative and Complementary Medicine, 12*(3), 281–290.

Jain, S., Shapiro, S. L., Swanick, S., Roesch, S. C., Mills, P. J., Bell, I., et al. (2007). A randomized controlled trial of mindfulness meditation versus relaxation training: Effects on distress, positive states of mind, rumination, and distraction. *Annals of Behavioral Medicine, 33*(1), 11–21.

Jellin, J. M., Gregory, P. J., Batz, F., & Bonakdar, K. (2002). *Pharmacist's letter/prescriber's letter natural medicines comprehensive database* (4th ed.). Stockton, CA: Therapeutic Research Faculty.

Kaplan, M., Mutlu, E. A., Benson, M., Fields, J. Z., Banan, A., & Keshavarzian, A. (2007). Use of herbal preparations in the treatment of oxidant-mediated inflammatory disorders. *Complementary Therapies in Medicine, 15*(3), 207–216.

Katz, P., & Lee, F. (2007). Racial/ethnic differences in the use of complementary and alternative medicine in patients with arthritis. *Journal of Clinical Rheumatology, 13*(1), 3–11.

Kelly, J. P., Kaufman, D. W., Kelley, K., Rosenberg, L., & Mitchell, A. A. (2006). Use of herbal/natural supplements according to racial/ethnic group. *Journal of Alternative and Complementary Medicine, 12*(6), 555–561.

Khalsa, D. S., & Stauth, C. (2001). *Meditation as medicine: Activate the power of your natural healing force*. New York: Simon & Schuster.

Krieger, D. (1979). *The therapeutic touch*. Upper Saddle River, NJ: Prentice Hall.

Krieger, D. (1993). *Accepting your power to heal*. Sante Fe, NM: Bear & Co.

Kshettry, V. R., Carole, L. F., Henly, S. J., Sendelbach, S., & Kummer, B. (2006). Complementary alternative medical therapies for heart surgery patients: Feasibility, safety, and impact. *Annals of Thoracic Surgery, 81*(1), 201–205.

Kwekkeboom, K. L., Bumpus, M., Wanta, B., & Serlin, R. C. (2007, October 22). Oncology nurses' use of nondrug pain interventions in practice. *Journal of Pain and Symptom Management*, Epub.

Labbé, E., Schmidt, N., Babin, J., & Pharr, M. (2007, October 27). Coping with stress: The effectiveness of different types of music. *Applied Psychophysiological Feedback*, Epub.

Lafferty, W. E., Downey, L., McCarty, R. L., Standish, L. J., & Patrick, D. L. (2006). Evaluating CAM treatment at the end of life: A review of clinical trials for massage and meditation. *Complementary Therapies in Medicine, 14*(2), 100–112.

Lang, E. V., Berbaum, K. S., Faintuch, S., Hatsiopoulou, O., Halsey, N., Li, X., et al. (2006). Adjunctive self-hypnotic relaxation for outpatient medical procedures: A prospective randomized trial with women undergoing large core breast biopsy. *Pain, 126*(1), 3–4.

Liu, R. W., Mehta, P., Fortuna, S., Armstrong, D. G., Cooperman, D. R., Thompson, G. H., et al. (2007). A randomized prospective study of music therapy for reducing anxiety during cast room procedures. *Journal of Pediatric Orthopedics, 27*(7), 831–833.

Margolin, A., Kleber, H. D., Avants, S. K., Konefal, J., Gawin, F., Stark, E., et al. (2002). Acupuncture for the treatment of cocaine addiction: A randomized controlled trial. *Journal of the American Medical Association, 287*(1), 55–63.

Matthews, A. K., Sellergren, S. A., Huo, D., List, M., & Fleming, G. (2007). Complementary and alternative medicine use among breast cancer survivors. *Journal of Alternative and Complementary Medicine, 13*(5), 555–562.

Mehta, D. H., Phillips, R. S., Davis, R. B., & McCarthy, E. P. (2007). Use of complementary and alternative therapies by Asian Americans. Results from the National Health Interview Survey. *Journal of General and Internal Medicine, 22*(6), 762–767.

Myklebust, M., Colson, J., Kaufman, J., Winsauer, J., Zhang, Y. Q., & Harris, R. E. (2006). Policy for therapeutic acupuncture in an academic health center: A model for standard policy development. *Journal of Alternative and Complementary Medicine, 12*(10), 1035–1039.

Myklebust, M., & Iler, J. (2007). Policy for therapeutic massage in an academic health center: A model for standard policy development. *Journal of Alternative and Complementary Medicine, 13*(4), 471–475.

National Institutes of Health Consensus Panel. (1997). *Acupuncture: National Institutes of Health consensus development statement*. Bethesda, MD: National Institutes of Health.

Nedrow, A. (2006). Status of credentialing alternative providers within a subset of U.S. academic health centers. *Journal of Alternative and Complementary Medicine, 12*(3), 329–335.

Owen-Smith, A., Diclemente, R., & Wingood, G. (2007). Complementary and alternative medicine use decreases adherence to HAART in HIV-positive women. *AIDS Care, 19*(5), 589–593.

Pagnoni, G., & Cekic, M. (2007). Age effects on graymatter volume and attentional performance in Zen meditation. *Neurobiology and Aging, 28*(10), 1623–1627.

Paul, G., Elam, B., & Verhulst, S. J. (2007). A longitudinal study of students' perceptions of using deep breathing meditation to reduce testing stresses. *Teaching and Learning Medicine, 19*(3), 287–292.

Pearson, N. J., Johnson, L. L., & Nahin, R. L. (2006). Insomnia, trouble sleeping, and complementary and alternative medicine: Analysis of the 2002 National Health Interview Survey data. *Archives of Internal Medicine, 166*(16), 1775–1782.

Reed, T. (2007). Imagery in the clinical setting: A tool for healing. *Nursing Clinics of North America, 42*(2), 261–277.

Rossini, P. M., & Rossi, S. (2007). Transcranial magnetic stimulation: Diagnostic, therapeutic, and research potential. *Neurology, 68*(7), 484–488.

Scharff, L., Marcus, D. A., & Masek, B. J. (2002). A controlled study of minimal-contact thermal biofeedback treatment in children with migraine. *Journal of Pediatric Psychology, 27*(2), 109–119.

Smallwood, J., Brown, R., Coulter, F., Irvine, E., & Copland, C. (2001). Aromatherapy and behavior disturbances in dementia: A randomized controlled trial. *International Journal of Geriatric Psychiatry, 16*(10), 1010–1013.

Smith, A., Graham, L., & Senthinathan, S. (2007). Mindfulness-based cognitive therapy for recurring depression in older people: A qualitative study. *Aging and Mental Health, 11*(3), 346–357.

Stephen, J. E., Mackenzie, G., Sample, S., & Macdonald, J. (2007). Twenty years of therapeutic touch in a Canadian cancer agency: Lessons learned from a case study of integrative oncology practice. *Supportive Care for Cancer, 15*(8), 993–998.

Stickgold, R. (2002). EMDR: A putative neurobiological mechanism of action. *Journal of Clinical Psychology, 58*(1), 61–75.

Taylor, D. M., Walsham, N., Taylor, S. E., & Wong, L. (2006a). Complementary and alternative medicines versus prescription drugs: Perceptions of emergency department patients. *Emergency Medicine Journal, 23*(4), 266–268.

Taylor, D. M., Walsham, N., Taylor, S. E., & Wong, L. (2006b). Potential interactions between prescription drugs and complementary and alternative medicines among patients in the emergency department. *Pharmacotherapy, 26*(5), 634–640.

van der Kolk, B. A., Spinazzola, J., Blaustein, M. E., Hopper, J. W., Hopper, E. K., Korn, D. L., et al. (2007). A randomized clinical trial of eye movement desensitization and reprocessing (EMDR), fluoxetine, and pill placebo in the treatment of posttraumatic stress disorder: Treatment effects and long-term maintenance. *Journal of Clinical Psychiatry, 68*(1), 37–46.

Wettstein, A. (2000). Cholinesterase inhibitors and ginkgo extracts—are they comparable in the treatment of dementia? Comparison of published placebo-controlled efficacy studies of at least six months' duration. *Phyto-Medicine, 6*, 393–401.

Wong, H. H., & Smith, R. G. (2006). Patterns of complementary and alternative medical therapy use in children diagnosed with autism spectrum disorders. *Journal of Autism and Developmental Disorders, 36*(7), 901–909.

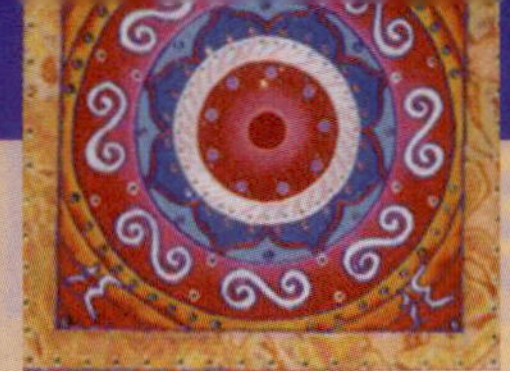

CHAPTER

34

Crisis Intervention

CAROL REN KNEISL

KEY TERMS

anticipatory guidance *904*
crisis *893*
crisis intervention *894*
critical incident stress management *904*
maturational crisis *898*
resilience *895*
situational crisis *897*
vicarious traumatization *908*

LEARNING OUTCOMES

After completing this chapter, you will be able to:

1. Describe the types of maturational and situational crises a person can experience.
2. Explain why a crisis is a turning point in a person's life.
3. Trace the sequence of a crisis and determine its significance for the nursing care of a client in crisis.
4. Incorporate an understanding of the origins of a crisis, risk factors, and balancing factors during the assessment phase of crisis management.
5. Identify three possible crisis intervention modalities for a person in crisis.
6. Incorporate the ABCs of crisis counseling in a plan of care for a client in crisis.
7. Provide psychoeducation for clients and families who are disaster victims.
8. Analyze personal feelings and attitudes that may affect professional practice when caring for clients in crisis.

CRITICAL THINKING CHALLENGE

Katrinka V., a 43-year-old nurse, is a survivor of domestic violence. She and John, her husband of 15 years, have two children. Last night after a long period of drinking, John threatened Katrinka and the children with a gun. Katrinka managed to get herself and the children out of the house and into her car, where they spent the night. In the morning, Katrinka, distraught, highly anxious, and in crisis, arrived at the psychiatric emergency room. She said, "I can't think of what to do. I've got to get to my job and the kids have to go to school. It's not safe for any of us at either place. What should I do?"

1. How do you understand her current situation?
2. What critical areas do you need to assess?
3. What interventions would be helpful?

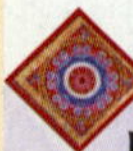

MEDIALINK 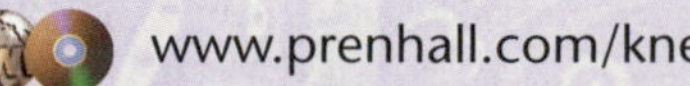

Go to the Pearson Health MediaLink CD-ROM and the Companion Website at www.prenhall.com/kneisl for interactive resources for this chapter.

On September 11, 2001, in the most devastating terrorist onslaught ever waged against the United States, knife-wielding hijackers crashed two airliners into New York City's World Trade Center, toppling its twin 110-story towers.

The deadly calamity was witnessed on television screens across the world as a third plane slammed into the Pentagon, and a fourth crashed outside Pittsburgh. The death toll, believed to number almost 3,000, also included firefighters, police officers, and medical personnel killed while attempting to rescue victims. The impact on New York City was horrific. Many people lost their jobs because businesses were demolished and tourists stayed away. Even the usual winter holiday festivities for which New York City is famous were conducted with an air of great sadness. The impact on the rest of the country—survivors, citizens, and visitors alike—and around the world was tremendous, as these clinical examples illustrate.

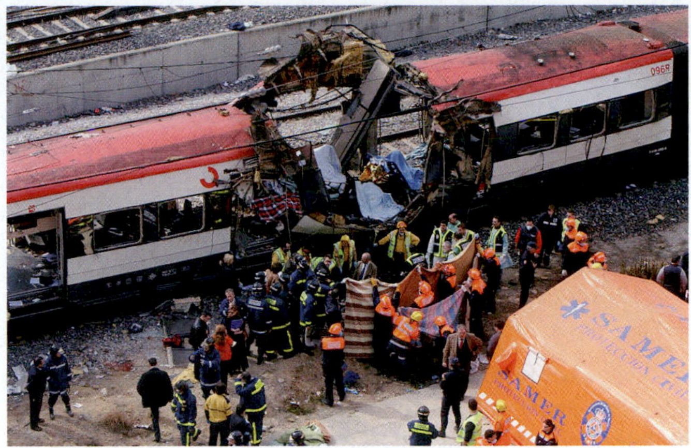

FIGURE 34-1 ■ Rescue workers cover up bodies near a bomb-damaged train in Madrid, Spain. The explosion killed more than 170 rush-hour commuters and wounded more than 500.

Source: AP Wide World Photos, Paul White.

CLINICAL EXAMPLE

Nguyen, a visitor from Malaysia, was walking across the Brooklyn Bridge, admiring the view of lower Manhattan, when he saw the plane hit the first tower. He stood on the bridge in horror, watching the fireball as people jumped from the buildings. Although he has long since returned to Malaysia, he has nightmares in which he relives the experience over and over.

Two teenagers were at home in Arizona watching TV while getting ready for school when they saw the news. First they experienced sadness, then disbelief, confusion, anger, and, finally, fear. One said, "Now I know that terrorism isn't just something you see on the evening news that happens on the other side of the world. My life has been changed forever."

Alistair works at an airport outside of Liverpool, England. People were gathered around him, chatting about the disaster, crying, and praying. Alistair left work sick that day. He told his supervisor that he felt nauseated and weak in the knees at the thought that airplanes at his airport could be targeted and that life was so fragile.

The research literature suggests that more people need treatment for mental health difficulties than for physical symptoms directly stemming from an injury-causing agent or event (Parker, Barnett, Everly, & Links, 2006): not only posttraumatic stress disorder (PTSD), but also acute stress disorder, depression, complicated bereavement reactions, substance use disorders, fear, anxiety, somatization, anger control, and arrest or regression of childhood developmental progression (Murthy, 2007). Communities face an acute "mental health surge" that can overwhelm available community mental health resources.

Do you remember how you felt on Tuesday, September 11, 2001? Did you feel helpless? Did you know what to do or say to others? Did you believe you were in danger? Did you call anyone? Did you talk about the event with others? Did you want it all to go away? If you answered "yes" to any of these questions, you know what a crisis feels like. Chances are that you, your family, and your community were in crisis, along with many other individuals, families, and communities.

A **crisis** is an acute, time-limited state of disequilibrium resulting from situational, developmental, or societal sources of stress such as that illustrated in FIGURE 34-1 ■. An individual can be said to be in crisis when that person is in a situation in which usual problem-solving or adaptive methods are inadequate to resolve a problem or conflict, causing a state of disequilibrium. People involved in these incidents may be unable to effectively manage stressful events or environmental changes. They may be unable to function and may feel paralyzed and powerless.

It is likely that the terrorist attack (and other large-scale crisis events) will continue to have effects such as PTSD far into the future (Laugharne, Janca, & Widiger, 2007). Five years after the event, children were sad and tearful, anxious and fearful, irritable and angry, having intrusive thoughts and images, and having difficulty concentrating and sleeping (Covell et al., 2006). This same study found that older children, 12 to 17 years of age, were more likely to use drugs, corroborating the prediction made by Baker (2002) shortly after the attack and the findings of Vlahov and associates (2002). Those who study the survivors of hurricanes and other natural disasters find similar disruptions of psychosocial health (King & Steinmann, 2007). A study of Canadian military personnel who have been exposed to combat operations or have witnessed atrocities or massacres reported a 15% prevalence of a DSM-IV-TR mental disorder (Sareen et al., 2007). This was the first study to use a representative sample of 8,441 currently active military personnel to examine the relationship between deployment-related experiences and mental health problems.

Other examples of situations that have caused a crisis on a more limited scale are discussed in the following clinical example.

CLINICAL EXAMPLE

An ex-employee comes into an office building and shoots 15 people; a tragic school bus accident claims five 6-year-olds and their teacher; two teenagers from the same high school commit suicide the same week; a 66-year-old man retires and feels useless and considers suicide; a 23-year-old woman finds out that she has a fatal illness; a premature baby is born; a 12-year-old is kidnapped while walking home from school.

Nurses are intimately connected with crises. We often interact with people who are faced with new, frightening, and troublesome situations. Because of who we are, where we work, and our accessibility to individuals and families, we are in a position to offer supportive and therapeutic interventions that can change people's lives. You can help if you understand how to effectively intervene, that is, if you understand how to implement crisis intervention skills. **Crisis intervention** is a conceptual framework for intervention that calls for short-term, action-oriented assistance focused on problem solving, with a goal of restoring the individual's equilibrium. Effective crisis intervention will call for all the skills that a well-prepared nurse can muster.

Crisis intervention is not the specialty of any one professional group. People who intervene in crises come from the fields of nursing, medicine, psychology, social work, and theology. Police officers, teachers, school guidance counselors, rescue workers, and bartenders, among others, are often on-the-spot crisis intervenors. Obviously, crisis intervention can be the business of many different people. The Association of Traumatic Stress Specialists provides training programs and board certification for qualified intervenors. The association represents those who serve victims of crime, veterans, refugees, survivors of natural disasters and terrorist attacks, holocaust survivors, persons with line-of-duty-related injuries, individuals coping with a death, victims of school and workplace violence, victims of political persecution, and others who have experienced traumatic stress. The association can be accessed through the Companion Website for this book.

MEDIALINK Association of Traumatic Stress Specialists

CRISIS AS A TURNING POINT

The word *crisis* stems from the Greek *krinein*, "to decide." In Chinese, two characters are used to write the word; one is the character for danger and the other the character for opportunity. The interaction between *danger* and *opportunity* will become clearer as you read this chapter.

Crisis situations are turning points or junctures in a person's life that result in a new equilibrium. The new equilibrium may be close to that of the precrisis state, or it may be a more positive or more negative state. If the new equilibrium is more positive, the person experiences personal growth, increased competence, a better social network, newfound problem-solving abilities, or an improved self-image. If the new equilibrium is more negative, the individual may lose skills, regress to an earlier developmental stage, develop socially unacceptable behaviors, or develop a mental disorder. Unsuccessful negotiation of a crisis leaves the person feeling anxious, threatened, and ineffective. Individuals may also respond to a crisis event with disturbed personal coping or with frankly psychotic behavior. This process is illustrated in FIGURE 34-2 ■.

Because a state of disequilibrium is so uncomfortable, a crisis is self-limiting. That is, even without intervention, a crisis will resolve itself with either a favorable or unfavorable conclusion. However, a person experiencing a crisis alone is more vulnerable to unsuccessful negotiation than a person working through a crisis with help. Working with another person increases the likelihood that the person in crisis will resolve it in a positive way. This is why crisis intervention is sometimes referred to as *primary prevention for PTSD* (refer

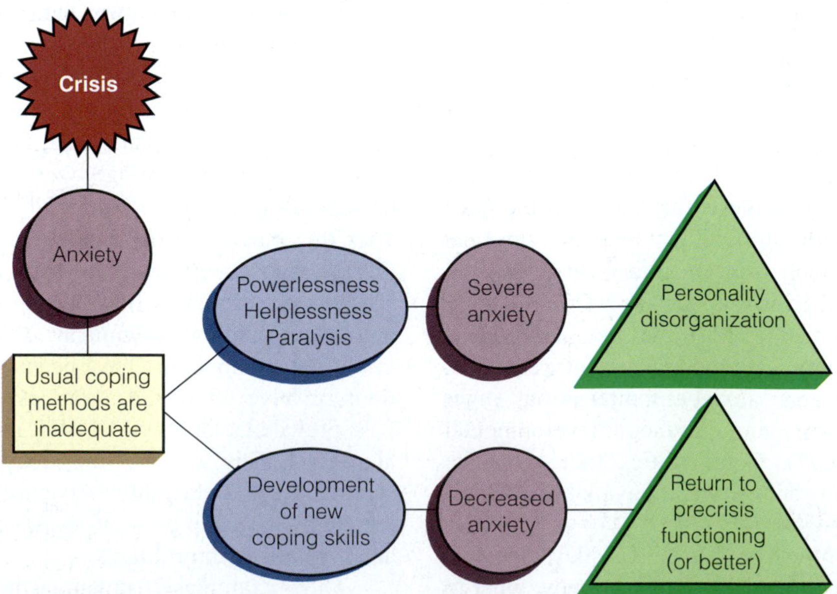

FIGURE 34-2 ■ The progression of a crisis to either successful or unsuccessful resolution depends on what people do when they discover that their usual coping mechanisms are ineffective.

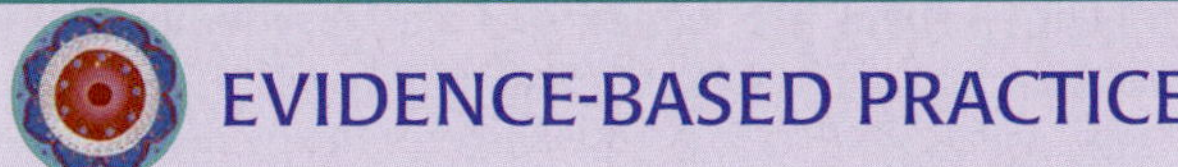

TANGIBLE SUPPORT FOR A CLIENT IN CRISIS

Mrs. Blankenship, a middle-age African-American woman, has been admitted for a crisis evaluation and brief stay at the behavioral unit in the general hospital in which you work. She has requested that a female perform her admission interview. In reviewing her records, you note that she has had multiple hospitalizations for crisis-type episodes, severe anxiety, and obsessive–compulsive disorder.

She is tearful and anxious, as well as depressed, and asks you to leave the door open and not to sit in front of it. Mrs. Blankenship connects most of her anxiety to the fact that she lives in a housing project in which stealing and drugs are rampant. Her greatest fear is for her own safety and the safety of her grandchildren. She is articulate and without ideas of suicide or homicide. She is not psychotic.

You are working the full week, and Mrs. Blankenship will be your client for the next 5 days. On the third day she tells you of a time when she was held captive for 6 hours and brutally raped by a man who lived in her building, sharing her fear that she is "going crazy." You implement the following interventions:

- Explain to Mrs. Blankenship that many of her problems could be related to the attack.
- Explore with her the coping styles that emerged from this event.
- Encourage her to make connections between the event and her current situation.
- Provide tangible support by helping her select an outpatient therapist who is competent to treat trauma victims and arrange for her to meet the therapist while she is still in the hospital.

Your interventions are based on your understanding of the following research studies that indicate that many individuals who seek psychiatric help have been traumatized and the trauma has not been recognized or adequately treated.

Glass, N., Perrin, N., Campbell, J. C., & Soeken, K. (2007). The protective role of tangible support on post-traumatic stress disorder symptoms in urban women survivors of violence. *Research in Nursing and Health, 30*(5), 558–568.

Scott, S. T. (2007). Multiple traumatic experiences and the development of posttraumatic stress disorder. *Journal of Interpersonal Violence, 22*(7), 932–938.

CRITICAL THINKING APPLICATION

1. In what ways can racist and sexist stereotypes influence rape blame attribution—that is, how do the victim, family and friends, and even health care providers attribute blame?
2. How is it possible that all of Mrs. Blankenship's symptoms can be explained by a diagnosis of PTSD?

to Chapter 18). The Evidence-Based Practice feature discusses the effects on a client of experiencing a crisis alone.

Common Characteristics of Crises

To understand the concept of crisis fully and to appreciate the interaction of risk factors, we must differentiate among levels of distress to illustrate what a crisis is not. Stress is not crisis. Everyone feels stress at various times, in a variety of forms (see the discussion in Chapter 8). Stress is pressure and tension. Stressful situations may demand our attention and may be exhausting, but they are not crises. An emergency is a situation that often demands an immediate response to ensure the survival of an individual. Although neither stress nor an emergency are themselves a crisis, stress or an emergency can ultimately precipitate a crisis. A crisis is not a mental disorder. A crisis can happen to someone who has never had a mental disorder or to someone who is currently experiencing a mental disorder. Common characteristics of crises are discussed in Box 34-1.

Resilience, Risk Factors, and Balancing Factors

Why do some people effectively manage disequilibrium while others go into crisis? This capacity is called **resilience**. Resilience is the ability not only to survive and bounce back from difficult and traumatic experiences, but also to continue to grow and develop emotionally and psychologically. The notion of resilience encompasses the biological and psychological characteristics intrinsic to an individual, such as personality style and quality of interpersonal relationships, that confer protection against the development of psychopathology (Hoge, Austin, & Pollack, 2007). Resilience probably

Box 34-1 Common Characteristics of Crises

- Many situational crises are experienced as sudden. The person is usually not aware of a warning signal, whether or not others could "see it coming." The individual or family may feel they have had little or no preparation for the event or trauma.
- The crisis may be experienced as ultimately life threatening, whether this perception is realistic or not.
- Communication with significant others is often reduced or cut off.
- There may be perceived or real displacement from familiar surroundings or significant loved ones.
- All crises have an aspect of loss, whether actual or perceived. The losses can include an object, a person, a hope, a dream, or any significant factor for that individual.

Box 34-2 Risk Factors for Crisis

- Intensity of exposure to the situation
- Preexisting psychiatric symptoms and diagnosis
- Prior history of traumatic exposure
- Family history of psychiatric problems, anxiety, and/or antisocial behavior
- Early separation from parents
- Childhood abuse
- Poverty
- Cultural expectations that prohibit asking others for help
- Degree of threat to life (being on a plane that crashes versus watching a plane crash from a distance)

explains why not all maltreated children experience mental health problems as adults (Collishaw et al., 2007). Researchers and clinicians alike have been surprised by the prevalence of the capacity for resilience (Mancini & Bonanno, 2006), and clinicians are beginning to focus on uncovering and energizing pathways to resilience in their clients.

There are several risk factors, in addition to the nature of the trauma or experience, that place individuals at high risk for crisis. These factors are identified in Box 34-2.

In addition to these risk factors, Aguilera (1998) indicates that these three balancing factors are important to the successful resolution of disequilibrium:

1. *Perception of the event:* How individuals perceive and understand the event/crisis in their lives. Are they being punished? Is this happening only to them and never to anyone else? How will the event affect their future? Do they see the situation realistically, or is it distorted?
2. *Situational supports:* The availability of people who can help individuals in crisis solve the problem. Meaningful relationships with others give support and assistance during the crisis. Individuals with inadequate support are likely to experience a decrease in self-esteem. In turn, lowered self-esteem may make an event appear more threatening.
3. *Coping mechanisms:* All people use mechanisms to cope with anxiety and tension. Because the individual has used these coping mechanisms with success in the past, they become part of the coping repertoire. These tension-relieving mechanisms can be obvious or subtle (see the discussion in Chapter 8 ∞).

If all these balancing factors are present when an individual experiences a state of disequilibrium—a realistic perception of the event, adequate situational support, adequate coping mechanisms—the problem will be resolved and equilibrium will be regained, making it unlikely that a crisis will result. If, however, one or more balancing factors are absent, the problem is likely to be unresolved, disequilibrium is likely to continue, and a state of crisis will result.

BIOPSYCHOSOCIAL THEORIES OF CRISIS

The recognition of crisis has a long history. As long ago as 400 BCE, physicians understood that a crisis was a hazardous life event. It was not until the 20th century, however, that strategies for helping people to cope with crisis were developed. Theories of crisis and crisis intervention resulted from early research studies that are now classics, as well as more recent events in the field of mental health. Some of these are described below.

- Lindemann's (1944) landmark study of the survivors of the tragic Coconut Grove nightclub fire in Boston identified symptoms common to individuals experiencing acute grief. Lindemann determined that if grieving was delayed or absent, the crisis resulted in negative outcomes.
- The observations of, and treatment by, military psychiatrists of World War II battle-weary and emotionally upset soldiers at the front lines allowed the soldiers to return to duty rather than having to be sent to inpatient psychiatric facilities.
- Tyhurst's (1957) studies of the stages individuals go through when experiencing transition states such as migration, retirement, and civilian disasters led to the identification of three phases—a period of impact, a period of recoil, and a posttraumatic period of recovery.
- Federal funding was made available in 1961 for community-based mental health programs such as suicide prevention and crisis services, including crisis telephone counseling services, known popularly as hot lines.
- Caplan's (1964) work in preventive psychiatry and anticipatory guidance in the early days of the Peace Corps expanded on Lindemann's work. Caplan studied developmental crises and accidental crises. He determined that successfully navigating the stages of a crisis required using new coping skills.
- The publication by the American Psychiatric Association of the *Diagnostic and Statistical Manual of Mental Disorders* in 1980 provided, for the first time, a system to measure the severity of psychosocial stressors and to reflect that severity with the psychiatric diagnosis via Axis IV (see Chapter 11 ∞).
- More contemporary methods of crisis intervention include Roberts' seven-stage crisis intervention model for frontline crisis workers (Roberts, 2005).

The etiology, psychobiology, epidemiology, comorbidity, and treatment of crisis and its sequelae are complicated. Some theories that attempt to explain what happens in a crisis and how to intervene in a crisis are described next.

Tyhurst's Stages of Disaster

Tyhurst (1957) identified three overlapping stages in response to a disaster. They are:

1. Impact
2. Recoil
3. Posttrauma

These stages are as relevant today as they were then, and they help mental health care workers understand the experiences of the victims of hurricanes, floods, fires, terrorist attacks, and other disasters as well as the people who experienced the disaster by watching it at home on their television sets.

Impact

The first stage, *impact*, is stimulated by the catastrophe. The victims recognize what is happening to them and are concerned mainly with the present. During this acute phase, the victim's major concern may be staying alive. According to Tyhurst, about 75% of the victims experience shock and confusion. Although they appear dazed, they also exhibit the physical signs of fear. Another group of people, up to 25%, remain coherent. They logically and rationally assess the situation and develop and implement a plan for dealing with the immediate problems brought on by the catastrophe. A third group, also up to 25%, may panic or become immobilized with fear. They may behave hysterically, or they may be overlooked because they sit and silently stare into space.

Recoil

In *recoil*, the second stage, the initial stress of the disaster has passed, and victims may no longer find their lives in immediate danger, although injuries and other discomforts come to their awareness. Emergency shelter, food, and clothing become available. The victims' behavior is usually dependent—they want to be taken care of. Weeping is common as survivors begin to realize all that has happened to them.

Posttrauma

The full impact of the losses the victims have experienced comes in the third, or *posttrauma*, period. Grief is a predominant response to the losses in their lives. Disturbed and psychotic responses may occur.

Caplan's Stages of a Crisis Reaction

Caplan (1964) studied various developmental crisis reactions to premature births, infancy, childhood, and adolescence, as well as accidental crises such as illness and death. Caplan built upon Tyhurst's work with disaster victims. According to him, the four stages of a crisis reaction are:

1. *Phase 1:* The individual experiences an initial increase in tension because of the emotionally hazardous crisis-precipitating event.
2. *Phase 2:* When the individual is unable to resolve the crisis quickly, tension and disruption of daily living increase.
3. *Phase 3:* If the individual attempts but fails to resolve the crisis by the usual problem-solving techniques, tension increases to such a level that the individual may become depressed.
4. *Phase 4:* At the final stage, the person may partly resolve the crisis by using new coping skills. Mental disruption or disorder may occur if the person does not develop new coping skills to manage the crisis.

Roberts' Model of Crisis Intervention

Roberts' seven-stage model of crisis intervention (2005) has been used to help people in acute psychologic crisis and acute situational crisis, persons in high-risk populations such as suicidal juvenile offenders (Roberts & Bender, 2006), and persons diagnosed with acute stress disorder. The seven stages are:

1. Plan and conduct a thorough assessment (including lethality assessment [refer to Chapter 23 ∞], assessment of dangerousness to self or others, and assessment of immediate psychosocial needs).
2. Make interpersonal contact, establish rapport, and rapidly establish the relationship (conveying genuine regard and respect for the client, acceptance, reassurance, and a nonjudgmental attitude; refer to Chapters 3 and 29 ∞).
3. Examine the dimensions of the problem in order to define it (including the "last straw" of the precipitating event).
4. Encourage an exploration of feelings and emotions through active listening (refer to Chapter 10 ∞).
5. Explore and assess past coping attempts and generate and explore alternatives and previously untried coping methods or solutions.
6. Restore cognitive functioning through the implementation of an action plan based on cognitive mastery (refer to Chapter 31 ∞).
7. Follow up with the client and leave the door open for future contact, especially around the time of the anniversary of the event (exactly 1 month or 1 year after the victimization).

FIGURE 34-3 ■ on page 898 illustrates Roberts' seven-step model.

Roberts' seven-step model is integrated throughout the Nursing Process section later in this chapter.

TYPES OF CRISES

In the contemporary view, the origin of a crisis is as important as the type of crisis. Roberts (2005) points out that if we know how the crisis began, we have a better opportunity to intervene effectively. Two general categories of crisis origins are situational and maturational.

Situational Crisis

A **situational crisis** can originate from three sources: material or environmental (fire, natural disaster, man-made biohazards, terrorist attacks); personal or physical (heart attack,

MEDIALINK Case Study: Reaction to Trauma

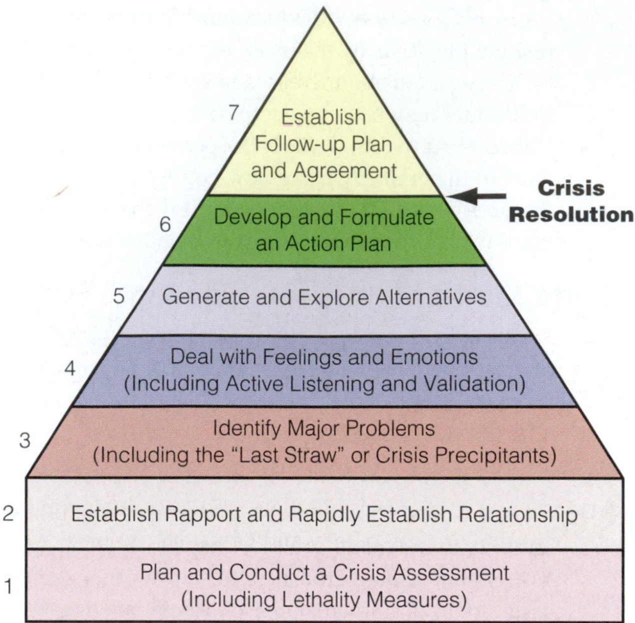

FIGURE 34-3 Roberts' seven-stage model of crisis intervention.

Source: Roberts, A. R. (Ed.). (2005). *Crisis intervention handbook: Assessment, treatment, and research* (2nd ed.) (Figure 1, p. 16). New York: Oxford University Press. Used by permission of Oxford University Press, Inc.

diagnosis of fatal illness, bodily disfigurement); and interpersonal or social (death of a loved one or divorce). Often, these life-threatening events motivate people to take significant action in their close relationships that alter their life course.

Because the event leading to the situational crisis is usually unanticipated, one generally cannot do anything directly to prevent it. In a more indirect sense, an individual can attempt to keep healthy and focus on the most effective methods of interacting with others. However, the complexity of the experience influences the ability of the individual to resolve the trauma. For instance, a person coping with one traumatic incident is more likely to resolve the experience than someone faced with multiple traumas or factors (Scott, 2007). An example of a situational crisis (in which the origin of the crisis is the husband's diagnosis of terminal cancer) follows.

CLINICAL EXAMPLE

Jessie, age 52, is a social worker at a local mental health clinic who is feeling increasingly less able to function since she learned that her husband has a terminal, inoperable form of cancer. Many arrangements need to be made, including finding adequate medical treatment and doing appropriate evaluations of her husband.

Jessie has been unable to work for 2 to 3 days and now tells a psychiatric–mental health nurse that she can no longer function—she has been unable to make any of the required phone calls, despite knowing she is the person who must coordinate everything. Jessie speaks of feeling overwhelmed, shakes her head, and says, "Can you believe it? I do this all the time for others, but I can't do it now. Isn't that a joke?"

Maturational Crisis

A **maturational crisis** involves life cycle changes or normal transitions of human development. These are the traditional stages of human development that include infancy, childhood, puberty, adolescence, adulthood, middle age, and old age. During each stage, the individual is subject to unique stressors. Each stage of development is characterized by developmental tasks the individual must accomplish in order to progress to the next level. A failure at any one level compromises the next stage of development.

Maturational crises also include such changes as marriage, retirement, and the transition from student to worker. Crises associated with these states arise when the individual enters a new area of development or functioning and cannot adapt to functioning at that level. If the person experiences additional trauma or change, the risk for experiencing a crisis increases. Whenever people experience more than two life changes or traumatic events, their coping capacity may be strained, and the potential for crisis becomes greater.

An example of a maturational crisis, in which the origin of the crisis is a decision to divorce complicated by multiple stressors, follows.

CLINICAL EXAMPLE

Bernie is a 62-year-old man who has been hospitalized several times for paranoid schizophrenia over the past 40 years. Bernie's wife Alice moved out of their apartment and told Bernie that she has decided to seek a divorce. After Alice moved out, the apartment caught fire and burned. Bernie moved to a boardinghouse and has become depressed and stopped taking his medication. He began to have auditory hallucinations. Bernie has come to the crisis center accompanied by the police, who found him on the street crying, sobbing, and mumbling incoherently.

NURSING SELF-AWARENESS

It is important that you develop increased awareness of yourself and are able to handle your feelings so that you can intervene in a crisis situation. It will help you to reflect upon your answers to the questions posed in the Your Self-Awareness feature at the top of page 899.

To remain effective in crisis work, and to continue to grow personally and professionally, you should practice these important behaviors:

- Respect and believe in a person's capacity to grow and change.
- Be aware of the impact on yourself of repeatedly listening to horrible stories.
- Formulate your own outlets for stress, frustration, and anger.

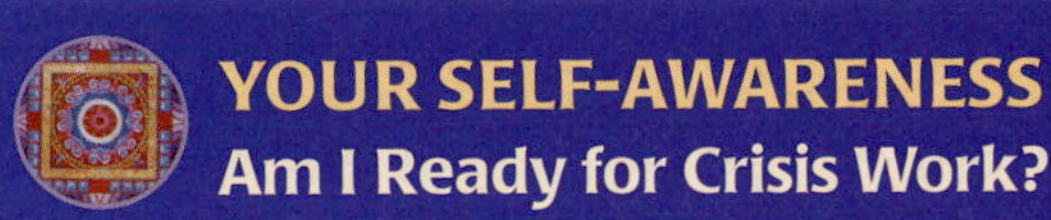

YOUR SELF-AWARENESS
Am I Ready for Crisis Work?

Thoughtfully consider and reflect on your answers to the following questions:

- Do I believe that people who are in crisis are helpless?
- Can I contain my own anxiety when I am working with someone who is severely anxious?
- How do I feel when I'm not in control in certain situations?
- How do I react to people who are frightened?
- How do I react to people who are angry?
- How do I react to people who threaten me?
- Do I have ideas that will hinder my ability to help others? For example, do I believe any of the following: Women who are raped are asking for it; men should be strong and not show emotions; children should be seen and not heard?

- Deal with your own fears about violence and your own vulnerability to stress and conflict.
- Develop realistic expectations about what you can do for others.
- Respect each person's own unique timetable for crisis resolution.
- Collaborate with other crisis intervenors and community groups.

You will become more skilled as you incorporate each of these behaviors into your professional repertoire.

Some additional activities that you can undertake to take care of yourself and lessen the personal impact of disaster and crises involves self-nurturance. Focus on what you did right every day, monitor your own reactions, keep a journal in which you write your personal thoughts and feelings, and practice the self-care tips in the Your Self-Awareness feature, "Self-Care Tips for Emergency and Disaster Response Workers." People in crisis will expect you to help them regain control of themselves, not to control them. Being self-assured and composed will help your clients to regain control.

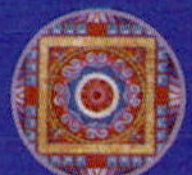

YOUR SELF-AWARENESS
Self-Care Tips for Emergency and Disaster Response Workers

Normal Reactions to a Disaster Event

- No one who responds to a mass casualty event is untouched by it.
- Profound sadness, grief, and anger are normal reactions to an abnormal event.
- You may not want to leave the scene until the work is finished.
- You will likely try to override stress and fatigue with dedication and commitment.
- You may deny the need for rest and recovery time.

Signs That You May Need Stress Management Assistance

- Difficulty communicating thoughts
- Difficulty remembering instructions
- Difficulty maintaining balance
- Uncharacteristic argumentativeness
- Difficulty making decisions
- Limited attention span
- Unnecessary risk taking
- Tremors/headaches/nausea
- Tunnel vision/muffled hearing
- Colds or flulike symptoms
- Disorientation or confusion
- Difficulty concentrating
- Loss of objectivity
- Greater tendency toward feeling easily frustrated
- Inability to engage in problem solving
- Inability to let down when off duty
- Refusal to follow orders
- Refusal to leave the scene
- Increased use of drugs/alcohol
- Unusual clumsiness

Ways to Help Manage Your Stress

- Limit on-duty work hours to no more than 12 hours per day.
- Make work rotations from high-stress to lower-stress functions.
- Make work rotations from the scene to routine assignments as feasible.
- Use counseling assistance programs available through your agency.
- Drink plenty of water and eat healthy snacks like fresh fruit or dried fruit, nuts, trail mix, whole grain breads, and other energy foods at the scene.
- Keep yourself hydrated with water, mineral water, decaffeinated coffee or tea, juice, and electrolyte supplements.
- If you are able to, take calcium supplements, which can counteract high levels of lactic acid produced by tension, and vitamin C, which may help you to maintain alertness.
- Take frequent, brief breaks from the scene as feasible.
- Talk about your emotions to process what you have seen and done.
- Stay in touch with your family and friends.
- Participate in memorials, rituals, and use of symbols as a way to express feelings.
- Pair up with another responder so that you may monitor one another's stress.

Source: Adapted from USDHHS Substance Abuse and Mental Health Services Administration. (2002). *Self-care tips for emergency and disaster response workers*. Retrieved November 27, 2007, from http://www.samhsa.gov.

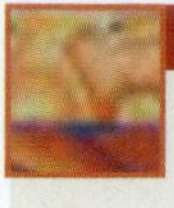

NURSING PROCESS
Clients in Crisis

Crisis intervention as a therapeutic strategy is strongly humanistic. People are viewed as capable of personal growth and as having the ability to influence and control their own lives. According to these concepts, the task of the intervenor is to help the individual in crisis understand the combination of events that led to the crisis and guide the individual, prior to a maladaptive response, toward a resolution that will meet the person's unique needs and foster future growth and strength. Especially during the acute phase, the goal of crisis intervention is to restore the person to the pretrauma level of functioning as quickly as possible.

In addition to the interventions discussed in this section, other strategies that are employed with clients in crisis can be found in other chapters. They are cognitive behavioral therapy interventions (Chapter 31), pharmacologic interventions (Chapters 7 and 32), and stress management techniques (Chapter 33). Providing psychoeducation for survivors of trauma helps them to better understand their own stress responses. Learning coping strategies provides a sense of control over these responses (Phoenix, 2007).

It is equally important that in this era of heightened security brought on by terrorist concerns that nurses also are educated and prepared to respond to crisis and disasters. Disaster preparedness plans are created by individual health care facilities, and most nurses undergo a program of continuing education training in their agency. However, it would be an effective primary prevention strategy to prepare nursing students for just such contingencies. For example, simulations have been effectively used as a teaching strategy to present bioterrorism interventions (Doran & Mulhall, 2007).

MediaLink Critical Thinking Exercise: Assessing a Victim of Violence

Assessment

Assessment takes place on three levels: individual, family, and sociocultural.

Individual Assessment

Assessment of the individual is the first phase of crisis intervention. The nurse or helper must focus on assessing the following elements that relate to the person and the problem. Collect data about:

- The client's resilience
- The client's coping style
- The precipitating event
- The situational supports
- The client's perception of the crisis
- Any guilt a disaster survivor may feel about having survived or about actions taken in order to survive
- The client's ability to handle the problem

The following Rx Communication feature shows an example of assessing a client's coping style.

Assessment is an essential and critical step of crisis intervention and the basis for later decisions about how and when to intervene, and whom to call (the first step of Roberts' model).

Also assess and evaluate the client's suicide potential. (See Chapter 23 for lethality assessment.) During this time, a client may need to be hospitalized to ensure safety, and a referral to a therapist or an emergency room in a general hospital or a psychiatric emergency room may be necessary. Part of the overall assessment is to determine what is necessary to return this client to a state of equilibrium; this may be different from what is necessary to solve the problem.

Family Assessment

Family assessment is important when an individual has been traumatized, because trauma reverberates through an entire family (Wells, 2006), as well as when a crisis involves all or several members within a family. Meet with as many family members as possible to assess family resilience, family resources, coping skills, and interpersonal styles. Crises often accompany role changes in families or increased stresses in families that do not have the resources to meet the challenge.

Some common family crises are the death of a family member, the terminal illness of a family member, single par-

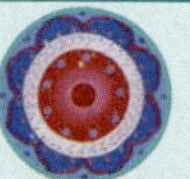

RX COMMUNICATION

CLIENT IN CRISIS

CLIENT: "How will I ever be able to get my son back from the foster home that child services put him in? I never seem to do anything right with him."

NURSE RESPONSE 1: "Jim, if you could rank yourself as a Dad on a scale of 1 to 10, with 10 meaning always doing everything 'right' and 1 meaning never doing anything 'right,' where would you rank yourself?"

RATIONALE: Using a scaling question will open the door to discussing with Jim the skills and competencies that are within his control and need to be worked on.

NURSE RESPONSE 2: "Let's talk about what you have been doing with Jimmy that is 'right.'"

RATIONALE: This intervention has two goals: eliciting a behavioral description of the interaction between father and son and helping the client identify his parenting strengths.

enting, divorce, drug/alcohol dependence, family violence, infidelity, remarriage, mental illness, incest, and "empty nest syndrome."

Sociocultural Assessment

A critically important source of the meaning of an individual's response to stress or trauma is the broader sociocultural context in which the person lives. A client's culture influences the sources of distress a client experiences, as well as the client's symptomatology, interpretation of symptoms, and methods of coping. For some examples, see Box 9-1 on culture-bound syndromes on page 189.

How one is raised influences how one experiences distress, whether or not one seeks help, and whether or not one allows oneself to be disabled by a mental health problem. For example, in some cultures, anxiety is considered a problem of individual strength or moral code, as opposed to a mental health problem. In some cultures it may be more acceptable to have a physical problem than an emotional problem.

Cultural competence requires knowledge about other cultures and sensitivity to the culture of your clients in order to select the interventions that will likely be most helpful. Cultural sensitivity involves much more than simply identifying a family's ethnic origins or health practices. Think about developing a culturagram as an aid to assessing culturally diverse families. The culturagram is discussed in Chapter 30 as it applies to family-based interventions. It is just as relevant a tool for working with culturally diverse families in crisis.

To be effective in sociocultural assessment, you must also become aware of the influences and beliefs from your own experiences. If you are not familiar with a client's culture, ask respectful questions to help the client fully express his or her distress. For example, "I want to understand how all of this might affect you. Can you tell me more about how you feel about this situation? Tell me how your neighbors (your friends/your family) might feel about it."

Disaster Assessment

Nurses as citizens are often at the scene of natural disasters or may be called on to help. Nurses can be particularly helpful during the initial stage of a disaster because, in addition to having the ability to provide care to the injured, they have the skills needed to perform physical assessments and assess psychologic distress. The Red Cross trains health care professionals as responders in disasters. Their website can be accessed via a direct link on the Companion Website for this book and provides information on the different training programs available.

Nursing Diagnosis: NANDA

People in crisis may have a variety of problems and symptoms. They may appear overwhelmed, calm, or agitated. They may speak clearly or they may ramble. Some appear rational, others psychotic. An individual's personal response and perception of the event will guide you toward determining the nursing diagnoses. The most common nursing diagnoses for people in crisis are:

- Ineffective Coping
- Interrupted Family Processes
- Risk for Self-Directed Violence
- Anxiety
- Acute Confusion
- Spiritual Distress
- Sleep Deprivation
- Risk for Post-Trauma Syndrome
- Complicated Grieving
- Impaired Social Interaction

Outcome Identification: NOC

Outcome criteria for clients in crisis should be determined in collaboration with the client to avoid irrelevant goals and unworkable solutions. Consider the following as possible outcome criteria for a client in crisis:

- The client will be able to identify effective, as well as ineffective, coping patterns.
- The client will be able to employ effective coping strategies.
- The client will ask for help when necessary.
- The client will use available social support.
- The client will report an increase in psychological comfort and a decrease in negative feelings.

Planning and Implementation: NIC

Effective planning for crisis intervention must be:

- Based on careful assessment and an understanding of human dependence needs
- Developed in active collaboration with the person in crisis and the significant people in that person's life
- Focused on immediate, concrete, contributing problems
- Appropriate to the person's level of thinking, feeling, and behaving
- Consistent with the person's lifestyle and culture
- Time limited, concrete, and realistic
- Mutually negotiated and renegotiated
- Organized to provide for follow-up

MediaLink 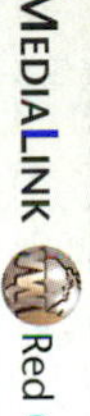 Red Cross

MediaLink Care Plan: Care of a Client in Crisis

Many of these principles form the basis for the therapeutic communication strategies in the Rx Communication feature on page 900.

Effective intervention is based on the ability to implement the second step of Roberts' model—make interpersonal contact, establish rapport, and rapidly establish the relationship (conveying genuine regard and respect for the client, acceptance, reassurance, and a nonjudgmental attitude). One–to–one interventions to make interpersonal contact, establish rapport, and establish the relationship are important to an individual in crisis. However, nurses who work with people in crisis often need to use many nontraditional interventions, which can be as important as any verbal interventions. Working successfully with people in crisis is based on having a flexible, open view of what may be therapeutic with different individuals. You must

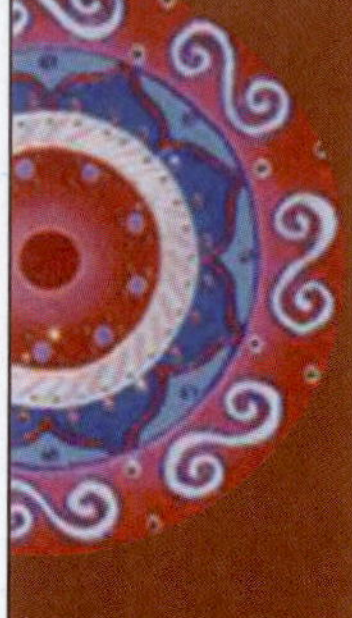

CARING FOR THE SPIRIT

Helping Clients to Recuperate from Crisis

It is important for people who have experienced a crisis or trauma to stay grounded. Suggest the following exercises to someone who is feeling confused, upset, in disbelief, or hopeless.

1. Sit on a chair, feel your feet on the ground, press on your thighs, feel your behind on the seat and your back supported by the chair. Look around you and pick six objects that have red or blue in them. This should allow you to feel in the present, more grounded, and in your body. Notice how your breath gets deeper and calmer. You may want to go outdoors and find a peaceful place to sit on the grass. As you do, feel how your body is held and supported by the ground.
2. Gently pat the different parts of your body with your hand, with a loose wrist. Your body may feel more tingling, more alive, sharp, and you may feel more connected to your feelings.
3. Tense your muscles, each group at a time. Hold your shoulders with your arms across your chest, tighten your grip, and pat your arms up and down. Do the same with your legs, tighten them and hold them from the outside, patting through their length. Tighten your back, tighten your front, then gently release the tension. This may help you to feel more balanced.
4. If you believe in prayer or in a greater power, pray for the rest of the souls of the dead, for the healing of the wounded, and for the consolation of the grieving. Pray for peace, understanding, wisdom, and for the forces of good to prevail. Do not give up faith in the ultimate goodness of being and keep your trust in humanity.

Take comfort in knowing that we humans are extremely resilient and have been able to recuperate from the most horrendous tragedies.

Source: Adapted from USDHHS Substance Abuse and Mental Health Services Administration. *After a disaster: Self-care tips for dealing with stress.* Retrieved November 27, 2007, from http://www.samhsa.gov.

have a full repertoire of skills and interventions that can be individualized to help all types of clients in crisis, including the ability to assist with spiritual needs. The Caring for the Spirit feature offers suggestions that integrate body, mind, and spirit.

Several different types of crisis intervention are discussed next.

Crisis Counseling

Crisis counseling is a type of brief, solution-focused therapy. Unlike therapies that focus on bringing about major personality change, crisis counseling focuses on strengths and solving immediate problems. Focusing on strengths is a resilience-oriented approach (Walsh, 2007).

Crisis counseling usually lasts for five or six sessions and involves individuals, groups, or families. The following techniques are used:

- Listening actively and with concern (The Your Intervention Strategies features on page 903 discuss communication strategies specific to working with a person in crisis.)
- Exploring the dimension of the problem, including the "last straw," in order to define it (Roberts' third step)
- Encouraging the open expression of feelings (Roberts' fourth step)
- Helping the client gradually accept reality
- Assessing past coping attempts and helping the client explore new ways of coping with problems (Roberts' fifth step)
- Linking the client to a social network
- Engaging in decision counseling or problem solving with the client, thus restoring cognitive mastery (Roberts' sixth step)
- Reinforcing newly learned coping devices
- Following up on the case after resolution of the crisis and leaving the door open for future contact, especially around the time of the anniversary of the event (Roberts' seventh step)

The second Your Intervention Strategies feature on page 903 summarizes the ABCs of crisis counseling.

Telephone Counseling

Suicide prevention and crisis intervention centers rely heavily on telephone counseling by volunteers who have professional consultation available to them. Also known as hotlines and often available around the clock, they allow callers to remain anonymous and test what it feels like to ask for assistance. No appointment, travel time, or money is necessary, and help is immediately available. The volunteers usually work within a protocol that indicates what information they need from the client to assess the crisis. Their goal is to plan steps to provide immediate relief and then long-term follow-up, if necessary.

The calls made to a hotline usually fall into one of four categories: crisis calls, ventilation calls (getting a problem "off one's chest"), combinations of ventilation and informa-

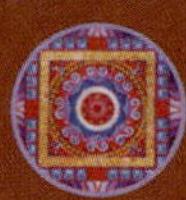

YOUR INTERVENTION STRATEGIES
Communication Strategies in Crisis Work

- Use silence—this gives the person time to reflect and become more aware of feelings. Silence can prompt elaboration. Simply being with the person is supportive.
- Use nonverbal communication—maintaining eye contact, head nodding, caring facial expressions, and occasional "uh-huhs" lets the person know that you are in tune.
- Paraphrase—understanding, empathy, and interest are conveyed by repeating portions of what the person said. Paraphrasing also checks for accuracy, clarifies misunderstandings, and lets people know they have been heard. You could say, "So, you are saying that . . ." or "I have heard you say that . . . ."
- Reflect feelings—this helps the person identify and articulate emotions. You could say, "You sound angry, scared, etc. Does that fit for you?"
- Allow the expression of emotions—this is an important part of healing. Venting often helps the person work through feelings in order to better engage in constructive problem solving.

Some Do's and Don'ts

Do Say:

- "These are normal reactions to an abnormal situation."
- "It is understandable that you feel this way."
- "It wasn't your fault; you did the best you could."
- "I am sorry that this happened."
- "Things will get better, and you will feel better, although they may never be the same again."

Don't Say:

- "It could have been worse."
- "You can always get another pet/car/house or have another child."
- "It's best if you just stay busy."
- "I know just how you feel."
- "You need to get on with your life."

Source: Adapted from USDHHS Substance Abuse and Mental Health Services Administration. *Disaster counseling.* Retrieved November 27, 2007, from http://www.samhsa.gov.

tion calls, or information-only calls. Calls that request information and ventilation are handled by supportive listening and giving information. Crisis calls need special techniques. Workers in crisis intervention centers generally follow a step-by-step agency protocol. For more information on suicide prevention hotlines, refer to Chapter 23.

Assisting with Environmental Changes

Working with an individual or a family in crisis may require taking steps to provide shelter. It may be necessary to find shelter for a homeless person, to obtain shelter in a safe house for an abused woman and her children, or to arrange for in-home health care.

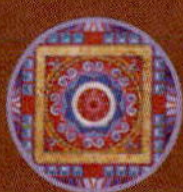

YOUR INTERVENTION STRATEGIES
ABCs of Crisis Counseling

Achieve Contact (Safety and Security)

- Introduce yourself, your name, role, and purpose.
- Ensure the physical and emotional safety of the victim.
- Ask the victim how he or she would like to be addressed.
- As appropriate, collect information regarding residency and health conditions for contacting family members, any support systems, or friends.
- Assess if the victim takes or needs medication.
- Identify the victim's feelings, reactions, and perceptions of the event.

Boil Down the Problem (Ventilate and Validate)

- Ask the victim to briefly describe what has just happened.
- Encourage the victim to talk about the present.
- Ask what is the most pressing problem (one at a time).
- Review and clarify what you heard as the primary and most immediate problem.
- Ask if the victim has ever experienced a similar situation or crisis in the past.
- How was it handled? Consider how the victim can regain control.

Cope with the Problem (Predict and Prepare)

- What does the victim want to happen? (Give additional options that may be more realistic.)
- What is the most important need?
- Explore what the victim feels is the best solution.
- Help the victim formulate a plan of action with resources, activities, and a timeline for accomplishing the plan.
- Reaffirm the future and talk in hopeful terms of a "new normal" or a "new reality."
- Arrange for follow-up contact or visit with the victim.
- Connect the victim to resources that offer longer-term support.

Source: ABCD tip card was developed by the Association of Traumatic Stress Specialists, *"Recognizing Standards of Excellence in Response, Treatment & Service,"* PO Box 2747, Georgetown, TX, 78627, 512-868-3677, 512-868-3678 fax, admin@atss-hq.com, www.atss-hq.com, © 2002 ATSS. The ABCD Model of Crisis Intervention was created by Romaine Edwards and Warren Jones; revisions by David Lowenberg, Paul Forgach, Carol Hacker, PhD, Jayne Crisp, CTS, CVAS, Paul Hamilton, MDiv. Retrieved November 27, 2007, from http://www.atss.com.

MEDIALINK National Alliance on Mental Illness

Anticipatory Guidance

Anticipatory guidance is providing assistance in anticipation of the potential for crisis, thus averting it. These are some examples of anticipatory guidance: discussing methods of contraception with adolescents or young adults, preparing a child and the family for a tonsillectomy, arranging for a volunteer from the Reach for Recovery Program to visit a woman who has had a mastectomy, and preparing a list of helpful phone numbers for the newly discharged schizophrenic client.

Helping Develop Social Supports

Immediate and tangible social support is crucial for clients in crisis because it may counteract or negate long-term adverse effects (Glass, Perrin, Campbell, & Soeken, 2007). Many people in crisis have limited social supports and are not always sure about how to access supports or develop them. You can help a client develop tangible social supports by: introducing a woman whose husband is an alcoholic to Al-Anon groups in her community, referring a family with a terminally ill member to a local hospice, giving a rape victim the telephone number of the rape crisis hotline, informing the newly discharged client with bipolar disorder and his family of the National Alliance on Mental Illness (NAMI) local group or national website (www.nami.org).

Critical Incident Stress Management

Critical incident stress management (CISM) is a comprehensive, integrative, and multifaceted approach to crisis intervention that spans the time sequence of a crisis. It is based on the notion that no single intervention alone is effective in crisis work. CISM consists of multiple components that can be applied to individuals, families, small groups, large groups, communities, and organizations. It can be best understood as a strategic delivery platform for primary, secondary, and tertiary prevention programs in the wake of large and small critical incidents (crises) rather than simply a crisis intervention treatment (Mitchell & Mitchell, 2006). TABLE 34-1 ■ describes the elements of CISM described by Everly and Mitchell (2008) and their intents.

The term CISM replaces the term critical incident stress debriefing (CISD) to describe this approach. CISD was originally formulated in the 1980s by Mitchell and Everly (1996) in response to an air disaster in Washington, DC. The original approach, known as critical incident stress debriefing, was intended to include four major elements—on-scene crisis intervention; post-incident small group discussion (known as defusing); a more formalized several-phase group discussion, which included debriefing; and follow-up support services. In practice, however, only one element, the group discussion, often to the exclusion of the others, became the focus of disaster mental health intervention. Its ease of use and the perception that it prevented PTSD led to its popularity. Although the small group meeting has both psychologic and psychoeducation elements, described later in this section, it should not by itself be considered psychotherapy or—according to the criticisms voiced in recent research (Levenson, 2006) and by its developers, Everly and Mitchell (2008)—a singular stand-alone crisis intervention or an effective way to prevent PTSD. Its most effective use appears to be in mitigating (decreasing, but not preventing) PTSD in soldiers and emergency services personnel. CISM is a more contemporary and broader approach and includes debriefing as one of its several components.

The debriefing process remains a valuable crisis intervention. The debriefing process offers an opportunity for individuals affected by a traumatic event to share their thoughts and feelings in a safe and controlled environment. Box 34-3 discusses the phases of the small group debriefing process in detail.

The typical settings in which debriefing as a component of CISM is used are: with staff on an inpatient unit after a suicide, with inmates after a murder in a jail, with military medical teams (Knobler, Nachshoni, Jaffe, Peretz, & Yehuda, 2007), with crisis line volunteers, with schoolchildren and school personnel after a multiple shooting in a school, with law enforcement personnel (Miller, 2006), as well as with rescue and health care workers after natural disasters (Johnstone, 2007) or terrorist attacks (Everly & Mitchell, 2008). In

TABLE 34-1 ■ Components of Critical Incident Stress Management (CISM)

Component	Intent
1. Pre-event planning and preparation	To provide anticipatory guidance and foster resilience
2. Assessment	To determine the need for intervention for those directly and indirectly exposed
3. Strategic planning	To improve the crisis response
4. Individual crisis intervention	To provide psychological first aid to individuals
5. Large group crisis intervention	To provide large group psychological first aid
6. Small group crisis intervention	To provide small group psychological first aid and powerful event group support
7. Family crisis intervention	To provide psychological first aid to families
8. Organizational and community intervention	To deliver services to organizations and communities and to improve preparedness
9. Pastoral crisis intervention	To provide faith-based support
10. Follow-up and referral	To ensure continuity of care for those directly and indirectly exposed

Box 34-3 **The Small Group Debriefing Process**

Introduction Phase (Setting the Tone for the Subsequent Phases)

- Explain the purpose of the meeting.
- Explain and give an overview of the process.
- Motivate the participants.
- Assure confidentiality.
- Explain the guidelines.
- Identify the team members.
- Answer questions or concerns.

Fact Phase (Imparting Power to the Participants Through Giving Information)

- Assist the participants to discuss the facts of the incident.
- Ask the participants to tell who they are.
- Ask the participants to tell how they were involved in the incident.
- Ask the participants to tell what happened from their perspective.

Thought Phase (Transitioning Between Impersonal Outside Facts and That Which Is Internal, Close, and Personal)

- Ask each participant to discuss his or her first thoughts or most prominent thoughts about the traumatic event.
- Expect to hear emotional comments.

Reaction Phase (Ventilating with a Potential for Emotional Abreaction)

- Most of the discussing is done by the participants.
- Discussion is freewheeling.
- Ask participants what the worst thing was about the situation, what they would choose to erase, and what aspect of the situation causes the most pain.

Symptom Phase (Normalizing and Attacking the Myth of Unique Weakness or Vulnerability)

- Move the group toward more cognitively oriented material.
- Ask participants to describe any cognitive, physical, emotional, or behavioral experiences they encountered at the scene of the incident.
- Ask about any symptoms that followed subsequently.

Teaching Phase (Moving Further Away from the Emotional Content of the Reaction Phase)

- Acknowledge symptoms described in the symptom phase.
- Reaffirm that symptoms are normal, typical, or predictable after what they've been through.
- Forewarn the group about possible symptoms they might experience in the future.
- Involve the participants in stress management activities.

Reentry Phase (Identifying Homogenizing Themes That May Be Used to Facilitate Closure and Provide a Psychological Uplift)

Participant Roles

- Introduce any new material they wish to discuss.
- Review old material already discussed.
- Ask any questions.
- Discuss whatever would help them to bring closure to the debriefing.

Debriefing Team Roles

- Answer any questions.
- Inform and reassure.
- Provide appropriate handouts and other written material.
- Provide referral sources for assessment, therapy, and so on.
- Summarize the debriefing experience with words of respect, encouragement, appreciation, support, and direction.

2007, the United Nations endorsed CISM as a "best practices" approach to staff support of its own field personnel.

Despite its apparent benefits, CISM is not universally implemented. A study of emergency room nurses after the Hurricane Katrina disaster indicated that none had been offered CISM (Battles, 2007).

Disaster Assistance

The type of help needed by victims of a disaster changes as the disaster unfolds. Initially, people need information about evacuation plans, rescue efforts, and the location of food, shelter, and medical care. The media can provide this information, especially when there is time to plan and anticipate need (as with floods or hurricanes).

After acute needs are met at the disaster scene, in makeshift hospitals, or in emergency rooms, morgues, and shelters, more far-reaching interventions are necessary. People need housing, jobs, and help in reconstructing their emotional lives. Two federal agencies assist with meeting the needs of both survivors and responders. The Federal Emergency Management Agency (FEMA) has a crisis counseling assistance and training program that provides mental health services to all individuals affected by a disaster (http://www.fema.gov). The Substance Abuse and Mental Health Services Administration (SAMHSA) of the Department of Health and Human Services also meets the mental health needs of survivors and responders (http://www.mentalhealth.samhsa.gov). Such data can be accessed on the Companion Website for this book.

These are the psychologic needs of victims both during and after a disaster:

- Talking about the experience and expressing their feelings of fear, panic, loss, and grief
- Becoming fully aware and accepting of what has happened to them

MediaLink Disaster Assistance

MediaLink Application: Mental Health and Psychosocial Education

- Resuming concrete activities and reconstructing their lives with the social, physical, and emotional resources available

To guide victims and their families through the crisis, crisis workers should:

- Listen with concern and sympathy, and ease the way for them to tell their tragic story, weep, and express feelings of anger, loss, frustration, and despair.
- Help them accept in small doses the tragic reality of what has happened. This means staying with them during the initial stages of shock and denial. It also may mean accompanying them back to the scene of the tragedy and being available for support when they are faced with the full impact of their loss.
- Help them make contact with relatives, friends, and other resources required for beginning the process of social and physical reconstruction. This could mean making telephone calls to locate relatives, accompanying someone to apply for financial aid, or giving information about social and mental health care agencies for follow-up services.

People who are panicked should receive prompt attention to minimize the potential for contagious panic that sometimes occurs in large groups. One strategy to help a panic-stricken person is to give the person a small, structured task that focuses energies constructively. Remember, however, that assigning tasks beyond the person's capabilities will add to the person's anxiety and feeling of helplessness. When in a disaster situation, remember to also incorporate concepts and intervention strategies related to death and loss such as those described in Chapter 17.

The effects of a disaster are felt long after the disaster is over. Provide anticipatory guidance that includes self-care tips to victims and their families so that they can mange their postdisaster experiences. Self-care tips are in the Partnering with Clients and Families feature below.

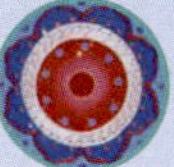

PARTNERING WITH CLIENTS AND FAMILIES

SELF-CARE TIPS AFTER A DISASTER

Things to Remember When Trying to Understand Disaster Events

- No one who sees a disaster is untouched by it.
- It is normal to feel anxious about your and your family's safety.
- Profound sadness, grief, and anger are normal reactions to an abnormal event.
- Acknowledging your feelings helps you to recover.
- Focusing on your strengths and abilities will help you to heal.
- Accepting help from community programs and resources is healthy.
- Everyone has different needs and different ways of coping.
- It is common to want to strike back at people who have caused great pain. However, nothing good is accomplished by hateful language or actions.

Signs That Adults Need Stress Management Assistance

- Difficulty communicating thoughts
- Difficulty sleeping
- Difficulty maintaining balance
- Easily frustrated
- Increased use of drugs/alcohol
- Limited attention span
- Poor work performance
- Headaches/stomach problems
- Tunnel vision/muffled hearing
- Colds or flulike symptoms
- Disorientation or confusion
- Difficulty concentrating
- Reluctance to leave home
- Depression, sadness
- Feelings of hopelessness
- Mood swings
- Crying easily
- Overwhelming guilt and self-doubt
- Fear of crowds, strangers, or being alone

Ways to Ease the Stress

- Talk with someone about your feelings—anger, sorrow, and other emotions—even though it may be difficult.
- Encourage others, as well as yourself, not to tell your stories in a repetitive way—this ultimately deepens the trauma. Instead, support and hear one another, but with breaks and interruptions of the story from beginning to end.
- Don't hold yourself directly responsible for the disastrous event or be frustrated because you feel that you cannot help directly in the rescue work.
- Take steps to promote your own physical and emotional healing by staying active in your daily life patterns or by adjusting them (i.e., healthy eating, rest, exercise, relaxation, meditation). This healthy outlook will help you and your family.
- Maintain a normal household and daily routine, limiting demanding responsibilities for yourself and your family.
- Spend time with family and friends.
- Participate in memorials, rituals, and use of symbols as a way to express feelings.
- Use existing support groups of family, friends, and house of worship.
- Establish a family emergency plan—this can be very comforting.
- Seek outside professional assistance if these self-help strategies are not helping you or you find that you are using drugs/alcohol in order to cope.

Source: Adapted from USDHHS Substance Abuse and Mental Health Services Administration. *After a disaster: Self-care tips for dealing with stress.* Retrieved November 27, 2007, from http://www.samhsa.gov.org.

Evaluation

Nurses in acute care or short-term settings may not see the long-term effects of their interventions. Typically, nurses in these settings need to evaluate the crisis, set up the plan, and begin implementing it.

In long-term settings, you can evaluate the client or family response to the intervention by determining whether clients have resumed their precrisis level of functioning or show evidence of increased functioning (growth). A nurse in either a long-term or short-term setting may also have an opportunity to evaluate whether a similar problem might lead to another crisis for the client.

It is difficult to evaluate the effectiveness of disaster intervention because of the large numbers of people involved and the disruptive nature of a disaster. Evaluation can take place at many different levels. Nurses can evaluate their work with individual clients; mental health care agencies can monitor statistics on groups of clients; government agencies can assess the numbers of unemployed and homeless; public health departments can measure the extent of disease and disability.

The most important aspect of evaluation is to review how the interventions were implemented and the effectiveness of the relief work. Disaster preparedness is needed to effectively intervene when the unthinkable—a disaster—occurs. Many hospitals and clinics have ongoing drills to prepare for the possibility of a disaster. It is important that you understand your role and the tasks and functions for which you are responsible.

CASE MANAGEMENT

Case management services for crisis may include any one or several activities. Arranging for crisis intervention or forensic intervention services may be necessary. In disaster situations, triaging—e.g., rapid medical and psychological evaluation—and hospitalization, if necessary, may be a case management activity. The case manager in all crisis situations will mobilize necessary mental health resources and monitor outcomes for clients. Referral for vocational training, family crisis intervention services, or grief counseling may be called for. Case managers for clients with prolonged postdisaster distress may refer clients for cognitive behavioral therapy, implemented no sooner than 60 days postdisaster (Hamblen, Gibson, Mueser, & Norris, 2006). This can function as an intermediate step between traditional crisis counseling and longer-term mental health treatments.

COMMUNITY-BASED CARE

Most communities have a wealth of community-based services, such as hotlines (see Chapter 23∞) or crisis centers appropriate for persons in crisis. After disasters, local communities and various government agencies band together to provide additional services to meet the expected surge in the need for mental health services.

Mobile crisis units (MCUs) are community-based programs that are designed to deliver crisis services to any location in the community. MCUs are staffed by teams that may include psychiatrists, psychiatric–mental health nurses, substance abuse counselors, psychologists, psychiatric social workers, child welfare workers, or other trained professionals. The specific functions of MCUs vary by community. The typical advantages that MCUs provide are:

- Intervening in crisis situations without delay
- Providing increased community access to services
- Assessing clients in their own community environment
- Avoiding unnecessary hospitalizations
- Facilitating hospitalization or detoxification when needed
- Avoiding unnecessary arrests
- Consulting to law enforcement

MCUs are thought to reduce the costs of mental health treatment as well as the number of inpatient admissions to psychiatric facilities. In fact, community-based mobile crisis services resulted in 8% fewer hospitalizations than hospital-based interventions (Guo, Biegel, Johnsen, & Dyches, 2001). The use of MCUs has also decreased psychiatric symptomatology, reduced homelessness, and increased global functioning in a population of homeless severely mentally ill persons (Morris & Warnock, 2001).

HOME CARE

Home visits are made when telephone counseling does not suffice or when the crisis workers need to obtain additional information by direct observation or to reach a client who is unobtainable by telephone. Home visits are appropriate when crisis workers need to initiate contact rather than waiting for clients to come to them—for example, when a telephone caller is assessed to be highly suicidal or when a concerned family member, neighbor, physician, or clergyman informs the agency of clients in potential crisis. Home crisis visits are also an effective intervention for persons with serious mental illnesses (Joy, Adams, & Rice, 2006), helping to keep them functioning in the community.

Often, clients in crisis are too disorganized or distraught to seek help by themselves. The police may arrange for a home crisis visit to avoid imprisoning or hospitalizing a client. Problems for which home crisis visits are usually instituted are spousal abuse, child abuse, psychiatric emergencies (such as drug overdose, suicide attempt or other life-threatening self-abuse, stalking, assault, rape, and homicide), and medical emergencies.

In many agencies, the crisis team often consists of a man and a woman who are highly skilled and experienced in crisis intervention. The male–female team is generally perceived as less threatening than two men, two women, or a single person. Their goal is to defuse the situation with as little disruption and violence as possible and to engage the client in longer-term treatment. They may also be members of mobile crisis units (discussed in the previous section).

There are others who intervene in community crises as well. The public health nurse is in an excellent position to identify, assess, and intervene with clients experiencing a life crisis.

Public health nurses often have access to community resources as well as informal communication lines, and they usually maintain contact with families and clients for longer periods of time than nurses in other settings. They are often recognized by the community as knowledgeable experts who are available for immediate assistance, as in the following clinical example.

CLINICAL EXAMPLE

Emily, age 78, and her sister Frances, age 84, lived in a run-down part of town. Frances became seriously ill with pneumonia and became progressively weaker. Emily's anxiety about Frances's health grew when her sister refused to see a doctor. Emily feared that her sister would die or need to go to a nursing home. Emily felt paralyzed and didn't know what to do. When the visiting nurse came by to visit Emily's neighbor, Emily asked the nurse to see Frances. Together, they were able to persuade Frances to get medical care so that she could stay home.

VICARIOUS TRAUMATIZATION

Disasters and traumatic experiences shake the foundations of our beliefs about how other people behave toward one another, and can shatter our assumption that the world is a safe place. In evaluating the aftereffects of a disaster, remember that there may be an impact on those who are not direct victims.

CLINICAL EXAMPLE

Matilda worked as a short-order cook in a restaurant in Wichita, Kansas. On Monday morning, Matilda decided to call in sick, although she was well. Matilda's fiancé, a waiter at the same restaurant, was killed along with several others when a propane gas talk in the restaurant's storage area exploded. Matilda now has vivid nightmares. She alternates between feeling sad and angry. She refuses to attend church anymore, asking God, over and over, why He spared her and not the others at the restaurant.

Janelle frantically pressed the redial button on her cell phone, trying to reach her mother, who lived in an area of southern California plagued by wildfires. After 3 hours of frantic but unsuccessful activity, Janelle, exhausted, sat down on a curb and sobbed. When her cell phone finally rang, it was Janelle's mother calling from a fire station that had evacuated residents threatened by the wildfires. She was dirty and scared, but okay. Despite this good news, Janelle couldn't stop crying. Months later, she still feels anxious.

A disaster can affect the mental health of various groups—a condition known as **vicarious traumatization**. Also known as *secondary trauma response*, vicarious traumatization is a condition in which psychological aftereffects are experienced by those who are not direct victims of the traumatic event. The groups most commonly at increased risk are identified in the following list. Those individuals who are most affected are listed first.

1. Next-of-kin
2. Injured survivors and their close ones
3. Uninjured survivors
4. Onlookers (the helpless helpers, who are at particularly high risk)
5. Rescuers
6. Body handlers
7. Health personnel (many mass injury situations may demand difficult prioritizing)
8. People responsible for the disaster
9. Coworkers in workplace disasters
10. Evacuees

The World Trade Center attack has focused a great deal of attention on the responses of rescue workers and their families in the posttrauma period. The impact of the event has resonated deeply with the families and children of the firefighters and policemen who gave their lives and also with those who survived (Menendez, Molloy, & Magaldi, 2006). They report a recurring theme—the need to be constantly vigilant in helping their families cope. The overall prevalence of PTSD among rescue and recovery workers was 12.4% (Perrin et al., 2007). Those at greatest risk for PTSD were workers and volunteers least likely to have had disaster training or experience, who performed tasks not common for their occupation, and who worked at the disaster site for long periods of time. This suggests the need for disaster preparedness training and shift and personnel rotations to enable shorter duration of service at disaster sites.

Nurses and other crisis workers are routinely exposed to victim suffering and to the aftereffects of inhumane acts (see FIGURE 34-4 ■). They are at risk for becoming what has been called "wounded healers." After Hurricane Katrina on August 29, 2005, a study of emergency department nurses who worked during the hurricane identified 20% as having PTSD (Battles, 2007). A debriefing for medical and rescue workers after the event can serve as a preventive intervention (Knobler et al., 2007). However, fully 100% of the nurses in the Battles study (2007) reported that CISM was not offered to them. Critical incident stress management has been discussed earlier in this chapter. The following

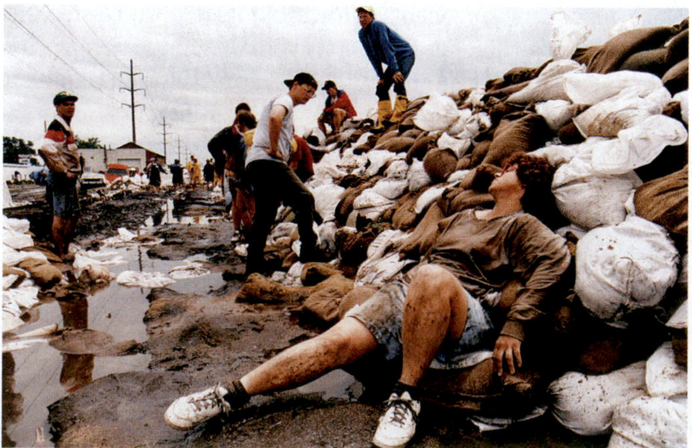

FIGURE 34-4 ■ Exhausted nurses and other crisis workers.

Source: AP Wide World Photos, Jeff Beiermann.

clinical example illustrates how vicarious traumatization can affect rescue workers.

CLINICAL EXAMPLE

Brian is a police officer from Buffalo, New York, who volunteered to assist the New York City Police Department in the days immediately after the terrorist attack at the World Trade Center. He was on a team looking for people who might still be alive in the rubble. Although Brian considered himself "tough" and had a macho image among his fellow officers, he burst into tears and had to be led away from the site to meet with a mental health counselor. Brian acts tougher than ever, but still occasionally bursts into tears and has difficulty controlling his emotions.

Sheila was a mental health nurse at a hospital in Gulfport, Mississippi, located only a few blocks from the Gulf of Mexico. She was also a volunteer who assisted survivors of Hurricane Katrina and first responders (firefighters, police officers, paramedics) and counseled them for several weeks. Sheila became preoccupied with the stories of her clients. Her insomnia and angry outbursts at home prompted Sheila to seek counseling for herself.

You should expect to be vulnerable to this condition if you work with clients in the highly disorganized crisis period; with those who are victims of sexual assault (Ghahramanlou & Brodbeck, 2000), violence, or disaster; or with those, such as sexual offenders, who traumatize others (Moulden & Firestone, 2007). Vicarious traumatization can also affect your own physical health by inducing gastrointestinal problems (such as gastritis or peptic ulcer), hypertension, and fatigue. In the home or the workplace, you could experience:

- An increase in the number of sick days
- Indecision or difficulty with problem solving
- Isolation or withdrawal
- Behavioral outbursts

Should this happen, seek additional support, supervision, and referral for professional assistance.

The opposite of vicarious traumatization, *vicarious resilience*, is an emerging topic for study. Vicarious resilience is a new concept put forth by Hernandez, Gangsei, and Engstrom (2007) that addresses the question of how psychotherapists who work with survivors of political violence or kidnapping are affected by their clients' stories of resilience. Their study illustrates, yet again, that therapists are affected by their clients' stories (this time positively) and that stories of resilience and constructive coping with adversity can contribute to sustaining and empowering trauma therapists.

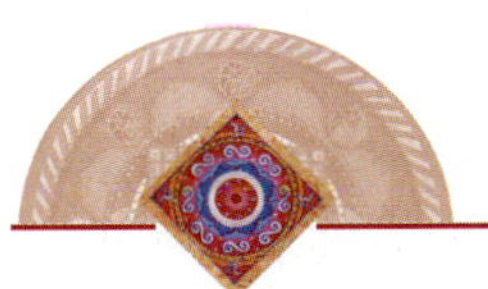

EXPLORE MEDIALINK 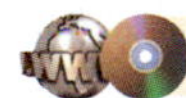 www.prenhall.com/kneisl

For NCLEX-RN® review questions, case studies, and other resources for this chapter see the Pearson Health MediaLink CD-ROM that accompanies this book and the Companion Website at www.prenhall.com/kneisl.

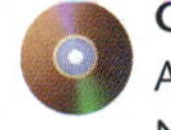

CD-ROM
Audio Glossary
NCLEX-RN® Review Questions

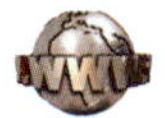

Companion Website
Audio Glossary
NCLEX-RN® Review Questions
Critical Thinking Exercise
- *Assessing a Victim of Violence*

Case Study
- *Reaction to Trauma*

Care Plan
- *Care of a Client in Crisis*

MediaLinks
MediaLink Application
- *Mental Health and Psychosocial Education*

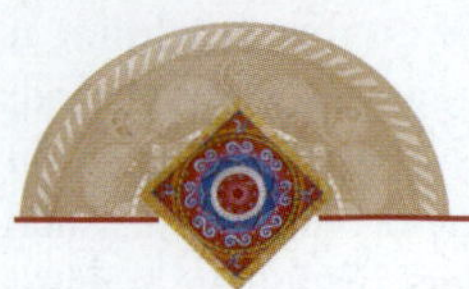

NCLEX-RN® REVIEW QUESTIONS

1. An important difference between a situational crisis and maturational crisis is that the onset of the maturational crisis is:
1. Foreseeable.
2. Complicated by the experience of multiple traumas.
3. Validated by other people.
4. Associated with personal growth.

2. Which of the following client statements best reflects the client's recognition of the nature of crisis?
1. "This is just like any other emergency."
2. "This must be what people with chronic illness feel like—never knowing what is coming next."
3. "Within 6 weeks, for better or worse, we will be past this place."
4. "I feel numb—like this is not really happening to me."

3. During which point in a crisis should the nurse anticipate providing survivors with the most intense nurturing?
1. Impact
2. Recoil
3. Posttrauma
4. Anniversary date

4. A peer in nursing school is going through a divorce. Most of her family is overseas. When you offer assistance, she smiles and states, "I handle things myself. I always have." Then she changes the subject. Which of the following statements from your peer provides you with the greatest assurance that she has what she needs?
1. "I will ask for help if I need it."
2. "I'll use the student health service if I need it."
3. "I know where to get help if I need it."
4. "My brother and I were always there for each other when we were children. I will ask him for help if I need it."

5. Identical twin adolescents experience the same crisis. The older twin reports the experience as one associated with personal growth, while the younger twin never regains the precrisis level of functioning. Their mother asks the nurse, "They have had the same life experiences. How could they react so differently?" Which of the following statements by the nurse best describes resilience?
1. "Perhaps the younger twin had an undiagnosed psychiatric problem prior to the crisis."
2. "Coping style, as well as number and depth of supportive relationships, may explain the difference."
3. "The twins probably perceived the crisis differently."
4. "The younger twin may feel inferior to the older twin."

6. Which of the following interventions are most appropriate for individuals experiencing a crisis? (Select all that apply.)
1. Pharmacological interventions
2. Self-help support groups
3. Stress management techniques
4. Cognitive behavioral interventions
5. Insight-oriented group psychotherapy

7. Which of the following nursing interventions is inconsistent with the ABCs of crisis counseling?
1. "That must bring up a lot of thoughts and fears from your past. For this session, let's focus on your childhood."
2. "What kind of resolution were you hoping for?"
3. "Let me see if I understand: Your chief concerns are for temporary housing and employment. Is that what you need?"
4. "Do you feel comfortable enough with me to share what has been happening to you?"

8. During a statewide environmental disaster, the most up-to-date and accurate psychoeducational resources most often include:
1. Other victims of the crisis.
2. Family members.
3. Local mental health professionals.
4. Mass media.

9. Which of the following behaviors in yourself would alert you to the need to reassess your behaviors and interventions in a crisis situation? (Select all that apply.)
1. Expressing doubt regarding the client's capacity to function
2. Supporting the client's dependent behavior
3. Addressing termination issues
4. Augmenting continuously the client's problem list
5. Thinking about clients during leisure time

10. Following a natural disaster, which health care worker statement suggests the need to assess for vicarious traumatization?
1. "After a while, you become accustomed to hearing the same stories over and over and you develop numbness."
2. "Usually I work alone, but in a disaster I have to work with other caregivers."
3. "Every night when I leave the site, I eat well and go straight to bed."
4. "There are lots of things you cannot change, and we all want to help everybody even more. You do the best you can."

See Appendix C for answers.

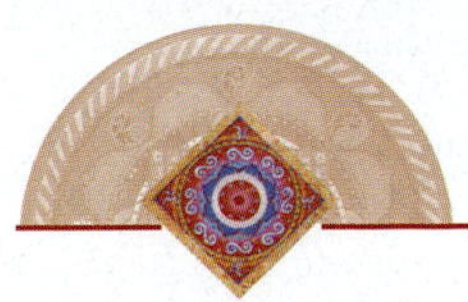

REFERENCES

Aguilera, D. C. (1998). *Crisis intervention: Theory and methodology*. St. Louis, MO: Mosby.

Baker, D. R. (2002). A public health approach to the needs of children affected by terrorism. *Journal of the American Medical Women's Association, 57*(2), 117–118, 121.

Battles, E. D. (2007). An exploration of post-traumatic stress disorder in emergency nurses following Hurricane Katrina. *Journal of Emergency Nursing, 33*(4), 314–319.

Caplan, G. (1964). *Principles of preventive psychiatry*. New York: Basic Books.

Collishaw, S., Pickles, A., Messer, J., Rutter, M., Shearer, C., & Maugham, B. (2007). Resilience to adult psychopathology following childhood maltreatment: Evidence from a community sample. *Child Abuse and Neglect, 31*(3), 211–229.

Covell, N. H., Allen G., Essock, S. M., Pease, S. A., Felton, C. J., Lanzara, C. B., et al. (2006). Service utilization and event reaction patterns among children who received Project Liberty counseling services. *Psychiatric Services, 57*(9), 1277–1282.

Doran, A. J., & Mulhall, M. (2007). Bioterrorism in the simulation laboratory: Preparing students for the unexpected. *Journal of Nursing Education, 46*(6), 292.

Everly, G. S., & Mitchell, J. T. (2008). *Integrative crisis intervention and disaster mental health*. Ellicot City, MD: Chevron Publishing Corporation.

Ghahramanlou, M., & Brodbeck, C. (2000). Predictors of secondary trauma in sexual assault trauma counselors. *International Journal of Emergency Mental Health, 2*(4), 229–240.

Glass, N., Perrin, N., Campbell, J. C., & Soeken, K. (2007). The protective role of tangible support on post-traumatic stress disorder symptoms in urban women survivors of violence. *Research in Nursing and Health, 30*(5), 558–568.

Guo, S., Biegel, D. E., Johnsen, J. A., & Dyches, H. (2001). Assessing the impact of community-based mobile crisis services on preventing hospitalization. *Psychiatric Services, 52*(2), 223–228.

Hamblen, J. L., Gibson, L. E., Mueser, K. T., & Norris, F. H. (2006). Cognitive–behavioral therapy for prolonged postdisaster distress. *Journal of Clinical Psychology, 62*(8), 1043–1052.

Hernandez, P., Gangsei, D., & Engstrom, D. (2007). Vicarious resilience: A new concept in work with those who survive trauma. *Family Process, 46*(2), 229–241.

Hoge, E. A., Austin, E. D., & Pollack, M. H. (2007). Resilience: Research evidence and conceptual considerations for posttraumatic stress disorder. *Depression and Anxiety, 24*(2), 139–152.

Johnstone, M. (2007). Disaster response and group self-care. *Perspectives in Psychiatric Care, 43*(1), 38–40.

Joy, C. B., Adams, C. E., & Rice, K. (2006). Crisis intervention for people with severe mental illnesses. *Cochrane Database Systems Review, 4*, CD001087.

King, F., 4th, & Steinmann, W. C. (2007). Why current medical management is failing victims of Hurricane Katrina: A review of past successes and failures in postdisaster psychosocial treatment. *Southern Medical Journal, 100*(10), 991–998.

Knobler, H. Y., Nachshoni, T., Jaffe, E., Peretz, G., & Yehuda, Y. B. (2007). Psychological guidelines for a medical team debriefing after a stressful event. *Military Medicine, 172*(6), 581–585.

Laugharne, J., Janca, A., & Widiger, T. (2007). Posttraumatic stress disorder and terrorism: Five years after 9/11. *Current Opinions in Psychiatry, 20*(1), 36–41.

Levenson, R. L., Jr. (2006). Internal affairs: Current problematic issues in Critical Incident Stress Management for emergency services. *International Journal of Emergency Mental Health, 8*(3), 153–155.

Lindemann, E. (1944). Symptomatology and management of acute grief. *American Journal of Psychiatry, 101*, 141–148.

Mancini, A. D., & Bonanno, G. A. (2006). Resilience in the face of potential trauma: Clinical practices and illustrations. *Journal of Clinical Psychology, 62*(8), 971–985.

Menendez, A. M., Molloy, J., & Magaldi, M. C. (2006). Health responses of New York City firefighter spouses and their families post-September 11, 2001 terrorist attacks. *Issues in Mental Health Nursing, 27*(8), 905–917.

Miller, L. (2006). Critical incident stress debriefing for law enforcement: Practical models and special applications. *International Journal of Emergency Mental Health, 8*(3), 189–201.

Mitchell, J. T., & Everly, G. S., Jr. (1996). *Critical incident stress debriefing: An operations manual*. Ellicott City, MD: Chevron Publishing.

Mitchell, S. G., & Mitchell, J. T. (2006). Caplan, community, and Critical Incident Stress Management. *International Journal of Emergency Mental Health, 8*(1), 5–14.

Morris, D. W., & Warnock, J. K. (2001). Effectiveness of a mobile outreach and crisis services unit in reducing psychiatric symptoms in a population of homeless persons with severe mental illness. *Journal of the Oklahoma State Medical Association, 94*(8), 343–346.

Moulden, H. M., & Firestone, P. (2007). Vicarious traumatization: The impact on therapists who work with sexual offenders. *Trauma, Violence, and Abuse, 8*(1), 67–83.

Murthy, R. S. (2007). Mass violence and mental health—Recent epidemiological findings. *International Review of Psychiatry, 19*(3), 183–192.

Parker, C. L., Barnett, D. J., Everly, G. S., Jr., & Links, J. M. (2006). Expanding disaster mental health response: A conceptual training framework for public health professionals. *International Journal of Emergent Mental Health, 8*(2), 101–109.

Perrin, M. A., DiGrande, L., Wheeler, K., Thorpe, L., Farfel, M., & Brackbill, R. (2007). Differences in PTSD prevalence and associated risk factors among World Trade Center disaster rescue and recovery workers. *American Journal of Psychiatry, 164*(9), 1385–1394.

Phoenix, B. (2007). Psychoeducation for survivors of trauma. *Perspectives in Psychiatric Care, 43*(3), 123–131.

Roberts, A. R. (Ed.). (2005). *Crisis intervention handbook: Assessment, treatment, and research* (3rd ed.). New York: Oxford University Press.

Roberts, A. R., & Bender, K. (2006). Juvenile offender suicide: Prevalence, risk factors, assessment, and crisis intervention protocols. *International Journal of Emergency Mental Health, 8*(4), 255–265.

Sareen, J., Cox, B. J., Afifi, T. O., Stein, M. B., Belik, S. L., Meadows, G., et al. (2007). Combat and peacekeeping operations in relation to prevalence of mental disorders and perceived need for mental health care: Findings from a large representative sample of military personnel. *Archives of General Psychiatry, 64*(7), 843–852.

Scott, S. T. (2007). Multiple traumatic experiences and the development of posttraumatic stress disorder. *Journal of Interpersonal Violence, 22*(7), 932–938.

Tyhurst, J. S. (1957). The role of transition states—including disasters—in mental illness. In *Symposium on preventive and social psychiatry* (pp. 1–23). Washington, DC: Walter Reed Army Institute of Research.

Vlahov, D., Galea, S., Resnick, H., Ahern, J., Boscarino, J. A., Bucuvalas, M., et al. (2002). Increased use of cigarettes, alcohol, and marijuana among Manhattan, New York, residents after the September 11th terrorist attacks. *American Journal of Epidemiology, 155*(11), 988–996.

Walsh, F. (2007). Traumatic loss and major disasters: Strengthening family and community resilience. *Family Process, 46*(2), 207–227.

Wells, M. E. (2006). Psychotherapy for families in the aftermath of a disaster. *Journal of Clinical Psychology, 62*(8), 1017–1027.

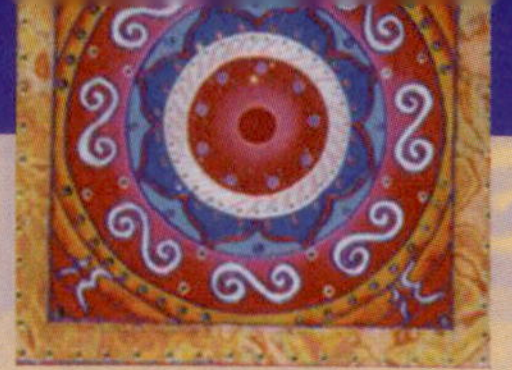

CHAPTER

35

Intervening in Violence in the Psychiatric Setting

SUE C. DELAUNE

KEY TERMS

dangerousness *917*
restraint *925*
seclusion *925*

LEARNING OUTCOMES

After completing this chapter, you will be able to:

1. Describe theoretical perspectives that are useful in understanding violence.
2. Determine the presence of behavioral and verbal cues that indicate impending violence.
3. Identify risk factors that contribute to violent behavior.
4. Describe nursing measures to de-escalate potentially violent behavior within the context of the principle of least restrictiveness.
5. Balance the issue of safety maintenance with the need to ensure the individual freedom of the aggressive client.
6. Implement a variety of nonpharmacological nursing strategies for intervening with violent clients.
7. Describe common staff responses to violence.
8. Analyze personal feelings and attitudes that may affect professional practice when caring for clients with aggressive behaviors.

CRITICAL THINKING CHALLENGE

Harold, an 80-year-old retired jeweler, was admitted to the inpatient unit after striking a nurse's aide at the extended care facility where he has resided for 10 years. On admission he is mute, does not eat, wanders in and out of other clients' rooms, and is easily frustrated. He has started to strike out at the nursing staff when they attempt to assist him with routine self-care activities. The staff has requested a case conference to develop a new approach to his care.

1. How do you rate Harold's potential for violence?
2. What primary need should Harold's treatment team address?
3. What are some specific measures staff members could implement to increase safety for Harold, other clients, and care providers?

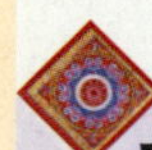

MEDIALINK 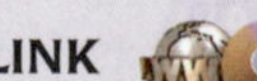 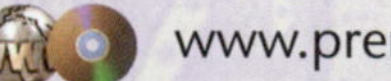 www.prenhall.com/kneisl

Go to the Pearson Health MediaLink CD-ROM and the Companion Website at www.prenhall.com/kneisl for interactive resources for this chapter.

AN OPEN LETTER TO THE STUDENT

Does the title of this chapter make your heart beat a little faster or cause you to become somewhat fearful? If your philosophy is "Don't tell me about danger," then certain sections of this chapter may cause you some discomfort. However, if you understand that our imaginations can be the fertile ground in which worry and anxiety grow, then you also understand that you have a choice. You can choose to worry about something, or you can take precautions and take action to find solutions. Taking precautions is constructive; remaining in a state of fear or worry is destructive.

The truth is that most psychiatric–mental health nurses live their professional lives without being victims of violence by mental health clients. The distorted and sensationalist views in the media—striking visuals and excited news anchors—combine to add to our fears of the people who happen to be our clients in the mental health settings in which we practice.

Whether you realize it or not, you use your ability to predict behavior in everyday life. You often know when a car will edge over into your lane without signaling. We often refer to that as our "intuition." The root of the word intuition *means to guard or protect. Don't dismiss it. It is a cognitive process that tells us it is time to call on our better judgment skills. The great scientist Albert Einstein once said that when you follow your intuition the solutions come to you and you don't know why or how. Many great discoveries have followed on the heels of a hunch, an intuition. You need to know how to harness your intuition by developing your assessment skills.*

In this chapter we will show you how your assessment skills will help you to predict and avoid violence and how specific nursing strategies can be used to de-escalate aggressive behavior if it occurs. Our goal is to help you to become safer and more comfortable, and reduce your fear, while acknowledging that a certain element of danger does exist in mental health settings.

Gavin de Becker, an expert on predicting violent behavior who has successfully proposed new laws to help manage violence, identifies three ways in which we can use our fears to improve our lives:

1. *When you feel fear, listen.*
2. *When you don't feel fear, don't manufacture it.*
3. *If you find yourself creating worry, explore and discover why (de Becker, 1997).*

We intend that this chapter will help you to avoid unwarranted fear and harness and respect your ability to recognize, prevent, and de-escalate aggressive behavior.

Carol Ren Kneisl and Eileen Trigoboff

Society in general, and nursing in particular, increasingly recognize that violence is a significant health problem. Violence is also an ever-increasing problem in health care environments. According to the National Institute for Occupational Safety and Health (NIOSH) (2002), hospital workers are at high risk for experiencing violence in the workplace. Health care providers in every setting are potential targets of violent behavior. Additional NIOSH data can be accessed through a direct resource link on the Companion Website for this book (http://www.cdc.gov/NIOSH).

Nurses are physically assaulted, threatened, and verbally abused more often than other professionals. One study conducted with individuals caring for elderly clients showed that 65% of nurses had experienced an incident of violence as compared to 42% of occupational therapists and 27% of physiotherapists (Mullan & Badger, 2007).

Nurses in every practice area encounter clients and family members who may be potentially violent. Factors that have contributed to the increasing violence in health care facilities include:

- Downsizing of staff
- Change in skill level of staff members, who now include greater numbers of paraprofessionals
- Increased client acuity levels
- Absence of workplace violence prevention programs

One other factor that contributes to aggression toward nurses is the mistaken belief that violence "is part of the job" (McPhaul & Lipscomb, 2004). These factors, and the fact that nurses are the most frequent victims of assault in health care facilities, magnify the need for psychiatric–mental health nurses to learn to accurately assess and intervene with clients in order to maintain safety.

This chapter provides theoretic perspectives for understanding aggressive and violent behavior. It also describes successful preventive measures such as exploring potential causative factors, recognizing warning signs of violence, nursing interventions, and client and staff education. The Evidence-Based Practice feature on page 914 illustrates the steps that can be taken to avoid the escalation of aggressive behavior.

NURSING SELF-AWARENESS

Not every nurse can work with angry, aggressive, or violent mentally ill clients. Since such work can be frightening and upsetting, it is important to take the time for self-reflection and to examine your reactions to others. This is particularly important when working with violent clients, since your own stress and anxiety can greatly interfere with your ability to attend to subtle cues and to initiate sensitive interventions in a timely manner. The Your Self-Awareness feature on page 914 lists some areas for you to consider when you work with violent clients.

Self-awareness is a process that helps you to avoid personalizing client comments and behaviors. Whenever we "take it personally," objectivity is lost and therapeutic effectiveness decreases. Often our responses to client aggressiveness reflect the beliefs that we incorporated as children. For example, as young children, some of us learned that anger was something to be feared and avoided at all costs. Others of us may have learned that aggressive expression of anger is powerful. These beliefs adopted in childhood often govern our behavior as adults. Self-reflection helps us to determine how our own beliefs influence our responses to clients.

MEDIALINK National Institute for Occupational Safety and Health

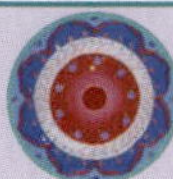

EVIDENCE-BASED PRACTICE

DE-ESCALATING STRATEGIES FOR AGGRESSION

Marty, a 42-year-old client on an inpatient unit, is becoming more aggressive toward staff and other clients. He paces in the hall and mutters to himself. When approached by the nursing staff, he shouts and curses at them. You recognize these behaviors as indicators of escalation of aggressive behavior.

In an attempt to avoid using seclusion and restraints, the nursing staff decides to use the following interventions aimed at de-escalating Marty's behavior:

- Identify the intensity of Marty's behavior.
- Make a personal connection with Marty by having a one-to-one interaction.
- Determine the meaning of Marty's behavior (i.e., understand what he needs).

Additional approaches that may be useful in helping Marty calm down are deep breathing, distraction, and the therapeutic use of music, dance, and movement therapy. Also, after Marty's behavior has stabilized, teaching him anger management techniques may be very useful.

These intervention approaches are based on the following research:

Bisconer, S. W., Green, M., Mallon-Cazjka, J., & Johnson, J. S. (2006). Managing aggression in a psychiatric hospital using a behaviour plan: A case study. *Journal of Psychiatric and Mental Health Services, 13*(5), 515–521.

Burke, J. (2005). Educating the staff at a homeless shelter about mental illness and anger management. *Journal of Community Health Nursing, 22*(2), 65–76.

Lundy, H., & McGuffin, P. (2005). Using dance/movement therapy to augment the effectiveness of therapeutic holding with children. *Journal of Child & Adolescent Psychiatric Nursing, 18*(3), 135–145.

CRITICAL THINKING APPLICATION

1. What is the basis for the belief that anger management can be taught successfully?
2. What is the rationale for adding deep breathing and distraction?
3. Why would music, dance, and movement therapy be helpful?

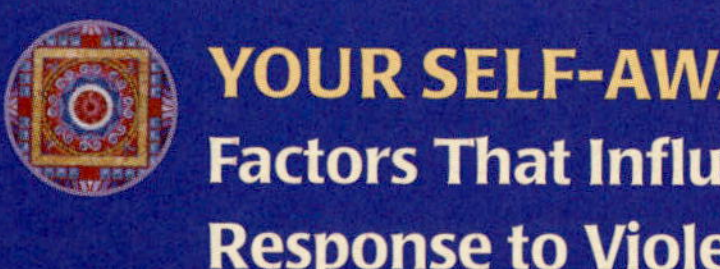

YOUR SELF-AWARENESS
Factors That Influence Your Response to Violence

When working with violent clients, be sure to monitor yourself for the following:

- Ability to use anger constructively and not to take clients' anger personally
- Capacity for clear verbal communication
- Ability to listen actively and nonjudgmentally
- Capacity to both establish and maintain empathic linkages with clients and to disengage
- Willingness to understand your fears and anxieties about violence
- Belief that violent clients are amenable to treatment

BIOPSYCHOSOCIAL THEORIES OF AGGRESSIVE BEHAVIORS

The ongoing debate in psychiatry of "nature versus nurture" (what we are born with versus what we learn) extends into the study of the causes of violence. The expression of aggressive behavior is affected by a complex interaction of biologic and psychosocial factors. Therefore, there is no simple answer for the etiology of violent behavior, and no single theoretic framework can sufficiently explain or predict violence. There is wide diversity among individuals and the situations in which they live. It is, therefore, more valuable to consider violence from a variety of perspectives.

Biologic Factors

Current research is exploring the biologic basis of aggression. While it is likely that violence may be influenced by many biologic variables—genetic factors, hormonal factors, neurotransmitters, and neurophysiologic factors—the exact relationship remains uncertain.

Physiologic changes within the brain may result in violent behavior. Trauma and other disturbances that produce anoxia (e.g., cardiorespiratory arrest) are likely culprits in the development of aggression in some individuals. For example, some people who experience brain tumors or cerebral vascular accidents (strokes) demonstrate violent behavior. Physiologic disorders such as severe hypoglycemia and other metabolic disorders, encephalitis, and dementia may also lead to violence.

In order to understand the underpinnings of violence, it is important for nurses to understand the structures of the brain and their effects on emotion and behavior:

- The serotonergic system (5-HT) and the hypothalamic-pituitary-adrenal axis (HPA) system may contribute to the development of impulsive aggression in some individuals (Gollan, Lee, & Coccaro, 2005).
- The amygdala, located in the lateral temporal lobe, directs emotional responses, including the aggressive expression of anger.

- The hippocampus regulates the recall of recent experiences and new information. Impairment in this area interferes with learning from past experiences, as is often demonstrated by individuals with impulsive behavior.
- The hypothalamus, which serves as a relay between the cerebral cortex and the lower autonomic centers and the spinal cord somatic centers, is the route through which the mind influences bodily function.
- Temporal lobe dysfunction (which occurs with seizures) may cause some people to become aggressive. It is not unusual for some individuals to become violent in the postictal phase of a seizure.
- The frontal lobe, the area in which reason and emotion interact, regulates the ability to problem solve, plan ahead, and restrain impulses. This structure mediates both purposeful behavior and thought and affects limbic system functioning. Damage to the frontal lobe, which often occurs with head trauma, impairs judgment and can cause personality changes and aggressive outbursts (Brower & Price, 2001). These outbursts may be triggered by minor environmental stimuli.
- The limbic system (a functional grouping rather than an anatomic one; includes nuclei, tracts, and structures along the border between the cerebrum and the diencephalon) mediates primitive emotions and basic drives, such as appetite, sexual urges, and aggression. Dysfunction of the limbic system may result in an increase or decrease in aggressive behavior. These structures of the brain are illustrated in Figure 35-1 ■.

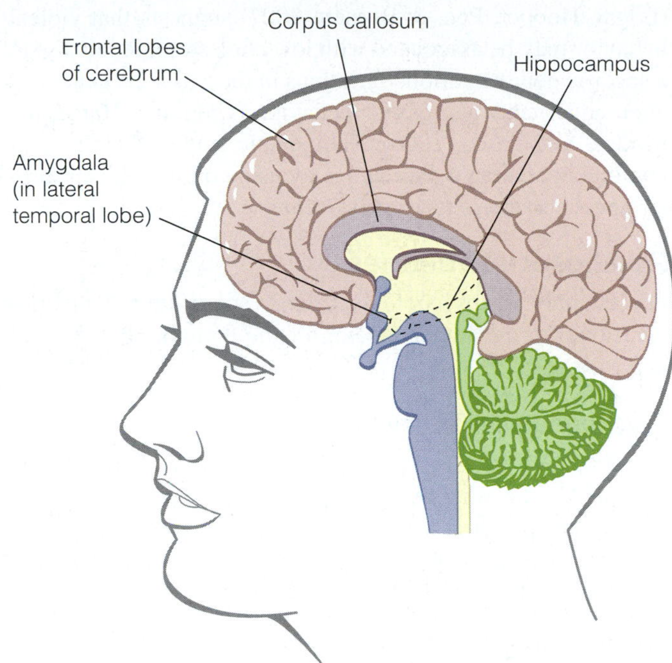

Figure 35-1 ■ Brain structures associated with aggressive behavior.

Numerous research studies substantiate that neurotransmitters, hormones, enzymes, and signaling molecules influence aggression (Chen, Tien, Juan, Tzeng, & Hung, 2005; Herrmann, Lanctot, Eryavec, Van Reekum, & Khan, 2004; Hibbeln, Ferguson, & Blasbalg, 2006). Table 35-1 ■ provides an overview of the effects of selected neurotransmitters on aggression.

Genetic Theories

No one gene or variant thereof has yet been identified as the causative factor of aggressive behavior. However, one study (van der Flier et al., 2007) showed that the apolipoprotein E genotype influences the severity of aggressive behavior in people with dementia of the Alzheimer's type. Another study

Table 35-1 ■ **Role of Neurotransmitters in Aggression**

Transmitter	Function	Description
Acetylcholine	Exerts excitatory effect Facilitates transmission of nerve impulses across myoneural junction	A deficiency (such as that occurring in dementia of the Alzheimer's type) may increase aggressive behavior by lowering the threshold for confusion and impairing memory.
Dopamine	Regulates emotional responses and movement	Increased levels heighten sexual activity, aggressive behavior, and vigilance.
Gamma-aminobutyric acid (GABA)	Exerts inhibitory response on brain activity	Exerts a regulatory effect on violence
Norepinephrine	Exerts excitatory response Is inactivated by monoamine oxidase (MAO)	May increase vigilance and aggression
Serotonin (5-HT)	Influences the processing of information Modulates sleep, sensory responses, and mood	Variations in 5-HT levels lead to misperception of stimuli, which may result in aggressive behavior.

Source: Data from Sadock, B. J., & Sadock, V. A. (2005). *Kaplan & Sadock's pocket handbook of clinical psychiatry* (4th ed.). Philadelphia: Lippincott Williams & Wilkins.

(Edgar, Hooper, Poa, & Burnett, 2007) suggests that violent behavior may be associated with low cholesterol levels due to a specific gene mutation. Variations in the 5-HT-2A gene may alter anger and aggressive behavior (Giegling, Hartmann, Moller, & Rujescu, 2006). The genetic study of violence is continuing at a rapid pace and is focusing on specific molecular genetic markers for aggressiveness.

Psychosocial Theories

Psychoanalytic, psychological, and sociocultural theories contribute to our understanding of the complex behavior of aggression.

Psychoanalytic Theory

Freud (1989) theorized that aggression is one of the two innate drives, the other being the pleasure principle. This viewpoint states that it is instinctive for humans to express anger in aggressive ways. When aggression is directed inward, depression results.

Psychological Theory

Aggression may be viewed as a direct result of unmet needs and wants. Whenever an individual's basic needs are unmet, the resulting threat to his or her existence may cause the person to respond in an aggressive manner. The frustration that arises from unmet needs may escalate to aggressiveness.

There are some mental disorders in which aggressiveness is more likely to occur. Box 35-1 lists some of the mental disorders in which aggressive behavior is prominent; note that the list is not inclusive.

It is also important to note that the diagnosis alone does not make the client violence prone. Rather, clients who have these disorders are likely to experience impairments in impulse control, sensory–perceptual functioning, cognitive functioning, and social skills. Individuals who have poor coping skills and feelings of helplessness and powerlessness are at high risk of exhibiting violent behavior.

Sociocultural Theory

There are numerous psychosocial variables that influence the development and expression of violent behavior. Current research is examining the effects of child abuse, emotional rejection in childhood, and parenting styles as precursors to the development of violence (Gibb, McGeary, Beevers, & Miller, 2006; Guttman, Mowder, & Yasik, 2006; Widom, Schuck, & White, 2006). Dysfunctional family dynamics and negative factors in the childhood home may contribute to violence. Many violent individuals had childhood experiences of abuse.

Sometimes people make the assumption that males are more likely to be involved in assaults than females. However, the differences in gender are insignificant in relation to assaults, with only a slightly higher frequency and intensity of verbal aggressive behaviors in males (Grube, 2007). Studies do show that staff are at increased risk for same-gender assault in both inpatient and community settings (Flannery, Marks, Laudani, & Walker, 2007)—that is, males are more likely to assault males, and females are more likely to assault females.

It is critical that you be culturally sensitive when interacting with clients, especially those demonstrating the potential for violence. Since the expression of aggressive behavior is significantly influenced by culture, there is a real potential for gender and racial discrimination unless you are culturally sensitive when assessing the onset of violence.

Box 35-1 Mental Disorders in Which Aggressiveness Often Occurs

- Antisocial personality disorder
- Borderline personality disorder
- Conduct disorder
- Delusional disorder
- Dementia of the Alzheimer's type
- Intermittent explosive disorder
- Schizophrenia
- Substance-related disorders

Behavioral Theory

Is aggressive behavior learned by witnessing violence? There is ongoing debate about the impact on children of viewing violence as portrayed in media such as television, movies, music, and video games. According to Mathiak and Weber (2006), video gameplay significantly activates the anterior cingulate and the amygdala (areas of the brain that affect emotions). Popular songs with aggressive lyrics influence the behavior of listeners (Fischer & Greitemeyer, 2006), and exposure to media violence brings about short-term and long-term effects in children and adults (Bushman & Huesman, 2006). Children who witness domestic violence are at risk for developing numerous problems, such as depression, anxiety, and violence directed at peers.

Humanistic Theories

Being valued as a person and judged to be worthy affects one's self-esteem, a basic need (Maslow, 1970). Valuing oneself as a significant person with something to contribute is part of self-esteem. When individuals feel they are inadequate, they begin to feel hopeless—for themselves and the future. If a person feels undervalued, unneeded, or insignificant, self-esteem becomes threatened. One response to such an existential threat may be aggressiveness. Acting out in an aggressive manner may be an individual's attempt to communicate self-importance.

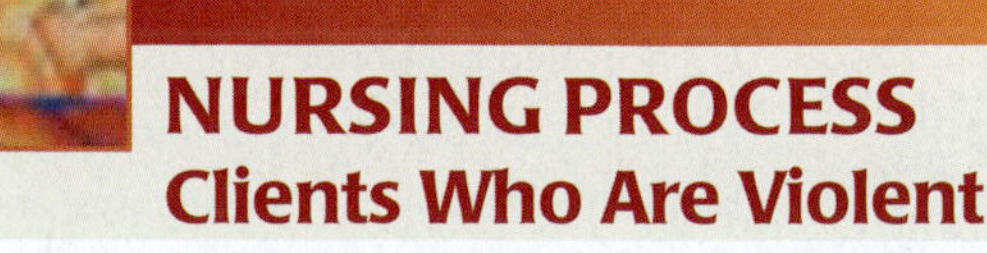

NURSING PROCESS
Clients Who Are Violent

Using the nursing process as the framework for delivery of care to violent clients results in continuity of care, which improves the quality of care.

Assessment

Assessing psychiatric clients for their violence potential is an ongoing process and occurs across the continuum of care (in both inpatient and community-based settings). The prediction of who in a given setting poses a risk for violence, and the perception that someone is more likely to be violent, is known as **dangerousness**. An assessment that someone is dangerous determines fundamental decisions about the need for hospitalization, special supervision, emergency psychopharmacologic intervention, and community placement options. The prediction of danger is the result of an assessment and is essential for guiding treatment decisions.

An increased risk for violence among acutely disturbed clients is associated with the following variables:

- History of violence
- Severity of psychopathology
- Higher levels of hostility–suspiciousness, thinking disturbance, and agitation–excitement (as measured on the Brief Psychiatric Rating Scale [BPRS])
- Length of time in the hospital
- Early age of onset of psychiatric symptoms
- Frequency of admission to psychiatric hospitals

In the following clinical example, Theodore meets almost all of these criteria.

CLINICAL EXAMPLE

Theodore, a 40-year-old single man, was brought to the psychiatric emergency room by the police in response to a call from his mother. He had been pounding on the door of his mother's home, screaming obscenities and wielding a knife. She was terrified. The staff recognized Theodore immediately—he had been hospitalized there more than 20 times over the past several years. He was diagnosed with paranoid schizophrenia at age 18. Early in his illness, he responded well to the supportive hospital environment and medications but did not follow up with day treatment, residential care, or medication when released from the inpatient setting.

It is important to begin your assessment by taking a comprehensive violence history on admission. The goal of history taking is to find patterns or trends in violent behaviors in order to identify the conditions under which an individual is likely to act violently.

Clients and significant others are important sources of information. Interview questions about the violent client's history should be open and direct, as if you were questioning a suicidal individual. Ask, "How much have you thought about violence?" "What have you done about it?" "What is the most violent thing you have done?" Do not, however, rely on client responses as the sole basis for your assessment. Also review the client's history and past records.

Managing and reducing the risk of violence is based on careful assessment of client behaviors. In addition to interviewing, observation is a tool most useful for gathering data about client aggressiveness. See the Your Assessment Approach box below for a listing of behavioral and verbal clues that indicate violence. Predicting the potential for violence helps one to anticipate and prevent aggressive outbursts. However, it is important to understand that while the risk cues clinicians use are useful, they lack consistent predictive power (Odeh, Zeiss, & Huss, 2006). Figure 35-2 ■ on pages 918–919 is a violence assessment tool that can be helpful in predicting danger.

Substance abuse increases the potential for aggressive behavior. Determine whether the client is under the influence of drugs including CNS depressants (e.g., alcohol, benzodiazepines), stimulants (e.g., cocaine, amphetamines), hallucinogens (e.g., PCP, LSD), and narcotics (e.g., morphine, oxycodone).

A thorough assessment also collects data about the client's sleep pattern (discussed later in this chapter), nutritional status, and history of medical problems such as temporal lobe epilepsy. The client's ability to solve problems and cope with stressors should also be noted.

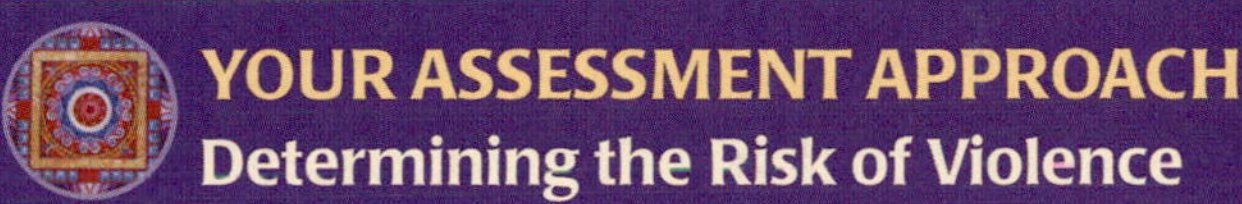

YOUR ASSESSMENT APPROACH
Determining the Risk of Violence

To help determine the risk of violence, you might ask the client the following questions:

- How do you know when you are getting angry at others? At yourself?
- On a scale of 1 to 10, with 1 meaning not angry to 10 meaning extremely angry, how would you rate your anger right now?
- Have you had a problem with anger in the past?
- What types of things trigger anger in you?
- When you become angry, what do you usually do?
- What do you do to help decrease your feelings of anger?

To help determine the risk of violence, you might observe the client for the following behaviors:

- Clenched jaws and fists
- Dilated pupils
- Intense staring
- Flushing of face and neck
- Frowning, glaring, or smirking
- Pacing
- Increased vigilance

To help determine the risk of violence, you might observe the client for the following verbal clues:

- Threatening harm
- A loud, demanding tone of voice
- Abrupt silence
- Sarcastic remarks
- Pressured speech
- Illogical responses
- Yelling, screaming
- Statements of fear
- Statements of suspicion

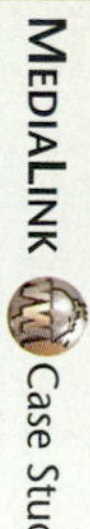

I. Clinical history

A. Diagnosis at discharge
Axis I: ________________
____
Axis II: ________________
____

B. Age: ________________

C. Sex: ____ M ____ F

D. Admitting status
____ 72-HR hold ____ Vol.
____ 14-DAY cert. ____ Other
____ Noncontested

E. Use of self-soothers (e.g., comfort wrap)?
Time out or quiet time?
____
____
____
____ Yes ____ No

F. Age at onset: ________________

G. Psychotropic medications:
____ Taking prior to admission
____ Not taking prior to admission

Medications:
____
____
____

H. Previous criminal history
____ Yes ____ No
____
____

I. Use of ETOH/street drugs
____ Yes ____ No
____
____
____

II. Violence history

A. Previous institutional violence ____ Yes ____ No

Type of institution: ________________ Date(s): ______ ______
Number of incidents: ________________ ______ ______

Type of violence:				
	Against person	____ Yes	____ No	Date ________
	Family	____ Yes	____ No	Date ________
	Stranger	____ Yes	____ No	Date ________
	Inmate/client	____ Yes	____ No	Date ________
	RN/LPT/MD	____ Yes	____ No	Date ________
	Other	____ Yes	____ No	Date ________
				Who ________
	Weapon used	____ Yes	____ No	Date ________
	Against property	____ Yes	____ No	Date ________
	Type	________		
	Verbal threat (only)	____ Yes	____ No	Date ________
Situational factors:	Time of day	________		
	Location	________		
	Engaged in therapeutic activity	____ Yes	____ No	
	Type of activity	________		

Other factors ________________
____
____
____

Interactional factors: Engaged in interaction with victim:
Type of interaction ________________
____
With whom: ________________
Content of conversation, request:
____
____

FIGURE 35-2 ■ A violence assessment tool.

(continued on page 919)

MEDIALINK Application: Assessing Risk of Violence

Nursing Diagnosis: NANDA

Clients who are violent usually have numerous problems, including poor impulse control, low self-esteem, and dysfunctional interpersonal relationships. The relevant nursing diagnoses for clients exhibiting violence are:

- Risk for Other-Directed Violence
- Risk for Self-Directed Violence
- Anxiety
- Ineffective Coping
- Chronic Low Self-Esteem, and Situational Low Self-Esteem

Outcome Identification: NOC

Clients who demonstrate violent behaviors challenge the entire treatment team. It is imperative that team members agree on the expected client outcomes. Following are some outcomes that apply to clients with aggressive behavior.

- Identifies precipitating events prior to losing control
- Refrains from self-injury and from injuring others
- Identifies alternative methods for expressing anger
- Refrains from impulsive behavior

Response to violence: Medications ____ Yes ____ No
Type and dose: ____________________

Seclusion only ____ Yes ____ No
Seclusion/restraint ____ Yes ____ No
Milieu management ____ Yes ____ No
Combination ____ Yes ____ No
(list) ____________________

Client's response to intervention(s): ____________________

B. Community violence
Previous violence: ____ Yes ____ No
Number of incidents: ______ Date(s): ______ ______

Type of violence: Against person ____ Yes ____ No Date ______
Family ____ Yes ____ No Date ______
Stranger ____ Yes ____ No Date ______
Inmate/client ____ Yes ____ No Date ______
RN/LPT/MD ____ Yes ____ No Date ______
Other ____ Yes ____ No Date ______
Who ______
Weapon used ____ Yes ____ No Date ______
Against property ____ Yes ____ No Date ______
Type ______
Verbal threat (only) ____ Yes ____ No Date ______
Situational factors: ETOH ____ Yes ____ No Amount ______
Street drugs ____ Yes ____ No
Type ______

Time of day ______ Activity ______

Location ______
Other factors ______

Interactional factors: Engaged in interaction with victim: ____ Yes ____ No
Type of interaction: ______

Others present: ______

Content of conversation, request, argument, or dispute: ______

FIGURE 35-2 ■ *(continued)*

Even though we have provided a list of suggested outcomes, remember that each client, violent or not, is an individual who has unique needs.

Planning and Implementation: NIC

The major goal for all clients is maintenance of safety; this is especially true for those who are at risk for violence. Protecting the client and others from harm is the primary goal for all health care providers in every setting, not only psychiatric settings. The feature What Every Emergency Department Nurse Should Know on page 920 suggests strategies for the emergency department.

Balance the issue of safety maintenance with the need for ensuring the violent client's individual freedom. Providing treatment in the least restrictive environment, while maintaining safety, is of paramount importance. Chapter 13 discusses the legal and ethical ramifications of the least restrictive environment.

Working successfully with clients who demonstrate violence, or the potential for violence, calls for teamwork, critical thinking, and creativity on the part of the entire treatment team. FIGURE 35-3 ■ on page 921 provides a model for analyzing the risks versus the benefits of several different interventions for a violent client. You may employ a

MEDIALINK Care Plan: Warning: May Contain Explosives

WHAT EVERY EMERGENCY DEPARTMENT NURSE SHOULD KNOW

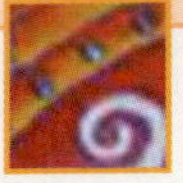

Assessing Anger and Preventing Violence

- Remember that there is a difference between anger (a subjective feeling) and aggression (a harmful behavior).
- When clients enter your emergency department, it is important to assess their level of anger—just as you assess every client's vital signs and pain level.
- Knowing how angry your client is will help determine your next action.
- Approach each client with a calm, reassuring manner. This will help the client feel less threatened and more secure.
- Involve clients in their own care as much as possible. This will increase their sense of control, which helps decrease anger.
- When a client's aggression is escalating, you must protect the safety of that client, other clients, yourself, and other staff.
- Call for help immediately if your interventions have not de-escalated the client's aggressive behavior.

variety of methods, including developing a therapeutic relationship, milieu management, limit setting, pharmacologic agents, behavioral interventions, restrictive measures, and client education.

Therapeutic Relationship

Establishing rapport with the client helps reduce suspiciousness by building trust. When clients feel that they are in a supportive, trusting relationship, there is less need to respond aggressively. Safety maintenance is a key element of a therapeutic relationship. Safety refers not only to physical but also to psychological factors; the environment must be one in which the client feels safe to express feelings and risk learning new behaviors.

A therapeutic nurse–client relationship also involves the nurse's demonstration of compassion and caring, which is actualized through presence, or therapeutic use of self. Be aware of the need to help clients learn to enhance self-esteem. Avoid labeling aggressive behavior as "attention-seeking" without doing a complete assessment to determine the precipitating events that led to the aggressive outburst.

Active listening is essential when working with violent clients or those who are at risk for becoming violent. Listen for the expression of unmet needs (such as control and dependency) and for the expression of the ability to regain/maintain control. (Active listening, or mindful listening, is a communication technique discussed in Chapter 10∞.) When interacting with violent clients, it is important that you constantly assess the potential for aggressive behavior. A list of factors that may predispose individuals to violence is in the Your Assessment Approach feature at right.

Milieu Management

Mental health care environments can be dehumanizing and depersonalizing. When clients feel devalued, aggressiveness usually escalates. Environmental elements contributing to violence in mental health settings include space and location, time of day, architectural design, staffing patterns, activity levels, and client population composition.

Space and Location Space and location factors include territoriality, privacy, and overcrowding. The concept of territoriality involves defending physical objects or the space a client has identified or "staked out" as personal space. For example, a client often "claims" a special chair on the unit, and a new client comes along and sits in it. The resulting conflicts over special territory also raise the issue of privacy.

Overcrowding is also related to the issue of privacy. Clients who are suspicious or have been abused as children often have difficulty tolerating people near them or touching them.

Architectural Design Architectural designs that create blind spots and opportunities for nonobservation can also increase the risk of violence. Mirrors have been used effectively to cope with particular architectural design problems in psychiatric units. Assess the environment for structures that lend themselves to frustration or blind spots. Sometimes the simple installation of one additional client telephone or a minor structural alteration on a unit can significantly reduce the number of violent incidents.

How an inpatient unit and its staff choose to handle potentially dangerous items such as glass, belts, and matches is complex and is related not only to institutional policy and unit philosophy but also to individual clinical judgment. On many units, staff members monitor these items, by using sign-up procedures or by locking them up and distributing them at the discretion of a member of the staff or a member of the client government.

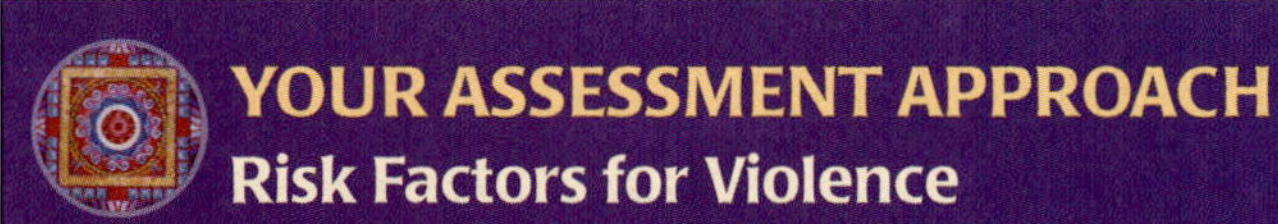

YOUR ASSESSMENT APPROACH
Risk Factors for Violence

Look for the presence of these factors when assessing clients for potential aggressive behavior:

- Availability of and/or possession of weapons
- Cognitive impairment
- Cruelty to animals
- Fire setting
- History of childhood abuse
- History of drug/alcohol abuse
- History of medication nonadherence
- History of violence directed toward others
- History of witnessing family violence
- Impulsivity
- Psychotic symptoms (e.g., hallucinations, paranoid delusions)
- Suicidal behavior

Jason is a voluntary client hospitalized on an open unit who punched another client, fracturing his jaw. You assess Jason after he hit his peer and find him very calm. You place him on 1:1 supervision with staff until you can decide on a course of action. You review his record and discover that he has been in prison for assault and battery. While hospitalized he has not engaged in any violence before today. You call the doctor, the nursing supervisor, the social worker and security; you also call in extra staff to maintain safety.

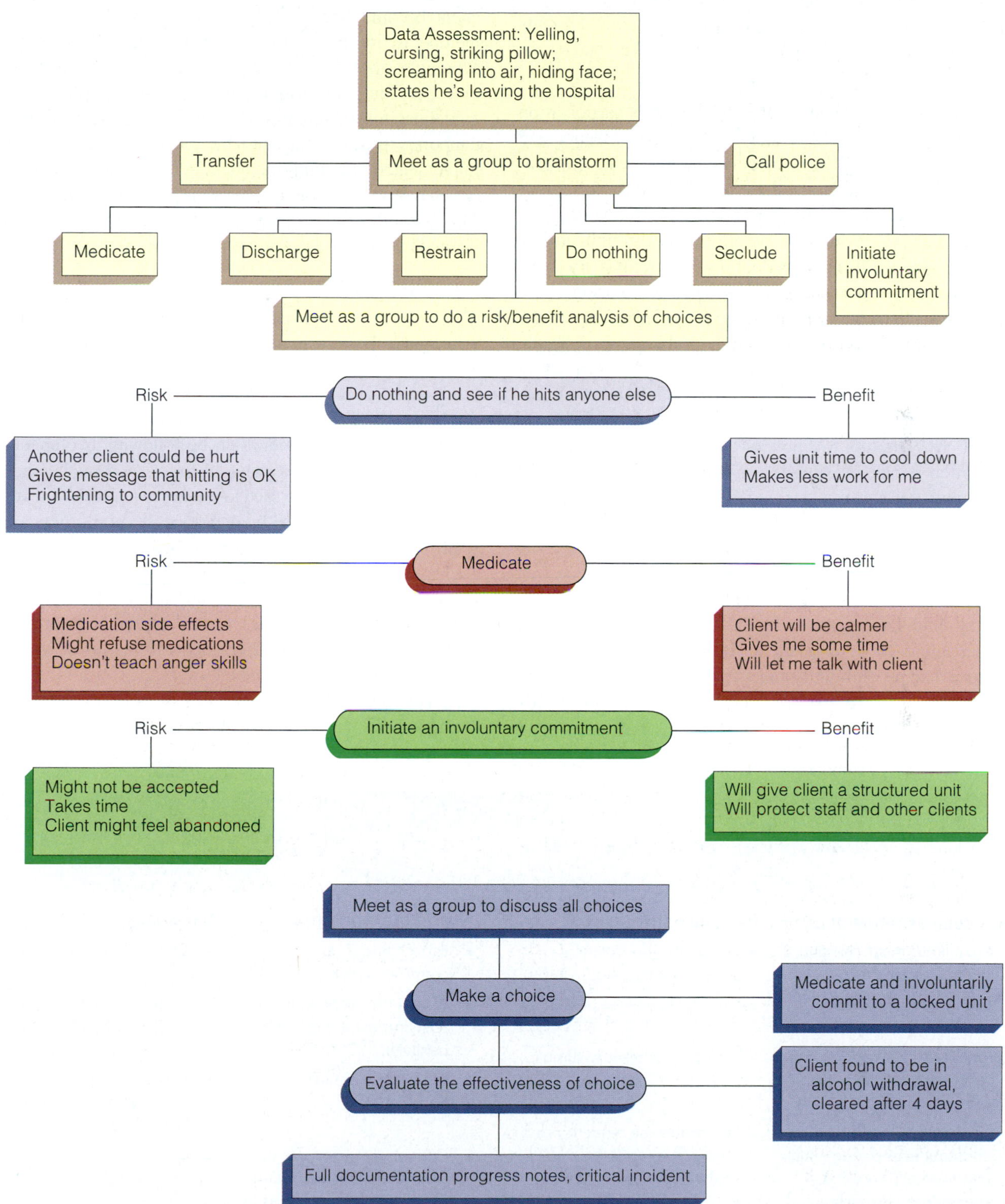

FIGURE 35-3 ■ Risk/benefit analysis as a means of making decisions about the treatment of a violent client.

Staffing Patterns The relationship between staffing patterns and violence is not well understood. Optimal staffing, often cited as a prerequisite for achieving treatment objectives, is being rigorously studied by the American Nurses Association and other professional groups. Whether a given health care facility has sufficient staff to manage potentially violent clients depends on the amount of care required by the total client population at that time.

Activity Level Activity level refers to the client's participation in therapeutic activities. Peak times for violent incidents tend to be mealtimes and periods of concentrated treatment programming. In both situations, there is a high concentration of clients, and performance and participation are demanded.

Peak activity levels can be modified through adjustments such as scheduling, coordinating, and temporary withdrawal. Scheduling staff breaks and mealtimes during client meals can create a situation of temporary understaffing on the unit. Staggering mealtimes for clients and staff is a simple mechanism that may prevent violent behavior. Coordinating client activities with the nursing staff schedule is an important consideration.

Staff who attempt to cajole or coerce clients into participation often create a situation in which the client feels trapped, and striking out becomes the only defense. Sometimes the most valuable intervention with any client—but particularly with one who is agitated, angry, or frightened—is temporary withdrawal. This allows the client quiet time free from the anxiety of interpersonal demands. Making frequent, brief, individualized contact with the client is more reassuring and does more to de-escalate a situation than forcing the client to attend a community meeting or other activity where the client's behavior is likely to be the focal point of discussion. Individualizing the milieu activities of clients may be as important to advancing their treatment and preventing violence as the proper medication regimen.

Limit Setting

Setting limits on inappropriate behavior is necessary when the client becomes increasingly agitated and aggressive. But remember to use limit setting as a therapeutic intervention, not as a punitive tool. The intent of limit setting is not to control the client but rather to provide consistent expectations and guidelines for self-control. Setting limits must be viewed as a temporary process to protect the client and others. Limits are implemented only until the client demonstrates, either verbally or behaviorally, the ability to establish and maintain self-control. The rationales and recommendations for setting limits are explained in the Your Intervention Strategies feature that follows.

Pharmacologic Interventions

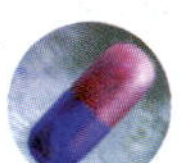

Many pharmacologic agents are currently used to reduce aggressiveness. Some medications frequently used are haloperidol (Haldol) and olanzapine (Zyprexa). Long-acting injectables such as risperidone (Risperdal Consta), fluphenazine (Prolixin), and haloperidol are used with clients discharged to the community to be followed as outpatients, as well as with clients who have histories of nonadherence. Trazodone (Desyrel) is also used to minimize aggressiveness.

In addition to these medications, several others are used specifically to minimize aggressiveness in older clients. They are the anticholinesterase inhibitors donepezil (Aricept), rivastigmine (Exelon), and galantamine (Reminyl), along with memantine (Namenda), which targets the brain chemical glutamate. These and other medications used with older clients are discussed in Chapter 14.

The second-generation antipsychotic agents such as clozapine (Clozaril) and risperidone (Risperdal) reduce the

YOUR INTERVENTION STRATEGIES
Limit Setting

Nursing Intervention	Rationale
State limits in specific and direct language.	Decreases possibility of misunderstanding
Use a calm, unhurried approach.	Promotes a sense of security
Offer time-out periods/one–to–one sessions in a quiet area.	Diminishes sensory stimuli
Explain the limits and consequences during initial interactions (i.e., tell the client what is expected and the related outcomes).	Promotes the tendency to behave according to expectations
Assure client that the staff will not allow client to hurt self and/or others.	Promotes a sense of safety and conveys external controls
Expect all staff to consistently reinforce limits.	Promotes behavior shaping
Accept the client while rejecting the inappropriate behavior.	Protects self-esteem and reinforces behavioral limits
Reward the desirable behavior(s).	Promotes continued demonstration of expected behavior(s)
Continuously evaluate the need for limits; discontinue external limits as soon as the client is able to self-regulate.	Empowers client to exercise self-control

symptoms of agitation and aggression while producing fewer extrapyramidal side effects than conventional antipsychotics. An anticonvulsant agent, valproic acid (Depakene), potentiates GABA-induced inhibition and thus leads to decreased aggressiveness in many individuals (Sadock & Sadock, 2005). The selective serotonin reuptake inhibitors (SSRIs), such as fluoxetine (Prozac) and paroxetine (Paxil), are often effective in decreasing aggressive behaviors in some clients. TABLE 35-2 ■ lists pharmacologic agents commonly used in reducing aggression. Refer to Chapters 7 and 32 for a thorough discussion of these medications.

Although medication is the most widely used treatment for the control of violent behavior in institutional settings, it is important to recognize that pharmacologic agents alone are not the answer to violence. Psychotropic medications must be used with greater caution in older clients as discussed in Chapter 14. Nonpharmacologic interventions with elders, and their rationales, are discussed in the What Every Geriatric Nurse Should Know feature.

Educating Clients

Education is an important intervention for clients who have a history of violence or who are at risk of becoming violent. Client teaching focuses on empowering the client by providing tools for increasing self-responsibility. Some specific topics appropriate for teaching aggressive clients are:

- Anger management
- Social skills training (discussed in Chapter 30)
- Problem solving
- Communication skills (discussed in Chapter 10)
- Assertiveness training (discussed in Chapter 3)
- Relaxation skills (discussed in Chapter 33)

TABLE 35-2 ■ Psychopharmacologic Agents Commonly Used to Reduce Aggression

Classification	Generic Name	Trade Name
Anticonvulsant	Carbamazepine	Tegretol
	Lomotrigine	Lamictal
	Valproic acid	Depakene
Anxiolytic	Buspirone	BuSpar
Benzodiazepine	Clonazepam	Klonopin
	Lorazepam	Ativan
Beta blocker	Propranolol	Inderal
Mood stabilizer	Lithium	Eskalith, Lithane, Lithobid
Neuroleptic	Clozapine	Clozaril
	Fluphenazine	Prolixin
	Haloperidol	Haldol
	Risperidone	Risperdal
Selective serotonin reuptake inhibitor (SSRI)	Fluoxetine	Prozac
	Paroxetine	Paxil

WHAT EVERY GERIATRIC NURSE SHOULD KNOW

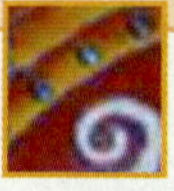

Avoiding Violence by Elders Through Nonpharmacologic Interventions

- Be aware of your own biases about older adults. *Negative biases influence your attitude and approach and may engender anger.*
- Do not expect all elders to be kindly and docile. *It is a myth that all elders are docile; their personalities and behavior may be exaggerated with increasing age. An angry young adult may become an even angrier older adult.*
- Assess mental status, including orientation level. *Confusion and disorientation can be frightening and may lead to impulsive or aggressively self-protective behavior.*
- Avoid touching confused elders, as your touch may be frightening or misinterpreted as an attack. *Touch should always be used judiciously after assessing that it is appropriate.*
- Use a calm approach to decrease anxiety level. *Just as anxiety can be interpersonally communicated, so can calmness and a sense of peace.*
- Establish rapport to lessen the older adult's sense of alienation. *Establishing rapport builds trust and helps the elder to feel connected to another.*
- Include the elder in decision-making that affects his or her interests. *Including the elder avoids dehumanization and provides the elder with a sense of control.*

An outline for a five-session anger management class that includes these topics is in the Partnering with Clients and Families feature on page 924. The classes can be modified as needed.

Calming the Escalating Client

Avoiding client injury that can occur with the use of seclusion and restraints requires an attempt to use alternative methods to calm clients whose anger is escalating. It is imperative that you fully attend to the client in order to determine where the client's behavior falls on the continuum of aggression. You also need to be able to understand the meaning underlying the client's behavior in order to intervene appropriately. Some strategies for reducing escalation and averting a crisis are given in the Your Intervention Strategies feature on page 924. The techniques listed are directed at de-escalating anger and aggressive behavior and should be used before the client becomes out of control.

Restrictive Measures: Verbal Interventions

All interventions must be considered within the context of the principle of least restrictiveness, discussed in Chapter 13. This principle requires staff to use less restrictive measures of control before resorting to more restrictive interventions. Staff members must document their efforts to intervene with a client using verbal strategies before they intervene physically.

MEDIALINK Critical Thinking Exercise: The Out-of-Control Client

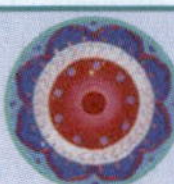

PARTNERING WITH CLIENTS AND FAMILIES

TEACHING ABOUT ANGER MANAGEMENT

Session 1: What Is Anger?
- Signs and symptoms
- Causes: just or unjust anger
- Responses: thoughts, feelings, and actions

Session 2: Managing Anger Through Relaxation
- Importance and advantages
- The relaxation response
- Demonstration and practice

Session 3: Managing Anger Through Communication
- Importance and advantages
- Communication process
- Assertive communication
- Demonstration, role play, practice

Session 4: Problem Solving
- Importance and advantages
- Process of problem solving
- Demonstration and practice

Session 5: Closure: Putting It All Together
- Review of processes
- Exercise: responding to a situation
- Self-evaluation

Forming a therapeutic relationship with the potentially violent client is often the first step to containing the violent behavior. It is important to convey control in the situation by using clear, calm statements and a confident physical stance rather than through remarks or cues that can be interpreted as challenging. A confrontational, aggressive, or threatening manner or a tendency to overidentify with the client's experience can make the staff member a target of violence and can actually precipitate it. The Rx Communication feature illustrates nonconfrontational verbal interventions that can be useful with angry clients.

Some violent behavior occurs impulsively and without warning. Most episodes, however, involve an escalation of behavior and are therefore more appropriate for verbal intervention. Establishing quick rapport and an alliance with the potentially violent client is essential. Examples of verbal interventions and positional strategies for working with potentially violent clients are provided in the following Your Intervention Strategies feature on page 925. The overall goal is to protect the client's already damaged self-esteem as much as possible in order to decrease the potential for violent behavior. Clinical judgment and the situation itself must dictate the appropriateness of their use.

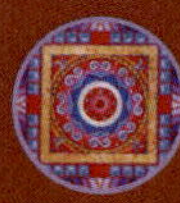

YOUR INTERVENTION STRATEGIES
De-Escalation Strategies for Angry or Aggressive Clients

- Diversion
- Exercise
- Change of surroundings
- Release from schedule or "demands"
- Relaxation
- Music
- Quiet periods
- Being read to or talked to by staff
- A quiet walk
- Reciting phrases or counting
- Thought stopping (a cognitive behavioral technique in which the client examines angry thoughts and feelings that drive action; see Chapter 31)

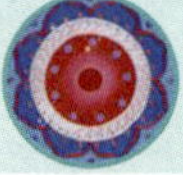

RX COMMUNICATION

COMMUNICATING WITH THE ANGRY, NONVERBAL CLIENT

CLIENT: Flares his nostrils and glares at the nurse.

NURSE RESPONSE 1: "Steven, you look angry today."

RATIONALE: Stating an observation, such as how the client appears, as well as using a feeling word, encourages communication. Talking about feeling angry may decrease the need to act out anger.

NURSE RESPONSE 2: "Steven, I can tell that you are upset. What's going on with you?"

RATIONALE: When you know a client is upset, this direct approach creates an opportunity for the client to discuss the feelings and thoughts with you.

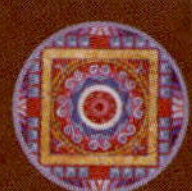

YOUR INTERVENTION STRATEGIES
Verbal Interventions and Positional Strategies

Technique	Rationale
■ Approach the client from the side. Do not stand face–to–face with a potentially violent person.	■ Decreases the tendency of the violent person to project and externalize the assault
■ Leave plenty of space between yourself and the client.	■ Reduces anxiety and the opportunity for assault
■ Speak slowly, directly, in a normal tone of voice, using simple statements such as "Mr. Jones, put the chair down," or "Mrs. Clark, let's sit down and talk about what's bothering you." Encourage the client to sit down. If the client is pacing and can't sit down, pace with the client.	■ Reduces anxiety, communicates control, increases the client's self-esteem, and models negotiation
■ Center your statements on the issues concerning the client. For example, if the client states, "The nurse said I'm too sick to leave the hospital," a response such as, "You're upset at this big disappointment" will likely be more effective than "I can see how you must be upset by that."	■ Deflects attention away from the staff member who has become the target for the violent behavior
■ When responding to the client's anger at not being allowed to leave, try saying, "I'm interested in understanding how terrible that is for you, Mr. Lewis."	■ Avoids challenging the client and expresses interest in the client's perspective
■ Express clear expectations of control. For example, "I expect you can control yourself." Resist touching clients when they are upset and posing an immediate danger.	■ Communicates clarity and emphasizes the client's ability to control own behavior; communicates respect for the client and maintains a comfortable distance, thereby reducing the client's sense of threat
■ Acknowledge nonviolent behavior. When the client sits down to talk, try saying, "Thank you for sitting with me. I can listen better this way."	■ Focuses on the client's strength and maintains the client's self-esteem

Sometimes verbal interventions are insufficient to contain the situation, particularly when the violent behavior occurs impulsively. In these instances, additional interventions—including medications, behavioral techniques, and seclusion and restraint—can be used with or instead of the verbal strategies.

Restrictive Measures: Seclusion and Restraint

Various behavioral strategies established around the principle of progressive isolation are often attempted before initiating seclusion and restraint. The therapeutic intent is to reduce disruptive stimulation and provide the client with a contained, well-defined space for reassurance and protection. Depending on unit construction, the client can be encouraged to seek quiet refuge at the back of the unit or in a private room. Isolation can progress from the back of the unit to the client's room to open seclusion or a quiet room as indicated. These strategies are typically used in conjunction with medications to avoid the more restrictive procedures of seclusion and restraint. The ethics of seclusion and restraint are discussed in Chapter 13∞.

When efforts to contain the client's behavior using verbal techniques or administering medications and behavioral techniques do not prevent the violent behavior, or if an assault occurs without warning, staff members must intervene to seclude or mechanically restrain the client in order to protect the client and others. **Seclusion** consists of confining a person to a room or area where the person is physically prevented from leaving. If seclusion is not effective in helping the individual regain behavioral control, then restraints may be instituted. A **restraint** is any device attached to a person's body that cannot be easily removed by the person; the device restricts the individual's freedom of movement.

Client Rights In the past few years, there has been a concerted effort by federal and state agencies, professional associations, and health care facilities to reduce the use of seclusion and restraint. Client safety is the primary reason for the trend toward eliminating seclusion and restraint in health care settings. According to the National Mental Health Association (NMHA) (2005), many people die every year from the improper use of restraints. Asphyxiation and cardiac arrest are the causes of most deaths associated with restraints used in psychiatric and geriatric settings.

The NMHA supports proposed federal legislation requiring improved staff training in crisis de-escalation techniques and advocates for improved access to medication and community-based treatment for individuals with severe mental illness. The Children's Health Act of 2000 enacted by the 104th Congress requires any public or health care facility that receives federal funding to protect and promote the rights of each resident with regard to restraints or involuntary seclusion. This act also mandates that restraints and seclusion may be imposed only to ensure physical safety and only on the written order of a physician or other licensed practitioner. Another significant part of this legislation is implementing regulations for appropriate staffing levels and training.

The movement toward a restraint-free environment of care is the exemplification of least restrictive measures. *Seclusion and restraint are to be used only in the case of behavioral emergency.* (The client's right to treatment in the least restrictive setting is explored in Chapter 13.) The following clinical example, which continues the story of Theodore, first described on page 917, illustrates a situation in which seclusion may be therapeutic.

CLINICAL EXAMPLE

Upon Theodore's admission to the psychiatric emergency room, he is disheveled, unable to cooperate with the staff, and is screaming and flailing. He is tormented with delusions and hallucinations that frighten him and lead him to strike out at others in the belief that they are trying to hurt him. He has a history of assaults against his mother and the nursing staff. The staff assess Theodore's risk for imminent violence to be high and administer haloperidol IM and place him in a seclusion room where they hope he will rest and feel safer.

MEDIALINK Seclusion and Restraint Guidelines

The American Psychiatric Nurses Association (APNA) has developed a position statement on the use of seclusion and restraint. Box 35-2 provides an overview of these principles (APNA, 2007). Additional data from APNA (http://www.apna.org), NMHA (http://www.nmha.org), the Health Care Financing Administration (HCFA) (http://www.cms.hhs.gov), and the Joint Commission on Accreditation of Health Care Organizations (JCAHO) (http://www.jcaho.org) can be accessed through direct resource links on the Companion Website for this book. Be sure to make yourself familiar with the policies of your agency and your state mental health code.

Box 35-2 Summary of the American Psychiatric Nurses Association Position Statement on the Use of Seclusion and Restraint

- Emphasizes prevention and reduction of the use of seclusion and restraint
- Calls for their use only in behavioral emergencies that pose an immediate risk of harm to a client or others
- Calls on psychiatric–mental health nurses to provide leadership in establishing a treatment environment that is client focused and noncoercive
- Urges working within a collaborative relationship with the client and family
- Focuses on the need for an individualized treatment plan that promotes the client's self-management

Source: American Psychiatric Nurses Association. (2007). *Position statement on the use of seclusion and restraint.* Retrieved April 6, 2007, from http://www.apna.org.

Several intervention approaches are being used in an attempt to reduce the use of restraints. Some of these approaches include improved staff–client ratios, crisis response teams, and second-generation antipsychotic medication (Smith et al., 2005). Facilities using seclusion and restraint require staff attendance at assault training programs. These programs teach policies and procedures for dealing with assaultive clients, including assessment, prevention of escalating aggressiveness, and legal and clinical documentation requirements, as well as appropriate physical contact for use with violent clients.

At no time should students or other untrained personnel intervene using these techniques, because they involve actual physical contact with clients, thereby increasing the risk of personal injury.

Care of the Client in Seclusion and Restraint Psychiatric–mental health nurses have a major responsibility in the decision to isolate and restrain as well as in caring for the client while in seclusion and restraints. Once the decision has been made to seclude and restrain a potentially violent client, a leader is chosen from among the available staff. The leader is responsible for designating roles to be performed by the remaining staff and for directing the steps in the seclusion and restraint procedure. Choice of the leader is important and can be based on various factors, one of which is familiarity with the client. Remember that the goal is to gain maximum cooperation from the client and minimize violence.

After a leader is chosen, a sufficient number of personnel must be gathered. This support staff should convey confidence and calm, reflecting a detached, professional approach to a familiar procedure. Avoid intimidating language and physical stances, since these behaviors may provoke the client's potential for violence. It is often sufficient to have the support staff gather around the leader the first time the client is approached. This show of force may be enough, and the client may comply without further intervention.

One staff member is assigned responsibility for managing the unit environment and other clients. This person is responsible for supporting and calming the other clients, who may become anxious during the procedure. In addition, the area near the seclusion room must be cleared of clients or physical obstructions to minimize the potential for injury.

Once the unit environment is safe, the team approaches the violent client. The leader offers a clear, brief statement of the purpose and rationale for seclusion or restraint. For example, the client is told that his or her behavior is out of control and that time in seclusion is required to help him or her regain control. The other team members position themselves around the client for easy access to the client's limbs. The leader then asks the client to walk into the seclusion room accompanied by staff. At this point, further discussion or negotiation should be avoided as it frequently aggravates the situation. The behavioral options given to the client must be kept simple, clear, and minimal. Specific procedures for placing a client in restraints should follow governmental regulations, professional association standards, and agency policies.

Once a client is placed in seclusion or restraint, nursing observations of the client's behavior are required every 15 minutes. These checks include a description of the client's behavior, as well as routine care activities, including meals, circulation checks, and toileting. These observations should be conducted by nursing staff entering the seclusion room and participating in a verbal exchange with the client. Document the content of these dialogues, paying particular attention to a reduction in the client's symptoms, responsiveness to limits, capacity to discuss options, and increased capacity to tolerate frustration. Documentation of these behavioral checks and routine physical care activities is required.

Release from Seclusion and Restraint The client may be released from seclusion and restraint when his or her behavior is under control and no longer poses a danger to self or others. The decision to release a client from seclusion or remove restraints is based on an assessment of data gathered while the client is in seclusion. The ability of the client to control his or her behavior has been observed many times during the course of seclusion or restraint and is the basis for the decision to release.

Professional Education

Education about the reduction of violence in the workplace, especially the de-escalation of violence, should be ongoing. The focus of the staff must be on the prevention, rather than the management, of aggressive behavior. The educational programs are designed to help nurses:

- Understand the ways in which they increase their own vulnerability to assault
- Develop provocation profiles (recognizing one's own personal triggers for aggression: refer back to the Your Self-Awareness feature on page 914) of themselves to increase their sensitivity and awareness
- Role-play conversations with violent clients
- Practice teamwork for physical restraint procedures
- Promote a safe, nonblaming environment to discuss their experiences of working with violent clients
- Develop sensitivity to the effects their own experiences of violence have in their daily work

Resistance to restraint reduction may exist despite the strong stances taken by professional organizations, regulating agencies, and mental health facility administrators. It is important to acknowledge the emotional responses of individual staff members and the culture of the mental health setting (Curran, 2007). Along with providing information to staff members, an educational program must identify barriers to restraint reduction such as concern for personal safety, lack of practice using alternate de-escalation skills, and fear of disrupting the therapeutic milieu.

Collegial Support

Nurses and other staff members who have been assaulted by clients need the support of their coworkers in a safe, supportive environment. An initial approach is to encourage nurses who have been attacked to discuss their feelings and experiences. Critical incident stress debriefing (CISD) is often used to help staff members come to terms with violent assaults. CISD is an interaction facilitated by mental health clinicians to allow personnel to talk about their thoughts, feelings, and reactions to a stressful event. CISD came under intense scrutiny in 2003–2004 when some studies reported that CISD could be harmful rather than helpful. These studies have since been criticized for their methodology (Wagner, 2005). Essentially, CISD has been found to be more beneficial for mitigating PTSD (posttraumatic stress disorder) symptoms in "secondary" victims of trauma (the nurses and staff members we discuss here) and less helpful, but not harmful, for primary victims of trauma (Jacobs, Horne-Moyer, & Jones, 2004). Refer to Chapter 34 ∞ for a complete explanation of CISD. Providing supportive crisis intervention for the staff may decrease the potential for retaliation and long-term negative consequences (Kindy, Petersen, & Parkhurst, 2005).

Evaluation

There are many elements to consider in evaluating the effectiveness of strategies for violence management. Individual characteristics, biologic factors, conditions in the social environment, and the interpersonal styles of both clients and staff contribute to violent behavior. Despite our theoretic understanding of violent behavior and efforts to implement management strategies to decrease the likelihood of its occurrence, we are not yet able to predict with absolute certainty when someone will act in a violent manner. We can, however, use the information presented earlier in this chapter to help predict based on:

- Identifying persons with mental disorders in which aggressiveness often occurs (see Box 35-1 on page 916)
- Assessing a client's risk factors for violence (see Your Assessment Approach feature on page 920)
- Assessing clients for indicators of impending violence (see the Your Assessment Approach feature on page 917)
- Determining a client's violence history (see Figure 35-2 on pages 918–919)

The fact remains: violence occurs in health care settings, and psychiatric–mental health nurses are at risk for assault from psychiatric clients.

Specific criteria to be considered when evaluating violent clients are listed below. Determine whether the client is able to:

- Refrain from verbal outbursts.
- Refrain from striking others.
- Refrain from violating others' personal space.
- Identify factors that precipitate violent behaviors.
- Identify feelings when angry or frustrated.
- Vent negative feelings appropriately.
- Identify alternative ways to cope with problems.

CASE MANAGEMENT

The concept of least restrictive environment is used to guide the planning of nursing care for all clients. However, when aggressive behavior begins to intensify, the safety of everyone involved—client, staff, and others in the community—overrides the client's right to freedom. Therefore, the case manager's role is often very challenging when coordinating care for the aggressive client in community settings. When referring clients with a history of violence to care providers, the case manager functions as an educator and an advocate. It is also important that the case manager assesses the client's adherence to the medication regimen and follow-up appointments as prescribed.

COMMUNITY-BASED CARE

Milieu management is not limited to inpatient treatment settings. When working in outpatient areas, such as clinics and offices, be aware of the relationship between the physical environment and the potential for violence. For example, a safe office arrangement calls for the furniture to be arranged in such a way that you can exit without being trapped. Having easy access to an emergency call system is also essential in maintaining the safety of both staff and clients.

HOME CARE

In order to assist aggressive clients to function in the home, it may be helpful to teach family members, friends, and significant others specific techniques for defusing violence. Refer to the de-escalating strategies in the Your Intervention Strategies feature on page 924. You can teach these same strategies to family members, friends, and significant others, as well as the indicators for impending violence identified in the Your Assessment Approach feature on page 917. Prior to discharge to the home, encourage the client to use anger management and relaxation skills as needed. Also, review the section on home care in Chapter 12.

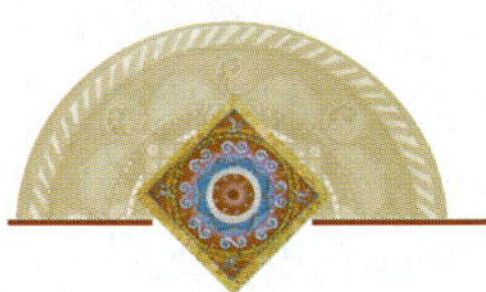

EXPLORE MEDIALINK

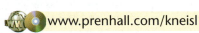

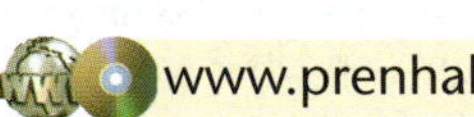

For NCLEX-RN® review questions, case studies, and other resources for this chapter see the Pearson Health MediaLink CD-ROM that accompanies this book and the Companion Website at www.prenhall.com/kneisl.

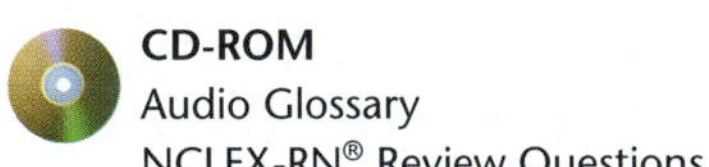

CD-ROM
Audio Glossary
NCLEX-RN® Review Questions

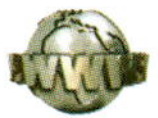

Companion Website
Audio Glossary
NCLEX-RN® Review Questions
Critical Thinking Exercise
- *The Out-of-Control Client*

Case Study
- *Pervasively Aggressive*

Care Plan
- *Warning: May Contain Explosives*

MediaLinks
MediaLink Application
- *Assessing Risk of Violence*

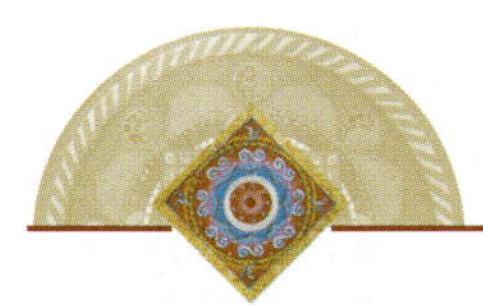

NCLEX-RN® REVIEW QUESTIONS

1. A family member states, "I do not understand why my family member recently developed violent behavior. How does it start?" Which of the following statements is an appropriate initial nursing response?
   1. "Aggression is regressed behavior and reflects dysfunction of the limbic system, a very primitive part of the brain."
   2. "Violent behavior often results from an injury associated with decreased oxygen to the brain."
   3. "No single theory consistently explains or predicts violent behavior."
   4. "Genetic factors may increase aggressive behavior in previously nonviolent individuals."

2. During the initial inpatient nursing assessment, the nurse asks, "Are you thinking about hurting anyone right now?" Which of the following client responses indicates that the nurse should anticipate imminent violence?
   1. The client glares at the nurse and is unable to respond verbally.
   2. "I keep thinking about poisoning my neighbor."
   3. "I'm not thinking about hurting anyone right now."
   4. "The voices never tell me to hurt people. They just keep me company."

3. Which of the following questions by a nurse reflect an understanding of the risk factors associated with violent behavior? (Select all that apply.)
1. "Do you understand that the staff has to care for other clients besides you?"
2. "If you are frightened or fearful, what do you do?"
3. "What do you usually do to relax?"
4. "In the past, have you ever acted on your thoughts of violence?"
5. "Can you wait 30 minutes until we are done with report?"

4. As you walk and talk with a pacing client, he indicates that he is feeling increasingly agitated. Which nursing statements assist in de-escalating violent behavior within the context of the least restrictive environment? (Select all that apply.)
1. "How can the staff and I help you maintain control?"
2. "Your PRN medication helped you cope with stress 2 days ago. Would you be willing to take that medication now?"
3. "I can offer you your medication. Do you want it by mouth or by injection?"
4. "You need to take some time out in the quiet room or we may have to seclude you."
5. "As we are walking around together, is the walking helping you?"

5. Which statement by a nurse reflects an understanding of the balance of safety with individual freedom?
1. "What happened last time when you could not follow the rules?"
2. "The sign next to the telephone says '10-minute limit.'"
3. "You can have an additional 10 minutes because you had such a hard time this morning."
4. "If you need more time on the telephone, let's identify a time when other clients aren't waiting to use the phone."

6. Which of the following nursing interventions is therapeutic for the aggressive client?
1. Ignore the client's behavior in order to defuse the aggressive situation.
2. Assist the client to consider alternative responses to angry feelings.
3. Ask the client why she feels the way she does.
4. Encourage the client to remain quiet and alone when she feels aggressive.

7. A client on an inpatient unit is observed pacing, agitated and hostile, toward other clients on the unit. What is the priority intervention by the nurse?
1. Provide safety for the other clients on the unit.
2. Remove the agitated client to a seclusion room.
3. Provide safety for the agitated client and other clients.
4. Ignore the agitated client's behavior until he can calm down.

8. A charge nurse develops a formal policy and procedure for conducting critical incident stress debriefing within 2 hours of any violent incident on the inpatient psychiatric unit. Which of the following are the best rationales for this development? (Select all that apply.)
1. The staff members will have an opportunity for team-building.
2. Formal crisis debriefing may improve risk management outcomes.
3. The debriefing session provides an opportunity for staff members to identify and ventilate their feelings.
4. Staff members need encouragement and a structured format for support in discussing their thoughts, feelings, and reactions to a violent incident.
5. It is important to review the incident so that the clients and/or staff receive consequences.

9. After a psychoeducational group session, a nursing student's client becomes violent. Which of the following is the best response by the nursing student to the client's violent behavior?
1. Remain with the other clients and staff who are physically removed from the violent client.
2. Participate in physical crisis intervention with the staff.
3. Assume the leadership role and designate the roles for other nursing staff.
4. Document the interventions of other staff as well as the client's response.

10. A hospital provides a workshop designed to decrease violence in the workplace. Which participant statements indicate that the educational program was effective? (Select all that apply.)
1. "I had never before considered psychiatric hospitalization from the client's perspective."
2. "My coworkers and I now know how to restrain an out-of-control visitor."
3. "I learned that I tend to smile when I am nervous, and this is an effective way to defuse a potentially threatening situation."
4. "Our team members are less likely to blame each other when a violent episode occurs."
5. "The role-playing exercise gave me a variety of facilitative statements."

See Appendix C for answers.

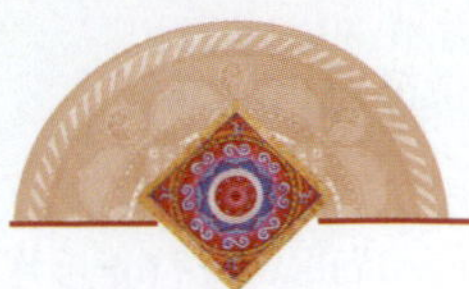

REFERENCES

American Psychiatric Nurses Association. (2007). *Position statement on the use of seclusion and restraint*. Retrieved April 6, 2007, from http://www.apna.org.

Bisconer, S. W., Green, M., Mallon-Cazjka, J., & Johnson, J. S. (2006). Managing aggression in a psychiatric hospital using a behaviour plan: A case study. *Journal of Psychiatric and Mental Health Services, 13*(5), 515–521.

Brower, M. C., & Price, B. H. (2001). Neuropsychiatry of frontal lobe dysfunction in violent and criminal behavior: A critical review. *Journal of Neurology and Neurosurgery in Psychiatry, 71*(6), 720–726.

Burke, J. (2005). Educating the staff at a homeless shelter about mental illness and anger management. *Journal of Community Health Nursing, 22*(2), 65–76.

Bushman, B. J., & Huesman, L. R. (2006). Short-term and long-term effects of violent media on aggression in children and adults. *Archives of Pediatric & Adolescent Medicine, 160*(4), 348–352.

Chen, C. Y., Tien, Y. M., Juan, C. H., Tzeng, O. J., & Hung, D. L. (2005). Neural correlates of impulsive-violent behavior: An event-related potential study. *Neuroreport, 16*(11), 1213–1216.

Curran, S. S. (2007). Staff resistance to restraint reduction: Identifying and overcoming barriers. *Journal of Psychosocial Nursing and Mental Health Services, 45*(5), 45–50.

de Becker, G. (1997). *The gift of fear: Survival signals that protect us from violence*. Boston: Little, Brown and Company.

Edgar, P. F., Hooper, A. J., Poa, N. R., & Burnett, J. R. (2007). Violent behavior associated with hypocholesterolemia due to a novel APOB gene mutation. *Molecular Psychiatry, 12*(3), 258–263.

Fischer, P., & Greitemeyer, T. (2006). Music and aggression: The impact of sexual-aggressive song lyrics on aggression-related thoughts, emotions, and behavior toward the same and the opposite sex. *Personality and Social Psychology Bulletin, 32*(9), 1165–1176.

Flannery, R. B. Jr., Marks, L., Laudani, L., & Walker, A. P. (2007). Psychiatric patient assault and staff victim gender: Fifteen-year analysis of the Assaulted Staff Action Program (ASAP). *Psychiatric Quarterly, 78*(2), 83–90.

Freud, S. (1989). *Civilization and its discontents* (J. Strachey, Ed.). New York: Norton. (Original work published 1930.)

Gibb, B. E., McGeary, J. E., Beevers, C. G., & Miller, I. W. (2006). Serotonin transporter (5-HTTLPR) genotype, childhood abuse, and suicide attempts in adult psychiatric inpatients. *Suicide and Life-Threatening Behavior, 36*(6), 687–693.

Giegling, I., Hartmann, A. M., Moller, H. J., & Rujescu, D. (2006). Anger- and aggression-related traits are associated with polymorphisms in the 5-HT-2A gene. *Journal of Affective Disorders, 96*(1–2), 75–81.

Gollan, J. K., Lee, R. I, & Coccaro, E. F. (2005). Developmental psychopathology and neurobiology of aggression. *Developmental Psychopathology, 17*(4), 1151–1171.

Grube, M. (2007). Gender differences in aggressive behavior at admission to a psychiatric hospital. *Aggressive Behavior, 33*(2), 97–103.

Guttman, M., Mowder, B., & Yasik, A. (2006). Early violence prevention programs: Implications for violence prevention against girls and women. *Annals of New York Academy of Scientists, 1087*, 90–102.

Herrmann, N., Lanctot, K. L., Eryavec, G., Van Reekum, R., & Khan, L. R. (2004). Growth hormone response to clonidine predicts aggression in Alzheimer's disease. *Psychoneuroendocrinology, 29*(9), 1192–1197.

Hibbeln, J. R., Ferguson, T. A., & Blasbalg, T. L. (2006). Omega-3 fatty acid deficiencies in neurodevelopment, aggression and autonomic dysregulation: Opportunities for intervention. *International Review of Psychiatry, 18*(2), 107–118.

Jacobs, J., Horne-Moyer, H. L., & Jones, R. (2004). The effectiveness of critical incident stress debriefing with primary and secondary trauma victims. *International Journal of Emergency Mental Health, 6*(1), 5–14.

Kindy, D., Petersen, S., & Parkhurst, D. (2005). Perilous work: Nurses' experiences in psychiatric units with high risks of assault. *Archives of Psychiatric Nursing, 19*(4), 169–175.

Lundy, H., & McGuffin, P. (2005). Using dance/movement therapy to augment the effectiveness of therapeutic holding with children. *Journal of Child & Adolescent Psychiatric Nursing, 18*(3), 135–145.

Maslow, A. (1970). *Motivation and personality* (2nd ed.). New York: Harper & Row.

Mathiak, K., & Weber, R. (2006). Toward brain correlates of natural behavior: fMRI during violent video games. *Human Brain Mapping, 27*(12), 948–956.

McPhaul, K., & Lipscomb, J. (2004). Workplace violence in health care: Recognized but not regulated. *Online Journal of Issues in Nursing, 9*(3). Retrieved August 6, 2007, from www.nursingworld.org/ojin/topic25/tpc24_6.htm.

Mullan, B., & Badger, F. (2007). Aggression and violence towards staff working with older patients. *Nursing Standard, 21*(27), 35–38.

National Mental Health Association. (2005 Rev). NMHA position statement: The use of restraining techniques and seclusion for persons with mental or emotional disorders. NMHA Program Policy P-41. Retrieved August 9, 2007, from http://mentalhealthamerica.net.

National Institute for Occupational Safety and Health. (2002). Violence: Occupational hazards in hospitals. DHH (NIOS) Publication No. 2002-101. Retrieved August 9, 2007, from http://www.cdc.gov/niosh.

Odeh, M. S., Zeiss, R. A., & Huss, M. T. (2006). Cues they use: Clinicians' endorsement of risk cues in predictions of dangerousness. *Behavioral Science Law, 24*(2), 147–156.

Sadock, B. J., & Sadock, V. A. (2005). *Kaplan & Sadock's pocket handbook of clinical psychiatry* (4th ed.). Philadelphia: Lippincott Williams & Wilkins.

Smith, G. M., Davis, R. H., Bixler, E. O., Lin, H. M., Altenor, R. J., Hardentstine, B. D., et al. (2005). Pennsylvania State Hospital system's seclusion and restraint reduction program. *Psychiatric Services, 56*(9), 1115–1122.

van der Flier, W. M., Staekenborg, S., Pijnenburg, Y. A., Gillissen, F., Romkes, R., Kok, A., et al. (2007). Apolipoprotein E genotype influence presence and severity of delusions and aggressive behavior in Alzheimer disease. *Dementia & Geriatric Cognitive Disorders, 23*(1), 42–46.

Wagner, S. L. (2005). Emergency response service personnel and the critical incident stress debriefing debate. *International Journal of Emergency Mental Health, 7*(1), 33–41.

Widom, C. S., Schuck, A. M., & White, H. R. (2006). An examination of pathways from childhood victimization to violence: The role of early aggression and problematic alcohol use. *Violence and Victimology, 21*(6), 675–690.

APPENDIX A

DSM-IV-TR CLASSIFICATION

NOS = Not Otherwise Specified

An *x* appearing in a diagnostic code indicates that a specific code number is required.

An ellipsis (. . .) is used in the names of certain disorders to indicate that the name of a specific mental disorder or general medical condition should be inserted when recording the name (e.g., 293.0 Delirium Due to Hypothyroidism).

If criteria are currently met, one of the following severity specifiers may be noted after the diagnosis:

Mild

Moderate

Severe

If criteria are no longer met, one of the following specifiers may be noted:

In Partial Remission

In Full Remission

Prior History

DISORDERS USUALLY FIRST DIAGNOSED IN INFANCY, CHILDHOOD, OR ADOLESCENCE

Mental Retardation

Note: *These are coded on Axis II.*

317 Mild Mental Retardation
318.0 Moderate Mental Retardation
318.1 Severe Mental Retardation
318.2 Profound Mental Retardation
319 Mental Retardation, Severity Unspecified

Learning Disorders

315.00 Reading Disorder
315.1 Mathematics Disorder
315.2 Disorder of Written Expression
315.9 Learning Disorder NOS

Motor Skills Disorder

315.4 Developmental Coordination Disorder

Communication Disorders

315.31 Expressive Language Disorder
315.32 Mixed Receptive-Expressive Language Disorder
315.39 Phonological Disorder
307.0 Stuttering
307.9 Communication Disorder NOS

Pervasive Developmental Disorders

299.00 Autistic Disorder
299.80 Rett's Disorder
299.10 Childhood Disintegrative Disorder
299.80 Asperger's Disorder
299.80 Pervasive Developmental Disorder NOS

Attention-Deficit and Disruptive Behavior Disorders

314.xx Attention-Deficit/Hyperactivity Disorder
  .01 Combined Type
  .00 Predominantly Inattentive Type
  .01 Predominantly Hyperactive-Impulsive Type
314.9 Attention-Deficit/Hyperactivity Disorder NOS
312.xx Conduct Disorder
  .81 Childhood-Onset Type
  .82 Adolescent-Onset Type
  .89 Unspecified Onset
313.81 Oppositional Defiant Disorder
312.9 Disruptive Behavior Disorder NOS

Feeding and Eating Disorders of Infancy or Early Childhood

307.52 Pica
307.53 Rumination Disorder
307.59 Feeding Disorder of Infancy or Early Childhood

Tic Disorders

307.23 Tourette's Disorder
307.22 Chronic Motor or Vocal Tic Disorder
307.21 Transient Tic Disorder
  Specify if: Single Episode/Recurrent
307.20 Tic Disorder NOS

Elimination Disorders

___.__ Encopresis
787.6 With Constipation and Overflow Incontinence
307.7 Without Constipation and Overflow Incontinence
307.6 Enuresis (Not Due to a General Medical Condition)
  Specify type: Nocturnal Only/Diurnal Only/Nocturnal and Diurnal

Other Disorders of Infancy, Childhood, or Adolescence

309.21 Separation Anxiety Disorder
  Specify if: Early Onset
313.23 Selective Mutism

313.89 Reactive Attachment Disorder of Infancy or Early Childhood
 Specify type: Inhibited Type/Disinhibited Type
307.3 Stereotypic Movement Disorder
 Specify if: With Self-Injurious Behavior
313.9 Disorder of Infancy, Childhood, or Adolescence NOS

DELIRIUM, DEMENTIA, AND AMNESTIC AND OTHER COGNITIVE DISORDERS

Delirium

293.0 Delirium Due to . . . *[Indicate the General Medical Condition]*
____.__ Substance Intoxication Delirium *(refer to Substance-Related Disorders for substance-specific codes)*
____.__ Substance Withdrawal Delirium *(refer to Substance-Related Disorders for substance-specific codes)*
____.__ Delirium Due to Multiple Etiologies *(code each of the specific etiologies)*
780.09 Delirium NOS

Dementia

294.xx Dementia of the Alzheimer's Type, With Early Onset *(also code 331.0 Alzheimer's disease on Axis III)*
 .10 Without Behavioral Disturbance
 .11 With Behavioral Disturbance
294.xx Dementia of the Alzheimer's Type, With Late Onset *(also code 331.0 Alzheimer's disease on Axis III)*
 .10 Without Behavioral Disturbance
 .11 With Behavioral Disturbance
290.xx Vascular Dementia
 .40 Uncomplicated
 .41 With Delirium
 .42 With Delusions
 .43 With Depressed Mood
 Specify if: With Behavioral Disturbance
Code presence or absence of a behavioral disturbance in the fifth digit for Dementia Due to a General Medical Condition:
0 = Without Behavioral Disturbance
1 = With Behavioral Disturbance
294.1x Dementia Due to HIV Disease *(also code 042 HIV on Axis III)*
294.1x Dementia Due to Head Trauma *(also code 042 HIV on Axis III)*
294.1x Dementia Due to Head Trauma *(also code 854.00 head injury on Axis III)*
294.1x Dementia Due to Parkinson's Disease *(also code 332.0 Parkinson's disease on Axis III)*
294.1x Dementia Due to Huntington's Disease *(also code 333.4 Huntington's disease on Axis III)*
294.1x Dementia Due to Pick's Disease *(also code 331.1 Pick's disease on Axis III)*
294.1x Dementia Due to Creutzfeldt–Jakob Disease *(also code 046.1 Creutzfeldt–Jakob disease on Axis III)*

ICD-9-CM code valid after October 1, 2000.

294.1x Dementia Due to . . . *[Indicate the General Medical Condition not listed above] (also code the general medical condition on Axis III)*
____.__ Substance-Induced Persisting Dementia *(refer to Substance-Related Disorders for substance-specific codes)*
____.__ Dementia Due to Multiple Etiologies *(code each of the specific etiologies)*
294.8 Dementia NOS

Amnestic Disorders

294.0 Amnestic Disorder Due to . . . *[Indicate the General Medical Condition]*
 Specify if: Transient/Chronic
____.__ Substance-Induced Persisting Amnestic Disorder *(refer to Substance-Related Disorders for substance-specific codes)*
294.8 Amnestic Disorder NOS

Other Cognitive Disorders

294.9 Cognitive Disorder NOS

MENTAL DISORDERS DUE TO A GENERAL MEDICAL CONDITION NOT ELSEWHERE CLASSIFIED

293.89 Catatonic Disorder Due to . . . *[Indicate the General Medical Condition]*
310.1 Personality Change Due to . . . *[Indicate the General Medical Condition]*
 Specify type: Labile Type/Disinhibited Type/Aggressive Type/Apathetic Type/Paranoid Type/Other Type/Combined Type/Unspecified Type
293.9 Mental Disorder NOS Due to . . . *[Indicate the General Medical Condition]*

SUBSTANCE-RELATED DISORDERS

The following specifiers apply to Substance Dependence as noted:
[a]With Physiological Dependence/Without Physiological Dependence
[b]Early Full Remission/Early Partial Remission/Sustained Full Remission/Sustained Partial Remission
[c]In a Controlled Environment
[d]On Agonist Therapy
The following specifiers apply to Substance-Induced Disorders as noted:
[I]With Onset During Intoxication/[W]With Onset During Withdrawal

Alcohol-Related Disorders

Alcohol Use Disorders

303.90 Alcohol Dependence[a,b,c]
305.00 Alcohol Abuse

Alcohol-Induced Disorders

303.00 Alcohol Intoxication
291.81 Alcohol Withdrawal
 Specify if: With Perceptual Disturbances
291.0 Alcohol Intoxication Delirium

291.0 Alcohol Withdrawal Delirium
291.2 Alcohol-Induced Persisting Dementia
291.1 Alcohol-Induced Persisting Amnestic Disorder
291.x Alcohol-Induced Psychotic Disorder
.5 With Delusions[I,W]
.3 With Hallucinations[I,W]
291.89 Alcohol-Induced Mood Disorder[I,W]
291.89 Alcohol-Induced Anxiety Disorder[I,W]
291.89 Alcohol-Induced Sexual Dysfunction[I]
291.89 Alcohol-Induced Sleep Disorder[I,W]
291.9 Alcohol-Related Disorder NOS

Amphetamine (or Amphetamine-Like)–Related Disorders

Amphetamine Use Disorders

304.40 Amphetamine Dependence[a,b,c]
305.70 Amphetamine Abuse

Amphetamine-Induced Disorders

292.89 Amphetamine Intoxication
Specify if: With Perceptual Disturbances
292.0 Amphetamine Withdrawal
292.81 Amphetamine Intoxication Delirium
292.xx Amphetamine-Induced Psychotic Disorder
.11 With Delusions[I]
.12 With Hallucinations[I]
292.84 Amphetamine-Induced Mood Disorder[I,W]
292.89 Amphetamine-Induced Anxiety Disorder[I]
292.89 Amphetamine-Induced Sexual Dysfunction[I]
292.89 Amphetamine-Induced Sleep Disorder[I,W]
292.9 Amphetamine-Related Disorder NOS

Caffeine-Related Disorders

Caffeine-Induced Disorders

305.90 Caffeine Intoxication
292.89 Caffeine-Induced Anxiety Disorder[I]
292.89 Caffeine-Induced Sleep Disorder[I]
292.9 Caffeine-Related Disorder NOS

Cannabis-Related Disorders

Cannabis Use Disorders

304.30 Cannabis Dependence[a,b,c]
305.20 Cannabis Abuse

Cannabis-Induced Disorders

292.89 Cannabis Intoxication
Specify if: With Perceptual Disturbance
292.81 Cannabis Intoxication Delirium
292.xx Cannabis-Induced Psychotic Disorder
.11 With Delusions[I]
.12 With Hallucinations[I]
292.89 Cannabis-Induced Anxiety Disorder[I]
292.9 Cannabis-Related Disorder NOS

Cocaine-Related Disorders

Cocaine Use Disorders

304.20 Cocaine Dependence[a,b,c]
305.60 Cocaine Abuse

Cocaine-Induced Disorders

292.89 Cocaine Intoxication
Specify if: With Perceptual Disturbances
292.0 Cocaine Withdrawal
292.81 Cocaine Intoxication Delirium
292.xx Cocaine-Induced Psychotic Disorder
.11 With Delusions[I]
.12 With Hallucinations[I]
292.84 Cocaine-Induced Mood Disorder[I,W]
292.89 Cocaine-Induced Anxiety Disorder[I,W]
292.89 Cocaine-Induced Sexual Dysfunction[I]
292.89 Cocaine-Induced Sleep Disorder[I,W]
292.9 Cocaine-Related Disorder NOS

Hallucinogen-Related Disorders

Hallucinogen Use Disorders

304.50 Hallucinogen Dependence[b,c]
305.30 Hallucinogen Abuse

Hallucinogen-Induced Disorders

292.89 Hallucinogen Intoxication
292.89 Hallucinogen Persisting Perception Disorder (Flashbacks)
292.81 Hallucinogen Intoxication Delirium
292.xx Hallucinogen-Induced Psychotic Disorder
.11 With Delusions[I]
.12 With Hallucinations[I]
292.84 Hallucinogen-Induced Mood Disorder[I]
292.89 Hallucinogen-Induced Anxiety Disorder[I]
292.9 Hallucinogen-Related Disorder NOS

Inhalant-Related Disorders

Inhalant Use Disorders

304.60 Inhalant Dependence[b,c]
305.90 Inhalant Abuse

Inhalant-Induced Disorders

292.89 Inhalant Intoxication
292.81 Inhalant Intoxication Delirium
292.82 Inhalant-Induced Persisting Dementia
292.xx Inhalant-Induced Psychotic Disorder
.11 With Delusions[I]
.12 With Hallucinations[I]
292.84 Inhalant-Induced Mood Disorder[I]
292.89 Inhalant-Induced Anxiety Disorder[I]
292.9 Inhalant-Related Disorder NOS

Nicotine-Related Disorders

Nicotine Use Disorder

305.1 Nicotine Dependence[a,b]

Nicotine-Induced Disorder

292.0 Nicotine Withdrawal
292.9 Nicotine-Related Disorder NOS

Opioid-Related Disorders

Opioid Use Disorders

304.00 Opioid Dependence[a,b,c,d]
305.50 Opioid Abuse

Opioid-Induced Disorders

292.89 Opioid Intoxication
Specify if: With Perceptual Disturbances
292.0 Opioid Withdrawal
292.81 Opioid Intoxication Delirium
292.xx Opioid-Induced Psychotic Disorder
.11 With Delusions[I]
.12 With Hallucinations[I]
292.84 Opioid-Induced Mood Disorder[I]
292.89 Opioid-Induced Sexual Dysfunction[I]
292.89 Opioid-Induced Sleep Disorder[I,W]
292.9 Opioid-Related Disorder NOS

Phencyclidine (or Phencyclidine-Like)–Related Disorders

Phencyclidine Use Disorders

304.60 Phencyclidine Dependence[b,c]
305.90 Phencyclidine Abuse

Phencyclidine-Induced Disorders

292.89 Phencyclidine Intoxication
Specify if: With Perceptual Disturbances
292.81 Phencyclidine Intoxication Delirium
292.xx Phencyclidine-Induced Psychotic Disorder
.11 With Delusions[I]
.12 With Hallucinations[I]
292.84 Phencyclidine-Induced Mood Disorder[I]
292.89 Phencyclidine-Induced Anxiety Disorder[I]
292.9 Phencyclidine-Related Disorder NOS

Sedative-, Hypnotic-, or Anxiolytic-Related Disorders

Sedative, Hypnotic, or Anxiolytic Use Disorders

304.10 Sedative, Hypnotic, or Anxiolytic Dependence[a,b,c]
305.40 Sedative, Hypnotic, or Anxiolytic Abuse

Sedative-, Hypnotic-, or Anxiolytic-Induced Disorders

292.89 Sedative, Hypnotic, or Anxiolytic Intoxication
292.0 Sedative, Hypnotic, or Anxiolytic Withdrawal
Specify if: With Perceptual Disturbances
292.81 Sedative, Hypnotic, or Anxiolytic Intoxication Delirium
292.81 Sedative, Hypnotic, or Anxiolytic Withdrawal Delirium
292.82 Sedative, Hypnotic, or Anxiolytic-Induced Persisting Dementia
292.83 Sedative-, Hypnotic-, or Anxiolytic-Induced Persisting Amnestic Disorder
292.xx Sedative-, Hypnotic-, or Anxiolytic-Induced Psychotic Disorder
.11 With Delusions[I,W]
.12 With Hallucinations[I,W]
292.84 Sedative-, Hypnotic-, or Anxiolytic-Induced Mood Disorder[I,W]
292.89 Sedative-, Hypnotic-, or Anxiolytic-Induced Anxiety Disorder[W]
292.89 Sedative-, Hypnotic-, or Anxiolytic-Induced Sexual Dysfunction[I]
292.89 Sedative-, Hypnotic-, or Anxiolytic-Induced Sleep Disorder[I,W]
292.9 Sedative-, Hypnotic-, or Anxiolytic-Related Disorder NOS

Polysubstance-Related Disorder

304.80 Polysubstance Dependence[a,b,c,d]

Other (or Unknown) Substance-Related Disorders

Other (or Unknown) Substance Use Disorders

304.90 Other (or Unknown) Substance Dependence[a,b,c,d]
305.90 Other (or Unknown) Substance Abuse

Other (or Unknown) Substance-Induced Disorders

292.89 Other (or Unknown) Substance Intoxication
Specify if: With Perceptual Disturbances
292.0 Other (or Unknown) Substance Withdrawal
Specify if: With Perceptual Disturbances
292.81 Other (or Unknown) Substance-Induced Delirium
292.82 Other (or Unknown) Substance-Induced Persisting Dementia
292.83 Other (or Unknown) Substance-Induced Persisting Amnestic Disorder
292.xx Other (or Unknown) Substance-Induced Psychotic Disorder
.11 With Delusions[I,W]
.12 With Hallucinations[I,W]
292.84 Other (or Unknown) Substance-Induced Mood Disorder[I,W]
292.89 Other (or Unknown) Substance-Induced Anxiety Disorder[I,W]
292.89 Other (or Unknown) Substance-Induced Sexual Dysfunction[I]
292.89 Other (or Unknown) Substance-Induced Sleep Disorder[I,W]
292.9 Other (or Unknown) Substance-Related Disorder NOS

Polysubstance-Related Disorder

304.80 Polysubstance Dependence[a,b,c,d]

Other (or Unknown) Substance-Related Disorders

Other (or Unknown) Substance Use Disorders

304.90 Other (or Unknown) Substance Dependence[a,b,c,d]
305.90 Other (or Unknown) Substance Abuse

Other (or Unknown) Substance-Induced Disorders

292.89 Other (or Unknown) Substance Intoxication
Specify if: With Perceptual Disturbances
292.0 Other (or Unknown) Substance Withdrawal
Specify if: With Perceptual Disturbances
292.81 Other (or Unknown) Substance-Induced Delirium
292.82 Other (or Unknown) Substance-Induced Persisting Dementia
292.83 Other (or Unknown) Substance-Induced Persisting Amnestic Disorder
292.xx Other (or Unknown) Substance-Induced Psychotic Disorder
.11 With Delusions[I,W]

.12 With Hallucinations[I,W]
292.84 Other (or Unknown) Substance-Induced Mood Disorder[I,W]
292.89 Other (or Unknown) Substance-Induced Anxiety Disorder[I,W]
292.89 Other (or Unknown) Substance-Induced Sexual Dysfunction[I]
292.89 Other (or Unknown) Substance-Induced Sleep Disorder[I,W]
292.9 Other (or Unknown) Substance-Related Disorder NOS

SCHIZOPHRENIA AND OTHER PSYCHOTIC DISORDERS

295.xx Schizophrenia
The following Classification of Longitudinal Course applies to all subtypes of Schizophrenia:
Episodic With Interepisode Residual Symptoms (*Specify if:* With Prominent Negative Symptoms)/Episodic With No Interepisode Residual Symptoms
Continuous (*Specify if:* With Prominent Negative Symptoms)
Single Episode in Partial Remission (*Specify if:* With Prominent Negative Symptoms)/Single Episode in Full Remission
Other or Unspecified Pattern
.30 Paranoid Type
.10 Disorganized Type
.20 Catatonic Type
.90 Undifferentiated Type
.60 Residual Type
295.40 Schizophreniform Disorder
Specify if: Without Good Prognostic Features/With Good Prognostic Features
295.70 Schizoaffective Disorder
Specify type: Bipolar Type/Depressive Type
297.1 Delusional Disorder
Specify type: Erotomanic Type/Grandiose Type/Jealous Type/Persecutory Type/Somatic Type/Mixed Type/Unspecified Type
298.8 Brief Psychotic Disorder
Specify if: With Marked Stressor(s)/Without Marked Stressor(s)/With Postpartum Onset
297.3 Shared Psychotic Disorder
293.xx Psychotic Disorder Due to . . . *[Indicate the General Medical Condition]*
.81 With Delusions
.82 With Hallucinations
____.__ Substance-Induced Psychotic Disorder *(refer to Substance-Related Disorders for substance-specific codes)*
Specify if: With Onset During Intoxication/With Onset During Withdrawal
298.9 Psychotic Disorder NOS

MOOD DISORDERS

Code current state of Major Depressive Disorder or Bipolar I Disorder in fifth digit:
1 = Mild
2 = Moderate
3 = Severe Without Psychotic Features
4 = Severe With Psychotic Features
Specify: Mood-Congruent Psychotic Features/Mood-Incongruent Psychotic Features
5 = In Partial Remission
6 = In Full Remission
0 = Unspecified
The following specifiers apply (for current or most recent episode) to Mood Disorders as noted:
[a]Severity/Psychotic/Remission Specifiers/[b]Chronic/[c]With Catatonic Features/[d]With Melancholic Features/[e]With Atypical Features/[f]With Postpartum Onset
The following specifiers apply to Mood Disorders as noted:
[g]With or Without Full Interepisode Recovery/[h]With Seasonal Pattern/[i]With Rapid Cycling

Depressive Disorders

296.xx Major Depressive Disorder
.2x Single Episode[a,b,c,d,e,f]
.3x Recurrent[a,b,c,d,e,f,g,h]
300.4 Dysthymic Disorder
Specify if: Early Onset/Late Onset
Specify if: With Atypical Features
311 Depressive Disorder NOS

Bipolar Disorders

296.xx Bipolar I Disorder
.0x Single Manic Episode[a,c,f]
Specify if: Mixed
.40 Most Recent Episode Hypomanic[g,h,i]
.4x Most Recent Episode Manic[a,c,f,g,h,i]
.6x Most Recent Episode Mixed[a,c,f,g,h,i]
.5x Most Recent Episode Depressed[a,b,c,d,e,f,g,h,i]
.7 Most Recent Episode Unspecified[g,h,i]
296.89 Bipolar II Disorder[a,b,c,d,e,f,g,h,i]
Specify (current or most recent episode): Hypomanic/Depressed
301.13 Cyclothymic Disorder
296.80 Bipolar Disorder NOS
293.83 Mood Disorder Due to . . . *[Indicate the General Medical Condition]*
Specify type: With Depressive Features/With Major Depressive-Like Episode/With Manic Features/With Mixed Features
____.__ Substance-Induced Mood Disorder *(refer to Substance-Related Disorders for substance-specific codes)*
Specify type: With Depressive Features/With Manic Features/With Mixed Features
Specify if: With Onset During Intoxication/With Onset During Withdrawal
296.90 Mood Disorder NOS

Anxiety Disorders

300.01 Panic Disorder Without Agoraphobia
300.21 Panic Disorder With Agoraphobia
300.22 Agoraphobia Without History of Panic Disorder

300.29 Specific Phobia
Specify type: Animal Type/Natural Environment Type/ Blood-Injection-Injury Type/Situational Type/ Other Type
300.23 Social Phobia
Specify if: Generalized
300.3 Obsessive-Compulsive Disorder
Specify if: With Poor Insight
309.81 Posttraumatic Stress Disorder
Specify if: Acute/Chronic
Specify if: With Delayed Onset
308.3 Acute Stress Disorder
300.02 Generalized Anxiety Disorder
293.84 Anxiety Disorder Due to . . . *[Indicate the General Medical Condition]*
Specify if: With Generalized Anxiety/With Panic Attacks/With Obsessive-Compulsive Symptoms
____.__ Substance-Induced Anxiety Disorder *(refer to Substance-Related Disorders for substance-specific codes)*
Specify if: With Generalized Anxiety/With Panic Attacks/ With Obsessive-Compulsive Symptoms/With Phobic Symptoms
Specify if: With Onset During Intoxication/With Onset During Withdrawal
300.00 Anxiety Disorder NOS

SOMATOFORM DISORDERS

300.81 Somatization Disorder
300.82 Undifferentiated Somatoform Disorder
300.11 Conversion Disorder
Specify type: With Motor Symptom or Deficit/With Sensory Symptom or Deficit/With Seizures or Convulsions/With Mixed Presentation
307.xx Pain Disorder
.80 Associated With Psychological Factors
.89 Associated With Both Psychological Factors and a General Medical Condition
Specify if: Acute/Chronic
300.7 Hypochondriasis
Specify if: With Poor Insight
300.7 Body Dysmorphic Disorder
300.82 Somatoform Disorder NOS

Factitious Disorders

300.xx Factitious Disorder
.16 With Predominantly Psychological Signs and Symptoms
.19 With Predominantly Physical Signs and Symptoms
.19 With Combined Psychological and Physical Signs and Symptoms
300.19 Factitious Disorder NOS

Dissociative Disorders

300.12 Dissociative Amnesia
300.13 Dissociative Fugue
300.14 Dissociative Identity Disorder
300.6 Depersonalization Disorder
300.15 Dissociative Disorder NOS

Sexual and Gender Identity Disorders

Sexual Dysfunctions

The following specifiers apply to all primary Sexual Dysfunctions:
Lifelong Type/Acquired Type
Generalized Type/Situational Type
Due to Psychological Factors/Due to Combined Factors

Sexual Desire Disorders

302.71 Hypoactive Sexual Desire Disorder
302.79 Sexual Aversion Disorder

Sexual Arousal Disorders

302.72 Female Sexual Arousal Disorder
302.72 Male Erectile Disorder

Orgasmic Disorders

302.73 Female Orgasmic Disorder
302.74 Male Orgasmic Disorder
302.75 Premature Ejaculation

Sexual Pain Disorders

302.76 Dyspareunia (Not Due to a General Medical Condition)
306.51 Vaginismus (Not Due to a General Medical Condition)

Sexual Dysfunction Due to a General Medical Condition

625.8 Female Hypoactive Sexual Desire Disorder Due to . . . *[Indicate the General Medical Condition]*
608.89 Male Hypoactive Sexual Desire Disorder Due to . . . *[Indicate the General Medical Condition]*
607.84 Male Erectile Disorder Due to . . . *[Indicate the General Medical Condition]*
625.0 Female Dyspareunia Due to . . . *[Indicate the General Medical Condition]*
608.89 Male Dyspareunia Due to . . . *[Indicate the General Medical Condition]*
625.8 Other Female Sexual Dysfunction Due to . . . *[Indicate the General Medical Condition]*
608.89 Other Male Sexual Dysfunction Due to . . . *[Indicate the General Medical Condition]*
____.__ Substance-Induced Sexual Dysfunction *(refer to Substance-Related Disorders for substance-specific codes)*
Specify if: With Impaired Desire/With Impaired Arousal/With Impaired Orgasm/With Sexual Pain
Specify if: With Onset During Intoxication
302.70 Sexual Dysfunction NOS

Paraphilias

302.4 Exhibitionism
302.81 Fetishism
302.89 Frotteurism
302.2 Pedophilia
Specify if: Sexually Attracted to Males/Sexually Attracted to Females/Sexually Attracted to Both
Specify if: Limited to Incest
Specify type: Exclusive Type/Nonexclusive Type
302.83 Sexual Masochism
302.84 Sexual Sadism

302.3 Transvestic Fetishism
Specify if: With Gender Dysphoria
302.82 Voyeurism
302.9 Paraphilia NOS

Gender Identity Disorders

302.xx Gender Identity Disorder
.6 in Children
.85 in Adolescents or Adults
Specify if: Sexually Attracted to Males/Sexually Attracted to Females/Sexually Attracted to Both/ Sexually Attracted to Neither
302.6 Gender Identity Disorder NOS
302.9 Sexual Disorder NOS

EATING DISORDERS

307.1 Anorexia Nervosa
Specify type: Restricting Type; Binge-Eating/Purging Type
307.51 Bulimia Nervosa
Specify type: Purging Type/Nonpurging Type
307.50 Eating Disorder NOS

SLEEP DISORDERS

Primary Sleep Disorders

Dyssomnias

307.42 Primary Insomnia
307.44 Primary Hypersomnia
Specify if: Recurrent
347 Narcolepsy
780.59 Breathing-Related Sleep Disorder
307.45 Circadian Rhythm Sleep Disorder
Specify type: Delayed Sleep Phase Type/Jet Lag Type/ Shift Work Type/Unspecified Type
307.47 Dyssomnia NOS

Parasomnias

307.47 Nightmare Disorder
307.46 Sleep Terror Disorder
307.46 Sleepwalking Disorder
307.47 Parasomnia NOS

Sleep Disorders Related to Another Mental Disorder

307.42 Insomnia Related to . . . *[Indicate the Axis I or Axis II Disorder]*
307.44 Hypersomnia Related to . . . *[Indicate the Axis I or Axis II Disorder]*

Other Sleep Disorders

780.xx Sleep Disorder Due to . . . *[Indicate the General Medical Condition]*
.52 Insomnia Type
.54 Hypersomnia Type
.59 Parasomnia Type
.59 Mixed Type
____.__ Substance-Induced Sleep Disorder *(refer to Substance-Related Disorders for substance-specific codes)*
Specify type: Insomnia Type/Hypersomnia Type/ Parasomnia Type/Mixed Type
Specify if: With Onset During Intoxication/With Onset During Withdrawal

IMPULSE-CONTROL DISORDERS NOT ELSEWHERE CLASSIFIED

312.34 Intermittent Explosive Disorder
312.32 Kleptomania
312.33 Pyromania
312.31 Pathological Gambling
312.39 Trichotillomania
312.30 Impulse-Control Disorder NOS

ADJUSTMENT DISORDERS

309.xx Adjustment Disorder
.0 With Depressed Mood
.24 With Anxiety
.28 With Mixed Anxiety and Depressed Mood
.3 With Disturbance of Conduct
.4 With Mixed Disturbance of Emotions and Conduct
.9 Unspecified
Specify if: Acute/Chronic

PERSONALITY DISORDERS

Note: *These are coded on Axis II.*
301.0 Paranoid Personality Disorder
301.20 Schizoid Personality Disorder
301.22 Schizotypal Personality Disorder
301.7 Antisocial Personality Disorder
301.83 Borderline Personality Disorder
301.50 Histrionic Personality Disorder
301.81 Narcissistic Personality Disorder
301.82 Avoidant Personality Disorder
301.6 Dependent Personality Disorder
301.4 Obsessive-Compulsive Personality Disorder
301.9 Personality Disorder NOS

OTHER CONDITIONS THAT MAY BE A FOCUS OF CLINICAL ATTENTION

Psychological Factors Affecting Medical Condition

316 . . . *[Specified Psychological Factor] Affecting . . . [Indicate the General Medical Condition]*
Choose name based on nature of factors:
Mental Disorder Affecting Medical Condition
Psychological Symptoms Affecting Medical Condition
Personality Traits or Coping Style Affecting Medical Condition
Maladaptive Health Behaviors Affecting Medical Condition
Stress-Related Physiological Response Affecting Medical Condition
Other or Unspecified Psychological Factors Affecting Medical Condition

Medication-Induced Movement Disorders

332.1 Neuroleptic-Induced Parkinsonism
333.92 Neuroleptic Malignant Syndrome

333.7 Neuroleptic-Induced Acute Dystonia
333.99 Neuroleptic-Induced Acute Akathisia
333.82 Neuroleptic-Induced Tardive Dyskinesia
333.1 Medication-Induced Postural Tremor
333.90 Medication-Induced Movement Disorder NOS

Other Medication-Induced Disorder

995.2 Adverse Effects of Medication NOS

Relational Problems

V61.9 Relational Problem Related to a Mental Disorder or General Medical Condition
V61.20 Parent–Child Relational Problem
V61.10 Partner Relational Problem
V61.8 Sibling Relational Problem
V62.81 Relational Problem NOS

Problems Related to Abuse or Neglect

V61.21 Physical Abuse of Child
(code 995.54 if focus of attention is on victim)
V61.21 Sexual Abuse of Child
(code 995.53 if focus of attention is on victim)
V61.21 Neglect of Child
(code 995.52 if focus of attention is on victim)
____.__ Physical Abuse of Adult
V61.12 (if by partner)
V62.83 (if by person other than partner) *(code 995.81 if focus of attention is on victim)*
____.__ Sexual Abuse of Adult
V61.12 (if by partner)
V62.83 (if by person other than partner) *(code 995.83 if focus of attention is on victim)*

Additional Conditions That May Be a Focus of Clinical Attention

V15.81 Noncomplicance With Treatment
V65.2 Malingering
V71.01 Adult Antisocial Behavior
V71.02 Child or Adolescent Antisocial Behavior
V62.89 Borderline Intellectual Functioning
Note: *This is coded on Axis II.*
780.9 Age-Related Cognitive Decline
V62.82 Bereavement
V62.3 Academic Problem
V62.2 Occupational Problem
313.82 Identity Problem
V62.89 Religious or Spiritual Problem
V62.4 Acculturation Problem
V62.89 Phase of Life Problem

ADDITIONAL CODES

300.9 Unspecified Mental Disorder (nonpsychotic)
V71.09 No Diagnosis or Condition on Axis I
799.9 Diagnosis or Condition Deferred on Axis I
V71.09 No Diagnosis on Axis II
799.9 Diagnosis Deferred on Axis II

MULTIAXIAL SYSTEM

Axis I Clinical Disorders
Other Conditions That May Be a Focus of Clinical Attention
Axis II Personality Disorders
Mental Retardation
Axis III General Medical Conditions
Axis IV Psychosocial and Environmental Problems
Axis V Global Assessment of Functioning

MULTIAXIAL ASSESSMENT

A multiaxial system involves an assessment on several axes, each of which refers to a different domain of information that may help the clinician plan treatment and predict outcome. There are five axes included in the DSM-IV multiaxial classification:

Axis I	Clinical Disorders Other Conditions That May Be a Focus of Clinical Attention
Axis II	Personality Disorders Mental Retardation
Axis III	General Medical Conditions
Axis IV	Psychosocial and Environmental Problems
Axis V	Global Assessment of Functioning

The use of the multiaxial system facilitates comprehensive and systematic evaluation with attention to the various mental disorders and general medical conditions, psychosocial and environmental problems, and level of functioning that might be overlooked if the focus were on assessing a single presenting problem. A multiaxial system provides a convenient format for organizing and communicating clinical information, for capturing the complexity of clinical situations, and for describing the heterogeneity of individuals presenting with the same diagnosis. In addition, the multiaxial system promotes the application of the biopsychosocial model in clinical, educational, and research settings.

The rest of this section provides a description of each of the DSM-IV axes. In some settings or situations, clinicians may prefer not to use the multiaxial system. For this reason, guidelines for reporting the results of a DSM-IV assessment without applying the formal multiaxial system are provided at the end of this section.

AXIS I: CLINICAL DISORDERS—OTHER CONDITIONS THAT MAY BE A FOCUS OF CLINICAL ATTENTION

Axis I is for reporting all the various disorders or conditions in the Classification except for the Personality Disorders and Men-

AXIS I	Clinical Disorders

Other Conditions That May Be a Focus of Clinical Attention

Disorders Usually First Diagnosed in Infancy, Childhood, or Adolescence (*excluding Mental Retardation, which is diagnosed on Axis II*)
Delirium, Dementia, and Amnestic and Other Cognitive Disorders
Mental Disorders Due to a General Medical Condition
Substance-Related Disorders
Schizophrenia and Other Psychotic Disorders
Mood Disorders
Anxiety Disorders
Somatoform Disorders
Factitious Disorders
Dissociative Disorders
Sexual and Gender Identity Disorders
Eating Disorders
Sleep Disorders
Impulse-Control Disorders Not Elsewhere Classified
Adjustment Disorders
Other Conditions That May Be a Focus of Clinical Attention

tal Retardation (which are reported on Axis II). The major groups of disorders to be reported on Axis I are listed in the box above. Also reported on Axis I are Other Conditions That May Be a Focus of Clinical Attention.

When an individual has more than one Axis I disorder, all of these should be reported. If more than one Axis I disorder is present, the principal diagnosis or the reason for visit should be indicated by listing it first. When an individual has both an Axis I and an Axis II disorder, the principal diagnosis or the reason for visit will be assumed to be on Axis I unless the Axis II diagnosis is followed by the qualifying phrase "(Principal Diagnosis)" or "(Reason for Visit)." If no Axis I disorder is present, this should be coded as V71.09. If an Axis I diagnosis is deferred, pending the gathering of additional information, this should be coded as 799.9.

AXIS II: PERSONALITY DISORDERS AND MENTAL RETARDATION

Axis II is for reporting Personality Disorders and Mental Retardation. It may also be used for noting prominent maladaptive personality features and defense mechanisms. The listing of Personality Disorders and Mental Retardation on a separate axis ensures that consideration will be given to the possible presence of Personality Disorders and Mental Retardation that might otherwise be overlooked when attention is directed to the usually more florid Axis I disorders. The coding of Personality Disorders on Axis II should not be taken to imply that their pathogenesis or range of appropriate treatment is fundamentally different from that for the disorders coded on Axis I. The disorders to be reported on Axis II are listed in the box at right above.

AXIS II	Personality Disorders

Mental Retardation

Paranoid Personality Disorder
Schizoid Personality Disorder
Schizotypal Personality Disorder
Antisocial Personality Disorder
Borderline Personality Disorder
Histrionic Personality Disorder
Narcissistic Personality Disorder
Avoidant Personality Disorder
Dependent Personality Disorder
Obsessive-Compulsive Personality Disorder
Personality Disorder Not Otherwise Specified
Mental Retardation

In the common situation in which an individual has more than one Axis II diagnosis, all should be reported. When an individual has both an Axis I and an Axis II diagnosis and the Axis II diagnosis is the principal diagnosis or the reason for visit, this should be indicated by adding the qualifying phrase "(Principal Diagnosis)" or "(Reason for Visit)" after the Axis II diagnosis. If no Axis II disorder is present, this should be coded as V71.09. If an Axis II diagnosis is deferred, pending the gathering of additional information, this should be coded as 799.9.

Axis II may also be used to indicate prominent maladaptive personality features that do not meet the threshold for a Personality Disorder (in such instances, no code number should be used). The habitual use of maladaptive defense mechanisms may also be indicated on Axis II.

AXIS III: GENERAL MEDICAL CONDITIONS

Axis III is for reporting current general medical conditions that are potentially relevant to the understanding or management of the individual's mental disorder. These conditions are classified outside the "Mental Disorders" chapter of ICD-9-CM (and outside Chapter V of ICD-10). A listing of the broad categories of general medical conditions is given in the box on page 940.

As discussed in the "Introduction," the multiaxial distinction among Axis I, Axis II, and Axis III disorders does not imply that there are fundamental differences in their conceptualization, that mental disorders are unrelated to physical or biological factors or processes, or that general medical conditions are unrelated to behavioral or psychosocial factors or processes. The purpose of distinguishing general medical conditions is to encourage thoroughness in evaluation and to enhance communication among health care providers.

General medical conditions can be related to mental disorders in a variety of ways. In some cases it is clear that the general medical condition is directly etiological to the development or worsening of mental symptoms and that the mechanism for this effect is physiological. When a mental disorder is judged to be a direct physiological consequence of the general medical condition, a Mental Disorder Due to a General Medical Condition should be diagnosed on Axis I and the general medical condition should be recorded on both Axis I

AXIS III General Medical Conditions (with ICD-9-CM codes)

Infectious and Parasitic Diseases (001–139)
Neoplasms (140–239)
Endocrine, Nutritional, and Metabolic Diseases and Immunity Disorders (240–279)
Diseases of the Blood and Blood-Forming Organs (280–289)
Diseases of the Nervous System and Sense Organs (320–389)
Diseases of the Circulatory System (390–459)
Diseases of the Respiratory System (460–519)
Diseases of the Digestive System (520–579)
Diseases of the Genitourinary System (580–629)
Complications of Pregnancy, Childbirth, and the Puerperium (630–676)
Diseases of the Skin and Subcutaneous Tissue (680–709)
Diseases of the Musculoskeletal System and Connective Tissue (710–739)
Congenital Anomalies (740–759)
Certain Conditions Originating in the Perinatal Period (760–779)
Symptoms, Signs, and Ill-Defined Conditions (780–799)
Injury and Poisoning (800–999)

and Axis III. For example, when hypothyroidism is a direct cause of depressive symptoms, the designation on Axis I is 293.83 Mood Disorder Due to Hypothyroidism, With Depressive Features, and the hypothyroidism is listed again and coded on Axis III as 244.9.

In those instances in which the etiological relationship between the general medical condition and the mental symptoms is insufficiently clear to warrant an Axis I diagnosis of Mental Disorder Due to a General Medical Condition, the appropriate mental disorder (e.g., Major Depressive Disorder) should be listed and coded on Axis I; the general medical condition should be coded only on Axis III.

There are other situations in which general medical conditions are recorded on Axis III because of their importance to the overall understanding or treatment of the individual with the mental disorder. An Axis I disorder may be a psychological reaction to an Axis III general medical condition (e.g., the development of 309.0 Adjustment Disorder With Depressed Mood as a reaction to the diagnosis of carcinoma of the breast). Some general medical conditions may not be directly related to the mental disorder but nonetheless have important prognostic or treatment implications (e.g., when the diagnosis on Axis I is 296.30 Major Depressive Disorder, Recurrent, and on Axis III is 427.9 Arrhythmia, the choice of pharmacotherapy is influenced by the general medical condition; or when a person with diabetes mellitus is admitted to the hospital for an exacerbation of Schizophrenia and insulin management must be monitored).

When an individual has more than one clinically relevant Axis III diagnosis, all should be reported. If no Axis III disorder is present, this should be indicated by the notation "Axis III: None." If an Axis III diagnosis is deferred, pending the gathering of additional information, this should be indicated by the notation "Axis III: Deferred."

AXIS IV: PSYCHOSOCIAL AND ENVIRONMENTAL PROBLEMS

Axis IV is for reporting psychosocial and environmental problems that may affect the diagnosis, treatment, and prognosis of mental disorders (Axes I and II). A psychosocial or environmental problem may be a negative life event, an environmental difficulty or deficiency, a familial or other interpersonal stress, an inadequacy of social support or personal resources, or other problem relating to the context in which a person's difficulties have developed. So-called positive stressors, such as job promotion, should be listed only if they constitute or lead to a problem, as when a person has difficulty adapting to the new situation. In addition to playing a role in the initiation or exacerbation of a mental disorder, psychosocial problems may also develop as a consequence of a person's psychopathology or may constitute problems that should be considered in the overall management plan.

When an individual has multiple psychosocial or environmental problems, the clinician may note as many as are judged to be relevant. In general, the clinician should note only those psychosocial and environmental problems that have been present during the year preceding the current evaluation. However, the clinician may choose to note psychosocial and environmental problems occurring prior to the previous year if these clearly contribute to the mental disorder or have become a focus of treatment—for example, previous combat experiences leading to Posttraumatic Stress Disorder.

In practice, most psychosocial and environmental problems will be indicated on Axis IV. However, when a psychosocial or environmental problem is the primary focus of clinical attention, it should also be recorded on Axis I, with a code derived from the section "Other Conditions That May Be a Focus of Clinical Attention."

For convenience, the problems are grouped together in the following categories:

- **Problems with primary support group**—e.g., death of a family member; health problems in family; disruption of

AXIS IV Psychosocial and Environmental Problems

Problems with primary support group
Problems related to the social environment
Educational problems
Occupational problems
Housing problems
Economic problems
Problems with access to health care services
Problems related to interaction with the legal system/crime
Other psychosocial and environmental problems

family by separation, divorce, or estrangement; removal from the home; remarriage of parent; sexual or physical abuse; parental overprotection; neglect of child; inadequate discipline; discord with siblings; birth of a sibling

- **Problems related to the social environment**—e.g., death or loss of friend; inadequate social support; living alone; difficulty with acculturation; discrimination; adjustment of life-cycle transition (such as retirement)
- **Educational problems**—e.g., illiteracy; academic problems; discord with teachers or classmates; inadequate school environment
- **Occupational problems**—e.g., unemployment; threat of job loss; stressful work schedule; difficult work conditions; job dissatisfaction; job change; discord with boss or co-workers
- **Housing problems**—e.g., homelessness; inadequate housing; unsafe neighborhood; discord with neighbors or landlord
- **Economic problems**—e.g., extreme poverty; inadequate finances; insufficient welfare support
- **Problems with access to health care services**—e.g., inadequate health care services; transportation to health care facilities unavailable; inadequate health insurance
- **Problems related to interaction with the legal system/crime**—e.g., arrest; incarceration; litigation; victim of crime
- **Other psychosocial and environmental problems**—e.g., exposure to disasters, war, other hostilities; discord with nonfamily caregivers such as counselor, social worker, or physician; unavailability of social service agencies

When using the Multiaxial Evaluation Report Form, the clinician should identify the relevant categories of psychosocial and environmental problems and indicate the specific factors involved. If a recording form with a checklist of problem categories is not used, the clinician may simply list the specific problems on Axis IV.

AXIS V: GLOBAL ASSESSMENT OF FUNCTIONING

Axis V is for reporting the clinician's judgment of the individual's overall level of functioning. This information is useful in planning treatment and measuring its impact, and in predicting outcome.

The reporting of overall functioning on Axis V can be done using the Global Assessment of Functioning (GAF) Scale. The GAF Scale may be particularly useful in tracking the clinical progress of individuals in global terms, using a single measure. The GAF Scale is to be rated with respect only to psychological, social, and occupational functioning. The instructions specify, "Do not include impairment in functioning due to physical (or environmental) limitations."

The GAF scale is divided into 10 ranges of functioning. Making a GAF rating involves picking a single value that best reflects the individual's overall level of functioning. The description of each 10-point range in the GAF scale has two components: the first part covers symptom severity, and the second part covers functioning. The GAF rating is within a particular decile if **either** the symptom severity **or** the level of functioning falls within the range. For example, the first part of the range 41–50 describes "serious symptoms (e.g., suicidal ideation, severe obsessional rituals, frequent shoplifting)" and the second part includes "any serious impairment in social, occupational, or school functioning (e.g., no friends, unable to keep a job)." It should be noted that in situations where the individual's symptom severity and level of functioning are discordant, the final GAF rating always reflects the worse of the two. For example, the GAF rating for an individual who is a significant danger to self but is otherwise functioning well would be below 20. Similarly, the GAF rating for an individual with minimal psychological symptomatology but significant impairment in functioning (e.g., an individual whose excessive preoccupation with substance use has resulted in loss of job and friends but no other psychopathology) would be 40 or lower.

In most instances, ratings on the GAF Scale should be for the current period (i.e., the level of functioning at the time of the evaluation) because ratings of current functioning will generally reflect the need for treatment or care. In order to account for day-to-day variability in functioning, the GAF rating for the "current period" is sometimes operationalized as the lowest level of functioning for the past week. In some settings, it may be useful to note the GAF Scale rating both at time of admission and at time of discharge. The GAF Scale may also be rated for other time periods (e.g., the highest level of functioning for at least a few months during the past year). The GAF Scale is reported on Axis V as follows: "GAF =," followed by the GAF rating from 0 to 100, followed by the time period reflected by the rating in parentheses—for example, "(current)," "(highest level in past year)," "(at discharge)."

In order to ensure that no elements of the GAF Scale are overlooked when a GAF rating is being made, the following method for determining a GAF rating may be applied:

STEP 1: Starting at the top level, evaluate each range by asking "is either the individual's symptom severity OR level of functioning worse than what is indicated in the range description?"
STEP 2: Keep moving down the scale until the range that best matches the individual's symptom severity OR the level of functioning is reached, **whichever is worse.**
STEP 3: Look at the next lower range as a double-check against having stopped prematurely. This range should be too severe on **both** symptom severity **and** level of functioning. If it is, the appropriate range has been reached (continue with step 4). If not, go back to step 2 and continue moving down the scale.
STEP 4: To determine the specific GAF rating within the selected 10-point range, consider whether the individual is functioning at the higher or lower end of the 10-point range. For example, consider an individual who hears voices that do not influence his behavior (e.g., someone with long-standing Schizophrenia who

accepts his hallucinations as part of his illness). If the voices occur relatively infrequently (once a week or less), a rating of 39 or 40 might be most appropriate. In contrast, if the individual hears voices almost continuously, a rating of 31 or 32 would be more appropriate.

In some settings, it may be useful to assess social and occupational disability and to track progress in rehabilitation independent of the severity of the psychological symptoms.

GLOBAL ASSESSMENT OF FUNCTIONING (GAF) SCALE

Consider psychological, social, and occupational functioning on a hypothetical continuum of mental health illness. Do not include impairment in functioning due to physical (or environmental) limitations.

Global Assessment of Functioning (GAF) Scale

Code	(Note: Use intermediate codes when appropriate, e.g., 45, 68, 72.)
100/91	Superior functioning in a wide range of activities, life's problems never seem to get out of hand, is sought out by others because of his or her many positive qualities. No symptoms.
90/81	Absent or minimal symptoms (e.g., mild anxiety before an exam), good functioning in all areas, interested and involved in a wide range of activities, socially effective, generally satisfied with life, no more than everyday problems or concerns (e.g., an occasional argument with family members).
80/71	If symptoms are present, they are transient and expectable reactions to psychosocial stressors (e.g., difficulty concentrating after family argument), no more than slight impairment in social, occupational, or school functioning (e.g., temporarily falling behind in schoolwork).
70/61	Some mild symptoms (e.g., depressed mood and mild insomnia) OR some difficulty in social, occupational, or school functioning (e.g., occasional truancy, or theft within the household), but generally functioning pretty well, has some meaningful interpersonal relationships.
60/51	Moderate symptoms (e.g., flat affect and circumstantial speech, occasional panic attacks) OR moderate difficulty in social, occupational, or school functioning (e.g., few friends, conflicts with peers or co-workers).
50/41	Serious symptoms (e.g., suicidal ideation; severe obsessional rituals, frequent shoplifting) OR any serious impairment in social, occupational, or school functioning (e.g., no friends, unable to keep a job).
40/31	Some impairment in reality testing or communication (e.g., speech is at times illogical, obscure, or irrelevant) OR major impairment in several areas, such as work or school, family relations, judgment, thinking, or mood (e.g., depressed man avoids friends, neglects family, and is unable to work; child frequently beats up younger children, is defiant at home, and is failing at school).
30/21	Behavior is considerably influenced by delusions or hallucinations OR serious impairment in communication or judgment (e.g., sometimes incoherent, acts grossly inappropriately, suicidal preoccupation) OR inability to function in almost all areas (e.g., stays in bed all day; no job, home, or friends).
20/11	Some danger of hurting self or others (e.g., suicide attempts without clear expectation of death; frequently violent; manic excitement) OR occasionally fails to maintain minimal personal hygiene (e.g., smears feces) OR gross impairment in communication (e.g., largely incoherent or mute).
10/1	Persistent danger of severely hurting self or others (e.g., recurrent violence) OR persistent inability to maintain minimal personal hygiene OR serious suicidal act with clear expectation of death.
0	Inadequate information.

The rating of overall psychological functioning on a scale of 0–100 was operationalized by Luborsky in the Health-Sickness Rating Scale (Luborsky L: "Clinicians' Judgments of Mental Health." *Archives of General Psychiatry* 7:407–417, 1962). Spitzer and colleagues developed a revision of the Health-Sickness Rating Scale called the Global Assessment Scale (GAS) (Endicott J, Spitzer RI, Fleiss JI, Cohen J: "The Global Assessment Scale: A Procedure for Measuring Overall Severity of Psychiatric Disturbance." *Archives of General Psychiatry* 33:766–771, 1976). A modified version of the GAS was included in DSM-ILL-R as the Global Assessment of Functioning (GAF) Scale.

APPENDIX B

2007–2008 NANDA INTERNATIONAL–APPROVED NURSING DIAGNOSES

Grouped by Gordon's Functional Health Patterns

NUTRITIONAL/METABOLIC

Autonomic Dysreflexia, Risk for
Blood Glucose, Risk for Unstable
Body Temperature, Risk for Imbalanced
Breastfeeding, Effective
Breastfeeding, Ineffective
Breastfeeding, Interrupted
Dentition, Impaired
Dysreflexia, Autonomic
Dysreflexia, Autonomic, Risk for
Failure to Thrive, Adult
Fluid Balance, Readiness for Enhanced
Fluid Volume, Deficient
Fluid Volume, Deficient, Risk for
Fluid Volume, Risk for Imbalance
Fluid Volume Excess
Fluid Volume Imbalance, Risk for
Growth, Risk for Disproportionate
Hyperthermia
Hypothermia
Infant Feeding Pattern, Ineffective
Nutrition, Imbalanced: Less than Body Requirements
Nutrition, Imbalanced: More than Body Requirements
Nutrition, Imbalanced: More than Body Requirements, Risk for
Nutrition, Readiness for Enhanced
Oral Mucous Membrane, Impaired
Skin Integrity, Impaired
Skin Integrity, Risk for Impaired
Sudden Infant Death Syndrome, Risk for
Swallowing, Impaired
Thermoregulation, Ineffective
Tissue Integrity, Impaired

HEALTH PERCEPTION/HEALTH MANAGEMENT

Aspiration, Risk for
Contamination
Contamination, Risk for
Denial, Ineffective
Falls, Risk for
Health Behavior, Risk Prone
Health Maintenance, Ineffective
Health Seeking Behaviors (Specify)
Immunization Status, Readiness for Enhanced
Infection, Risk for
Injury, Risk for
Latex Allergy Response
Latex Allergy Response, Risk for
Management of Therapeutic Regimen, Effective
Management of Therapeutic Regimen: Community, Ineffective
Management of Therapeutic Regimen: Family, Ineffective
Management of Therapeutic Regimen, Ineffective
Management of Therapeutic Regimen, Readiness for Enhanced
Noncompliance (Specify)
Poisoning, Risk for
Protection, Ineffective
Sudden Infant Death Syndrome, Risk for
Suffocation, Risk for
Surgical Recovery, Delayed
Trauma, Risk for

SLEEP/REST

Insomnia
Sleep Deprivation
Sleep, Readiness for Enhanced

ACTIVITY/EXERCISE

Activity Intolerance
Activity Intolerance, Risk for
Adaptive Capacity: Intracranial, Decreased
Airway Clearance, Ineffective
Breathing Pattern, Ineffective
Cardiac Output, Decreased
Development, Risk for Delayed
Disorganized Infant Behavior
Disorganized Infant Behavior, Risk for
Disuse Syndrome, Risk for
Diversional Activity, Deficient
Energy Field, Disturbed
Fatigue
Gas Exchange, Impaired
Home Maintenance, Impaired
Mobility: Bed, Impaired
Mobility: Physical, Impaired
Mobility: Wheelchair, Impaired
Organized Infant Behavior, Readiness for Enhanced
Perioperative Positioning Injury, Risk for
Peripheral Neurovascular Dysfunction, Risk for
Self-Care Deficit: Bathing and Hygiene, Dressing and Grooming, Feeding, Toileting, Total
Self-Care, Readiness for Enhanced
Spontaneous Ventilation, Impaired
Tissue Perfusion, Ineffective (Specify): Cardiopulmonary, Cerebral, Gastrointestinal, Peripheral, Renal
Transfer Ability, Impaired
Ventilatory Weaning Response, Dysfunctional
Walking, Impaired

Used by permission of NANDA International. Adapted from Functional Health Patterns, Gordon, M. (1994). *Nursing diagnosis: Process and application,* 3rd ed. St. Louis: Mosby.

ELIMINATION

Constipation
Constipation, Perceived
Constipation, Risk for
Diarrhea
Incontinence: Bowel
Incontinence: Urinary, Functional
Incontinence: Urinary, Overflow
Incontinence: Urinary, Reflex
Incontinence: Urinary, Stress
Incontinence: Urinary, Total
Incontinence: Urinary, Urge
Incontinence: Urinary, Urge, Risk for
Liver Function, Risk for Impaired
Urinary Elimination, Impaired
Urinary Elimination, Readiness for Enhanced
Urinary Retention

VALUE/BELIEF

Decision Making, Readiness for Enhanced
Decisional Conflict (Specify)
Grieving, Complicated
Grieving, Complicated, Risk for
Grieving, Dysfunctional
Human Dignity, Risk for Compromised
Moral Distress
Sorrow, Chronic
Spiritual Distress
Spiritual Distress, Risk for
Spiritual Well-Being, Readiness for Enhanced

SEXUALITY–REPRODUCTIVITY

Sexual Dysfunction
Sexuality Pattern, Ineffective

SELF-PERCEPTION/SELF-CONCEPT

Anxiety
Anxiety, Death
Body Image, Disturbed
Environmental Interpretation Syndrome, Impaired
Fear
Hope, Readiness for Enhanced
Hopelessness
Personal Identity, Disturbed
Power, Readiness for Enhanced
Powerlessness
Powerlessness, Risk for
Self-Concept, Readiness for Enhanced
Self-Esteem, Chronic Low
Self-Esteem, Risk for Situational Low
Self-Esteem, Situational Low

COGNITIVE/PERCEPTUAL

Comfort, Readiness for Enhanced
Communication, Impaired Verbal
Communication, Readiness for Enhanced
Confusion, Acute
Confusion, Acute, Risk for
Confusion, Chronic
Knowledge, Deficient (Specify)
Knowledge of (Specify), Readiness for Enhanced
Memory, Impaired
Nausea
Pain, Acute
Pain, Chronic
Sensory Perception, Disturbed (Specify): Auditory, Gustatory, Kinesthetic, Olfactory, Tactile, Visual
Thought Processes, Disturbed
Wandering
Unilateral Neglect

COPING/STRESS TOLERANCE

Coping: Community, Ineffective
Coping: Community, Readiness for Enhanced
Coping, Defensive
Coping: Family, Compromised
Coping: Family, Disabled
Coping: Family, Readiness for Enhanced
Coping: Individual, Readiness for Enhanced
Coping, Ineffective
Denial, Ineffective
Post-Trauma Syndrome
Post-Trauma Syndrome, Risk for
Rape-Trauma Syndrome
Rape-Trauma Syndrome, Compound Reaction
Rape-Trauma Syndrome, Silent Reaction
Relocation Stress Syndrome
Relocation Stress Syndrome, Risk for
Self-Mutilation
Self-Mutilation, Risk for
Stress Overload
Suicide, Risk for
Violence, Risk for Self-Directed

ROLE-RELATIONSHIP

Caregiver Role Strain
Caregiver Role Strain, Risk for
Family Processes, Interrupted
Family Processes, Dysfunctional: Alcoholism
Family Processes, Readiness for Enhanced
Home Maintenance, Impaired
Loneliness, Risk for
Parent/Infant/Child Attachment, Risk for Impaired
Parenting, Impaired
Parenting, Readiness for Enhanced
Parenting, Risk for Impaired
Role Conflict, Parental
Role Performance, Ineffective
Social Interaction, Impaired
Social Isolation
Violence, Risk for Other-Directed

Note: *The diagnoses Risk for Delayed Development, Delayed Growth and Development, and Risk for Disproportionate Growth can occur in any of the Functional Health Patterns.*

APPENDIX C

ANSWERS TO NCLEX-RN® REVIEW QUESTIONS

CHAPTER 1

1. Correct Answer: 3. A response that is other than that expected and culturally accepted to an event. **Rationale:** This characteristic distinguishes mental disorders from other disorders that nurses may encounter.

2. Correct Answers: 1. Historical and social norms. **Rationale:** Today, the "ship of fools" would be described as mass murder. 2. Situational context. **Rationale:** The man on the street corner who calls himself Napoleon is deviant, yet the man at the masquerade who calls himself Napoleon is ordinary. 4. Understanding of human behavior. **Rationale:** Homosexuality was voted out of the DSM-III in 1973. 5. Political norms. **Rationale:** Soviet dissidents were diagnosed and institutionalized for deviant behavior labeled as mental illness. "Delusions of societal reform" was a common medical diagnosis in the 1950s.

3. Correct Answer: 1. Has a pejorative connotation. **Rationale:** It is challenging to describe behavior that deviates from the norm with nonjudgmental, value-neutral language.

4. Correct Answer: 3. Incurable and dangerous. **Rationale:** In the early 19th century the emphasis was on the classification of symptoms of mental disorders. The mentally ill were seen as dangerous and incurable.

5. Correct Answer: 4. Rush. **Rationale:** Rush, the father of American psychiatry, viewed mental illness as a neurophysiological disorder.

6. Correct Answer: 1. Current medications and recent stressors. **Rationale:** Asking about current medications will elicit information about any current psychotropic drugs that treat mental illness from a biochemical perspective. Asking about recent stressors will elicit information from the social dimension. These areas reflect contemporary thinking related to mental illness.

7. Correct Answers: 3. Bipolar affective disorder. **Rationale:** Bipolar affective disorder is one of the mental disorders among the top ten causes of disability worldwide. 5. Schizophrenia. **Rationale:** Schizophrenia is one of the mental disorders among the top ten causes of disability worldwide.

8. Correct Answer: 1. Depression. **Rationale:** Depression ranks first among the top ten causes of disability worldwide.

9. Correct Answers: 1. A primary diagnosis of chemical dependency. **Rationale:** Only bullet 8 includes people who abuse substances (as individuals with co-occurring substance abuse and mental disorders). 2. PTSD. **Rationale:** As veterans return from abroad, incidence and prevalence of PTSD will increase. 5. Co-occurring mental disorders and traumatic brain injury. **Rationale:** As veterans return from abroad, incidence and prevalence of co-occurring mental disorders and traumatic brain injury will increase.

10. Correct Answers: 2. Availability of secondary care. **Rationale:** Bullets 5, 7, 8, 10, and 11 pertain to treatment of individuals with identified mental disorders. 3. Stigma associated with mental disorders. **Rationale:** The theme of "individuals with identified mental disorders who do not receive treatment," coupled with bullet 10 (cultural competence), suggests that stigma may interfere with treatment. 4. Availability of primary care (illness prevention and identification of at-risk populations). **Rationale:** Bullets 1, 4, 10, 11, and 12 involve screening and identification of at-risk individuals.

CHAPTER 2

1. Correct Answer: 1. Continued development of the multifaceted role of the nurse. **Rationale:** Promotion of self-care and psychobiological interventions are associated with custodial care. However, the inclusion of counseling, milieu management, health teaching, case management, and health promotion and maintenance extend the nurse's role.

2. Correct Answers: 1. Flexibility and variety within settings based on education and experience (as laws and regulations permit). **Rationale:** A health care team with healthy dynamics may utilize individuals' strengths to their full potential. 3. Rivalist behavior. **Rationale:** Blurring of roles within a dysfunctional group may lead to competitive, individual-centered behavior that does not regard the client as the central focus. 4. Increased cohesiveness of the health care team. **Rationale:** If the team members can flex with the needs of the clients and the institution and all the work gets done, members may experience greater job satisfaction. 5. Frustration and burnout. **Rationale:** If the team members do not work well together, they may experience decreased productivity along with job dissatisfaction.

3. Correct Answer: 4. Teaching and counseling. **Rationale:** Each health care team member performs teaching (formal or informal) and counseling (reflection on or analysis of behavior, thoughts, or feelings).

4. Correct Answers: 1. A cooperative, integral member. **Rationale:** Client partnering and advocacy are central to the mental health care team, of which the client is an active participant. 2. A team member who can influence others to cooperate. **Rationale:** A cooperator with leadership skills may influence maximizers and rivalists to work together. 4. A leader. **Rationale:** A team member who consistently brings focus to the client's needs may emerge as a leader (someone who guides or directs others).

5. Correct Answers: 1. Influx of World War II veterans with psychiatric disabilities. **Rationale:** The numbers of veterans compared to the numbers of psychiatric nurses encouraged the innovation of group therapy as a treatment modality. 2. The development of milieu therapy as a treatment modality. **Rationale:** Because of their continuous presence on inpatient units, nurses were responsible for development and maintenance of the therapeutic milieu. 4. Psychiatric nursing textbooks and journals. **Rationale:** Prior to 1920, psychiatric textbooks were written by psychiatrists who devoted only a few pages to the instruction of nurses. As psychiatric nursing knowledge was collected and disseminated, the number and scope of nursing interventions increased, contributing to improved care of clients in both psychiatric and nonpsychiatric settings. 5. Discovery of new psychopharmacological agents. **Rationale:** As the variety of agents increased, the nurse's role in clinical assessment and evaluation of the efficacy of a particular pharmacological regimen became more critical.

6. Correct Answer: 2. Prescriptive privileges for nursing. **Rationale:** This role change was not a consequence of the National Mental Health Act.

7. Correct Answer: 3. Demonstrated that psychiatric–mental health nursing strategies could be articulated and taught to other practitioners. **Rationale:** The publication of these interventions spurred further identification and dissemination of psychiatric nursing strategies.

8. Correct Answer: 1. Peplau's humanistic approach and existential values influencing general nursing theory. **Rationale:** Many theorists, including Roy, have revised their models to incorporate Peplau's values.

9. Correct Answer: 2. Attention to the nurse–client interaction. **Rationale:** The quality of this interaction is the focus of psychiatric nursing theory.

10. Correct Answer: 4. Resources, limitations, and client needs. **Rationale:** Theories may be used in combination, and a combined or eclectic approach demands that you be capable of functioning according to all theories of care.

CHAPTER 3

1. Correct Answer: 3. People cause their own problems. **Rationale:** The concept of blame infers that individuals cause their own problems.

2. Correct Answer: 2. Emotionally distances himself or herself in order to help others. **Rationale:** To maintain professional boundaries and prevent burnout, nurses emotionally distance themselves from clients in order to care for them and remain objective.

3. Correct Answer: 1. People create their own problems but need to rely on others to solve them. **Rationale:** The concept that people do create their problems but seek assistance from others to solve them is inherent in the Enlightenment Model.

4. Correct Answer: 3. Ask clients what cultural issues are important to them. **Rationale:** Asking clients about their cultural needs demonstrates respect and concern.

5. Correct Answer: 3. Recognizing and responding to his or her own internal stress signals. **Rationale:** Being aware of your own feelings and stress factors will help to decrease the rate of burnout.

6. Correct Answer: 4. The ability to ask for what you want while respecting other people. **Rationale:** Assertiveness is the ability to express your needs while still respecting others' needs.

7. Correct Answer: 3. Accountability. **Rationale:** Being an accountable nurse requires that you maintain a current knowledge base and standards to maintain quality care.

8. Correct Answer: 2. "I want to make sure I understood what you said." **Rationale:** Clarifying a client's feelings reflects a respect for the dignity of the client.

9. Correct Answer: 3. "I don't know how you feel, but I hear what you are saying." **Rationale:** We cannot know what or how our clients feel and it is appropriate to acknowledge that and let them know you hear them.

10. Correct Answer: 1. The significance of religious practices and rituals in the client's life. **Rationale:** Understanding the importance of religion and religious rituals in a client's life enables the nurse to plan care that meets the client's spiritual needs.

CHAPTER 4

1. Correct Answer: 2. Clinical research and practice. **Rationale:** Clinical research is the basis for evidence-based practice.

2. Correct Answer: 1. Practice guidelines. **Rationale:** Based on clinical research and clinical practice, nurses can develop clinical guidelines for nursing care.

3. Correct Answer: 3. Integrating personal experiences and beliefs into the process. **Rationale:** Including personal experiences and beliefs will inhibit one's ability to remain objective.

4. Correct Answer: 2. Reflect client outcomes based on nursing interventions. **Rationale:** Critical pathways integrate nursing interventions to achieve client outcomes.

5. Correct Answer: 1. Assessment. **Rationale:** In order to make a change, an assessment of the need to change is needed.

6. Correct Answer: 4. Review current nursing research. **Rationale:** Reviewing current nursing research will assist the nurse in maintaining an evidence-based model of care.

7. Correct Answer: 1. Identify what research questions to pursue. **Rationale:** The first step in any research project is to establish the research questions that the study will try to answer.

8. Correct Answer: 2. Identify resources needed to access evidence-based information. **Rationale:** Determining availability of resources to assist in the change to evidence-based practice will support the change process.

9. Correct Answer: 4. Establish criteria to be used in the evaluation process. **Rationale:** Decide what criteria you will use to evaluate this study's value to clients in your clinical area.

10. Correct Answer: 2. Outcomes of a research project. **Rationale:** Outcomes of research will reveal evidence to support clinical practice.

CHAPTER 5

1. Correct Answer: 3. Interactionism. **Rationale:** The belief that individuals control their own lives and events is the basis of interactionism.

2. Correct Answer: 3. Humanism. **Rationale:** Humanism focuses on humanity, science, and democracy.

3. Correct Answers: 1. The biological aspect of illness is considered. **Rationale:** A holistic approach to psychiatric–mental health nursing care examines how physiologic changes that occur with an illness affect emotional well-being. 2. Physical symptoms are interrelated with mental factors. **Rationale:** Physical symptoms can directly impact a client's emotional well-being and mental health. 4. The client's socioeconomic status is considered in planning care. **Rationale:** A client's socioeconomic status can directly affect a client's ability to access health care.

4. Correct Answer: 3. All behavior has meaning. **Rationale:** The belief that behavior has different meanings for different people reflects interactionism.

5. Correct Answer: 3. Moral behavior. **Rationale:** The superego focuses on moral behavior.

6. Correct Answer: 1. Participating in political systems to promote a holistic approach to mental health care. **Rationale:** The humanistic interactional model promotes a holistic approach to mental health care.

7. Correct Answer: 3. Cognitive behavioral. **Rationale:** Cognitive behavioral interventions focus on what the client thinks and feels and identifies the meaning of behavior.

8. Correct Answer: 2. Reinforcement. **Rationale:** Reinforcement rewards desired behaviors.

9. Correct Answer: 4. Psychobiology. **Rationale:** Psychobiology focuses on the disease process and how it impacts mental health.

10. Correct Answer: 4. A holistic approach to care includes the client system. **Rationale:** General systems theory looks at the whole being, including the family structure, and is a holistic approach.

CHAPTER 6

1. Correct Answer: 4. Parietal lobe. **Rationale:** The parietal lobe is involved with mathematical ability, as well as spelling, visual and spatial balance, and (with input from the thalamus) somatosensory integration.

2. Correct Answer: 4. Extrapyramidal system. **Rationale:** The extrapyramidal system includes motor neurons that affect gross motor movements and facial expressions associated with emotional responses.

3. Correct Answer: 1. Norepinephrine. **Rationale:** Norepinephrine mediates mood and anxiety, and the second client may have more available norepinephrine than the first client.

4. Correct Answers: 2. Excessive fluid intake associated with water intoxication. **Rationale:** Excessive hypothalamic dopamine may result in disrupted endocrine function and excessive fluid intake. 3. Bizarre behavior. **Rationale:** Decreased inhibition and decreased social awareness are associated with dopamine in the frontal cortex pathway. In addition, delusions and hallucinations correlate with increased availability of dopamine, and these breaks in reality are often associated with bizarre behavior. 5. Hallucinations. **Rationale:** Hallucinations and delusions correlate with increased availability of dopamine.

5. Correct Answer: 3. "Individuals with schizophrenia are born with schizophrenia genes that are activated by stress." **Rationale:** Some interventions with schizophrenia are based on the stress–diathesis model.

6. Correct Answers: 1. "Your illness is associated with a biochemical imbalance." **Rationale:** This statement is part of a comprehensive, accurate answer. 3. "Stress management early in the course of the illness can lead to fewer illness episodes." **Rationale:** This statement is part of a comprehensive, accurate answer. 5. "Medications help to correct the chemical imbalance." **Rationale:** This statement is part of a comprehensive, accurate answer.

7. Correct Answer: 4. The client's level of functioning increases further, as substance P has a different action on the neuronal pathway than traditional monoamine receptor–based pharmacotherapy. **Rationale:** Substance P, theoretically synthesized as part of a neurogenic inflammatory response to stress, has a different action on the neuronal pathway than traditional monoamine receptor–based pharmacotherapy. In the future, the client may realistically hope for full recovery from a major mental illness.

8. Correct Answer: 1. To assess the hypothalamic–pituitary–adrenal (HPA) axis. **Rationale:** Nonsuppression suggests pathology in the HPA axis function.

9. Correct Answer: 2. Kindling. **Rationale:** When subjected to repeated stress, the neuron may become sensitized, rendering the individual more vulnerable to stress and further episodes.

10. Correct Answers: 2. Decrease in shame and stigma. **Rationale:** As clients and families are able to describe mental illness as biologically based, they experience less shame, and stigma decreases over time. 3. Acceptance of client responsibility for treatment. **Rationale:** Participation in the treatment plan and selecting treatments of choice are empowering for the client and internalize the client's locus of control. 4. Informed family planning. **Rationale:** With genetic markers and identified predispositions, individuals and families are able to make informed choices associated with family planning. 5. Instillation of hope. **Rationale:** With increased knowledge of neurobiology, there is potential for more specific and varied interventions for particular disorders.

CHAPTER 7

1. Correct Answers: 2. "Pharmacologic intervention makes other therapies possible." **Rationale:** Psychiatric medications form the primary treatment for many psychiatric diagnoses. One might say that chlorpromazine gave birth to the modern notions of psychiatric treatment—unlocked wards, milieu treatment, occupational and recreational therapy, psychiatric rehabilitation, and supervised living environments. The entire field of community mental health is ultimately linked to its discovery. 3. "The psychiatric–mental health nurse's responsibilities include pharmacologic expertise." **Rationale:** The area of psychopharmacology continues to grow as a result of research and clinical expertise. Psychiatric–mental health nursing has similarly grown, and our responsibilities to recipients of mental health services involve, to a large degree, psychopharmacologic expertise. 5. "We consider the client holistically when prescribing a pharmaceutical regimen." **Rationale:** Ours is a holistic function, incorporating the client's life, likes, and activities along with symptomatology into a comprehensive view of treatment.

2. Correct Answer: 2. Less-comprehensive to more-comprehensive symptom relief. **Rationale:** This trend is evident in antipsychotic, antidepressant, and mood stabilization therapy.

3. Correct Answer: 1. Client 1 has always required more medication than Client 2 to achieve the same therapeutic effect, and the clients belong to different ethnic groups. **Rationale:** Distinct ethnic groups demonstrate variances in metabolic rates, and the variances explain their differences in clinical response.

4. Correct Answers: 3. "The lithium has removed the big highs and lows, so that he is on a more 'even keel.' " **Rationale:** This is a common description of the observable effect of lithium and other mood stabilizers. 5. "The medication has helped his hallucinations and unrealistic thoughts, but now he just stays in bed all day and doesn't want to do anything." **Rationale:** This statement reflects improvement of the positive symptoms of a thought disorder. However, it may also reflect absence of improvement regarding the negative symptoms of apathy and avolition.

5. Correct Answers: 1. "I feel just like I did before I was hospitalized. I'm getting back to my life like this was all a bad dream." **Rationale:** This statement may reflect "flight into health." The client's return to the premorbid life situation without further modification may lead to relapse. 3. "I feel like myself again. Maybe I don't really need to take this medication anymore." **Rationale:** Although medications may successfully treat the client's symptoms, they do not affect insight, and the symptom-free client may stop taking medication. 4. "My therapist wants me to take coping skills and stress management classes, but the medication is enough. I don't need classes." **Rationale:** If antianxiety medications are given without regard for the actual anxiety level and the individual's need to learn coping skills, it is possible to obliterate the need to learn to cope. 5. "I still think about death, but at least I don't lie in bed all day." **Rationale:** Increased energy before improved depression may result in the client's successful suicide.

6. Correct Answer: 1. The health care team must address your individual client's concerns. **Rationale:** The data presented in this study would have little meaning unless each individual client's concerns were heard and addressed. Participants would not have changed medications; they would have stopped participating in the study.

7. Correct Answer: 1. Alcohol withdrawal and anxiety disorders. **Rationale:** Benzodiazepines are used to treat anxiety disorders, sleep disorders, mood disorders, and alcohol withdrawal.

8. Correct Answer: 3. They alter the availability of specific neurotransmitters in the synaptic cleft. **Rationale:** These medications either increase or decrease availability of the neurotransmitters in a variety of ways.

9. Correct Answer: 4. "This new medication doesn't slow down my thinking or relax me as much as the benzodiazepine did." **Rationale:** Because the nonbenzodiazepine sedative–hypnotic medications bind only to the Type 1 benzodiazepine receptors, they induce sleep. The nonbenzodiazepine sedative–hypnotic medications do not bind to the Type 2 benzodiazepine receptors; therefore, these medications do not exert effects on cognition, memory, and psychomotor functioning (to which the client familiar with benzodiazepines is accustomed).

10. Correct Answer: 2. "He should experience fewer of the deficit symptoms of the disease." **Rationale:** This effect on the negative symptoms is a function of the atypical antipsychotics' reduced affinity for D_2 receptors.

CHAPTER 8

1. Correct Answer: 3. Process of cognitive appraisal. **Rationale:** The steps of primary appraisal, secondary appraisal, coping, and reappraisal may be equated with assessment, planning, implementation, and evaluation.

2. Correct Answer: 1. Insomnia related to anticipation of threat to basic needs and security. **Rationale:** The sleep pattern disturbance of insomnia is the client's presenting problem. The etiology relates to potential threat. Either actual interference with basic needs or anticipation of interference with basic needs may cause anxiety.

3. Correct Answer: 4. Your friend informs you that when she is stressed, she copes with massages, manicures, and cosmetic makeovers. "When my body looks better and feels better, it makes me feel emotionally grounded, like the outside mirrors the inside." **Rationale:** For this individual, physical appearance and comfort are a symbolic substitute for management of emotional tension.

4. Correct Answer: 4. Lazarus's secondary appraisal results. **Rationale:** Generalized resistance resources (factors in the person, group, or organization that help in managing tension) equate to secondary appraisal results (coping resources and options).

5. Correct Answer: 1. Repression. **Rationale:** Repression is the basis of all defense mechanisms and refers to the unconscious exclusion of distressing thoughts and feelings from awareness. Clients experiencing delirium may verbalize feelings such as guilt that were previously repressed.

6. Correct Answer: 2. Dissociation is functional for adults. **Rationale:** Dissociation is often disruptive for adults when they act without conscious awareness and have periods of time for which they cannot account. Dissociation serves an important purpose for a child in a traumatic situation, keeping the trauma from conscious awareness.

7. Correct Answer: 4. Create a safe interpersonal environment so that the client can explore precipitating events. **Rationale:** A safe interpersonal environment reduces anxiety. If the client perceives decreased anxiety, the client will experience decreased threat and increased ability to work with the nurse.

8. Correct Answer: 1. Gather data about family circumstances prior to the illness exacerbation. **Rationale:** An accurate assessment of family circumstances and the client's perception is the basis on which interventions are built.

9. Correct Answer: 3. Gather more data regarding his mental status and suicidality. **Rationale:** You need more data regarding the nature of "this horrible disease." (He may not be referring to schizophrenia.) If the disease to which he refers is schizophrenia, denial has been protecting him from anxiety. He may experience increased disorganization and may harm himself.

10. Correct Answer: 4. Demonstrate involvement of the neurological, endocrine, and immunological systems. **Rationale:** The emotional centers of the brain—the cerebral cortex and limbic system—are intimately tied to the endocrine organs, through the axis of the hypothalamus and the anterior pituitary.

CHAPTER 9

1. Correct Answer: 4. Pathological changes. **Rationale:** Pathological changes begin to occur in the presymptomatic stage, even though the client may be asymptomatic.

2. Correct Answer: 3. Professional awareness of the significance of cultural factors in the delivery of health care. **Rationale:** Cultural sensitivity is a professional awareness of the significance of cultural factors in the delivery of health care.

3. Correct Answers: 1. Disseminating information. **Rationale:** The nurse acts as a broker of information related to health care for a culturally diverse group. 2. Conflict resolution with a culturally diverse nursing staff. **Rationale:** As a nurse culture broker, the nurse may intervene if conflict occurs among a culturally diverse staff. 4. Facilitating acquisition of health care for clients. **Rationale:** The nurse as a culture broker serves as facilitator between clients and the health care system in obtaining care.

4. Correct Answer: 1. Religious practices that are relevant to the client. **Rationale:** Cultural competence includes the ability to incorporate the client's religious practices and beliefs into nursing care.

5. Correct Answer: 3. Include individual lifestyle habits. **Rationale:** Lifestyle habits influence expression, reporting, and evaluation of mental disorders.

6. Correct Answer: 4. Multifactorial causation. **Rationale:** Multifactorial causation is a combination of causes or factors needed to produce a disorder.

7. Correct Answer: 4. Involve those affected by the problem in the planning process. **Rationale:** When planning a program, it is important to involve those affected by the problem. This will better serve to meet the group's needs.

8. Correct Answer: 3. Learn about traditional healers within the community. **Rationale:** Learning about traditional healers and their practices within the community provides the nurse with a resource for the members of the cultural group. This is the only option that enhances the nurse's understanding of a specific cultural group.

9. Correct Answer: 2. Ethnicity. **Rationale:** Ethnicity is one's sense of identity, social belonging, and loyalty to a particular reference group within society.

10. Correct Answer: 4. Perception. **Rationale:** In the perception stage, the nurse assesses the impact of conflict or breakdown in health care interaction. There is a perceived need for brokering.

CHAPTER 10

1. Correct Answer: 2. The communication needs to be efficient, appropriate, flexible, and include feedback. **Rationale:** The formal criteria for successful communication are efficiency, appropriateness, flexibility, and feedback.

2. Correct Answer: 3. Facial expressions. **Rationale:** Facial expressions communicate emotions and are the single most important source of nonverbal communication.

3. Correct Answer: 4. It is mutually negotiated between the individuals involved in the interaction. **Rationale:** The meaning of the message is mutually agreed upon between the individuals involved in the process.

4. Correct Answer: 2. Overload. **Rationale:** Overload results from sensory input exceeding the tolerance level of the receiver.

5. Correct Answer: 2. The client processing auditory information. **Rationale:** An individual processing auditory information usually moves the eyes from side to side.

6. Correct Answer: 4. Make sure the client can see her lips move when she is speaking. **Rationale:** Clients who are hard of hearing may need to see the other person's lips moving to know they are speaking. They may also read lips in an attempt to understand what is being said.

7. Correct Answer: 4. "You've been feeling like a failure your entire life?" **Rationale:** This response restates what the client said and in doing so encourages the client to continue talking.

8. Correct Answer: 3. "I know some of these questions are difficult for you." **Rationale:** This statement is empathic and acknowledges the client's feelings.

9. Correct Answer: 2. The present and not the past. **Rationale:** Focusing on the here and now makes the feedback more meaningful. Feedback should be given as soon as it is appropriate to do so.

10. Correct Answer: 3. Emotions. **Rationale:** Facial expressions are the most important nonverbal communication and convey emotions.

CHAPTER 11

1. Correct Answers: 2. If data from different sources conflict, document all versions of the event(s), clearly identifying the sources of information. **Rationale:** Another clinician who reads your assessment receives the same data as you did. 3. Document, using the client's own words. **Rationale:** Descriptors such as "disorganized," "profane," and "threatening" are conclusions. If you include direct quotations, a clinician reading your documentation has the data at his/her disposal. 4. Identify the client's strengths. **Rationale:** Identifying and documenting the client's strengths contributes to a holistic and accurate psychiatric–mental health assessment. 5. Maintain self-awareness throughout the assessment process. **Rationale:** This principle enables the nurse to be receptive and nonjudgmental, so that the client is comfortable sharing truthfully.

2. Correct Answer: 1. The nursing process. **Rationale:** The psychiatric–mental health assessment is ongoing and subject to augmentation as additional data become available.

3. Correct Answer: 2, 3, 4, 1. 2. **Rationale:** (Step 1.) Encourage the client to share his story. The client's perspective and major concerns will be evident, and this demonstrates respect, forming a basis for trust. Clarify facts and the chronological sequence of events as necessary. 3. **Rationale:** (Step 2.) Review the admission assessment form with the client and ask direct questions. In this manner, you can complete the psychiatric history regarding the areas the client did not address. 4. **Rationale:** (Step 3.) Document your findings. If you document the data obtained up to this point, you will be able to remain clear regarding who the historian was for the data collected up to this point. 1. **Rationale:** (Step 4.) Meet with family members, noting relationships to client, and encourage them to share their stories and concerns. This step allows the nurse to ask specific questions where client's history may not be comprehensive. (This step assumes you have client's consent to interact with family.) Be sure to document this additional information along with the source.

4. Correct Answer: 3, 4, 2, 1. 3. **Rationale:** (Step 1.) General appearance and behavior. This assessment component begins the moment the nurse observes the client. It continues throughout the assessment, and the assessment is ongoing throughout hospitalization. 4. **Rationale:** (Step 2.) Orientation and memory. Many clinicians begin the MSE with orientation questions because disorientation should cause the examiner to question the validity and reliability of data obtained subsequently. Memory difficulties may indicate that subsequent information should be validated. 2. **Rationale:** (Step 3.) Characteristics of speech. These will be evident as the client answers initial questions and relaxes with the clinician. 1. **Rationale:** (Step 4.) Content of thought. Assessment of thought content may be perceived as very personal by the client. Some rapport should be established with the client before the clinician inquires about hallucinations, delusional thinking, suicidal ideation, and homicidal ideation.

5. Correct Answer: 3. The Mental State Examination assists the clinician in identifying risks for harm of self and others. **Rationale:** In addition, it provides the clinician with information regarding the client's orientation, memory, concentration emotional state, level of organization, and defects in reality testing, insight, and judgment.

6. Correct Answer: 2. "I did not have time to complete a full Mental State Examination." **Rationale:** If there is insufficient time to complete a full MSE, it is possible to fairly accurately assess and evaluate a client's functioning in a streamlined manner.

7. Correct Answer: 1. Physiologic assessment. **Rationale:** A general health history and physical examination are essential data for holistic physiologic assessment.

8. Correct Answer: 3. External (nonpsychological) psychosocial stressors. **Rationale:** Axis IV includes social, legal, and economic problems.

9. Correct Answer: 4. Axis V. **Rationale:** The GAF is reflective of impairment of functioning and severity of symptoms.

10. Correct Answer: 1. The quality of treatment plans and the appropriateness of subsequent interventions depend upon the quality of the assessment. **Rationale:** If the assessment of a client is based on incomplete, misinterpreted, or inaccurate information, the psychiatric diagnosis, prognosis, and treatment plans may be faulty.

CHAPTER 12

1. Correct Answer: 3. Assertive community mental health outreach. **Rationale:** Assertive mobile outreach units extend services to underserved individuals in the community who are unaware of services, or who are too disorganized to request them.

2. Correct Answers: 1. Autonomy versus beneficence. **Rationale:** To make housing contingent upon treatment plan adherence may be considered coercive. 2. Justice versus beneficence/nonmaleficence. **Rationale:** It could be argued that "doing what is right" means giving the housing to a more cooperative individual conflicts with "doing good" or "doing no harm" to your uncooperative client. 4. Fidelity versus autonomy. **Rationale:** This conflict exists if the client received housing without obligation to adhere to the treatment plan. Revoking his housing would constitute the rescinding of an agreement. 5. Veracity versus beneficence. **Rationale:** This conflict exists if the housing is not, in fact, contingent upon the client's treatment adherence.

3. Correct Answer: 1. The client's ambivalence about in-home assessment. **Rationale:** The client's ambivalence (and possible mistrust of home health care providers) is encountered more often in psychiatric–mental health home nursing than with other home health nursing situations.

4. Correct Answer: 4. "It may present a challenge, but it is a change in the best interest of both the clients and the mental health center staff." **Rationale:** The team structure is believed to reduce stress and burnout of individual case managers by sharing the load of difficult clients.

5. Correct Answer: 2. Increased continuity of care between inpatient and outpatient services. **Rationale:** One of the benefits of MCOs is increased continuity of care because it is cost effective to the organization. Quality improvement programs focus on this outcome.

6. Correct Answers: 2. Case manager. **Rationale:** You creatively facilitated appropriate treatment in the least restrictive setting. 3. Gatekeeper. In this example, you facilitated the client's access to innovative, out-of-plan benefits. 4. Client advocate. **Rationale:** If you worked to modify benefits to meet client's needs, you advocated for the client in this system.

7. Correct Answer: 4. The potential for blurring of professional boundaries as the case manager provides social support. **Rationale:** Case managers often find they are fulfilling many roles for their clients that have not been satisfied by other clinical resources, including a sense of social support. This blurring of boundaries is less likely within the inpatient setting, as relationships are, by their nature, time-limited.

8. Correct Answer: 1. "We provide the least restrictive safe environment. Clients participate in their treatment and aftercare planning." **Rationale:** These statements identify the unique characteristics of milieu therapy: the least restrictive environment and utilization of the client's strengths to move toward wellness.

9. Correct Answer: 2. The only commonality in this population is the presence of psychiatric disability. **Rationale:** The core feature of a severe and persistent disorder is not diagnosis or prognosis, but the experience of psychiatric disability. Since each client's needs are unique, flexibility and individualization are absolutely necessary.

10. Correct Answer: 1. Readmission is equated with failure of the current treatment intervention(s). **Rationale:** Health care providers are likely to favor intervention with a client who has not yet received any intervention over intervention with a recidivist client.

CHAPTER 13

1. Correct Answer: 2. Beneficence. **Rationale:** Protecting clients from harm because of their thoughts, feelings, and behaviors is an example of beneficence. An involuntary commitment is necessary to protect the client from harming self or others.

2. Correct Answer: 2. Explaining the exact limits of confidentiality in the exchange between the client and the nurse. **Rationale:** Client education regarding the exact limits of confidentiality empowers the client.

3. Correct Answer: 3. The client is unable to provide for basic needs. **Rationale:** If a client is unable to provide for basic needs—i.e., food, water, medications, etc.—the client can be involuntarily committed for treatment.

4. Correct Answer: 1. Enable the client's treatment team to plan appropriate and comprehensive care. **Rationale:** A psychiatric diagnosis or diagnostic label enables the health care team to plan appropriate care for the client.

5. Correct Answers: 2. Competency therapist. **Rationale:** The psychiatric forensic nurse acts a competency therapist, conducting forensic interviews, assessing competence and mental disorder, administering assessment tests, and completing formal reports to the court. 3. Expert witness. **Rationale:** When called upon as an expert witness, the court recognizes the nurse as having a high level of skill in a designated area and the ability to render an opinion on a legal matter.

6. Correct Answer: 3. Provides clients with some control over their treatment and empowers them. **Rationale:** The psychiatric advance directive is a tool to empower clients and allows for self-determination of care.

7. Correct Answer: 3. The client cannot be under the influence of medication that may alter cognition. **Rationale:** Clients cannot be under the influence of medications that alter cognition or level of consciousness when signing an informed consent form.

8. Correct Answer: 2. False imprisonment. **Rationale:** False imprisonment is an example of a tort, a wrongful act. The nurse can be held liable for his or her actions.

9. Correct Answer: 3. Discuss her concerns with the nurse manager. **Rationale:** The nurse has a responsibility to discuss her concerns with the nurse manager.

10. Correct Answer: 2. 3 to 5 days. **Rationale:** A client admitted as an emergency involuntary admission will be detained for a minimum of 3 to 5 days to allow for stabilization of symptoms.

CHAPTER 14

1. Correct Answer: 2. Delirium. **Rationale:** Delirium presents with the abrupt onset of a confusional state. The client experiences prominent disorientation, disorders of perception, terrifying hallucinations with vivid dreams, agitation, and insomnia.

2. Correct Answer: 3. Agoraphobia. **Rationale:** Agnosia, the loss of ability to recognize common everyday objects, is associated with DAT.

3. Correct Answer: 3. "These clients do not have any idea what is going on." **Rationale:** Clients with cognitive impairments do have an understanding, however limited, of their environment. The nurse's response is of concern because it reflects a lack of knowledge and understanding of the needs of the cognitively challenged client.

4. Correct Answer: 2. "I will put notes on the different rooms of the house so my father remembers what room he is in." **Rationale:** Posting notes on rooms and key locations throughout the house will remind the client of where things are or what needs to be done.

5. Correct Answer: 3. Have fluctuating consciousness. **Rationale:** Clients with delirium experience fluctuating consciousness due to the pathophysiology associated with the delirium.

6. Correct Answer: 1. An infection. **Rationale:** Delirium can frequently be precipitated by an infectious process and the demands the infection places on the body.

7. Correct Answer: 1. Risk for Injury. **Rationale:** Due to the client's altered perception and acute confusion, the client is at immediate risk for injury. Client safety is the highest priority.

8. Correct Answer: 4. Donepezil (Aricept). **Rationale:** Donepezil (Aricept) is an anticholinesterase inhibitor used to improve cognitive functioning.

9. Correct Answer: 3. Unknown. **Rationale:** There is no known cause for dementia associated with dementia of the Alzheimer's type. Researchers are trying to identify the exact cause of this dementia and research is indicating a multicausal relationship for this disorder.

10. Correct Answer: 2. Purchasing a MedicAlert® bracelet, identifying the client as having DAT. **Rationale:** Wearing a MedicAlert® bracelet that indicates the client has dementia of the Alzheimer's type will assist in emergency interventions if the client wanders from the home.

CHAPTER 15

1. Correct Answers: 1. Low self-esteem. **Rationale:** Clients have a diminished sense of self-worth and value. Alcohol can numb these feelings and clients perceive themselves as more social, more relaxed, and enjoying life more. 2. Difficulty dealing with intimacy. **Rationale:** The client may feel inadequate, insecure, and have low self-esteem. Personal intimacy threatens the alcoholic's sense of self. Alcohol is thought to be an avenue to alleviate anxiety and feelings of inadequacy. 4. Poor impulse control. **Rationale:** The need for immediate gratification can drive alcohol and drug abuse, which is perceived by the client as a path to feel good immediately. 5. Narcissistic behaviors. **Rationale:** The narcissistic person tends to feel unique or superior to others and is in control of the situation, including behaviors involving substance consumption.

2. Correct Answer: 3. Tachycardia, severe diaphoresis. **Rationale:** Tachycardia and severe diaphoresis are associated with major withdrawal from alcohol.

3. Correct Answer: 3. Risk for Injury. **Rationale:** The client experiencing delirium tremens may be confused, disoriented, and have altered sensory perceptions and seizures. Nursing interventions should be aimed at protecting the client from injury during a seizure or periods of disorientation and confusion.

4. Correct Answer: 3. Naloxone (Narcan). **Rationale:** Naloxone (Narcan) is a narcotic antagonist that reverses the central nervous system depression and respiratory depression associated with opioid overdoses. The client ingested an unknown amount of a narcotic.

5. Correct Answer: 1. "These clients have more excuses for their problems than anyone I know." **Rationale:** MICA clients are at risk for frequent relapses and setbacks. Chronic mental illness often impairs their judgment and insight, limiting their ability to acknowledge their problems or solve them. The nurse's response reflects her lack of understanding of the complexity of mental illnesses and substance use.

6. Correct Answer: 4. High school graduate. **Rationale:** Statistically, more education increases knowledge of the health and emotional risks of substance abuse; increases opportunities to function well in the community, thereby reducing stressors; and decreases the risk of developing drug dependence.

7. Correct Answer: 2. Rationalization. **Rationale:** Substituting acceptable reasons or explanations for real or actual problems that motivate a client's behavior is rationalization. The client is rationalizing his drinking by justifying why he needs to drink.

8. Correct Answers: 1. Individual therapy. **Rationale:** Individual therapy provides the client with the opportunity to work with a health care provider to address psychological issues. This is especially important for the client who is trying to maintain sobriety and prevent relapse. Through treatment the client will learn effective coping skills and identify triggers to relapse and treatment prevention. 2. Self-help groups. **Rationale:** Participants in self-help groups have similar problems and help one another by sharing their individual experiences and treatment strategies, and by educating one another. This is a very effective aspect of relapse prevention. 3. Twelve-step program. **Rationale:** The twelve-step programs are typically spiritual programs based on fellowship among members. Groups meet daily or more often. Participants acknowledge they are powerless over chemicals and live "one day at a time." 4. Lifestyle changes. **Rationale:** Clients learn to identify different coping strategies and discover new interests and capabilities within themselves. Clients learn that hanging out with previous friends who continue to abuse drugs or alcohol places them at greater risk of relapse.

9. Correct Answer: 3. "I have not used Demerol in 2 days since I started using relaxation exercises." **Rationale:** This response reflects the client's adaptation of coping mechanisms that are effective. Not using for 2 days is a measurable outcome.

10. Correct Answer: 2. Increased psychiatric symptoms. **Rationale:** The side effects of cocaine abuse increase the client's psychiatric symptomatology. Clients may also be nonadherent with psychotropic medications during periods of cocaine abuse, thus increasing symptomatology.

CHAPTER 16

1. Correct Answer: 2. "You can read my mind. This light of mine will shine, fine; blinding world will end at nine." **Rationale:** The speaker demonstrates some delusional thinking as well as clanging speech.

2. Correct Answer: 1. The many differences in the presentation of schizophrenia. **Rationale:** There are many different symptoms of schizophrenia. Even in the same family there are likely to be differences in the subtype of schizophrenia, the symptoms, and the stage of the family member's illness.

3. Correct Answers: 1. "I'm going to help my family member figure out what to tell other family members, friends, and business associates about why he's been on medical leave." **Rationale:** The client may feel shame or may be concerned about the social stigma of mental illness. This statement indicates the need to anticipate the questions of friends and acquaintances. 4. "I'll attend a support group, but I'm afraid my family member will not go . . . s/he would rather try to 'pass' as not mentally ill." **Rationale:** Because mental illness is not a readily visible disability, clients are more likely to avoid group affiliation and identification. 5. "It would be great if my family member could identify somebody to trust and believe when that person says, 'Your symptoms are worse. Let's go to the psychiatrist.' " **Rationale:** It is often difficult for a client to accept feedback from multiple others who observe the client's deterioration. When the client is able to identify a significant other whose judgment is trusted, the client may be able to receive the feedback more readily and be more amenable to early intervention. The selection of that individual may also be personally empowering for the client.

4. Correct Answers: 2. "I'm going to look for a job where I can use my college degree but have less day-to-day stress." **Rationale:** This statement reflects the recognition of a need for structure and meaningful work, as well as the need to manage job-related stressors that might contribute to exacerbation of symptoms and relapse. 4. "If I can't stand the side effects, how will I ask my prescriber to change my medication?" **Rationale:** This question implies recognition of the need to work with the prescriber rather than adjusting or discontinuing the medication independently. In addition, it implies recognition of the need for communication and assertiveness skills. 5. "I have designed a weekly schedule so that I can get tasks done and have planned time to relax." **Rationale:** The client has identified the need for a routine regarding work and leisure time.

5. Correct Answer: 3. "What might get in the way of your taking your medications?" **Rationale:** This proactive question engages the client in anticipating difficulty and is an open-ended question, which encourages elaboration.

6. Correct Answer: 1. An accurate description of the medication regimen with a specific plan for obtaining refills. **Rationale:** Relapse is largely dependent on medication adherence.

7. Correct Answer: 2. Reflecting on your behavior. **Rationale:** This response increases your self-awareness and may bring thoughts into focus that contribute to the situation.

8. Correct Answers: 1. "He may be demonstrating flattening of affect and anhedonia." **Rationale:** Flat affect and anhedonia are two of the negative symptoms of schizophrenia. 3. "Maybe he's depressed about having a chronic illness." **Rationale:** Depression is a common response to facing the prognosis associated with schizophrenia. Twenty-five percent of clients with schizophrenia attempt suicide, and 10% succeed. 5. "He may have sedation or masked facial expressions from his medications." **Rationale:** Sedation is a common side effect that typically decreases within 2 weeks of consistent dosing. Masked facial expressions are associated with parkinsonism, an extrapyramidal side effect of antipsychotic medications.

9. Correct Answer: 4. "If you can increase your self-assessment skills, you'll be able to tell when you're getting more stressed." **Rationale:** This statement relates to self-monitoring for symptoms and is most useful for preventing relapse.

10. Correct Answer: 1. "Your support group encourages you to make healthy choices. Taking your meds is a healthy thing you can do every day, just like brushing your teeth." **Rationale:** This statement reinforces the behavior as a self-care action for which the client can take responsibility.

CHAPTER 17

1. Correct Answer: 3. "You and your family stated you did not sleep at all last night. That can be tough on your system." **Rationale:** This response makes an observation, gives some health information, and allows the client to choose.

2. Correct Answer: 4. "Often, individuals with bipolar disorder can feel elated, are productive, and do not think there is anything wrong when they have manic feelings." **Rationale:** Clients with bipolar disorder frequently report that they enjoy the "highs" of mania. Mood stabilizers mediate this elation and many clients report this therapeutic impact as a reason for nonadherence to the treatment regimen. In contrast, clients with major depression report feeling "bad," even if they do not describe themselves as having a mood disorder.

3. Correct Answers: 3. "There are probably several genetic or biologic abnormalities associated with depression." **Rationale:** Families may have a number of individuals with various psychiatric disorders, but disruption in the experience of moods can indicate a genetic predisposition. 4. "Heredity does seem to play a role in mood disorders. You and your family members may have the same biologic predisposition." **Rationale:** The incidence of depression is higher among relatives of depressed individuals than in the general population.

4. Correct Answer: 1. "Although some abnormal results are found in individuals with mood disorders, there are no diagnostic lab tests specific to mood disorders at this time." **Rationale:** While there are no laboratory studies that definitively diagnose mood disorders, some abnormal findings are noted more often in mood-disordered individuals when symptoms are present than in control subjects.

5. Correct Answers: 2. "In addition, we are going to assist you in regulating your circadian rhythms, which should improve your depression." **Rationale:** Disturbed circadian rhythms can explain a number of mood disorder symptoms, and establishing a structured day with regular activities and rest can decrease those symptoms. 3. "It should help your depression, and you should feel the full therapeutic effect in 2 to 3 weeks." **Rationale:** This statement frames positively the fact that the client will not experience the therapeutic effect immediately but the depression will be ultimately addressed. 4. "This medication should increase the availability of neurotransmitters in your brain." **Rationale:** Although this is the antidepressant's expected mechanism of action, depending on the client's understanding of the physical and chemical processes, this may not be the first statement you make.

6. Correct Answer: 2. Antidepressants and mood stabilizers can help restore circadian rhythms. **Rationale:** Animal studies have demonstrated that alcohol and antimanic drugs, such as lithium, slow the biological clock, while estrogen and tricyclic antidepressants accelerate it or restore normal rhythms.

7. Correct Answer: 1. Ask about depression and suicidal ideation directly. **Rationale:** One out of every six people going to a medical office is depressed. One out of every six of those people is diagnosed and treated for depression. In addition, it is estimated that 50% of individuals who succeed in suicide had visited a health care practitioner within 24 hours of their suicide. Although clients may not offer this information, you should ask about suicidal ideation.

8. Correct Answer: 3. The client may have enough energy to plan and complete a suicide attempt. **Rationale:** Be aware that the risk of suicide increases as the severest stage of depression is alleviated, because clients then have sufficient energy and cognitive ability to plan and successfully implement a suicide plan.

9. Correct Answer: 4. "It can be frustrating to care for chronically ill clients." **Rationale:** An empathic response implies that you responded to the thought and feeling, which may be validating for your colleague.

10. Correct Answers: 1. Emotional contagion. **Rationale:** Recognize that working with depressed people may eventually lower your mood and make you feel "down" yourself. 2. Frustration with continued depression. **Rationale:** Many health care providers become frustrated with the depressed client's lack of initiative or discernible progress. 4. Rescue fantasy with a depressed client. **Rationale:** Review the limits of the therapeutic relationship and have your altruistic needs met elsewhere. 5. Anger at help-rejecting behavior. **Rationale:** Part of depression is help-rejecting behavior and keeping others at a distance. This client response can be hurtful, particularly to novice practitioners.

CHAPTER 18

1. Correct Answer: 4. Childhood obsessive–compulsive disorder. **Rationale:** There is an alteration in serotonin synthesis in the brains of children and adolescents who develop OCD.

2. Correct Answer: 2. "It is possible that progesterone metabolites are actually helping her to relax." **Rationale:** Some women with panic disorder have a reduction in their symptoms during pregnancy as a result of increased levels of progesterone. The metabolism of progesterone results in by-products that exert BZD-like effects, thus calming the panicked woman. You may hypothesize that in the pregnant woman with generalized anxiety disorder, the effect is decreased baseline anxiety.

3. Correct Answer: 1. "Anxiety disrupts your ability to function. It's the same for your loved one, who defends against anxiety by separating thoughts from feelings." **Rationale:** This statement imparts information and promotes recognition of the commonality between the disorders.

4. Correct Answers: 1. Markedly different presentations over time. **Rationale:** Many clients with dissociative disorders have received a variety of psychiatric diagnoses, depending on their level of conscious awareness, memory, or perceptual problems. 3. Need for long-term treatment with guarded prognosis. **Rationale:** Pharmacotherapy and cognitive behavioral therapy along with long-term individual therapy (focused on decreasing the need to dissociate) are indicated for clients with dissociative disorders. Clients with anxiety disorders more often have a good prognosis with pharmacologic intervention and short-term psychotherapy. 4. Psychosocial history with "missing" blocks of time. **Rationale:** Impaired memory and blocks of time that are "unaccounted for" are characteristic of clients with dissociative disorders.

5. Correct Answer: 4. "In dissociative disorders, an unconscious memory spontaneously enters conscious awareness, triggering the development of dissociation." **Rationale:** This phenomenon, the defense mechanism of dissociation, is characteristic of each of the dissociative disorders; it is not characteristic of panic attacks.

6. Correct Answer: 3. Within 1 month, the client will experience decreased frequency of episodes. **Rationale:** This outcome may not occur, but it is realistic. Within 1 month, with intervention, the client may experience a decrease in symptoms.

7. Correct Answer: 1. "Dissociation helps decrease anxiety by isolating the thoughts from the feelings about the experience and keeps the person from being completely overwhelmed." **Rationale:** Dissociation may include a sense of detachment or numbing, depersonalization, derealization, dissociative amnesia, or decreased awareness of surroundings. It is an extreme example of the defense mechanism of isolation of thought from affect.

8. Correct Answers: 1. Comorbidity with other anxiety disorders. **Rationale:** It is relatively common for a person to have one anxiety disorder coexisting with another. 3. Individuals who succeed in avoidance behavior may not demonstrate anxiety despite significant disabling effects on occupational and social functioning. **Rationale:** For such individuals, the problems with daily living may be identified only through active listening regarding patterns of daily living. 4. Anxiety may express itself indirectly through nonspecific somatic symptoms. **Rationale:** Anxiety may express itself through relatively mild somatic symptoms in which the existence of underlying anxiety is overlooked. 5. Clients with panic disorder often appear asymptomatic. **Rationale:** Unless they are in the throes of a panic attack, clients with panic disorder may not exhibit anxiety.

9. Correct Answer: 3. "Anyone I have ever cared for with a dissociative disorder is a pathological liar." **Rationale:** Clients with dissociative disorders are often accused of lying as a result of their inability to remember past events.

10. Correct Answers: 1. "I'm not sure I believe there is such a thing as dissociative identity disorder, but I can certainly think of these clients as having immobilizing anxiety." **Rationale:** This statement indicates that the nurse can empathize with the client's feelings. 2. "Whenever a client starts causing me stress, I take some slow, deep breaths." **Rationale:** This statement indicates the nurse's awareness that her own anxiety will interfere with communication and may escalate the client's own anxiety. 3. "Most of my clients with OCD find fault with something, but they appear less anxious if you give them some choices." **Rationale:** This statement reflects the understanding of the client's need for some control. 4. "When all the emergency room tests come back as unremarkable, we give the clients a brochure about panic disorder. It discusses the disorder as a legitimate medical disorder and gives them hope for recovery with treatment." **Rationale:** This intervention validates the legitimacy of the client's distress and instills hope.

CHAPTER 19

1. Correct Answer: 3. Lack appropriate coping skills. **Rationale:** Communication theorists believe the symptoms of somatization disorders are nonverbal body language intended to communicate a message to a significant other. The primary and secondary gains associated with the symptomatology result in attention and sympathy.

2. Correct Answer: 2. Conversion disorder. **Rationale:** A conversion disorder is an impairment or loss of physical function that is not caused by pathophysiological factors. The conversion disorder is believed to be an expression of a psychological need. The client may perceive the recital to be distressing and avoids it because of the paralysis.

3. Correct Answer: 3. "I will make a note of what you said." **Rationale:** Responding to the client's complaints in a matter-of-fact manner, without elaborating on the symptoms, will prevent or reduce secondary gain.

4. Correct Answers: 2. Presented in excessive detail. **Rationale:** An overdramatization of physical symptomatology is not uncommon in the client who has a somatization disorder. Clients present their health history with excessive detail, even though the information does not specifically describe the actual physical symptoms. 3. Related to how the symptoms impact relationships. **Rationale:** Clients frequently relate their physical symptoms to the impact the symptoms have had on their personal, social, and occupational relationships. 4. Lacking in a specific description of the nature, character, location, onset, and duration of symptoms. **Rationale:** Clients with somatization disorders have difficulty describing specific facts related to previous medical and surgical care. They are unable to focus on specific symptomatology.

5. Correct Answer: 1. Assisting the client in identifying stressful situations that precipitate physiological symptoms. **Rationale:** Working with the client to identify the cause-and-effect relationship of triggers and associated symptoms provides the client with insight and direction in learning to cope with triggers.

6. Correct Answer: 3. Decreased metabolic rate. **Rationale:** An increased metabolic rate is associated with primary insomnia. A decreased metabolic rate results in decreased energy production, which is favorable for sleep.

7. Correct Answer: 4. 24-hour food diary. **Rationale:** Caffeine consumption can interfere with sleep patterns; however, a 24-hour recall of the client's diet is not included in the basic sleep pattern assessment.

8. Correct Answer: 2. Communication. **Rationale:** Communication theorists believe somatization symptomatology to be nonverbal communication intended to express a message to significant others.

9. Correct Answer: 3. Fragmented, restless sleep with bizarre dreams. **Rationale:** With acute alcohol intoxication clients experience increased sleepiness for 3–4 hours. They may also experience

REM suppression. Sleep tends to be very fragmented and clients report bizarre dreams.

10. Correct Answer: 2. Increasing physical exercise during the day. **Rationale:** Increasing physical activity during the day can result in physical tiredness and less boredom. The client may be more tired when it is time to go to sleep.

CHAPTER 20

1. Correct Answer: 4. An individual's personal or private sense of identity as male or female. **Rationale:** A person's gender identity reflects the individual's personal and private sense of identity and is imposed by others at birth, is influenced by biology, and develops over time as self-identity.

2. Correct Answer: 4. Proficiency in the use of the nursing process and ability to assess the client's sexual health. **Rationale:** The generalist nurse needs to be proficient in the use of the nursing process to accurately assess the client's sexual health and sexual concerns.

3. Correct Answer: 2. Frotteurism. **Rationale:** Frotteurs rub up against others in an attempt to experience sexual arousal. No attempt is made to engage in sex with the victim.

4. Correct Answer: 3. Obscene phone calling. **Rationale:** A coercive paraphilia occurs when the individual includes nonconsenting persons in sexual acts. The victim of an obscene phone call is a nonconsenting person and may be harmed by the caller's behaviors.

5. Correct Answer: 1. The child being rewarded for adopting behaviors of the other sex. **Rationale:** Behaviorists believe gender dysphoria is a result of social learning. Rewarding the child for adopting behaviors of the other sex reinforces the behavior, although the child's natural responses are repressed. At some point the discomfort with the behavior that has been reinforced overwhelms the individual.

6. Correct Answer: 3. "How has your religion influenced your sexual values and behaviors?" **Rationale:** The cognitive domain of the assessment focuses on thinking and thought processes. The client's thoughts on the influence of religion and sexual values are reflected in the cognitive assessment.

7. Correct Answers: 1. Preoccupation. **Rationale:** The individual thinks about sex to the exclusion of other thoughts, resulting in a sexual high. The addiction supplants appropriate behaviors. 2. Ritualization. **Rationale:** Ritualistic behaviors are a pattern of sexual addiction. The rituals may control the sexual addict's anxiety. Addicts are usually unable to abandon a ritual without suffering tremendous emotional consequences until they learn how to cope with their anxiety. 3. Compulsivity. **Rationale:** The individual is unable to control sexual behavior, which has become the most important factor of his or her life. Other behaviors such as work, education, and hobbies are nonexistent or greatly minimized. 5. Despair. **Rationale:** Once the sexual act has been completed, the person experiences guilt and shame for the loss of control. The feelings of guilt and pain associated with the despair create anxiety and the need to begin the cycle all over again.

8. Correct Answer: 2. The nurse conveys the attitude to the clients that sexual thoughts and fantasies between consenting adults are allowed. **Rationale:** The nurse gives permission when he or she, by word or attitude, conveys to the clients that sexual fantasies, behaviors, and thoughts are acceptable between two consenting adults. Acknowledging the clients' verbal or nonverbal concerns conveys that these issues are important to the nurse.

9. Correct Answer: 2. Community education and awareness. **Rationale:** Education regarding this practice is needed to alert individuals of the risk of accidental death. Parents need to be aware of physical signs of trauma to the neck, including abrasions, pressure marks, or rope burns. Once signs are seen, a discussion about the risks involved could save lives.

10. Correct Answer. 2. The ability to explore personal values and attitudes related to sexual health. **Rationale:** The nurse needs to be aware of personal values and attitudes related to sexual health and how this affects treatment. The nurse must be able to separate these values from those of the client.

CHAPTER 21

1. Correct Answer: 2. There is a strong emphasis on low body weight justifying high self-esteem. **Rationale:** An individual's identity and self-esteem are linked to body weight.

2. Correct Answers: 1. Unclear boundaries between family members. **Rationale:** The family systems theory believes that in families that become enmeshed, there are no clear boundaries between family members. This family environment contributes to the development of an eating disorder. 3. Family members' preoccupation with food and eating. **Rationale:** The entire family of an individual with anorexia is overly involved and preoccupied with eating, foods, and rituals associated with meals. This atmosphere makes food and relevant activities the main focus of life.

3. Correct Answer: 4. Depression. **Rationale:** Depression is the most common disorder associated with anorexia and bulimia. It is unclear if the eating disorder is the primary disorder resulting in depression (a secondary depression) or if depression is primary and the eating disorder is a coping method.

4. Correct Answer: 3. Increased risk of mortality. **Rationale:** The most serious complication of anorexia nervosa is the risk of death due to the severe physiological changes and the risk of suicide.

5. Correct Answer: 1. Osteoporosis. **Rationale:** Clients with anorexia have low estrogen levels and are at high risk for developing osteopenia and osteoporosis. This is an objective finding.

6. Correct Answer: 3. Monitoring the client for at least 1 hour after meals. **Rationale:** Clients with bulimia need to be monitored for at least 1 hour after meals to prevent purging.

7. Correct Answer: 4. Expressing love and affection both verbally and physically. **Rationale:** Clients in treatment are learning how to feel good about themselves without the use of food. Underlying issues related to family relationships can contribute to an eating disorder. Clients need to feel accepted and loved for who they are.

8. Correct Answer: 3. Interrupt the behavior and offer to walk with the client. **Rationale:** The nurse should interrupt behavior and offer to walk with the client. This allows the nurse to set the pace of the walk and offer the client an opportunity to discuss feelings.

9. Correct Answer: 2. Blood pressure of 80/40 mm Hg. **Rationale:** A decreased blood pressure is indicative of impaired cardiac and tissue perfusion. The dropping blood pressure, if not corrected, will impair vital organs. The health care provider should be alerted to this finding.

10. Correct Answer: 1. Provide flexibility in activities of daily living. **Rationale:** Allowing the client the ability to determine daily activities encourages autonomy and increases the client's sense of responsibility.

CHAPTER 22

1. Correct Answer: 1. Interfere with role functioning. **Rationale:** A PD is a lifelong maladaptive pattern of perceiving, thinking, and relating that impairs social or occupational functioning and can be traced back to at least adolescence or early adulthood.

2. Correct Answers: 2. Lack of insight. **Rationale:** In this example, the student does not demonstrate understanding of the impact of her choice of subject matter for the thesis. 3. External response to stress. **Rationale:** The student deals with the stress by finding fault with the professor and attempting to alter the grade through the department chair. 5. Failure to accept consequences. **Rationale:** The student chooses to debate the grade and attempts to manipulate the department chair rather than learn from the outcome.

3. Correct Answer: 2. Cluster B personality disorders. **Rationale:** Increased levels of testosterone, 17-estradiol, and estrone have been observed in people with impulse control problems. The serotonin metabolite 5-HIAA has been shown to be low in people who attempt suicide and in those with aggression and impulse control problems. Impulse control is associated with the personality disorders grouped together in Cluster B.

4. Correct Answer: 2. Obsessive–compulsive personality disorder. **Rationale:** People with the dopamine D_3 receptor gene variant are approximately 2.5 times more likely to be diagnosed with obsessive–compulsive personality disorder.

5. Correct Answer: 3. Reinforce the client's sense of mastery by pointing out previous success. **Rationale:** The nurse attempts to reinforce the client's sense of mastery by pointing out previous success.

6. Correct Answer: 1. Demonstrate honesty and sincerity in all interactions with the client. **Rationale:** Establishing a therapeutic relationship with personality-disordered individuals is challenging because it goes against the basic nature of most personality-disordered clients to trust others and express their true feelings. Without the foundation for trust, including clear and open communication, other interventions are likely to be ineffective.

7. Correct Answer: 2. "What are you experiencing right now?" **Rationale:** Encouraging the client to identify thoughts and feelings is the approach most likely to increase the client's self-awareness.

8. Correct Answers: 1. Consistency minimizes the opportunity for the client to split staff. **Rationale:** The staff members can focus on the unique needs of this client and the needs of other clients when the staff is unified. 4. Staff members are more likely to detect subtle changes in the client's behavior. **Rationale:** The staff members are also better positioned to point out these changes to the client. 5. Predictability may increase the client's sense of trust and security. **Rationale:** Trust is generally difficult for these clients. A smaller group of staff members increases the potential for trust to develop.

9. Correct Answer: 4. "I wish we could identify what she needs and provide it before she acts out on the unit." **Rationale:** This statement approaches the client as a person with unique needs and suggests an approach to positively affect her treatment.

10. Correct Answer: 2. "It is frustrating to care for people with persistent behaviors." **Rationale:** This response demonstrates empathy for your coworker. In addition, it encourages her to continue sharing her thoughts and feelings without seeming judgmental of her. As the dialogue continues, you may be able to identify effective treatment interventions for the client. Approaching the client as a united team is most likely to ensure consistency and minimize the potential for splitting of staff.

CHAPTER 23

1. Correct Answers: 1. Presence of psychiatric illness. **Rationale:** Over 90% of people who commit suicide have a psychiatric illness. 2. Receiving psychiatric–mental health care. **Rationale:** Over 50% of people who commit suicide are under active psychiatric–mental health care. 3. History of self-injurious behavior. **Rationale:** Of those individuals reporting self-injurious behavior, 40.3% also reported suicidal ideation. 5. Use of alcohol. **Rationale:** Alcohol consumption is estimated to cause adolescent males to be up to 17 times more likely to attempt suicide, and females 3 times more likely. This factor may be the single greatest predictive factor for suicidal behavior.

2. Correct Answer: 1. "I just had to succeed in school. When I failed, I could think of no other answer to my situation." **Rationale:** The common purpose for suicide is to seek a solution to what appears to be an otherwise insoluble problem.

3. Correct Answer: 3. Decreased constriction in thought. **Rationale:** The thought processing of suicidal clients is generally constricted; that is, people who are suicidal have great difficulty (if they can do it at all) considering alternatives to their current dilemma. The ability to envisage alternatives is a factor that could change during the course of a telephone intervention.

4. Correct Answers: 1. Reduced serotonin activity in the frontal cortex. **Rationale:** This part of the brain is thought to be associated with controlling impulsive behavior. 2. Dichotomous thinking. **Rationale:** Suicidal individuals often believe that there is an either/or choice rather than a range of options. 5. Dysfunction of the hypothalamic–pituitary–adrenocorticoid axis. **Rationale:** Some researchers report that dysfunction of the hypothalamic–pituitary–adrenocorticoid axis is associated with suicidal behavior.

5. Correct Answer: 4. Very high risk of imminent suicide. **Rationale:** The client is in a high-risk demographic group (55 years old, white, non-Hispanic, widowed, and male). He has a history of suicide attempts using a mixture of alcohol and opiates, a highly lethal means. In addition, he is cut off from resources and has just experienced forced retirement, a serious loss. This client is best characterized as being at very high risk of imminent suicide.

6. Correct Answer: 1. Remain with the client. **Rationale:** One-to-one staffing provides the greatest physical safety for the client.

7. Correct Answers: 3. "Tell me more about your thoughts." **Rationale:** Encouraging the client to elaborate gives the client an opportunity to explore and ventilate feelings, which will decrease anxiety. 4. "Sometimes clients who feel hopeless think about killing themselves. Have you had any thoughts about killing yourself?" **Rationale:** Although the client denied he would hurt himself, consider asking about suicide directly, in case the client has framed death as nonhurtful and beneficial. 5. "You have told me that you have not had thoughts about hurting yourself. If you start having these thoughts, can you tell me or another staff member before you act on them?" **Rationale:** This question is the basis for a no-self-harm/no-suicide contract.

8. Correct Answer: 1. "It is important for you to get what you need. What do you need for yourself at this time?" **Rationale:** The family members are experiencing stress. Use active listening and remain nonjudgmental as you indicate to them that you know they are in distress.

9. Correct Answers: 1. Consider whether you need an opinion from another clinician. **Rationale:** If you are concerned that your feelings were perceived by the client or otherwise interfere with the assessment, a second opinion from another nurse or clinician is a reasonable and prudent option. 2. Allow time for yourself to explore the thoughts behind your emotional response to this situation. **Rationale:** It is essential that you inventory your response to this client so that you develop self-awareness without acting out your feelings. 3. Examine the ethical conflict of autonomy versus beneficence/nonmaleficence. **Rationale:** The interaction may have revealed an ethical dilemma for you. 5. Consider the issues of control and responsibility in the interaction with this client. **Rationale:** Clients who appear to reject values of health and preservation of life may elicit frustration in health care providers.

10. Correct Answers: 2. The belief that health care providers should wait for family members to approach them. **Rationale:** Survivors rarely seek assistance from mental health professionals. Therefore, health care providers should be prepared to offer assistance. 3. Fear of being blamed for the client's suicide. **Rationale:** Family members' blame of the health care team is a common response. If this response is anticipated, offers of support to the family may be made through pastoral care or volunteer services. 4. The belief that family members will receive adequate support from their own support network. **Rationale:** Families and friends may not receive the same degree of support as bereaved people whose loved ones died because of illness or accident. Therefore, offers of additional support (such as connection to a survivors-of-suicide support group) may be welcomed. 5. Concerns about litigation, with management directives not to interact with family members. **Rationale:** This is a legitimate concern. If this response is anticipated, offers of support to the family may be made through nonclinical support services (pastoral care or volunteer services) or a designated administrator.

CHAPTER 24

1. Correct Answer: 2. None of the contributing factors consistently results in or is predictive of rape or intrafamily abuse. **Rationale:** Although a genetic predisposition may make certain behaviors more likely, it does not make them inevitable.

2. Correct Answer: 1. Fluid boundaries. **Rationale:** An adult may move "down" in the structure or a child may move up in terms of roles and influence (boundaries). If the father moves downward, he assumes a childlike role and is cared for and nurtured like a child in the family. In this position, the father assumes little parental responsibility. He may then turn to the daughter as a "peer" for sexual and emotional gratification.

3. Correct Answer: 4. Client in the emergency room immediately after the rape. **Rationale:** The immediate goals for this client include "Client will make choices regarding care" and "Client will identify feelings."

4. Correct Answers: 2. Family's immigrant or refugee status. **Rationale:** Abrupt relocation to an unfamiliar place contributes to individual and family perception of isolation, a common dynamic in families of abuse. 3. Family's primary language other than community's dominant language. **Rationale:** Inability to communicate in the dominant language contributes to isolation, a common dynamic in families of abuse. 4. Breadwinner's active military status. **Rationale:** If the breadwinner is absent from the household, the remaining parent has fewer resources and may experience isolation. The multiple moves that military families experience decrease social connections. Such isolation is a common dynamic in families of abuse. Support systems available to these families may offer assistance for more universally experienced stressors and may not actively seek out families at risk for abuse.

5. Correct Answers: 1. Identify areas of control. **Rationale:** This intervention empowers the client. 3. Support the client in the decisions he/she makes. **Rationale:** This intervention empowers the client and enhances the client's current problem-solving ability. 5. Establish trust and rapport. **Rationale:** This intervention provides the client with an ally.

6. Correct Answer: 1. "I am required by law to report suspected abuse." **Rationale:** It is best to be honest and direct.

7. Correct Answer: 3. Isolation. **Rationale:** Spirituality includes a sense of connectedness to others. Survivors must begin the long journey of developing trusting relationships.

8. Correct Answers: 1. You role-model self-respect in the workplace. **Rationale:** This behavior decreases the potential for sexual harassment. 2. You confront sexual harassment among pre-adolescents and adolescents. **Rationale:** This behavior forces them to consider gender stereotypes as negative events and offers them an alternative. 4. During your assessment, you inquire about parenting challenges and interventions. **Rationale:** If parents report distress, you have an opportunity to connect them with available resources. 5. Your community association assists new residents to develop social support networks. **Rationale:** Connecting socially with others decreases the isolation that is characteristic of dysfunctional families.

9. Correct Answers: 2. The nurse may assume the perpetrator was a stranger. **Rationale:** As members of society, nurses are affected by misperceptions and myths. This assumption may result in unsafe plans for the client's aftercare. 3. The perpetrator's safety may be jeopardized. **Rationale:** If the nurse does not inquire about the perpetrator's identity or the client's immediate plan for safety, the client may harm the perpetrator. Furthermore, the client would have to contend with the legal system as a consequence of taking violent action against the perpetrator. 4. The nurse may "normalize" behavior the client perceives as violent. **Rationale:** The client may not be communicating clearly or appropriately, and the nurse may misinterpret that a controlled, emotionless account of the violence means the event was nonthreatening or insignificant. 5. The client may feel obligated to defend the perpetrator. **Rationale:** The nurse's communicated rage toward a perpetrator of incest or rape may result in the victim defending the perpetrator from the nurse.

10. Correct Answer: 2. "Perpetrators often present as pleasant, concerned individuals." **Rationale:** Making the assumption that the perpetrator will announce undercurrents of criminal behavior in some way runs counter to the facts concerning sexual and physical abusers.

CHAPTER 25

1. Correct Answers: 2. Deficits in problem-solving skills. **Rationale:** Individuals with serious mental illness often exhibit impaired judgment and reasoning secondary to disease pathology, nonadherence with treatment and medications, and lack of formal knowledge. This combination of behaviors increases the individual's risk factors for exposure to HIV/AIDS. 3. Limited impulse control. **Rationale:** Individuals with serious mental illness often exhibit impaired judgment and reasoning secondary to disease pathology, and nonadherence with treatment and medication. Impaired impulse control is a symptom of many chronic mental illnesses. This combination of behaviors increases the individual's risk factors for exposure to HIV/AIDS. 5. Impaired judgment. **Rationale:** Individuals with serious mental illness often exhibit impaired judgment and reasoning secondary to disease pathology, nonadherence with treatment and medications, and lack of formal knowledge. This combination of behaviors increases the individual's risk factors for exposure to HIV/AIDS.

2. Correct Answers: 2. The side effects of the pharmacological treatment. **Rationale:** The antiviral medications and medications used to treat the opportunistic infections cause several neurological side effects, resulting in behavioral and neurological changes. 5. A viral invasion of the central nervous system (CNS). **Rationale:** The neuropsychiatric changes associated with HIV result from viral invasion of the central nervous system (CNS), resulting in opportunistic infections or neoplasms.

3. Correct Answer: 1. Risk for Injury. **Rationale:** The client with HIV dementia experiences cognitive dysfunction, declining motor performance, behavioral changes, and headaches or seizures. These changes place the client at increased risk for injury. Maintaining the client's physical, biological, and psychosocial safety is the priority focus.

4. Correct Answer: 4. Slowness of thought. **Rationale:** Changes in thought processes, slowed thoughts, and loss of concentration are examples of cognitive changes associated with HIV dementia.

5. Correct Answer: 3. Using brief, direct statements. **Rationale:** The cognitive changes associated with HIV-related dementia result in impaired communication for the client. Making brief, direct statements enables the client to focus and follow directions.

6. Correct Answer: 1. "I can French-kiss my girlfriend and will not contract HIV." **Rationale:** Sexual activities that include the exchange of blood or body fluids are considered high-risk behaviors. Mucous membrane damage in the mouth (an open sore or bleeding gums, for example) involves the exchange of blood. The exchange of saliva is a possible risk factor, although it is not universally considered a risk factor by all researchers.

7. Correct Answer: 4. Protect the intravenous drug user (IDU) from contracting HIV and other life-threatening diseases. **Rationale:** Harm reduction works with intravenous drug users through harm reduction education in teaching these clients how to prevent contracting HIV or hepatitis C.

8. Correct Answer: 4. Support of others who have experienced a similar death. **Rationale:** Having support from individuals who have shared a similar loss provides the individual with an opportunity to share feelings and concerns. This is critical in assisting the survivors to work through their feelings.

9. Correct Answer: 1. "I can't touch the client or I will get HIV/AIDS." **Rationale:** Clients with HIV/AIDS and a psychiatric diagnosis require therapeutic touch just as any other client does. Appropriate universal precautions should be adhered to for all clients. The nursing student should wear gloves if there is contact with blood or body fluids or the student has impaired skin integrity on his/her hands.

10. Correct Answer: 3. Side effect of the antiretroviral medication. **Rationale:** Antiviral medications can cause neuropsychiatric side effects, including hallucinations, sleep disturbances, memory impairment, agitation, anxiety, confusion, irritability, delirium, and headache. The client's symptoms are consistent with medication side effects.

CHAPTER 26

1. Correct Answer: 3. Identifying psychiatric diagnoses. **Rationale:** The child psychiatric–mental health nurse develops and provides a nursing diagnosis. The child psychiatric–mental health nurse does *not* give a psychiatric diagnosis unless the nurse is an advanced-practice nurse (clinical nurse specialist or nurse practitioner).

2. Correct Answer: 4. Cognitive behavioral theory. **Rationale:** In cognitive behavioral theory, the child's environment has a major role in the child's psychological development. How the child thinks about and interprets the environment has a direct impact on the child's behavior.

3. Correct Answer: 2. There is no predictable set of risk factors. **Rationale:** Childhood responses, experiences, and perception of the environment contribute to the development of mental health well-being or mental disorder.

4. Correct Answer: 3. Family history of mental health well-being. **Rationale:** A family history of emotional well-being directly impacts upon how family members interact with one another. Healthy family interactions promote emotional well-being in children and other family members.

5. Correct Answer: 1. Experience no loss of previously acquired skills. **Rationale:** Children with Asperger's disorder have no loss of previously learned skills. Children with autism have deficits in normal development and experience losses in language, social skills, and play.

6. Correct Answer: 3. What do you believe to be the cause of your child's problem? **Rationale:** This question allows the family to explore their feelings and beliefs regarding the underlying cause(s) of the child's mental health problems. The nurse can identify the family's cultural beliefs and practices by expanding on this question, based on the family's response.

7. Correct Answer: 1. Relive past events and feelings through play. **Rationale:** Abreaction allows the child to gradually assimilate previous painful or traumatic experiences through the release of related emotions. The child is able to integrate feelings and emotions through play, which enables the child to gain mastery and control over the experience.

8. Correct Answer: 2. The child's behavior. **Rationale:** The child's behavior is one of the three components addressed in child–parent therapy. The nurse assists the child in identifying difficulties in behavior and developing more effective methods to deal with the behavior. The nurse strives to improve the child's interpersonal skills.

9. Correct Answer: 2. Risk for Aspiration. **Rationale:** Due to the seizures that can occur with lithium toxicity, the child is at risk for aspiration during a seizure. This can also occur if the child is comatose. Based on Maslow's hierarchy of needs, maintaining a patent airway is the priority nursing diagnosis.

10. Correct Answer: 4. "I know exactly how the child feels. I went through the same thing when I was that age." **Rationale:** This statement indicates the nurse is projecting personal feelings and experiences onto the child's situation. This prevents the nurse from remaining objective in the child's treatment. This issue would need to be addressed with the nurse.

CHAPTER 27

1. Correct Answer: 3. Explains the biochemical and physiological causes of obesity. **Rationale:** Identifying the biochemical and physiological causes of obesity challenges and may minimize societal biases and prejudices regarding obesity.

2. Correct Answers: 1. Hormonal changes. **Rationale:** The hormonal changes associated with adolescents directly influence psychosocial and physical well-being. An assessment of hormonal factors should be included in the assessment. 2. Chronic illnesses. **Rationale:** The impact of chronic illness on an adolescent's well-being directly affects all aspects of the client's life. Underlying medical conditions and chronic illness can result in depression and should be included in the assessment. 3. Immune function. **Rationale:** The overall status of the adolescent's immune system functioning is a reflection of the client's physical and psychosocial well-being. This area should be included in the assessment. 4. Growth spurts. **Rationale:** Hormonal changes directly influence an adolescent's growth spurts. The changes associated with growth spurts can affect an adolescent's sense of self and self-esteem. This area should be assessed.

3. Correct Answer: 2. The client's goals for retirement. **Rationale:** It is important to know the client's immediate and distant goals for the future. However, the adolescent is not likely to be able to verbalize retirement plans. This information is not needed for the treatment planning process.

4. Correct Answer: 3. Actively participate in curriculum development within the school. **Rationale:** Active participation in curriculum development and planning exposes the nurse to the different needs of the school and students and enables the nurse to interact with different faculty. This action is essential to establishing a working relationship with school officials and faculty and improving visibility within the school.

5. Correct Answer: 4. Identifying an effective way to resolve the problem. **Rationale:** By identifying an effective way to resolve the problem, the nurse acknowledges the significance of the adolescent's behavior and assists the client in identifying a resolution to the immediate problem. This is an effective solution.

6. Correct Answer: 2. Role-modeling socially acceptable behaviors. **Rationale:** By role-modeling socially acceptable behaviors, the nurse gives the client the opportunity to develop more effective coping and communication skills. The client is also given control over his/her actions as the decision to incorporate this new behavior is left up to the client. This is an effective intervention.

7. Correct Answer: 1. "I will not accept phone calls from my family while in the treatment program." **Rationale:** Maintaining contact with family members is an integral part of treatment, and family contact should be maintained.

8. Correct Answer: 1. "Don't you ever speak to me like that again." **Rationale:** This response challenges the client to test the limits the nurse is attempting to set and may result in escalating the client's negative behaviors.

9. Correct Answer: 2. Rescue the client who is being scapegoated from the group. **Rationale:** Attempting to rescue the client being scapegoated will exacerbate the other clients' behaviors and increase their anger and frustration. This intervention would have a negative impact on the behavior.

10. Correct Answer: 2. Accept and support all behaviors exhibited by clients without question. **Rationale:** It would be dishonest and nontherapeutic for a nurse to accept and support all clients' behaviors without question.

CHAPTER 28

1. Correct Answers: 2. Increased incidence of other chronic disabling conditions. **Rationale:** The old-old group tends to have the greatest incidence of depression, delirium, dementia, and other chronic and disabling conditions. 3. Increased numbers of chronically disabled individuals requiring assistance with activities of daily living. **Rationale:** Of those individuals with chronic disabling conditions, 49% have some limitation in their ability to perform activities of daily living. 4. Increased numbers of frail older adults (who consume many health care resources, maintenance services, and residential placements). **Rationale:** Although this group represents only 5% of the over-65 population, the number of individuals in this group is increasing. 5. Increased numbers of underfunctioning older adults due to inadequate intervention associated with stigma and ignorance. **Rationale:** Older adults are reluctant to seek mental health services. The reasons include: misidentification of mental illness symptoms as the expected changes of the aging process, stigma of seeking mental health treatment, cost of mental health services, ageism, and fear of institutionalization.

2. Correct Answer: 4. Wear-and-tear theory. **Rationale:** Even though this theory allows for variable rates of cell deterioration, the emphasis is one of loss and decline in later life.

3. Correct Answer: 2. Activity theory. **Rationale:** This theory proposes that the way to age successfully is to stay active and involved. Activity theory focuses on the current behavior of the older adult.

4. Correct Answer: 1. The clinical presentation of mental illness in older adults differs from that in other age groups. **Rationale:** Currently, there are few age-specific descriptors or criteria. However, research and identification of diagnostic criteria in children experiencing bipolar disorder is likely to appear in a future edition of the DSM, suggesting that specific criteria for older adults may appear in future editions as well.

5. Correct Answers: 1. "How did this current problem start?" **Rationale:** The onset of behavioral change (precipitating event, acute onset, or gradual onset) may assist in ruling out a medical, nonpsychiatric problem. 4. "What other changes have you experienced recently?" **Rationale:** The client and/or the daughter may have identified other changes or precipitating factors that they have not mentioned (that may be less troublesome but may indeed be clinically significant). 5. "What has it been like for you in the past when you experienced sadness and body complaints?" **Rationale:** It is noteworthy whether the client's past episodes of depression or somatic complaints bear any resemblance to the current presentation.

6. Correct Answer: 1. "Cognitive changes can be associated with depression, dementia, and other medical, nonpsychiatric conditions. Your parent may respond well to this intervention." **Rationale:** This response answers the question and provides accurate information.

7. Correct Answers: 2. Animal Afternoon, during which residents interact with certified therapy animals. **Rationale:** Animal therapy typically provides affection, attention, diversion, and relaxation to residents while placing few demands on the resident. 4. Music Night, during which a stage band plays requests from the residents. **Rationale:** This activity promotes reminiscence and routinely benefits individuals with short-term memory impairment.

8. Correct Answers: 2. "Attending an adult day care would give her something to anticipate each day and would provide a schedule with structure." **Rationale:** Both anticipation of the future and a defined routine are important for maintaining mental health. 3. "If you have a particular adult day care in mind, it might be worth scheduling a visit to see what it is like." **Rationale:** No amount of information can replace observing the actual setting on a typical day. The experience may decrease anxiety and dispel fear. 5. "She would have the opportunity to meet other people and engage in activities that you do not do at home." **Rationale:** Often, group activities (such as game tournaments) and outside visitors (such as entertainment or service organizations) provide stimulation that is unavailable in a private residence.

9. Correct Answer: 3. "Everyone ages a little differently, but there are very few changes to the mind that are associated with age alone." **Rationale:** This response answers the client's question and addresses what may very well be a genuine fear, without violating the confidentiality of other residents.

10. Correct Answer: 1. "That change has nothing to do with age. When the client changes that dramatically in a short period of time, there is something really wrong with that client." **Rationale:** This response conveys essential information: 1) that the client's presentation is not to be dismissed; and 2) that with rapid onset and severe deterioration, this is an emergency.

CHAPTER 29

1. Correct Answer: 2. "My nurse wants to focus on anger management techniques, and I want to examine my early childhood." **Rationale:** This statement reflects the absence of mutually defined goals and foci that characterize the functional one-to-one relationship.

2. Correct Answer: 1. "One of the goals you had set was to identify more self-actualizing coping strategies. You just identified a problem." **Rationale:** Relating the client's behavior to the established goals and giving positive reinforcement for identifying an area for exploration support the client's personal growth.

3. Correct Answer: 3. "You have been silent for long periods during the last 10 minutes." **Rationale:** This response addresses the client's behavior and encourages the client to share. If the client is demonstrating resistance, the behavior is addressed rather than ignored.

4. Correct Answer: 4. "I thought a lot about your situation this week. Last night, you were in my dream." **Rationale:** This response reflects the nurse's feelings about the client (countertransference) and does not provide a therapeutic platform for the client to reach stated goals. Avoid self-disclosure of countertransference to clients. Sharing these feelings may overwhelm clients and burden them in a destructive way.

5. Correct Answer: 1. "I feel safe enough with my nurse that I could share my thoughts and feelings." **Rationale:** In the orientation phase, establishing trust is essential for the therapeutic work to proceed.

6. Correct Answer: 2. "I did not accomplish everything I wanted to, but I will come back for more therapy when I am ready." **Rationale:** Complete resolution of all issues seldom occurs. Often, the client achieves more limited behavioral changes and agrees to return for future work or referral as necessary.

7. Correct Answers: 3. It is characteristic of the working phase. **Rationale:** During the working phase, the nurse has two general therapeutic goals: behavioral analysis and constructive change in behavior. 5. The nurse and client may reprioritize therapeutic goals. **Rationale:** The working phase is characterized by revising and updating therapeutic goals, and identifying this issue could change the original goals.

8. Correct Answer: 1. Experiencing the stressors associated with the termination phase. **Rationale:** The client's behaviors are typically associated with the termination phase, potentially the most difficult for clients because it arouses feelings associated with past losses of significant others.

9. Correct Answer: 4. A longer orientation phase. **Rationale:** You can predict that it will take the client longer to trust you.

10. Correct Answer: 3. "Whether or not that's true, I am right here with you. I will stay with you. You are not alone." **Rationale:** This reassures the client of the basis of the therapeutic alliance.

CHAPTER 30

1. Correct Answers: 1. Determine how to identify potential members. **Rationale:** This step is essential if the nurse is forming a group for a particular population. Often, the nurse controls for heterogeneity or homogeneity (of level of functioning, gender, or age). 4. At the first meeting, provide a basic list of group rules in writing. **Rationale:** Many clients with chronic mental illness demonstrate anxiety in interpersonal situations, and the basic ground rules about membership (open or closed), confidentiality, and duration of the group should be delineated concretely.

2. Correct Answer: 1. The group will meet weekly to discuss any current concerns of interest to the group members. **Rationale:** This is a realistic goal for clients with chronic mental illness. The nurse anticipates the presence of interpersonal anxiety. Trust may develop over time, after which participants may become more comfortable with sharing feelings, and interpersonal learning may occur.

3. Correct Answer: 3. "As other members give you feedback about the effect you have on others, you learn to see yourself differently." **Rationale:** This response paraphrases the idea that change in one quadrant inevitably leads to changes in each of the other quadrants of the Johari window.

4. Correct Answer: 2. "You have expressed hurt when people have interrupted you, but for the past 20 minutes you have talked without allowing others to share." **Rationale:** This statement focuses on the current behaviors, thus meeting the criteria for here-and-now activation.

5. Correct Answer: 1. Unsatisfactory role negotiation with disequilibrium. **Rationale:** When the matriarch was unable to lead, the family structure had no provision for leadership. Problem solving and decision making remain impaired, and the system is currently in disequilibrium.

6. Correct Answer: 2. A stable household, comprised of a married couple with two teenage children, is augmented when a family member with a chronic, debilitating illness moves into a spare room. **Rationale:** This scenario indicates that a family member with complex needs is entering a functional household. The change may go smoothly, but it presents a potential disruption of usual roles and may represent a crisis.

7. Correct Answer: 4. Both parents and two of the four siblings have active chemical dependency problems. **Rationale:** Families with chemical dependence are characteristically chaotic, enmeshed, and unpredictable.

8. Correct Answer: 4. The food preferences of each family member. **Rationale:** Food preferences of each family member are not critical to this assessment, as people's food preferences change throughout the life cycle.

9. Correct Answer: 4. Family members do not have a strong sense of self. **Rationale:** Individuals in an enmeshed family do not have a clearly differentiated sense of self. Family members are unable to define their own values and beliefs.

10. Correct Answer: 1. "Neither my siblings nor my father can deal with the burden I present. I have no options." **Rationale:** Recall the chapter on suicide. Clients who make serious attempts often feel as if they have no choice and see death as an escape from an unbearable situation.

CHAPTER 31

1. Correct Answers: 2. Attribution. **Rationale:** An individual's thoughts and behaviors lead to feelings. By labeling or assigning meaning to a situation or circumstance, we make attributions. If an individual consistently makes a negative attribution to a situation, subsequent feelings will reflect this negativity. 3. Self-efficacy. **Rationale:** The ability to feel effective through one's actions is self-efficacy. Individuals who perceive themselves to be successful in a given situation will gain self-confidence. Individuals who consistently perceive themselves in a negative manner will develop unrealistic and maladaptive thought patterns. 4. Modeling. **Rationale:** Imitating the actions and behaviors of another individual with the expectation that one will receive rewards is modeling. Individuals learn behaviors by modeling the behaviors of others.

2. Correct Answer: 2. Change maladaptive thoughts. **Rationale:** The goal of cognitive therapy is to change or alter maladaptive thoughts that result in maladaptive behaviors.

3. Correct Answer: 2. "What's the point of studying? I am never going to graduate." **Rationale:** This statement reflects negative self-efficacy. The maladaptive belief that the individual will not graduate reinforces the negative feelings related to studying.

4. Correct Answer: 2. Reinforcing positive behaviors that result in desired learning outcomes. **Rationale:** By reinforcing desired behaviors, an individual is likely to adopt the desired outcomes over maladaptive ones. Positive reinforcement of certain behaviors reinforces the desired behavior.

5. Correct Answer: 3. Client will identify three feelings associated with smoking. **Rationale:** Having the client identify feelings associated with smoking is the first step in changing cognitive behaviors. This goal is client-specific and appropriate to the smoking cessation.

6. Correct Answer: 4. To assist the student in identifying recent behaviors or activities that reflect the student's success. **Rationale:** This response interrupts the student's negative thought process and assists the student in identifying positive attributes and accomplishments.

7. Correct Answer: 1. Have the members of the treatment team develop the contract for the client. **Rationale:** When developing a behavioral contract, it is essential that the client is included in the planning process. The client needs to agree to the terms of the contract if there is any possibility of success. Developing a contract with only the members of the treatment team sets the client up for failure and lack of commitment.

8. Correct Answer: 3. Assist the client to identify feelings that trigger the impulsive behaviors. **Rationale:** Working with the client to identify feelings that trigger the behaviors is one of the first steps in helping the client learn to overcome the behaviors. By associating feelings with the behaviors, the client can begin to learn how to deal more effectively with the feelings.

9. Correct Answer: 2. "Why are we wasting our time with these people? They are never going to get any better." **Rationale:** This statement reflects the nurse's personal biased view of mentally ill clients. The nurse may associate a mental health diagnosis with failure. This comment by the nurse requires further investigation.

10. Correct Answer: 3. Think about being in control throughout a particular situation. **Rationale:** Mastery imagery shapes the individual's thoughts about being in control. This technique practices imagined successful behavior change.

CHAPTER 32

1. Correct Answers: 1. Elevated blood pressure. **Rationale:** An increase in blood pressure can be an adverse effect of the medication and requires careful follow-up. Many psychotropic medications can directly affect the cardiac cycle. 2. Increased agitation. **Rationale:** A change in the client's behavior requires ongoing assessment and monitoring. Increasing agitation may indicate the client's poor response to a medication or intolerance of the side effects. 3. Bradycardia. **Rationale:** A decreased or slowing heart rate requires follow-up and intervention. Left untreated, the long-term outcome could be heart block. 4. Increased thirst. **Rationale:** This side effect, although common with medications that have an anticholinergic effect, may also be a symptom of diabetes. The nurse should follow up on this symptom in addition to doing patient education.

2. Correct Answer: 4. Dystonia. **Rationale:** Dystonia is a severe muscle spasm occurring in the first days of treatment or even after a single dose of medication.

3. Correct Answer: 1. Maintain clear walkways throughout the house. **Rationale:** Clients with drug-induced parkinsonism experience rigidity, tremor, or rhythmic oscillations of the extremities, and a shuffling gait. They are at an increased risk for falls. Safety measures should be implemented to decrease the risk.

4. Correct Answer: 2. Suicidality. **Rationale:** Therapeutic effects of antidepressants can be felt within 2 weeks of starting treatment. During this time period, clients have increased energy and can still be actively depressed. Clients need to be monitored for suicidal and homicidal ideations, plan, or intent. This is the priority nursing assessment at this time in treatment.

5. Correct Answer: 3. When the client is stabilized and psychotic symptoms are manageable. **Rationale:** Once the client has been stabilized and is able to understand the information presented, the nurse would provide the education. The nurse applies the principles of teaching and learning when providing client education.

6. Correct Answer: 4. Difficulty achieving orgasms. **Rationale:** Hyperprolactinemia results from an increased production of the hormone prolactin, which results in difficulties with libido, arousal, excitation, orgasm, and male ejaculatory volume.

7. Correct Answer: 3. Insatiable thirst. **Rationale:** The client has a family history of diabetes. Antipsychotic medications typically cause weight gain, which increases the risk of diabetes and heart disease. Insatiable thirst may be an indicator of hyperglycemia and/or diabetes. The nurse must monitor the client's thirst level closely.

8. Correct Answer: 3. Repeatedly folding pages in a magazine. **Rationale:** Clomipramine (Anafranil), a tricyclic antidepressant, is used as an antiobsessional agent. The client's actions reflect compulsive behaviors.

9. Correct Answer: 3. Elevated body temperature. **Rationale:** Clozapine can cause agranulocytosis, which can result in a serious infection. An elevated body temperature may be an early indicator of an infection. The nurse should also monitor the client's white blood cell count.

10. Correct Answer: 2. Risk for Aspiration. **Rationale:** The client will have an altered level of consciousness, increased salivation, and difficulty swallowing. Maintaining the client's airway is the priority intervention.

CHAPTER 33

1. Correct Answer: 3. A client who is severely depressed and cannot focus on simple tasks. **Rationale:** Clients need to be able to focus on the CAM methods and follow simple and complex directions. A client with severe depression may have cognitive impairments due to the depression and will not be able to actively and effectively participate in CAM.

2. Correct Answer: 3. Massage. **Rationale:** This technique is performed by the caregiver and can result in decreased anxiety and emotional distress and increased relaxation for the client with DAT at any stage.

3. Correct Answer: 1. Muscle tension is the body's physiologic response to anxiety-provoking thoughts. **Rationale:** Progressive relaxation is based on the premise that muscle tension is the body's physiologic response to anxiety-provoking thoughts.

4. Correct Answers: 3. Client's interest in utilizing alternative medicine techniques. **Rationale:** If a client expresses an interest and motivation to participate in CAM, there is a greater likelihood the client will more actively participate in the activities and be successful. Clients who are not interested in CAM would not be appropriate for the techniques. 4. History of cardiac disease. **Rationale:** Many CAM techniques lower blood pressure and decrease heart rate. Clients with a history of cardiac disease may be at an increased risk for cardiac arrhythmias and would need to be monitored closely for possible complications. 5. Medications, herbs, or other nutraceuticals the client is currently taking. **Rationale:** The nurse needs to assess the medications (prescription and over-the-counter), herbs, and other nutraceuticals the client is taking, as some of these may have side effects that affect blood pressure and heart rate. These side effects in conjunction with the effects of certain CAM methods can cause hypotension and other serious complications.

5. Correct Answer: 2. "I will ask my friends for the name of a practitioner who is good." **Rationale:** Word of mouth may be helpful but should not be the only criterion for selecting a CAM technique or practitioner. Consumers need to be informed of the practices, benefits, and risks of treatment modalities.

6. Correct Answer: 1. Producing endorphins in the brain. **Rationale:** Soothing music produces endorphins, which are the "feel good" chemicals of the brain. The endorphins, in conjunction with deep breathing exercises, enhance the relaxing effect of the music, reduce stress, and promote relaxation.

7. Correct Answer: 2. There is an increased risk of liver failure with long-term use. **Rationale:** There is an increased risk of liver failure with long-term use of kava. A client with chronic alcohol abuse has compromised liver function due to the alcoholism and is at an increased risk of further liver damage with the use of kava.

8. Correct Answer: 3. Caffeine. **Rationale:** Clients taking clozapine (Clozaril) should avoid all forms of caffeine—tea, cocoa, coffee, and cola—because of the interactions between the medication and caffeine.

9. Correct Answer: 3. Nonadherence with the medications. **Rationale:** Failure to take medications as prescribed is not a drug interaction. Medication nonadherence is an issue that would be addressed in treatment.

10. Correct Answer: 3. "These techniques are appropriate for all clients." **Rationale:** Complementary and alternative medicine (CAM) is not indicated for all clients. Clients with a cardiac history, altered thought processes, and severe depression may be unable to participate in the exercises due to untoward side effects. Clients should be screened before beginning these techniques.

CHAPTER 34

1. Correct Answer: 1. Foreseeable. **Rationale:** The event leading to the situational crisis is usually unanticipated. Consequently, situational crises have the potential to disrupt equilibrium unexpectedly. A maturational crisis involves life cycle changes or normal transitions of human development; therefore, they are foreseeable.

2. Correct Answer: 3. "Within 6 weeks, for better or worse, we will be past this place." **Rationale:** This statement demonstrates the understanding that crisis is, by definition, both a watershed and a self-limiting event.

3. Correct Answer: 2. Recoil. **Rationale:** Survivors become more dependent during the recoil stage, and the nurse should anticipate caring for survivors and identifying additional resources for emergency shelter, food, and clothing.

4. Correct Answer: 4. "My brother and I were always there for each other when we were children. I will ask him for help if I need it." **Rationale:** This is a specific plan to call a particular individual. In addition, it is a plan that your peer has utilized in the past and that has been effective.

5. Correct Answer: 2. "Coping style, as well as the number and depth of supportive relationships, may explain the difference." **Rationale:** Resilience encompasses the biological and psychological characteristics intrinsic to an individual, such as personality style and quality of interpersonal relationships, that confer protection against the development of psychopathology.

6. Correct Answers: 1. Pharmacological interventions. **Rationale:** Clients in crisis often benefit from medications to treat anxiety, depression, and/or sleep disturbance. 3. Stress management techniques. **Rationale:** Increasing the client's repertoire of stress management techniques increases coping strategies and empowers the client. 4. Cognitive behavioral interventions. **Rationale:** These interventions alter the perception of the trauma and increase the client's repertoire of responses.

7. Correct Answer: 1. "That must bring up a lot of thoughts and fears from your past. For this session, let's focus on your childhood." **Rationale:** Crisis intervention focuses on the here-and-now. It is potentially countertherapeutic for the nurse to delve into long-standing issues when the goal is for the client to resume optimal functioning as soon as possible.

8. Correct Answer: 4. Mass media. **Rationale:** Public service announcements through mass media are likely to contain the most accurate information for individuals in need. It is essential for crisis workers to impart this information to victims, since victims are likely displaced and disconnected from communication networks.

9. Correct Answers: 1. Expressing doubt regarding the client's capacity to function. **Rationale:** The goal of crisis intervention is to restore the person to the pretrauma level as quickly as possible. A review of the outcome criteria for your client in crisis may reveal that the client has met the criteria and is able to resume responsibilities without further intervention. 4. Augmenting continuously the client's problem list. **Rationale:** Crisis intervention focuses on return to function rather than addressing all identified problems. 5. Thinking about clients during leisure time. **Rationale:** Preoccupation with clients is associated with caregiver stress and vicarious traumatization. Increased self-awareness and self-care is usually warranted.

10. Correct Answer: 1. "After a while, you become accustomed to hearing the same stories over and over and you develop numbness." **Rationale:** Profound sadness, grief, and anger are normal reactions to an abnormal event. Absence of response, or lack of awareness of a response, suggests the need for further assessment.

CHAPTER 35

1. Correct Answer: 3. "No single theory consistently explains or predicts violent behavior." **Rationale:** This statement offers a broad basis to augment with additional teaching. It may decrease shame and frustration on the part of the family member, who is unable to comprehend a change in the loved one's behavior.

2. Correct Answer: 1. The client glares at the nurse and is unable to respond verbally. **Rationale:** The client's inability to respond verbally may indicate that the client is unable to process information due to panic-level anxiety. The nurse should determine which measures are necessary to provide for the safety of the client, other clients, and staff members.

3. Correct Answers: 2. "If you are frightened or fearful, what do you do?" **Rationale:** Clients are most likely to become violent when they feel threatened. If the nurse is aware of past violent episodes, a good follow-up question might be, "In the past, when you have become violent, what was going on right before that happened?" 3. "What do you usually do to relax?" **Rationale:** Empowering the client by assisting with identifying usual coping strategies may decrease the client's distress and powerlessness. If the client's usual coping strategies are currently unavailable, this limited repertoire may contribute to violent behavior. 4. "In the past, have you ever acted on your thoughts of violence?" **Rationale:** A history of violent behavior is a strong predictor for future acts of violence. The nurse can utilize the client's history and reports of family members as additional sources of information.

4. Correct Answers: 1. "How can the staff and I help you maintain control?" **Rationale:** Engaging the client in the problem-solving process while offering assistance is empowering and consistent with the principle of least restrictiveness. 2. "Your PRN medication helped you cope with stress 2 days ago. Would you be willing to take that medication now?" **Rationale:** Identifying assistance that has worked in the past and offering the client a choice is empowering. Most clinicians believe that chemical assistance with behavior control is less restrictive than physical seclusion or restraint. 5. "As we are walking around together, is the walking helping you?" **Rationale:** Assisting the client to identify factors currently alleviating stress is empowering. Accompanying the client as he engages in gross motor activity may increase or decrease his distress; requesting his evaluation is respectful and consistent with the principle of least restrictiveness.

5. Correct Answer: 4. "If you need more time on the telephone, let's identify a time when other clients aren't waiting to use the phone." **Rationale:** This response provides for the freedom and needs of the individual client while providing for the physical and emotional safety (via predictability) of the other clients.

6. Correct Answer: 2. Assist the client to consider alternative responses to angry feelings. **Rationale:** This strategy is a problem-solving intervention, which is effective for many violent clients.

7. Correct Answer: 3. Provide safety for the agitated client and other clients. **Rationale:** The safety of *all* clients on the unit is the priority. Clients need a sense of comfort and safety.

8. Correct Answers: 2. Formal crisis debriefing may improve risk management outcomes. **Rationale:** Providing supportive crisis intervention for the staff may decrease the potential for retaliation and long-term negative consequences. 4. Staff members need encouragement and a structured format for support in discussing their thoughts, feelings, and reactions to a violent incident. **Rationale:** It is essential to debrief as a group after such an incident. At the same time, health care personnel may not want to put time and effort into a debriefing unless it is required by policy and procedure.

9. Correct Answer: 1. Remain with the other clients and staff who are physically removed from the violent client. **Rationale:** At no time should students or other untrained personnel intervene using crisis response techniques, because they involve actual physical contact with clients, thereby increasing the risk of personal injury. However, it is often beneficial for other staff and available students to remain with the rest of the clients. Seeing another individual out of control is frightening for uninvolved clients, and the presence of other staff and students is often very comforting.

10. Correct Answers: 1. "I had never before considered psychiatric hospitalization from the client's perspective." **Rationale:** This increased awareness from the client's perspective is beneficial in identifying precipitants to aggressive behavior. 4. "Our team members are less likely to blame each other when a violent episode occurs." **Rationale:** A nonblaming environment promotes honest feedback and improvement in quality of care. 5. "The role-playing exercise gave me a variety of facilitative statements." **Rationale:** Learning a variety of approaches and tools empowers the staff.

Find complete rationales on the CD-ROM that accompanies this textbook.

INDEX

Page numbers followed by *f* indicate figures and those followed by *t* indicate tables, boxes, or special features.

A

B

E

F

S